Oxford Textbook of Medicine

Infection

Oxford Textbook of Medicine
Infection

Selected and updated chapters from the Oxford Textbook of Medicine, Fifth Edition

Edited by

David A. Warrell
Emeritus Professor of Tropical Medicine, Nuffield Department of Clinical Medicine; Honorary Fellow, St Cross College, University of Oxford, Oxford, UK

Timothy M. Cox
Professor of Medicine, University of Cambridge; Honorary Consultant Physician, Addenbrooke's Hospital, Cambridge, UK

John D. Firth
Consultant Physician and Nephrologist, Addenbrooke's Hospital, Cambridge, UK

With guest editor

Estée Török
Senior Research Associate, University of Cambridge and Honorary Consultant in Infectious Diseases and Microbiology, Cambridge University Hospitals NHS Foundation Trust, Cambridge, UK

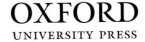

OXFORD
UNIVERSITY PRESS

OXFORD
UNIVERSITY PRESS

Great Clarendon Street, Oxford OX2 6DP
United Kingdom

Oxford University Press is a department of the University of Oxford.
It furthers the University's objective of excellence in research, scholarship,
and education by publishing worldwide. Oxford is a registered trade mark of
Oxford University Press in the UK and in certain other countries

© Oxford University Press 2012

The moral rights of the authors have been asserted

Oxford Textbook of Medicine: Infection 2012

Updated material from Oxford Textbook of Medicine, fifth edition, 2010

Impression: 1

British Library Cataloguing in Publication Data

Data available

Library of Congress Cataloging in Publication Data

Data available

ISBN 978–0–19–965213–6

Printed in China by
C&C Offset Printing Co., Ltd.

Foreword

It is a pleasure to be invited to write the Foreword for this selection of updated chapters on Infectious and Tropical Diseases from the *Oxford Textbook of Medicine*.

The *Oxford Textbook of Medicine* is one of the most comprehensive, respected, and widely read textbooks of medicine. Regularly updated, it has become ever larger since it was first published in 1983 as medical knowledge increased exponentially.

Wisely, a decision has been made to publish the infection section of the textbook, one of the largest, as a stand-alone volume—the *Oxford Textbook of Medicine: Infection*.

During a life-time of clinical practice I have seen infectious diseases develop from a 'behind closed doors' speciality, principally practised in isolation hospitals, to one of the most dynamic areas of medicine with major advances in the biology, pathogenesis, diagnosis, prevention, and treatment of microbial diseases. All of these aspects are dealt with in detail in this new book of over 800 pages.

The contents range from the classical infectious diseases of childhood to exotic infections originating in tropical countries. David Warrell's vast experience of medicine in developing countries is reflected in the authoritative coverage of tropical diseases. Recently recognised infections are described in detail and the sections on immunisation and antimicrobial therapy are comprehensive.

The *Oxford Textbook of Medicine: Infection*, with chapters written by authorities from around the world, encompasses all that a physician needs to know about infection.

It is difficult, as I know from personal experience, to edit chapters written by multiple contributors; the Editors have succeeded in doing so.

I greatly enjoyed reading the book and congratulate the Editors on their endeavours. I wish that this book had been available when I practised infectious diseases. The on-line version will be especially attractive.

Alasdair Geddes
Emeritus Professor of Infectious Diseases,
University of Birmingham.
Past-President, International Society for Infectious Diseases.

Preface

Infectious diseases command increasing concern and attention in western and tropical developing countries. The maintenance of global public health is challenged by uncontrolled population growth; emergence and spread of new, virulent, or multidrug resistant pathogens—and tectonic displacement and climatic extremes create humanitarian disasters. Global warming enhances the vectorial capacity of mosquitoes and other vectors and reservoirs and everywhere the problem of nosocomial and other healthcare-associated infections burgeons. Above all, it is the failures and derelictions by politicians and international organizations that hinder or disable attempts to meet these challenges by correcting inequities in the distribution of resources. A few examples will illustrate the highly unstable and dynamic state of the contest between pathogens and their human hosts in 2012.

Globalisation of disease

The unprecedented rise of international travel, for business, tourism, religious pilgrimage, adventure, and migration, has promoted the spread of pathogens far beyond their sites of origin and known endemic foci. Gram-negative Enterobacteriaceae with resistance to carbapenems conferred by the ^{bla}NDM-1 (New Delhi metallo-beta-lactamase) gene now pose a global threat. It is clear that many patients in the UK harbouring these strains had travelled to or been in hospital in India and Pakistan. NDM-1 producing organisms imported from the Indian subcontinent have also been reported in other European countries, North America, Japan, and Australia. Antibiotic resistant *Acinetobacter baumannii-calcoaceticus* complex bacteria were imported in military and civilian casualties from field hospitals in Iraq to USA and UK where they pose an increasing risk to immuno compromised or severely ill patients in intensive care units.

Modern plagues

Starting in May 2011, there was an outbreak of infections by an unusual Shiga-toxin-producing *Escherichia coli* 0104: H4 with extended-spectrum β lactamases in northern Germany. Almost 4000 people were affected, of whom 800 developed haemolytic uraemic syndrome and 43 died. Differences from previous enterohaemorrhagic *E. coli* epidemics included the higher proportion of young and middle-aged women and the higher incidence of severe acute kidney injury, neurological complications, and mortality.

In October 2010, ten months after the catastrophic Haitian earthquake (Richter magnitude scale M_w 7.0), a massive epidemic of cholera began, spreading rapidly throughout the country and to neighbouring Dominican Republic. By December 2011 a total of 543 767 cases and 7364 deaths had been reported.

Chikungunya virus appeared in western Indian Ocean islands in early 2005 causing hundreds of thousands of cases. Selection of the A226V mutation allowed transmission by *Aedes albopictus* mosquitoes conferred increased virulence. The pandemic spread to India (1.42 million reported cases), elsewhere in South Asia, Africa, and in rural Emilia-Romagna in Italy, where autochthonous transmission was established for a while in 2007.

Emerging and re-emerging pathogens

Human encroachments on the natural environment have caused ecologic chaos and degradation associated with the emergence of lethal pathogens including filoviruses, arenaviruses, henipaviruses/paramyxoviruses, rhabdoviruses, and coronaviruses. Growing evidence implicates distinctive mammalian vectors, many of which are bats, whose importance for human health is cause for increasing concern.

Nosocomial and other healthcare-associated infections

The term 'healthcare-associated infection' (HCAI) was coined to reflect the risk of iatrogenic infection acquired through medical procedures performed outside hospitals (in the home, general practice, and nursing home) as well as in hospitals (nosocomial infections). One in ten patients admitted to hospitals are affected by HCAI causing much morbidity and mortality. Since the mid-1980s the emergence and spread of epidemic strains of methicillin-resistant *Staphylococcus aureus* (MRSA) in UK hospitals prompted the Department of Health to institute a number of control measures, including screening, decolonisation, and mandatory reporting of MRSA bloodstream infections. Subsequently, MRSA bloodstream infections have declined but it is not clear whether this is attributable more to infection control measures rather than changes in circulating strains. MRSA has also become as an important pathogen in community settings—in the USA the emergence and spread of the USA 300 strain was characterised by outbreaks of skin and soft tissue infection, necrotising pneumonia, and severe sepsis. This strain has recently been reported in the UK potentially threatening the advances made in MRSA control.

In the early 2000s, the emergence and spread of a new hypervirulent strain of *Clostridium difficile* (B1/NAP1/027) resulted in dramatic increases in the incidence, severity and mortality of *C. difficile* disease. Again, the UK Department of Health responded by reinforcing implementation of infection control measures such as environmental cleaning and mandatory reporting of *C. difficile* disease, following which, incidence has decreased. There has also been progress in developing therapeutic antibodies and vaccines against *C. difficile* toxins. The dramatic success of the pigbel vaccination campaign in Papua New Guinea against endemic enteritis necroticans caused by the β-toxin of *Clostridium perfringens* should surely encourage these efforts.

Despite these improvements, understanding of the molecular epidemiology and transmission pathways of nosocomial pathogens at local, national and international levels remains incomplete, and this hampers efforts towards their control.

In developing countries, the emergence and spread of extensively drug resistant tuberculosis, particularly in hospitals, poses enormous difficulties for treatment and control that require substantial support from donor agencies and international organisations.

Facing the challenges

Application of molecular biology is revolutionizing the design of new vaccines and drugs, diagnostic methods, and surveillance techniques; treatment and prevention of infectious diseases, as well as the advice given to travellers and immunosuppressed patients, is already much improved. These advances are discussed fully in this freshly updated and revised edition of the infectious diseases section of the *Oxford Textbook of Medicine, Fifth Edition*. There is an urgent need to coordinate strategic efforts and safe and effective management of resources by improving communication between hospitals, politicians, academic institutions, donor agencies, and international organisations. In the interests of disseminating reliable and up-to-date information among our broad constituency of readers, we trust that this new book, with its electronic counterpart in the *Oxford Textbook of Medicine* online, will hit the mark.

David A. Warrell
Timothy M. Cox
John D. Firth
M. Estée Török

February 2012

Contents

Contributors

P. Aaby Bandim Health Project, National Institute of Health, Guinea-Bissau

5.6: Measles

Michael J. Aldape Assistant Research Scientist, Infectious Diseases Section, Veterans Affairs Medical Center, Boise, Idaho, USA

6.24: Botulism, gas gangrene, and clostridial gastrointestinal infections

Emmanouil Angelakis Faculté de Médecine et de Pharmacie, Université de la Méditerranée, Marseille Cedex, France

6.42: Bartonellas excluding B. bacilliformis

Gregory M. Anstead Associate Professor, Division of Infectious Diseases, Department of Medicine, University of Texas Health Science Center at San Antonio, and Medical Director, Immunosuppression and Infectious Diseases Clinics, South Texas Veterans Healthcare System, San Antonio, Texas, USA

7.3: Coccidioidomycosis

D. Barlow Consultant Physician, Department of Genitourinary Medicine, Guy's and St Thomas' Hospitals, London, UK

6.6: Neisseria gonorrhoeae

John G. Bartlett Professor of Medicine, Johns Hopkins University School of Medicine, Baltimore, Maryland, USA

6.23: Clostridium difficile

Buddha Basnyat Oxford University Clinical Research Unit, Patan Hospital, Nepal

6.8: Typhoid and paratyphoid fevers

Gordon R. Bernard Melinda Owen Bass Professor of Medicine, Division of Allergy, Pulmonary, and Critical Care Medicine; Associate Vice Chancellor for Research, Senior Associate Dean for Clinical Sciences, Vanderbilt University School of Medicine, Nashville, Tennessee, USA

1.2: Physiological changes, clinical features, and general management of infected patients

J.M. Best Emeritus Reader in Virology, King's College London, UK

5.13: Rubella

Delia B. Bethell Armed Forces Research Unit of Medical Sciences, Bangkok, Thailand (Clinical Trials Investigator); Oxford Radcliffe Hospital NHS Trust, Oxford, UK (Honorary Consultant Paediatrician)

6.1: Diphtheria

T.C. Boswell Consultant Medical Microbiologist, Nottingham University Hospitals, Nottingham, UK

6.38: Legionellosis and legionnaires' disease

I.C.J.W. Bowler Consultant Microbiologist and Clinical Lead, Department of Medical Microbiology, Oxford Radcliffe Hospitals NHS Trust, Oxford, UK

2.3: Nosocomial infections

Petter Brandtzaeg Department of Paediatrics, Oslo University Hospital, Oslo, Norway

6.5: Meningococcal infections

Philippe Brasseur Emeritus Professor of Parasitology, Faculty of Medicine of Rouen (France) and Research Unit (UMR 198), Institute of Research for Development, Dakar, Senegal

8.3: Babesiosis

Arthur E. Brown Colonel, U.S. Army, Armed Forces Research Institute of Medical Sciences, Bangkok, Thailand

6.20: Anthrax

Kevin E. Brown Consultant Medical Virologist, Virus Reference Department, Centres for Infection, Health Protection Agency, London, UK

5.20: Parvovirus B19

Michael Brown Senior Lecturer, Department of Infectious & Tropical Diseases, London School of Hygiene & Tropical Medicine, London, UK

9.4: Strongyloidiasis, hookworm, and other gut strongyloid nematodes

Amy E. Bryant Research Scientist, Infectious Diseases Section, Veterans Affairs Medical Center, Boise, Idaho; Affiliate Assistant Professor, University of Washington School of Medicine, Seattle, Washington, USA

6.24: Botulism, gas gangrene, and clostridial gastrointestinal infections

A.D.M. Bryceson London School of Hygiene and Tropical Medicine, London, UK

8.12: Leishmaniasis

Gilbert Burnham Co-Director of the Center for Refugee and Disaster Response, Johns Hopkins, Department of International Health, Baltimore, Maryland, USA

9.1: Cutaneous filariasis

Valai Bussaratid Assistant Professor of Tropical Medicine, Department of Clinical Tropical Medicine, Mahidol University, Bangkok, Thailand

9.7: Gnathostomiasis

Geoffrey A. Butcher The Malaria Centre, Department of Life Sciences, Imperial College London, London, UK

8.2: Malaria

S.M. Cacciò Department of Infectious, Parasitic and Immunomediated Diseases, Istituto Superiore di Sanità, Viale Regina Elena, Rome, Italy

8.5: Cryptosporidium and cryptosporidiosis

Richard E. Chaisson Professor of Medicine, Epidemiology and International Health, Johns Hopkins University School of Medicine and Bloomberg School of Public Health, Baltimore, Maryland, USA

6.25: Tuberculosis

J. Cohen Dean of Medicine and Professor of Infectious Diseases, Brighton & Sussex Medical School, Brighton, UK

2.4: Infection in the immunocompromised host

J. Collier Consultant in General Medicine, John Radcliffe Hospital, Oxford, UK

5.22: Hepatitis C

C.P. Conlon Reader in Infectious Diseases and Tropical Medicine, University of Oxford; Consultant Physician, John Radcliffe Hospitals, Nuffield Department of Medicine, John Radcliffe Hospital, Oxford, UK
4: Travel and expedition medicine; 5.23: HIV/AIDS

John E. Cooper The University of the West Indies, St Augustine, Trinidad & Tobago, West Indies; Department of Veterinary Medicine, University of Cambridge, Cambridge, UK
8.7: Sarcocystosis (sarcosporidiosis)

Derrick W. Crook Infectious Disease and Clinical Microbiology, Nuffield Department of Medicine, John Radcliffe Hospital, Oxford, UK
6.12: Haemophilus influenzae

Linda Dayan Senior Staff Specialist and Director of Sexual Health Services, Royal North Shore Hospital, Sydney; Clinical Lecturer, School of Public Health, University of Sydney, Sydney, Australia
6.36: Syphilis

Kevin M. De Cock Centers for Disease Control and Prevention, Nairobi, Kenya
5.24: HIV in the developing world

Ulrich Desselberger Director of Research, Department of Medicine, Addenbrooke's Hospital, Cambridge, UK
5.8: Enterovirus infections; 5.9: Virus infections causing diarrhoea and vomiting

Basil Donovan Professor of Sexual Health, National Centre in HIV Epidemiology and Clinical Research, University of New South Wales; Senior Staff Specialist, Sydney Sexual Health Centre, Sydney Hospital, Sydney, Australia
6.36: Syphilis

Philip Dormitzer Senior Director, Senior Project Leader, Viral Vaccine Research, Novartis Vaccines and Diagnostics, Cambridge, Massachusetts, USA
5.9: Virus infections causing diarrhoea and vomiting

D.W. Dunne Department of Pathology, University of Cambridge, Cambridge, UK
11.1: Schistosomiasis

Christopher J. Ellis Consultant Physician, Department of Infection and Tropical Medicine, Heartlands Hospital, Birmingham, UK
2.1: Clinical approach

M.A. Epstein Nuffield Department of Clinical Medicine, John Radcliffe Hospital, Oxford, UK
5.3: Epstein–Barr virus

Jeremy Farrar Oxford University Clinical Research Unit, Wellcome Trust Major Overseas Programme Vietnam; South East Asia Infectious Disease Clinical Research Network, Ho Chi Minh City, Vietnam
5.15: Dengue

R.G. Finch Professor of Infectious Diseases, Nottingham University Hospitals NHS Trust, Nottingham, UK
2.5: Antimicrobial chemotherapy

Hector H. Garcia Professor, Department of Microbiology, Universidad Peruana Cayetano Heredia, Lima, Peru; Head, Cysticercosis Unit, Instituto de Ciencias Neurológicas, Lima, Peru
10.1: Cystic hydatid disease (Echinococcus granulosus); 10.3: Cysticercosis

Robert H. Gilman Professor, Department of International Health, Johns Hopkins Bloomberg School of Hygiene and Public Health, Baltimore, Maryland, USA
10.3: Cysticercosis

D. Goldblatt Professor of Vaccinology and Immunology, Consultant in Paediatric Immunology, Head, Immunobiology Unit, Director, Clinical Research and Development and, Director, NIHR Biomedical Research Centre, Great Ormond Street Hospital for Children NHS Trust and Institute of Child Health, University College London, UK
3: Immunization

Armando E. Gonzalez Dean, School of Veterinary Medicine, Universidad Nacional Mayor de San Marcos, Lima, Peru
10.1: Cystic hydatid disease (Echinococcus granulosus)

Eduardo Gotuzzo Instituto de Medicina Tropical Alexander von Humboldt Universidad Peruana Cayetano Heredia Av. Honorio Delgado, San Martín de Porres, Lima, Peru
5.25: HTLV-1, HTLV-2, and associated diseases

P. Goulder Wellcome Senior Clinical Fellow & Honorary Consultant Paediatrician, University of Oxford, Oxford, UK
5.23: HIV/AIDS

Alison D. Grant Department of Paediatrics, University of Auckland, Auckland, New Zealand
5.24: HIV in the developing world

Cameron Grant Department of Paediatrics, University of Auckland, Auckland, New Zealand
6.14: Bordetella infection

John R. Graybill Professor Emeritus, Division of Infectious Diseases, Department of Medicine, University of Texas Health Science Center at San Antonio, San Antonio, Texas, USA
7.3: Coccidioidomycosis

David I. Grove Formerly Director of Clinical Microbiology and Infectious Diseases, The Queen Elizabeth Hospital, Woodville and Clinical Professor, University of Adelaide, South Australia, Australia
9.5: Gut and tissue nematode infections acquired by ingestion; 10.4: Diphyllobothriasis and sparganosis; 11.2: Liver fluke infections; 11.4: Intestinal trematode infections

D.J. Gubler Director, Program on Emerging Infectious Disease, Duke-NUS Graduate Medical School, Singapore; Asian Pacific Institute of Tropical Medicine and Infectious Diseases, University of Hawaii, Honolulu
5.12: Alphaviruses; 5.14: Flaviviruses (excluding dengue)

Richard L. Guerrant Hunter Professor of International Medicine, Division of Infectious Diseases and International Health; Director, Center for Global Health, University of Virginia, Charlottesville, Virginia, USA
6.11: Cholera

Roderick J. Hay Professor of Cutaneous Infection, Dermatology Department, King's College Hospital, London, UK
6.30: Nocardiosis; 7.1: Fungal infections

David W. Hecht The John W. Clarke Professor and Chairman, Department of Medicine, Loyola University Medical Center, Maywood, Illinois, USA
6.10: Anaerobic bacteria

Janet Hemingway Director, Liverpool School of Tropical Medicine, Liverpool, UK
8.2: Malaria

Martin F. Heyworth Staff Physician and Adjunct Professor of Medicine, VA Medical Center and University of Pennsylvania, Philadelphia, Pennsylvania, USA
8.8: Giardiasis, balantidiasis, isosporiasis, and microsporidiosis

Tran Tinh Hien Vice Director, Centre for Tropical Diseases (Cho Quan Hospital), Ho Chi Minh City, Vietnam
6.1: Diphtheria

Sharon Hillier Professor, Department of Obstetrics, Gynecology and Reproductive Sciences, University of Pittsburgh School of Medicine, Pittsburgh, Pennsylvania, USA
8.13: Trichomoniasis

H. Hof Labor Limbach, Heidelberg, Germany
6.37: Listeriosis

Bala Hota Division of Infectious Diseases, Department of Medicine, John H. Stroger Jr. Hospital of Cook County; Assistant Professor, Rush University Medical Center, Chicago, Illinois, USA
6.4: Staphylococci

Laurence Huang Professor of Medicine, University of California San Francisco; Chief, AIDS Chest Clinic, HIV/AIDS Division, San Francisco General Hospital, San Francisco, California, USA
7.5: Pneumocystis jirovecii

H.C. Hughes Specialty Registrar (Infectious diseases/Microbiology), University Hospital of Wales, UK
5.29: Newly discovered viruses

C. Ison Director, Sexually Transmitted Bacteria Reference Laboratory, Health Protection Agency Centre for Infections, London, UK
6.6: Neisseria gonorrhoeae

K.J.M. Jeffery Consultant Virologist, Oxford Radcliffe NHS Trust, John Radcliffe Hospital, Oxford, UK
5.22: Hepatitis C

Jørgen Skov Jensen Mycoplasma Laboratory, Copenhagen, Denmark
6.45: Mycoplasmas

Summerpal S. Kahlon Melbourne Internal Medicine Associates, Melbourne, Florida, USA
5.16: Bunyaviridae

Paul Klenerman Nuffield Department of Medicine, University of Oxford, Oxford, UK
5.22: Hepatitis C

Richard Knight Associate Professor of Parasitology (retired), Department of Microbiology, University of Nairobi, Kenya
8.1: Amoebic infections; 8.9: Blastocystis hominis infection; 9.2: Lymphatic filariasis; 9.3: Guinea worm disease (dracunculiasis); 9.6: Parastrongyliasis (angiostrongyliasis); 10.2: Cyclophyllidian gut tapeworms

Daniël Knockaert General Internal Medicine, University Hospital Gasthuisberg, Leuven, Belgium
2.2: Fever of unknown origin

G.C.K.W. Koh Honorary Specialist Registrar, Department of Medicine, University of Cambridge, Cambridge, UK
6.7.2: Pseudomonas aeruginosa

R. Lainson Ex Director, The Wellcome Parasitology Unit, and research-worker, Department of Parasitology, Instituto Evandro Chagas, Rodovia, Bairro Levilândia, Ananindeua, Pará, Brazil
8.6: Cyclospora and cyclosporiasis

J.W. LeDuc Professor, Microbiology and Immunology, Robert E. Shope M.D. and John S. Dunn Distinguished Chair in Global Health, Deputy Director, Galveston National Laboratory, University of Texas Medical Branch, Galveston, USA
5.16: Bunyaviridae

Oliver Liesenfeld Professor of Medical Microbiology and Infection Institute for Microbiology and Hygiene, Charité Medical School Berlin, Berlin, Germany
8.4: Toxoplasmosis

Aldo A.M. Lima Professor of Medicine and Pharmacology, Faculty of Medicine, Federal University of Ceará, Fortaleza, CE, Brazil
6.11; Cholera

A. Llanos-Cuentas School of Public Health & Administration and School of Medicine, Universidad Peruana Cayetano Heredia, Lima, Peru
6.43: Bartonella bacilliformis infection

Diana N.J. Lockwood Professor of Tropical Medicine, London School of Hygiene and Tropical Medicine, and Consultant Leprologist, Hospital for Tropical Diseases, London, UK
6.27: Leprosy (Hansen's disease); 8.12: Leishmaniasis

Graz A. Luzzi Consultant in Genitourinary Medicine and Honorary Senior Clinical Lecturer, University of Oxford, Wycombe Hospital, High Wycombe, UK
5.23: HIV/AIDS

David Mabey Professor of Communicable Diseases, Department of Infectious and Tropical Diseases, London School of Hygiene and Tropical Medicine, London, UK
6.44: Chlamydial infections

J.T. Macfarlane Lately Professor of Respiratory Medicine, University of Nottingham, and Consultant Respiratory Physician, Nottingham University Hospitals, Nottingham, UK
6.38: Legionellosis and legionnaires' disease

M. Monir Madkour‡ Consultant Physician, Military Hospital, Riyadh, Saudi Arabia
6.21: Brucellosis

‡ Deceased.

C. Maguiña-Vargas Instituto de Medicina Tropical Alexander von Humboldt, Universidad Peruana Cayetano Heredia, Lima, Peru
6.43: Bartonella bacilliformis infection

T.J. Marrie Dean, Faculty of Medicine, Dalhousie University, Clinical Research Centre, Halifax, Nova Scotia, Canada
6.41: Coxiella burnetii infections (Q fever)

Kevin Marsh Director, KEMRI Wellcome Research Programme, Kilifi, Kenya
8.2: Malaria

Duncan J. Maskell Head of Department and Marks & Spencer Professor of Farm Animal Health, Food Science & Food Safety, Department of Veterinary Medicine, University of Cambridge, Cambridge, UK
1.1: Biology of pathogenic microorganisms

J. ter Meulen Executive Director Vaccine Basic Research, Merck Research Laboratories, West Point, Pennsylvania, USA
5.17: Arenaviruses; 5.18: Filoviruses

Wayne M. Meyers Visiting Scientist, Department of Environmental and Infectious Disease Sciences, Armed Forces Institute of Pathology, Washington DC, USA
6.28: Buruli ulcer: Mycobacterium ulcerans infection

M.A. Miles Professor of Medical Protozoology, Pathogen Molecular Biology Unit, Department of Infectious and Tropical Diseases, London School of Hygiene and Tropical Medicine, London, UK
8.11: Chagas disease

Robert F. Miller Professor, Reader in Clinical Infection, Centre for Sexual Health and HIV Research, University College London, London, UK
7.5: Pneumocystis jirovecii

Philip Minor Division of Virology, National Institute for Biological Standards and Control, South Mimms, UK
5.8: Enterovirus infections

D.H. Molyneux Centre for Neglected Tropical Diseases, Liverpool School of Tropical Medicine, Pembroke Place, Liverpool, UK
9.2: Lymphatic filariasis

Marina S. Morgan Consultant Medical Microbiologist, Royal Devon & Exeter Foundation NHS Trust, UK
6.18: Pasteurella

Pedro L. Moro Immunization Safety Office, Centre for Disease Control and Prevention, Atlanta, Georgia, USA
10.1: Cystic hydatid disease (Echinococcus granulosus)

Jean B. Nachega Associate Scientist, Department of International Health, Johns Hopkins University, Bloomberg School of Public Health, Baltimore, Maryland, USA; Extraordinary Professor, Department of Medicine, and Director, Centre for Infectious Diseases, Stellenbosch University, Tygerberg, Cape Town, South Africa
6.25: Tuberculosis

Robert B. Nadelman Division of Infectious Diseases, Department of Medicine, New York Medical College, Valhalla, New York, USA
6.32: Lyme borreliosis

N.V. Naoumov Immunology and Infectious Diseases, Novartis Pharma AG, Basel, Switzerland, and Honorary Professor of Hepatology, University College London, UK
5.21: Hepatitis viruses (excluding hepatitis C virus)

John Nowakowski Division of Infectious Diseases, Department of Medicine, New York Medical College, Valhalla, New York, USA
6.32: Lyme borreliosis

E.E. Ooi Associate Professor and Program Director (Biological Defence), DSO National Laboratories, Singapore
5.12: Alphaviruses; 5.14: Flaviviruses (excluding dengue)

Petra C.F. Oyston Defence Science and Technology Laboratories in the Biomedical Sciences Department, Dstl Porton Down, Salisbury, UK; Chair at the University of Leicester in the Department of Infection, Immunity and Inflammation
6.19: Francisella tularensis infection

Nigel O'Farrell Consultant Physician, Ealing Hospital, London, UK
6.13: Haemophilus ducreyi and chancroid

Philippe Parola Unité de Recherche en Maladies Infectieuses et Tropicales Emergentes, WHO Collaborative Centre for Rickettsioses and other Arthropod borne Bacteria, Faculté de Médecine, Université de la Mediterranie, Marseilles, France
6.39: Rickettsioses

C.M. Parry Oxford University Clinical Research Unit, Hospital for Tropical Diseases, Ho Chi Minh City, Vietnam
6.8: Typhoid and paratyphoid fevers

J. Paul Regional Microbiologist, Health Protection Agency, South East Region, Regional Microbiologist's Office, Royal Sussex County Hospital, Brighton, UK
6.46: A check list of bacteria associated with infection in humans; 12: Nonvenomous arthropods

S.J. Peacock Professor of Clinical Microbiology, Department of Medicine, University of Cambridge Cambridge, UK
6.7.2: Pseudomonas aeruginosa; 6.15: Melioidosis and glanders

Malik Peiris Department of Microbiology, The University of Hong Kong, Queen Mary Hospital Pokfualm, Hong Kong SAR
5.1: Respiratory tract viruses

Hugh Pennington Emeritus Professor of Bacteriology, University of Aberdeen, UK
6.7.1: Enterobacteria and bacterial food poisoning

Eskild Petersen Department of Infectious Diseases, Aarhus University Hospital, Skejby, Aarhus, Denmark
8.4: Toxoplasmosis

L.R. Petersen Director, Division of Vector-borne Infectious Diseases, Centers for Disease Control and Prevention, Fort Collins, Colorado, USA
5.12: Alphaviruses; 5.14: Flaviviruses (excluding dengue)

T.E.A. Peto Professor of Infectious Diseases, University of Oxford; Consultant Physician, Oxford Radcliffe Hospitals, Nuffield Department of Medicine, John Radcliffe Hospital, Oxford, UK
5.23: HIV/AIDS

Kyle J. Popovich Assistant Professor, Rush University Medical Center - Infectious Disease, Chicago, Illinois, USA
6.4: Staphylococci

Françoise Portaels Mycobacteriology Unit, Department of Microbiology, Institute of Tropical Medicine Nationalestraat, Antwerpen, Belgium
6.28: Buruli ulcer: Mycobacterium ulcerans infection

William G. Powderly Professor of Medicine and Therapeutics, Dean of Medicine, UCD School of Medicine and Medical Sciences, University College Dublin, Dublin, Ireland
7.2: Cryptococcosis

Michael B. Prentice Professor of Medical Microbiology, Department of Microbiology, University College Cork, Cork, Ireland
6.16: Plague: Yersinia pestis; 6.17: Other yersinia infections: yersiniosis

M. Ramsay Consultant Epidemiologist, Immunisation, Hepatitis and Blood Safety Department, HPA Centre for Infections, London, UK
3: Immunization

Didier Raoult Faculté de Médecine et de Pharmacie, Université de la Méditerranée, Marseille Cedex, France
6.39: Rickettsioses; 6.42: Bartonellas excluding B. bacilliformis

Todd W. Rice Assistant Professor of Medicine, Division of Allergy, Pulmonary, and Critical Care Medicine, Vanderbilt University School of Medicine, Nashville, Tennessee, USA
1.2: Physiological changes, clinical features, and general management of infected patients

J. Richens Centre for Sexual Health and HIV Research, Research Department of Infection & Population Health, University College London, London, UK
6.9: Intracellular klebsiella infections (donovanosis and rhinoscleroma)

A.B. Rickinson Institute for Cancer Studies, University of Birmingham, Birmingham, UK
5.3: Epstein–Barr virus

B.K. Rima Deputy Head of the School of Medicine, Dentistry and Biomedical Sciences, Belfast, Ireland
5.5: Mumps: epidemic parotitis

Jean-Marc Rolain Faculté de Médecine et de Pharmacie, Université de la Méditerranée, Marseille Cedex, France
6.42: Bartonellas excluding B. bacilliformis

K.P. Schaal Emeritus Professor of Medical Microbiology; Member of the Expert Committee of the Federal Ministry of Labour and Social Affairs Institute for Medical Microbiology, Immunology and Parasitology, University Hospital, Bonn, Germany
6.29: Actinomycoses

Anthony Scott Wellcome Trust Senior Research Fellow in Clinical Science, KEMRI Wellcome Trust Research Programme, Kilifi, Kenya; Nuffield Department of Clinical Medicine, University of Oxford, Oxford, UK
6.3: Pneumococcal infections

Keerti V. Shah Department of Molecular Microbiology and Immunology, Johns Hopkins Bloomberg School of Public Health, Baltimore, Maryland, USA
5.19: Papillomaviruses and polyomaviruses

Jackie Sherrard Consultant in Genitourinary Medicine, Churchill Hospital, Oxford, UK
6.6: Neisseria gonorrhoeae

M.A. Shikanai-Yasuda Professor of Department of Infectious and Parasitic Diseases, Endemic Diseases Group/Infections in Immunosupressed Host Programme, Faculdade de Medicina, University of São Paulo, Brazil
7.4: Paracoccidioidomycosis

Udomsak Silachamroon Assistant Professor of Tropical Medicine, Department of Clinical Tropical Medicine, Faculty of Tropical Medicine, Mahidol University, Bangkok, Thailand
11.3: Lung flukes (paragonimiasis)

Robert E. Sinden The Malaria Centre, Department of Life Sciences, Imperial College London, London, UK
8.2: Malaria

Thira Sirisanthana Professor of Medicine, Chiang Mai University, Thailand
6.20: Anthrax; 7.6: Penicillium marneffei infection

J.G.P. Sissons Regius Professor of Physic, Director, Cambridge University Health Partners, School of Clinical Medicine, University of Cambridge, Cambridge, UK
5.2: Herpesviruses (excluding Epstein–Barr virus)

Geoffrey L. Smith Wellcome Principal Research Fellow, Section of Virology, Faculty of Medicine, Imperial College London, London, UK
5.4: Poxviruses

Robert W. Snow Head, Malaria Public Health Group, KEMRI/Wellcome Trust Programme and Advisor, National Malaria Control Programme, Ministry of Health, Nairobi, Kenya
8.2: Malaria

Dennis L. Stevens Chief, Infectious Diseases Section, Veterans Affairs Medical Center, Boise, Professor of Medicine, University of Washington School of Medicine, Seattle, Washington, USA
6.2: Streptococci and enterococci; 6.24: Botulism, gas gangrene, and clostridial gastrointestinal infections

August Stich Department of Tropical Medicine, Medical Mission Institute, Würzburg, Germany
8.10: Human African trypanosomiasis

Pravan Suntharasamai Mahidol University, Bangkok, Thailand
9.7: Gnathostomiasis

C.T. Tan Professor, Department of Medicine, University of Malaya, Kuala Lumpur, Malaysia
5.7: Nipah and Hendra virus encephalitides

David Taylor-Robinson Emeritus Professor of Genito-Microbiology and Medicine, Imperial College London, Division of Medicine, London, UK
6.44: Chlamydial infections; 6.45: Mycoplasmas

C.L. Thwaites Oxford University Clinical Research Unit, Ho Chi Minh City, Vietnam
6.22: Tetanus

P.A. Tookey Senior Lecturer, MRC Centre of Epidemiology for Child Health, UCL Institute of Child Health, London, UK
5.13: Rubella

Jakko van Ingen Clinician and Research Associate, Radboud University, Nijmegen Medical Centre, Department of Medical Microbiology, The Netherlands.
6.26: Disease caused by environmental mycobacteria

Steven Vanderschueren General Internal Medicine, University Hospital Gasthuisberg, Leuven, Belgium
2.2: Fever of unknown origin

Sirivan Vanijanonta Emeritus Professor of Tropical Medicine, Department of Clinical Tropical Medicine, Faculty of Tropical Medicine, Mahidol University, Bangkok, Thailand
11.3: Lung flukes (paragonimiasis)

B.J. Vennervald DBL-Centre for Health Research and Development, Faculty of Life Sciences University of Copenhagen, Thorvaldsensvej, Denmark
11.1: Schistosomiasis

Anilrudh A. Venugopal Division of Infectious Diseases, St. John Hospital and Medical Center; and Assistant Professor, Wayne State University School of Medicine, Detroit, Michigan, USA
6.10: Anaerobic bacteria

Kristien Verdonck Institute of Tropical Medicine Antwerp Nationalestraat, Antwerp, Belgium; Instituto de Medicina Tropical Alexander von Humboldt Universidad Peruana Cayetano Heredia Av. Honorio Delgado, San Martín de Porres Lima, Peru
5.25: HTLV-1, HTLV-2, and associated diseases

Raphael P. Viscidi Department of Pediatrics, Johns Hopkins University School of Medicine, Baltimore, Maryland, USA
5.19: Papillomaviruses and polyomaviruses

David A. Warrell Emeritus Professor of Tropical Medicine, Nuffield Department of Clinical Medicine; Honorary Fellow, St Cross College, University of Oxford, Oxford, UK
4: Travel and expedition medicine; 5.10: Rhabdoviruses: rabies and rabies-related lyssaviruses; 5.11: Colorado tick fever and other arthropod-borne reoviruses; 5.27: Orf; 5.28: Molluscum contagiosum; 6.31: Rat-bite fevers; 6.33: Relapsing fevers; 6.35: Nonvenereal endemic treponematoses: yaws, endemic syphilis (bejel), and pinta; 8.2: Malaria; 13: Pentastomiasis (porocephalosis, linguatulosis/linguatuliasis)

M. J. Warrell Oxford Vaccine Group, University of Oxford, Centre for Clinical Vaccinology & Tropical Medicine, Churchill Hospital, Oxford, UK
5.10: Rhabdoviruses: rabies and rabies-related lyssaviruses; 5.11: Colorado tick fever and other arthropod-borne reoviruses

George Watt Associate Professor of Medicine, University of Hawaii at Manoa, John A. Burns School of Medicine, Hawaii, USA
6.34: Leptospirosis; 6.40: Scrub typhus

Robert A. Weinstein The C. Anderson Hedberg Professor of Internal Medicine, Rush Medical College, Interim Chair, Department of Medicine, John H. Stroger Jr. Hospital of Cook County, Professor, Rush University Medical Center, Chicago, Illinois, USA
6.4: Staphylococci

R.A. Weiss Professor of Viral Oncology, Division of Infection and Immunity, University College London, London, UK
5.26: Viruses and cancer

H.C. Whittle Visiting Professor, London School of Hygiene and Tropical Medicine, MRC Laboratories, The Gambia, West Africa
5.6: Measles

Bridget Wills Hospital for Tropical Diseases, Oxford University Clinical Research Unit, Wellcome Trust Major Overseas Programme, Vietnam, Ho Chi Minh City, Vietnam
5.15: Dengue

Gary P. Wormser Division of Infectious Diseases, Department of Medicine, New York Medical College, Valhalla, New York, USA
6.32: Lyme borreliosis

Lam Minh Yen Hospital of Tropical Disease, Ho Chi Minh City, Vietnam
6.22: Tetanus

1

Pathogenic microorganisms and the host

Contents

1.1 Biology of pathogenic microorganisms

Duncan J. Maskell

Essentials

Microorganisms are present at most imaginable sites on the planet, and have evolved to occupy these ecological niches successfully. A host animal is simply another ecological niche to be occupied.

The ability to cause disease may in some cases be an accidental bystander event, or it may be the result of evolutionary processes that have led to specific mechanisms allowing the pathogen to exploit the rich source of nutrients present in the host, before moving on to another fresh host.

Pathogenicity often relies on a series of steps, with specific and often distinct mechanisms operating at each of them. Some types of pathogen must adapt to the host environment by altering gene expression, and all must retain the ability to be transmitted readily between hosts. Specific mechanisms have evolved in microorganisms for the exploitation of the host and for evasion or avoidance of the innate and acquired immune systems.

The advent and application of hyper-rapid and ultra-high throughput whole-genome scale sequencing technologies is providing a mass of information, which—when sensibly and carefully gathered and used—will change fundamentally our way of looking at infectious diseases and our understanding of how pathogens work. This should enable the development of new intervention strategies, especially vaccines and antimicrobials, but the complexity of some of the biological mechanisms involved may make this a difficult exercise. Furthermore, pathogens may vary and evolve rapidly, and thus are likely to remain one step ahead of these strategies.

We live in a rapidly changing world. New pathogens will emerge to exploit new circumstances presented by changes in society, and ancient scourges will remain and re-emerge to plague us. Many of the new infectious disease challenges will arise from animals, and will be zoonoses, at least in the early stages of their emergence. It is therefore probably more important in this field than in any other to develop the vision of "One Medicine", with medical and veterinary clinicians and basic scientists working together, if we are to give ourselves the best chance of success in warding off threats from global infectious diseases.

Introduction

Microorganisms occupy almost all imaginable ecological niches. Microbes have been isolated from deep-sea sites, where they survive very high pressures, from extremely cold and extremely hot regions, where hyperthermophiles grow optimally at temperatures well in excess of 100°C, and even from rocks, where they can exploit chemical substrates for energy generation. It is no wonder, then, that microorganisms should also exploit other living organisms as potential habitats, from viruses that use other microorganisms (e.g. bacteriophage) as hosts through to microorganisms that occupy various ecological niches within and upon the mammalian body, sometimes to the benefit and sometimes to the severe detriment of the host. Microorganisms have been supremely successful in evolutionary terms and they contain enormous untapped reserves of biodiversity, much of which is to be found in those that we can neither isolate nor grow and which make up the vast majority of microbes on the planet. Since microorganisms reproduce much more rapidly than their mammalian hosts and have several specialized mechanisms for horizontal gene transfer, it is not surprising that they are often able to evolve quickly to stay one step ahead of any mechanisms that exist, or are invented by humans, to control them.

The control of infectious diseases over the last century or so has been a major achievement, relying mainly on improved public health systems and social conditions, as well as on technological advances such as antimicrobial drugs and vaccines. A wave of overconfidence led the United States Surgeon General, William H Stewart, to announce in the 1960s that the war against infectious diseases had been won. This optimistic proclamation was bolstered by the eradication of smallpox in 1977, achieved by a monumental worldwide public health and vaccination programme. But, as Aldous Huxley wrote, "Hubris against the … order of Nature would be followed by its appropriate Nemesis", and so it is was that very soon afterwards we had to learn to cope with the global catastrophe that is AIDS, along with the resurgence of ancient killers such as tuberculosis, and the emergence of apparently new threats such as bovine spongiform encephalopathy (BSE) and West Nile fever. In 2009, the world found itself dealing with the long-predicted global pandemic of influenza which severely stretched and tested the ingenuity and organizational abilities of international human society in its attempts to control the spread and impact of the virus. That this pandemic had a relatively minor impact, despite rapid and widespread dissemination and transmission, was largely due to the generally mild nature of disease caused by this virus. Lessons for public health regarding control are still being learned from this incident.

Pathogenicity in stages

It is important to break down pathogenesis into different steps and stages. Most viral and bacterial pathogens enter the host via the mucosa of the respiratory, gastrointestinal, or genitourinary tracts, although some important pathogens are introduced by injection from insect vectors or through abraded or wounded skin. Most pathogens then have to stick to a surface and have evolved structures to do so; these are usually constructed from proteins and many of them are complex and specialized. In bacteria, these protein molecules are known as adhesins and are often but not always delivered at the end of long proteinaceous organelles called pili or fimbriae. The precise amino acid sequence of the adhesin, and hence its structure, can dictate which host and even which tissues within the host the bacterium sticks to and can, therefore, play a major role in dictating host range and tissue tropism. For example, enterotoxigenic *Escherichia coli* (ETEC) expressing K88 fimbriae will stick to piglet intestine and cause disease, those expressing K99 will stick to calf and lamb intestine, and those expressing colonization factor antigen (CFA) I and CFAII will stick to human intestine. Similarly, *E. coli* expressing P fimbriae (otherwise known as PAP pili) will stick efficiently to the human urinary tract and cause infection at that site. After initial loose adherence, enteropathogenic *E. coli* (EPEC) will stick more firmly to the intestinal surface via the nonfimbrial adhesin, intimin. The receptor for intimin on the host cell surface is a protein called Tir, which is itself an *E. coli* protein that has been translocated into the host cell via a specialized needle-like structure, a type 3 secretory system (T3SS), which is itself closely related to bacterial flagella. This complex, coordinated series gives an insight into the extraordinary sequences that have evolved to enable bacteria to exploit their hosts as ecological niches.

Viruses also rely on surface structures for host specificity. An example of current interest is influenza virus. Among several other mechanisms, the host range and molecule. On the respiratory epithelium, haemagglutinin binds to sialic acid which is linked to galactose on the host cell surface via either an α2,3 or an α2,6 linkage. Human influenza viruses bind preferentially to the α2,6-linked molecule, which is abundant on human tracheal epithelium, whereas avian influenza viruses bind preferentially to the α2,3-linked version, which is abundant on duck intestinal epithelium. The different binding capacities of the haemagglutinin molecules are also important in the transmissibility of the virus, which is clearly a major element in determining whether or not an epidemic will occur. Interestingly, pig trachea expresses plenty of both types of molecule, which may explain in part why pigs are susceptible to both avian and human influenza viruses, and why pigs may be a major source of reassorted virus that could jump species, including from avian to human. A caveat here is that a recent study suggests that the distribution of human and avian influenza viruses in the pig respiratory tract is such that they probably infect different cell types. For virus reassortment to occur, the same cell must be infected by both the avian and human types of virus, and therefore this observation may raise a serious problem for the dogma that the pig may be the 'mixing vessel'. A further recent observation indicates that the precise cell tropism in the human respiratory tract for viruses of different host origin may correlate with the type of disease caused, and possibly the amount of virus that can be shed, leading to different disease severities and potentially different transmission dynamics.

Once established at a surface, pathogens have a wide array of possible strategies. They can stay at that surface and cause very little damage, and indeed be carried without causing any clinical signs. Bacteria such as *Haemophilus influenzae* and *Neisseria meningitidis* are good examples of this. Only as a result of some unknown and rare set of circumstances will these bacteria move into the bloodstream to cause septicaemia and sometimes meningitis. To survive and spread in the blood, bacteria have evolved a range of molecular strategies to inhibit the activation and activity of complement, and to avoid or resist phagocytosis. Alternatively, the bacteria can stay at the mucosal surface and cause considerable damage—by direct invasion and destruction of the tissue, by inducing a damaging inflammatory response, or by elaborating a toxin. The precise pathology caused, and consequently the clinical signs, depends on the precise nature of the toxin and the site at which it has its effects. Thus ETEC makes labile toxin (LT) and stable toxin (ST) which will usually result in watery diarrhoea, whereas enterohaemorrhagic *E. coli* (EHEC) can make Shiga toxin, which is spread systemically and acts at a distance from the gut with severe consequences such as thrombocytopenia and kidney damage, leading to haemolytic uraemic syndrome (HUS). Other bacteria invade and spread systemically, finally lodging in particular tissues and causing direct pathology or inducing inflammatory responses that result in immunopathology (e.g. the lesions associated with systemic salmonella infections such as typhoid fever). These pathologies often result from the binding of host receptors (pattern recognition receptors, PRRs) to relatively invariant structures on the invading organisms (pathogen-associated molecular patterns, PAMPs), such as endotoxin, peptidoglycan, flagella, or in viruses double-stranded RNA, leading to expression of a range of cytokines that mediate the inflammatory response. If this process gets out of control, or happens at the wrong time and in the wrong place, severe pathology can result. An example of this is the systemic inflammation that leads to sepsis, with attendant tissue damage, circulatory collapse, and often death.

Each of the different stages of infection relies on the bacterial pathogen being able to adapt physiologically and metabolically to the different niches in which it finds itself, and having the appropriate structures to survive the onslaught of innate and adaptive immune responses. It is becoming increasingly apparent that many bacteria can adapt gene expression profiles rapidly, and have sophisticated molecular mechanisms for rapid switching of many of the structures that are required for virulence or are recognized by the immune system.

Virulence factors versus fitness factors

Almost any gene product that has been identified as being required for infection has been called a 'virulence factor' in the literature. However, this is imprecise and can be misleading. For bacteria, many of the genes required for host exploitation might be better considered as 'fitness factors', but are no less important in the consideration of infectious diseases and how to combat them. Bacteria can often grow outside their hosts and so not all their genes are necessarily required for fitness inside the host. Those that are include classic virulence factors such as adhesins and toxins, and also various metabolic genes and pathways that enable the bacterium to survive for long enough and grow in the host causing damage.

Viruses on the other hand are obligate host parasites. They tend (with notable exceptions such as herpesviruses and poxviruses with genomes of 100–200 kb) to have rather small genomes with few genes. Therefore, in most viruses, each gene is required for exploitation of the host in some way and is highly likely to be a fitness factor in the sense of evolutionary fitness. It may well be appropriate to consider them as virulence factors in pathogenesis.

In considering virulence vs fitness in evolution, we might ask, 'Why do pathogens cause damage rather than simply existing in harmony with their host?' This question might be framed better as, 'What evolutionary pathway has resulted in pathogens that cause damage to their hosts?' There are many possible answers. The pathogen might have evolved to exploit a particular ecological niche rather than a particular host, but has found itself by accident in a host, which it then damages almost as a bystander event. Another answer might be that by inducing a certain pathology the pathogen liberates more nutrients for itself and/or facilitates its transmission to another host (preferably in most cases before it kills its original host). Whatever the truth is behind these evolutionary pathways, it is essential that people working with infectious diseases should recognize that there is more to the evolution of a pathogen than the acquisition of a toxin or two.

Adaptation to the environment

A major shift in the minds of infectious disease researchers in recent years has been the realization that pathogens are far from the relatively static entities they were once thought to be. It is now clear, from many different examples, that bacterial pathogens sense the environment in which they live, and alter gene expression profiles accordingly to enable exploitation of and survival in that environment. For example, a food-poisoning bacterium such as *Salmonella enterica* might be living on a nutrient-rich piece of meat, but at a cold temperature. The meat might then be cooked, providing the bacterium with heat stress. If the meat is undercooked the salmonellae will survive the heat stress by expression of different heat-shock operons, which incidentally might also lead to the expression of genes required to survive subsequent assaults in the host. On entry into the mouth, defences such as lysozyme and IgA must be overcome, and on entry into the stomach, a very low pH is encountered. Gene expression will again change in the salmonellae such that genes for acid tolerance and acid resistance are now to the fore. Once the bacteria exit the stomach, the pH will change again and they will be assaulted by bile salts and many other defence mechanisms until they arrive at their point of attachment to the small intestine. Although there are very few experimental data about these phenomena in actual host animals, experiments *in vitro* and a few experiments in cells or in animal models are beginning to reveal the complex changes that must take place in gene expression for a bacterium to establish itself in a host animal.

Many of these changes are orchestrated through well-understood environmental sensory and signal transduction systems. One of the most common is the two-component sensory system. One component is a membrane protein that senses external environmental cues and the second is an intracellular protein that binds to DNA and either activates or represses the transcription and expression of sets of genes, usually called regulons. A signal is transmitted from the sensor to the activator/repressor when the environment changes. Signal transduction is achieved via histidine protein kinases. These two-component systems are very common in bacteria. Those bacteria that can live in numerous environments tend to have many more of them (e.g. *c.*90 in *Pseudomonas*), whereas those bacteria that have become adapted to a lifestyle in a particular host have very few (e.g. 2 in *Chlamydia*, 0 in *Mycoplasma*) and there is often a concomitant loss of genomic size. A better understanding of how bacteria behave and of the genes that are actually expressed inside the host will very likely lead to breakthroughs in the design of new antimicrobials and vaccines.

Interaction with the immune system: antigenic variation

The survival of pathogens in hosts is made particularly challenging by the existence of the immune system. Pathogens have responded to this challenge by evolving many specific mechanisms for the avoidance, evasion, or subversion of both innate and acquired host resistance mechanisms. For example, some viruses are inherently genetically unstable. The natures of the polymerases that replicate the RNA genomes of influenza virus and lentiviruses such as HIV result in errors being incorporated at a high rate. Many of these errors will be incompatible with the continued existence of the virus as an entity capable of self-reproduction. Consequently, many defective viruses can be detected, but often the base pair changes may not effectively alter the functionality of the viral protein affected other than to alter its antigenicity and this may confer fitness benefits in the face of population-level immunity, leading to selection of the variant viruses. In this way, over time, these viruses evade the immunity that develops in response to infection. Viruses such as influenza have evolved segmented genomes. If two viruses happen to be occupying the same host cell, different segments can reassort and a new virus can be assembled. An intriguing question is how the proper segments are gathered together and packaged into the assembled virion, given that segments from different viruses can reassort. This type of large-scale reassortment leads to the antigenic shifts that overcome even solid levels of herd immunity and allow epidemics of influenza to occur. At a different level, within-host antigenic variation is thought to be one mechanism that allows HIV to continue to be carried chronically in the face of what might appear to be a strong immune response. Many other pathogens may also escape the immune response by antigenic variation within the host. Bacteria such as *Haemophilus influenzae*, *Neisseria meningitidis*, and *Campylobacter jejuni* have evolved tracts of repetitive DNA in single base pair repeats or repeats of four or more base pairs. The number of these repeats can change, apparently randomly. This is a powerful mechanism that allows the existence of a population of bacteria with a number of different antigens that may be 'randomly' expressed or not expressed in individuals within the population. This may be a kind of altruistic evasion strategy whereby some members of the population are lacking a particular structure which is itself a target for the immune system, such that they will survive and thus continue the existence of that bacterial population. Other mechanisms involving recombination and gene conversion exist in other pathogens, leading to the expression of alternative antigenic versions of the same protein and underlying the cycling of different forms of, e.g. variant surface glycoprotein in trypanosomes and the opportunistic fungal pathogen *Pneumocystis jirovecii* or pili in neisseriae.

Pathogens have also evolved mechanisms to subvert the immune system by mimicking elements of the innate response. Good examples are herpes and poxviruses that encode chemokine homologues and/or chemokine receptor homologues or analogues.

Genomes

Many bacterial, viral, fungal, and protozoal genome sequences are now complete. New genome sequencing technologies that are currently coming on stream are increasing massively our ability to generate raw sequence data. The availability of genome-scale sequence data for these pathogens has revolutionized our understanding of their biology and has opened up completely new methods of study and ways of thinking about how they interact with their hosts. Immediate benefits of having complete genome sequences include the obvious knowledge of the complete gene set. This means that we now 'know' every conceivable target for the immune system and every conceivable target for novel antimicrobial development. The real challenge for researchers and infectious disease physicians is to sift and unravel the whole mass of information and to select from it that which is genuinely useful. Once complete genome information is available, it will be interesting to see whether current vaccine target antigens, which have been derived empirically, really are the best targets. For example, *Bordetella pertussis* pertactin is one of a family of proteins called autotransporters. It is a very important component of the acellular whooping cough vaccine, and was discovered through much experimentation by several groups over many years. The genome sequence of *B. pertussis* contains a large number of other autotransporters, any one of which might be a vaccine candidate, and could conceivably be better than pertactin. Much research needs to be done to clarify these questions.

It might be better to invent strategies to let the host biology and the genome itself indicate which genes and antigens are likely to be useful as vaccine targets. Some of these methods are now being published and a good example is 'reverse vaccinology'. Here, genes for outer membrane proteins from a pathogen of interest are selected using computer algorithms, cloned using the polymerase chain reaction (PCR) or synthesized *de novo*, and the encoded protein

expressed and purified. These proteins can then be used to interrogate sera from animals or humans that have been infected and are convalescent, to identify which of them is expressed as an antigen during infection, although this step is not essential. The proteins can subsequently be used to immunize animals with the intention of testing the resultant immune response for its ability to protect against virulent challenge in different infection models. The choice of readout and model is of course crucial if an effective vaccine for humans is to be designed. Despite many possible pitfalls, reverse vaccinology is an exciting technology platform with great promise for the exploitation of genomes to generate completely new candidate vaccines against bacteria. Indeed a new vaccine against group B meningococcus has been developed using this strategy and was reported in 2008 as already having been through a successful phase II clinical trial.

Another fascinating story, emerging from the availability of many genome sequences and coupled with technology such as microarrays, has been the recognition of diversity within bacterial species and the evolutionary relationships between bacteria that this implies. It is clear that many bacterial species share their DNA promiscuously and that this can lead to rapid evolution of drug resistance and altered pathogenicity. Many tried and trusted schemes for classifying and typing bacteria need to be reassessed in the light of genomic information. Classic typing schemes, such as Kaufman–White for salmonellae, based on recognition of antigens on the bacteria by standardized antibodies, are being replaced by DNA-based methods such as multilocus sequence typing, analysis of single nucleotide polymorphisms (SNPs), and microarray-based approaches, and even these methods will soon be replaced by the rapid and inexpensive acquisition of whole-genome sequence data for clinical isolates. DNA sequencing technology is improving at an astonishing rate, and ultra-high-throughput sequencing machines are now available that make the determination of a draft genome for a bacterium less expensive than a routine microbiological workup. Real-time whole-genome sequencing is already at a stage where it could be used to inform infection control measures. A study of *Staphylococcus aureus* in which 63 isolates of MRSA were sequenced gave clear-cut information about the geographic origin of the isolates and definitive information about person-to-person spread in the hospital environment. A similar study on *Streptococcus pneumoniae*, in which 240 genome sequences were determined, has been able to follow how the bacteria have adapted to clinical interventions, in the form of vaccines and antimicrobials, over very short time scales. This kind of approach will become routine in hospitals much sooner than we might think, and will revolutionize how we think about infections and their control.

Future challenges

Most infectious diseases are unlikely to be eradicated in the near future. Even if they were, new infectious agents would inevitably evolve to exploit the rich environments presented by host animals. Infectious disease biology and medicine are currently undergoing a renaissance, driven by the revolution in genome science, allied to the real and present dangers still presented by many pathogens. Infectious diseases still kill more people worldwide than any other class of disease. They have the capacity to deliver sudden severe global pandemics resulting in high global mortality. Emerging infections presenting acute public health problems are likely to be viral in nature, to have originated in an animal population and, therefore, at least initially, to be zoonoses, and to be spread quickly via air travel. Changing social conditions, e.g. increasing urbanization in certain parts of Africa, bring together animal and human populations that have rarely if ever been closely associated. This brings with it an increased chance for microorganisms to be shared between these species, with a resulting increased chance of new pathogens emerging. Even relatively minor changes in societal behaviour can lead to major disease problems. For example, changes to methods for preparing cattle feed led to the emergence of the BSE prion as a human disease problem in recent years in the United Kingdom and elsewhere.

This analysis does not take into account the added problem of possible biowarfare attacks, although the paranoia surrounding this subject is disproportionate to the threat.

To deal with these disease threats, the regulatory framework underlying the development and legal deployment of antimicrobials and vaccines will have to be adapted and evolved in step with the evolution of the diseases themselves. The pathogens are likely to win this race too! Artificial distinctions between 'human' and 'veterinary' medicine need to be removed. Most pathogens infect more than one species of host animal and certainly do not respect the anthropocentric division of research effort. The concept of 'One Medicine', introduced by Calvin Schwabe, is nowhere more pertinent than in consideration of infectious diseases and the biology of pathogens.

A concerted effort is needed to deal with pathogens in all parts of the world and not just in the developed world. Inexpensive but effective intervention strategies must be developed to defeat acute and chronic infectious diseases worldwide. The lives affected by pathogenic microorganisms in developing countries are just as valuable as those in more affluent areas, but are much more numerous. It is our task, whether from a medical, veterinary, or basic science background, to try to understand how pathogenic microorganisms work, and to harness that knowledge to defeat, wherever possible and by whatever means, these ever-adaptable scourges.

Further reading

Croucher NJ, *et al.* (2011). Rapid pneumococcal evolution in response to clinical interventions. *Science*, **331**, 430–4.

Dean P, Maresca M, Kenny B (2005). EPEC's weapons of mass subversion. *Curr Opin Microbiol*, **8**, 28–34.

Galan JE, Wolf-Watz H (2006). Protein delivery into eukaryotic cells by type III secretion machines. *Nature*, **444**, 567–73.

Harris SR, *et al.* (2010) Evolution of MRSA during hospital transmission and intercontinental spread. *Science*, **327**, 469–74.

Janeway CA, Medzhitov R (2002). Innate immune recognition. *Annu Rev Immunol*, **20**, 197–216.

Kuiken T, *et al.* (2006). Host species barriers to influenza virus infections. *Science*, **312**, 394–7.

Mora M, *et al.* (2006). Microbial genomes and vaccine design: refinements to the classical reverse vaccinology approach. *Curr Opin Microbiol*, **9**, 532–6.

Moxon R, Bayliss C, Hood D (2006). Bacterial contingency loci: the role of simple sequence DNA repeats in bacterial adaptation. *Annu Rev Genet*, **40**, 307–33.

Murphy PM (2001). Viral exploitation and subversion of the immune system through chemokine mimicry. *Nat Immunol*, **2**, 116–22.

Neumann G, Kawaoka Y (2006). Host range restriction and pathogenicity in the context of influenza pandemic. *Emerg Infect Dis*, **12**, 881–6.

Roumagnac P, *et al.* (2006). Evolutionary history of *Salmonella typhi*. *Science*, **314**, 1301–4.

van Riel D, *et al.* (2007). Human and avian influenza viruses target different cells in the lower respiratory tract of humans and other mammals. *Am J Pathol*, **171**, 1215–23.

1.2 Physiological changes, clinical features, and general management of infected patients

Todd W. Rice and Gordon R. Bernard

Essentials

Pathophysiological mechanisms

The host response to an infectious stimulus involves an intricate link between the inflammatory and coagulation systems, also mechanisms designed to limit damage to normal tissues. Key elements are: (1) the inflammatory cascade—antigens from infectious agents stimulate macrophages and monocytes (and other cells) via Toll-like receptors to release tumour necrosis factor α (TNFα), resulting in a cascade of pro-inflammatory cytokine release which is a vital component of the host's attempt to control and eradicate infection, but unfortunately can also result in damage to both infected and uninfected host tissues; inflammatory mediators with prolonged actions or appearing later in the course of sepsis are likely to play an important role in determining prognosis; (2) the anti-inflammatory cascade—a compensatory response involving anti-inflammatory cytokines, soluble receptors, and receptor antagonists directed against pro-inflammatory cytokines that is intended to localize and control the systemic proinflammatory response to the infection; (3) the coagulation cascade—activated in an attempt to contain infection locally and prevent spread to other parts of the body; platelets are activated, procoagulant pathways are initiated, and anticoagulant mediators are down-regulated; (4) the anticoagulation cascade—the coagulation response to sepsis is regulated via antithrombin, tissue factor pathway inhibitor (TFPI), activated protein C (APC), and fibrinolysis.

Clinical features

Definitions—(1) Systemic inflammatory response syndrome (SIRS)—which can occur as a result of an infectious or noninfectious insult—requires the presence of at least two of the following: (a) hyper- or hypothermia, (b) tachycardia, (c) tachypnoea or hyperventilation, (d) leucocytosis, leucopenia or left shift. (2) Sepsis—a suspected or confirmed infection plus criteria for SIRS. (3) Severe sepsis—sepsis resulting in the acute dysfunction of at least one organ system. (4) Septic shock—infection resulting in hypotension despite adequate fluid resuscitation.

Management—key elements are (1) antibiotics—often initiated empirically before culture results are available; (2) control of the source of infection—searching for the site of infection so that it can be eradicated should begin as soon as haemodynamic and respiratory status are stabilized; antibiotics without source control often fail; (3) early goal-directed resuscitation—requiring (a) crystalloid infusions to maintain central venous pressure, (b) vasopressors if arterial pressure remains low, and (c) transfusion of packed red blood cells and/or infusion of dobutamine if central venous oxygen saturation remains low; (4) consideration of other treatments—many specialists advocate recombinant APC for patients with severe sepsis who have a low risk of bleeding and a high risk of death.

Introduction

The term sepsis describes the physiological consequences of the activation of the systemic inflammatory cascade that occurs in infected patients. The cascade of events in response to infectious stimuli has been well characterized using both animal and human models. This response is the main focus of this chapter. Other aspects of sepsis, including epidemiology, clinical features, treatment, prognosis, and the controversial role of corticosteroids and tight glycaemic control will also be addressed.

Pathophysiology of infection

Initial investigations suggested that inflammatory cytokines mediated the physiological responses seen in patients with sepsis. However, information from studies of the coagulation system in sepsis and the subsequent examination of autopsy specimens demonstrated microthrombi in the arterioles and venules of various organs, suggesting that the coagulation system played at least some role in the pathophysiology. It is now clear that the inflammatory and coagulation systems are intricately linked and homeostasis of both is altered in infected patients.

Inflammatory cascade

Early phase

Sepsis syndrome describes the physiological effects of the systemic inflammatory cascade produced by the human body in response to any of a variety of infectious stimuli. Antigens from infectious agents stimulate macrophages and monocytes to release tumour necrosis factor-α (TNFα) resulting in a cascade of cytokine release. Numerous cell wall antigens are able to stimulate this response, including lipopolysaccharide (LPS) or endotoxin from Gram-negative bacteria, lipoteichoic acid from Gram-positive bacteria, peptidoglycan and flagellin from both Gram-negative and Gram-positive bacteria, and mannan from fungi. These antigens initiate an inflammatory response via type I transmembrane receptors called Toll-like receptors found on the surface of a variety of cell types including macrophages, neutrophils, fibroblasts, and some epithelial and endothelial cells. Numerous Toll-like receptors have been identified, but subtypes 2 (TLR2) and 4 (TLR4) appear to play a major role in mediating the inflammatory response to infectious stimuli. TLR2 binds both peptidoglycan and lipoteichoic acid from Gram-positive bacteria. On the other hand, TLR4 serves as the signal transduction component for LPS from Gram-negative bacteria. In macrophages and neutrophils, binding of LPS to TLR4 results in the release of TNFα via NF-κB, a eukaryotic transcription factor. Circulating TNFα stimulates the release of other proinflammatory cytokines from macrophages and neutrophils. These proinflammatory cytokines, especially interleukins 1 and 6 (IL-1, IL-6), trigger numerous additional proinflammatory events within endothelial cells and leucocytes (Fig. 1.2.1). TNFα acts in conjunction with IL-1 to produce the fever, tachycardia, and tachypnoea seen with systemic inflammation. In addition, their synergistic effects are probably responsible for the hypotension and resultant organ dysfunction seen early in the course of severe sepsis. The purpose of this proinflammatory response, which represents a vital component

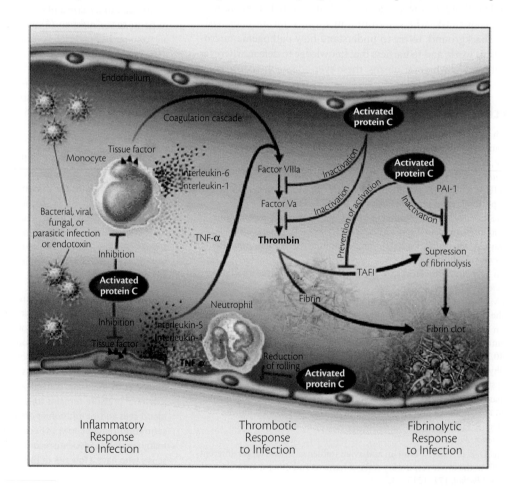

Fig. 1.2.1 The intricate link between the inflammatory and procoagulant response to infection with sites of action for activated protein C. PAI-1, plasminogen activator inhibitor type 1; TNF-α, tumour necrosis factor-α. (From Bernard GR, *et al.* (2001). Efficacy and safety of recombinant human activated protein C for severe sepsis. *N Engl J Med*, **344**, 699–709. Copyright © 2001 Massachusetts Medical Society. All rights reserved.)

of the host defence, is to control and eradicate the infection. Unfortunately, the response is often so exuberant and poorly controlled that it results in damage to both infected and uninfected host tissues.

Late phase

The symptoms of sepsis, specifically tachypnoea, tachycardia, fever, or hypotension, are what prompt most patients to seek medical attention. Unfortunately, these result from the early inflammatory cascade which is already well into its course by the time patients present for medical care. Administration of endotoxin to humans demonstrates that TNF is the primary protagonist of the inflammatory response as serum levels rise almost immediately. However, the presence of TNF in the serum is short-lived and the majority of patients with sepsis have undetectable levels at the time of presentation, even the most critically ill with organ failure or shock.

Many sepsis deaths occur later in the course, at least 48 to 72 h after the onset of symptoms. This has prompted many to speculate that inflammatory mediators with more prolonged actions or appearing later in the course of sepsis are likely to play an important role in determining prognosis. High-mobility group box protein 1 (HMGB1) is one such late mediator; it is a 30-kDa protein, named for its rapid migration on electrophoretic gels, which was purified along with histones from nuclei in the 1970s and is now classified as a nonhistone chromatin-associated protein. The critical role played by HMGB1 in gene transcription and DNA repair and replication has been known since shortly after its discovery. However, recent data suggest that HMGB1 also possesses inflammatory properties. Using nuclear pores, HMGB1 is able to move from the nucleus to the cytosol, making it available for extracellular secretion from macrophages when stimulated with LPS or TNF. Cell necrosis, but not apoptosis, results in the passive release of HMGB1 from all nucleated cells. Once outside the cell, HMGB1 functions as an important mediator of both inflammation and coagulation, stimulating the release of proinflammatory cytokines, including TNFα, IL-1, and IL-6 from endothelial cells and monocytes. HMGB1 also helps regulate coagulation by inducing the expression of adhesion molecules on endothelial cells, resulting in the secretion of plasminogen activator inhibitor type 1 (PAI-1) and tissue plasminogen activator.

Animal models of sepsis demonstrate that serum levels of HMGB1 increase after LPS administration. However, unlike TNF and IL-1 which peak early in the course of sepsis and become undetectable within a few hours, serum levels of HMGB1 remain undetectable until 8 h after LPS administration and continue to increase until they plateau 24 to 32 h later. Similar elevations in levels of HMGB1 can be detected in the serum of humans with severe sepsis or septic shock and in plasma and bronchoalveolar lavage fluid of patients with sepsis and acute lung injury. Serum levels of HMGB1 may also have prognostic significance as higher levels are associated with mortality.

Mice treated with sublethal doses of HMGB1 develop signs of endotoxaemia within 2 h and higher doses result in death within 18 to 36 h, even in mice resistant to the effects of LPS. Numerous animal models have also demonstrated that antagonizing the effects of HMGB1 improves survival in sepsis, even when the antagonism is considerably delayed. Anti-HMGB1 antibodies, ethyl pyruvate (a nontoxic food derivative that inhibits the release of HMGB1 from LPS-stimulated and TNF-stimulated macrophages), and

competitive inhibition of the HMGB1 binding site on macrophages all result in improved survival in animal models in which sepsis was induced with endotoxin and caecal ligation and puncture. However, treatment with these antagonists did not just extend the time to death, but allowed many of the animals to survive until necropsy and 'rescued' animals that already exhibited signs of severe sepsis.

Anti-inflammatory cascade

Although the initial inflammatory response in sepsis was originally believed to be largely uncontrolled, subsequent investigations have demonstrated that the body employs a compensatory anti-inflammatory response (CARS) in an attempt to maintain homeostasis. In addition to stimulating the release of other proinflammatory mediators, TNFα and IL-1 also stimulate leucocytes to release anti-inflammatory mediators, including IL-10, IL-13, and transforming growth factor β (TGFβ). These cytokines exert a direct anti-inflammatory effect on macrophages and endothelial cells and inhibit the synthesis of proinflammatory mediators. IL-10 and IL-13 also inhibit the ability of monocytes effectively to present antigens to other immune cells. Two new cytokines that might be therapeutic targets in the treatment of severe sepsis are IL-17 which promotes inflammation by triggering production of IL-1b, IL-6, and TNFα and macrophage migration inhibitory factor (MIF) which modulates TLR4. The inflammatory response is further controlled by the release of soluble receptors and receptor antagonists directed against proinflammatory cytokines. This compensatory anti-inflammatory response is intended to localize and control the systemic proinflammatory response to the infection. Unfortunately, the anti-inflammatory response often exceeds the proinflammatory response in the later phases of sepsis, resulting in a hyporesponsiveness of immune cells and an inability to mount an effective immune response to additional infectious insults. In a recent study, anti-CD3/anti-CD28- and lipopolysaccharide-stimulated splenocytes from patients dying of sepsis showed grossly impaired ability to secrete tumour necrosis factor, interferon, IL-6 and IL-10. Their spleens and lungs showed increased expression of inhibitory receptors and ligands and expansion of suppressor cell populations. Immunohistochemical staining showed extensive depletion of splenic CD4, CD8, and HLA-DR cells and expression of ligands for inhibitory receptors on lung epithelial cells. This lymphopenia and immunoparalysis late in the course of sepsis leads to delayed hypersensitivity, inability to clear infections, and an increased susceptibility to nosocomial infections, all of which contribute to the late morbidity and mortality in these patients.

Coagulation cascade

Earlier investigations implicated the inflammatory cascade in sepsis, but more recent work has demonstrated the involvement of the clotting and fibrinolytic systems which are intricately related to the inflammatory response (Fig. 1.2.1). As well as disrupting proinflammatory and anti-inflammatory homeostasis, sepsis also disturbs coagulation homeostasis. In response to infectious stimuli, the body rouses the coagulation cascade in an attempt to contain infection locally and prevent spread to other parts of the body. To accomplish this, platelets are activated, procoagulant pathways are initiated, and anticoagulant mediators are down-regulated. Unfortunately, this often results in a 'sepsis-associated coagulopathy', which may range from mild thrombocytopenia or increase in prothrombin time to overt disseminated intravascular coagulopathy. If the procoagulant response becomes too exuberant, microvascular thromboses can form resulting in local tissue hypoxia and subsequent organ dysfunction.

The activation of the coagulation response is intricately linked to the inflammatory response. TNFα and IL-1 both stimulate the release of tissue factor from monocytes and neutrophils and cause tissue factor normally present on endothelial cells, but not exposed to the circulation, to be 'unveiled' (Fig. 1.2.1). Tissue factor acts as the bridge between the inflammatory and coagulation pathways by activating the extrinsic clotting system and stimulating the formation of thrombin and fibrin clots. Specifically, the highly thrombogenic tissue factor (TF) combines with circulating factor VII to form a TF:VIIa complex. This complex activates factor X, which subsequently produces thrombin from prothrombin. Thrombin stimulates the formation of fibrin clots in the microcirculation with the aim of confining the infection to the local site. The disadvantage created by diffuse intravascular microthrombi is the creation of areas of regional hypoperfusion, resulting in tissue ischaemia, coagulation necrosis, and organ dysfunction.

Thrombin, TF:VIIa complex, and activated factor X also provide positive feedback to the inflammatory cascade. All three function as potent inflammatory mediators, stimulating neutrophil migration and release of additional proinflammatory cytokines. In turn, this positive feedback loop eventually fuels additional tissue factor release and more thrombin and fibrin clot formation.

Anticoagulation cascade

In similar fashion to its compensatory anti-inflammatory response, the body also regulates the coagulation response to sepsis. The anticoagulant response is mediated via four mechanisms: (1) antithrombin, (2) tissue factor pathway inhibitor (TFPI), (3) activated protein C (APC), and (4) fibrinolysis. Unfortunately, inflammation in sepsis suppresses many of these counter-regulatory measures, promoting a procoagulant environment. In sepsis, infection-induced inflammatory responses are procoagulant through tissue factor activation of factor VII and thence factor X and thrombin. This is enhanced by complement activation. Anticoagulant mechanisms such as protein C, antithrombin, and tissue factor pathway inhibitor are simultaneously impaired. Tissue factor, a transmembrane glycoprotein expressed by adventitial fibroblasts and vascular smooth muscle cells, comes into contact with blood through vascular damage, stimulation of mononuclear and endothelial cells by bacterial endotoxin or proinflammatory cytokines, or via microparticles shed from leucocytes, endothelial cells, vascular smooth muscle cells, and platelets. Neutrophils localize fibrin deposition to small blood vessels so limiting the spread of pathogens. Protease-activated receptors (PARs) 1–4 are activated by proteases such as thrombin, activated protein C, plasmin, trypsin, cathepsin-G, mast cell tryptase, leucocyte proteinase-3, and bacteria-derived enzymes. PARs increase vascular permeability via sphingosine 1 phosphate (S1P) receptors.

Antithrombin

Antithrombin is synthesized in the liver and secreted into the circulation. It occurs free in the plasma and attached to platelets and endothelial cells, where it functions as an inhibitor of the coagulation system. Antithrombin directly suppresses thrombin-induced fibrin formation, inhibits factors IXa, XIa, and XIIa of the intrinsic coagulation pathway, and decreases the activation of factor Xa which is common to both the intrinsic and extrinsic coagulation pathways. The serum half-life of antithrombin, normally 36 to 48 h, is reduced to 8 h or less in sepsis-associated coagulopathy, resulting in a rapid depletion of antithrombin and a shift towards a procoagulant microvascular environment. Despite data showing that low or falling antithrombin levels were associated with a worse outcome in severe sepsis, administration of exogenous antithrombin failed to improve the prognosis in these patients.

TFPI

Endothelial cells synthesize and secrete TFPI, which inhibits the TF:VIIa complex and activated factor X. This results in suppression of the extrinsic pathway of coagulation and decreases the formation of thrombin and fibrin clots. Sepsis results in a truncated form of TFPI, with reduced anticoagulant properties. Although overall TFPI levels are elevated in septic patients, their reduced anticoagulant effect still favours thrombin formation and fibrin deposition at the endothelium. Unfortunately, administration of a recombinant TFPI also failed to produce clinical benefit in a large trial of patients with severe sepsis.

APC

Protein C is synthesized in the liver through a vitamin K-dependent pathway and is secreted into the blood as an inactive zymogen. In the presence of endothelial protein C receptor (EPCR) and a properly functioning endothelium, protein C is converted to its active form by complexing with thrombin and endothelial cell thrombomodulin. APC inhibits PAI-1 and inactivates clotting factors Va and VIIIa (Fig. 1.2.1). These profibrinolytic and antithrombotic properties restore and maintain, respectively, microcirculatory blood flow which help re-establish coagulation homeostasis and preserve the microcirculation. APC also has anti-inflammatory properties, such as limiting the inflammatory response induced by thrombin and inhibiting TNF production (Fig. 1.2.1). Unfortunately, severe sepsis down-regulates EPCR causing it to be sloughed from the cell surface, resulting in endothelial dysfunction. Sepsis also decreases plasma concentrations of thrombomodulin. These changes impair the conversion of protein C to its active form, resulting in a deficiency of APC. Most patients with severe sepsis have low levels of protein C and lower levels are associated with poorer outcomes.

Fibrinolysis

Under normal homeostatic circumstances, dissolution of fibrin clots (fibrinolysis) serves as an additional counter-regulatory measure to the coagulation cascade. Plasminogen activators convert plasminogen to active plasmin which then mediates clot lysis by degrading the cross-linked fibrin present in the clot. This fibrinolytic response is controlled primarily by plasminogen activator inhibitors, predominantly PAI-1. The production of PAI-1 is stimulated by proinflammatory cytokines, resulting in elevated levels which decrease plasminogen and plasmin levels over time (Fig. 1.2.1). Some plasmin-induced fibrinolysis still occurs in this environment, but is often insufficient to maintain coagulation homeostasis.

Epidemiology

The incidence of sepsis is about 240 cases per 100 000 people per year. It is the second most common cause of death in critically ill patients, after cardiovascular events, resulting in the deaths of

225 000 out of almost 750 000 patients with sepsis each year in the United States of America alone where the overall cost of caring for these patients exceeds $17 billion annually. In recent years, the incidence of sepsis has risen by almost 9% each year and will continue to increase with the ageing population, growing antibiotic resistance, increasing immunocompromised state of patients, and the expanding use of invasive procedures.

Although many patients afflicted with severe sepsis have obvious risk factors, the syndrome is not limited to the old, debilitated, or immunocompromised. Sepsis can affect anyone, including healthy young people, and often has devastating consequences. Men are more commonly affected than women and nonwhite people are affected almost twice as often as white people. Respiratory infections are the most common cause, but genitourinary sources predominate in women. Gram-positive bacteria account for over one-half of all infections, Gram-negative bacteria for about one-third, and fungi for 5%.

Clinical features and criteria for diagnosis

Definitions of systemic inflammatory response syndrome (SIRS), sepsis, and severe sepsis are frequently confused. SIRS, which can occur as a result of an infectious or noninfectious insult, is defined by demonstrating at least two of the following four criteria: (1) hyperthermia or hypothermia (temperature $\geq 38°C$ or $\leq 36°C$), (2) tachycardia (heart rate > 90 beats/min), (3) tachypnoea or hyperventilation (> 30 respirations/min or $Paco_2 < 32$ mmHg), and (4) leucocytosis, leucopenia, or left shift (≥ 12 or $\leq 4 \times 10^9$ white blood cells/litre or $> 10\%$ immature neutrophils). Sepsis is defined as a suspected or confirmed infection plus at least two of the above SIRS criteria. Severe sepsis is used to describe sepsis resulting in the acute dysfunction of at least one organ system. When the infection results in hypotension despite adequate fluid resuscitation, the patient has septic shock.

Tachypnoea is usually the first detectable clinical sign and is so common in severe sepsis that its absence should make the diagnosis suspect. The cause of the rapid breathing is often multifactorial. The lung is the most frequent site of infection and acute lung injury resulting from nonpulmonary sources of infection and respiratory compensation for metabolic acidosis also contribute. Tachycardia is virtually universal unless prevented by a cardiac conduction defect or pharmacotherapy (e.g. β-blockers). Increasing heart rate is an important compensatory mechanism to respond to the hypermetabolic state of sepsis as well as to maintain perfusion in response to intravascular volume deficits, reduced cardiac contractility, and vasodilation.

Differential diagnosis and clinical investigation

The diagnosis of sepsis may be obvious in some patients, but making the diagnosis in most requires a high level of suspicion and a fair amount of investigation. Noninfectious conditions such as pancreatitis, trauma, severe haemorrhage, myocardial infarction, drug overdose, and even heat stroke can mimic sepsis and often need to be ruled out before the diagnosis of sepsis syndrome can be established.

Laboratory abnormalities are often present, but are not specific for infection. Although suspicious, leucocytosis, bandaemia, and leucopenia are neither sensitive nor specific for the diagnosis. The hallmark of sepsis is a positive culture from a normally sterile body site, such as blood, urine, or cerebrospinal fluid, but culture results often take 24 to 48 h to return and are negative in up to one-third of cases. Clinical investigations, such as radiographs, urinalysis, or cerebrospinal fluid examination may demonstrate the site of infection. Other suggestive, but nonspecific laboratory results that may aid diagnosis include: elevated arterial lactate, metabolic acidosis with reduced serum bicarbonate, blood urea nitrogen, creatinine, glucose, bilirubin, alkaline phosphatase, and aminotransferase measurements. An elevated serum procalcitonin level may be a reasonable marker of sepsis in patients with SIRS, but is usually not readily available.

Treatment of sepsis

Antibiotics

Early administration of properly chosen antibiotics reduces morbidity and mortality in patients with sepsis. In clinical trials, an appropriate antibiotic regimen is begun in a timely fashion in 85 to 95% of occasions, but failure to do so is associated with a 25% higher overall case fatality. Since culture results are not immediately available for most septic patients, clinicians must use antibiotics empirically. When initiating therapy, the suspected site of infection, patient's immune status, recent antibiotic use, local resistance patterns, location in which the patient acquired the infection (i.e. nosocomial vs community), and Gram's stain and culture results should all be considered. Unless the causative organism and susceptibility are known, initial antibiotic therapy should cover a broader spectrum of possibilities when the patient is critically ill. Once microbiological data are available, therapy should be tailored promptly to the narrowest spectrum, least toxic, and least expensive agent.

Source control

Searching for the site of infection should begin as soon as haemodynamic and respiratory status are stabilized. Effective management relies on eradicating the source of infection, as antibiotics without source control often fail. Any devitalized tissue or sizeable collection of pus should be resected or drained, either surgically or using less invasive percutaneous drainage techniques. All foreign bodies, including intravascular catheters, should be carefully examined and removed promptly if there is any suspicion of infection.

Early goal-directed resuscitation

The inflammatory cytokines released in sepsis decrease systemic resistance, reduce filling pressure, and depress myocardial contractility. Increased venous pooling, greater insensible losses from anorexia, sweating, vomiting and diarrhoea, and worsening microvascular permeability all contribute to decreased intravascular volume. Consequently, many septic patients rapidly develop cardiovascular insufficiency manifested as hypotension. Aggressive resuscitation, aimed at restoring and maintaining an adequate blood pressure, should be initiated early in the course of treatment. In adults of normal size, this resuscitation often requires large amounts of colloid or 6 to 10 litres isotonic crystalloid. Although the endpoint for discontinuing aggressive resuscitation and the optimal measure of adequate perfusion pressure remains ill-defined, early goal-directed resuscitation (EGDT) during the first 6 h has been shown to lower mortality in one single-centre study of patients with severe sepsis and lactic acidosis or septic shock. Intention-to-treat analysis demonstrated that patients receiving EGDT during the first 6 h of care had a 33% relative reduction and 16% absolute reduction in hospital mortality (30.5% vs 46.5%; $P = 0.009$), with improvement in mortality persisting to at least 60 days. The reduction in mortality was largely attributable to a decrease in late, sudden cardiovascular collapse in patients treated with EGDT.

Treatment of hypotension

The EGDT algorithm utilizes crystalloid infusions to maintain a central venous pressure of 8 to 12 mmHg. If mean arterial pressure remains below 65 mmHg, vasopressors are initiated. During resuscitation, central venous oxygen saturation ($Scvo_2$) is monitored continuously using a central venous catheter. If the patient has a central venous pressure and mean arterial pressure within the target ranges, but the $Scvo_2$ measurement remains below 70%, packed red blood cells are transfused to achieve a haematocrit of 30%. If the haematocrit is 30% or higher and the $Scvo_2$ is still below 70%, dobutamine is begun. Vasopressin, a stress hormone released in response to hypotension, stimulates a family of receptors: AVPR1a, AVPR1b, AVPR2, oxytocin receptors, and purinergic receptors. In septic shock, vasopressin secretion is inadequate. Low-dose vasopressin infusion improves blood pressure, decreases requirements for noradrenaline, improves renal function and, in the *Vasopressin and Septic Shock Trial* (VASST), low-dose vasopressin decreased mortality in patients with less severe septic shock (26% vs 36%, respectively, $P = 0.04$). Patients with 'less severe shock' were defined as those on modest doses of noradrenaline (5 to 14 μg/ minute) at randomization and with lower serum lactate concentrations. However, in the whole group of patients, there was no difference in 28-day mortality between those treated with vasopressin and with noradrenaline (35% vs 39%, respectively). Low-dose vasopressin infusion plus corticosteroids significantly decreased 28-day mortality compared with corticosteroids plus noradrenaline (44% vs 35%, respectively, $P = 0.03$; $P = 0.008$ interaction statistic).

Corticosteroid treatment

In one study, 54% of patients with septic shock who had adrenal insufficiency defined by basal plasma cortisol levels above 34 μg/dL, and cortisol response to short corticotrophin stimulation test below 9 μg/dL, had a higher mortality. Impairement of hypothalamo–pituitary–adrenal responses during critical illness may result from decreased production of corticotropin-releasing hormone (CRH), ACTH, and cortisol and dysfunction of their receptors such as CRH receptor 1 (CRHR1) and AVPR1b. Although corticosteroids possess a variety of anti-inflammatory actions, numerous studies have demonstrated that high doses, aimed at suppressing the inflammatory response to infection, confer no benefit to patients with severe sepsis or septic shock. Meta-analyses of these studies confirm the lack of efficacy and even suggest a trend towards harm. More recent data suggest that lower, more physiological doses, administered over a longer period of time, may benefit a subset of patients with septic shock and relative adrenal insufficiency. Unfortunately, a multinational double-blind placebo-controlled study investigating this 'replacement dose' strategy found no difference in 28-day all-cause mortality or shock-free days. Given the numerous negative studies, the routine use of corticosteroids in

patients with severe sepsis or septic shock cannot be recommended at this time. However, a recent systematic review suggested that low dose corticosteroid might improve survival in patients with severe sepsis.

Eritoran tetrasodium, anti-Toll-like receptor (TLR)-4

Unfortunately, the attempt to manipulate TLR4 signalling with the new anti-Toll-like receptor (TLR)-4 compound eritoran tetrasodium (Eisai) failed to demonstrate improvement in 28-day all-cause mortality in a cohort of 2000 patients with severe sepsis.

Drotrecogin alfa (activated) or recombinant human activated protein C

In late 2001, recombinant human activated protein C (rhAPC), or drotrecogin alfa (activated) (DAA), became the first drug approved for use in patients with a high risk of death from severe sepsis. A large phase III randomized blind placebo-controlled multinational trial was discontinued early, after 1690 of the planned 2280 patients were enrolled, because the predefined stopping boundary for efficacy was surpassed. rhAPC, administered as a continuous intravenous infusion of 24 μg/kg per h for 96 h, resulted in a 6% absolute and 19% relative reduction in 28-day all-cause mortality compared to placebo (24.7% vs 30.8%; $P = 0.005$). The survival difference became apparent shortly after initiation of the infusion, continued to increase for the duration of the study period, and persisted out to at least 1 year of long-term follow-up. Subsequent prospective data suggested that early treatment with rhAPC (i.e. within 24 h of organ dysfunction onset) resulted in better outcomes than delayed initiation. Although the criteria for high risk of death are hotly debated, patients with Acute Physiology and Chronic Health Evaluation II (APACHE II) scores of more than 25 or requiring vasopressors or mechanical ventilation are widely considered appropriate candidates for the drug.

Not unexpectedly given its anticoagulant properties, rhAPC increases the risk of bleeding. Although uncommon in both arms of the study, severe bleeding episodes were also almost twice as high in those receiving rhAPC compared to placebo (3.5% vs 2.0%; $P = 0.06$). These bleeding rates are similar to those seen with other forms of full systemic anticoagulation, such as full-dose heparin. Although patients at high risk of bleeding were excluded from the landmark study, those with either traumatic injury of a highly vascular organ or major blood vessel, ulcerations in the gastrointestinal system, meningitis, or markedly abnormal coagulation parameters (platelet counts <30 000/ml, INR >3, or activated partial thromboplastin time >120 s) had more bleeding.

Subsequent studies in adult patients with low risk of death (i.e. APACHE II <25, not on vasopressors, not in the intensive care unit) and children were stopped early because of inefficacy and side effects. Analysis of these data found that children with sepsis and postoperative patients with single-organ failure from sepsis did not derive benefit from administration of rhAPC, and both groups experienced higher bleeding rates. The drug is therefore not recommended for use in these populations.

Unfortunately, in October 2011, Eli Lilly announced withdrawal of drotrecogin alfa (Xigris) because of the failure of its PROWESS shock trial to demonstrate improved outcome. This was the only drug approved specifically for the treatment of severe sepsis.

Volume-limited and pressure-limited mechanical ventilation strategy

The vast majority of patients with severe sepsis require mechanical ventilation, many from sepsis-induced acute lung injury. Preventing undue distension of normally compliant segments of the injured lung, and subsequent release of inflammatory cytokines by using a volume-limited and pressure-limited ventilation strategy in patients with acute lung injury has been shown to decrease mortality and increase time alive and off the ventilator. To accomplish this, patients should be ventilated using volume-limited ventilation strategies with tidal volumes set at 6 ml/kg of predicted body weight. These tidal volumes should be titrated downwards as needed to maintain plateau pressure less than 30 cm H_2O. Ventilator weaning that is protocol-driven and employs daily spontaneous breathing trials results in earlier successful extubation.

Preventing complications and nosocomial infections

Since patients with severe sepsis possess multiple risk factors for deep venous thrombosis, prophylaxis for this complication should be nearly routine. Patients with low bleeding risk should receive a known effective dose of low molecular weight or unfractionated heparin, while intermittent compression devices should be used in patients at significant risk of bleeding. H_2-receptor antagonists have been shown to be superior to treatment with sucralfate in prevention of gastrointestinal bleeding for mechanically ventilated patients. Therefore, current therapy should almost always include an H_2-receptor blocker or a proton pump inhibitor.

The compensatory anti-inflammatory response and impaired host defence, along with numerous invasive procedures and broad-spectrum antibiotic exposure, predisposes patients with severe sepsis to nosocomial infections. Hand washing between patients and using barrier precautions (gloves and gowns) when examining patients colonized with resistant organisms should be universally employed. Likewise, inserting central lines using full barrier precautions, limiting the number of catheter manipulations, and utilizing closed infusion systems with minimal tubing changes can minimize vascular catheter infections. The risk of nosocomial pneumonia can be reduced by raising the head of the bed to 30 to 45 degrees in mechanically ventilated patients, especially those receiving enteral feedings. Draining the condensate from ventilator tubing and minimizing tubing changes also decreases the incidence of nosocomial pneumonia. If possible, all feeding and endotracheal tubes should be orally placed to reduce the incidence of sinusitis. If a tube must be placed through the nose, it should be small-bore and flexible to decrease the degree of sinus ostial obstruction.

Prognosis

Sepsis without organ dysfunction is a very serious condition, with in-hospital mortality rates ranging from 5 to 10%. However, once organ dysfunction is present, even with modern advances in the care of the critically ill, one-third to one-half of all patients with severe sepsis die before being discharged from hospital, and patients with septic shock have hospital mortality rates of 50 to 80%. Patients who survive their initial encounter with severe sepsis continue to have higher rates of death throughout the first year after hospital discharge for unknown reasons. The principal prognostic factors include age, severity of underlying diseases, number of organ system dysfunctions, severity of illness scores, hypothermia, neutropenia, thrombocytopenia, lactic acidosis, multisource of infection, positive blood culture, type of infecting organism, and blood concentrations of endotoxin and cytokines.

Areas of uncertainty

As with all diseases, areas of uncertainty exist in treating patients with severe sepsis. Corticosteroid treatment and tight glucose control with intensive insulin therapy represent two current areas of uncertainty. Although corticosteroids possess a variety of anti-inflammatory actions, numerous studies have demonstrated that high doses, aimed at suppressing the inflammatory response to infection, confer no benefit to patients with severe sepsis or septic shock. Meta-analyses of these studies confirm the lack of efficacy and even suggest a trend towards harm. More recent data suggest that lower, more physiological doses, administered over a longer period of time, may benefit a subset of patients with septic shock and relative adrenal insufficiency. Unfortunately, a multinational double-blind placebo-controlled study investigating this 'replacement dose' strategy found no difference in 28-day all-cause mortality or shock-free days. Given the numerous negative studies, the routine use of corticosteroids in patients with severe sepsis or septic shock cannot be recommended at this time.

The use of intensive insulin therapy, aimed at maintaining serum blood glucose levels between 80 and 110 mg/dL, also remains controversial. An initial study demonstrated that this tight glycaemic control improved survival, decreased bacteraemia, and reduced renal failure in cardiac surgery patients, regardless of a history of diabetes. A subsequent study in critically ill medical patients was unable to replicate the results, although some benefit was seen in patients requiring intensive care for longer than 72 h. Although hypoglycaemia is uncommon, patients who develop it have significantly higher mortality rates. Further research into this area will need to be undertaken to identify the optimal patient population and target glucose levels for intensive insulin treatment in patients with sepsis.

Further reading

Aird WC (2001). Vascular bed-specific hemostasis: role of endothelium in sepsis pathogenesis. *Crit Care Med*, **29** Suppl 7, 28–35.

Angus DC (2011). The search for effective therapy for sepsis: back to the drawing board? *JAMA*, **306**, 2614–15.

Annane D, *et al.* (2000). A 3-level prognostic classification in septic shock based on cortisol levels and cortisol response to corticotropin. *JAMA*, **283**, 1038–45.

Annane D, *et al.* (2002). Effect of treatment with low doses of hydrocortisone and fludrocortisone on mortality in patients with septic shock. *JAMA*, **288**, 862–71.

Annane D, *et al.* (2009). Corticosteroids in the treatment of severe sepsis and septic shock in adults: a systematic review. *JAMA*, **301**, 2362–75.

Bernard GR, *et al.* (2001). Efficacy and safety of recombinant human activated protein C for severe sepsis. *N Engl J Med*, **344**, 699–709.

Bone RC (1996). Sir Isaac Newton, sepsis, SIRS and CARS. *Crit Care Med*, **24**, 1125–8.

Boomer JS, *et al.* (2011). Immunosuppression in patients who die of sepsis and multiple organ failure. *JAMA*, **306**, 2594–605.

Cook DJ, *et al.* (1998). A comparison of sucralfate and ranitidine for the prevention of upper gastrointestinal bleeding in patients requiring mechanical ventilation. *N Engl J Med*, **338**, 791–7.

Dellinger RP, *et al.* (2004). Surviving Sepsis Campaign guidelines for management of severe sepsis and septic shock. *Crit Care Med*, **32**, 858–73.

Hotchkiss RS, Karl IE (2003). The pathophysiology and treatment of sepsis. *N Engl J Med*, **348**, 138–50.

Kollef MH, *et al.* (1999). Inadequate antimicrobial treatment of infections: a risk factor for hospital mortality among critically ill patients. *Chest*, **115**, 462–74.

Levi M, *et al.* (1993). Pathogenesis of disseminated intravascular coagulopathy in sepsis. *JAMA*, **270**, 975–9.

MacIntyre NR, *et al.* (2001). Evidence-based guidelines for weaning and discontinuing ventilatory support: a collective task force facilitated by the American College of Chest Physicians; the American Association for Respiratory Care; and the American College of Critical Care Medicine. *Chest*, **120** Suppl 6, S375–95.

Martin GS, *et al.* (2003). The epidemiology of sepsis in the United States from 1979 through 2000. *N Engl J Med*, **348**, 1546–54.

Mitka M (2011). Drug for severe sepsis is withdrawn from market, fails to reduce mortality. *JAMA*, **306**, 2439–40.

Rivers E, *et al.* (2001). Early goal-directed therapy in the treatment of severe sepsis and septic shock. *N Engl J Med*, **345**, 1368–77.

Russell JA, et al. (2008). Vasopressin versus norepinephrine infusion in patients with septic shock. *N Engl J Med*, **358**, 877–87.

Russell JA (2011). Bench-to-bedside review: Vasopressin in the management of septic shock. *Crit Care*, **15**, 226.

The Acute Respiratory Distress Syndrome Network (2000). Ventilation with lower tidal volumes as compared with traditional tidal volumes for acute lung injury and the acute respiratory distress syndrome. *N Engl J Med*, **342**, 1301–8.

Ulloa L, *et al.* (2002). Ethyl pyruvate prevents lethality in mice with established lethal sepsis and systemic inflammation. *Proc Natl Acad Sci U S A*, **99**, 12 351–6.

van den Berghe G, *et al.* (2001). Intensive insulin therapy in critically ill patients. *N Engl J Med*, **345**, 1359–67.

van den Berghe G, *et al.* (2006). Intensive insulin therapy in the medical ICU. *N Engl J Med*, **354**, 449–61.

van Deventer SJH, *et al.* (1990). Experimental endotoxemia in humans: analysis of cytokine release and coagulation, fibrinolytic and complement pathways. *Blood*, **76**, 2520–6.

Wang H, *et al.* (1999). HMG-1 as a late mediator of endotoxin lethality in mice. *Science*, **285**, 248–51.

Wiersinga WJ (2011). Current insights in sepsis: from pathogenesis to new treatment targets. *Curr Opin Crit Care*, **17**, 480–6.

Yang H, *et al.* (2004). Reversing established sepsis with antagonists of endogenous HMGB1. *Proc Natl Acad Sci U S A*, **101**, 296–301.

2

The patient with suspected infection

Contents

2.1 Clinical approach

Christopher J. Ellis

Essentials

Infection is most often suspected when patients present with pyrexia and is certainly the most common cause of this presentation, whether in hospitalized patients or those in the community. The other principal causes of fever are primary inflammatory conditions and malignancy, but infections are likely to be most rapidly progressive and acutely life threatening and hence must be the physician's first concern.

The clinical approach to patients with likely infection begins with a focused history, leading on to a clinical examination which assesses the extent of the physiological derangement and looks for a focus of infection. Standard physiological measures define likely sepsis (see Chapter 1.2), which is the commonest reason for their sudden derangement in hospitalized patients. Investigations should be phased and must not delay the start of potentially life-saving treatment, the response to which must be carefully followed, especially when treatment has to be started before a complete or certain diagnosis is possible, and compared with the likely speed of response for the putative condition being treated. There is increasing evidence that delays in initiating appropriate therapy, especially antimicrobial medication and circulatory support, increase mortality.

Introduction

No diagnostic challenge better illustrates the power of traditional clinical methods than the patient with possible infection; clinicians rarely find themselves in a situation where there is potentially so much urgency in establishing a working hypothesis and management plan.

It is vital to keep in mind that previously healthy people with life-threatening infections may have few symptoms other than malaise, and little in the way of abnormality on examination other than an altered body temperature and tachycardia. However, at this point only decisive intervention will prevent a rapid decline into circulatory collapse, coagulopathy, and multiple organ failure with a high risk of death.

What suggests that the patient's life is in danger?

Standard observations (vital signs) are usually valuable pointers to life-threatening situations and have been combined to define sepsis syndromes (Box 2.1.1).

Observations made routinely on hospitalized patients are now codified to produce early-warning track and trigger systems, such as the modified early warning score (MEWS), which highlight developing sepsis. In general hospitals, the development of sepsis is currently the most common single reason for patients' scores reaching the trigger point.

Although these alarm calls are important, they will not identify all patients in whom urgent treatment is vital. Table 2.1.1 lists

---

Box 2.1.1 Sepsis syndromes

Sepsis (systemic inflammatory response syndrome, SIRS)

Defined by two or more of:

- Temperature >38°C or <36°C
- Pulse rate >90/min
- Respiratory rate >20/min
- Leucocyte count >12 or $<4 \times 10^9$/litre

Severe sepsis

Sepsis with one or more of:

- Hypotension
- Confusion
- Oliguria
- Hypoxia
- Acidosis
- Disseminated intravascular coagulation (DIC)

Septic shock

- Severe sepsis with hypotension despite fluid resuscitation

---

some conditions that typically present in a bland and nonspecific manner although the patient may be only a day or two from death if not treated appropriately.

Infection may be mimicked by life-threatening noninfectious conditions. Primary vasculitic conditions commonly present with fever and skin infarcts identical to those seen in patients with endocarditis, while cerebral systemic lupus erythematosus (SLE) is clinically indistinguishable from an infective encephalitis. Conditions such as DRESS syndrome (drug reaction eosinophilia and systemic symptoms) may be precipitated by antibiotics and also mimic severe sepsis.

Management before diagnosis

Acute medicine has been described as 'the art of making sufficient conclusions on insufficient information'. When confronted with a patient who fulfils the criteria for severe sepsis, attention must be

Table 2.1.1 Conditions presenting in a nonspecific manner

Condition	Key clue
Malaria	Travel history
Early meningococcaemia	Early purpura
Bacteraemia	Rigor, i.e. visible shivering for at least 10 s
Fasciitis	Tenderness to pressure beyond apparent bounds of cellulitis
Toxic shock syndrome	The patient has fainted on standing (because of incipient shock); erythematous rash

paid to oxygenation, circulatory support, and intravenous antimicrobials, even if the clinician is still some way from a definitive diagnosis. In these fraught circumstances, organizational confusion can lead to vital actions being omitted or delayed. In particular, the prescriber should ensure the prompt administration of intravenous antimicrobials and deliver a fluid challenge to patients with hypovolaemia, bearing in mind that up to 40% of effective circulating volume can be lost, usually through vasodilatation, before vital signs register more than tachycardia. One litre of saline given over 30 min, and repeated if the pulse rate does not fall, is an appropriate prescription for an adult in this situation.

The history of the illness

Once immediate life-saving measures are in hand, if they are indicated, a thorough, focused history must include several questions that are not routinely asked (Table 2.1.2).

Clinical examination and chest radiograph

Examination of a patient with suspected infection can be both rapid and comprehensive. Having noted the vital signs, the clinician can proceed from head to toe. Temporal arteries should be examined in patients over the age of 50 years with fever and headaches; the mouth should be examined for poor dentition and oral candidiasis (a pointer to possible HIV infection), and the heart for murmur(s). A chest radiograph may reveal areas of consolidation in patients without any respiratory symptoms and hilar lymphadenopathy in patients without palpably enlarged nodes elsewhere. Conversely, a normal chest radiograph does not exclude early pneumonia. Examination of the abdomen should pay particular attention to liver enlargement and/or tenderness and include several firm blows over the ribs overlying the posterior surface of the liver which may elicit tenderness in patients with posterior liver abscesses. Tenderness in the right iliac fossa might indicate bowel-related sepsis, such as an appendix mass, while bimanual examination may reveal an enlarged or tender kidney. The patient's posture should be noted; flexion of the hip points to a possible psoas abscess. Examination of the perineum is mandatory in febrile neutropenic patients; it may reveal septic necrosis spreading from the rectum.

Enlarged lymph nodes should be carefully sought in the neck and in the axilla, where they are easily overlooked. The entire skin should be inspected for rash or for areas of inflammation. The spine should be palpated and percussed looking for angulation or tenderness. The nervous system should be examined if there is evidence of meningitis, encephalitis, or focal neurological symptoms.

Investigations

These should be phased in the interests of both time and money and to avoid misleading false-positives. Initial blood tests must include a specific test for malaria, if the patient has travelled to an endemic area. Blood samples for culture should be taken before antibiotics are started. Patients who have been started on antibiotics before investigation should have them stopped, provided it is judged safe to do so, and blood taken for culture 24 h later.

Table 2.1.2 Questions that must be asked concerning the history of the illness

Open question	Possible significance
Have you travelled?	All cases of falciparum malaria imported into nonendemic areas are in people who have visited malarial areas in the preceding 3 months; most are within 1 month. In the UK, 90% of these infections will have been acquired in sub-Saharan Africa
	Approximately one-half of the cases of Legionnaire's disease in the UK are in patients who have returned from Europe or Turkey in the preceding 2 weeks
Have you been sexually active?	Unprotected sex with a new partner (or a promiscuous regular partner) in the previous 2 months increases the probability of primary HIV and secondary syphilis
Have you been exposed to crowds of new social contacts (e.g. university freshers week, new military recruits, or large military deployments)?	Increased probability of meningococcal or pneumococcal infection
Have you been hospitalized or have you received medical attention recently?	Fever following the start of medication raises the possibility of drug fever (typically when a course of penicillin is extended beyond 1 week)
	Recent administration of antibacterial drugs predisposes to *Clostridium difficile* colitis
	Acquisition of a resistant strain of bacteria (e.g. extended-spectrum β-lactamase-producing or carbapenemase-producing bacteria)
	Dental work predisposes to endocarditis
	Previous splenectomy predisposes to fulminating pneumococcal septicaemia
	Infection of surgical wounds, retained surgical material, or prostheses
	Partial treatment of an abscess, most commonly intra-abdominal or retroperitoneal, including psoas abscess
Is the illness remittent?	Characteristically remittent conditions, including vivax malaria, systemic Still's disease, lymphoma
	Temporary improvement with antibacterial drugs suggests a possible 'collection', a concealed abscess

The chest radiograph should be inspected on admission. All patients should have a properly taken midstream or clean-catch urine sample sent for analysis.

Liaison with the microbiology laboratory is essential, and prompt delivery of specimens is a priority. Investigations involving cell counts, i.e. cerebrospinal fluid and urine microscopy, must be carried out on the day they were obtained.

Initial investigations are therefore:

◆ Background—full blood count, urea and electrolytes, liver function tests, C-reactive protein (CRP)

◆ Specific—blood culture, malaria test if indicated, urine analysis, chest radiograph

In assessing the results of these tests, the clinician must be aware of the significance of collateral effects, such as thrombocytopenia in disseminated intravascular coagulation (DIC) and malaria, and moderate elevations of transaminases in bacteraemia from any focus. The nature of bacteria isolated from blood culture often indicates the need for attention to a likely source, e.g. *Streptococcus viridans* to endocarditis, *Streptococcus milleri* to endocarditis or liver abscess, *Streptococcus bovis* to both endocarditis and neoplasm of the colon, while a mixture of gram-negative rods and anaerobes points to liver abscess or gut-related sepsis.

Second phase investigations

If the initial investigations do not point to a particular focus, imaging of the abdomen should be performed. Ultrasound examination is good for detecting fully liquefied liver abscesses and hydronephrosis and may point to focal sepsis or enlarged nodes. If ultrasound is negative, a CT scan should be considered.

Therapeutic trials

A therapeutic trial of an antibacterial may be indicated when, e.g. the patient reports temporary improvement following a previous course and the investigations outlined above have proved unhelpful. The spectrum covered by the previous antibiotic should be taken into consideration when selecting the trial agent. For example, a response to flucloxacillin suggests the need for a more protracted course of antistaphylococcal therapy. It is essential to compare the response to treatment with the response expected in the condition that has been provisionally diagnosed. In most bacterial infections pyrexia will settle within 48 h of starting appropriate antibacterial therapy, but there are notable exceptions, including typhoid fever, tuberculosis, melioidosis, any abscess with a volume of more than about 10 ml, and conditions in which there is a significant host response to the infection, such as the development of pleural effusion in patients with pneumococcal pneumonia.

A trial of antituberculosis chemotherapy is routine in patients in whom this infection is likely on clinical grounds, while awaiting culture results. It should also be considered when a tissue biopsy reveals granulomata.

Finally, when the history suggests the possibility of systemic Still's disease with criteria either fulfilled or approximated, or when a patient over the age of 50 has intermittent fever and symptoms consistent with giant cell arteritis, a trial of corticosteroids should be considered. This should not be delayed, but if the patient does not show clear improvement within 5 days of starting prednisolone 60 mg daily, the trial should be stopped. Such a course carries only a small risk of significant adverse effects and the likelihood of infection 'lighting up' is, in practice, very small.

2.2 Fever of unknown origin

Steven Vanderschueren and Daniël Knockaert

Essentials

Fever of unknown origin (FUO) refers to a prolonged febrile illness that persists without diagnosis after careful initial assessment. Although over 200 causes have been described, including rare diseases, most cases are due to familiar entities presenting in an atypical fashion.

Causes of FUO—The 'big three' are (1) infections—including tuberculosis, endocarditis, abdominal and hepatobiliary infections and abscesses, complicated genitourinary tract infections, pleuropulmonary infections, bone and joint infections, salmonellosis, cytomegalovirus, Epstein–Barr virus and HIV; (2) tumours—including lymphoma; and (3) multisystem inflammatory conditions—including connective tissue diseases, vasculitic syndromes and granulomatous disorders. A miscellaneous category including factitious fever, habitual hyperthermia, and drug fever deserves consideration early in a patient's workup, since timely recognition may avert invasive and expensive procedures.

Clinical approach to the patient with FUO—The clinician must rely on a very careful and thorough clinical history and examination that does not neglect any part of the body, followed by appropriately targeted investigations directed by knowledge of the broad spectrum of diseases and local epidemiology. As advocated by Sutton's law—'go where the money is'—the approach should follow any possible diagnostic clues, which may sometimes be subtle. If clues are absent or prove misleading, then screening imaging techniques can focus further investigation, but a rigid algorithm and a blind pursuit of increasingly complex tests are ill-advised. Likewise, therapeutic trials without firm foundation are rarely diagnostically rewarding. If the diagnosis in a stable patient remains elusive despite vigorous effort, a watchful waiting approach is warranted as most patients with fever of persistently unknown origin do well.

Definition

Original definition

Most fevers are readily explained or resolve rapidly. Fever with unclear cause or source at first sight should not be labelled fever (or pyrexia) of unknown (or undetermined) origin (FUO). Defined properly, true FUO is uncommon and is encountered once or twice a month at most teaching hospitals. A strict definition, which should not be changed too rapidly, is necessary for comparison of literature data and to guide clinicians faced with this rather rare clinical problem. The three criteria initially proposed by Petersdorf and Beeson in 1961 are: (1) an illness of at least 3 weeks' duration, (2) a fever (temperature more than 38.3 °C on at least three occasions), and (3) no established diagnosis after 1 week of hospital investigation. The first criterion eliminates acute, self-limiting, frequently viral diseases and the second eliminates habitual hyperthermia, an entity commonly diagnosed at that time.

Update of the initial definition

In 1991, Durack and Street suggested modification of the third criterion to an uncertain diagnosis after at least three outpatient visits or at least 3 days in hospital. This revision reflected trends in medical practice, including a shift towards outpatient management, advances in diagnostic techniques, and an accelerated pace of investigation. They also divided FUO into four groups: classic FUO, nosocomial FUO, neutropenic FUO, and HIV-associated FUO. In the last three groups the case mixture differs from that of classic FUO, and the predominance of nosocomial and opportunistic infections in these often frail patients frequently justifies early empirical antimicrobial therapy. The present chapter focuses on classic FUO in adults.

Contemporary definition of classic fever of unknown origin

Recently, it has been suggested that the third criterion should be changed from a quantitative to a qualitative one, specifying which particular examinations are necessary before an unsolved prolonged febrile illness classifies as FUO, rather than an arbitrary number of hospital days or outpatient visits. These minimum requirements (Box 2.2.1) should be adapted to regional, mainly infectious, epidemiological factors. Finally, a protracted unexplained febrile illness with fever below 38.3 °C but with persistently raised inflammatory markers should probably be approached similarly. These proposed changes culminated in a modern definition of classic FUO (Box 2.2.2) which can be used for the next few decades.

Causes

Diagnostic spectrum

The list of differential diagnoses is among the longest and most challenging in internal medicine, encompassing more than 200 entities. Common and uncommon causes of FUO in adults are listed in Boxes 2.2.3 and 2.2.4. These causes are conveniently classified into five categories: (1) infections, (2) malignancies, (3) noninfectious inflammatory diseases, (4) miscellaneous causes, and (5) undiagnosed cases. Infections predominated in earlier case series, in paediatric series, and in series from developing countries and from secondary care hospitals. In recent series from western European and Japanese referral centres, noninfectious inflammatory disease (comprising connective tissue disorders, vasculitides, and granulomatous disorders) surpassed infections as the most prevalent category. In spite of innovative rapid microbiological techniques, old and emerging infectious diseases will remain an important source of FUO, due to increasing global travel, migration, implantation of devices, and resistance of microorganisms. Somewhat counterintuitively, the proportion of undiagnosed cases is highest in referral centres and has risen over recent decades, amounting to 25 to 50% of cases. This apparent loss of diagnostic yield is partially attributable to the improved diagnostic armamentarium that reveals the aetiology or source well before a febrile illness turns into FUO. Yet the cause of some prolonged fevers remains unknown despite vigorous clinical efforts. In larger series, even autopsy failed to unravel the cause of the FUO in a substantial minority.

Subpopulations

The cause of FUO differs among subpopulations. The importance of geographical origin and the immune status of the host have

Box 2.2.1 Minimum diagnostic evaluation to qualify as fever of unknown origin

- Comprehensive history (including accompanying symptoms, travel history, sexual risk behaviour, profession, hobbies, contact with animals (pets, birds, insects) and ill persons, family history, use of medications and illicit drugs, past medical and surgical history, presence of foreign material)
- Meticulous physical examination (eyes, mucosal surfaces, temporal arteries, skin, hands and nails, lymph nodes, thyroid, heart, lungs, abdomen, rectal examination, musculoskeletal system, neurological examination, vascular examination)
- Erythrocyte sedimentation rate (ESR), C-reactive protein, serum protein electrophoresis
- Complete blood count, including differential and platelet count
- Routine blood chemistry, including creatinine, sodium, potassium, lactate dehydrogenase, bilirubin, liver enzymes, creatine kinase
- Antinuclear and antineutrophil cytoplasmic antibodies, angiotensin-converting enzyme
- Urinalysis, including microscopic examination
- Routine blood and urine cultures taken while not receiving antibiotics, cultures of other normally sterile fluids (e.g. from joints, pleura, or cerebrospinal space) whenever appropriate
- Tuberculin skin test, interferon-gamma release assay
- Chest radiograph
- Abdominal ultrasonography (including pelvis)
- Further evaluation of any abnormalities detected by above tests (e.g. HIV serology, hepatitis serology, echocardiography in case of cardiac murmur, blood smear for malaria in the traveller, Epstein–Barr virus and cytomegalovirus serology in case of reactive lymphocytosis)

already been alluded to, and age matters as well. In older people, giant cell arteritis, tuberculosis, malignancies, and drug fever are important considerations, while in younger adults, viral infections, particularly cytomegalovirus infection, adult-onset Still's disease, habitual hyperthermia, factitious fever, and undiagnosed cases are more prevalent. In recurrent or episodic FUO, defined as at least two episodes of fever with fever-free intervals of at least 2 weeks and seeming remission of the underlying illness, traditional causes

Box 2.2.2 Modern definition of classic fever of unknown origin

- Illness of more than 3 weeks duration
- Temperature of at least 38.3°C, or lower temperature with laboratory signs of inflammation, on at least three occasions
- No diagnosis or reasonable (eventually confirmed) diagnostic hypothesis after an initial diagnostic investigation[a]
- Exclusion of nosocomial fevers and severe immunocompromise

[a] See Box 2.2.1

Box 2.2.3 Common causes of classic fever of unknown origin in adults

Infections
- Tuberculosis
- Endocarditis
- Abdominal and hepatobiliary infections and abscesses
- Complicated genitourinary tract infections
- Pleuropulmonary infections
- Bone and joint infections
- Salmonellosis (including typhoid fever)
- Cytomegalovirus, Epstein–Barr virus, HIV

Neoplasms
- Haematological
  - Non-Hodgkin's lymphoma
  - Hodgkin's disease
  - Leukaemia
- Solid
  - Adenocarcinoma (e.g. colon, kidney)

Noninfectious inflammatory diseases
- Connective tissue diseases
  - Adult-onset Still's disease
  - Polymyalgia rheumatica
  - Rheumatoid arthritis
  - Sjögren's syndrome
  - Systemic lupus erythematosus
- Vasculitis syndromes
  - Giant cell arteritis
  - Polyarteritis nodosa
  - Wegener's granulomatosis
- Granulomatous disorders
  - Inflammatory bowel disease
  - Sarcoidosis

Miscellaneous
- Drug fever
- Habitual hyperthermia
- Factitious fever
- Subacute thyroiditis
- Venous thromboembolism
- Haematoma

Box 2.2.4 Rare causes of fever of unknown origin in adults

Infections

- Bartonellosis (including *Bartonella henselae*, *B. quintana*), brucellosis, campylobacteriosis, gonococcaemia, melioidosis, meningococcemia, listeriosis, tularaemia, yersiniosis
- Chlamydial infections (including psittacosis), ehrlichioses, rickettsioses, *Coxiella burnetii* (Q fever)
- Nontuberculous mycobacteria, leprosy
- Febris recurrens, leptospirosis, Lyme disease, rat-bite fever, syphilis
- Actinomycosis, nocardiosis, Whipple's disease
- Human herpesvirus type 8, parvovirus B19
- Aspergillosis, blastomycosis, candidiasis, coccidioidomycosis, cryptococcosis, histoplasmosis, mucormycosis, pneumocystosis, sporotrichosis
- Amoebiasis, babesiosis, echinococcosis, fascioliasis, malaria, leishmaniasis, schistosomiasis, toxocariasis, toxoplasmosis, trichinosis, trypanosomiasis
- Malakoplakia, xanthogranulomatous pyelonephritis
- Central nervous system infection, dental infection, upper respiratory tract infection, wound infection
- Intravenous catheter infection, infected vascular graft, mycotic aneurysm

Neoplasms and related conditions

- Haematological malignancies
  - Angioimmunoblastic T-cell lymphoma
  - Intravascular lymphoma
  - Amyloidosis
  - Hypereosinophilic syndrome
  - Multiple myeloma
  - Myelodysplastic syndromes
  - Myelofibrosis
- Solid tumours
  - Atrial myxoma
  - Hepatoma
  - Renal cell carcinoma
  - Other (more than 30 reported), with or without necrosis, with or without metastases

Noninfectious inflammatory diseases

- Connective tissue diseases
  - Acute rheumatic fever
  - Crystal-induced arthropathy
  - Eosinophilic fasciitis
  - Felty's syndrome
  - Mixed connective tissue disease

- Polymyositis, dermatomyositis
- Reactive arthritis, including Reiter's syndrome
- Relapsing polychondritis
- Seronegative spondylarthropathy
- Vasculitis syndromes
  - Behçet's disease
  - Henoch–Schönlein purpura
  - Mixed cryoglobulinaemia
  - Takayasu's arteritis
  - Urticarial vasculitis
- Granulomatous disorders
  - Granulomatous hepatitis

Miscellaneous

- Addison's disease, hyperparathyroidism, hyperthyroidism, hypothalamic hypopituitarism, phaeochromocytoma
- Erythema multiforme, erythema nodosum, linear IgA dermatosis, Sweet's disease
- Castleman's disease, inflammatory pseudotumour of lymph nodes, Kikuchi's disease
- Vogt–Koyanagi–Harada syndrome
- Giant haemangioma
- Dissecting aneurysm
- Retroperitoneal fibrosis
- Thrombophlebitis
- Cholesterol embolism, PTFE (Teflon) embolism, silicone embolism
- Antiphospholipid syndrome
- Cyclic neutropenia, haemolytic anaemia, haemoglobinopathies, macrophage activation (haemophagocytic) syndrome, vitamin B12 deficiency
- Schnitzler's syndrome
- Dressler's syndrome (postmyocardial infarction syndrome)
- Cerebrovascular accident, epilepsy
- Alcoholic hepatitis, autoimmune hepatitis, cirrhosis (with active necrosis), primary sclerosing cholangitis
- Extrinsic allergic alveolitis, hypersensitivity pneumonitis, interstitial pneumonia
- Hereditary periodic fever syndromes (familial Mediterranean fever, tumour necrosis factor receptor-1-associated periodic syndrome, hyper-IgD syndrome, Muckle–Wells syndrome, familial cold autoinflammatory syndrome)
- Gaucher's disease, Fabry's disease
- Hypertriglyceridaemia
- Erdheim–Chester disease

such as infections and malignancies are less frequently implicated. Recurrent FUO is especially challenging, as a final diagnosis is established in no more than one-half of the patients. As the duration of the fever increases, the likelihood of an infectious cause decreases.

Common diseases prevail

Although the possible aetiologies of FUO are myriad, a limited list of disorders (Box 2.2.3) accounted for the great majority of diagnoses in published series. Most patients do not have esoteric diseases, unfamiliar to the clinician, but rather are exhibiting a typical manifestations of common illnesses. A few examples may illustrate this point. The forms of tuberculosis that give rise to FUO are often disseminated disease, yet without the characteristic miliary pattern on chest radiograph, or extrapulmonary disease without clear localizing features; tuberculin skin tests and sputum smears are often negative. The forms of endocarditis that enter the FUO spectrum are frequently culture-negative or are caused by fastidious organisms; a new regurgitant murmur or signs of peripheral emboli are frequently absent. Leukaemia presents as an FUO characteristically in the aleukaemic phase. Giant cell arteritis may manifest with constitutional symptoms only (anorexia, weight loss, fever), without polymyalgia or arteritic signs and symptoms, and without a strikingly elevated ESR. Likewise, in subacute thyroiditis, localizing symptoms and signs may be subtle or nonexistent.

Approach to the adult with classic fever of unknown origin

Ruling out the 'little three'

For didactic and practical purposes, it is convenient to split the aetiologies into the 'big three' and the 'little three'. The 'big three' are infections, neoplasms, and noninfectious inflammatory diseases, which together represent the bulk of diagnoses. The 'little three' comprise factitious fever, habitual hyperthermia, and drug fever. While these three causes are numerically less important, considering them from the start may prevent painstaking and invasive investigations. For this reason, at an early stage, fever should be verified, temperature charts recorded, and an effort made to stop all nonessential medications and switch essential ones to unrelated alternatives.

Factitious fever

Due to either manipulation of the thermometer or self-induced disease (e.g. by self-injection of contaminated materials), this characteristically occurs in young women, often in health professionals. Discrepancy between symptoms and clinical and laboratory findings raises the suspicion of fraudulent fever. Unexplained polymicrobial bacteraemia, serial episodes of bacteraemia by different pathogens, or recurrent soft tissue infections suggest self-induced infection.

Habitual hyperthermia

This is also seen mainly in young women who complain of 'flu-like' and functional symptoms. In this syndrome, which overlaps with chronic fatigue syndrome and fibromyalgia, the diurnal variation in body temperature is maintained. Evening temperatures are on average 0.5°C higher than morning temperatures, body temperature rises especially following physical and intellectual activity, the response to antipyretics is poor, and temperatures only occasionally exceed 38.3°C. Laboratory evaluation, including acute-phase reactants, is entirely unremarkable.

Drug fever

Virtually any drug can cause fever, with the possible exceptions of digitalis and aminoglycosides. The mechanisms are multiple and often poorly understood, with hypersensitivity being most common. Examples of drugs causing FUO include anticonvulsants, antimicrobials (such as minocycline, β-lactams, vancomycin, sulphonamides, and nitrofurantoin), antihistamines, nonsteroidal anti-inflammatory drugs (including salicylates), antihypertensives (hydralazine, methyldopa), antiarrhythmics (quinidine, procainamide) and allopurinol. Patients may have been on the offending drug for prolonged periods. Fever is rarely the sole manifestation but may be accompanied by rash, urticaria, mucosal ulceration, eosinophilia and other haematological abnormalities, hepatic or renal dysfunction, or pulmonary involvement. Phenytoin and carbamazepine are notorious for inducing a pseudolymphoma syndrome. Some patients with drug fever look severely ill and toxic, while others look and feel surprisingly well. Withdrawal of the offending drug usually results in defervescence within 72 to 96 h. Rechallenge is generally safe unless organ damage (e.g. hepatitis or interstitial nephritis) has occurred, but is rarely performed in clinical practice. Formal allergy testing is sometimes used to confirm the diagnosis of drug allergy, particularly if the patient appears to have multiple drug allergies or is likely to require treatment with a particular drug or related drugs in the future.

Fever characteristics

While recording and monitoring of body temperature are imperative, fever height and pattern do not contribute much to diagnosis. The few entities that have a distinctive fever pattern (e.g. nonfalciparum malaria or cyclic neutropenia) are rare, as are fever patterns thought to be characteristic of other diseases, such as Pel–Ebstein fever (a relapsing fever that disappears and reappears at intervals of several days) in Hodgkin's disease. Other features that lack diagnostic discrimination among the numerous sources of FUO are the presence of night sweats, weight loss, chills, and relative bradycardia (a heart rate lower than expected for the degree of fever). The naproxen test was proposed on the assumption of a selective antipyretic activity against neoplastic fever, but in clinical practice the accuracy of this test too is too low to be discriminatory.

Go where the money is

The diagnostician confronted with FUO should keep in mind Sutton's law: 'go where the money is'. Possible diagnostic clues elicited from the history, physical examination, and the preliminary diagnostic evaluation (Box 2.2.1) should, of course, guide further investigation, but many cases become a FUO because these clues are misleading. Whenever possible, the clinician should strive to achieve microbiological or pathological confirmation. Any suspected focal abnormality that is accessible should be aspirated or biopsied. Close communication with the microbiologist and the pathologist will increase the diagnostic yield.

When diagnostic clues are either absent or misleading, an individualized approach is preferable. Indeed, there are no useful or evidence-based rigid algorithms.

Screening imaging techniques

Imaging is used primarily to localize abnormalities for further evaluation. Due to the higher spatial resolution compared with chest radiographs and ultrasound of the abdomen, CT scanning of thorax or abdomen is useful when looking for focal disease, mainly infectious or neoplastic. In the near future, the role of MRI in the work-up of FUO is anticipated to grow as its benefits relative to CT are demarcated. The choice between a whole variety of radiopharmaceuticals depends on local availability, cost, and skill. We do not advocate tracers that are more specific for infections, such as labelled leucocytes, because a wide range of inflammatory and neoplastic conditions enter the differential diagnosis, not just infections. In particular, ^{18}F-fluorodeoxyglucose positron emission tomography (FDG-PET) is a promising inflammation tracer technique in FUO, yielding the diagnosis in 25 to 40% of patients and performing at least as well as gallium scintigraphy. However, unlike gallium, fluorodeoxyglucose is taken up in vasculitic lesions in large blood vessels (giant cell arteritis and Takayasu's arteritis), which are classic causes of FUO.

Selective testing

The imaging studies may unmask hidden infectious, neoplastic, and inflammatory foci, but endoscopic techniques (e.g. gastrointestinal endoscopy, bronchoscopy), selective radiographs (e.g. of teeth, sinuses, sacroiliac joints), or contrast studies (e.g. gastrointestinal series, arteriography) should be ordered only when there is a well-founded and specific clinical suspicion. They should not be used as routine tests for FUO. This is even more the case for invasive procedures such as mediastinoscopy, thoracoscopy, or laparoscopy, techniques that are being replaced increasingly by less invasive ultrasound echoendoscopy, or CT-guided biopsy. Nowadays, exploratory laparoscopy is restricted to exceptional situations, e.g. when peritoneal carcinomatosis or tuberculosis are suspected and other tests have failed. Likewise, biopsies of lymph nodes, bone marrow, or liver, and lumbar puncture can be diagnostic, but should not be performed blindly, in the absence of firm suspicion of pathological involvement. The only biopsy that may be routinely performed is temporal artery biopsy in a patient over the age of 50 with a prolonged unexplained fever and vigorous acute-phase response, even in the absence of arteritic symptoms. Giant cell arteritis is one of the most frequent diagnoses in this age group and carries a serious risk of visual loss and other ischaemic complications.

Watchful waiting

An undirected pursuit of often increasingly costly and invasive tests is discouraged. Instead, when the diagnosis remains in doubt, all data including those from other hospitals should be critically reviewed and history taking, physical examination, and some basic tests (e.g. white blood cell count with differential, creatine kinase, urinalysis, chest radiograph) repeated in an effort to find clues that were previously overlooked or inapparent. There is no substitute for observing, talking to, and thinking about the patient. If the diagnosis cannot be established after intelligent thorough investigation, an expectant approach is justified if the patient's condition is stable. In published series, most patients with FUO who left hospital without a diagnosis did remarkably well.

Therapeutic trials

Therapeutic trials are seldom diagnostically rewarding and tend to obscure rather than illuminate. In contrast to the approach to fever in immunocompromised patients (Chapter 2.4), the general goal when dealing with classic FUO is to ascertain the diagnosis before starting therapy. Antipyretics, mainly nonsteroidal anti-inflammatory drugs, may be symptomatically useful but rarely aid diagnosis. Blind administration of corticosteroids is discouraged. Infections such as tuberculosis may seemingly respond initially, only to deteriorate thereafter. Most patients have already had a failed trial of antibiotics before referral to secondary or tertiary care. Defervescence following administration of an antimicrobial agent is rarely diagnostic as the spectrum generally involves more than a single microorganism. Moreover, fevers caused by infections such as disseminated tuberculosis or culture-negative endocarditis may wane only several days after starting appropriate therapy. Spontaneous resolution of fever may coincide with a therapeutic trial, which is another argument against its routine use. The exception to the rule of withholding empirical therapy in classic FUO is the severely deteriorating patient. In such situations, antituberculosis chemotherapy is warranted, since tuberculosis is probably the most common cause of avoidable death in adults with classic FUO. Corticosteroid treatment is the next step in case of further deterioration of the clinical condition.

Prognosis

Not surprisingly, the outcome of classic FUO is highly variable and depends on the underlying disease. In the series of Larson *et al.* from the 1980s, for instance, only 9% of patients with malignancies were long-term survivors, while 78% of patients with infections and 88% of patients with FUO in other categories were alive after 1 year. Older age carries a worse prognosis. In a series from the 1990s, haematological malignancies (especially non-Hodgkin's lymphoma), constituted 12% of diagnoses, but accounted for almost 60% of deaths. Treatable causes of death have included abdominal abscesses, endocarditis, vasculitis, pulmonary embolism, and especially tuberculosis.

Most patients who cannot be diagnosed do well and over two-thirds have no recurrence of symptoms. Among the rest, a subgroup have clinical features suggesting protracted noninfectious inflammatory conditions, without meeting accepted diagnostic criteria for any particular disease. Most of these fevers respond to corticosteroid therapy.

Further reading

Arnow PM, Flaherty JP (1997). Fever of unknown origin. *Lancet*, **350**, 575–80.

Cunha BA (2007). Fever of unknown origin: Clinical overview of classical and current concepts. *Infect Dis Clin N Am*, **21**, 867–915.

Durack DT, Street AC (1991). Fever of unknown origin: reexamined and redefined. *Curr Clin Top Infect Dis*, **11**, 35–51.

Hirschmann JV (1997). Fever of unknown origin in adults. *Clin Infect Dis*, **24**, 291–302.

Knockaert DC, Vanderschueren S, Blockmans D (2003). Fever of unknown origin in adults: 40 years on. *J Intern Med*, **253**, 263–75.

Knockaert DC, *et al.* (1992). Fever of unknown origin in the 1980s. An update of the diagnostic spectrum. *Arch Intern Med*, **152**, 51–5.

Larson EB, Featherstone HJ, Petersdorf RG (1982). Fever of undetermined origin: diagnosis and follow-up of 105 cases, 1970–1980. *Medicine*, **61**, 269–92.

Petersdorf RB, Beeson PB (1961). Fever of unexplained origin: report on 100 cases. *Medicine*, **40**, 1–30.

Vanderschueren S, *et al.* (2003). From prolonged febrile illness to fever of unknown origin. The challenge continues. *Arch Intern Med*, **163**, 1033–41.

2.3 Nosocomial infections

I.C.J.W. Bowler

Essentials

Hospital-acquired or nosocomial infections—defined for epidemiological studies as infections manifesting more than 48 hours after admission—are common. They affect 1.4 million people worldwide at any one time and involve between 5 and 25% of patients admitted to hospital, with considerable associated morbidity, mortality, and cost.

Clinical features—the most common sites of nosocomial infection are the urinary tract, surgical wounds, and the lower respiratory tract. Bacteria are the most important causes, including *Escherichia coli*, *Staphylococcus aureus* (including methicillin-resistant *Staphylococcus aureus*, MRSA), enterococci, *Pseudomonas aeruginosa*, and coagulase-negative staphylococci. The principal risk factors are extremes of age, the severity of underlying acute disease (e.g. neutropenia, organ system failure), and chronic medical conditions (especially diabetes, renal failure, and alcohol abuse).

Prevention—between 15 and 30% of nosocomial infections are preventable, and hospital practitioners have a duty of care to minimize the risk of infection for their patients. Systematic surveillance to assess the incidence and prevalence of such infections, together with a regularly audited organized programme to prevent or minimize their impact, should be an important part of every hospital's quality assurance system. Hospital managers must ensure appropriate staffing and resources to provide (1) access to advice from appropriately trained experts in infection control; (2) surveillance of infection with regular feedback of the data to staff; (3) isolation of patients with infections, with appropriate arrangements for their nursing and medical management; (4) appropriate arrangements for carrying out procedures likely to increase the risk of infection, e.g. insertion of central venous lines; and (5) policies for outbreak management. All staff should receive regular education to ensure that they recognize that infection control is 'everyone's business'.

Definitions

Nosocomial infections are distinct from community-acquired infections; they may affect patients and, less often, hospital staff. They can be usefully defined for epidemiological studies as infections manifesting more than 48 hours after admission to hospital. However, some nosocomial infections may not be so easily identified as hospital acquired, e.g. hospital-acquired hepatitis B infection may not become clinically apparent until months after the patient has been discharged because of the prolonged incubation period. These are therefore called healthcare-associated infections. Iatrogenic infections are acquired as the direct consequence of a therapeutic intervention (e.g. insertion of a urinary catheter). Opportunistic infections are caused by organisms that do not ordinarily harm healthy people; they occur in people with impaired defences. Endogenous (autogenous) infections are produced by the patient's normal flora, while exogenous infections result from transmission of organisms to the patient from elsewhere. Although in practice it may not always be possible to distinguish endogenous from exogenous infections, this differentiation must be attempted because of important implications for control.

Scale and costs of nosocomial infections

Rates of nosocomial infections between 6.9 and 25 per 100 admissions have been reported. The urinary tract, surgical wounds, and the lower respiratory tract are the most common sites, in that order (Table 2.3.1). In the United States of America it is estimated that 80 000 deaths are directly attributable to nosocomial infection each year, and in 2005 costs were estimated at $4.5 to $5.7 billion. In England in 2000 the costs were estimated at £1 billion annually, and were mainly attributed to delayed discharge from hospital of infected patients. In Mexico an estimated 450 000 cases of nosocomial infection cause 32 deaths per 100 000 inhabitants each year at a cost of US$1.5 billion (World Health Organization 2005). Rapid changes in health care provision mean the frequency and nature of nosocomial infection are also changing. The increasing trend to early discharge, particularly for surgical patients, can lead to an underassessment of the disease burden. New interventions provide new opportunities for infection. For instance, flexible endoscopes, which have revolutionized the investigation and management of a wide variety of diseases, can transmit hepatitis B between patients if the endoscopes are not decontaminated between procedures.

Host factors

The principal risk factors are extremes of age and the severity of the underlying disease (e.g. neutropenia, organ system failure). The rapidly ageing population of the more developed world has had a major impact on the prevalence of hospital-acquired infection in these countries. In multivariate analysis, several medical diagnoses on admission, especially diabetes mellitus, renal failure,

Table 2.3.1 Rates and sites of nosocomial infection in three countries

	USA (1996)	France (2001)	UK (2006)
Rates	9.8[a]	6.9[b]	7.6[b]
Sites (% of all infections)			
Urinary tract infection	34	40	20
Surgical wound infection	17	10	15
Lower respiratory tract infection	13	10	16
Other	36	40	49

[a] Cases/1000 patient days (incidence).
[b] Cases/100 admissions (prevalence).

or alcohol abuse, are most strongly associated with risk. Treatment itself may lower host defences, e.g. surgical incisions, bladder catheterization, mechanical ventilation, and neutropenia following cancer chemotherapy. Pathogens are able to form biofilms on the increasingly used prosthetic devices (e.g. intravascular catheters, cardiac valves and pacemakers, vascular grafts, and joint replacements) subverting normal host clearance mechanisms. Patients with similar clinical problems, who are likely to share similar risk factors for infection, tend to be nursed together for convenience, but the introduction of a microorganism into such a group can rapidly infect a number of patients. A good example is the rapid spread of norovirus gastroenteritis in geriatric wards. A poorly maintained hospital environment is a threat to vulnerable patients; for instance, in units caring for patients with solid organ transplants, outbreaks of legionellosis can result from defective air-conditioning and hot-water systems.

Microorganisms

Bacteria (*Escherichia coli*, *Staphylococcus aureus*, enterococci, *Pseudomonas aeruginosa*, and coagulase-negative staphylococci, in decreasing order of frequency) are the most important. Viruses, fungi, and protozoa play a minor part.

Whether endogenous or exogenous, the organisms causing nosocomial infection are usually part of a patient's colonizing flora. It may be difficult to distinguish infecting from colonizing organisms using bacteriological tests alone. The organisms are frequently multidrug resistant, since the widespread use of antibiotics in hospitals gives these strains a selective advantage. Empirical antibiotic therapy must accommodate the shift towards more resistant colonizing flora occurring in hospitals, particularly in burns and intensive care units. For example, *Escherichia coli*, *Klebsiella pneumoniae*, *Pseudomonas aeruginosa*, MRSA, and enterococci exhibit multidrug resistance to antimicrobials, thus making them difficult and expensive to treat. Increasing international travel means that organisms which are geographically restricted such as NDM *E. coli* and *K. pneumoniae* in India, which are resistant to nearly all antibiotics, including carbapenems, can spread when patients are transferred to hospitals in other countries. It is important that these organisms are detected by screening cultures when patients are transferred, so appropriate precautions to prevent their spread can be reinforced.

Principles of hospital infection control

The main aim of the hospital infection control programme is to prevent nosocomial infection. Infections must be identified as endemic or epidemic by clinical and epidemiological investigations. The identification and typing of isolates causing nosocomial infection allow recognition of organisms that are epidemiologically linked. Invasive multidrug-resistant organisms, such as MRSA, often require infection control measures to prevent their spread and so minimize the use of expensive, sometimes toxic, antibiotics required for their prophylaxis and treatment.

Epidemic infections account for less than 10% of the nosocomial disease burden but attract professional and media interest because they are unusual. They are amenable to measures that interrupt the spread of infection, such as the use of gowns and gloves,

and careful hand hygiene by those attending patients. Transfer of colonized or infected patients to a single room or an isolation ward is a physical means of preventing spread. Patients infected with the same organism can be grouped together (cohorted) and attended to by a group of nurses not involved with uninfected patients. Identification of additional carriers and elimination of colonization may be necessary for some epidemic outbreaks. Controlled trials demonstrating the efficacy of such measures have not been made, but many observational studies support their use.

Endemic nosocomial infections are more difficult to control. The size of the problem may not be apparent because attack rates in individual units may be low, or because some infection is seen as a normal consequence of certain interventions. It is important that information about endemic infections is collected systematically in a comprehensive surveillance programme, analysed, disseminated, and discussed so that preventive strategies can be improved. Control measures are applied to selected patients according to risk, e.g. correctly timed antimicrobial prophylaxis and meticulous sterile technique in prosthetic joint replacement surgery.

Site of nosocomial infections

Urinary tract

A bacterial count of at least 10^5 organisms/ml in freshly voided cultured urine indicates infection. However, counts as low as 10^2 organisms/ml are included by some classifications and any organisms grown from a urine sample taken from a urinary catheter may indicate infection. Most patients with catheter-related urinary tract infection remain asymptomatic, but 20 to 30% develop the symptoms of urinary tract infection and about 1 in 100 of these develop bacteraemia.

Indwelling urinary catheters account for 80% of nosocomial urinary tract infections; 80% of patients catheterized for longer than 7 to 10 days develop bacteriuria. Instrumentation of the urinary tract is also a risk factor for urinary tract infection. The main source of organisms is the periurethral flora, and *E. coli* is the dominant pathogen in all studies. Bacteria gain access to the bladder, usually by spreading up along the urinary catheter. Occasionally, infection is acquired exogenously during an epidemic of nosocomial infection. Most symptomatic or bacteraemic infections occur within 24 h of the organisms gaining access to the bladder. Treatment is with broad-spectrum antimicrobials administered empirically after obtaining appropriate cultures and later adjusted after receiving results of bacteriological studies. Asymptomatic patients need not be treated.

Since the important risk factor is the duration of catheterization, prevention is by avoiding catheterization or reducing the period of catheterization. Catheters should be inserted aseptically, and closed sterile drainage systems, uninterrupted gravity drainage, or intermittent or suprapubic catheterization employed. Some practitioners advocate a single prophylactic dose of antibiotic at the time of urinary catheter insertion or exchange in men to prevent bacteraemia. In other settings prophylactic antibiotics have not been shown to prevent infection for more than a few days. Catheters coated with antimicrobials such as silver have been shown to reduce infection rates in some patient groups, but their cost-effectiveness is disputed.

Surgical wound infection

One acceptable definition requires the presence of a purulent discharge in, or exuding from, a wound. Rates vary according to the definitions used. Internationally agreed definitions are used for high-quality epidemiological studies (Horan and Gaynes 2004).

Most wound infections follow direct inoculation of organisms into the wound at surgery or spread of bacteria to open wounds such as burns. The main risk factor is the degree of wound contamination at operation. Operations may be 'clean' (e.g. herniorrhaphy), 'clean–contaminated' (e.g. appendicectomy which requires incision of bowel), or 'contaminated' (e.g. gross spillage from the gastrointestinal tract during surgery). *S. aureus* causes most infections complicating clean surgery and rates below 2% are expected. 'Contaminated' surgery is associated with polymicrobial infections, especially with *E. coli* and mixed anaerobes originating from the patient's gastrointestinal tract, and rates of infection are 5 to 15%. Other risk factors include age, obesity, the duration of the operation, and a remote infection.

Wound infections present with local symptoms and signs (pain, erythema, pus, dehiscence) and with general features of infection, such as fever. Appropriate cultures, including blood cultures, are taken, pus is drained, and broad-spectrum antimicrobials are given empirically, directed at the likely flora but later adjusted according to bacteriological results.

Prevention is by meticulous aseptic surgical techniques. Prophylactic antimicrobials, given no more than 2 h before the surgical incision, have been shown to reduce wound infection rates by between two- and fivefold for clean–contaminated and contaminated procedures, and in clean surgery when a prosthesis is inserted (e.g. joint replacement, vascular graft insertion).

Nosocomial pneumonia

Pneumonia is defined clinically by the production of purulent sputum, signs of respiratory consolidation, a fall in arterial P_{O_2}, and the appearance of new infiltrates on the chest radiograph. Between 0.55 and 1.5% of patients admitted to hospital develop lower respiratory tract infections. Crude case fatality rates of between 20 and 30% are quoted, but death may occur as a result of underlying disease. Patients who are intubated and ventilated patients have a high risk of developing pneumonia as bacteria colonizing the upper respiratory and gastrointestinal and upper respiratory tracts may be aspirated. The organisms causing ventilator-associated pneumonia are usually acquired after admission to hospital and the bacteria are often more antibiotic-resistant than community-acquired organisms. Examples of organisms causing nosocomial pneumonia are listed in Table 2.3.2.

Culture of expectorated sputum or tracheal aspirate is poorly predictive of the bacterial cause of nosocomial pneumonia, which is best determined by quantitative culture of specimens obtained by sampling the terminal airways (e.g. by bronchoalveolar lavage). Initially, broad-spectrum antimicrobials appropriate for likely infecting flora should be given empirically. Once the susceptibility of the causative pathogen has been determined, specific antimicrobial treatment can be instituted.

The risks of nosocomial pneumonia can be reduced by a variety of strategies, including avoidance of intubation and the use of noninvasive ventilation techniques. For those who are intubated, continuous aspiration of subglottic secretions and nursing in the semirecumbent position have been shown to be effective in good-quality studies.

Table 2.3.2 Causative organisms identified in samples obtained at bronchoscopy by protected specimen brush (percentage of all pneumonias)

	France (2000)	Spain (2000)
Pseudomonas aeruginosa	22	33
Staphylococcus aureus including MRSA	17	26
Escherichia coli or 'coliform'	10	23
Streptococci	16	3
Haemophilus spp.	7	6
Acinetobacter spp.	5	0
Other species	23	9
Polymicrobial	12	0

MRSA, methicillin-resistant *Staphylococcus aureus*.

Selective decontamination of the digestive tract has reduced the occurrence of nosocomial pneumonia and mortality in ventilated patients, but has shown less benefit in units where there is a high prevalence of multidrug-resistant organisms. Short courses of antibiotics at the time of intubation have been shown to be effective in certain patient groups. Epidemic nosocomial pneumonia usually results from bacterial contamination of respiratory equipment, such as nebulizers, ventilators, or bronchoscopes, and can be prevented by ensuring that single-use respiratory devices are not reused, by cleaning and disinfecting equipment, and by hand hygiene before and after patient contact.

Intravascular device-associated infections

Bacteraemia is the most important intravascular device-associated infection; it varies in prevalence from about 0.04% for subcutaneous central venous ports to about 0.2% for peripheral intravenous cannulae and approximately 10% for temporary nontunnelled central venous haemodialysis catheters.

The duration of intravascular cannulation is the most significant risk factor. Bacteria usually gain access to the blood by direct spread from the skin surface along the subcutaneous catheter tunnel to its tip in the blood vessel. Bacteraemia from intraluminal bacteria results from contamination of connecting devices. This is particularly important in catheters with subcutaneous cuffs, such as Hickman catheters, where the periluminal route of infection is less likely. The organisms that most frequently cause intravenous device-related bacteraemia are *S. aureus*, pseudomonas, and candida. In patients with haematological malignancies, coagulase-negative staphylococci and enterococci are also frequently implicated.

Line-related sepsis presents with local inflammation or signs of thrombophlebitis often with features of bacteraemia and even thromboembolism. Blood cultures are obtained, the affected catheter is removed the catheter tip cultured, and empirical antimicrobials are given. Sometimes, long-term intravenous catheters, such as Hickman lines, can be 'sterilized' by administering parenteral antibiotics into the line and using 'antibiotic lock' therapy. Exit site infections involving these devices may be treated with antibiotics and line retention. Tunnel infections usually require line removal of the line.

Prevention of line-associated infections is by using aseptic techniques when inserting catheters, maintaining a high standards of line care, and removing catheters as soon as possible. Before insertion, the skin should be prepared with a reliable disinfectant such as an alcoholic solution of chlorhexidine. At insertion, the operators should wash their hands and, for long-line insertion, use a large sterile drape to isolate the insertion site and wear sterile gloves, gown, face mask, and hat. Central venous catheters are usually removed only if blocked or suspected as a source of sepsis. Peripheral intravascular devices should be removed or changed every 3 days. The skin at the exit site should be checked daily and the device removed if sepsis is suspected. Subcutaneous tunnelling, insertion of a subcutaneous cuff (Hickman line), burying them subcutaneously (e.g. portacaths), and incorporating antimicrobials onto the surface of the device can all reduce the infection rate significantly. Replacing the entire intravenous delivery set every 72 h is sufficient to reduce sepsis secondary to intraluminal contamination of 'giving' sets.

Prosthetic device-related infection

Infections of prosthetic devices such as heart valves, vascular grafts, cerebrospinal fluid shunts, artificial lenses, and joint replacements are usually caused by the normal skin flora. The devices become coated with a layer of host-derived macromolecules such as fibronectin and fibrin which have specific adhesion receptors for bacteria, particularly staphylococci. Once attached, these organisms multiply on the surface of the coated prosthesis forming a biofilm in a state physiologically different from rapidly dividing, 'free' microorganisms. They are inherently more resistant to antimicrobials, which explains the frequent failure of antimicrobial treatment. Bacteria gain access to prosthetic devices by direct inoculation, usually at surgery, or by settling on a prosthesis after haematogenous spread. Direct inoculation at surgery is responsible for prosthetic-device infections occurring more than 1 year after insertion since the organisms involved are usually skin commensals of low virulence, e.g. coagulase negative staphylococci. These infections are rarely cured with antimicrobial therapy alone and frequently require removal of the prosthetic device. In contrast artificial lens infections in the eye are often cured by antimicrobial treatment.

Prevention is by avoiding contamination of the wound at surgery and by using strict aseptic surgical techniques. In orthopaedic implant surgery, a large randomized controlled trial showed that an ultraclean air supply to the operating theatre is of benefit. Prophylactic antimicrobials given at the time of surgery have also been shown to reduce the risk of prosthetic joint infections.

Antibiotic-associated diarrhoea

Up to 30% of patients treated with antibiotics will develop diarrhoea as a result of the disturbance of the complex gut flora. In a few, loss of 'colonization resistance' predisposes to acquisition of *Clostridium difficile*. Faecal colonization by this organism is usually harmless, but in about one-third of patients, particularly older patients, the organism may overgrow and produce a cytotoxin resulting in colitis.

The clinical picture varies from mild diarrhoea with fever to fulminating colitis with dilatation of the colon (toxic megacolon) requiring colectomy. More severe disease and a greater likelihood of relapse can be the result of infection with a quinolone-resistant clone of *C. difficile*, prevalent in North America, the United Kingdom, and the Netherlands, which produces large amounts of toxin due to the deletion of a regulator gene *tcdC*. *C. difficile*-associated diarrhoea delays discharge from hospital by about 3 weeks. Since attack rates in older patients are around 5% and relapse can

occur in up to 30%, the disease can have a major impact on hospital resources. Diagnosis is by detection of the cytotoxin in a stool sample, but the test has poor specificity: toxin may be found in the stool of asymptomatic patients, and for many weeks after full recovery in those with symptoms. Patient management includes adequate rehydration, avoiding drugs which inhibit gut motility and proton pump inhibitors, and stopping the provoking antibiotics. Treatment is with oral metronidazole or vancomycin and surgical review is required for severe cases. The use of intravenous immunoglobulin in severe cases is controversial.

Prevention is by restricting the use of antibiotics according to agreed and audited protocols. Hand washing after patient contact, isolation of patients with diarrhoea, and cleaning the ward environment are employed on microbiological grounds, despite a lack of prospective studies showing their efficacy.

Nosocomial bacteraemia

Bacteraemia may occur secondarily to the infections mentioned above. The incidence is approximately 3 per 1000 hospital discharges. The case fatality is about 40%, but varies with the severity of the underlying disease, being as low as about 2% in obstetric patients. Most cases are related to a urinary catheter, intravascular catheter or postsurgical infection. The focus must be identified and, if possible, removed. Appropriate antimicrobials are given after obtaining blood and other relevant samples for microbiological culture.

Future developments

The increasing cost of healthcare will drive governments to impose mandatory surveillance and targets for reduction of selected nosocomial infections as these measures are highly cost effective. In the United Kingdom this is demonstrated by legislation ('The Health Act 2006: A code of practice for the prevention and control of healthcare associated infection') which mandates hospitals to have in place processes for the continuous improvement of infection rates. The United Kingdom government has published 'care bundles' of 'high impact interventions' outlining evidence-based practice for how this can be achieved. Coincident with the implementation of these measures since 2006, MRSA bacteraemia and *C. difficile* infection rates have declined significantly in the United Kingdom. Rapidly developing techniques of molecular biology are likely to reveal more clearly the relationship between hospital patients and the organisms which infect them, pointing the way to new risk-reducing strategies. The dissection of organisms by whole genome sequencing will improve our understanding of transmission pathways, virulence, and pathogenicity, enabling targeted interventions. Human genetic studies may also identify polymorphisms which predispose certain individuals or groups of individuals to infection.

Further reading

Bennett JV, Brachman PS (eds) (1998). *Hospital infections*, 4th edition. Lippincott-Raven, Philadelphia.

Edgeworth JD, *et al.* (2007). An outbreak in an intensive care unit of a strain of methicillin-resistant *Staphylococcus aureus* sequence type 239 associated with an increased rate of vascular access device-related bacteraemia. *Clin Infect Dis*, **44**, 493–501.

Flores C, *et al.* (2006). A CXCL2 tandem repeat promoter polymorphism is associated with susceptibility to severe sepsis in the Spanish population. *Genes Immun*, **7**, 141–9.

Harris SR, *et al.* (2010). Evolution of MRSA during hospital transmission and intercontinental spread. *Science* **327**(5964), 469–74.

Jarvis WR, (ed) (2007) *Bennett and Brachman's hospital infections*, 5th edition. Lippincott Williams & Wilkins, Philadelphia.

National Nosocomial Infections Surveillance (NNIS) System Report, data summary from January 1992 through June 2004, issued October 2004. *Am J Infect Control*, **32**, 470–85.

World Health Organization (2005). *Global patient safety challenge: 2005-6/world alliance for patient safety.* World Health Organization, Geneva.

Websites

New Delhi metallo-beta-lactamase 1 (NDM-1) http://en.wikipedia.org/wiki/New_Delhi_metallo-beta-lactamase_1

UK Department of Health. HCAI: Reducing healthcare associated infections http://hcai.dh.gov.uk/whatdoido/high-impact-interventions/ UK Health Act 2006 http://webarchive.nationalarchives.gov.uk/+/www.dh.gov.uk/en/Publicationsandstatistics/Publications/PublicationsPolicyAndGuidance/DH_4139336

2.4 Infection in the immunocompromised host

J. Cohen

Essentials

The term 'immunocompromised host' embraces a group of overlapping conditions in which the ability to respond normally to an infective challenge is in some way impaired. This includes patients with underlying conditions such as protein–calorie malnutrition and diabetes, as well as organ transplant recipients, those with haematological malignancies and others receiving therapeutic immunosuppression, and patients with HIV infection. Many patients have multiple risk factors that increase the risk of opportunistic infection.

General clinical approach

A high level of awareness is essential to the management of patients who are immunocompromised; infections can progress with frightening rapidity, the early physical signs are often muted, and the microbiology can be confusing. Aside from a full history and detailed physical examination, assessment should take account of risk factors such as the depth and duration of neutropenia, or the dose and duration of immunosuppressive therapies. It is particularly helpful to try to form a judgement of how quickly the condition is progressing. Patients must be reviewed frequently and will often require empirical antimicrobial therapy, but when possible it is better to try to establish the cause of the infection before starting treatment. This is partly because the differential diagnosis is wide and choosing the right treatment depends on knowing the causative organism, and partly because it is not uncommon for multiple organisms of different types to be involved.

Particular clinical syndromes

Fever of unknown origin—this is common in patients with neutropenia, with the risk of bacteraemia being most acute when the neutrophil count falls to less than 0.1×10^9/litre; in 50% of cases an organism is never identified. Empirical antibiotic therapy is vital and needs to be directed against both Gram-negative and Gram-positive organisms. The risk of invasive fungal infection rises if fever persists, in which case empirical antifungal therapy is justified.

Fever and new pulmonary infiltrates—this is a challenging problem with a wide range of potential causes depending on the clinical setting, including conventional respiratory pathogens, nosocomial pathogens, 'atypical' organisms, mycobacteria and related organisms, viruses, fungi, parasites, and also noninfectious causes such as pulmonary oedema, pulmonary haemorrhage, pulmonary emboli/infarction and drug toxicity. The clinical and radiological features are very rarely pathognomonic, hence a diagnostic procedure such as bronchoalveolar lavage should be performed whenever possible.

Acute neurological syndromes—these include both (1) meningoencephalitis—associated with conventional bacterial infections, listeriosis and tuberculosis, as well as fungi such as cryptococcus and candida; and (2) space-occupying lesions—caused by e.g. toxoplasma, aspergillus and nocardia. Once again there is a wide differential diagnosis and a low threshold of diagnostic suspicion is needed.

Gastrointestinal syndromes—these are frequent and include (1) stomatitis—the three commonest causes (candida, herpes simplex virus, and chemotherapy-induced mucositis) are clinically indistinguishable and can coexist; (2) diarrhoea—graft-versus-host disease is very difficult to distinguish from infective causes in bone marrow transplant recipients; (3) abnormalities of liver function tests—mild derangements are a common accompaniment to many systemic infections, but hepatitis is a particular feature of both toxoplasmosis and cytomegalovirus infection.

Prevention

This is an integral part of the management of patients who are immunosuppressed and, depending on context, comprises interventions such as nursing them in single rooms and chemoprophylaxis, e.g. co-trimoxazole to prevent pneumocystis and valganciclovir to prevent cytomegalovirus but, perhaps the single most important factor is being aware of the different and often subtle presentations of infection in this vulnerable group of patients.

Classification

The term 'immunocompromised host' has no formal definition but it embraces a group of overlapping conditions in which the ability to respond normally to an infective challenge is in some way impaired. It is helpful to think of such patients as falling into one of several distinct groups (Fig. 2.4.1).

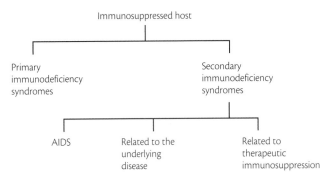

Fig. 2.4.1 A classification of the immunocompromised host.

Primary immunodeficiency syndromes

These are patients with congenital defects in immunity that render them more susceptible to infection. At the most extreme, children with severe combined immunodeficiency have virtually no functioning cellular or humoral immunity and, if unprotected, they will die from infection within a few months of birth. In contrast, some patients with chronic granulomatous disease, an inherited defect in neutrophil function, remain undiagnosed until early adult life. A complete description of the diagnosis and management of this group of disorders is given in Oxford Textbook of Medicine 5e Chapter 5.2.

AIDS

HIV causes AIDS which is a model for an acquired defect of cellular immunity leading to an increased risk of infection. Although there are inevitably parallels with other groups of immunocompromised patients, there are particular issues both in the diagnosis and management of infection in AIDS that warrant separate discussion (Chapters 5.23, 5.24).

Infection related to the underlying condition

The notion of opportunistic infection in the immunocompromised host is most familiar with haematological malignancy or organ transplantation, discussed in detail below. Less obvious, but probably more numerous, are the many physiological conditions and other diseases associated with an increased incidence of infection (Box 2.4.1). These immune defects are usually mixed and frequently poorly characterized. The susceptibility to infection varies considerably both in the pattern and severity of infection that occurs, but the clinical problem is real enough. For example, in malnutrition infection due to mycobacteria and *Salmonella* is more common, and *Pneumocystis* pneumonia was first described in children with protein-calorie malnutrition. There is extensive literature documenting multiple defects of host defence in association with

> **Box 2.4.1** Examples of conditions associated with impaired immune responses and an increased risk/severity of infection
>
> ◆ Alcohol abuse
> ◆ Burns
> ◆ Cushing's disease
> ◆ Diabetes mellitus
> ◆ Down's syndrome
> ◆ Extremes of age
> ◆ Haemochromatosis
> ◆ Haemodialysis
> ◆ Intravenous drug abuse
> ◆ Malnutrition
> ◆ Pregnancy
> ◆ Severe liver disease
> ◆ Spinal cord injury
> ◆ Splenectomy
> ◆ Trauma/surgery
> ◆ Uraemia

alcohol abuse; clinically, this is reflected in an excess of lower respiratory tract infections with *Streptococcus pneumoniae*, *Mycobacterium tuberculosis*, and *Klebsiella pneumoniae*. In Cushing's disease, the excess endogenous steroid production can result in a pattern of opportunist infections that mirrors that seen in patients receiving corticosteroid therapy (see below). Diabetes mellitus is a good example of a disease that is frequently complicated by infection, typically with staphylococcal skin abscesses, and in endemic countries, meiloiodosis.

Patients who have had their spleen removed or who have functional (or more rarely congenital) asplenia are at increased risk of certain infections caused by particular organisms, notably *S. pneumoniae* and *Haemophilus influenza*, and *Neisseria meningitidis*. The degree of risk is related to the underlying cause; overall, approximately 5% of patients will have a serious infection, but this varies from 1.5% following traumatic splenectomy to as high as 25% in patients with thalassaemia. Serious infections are most common during the first 5 years following splenectomy and particularly during the first year, but overwhelming postsplenectomy sepsis can occur decades after the surgery.

In myeloma and chronic lymphocytic leukaemia the primary defect is hypogammaglobulinaemia. This is manifested clinically by an excess of bacterial infections, typically those caused by encapsulated organisms such as *S. pneumoniae* and *H. influenzae*. These patients (and others, especially those with rheumatoid arthritis, systemic lupus erythematosus, or polyarteritis nodosa) all have impaired immunity as a consequence of their underlying disease, but because they also commonly receive treatment with immunosuppressive drugs it can be very difficult to attribute cause and effect.

Infection complicating therapeutic immunosuppression

In addition to the well-recognized risk groups, such as those with haematological malignancy or allograft recipients, infective complications of immunosuppression are now being recognized in a much broader range of patients. Conditions as diverse as severe skin disease, asthma, inflammatory bowel disease, rheumatoid arthritis are routinely treated with immunosuppressive drugs such as prednisolone, azathioprine, ciclosporin, cyclophosphamide, and anti-tumour necrosis factor (anti-TNF) drugs. These patients are not so profoundly immunosuppressed as a bone marrow transplant recipient, but they are certainly at risk of opportunistic infections; a good example of this is the recent recognition of the increased risk of mycobacterial infections in patients with rheumatoid arthritis receiving the anti-TNF agent Infliximab.

Immunosuppressed patients have multiple risk factors; a bone marrow transplant recipient may have been neutropenic, receiving corticosteroids and ciclosporin for management of graft-versus-host disease, and have an indwelling right atrial catheter for feeding purposes. Clearly each of these factors represents a substantial and very different type of risk factor for infection and it is important to remember that, in such patients, multiple pathogens can cause disease simultaneously.

Factors such as the precise nature and intensity of the immunosuppressive regimen, anatomical and/or surgical considerations, and the premorbid status of the patient will all have some influence on the pattern of opportunistic infections that occur. For instance, BK virus is a human polyoma virus that can cause renal allograft rejection but virtually never occurs in other organ recipients; liver transplantation is notable for the high incidence of invasive *Candida* infections, and toxoplasmosis is recognized to be a particular problem following cardiac transplantation. The recent introduction of the anti-CD20 monoclonal antibody rituximab has led to an increase in the incidence of opportunistic viral infections such as cytomegalovirus and hepatitis C. A detailed consideration of these differences is beyond the scope of this chapter. The following sections describe the management of some of the common clinical syndromes that present as infection in immunosuppressed patients.

Common clinical syndromes

A general approach to management

Infections in immunosuppressed patients can progress with frightening rapidity; the early physical signs are often muted and the microbiology can be confusing. Patients need to be reviewed frequently and will often need empirical therapy, but this need not be totally 'blind'; a structured and informed assessment will generally allow a logical response to what are the most likely pathogens. Most hospitals will have antimicrobial policies to guide empirical therapy in immunocompromised patients.

History

This may reveal exposure to community-acquired infections such as varicella zoster or tuberculosis, which can be particularly severe in the immunocompromised patient. Note should be made of any past history of infection; bronchiectasis, for instance, can be very troublesome in transplant recipients. A detailed travel history is important; patients who have visited certain parts of the United States of America may have been exposed to the systemic mycoses such as histoplasmosis or coccidioidomycosis, which are unfamiliar to many clinicians. Visitors to Central America or the Far East, even many years ago, may have acquired an asymptomatic infection with the helminth *Strongyloides stercoralis*; immunosuppression can lead to overt disease (the hyperinfection syndrome) with a high mortality (see below).

Physical examination

This may be unhelpful; as immunosuppressed patients often do not mount a good inflammatory response. Thus there may be only a low-grade fever, a thin serous exudate may suffice for pus, and mild abdominal tenderness can be the only sign of peritonitis. Nevertheless, careful, and if necessary repeated clinical examination is worthwhile, as signs of inflammation may become apparent only when immune function returns. Particular attention should be paid to the presence of new skin lesions. In neutropenic patients, bacteraemias may be accompanied by striking embolic lesions (Fig. 2.4.2); *Pseudomonas* infections (and less commonly *Klebsiella* and *Aeromonas*) can cause a focal necrotic cellulitis called ecthyma gangrenosum. Fungal infections present as indolent locally invasive lesions (Fig. 2.4.3); aspergillus infections often have a black eschar. The perianal area and the insertion sites of indwelling right atrial catheters repay careful examination. Aspiration and/or biopsy of any new skin lesion in immunosuppressed patients are well worthwhile, since they may quickly point to an otherwise inapparent diagnosis. Lymphadenopathy is always important and will usually require aspiration or biopsy. It may be a manifestation of a lymphoproliferative condition, post-transplant lymphoproliferative disease (PTLD), arising as a consequence of the intense immunosuppressive regimens now in widespread use. Although

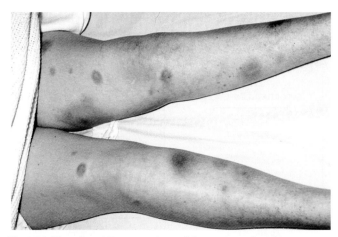

Fig. 2.4.2 Disseminated Gram-negative sepsis in a neutropenic patient.

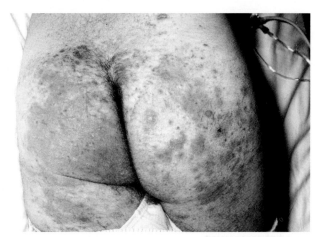

Fig. 2.4.3 Extensive dermatophyte infection in a bone marrow transplant recipient.

the precise pathogenesis of PTLD is still unclear, it is generally accepted that Epstein–Barr virus (EBV) infection or reactivation and intensive anti-T-lymphocyte regimens play a major role. PTLD is emerging as one of the major causes of late death following renal transplantation.

Underlying disease

This can provide valuable clues. Neutropenia is a major risk factor for infection and renders the patient susceptible to bacteraemia, particularly with Gram-negative organisms such as *Escherichia coli* and *Pseudomonas aeruginosa*. A patient with an obstructing bronchial neoplasm may develop a lung abscess due to inadequate drainage. Corticosteroids are used widely; when given in doses exceeding 15 to 20 mg daily for long periods they increase susceptibility to infections with viruses, fungi, parasites, and bacteria such as *Mycobacterium tuberculosis* and *Nocardia*, all organisms normally associated with cellular immune defences.

Duration of immunosuppression

This often has a profound effect on the type of infection that occurs, and is well illustrated by comparing the 'timetables' of infections in renal transplant recipients with patients receiving bone marrow transplants (Fig. 2.4.4). In the first 6 weeks after renal transplantation bacterial infections predominate, typically surgical

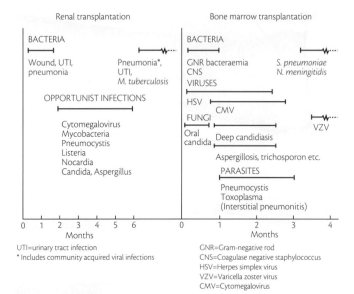

Fig. 2.4.4 Timetable for the development of infective complications in renal transplant and bone marrow transplant recipients.

complications of the procedure or urinary infections. Between 6 weeks and 6 months post-transplantation the patient is most at risk from the 'classic' opportunistic infections; as time continues and the intensity of immunosuppression declines, typical community-acquired infections become more common. In bone marrow transplantation, the initial period of neutropenia is characterized by bacterial infections; later, when many patients receive high-dose steroids for graft-versus-host disease, cytomegalovirus and fungal infections (candida and aspergillus) develop.

Speed of progression

An assessment of this is helpful in both differential diagnosis and in deciding on empirical therapy. In neutropenic patients, the onset of fever is usually an indication for immediate empirical antibiotic therapy (see below). In contrast, the response to a fever and new pulmonary infiltrates in a patient who is 8 months post renal transplantation will depend on the pace of the illness. Rapid deterioration over the space of a few hours will suggest a bacterial infection or a noninfectious cause, and will need urgent therapy; a more indolent presentation would point to a fungal or mycobacterial aetiology, and treatment can be delayed for a short period to try and establish the diagnosis.

Investigations

It is important that the diagnostic laboratories be made aware of the clinical problem since handling of specimens from immuno-suppressed patients—and interpretation of the results—will often differ substantially from routine procedures.

Fever of unknown origin

In neutropenic patients, fever is often the first and only sign of bacteraemia, and prompt action is necessary. In this setting, a fever of unknown origin is defined as a fever of over 38 °C sustained for 2 h and not obviously due to an identifiable cause such as concomitant blood transfusion.

The risk of bacteraemia is directly related to the depth of the neutropenia; the incidence of infection rises when the neutrophil

count falls to below 0.5×10^9/L, and is particularly severe when the count falls to less than 0.1×10^9/L (Fig. 2.4.5). Some years ago, the commonest bloodstream isolates were Gram-negative bacteria such as *E. coli* and klebsiella, generally derived from the patient's gut flora, and *P. aeruginosa*, a common environmental pathogen. Gram-negative bacteraemia in neutropenic patients carried a very high mortality and led to the introduction of several preventative strategies such as the use of prophylactic antibiotics and colony-stimulating factors. Although these approaches have not been entirely successful, the incidence of Gram-negative bacteraemias has declined substantially, and in most units Gram-positive organisms, notably coagulase-negative staphylococci (*Staphylococcus epidermidis*) are now the most common isolates. Importantly though, tissue-based infections such as pneumonia continue to be caused predominantly by Gram-negative bacteria.

Clinical features are frequently unhelpful. Sometimes a focus will be suggested by erythema around the point of entry of an indwelling catheter, a finding often associated with staphylococcal infection. Septic shock is infrequent, although it can be associated with viridans streptococci; interestingly, endocarditis is rare.

Blood cultures should be drawn before treatment is begun. Ideally two sets should be obtained, at least one of which should be from a peripheral vein (rather than an indwelling catheter), although this is not always possible. Culturing larger volumes of blood (e.g. 30 ml compared to the more conventional 10 ml) will increase the yield. Appropriate samples must also be taken from other potential foci of infection. Nevertheless, it has been one of the enduring frustrations of this subject that even the most rigorous of microbiological investigations in the febrile neutropenic patient will yield only 40 to 50% of positive cultures. The explanation for this is unknown; some studies have suggested that it is due to endotoxaemia in the absence of bacteraemia, but the data are inconclusive. What is clear, however, is that treatment must begin

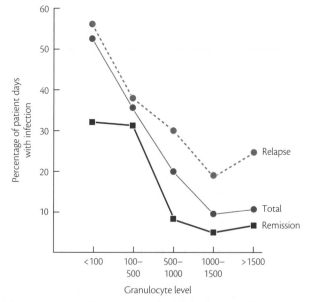

Fig. 2.4.5 Relationship between neutrophil count and the risk of invasive Gram-negative infection.
(From Bodey GP, *et al.* (1966). Quantitative relationships between circulating leukocytes and infection in patients with acute leukemia. *Ann Intern Med*, **64**, 328–40, with permission.)

before the results of the cultures are available; delay will lead to unacceptable fatalities.

The choice of the initial empirical antibiotic regimen for the febrile neutropenic patient has been the subject of intense investigation. The ideal regimen will be safe and have good bactericidal activity against all the common pathogens. No single regimen is perfect; much will depend on the availability (and cost) of antibiotics in a given institution, and on local patterns of antibiotic susceptibility. The Infectious Diseases Society of America has published helpful guidelines on the management of these patients (see Further reading).

An important recent development in practice has been the risk assessment of febrile neutropenic patients. The goal is to distinguish those high-risk patients that need hospital admission and parenteral antibiotics, from a low-risk group (<5% risk of complications) who can be managed as outpatients with oral therapy. Well-validated hospital-based regimens include the combination of an antipseudomonal penicillin plus an aminoglycoside or the use of single agents such as a third- or fourth-generation cephalosporin (e.g. ceftazidime or cefepime), a carbapenem such as meropenem, or a β-lactam/β-lactamase inhibitor combination (e.g. piperacillin–tazobactam). A meta-analysis concluded that monotherapy was on balance at least as effective as and probably safer than combination therapy.

All these regimens are very active against the common Gram-negative organisms, but are relatively ineffective at treating-antimicrobial resistant Gram-positive bacteria, such as coagulase-negative staphylococci or meticillin (methicillin)-resistant *Staphylococcus aureus* (MRSA), that are nowadays common problems in many units. Unfortunately, there are only a very limited number of drugs that are reliably active against these organisms, notably glycopeptides such as vancomycin and teicoplanin, and more recently linezolid. Some clinicians have advocated adding an anti-Gram-positive agent to the initial empirical regimen; one disadvantage of this approach is the toxicity (and cost) of vancomycin which may not be justified, particularly because coagulase-negative staphylococci rarely cause death. Several prospective clinical trials have concluded that unless there are strong grounds for considering MRSA infection, vancomycin can usually be withheld until the results of blood cultures are known. A randomized controlled trial in febrile neutropenic patients concluded that linezolid was not inferior to vancomycin in either safety or efficacy.

Patients who are assessed as being in a low-risk group may be managed either with a brief period of inpatient parenteral therapy followed by rapid conversion to oral agents, or by oral therapy from the outset. A typical oral regimen is a combination of a quinolone plus amoxicillin/clavulanate.

In patients who respond to the initial regimen, the treatment should be continued for at least 7 days, and ideally until the neutrophil count has returned to over 0.5×10^9/L. Sometimes this is not possible; the patient may have a persistent or unresponsive neutropenia (e.g. aplastic anaemia, or following bone marrow transplantation). In these patients, treatment is usually cautiously stopped after an arbitrary period such as 14 days; rebound bacteraemias can occur and will need further treatment.

A common problem is the patient who continues to have high swinging fevers after 48 to 72 h of broad-spectrum antibacterial antibiotics. The patient must be carefully re-evaluated: Has some new clinical sign appeared? Could there be a resistant organism or an occult source of the sepsis? Simply changing the antibiotic

regimen or adding vancomycin in the absence of any evidence to support these moves is not supported by clinical trial data. In this situation, invasive fungal infection becomes more likely. Randomized clinical trials have demonstrated that empirical addition of an antifungal agent, either an amphotericin B formulation or an antifungal triazole such as voriconazole is associated with a response rate of approximately 30%.

Fever of unknown origin in the non-neutropenic immunosuppressed patient presents as a completely different problem. Fever in this setting is rarely immediately life-threatening, and the wide differential diagnosis means that it is generally better to pursue the cause rather than embark on empirical therapy.

Fever and new pulmonary infiltrates

The development of fever and new pulmonary infiltrates is one of the most challenging clinical problems in this group of patients. Pneumonia is the commonest infective cause of death in immunocompromised patients. In the presence of diffuse airspace disease, the mortality approaches 50% irrespective of the underlying defect in host defence, although the epidemiology varies both between different patient groups and at different times reflecting the intensity of the immunosuppression (Table 2.4.1).

The condition can progress extremely quickly, and conventional diagnostic procedures may be unhelpful. The list of possible causes is so daunting (Box 2.4.2) that clinicians may be tempted to use multiple empirical antimicrobial agents, sometimes to the patient's detriment. It is often not possible to 'guess' with any certainty the precise cause of the problem (indeed, it can be dangerous to do so, since it is not uncommon for multiple causes to be present simultaneously), but by considering the available information one can construct a 'short list' which will guide further investigation and treatment.

Table 2.4.1 Aetiology of the 'febrile pneumonitis' syndrome in different patient groups

	Renal transplantation	Bone marrow transplantation
Less than 1 month	Aspiration Nosocomial LRTI	Aspiration Nosocomial LRTI Aspergillus
1–3 months[a]	Cytomegalovirus Pneumocystis Aspergillus Nocardia Mycobacteria Mucor	Cytomegalovirus Pneumocystis Aspergillus Respiratory syncytial virus Mycobacteria Mucor Noninfective causes[b]
More than 3 months[a]	Influenza Legionella Common respiratory bacteria	Varicella zoster GVHD Common respiratory bacteria and viruses

GVHD, graft-versus-host disease; LRTI, lower respiratory tract infection.
[a] Six months in renal transplant recipients.
[b] Includes idiopathic interstitial pneumonitis in bone marrow transplant recipients.
Modified from Wilson WR, Cockerill FR 3rd, Rosenow EC 3rd (1985). Pulmonary disease in the immunocompromised host (2). *Mayo Clin Proc*, **60**, 610–31.

Box 2.4.2 Causes of fever and new pulmonary infiltrates in the immunocompromised host

Infections

Bacterial

- Conventional respiratory pathogens
  - *S. pneumoniae, H. influenzae, Klebsiella*
- Nosocomial pathogens
  - *E. coli, Pseudomonas, Legionella*
- 'Atypical' organisms
  - *Chlamydia psittaci, C. pneumoniae*, mycoplasma
- Mycobacteria and related organisms
  - *M. tuberculosis*, nontuberculous mycobacteria, nocardia.

Viral

- Herpes viruses
  - Cytomegalovirus, herpes simplex virus, varicella zoster virus
- Respiratory viruses
  - Respiratory syncytial virus, influenza and parainfluenza viruses, adenovirus, measles

Fungi

- Systemic mycoses
  - Blastomycosis, histoplasmosis, coccidioidomycosis
- Opportunist mycoses
  - Candida, aspergillus, mucor, cryptococcus
- Other rare fungi
  - *Trichosporon, Pseudallescheria boydii*

Parasites

- *Pneumocystis jirovecii, Strongyloides stercoralis, Toxoplasma gondii*

Noninfective causes

Pulmonary pathology

- Pulmonary oedema, pulmonary infarction/emboli, pulmonary haemorrhage
- Primary or secondary malignancy

Other causes

- Drugs (e.g. sulphonamides, methotrexate, bleomycin, procarbazine, cyclophosphamide, sirolimus)
- Activity of the underlying disease (e.g. systemic lupus erythematosus)
- Radiation pneumonitis

The initial evaluation should follow the approach outlined above, in particular making an assessment of the intensity of the immunosuppression and the speed of progression of the pulmonary disease. The main purpose of this is to determine the need for empirical therapy, either because the clinical picture is suggestive of a 'simple' bacterial pneumonia or because of a potentially more serious progressive cause of uncertain aetiology. Factors that would favour a bacterial aetiology include the presence of neutropenia, a rapidly developing clinical evolution (e.g. deterioration over a period of 12 h), progressive hypoxia, a sputum Gram stain showing a marked predominance of a single bacterial morphology (even in the absence of neutrophils), or a chest radiographic appearance that has worsened significantly over a short period. High fever is not necessarily a part of this syndrome; indeed, it is important to emphasize that this rapidly evolving clinical picture is not inevitably due to infection. Noninfective causes such as acute lung haemorrhage or pulmonary oedema can present in an identical fashion, and the most appropriate therapy may be diuretics rather than antimicrobials. However, antimicrobials will often need to be given as well because of what has been termed 'infection-provoked relapse'. In immunologically mediated diseases such as systemic lupus erythematosus or anti-glomerular basement membrane (GBM) disease (Goodpasture's syndrome) infection can precipitate a relapse of the underlying disease. Thus, the development of fever and new pulmonary shadows in a patient with anti-GBM disease may be primarily due to lung haemorrhage associated with a rise in anti-GBM antibodies, but this in turn can be precipitated by an infection that need not necessarily be in the lung. Treatment must be directed both towards improving oxygenation and the underlying infection.

Blood cultures should always be obtained, and sputum obtained if it is available. A chest radiograph and arterial blood gas analysis are essential. The initial treatment will be dictated by the clinical circumstances, but the temptation to use a complex regimen to provide very broad spectrum cover is best avoided. Rapid clinical deterioration is usually caused by bacterial infections; a combination of piperacillin–tazobactam plus erythromycin will be appropriate. The addition of vancomycin may be necessary if there are clinical or epidemiological grounds to be concerned about MRSA infection. Unusual ('opportunistic') organisms such as mycobacteria, nocardia, or cytomegalovirus rarely cause such a rapid clinical deterioration and it is extremely difficult to distinguish them on clinical grounds alone. For these reasons, the addition of further empirical agents is usually not warranted.

In patients in whom immediate empirical therapy is not necessary, additional diagnostic procedures can be done. These should include serological tests for atypical organisms (including histoplasma and coccidioides in patients who have been in endemic areas), and examination of blood for cytomegalovirus DNA. The chest radiograph should be repeated, but it is not as sensitive as arterial blood gas measurements, which should be done twice daily. The radiographic appearances are rarely sufficiently specific as to suggest a precise diagnosis, although they can provide helpful pointers. Thus a bilateral interstitial midzone infiltrate associated with marked hypoxia is typical of pneumonia due to *Pneumocystis jirovecii* (previously called *P. carinii*), and a pleura-based infarct is suggestive of aspergillus. However, there are pitfalls in relying on the radiographic appearance alone in guiding the choice of therapy. First, no radiographic appearance is pathognomonic of any single pathological process; e.g. cytomegalovirus or pulmonary oedema can mimic *Pneumocystis*, and *Legionella* pneumonia cannot be distinguished from *Aspergillus*. Second, multiple agents can be present simultaneously, and each may require separate treatment. Other imaging techniques such as high-resolution CT can often provide useful additional information on the extent of the process, and will sometimes point to the cause (e.g. the 'halo sign' associated with invasive aspergillosis).

If the condition does not resolve and initial investigations are unhelpful it is often appropriate to try to make a specific diagnosis by obtaining material directly from the bronchial tree. In most cases the method of choice is bronchoscopy with bronchoalveolar lavage. This will provide adequate material without incurring a serious risk of bleeding (many such patients are thrombocytopenic). In most series, bronchial brush or transbronchial biopsy specimens produce only a marginal increase in the diagnostic yield, and are usually not done unless the clinical picture is suggestive of a non-infective process such as an infiltrating tumour. Close liaison with the microbiology laboratory is very important because additional diagnostic procedures will need to be performed.

Acute neurological syndromes

A large number of conventional and opportunistic pathogens can lead to neurological infection in immunocompromised patients. Although there is some degree of overlap, the underlying defect in host defence is often a good indicator of the likely cause (Table 2.4.2).

The clinical features may help suggest the diagnosis. Meningitic syndromes are more likely to be associated with conventional bacterial infections, listeriosis, and tuberculosis, as well as fungi such as cryptococcus and candida. In contrast, infections with *Toxoplasma*, *Aspergillus*, or *Nocardia* more commonly present as space-occupying lesions. Pure encephalitic syndromes are less common, but can occur with herpes simplex virus. Rhinocerebral mucormycosis is a progressive, destructive infection caused by mucor and related moulds that usually begins in the paranasal sinuses and spreads caudally to involve the orbits or the frontal lobes of the brain (Fig. 2.4.6). It is seen particularly in patients with uncontrolled diabetes mellitus or as a complication of neutropenia. Progressive multifocal leukoencephalitis (PML) is a subacute neurological disease caused by the JC polyomavirus. PML presents with the insidious onset of impairment of speech, vision, and higher functions without evidence of raised intracranial pressure. The condition progresses inexorably, usually leading to death in about 6 months.

Bacterial infections generally proceed rapidly, while fungi and parasites pursue a more indolent course. However, exceptions to this are common and there is no substitute for obtaining a precise diagnosis. Examination of the skin (see below) and fundoscopy may be valuable. Retinitis is not usually a feature of systemic

Table 2.4.2 Organisms causing neurological infections in different patient groups

	Bacteria	**Fungi**	**Parasites**	**Viruses**
Neutropenia	Gram-negative Enterobacteriaceae	Candida		
		Aspergillus		
		Mucor		
T cell/ monocyte defect	Listeria	Cryptococcus	Toxoplasma	Varicella zoster
	Legionella	Aspergillus	Strongyloides	Herpes simplex
	Nocardia	Mucor		Polyomavirus
	Mycobacteria	Coccidioides		
Splenectomy	S. pneumoniae			
	H. influenzae			
	Neisseria			

infection with toxoplasma or cytomegalovirus; in contrast, candida endophthalmitis may be the only manifestation of deep-seated infection (Fig. 2.4.7).

Examination of the cerebrospinal fluid is mandatory. A high index of suspicion is necessary, since the clinical features of meningitis are often muted in these patients. An unexplained low-grade fever and mild headache may be the only clues; frank meningism, photophobia, or focal neurological signs occur late. Examination of the cerebrospinal fluid should include direct microscopy and culture for bacteria, mycobacteria, and fungi, a cryptococcal latex agglutination test, antigen tests for *S. pneumoniae*, and the demonstration of specific antibody production or DNA sequences by the polymerase chain reaction (e.g. for herpes simplex, polyomaviruses).

Certain organisms are notable for their absence on direct microscopy: mycobacteria are seen in less than 10% of cases, and

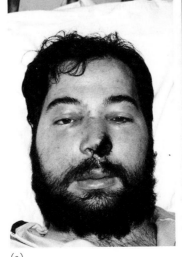

Fig. 2.4.6 Invasive mucormycosis. (a) Clinical appearances. (b) CT scan showing extensive sinus involvement.

(a)

(b)

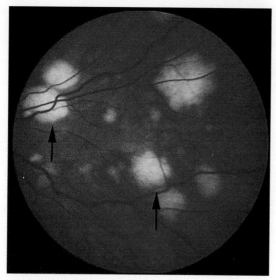

Fig. 2.4.7 Candida endophthalmitis.

Nocardia and *Aspergillus* only very rarely. A predominance of lymphocytes suggests partially treated bacterial infection, tuberculosis, or a viral aetiology, but not infection with listeria, despite its name. A low cerebrospinal fluid glucose points to bacterial meningitis or tuberculosis but is not specific. Sometimes the only abnormality is a modest elevation of the cerebrospinal fluid protein; this should never be ignored, even in the seeming absence of other features of neurological infection. Where appropriate, cytological examination of the cerebrospinal fluid should be done to exclude carcinomatous or leukaemic meningitis, which can mimic an acute infective presentation.

Certain neurological infections are often associated with pulmonary disease; these include *Legionella*, tuberculosis, *Aspergillus*, *Mucor*, and *Nocardia*. A contrast-enhanced CT brain scan should be performed. Focal, usually enhancing lesions are particularly associated with pyogenic abscesses and toxoplasmosis. Tuberculomas can appear as single lesions. MRI is superior to CT scanning particularly for abnormalities of the brain stem (e.g. the basal meningitis associated with cryptococcal infection), and frequently reveals lesions in toxoplasmosis that are not seen on CT scans. It may be particularly helpful in avoiding a brain biopsy when a diagnosis of PML is considered.

Any new skin lesions should be biopsied, and a nasal biopsy may reveal *Mucor*. An electroencephalogram is rarely helpful. Brain biopsy is done very rarely; it should not be considered unless empirical therapy has failed and there is a real prospect of therapeutic benefit to the patient.

If the cerebrospinal fluid is nondiagnostic but bacterial infection cannot be excluded, empirical antibiotics should be given immediately. Ceftriaxone is used first-line but a carbapenem such as meropenem should be considered in patients who have recently received broad-spectrum antibacterials or in whom *Nocardia* is a possibility. Serological tests for toxoplasmosis are not specific in this setting, and if the infection is suspected it is better to start empirical therapy with pyrimethamine and sulfdiazine or cotrimoxazole. Cerebral aspergillosis and mucormycosis have a very poor prognosis; treatment should be begun with high-dose amphotericin B, and surgical debridement considered if possible. There is no effective treatment for PML.

Acute gastrointestinal syndromes

The organisms associated with specific gastrointestinal syndromes in immunocompromised patients are shown in Table 2.4.3.

Severe stomatitis is a common complaint in immunosuppressed patients. The three most common causes *Candida*, herpes simplex virus, and chemotherapy-induced mucositis are clinically indistinguishable and can indeed coexist. For these reasons, the diagnosis should always be confirmed by microscopy and culture. Herpetic stomatitis in particular can be atypical in these patients; the classic appearance of groups of small vesicles is unusual, and a more common presentation is ulceration, which can be extensive (Fig. 2.4.8). In profoundly immunosuppressed patients such as bone marrow transplant recipients oral candidiasis is very common, and in patients who are seropositive before transplantation, reactivation of herpes simplex is almost universal. For these reasons, antiviral prophylaxis is usually given. Both herpes simplex virus and candida can cause oesophagitis, generally (but not exclusively) as an extension of oral disease. If necessary, oesophagoscopy with brush cytology and/or biopsy is the investigation of choice. Proven oesophageal candidiasis should be regarded as 'invasive' disease and treated with systemic antifungals (amphotericin B or fluconazole).

A large number of organisms can cause acute diarrhoeal syndromes; in addition, noninfective conditions such as radiation enteritis, drugs, and graft-versus-host disease must be included in the differential diagnosis. There are no distinguishing clinical features of note, and diagnosis depends on microbiological examination of the faeces.

The diarrhoea due to *Clostridium difficile* is usually caused by a cytotoxin resulting in pseudomembranous colitis. However, patients with leukaemia or aplastic anaemia may develop neutropenic enterocolitis (previously called typhlitis), a fulminating invasive colitis characterized by diffuse dilation and oedema of the bowel walls, haemorrhage, ulceration, and a high mortality.

Table 2.4.3 Gastrointestinal syndromes in the immunocompromised host

	Bacteria	Fungi	Parasites	Viruses
Oral infection		Candida		Herpes simplex virus
Diarrhoeal syndromes	Neutropenic enterocolitis	Candida	Giardia lamblia	Enterovirus
	C. difficile		Isospora belli	Adenovirus
	Salmonella Shigella Campylobacter E. coli 0157		Cryptosporidium	Cytomegalovirus
	Nontuberculous mycobacteria		Microsporidium	Rotavirus
Hepatic syndromes		Candida	Toxoplasma gondii	Cytomegalovirus
				Hepatitis B, C, and E viruses
				Herpes simplex virus
				Varicella zoster virus
				Epstein–Barr virus

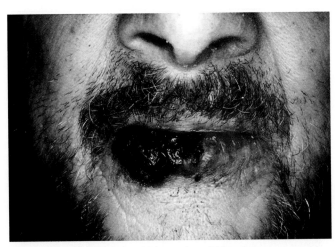

Fig. 2.4.8 Severe herpetic stomatitis in a patient with lymphoma.

Classically this has been associated with clostridial bacteraemia, in particular *Clostridium septicum*, but other clostridia, including *C. difficile*, and even Gram-negative bacteria can also be found.

Strongyloides stercoralis is a nematode that can be carried asymptomatically for many years after exposure. Strongyloidiasis has been recognized as a complication of human T-lymphotropic virus 1 (HTLV-1) infection, and also occurs secondary to immunosuppression (typically with high-dose corticosteroids and in solid organ transplant recipients). A rise in the worm burden results in the hyperinfection syndrome, which may present as pneumonitis or intermittent intestinal obstruction. The movement of the worms through the gut wall can carry with them enteric bacteria, resulting in polymicrobial bacteraemias and Gram-negative meningitis when the worms penetrate the blood–brain barrier.

Giardiasis is particularly associated with hypogammaglobulinaemia, and curiously is rarely seen in other groups. Cryptosporidia, Microsporidia, and Isospora are now well-recognized causes of severe and sometimes chronic diarrhoea in AIDS patients, but may also occur in other less severely immunocompromised patients. Among the viruses the most problematic is cytomegalovirus. Cytomegalovirus can cause a severe colitis, and in these cases ganciclovir is beneficial. Ideally the diagnosis should be confirmed by biopsy, but ultimately may depend on the result of a therapeutic trial since demonstration of the organism does not necessarily indicate that it is causing disease.

Mild abnormalities of liver function tests are a common accompaniment to many systemic infections, but hepatitis is a particular feature of both toxoplasmosis and cytomegalovirus infection. An increased prevalence of hepatitis B has been found in patients on chronic haemodialysis (10%) and those with Hodgkin's disease (8%) and lepromatous leprosy (20%). The acute hepatitic episode is mild, often anicteric, and may pass unnoticed. However, persistent viral replication and the development of complications associated with chronic infection are more likely. Cirrhosis secondary to hepatitis C is currently the commonest indication for liver transplantation; recurrence of infection post-transplantation is almost inevitable and requires specific approaches to prevention and treatment. Other immunosuppressed patients are at risk of infection and nosocomial spread of hepatitis C among hospitalized patients being treated for cancer has been reported. Chronic hepatitis E virus infection has also been reported in solid organ transplant recipients. Epstein–Barr virus replication may detected in 20 to 30% of solid organ transplant recipients and up to 80% of those who receive antithymocyte globulin and high doses of immunosuppressants. Clinical manifestations range from a benign mononucleosis syndrome to hepatitis to post-transplant lymphoproliferative disorder.

Table 2.4.4 Infection prevention strategies in organ transplant recipients and patients with neutropenia[a]

	Strategy	Comment
Bacterial infections		
Bacterial sepsis in neutropenia	Oral quinolones	Re-emerging following earlier concerns with efficacy and risk of resistance
	High-efficiency particulate air (HEPA)-filtered rooms	Very expensive and no clear advantage in survival
Overwhelming postsplenectomy sepsis	Immunization (pneumococcal, Hib, and meningococcal) and oral penicillin	
Tuberculosis	Isoniazid	In exposed or high-risk patients, especially if receiving prolonged high-dose corticosteroids
Viral infections		
Herpes simplex, cytomegalovirus	Aciclovir, ganciclovir, valganciclovir	Dose and drug varies depending on specific indication
Influenza	Immunization	Not routine except in high-risk groups
Fungal infections		
Candida, Aspergillus	Fluconazole, itraconazole, voriconazole, and liposomal amphotericin B	Choice and duration of drug depends on type of transplant
Pneumocystis jirovecii	Co-trimoxazole	Used for both bone marrow transplantations and in some solid organ transplantations

[a] Excludes post-exposure prophylaxis.

A particular form of systemic candidiasis has been called chronic hepatosplenic candidiasis, but the syndrome is better referred to as chronic disseminated candidiasis (CDC). Approximately 85% of the patients with CDC and underlying acute leukaemia are in remission at the time of diagnosis. The most common manifestation of CDC is persistent fever not responsive to conventional antibiotics. There is often abdominal pain; palpable hepatomegaly is unusual. The liver function tests show a markedly raised alkaline phosphatase and there may be hyperbilirubinaemia, but microbiological investigations (including fungal blood cultures) are frequently negative. Characteristic lesions are seen on MRI. Large doses of amphotericin B formulations are required to treat the infection and prevent further relapses.

Prevention of infection

Approaches designed to prevent infection in immunosuppressed patients have assumed increasing importance. For profoundly neutropenic patients, measures including nursing them in single rooms and taking great care to avoid nosocomial acquisition of infection from staff, visitors, or other patients is simple but effective. Chemoprophylaxis for a wide range of bacterial, viral, and fungal pathogens has had a major impact (Table 2.4.4). Immunization has only a limited role at present, although when feasible (e.g. providing pneumococcal vaccination before an elective splenectomy) it is worthwhile. In addition, routine screening of transplant recipients and donors should include serological tests for cytomegalovirus, hepatitis B, and HIV.

Further reading

Bucaneve G, et al. (2005). Levofloxacin to prevent bacterial infection in patients with cancer and neutropenia. N Engl J Med, 353, 977–87.

Davies JM, Barnes R, Milligan D (2002). Update of guidelines for the prevention and treatment of infection in patients with an absent or dysfunctional spleen. Clin Med, 2, 440–3.

Fischer SA (2006). Infections complicating solid organ transplantation. Surg Clin North Am, 86, 1127–45.

Freifeld AG, et al. (2011). Clinical practice guideline for the use of antimicrobial agents in neutropenic patients with cancer: 2010 update by the Infectious Diseases Society of America. Clin Infect Dis, 52, e56–93.

Jaksic B, et al. (2006). Efficacy and safety of linezolid compared with vancomycin in a randomized, double-blind study of febrile neutropenic patients with cancer. Clin Infect Dis, 42, 597–607.

Paul M, Soares-Weiser K, Leibovici L (2003). β lactam monotherapy versus β lactam-aminoglycoside combination therapy for fever with neutropenia: systematic review and meta-analysis. BMJ, 326, 1111–19.

Pfaller MA, Pappas PG, Wingard JR (2006). Invasive fungal pathogens: current epidemiological trends. Clin Infect Dis, 43 Suppl 1, S3–14.

Richardson MD (2005). Changing patterns and trends in systemic fungal infections. J Antimicrob Chemother, 56 Suppl 1, i5–11.

Sipsas NV, Bodey GP, Kontoyiannis DP (2005). Perspectives for the management of febrile neutropenic patients with cancer in the 21st century. Cancer, 103, 1103–13.

Viscoli C, Varnier O, Machetti M (2005). Infections in patients with febrile neutropenia: epidemiology, microbiology and risk stratification. Clin Infect Dis, 40 Suppl 4, S240–5.

Walsh TJ, et al. (2002). Voriconazole compared with liposomal amphotericin B for empirical antifungal therapy in patients with neutropenia and persistent fever. N Engl J Med, 346, 225–34.

2.5 Antimicrobial chemotherapy

R.G. Finch

Essentials

The practice of medicine changed dramatically with the availability of effective antimicrobial agents. Fatal diseases such as bacterial meningitis and endocarditis became treatable; much minor community infectious morbidity became readily controlled; many surgical procedures became much safer, and developments in solid organ and bone marrow transplantation became possible. However, the very success of antimicrobial chemotherapy has led to overuse, misuse and inappropriate pressures from the public to prescribe. In many countries, antibiotics are freely available to the public for purchase 'over the counter', with few controls or guidance to ensure their safe and effective use. The emergence and spread of antimicrobial resistance worldwide and the decline in development and licensing of new antimicrobials threaten the future successful treatment of bacterial infections.

Antimicrobial drugs

Pharmacological characteristics and antimicrobial spectrum—antibacterial drugs can be divided according to their mode of action into those that (1) inhibit cell wall synthesis—e.g. penicillins and cephalosporins; (2) interfere with protein synthesis—e.g. tetracyclines, aminoglycosides; (3) inhibit bacterial nucleic acid synthesis—e.g. fluoroquinolones; and (4) act on metabolic pathways—e.g. sulphonamides and trimethoprin. The antimicrobial spectrum of a drug is determined by the mode of action and ability to reach the relevant target site. Antibiotics active against a few particular bacteria are considered narrow spectrum (e.g. vancomycin), while others are active against many bacteria and are labelled broad spectrum (e.g. meropenem). Some antimicrobials are only active against anaerobically dividing bacteria (e.g. metronidazole).

Clinical effectiveness—to be effective clinically, sufficient drug must reach the infection site. The pharmacokinetic characteristics of absorption, distribution, metabolism and excretion are critical to defining dose, efficacy and often safety. Poorly absorbed agents are often administered parenterally, some topically. Hydrophobicity and hydrophilicity are important in defining tissue and extracellular fluid concentrations, as are factors such as molecular size and pH. Highly protein-bound drugs such as flucloxacillin may achieve lower tissue concentrations in selected body sites.

Excretion, metabolism and drug monitoring—many drugs are metabolically degraded in the liver and/or excreted by the kidney via glomerular filtration or tubular secretion. It should therefore be anticipated that dose modification may be necessary to avoid toxicity in patients with compromised hepatic or renal function. Therapeutic drug monitoring is important in ensuring therapeutic and nontoxic concentrations of some drugs, e.g. gentamicin and vancomycin.

Antiviral, antifungal, and antiparasitic drugs—the availability of drugs to treat herpesvirus infections (herpes simplex, varicella–zoster, and cytomegalovirus), and the development of new drugs active against hepatitis viruses, influenza viruses, and HIV have revolutionized the treatment of viral infections. Advances in the management of invasive fungal disease have been slower: the reliance on polyenes, e.g. amphotericin, has only recently been eclipsed with the availability of potent azoles and triazoles and echinocandins. In the case of many parasitic diseases, advances have been extremely slow, but the importance of malaria has led to new compounds being developed (e.g. the artemisin derivatives), also new ways of using established drugs in combination.

Resistance to antimicrobial drugs

Resistance mechanisms—loss of efficacy through resistance mechanisms is unique to antimicrobial drugs. There are four main types: (1) drug inactivation or destruction, (2) target site alteration, (3) reduced cell wall permeability (porin mutation) or increased removal from the cell (efflux resistance); and (4) inhibition as a result of metabolic bypass. Individual drugs can be subject to one or more mechanisms of resistance, which may vary by infecting microorganism.

Spread of resistance—genetic mutations that confer resistance do not just affect the target pathogen in the treated individual. They can disseminate both horizontally and vertically as a result of person-to-person or indirect spread of the pathogen. Spread through genetic mechanisms via plasmids, transposons, integrons, and phages between bacteria of the same and different species are common, as is spread between genera. Likewise, resistance mechanisms can spread to organisms making up the normal flora of the gut and skin.

Clinical impact—antibiotic resistance is of increasing medical and public concern, and affects all aspects of medicine. Infections become unresponsive to initial therapy, sometimes with fatal consequences in the seriously ill. In others, reassessment and alternative therapy with agents are often more toxic and more expensive are required, leading to increased morbidity and increased costs through prolonged hospitalization. The spread of resistant pathogens within hospitals, nursing homes and the community is a very significant concern. High rates of meticillin-resistant Staphylococcus aureus (MRSA) infections are present in many countries, including the United States of America, the United Kingdom, and southern Europe. Public confidence in health care has been eroded, leading to major government initiatives in the European Union, North America, and Australia in efforts to contain these resistant pathogens.

Prescribing of antimicrobial drugs

A set of principles has emerged to support safe and effective prescribing, covering issues of choice of drug, dose and route of administration, duration of therapy, strategies to minimize adverse reactions, and what factors need to be considered should initial treatment fail. The complexity of modern therapeutics has led to the development of formularies and practice guidelines, the latter increasingly being evidence based, with the twin goals of supporting cost-effective safe prescribing whilst minimizing the risks of emergence of antibiotic resistance.

Introduction

The discovery and clinical application of antibiotics and antimicrobial chemotherapeutic agents is one of the major achievements in medicine. Life-threatening infections such as meningitis, endocarditis, and typhoid fever are now treatable, whereas before they were generally fatal. Likewise, the morbidity associated with many infectious diseases of a less life-threatening nature, such as urinary tract infections, skin and soft tissue infections, and bone and joint sepsis, has been substantially reduced. Major advances in medicine, such as solid organ and especially bone marrow transplantation, as well as the use of cancer chemotherapy, have become safer because of the availability of effective antimicrobial agents. In the field of surgery, perioperative prophylactic use of antibiotics has reduced the risk of infections complicating procedures such as large bowel and gall bladder surgery, vaginal hysterectomy, and implant surgery such as the insertion of prosthetic heart valves, joints, and neurosurgical shunting devices.

Antimicrobial chemotherapy is the use of antibiotics and chemotherapeutic substances to control infectious disease. The term 'antibiotic' was coined by Waksman to describe a substance derived from naturally occurring microorganisms and possessing antimicrobial activity in high dilution. The latter characteristic is essential in defining its selective toxicity to other microorganisms. True antibiotics include penicillin, derived from the mould Penicillium notatum, streptomycin from Streptomyces griseus, and the cephalosporins from Cephalosporium spp. Many chemotherapeutic substances with antimicrobial activity have been artificially synthesized, such as the sulphonamides, quinolones, and isoniazid. However, the term 'antibiotic' is loosely applied to both the true antibiotics and other antimicrobial agents.

Antibiotics are among the most widely prescribed drugs, accounting for an international expenditure of $33 billion. In the United Kingdom, around 80% of all prescribing is in the community where the emphasis is largely on oral agents; the remainder are used in hospitals where there is a greater emphasis on injectable drugs. More than 125 different antibiotics are available, but a relatively small number are necessary to deal with most prescribing needs. It is important that clinicians who prescribe these drugs are familiar with the principles of antimicrobial chemotherapy and that they adopt a continuous learning approach throughout their professional lives to ensure safe and effective prescribing. Table 2.5.1 summarizes the agents available for the treatment of bacterial, mycobacterial, fungal, viral, protozoal, and helminthic infections. More agents have been developed for the treatment of bacterial infections, but globally viral, fungal, and parasitic infections predominate. In recent years, there have been major advances in the availability of antiviral drugs particularly for the treatment of viral infections. Likewise, safe and effective systemic antifungal agents have resulted from the discovery of azoles, triazoles, and echinocandins.

The very success of antimicrobial chemotherapy has led to widespread and often excessive use, particularly in community practice where prescribing is largely empirical and clinical distinction between viral and bacterial infections is difficult. Antibiotics are used extensively in animal husbandry both for the treatment and prevention of infectious disease and, more controversially, in some countries as growth-enhancing agents among commercially raised poultry and swine. This has raised concerns about the emergence and spread of antibiotic resistance, which affects many classes of antibiotic, may be intrinsic to a particular pathogen, or may result from genetic mutation, and in 2006 led to the European Union banning the use of all such agents as growth promoters. Resistance may be caused by enzymatic inactivation (β-lactamase), failure of drug penetration into the bacterial cell (porin mutation),

Table 2.5.1 Antimicrobial agents available by class or indication effective against bacterial, fungal, viral, protozoal, and helminthic infection (indicative number of agents available[a])

Antibacterial (68)	Antifungal (14)	Antiviral (37)	Antiprotozoal (9)	Anthelminthics (15)
Penicillins	Polyenes	Hepatitis B & C agents	Antimalarials	Anticutaneous larva migrans
Cephalosporins	Caspofungin	Herpesvirus agents	Amoebicides	Antihydatid agents
Carbapenems	Echinocandin	HIV nucleoside analogues	Trichomonacides	Antistrongyloidiasis
Monobactams	Flucytosine	HIV non-nucleoside agents	Antigiardials	Antithreadworm/hookworm
Tetracyclines	Griseofulvin	HIV protease inhibitors	Leishmaniacides	Ascaricides
Aminoglycosides	Azoles	HIV fusion entry inhibitor	Trypanocides	Filaricides
Macrolides	Triazoles	Ribavirin	Antipneumocystis agents	Schistosomicides
Ketolides	Terbinafine	Amantadine/rimantadine		Taeniacides
Lincosamides		Foscarnet		
Chloramphenicol		Neuraminidase inhibitors		
Sodium fusidate				
Glycopeptides				
Linezolid				
Quinupristin/dalfopristin				
Colistin				
Sulphonamides				
Trimethoprim				
Antituberculous				
Antileprotic				
Nitroimidazoles				
Quinolones				
Urinary antiseptics				

[a] Based on agents listed in the British National Formulary (www.bnf.org)

alteration of the target binding site (e.g. penicillin-binding protein alteration in penicillin-resistant *Streptococcus pneumoniae*), or from efflux resistance whereby the drug is extruded from the bacterial cell (e.g. chloroquine-resistant *Plasmodium falciparum*). Organisms can also develop alternative metabolic pathways which bypass drug inactivation.

Resistance may be transferable between the same species or genera but may also spread between genera. Coding for multiple antibiotic resistance has been increasingly observed and results from several mechanisms, in particular plasmid transfer.

Despite the advances in antimicrobial chemotherapy, fresh challenges remain. These include the treatment of viral causes of enteric infection, hepatitis A and E, and viral meningitis, all of which are still without effective chemotherapy. Tuberculosis and malaria are among the world's major infectious disease killers and here problems of antibiotic resistance have escalated. In the case of tuberculosis, the continuing reliance on lengthy and complex regimens continue to frustrate disease management as a result of cost, toxicity, and patient compliance with these regimens. Recent advances include the development of new agents with novel mechanisms of action: for example, TMC 207 (a mycobacterial ATP

synthase inhibitor) and PA 824 (a nitroimidazole), both of which look promising in early clinical trials.

Among the more worrying trends in antibiotic resistance is the emergence within hospitals of meticillin-resistant *Staphylococcus aureus* (MRSA) and vancomycin-resistant enterococci (VRE). Hospital-acquired MRSA has now spread into the community, largely among nursing home residents. Furthermore, more virulent strains of MRSA have recently arisen in the community in the United States of America and Australia. *Streptococcus pneumoniae* is another community pathogen which has rapidly become less sensitive to penicillin causing clinical failures when causing meningitis or otitis media. Internationally, multidrug-resistant (MDR) and extensively drug-resistant (XDR) tuberculosis and multidrug-resistant salmonellae, including *Salmonella typhi*, are of major concern.

Resistance is not confined to bacteria. Fungal resistance is increasing (e.g. *Candida albicans* and *C. krusei* to fluconazole). Resistance of the HIV to the nucleoside, non-nucleoside, and protease inhibitors is rapidly emerging with many treatment-naive patients acquiring virus resistant to one or more agents. Antiviral resistance resulting in virological treatment failure is now a major factor responsible for progression of HIV disease.

Pharmacology

Mode of action

Knowledge of the pharmacological mode of action of an antimicrobial agent permits an understanding of the diverse mechanisms of microbial inhibition and the opportunities for drug resistance. This is best established for antibacterial and antiviral agents. In the case of antifungal and especially antiparasitic agents the modes of action are less well defined. This reflects the process of drug discovery whereby an understanding of the biochemical and molecular action of agents derived from natural or chemical sources has not always been a priority in establishing efficacy and safety, especially with regard to older agents.

Antibacterial drugs

Antibacterial agents may affect cell wall or protein synthesis, nucleic acid formation, or may act on critical metabolic pathways (Table 2.5.2).

The β-lactams (penicillins, cephalosporins, carbapenems, and monobactams (aztreonam)) and the glycopeptides (vancomycin and teicoplanin), inhibit cell wall synthesis. The β-lactams, which share the common β-lactam ring, act on cell wall transpeptidases to inhibit cross-linking of peptidoglycan. The glycopeptide antibiotics act at an earlier stage of cell wall synthesis by binding to acyl-D-alanyl-D-alanine. Despite their similar mode of action, the glycopeptides are less efficient bactericidal agents than the β-lactams.

Inhibitors of protein synthesis

Antibacterial agents that inhibit protein synthesis act on the 30S ribosomal subunit responsible for binding mRNA, or the 50S subunit which binds aminoacyl tRNA. The aminoglycosides, tetracy-clines, and macrolide antibiotics are the most widely used inhibitors of protein synthesis. Chloramphenicol, clindamycin, and the recently introduced agent linezolid also act at this site.

Inhibitors of nucleic acid

Nucleic acid synthesis is targeted by quinolones, metronidazole, and rifampicin. The bacterial DNA gyrase is essential for the super-coiling of bacterial DNA. This, together with the enzyme topoisomerase IV, are the major targets for the quinolones. These enzymes are absent in humans, explaining the selective activity of these drugs. Rifampicin and other rifamycins interfere with DNA-dependent RNA polymerase, preventing chain initiation.

Metabolic inhibitors

The best known metabolic inhibitors are the sulphonamides and trimethoprim which interfere with folic acid synthesis by sequentially inhibiting the enzymes dihydropteroic acid synthetase (EC 2.5.1.15) and dihydrofolate reductase (EC 1.5.1.3). The two drugs act sequentially on the metabolic pathway, resulting in a combined antibiotic effect. The selective activity of these compounds is dependent on the fact that humans are unable to synthesize folic acid and require preformed folic acid in their diet.

Antiviral agents

Viruses live and replicate within the host cell. Antiviral chemotherapy therefore presents a particular challenge if it is to be selectively toxic. The cycle of viral replication provides several opportunities for therapeutic intervention. Most available antiviral agents are nucleoside analogues, largely used in the treatment of HIV or herpesvirus infections (Table 2.5.3). The recent growth in numbers of antiviral agents has benefited greatly from HIV-related research through the identification of new drug targets (Fig. 2.5.1). Interference with cell surface attachment through ligand blockade of surface receptors provides a theoretical, but so far unfulfilled, target. Penetration into the host cell may be through a process of translocation or direct fusion between the outer lipid membrane of the virus and the cell membrane, before uncoating and release of viral nucleic acid. Replication differs among viruses, thereby providing several therapeutic options. Viral mRNA becomes translated into multiple copies of viral proteins encoded by the viral genome either as a result of virus-specific enzymes or by co-opting host-derived protein. For example, HIV employs its own reverse transcriptase to convert RNA to DNA before integration into the host cell chromosome. Transcription and translation follow. Before the virus can be released, new viral particles must be assembled for which host cell proteins and mechanisms of phosphorylation and glycosylation may be recruited. The protease inhibitors act at this stage and have been particularly successful. Virus release is the result of either transportation and budding or host cell lysis.

Antifungal agents

The polyene antifungals (amphotericin B and nystatin) act on ergosterol within the fungal cell membrane. Ergosterol is largely absent from bacteria and humans, explaining the selective toxicity of these agents. The azole antifungals include the imidazoles (e.g. clotrimazole, miconazole, and ketoconazole) and the triazoles (fluconazole, itraconazole, and voriconazole) which bind preferentially to fungal cytochrome P450 to inhibit 14-α-methylsterol demethylation to ergosterol. The echinocandins (e.g. caspofungin, micafungin, and anidulafungin) act on fungal cell wall β(1-3)D-glycan to inhibit growth.

Table 2.5.2 Microbial site of action and targets for selected antibacterial drugs

Site of action	Drugs	Target
Cell wall peptidoglycan	Penicillins	Transpeptidase
	Cephalosporins	Transpeptidase
	Vancomycin	Acyl-D-alanyl-D-alanine
	Teicoplanin	Acyl-D-alanyl-D-alanine
	Daptomycin	Binds to bacterial membranes
Ribosome	Chloramphenicol	Peptidyl transferase of 50S subunit
	Clindamycin	50S ribosomal subunit transpeptidation
	Linezolid	Blocks initiation phase
	Macrolides	50S ribosomal subunit
	Tetracyclines	Ribosomal A site
	Aminoglycosides	Initiation complex and translation
	Fusidic acid	Elongation factor G
Nucleic acid	Quinolones	DNA gyrase
	Metronidazole	DNA strands
	Rifampicin	RNA polymerase
Folic acid synthesis	Sulphonamides	Pteroic acid synthetase
	Trimethoprim	Dihydrofolate reductase

Table 2.5.3 Mode of action of selected antiviral drugs

Drug	Target virus	Antiviral activity
Aciclovir	HSV, VZV	Nucleoside analogue
Cidofovir	CMV	Nucleoside analogue
Famciclovir	HSV and VZV	Nucleoside analogue
Foscarnet	CMV	Inhibits DNA polymerase
Ganciclovir	CMV	Nucleoside analogue
Valaciclovir	HSV, VZV	Valyl ester of aciclovir
Valganciclovir	CMV	Valyl ester of ganciclovir
Interferon	HBV, HCV	Induce interferon stimulated genes and block viral protein synthesis
Adefovir	HBV	Nucleotide reverse transcriptase inhibitor
Entecavir	HBV	Nucleoside analogue
Telbivudine	HBV	Nucleoside analogue
Ribavirin	HCV, RSV	Inhibits replication of DNA and RNA viruses, inhibits initiation and elongation of RNA fragments
Boceprevir	HCV	Binds to NS3 serine protease of HCV
Telaprevir	HCV	Binds to NS3 serine protease of HCV
Oseltamivir	Influenza A and B	Inhibits viral neuraminidase
Zanamivir	Influenza A and B	Inhibits viral neuraminidase
Amantadine	Influenza A	Uncoating and assembly
Rimantadine	Influenza A	Uncoating and assembly
Abacavir	HIV	Nucleoside reverse transcriptase inhibitor
Didanosine	HIV	Nucleoside reverse transcriptase inhibitor
Emtricitabine	HIV	Nucleoside reverse transcriptase inhibitor
Lamivudine	HIV, HBV	Nucleoside reverse transcriptase inhibitor
Stavudine	HIV	Nucleoside reverse transcriptase inhibitor
Tenofovir	HIV	Nucleotide reverse transcriptase inhibitor
Zalcitabine	HIV	Nucleoside reverse transcriptase inhibitor
Zidovudine	HIV	Nucleoside reverse transcriptase inhibitor
Delaviridine	HIV	Non-nucleoside reverse transcriptase inhibitor
Efavirenz	HIV	Non-nucleoside reverse transcriptase inhibitor
Etravirine	HIV	Non-nucleoside reverse transcriptase inhibitor
Nevirapine	HIV	Non-nucleoside reverse transcriptase inhibitor
Rilpivirine	HIV	Non-nucleoside reverse transcriptase inhibitor
Amprenavir	HIV	Protease inhibitor
Atazanavir	HIV	Protease inhibitor
Darunavir	HIV	Protease inhibitor
Indinavir	HIV	Protease inhibitor
Fosamprenavir	HIV	Protease inhibitor
Lopinavir	HIV	Protease inhibitor
Nelfinavir	HIV	Protease inhibitor
Ritonavir	HIV	Protease inhibitor
Saquinavir	HIV	Protease inhibitor
Tipranavir	HIV	Protease inhibitor
Enfurvitide	HIV	Fusion entry inhibitor
Raltegravir	HIV	Integrase inhibitor
Maraviroc	HIV	CCR5 antagonist

CMV, cytomegalovirus; HBV, hepatitis B virus; HCV, hepatitis C virus; HSV, herpes simplex virus; RSV, respiratory syncytial virus; VZV, varicella zoster virus

Antiparasitic agents

The mechanism of action of many antiparasitic drugs is only partially known. Among the antimalarials, chloroquine interferes with the metabolism and utilization of haemoglobin by malaria parasites. It also concentrates within parasite acid vesicles and raises internal pH, inhibiting parasite growth. Amodiaquine is similar in structure to chloroquine and there is cross-resistance between the two drugs.

Quinine acts by depressing oxygen uptake and carbohydrate metabolism and by intercalating into DNA, disrupting parasite replication and transcription. Mefloquine is a quinolone methanol compound structurally similar to quinine. Primaquine disrupts mitochondria, disrupts DNA, and eliminates the tissue exoerythrocytic forms of *Plasmodium falciparum*. The exact mechanism of action of lumefantrine is unknown but it may inhibit the formation of β-haematin by complexing with haemin.

Sulfadoxine–pyrimethamine inhibits tetrohydrofolic acid synthesis. Atovaquone inhibits parasite electron transport in mitochondria, resulting in inhibition of ATP and nucleic acid synthesis. Proguanil inhibits dihyrofolate reductase. Together, atovaquone and proguanil affect the erythrocytic and exoerythrocytic stages of parasite development.

Artemisin derivatives include artemether, arteether, dihydroartemisinin, and artesunate. They appear to act by binding iron, breaking down peroxide bridges leading to the generation of free radicals that damage parasite proteins. They kill all blood stages of Plasmodium spp. and have the fastest parasite clearance times of any antimalarial.

Metronidazole is active against several protozoa such as *Entamoeba histolytica* and *Giardia lamblia* as well as anaerobic bacteria. It acts as an electron sink, by reduction of its 5-nitro group activated by nitroreductase within the target pathogen, thus interrupting DNA synthesis.

Among the anthelmintic drugs, piperazine and praziquantel act by selectively inducing muscle paralysis in the target helminth. Others, such as thiabendazole, inhibit parasitic ATP synthesis and energy production.

Antimicrobial spectrum of activity

The antimicrobial spectrum of an agent is dependent on target site susceptibility among pathogenic organisms at clinically achievable drug concentrations. Some microorganisms are intrinsically resistant to certain antibiotics. For example, the aminoglycosides are inactive against anaerobic bacteria because cell entry is an energy-dependent process relying on respiratory quinones, which are absent in anaerobic bacteria. Certain strains of *Pseudomonas aeruginosa* are resistant to the aminoglycosides as a result of altered protein porin channels, which inhibit antibiotic penetration.

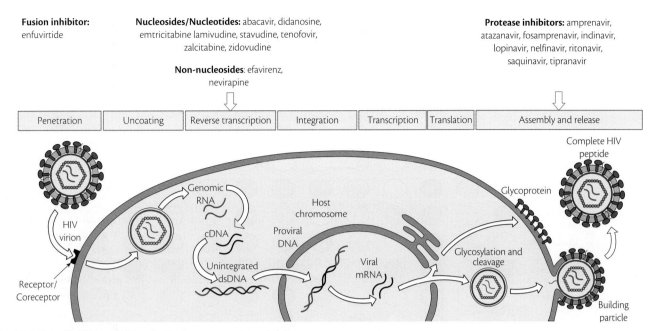

Fusion inhibitor: enfuvirtide

Nucleosides/Nucleotides: abacavir, didanosine, emtricitabine lamivudine, stavudine, tenofovir, zalcitabine, zidovudine

Non-nucleosides: efavirenz, nevirapine

Protease inhibitors: amprenavir, atazanavir, fosamprenavir, indinavir, lopinavir, nelfinavir, ritonavir, saquinavir, tipranavir

Fig. 2.5.1 Sites of inhibition of HIV replication by current antiretroviral drugs.

The antimicrobial spectrum of a drug in part dictates its clinical indications. While information on this spectrum is more easily determined *in vitro*, *in vivo* efficacy can only be confirmed through clinical use, which can be supported by animal model data during drug development. For example, *in vitro Salmonella typhi* is susceptible to gentamicin, but the drug is not effective clinically.

Narrow-spectrum and broad-spectrum agents

There are few truly narrow-spectrum agents. Fusidic acid, mupirocin, the glycopeptides (vancomycin and teicoplanin), and linezolid target specific pathogens and are mainly used to treat microbiologically confirmed infections.

Broad-spectrum agents, such as the quinolone antibiotics and the parenteral cephalosporins such as cefotaxime and ceftriaxone, are active against many Gram-positive and Gram-negative pathogens. Metronidazole has activity against a large number of anaerobic bacteria and, because of this restricted activity, is considered to have a narrow spectrum. The aminoglycosides, although active against staphylococci and aerobic Gram-negative bacilli are inactive against streptococci and anaerobes and are, therefore, frequently prescribed in combination. The carbapenems (imipenem, meropenem, and ertapenem) possess the broadest spectrum of activity which includes most aerobic and anaerobic bacterial pathogens. Ertapenem differs from the other carbapenems in its lack of activity against *Pseudomonas*. Broad-spectrum agents are often used empirically in the initial management of severe infection. However, they frequently affect the normal flora so that superinfection with *Clostridium difficile* and yeasts are more likely to arise.

Susceptibility testing

Antibiotic susceptibility testing of clinical isolates is important for appropriate prescribing and for gathering epidemiological data. It is determined *in vitro* by using either broth-based or agar-based methods. Pathogens are exposed to known concentrations of an antibiotic and their degree of inhibition compared to a standard control. Disc susceptibility testing is the most widely used method. Zones of inhibition around the antibiotic-containing disc are measured, compared to a standard, and the pathogen designated sensitive, resistant, or of intermediate susceptibility to the drug. Currently, such methods require the isolate to be tested in pure culture. It is, therefore, difficult to obtain information on the susceptibility of a pathogen in less than 36 to 48 h from sample collection.

The minimum inhibitory concentration (MIC) in milligrams per litre provides more precise *in vitro* information on the activity of a drug against a bacterial pathogen. It is more time consuming and costly to determine, although automated systems and commercial strip tests are available (Fig. 2.5.2). Defining susceptibility by MIC determination permits greater predictive benefit in the treatment of certain infections such as gonorrhoea, bacterial endocarditis, and pneumococcal meningitis. Knowledge of the *in*

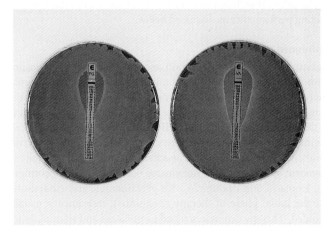

Fig. 2.5.2 *S. aureus* resistant to penicillin (MIC 8 mg/litre) on the left and sensitive to vancomycin (MIC 1.0 mg/litre) on the right, as demonstrated by a commercial strip test.

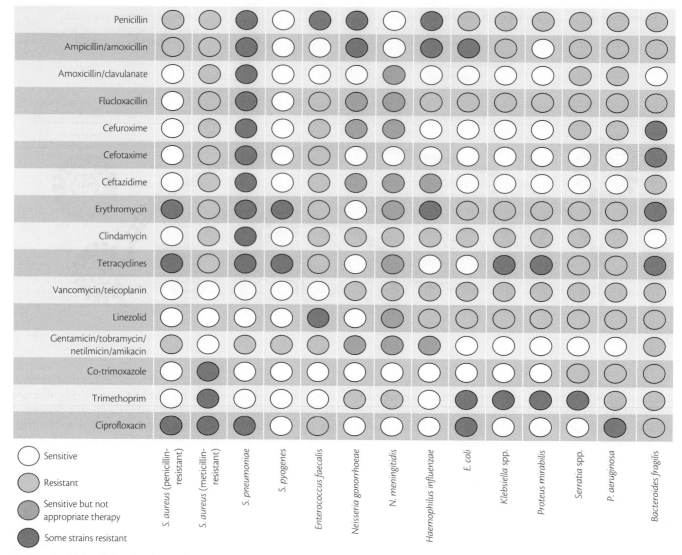

Fig. 2.5.3 Sensitivity of selected pathogenic bacteria to some common antibacterial agents.

vitro susceptibility of common pathogens to antimicrobial agents (Fig. 2.5.3) is helpful in selecting drug therapy but is only relevant to the achievable drug concentrations, which is important in predicting performance as discussed below.

Combined drug therapy

In hospital practice, it is common to combine agents when dealing with mixed infections or where initial broad-spectrum empirical therapy is required. Another important reason for combining drugs is to prevent the emergence of antibiotic resistance, such as in the treatment of tuberculosis, HIV, and malaria. Antituberculosis regimens have been developed to ensure that naturally occurring minority populations of *Mycobacterium tuberculosis* resistant to isoniazid or rifampicin do not emerge during therapy. By combining isoniazid and rifampicin with pyrazinamide and ethambutol for the initial phase of therapy (2 months), resistance is usually avoided. Therapy can be restricted to isoniazid and rifampicin for the continuation phase (4 months). The regimen is extended in those patients unable to tolerate pyrazinamide and in the treatment of tuberculous meningitis (Box 2.5.1).

HIV infection is treated with multidrug regimens. The success of highly active antiretroviral therapy, in which nucleoside/nucleotide analogues and protease inhibitors are combined in a three-drug regimen, is not only based on greater efficacy of the combined regimen but also on its ability to slow the emergence of drug-resistant mutants. The non-nucleoside reverse transcriptase inhibitors, such as efavirenz, appear to be equally effective in combination with nucleoside analogues but have a lower barrier to resistance. The options for treating HIV infection are summarized in Box 2.5.2 (see also Chapter 5.23).

Occasionally, drugs are combined for the purpose of achieving a synergistic effect based on evidence that the *in vitro* activity of the combination is shown to be greater than the sum of the activity of the individual agents. Most drugs in combination will simply be additive in effect. One of the more frequently prescribed synergistic combinations is that of penicillin (or ampicillin) and streptomycin (or gentamicin) in the treatment of endocarditis caused by *Enterococcus* spp. The aminoglycoside alone is generally inactive against enterococci but in combination with ampicillin achieves synergistic killing (Fig. 2.5.4). A similar effect is employed in the treatment of viridans streptococcal endocarditis with this combination.

Box 2.5.1 Tuberculosis treatment regimens for pulmonary and extrapulmonary[a] tuberculous infection caused by *Mycobacterium tuberculosis*

Initial phase (2 months)

- Isoniazid
- Rifampicin
- Pyrazinamide
- Ethambutol

Continuation phase (4 months)

- Isoniazid
- Rifampicin

[a] Central nervous system and disseminated tuberculosis should be treated for 10 months after the initial phase of four drugs.

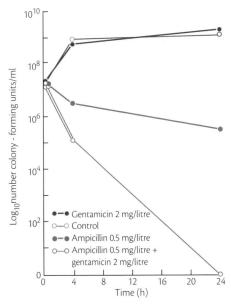

Fig. 2.5.4 Effects of ampicillin (0.5 mg/litre) and gentamicin (2 mg/litre) alone and in combination on a strain of *Enterococcus faecalis* from a patient with infective endocarditis. A synergistic effect is observed with the combined agents.

Box 2.5.2 HIV infection: initial treatment regimens for antiretroviral-naive patients[a]

- Two nucleoside/nucleotide reverse transcriptase inhibitors[b] + non-nucleoside reverse transcriptase inhibitor[c]
- Two nucleoside/nucleotide reverse transcriptase inhibitors + boosted protease inhibitor[d]
- Two nucleoside/nucleotide reverse transcriptase inhibitors + raltegravir

[a] See Table 2.5.3 for agents available.

[b] The recommended NRTI conformulation is tenofovir and emtricitabine

[c] The recommended NNRTI is efavirenz

[d] The recommended boosted PI combinations are atazanavir + ritonavir or darunavir + ritonavir

Another widely used example of synergistic inhibition is the combined effects of an antipseudomonal β-lactam, such as ceftazidime or piperacillin, and an aminoglycoside, such as gentamicin, tobramycin, or amikacin. This combination is used to treat documented or suspected *P. aeruginosa* infections occurring in neutropenic states complicating bone marrow transplantation, cytotoxic chemotherapy, and burn wound infections.

Antibiotic resistance

General considerations

Antibiotic resistance has been recognized since the introduction of effective antibiotics. For example, penicillin-resistant strains of *S. aureus* became widespread shortly after the introduction of this agent; penicillin-sensitive strains are now uncommon. Resistant strains of Gram-negative bacteria, such as *Klebsiella*, *Enterobacter*, *Acinetobacter*, and *Pseudomonas* are commonly found in high-dependency units where they may cause epidemics. The international emergence of epidemic MRSA infections, initially within hospitals

but increasingly in the community, is worrying. Conventional approaches to controlling these infections have been largely unsuccessful. The emergence of MRSA together with multiple-antibiotic-resistant coagulase-negative staphylococci has rapidly increased the use of vancomycin. Vancomycin-resistant enterococci have emerged in specialist hospital facilities such as dialysis and haematology units; therapeutic options are limited. Vancomycin intermediate sensitivity *S. aureus* (VISA) and vancomycin resistant *S. aureus* (VRSA) have also been reported. Other problems include the emergence of penicillin-resistant pneumococci and β-lactamase-producing *Haemophilus influenza,* and carbapenemase-producing Enterobacteriaceae.

At present, there is great international concern among professionals, politicians, and, increasingly, the public about antibiotic resistance. In the United Kingdom, the House of Lords published an influential document in 1998 reviewing the issues surrounding this problem. This led to several initiatives including: (1) reducing the use of antibiotics, particularly in the treatment of minor upper respiratory tract infections in the community, (2) education strategies for prescribers and the public, and (3) better enforcement of infection control policies. Within the European Union, similar measures have been proposed together with a ban on the use of antibiotics as growth promoters in livestock animals. However, antibiotic resistance is a global problem. An increasing number of multidrug-resistant infections caused by *Salmonella* spp. and *Mycobacterium tuberculosis* are being imported from developing countries where the availability or prescribing of antibiotics is less controlled. The recent emergence of XDR TB is a major cause for concern.

Antibiotic resistance drives changes in patterns of prescribing and is a major impetus to the pharmaceutical industry in its search for new therapies. Microorganisms differ in their ability to develop resistance, which may affect a particular drug, a class, or multiple classes of antibiotics. Genetic mutations select for antibiotic resistance, which frequently occurs under the influence of antibiotic

Table 2.5.4 Examples of resistance mechanisms for selected antibiotics

Enzymatic/inactivation	Altered target site	Altered permeability	Efflux	Metabolic bypass
Aminoglycosides	Erythromycin	β-Lactams	Tetracycline	Sulphonamides
β-Lactams	Chloramphenicol	Quinolones	Quinolones	Trimethoprim
Chloramphenicol	Fusidic acid		β-Lactams	
	Streptomycin			

pressure. The major mechanisms of resistance are summarized in Table 2.5.4. Resistance to single or multiple antibiotics may be either chromosomally or plasmid mediated, or both. In turn, genes may code for resistance to a single or multiple antibiotics. In addition to plasmid-mediated resistance, other transposable genetic elements (transposons) and insertion sequences (integrons) incapable of self-replication may exist within a chromosome, plasmid, or bacteriophage.

Resistance genes are most frequently transferred between organisms by conjugation. This occurs between the same or different species of bacteria and also between different genera. Other mechanisms of transferring resistance include transduction via a bacteriophage and, less commonly, transformation in which naked DNA released during cell lysis is taken up by other bacteria.

Transposon-mediated resistance reflects transfer of discreet sequences of DNA between chromosomes or plasmids whereby individual or groups of genes can be inserted into the host bacterial cell. Integrons may contain one or more gene cassettes which carry determinants of combinations of resistance genes within the bacterial chromosome, plasmid, or transposons. The antibiotic resistance genes are bound on each side by conserved segments of DNA. These individual resistance genes can be inserted or removed between the conserved structures and act as expression vectors for antibiotic resistance genes.

While the molecular mechanisms of antibiotic resistance are legion, the ability of drug-resistant microorganisms to survive, disseminate, and cause disease varies widely. In many instances, antibiotic resistance may give a survival advantage only in the presence of continued antibiotic exposure to such agents. This is reflected in the occurrence of epidemic infections in high-dependency units such as intensive care facilities where antibiotic usage is often high. However, it is also clear that once the genetic mechanism for evading antimicrobial activity has been acquired, it is rarely lost and adds to the continuously expanding genetic memory that has steadily eroded the efficacy of many antimicrobial drugs.

Enzymatic inactivation

Aminoglycoside-modifying enzymes include adenylating, acetylating, and phosphorylating enzymes. Gentamicin is the most susceptible and amikacin the least susceptible to such inactivation. However, the largest group of inactivating enzymes are the β-lactamases (E.C. 3.5.2.6) which hydrolyse the β-lactam ring common to all penicillins and cephalosporins. Penicillinase was the first β-lactamase to be identified and is the reason why most strains of *S. aureus* are resistant to this drug. Another important β-lactamase is TEM-1, which is responsible for resistance to ampicillin by *Haemophilus influenzae*. The major impetus to the development of the broad-spectrum penicillins and cephalosporins was to extend

their activity by resisting inactivation by β-lactamases present in many aerobic Gram-negative bacilli. However, new inactivating enzymes continue to emerge, including the extended-spectrum β-lactamases, which are now limiting the clinical utility of third-generation cephalosporins. A further example is the carbapenemase group of β-lactamases which hydrolyse imipenem, meropenem, and ertapenem.

Impermeability resistance

Drug uptake of antibiotics such as the penicillins, tetracyclines, and quinolone antibiotics by bacteria is through protein channels (porins) which cross the outer membrane. Alterations in the permeability of the outer membrane of Gram-negative bacteria is an increasingly important mechanism of drug resistance. Mutations in porin structure are responsible for resistance among pathogens such as *P. aeruginosa* and *Serratia marcescens*.

Alterations in target site

Another important mechanism of resistance is mutational modification of drug binding sites. This affects susceptibility to β-lactams, erythromycin, chloramphenicol, and rifampicin. Erythromycin and chloramphenicol bind to the bacterial 50S ribosomal subunit which is subject to genetic mutation. In contrast, the quinolones target DNA gyrase which is subject to subunit structure alteration resulting in one variety of resistance to drugs such as ciprofloxacin. The increasing resistance to penicillin among *S. pneumoniae* is the result of reduced binding of penicillin to several binding proteins (PBP2a and PBP2x). *S. aureus* resistance to meticillin is due to the presence of penicillin binding protein (PBP2a) which has reduced affinity for meticillin and other β-lactams and is encoded by the *mecA* gene.

The problem of vancomycin-resistant enterococci, which largely affects *Enterococcus faecium*, is the result of the production of enzymes (ligases) which permit continued cell wall synthesis despite the presence of vancomycin. To date, five different genes have been found responsible for this phenomenon (*vanA* to *vanE*) which result in different phenotypic patterns of resistance to the glycopeptides vancomycin and teicoplanin. The transfer of the vanA gene from *E. faecium* to *S. aureus* has resulted in the emergence of VRSA, of which 11 cases have been reported to date.

Metabolic bypass resistance

Bacteria must synthesize folic acid from the precursor *p*-aminobenzoic acid. The sulphonamide antibiotics competitively inhibit the enzyme dihydropteroate synthetase. Trimethoprim acts on the same metabolic pathway by inhibiting dihydrofolate reductase. The sequential inhibitory effects of trimethoprim and sulfamethoxazole (co-trimoxazole) result in synergistic bactericidal activity against many pathogens. Resistant organisms are able to synthesize their own enzymes thereby evading such competitive inhibition.

Surveillance of antibiotic resistance

Information on the susceptibility of pathogenic microorganisms is important. Such data can provide information on the relative frequency of pathogens and the pattern of susceptibility to prescribed agents. Surveillance, therefore, has a role in guiding prescribing, in developing prescribing policies, and in identifying and monitoring organisms that are subject to infection control measures. On a broader front, surveillance is also of value in alerting industry and health care planners to the need for new drug and vaccine strategies for disease control.

To be of maximum benefit, surveillance needs to be sensitive to a defined geographical base, which may simply reflect the catchment area of specimens submitted to a particular laboratory, providing information on the trends in community and hospital isolates. Within hospitals, more specific information can be provided about susceptibility patterns in high-dependency units, where antibiotic consumption is often greater, and more resistant pathogens such as *Klebsiella*, *Serratia*, *Enterobacter*, and *Acinetobacter* spp. and *P. aeruginosa* are found. Among Gram-positive pathogens, enterococci and, especially, *S. aureus* present an increasing challenge to prescribing and infection control practice.

National networks of surveillance often vary in their focus and include data on Gram-negative pathogens such as *Escherichia coli* and *P. aeruginosa*, *S. aureus*, penicillin resistance among pneumococci, and, more recently, vancomycin-resistant enterococci. There are important international networks which collect information on such pathogens as *Legionella pneumophila* and *Mycobacterium tuberculosis*. Drug-resistant tuberculosis is increasingly prevalent in the United Kingdom and elsewhere.

Surveillance of resistance to antiviral agents is largely confined to HIV in a few countries. Patient-specific data are increasingly sought in those with HIV infection to assess drug failure, guide change in management, and direct primary therapy in selected cases of person-to-person and mother-to-infant transmission. Determination of phenotypic resistance is still costly and time consuming, and most data relate to genotypic patterns of resistance to antiretroviral drugs among HIV isolates.

Pharmacokinetics

To be effective, antimicrobial agents must achieve therapeutic concentrations at the site of the target infection. This may be localized to a single anatomical site, such as the bladder or the cerebrospinal fluid, or involve major organs, such as the lung. Infections may also be generalized and affect many body sites. Drug selection must also take into consideration the fact that pathogens such as *Mycobacterium tuberculosis*, *Legionella pneumophila*, and *Salmonella typhi* replicate intracellularly. Antimicrobial drugs may be administered parenterally, orally, or topically to the skin, oral and genital mucosae, external auditory meatus, conjunctiva, and by intraocular application. In the case of systemically active agents, the effective drug concentrations are determined by the standard pharmacokinetic parameters of absorption, distribution, metabolism, and elimination. Since selective toxicity is crucial to safe prescribing, the dose regimen for each agent aims to avoid concentrations toxic to the host but inhibitory to the microorganism. This 'therapeutic window' varies by drug.

Bioavailability

The rate and degree of absorption from the gastrointestinal tract is not only important for plasma concentrations reflected in the pharmacokinetic parameters of C_{max} and T_{max} of a drug, but also for potential adverse effects on the bowel (Table 2.5.5). For example, ampicillin, the first of the aminopenicillins, commonly caused gastrointestinal side effects, most notably diarrhoea. These effects have been reduced by increasing the bioavailability of the active drug through the introduction of hydroxyampicillin (amoxicillin) and various esters and prodrugs of ampicillin.

Some agents such as cefalexin, doxycycline, and several quinolone antibiotics are extremely well absorbed, achieving 80 to 100% bioavailability. In the case of some recent quinolones, the excellent bioavailability has raised the possibility of treating with oral antibiotics some severely ill patients who might normally require parenteral therapy. In contrast, drugs which are poorly bioavailable, such as cefixime and cefuroxime axetil, not only have a higher incidence of gastrointestinal side effects but also are more likely (although not uniquely) to select for *C. difficile*-associated disease.

Table 2.5.5 Bioavailability and intestinal elimination of some commonly prescribed antibacterial drugs after oral administration

Drug	Bioavailability (%)	Intestinal elimination
Penicillins		
Amoxicillin	80–90	Concentrated up to 10-fold in bile
Ampicillin	50	Concentrated up to 10-fold in bile
Flucloxacillin	80–90	Negligible
Cephalosporins		
Cefalexin	80–100	Concentrated up to 3-fold in bile
Cefixime	40–50	Concentrated up to 50-fold in bile
Cefuroxime axetil	30–40	Bile concentrations of up to 80% of serum
Quinolones		
Ciprofloxacin	70–85	Concentrated up to 10-fold in bile
Nalidixic acid	90–100	Biliary concentrations similar to serum
Other antibacterials		
Erythromycin	18–45	Concentrated up to 300-fold in bile
Metronidazole	80–95	Concentrations in bile similar to serum
Rifampicin	90–100	Concentrated up to 1000-fold in bile
Sulfamethoxazole	70–90	Concentrations in bile 40–70% of serum
Tetracycline	75	Concentrated up to 10-fold in bile
Trimethoprim	80–90	Concentrated up to 2-fold in bile

Note that drugs which are well absorbed may still achieve high concentrations in the faeces because of secretion into bile or other enteral secretions.

Distribution

Most drugs are distributed in the blood via the plasma before gaining access to the extracellular fluid. Tissue concentrations of a particular agent are affected by pH, drug ionizability, lipid solubility, and the presence of an inflammatory reaction whereby the capillary fenestrations are increased in size. In the case of agents administered intravenously by infusion or by bolus injection, the distribution phase is rapid in comparison with orally, rectally, or intramuscularly administered drugs. Drugs which are poorly lipophilic, such as the β-lactams and aminoglycosides, achieve low concentrations in tissues such as the brain. However, the β-lactams achieve therapeutic concentrations in the cerebrospinal fluid as a result of the inflammatory reaction which accompanies meningitis.

Drugs may also be taken up intracellularly, as in the case of macrolides and quinolones, resulting in a large volume of distribution compared to drugs confined to the extracellular space, such as the β-lactams and aminoglycosides. This is important in relation to the treatment of intracellular pathogens such as *Mycoplasma pneumoniae*, *Legionella pneumophila*, and *Mycobacterium tuberculosis* which can only be effectively treated by drugs that are concentrated and remain biologically active within the cell.

The plasma half-life ($T_{1/2}$), which is the time required for the concentration of a drug in the plasma to fall by one-half, is affected by drug distribution and, in particular, its rate of elimination as a result of metabolism and excretion. This in turn affects the time taken to reach steady state. In the treatment of life-threatening infections, it is important that steady state kinetics are achieved rapidly and the administration of a loading dose may be required. This applies to the use of agents such as intravenous quinine in the case of life-threatening malaria and gentamicin for the treatment of serious Gram-negative infections where the pharmacokinetic behaviour can be altered by the severity of the disease in comparison with healthy subjects (Fig. 2.5.5).

Drugs are commonly distributed in the blood and tissues bound to plasma proteins, mostly albumin, and they vary in their degree of protein binding. With agents such as flucloxacillin and ceftazidime it exceeds 95%. The importance of protein binding lies in the fact that the active moiety is the unbound drug. Dissociation from the bound to the unbound state is usually rapid, but this equilibrium may affect drug performance at certain sites such as the joints. The relationship between protein binding and drug performance has been emphasized from studies of the pharmacodynamics of drug activity (see below).

Metabolism

Antibiotics, like other drugs, are degraded at various sites in the body but predominantly within the liver. Degradation involves conjugation, hydrolysis, oxidation, glucuronidation, or dealkylation, according to the particular drug. Members of the hepatic cytochrome P450 group of enzymes play a dominant role in this process. Drug metabolites are usually but not always biologically inactive. For example, cefotaxime is degraded to desacetylcefotaxime and clarithromycin to hydroxyclarithromycin, both of which are biologically active and contribute to the overall antibacterial activity of these agents.

Excretion

Most drugs are excreted in the urine by glomerular filtration, tubular secretion, or a combination of these mechanisms. Thus high concentrations of drug will often be present in the urine; this has therapeutic importance in the treatment of urinary tract infections. Urinary pH affects the biological activity of many drugs; e.g. the activity of ciprofloxacin is markedly reduced at pH 5.5. Tubular excretion can be blocked by probenecid. This was formerly used to ensure higher plasma concentrations of penicillin and is still recommended in alternative treatment regimens for gonorrhoea when single doses of amoxicillin are prescribed. It is also important to note that any reduction in glomerular filtration rate will affect not only urinary concentrations of drug but also the plasma half-life and, in turn, serum concentrations of drugs which are primarily excreted by this route. In the case of antibiotics such as the aminoglycosides and vancomycin, the dose must be reduced in renal failure.

Biliary excretion is another important route for drug elimination either as the active compound or as a microbiologically active or inactive metabolite. Reabsorption from the gastrointestinal tract can result in enterohepatic recirculation, which in turn may affect plasma half-life. Drugs which achieve high concentrations in the bile are effective in the treatment of infections at this site such as cholecystitis. However, biliary obstruction or hepatic impairment may reduce therapeutic efficacy and require dose reduction to avoid toxic effects. Examples include clindamycin, efavirenz, mefloquine, and tetracyclines.

Therapeutic drug monitoring of some antibiotics is essential in order to ensure therapeutic yet nontoxic concentrations. This applies particularly to aminoglycosides which have a relatively narrow therapeutic index. Trough concentrations of gentamicin in excess of 2 mg/litre, if sustained, can result in nephrotoxicity and ototoxicity. The target cells for such toxicities are the renal tubular lining cells and the cochlear hair cells of the inner ear, respectively. Vancomycin is also frequently monitored, particularly in patients with impaired renal function.

Pharmacodynamics

The inter-relationship between drug, microorganism, and the infected host creates an important pharmacological dynamic.

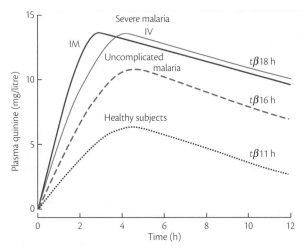

Fig. 2.5.5 Average plasma quinine concentrations following administration of a loading dose of 20 mg (salt)/kg to patients with severe and uncomplicated malaria, compared with those predicted to occur in normal subjects. (From White NJ (1992). Antimalarial pharmacokinetics and treatment regimens. *Br J Clin Pharmacol*, **34**, 1–10, with permission.)

Table 2.5.6 Effect of macrolides on bacterial virulence at subinhibitory concentrations

Factor	Effect	Factor	Effect
Adhesins (pili, fimbriae)	↓	Exoenzyme production:	
Fibronectin binding	↓	Elastase	↓
Alginate production	↓	Protease	↓
Exotoxin A production	↓	DNAse	↓
β-Haemolysin activity	↓	Coagulase	↓
Serum susceptibility	↑	Leukocidin	↓
Flagellar function	↓		

From Shyrock TR, Mortensen JE, Baumholtz M (1998). The effects of macrolides on the expression of bacterial virulence mechanisms. *J Antimicrob Chemother*, **41**, 505–12.

Antibiotics are unique in therapeutics in that they are targeted at an invading microorganism which may be present at a particular site or be more widely distributed in the body. The host's response to infection may modify the pharmacokinetic handling of a drug. Many antibiotics have a measurable effect on a variety of bacterial and host cell functions, even at subinhibitory concentrations. It is difficult to establish the exact role that these factors play clinically, but they are likely to contribute to the overall effect of an antibiotic. Macrolides such as erythromycin illustrate this point since they affect a variety of virulence characteristics (Table 2.5.6) as well as affecting the host's response to infection.

Exposure of microorganisms to sublethal concentrations of an antibiotic may temporarily inhibit growth which recommences following removal of the drug. The time to recovery is known as the post-antibiotic effect. This varies with the drug and the microorganism; e.g. the quinolones have a longer postantibiotic effect than β-lactams (Table 2.5.7). The relevance of this observation to the *in vivo* situation, where plasma drug concentrations are often well above the inhibitory concentration and are sustained through repeat doses, remains uncertain. It may have greater relevance to tissue concentrations, which tend to be lower than plasma concentrations. The postantibiotic effect certainly contributes to the effects of agents that are administered once daily, such as gentamicin.

The relationship between the pharmacokinetic characteristics of a drug and bacterial inhibition is critical to therapeutic outcome

Table 2.5.7 Postantibiotic effects (h) of selected drugs against *S. aureus*, *E. coli*, and *P. aeruginosa*

Drug	S. aureus	E. coli	P. aeruginosa
Ampicillin	1.7	0.1	NT
Cefotaxime	1.4	0.2	0.3
Ciprofloxacin	2.0	2.1	2.4
Erythromycin	3.1	NT	NT
Gentamicin	2.0	1.8	2.2
Imipenem	2.6	0.5	1.5
Rifampicin	2.8	4.2	NT
Vancomycin	2.2	NT	NT

NT, not tested.

(Table 2.5.8). In the case of agents such as penicillins and cephalosporins, the time that drug concentrations are maintained above the MIC predicts the response. This contrasts with agents such as the quinolones and aminoglycosides, where it is more important to achieve high C_{max} to MIC ratios. Modelling the MIC of a particular organism against the dose response curve for a drug (Fig. 2.5.6) has established several important pharmacodynamic parameters, which have been supported by studies in animal models and man. For example, dosage regimens of quinolones such as ciprofloxacin and levofloxacin have been based on pharmacodynamic data. The ratio of C_{max} to MIC has been refined in the parameter area under the inhibitory concentration, which is the ratio of the area under the time curve (AUC) to MIC. This is more predictive of outcome. The importance of protein binding for drug performance has also emerged as an important modifying factor in this modelling. The AUC to MIC ratio of the free drug is the most sensitive predictor of response. The manner in which these ratios differ for selected quinolones is shown in Table 2.5.9.

Principles of use

In comparison with many other classes of drugs, antimicrobial agents are usually prescribed in short courses ranging from a single dose to a few days. Prolonged therapy is required for certain infections such as tuberculosis and bone and joint infections, and for HIV infection treatment is lifelong.

Most antibiotic prescribing, especially within community practice, is empirical. Even among patients in hospital, where there are greater opportunities for diagnostic precision based on laboratory investigations, the exact nature of the infection is established in only a minority of cases. Most therapeutic prescribing requires a presumptive clinical diagnosis that, in turn, is linked to a presumptive microbiological diagnosis based on knowledge of the usual microbial causes of such infections. Among the most widely treated infections are those affecting the upper and lower respiratory tracts, the urinary tract, and skin and soft tissues for which the likely microbial aetiology is restricted. For example, urinary tract infections arising in the community are usually caused by *E. coli* and other Gram-negative enteric pathogens and, less commonly, by enterococci or *Staphylococcus saprophyticus*. Local knowledge of the susceptibility of these pathogens to commonly used agents such as trimethoprim, ampicillin, and a quinolone such as ciprofloxacin is helpful in recommending initial empirical antibiotic management.

In more severe infections, such as community-acquired pneumonia, prompt empirical therapy is essential. Although the range of possible pathogens is more extensive (Table 2.5.10), *S. pneumoniae* predominates and must always be targeted. Assessment of severity, based on validated criteria, assists in defining the initial empirical antibiotic regimen. This is illustrated by the British Thoracic Society's recommendations for the initial empirical antibiotic management of community-acquired pneumonia (Table 2.5.11).

The use of empirical therapy depends on the ease with which a clinical diagnosis can be made, as well as disease severity and drug toxicity. In the case of herpesvirus infections, the empirical use of aciclovir for the treatment of mucocutaneous herpes simplex infections or of shingles in older people is now common. However, it would be inappropriate to start treatment for HIV or cytomegalovirus infections without laboratory support for these diagnoses in view of the toxicity and cost of the antiviral agents used to treat these infections.

Table 2.5.8 Summary of major pharmacodynamic differences between aminoglycosides and β-lactams

Pharmacodynamic measurement	Aminoglycosides	β-Lactam
Rate of bacterial killing	Rapid and dose related	Slower with little or no increase at higher doses
Number of bacteria killed per dose administered	Concentration-dependent over a wide concentration range	Little increase in degree or rate of killing at concentrations above minimum bactericidal concentration (MBC)
Post-antibiotic effect	Concentration-dependent over a wide concentration range for Gram-positive and Gram-negative pathogens	Unpredictable in Gram-negative bacteria, always short with little or no increase related to concentration
Experimental models	Large, infrequent doses more effective than smaller, more frequent doses which supports once-daily dosing for Gram-negative infections	Frequent (hourly) injection or constant infusion most effective
Clinical trials	High peak serum concentration to *in vitro* minimum inhibitory concentration (MIC) ratio is strongly related to treatment outcome for Gram-negative bacteraemia or pneumonia	Limited supportive data in patients with neutropenia or nosocomial pneumonia with dosing regimens that keep serum concentrations above the MIC throughout therapy
	Clinical trials with amikacin, gentamicin, and netilmicin have shown single daily dosing to be effective	

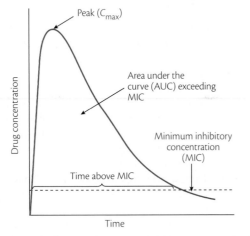

Fig. 2.5.6 Relationship between the minimum inhibitory concentration (MIC) of a drug and its pharmacokinetic profile.

Antibiotic prophylaxis

Antibiotics are used widely in the prevention of infection, in association with surgery, and in a range of medical conditions (see above). Antibiotic prophylaxis is used for selected surgical procedures where the risk of infection, although relatively low, is of serious import should it occur. Examples include prosthetic joint implantation and cardiac surgery in which prosthetic valves and intracardiac patches are inserted. The principles of antibiotic prophylaxis are based on the selection of an agent active against the known potential target pathogen(s). The drug should be present in high concentrations at the site and time of surgery and be relatively free from adverse reactions. One or two doses are generally effective depending on the length of the procedure. No regimen can be effective against all potential pathogens, hence the importance of postoperative follow-up.

A previously important medical indication for the use of prophylactic antibiotics was the prevention of bacterial endocarditis in adults and children with structural cardiac conditions (acquired valvular hear disease, valve replacement, structural congenital heart disease, hypertrophic cardiomyopathy, previous infective endocarditis). However, in 2008 the United Kingdom National Institute for Health and Clinical Excellence recommended that routine antibiotic prophylaxis should no longer be given to those at risk of endocarditis undergoing dental procedures or nondental procedures of the gastrointestinal, genitourinary, and respiratory tracts. Another example of prophylaxis is the use of low-dose suppressive therapy to prevent *Pneumocystis jiroveci (carinii)* pneumonia in those with advanced HIV infection. Co-trimoxazole is the preferred agent; dapsone, atovaquone, or inhaled pentamidine are also used.

Anatomical or functional asplenia is associated with a 12.6-fold increased incidence of severe sepsis compared with the general population. This risk is related to the patient's age and, in those splenectomized, the reason for surgery and the period of time that has elapsed. Young children are particularly at risk, but this declines substantially after the age of 16 years. Hence the recommendation that immunization be supplemented with prophylactic oral penicillin (erythromycin for the intolerant) to prevent

Table 2.5.9 Pharmacokinetic and pharmacodynamic parameters of some recent quinolone antibacterial drugs

Drug (dose mg)	Protein binding (%)	MIC₉₀ S. pneumoniae	AUC total (mg/h per litre)	AUC free (mg/h per litre)	AUIC (total drug)	AUIC (free drug)
Gatifloxacin (400)	20	0.5	51.3	41.0	102.6	82
Levofloxacin (500)	25	2.0	72.5	54.4	36.2	27.2
Moxifloxacin (400)	48	0.25	26.9	14.0	107.6	56.0

AUC, area under the concentration curve; AUIC, AUC to MIC ratio or area under the inhibitory concentration of total and free (unbound) drugs; MIC₉₀, minimum inhibitory concentration active against 90% of isolates tested.

Table 2.5.10 Microbiological aetiology (%) of adult community-acquired pneumonia in the United Kingdom

Pathogens	Community (n=236)	Hospital (n=1137)	ICU (n=185)
S. pneumoniae	36.0	39.0	21.6
Haemophilus influenzae	10.2	5.2	3.8
Legionella spp.	0.4	3.6	17.8
S. aureus	0.8	1.9	8.7
Moraxella catarrhalis	?	1.9	?
Enterobacteriaceae	1.3	1.0	1.6
Mycoplasma pneumoniae	1.3	10.8	2.7
Chlamydophila pneumoniae	?	13.1	?
Chlamydophila psittaci	1.3	2.6	2.2
Coxiella burnetii	0	1.2	0
Viruses	13.1	12.8	9.7
Influenza A and B	8.1	10.7	5.4
Mixed	11.0	14.2	6.0
Other	1.7	2.0	4.9
None	45.3	30.8	4.0

ICU, intensive care unit.

From Lim WS, et al. (2009). The British Thoracic Society guidelines for the management of community-acquired pneumonia in adults. *Thorax*, **64** Suppl III, 1–61.

fulminant pneumococcal sepsis which predominates. Other recommended vaccines include *Haemophilus influenzae* type b (Hib) and meningococcal group C conjugate. Apart from good evidence for the benefit of prophylaxis in children with sickle cell disease, there is poor support for efficacy in other populations of splenectomized patients. There remain, therefore, differences of opinion about the recommendation for the continued use of chemoprophylaxis in adults, although some recommend that a period of 2 years is appropriate. Issues of cost, compliance, and drug-resistant pathogens add further fuel to the debate. What is clear is that the patient or legal guardian(s) should be educated concerning this risk.

Dose selection

Few antibacterial drugs are specific to a single pathogen, hence the dosage regimen must capture a range of susceptibilities of the various target microorganisms to ensure a successful response. The dosage regimen is determined initially by pharmacokinetic studies in healthy volunteers. This is supplemented by information from standardized animal models that simulate infections such as peritonitis, endocarditis, meningitis, thigh abscess, otitis media, pneumonia, and sepsis complicating neutropenia. In man, information on drug penetration into the cerebrospinal fluid, bile, joint fluid, and cutaneous blisters can be supplemented by data from biopsy specimens from sites such as tonsils, bronchus, and prostate. The role of pharmacodynamic assessment is of increasing importance in defining dose and predicting outcome as discussed earlier.

Table 2.5.11 Preferred and alternative initial empirical treatment regimens for community-acquired pneumonia as recommended by the British Thoracic Society

Pneumonia severity (based on clinical judgement supported by CURB65 severity score)	Treatment site	Preferred treatment	Alternative treatment
Low severity (e.g. CURB65 = 0–1 or CRB65 score = 0, < 3% mortality)	Home	Amoxicillin 500 mg tds orally	Doxycycline 200 mg loading dose then 100 mg orally *or* clarithromycin 500 mg bd orally
Low severity (eg, CURB65 = 0–1, < 3% mortality) but admission indicated for reasons other than pneumonia severity (e.g. social reasons/unstable comorbid illness)	Hospital	Amoxicillin 500 mg tds orally. If oral administration not possible: amoxicillin 500 mg tds IV	Doxycycline 200 mg loading dose then 100 mg od orally *or* clarithromycin 500 mg bd orally
Moderate severity (e.g. CURB65 = 2, 9% mortality)	Hospital	Amoxicillin 500 mg–1.0 g tds orally *plus* clarithromycin 500 mg bd orally. If oral administration not possible: amoxicillin 500 mg tds IV *or* benzylpenicillin 1.2 g qds IV *plus* clarithromycin 500 mg bd IV	Doxycycline 200 mg loading dose then 100 mg orally *or* levofloxacin 500 mg od orally *or* moxifloxacin 400 mg od orally*
High severity (e.g. CURB65 = 3–5, 15–40% mortality)	Hospital (consider critical care review)	**Antibiotics given as soon as possible** Co-amoxiclav 1.2 g tds IV *plus* clarithromycin 500 mg bd IV (If legionella strongly suspected, consider adding levofloxacin†)	Benzylpenicillin 1.2 g qds IV *plus* either levofloxacin 500 mg bd IV *or* ciprofloxacin 400 mg bd IV **OR** Cefuroxime 1.5 g tds IV *or* cefotaxime 1 g tds IV *or* ceftriaxone 2 g od IV, *plus* clarithromycin 500 mg bd IV (If legionella strongly suspected, consider adding levofloxacin†)

bd, twice daily; IV, intravenous; od, once daily; qds, four times daily; tds, three times daily.

* Following reports of an increased risk of adverse hepatic reactions associated with oral moxifloxacin, in October 2008 the European Medicines Agency (EMEA) recommended that moxifloxacin "should be used only when it is considered inappropriate to use antibacterial agents that are commonly recommended for the initial treatment of this infection".

† Caution – risk of QT prolongation with macrolide-quinolone combination.

From Lim WS, et al. (2009). The British Thoracic Society guidelines for the management of community-acquired pneumonia in adults. *Thorax*, **64** Suppl III, 1–61.

Despite all this information, the definitive dosage regimen still requires support from large clinical trials in which the endpoints of response are precisely determined.

Bactericidal versus bacteriostatic agents

In the treatment of many common community infections which are usually of mild or moderate severity, the choice of either a bacteriostatic or a bactericidal antibiotic is of limited importance. However, in patients with severe infection, particularly when complicating an immunocompromised state, a bactericidal agent must be used. This applies particularly to those with severe granulocytopenia which is a common accompaniment of cytotoxic chemotherapy, especially in the treatment of haematological malignancies and following bone marrow transplantation. Another important indication for selecting a bactericidal regimen is in the treatment of infective endocarditis; although the infected vegetations are in the bloodstream, they are relatively protected from host phagocytic control. Effective penetration into the fibrin–platelet mass requires high concentrations of a bactericidal drug to sterilize the infected vegetations.

Duration of treatment

The duration of therapy for many common infections has not been rigorously determined. The treatment of many common conditions is based on custom and practice and often varies internationally. The duration of treatment has been more thoroughly determined in the following cases:

◆ Gonococcal urethritis responds promptly to single-dose treatment with agents such as ceftriaxone, or a quinolone antibiotic such as ciprofloxacin or ofloxacin.

◆ Uncomplicated urinary tract infection, particularly when affecting women of child-bearing years, responds promptly to selected agents such as trimethoprim and norfloxacin. Although bacteriuria can be eliminated with a single dose, the symptoms of dysuria and frequency take longer to subside, hence a 3-day course is preferred.

◆ Pharyngitis caused by *Streptococcus pyogenes* improves symptomatically within a few days of antibiotics such as penicillin, but eradication of the infecting organism from the throat often takes up to 10 days. It is acknowledged that this presents major difficulties with regard to drug compliance.

◆ For pulmonary tuberculosis the current recommendation of an initial 2-month treatment with rifampicin, isoniazid, pyrazinamide, and ethambutol, reducing to isoniazid and rifampicin for a further 4 months provided the isolate is confirmed to be susceptible, is based on extensive clinical trials (Box 2.5.1).

◆ In cases of bacterial endocarditis, knowledge of the *in vitro* susceptibility of the infecting organism is crucial in determining dose, duration, and outcome of therapy. Highly penicillin-sensitive strains (MIC ≤0.1 mg/litre) of viridans streptococci are treated effectively with a 2-week regimen of parenteral penicillin and gentamicin or 4 weeks parenteral penicillin alone. Less sensitive strains should be treated with parenteral penicillin for a total of 4 weeks. If the infecting organism is an enterococcus, a minimum of 4 weeks' treatment with parenteral penicillin (or ampicillin) and aminoglycoside is essential.

Infections caused by *S. aureus* are a particular challenge since the severity is highly variable and yet the potential for metastatic infection and chronicity, as in the case of osteomyelitis, must be kept in mind. The isoxazolyl penicillins such as flucloxacillin are preferred with or without the addition of fusidic acid. Clindamycin and linezolid are useful alternative agents. Many *S. aureus* infections of the skin and soft tissues respond promptly to 7 to 14 days oral therapy. Where there is a severe systemic response to infection, parenteral therapy is appropriate initially. Where there is evidence of dissemination, treatment should be extended for periods of up to 4 weeks.

In the case of septic arthritis, antibiotics should be given promptly and joint aspiration carried out, sometimes repeatedly, to avoid damage to the articular cartilage. The duration of therapy has not been rigorously determined. Most infections will resolve in 2 to 3 weeks. One of the most challenging infections is staphylococcal osteomyelitis. To avoid chronicity, it is customary to treat for 4 to 6 weeks. Treatment is generally administered parenterally. In centres where skill, experience, and administrative support exist, patients are increasingly being managed in the community by parenteral administration through peripherally inserted venous catheters. Under these circumstances, a glycopeptide such as teicoplanin is convenient since it is administered once daily.

For most infections, the duration of therapy remains uncertain. However, many mild to moderate uncomplicated infections will defervesce within a 3- to 5-day period suggesting that 5 to 7 days of treatment is usually adequate. There is little evidence to suggest that treatment periods of 7 to 14 days, or longer, are any more effective. They are also likely to be associated with an increased risk of side effects, superinfection, and the selection of antibiotic-resistant organisms, as well as being more costly.

The parenteral administration of antibiotics is appropriate in the management of severe life-threatening infections and when oral therapy is contraindicated, such as in the postoperative period, if the patient is vomiting, or where gastrointestinal absorption cannot be relied on. However, the need for continued parenteral therapy should be reviewed regularly. In the treatment of many common infections, the acute features of infection such as temperature, tachycardia, and an elevated circulating neutrophil count usually improve within a period of 48 to 72h. Provided there is no contraindication to oral therapy, this should be considered early in the course of patient management. The advantages are not just in the reduced cost of medication; the risk of intravenous line associated complications, such as infection, is also eliminated and discharge from hospital may be hastened.

Adverse drug reactions

Overall, antimicrobial agents have an outstanding record of safety. Nonetheless, no drug is without the potential for side effects. The risk varies by agent and sometimes by dose, while host genetic factors and pathophysiological status can also be important.

Oral antibiotics are largely used in the community where they are generally well tolerated and used in the treatment of minor infections in large populations. Injectable agents selected for short-course perioperative prophylaxis have a well-established safety record. However, agents such as the antiretroviral drugs and amphotericin B carry a higher risk of more serious adverse drug reactions, which must be balanced against the life-threatening nature of their target infections.

While drug safety is assessed during drug development, the full repertoire of adverse reactions becomes apparent only during widespread clinical use, hence, the importance of adverse drug reaction reporting systems. In the United Kingdom, the 'yellow card' system has been very successful and relies on voluntary reporting of possible adverse drug events to the Medicines & Healthcare Products Regulatory Agency (MHRA, www.mhra.gov.uk) by doctors, dentists, coroners, pharmacists, nurses (including midwives and health visitors), radiographers, optometrists, and, most recently, patients. It is important to distinguish between adverse event reporting and adverse drug reaction reporting. The latter is more difficult to establish with certainty and may require rechallenge, which raises medical and ethical concerns.

It is essential to enquire about previous drug reactions as well as other forms of drug toxicities before prescribing. The relationship to a previously prescribed drug requires careful assessment. Hypersensitivity is among the more common of drug reactions and, in the case of β-lactam drugs, appears to be more a function of the five-membered thiazolidine ring (Fig. 2.5.7) of the penicillin molecule, since hypersensitivity reactions are less common with the cephalosporins which have a six-membered dihydrothiazine ring. The monobactam aztreonam has neither ring structure and hypersensitivity reactions appear to be rare. However, it is important to note that accelerated systemic hypersensitivity reactions (anaphylaxis) can be life-threatening such that any previous association

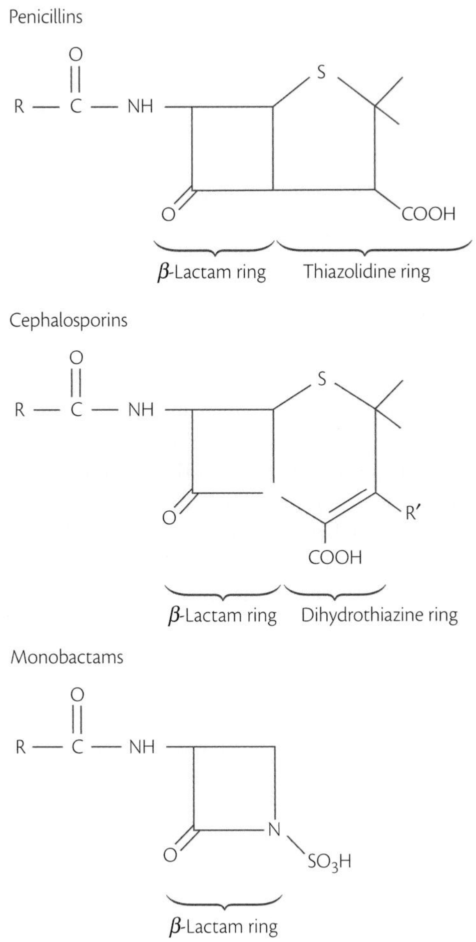

Fig. 2.5.7 Chemical structure of the β-lactam antibiotics (penicillins, cephalosporins, and monobactams) identifying the common β-lactam ring component which is subject to hydrolysis by β-lactamases.

with a β-lactam drug is an absolute contraindication to the use of all β-lactams.

Some drug toxicities are genetically determined. For example, people who are genetically slow acetylators of isoniazid are more at risk of side effects such as peripheral neuropathy. Those genetically deficient in the enzyme glucose-6-phosphate dehydrogenase (EC 1.1.1.49) are at risk of drug-induced haemolysis. This risk is more common in those of African, Mediterranean, or Far Eastern descent. Hence, it is important to screen for this red cell enzyme deficiency before the administration of oxidant drugs such as primaquine.

Adverse drug reactions may not always be acute in their presentation but reveal themselves after prolonged drug exposure. Oral flucloxacillin and co-amoxiclav when administered for several weeks, particularly in older patients, are more likely to induce drug-associated hepatotoxicity. Likewise, parenteral formulations of selected drugs may be more toxic than their oral formulation, as is the case with fusidic acid where prolonged parenteral administration frequently gives rise to hepatotoxicity.

Concentration-dependent adverse reactions (Table 2.5.12) are more likely to occur in the presence of organ system failure. Aminoglycoside toxicity is more common in older people, in those with preexisting renal failure, and after repeated aminoglycoside doses or other nephrotoxic drugs. Concentration-dependent bone marrow suppression characterizes the use of chloramphenicol whereby pancytopenia arises when plasma concentrations are in excess of 25 mg/litre. This is to be distinguished from the idiopathic aplastic anaemia that is a rare accompaniment of chloramphenicol use, but unfortunately is rarely reversible.

Much has been learned about the structure–activity determinants of drug toxicity. For example, the quinolone antibiotics as a class have the potential to induce phototoxicity, arthrotoxicity, central nervous system (CNS) toxicity, cardiotoxicity, and interact with agents such as caffeine, theophylline, and nonsteroidal anti-inflammatory drugs (Fig. 2.5.8). Knowledge of such predictors has lead to the selection of agents with safer structural profiles. Despite this, adverse drug reactions have led to the withdrawal or modification of the licensed indications for several quinolones, notably temafloxacin, trovafloxacin and sparfloxacin, emphasizing the importance of clinical recognition and reporting of adverse events.

Few infectious conditions require lifelong therapy. The management of HIV infection has challenged this tenet. To date, drugs directed at the causative viruses or complicating opportunistic infections are suppressive rather than achieving eradication. It is also important to note that the drugs used in the treatment of HIV and AIDS are often licensed with limited information concerning their long-term safety. The potential for adverse reactions and especially interactions is considerable and requires careful attention to their detection and management. This has become an increasingly important challenge as life expectancy for those with HIV infection improves. It is important to balance drug safety while encouraging compliance and the maintenance of a reasonable state of health.

Failure of antibiotic therapy

Antimicrobial therapy may fail for several reasons. The agent selected may be inappropriate for the particular infection and fail to inhibit the target organism, or fail to reach the site of infection in sufficient concentration. For example, drugs such as nitrofurantoin and norfloxacin, while achieving high urinary concentrations,

Table 2.5.12 Dose-related adverse effects of selected antimicrobials

Drug	Adverse effect	Comment
Antibacterial drugs		
General	Superinfection by yeasts or *C. difficile*; selection of drug-resistant bacteria from the normal flora	These are universal adverse effects of antibacterial drugs and are generally related to the duration of exposure
β-Lactams	Myelosuppression	Neutropenia may occur after 1–2 weeks of high-dose IV therapy
	Drug fever	Occurs during prolonged (>1 week), high-dose IV therapy (e.g. endocarditis)
	Central nervous stimulation/convulsions	Can occur with overdose in renal failure
Aminoglycosides	Nephrotoxicity; ototoxicity	Monitoring of serum concentrations minimizes but does not avoid toxicity; risk of toxicity is related to the duration of the dose and concomitant therapy
Vancomycin	Nephrotoxicity; ototoxicity	May potentiate aminoglycoside nephrotoxicity
Macrolides (e.g. erythromycin)	Gastrointestinal stimulation	This is a prokinetic effect of erythromycin which does not occur with all macrolides
	Ototoxicity; cardiac arrhythmias	Only with high-dose IV therapy
	Drug interactions	Increased serum concentrations of theophylline and ciclosporin
Quinolones (e.g. ciprofloxacin)	Central nervous stimulation	Quinolones are weak GABA antagonists; this effect is potentiated by coadministration with NSAIDs, especially fenbufen
	Drug interactions	May inhibit metabolism of theophylline
Oxazolidinone (e.g. linezolid)	Anaemia, neutropenia, thrombocytopenia; neuropathy; lactic acidosis	Limit treatment to 28 days to reduce risk of haematological toxicity
Antifungal/antiprotozoal/ antiviral drugs		
Amphotericin B	Nephrotoxicity	Decreased creatinine clearance and renal potassium wasting are universal at clinically effective doses
	Rigors/hyperthermia/hypotension	Related to the rate of infusion
Ketoconazole	Inhibition of steroid synthesis	Occurs with prolonged (>1 week) high-dose therapy
Aciclovir	Central nervous adverse effects; crystalluria	Rare except with high-dose IV therapy
Quinine	Hypoglycaemia	

GABA, γ-aminobutyric acid; NSAID, nonsteroidal anti-inflammatory drug.

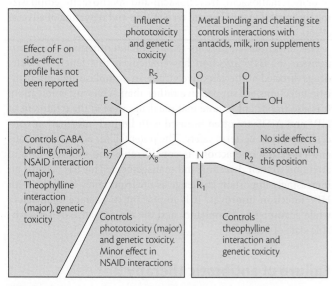

Fig. 2.5.8 Structure–activity side-effect relationships of the fluoroquinolone antibacterial drugs. GABA, γ-aminobutyric acid; NSAID, nonsteroidal anti-inflammatory drug.
(Redrawn from Domagala JM (1994). Structure–activity and structure–side-effect relationships for the quinolone antibacterials. *J Antimicrob Chemother*, **33**, 685–706.)

fail to deal adequately with parenchymatous infection of the kidney or bacteraemia which may complicate acute pyelonephritis.

The prostate also presents a chemotherapeutic challenge owing to the relatively low pH (*c*.6.4) in chronic bacterial prostatitis. Drugs which are weak bases, such as trimethoprim either alone or in combination with sulfamethoxazole (co-trimoxazole), are preferred, especially since they are also lipid soluble. Ciprofloxacin has similar characteristics and has also produced favourable results. However, treatment of acute bacterial prostatitis sometimes needs to be prolonged (4–6 weeks and occasionally longer), especially if there is a history of chronic relapsing infection.

The drug may be appropriate, but the dose selected may be inadequate. This may apply to such conditions as unsuspected bacterial endocarditis where high-dose parenteral antibiotic is required. Likewise, the concentration of penicillin required to deal with pneumococcal meningitis greatly exceeds that effective in the treatment of pneumococcal pneumonia; occasionally the two diseases may coexist. Infections caused by *Legionella pneumophila* and *Chlamydia* spp. require drugs that achieve high intracellular concentrations such as the macrolides, tetracyclines, or quinolones.

Resistance emerging during treatment is an uncommon cause of clinical failure but should be considered. Drug-resistant

Table 2.5.13 The World Health Organization (2007) model list of essential drugs (anti-infectives)

Anthelmintics	Antibacterials	Antituberculosis medicines	Antifungals	Antivirals	Antiprotozoals
Albendazole	Amoxicillin	Ethambutol	Amphotericin B	Abacavir	Amodiaquine
Levamisole	Ampicillin	Isoniazid	Flucytosine	Aciclovir	Diloxanide
Mebendazole	Benzathine benzylpenicillin	Isoniazid + ethambutol	Potassium iodide	Didanosine	Metronidazole
Niclosamide	Benzylpenicillin	Pyrazinamide	Nystatin	Emtricitabine	Meglamine
Praziquantel	Cloxacillin	Rifampicin	Clotrimazole	Emtricitabine + Tenofovir	Pentamidine
Pyrantel	Phenoxymethylpenicillin	Rifampicin + isoniazid	Fluconazole	Lamivudine	Amphotericin B
Ivermectin	Procaine benzylpenicillin	Rifampicin + isoniazid + pyrazinamide	Griseofulvin	Stavudine	Amodiaquine
Praziquantel	Amoxicillin + clavulanic acid	Rifampicin + isoniazid + pyrazinamide + ethambutol		Stavudine + Lamivudine + Nevirapine	Artemether + Lumefantrin
Triclabendazole	Cefazolin	Streptomycin		Tenofovir	Chloroquine
Oxamniquine	Cefixime	Amikacin		Efavirenz	Primaquine
	Ceftazidime	p-Aminosalicylic acid		Efavirenz + Emtricitabine + Tenofovir	Doxycycline
	Ceftriaxone	Capreomycin		Nevirapine	Mefloquine
	Imipenem + cilastatin	Cycloserine		Ribavirin	Sulfadoxine + Pyrimethamine
	Azithromycin	Ethionamide		Ritonavir	Artemether
	Chloramphenicol	Kanamycin		Lopinavir + Ritonavir	Artesunate
	Ciprofloxacin tablet	Ofloxacin		Nelfinavir	Mefloquine
	Doxycycline			Saquinavir	Paromomycin
	Erythromycin			Zidovudine	Proguanil
	Gentamicin			Zidovudine + Lamivudine	Pentamidine
	Metronidazole			Zidovudine + Lamivudine + Nevirapine	Pyrimethamine
	Nitrofurantoin				Sulfamethoxazole + Trimethoprim
	Spectinomycin				Melarsoprol
	Sulfadiazine				Pentamidine
	Sulfamethoxazole + trimethoprim				Suramin sodium
	Trimethoprim				Eflornithine
	Clindamycin				Benznidazole
	Vancomycin				Nifurtimox
	Clofazimine				
	Dapsone				
	Rifampicin				

Mycobacterium tuberculosis can develop on therapy as a result of the emergence of minority populations of organisms resistant to such first-line drugs as rifampicin and isoniazid. The current multidrug regimens are, in part, designed to avoid this occurrence. Likewise, in those with HIV infection, drug-resistant virus is an increasingly important cause of treatment failure and requires good compliance with multidrug regimens to slow its rate of emergence.

Mixed infections are commonly associated with intra-abdominal sepsis and occasionally with infections of the lung. They may fail to respond to treatment unless the regimen covers the full range of bacterial pathogens. In the case of intra-abdominal sepsis, the regimen should be active against anaerobic as well as aerobic bacterial pathogens.

Another important cause of antibiotic failure is the continued presence of a focus of infection. This may be an abscess that requires surgical drainage or the removal of an implanted medical device such as an intravascular catheter. Much more serious is infection of a prosthetic heart valve, hip joint, or CNS shunt where revision surgery carries significant risks. Many antibiotics fail to achieve therapeutic concentrations within abscess cavities, or are pH sensitive. Implant-associated infections present a similar challenge since bacteria often replicate slowly within a biofilm that is protective against normal host defences.

Finally, it should be remembered that a persistently elevated temperature in the presence of what appears to be adequate antibiotic treatment can reflect drug fever or indeed fever complicating a nonmicrobial diagnosis. This emphasizes the importance of monitoring the response to treatment and repeated patient assessment.

Practice guidelines and formularies

The plethora of therapeutic agents currently available presents a considerable challenge to the prescriber. Guidance on the choice of agent and the management of disease is becoming increasingly important. This is not only to ensure that the selection of treatment is appropriate for the target infection and consistent with current patterns of antimicrobial susceptibility but also that it reflects an acceptable safety profile as well as being sensitive to the appropriate use of health care resources. Such guidance is increasingly provided within formularies designed for local use, within either a hospital or a community practice. These frequently offer information on preferred and alternative regimens for particular infections. Formularies should include drugs currently tested by the diagnostic laboratory, since changing patterns of susceptibility may require modification of recommended drugs.

Within hospital practice, it is common for such formularies to identify drugs which may be prescribed freely according to specific indications and those for which expert advice from a clinical microbiologist or infectious disease specialist should be sought. The latter applies particularly to drugs that require specific skill and experience in their use, need drug levels to be monitored, or are expensive. For example, the treatment of deep-seated fungal infections with amphotericin B requires careful clinical assessment and guidance on dosage and monitoring. Likewise, the treatment of HIV infection is increasingly a specialist area. Antibiotics which are expensive to prescribe such as parenteral quinolones, third-generation cephalosporins, and the carbapenems may be restricted. The policy may also have recommendations for the timing of transfer from parenteral to oral therapy in order to minimize the use of injectable agents.

Formularies are educational and allow the prescriber to become familiar with indications and safety of the most commonly used agents. Their use should be supported by educational activities both at undergraduate and postgraduate level. Ideally, the selection of agents for inclusion in the formulary should be based on sound evidence of efficacy, safety, and economic benefit. However, such evidence-based medicine is often lacking or incomplete for commonly treated infections, since clinical trials of antibiotics, although increasingly robust in their design, are largely conducted to support licensing requirements rather than to address clinical use. They generally demonstrate the equivalence (or noninferiority) of a new agent in comparison with existing therapies. As a result, the recommendations of formularies and practice guidelines are based on a matrix of information derived from knowledge of the *in vitro* profile of an agent, its pharmacokinetic parameters, its clinical and microbiological efficacy, and its safety profile. This, in turn, is modified by custom and practice which explains why there is local and, sometimes, national and international variation in recommendations for some common indications such as community-acquired pneumonia and bacterial meningitis.

In developing countries, where medical resources are much more limited, greater reliance is placed on low-cost agents. The World Health Organization regularly updates its list of recommended essential drugs which includes anti-infective agents (Table 2.5.13). Despite the emphasis on low-cost agents, the drugs offered cover the majority of infections and prescribing needs of developing countries. The agents available in individual countries often vary according to local interpretation of the needs for these 'essential' drugs.

Recent developments in economically advanced countries have included an assessment of health care technologies for current management, national need, and the resources available. In the United Kingdom, the National Institute for Health and Clinical Excellence (NICE, www.nice.org.uk) was established in 1999 to assess a variety of health care technologies including procedures as well as new therapies. Such assessments place greater emphasis on ensuring that new technologies are evaluated in a manner that more closely resembles clinical practice as well as demonstrating economic benefit, in contrast to drug licensing which addresses the quality, safety, and efficacy of new therapies. This new emphasis is likely to require a greater partnership between health care systems and pharmaceutical companies to ensure that the place of new technologies is rapidly assessed and that their use is consistent with health care strategies.

Further reading

American Thoracic Society, Centers for Disease Control and Infectious Diseases Society of America (2003). *Treatment of tuberculosis.* www.cdc.gov/mmwr/preview/mmwrhtml/rr5211a1.htm#top

Bennett WM, *et al.* (1994). *Drug prescribing in renal failure: Dosing guidelines for adults*, 3rd edition. American College of Physicians, Philadelphia.

Davies JM, Barnes R, Milligan D (2002). Update of guidelines for the prevention and treatment of infection in patients with an absent or dysfunctional spleen. *Clin Med*, **2**, 440–3.

Domagala JM (1994). Structure–activity and structure–side-effect relationships for the quinolone antibacterials. *J Antimicrob Chemother*, **33**, 685–706.

Elliott TSJ, Foweraker J, Gould FK (2004). Guidelines for the antibiotic treatment of endocarditis in adults: report of the Working Party of the British Society for Antimicrobial Chemotherapy. *J Antimicrob Chemother*, **54**, 971–81.

Finch RG, Williams RJ (1999). *Baillière's clinical infectious diseases: antibiotic resistance*. Baillière Tindall, London.

Finch RG, *et al.* (2003). *Antibiotic and chemotherapy*, 8th edition. Churchill Livingstone, Edinburgh.

Gould FK, Elliott TSJ, Foweraker J (2006). Guidelines for the prevention of endocarditis: report of the Working Party of the British Society for Antimicrobial Chemotherapy. *J Antimicrob Chemother*, **57**, 1035–42.

Hughes WT, *et al.* (2002). Infectious Diseases Society of America 2002 guidelines for the use of antimicrobial agents in neutropenic patients with cancer. *Clin Infect Dis*, **34**, 730–51.

Joint Tuberculosis Committee of the British Thoracic Society (1998). Chemotherapy and management of tuberculosis: recommendations. *Thorax*, **53**, 536–48.

Kerr KG (1999). The prophylaxis of bacterial infections in neutropenic patients. *J Antimicrob Chemother*, **44**, 587–91.

Kucers A, *et al.* (1997). *The use of antibiotics*, 5th edition. Butterworth Heinemann, Oxford.

Lim WS, *et al.* (2009). The British Thoracic Society guidelines for the management of community acquired pneumonia in adults. *Thorax*, **64** Suppl III, 1–61.

NICE Short Clinical Guidelines Technical Team (2008). *Prophylaxis against infective endocarditis: antimicrobial prophylaxis against infective endocarditis in adults and children undergoing interventional procedures*. National Institute for Health and Clinical Excellence, London.

NICE *Tuberculosis: clinical diagnosis and management of tuberculosis, and measures for its prevention and control*. Clinical Guidelines 33 www.nice.org.uk/CG033 (accessed 22.10.09).

Russell AD, Chopra I (1996). *Understanding antibacterial action and resistance*, 2nd edition. Ellis Horwood, London.

Shyrock TR, Mortensen JE, Baumholtz M (1998). The effects of macrolides on the expression of bacterial virulence mechanisms. *J Antimicrob Chemother*, **41**, 505–12.

Standing Medical Advisory Committee Subgroup on Antimicrobial Resistance (1998). *The path of least resistance*. Department of Health, London.

White NJ (1992). Antimalarial pharmacokinetics and treatment regimens. *Br J Clin Pharmacol*, **34**, 1–10.

Wise R, Honeybourne D (1999). Pharmacokinetics and pharmacodynamics of fluoroquinolones in the respiratory tract. *Eur Respir J*, **14**, 221–9.

World Health Organization (2007) Model list of essential medicines (15th edition) http://www.who.int/medicines/publications/essentialmedicines/eu

3

Immunization

D. Goldblatt and M. Ramsay

Essentials

Immunization is one of the most successful medical interventions ever developed: it prevents infectious diseases worldwide.

Mechanism of effect—the basis for the success of immunization is that the human immune system is able to respond to vaccines by producing pathogen-specific antibody and memory cells (both B and T cells) which protect the body should the pathogen be encountered.

Clinical practicalities—most currently licensed vaccines contain live or killed bacterial or viral constituents, bacterial polysaccharides, or bacterial toxoids, while new types of vaccines are being developed that contain DNA. Most vaccines are delivered directly into skin or muscle via needles, or they are administered orally. New edible vaccines and vaccines delivered via the skin without the use of needles are being developed.

Who should be immunized?—vaccines can be used in a targeted way, i.e. only for those at high risk, or they can be recommended for mass immunization of whole populations. The latter approach may eventually lead to complete eradication of an infectious disease, as was the case with smallpox: polio eradication is the next global challenge. Vaccines that are able to interrupt the transmission of a pathogen between individuals are able to provide indirect protection, with the benefit of vaccination extending beyond the vaccinated population, e.g. infant immunization with pneumococcal vaccine has reduced the burden of disease in adults.

Global perspective—the Expanded Program on Immunization, set up by the World Health Organization to define which vaccines should be delivered in resource poor countries, has done much to increase coverage of vaccination amongst infants most at risk of infectious diseases. The evaluation of immunization programmes includes measurement of vaccine coverage, continuing surveillance for vaccine preventable infections, seroprevalence studies to assess population immunity, and systems for monitoring and reporting adverse events.

Introduction

Infectious diseases remain a major cause of mortality and morbidity worldwide. The prevention of certain infectious diseases by effective immunization programmes is one of the major triumphs of 20th century medicine. Most of this was achieved in the final third of that century, during which rapid strides in the understanding of the biology and pathogenicity of infectious agents or their components, and improved techniques for their purification, led to the development of safe and effective vaccines. The greatest triumph in the field of immunization was the eradication of smallpox. In 1959 the World Health Organization (WHO) declared its intention to eradicate smallpox, and in 1966 began to allocate sufficient resources to accomplish this ambitious goal. Thirteen years later, in 1979, the global eradication of smallpox was officially declared. Effective vaccines can eliminate infectious diseases, but to do this they must be implemented and used appropriately. Of the more than 12 million children under the age of 5 years who die annually, 2.4 million die of diseases that could be prevented by vaccines already available through the WHO's Expanded Program on Immunization (EPI). While rapid advances in vaccine science have introduced new techniques such as DNA vaccines, delivering vaccines to those most at risk must remain a priority.

Immunology of active immunization

Both nonspecific (innate) and specific (adaptive or acquired) immune systems are responsible for protecting humans against infectious diseases. The ability of the adaptive immune system to refine its antigen-recognition domains and establish immunological memory is the basis of successful active immunization. The antigen-specific component of the immune system contains both cellular and humoral elements (secreted antibody), whose relative importance differs depending on the nature of the infecting organism. The global eradication of type 2 poliovirus was achieved in 1999. In 2005, new monovalent vaccines targeting type-specific polio were developed and used for the first time. By 2008, however, poliovirus transmission continues in the four endemic countries, with importation into neighbouring countries and cases returning to 1999 levels. By 2009, polio eradication tools will be optimized with the availability of bivalent OPV against type 1 and type 3, as part of the framework for intensifying eradication efforts in 2010–2012.

Cellular responses are induced when antigen-presenting cells, such as dendritic cells, present antigens to T cells. T cells do not respond to soluble, unmodified antigens, and only recognize peptide antigens in association with major histocompatability complex (MHC) molecules. Two major forms of MHC molecules exist. Most nucleated cells produce MHC class I molecules, which stimulate a subset of T cells that produce the CD8 differentiation antigen. These T cells recognize and lyse infected target cells, hence their designation as cytotoxic T lymphocytes. By contrast, MHC class II molecules are produced by cells that participate in the immune response, and are recognized via a subset of T cells producing the CD4 differentiation antigen. A major role of such T cells is to augment the immune response, and so they are known as T helper cells. Several subsets of T helper cells have been described: T helper 1 cells are involved in cytotoxic and delayed-type hypersensitivity responses, T helper 2 cells support antibody production, follicular helper T cells provide help to B cells enabling them to develop into antibody-secreting plasma cells, while Th17 cells are important for protection against bacteria and fungi at mucosal surfaces.

Immunoglobulin receptors on the surface of B cells are able to recognize soluble antigens, and so initiate the process of B-cell activation and differentiation. During differentiation, naive B cells become antibody-secreting plasma cells. In addition, B cells endocytose antigen bound to their surface immunoglobulins, and re-express it in the form of small peptides on the surface of the B cell in the context of MHC class II molecules. Thus B cells act as antigen-presenting cells and recruit T-cell help. The signals and soluble factors that result from such T-cell help drive the B-cell process of affinity maturation and memory formation. This takes place in the germinal centres of lymph nodes, where there is intimate contact between B cells, T cells, and dendritic cells. It is here that memory B cells are formed and then migrate to the bone marrow, spleen, and the submucosa of the respiratory tract and gut. On re-encountering the antigen, memory B cells undergo rapid activation and differentiation into plasma cells, and secrete large amounts of switched, high-affinity antibody.

Thus the ideal vaccine antigen will lead to the activation, replication, and differentiation of T and B lymphocytes. Ideally the antigen will persist in lymphoid tissue, conformationally intact, to allow the continuing production of cells that secrete high-affinity antibody, and the generation of memory cells.

Vaccine antigens

The ideal vaccine antigen is safe, with minimal side-effects, promotes effective resistance to the disease (although it does not necessarily prevent infection), and promotes lifelong immunity. It needs to be stable and remain potent during storage and shipping, and also has to be affordable to allow widespread use. Most currently licensed vaccines contain live or killed bacterial or viral constituents, bacterial polysaccharides, or bacterial toxoids (Table 3.1).

Live vaccines are ideal for certain diseases, as replication in the body mimics natural infection, thereby inducing appropriate and site-specific immunity. Live vaccines must be attenuated to remove the danger of clinical disease, but retain the beneficial effects of inducing immunity. Some live vaccines may be spread from person to person, and thus enhance herd immunity, although such spread may endanger immunocompromised individuals, in whom live vaccines should be avoided. Live vaccines are inherently less stable than killed vaccines, and the possibility of reversion of vaccine virus to the wild type exists (as in polio). Killed vaccines do not carry the risk associated with person-to-person spread, and are inherently

Table 3.1 Currently licensed vaccines for use in humans

Vaccine type	Live vaccines	Killed/subunit vaccines
Viral	Rubella	Poliomyelitis (Salk)
	Measles	Influenza
	Poliomyelitis (Sabin)	Rabies (human diploid cell)
	Yellow fever	Hepatitis A
	Mumps	Hepatitis B
	Varicella zoster	Japanese encephalitis
	Rotavirus	Human papillomavirus
		Tick-borne encephalitis
Bacterial	Bacillus Calmette–Guérin	Cholera
		Neisseria meningitidis group B
	Typhoid	Typhoid
	Cholera	Pertussis
		Borrelia burgdorferi
		Anthrax
		Plague
Bacterial polysaccharides		*Haemophilus influenzae* type b
		Neisseria meningitidis group A , Y, W135
		Streptococcus pneumoniae
Rickettsial		Typhus
Bacterial toxoid		Diphtheria
		Tetanus

more stable, but often require two or three doses to induce optimal immunity, especially when used in the first year of life.

New developments in vaccine antigens

Developments in molecular biology have begun to revolutionize the field of vaccine science, and provide a glimpse of the future, when the traditional reliance on live attenuated viral vaccines or purified bacterial or viral products as vaccine antigens may be reduced. The first licensed vaccine to contain recombinant genetic material was the hepatitis B vaccine. Despite the licensing of highly effective plasma-derived hepatitis B vaccines in the early 1980s, fears about safety, and their high cost, led to the search for other hepatitis B vaccines.

Several vaccine manufacturers used recombinant DNA technology to express hepatitis B surface antigen in other organisms, which led to the development of new vaccines.

DNA itself has also attracted interest as a vaccine antigen. The potential of this approach as a vaccine antigen was discovered by chance in 1989 during a gene therapy experiment, when it was shown that a gene inserted directly into a mammalian cell could induce the cell to manufacture the protein encoded by that gene. In early experiments, DNA was injected directly into muscle, and the resulting immune response was measured.

DNA vaccines can induce protective immunity to a variety of pathogens in animals, but data in humans are limited. As DNA has the theoretical potential to be incorporated into the host genetic make-up and subvert the genetic working of cells, safety concerns have delayed studies in humans. Phase I studies, however, have assessed DNA vaccines designed to protect against hepatitis B, herpes simplex type 1 and 2, HIV, influenza, and malaria. So far clinical trials have proved disappointing, either because the level of the response was inadequate or because excessive doses of DNA were required to achieve an adequate response. This poor immunogenicity of DNA vaccines remains a major hurdle. Prime boost strategies where the immune system is primed with a vector coding for one antigen and then subsequently boosted with a different vector or the antigen itself has been the one area of promise in this field and has been applied to malaria, HIV, and new TB vaccines.

The abundant information now available about the genomic make-up of pathogens has ushered in a new era that has been termed 'reverse vaccinology'. Using information from the pathogen genome, sequences coding for likely protective antigens have been cloned into expression systems, expressed and screened as vaccine antigens using animal models. The first vaccine developed in this way, a protein-based serogroup B meningococcal vaccine, is close to being licensed. A related but alternative technique involves highly representative small-fragment genomic libraries that are expressed to display frame-selected epitope-size peptides on a bacterial cell surface. These are then screened with disease-relevant high-titre sera and the candidate antigens recognized are assessed further for their potential as vaccine antigens. This experimental approach has been described for a number of bacteria including *Staphylococcus aureus* and *epidermidis*; *Streptococcus pyogenes*, *agalactiae*, and *pneumoniae*; *Enterococcus faecalis*; *Helicobacter pylori*; *Chlamydia pneumoniae*; the enterotoxigenic *Escherichia coli*; and *Campylobacter jejuni*.

Despite these new technologies, vaccines for some pathogens are proving difficult to develop. Vaccines for HIV remain a major health priority but phase III clinical trials to date have proved disappointing. The RV144 HIV vaccine trial is the only phase III vaccine trial that has shown a modest protection (31%) against HIV infection. It was conducted in Thailand where more than 16 000 participants received a four priming injections of a recombinant canarypox vector vaccine plus two booster injections of a recombinant glycoprotein 120 subunit vaccine. Despite the relatively modest effect of the vaccine, the large study size will permit the evaluation of correlates of protection which are vital for the ongoing effort to find a safe and effective vaccine.

Improved vaccines for TB are a priority as the BCG vaccine provides imperfect protection. Several recombinant BCG constructs have entered clinical trials and a number of new subunit vaccines, formulated as adjuvanted or viral vectored vaccines and designed to be used with BCG in a 'prime-boost' approach are currently in clinical trials. The absence of true biomarkers that can predict the clinical outcome of TB disease and be utilized as correlates of protection for vaccine assessment are hampering the discovery and evaluation of new TB vaccines.

New developments in vaccine delivery

Research into different routes of vaccine delivery has been driven by the limitations of the parenteral route. These include the difficulty associated with the use of live viral vaccines in the first 6 to 9 months of life (because of the neutralizing effect of passively transferred maternal antibody) and the difficulty and expense of delivering mass immunization by injection. Mucosal delivery of vaccine via the intranasal route has been studied for a number of antigens, including measles, influenza, rubella, varicella, and *Streptococcus*

pneumoniae. The induction of local immunity for pathogens that either enter the body via the nasopharynx (measles, influenza) or are commonly carried in the nasopharynx (*S. pneumoniae*) is attractive.

Edible vaccines are attracting increasing attention, providing as they do both a means of antigen production and delivery. Studies in animals, and phase I studies in humans, have demonstrated their potential. Mice fed with potatoes expressing a nontoxic fragment of the cholera toxin developed mucosal antibodies to the toxin, which reduced diarrhoea on challenge with whole cholera toxin. Humans fed raw potatoes expressing the B subunit of enterotoxigenic *Escherichia coli* also showed mucosal immune responses and an increase in neutralizing antibody levels. There are some problems with stability, but edible vaccines are a potentially simple and convenient method of vaccine delivery on a wide scale.

The requirement for increased immunogenicity of existing vaccines has driven the search for better adjuvants. Until recently the only adjuvants in widespread use have been aluminium salts. New, safe adjuvants with acceptable safety profiles are finally appearing in vaccines and include oil in water emulsions such as ASO4 and a combination of aluminum hydroxide and monophosphoryl lipid A, part of a licensed human papillomavirus vaccine.Experience with H1N1 influenza vaccines, containing another oil in water adjuvant (MF-59), have demonstrated good immune response to a novel strain of influenza with only a single dose, thus enabling vaccine to provide protection earlier than expected in the recent pandemic.

The aim of immunization programmes

Once a vaccine has been developed and shown to be effective it can be used in different ways. Many vaccines are used selectively in groups of the population who are at increased risk of infection (e.g. because of occupation or travel) or of severe consequences of the disease (e.g. because of an underlying medical condition). Other vaccines are employed for mass immunization targeting the whole population. Mass immunization can eradicate, eliminate, or control an infectious disease. Eradication, the state where a disease and its causal agent have been removed from the natural environment, has been achieved only for smallpox. Once eradication has been certified, mass immunization programmes can cease, and resources can be transferred to other programmes.

The next target for the WHO is the global eradication of poliomyelitis. Characteristics that favour eradication are the absence of an animal host, the absence of a carrier state, and lifelong protection given by vaccination. The polio eradication campaign has involved the use of National Immunization Days (NIDs), on which live attenuated polio vaccine is delivered to a high proportion of the childhood population on a single day. Millions of children have been immunized with trivalent oral polio vaccine (against types 1, 2, and 3) during NIDs. This had led to the successful interruption of poliovirus transmission in many previously endemic countries. The global eradication of type 2 poliovirus was achieved in 1999, and type 3 is now largely confined to northern Nigeria. In 2005, new monovalent vaccines targeting type-specific polio were developed and used for the first time . In 2011, however, poliovirus transmission continues in the four endemic countries (India, Pakistan, Nigeria, and Afghanistan), with imported polio types 1 and 3 occurring in several African countries and reintroduction of type 1 virus into the central Asian republics in the European region.

For some infections, eradication by immunization is not possible. A good example is tetanus, where the agent is distributed widely in the environment. For these programmes the aim is to control infection to the point where it no longer constitutes a public health burden. To maintain control, immunization must be continued indefinitely.

For diseases that are transmitted from person to person, a good immunization programme provides protection by conferring both individual and herd immunity. For many vaccines, herd immunity can be achieved by vaccinating a high proportion of the childhood population; older individuals are generally immune as a result of previous natural infection. If such a situation can be sustained, transmission of the infection may be interrupted, and elimination or eradication becomes possible. If vaccine coverage or efficacy is suboptimal, however, then, in the absence of natural transmission, the number of susceptible people will gradually increase. Eventually, the proportion of susceptible people (those who did not receive vaccine or who failed to respond to it) may reach a level sufficient to support an epidemic. Although the size of these epidemics may be small by prevaccine standards, the average age of those infected will be higher than in the prevaccine era. For infections that have more severe consequences in older individuals the morbidity associated with such outbreaks can be substantial. A tragic example of this has recently been observed in Greece, where mass vaccination against rubella in childhood has been recommended since 1975. Implementation was poor, however, and during the 1980s coverage was below 50%. The low level of coverage was sufficient to interrupt transmission for several years, but by the time rubella infection recurred in 1993, a high proportion of pregnant women were susceptible to rubella and an epidemic of congenital rubella syndrome occurred.

Other potential negative consequences of achieving high vaccine coverage, and therefore high herd immunity, have been described. One negative impact may be that pressure is created on an organism to mutate, or that other strains may expand to fill an ecological niche left, for example by eradicating nasopharyngeal carriage. The introduction of a 7-valent pneumococcal conjugate vaccine into the routine infant immunization programme of the United States of America, and the associated surveillance for invasive pneumococcal disease, has revealed not only the direct impact of the vaccine in reducing disease in vaccinated children, but also a huge indirect effect, which has resulted in the reduction of invasive pneumococcal disease in unvaccinated adults. A similar experience, however, has been followed by a increase in serotypes not covered by the vaccine in several countries. Vaccines with higher valencies (covering 10 or 13 serotypes) are now being employed; long-term surveillance to monitor whether these too lead to replacement is essential. Another negative impact of the introduction of vaccination may be disruption of asymptomatic transmission and reduction in natural boosting of immunity. This can result in protection from vaccine waning earlier than expected, and therefore in resurgences in disease in older individuals. This may partially explain some of the recent outbreaks of mumps described in several countries with high vaccine coverage. Although it is clear that morbidity associated with mumps in vaccinated individuals is substantially reduced, waning immunity may prevent the long-term elimination of mumps infection.

The Expanded Program on Immunization

In 1974 the WHO launched the EPI, in recognition of the major contribution of vaccines to public health. At the start of the programme fewer than 5% of the world's infants were immunized against the six target diseases—diphtheria, tetanus, whooping cough, polio, measles, and tuberculosis. Between 1990 and 1997, around 80% of the 130 million children born each year were immunized by their first birthday, preventing around 3 million deaths each year. Each year, more than 500 million immunization contacts occur with children, and these have provided an opportunity for the delivery of other primary health care interventions.

During the 1990s the EPI added immunization against yellow fever and hepatitis B to its target diseases (Table 3.2). The introduction of these vaccines, however, has been less impressive, particularly in the poorest countries in greatest need. Of 33 African countries at risk of yellow fever, only 17 have included the vaccine in the childhood schedule. By 1998, hepatitis B vaccine had been incorporated into the national programmes of 90 countries, but it is estimated that 70% of the world's hepatitis B carriers live in countries without programmes. The major barrier to using new vaccines in the developing world is likely to be sustainable funding.

Delivery of immunization programmes

For mass immunization to achieve its aims, high and uniform coverage of immunization must be reached and sustained. The level of coverage of immunization is associated with a variety of factors, including the sociodemographic characteristics of the population, the organization of health services, knowledge among health professionals, and parental attitudes.

Sociodemographic factors that may influence vaccine coverage include deprivation, maternal education, and family size. Centrally coordinated health services with few barriers to access, and standard record systems with facilities for call and recall are likely to achieve higher vaccine coverage. Health professionals with accurate knowledge of the indications and true contraindications to immunization are important. Excessive lists of contraindications for diphtheria–tetanus–pertussis immunization in the newly independent states of the former Soviet Union contributed to a massive resurgence of diphtheria in the early 1990s. The number of cases rose from 2000 in 1990 to over 47 000 in 1994; 2500 deaths from diphtheria occurred between 1990 and 1995.

Table 3.2 Immunization schedule for infants, recommended by the WHO Expanded Program on Immunization

Age	Vaccines	Hepatitis B[a]	
		Scheme A	Scheme B
Birth	BCG, OPV	HB1	
6 weeks	DTP1, Hib1, OPV1	HB2	HB1
10 weeks	DTP2, Hib2, OPV2		HB2
14 weeks	DTP3, Hib3, OPV3	HB3	HB3
9 months	Measles		
	Yellow fever[b]		

BCG, Bacillus Calmette–Guérin; DTP, diphtheria, tetanus, pertussis; HB, hepatitis B; Hib, *Haemophilus influenza* type b; OPV, oral polio vaccine.

[a] Scheme A is recommended where perinatal transmission is frequent (e.g. in Southeast Asia); scheme B may be used where perinatal transmission is less frequent (e.g. in sub-Saharan Africa).

[b] In countries where yellow fever poses a risk.

Whether or not parents decide to have their children vaccinated depends on their perceptions of the severity of the disease and of the safety and effectiveness of the vaccine. Knowledge of parental perceptions can be used successfully to target health promotion campaigns. When coverage is high, the incidence of vaccine-preventable disease declines, and parental perception of the severity of that disease may decrease. In this situation, concerns about the safety of the vaccine become paramount and can lead to a decline in vaccine coverage. Such a situation arose in the United Kingdom in the early 1970s, when concern about the safety of pertussis vaccine led to a fall in coverage. This resulted in resurgence of the disease, with consequent mortality and morbidity (Fig. 3.1). Over the next decade vaccine coverage improved again, and the incidence of the disease fell to the lowest levels ever.

In 2003–4, concern about the safety of the polio vaccine led to the suspension of the programme in northern Nigeria. This led to an outbreak of polio in west and central Africa and the reintroduction of poliovirus into 22 previously polio-free countries. By 2005, after massive efforts from the international community, successful campaigns were launched to stop these outbreaks and transmission was contained in all but six of these countries. In 2008, a further polio outbreak occurred in Nigeria, leading to persistent importations into neighbouring countries and re-established transmission in Angola, Chad, the eastern part of Democratic Republic of Congo, and southern Sudan. This experience illustrates the major global implications of failure to sustain confidence in vaccination.

Other potential negative consequences of achieving high vaccine coverage, and therefore high herd immunity, have been described. One negative impact may be that pressure is created on an organism to mutate, or that other strains may expand to fill an ecological niche left, for example by eradicating nasopharyngeal carriage. The introduction of a 7-valent pneumococcal conjugate vaccine into the routine infant immunization programme of the United States of America, and the associated surveillance for invasive pneumococcal disease, has revealed not only the direct impact of the vaccine in reducing disease in vaccinated children, but also a huge indirect effect, which has resulted in the reduction of invasive pneumococcal disease in unvaccinated adults. A similar experience, however, has been followed by a increase in serotypes not covered by the vaccine in several countries. Vaccines with higher valencies (covering 10 or 13 serotypes) are now being employed; long-term surveillance to monitor whether these too lead to replacement is essential. Another negative impact of the introduction of vaccination may be disruption of asymptomatic transmission and reduction in natural boosting of immunity. This can result in protection from vaccine waning earlier than expected, and therefore in resurgences in disease in older individuals. This may partially explain some of the recent outbreaks of mumps described in several countries with high vaccine coverage. Although it is clear that morbidity associated with mumps in vaccinated individuals is substantially reduced, waning immunity may prevent the long-term elimination of mumps infection.

Evaluation of immunization programmes

Evaluation of an immunization programme may include the measurement of vaccine coverage, surveillance of disease incidence, assessment of prevalence of immunity, and the monitoring of adverse events.

Vaccine coverage

Timely measurement is important for monitoring trends in vaccine coverage and identifying pockets of low coverage. Low coverage may be apparent before any increase in disease incidence is observed. Since the late 1970s, three outbreaks of poliomyelitis have been observed among groups in the Netherlands with religious objections to immunization. Despite national coverage of 96% for MMR vaccine, the same group has recently been the focus of a large epidemic of measles. Between April and December 1999, 1750 cases of measles occurred in the Netherlands, compared with only 9 in the whole of 1998.

Disease surveillance

Once an immunization programme has been implemented, disease incidence data can be used to monitor the effectiveness of the strategy. For example, the dramatic decline in the incidence of invasive *Haemophilus influenzae* infection described in both the Netherlands and the United Kingdom can be used to demonstrate the impact of conjugate vaccination. The age distribution of infection may change, as children above or below the target age form an increasing proportion of those infected. Various epidemiological methods, including case–control studies, cohort studies, and the screening method can be used to estimate the efficacy of the vaccine in the field. The impact of vaccines should be monitored in age groups other thanthose targeted by vaccination, to determine the effect of herd immunity. *Neisseria meningitidis* Group C (Men C) polysaccharide-conjugate vaccine was introduced into the United Kingdom in 1999 and by 2002 all under the age of 25 years in the population had been offered the vaccine. The effect of invasive Men C disease reduction was, however, seen in all ages, both those directly immunized and those protected by reduced transmission of the bacterium from the nasopharynx in vaccinated individuals to the rest of the population (Fig. 3.2).

Seroprevalence studies

Seroprevalence studies are used to assess population immunity to infection. Such immunity results either from immunization or from natural infection. This can detect groups that include a high

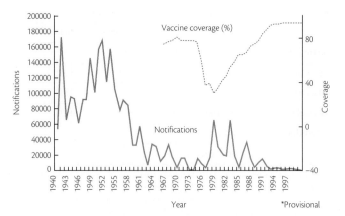

Fig. 3.1 Whooping cough cases and vaccine coverage in England and Wales between 1940 and 1998.

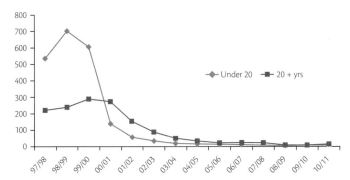

Fig. 3.2 Group C meningococcal infection in England and Wales in those below or above the age of 20 year from 1997/8–2010/1 (data from the Health Protection Agency).

proportion of susceptible individuals, who may be the focus of future outbreaks. In 1991, seroprevalence studies in the United Kingdom identified that a large proportion of school-age children was susceptible to measles, and therefore that an epidemic of measles was likely. A large campaign was mounted in November 1994 to immunize children from 5 to 16 years of age. The number of cases of measles fell rapidly and remained at low levels over the next 5 years.

Adverse events

The monitoring of adverse events is important for maintaining public confidence in an immunization programme and for detecting rare events that could not be identified before licensing the vaccine. The detection of such events may lead to the withdrawal of certain vaccines. In August 1998, a quadrivalent vaccine using reassortant rhesus rotavirus strains was licensed for use in the United States of America and recommended for the mass immunization of infants. During prelicensing studies, five cases of intussusception had been reported in around 10 000 recipients, compared with only

1 in almost 5000 controls; this difference was not statistically significant. During postlicensure surveillance, however, 15 cases were reported to the Vaccine Adverse Event Reporting System. On 22 October 1999, a review of scientific data concluded that there was an increased frequency of intussusception in the 1 to 2 weeks after vaccination, which led to withdrawal of the first licensed vaccine. New rotavirus vaccines that appear to be less likely to produce intussusception are now licensed. Adverse events may be linked to the active antigen or to other contents of the vaccine. Concerns in Finland about an observed excess of cases of narcolepsy occurring after the adjuvanted pandemic influenza vaccine suggest that the novel adjuvant MF-59 may be a trigger.

Further reading

Chen RT (1999). Vaccine risks: real, perceived and unknown. *Vaccine*, **17**, S41–46.

Czerkinsky C, *et al.* (1999). Mucosal immunity and tolerance: relevance to vaccine development. *Immunol Rev*, **170**, 197–222.

Lehtinen M, *et al.* (2012). Overall efficacy of HPV-16/18 AS04-adjuvanted vaccine against grade 3 or greater cervical intraepithelial neoplasia: 4-year end-of-study analysis of the randomised, double-blind PATRICIA trial. *Lancet Oncol*, **13**, 89–99.

Orenstein WA, Bernier RH, Hinman AR (1988). Assessing vaccine efficacy in the field. Further observations. *Epidemiol Rev*, **10**, 212–41.

Pilishvili T, *et al.* (2010). Active Bacterial Core Surveillance/Emerging Infections Program Network. Sustained reductions in invasive pneumococcal disease in the era of conjugate vaccine. *J Infect Dis*, **201**, 32–41.

Rappuoli R, Black S, Lambert PH. (2011) Vaccine discovery and translation of new vaccine technology. *Lancet*, **378**(9788), 360–8.

Rerks-Ngarm S, *et al.* (2009). Vaccination with ALVAC and AIDSVAX to prevent HIV-1 infection in Thailand. *N Engl J Med*, **361**, 2209–20.

Tacket CO, *et al.* (1998). Immunogenicity in humans of a recombinant bacterial antigen delivered in a transgenic potato. *Nat Med*, **4**, 607–9.

Travel and expedition medicine

C.P. Conlon and David A. Warrell

Essentials

Tourists, business people, pilgrims, and visitors to friends and relatives are making increasing numbers of trips to tropical and developing parts of the world, where the risk and range of infectious and environmental diseases and injuries may be much higher than in Western countries. The aim of travel and expedition medicine is to reduce risk through education, appropriate immunizations and other medical advice, hence enhancing the enjoyment and achievements of travelling abroad. Explorers, expeditioners, and wilderness travellers face the greatest health challenges, but risk can be minimized by technical competence, careful planning, training in practical medical skills, and rehearsing emergency evacuation.

Pretravel advice—this requires precise information about the mode of travel, geographical itinerary and the purpose of the visit, and must take into account the age, background health and immunocompetence of the traveller. Important provisions are (1) a first-aid kit, (2) sun-block, (3) insect repellent, (4) treatments for motion sickness, jet lag and high altitude sickness, (5) supplies of regular medications for chronic medical conditions, and (6) generous, comprehensive travel insurance.

Pre-travel immunization—this involves (1) boosting childhood vaccinations—e.g. tetanus, poliomyelitis, and diphtheria; (2) adding protection against hepatitis A (and B in those at risk of parenteral or sexual exposure) and infections endemic in the areas to be visited, e.g. yellow fever in equatorial Africa and South America, Japanese encephalitis in South-East Asia, tick-borne encephalitis in northern Europe and Asia, *Neisseria meningitidis* in the meningitis belt of Africa, typhoid in South Asia, and rabies in most parts of the world. Pregnancy and immunocompromise present particular problems of vulnerability to infections and restrict the use of live vaccines.

Reducing the risk of infections—food and water hygiene are crucial for prevention of travellers' diarrhoea, the commonest medical problem likely to be encountered. Avoidance of bites by disease vectors such as mosquitoes and ticks and use of appropriate prophylactic drugs reduces the risk of malaria and many other tropical infections.

Other medical hazards of travel—long flights can lead to deep vein thrombosis and respiratory infection. Underestimated hazards of travel include sexually transmitted infections, schistosomiasis, drowning and road traffic accidents.

Introduction

International tourism has grown prodigiously over the last few years. During 2010 and 2011, international tourist arrivals continued to increase by about 4 to 7% each year to a total exceeding 700 million. Approximately 30% of which were to tropical or subtropical developing countries. United Kingdom citizens make 56 million visits abroad each year, 8% of these to developing countries, which carry a higher risk of illness (600-fold increased risk in Mexico, 1835-fold in the Indian subcontinent) than travel to European countries such as France. It has been estimated that 50 to 75% of short-term travellers to tropical or subtropical countries become unwell, usually because of an infection. Those travelling outside Europe need to be provided with adequate medical advice to minimize the risks of their journeys, while back at home, admitting physicians should consider a broader range of differential diagnoses, diagnostic tests, and specific treatments. Among the more common infectious disease health risks faced by travellers to developing countries are traveller's diarrhoea, malaria, dengue fever, acute lower respiratory tract infection, hepatitis A, gonorrhoea, and animal bites with rabies risk (Table 4.1).

Pretravel advice

This can be obtained from a variety of sources, but ideally should be sought from medical practitioners and clinics with a special interest in travel medicine. Other sources include the embassies of the countries to be visited, travel agencies, and, increasingly, the internet (see 'Further reading' below). People travel for a variety of reasons: business travel, pilgrimage, gap-year and educational travel, and tourism are all increasing. Many members of the immigrant communities of Western countries travel to visit their friends and relatives abroad (VFRs); such travellers are less likely to seek pretravel advice, and yet may be more vulnerable to endemic

Table 4.1 Immunizations

Vaccine	Type	Route	Primary course	Booster
Routine				
Diphtheria	Adsorbed toxoid	IM/SC	Three doses at monthly intervals	Single low dose if under 10 years old
Polio (Salk)	Killed virus	IM/SC	Three doses at monthly intervals	10 years
Tetanus	Adsorbed toxoid	IM/SC	Three doses at monthly intervals	10 years (maximum 5 doses)
Combined tetanus, polio, diphtheria	–	IM/SC	Three doses at monthly intervals	10 years (maximum 5 total doses)
Haemophilus influenzae [b]	Conjugated polysaccharide	IM	Two to three doses, 2 months apart	Single dose
Influenza	Killed virus	IM	Single dose	Yearly
Pneumococcal	23-valent polysaccharide	IM/SC	Single dose	Repeat in those at high risk
Pneumococcal	7-valent conjugate polysaccharide	IM/SC	Three doses at 2, 4, and 13 months (not licensed for adults)	Repeat in those at high risk
Travel				
Hepatitis A [a]	Killed virus, Vero cell vaccine	IM	Two doses, 6–12 months apart	Probably not required
Hepatitis B	Adsorbed	IM [b]	Three doses at 0, 1, and 6 months	Single booster at 5 years (may not be required)
Japanese B encephalitis	Killed virus, Vero cell vaccine	SC	Two doses on days 0 and 28	One year, later boosting uncertain
Meningococcal	Conjugate (ACYW135–Menactra)	IM	Single 0.5-ml dose	Every 3–5 years. Those previously immunized with polysaccharide vaccines should be boosted with conjugate vaccine
Rabies	Killed virus	IM [b]/ID [b,c] 0.1 ml	Three doses on days 0, 7, and 28	Once, after 1–2 years
Tick-borne encephalitis	Killed virus	IM	Two doses 4 weeks apart, then at 9–12 months	Every 3 years.
Tuberculosis: BCG	Attenuated	ID	Single dose	None
Cholera	Inactivated O1 strain plus recombinant B toxin subunit	PO	Two doses 1 week apart	6 months
Typhoid	Live Ty21a strain (attenuated)	PO	Three doses on alternate days	Every 5 years
Typhoid [a]	Capsular Vi polysaccharide	IM	Single dose	Every 3 years
Yellow fever	Live virus (attenuated)	SC	Single dose	Every 10 years

ID, intradermal; IM, intramuscular; PO, oral; SC, subcutaneous.
[a] Combined hepatitis A and typhoid vaccines are available.
[b] Should not be given into the buttock; deltoid or anterior thigh preferred. Double the dose for immunocompromised patients, or those on dialysis.
[c] Efficacy reduced if given with chloroquine antimalarial prophylaxis.

diseases in the tropics because of the living conditions at their destination.

At the pretravel clinic, the clinician elicits details about the proposed journey and the individual traveller's previous health and requirements. Such discussions allow a proper risk assessment to be made, so that advice and immunizations can be appropriately tailored. Issues that should be considered include general health advice, an assessment of the problems posed by different climates or environments, and the route, type, and duration of travel. Specific advice will include details of the necessary immunizations, and protection against malaria and other relevant diseases. It is important to discuss what might be done if the traveller were to fall ill while abroad or become unwell after their return. Travellers should be encouraged to take out generous and specific travel and health insurance including cost of repatriation in case of serious illness or accident.

General advice about health

First-aid kit

Travellers should carry a basic first-aid kit that should include a topical antiseptic solution; bandages; plasters; proprietary drugs for pain relief, diarrhoea, constipation, dyspepsia, allergy, and itch; sunscreen preparations; water purification tablets; and insect repellents.

Motion sickness

Antiemetic drugs such as cyclizine are effective, but they may cause sedation and a dry mouth. Long-acting transdermal skin patches containing scopolamine or antiemetics that can be absorbed through the buccal mucosa are preferable.

Air travel and jet lag

Long-haul air flights lead to jet lag: sleep disturbance, fatigue, a feeling of lightheadedness and unreality, and poor concentration.

These symptoms may be attributable to a hangover if excessive alcohol has been drunk on the flight. A short-acting benzodiazepine such as temazepam, taken for the first couple of nights after flying, helps to re-establish a regular sleeping pattern. Some travellers have found that melatonin is helpful (Oxford Textbook of Medicine 5e Chapter 13.13), but obtaining products with the active ingredient can be a problem. The appropriate timing of exposure to daylight and meals can speed up the adjustment of circadian rhythms. People with diabetes may need advice on adjusting their insulin regimen or diet for changes in time zones, as may patients taking other regular medications. The closed recirculation of cabin air can spread respiratory pathogens. The risk of deep vein thrombosis from prolonged immobility and dehydration can be reduced by wearing tailored elastic stockings, moving about as much as possible, and frequently drinking water.

Regular medications

Patients with chronic illnesses such as diabetes or asthma should take plenty of their current medications, as these may not be available abroad. It is a good idea to divide the supplies among several bags in case one is lost or stolen. Patients should carry a letter from their physician outlining the condition and itemizing the medications to be carried.

Food and water hygiene

Strict food and water hygiene are important in countries with relatively poor sanitation. 'Boil it, peel it, or forget it' is a useful adage for the traveller, but is sometimes difficult to implement without causing offence when receiving hospitality. Foods to be avoided are raw or rare meat, fish and other seafood (but see below), food that has been stored unrefrigerated since it was cooked, 'street food' unless freshly boiled or fried, unpasteurized dairy products, cold sauces and dressings, raw salads and vegetables, and unpeeled fruits or even peeled tomatoes. Water purification tablets and many types of portable water filters are available. Beverages made with boiled water are generally safe, whereas bottled water and especially ice cubes are unreliable. Treated water should always be used, even for tooth cleaning and washing fruit. Unfortunately, marine toxins are not destroyed by heat and so high-risk seafoods, such as puffer fish, large reef fish, and shellfish gathered while there is a 'red tide', should be avoided.

Climatic and environmental extremes

Sun and heat

Travellers should be reminded of the risks of sun exposure, and encouraged to dress and behave appropriately, to use sunscreen, and to wear a hat or other head protection in the sun. They must keep adequately hydrated and be aware of the risk of heatstroke. Several days of relative inactivity are needed to acclimatize safely to hot climates.

Swimming

Apart from the risk of drowning (Oxford Textbook of Medicine 5e Chapter 9.5.3), or being bitten, stung, or attacked by aquatic animals (Oxford Textbook of Medicine 5e Chapter 9.2), swimmers and bathers can be exposed to waterborne diseases such as schistosomiasis and leptospirosis in fresh water, together with the possibility of ingesting water and contracting gastrointestinal illnesses, even in swimming pools. Generally, swimming in chlorinated water is to be preferred. Schistosomiasis (bilharzia) occurs in Africa

(including Madagascar), the Middle East, eastern South America, China and South-East Asia (Fig. 11.1). Infection is acquired by both bathing and washing with fresh water in lakes and sluggish rivers. Many United Kingdom cases are from scuba-diving schools in Lake Malawi, which has been erroneously declared 'bilharzia-free'. Travellers usually present weeks or months later with haematuria and, rarely, ascending flaccid paralysis.

Vector-borne diseases

Travellers should be warned about the risk of diseases transmitted by the bites of mosquitoes (e.g. malaria, dengue fever, chikungunya, Japanese encephalitis) and ticks (e.g. tick-borne encephalitis, Lyme disease, rickettsioses) and advised how to avoid bites.

High altitude

At high altitudes, snow blindness and severe sunburn can occur under clear skies, even at very low ambient temperatures. Those going to high altitudes should acclimatize slowly and build up their level of physical activity gradually (see Oxford Textbook of Medicine 5e Chapter 9.5.4). They should be aware of the symptoms and signs of altitude sickness. Acetazolamide (Diamox) in an adult dose of 250 mg twice a day, starting 12 h before starting the ascent, is effective prophylaxis for mild mountain sickness, especially if the traveller has to ascend rapidly (e.g. flying from sea level to more than 3 000 m). But gradual ascent allowing acclimatization is preferable, and if severe symptoms develop there is no substitute for rapid descent. In the tropics, heat, dehydration, and salt depletion may cause additional problems.

Wilderness, game parks, and safaris

Careful planning should include provision of navigational aids to avoid getting lost; appropriate clothing, equipment, and vehicle; and adequate food and drink. Wilderness travellers may be exposed to a variety of environmental dangers including unpredictable meteorological extremes. These might include flash floods and lightning strikes, unfriendly local inhabitants, and attacks by large wild animals.

Blood-borne and parenteral infections

In many developing countries, blood-borne pathogens such as hepatitis B and C viruses, HIV, human T-cell leukaemia/lymphoma virus type 1, and, in some areas, malaria, trypanosomiasis, and other infections are prevalent. Screening of donated blood may not be rigorous, and needles are commonly reused, sometimes without adequate sterilization. As a result, travellers have been advised to take AIDS kits, usually containing needles, cannulas, intravenous giving sets, syringes, and artificial plasma expanders. These are too bulky and expensive for most travellers, but it is worth taking a few 21-gauge needles and 10-ml syringes in case blood must be taken for a laboratory test, or an injectable drug is needed. A covering letter from a doctor may allay the suspicion of customs officials that they are to be used for drug abuse.

Sexually transmitted infections

Surveys indicate that 4 to 19% of travellers have casual sex while abroad, and that these acts are unprotected on 50% of occasions. One result is about 7 new cases of HIV per 100 000 travellers per year. For United Kingdom residents, the risk of acquiring HIV is 300 times greater while travelling abroad than at home. Between 14 and 25% of cases of gonorrhoea and syphilis diagnosed in Europe are imported. Travellers are clearly more likely than usual to engage in unprotected sexual activity, especially when disinhibited by alcohol or other recreational drugs. Since sexually transmitted diseases, including HIV, are highly prevalent in many holiday resorts (not only in prostitutes), good-quality condoms, often not available when travelling, should be carried and used. Pretravel advice should include a discussion of the risks of unsafe sex.

Immunizations

Childhood vaccinations

The traveller's record of childhood immunizations should be reviewed (Chapter 3). Many adults will require booster doses for tetanus, polio, and diphtheria and may not have been adequately immunized against measles or mumps. Over the past few years, outbreaks of mumps and measles have occurred in many countries.

Since 1990 there has been an epidemic of diphtheria in the newly independent states of the former USSR. There were more than 150 000 cases and 5000 deaths reported from these states until 1998, but since then, widespread immunization campaigns have largely controlled the epidemic, although cases of diphtheria continue to be reported rarely in tourists and travellers to this region.

Previous travel immunizations should be noted, so that they are neither repeated unnecessarily nor allowed to lapse.

Hepatitis A

The incidence of hepatitis A in developing countries ranges from 300 to 2000 cases per 100 000 unprotected travellers per month of stay. Active immunization is safe, effective, and durable. Those who have received a full course of immunization will probably not need any further boosting doses (see Chapter 3).

Hepatitis B

This is a risk to medical or laboratory staff whose work involves contact with human blood and to those staying for prolonged periods, such that there is a possibility of receiving unscreened blood transfusions (see Oxford Textbook of Medicine 5e Chapter 15.21). It is also a risk of unprotected sexual activity. Vaccination in these circumstances is sensible.

Yellow fever

This is the only vaccination for which an internationally valid certificate is statutorily required for entry into countries where the disease is endemic, and for travellers returning from those places. Yellow fever is only endemic in tropical Africa and South America, not in Asia (see 5.14.4). Recently, the World Health Organization (WHO) reduced the extent of geographical areas in which vaccination is recommended (Fig. 4.1). Recently, there have been outbreaks of the disease in South America (Brazil, Peru) and sub-Saharan Africa (Cameroon, Côte d'Ivoire, Ghana, Sierra Leone, Senegal, Uganda). There have been worrying reports of adverse events associated with yellow fever vaccine, particularly in older people. Such reactions may be more common in those with thymic dysfunction or with other types of immune defect.

Cholera

Vaccination is no longer required by international regulations. Earlier vaccines were of little use, and although there is now a licensed oral vaccine, it is really only necessary for those, like aid workers in refugee camps, who have a high risk of exposure.

Typhoid

This potentially serious infection remains prevalent in Pakistan, India, Bangladesh, Indonesia, and Nepal, where the incidence of infection is approximately 1 in 3000 per month of stay. Those staying for long periods in rural areas, and especially those visiting friends and relatives abroad, are at greatest need of vaccination.

Meningococcal disease

In the meningitis belt of sub-Sahelian Africa (see Fig. 6.5.3), from Senegal to Sudan, and in some other areas, cool, dry-season meningococcal meningitis outbreaks are so predictable that immunization is recommended. The quadrivalent meningococcal vaccine (covering serogroups A, C, W135, and Y) is recommended. The new conjugate meningococcal vaccine (ACYW135—Menactra) has proved safe and immunogenic in all age groups including infants. The quantity and quality of the antibody response is superior to that produced by polysaccharide vaccines and their use reduces meningococcal carriage, reducing transmission. Following outbreaks associated with the Hajj over the past few years, pilgrims to Mecca are required to be immunized and provide proof.

Rabies

Pre-exposure rabies vaccination is increasingly being used (see Chapter 5.10). Although the risk of transmission is fairly low, the lack of effective treatment for rabies encephalitis, and the fear engendered by bites by dogs, and in many parts of the world, by bats, justifies considering immunization. It is wrong to assume that the essential vaccine and rabies immune globulin will be immediately available when and where it is urgently needed after a potentially rabid bite overseas.

Other encephalitides

Vaccination against Japanese encephalitis (see Fig. 5.14.2) and tick-borne encephalitis (see Fig. 5.14.5) may be considered after reviewing the travel itinerary and risk of exposure (Table 4.1). A new Vero cell-derived vaccine against Japanese encephalitis (IXIARO) was licensed in 2009.

Prevention of malaria

Both travellers and nonspecialist physicians must be educated about the prevention and recognition of malaria (see Chapter 8.2). It is important to be aware of the need to prevent mosquito bites by all possible means: wearing appropriate clothing, application of insect repellents to exposed skin and clothing, and the use of insecticide-impregnated bed nets and insecticide sprays or vaporizers in the sleeping quarters. Guidelines for antimalarial chemoprophylaxis are regularly updated (see 'Further reading: internet sites' below) and for travel to areas where the risk of malaria, although finite, is low, standby antimalarial treatment rather than prophylaxis is increasingly recommended. In areas of low incidence (less than 10 cases of malaria per 1000 of the local population per year) such as Central America and South East Asia, the risk of taking antimalarial drugs outweighs the risk of infection and so reliance is placed on antimosquito measures and carrying a course of standby emergency treatment to be taken if the traveller develops symptoms suggestive

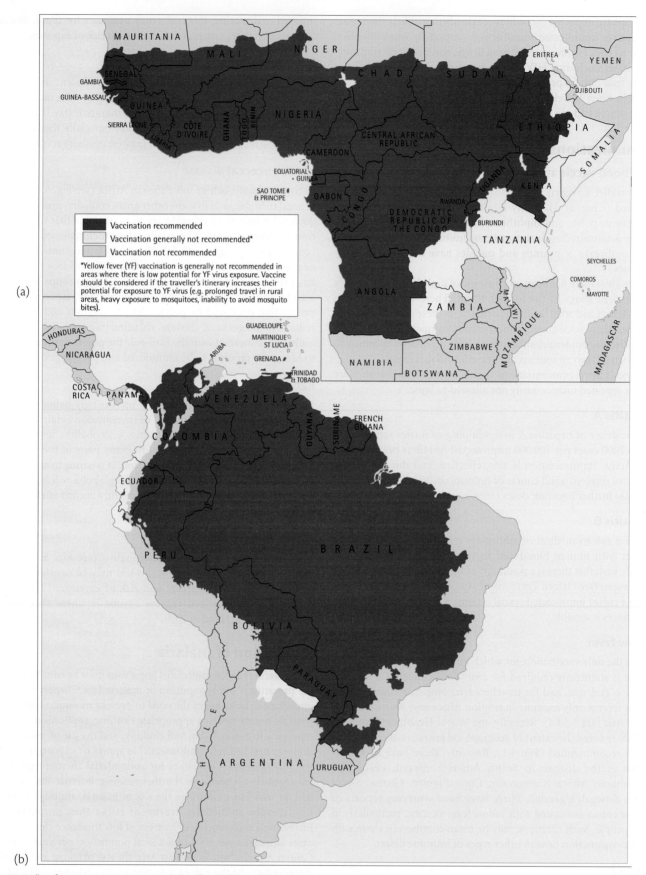

Fig. 4.1 Yellow fever vaccination recommendations for a) Africa and b) South America from http://www.nathnac.org/pro/factsheets/yellow.htmand http://www.nathnac.org/pro/factsheets/yellow.htm and WHO (2011) http://www.who.int/ith/en/.

of malaria while out of reach of medical care (see http://www.dtg.org/ for map).

Between May and September 2011, 20 autochthonous cases of *Plasmodium vivax* malaria were identified in southern Greece, especially in Evrotas, Lakonia. This led the United States Centers for Diease Control temporarily to recommend malarial chemoprophylaxis for travellers visiting this district.

Prevention and management of travellers' diarrhoea

Box 4.1 Some causes of travellers' diarrhoea
Bacteria
Enterotoxigenic and enteroaggregative *Escherichia coli* (*c.*15–80%)
Aeromonas spp., *Plesiomonas* spp.
Campylobacter jejuni
Salmonella typhi
Other *Salmonella* spp.
Shigella spp.
Vibrio parahaemolyticus
Protozoa
Cryptosporidium parvum
Cyclospora cayetanensis
Entamoeba histolytica
Giardia intestinalis
Plasmodium falciparum
Other
Rotavirus/norovirus
Schistosoma mansoni
Strongyloides stercoralis
Irritable and inflammatory bowel disease
Tropical sprue
Food allergy
Drug side effects,
Clostridium difficile toxin, fish/shellfish toxins

Diarrhoea is the most common health problem of travellers. Symptoms are usually mild, lasting only about 3 to 5 days, but holiday and business plans may be disrupted. The most common cause is enterotoxigenic *Escherichia coli* (ETEC). *Salmonella* spp., *Campylobacter* spp., *Shigella* spp., and other pathogenic *E. coli* are also common. Protozoan pathogens, such as *Giardia intestinalis*, *Entamoeba histolytica*, *Cryptosporidium parvum*, *Cyclospora cayetanensis* and viruses are less common causes. Fish and shellfish poisoning cause similar symptoms, starting within minutes or hours of exposure (Oxford Textbook of Medicine 5e Chapter 9.2).

Strict food and water hygiene reduce the risk of gastroenteritis. Heating water to 100°C will kill most pathogens, as will chemical treatment with chlorine or iodine (iodine is contraindicated in pregnant women and some patients with thyroid disease). Water filters are also effective. Antimicrobials such as fluoroquinolones, azithromycin (for fluoroquinolone-resistant campylobacter in South and South East Asia) or rifaximin, a poorly absorbed rifamycin derivative (for ETEC in Latin America and Africa) provide some protection, but are not cheap, may cause side effects, cannot be taken for prolonged periods, and may encourage antimicrobial resistance. Colloidal bismuth salts are cheaper, safer, and reasonably effective, but the large volumes are inconvenient. An experimental transcutaneous heat-labile enterotoxin vaccine reduced the frequency and severity of travellers' diarrhoea but oral killed *Vibrio cholerae* vaccine had little effect despite inducing crossimmunity to ETEC.

Treatment involves maintaining an adequate fluid intake and using sachets of oral rehydration salts that can be made up with boiled water. Eating solid food may stimulate bowel action by the gastrocolic reflex. Antidiarrhoeal agents such as codeine phosphate and loperamide often relieve symptoms sufficiently to allow normal activities to continue. Short courses of empirical antimicrobials, e.g. ciprofloxacin (500 mg for 3 days, adults only), azithromycin, or rifaximin can be useful, particularly for patients with underlying diseases. Combination of an antimicrobial such as rifaximin with loperamide has proved more effective symptomatically. Localized abdominal pain, high fever, and bloody diarrhoea are indications for seeking medical help immediately.

Special groups of travellers

Immunocompromised travellers

Except for asplenic patients, immunocompromised travellers—including those who have recently received chemotherapy or radiotherapy—should not be given live vaccines such as yellow fever, oral polio, and oral typhoid. Killed or synthetic vaccines are safe. Those patients with mild to moderate immune suppression will probably make a reasonable response to immunization; those with more severe immunosuppression may still make a useful, though less durable, response. Influenza, pneumococcal, and *Haemophilus influenzae* b conjugate vaccines are recommended, as these patients' risk of respiratory infection and bacteraemia is increased. Studies show that immunosuppressed patients can make a response to hepatitis A immunizations, although the durability of this response is again uncertain. People with HIV will often make a good response if they are on antiretroviral medication and have made a good CD4 response. Asplenic individuals should be on prophylactic antibiotics, such as amoxicillin, particularly if travelling, and should be dissuaded from travelling to areas with high rates of malaria transmission, as they are more likely to get severe disease if infected.

Immunocompromised patients should carry antimicrobials with them for treating respiratory or gastrointestinal infections, should seek medical help when abroad, and should carry a letter from their physician outlining their condition and medication.

Pregnant travellers

Commercial airlines will not normally convey a woman who is 36 weeks or more pregnant, without a covering letter from her physician. Insurance to cover the cost of delivery abroad should be considered. If possible, pregnant women should avoid travelling to areas where diseases are prevalent that pose a special risk in their condition, such as malaria and viral hepatitis E.

The risk–benefit assessment of immunizations and chemoprophylaxis is of particular importance for the pregnant woman and the fetus. Live vaccines should be avoided, but if there is a genuine risk of yellow fever the vaccine should be given, as there is no recognized associated teratogenicity. Inactivated polio vaccine may be given parenterally, and tetanus immunization is safe. Heat-killed typhoid vaccine is best avoided, as it might cause a febrile reaction and stimulate premature labour. However, the modern polysaccharide capsular Vi vaccine should be safe. Pneumococcal, meningococcal, and hepatitis B vaccines are safe in pregnancy, as is gamma globulin.

Malaria is especially dangerous in pregnant women (see Chapter 8.2). Chloroquine and proguanil are safe prophylactic drugs, and quinine in normal therapeutic doses is safe for treatment. Mefloquine is best avoided in the first trimester of pregnancy. Pregnant women should take special care with food and drink when abroad, as dehydration may threaten the fetus. There are concerns about congenital goitre when pregnant women use iodine to purify water; the maximum recommended daily intake is 175 μg. Loperamide as an antidiarrhoeal agent is safe, but antimicrobials such as tetracyclines and quinolones should be avoided.

Extremes of age

Young children should have completed their routine immunizations before travelling. Malaria chemoprophylaxis is recommended for all ages. Yellow fever vaccine should be given only to children older than 9 months, as a few cases of vaccine-associated encephalitis have occurred in younger children. Most other vaccines, including rabies, are safe. Hepatitis A is rarely symptomatic in children under 5 years old. Families planning to live in developing countries should be offered BCG vaccination for their children to reduce the risk of tuberculous meningitis.

Older people should have the same immunizations as younger adults, and should take antimalarial drugs. They are more prone to respiratory infection, and should therefore be given influenza, pneumococcal, and *Haemophilus influenzae* vaccines. Jet lag and changes in time zones may be very disturbing. Older people are more likely to have an underlying medical condition requiring medication; it is important that sufficient supplies of medicines are taken abroad and that the patient has a detailed list of these medicines and their dosages in case the tablets are lost or stolen. They should carry the name and contact address of their home physician, in case of emergency.

Explorers and expeditions

Because of their adventurous aims, expeditions are likely to involve exposure to greater environmental extremes and hazards than ordinary travel. Expeditions usually take place in areas remote from even rural health centres, and so a greater responsibility for dealing with medical problems will devolve to the expedition members. The explorer's greatest fear may be to fall victim to a lethal tropical disease or an attack by a wild animal, but the reality is much more mundane: road traffic accidents, mountaineering disasters, drowning, and attacks by humans claim most lives.

The prevention and treatment of medical problems must be planned well in advance. Detailed advice and information can be obtained from a number of organizations, such as the Expedition Advisory Centre (Geography Outdoors) of the Royal Geographical Society in London, from clubs specializing in mountaineering, cave exploring, diving, and other activities, and from books, journals, and websites. All expeditions should have a designated medical officer, and all their members should receive first-aid training aimed at the particular needs of the expedition. The basics are clearing the airway, controlling bleeding, treating shock, relieving pain, and moving the injured person without causing further damage. Expedition medical kits should be more comprehensive than those carried by ordinary tourists and travellers. Lists of essential drugs are given in Johnson *et al.* (2008). Scissors, a generous supply of large triangular and crêpe bandages, adhesive plasters, and an AIDS kit (to reduce the risk of infection from dirty needles and intravenous fluids) are important. Lightweight emergency insulation must be taken if there is any risk of exposure in severe weather conditions; a lightweight collapsible stretcher should be taken for mountaineering, and an adequate water supply must be assured or taken if the expedition is into desert areas.

A covering letter on official notepaper, signed by a doctor, may be helpful in allowing drugs, even apparently innocuous ones such as codeine, through customs (e.g. the Russian Federation) and explaining the need for needles and syringes. The medical facilities nearest to the site of the expedition must be identified and contacted in advance. An emergency plan must be drawn up for the first-aid treatment and evacuation of severely ill or injured expedition members. In some areas, flying doctor and air evacuation services (such as AMREF in East Africa) are available. Medical insurance must be generous and comprehensive, and include repatriation of the injured. Before leaving their home country, expedition members should have a thorough dental check and treatment for any outstanding medical or surgical problems. Control of chronic medical problems such as diabetes mellitus, hypertension, and asthma should be stabilized. In selecting members for an expedition, the most important attributes are experience, possession of the necessary technical skills (e.g. diving and mountaineering), physical fitness, and proven psychological stability under stress. It is advisable always to appoint a reliable local agent in the country where the expedition will take place.

Illness in returning travellers

Details are needed about the countries visited, the activities undertaken while travelling, immunizations, and antimalarials taken. Common problems are fever, rash, diarrhoea, and eosinophilia (Tables 4.2 and 4.3, and Box 4.2).

The most important diagnosis to exclude in a traveller from the tropics with a fever is malaria. In travellers with acute diarrhoea, a dietary history, assessment of hydration state, stool microscopy and culture, abdominal films, and sigmoidoscopy may be needed. There are many possible causes (see Box 4.1). Patients with chronic diarrhoea may be infected with *Giardia* spp., *Cryptosporidium* spp., *Entamoeba histolytica*, shigellae, or salmonellae. Investigations should include a search for *Clostridium difficile* and its toxin, especially if the patient took antimicrobials while abroad. A minority of patients may develop postinfective enteropathy, the most common problem being secondary lactose intolerance. Rarely, bacterial overgrowth or tropical sprue develops.

The most common causes of eosinophilia are allergy, drug reactions, and helminths (Box 4.2).

Table 4.2 Causes of fever in returned travellers

Tropical infections	Other infections	Noninfective causes
Short incubation; <3 weeks	Endocarditis	Connective tissue disease
African trypanosomiasis	Pneumonia	Drug reaction
Brucellosis	Prostatitis	Factitious inflammatory bowel disease
Dengue fever	Sexually transmitted disease	
Haemorrhagic fevers (e.g. Lassa)	Sinusitis	Malignancy
Hepatitis A	Urinary tract infection	
Malaria		
Relapsing fevers		
Tick/scrub typhus		
Typhoid		
Leptospirosis		
Malaria		
Long incubation; >3 weeks		
Amoebic abscess		
Brucellosis		
Coccidiomycosis		
Filariasis		
Hepatitis A, B, or C		
HIV (?incubation)		
Leishmaniasis		
Malaria		
Schistosomiasis (Katayama fever)		
Tuberculosis		
Typhoid		

Table 4.3 Causes of rash in returning travellers

Infective	Non-infective
Cutaneous larva migrans; myiasis	Contact allergy
Cutaneous leishmaniasis	Drug reaction
Dengue fever	Erythema multiforme
Dermatophytes	Insect bites
Lyme disease	Sunburn
Meningococcal illness	
Mycobacteria	
Scabies/lice	
Sexually transmitted infections	
Tick/scrub typhus	
Tinea versicolor	
Typhoid/paratyphoid	

Box 4.2 Infective causes of eosinophilia in travellers

Angiostrongylus (Parastrongylus) spp.

Ascaris spp.

Echinococcus spp.

Filariasis (onchocerciasis)

Gnathostoma spp.

Hookworm and other gut nematodes

Pulmonary eosinophilia

Schistosomiasis

Strongyloides spp.

Trichinosis

Trichuris spp.

Visceral larva migrans

Further reading

Auerbach PS (ed) (2012). *Wilderness medicine*, 6th edition. Mosby Elsevier, Philadelphia.

Backer HD, *et al.* (eds) (1998). *Wilderness first aid: emergency care for remote locations*. Jones and Barlett, Boston.

Barwick R (2004). History of thymoma and yellow fever vaccination. *Lancet*, **364**, 936.

Chen LH, *et al.* (2011). Vaccination of travelers: how far have we come and where are we going? *Expert Rev Vaccines*, **10**, 1609–20.

Conlon CP (2001). The immunocompromised traveler. In: DuPont HL, Steffen R (eds) *Textbook of travel medicine and health*, 2nd edition. BC Becker, London.

Dawood R (2002). *Travellers' health: how to stay healthy abroad*. Oxford University Press, Oxford.

Deutsche Gesellschaft für Tropenmedizin und Internationale Gesundheit (DTG) (2011). *Empfehlungen zur Malariavorbeugung* (map, p. 21) http://www.dtg.org/

Forgey WW (2000). *Wilderness medicine: beyond first aid*, 5th edition. Globe Pequot Press, Guilford, Connecticut.

Hill DR, Ford L, Lalloo DG (2006). Oral cholera vaccines: use in clinical practice. *Lancet Infect Dis*, **6**, 361–72.

Johnson C, *et al.* (eds) (2008). *Oxford handbook of expedition and wilderness medicine*. Oxford University Press, Oxford.

Johnston V *et al.* (2009). Fever in returned travellers presenting in the United Kingdom: recommendations for investigation and initial management. *J Infect.* **59**, 1–18.

Khatami A, Pollard AJ (2010). The epidemiology of meningococcal disease and the impact of vaccines. *Expert Rev Vaccines*, **9**, 285–98.

Layer P, Andresen V. (2010). Review article: rifaximin, a minimally absorbed oral antibacterial, for the treatment of travellers' diarrhoea. *Aliment Pharmacol Ther*, **31**, 1155–64.

Monath TP, Modlin JF (2002). Prevention of yellow fever in persons traveling to the tropics. *Clin Infect Dis*, **34**, 1369–78.

Potter SA (ed.) (1992). *ANARE Antarctic field manual*, 4th edition. Australian Antarctic Division, Kingston, Tasmania.

Steedman DJ (1994). *Environmental medical emergencies*. Oxford University Press, Oxford.

The Voluntary Aid Societies, St. John Ambulance, St. Andrew's Ambulance Associate and the British Red Cross (2006). *First aid manual*. Dorling Kindersley, London.

Ward MP, Milledge JS, West JB (2000). *High altitude medicine and physiology*, 3rd edition. Arnold, London.

WHO (2011). *International travel and health, 2011 edition*. http://www.who.int/ith/en/

Wilderness & Environmental Medicine (formerly Journal of Wilderness Medicine) (1990–). Published for the Wilderness Medical Society by Elsevier. http://wemjournal.org/

Zuckerman JN, Connor BA, von Sonnenburg F (2005). *Hepatitis A and B booster recommendations: implications for travelers. Clin Infect Dis*, **41**, 1020–26.

Websites

General travel advice

Centers for Disease Control and Prevention. *Travelers' Health.* http://wwwn.cdc.gov/travel/

Health Protection Agency. http://www.hpa.org.uk/ http://www.hpa.org.uk/HPA/Topics/InfectiousDiseases/InfectionsAZ/1191942149486/

National Travel Health Network and Centre (NaTHNaC). *Protecting the Health of British Travellers.* http://www.nathnac.org

National Travel Health Network and Centre. *The Yellow Book.* http://www.nathnac.org/yellow_book/01.htm

Royal Geographical Society, Expedition Advisory Centre. http://www.rgs.org/OurWork/Fieldwork+and+Expeditions/Specialist+Advice/Medical+Cell/Expedition+Medical+Cell.htm

The International Society of Travel Medicine. http://www.istm.org

World Health Organization. *International Travel and Health.* http://www.who.int/ith/

Malaria

Centers for Disease Control and Prevention. *Malaria.* http://www.cdc.gov/malaria/index.htm

Health Protection Agency. *Malaria.* http://www.hpa.org.uk/webw/HPAweb&Page&HPAwebAutoListName/Page/1191942128239?p=1191942128239

World Health Organization (2006). *Guidelines for the treatment of malaria.* http://www.who.int/malaria/docs/TreatmentGuidelines2006.pdf

5

Viruses

Contents

5.1 Respiratory tract viruses

Malik Peiris

Essentials

Viral respiratory infections, including rhinovirus, coronavirus, adenovirus, respiratory syncytial virus, human metapneumovirus, parainfluenza viruses, and influenza viruses, are a substantial cause of morbidity worldwide. Transmission occurs through direct contact, contaminated fomites, and large airborne droplets, with long-range transmission by small particle aerosols reported in at least some instances of influenza and severe acute respiratory syndrome (SARS).

Clinical syndromes affect the upper and/or lower respiratory tract, including coryza, pharyngitis, croup, bronchiolitis, and pneumonia. Each syndrome can potentially be caused by a number of viruses, and each respiratory virus can be associated with different clinical syndromes. Measles is a major cause of lower respiratory tract infections and fatality in tropical countries.

Diagnosis—nasopharyngeal aspirates, washes and swabs are superior to throat and nose swabs for diagnosis, with virus detected by culture or detection of antigen or nucleic acid (e.g. PCR-based methods). New respiratory viruses continue to be discovered, but some acute respiratory infections have no identifiable aetiology, and some patients have multiple respiratory viruses detectable in the respiratory tract in association with their disease—whether these have a synergistic role in pathogenesis remains unclear.

Particular respiratory tract viruses

Influenza—types A and B are clinically important causes of human disease; the viral envelope contains two glycoproteins, haemagglutinin (H) and neuraminidase (N), which are critical in host immunity and used to designate viral subtype, e.g. H1N1. Potential to cause pandemics makes influenza type A a unique challenge for global public health. Typically causes an illness associated with fever, chills, headache, sore throat, coryza, nonproductive cough, myalgia, and sometimes prostration. Can cause pneumonia directly or by secondary bacterial infections. Oseltamivir and zanamivir result in a reduction of 1 to 2 days in the time to alleviation of symptoms when administered within the first 48 h of illness, but even later commencement of therapy may still confer clinical benefit in severe influenza illness. Can be prevented by influenza vaccine, which contains antigens from the two subtypes of human influenza A (H3N2 and H1N1) and B viruses, but the composition of the vaccine must be updated on an annual basis to keep abreast of change in the surface antigens of the virus, and annual reimmunization is required. Synergistic interaction with *Streptococcus pneumoniae* enhances pathogenesis, and pneumococcal conjugate vaccine reduces hospitalization associated with respiratory viruses.

Respiratory syncytial virus (RSV)—a major cause of bronchiolitis and pneumonia in infants. Infection in adults is often asymptomatic, but during the RSV season (winter months in temperate regions) it is an important cause of lower respiratory tract infection in adults, particularly elderly people. May be lethal (as can other respiratory viruses) in patients immunocompromised following organ or blood and marrow transplants (but is not a significant problem in patients with AIDS).

Severe acute respiratory syndrome (SARS)—this novel coronavirus of animals adapted to efficient human transmission and spread worldwide, causing a global outbreak in 2003 of an illness characterized by lower respiratory tract manifestations, severe respiratory failure, and death in about 10% of cases. Public health interventions interrupted viral transmission and it is no longer transmitting within humans, but the precursor virus remains in the animal reservoir (bats, *Rhinolophus* spp.) and may readapt to cause human disease in the future.

Introduction

Viral respiratory infections are one of the most common afflictions of humankind. They are the most frequent reasons for medical consultations, are believed to account for 30% of work absences and school absenteeism, and are a major reason for antibiotic prescriptions. Longitudinal family studies suggest that a person has on average 2.4 respiratory viral infections per year, a quarter of them leading to a medical consultation. The synergistic interaction between viruses and bacteria in pathogenesis are being increasingly recognized, for example that between influenza virus and *Streptococcus pneumoniae* and *Staphylococcus aureus*. With the exception of influenza in elderly people, these viral infections are not a major cause of mortality in otherwise healthy people in the developed world, but it is estimated that they contribute to over 1 million deaths annually in the developing world.

The term 'respiratory virus' for the purpose of this discussion will include those that have the respiratory tract as their primary site of clinically relevant pathology. Taxonomically, they belong to six virus families (Table 5.1.1) and are global in distribution. Other viruses cause systemic disease with respiratory tract involvement as part of an overall disseminated disease process in patients who are immunocompetent (e.g. measles, Hantavirus pulmonary syndrome) or immunocompromised (e.g. cytomegalovirus). These are dealt with elsewhere.

A respiratory virus may cause a range of clinical syndromes. Conversely, a respiratory syndrome may be caused by more than one virus. The major viral respiratory syndromes and their common aetiological agents are shown in Table 5.1.2. Although seasonality may differ, the patterns of disease seen in tropical countries are similar; but a notable difference is the role of measles as a major cause of lower respiratory tract infections and fatality in the tropics.

The anatomical demarcation between upper (URTI) and lower respiratory tract infections (LRTI) is the larynx. Influenza, respiratory syncytial virus, parainfluenza virus and adenoviruses are well-recognized causes of LRTI in adults as well as in children, although many other respiratory viruses may do so occasionally. Severe acute respiratory syndrome coronavirus (SARS CoV) and avian influenza H5N1 are unusual in that lower respiratory manifestations predominate over the involvement of the upper respiratory tract.

With newer molecular-based approaches to pathogen discovery, new respiratory viruses continue to be recognized. Some recently recognized viruses have been long endemic in humans (e.g. human

Table 5.1.1 Respiratory tract viruses: summary of classification, incubation period, duration of infectivity, and diagnostic options

Virus	Classification (virus family) and composition of virus	Subgroups, serotypes, and subtypes	Incubation period (days)	Duration of virus shedding in immunocompetent patients (days)	Options for laboratory diagnosis[a]
Rhinovirus	Picornaviridae Nonenveloped RNA viruses	>102 serotypes phylo-genetically divided into 3 groups A, B and C	1–2 days	5–6 days by culture; 50% remain positive by RT-PCR 2 weeks later	RT-PCR or viral culture (less sensitive)
Enterovirus	Picornaviridae Nonenveloped RNA viruses	65 serotypes	Few days	Up to 2 weeks from respiratory tract, much longer in faeces	RT-PCR. Viral culture less sensitive and not possible for some types unless animal inoculation is used
Coronavirus	Coronaviridae. Enveloped RNA viruses	5 types (OC43, 229E, NL-63, HKU-1, SARS CoV	4–5 days	5–8 days	RT-PCR
Respiratory syncytial virus (RSV)	Paramyxoviridae Enveloped RNA virus	Subgroup A and B	5 days	6–7 days	Culture Rapid antigen detection,[a] RT-PCR Serology: useful in adults but less so in infants
Human metapneumovirus	Paramyxoviridae Enveloped RNA virus	Serotypes A and B	ND	ND	RT-PCR Viral antigen detection
Parainfluenza	Paramyxoviridae Enveloped RNA virus	Type 1, 2, 3, 4a, 4b	3–6 days	7 days	Culture Rapid antigen detection,[a] RT-PCR Serology: useful in adults but less so in infants
Influenza	Orthomyxoviridae Enveloped RNA virus	Types A, B, C Human influenza A subtypes currently in circulation are H1N1 and H3N2	Average 2–3 (range 1–7)	c.5 days in adults c.7 days in children	Culture Rapid antigen detection[2], RT-PCR Serology
Adenovirus	Adenoviridae Nonenveloped DNA virus	Subgroups A–F Types 1–51	Average 10 (range 2–15)	Days–weeks (from respiratory tract), weeks–months (in faeces)	Culture Rapid antigen detection,[a] RT-PCR, Serology
Bocavirus	Parvoviridae Nonenveloped DNA virus	One phylogenetic group	ND	ND	RT-PCR

ND, not defined.

[a] Best sensitivity from nasopharyngeal aspirates or nasopharyngeal swabs (in that order). Throat swabs give lower sensitivity.

Table 5.1.2 Viral aetiology of common respiratory syndromes

Virus	Coryza	Pharyngitis	Croup	Bronchiolitis	Pneumonia
Rhinovirus	+++[a]	++	+	+	Rare
Coronavirus	++	+	+ (NL-63)		SARS CoV, HKU-1
Adenoviruses	(+)	++	++	++	++ (all ages)
RSV	++	+	++	+++	+++ (children); + (elderly)
Human metapneumovirus	+	+	+	++	++ (children)
Parainfluenza 1	+	++	+++	+	
Parainfluenza 2	+	++	++	+	
Parainfluenza 3	+	++	++	++	++ (children)
Influenza A/B	+	++	++	+	++ (all ages)

[a] Frequency of cases caused by the virus: +++ the major cause (>25%); ++ a common cause (5–25%); + an occasional cause; blank, rare cause or not reported.
(Data adapted from Treanor 2009).

metapneumovirus, coronaviruses NL-63 and HKU1, bocavirus) while others are novel pathogens, newly emergent as causes of human infections such as SARS and avian flu H5N1.

Transmission

The routes of respiratory virus transmission are through direct contact, contaminated fomites, and large airborne droplets (mean diameter >5 μm, range of transmission <1 m). There remains controversy over the potential for the spread of viruses such as influenza over longer distances by small particle aerosol (mean diameter <5 μm), but even here, large droplets, direct contact, and fomites are probably more important. Occasionally, SARS CoV appears to have spread by small particle aerosols, although droplets and fomites probably contributed to the major part of the transmission of this disease. Adenoviruses are transmitted by the faeco-oral route as well as by direct contact and large droplets.

Factors increasing transmission of respiratory viruses include the time of exposure, close contact (e.g. spouse, mother), crowding, family size, and lack of pre-existing immunity (including lack of breastfeeding). School-age children often introduce an infection into the family and the beginning of school term may affect transmission patterns in the community. Infected children shed higher titres of viruses than adults. The duration of virus excretion is shown in Table 5.1.1. Infectivity usually precedes the onset of clinical symptoms. Immunocompromised patients shed virus for a longer time.

Seasonality

Some respiratory viruses have a predictable seasonality, which varies regionally. For example, influenza A is a typically winter disease in temperate regions, a spring/summer disease in the subtropics (e.g. Hong Kong) and occurs all year round (e.g. Singapore) or predominantly in the rainy season (e.g. Thailand) in the tropics. The basis for such seasonality is unclear, but climatic factors such as high humidity and temperature may help virus survival in small particle aerosols or droplets, and on contaminated surfaces. Factors affecting population congregation such as commencement of school term and seasonal effects on social behaviour may also play a role.

Laboratory diagnosis

A well-collected specimen is the first and often most important determinant in successful laboratory diagnosis. Nasopharyngeal aspirates (secretions aspirated from the back of the nose into a mucus trap), nasopharyngeal washes, and nasopharyngeal swabs are superior to throat and nose swabs for the diagnosis of many respiratory viruses. They offer the advantage that rapid ('same day') diagnosis for a number of viruses is possible provided the appropriate methods are available. Swabs for viral culture are placed in viral transport medium immediately upon collection and kept cool (around 4°C) until processed. More invasive specimens such as endotracheal aspirates, bronchoalveolar lavage, or lung biopsy, when available, usually provide better information. For example, in patients with influenza pneumonia during the 2009 pandemic, endotracheal aspirate specimens sometimes provided positive results even when the upper respiratory tract specimens were negative. However, the likely site of pathology must be kept in mind—the more invasive specimen is not always better.

Laboratory methods used for detecting a virus in clinical specimen/s are viral culture, antigen detection, and, more recently, nucleic acid detection (e.g. polymerase chain reaction (PCR)-based methods). The widespread use of molecular methods for viral detection has led to recognition that some viruses that are difficult to culture (e.g. coronaviruses and some rhinoviruses and enteroviruses) are found more often in patients with acute respiratory disease than previously recognized. Similarly, these methods have allowed the discovery of novel viruses associated with respiratory disease (e.g. coronaviruses NL-63, HKU1, bocavirus). They have also revealed that infection with multiple viruses is relatively common. These findings necessitate a reassessment of the clinical relevance of positive PCR results. Relevant questions include how commonly these viruses are detectable by these methods in age-matched healthy controls and how long viruses remain detectable after infection. It is important to understand the relevance of detection of multiple pathogens in a respiratory specimen. Are these viruses synergistic in pathogenesis or is one more important than another? Many of these questions remain to be resolved.

Demonstration of rising antibody titres in paired sera is used to diagnose some respiratory virus diseases, but serology is impracticable for others such as rhinoviruses where the large number of antigenically distinct serotypes have no common immunodominant antigen(s). However, adenoviruses and influenza viruses, though having many antigenic types or variants, have common antigen(s) and a single antigen can detect serological responses to many of them. IgM assays are not routinely available for diagnosis of respiratory viral diseases. Serology is also helpful in assessing the clinical relevance of a virus detected in a respiratory specimen (see above) by helping differentiating recent infection from more remote events.

'Near patient testing' is becoming a reality for some viruses (e.g. influenza, RSV) with availability of tests that can be performed in a general practice setting. These become more relevant with the greater availability of antiviral drugs.

Rhinoviruses

Rhinoviruses belong to the Picornavirus family and are adapted to replicate at temperatures of 33–35°C, as found in the external airways. Until recently, more than 150 serotypes of rhinoviruses were recognized phylogenetically clustered into groups A, B, and C; group C viruses are noncultivable and recently discovered by molecular methods. A number of rhinovirus types will circulate in a region at any given time.

Epidemiology

Rhinoviruses remain one of the commonest infections of humans: 0.5 infections per person per year is a conservative estimate. Secondary attack rates in families may be around 50% overall and 70% in those who are antibody negative. They were thought to cause mainly mild community infections, but are being recognized increasingly as the commonest viral agent detected by RT-PCR in children hospitalized with acute respiratory illness. Many of these represent coinfections with other potential respiratory pathogens. As rhinoviruses are often detectable by RT-PCR for weeks after initial infection (50% remain positive at 2 weeks), the aetiological significance of this finding is unresolved and more studies with relevant control populations are needed.

Immunity

In experimental challenges, immunity is serotype specific. Homologous type specific protection lasts for at least 1 year and correlates with serum IgA, IgG, and secretory IgA antibody levels.

Pathogenesis

Viral replication occurs predominantly in the ciliated epithelial cells of the nasopharynx. The structure of the epithelium is preserved. Mucosal secretions associated with coryza appear to be due to the release of inflammatory mediators and neurogenic reflexes.

It was thought that the preference of the virus for a lower temperature for replication restricted it to the upper respiratory tract. However, this is not strictly true. The virus has been isolated from the lower respiratory tract (including bronchial brushings) and viral RNA has been demonstrated by *in situ* hybridization in bronchial epithelial cells. Rarely, the virus has been isolated post-mortem from lungs of immunocompromised patients.

Clinical manifestations

Rhinorrhoea, nasal obstruction, pharyngitis, and a cough are common features of rhinovirus infections. Fever and systemic symptoms are rare, but more common in the elderly in whom disease can be more severe. Rhinoviruses are a major cause of exacerbations of asthma and chronic obstructive respiratory disease in adults. Lower respiratory tract symptoms are uncommon in healthy young adults, but may occur in children (bronchiolitis), the immunocompromised, and the elderly. Rhinovirus infections associated with wheezing in the first 3 years of life is predictive of asthma in later childhood.

Treatment and prevention

There are no established antiviral drugs for treatment and management is symptomatic. Topical interferon-α prevents symptoms if given before onset of disease, but cannot be used for prophylaxis over prolonged periods because of side effects. Pleconaril is a viral capsid-binding agent that blocks viral attachment and uncoating and has had modest benefit in clinical trials, but concerns over side effects have prevented its licensing. Antibiotics are ineffective in preventing bacterial complications of the common cold. Mucopurulent discharges are part of the natural course of the common cold and are not an indication for antimicrobial treatment, unless it persists (e.g. >10 days). Given the large number of rhinovirus serotypes, vaccination is not an option.

Enteroviruses

Enteroviruses and rhinoviruses (see above) are genera within the family Picornaviridae. Enteroviruses have long been known as causes of central nervous system infections, myocarditis, or exanthema rather than as a respiratory pathogen, the latter role being assigned to rhinoviruses. As many enteroviruses fail to replicate in cell culture, the wider use of molecular diagnosis has revealed an increased role of enteroviruses in acute respiratory infections. Clinically, patients present with rhinitis, cough, fever, sore throat, or otitis media. There remains a need for studies of age-matched controls to better establish the clinical relevance of these molecular tests. In comparative studies done on the duration of shedding of enteroviruses and rhinoviruses, fewer enterovirus infected children continue to shed virus for longer than 2 weeks while 50% of rhinovirus infections do. This suggests that a positive enterovirus RT-PCR result in the respiratory tract is probably more likely to be clinically relevant than one for rhinovirus.

Coronaviruses

Five human coronaviruses are currently known, three of them being new viruses discovered since the SARS outbreak in 2003. Coronaviruses are taxonomically subdivided into three groups and the human coronaviruses 229E and NL-63 belong to group 1 while OC43, HKU1, and SARS CoV belong to group 2. There are no known human group 3 coronaviruses. Human coronaviruses OC43 and 229E have long been recognized as important causes of the common cold but coronaviruses cause a range of respiratory illnesses. SARS CoV is a newly emerged pathogen. Human coronaviruses are difficult to culture from clinical specimens and laboratory diagnosis largely relies on molecular methods.

Epidemiology

Infection with OC43 and 229E occur in early childhood and 85 to 100% of adults have antibody to both virus types. NL-63 has a similar epidemiology but less is presently known of HKU1. SARS CoV emerged from an animal reservoir, adapted to human transmission and caused a global outbreak in 2003 that affected 29 countries across 5 continents. However, determined public health interventions interrupted transmission of this virus and it is no longer transmitting within humans. However, the precursor virus remains in the animal reservoir (bats, *Rhinolophus* spp.) and these may at some future date, readapt to cause human disease.

Immunity

Volunteer reinfection studies with 229E show that 1 year after initial infection, protection from reinfection and illness following a challenge from the homologous virus is incomplete. Comparable data are not available for the newly recognized NL-63, HKU1, or SARS CoV.

Pathogenesis

In common with rhinoviruses, coronaviruses 229E induce little or no damage to the respiratory mucosa. The mucosal discharge is caused by the release of mediators from affected host cells. SARS CoV had a predilection to involve alveolar pneumocytes in the lower respiratory tract and consequently caused a severe viral pneumonia. Disease severity of SARS was markedly age related. Children had mild disease whereas those over 50 years had a poor prognosis. The basis for this age-related pathogenesis is unknown. The virus receptor for 229E is CD13, while both SARS CoV and NL-63 utilize the human ACE-2 molecule for virus entry.

Clinical findings

Coronaviruses 229E and OC43 typically cause URTI and the common cold but also cause a range of other respiratory manifestations and are significant pathogens in elderly people. NL-63 and HKU1 cause both upper and lower respiratory disease. NL-63 appears to be an important cause of croup, bronchiolitis, and pneumonia. HKU1 appears to be an important pathogen particularly in those with underlying respiratory complications.

SARS typically presented with lower respiratory tract manifestations and radiological changes with minimum involvement of the upper respiratory tract. Many patients had diarrhoea resulting from viral replication in the gastrointestinal tract. Overall case fatality was 9.6%. Terminal events were severe respiratory failure associated with acute respiratory distress syndrome (ARDS) and multiple organ failure. Autopsies showed diffuse alveolar damage corresponding to the clinical presentation of acute respiratory distress syndrome. Age, comorbidities, and viral load in the nasopharynx and serum during the first 5 days of illness correlated with an adverse prognosis.

Treatment and prevention

There are presently no clinically validated antiviral treatments for human coronaviruses disease, although a number of drugs have been documented to have *in vitro* activity against SARS CoV. A number of experimental vaccines were developed for SARS, but with its disappearance from the human population, the incentive to take these forward to human clinical trials and licensing has waned.

Adenoviruses

Currently there are 51 adenovirus types classified in six groups (A–F); four additional noncultivable adenovirus types 52 to 55 have been reported, but their taxonomic status remains to be confirmed. Adenoviruses in subgroups A to D cause respiratory, ocular, hepatic, genitourinary, or gastrointestinal system disease in immunocompetent or immunocompromised individuals. Only respiratory diseases are considered here.

Productive replication and excretion of infectious virus can occur for a prolonged period (see below). In addition, adenoviruses can establish chronic persistence or 'latency', the virological basis and clinical significance of which is poorly understood.

Epidemiology

Adenovirus infections are common during childhood (usually serotypes 1, 2, 5 in early childhood, 3 and 7 during school years or later), but continue to occur throughout life. Reinfection with the same serotype occurs but is usually asymptomatic. Serotypes 1, 2, 5, and 6 are typically endemic, types 4 and 7 more typically associated with outbreaks, and type 3 can occur in either situation. Recently, adenovirus 14p1 (previously designated 14a) has been spreading in the United States of America and elsewhere and is associated with more severe disease.

Clinical features

Adenovirus respiratory illness often leads to URTI with coryza and sore throat. Fever may last up to 2 weeks. The sore throat may be exudative and clinically difficult to differentiate from streptococcal infection. Adenoviral infection may present as pharyngoconjunctival fever. Otitis media is a complication in children. Unlike other respiratory viral infections, adenoviruses may be associated with elevated white blood cell counts (exceeding 15×10^9/litre), C-reactive protein, or ESR and thus more easily confused with bacterial diseases.

Though uncommon, pneumonia may occur sporadically or in epidemics (e.g. caused by serotypes 4 and 7), particularly in closed communities such as the military where stress and physical exertion may predispose to lower respiratory tract involvement. Community outbreaks of adenoviral pneumonia have been reported. Radiological appearance varies from diffuse to patchy interstitial infiltrates and pleural effusion may be present. Adenovirus type 7 pneumonia can lead to permanent lung damage, including bronchiectasis, bronchiolitis obliterans, and unilateral hyperlucent lung syndrome.

Adenoviral infection may disseminate and present as 'septic shock' in neonates. Manifestations in immunocompromised patients include hepatitis (especially in liver transplant recipients), colitis, and haemorrhagic cystitis (in renal and bone marrow transplant recipients) in addition to pneumonia. The serotypes associated with disease in these patients may differ from those typically found in the immunocompetent patient, and include the subgroup B2 serotypes 11, 34, and 35. With improving control of other common viral diseases of immunocompromised patients (e.g. cytomegalovirus), the role of adenovirus infections is being increasingly appreciated.

Isolation of an adenovirus from a clinical specimen presents a challenge in interpretation. Adenoviruses are excreted for a prolonged period after initial infection, especially, but not exclusively, from faeces. In children, one-third of patients shed viruses for longer than 1 month and 14% longer than 1 year. The clinical significance of a positive result depends on the specimen, the method, and the serotype. Isolation of viruses from the respiratory tract carries greater significance than that from faeces. Patients who have symptomatic adenoviral diseases have higher viral loads than those with asymptomatic carriage. Thus, a rapidly growing virus, a positive antigen detection test from a respiratory specimen (both reflecting higher virus load), or a detectable serological response all point to greater clinical significance.

Immunocompromised patients may be infected with unusual serotypes. The detection of the virus in the peripheral blood or in multiple body sites suggests greater clinical significance and is an indication that therapeutic intervention needs to be considered.

Treatment and prevention

Most adenoviral infections in immunocompetent patients are self-limited and require no specific therapy; however, some infections, especially but not exclusively in immunocompromised patients, are severe and life threatening. Ribavirin, vidarabine, cidofovir, and ganciclovir are active against adenoviruses *in vitro*. Although there are anecdotal reports of the therapeutic use of each of these drugs with variable success, on the basis of limited clinical studies cidofovir appears to be the antiviral of choice.

Live attenuated oral vaccines containing serotypes 4 and 7 (associated with outbreaks in military conscripts) are safe and effective, but not licensed for general use.

Respiratory syncytial virus

Respiratory syncytial virus (RSV) infects human and nonhuman primates and was first isolated from a chimpanzee with a 'cold'. The virus has two surface glycoproteins on its envelope (G and F) and the immune responses to them correlate with protection. Two subgroups (A and B) are recognized on the basis of antigenic differences of the G glycoprotein.

Epidemiology

Over two-thirds of infants acquire RSV infection during the first year of life. Of patients hospitalized with RSV disease, 75% are younger than 5 months. The peak of morbidity occurs around 2 to

4 months of age, a time when passive maternal antibodies protect against most other viral infections. Primary infection does not lead to solid immunity and reinfection is common. The first reinfection can still be associated with lower respiratory tract involvement. Subsequent reinfection occurs throughout life leading to asymptomatic or URTI. However, significant diseases may result in the immunocompromised or elderly.

Immunity

Both antibody and cell mediated immunity are important in protection. Antibody to the G protein prevents attachment of viruses to the cellular receptor, but immunity to the F protein is required to prevent cell to cell spread via fusion of virally infected cells. Cell mediated immunity is important in eliminating established viral infection.

Pathogenesis

The virus leads to a ballooning degeneration of the ciliated epithelial cells, lymphocytic infiltration, and necrosis of the epithelium. There is oedema and increased secretion from the mucous cells and the formation of plugs of mucous and cellular debris in the bronchioles. This results in obstruction and air trapping leading to collapse or over-distension of the distal alveoli. Cells throughout the respiratory tract are affected but the alveoli are spared unless there is RSV pneumonia. The pathogenesis of RSV bronchiolitis still remains controversial.

Severe RSV bronchiolitis is strongly associated with subsequent childhood asthma. RSV appears to promote type 1 hypersensitivity responses following subsequent exposure to unrelated antigens.

Clinical features

RSV infections of infants may lead to bronchiolitis and pneumonia. Bronchiolitis in infants is associated with expiratory wheeze, subcostal recession, hyperinflation of the chest, nasal flaring, and hypoxia with or without cyanosis. Fever is not prominent in one-half of the patients. Complete obstruction of a small airway leads to subsegmental atelectasis. Apnoea may occur (particularly in premature infants or in those <3 months of age) and may precede the development of bronchiolitis. Interstitial pneumonitis is uncommon but carries a bad prognosis. Otitis media is a common complication of RSV infection in children. Infants at highest risk from severe RSV disease are those <6 months, those with pre-existing congenital heart disease, chronic lung diseases (e.g. bronchopulmonary dysplasia), and those born premature.

Infection in adults is often asymptomatic or leads to URTI. However, during the RSV season, it is an important cause of LRTI in adults and elderly people and it is estimated to cause 2 to 9% of the hospitalizations and deaths associated with pneumonia in elderly individuals. Much of this morbidity is clinically indistinguishable from influenza.

RSV (as well as parainfluenza and influenza) infections in the immunocompromised patient can be life threatening. They usually occur during community outbreaks, but a significant proportion are nosocomially acquired. The disease typically commences as an URTI but may progress to involve the lower respiratory tract with more serious consequences. Factors that increase risk of disease progression appear to include bone marrow transplant recipients who acquire the infection in the period prior to engraftment and oncology patients with neutrophil counts less than 0.5×10^9/litre.

Those immunocompromised by HIV appear to tolerate community acquired respiratory viruses better than oncology patients and transplant recipients.

Treatment and prevention

Ribavirin has activity against RSV *in vitro*. Administration of small particle aerosols via a mist tent, mask, oxygen hood, or ventilator has been recommended because it results in much higher concentrations in the respiratory tract than can be achieved by intravenous administration. There seems little therapeutic benefit of ribavirin therapy in RSV disease in immunocompetent children or adults. However, in patients at high risk for severe RSV disease such as adult bone marrow transplant recipients, an uncontrolled study of ribavirin together with intravenous immune globulin (selected batches with high neutralizing antibody titre) appeared to be beneficial when compared to historical controls. More information is required for deciding the best management strategy.

Monthly intravenous administration of a polyclonal immune globulin enriched in neutralizing antibodies to RSV (RespiGam) or a humanized monoclonal antibody to RSV (palivizumab) during the RSV season protects against disease of the lower respiratory tract and otitis media in children with pre-existing risk factors. Palivizumab appears to be more effective than RespiGam and there is less of a problem with fluid overload in children with chronic heart disease. High-titre RSV intravenous immunoglobulin by itself is ineffective in treatment of established RSV disease.

Candidate vaccines for RSV are undergoing clinical trials at present but none is yet available for routine use. Experience of early trials with inactivated RSV vaccines that led to enhanced RSV disease, rather than protection continues to haunt the field.

Parainfluenza virus

Parainfluenza viruses, despite their name, are not related to influenza viruses, and are more akin to respiratory syncytial virus with which they are classified (Table 5.1.1). They carry two envelope glycoproteins: HN containing both haemagglutinin and neuraminidase activity and F carrying fusion activity.

Epidemiology

The total impact on hospitalization of children by all four types of parainfluenza viruses taken together is similar to that of RSV but, in contrast to RSV, their impact is in later infancy and childhood. In temperate countries, parainfluenza virus type 3 occurs annually and infects two-thirds of all infants in their first year of life. Parainfluenza types 1 and 2 tend to occur in alternate years and infection is acquired more slowly over childhood. Reinfection with parainfluenza viruses occurs, but rarely leads to LRTI.

Pathogenesis

The virus is confined to the respiratory epithelial cells, macrophages, and dendritic cells within the respiratory tract. Dissemination is rarely documented even in immunocompromised patients.

Immunity

Reinfection with parainfluenza viruses continues throughout life. Presence of virus-specific IgE in nasopharyngeal secretions has been implicated in the development of parainfluenza croup or bronchiolitis.

Clinical features

Parainfluenza type 1 predominantly causes croup, while types 2 and 3 also cause bronchiolitis and pneumonia. Croup (or laryngotracheobronchitis) in children is associated with fever, hoarseness, and a barking cough and may progress to inspiratory stridor due to narrowing of the subglottic area of the trachea. The differential diagnosis is epiglottitis due to *Haemophilus influenzae* type b. Parainfluenza type 4 infection is less common, but causes bronchiolitis and pneumonia in children, often in those with underlying disease.

Reinfection in adults, when symptomatic, is a coryzal illness with hoarseness being prominent. Parainfluenza viruses (type 3 in particular) are significant causes of LRTI in adults when the virus is active in the community.

As with RSV, parainfluenza viruses cause problems in immunocompromised patients. Lower respiratory tract involvement is associated with wheezing, rales, dyspnoea, and diffuse interstitial infiltrates, and a fatal outcome in one-third of patients with allogenic bone marrow transplants. When pneumonia occurs, the histological appearance of the lung is that of a giant cell or an interstitial pneumonia.

Treatment and prevention

The need for specific antiviral therapy arises, particularly in the immunocompromised. Ribavirin is effective *in vitro* and was associated with a reduction of viral replication *in vivo* in anecdotal cases but there are no controlled trials documenting its clinical efficacy.

There are no options for prevention at present, either using vaccines or passive immunization. A live attenuated bovine-derived vaccine strain is currently undergoing clinical trials.

Human metapneumovirus

Human metapneumovirus (HMPV) belongs to the genus Metapneumovirus within the virus family Paramyxoviridae, subfamily Pneumovirinae. It closest known relative is the avian pneumovirus, an upper respiratory tract disease of turkeys and among human viruses is RSV which also belongs to the subfamily Pneumovirinae. It was first recognized in 2001 but is a virus that has circulated unrecognized in humans for many decades. There are at least two serotypes A and B which are antigenically distinct and appear to provide partial cross-protection.

Epidemiology

The virus is ubiquitous and most children have been infected with one or both serotypes by the age of 5 years. Symptomatic reinfection is common through life. Infection is commonest in the winter months in temperate regions and in late spring or summer in subtropical areas.

Clinical manifestations

HMPV is one of the common causes of hospitalization of children under 5 years of age and accounted for 12% of all LRTI hospitalization in one long-term study. However, the incidence in any given year may vary widely. The peak age for HMPV morbidity is between 6 and 12 months, which is later than that for RSV (2–4 months).

Clinical features of HMPV are similar to that of RSV and range from URTI to bronchiolitis and pneumonia. In common with rhinovirus and RSV, HMPV appears to trigger exacerbations of asthma. Diarrhoea, vomiting, rash, febrile seizures, conjunctivitis, and otitis media have been reported. HMPV has on one occasion been isolated as the sole pathogen from the brain in a patient with encephalitis.

HMPV can cause respiratory disease in elderly or immunocompromised individuals, and those with underlying conditions at any age.

Since HMPV is difficult to grow *in vitro*, laboratory diagnosis is reliant on the detection of viral RNA in clinical specimens by molecular methods.

Treatment and prevention

There are currently no available vaccines. As with RSV, the F and G proteins are the main targets of the neutralizing antibody response and while the former is antigenically conserved, the latter is more variable. Thus the F protein has been the focus of vaccine development. Ribavirin has comparable *in vitro* activity against HMPV as against RSV but there is no clinical trial data that demonstrates therapeutic efficacy.

Influenza viruses

Influenza viruses contain a segmented RNA genome. Types A, B, and C are antigenically distinct; of these, types A and B are clinically important causes of human disease. The viral envelope contains two glycoproteins, the haemagglutinin (H) and neuraminidase (N) which are critical in host immunity. The M2 transmembrane protein is also found on the virion surface and can provide broadly cross-reactive immunity following experimental immunization but does not appear to elicit a significantly protective host response following natural infection. Human influenza viruses are designated by the virus type, place of isolation, strain designation, year of isolation, and the H and N antigen subtype, e.g. A/Sydney/5/1995 (H3N2).

Epidemiology

The H and N genes of influenza types A and B undergo mutational change resulting in the emergence of antigenic variants ('antigenic drift'). Every few years, a variant successful in evading the prior immunity of the human population emerges, to cause a global epidemic. Influenza viruses have a marked winter seasonality in temperate regions, making the disease burden of the virus more obvious. The more diffuse seasonality in tropical and subtropical regions leads to an obscuring of the clinical impact of the virus, leading to the illusion in some quarters that influenza is less significant in warmer climates. However, careful epidemiological studies demonstrate that the burden of mortality and morbidity in temperate and tropical regions are very similar. In those 65 years or older, influenza is associated with approximately 1 excess death per 1000 population annually in both the temperate and tropical regions.

In aquatic birds, the natural reservoir of the virus, 16 H and 9 N subtypes of influenza A are found. From 1918 till 1957, human influenza A viruses carried H1N1 surface antigens. In 1957, this virus acquired the novel H, N, and additional polymerase gene (PB1) from an avian influenza virus through genetic reassortment of its segmented genome giving rise to the H2N2 subtype virus ('antigenic shift'). As the human population lacked immunity to these novel viral antigens, this led to the 'Asian flu' pandemic. A similar reassortment event gave rise to the H3N2 virus and the 'Hong Kong influenza' pandemic of 1968. In contrast, the pandemic of 1918 is believed to have arisen by the direct adaptation of an avian influenza virus without reassortment with the pre-existing human influenza virus. Although all three influenza pandemics of the 20th century resulted in significant morbidity and mortality, the toll exacted by the 'Spanish flu' of 1918 was particularly horrendous—over 40 million deaths, greater than that of both World Wars combined. Since influenza B (and C) have no significant zoonotic reservoirs, antigenic shift and pandemics do not occur.

In early 2009, a novel H1N1 virus of swine-origin gave rise to the first pandemic of the 21st century. The pandemic arose in Mexico and rapidly spread worldwide along routes of air-travel. Unlike the two previous pandemics (1957, 1968) that arose through genetic reassortment of an avian virus with the prevailing human seasonal influenza virus, the pandemic virus of 2009 arose through reassortment between swine viruses previously documented in North America (so called 'triple reassortant' swine viruses that contained virus gene segments of swine, avian and human origin) and 'Eurasian-swine' viruses. Although the H1 haemagglutinin of both human and swine influenza viruses was originally derived from the 1918 'Spanish flu' H1N1 virus, they had antigenically diverged during their subsequent evolution in these two hosts so that the contemporary seasonal human H1N1 virus offered little cross-protection against the pandemic H1N1 virus of swine-origin. However, people born prior to the 1950s had substantial cross-protection against the novel pandemic virus, presumably derived by infection with H1N1 viruses circulating in the first half of the 20th century. Thus the pandemic was associated with explosive outbreaks in children and young adults while there was less infection in older adults. When infection did occur, severity of disease in older adults was much more severe than that in children. Overall, the disease was largely a mild-influenza-like illness comparable with seasonal influenza, sometimes associated with gastrointestinal symptoms of diarrhoea and vomiting. However, complications, severe illness, and fatalities did occur, especially in those who were pregnant or with underlying comorbidities including asthma and other lung disease, cardiovascular diseases, diabetes, neurological disorders, autoimmune disorders, and morbid obesity. While some of those with severe disease had secondary bacterial infections, others developed a primary viral pneumonia leading to acute respiratory distress syndrome.

Avian viruses (e.g. subtype H5N1, H9N2, H7N7) can zoonotically infect humans occasionally without undergoing prior reassortment with existing human strains. Currently, an H5N1 virus that is highly pathogenic for chickens has become entrenched in poultry flocks in a number of Asian and African countries and continues to zoonotically transmit to humans, often causing severe disease and pandemic concern. Such transmission has so far not led to sustained human-to-human transmission which is the prerequisite for the generation of a new pandemic. However, recent studies with experimentally mutated H5N1 viruses have shown that these viruses can acquire droplet transmission capacity in ferrets, the best available surrogate for viruses with human transmission potential.

Pathogenesis

Viral replication occurs in the columnar epithelial cells leading to its desquamation down to the basal cell layer. The pathology typically involves the upper respiratory tract and the tracheobronchial tree. Infection results in decreased ciliary clearance, impaired phagocyte function, and increased adherence of bacteria to viral infected cells, all of which promote the occurrence of secondary bacterial infection.

While there may be differences in viral virulence, pre-existing cross-reactive immunity is a major determinant in reducing disease severity. Virus dissemination outside the respiratory tract is uncommon with human influenza viruses. However, zoonotic infections with the avian H5N1 virus may disseminate, and virus has been often detected in the gastrointestinal tract and occasionally in the central nervous system.

Immunity

Infection by an influenza virus results in long-lived immunity to homologous reinfection. However, the continued antigenic change in the virus allows it to keep ahead of the host immune response. Cross-immunity to 'drifted' strains within the same H or N subtype may provide partial protection, but there is believed to be little cross protection between different subtypes. Local and systemic antibody responses and cytotoxic T cells contribute to host protection.

Clinical features

The severity of influenzal disease ranges from asymptomatic infection, through the typical influenza syndrome, to the complications of influenza. Although it cannot always be distinguished from other viral infections on clinical grounds, the typical influenza syndrome is relatively characteristic in the adult. It is associated with fever, chills, headache, sore throat, coryza, nonproductive cough, myalgia, and sometimes prostration. The onset of illness is abrupt and the fever lasts 1 to 5 days. The pharynx is hyperaemic but has no exudate. Cervical lymphadenopathy is often present and crackles or wheezing are heard in around 10% of patients. While the acute illness usually resolves in 4 to 5 days, cough and fatigue may persist for weeks thereafter.

Common (>10% of symptomatic patients) complications of influenza include otitis media (in children) and exacerbation of asthma, chronic airways obstruction, and cystic fibrosis. Less common complications are acute bronchitis, primary (viral) and secondary (bacterial) pneumonia, myocarditis, febrile convulsions, encephalopathy, encephalitis, and myositis (especially in patients with influenza B infection). Age, prior immunity, virus strain, the presence of underlying diseases, pregnancy, and smoking all influence morbidity and severity.

Treatment and prevention
Antiviral therapy

Antiviral drugs with proven clinical efficacy for treatment of influenza A are the ion channel (M2) blockers that interfere with viral uncoating (amantadine, rimantadine) and the neuraminidase inhibitors (e.g. zanamivir, oseltamivir) which block virus release from infected cells. The neuraminidase inhibitors are also active against influenza B, while amantadine and rimantadine are only active against influenza A.

Since 2003, seasonal H3N2 and H1N1 viruses increasingly acquired resistance to amantadine and rimantadine and the 2009 pandemic H1N1 virus is also resistant to these drugs. Thus they are no longer drugs of choice in the treatment or prophylaxis of human influenza. Oseltamivir resistance to seasonal H1N1 viruses emerged in early 2008 and spread worldwide but this strain has largely been replaced by the pandemic H1N1 that emerged in 2009. Thus the influenza A (pandemic H1N1 virus and seasonal H3N2 viruses) and influenza B viruses remain sensitive to oseltamivir. Although resistant pandemic H1N1 viruses have been occasionally reported, these have not so far become dominant within the human population. Zanamivir remains uniformly effective against seasonal and pandemic influenza viruses.

Zanamivir is administered by inhalation and oseltamivir orally. Inhaled zanamivir may occasionally cause bronchospasm in those with underlying airways disease or asthma. In patients infected with viruses sensitive to these drugs, zanamivir or oseltamivir treatment commenced within the first 48 h of disease onset leads to a 1 to 2 days reduction in the time to alleviation of clinical symptoms and also reduces incidence of influenza associated complications. Some studies have indicated benefit in reducing the complications of influenza even for patients in whom treatment commenced after the second day of clinical illness.

However, the sooner the drugs are used, the better the chance of clinical benefit. With a virus such as the highly pathogenic H5N1 virus which can disseminate beyond the respiratory tract, a systemically administered drug (oseltamivir) is likely to be superior to one administered by inhalation (zanamivir). However, oseltamivir has had variable success in the treatment of H5N1 influenza and although therapeutic failure may be partly due to late commencement of therapy, poor drug bioavailability in a severely ill patient and emergence of resistance may also contribute. Options for parenteral therapy (i.v peramivir or zanamivir) may result in more reliable and higher blood levels of drug for such patients and are currently undergoing clinical trials. Peramivir is presently licensed for clinical use in Japan and South Korea.

Aspirin should be avoided in children with influenza because of the increased risk of Reye's syndrome.

Vaccines

Influenza vaccine is a trivalent vaccine containing antigens from the two subtypes of human influenza A (H3N2 and N1N1) and B viruses. To keep abreast of change in the surface antigens of the virus, its composition must be modified on an annual basis and annual reimmunization is required. This updating of the vaccine is achieved through a collaborative effort of the global influenza virus surveillance network coordinated effort by the World Health Organization (WHO). As a result of this surveillance, the WHO makes recommendations of candidate vaccine viruses twice annually for vaccine production for the northern and southern hemispheres.

Vaccines currently in use are based on antigen derived from viruses grown in embryonated eggs or (less commonly) cell cultures and contain detergent-treated virus (split virus vaccines) or purified surface antigens (subunit of surface antigen vaccines). These vaccines have less side effects than killed vaccines containing the whole virus which were used in the past and are licensed for use in anyone 6 months of age or older. Previously unvaccinated children require two doses at least 1 month apart, whereas a single dose appears adequate for adults. These vaccines are generally safe, the most common side effect being soreness at the injection site lasting a few days. Vaccine efficacy is best when there is a good antigenic match between the vaccine and outbreak virus.

An intranasally administered, cold-adapted, live attenuated vaccine is now also licensed for use in those aged 2 to 49 years and offers the advantages of broader cross-protection across antigenic drifted viruses as well as easier administration and greater patient acceptability.

Inactivated and cold-adapted live attenuated monovalent vaccines containing the pandemic H1N1 were rapidly developed and used in 2009 in response to the pandemic. Some of these inactivated vaccines had adjuvents (MF59; AS03) added to enhance immune response. Since 2010 the 'pandemic H1N1' virus is included as one component of the seasonal influenza vaccine, together with the prevailing H3N2 and influenza B virus. The previous seasonal H1N1 viruses appear to have been largely replaced by the pandemic H1N1.

Immunogenicity and clinical protection are better in healthy young adults compared to patients with chronic renal failure and immunocompromised or elderly patients (all groups most at need of the vaccine). However, the vaccine is still effective in reducing influenza and pneumonia-related hospitalization and mortality in elderly people and is cost-saving. An additional option for protecting such high-risk individuals is the immunization of children and caregivers in contact with these individuals. In young adults, vaccination is associated with decreased absenteeism from work. The duration of protection is limited and therefore vaccine administration should be timed to precede the expected peak of influenza activity.

Influenza vaccine recommendations vary from country to country. In general, vaccine is recommended to those groups at highest risk of influenza related complications including (1) those aged 6 months to 5 years of age; (2) those aged 65 years or older (in the United States of America all those over 50 are recommended for vaccination); (3) pregnant women who will be in the second or third trimester during the influenza season; and (4) those with chronic medical conditions including persons with chronic disorders of pulmonary or cardiovascular systems (except hypertension), those with renal dysfunction, haemoglobinopathies, metabolic disorders, or immunodeficiency and those aged 6 months to 18 years who are on long-term aspirin therapy. Furthermore, vaccine is also recommended for health care workers and for persons living or caring for those at high risk, who may transmit influenza to such high-risk individuals.

Bocavirus and polyomavirus KI and WU

Human bocavirus is a member within a newly discovered genus Bocavirus within the family Parvoviridae. As with other parvoviruses, they are relatively resistant to inactivation by acid or alkaline pH or moderate heat (e.g. 56°C). Molecular detection by PCR in respiratory clinical specimens is the main option for diagnosis. The virus can also be sometimes detected in serum. Using these methods, it is one of the five most commonly detected viral agents in respiratory specimens from children with acute respiratory disease. However, relatively few studies have included age-matched healthy controls to assess the clinical relevance of the detection of these agents and the available data is at present contradictory. The peak age of detection is in children aged 6 months to 2 years and occasionally in adults. These patients presented with rhinitis, a cough that is often paroxysmal or 'pertussis-like', and wheezing and were categorized as bronchiolitis, pneumonia, or asthma. Some patients also had diarrhoea, vomiting, and a skin rash. The virus has been detected worldwide and is likely to have been long endemic in humans. Reliable tests to study the seroepidemiology of this infection are still awaited.

KI and WU are two novel polyomaviruses recently discovered in the respiratory tract of patients with acute respiratory infections. There are found in a proportion of children and adults with acute respiratory infection but often found as coinfections with other known respiratory pathogens. Their contribution to disease causation is still unclear.

Nosocomial infection

Respiratory viruses are efficient nosocomial pathogens. Though paediatric units face the brunt of the problem, adult wards are not exempt. Transmission may occur from patient to patient, patient to staff, and staff to patient, with visitors making their own contribution. Although influenza and RSV are the most notorious among the endemic respiratory viruses, even rhinoviruses cause problems when transmitted to immunocompromised patients. Once infected, immunocompromised patients have a prolonged period of viral shedding and pose a significant risk of transmission to other high-risk patients.

Transmission of many respiratory virus infections occurs by large respiratory droplets gaining access to the mucosa of a susceptible individual. Large respiratory droplets have a relatively short dispersal range (<1 m). On the other hand, direct hand contact is an important means of transmission within health care settings and adherence to strict hand-washing is the most critical preventive measure. Gloves are useful in reinforcing the 'hand-washing message', but will only be effective if they are changed between patients. Cohorting infected patients, either by symptoms (during the outbreak season) or by rapid viral diagnostic results, is useful. Influenza A vaccination of health care workers, especially those caring for high-risk children, is to be recommended. Staff education is vital, including awareness of the fact that some of these viruses manifest themselves as a mild 'cold' in adults, and that infected staff members can transmit to patients under their care.

The most dramatic example of the impact of nosocomial transmission with a respiratory virus occurred with SARS where health care facilities served as a major hub of virus transmission and health care workers accounted for one-fifth of all documented cases. Much of this transmission was preventable by basic (large) droplet and contact precautions, although protection from small particle aerosols was important when carrying out aerosol-generating procedures such as intubation.

Further reading

Abed Y, Boivin G (2006). Treatment of respiratory virus infections. *Antiviral Res*, **70**, 1–16. [Reviews role of antiviral therapy for respiratory virus infections.]

Centers for Disease Control and Prevention (2010). *Prevention and control of influenza with vaccines: recommendations of the Advisory Committee on Immunisation Practices (ACIP)*. *MMWR*, **59**, RR-8, 1–61. Atlanta, GA. [Reviews the disease burden of influenza and the use of influenza vaccines.]

Dolin R, Wright PF (eds) (1999). *Viral infections of the respiratory tract*. Marcel Dekker, Basel, pp. 1–432. [Comprehensive monograph with chapters on each of the respiratory viruses, antiviral therapy, and on infections in immunocompromised patients.]

Dowell SF (ed.) (1998). Principles of judicious use of antimicrobial agents for pediatric upper respiratory tract infections. *Pediatrics*, **101** Suppl, 163–84. [Journal supplement reviewing the use and abuse of antibiotics in upper respiratory tract infections.]

Falsey AR, Walsh EE (2006). Viral pneumonia in older adults. *Clin Infect Dis*, **42**, 518–24. [Reviews role of virus in lower respiratory tract disease of adults.]

Gern JE, (2010). The ABCs of rhinoviruses, wheezing, and asthma. *J Virol*, **84**, 7418–26.

Ison MG, Lee N (2011). Influenza 2010–11: Lessons from the 2009 pandemic. *Cleveland Clinic J Med*, **77**, 812–20. [Reviews clinical experience with the 2009 pandemic.]

Kim YJ, Boeckh M, Englund JA (2007). Community respiratory virus infections in immunocompromised patients: hematopoietic stem cell and solid organ transplant recipients, and individuals with human immunodeficiency virus infection. *Semin Respir Crit Care Med*, **28**, 222–42. [Reviews the management of respiratory viral infections in the immunocompromised patient.]

Madeley CR, Peiris JSM, McQuillin J (1996). Adenoviruses. In: Myint S, Taylor-Robinson D (eds) *Viral and other infections of the human respiratory tract*, pp. 169–90. Chapman & Hall, London. [Reviews the adenoviral respiratory disease and laboratory diagnosis.]

Mallia P, Johnston SL (2006). How viral infections cause exacerbation of airway diseases. *Chest*, **130**, 1203–10.

Nicholson KG, Webster RG, Hay AJ (eds) (1998). *Textbook of influenza*. Blackwell Scientific, Oxford. [Comprehensive review of the ecology, clinical features, and control of influenza.]

Peiris JSM, De Jong MD, Guan Y (2007). Avian influenza virus (H5N1): a threat to human health. *Clin Microbiol Rev*, **20**, 243–67. [Reviews the threat from emerging zoonotic and potentially pandemic influenza viruses.]

Peiris JSM, *et al.* (2006). Severe acute respiratory syndrome (SARS). In Scheld WM, Hooper DC, Hughes JM (eds) *Emerging infections 7*, pp. 23–50. ASM Press, Washington DC. [Reviews the epidemiology, clinical features, pathogenesis and management of SARS.]

Siddell S, Myint S (1996). Coronaviruses. In: Myint S, Taylor-Robinson D (eds) *Viral and other infections of the human respiratory tract*, pp. 141–67. Chapman & Hall, London.

Treanor J (2009). Respiratory infections. In: Richmond DD, Whitley RJ, Hayden FG (eds) *Clinical Virology*, 3rd edition, pp. 7–27. ASM Press, Washington, DC. [Reviews viral respiratory infections.]

van den Hoogen BG, Osterhaus ADME, Fouchier RAM. (2006). Human metapneumovirus. In: Scheld WM, Hooper DC, Hughes JM (eds) *Emerging Infections 7*. pp. 51–68, ASM Press, Washington, DC.

Writing Committee of the WHO Consultation on Clinical Aspects of Pandemic (H1N1) 2009 Influenza (2010). Clinical aspects of pandemic 2009 influenza A (H1N1) virus infection. *N Engl J Med*, **362**, 1708–19. [Reviews clinical aspects of pandemic H1N1 2009.]

5.2 Herpesviruses (excluding Epstein–Barr virus)

J.G.P. Sissons

Essentials

Eight human herpesviruses, all with a linear double-stranded DNA genome and divided into alpha-, beta-, and gamma-subfamilies on the basis of genomic and biological properties, share the capacity to produce latent infection. The diseases they cause may result from primary infection, or reactivation of the virus from latency, and tend to be more severe in immunosuppressed patients. Diagnosis of the various herpesvirus infections may be made on clinical grounds alone, by culture or demonstration of viral particles by electron microscopy of relevant samples, by serological testing, or (increasingly) by PCR-based tests.

Herpes simplex viruses (HSV)

These two alpha-herpesviruses infect epithelial cells and become latent in the central nervous system. (1) HSV-1—transmitted by direct contact with infected secretions from a carrier; predominantly causes orofacial infections; becomes latent in the trigeminal ganglion; reactivation may give rise to recurrent orolabial mucosal ulcers ('cold sores') on the lips or skin around the mouth; is the commonest identified cause of acute sporadic encephalitis occurring in immunocompetent subjects in Western countries. (2) HSV-2—usually acquired through sexual contact and is the predominant cause of genital HSV infection, which may also be recurrent.

Treatment of both HSV-1 and HSV-2 is with aciclovir, which is preferentially phosphorylated in HSV-infected cells, or other newer related drugs (famciclovir and valaciclovir). Oral treatment is used in immunocompetent patients, but intravenous therapy is indicated in severe infections, encephalitis and in immunosuppressed patients.

Varicella zoster virus (VZV)

This alpha-herpesvirus is presumed to spread by the respiratory route and after an incubation period of 10 to 20 days causes varicella (chickenpox), predominantly an exanthematous disease of childhood, but which may be complicated in adults by pneumonitis and encephalitis. The virus becomes latent in dorsal root ganglia after primary infection, whence it can reactivate to cause herpes zoster (shingles), with pain, erythema, and vesicular lesions occurring in a dermatomal distribution, particularly in elderly and immunosuppressed individuals. Treatment of severe varicella or herpes zoster is with aciclovir, with higher doses being required than for HSV. A live attenuated VZV vaccine is available: this induces 90% protection from natural varicella in children, and also diminishes the incidence of zoster and postherpetic neuralgia when given to older age groups.

Human cytomegalovirus (HCMV)

This beta-herpesvirus is the largest human herpesvirus. Infection is spread by close contact with body fluids of infected individuals: from 50 to 100% of adults are seropositive, depending on socioeco-nomic and sexual risk, with myeloid lineage cells being a principal site of HCMV latency. Primary infection in children and adults is usually asymptomatic, but infectious mononucleosis clinically indistinguishable from that caused by primary Epstein–Barr virus (EBV) infection can be produced (see Chapter 5.3), and HCMV can produce severe disease in two particular situations. (1) Fetal infection—congenital HCMV infection occurs in around 0.5 to 1% of live births in developed countries; most infected babies are asymptomatic, but classical 'cytomegalic inclusion disease' has a high mortality and surviving infants have mental, visual, and hearing impairment. (2) Infection in patients who are immunosuppressed patients—the most serious forms are pneumonitis in bone marrow transplant recipients and retinitis in HIV/AIDS patients. Specific treatment for HCMV is usually with ganciclovir, which requires intravenous administration and has limiting side effects including myelotoxicity; valganciclovir has higher oral bioavailability and is particularly used for prophylaxis.

Human herpesvirus 6 and 7 (HHV-6 and 7)

These are beta-herpesviruses, most probably transmitted via maternal saliva. Primary infection with HHV-6 in young children is associated with roseola infantum (exanthem subitum, sixth disease), and also with a febrile illness without rash. More than 90% of children are seropositive for HHV-6 by 2 years of age. HHV-6 reactivation may occur in immunosuppressed solid-organ and bone marrow transplant recipients, but it is not clear that HHV-6 causes disease in these patients. HHV-6 sensitivity to antiviral drugs corresponds with that of HCMV, but no treatment is usually required. HHV-7 has been associated with some cases of roseola, but there is no other evidence for its being pathogenic.

Human herpesvirus-8 (HHV-8)

This member of the rhadinovirus (gamma 2-herpesvirus) family is the most recently discovered human herpesviruses, having been isolated from Kaposi's sarcoma tissue in 1994. The mechanism of transmission is probably by saliva and sexual contact; reported seroprevalence is around 50% or more in many African adult populations, but 5% or less in blood donors in the United Kingdom and the United States of America, with intermediate rates in Italy and other Mediterranean countries.

HHV-8 (as other gamma-herpesviruses such as EBV) is potentially oncogenic: it is clearly associated with (1) Kaposi's sarcoma—HHV-8 can be detected by PCR in the blood of nearly all cases. Manifests clinically as purplish brown macules, papules and plaques, and is described in four clinical settings: (a) the classic form—typically presents in elderly Mediterranean or Jewish men with lesions on the extremities and an indolent course; (b) the endemic African form—accounts for 10% of cancer in equatorial Africa and is similar clinically to the classic form of the disease; (c) in patients with immunodeficiency states such as transplant recipients—lesions are more widespread and rapidly progressive, but visceral involvement is unusual; and (d) the AIDS-associated form—with widespread cutaneous lesions, involvement of the oral mucosa, visceral lesions in the lungs or gastrointestinal tract, and sometimes rapid progression. Kaposi's sarcoma lesions may regress with antiretroviral treatment, withdrawal of immunosuppression, and the disease can also be treated with radiation therapy and (for widespread cutaneous or visceral disease) with chemotherapy. (2) Primary effusion lymphoma—HHV-8 is present in the tumour cells of all cases of this rare and aggressive type of B cell lymphoma that presents in patients with AIDS. (3) Multicentric Castleman's disease (angiofollicular lymph node hyperplasia)—HHV-8 is present in most cases of this condition, especially those associated with HIV.

Cercopithecine herpesvirus 1

This alpha-herpesvirus (formerly named herpes B virus) is closely related to HSV, and found in Old World monkeys, its natural host. Transmission to humans from monkey bites results in a high incidence of severe disease, with progressive encephalitis. Treatment is with aciclovir or ganciclovir, but morbidity and mortality are high.

Human herpesviruses

The Herpesviridae family is widely distributed in the animal kingdom. More than 100 have been isolated from humans, primates, and other mammals, and from reptiles and fish. Comparative sequence analysis suggests they have been coevolving with their individual hosts for millions of years. Eight human herpesviruses have been identified to date (Table 5.2.1). Shared genomic and biological properties divide the herpesviruses into three subfamilies, the alpha-, beta-, and gamma-herpesvirinae.

All the herpesviruses have a linear double-stranded DNA genome contained inside an icosahedral capsid that is surrounded by a protein tegument. The outer lipid envelope contains virus glycoprotein spikes. These large viruses have genomes consisting of unique segments of DNA flanked by inverted repeats, and encode most of the proteins needed for replication. All herpesviruses share an important biological feature, their capacity to produce latent infection in their natural host, during which the viral genome persists in cells, usually as a closed circle (episome), expressing only a limited subset of virus genes. This property results in their ability to produce lifelong infection in different types of cell, depending on the individual virus, and thus to persist in the population. Herpesvirus disease may result from primary infection, or reactivation of the virus from latency, and tends to be more severe in immunosuppressed patients. The gamma-herpesviruses can induce cell transformation, and are associated with specific tumours.

Herpes simplex virus infections

Historical background

'Herpes' derives from the Greek, meaning to creep or crawl, apparently used since antiquity to describe the evolution of the skin lesions caused by herpes simplex virus (HSV) and varicella–zoster virus. HSV was the first of the herpesviruses to be isolated, in the 1930s, although the transmission of infection to animals had been demonstrated in 1919. The serological distinction between the two types, HSV-1 and HSV-2, and the association of HSV-2 with genital herpes, was made in the 1960s. HSVs are now some of the most intensively studied human viruses.

Aetiology

HSV has a genome size of 150 kbp, and codes for about 80 proteins. The genomes of HSV-1 and HSV-2 are largely colinear, but have different restriction endonuclease sites. Gene expression occurs in three temporally regulated phases: immediate early, early, and late. Immediate-early proteins are largely regulatory proteins that prepare the cell to produce further virus. The early genes code particularly for enzymes involved in the replication of virus DNA, and the late genes for the structural proteins of the virion. Antigenic differences in the surface glycoprotein G are used to distinguish between HSV-1 and HSV-2. The release of progeny virus is normally accompanied by cell death, i.e. the infection is lytic. The virus infects a relatively wide range of cells *in vitro*, and can also infect experimental animals, allowing studies of its pathogenesis.

Epidemiology

HSV is a ubiquitous virus, widely distributed in populations throughout the world. Although animals can be infected experimentally, there are no natural animal hosts, and humans are the only reservoir. Transmission occurs when a susceptible person has direct contact with infected secretions from an HSV carrier, usually from oral, genital, or skin lesions, to mucous membranes or abraded skin of the recipient. HSV carriers can excrete virus asymptomatically, and 1 to 15% of adult carriers excrete HSV at any one time. Conventionally, the prevalence of infection is assessed by demonstrating antibody to HSV-1 or HSV-2. The prevalence of HSV-1 increases with age, although the time of acquisition of HSV-1 antibody varies depending on socioeconomic factors. Seroprevalence in early life is higher among lower socioeconomic groups, 70 to 90% of children having antibodies by the age of 10, whereas only about 30%

Table 5.2.1 The human herpesviruses

Common name	Designation	Subfamily	Genome size (kbp)	Site of latency and persistence
Herpes simplex virus 1	Human herpesvirus 1	α	152	Neurons (sensory ganglia)
Herpes simplex virus 2	Human herpesvirus 2	α	152	Neurons (sensory ganglia)
Varicella zoster virus	Human herpesvirus 3	α	125	Neurons (sensory ganglia)
Epstein–Barr virus	Human herpesvirus 4	γ	172	B lymphocytes (oropharyngeal epithelium)
Human cytomegalovirus	Human herpesvirus 5	β	235	Blood monocytes (and possibly epithelial cells)
HHV6	Human herpesvirus 6	β	170	Monocytes, T lymphocytes
HHV7	Human herpesvirus 7	β	145	–
Kaposi's sarcoma-associated herpesvirus	Human herpesvirus 8	γ	230	Uncertain

of children in higher socioeconomic groups have antibodies by this time. By mid life, 80 to 90% of people are HSV-1 seropositive.

HSV-2 infection is usually acquired through sexual contact; consequently, seroconversion correlates with the onset of sexual activity, and a progressive increase in seroprevalence to HSV-2 begins in adolescence. The number of sexual contacts is a major risk factor for the acquisition of HSV-2. Cumulative seroprevalence rates in adults vary from 10 to 80%, depending on the population and risk factors.

HSV can be transmitted to neonates by infection (usually HSV-2) from maternal genital secretions at the time of delivery. The mothers are most often asymptomatic excretors of the virus who have no history of genital herpes.

Pathogenesis

HSV infects and replicates in epithelial cells at the site of inoculation onto mucous membranes or abraded skin, with an incubation period of 4 to 6 days before clinical lesions appear. There is a marked local inflammatory response, but viraemia and dissemination may occur in the immunocompromised host. Following local epithelial replication, HSV enters the peripheral sensory nerves innervating the site of replication, and ascends the axons by retrograde transport to reach the dorsal root ganglia, or the trigeminal ganglion in the case of oral or conjunctival inoculation. The virus then becomes latent in the sensory ganglia, but despite extensive study, the mechanism of virus latency remains uncertain.

Latent HSV DNA is in an inactive state, with minimal gene expression. RNA species called latency-associated transcripts are the only detectable transcripts. These have no detectable protein product, and their deletion from the genome does not prevent the establishment of latency, although reactivation is impaired. Latent HSV is carried for the lifetime of the host, but may be reactivated in response to certain stimuli, including stress, menstruation, ultraviolet light, and immunosuppression. Upon reactivation, infectious virus is produced, travels down the peripheral nerves by anterograde axonal transport, and replicates in the epithelial cells at the nerve ending.

The neuronal latency of HSV and varicella–zoster virus is an extremely effective method of virus persistence. Latent virus in neuronal cells appears to be inaccessible to the immune response, and as it does not replicate is not susceptible to the action of antiviral drugs. In normal HSV carriers, reactivation at local sites is thought to be controlled by a specific effector T-lymphocyte response. However, HSV DNA encodes proteins that interfere with antigen processing by the class I MHC pathway, and are presumed to help the virus evade the T-cell immune response. There is no good evidence that the immune response to HSV of people who have symptomatic reactivation episodes differs from that of asymptomatic carriers.

Clinical features

Primary infection with HSV is often asymptomatic; among sexually active subjects, only 60% of primary infections with HSV-1, and 40% with HSV-2, are symptomatic. HSV-1 is the predominant cause of orofacial infections, whereas HSV-2 is the usual cause of genital HSV infection, but the clinical manifestations overlap.

Gingivostomatitis

This is the most common clinical form of primary infection with HSV-1. It is most often seen in children, following an incubation period of 2 to 12 days. Primary infection may be associated with a

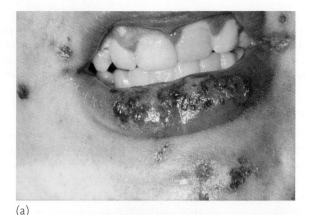

(a)

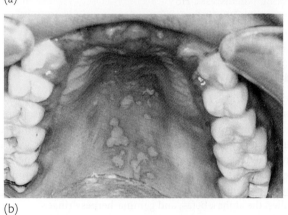

(b)

Fig. 5.2.1 Herpes simplex gingivostomatitis: (a) and (b).

considerable systemic reaction, involving fever, sore throat, pharyngeal oedema, and redness. Painful vesicles appear a few days later on the pharynx and oral mucosa, the lips, and the skin around the mouth (Fig. 5.2.1). There may be cervical lymphadenopathy. Affected patients may have difficulty in eating, and the lesions last from 3 days to 2 weeks. The differential diagnosis includes other causes of pharyngitis, including bacterial pharyngitis and herpangina (from Coxsackie A virus infection) (Fig. 8.5.3). Anterior vesicles and ulceration affecting the lips and skin around the mouth are more suggestive of HSV infection. Stevens–Johnson syndrome and severe aphthous ulceration may appear similar, and staphylococcal impetigo affects the skin around the mouth, but is not associated with oral ulceration.

Reactivation of HSV may give rise to recurrent orolabial lesions, appearing as intraoral mucosal ulcers, but more frequently as the classical cold sore on the lips or skin around the mouth. A tingling sensation in the area of impending ulceration may precede the appearance of vesicles by 1 to 2 days. The lesions usually recur at the same site in individual patients. Around 25% of HSV-1 seropositive people develop recurrent orolabial lesions. The majority have only one or two reactivation episodes per year, although a minority (<10%) have more than one attack per month. The episodes are not associated with systemic symptoms, and diagnosis is usually straightforward.

Infection at other cutaneous sites
Herpetic whitlow

HSV infection of the finger, herpetic whitlow, may complicate primary oral or genital herpes by autoinoculation of virus, or may occur through occupational exposure (e.g. in nursing, medical, and dental staff). There is oedema, erythema, and local tenderness of the infected finger (Fig. 5.27.4). Lesions at the fingertip may be confused with pyogenic bacterial paronychias and incised, which is contraindicated for herpetic whitlow, and may even spread infection.

Herpes gladiatorum

This is mucocutaneous HSV infection occurring by transmission of virus via skin trauma resulting from wrestling or other contact sports.

Eczema herpeticum

HSV infections of the skin are more severe in patients with pre-existing skin disease. In patients with eczema, burns, or other blistering skin diseases, HSV infection may become disseminated.

Cutaneous HSV infection can be confused with herpes zoster, although the latter is usually easy to diagnose by its unilateral dermatomal distribution.

Herpes simplex and erythema multiforme

About 15% of all cases of erythema multiforme are preceded by a symptomatic attack of recurrent herpes simplex, and in susceptible people the characteristic rash can be induced by the intradermal inoculation of inactivated herpes simplex virus antigen. The rash of erythema multiforme starts several days after the onset of the herpetic vesicles, and in severe cases can involve the mucous membranes (Stevens–Johnson syndrome). The frequency of these attacks can be reduced by aciclovir prophylaxis.

Keratitis

HSV keratitis is characterized by the acute onset of pain, blurred vision, conjunctival injection, and dendritic ulceration of the cornea (Fig. 5.2.2). It can cause corneal blindness, and treatment is urgent. Topical aciclovir is the drug of choice; topical steroids may make the infection worse. HSV can also cause an acute necrotizing retinitis, usually only seen in immunosuppressed people, including those with HIV infection.

Genital herpes

Primary genital HSV infection is sexually transmitted, and may be associated with systemic symptoms such as fever, headache, and myalgias. Symptoms tend to be more severe in women than men. There is local pain and itching, dysuria, vaginal discharge, and inguinal lymphadenopathy, with vesicles and ulcers on the vulva, perineum, vagina, and cervix, and sometimes on the skin of the buttocks (Fig. 5.2.3). In males, primary HSV lesions are vesicles on the shaft or glans of the penis, and there may be associated urethritis. HSV-2 causes most genital infections, with a variable smaller proportion resulting from HSV-1. Only 40% of primary HSV-2 genital infections are symptomatic. In patients who have had prior HSV-1 infection, the symptoms of primary genital herpes tend to be less severe. HSV has been isolated from the urethra in 5% of women with urethral syndrome, in the absence of obvious genital lesions. Other manifestations of genital tract disease resulting from primary HSV infection are, rarely, endometritis and salpingitis in women, and prostatitis in men.

HSV proctitis may follow rectal intercourse. There is anorectal pain and discharge, with ulcerative lesions visible on sigmoidoscopy. Perianal lesions are seen in immunosuppressed patients, and

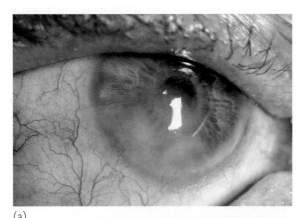

(a)

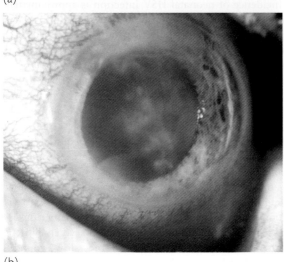

(b)

Fig. 5.2.2 Herpes simplex keratitis: (a) disciform, and (b) dendritic.
(Courtesy of the late Dr B E Juel-Jensen.)

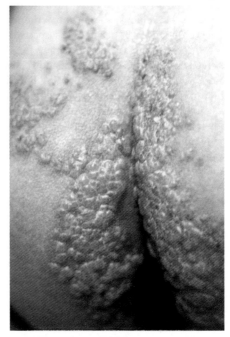

Fig. 5.2.3 Genital herpes in the natal cleft.
(Courtesy of the late Dr B E Juel-Jensen.)

spreading perianal HSV infection and HSV proctitis occur in HIV-infected patients.

Recurrent genital herpes is frequent in the first year after primary genital disease (90% for HSV-2 and 55% for HSV-1). Thereafter, the recurrence rate tends to decrease with time, to around three to four attacks per year for HSV-2, but fewer for HSV-1. Severe recurrent genital herpes is particularly troublesome to women.

The complications of primary genital HSV infection include sacral radiculomyelitis, with urinary retention and hyperaesthesia of the perineal area, which usually resolves over several weeks. Aseptic meningitis requiring admission to hospital occurs in up to 7% of women and 2% of men, although suggestive symptoms are more common. Occasionally, and more seriously, transverse myelitis may occur.

HSV encephalitis (see also Oxford Textbook of Medicine 5e Chapter 24.11.2)

Encephalitis is the most serious type of disease produced by HSV in the immunocompetent host, and has an estimated annual incidence of two to three cases per million. It is the most commonly identified cause of acute sporadic encephalitis in Western countries. The great majority of cases are caused by HSV-1. A biphasic age incidence is reported, with higher rates between the ages of 5 and 30 years, and in those older than 50 years. The clinical features are of focal encephalitis, with acute onset of fever, confusion, and unusual behaviour, impaired consciousness, and possibly focal neurological abnormalities. However, there are no specific features, and the diagnosis of HSV should be considered in any patient with possible encephalitis.

The cerebrospinal fluid shows lymphocytic pleocytosis, although neutrophils and red cells may also be present, with a raised protein level. CT scans of the brain may show changes in the temporal lobe; MRI is a more sensitive method of detection. The electroencephalogram classically shows spike and slow-wave activity localized in the temporal lobes. The definitive way of establishing the diagnosis is brain biopsy. In the original trial of aciclovir for the treatment of HSV encephalitis, brain biopsy was an entry criterion, but confirmed the diagnosis in only 50% of clinically suspected cases. Since the advent of effective nontoxic chemotherapy for HSV, brain biopsy is very rarely used. There is good correlation between a positive polymerase chain reaction (PCR) test for HSV DNA in the cerebrospinal fluid, and a diagnosis of HSV encephalitis by brain biopsy and virus isolation. Evidence of intrathecal production of specific HSV antibody is also diagnostic, but as it is usually not detectable until 1 week after onset, PCR-based diagnosis is more useful. Serum or cerebrospinal fluid titres of antibodies to HSV do not usually increase in the first week of the illness. In practice, the diagnosis is established by a compatible clinical picture, evidence of characteristic temporal lobe involvement on CT or MRI, and EEG, and by PCR-based detection of HSV DNA in the cerebrospinal fluid.

The pathological features are of focal haemorrhagic necrotizing encephalitis affecting the temporal lobes. The pathogenesis of HSV encephalitis remains uncertain. Up to one-half of patients have primary infection, and in the rest the disease is presumed to result from reactivation. However, where HSV has been isolated from the brain and mouth simultaneously in the same patient, the two isolates differ by restriction endonuclease analysis in about 30% of cases, suggesting a new exogenous virus infection in an already seropositive patient. HSV DNA can be detected at autopsy in the brains of nor-mal virus carriers, and the factors precipitating HSV encephalitis are not known. Immunosuppression is not usually associated with HSV encephalitis, which predominantly affects apparently immunocompetent adults, and very rarely patients with advanced HIV infection. However, rare mutations affecting the Toll-like receptor 3 signalling pathway causing autosomal recessive UNC-93B and TLR3 deficiencies and autosomal dominant TLR3 and TRAF3 deficiencies have been associated with primary HSV encephalitis in children.

Treatment with intravenous aciclovir should be started immediately if HSV encephalitis is clinically suspected, without waiting for confirmation of the diagnosis (in doses as below; see 'CNS infections'). The untreated mortality from HSV encephalitis is more than 70%, and very few survivors make a full neurological recovery. Intravenous aciclovir was established to be more effective than the previous best therapy of vidarabine in a randomized trial reported in 1986. Mortality in the aciclovir-treated group was 28%, although a lower Glasgow coma score on entry carried a higher risk of mortality. However, only 38% of those who received aciclovir had fully recovered at 6 months. There is still a high incidence of permanent neurological sequelae, particularly seizures, defects of memory, and personality changes, and the prognosis of HSV encephalitis remains poor.

Meningitis

HSV can cause aseptic meningitis, which is quite independent of, and not associated with progression to, HSV encephalitis. It is most commonly associated with primary genital HSV-2 infection, in which the incidence of proven HSV meningitis is 7% in women and 2% in men. There is pleocytosis, usually lymphocytic, but neutrophils may predominate in early meningitis. HSV may be isolated from the cerebrospinal fluid by culture, but is now more reliably detected by PCR for HSV DNA. In a high proportion of patients with Mollaret's meningitis (recurrent aseptic meningitis of unknown aetiology; Oxford Textbook of Medicine 5e Chapter 24.11.2), HSV DNA is reported to be detectable in the cerebrospinal fluid by PCR. The role of HSV in this syndrome remains uncertain.

Neonatal HSV infection and pregnancy

The incidence of neonatal HSV infection is approximately 1 in 3500 deliveries per annum in the United States of America, but appears to be lower in the United Kingdom, at 1 in 6600 live births. About 70% of cases are caused by HSV-2, and result from fetal acquisition of HSV-2 from maternal genital secretions during delivery. Most infants with neonatal HSV are born to mothers without clinically evident HSV infection. The risk of transmission from women with symptomatic primary HSV or clinically evident recurrent HSV-2 infection is about 50 and 20%, respectively. A small proportion (c.10%) of infections is acquired postnatally through contact with people with active lesions.

Neonatal HSV infection may appear as lesions on the skin, eye, and mouth, or as encephalitis or disseminated visceral infection. Although initial superficial infection may progress to visceral infection, visceral infection can present without cutaneous lesions, and the diagnosis should be considered in severely ill neonates. Untreated, visceral infection has a high mortality (around 60%). Primary infection in early pregnancy can lead to congenital HSV infection, which is rare, but can produce serious congenital abnormalities.

HSV in immunosuppressed patients

HSV infections in immunosuppressed people are usually because of reactivation, rather than primary infection. They tend to be more severe, are more likely to progress, and take longer to heal than in the immunocompetent host. Clinical manifestations in patients with HIV infection include severe perineal, orofacial, and oesophageal infection. HSV pneumonitis, hepatitis, and colitis are also described in immunosuppressed patients.

Pathology

The histological appearance of HSV infection remains the same, whether it is primary or recurrent. There is ballooning of infected cells, with condensed chromatin in the cell nuclei; intranuclear inclusion bodies (Cowdry type A bodies) may be seen; and multi-nucleated giant cells form. Varicella–zoster virus produces a similar appearance.

Laboratory diagnosis

Definitive diagnosis is made by virus isolation. Swabs from vesicular fluid or other body fluids in virus transport medium can be inoculated into tissue culture, producing typical cytopathic effects. Electron microscopy of negatively stained vesicle fluid is rapid, but will not differentiate HSV from varicella–zoster virus. The use of PCR-based techniques to detect viral DNA is becoming more widespread. It is particularly applicable to the detection of HSV DNA in cerebrospinal fluid.

Serological tests for antibody to HSV are useful only for making a retrospective diagnosis. Seroconversion provides proof of primary infection, and the absence of antibody to HSV-1 or HSV-2 rules out a diagnosis of recurrent HSV infection. However, making a diagnosis of reactivation by demonstrating rising antibody titres is of limited value.

Treatment

The introduction of aciclovir heralded a new era of specific antiviral drugs, and superseded the drugs previously used for the treatment of HSV infections, such as vidarabine and idoxuridine. Aciclovir is an acyclic nucleoside that is preferentially phosphorylated to the monophosphate in HSV-infected cells by the virus-encoded thymidine kinase. Cellular kinases then phosphorylate the monophosphate to the triphosphate, which is incorporated into nascent HSV DNA, where it acts as a chain terminator; aciclovir also directly inactivates the HSV DNA polymerase. Two newer, related drugs with the same mechanism of action are famciclovir, a prodrug of penciclovir, and valaciclovir, the valyl ester of aciclovir, which has greater bioavailability and less frequent dosage. All these drugs are relatively free of side effects, although intravenous aciclovir can crystallize in the renal parenchyma and produce renal impairment; it should be given by infusion over an hour, and patients should be adequately hydrated. The doses should be reduced in patients with renal impairment.

Primary mucocutaneous infection

In primary oral and genital infection, aciclovir 200 mg 5 times daily given orally for 10 to 14 days from the onset reduces the severity of infection, the duration of symptoms, and the duration of viral shedding. There is little evidence that the treatment of primary infection reduces the incidence of subsequent symptomatic reactivation episodes. If swallowing is difficult, intravenous aciclovir

(5 mg/kg 8 hourly) may need to be given. Famciclovir 250 mg 3 times daily or valaciclovir 500 mg twice daily are alternatives.

Symptomatic reactivation of mucocutaneous infection

The treatment of recurrent infections in immunocompetent hosts is often unnecessary, as the symptoms are usually very mild. However, aciclovir can shorten the duration of symptoms if it is given very early in the course of the recurrence, preferably during the prodrome before vesicles appear. Oral aciclovir is effective, and anecdotal reports suggest that topical aciclovir is effective symptomatically. The same dosage as above for primary infection can be given for 5 days. Patient-initiated courses of single-day famciclovir (1 g twice daily) or 3-day valaciclovir (500 mg twice daily) have been shown to be effective for recurrent genital HSV.

Long-term suppressive therapy

This can be considered in immunocompetent patients with genital herpes who have frequent reactivation episodes. Trials of aciclovir in recurrent genital herpes have shown that a dose of 400 mg twice daily significantly reduces the frequency of attacks. However, patients may be able to find a lower effective dose, and in some, 200 mg daily prevents attacks. Because there is some evidence that resistant virus is a problem in this population, it is advisable to stop treatment for a month every 6 to 12 months. Valaciclovir 500 mg daily or famciclovir 250 mg twice daily are alternatives.

CNS infections

For HSV encephalitis, intravenous aciclovir (10 mg/kg 8 hourly for 10–14 days) should be given to any patient in whom the diagnosis is clinically suspected (see 'HSV encephalitis' above). For HSV meningitis, intravenous aciclovir 5 mg/kg 8 hourly can be used, with conversion to oral valaciclovir 1 g twice daily when improvement occurs, for a total of 10 days.

Systemic infection in the immunosuppressed

Oral treatment, as for primary HSV, can be used for mild mucocutaneous infection, but for more severe and for visceral involvement, intravenous aciclovir 5 mg/kg 8 hourly should be used. After resolution, continued prophylaxis is usually necessary until immunocompetence is restored, particularly in patients with HIV.

Aciclovir resistance

Resistance of HSV to aciclovir develops readily *in vitro*, but is clinically rare; it results from mutations in the HSV thymidine kinase or DNA polymerase genes. It is seen almost exclusively in immunocompromised patients who have received prolonged aciclovir prophylaxis, especially those with HIV infection, and is manifest as unresponsive or worsening HSV disease despite treatment with aciclovir. There is usually cross-resistance to famciclovir and valaciclovir, and intravenous foscarnet is the most useful alternative drug in severe infection caused by resistant HSV, although it is more usually used for human cytomegalovirus (see 'Human cytomegalovirus' below).

Prevention and control

No vaccine is licenced for HSV, although a gD (glycoprotein D) based vaccine reduced new HSV2 infection in seronegative women, and other candidates are approaching phase III trials. There is particular interest in the use of vaccines for postinfective immunization to reduce the frequency of recurrent genital HSV attacks. This has proved possible in guinea pigs.

Special problems in pregnant women

Prevention of neonatal HSV infection is best achieved by preventing genital HSV infection late in pregnancy. There is no reason to give aciclovir prophylactically to women with a history of recurrent genital herpes who are asymptomatic, as the incidence of neonatal HSV infection is low in their children. However, women with clinically apparent genital herpes in the last trimester (and probably at any other time in pregnancy) can be treated with aciclovir, although the drug is not licensed for treatment in pregnancy. Women with no clinical lesions may have a vaginal delivery, but the presence of active lesions at the time of labour is an indication for Caesarean section. Babies born to mothers with clinically apparent genital HSV infection, or with a history of recurrent genital HSV infection, should be screened for HSV by cultures from the nasopharynx and eyes after birth.

Proven neonatal HSV infection should be treated with high-dose intravenous aciclovir (20 mg/kg per day every 8 h for 21 days).

Varicella–zoster virus infection

Historical background

There are clinical descriptions of varicella (chickenpox) and herpes zoster (shingles) in very early medical literature, although the skin lesions of herpes simplex and herpes zoster were grouped together under the term herpes. The similarities between the exanthematous rashes associated with smallpox and varicella meant they were not distinguished until the late 19th century. The characteristic clinical appearance of shingles, in a dermatomal distribution, was recognized as a discrete entity in the early Greek literature. The term zoster is derived from the Greek word for a girdle, and shingles from the Latin cingere meaning to encircle.

In 1892 von Bocquet observed that children developed varicella after contact with adults with herpes zoster, and in 1925 it was shown that vesicular fluid from patients with zoster, inoculated into susceptible people, produced chickenpox. The idea that zoster resulted from the reactivation of latent virus remaining in the tissues following childhood varicella was put forward by Garland in 1943, and strengthened by the work of Hope-Simpson, a British general practitioner. Varicella–zoster virus (VZV) was isolated in 1958, and Weller and colleagues showed the similarity between viral isolates from varicella and zoster patients. Restriction endonuclease analysis showed that the isolates from chickenpox and from later zoster in the same immunocompromised patient were identical. The long interval between the two illnesses has prevented such studies in immunocompetent people.

Aetiology

VZV is structurally similar to other members of the herpesvirus family. The genome is a linear double-stranded DNA of 125 kbp. VZV is an alpha-herpesvirus, and encodes sets of genes that are largely colinear to those of HSV, and are also expressed in immediate-early, early, and late phases. The virus is closely cell associated, and spreads from cell to cell in tissue culture.

Epidemiology

VZV infects only humans, which are thus the only reservoir. The virus is presumed to spread by the respiratory route. Varicella is predominantly a disease of childhood, affecting both sexes and 90% of cases occur in children under the age of 13 years. The incubation period is about 2 weeks (with a range of 10–20 days); patients are infectious for about 48 h before the vesicles appear, and remain so for 4 to 5 days afterwards, until all the vesicles have crusted over. The secondary attack rate in susceptible contacts with an index case in the household is 70 to 90%. The prevalence of VZV varies in different ethnic groups. In Europe, about 10% of the population over 15 years old is seronegative, and consequently susceptible to infection, although in tropical countries only 50% of young adults may be seropositive. Varicella in adults is uncommon in Europe, and less than 2% of all cases occur in patients older than 20 years. Subclinical infection is unusual, and accounts for less than 5% of all infections, but the disease may be mild, and in some surveys only 10% of people with a negative history were in fact seronegative for VZV. One attack of chickenpox usually confers lifelong immunity.

After primary infection, VZV becomes latent in dorsal root ganglia. Reactivation appears clinically as herpes zoster, which is a common disease affecting all age groups, but particularly older and immunosuppressed people; about 20% of the population will experience an attack. There is no evidence that exposure to people with active VZV infection predisposes to herpes zoster in their contacts, but a seronegative person may catch varicella from contact with the vesicles of a patient with shingles. Nosocomial varicella infection is well recognized, and the isolation of patients with varicella, and immunocompromised patients with herpes zoster, should be ensured in hospitals. Local unidermatomal zoster is less likely to cause infection, and consequently to need isolation.

Pathogenesis

During primary infection, initial virus replication probably occurs in the epithelial cells of the upper respiratory tract mucosa, followed by a phase of viraemia during which VZV can be isolated from leucocytes, and the disseminated rash appears. In the skin, the virus infects capillary endothelial cells, and adjacent fibroblasts and epithelial cells. During the viraemic phase, virus may spread to visceral organs, including alveolar epithelial cells, and transient subclinical hepatitis is probably a normal feature of varicella. VZV encephalitis may be a feature of primary infection, particularly affecting the cerebellum. Patients usually recover completely from encephalitis (unlike that associated with HSV), and it has been suggested its pathogenesis may be immune mediated. Following recovery from primary infection, the virus persists for life in a latent state in dorsal root ganglia. VZV reaches the ganglia by retrograde axonal transport from the skin lesions during primary infection, and all dorsal root ganglia and the trigeminal ganglion can potentially carry latent VZV in neurones and possibly in satellite cells.

As with other herpesviruses, the host response is critical in containing the initial infection. Cellular immunity is important, since varicella may be progressive in patients with severely impaired T-cell immunity. Both CD4 and CD8 cytotoxic T lymphocytes specific for VZV are present in normal people carrying latent VZV. The cellular immune response presumably plays a part in controlling reactivation, since impaired T-cell immunity increases the risk of developing zoster, and of having vesicles in multiple dermatomes, and cutaneous dissemination of reactivated virus. The increasing incidence of herpes zoster with age may reflect waning cellular immunity to VZV.

Clinical features

Primary infection and varicella

The most striking feature of varicella is the rash, which is centripetal (mainly on the trunk). The lesions are initially present on the face and scalp, before progressing to the trunk and later to the limbs (Fig. 5.2.4). A macular erythematous rash, papules, and vesicles may all be present together. Individual lesions progress from being papules to vesicles to pustules, and then crust over. The scabs normally separate after 10 days, without scarring. The systemic symptoms associated with varicella vary considerably. In most children there is a mild illness with fever. Adults characteristically have a more severe illness, with myalgia, headache, arthralgia, malaise, and higher fever, with the complications listed below. Symptoms may precede the rash by 1 to 2 days.

Complications of varicella

The principal complications of varicella in immunocompetent patients are pneumonitis and encephalitis.

Pneumonitis In a prospective study, 6% of young adults with chickenpox had respiratory symptoms, although 16% had changes on chest radiography, but the rate of admission to hospital for pneumonia in adults with varicella is only about 0.3%. Patients present with dyspnoea, cough, hypoxia, and bilateral infiltrates on the chest radiograph, occurring 1 to 6 days after the appearance of the rash. Hypoxia may be more severe than expected from the physical signs or the chest radiograph. The interstitial pneumonitis can progress to respiratory failure requiring artificial ventilation and intensive care (Fig. 5.2.4a), but it is more commonly transient, resolving completely within 2 to 3 days. Varicella pneumonia is said to be more common in smokers. Fatalities are rare, and VZV pneumonia is not associated with long-term respiratory problems. Benign nodular calcification throughout the lung occasionally follows.

Encephalitis Central nervous system involvement during varicella most commonly presents as acute cerebellar ataxia within 1 week of onset of the rash, although it may appear up to 21 days after the rash. It resolves completely over 2 to 4 weeks. A frequency of 1 in 4000 children aged less than 15 years has been quoted. The cerebrospinal fluid of these patients shows lymphocytosis and elevated protein concentration.

More serious encephalitis can occur in 0.1 to 0.2% of cases of varicella. This begins earlier in the course of infection than cerebellar ataxia, with headache, vomiting, confusion, and impaired consciousness. There is evidence of diffuse cerebral oedema, but no defined pattern of CT or MRI abnormality. The encephalitis may be progressive, and the mortality is between 5 and 20%, with neurological sequelae in up to 1% of survivors.

Varicella meningitis can occur. Other rarely reported neurological complications include optic neuritis, transverse myelitis, and Reye's syndrome.

Other complications Primary VZV infection may be complicated by acute thrombocytopenia, with petechiae, purpura, haemorrhage into vesicles, and other haemorrhagic manifestations. The platelet count can remain low for weeks after the illness has resolved. Secondary infection of the skin lesions with *Staphylococcus aureus* or *Streptococcus pyogenes* may occur. Purpura fulminans is a rare complication associated with arterial thrombosis and haemorrhagic gangrene (Fig. 5.2.5). Nephritis and arthritis have been reported as occasional complications, and myocarditis, pericarditis, pancreatitis, and orchitis are even more rare.

Special problems in pregnant women Varicella in pregnant women can be severe, with a maternal mortality of 1%. Varicella in

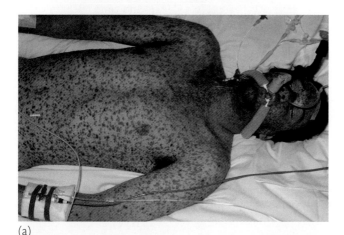

(a)

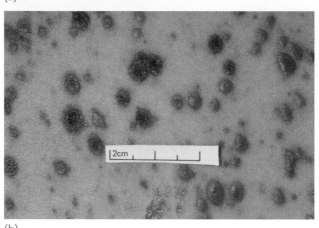

(b)

Fig. 5.2.4 Severe chickenpox: (a) and (b).
(Copyright D A Warrell.)

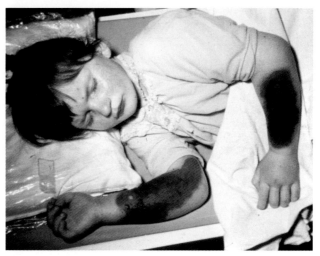

Fig. 5.2.5 Varicella purpura fulminans.
(Courtesy of the late Dr B E Juel-Jensen.)

the first trimester can cause varicella embryopathy. Affected infants may have a scarred, atrophic limb, microcephaly, cortical atrophy, and eye defects including chorioretinitis, microophthalmia, and cataracts. The autonomic nervous system may be damaged. Varicella embryopathy is rare; in recent reported series the risk was about 1 to 2% in mothers with varicella in the first 20 weeks of pregnancy. Varicella–zoster immunoglobulin should be considered for pregnant women in contact with varicella, and varicella in pregnancy should be treated with aciclovir on a named-patient basis. Neonatal varicella occurs in babies whose mothers contract varicella just before or after delivery, and is most severe when maternal disease appears from 2 to 7 days after delivery.

Herpes zoster

The clinical syndrome caused by the reactivation of VZV from sensory ganglia is herpes zoster. Typical prodromal localized pain or paraesthesia is followed by erythema and vesicular lesions occurring in a dermatomal distribution. The thoracic dermatomes, especially T4 to T12, are involved in about 50% of cases (Fig. 5.2.6); the lumbosacral dermatomes in about 16%; and the cranial nerves (mainly the Vth) in 14 to 20% of patients (Fig. 5.2.7a). The first symptoms are usually paraesthesia and shooting pains in the affected dermatome, which precede the eruption of vesicles by several days, occasionally 1 week or more. Erythematous maculopapular lesions then appear and quickly evolve into a vesicular rash, nearly always in a unilateral dermatome, with no vesicles beyond the midline. The vesicles usually form scabs after 3 to 7 days, and these separate after 2 weeks or so, but there is sometimes a more severe locally necrotic reaction (Fig. 5.2.8). There is a risk of secondary infection, particularly with *Staphylococcus aureus*. There may be malaise and low-grade fever, but laboratory investigations usually show no abnormalities, although up to 40% of patients with uncomplicated zoster may have lymphocytes and elevated protein in the cerebrospinal fluid. Involvement of the mandibular branch of the Vth cranial nerve can give intraoral lesions on the palate (Fig. 5.2.7b), floor of the mouth, and tongue. Involvement of the geniculate ganglion results in Ramsay Hunt syndrome, with pain and vesicles in the external auditory meatus, a loss of taste in the anterior two-thirds of the tongue, and a lower motor neurone VIIth cranial nerve palsy.

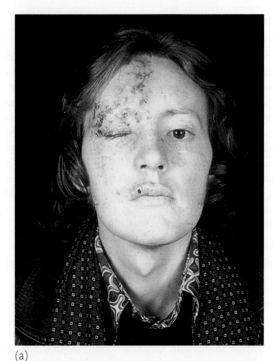

(a)

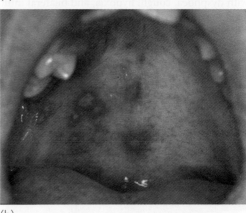

(b)

Fig. 5.2.7 Herpes zoster of the Vth cranial nerve: (a) ophthalmic division, and (b) lesions on the palate.
(Courtesy of the late Dr B E Juel-Jensen.)

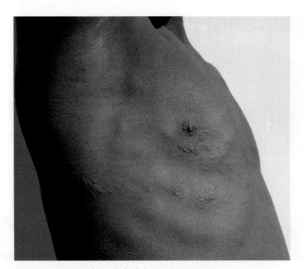

Fig. 5.2.6 Herpes zoster (shingles) of the T4 dermatome.
(Copyright D A Warrell.)

Complications of zoster

Ophthalmic zoster VZV reactivation from the trigeminal ganglion can affect the ophthalmic division of the trigeminal nerve, resulting in ophthalmic zoster (Fig. 5.2.7a). The features include conjunctivitis, anterior uveitis, keratitis, and sometimes iridocyclitis, with secondary glaucoma and panophthalmitis. However, these latter sight-threatening complications of ophthalmic zoster are unusual. A rare association with ophthalmic zoster is granulomatous cerebral angiitis, which can be associated with arterial thrombosis; cerebral angiography shows segmental narrowing in the cerebral arteries on the side of the ophthalmic zoster occurring weeks after the rash. CT may show cerebral infarcts, particularly in the middle cerebral artery territory, and contralateral hemiparesis can occur.

Motor zoster Weakness or paralysis can sometimes be associated with zoster, and results from the involvement of the anterior horn

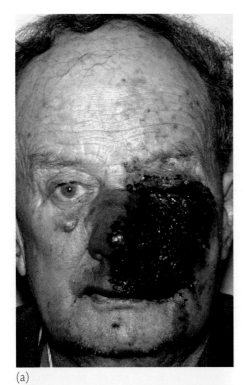

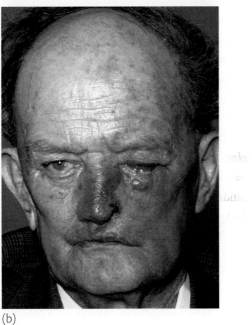

Fig. 5.2.8 Herpes zoster of the Vth cranial nerve, showing severe necrotic effects: (a) acutely, and (b) after recovery.
(Courtesy of the late Dr B E Juel-Jensen.)

cells in the same segment of the spinal cord as the involved dorsal root ganglion. Depending on the segment involved, this can lead to a monoparesis affecting the upper or lower limb, or to diaphragmatic palsy (with the involvement of C5/6). Paralysis usually recovers completely, although the outlook for the recovery of facial nerve palsy is more variable. It is suggested VZV may be responsible for some cases of idiopathic VIIth nerve (Bell's) palsy.

Autonomic zoster Lumbosacral herpes zoster can be associated with neurogenic bladder, and acute retention of urine. This may be accompanied by haemorrhagic cystitis resulting from vesicles on the bladder wall. Intestinal ileus and obstruction may occur.

Zoster meningoencephalitis Meningoencephalitis may accompany zoster at any site, and is heralded by impaired consciousness, headache, photophobia, and meningism. The interval from the onset of skin lesions to symptoms is around 9 days, but may be as long as 6 weeks. Symptomatic encephalitis usually lasts around 2 weeks, and is nearly always followed by full recovery without neurological sequelae.

Transverse myelitis, although rare, can occur at any level of the spinal cord.

Postherpetic neuralgia The incidence of postherpetic neuralgia rises with the increasing age of the patient. It is uncommon in young people, but can occur in 50% of patients older than 50 years. It is characterized by pain in the affected dermatome persisting for 1 month or more after the acute attack of zoster has resolved. The pain may be steady and burning, or paroxysmal and stabbing in nature; it may occur spontaneously, or be triggered by stimuli such as temperature or touch.

Zoster sine herpete This term refers to radicular pain similar to that experienced in zoster, but without the antecedent skin lesions of zoster. It was originally applied to patients who did have obvious zoster, but had dermatomal pain in areas distinct from those where there was rash. However, it is more commonly applied to patients with radicular pain and no rash at all. There have been reports describing the use of PCR testing for the detection of VZV DNA in the cerebrospinal fluid of patients with presumed zoster sine herpete. The literature is anecdotal, and it is difficult to regard zoster sine herpete as a diagnostic entity unless there is good evidence for VZV involvement, e.g. by the detection of VZV DNA in cerebrospinal fluid and/or blood mononuclear cells. It should be included in the differential diagnosis of radicular pain of unknown cause. Any possible mechanism is speculative.

VZV infection in immunosuppressed patients In patients with immunosuppression, particularly of cellular immunity, varicella can be much more severe. The skin lesions are more diffuse (Fig. 5.2.9), and can take up to 3 times as long to heal. There may be visceral dissemination to the lungs, liver and central nervous system. Patients with lymphoma undergoing chemotherapy are particularly susceptible.

Herpes zoster in immunosuppressed patients is also more severe than in healthy subjects. Before effective antiviral therapy was available, skin lesions were more extensive and could take several weeks longer to heal. Dissemination, presumably because of viraemic spread, with widespread skin lesions as in varicella, occurs in 10 to 40% of patients. Cutaneous dissemination is more likely to be associated with visceral dissemination to the same sites as those associated with varicella.

Patients with HIV infection or AIDS are prone to multidermatomal zoster, which can be one of the defining features of AIDS.

VZV retinitis This is a combination of pain and blurred vision in one eye, with progressive necrotizing retinitis seen on ophthalmoscopy. Adjacent cutaneous zoster indicates the diagnosis, but occasionally VZV retinitis occurs in immunocompetent patients as the sole manifestation of VZV reactivation. VZV retinitis may be difficult to distinguish from CMV retinitis. A severe form of the disease, seen particularly in patients with HIV infection, and named

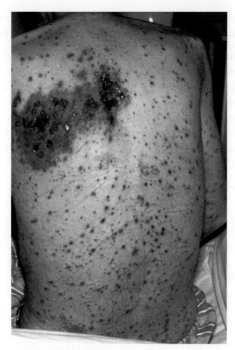

Fig. 5.2.9 Herpes zoster varicelliformis.
(Courtesy of the late Dr B E Juel-Jensen.)

progressive outer retinal necrosis, is associated with a high incidence of retinal detachment, and may require treatment with ganciclovir, as aciclovir is often ineffective.

Differential diagnosis

Varicella is usually recognized relatively easily. Other causes of a vesicular rash are generalized herpes simplex in the immunosuppressed patient, and enteroviral disease, particularly hand, foot, and mouth disease caused by Coxsackie virus infection, but the rash on the hands and feet is unlike that of varicella, which has a centripetal distribution (Chapter 5.8). Human cases of infection with animal pox viruses (monkey pox and camel pox) have rarely been described (Chapter 5.4). Localized pain before the appearance of shingles or in zoster sine herpete may be severe enough to suggest myocardial ischaemia, or lung or intra-abdominal pathology if it involves the thoracic dermatomes.

Pathology

The histological appearance of VZV infection is similar or indistinguishable from that of HSV infection.

Laboratory diagnosis

The diagnosis of varicella and herpes zoster is usually made on clinical criteria alone. Virus can be seen in vesicular fluid by electron microscopy, or isolated in culture. A serological diagnosis of varicella can be made by demonstrating seroconversion or VZV IgM antibody. Urgent serology is needed to confirm the seronegative status of contacts at risk of severe VZV infection, to determine the need for VZV immunoglobulin (see 'Prevention and control' below). PCR-based tests for the detection of VZV DNA are available, and are of most use in testing cerebrospinal fluid in cases of suspected central nervous system disease.

Treatment

Pruritus may be alleviated by calamine lotion and antihistamines in patients with chickenpox. Fingernails should be closely cut to minimize scratching. Skin care is important to prevent secondary bacterial infection in patients with varicella and zoster. Aspirin should be avoided in children with chickenpox because of the risk of Reye's syndrome. Strong analgesia may be needed in patients with zoster.

VZV is sensitive to the nucleoside analogues aciclovir, famciclovir, and valaciclovir; as for HSV, VZV encodes a thymidine kinase that preferentially phosphorylates these drugs in infected cells. The median 50% inhibitory concentration of aciclovir against HSV is 0.1 μM, but is 2.6 μM against VZV, so 800 mg orally is necessary to achieve inhibitory concentrations.

The treatment recommendations for varicella and herpes zoster are summarized in Box 5.2.1.

Varicella

Whether to treat normal children with varicella (who are the great majority of patients) has been much debated; the argument can be made that the disease is not always mild and it is not possible to

---

Box 5.2.1 The use of aciclovir in varicella–zoster infections

Indications for intravenous aciclovir (10 mg/kg 8 hourly)

Chickenpox:

◆ Immunocompromised patients

◆ Neonatal chickenpox

◆ Chickenpox with systemic complications

◆ Severe chickenpox in adults and in pregnancy (5 mg/kg 8 hourly)

Shingles:

◆ Severe shingles in immunocompromised patients

◆ Multidermatomal shingles

◆ Shingles complicated by ocular, motor, autonomic, or systemic involvement

◆ VZV retinitis (severe forms in AIDS may require foscarnet or ganciclovir)

Indications for oral aciclovir (800 mg 5 times daily)

◆ Uncomplicated chickenpox (except for mild chickenpox in children)

◆ Uncomplicated shingles in patients over 45 years

◆ Uncomplicated shingles in immunosuppressed patients

◆ Shingles presenting with severe pain

Infections not requiring active antiviral treatment

◆ Uncomplicated mild chickenpox in children

◆ Patients presenting more than 48 h after the appearance of the last lesion, or when all lesions have crusted

◆ Uncomplicated shingles in patients under 45 years

◆ Postherpetic neuralgia

predict which child may have a severe case. Therapy with aciclovir is safe, and although it has been suggested that widespread treatment with antivirals might result in viral resistance, or failure to develop normal immune responses, there is no evidence of this in controlled trials. Treatment with aciclovir begun within 24 h of the onset of the rash leads to a 25% decrease in the duration and severity of chickenpox. The argument for treating all adolescents and adults is easier, as chickenpox is more severe for them than it is for young children. Chickenpox in neonates, children with leukaemia, and transplant recipients should always be treated with aciclovir. Intravenous aciclovir limits the visceral spread of the virus if given immediately on diagnosis. Treatment in these immunosuppressed patients can be changed from intravenous to oral aciclovir once the fever has settled, if there is no evidence of visceral varicella.

Herpes zoster

The major justification for the antiviral treatment of herpes zoster in immunocompetent patients has been to limit postherpetic neuralgia. Although there are difficulties in accurately and objectively quantifying the pain of postherpetic neuralgia, trial data indicate that aciclovir, valaciclovir, and famciclovir can limit the duration of zoster-associated pain, and that valaciclovir is slightly more effective. All three drugs accelerate the healing of cutaneous lesions by 2 days over placebo; valaciclovir and famciclovir have the advantage of more convenient dosage, as well as probably being slightly more effective.

Patients over the age of 50 years with zoster have the highest risk of postherpetic neuralgia, and so should be offered antiviral treatment. Younger patients may warrant treatment if they have marked pain. All patients with ophthalmic zoster should be treated urgently with antivirals, even if they present relatively late, as aciclovir reduces the incidence of keratitis. Immunosuppressed patients with herpes zoster should receive intravenous aciclovir to prevent cutaneous and visceral dissemination. Valaciclovir and famciclovir may be used if zoster presents in a localized form in less severely immunosuppressed patients.

Corticosteroids have been advocated in patients with herpes zoster, in order to reduce the severity of postherpetic neuralgia. However, the addition of oral prednisone to aciclovir slightly increases the rate of healing of skin lesions, but does not affect the incidence of postherpetic neuralgia; a role for corticosteroids thus remains unproven. Established postherpetic neuralgia can be managed with analgesics, tricyclic antidepressants, and other agents used for neuropathic pain, such as gabapentin and pregabalin, which were effective for the treatment of postherpetic neuralgia in large placebo-controlled trials. Although the use of opioids for the treatment of neuropathic pain is controversial, several studies support their efficacy and safety; oxycodone and tramadol have been shown to be superior to placebo for the treatment of postherpetic neuralgia. Topical agents such as lidocaine 5% patches and topical capsaicin have been useful in ameliorating postherpetic neuralgia, but are unsatisfactory for use as sole agents (see also Oxford Textbook of Medicine 5e Chapter 24.12).

Prevention and control

Varicella–zoster immune globulin, prepared from high-titre immune human serum, has been shown to prevent or ameliorate varicella in seronegative people at high risk, such as immunocompromised people and pregnant women. It should be given to seronegative immu-nodeficient patients (including those on high-dose corticosteroid treatment), and pregnant women with definite contact with varicella. It should be administered within 10 days (preferably 2–4 days) of exposure. Neonates whose mothers have had varicella less than 1 week before delivery, or within 28 days after delivery are also recommended to receive varicella–zoster immune globulin.

A VZV vaccine is available; a live attenuated vaccine containing the Oka strain of VZV. It confers 90% protection from natural varicella when administered to susceptible immunosuppressed people (such as patients with leukaemia and lymphoma receiving chemotherapy), but it produces rash in up to 40% of these recipients. In immunized healthy children the risk of subsequent varicella after community exposure is reduced to less than 5%, and the vaccine-induced rash is much less common (about 5% of recipients). This vaccine is licensed in Japan, some European countries, and the United States of America, where it is recommended for the routine immunization of children aged 12 to 18 months. However, in the United Kingdom it is recommended only for use in seronegative health care workers and children over 1 year in contact with individuals at high risk of severe varicella. Trials have shown that the postinfective immunization of subjects aged 60 years or over diminishes the incidence of zoster and postherpetic neuralgia, and the vaccine is now licensed in the United States of America for the prevention of herpes zoster in this age group.

The nosocomial transmission of VZV by patients with varicella requiring admission to hospital is a significant risk, as 10% of adults are seronegative. Nursing and managing patients with varicella in hospital should be restricted to those staff known to be seropositive for VZV. Patients with varicella in hospital should ideally be isolated in negative-pressure rooms to prevent airborne transmission.

Human cytomegalovirus infection

Historical background

The syndrome of congenital cytomegalovirus infection, cytomegalic inclusion disease, was described in children with fatal infection in 1904, but the intranuclear inclusions were attributed to a protozoan parasite. In 1921, the pathologist Goodpasture suggested that the inclusions in the parotid glands of infants were caused by a virus, because a filterable agent produced similar histology in guinea pig salivary glands, and the lesions were attributed in 1926 to 'salivary gland virus'. Human cytomegalovirus (HCMV) was finally isolated in 1956, and so named by Weller for the characteristic owl's-eye, or cytomegalic inclusions it produces in the nuclei of infected cells.

HCMV produces little morbidity in immunocompetent people, but can produce severe disease in the fetus if infection is acquired *in utero*, and in immunosuppressed patients.

Aetiology

HCMV is the largest human herpesvirus, with a linear double-stranded DNA genome of 250 kb encoding more than 200 proteins. Mammalian cytomegaloviruses are species specific, and so HCMV cannot be studied in animal models. The most widely studied laboratory strain, AD169, shows significant genomic variation from recent clinical isolates, which possess an additional 15 kb of DNA. HCMV replicates slowly compared with other herpesviruses, and gene expression occurs sequentially in immediate-early, early, and late phases.

Epidemiology

Following primary infection, HCMV persists for life as a latent infection, with periodic asymptomatic excretion of virus in saliva, breast milk, urine, semen, and cervical secretions. Infection is spread by close contact with these body fluids. In developing countries, HCMV is usually acquired in childhood, and nearly 100% of young adults are seropositive. In developed countries, seroconversion progresses with age, but seroprevalence is higher in lower socioeconomic groups. Overall, about 50% of adults are seropositive. In childhood, HCMV is acquired from breast milk or contact with infected children excreting virus in their saliva or urine. Children in day nurseries transmit the virus to each other, and to susceptible adult carers. Later, sexual transmission becomes a major route of infection, and seroprevalence approaches 100% in homosexual men, and sex workers.

Blood and blood products from normal seropositive donors can transmit HCMV. Transfusion recipients at risk of HCMV disease now usually receive screened seronegative blood; otherwise the risk of transfusion-related HCMV infection is 2.5% per unit of blood. The virus is carried in leucocytes, and leukodepletion of blood greatly reduces the risk of HCMV transmission. The technique is also being widely adopted as a preventive measure against transmissible spongiform encephalopathies. Finally, solid organ and bone marrow transplants from seropositive donors can transmit HCMV, producing particularly severe disease in seronegative recipients.

Pathogenesis

Current evidence suggests myeloid-lineage cells are a principal site of HCMV latency, and that virus may be reactivated from dendritic cells and monocytes as they differentiate. Endothelial cells, possibly epithelial and other cells, may also be sites of latency.

The immune response is critical for controlling infection in the normal host. Normal immunocompetent individuals infected with HCMV mount a strong T-cell response, with very high frequencies of cytotoxic (CD8+) T lymphocytes in the peripheral blood targeted particularly at the HCMV major tegument protein pp65, and the major immediate-early protein IE1. Impairment of this response is associated with the risk of disseminated infection. HCMV possesses multiple immune-evasion genes, whose products interfere with the class I MHC antigen-processing pathway, and recognition by natural killer (NK) cells, which may help the virus reactivate by delaying T- and NK-cell recognition of infected cells. Antibody probably limits blood-borne dissemination of HCMV, as maternal IgG appears to be especially important in preventing viral transmission to the fetus.

Subclinical reactivation occurs frequently in the normal host, but is controlled by the immune response. Immune deficiency, particularly of the T-cell response, such as iatrogenic or disease-induced immunosuppression, may allow uncontrolled replication and result in HCMV disease. Pathology is presumably produced by the direct cytopathic effects of the virus, although indirect effects produced by soluble virus-encoded proteins or the host response are also possible. The presence of HCMV in a diseased organ does not necessarily implicate the virus as a cause; reactivation of the virus can sometimes be nonpathogenic, and reflects its being a bystander, coexisting with another pathogenic process.

Clinical features of HCMV disease
Primary infection in immunocompetent subjects

Primary infection in children and adults is asymptomatic in most cases, but HCMV can produce an illness clinically indistinguishable from infectious mononucleosis caused by primary Epstein–Barr virus (EBV) infection, typically with fever, myalgia, cervical lymphadenopathy, and mild hepatitis. Tonsillopharyngitis is much less common than in primary EBV infection, and lymphadenopathy and splenic enlargement are less prominent features. The fever lasts 2 to 3 weeks, but can persist for up to 5 weeks. In developed countries an increasing proportion of HCMV seroconversion illness is seen in older adults, and the diagnosis should still be considered in patients aged over 50 years. Myocarditis, pneumonitis, and aseptic meningitis are rare complications. A proportion (5–10%) of patients with Guillain–Barré syndrome show serological evidence of primary HCMV infection; they are more likely to have antibodies to the GM2 ganglioside than other patients with Guillain–Barré syndrome, and a causal relationship has been postulated.

Primary HCMV infection acquired from blood transfusion results in a similar clinical picture occurring 3 to 6 weeks after transfusion, and is usually self limiting in the normal host. To distinguish between primary HCMV infection and other causes of mononucleosis syndromes, such as EBV and toxoplasmosis, requires serological testing (the Paul–Bunnell and monospot tests are negative in HCMV mononucleosis).

HCMV disease in immunosuppressed patients

HCMV infection is most severe in immunosuppressed patients, particularly solid organ and bone marrow transplant recipients, and those with AIDS, all of whom have impaired T-lymphocyte function. This strongly supports the importance of T cells in controlling infection.

Solid organ transplant recipients

The risk of HCMV disease is 3 to 5 times greater in a seronegative recipient receiving a graft from a seropositive donor, and it causes much more severe infection than in a seropositive recipient who has a reinfection or reactivation of latent virus. Many centres pair seronegative donors with seronegative recipients, although this is often thwarted by organ shortage. Clinically, there may be specific organ involvement, which is not seen in normal patients. Interstitial pneumonitis caused by HCMV is rare, except in bone marrow transplant recipients, and carries a poor prognosis; gastrointestinal disease includes oesophagitis, gastritis and peptic ulceration, and colitis; and HCMV retinitis may occur in severely immunosuppressed patients. HCMV has been reported to be associated with increased graft rejection and renal artery stenosis in renal transplant recipients; with accelerated coronary artery stenosis in heart transplant recipients; and with vanishing bile duct syndrome in liver transplant recipients. However, none of these associations is definitively established as causal.

Bone marrow transplant recipients

HCMV disease is a major problem in allogeneic bone marrow transplant recipients, with a 30 to 50% incidence of clinically significant infection. It is a lesser problem in autologous bone marrow transplant. If the donor and/or recipient is seropositive there is a risk of HCMV disease, but if both donor and recipient are seronegative, infection can be prevented if solely HCMV-seronegative blood products are used to support the patient. Pneumonitis is the most serious manifestation of HCMV infection after bone marrow transplant, occurring in 10 to 15% of allogeneic bone marrow transplant recipients, with a mortality of 80% without antiviral therapy. The clinical presentation is interstitial pneumonitis in the absence of any other identifiable pathogen, with increasing arterial hypoxaemia, and progression to respiratory failure. It is suggested that graft versus host disease may contribute to the lung injury in HCMV pneumonitis in bone marrow transplant recipients. The relationship between HCMV and graft versus host disease is controversial, with suggestions that HCMV may predispose to graft versus host disease, and vice versa.

Patients with AIDS

HCMV disease is one of the most frequent opportunistic infections in patients with advanced HIV infection, of whom 40% develop sight- or life-threatening HCMV disease. A CD4 count of less than 50/µl carries a high risk of disease, although the widespread use of antiretroviral therapy in developed countries means that relatively few patients now have such low CD4 counts, and the incidence of HCMV disease in patients with AIDS has declined significantly.

HCMV retinitis has been seen in up to 25% of patients with AIDS not receiving effective antiretroviral therapy. Haemorrhagic retinal necrosis spreads along retinal vessels, and threatens sight when disease encroaches on the macula (Fig. 5.2.10). The clinical effect is visual impairment, and the risk of retinal detachment and haemorrhage is increased, hence those with low CD4 counts should have regular optic fundoscopy to detect retinitis before it becomes symptomatic. Diagnosis is made by the ophthalmological detection of typical retinal changes, preferably with accompanying evidence of HCMV viraemia. In the absence of treatment, HCMV retinitis almost invariably progresses to affect both eyes and destroy vision.

HCMV is reported to produce diffuse encephalitis in AIDS patients, but although the virus is sometimes seen in neuronal cells at autopsy, encephalitis attributable to HCMV is relatively rare in clinical practice by comparison with the other causes of encephalitis in AIDS. HCMV can also produce a progressive radiculopathy, causing low-back pain that radiates to the area supplied by the affected spinal nerve root, and the development of flaccid paraparesis.

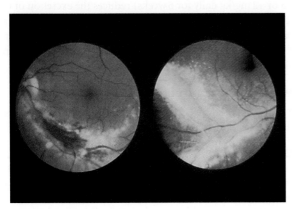

Fig. 5.2.10 CMV retinitis.

In the gastrointestinal tract, HCMV is associated with oesophagitis, gastritis, and enterocolitis, and virus can be seen in biopsies from these sites, usually in shallow ulcers. HCMV pneumonitis is rare in patients with AIDS, suggesting that there must be additional factors to account for its frequency in bone marrow transplant recipients.

Congenital and neonatal HCMV infection

HCMV infection of the neonate may be congenital from intrauterine infection, perinatal from transmission during birth, or postnatal from breast milk. The frequency of congenital HCMV infection in developed countries is around 0.5 to 1% of live births, resulting from either primary maternal infection in pregnancy, or from reactivation of HCMV in a previously infected mother during pregnancy. The risk of primary maternal infection in pregnancy is about 1%, and it carries a 40% risk of congenital infection. Fetal infection is more likely to be severe following primary infection in early pregnancy, whereas the risk of symptomatic congenital infection is much lower, although not absent, from reactivation of maternal HCMV. Pre-existing maternal immunity limits spread to the fetus.

Approximately 5 to 20% of congenitally infected babies are symptomatic at birth. In its most severe form, usually in babies of mothers with primary maternal infection, the clinical features of congenital HCMV are: microcephaly; chorioretinitis; nerve deafness; hepatitis with jaundice and hepatosplenomegaly; and thrombocytopenia with petechiae. This classical cytomegalic inclusion disease has a high mortality, and 80% of all infants symptomatic at birth who survive have serious sequelae, such as learning, visual, and hearing impairment. However, most congenitally infected babies are asymptomatic at birth, and only 5 to 15% of these subsequently develop sequelae on long-term follow up, the most common being sensorineural deafness, which also occurs in isolation in otherwise normal babies.

Perinatally or postnatally acquired HCMV infection is rarely symptomatic or associated with long-term sequelae, if the mother is seropositive.

Pathology

On light microscopy, typical HCMV-infected cells appear large, with a relative reduction in cytoplasm, and nuclei that contain prominent inclusions surrounded by a clear halo (described as owl's-eye inclusions). These cells contain replicating virus, and are associated with active infection and disease; they are diagnostic when seen in biopsies of affected organs. In patients dying of severe disease, histological evidence of HCMV involvement can be found in most organs, whereas it infects a restricted range of cells *in vitro*.

Malignancy

Although associations between HCMV and malignancy have been postulated in the past, there is currently no good evidence to associate the virus with any human malignancy.

Laboratory diagnosis

Primary infection is usually diagnosed by the detection of IgM antibody to HCMV in the absence of IgG antibody; there is a marked atypical lymphocytosis (mainly increased CD8+ T cells), but heterophile antibody (as detected in primary EBV infection by the monospot or Paul–Bunnell tests) is absent. IgG antibody is a useful marker of HCMV carriage, but titres do not rise reliably in disease; IgM antibody, a marker of primary infection, is also sometimes found with reactivation in immunosuppressed patients, and serology is of limited use in confirming HCMV disease in these patients. Culture of virus from urine may only indicate asymptomatic reactivation, but culture from the blood buffy coat suggests HCMV disease. The virus can never be cultured from the blood of normal HCMV carriers, and culture from an organ site (such as bronchoalveolar lavage fluid) may indicate locally active infection.

Rapid culture methods such as DEAFF (detection of early antigen fluorescent foci), which uses a monoclonal antibody against an immediate-early viral protein, or shell vial tests (centrifuging samples onto cell cultures) are now used less often. PCR techniques are increasingly used to detect and quantify the HCMV load in blood or plasma, and this is now the standard assay for detecting HCMV in most laboratories. As virus can never be detected in plasma (as opposed to leucocytes) in normal carriers, the presence of HCMV DNA in plasma indicates active viral replication. Detection of virus in biopsy specimens by histological and immunohistological techniques implies active HCMV infection in the relevant tissue.

In practice, HCMV disease is usually diagnosed by the combination of an appropriate clinical syndrome, and detection of HCMV DNA by quantitative PCR above a threshold level in blood or plasma, or in biopsies from involved organs, in the absence of any other likely causal microbial pathogen.

Treatment

Several drugs are now available for the treatment of HCMV disease. Aciclovir has little *in vitro* activity against HCMV, which does not possess a thymidine kinase (see 'Herpes simplex virus infections' above), and has no place in therapy (although valaciclovir is used in prophylaxis; see 'Antiviral prophylaxis' below).

Ganciclovir, another nucleoside analogue, is monophosphorylated in infected cells by the *UL97* gene product of HCMV, and is active against HCMV; its most limiting side effect is myelotoxicity, with leukopenia and thrombocytopenia, but it has many other potential side effects, including azoospermia, and intravenous administration is necessary. Valganciclovir, a valyl ester prodrug of ganciclovir, has much higher oral bioavailability, and produces equivalent plasma concentrations to intravenous ganciclovir; it is thus useful for prophylaxis. Resistance to ganciclovir results from a mutation in the HCMV DNA polymerase, or in the *UL97* gene, and is seen mainly in immunosuppressed patients in whom prolonged use is necessary.

An alternative drug to ganciclovir is foscarnet, a competitive inhibitor of the viral DNA polymerase, which shows no cross-resistance with ganciclovir. This also must be given intravenously, and its side effects include renal impairment and hypocalcaemia. Cidofovir, a nucleotide analogue acting on the viral DNA polymerase, is highly nephrotoxic (probenecid must be given concurrently to prevent irreversible renal damage), and therefore relatively infrequently used. Ganciclovir resistance remains a significant problem, and hence other drugs with *in vitro* activity against HCMV are currently being studied, and have been used in initial small clinical trials, although none is yet licensed for HCMV infection: these include maribavir, leflunomide, and artesunate.

Primary infection

In the immunocompetent host this usually requires no specific antiviral treatment, although occasionally, severe primary infection may lead to hospitalization and require treatment.

HCMV disease in immunosuppressed patients

Whether due to primary or secondary infection, or reactivation, this is usually treated with ganciclovir or foscarnet for 2 to 3 weeks, with full-dose induction intravenous therapy; for ganciclovir this is 5 mg/kg every 12 h and for foscarnet 60 mg/kg every 8 h. Oral valganciclovir 900 mg twice daily is an equivalent dose to intravenous ganciclovir. Secondary prophylaxis may well be needed if immunosuppression persists (see 'Prevention and control' below).

HCMV pneumonitis in bone marrow transplant recipients

This responds poorly to ganciclovir or foscarnet alone, but the combination of full-dose ganciclovir with intravenous immunoglobulin has been reported to reduce mortality. Specific anti-CMV immunoglobulin was initially used, then other trials suggest normal pooled intravenous immunoglobulin was equally effective, and recent reports question whether IVIg confers any additional benefit. Many centres monitor bone marrow transplant recipients, especially of allogeneic grafts, for CMV viraemia, and commence preemptive therapy with ganciclovir if viraemia is detected before the development of symptomatic or obvious organ disease.

HCMV retinitis in AIDS

This is treated with an induction course of ganciclovir or foscarnet (both drugs have also been used in combination) or valganciclovir 900 mg twice daily for 21 days. Continued prophylaxis is needed to prevent relapse until significant recovery of the CD4 count can be induced with antiretroviral therapy; valganciclovir 900 mg daily is most convenient. Implantable intraocular devices providing sustained release of ganciclovir into the vitreous humour have also been used. The use of combination antiretroviral therapy in HIV-infected patients is associated with much improved long-term control of HCMV infection. However, the syndrome of immune-recovery vitritis, characterized by posterior segment inflammation, can occur in patients with previously treated CMV retinitis when their CD4 count reconstitutes on antiretroviral therapy.

Congenital HCMV infection

Treating symptomatic congenital HCMV infection with ganciclovir (8 or 12 mg/kg daily for 6 weeks) reduces the excretion of CMV in the urine, but viruria returns to near pretreatment levels after cessation of therapy. Hearing improvement may occur, but the role of antiviral therapy in congenital HCMV infection remains to be established.

Prevention and control

The problem posed by HCMV in immunosuppressed patients has led to several approaches to prophylaxis.

Antiviral prophylaxis

There is a definite case for primary prophylaxis in solid organ and bone marrow transplant recipients at high risk of disease (seronegative recipients of a seropositive graft, or seropositive recipients), and in AIDS patients with fewer than 100 CD4 cells/μl. Ganciclovir has been widely used, and valganciclovir 900 mg daily is effective in many of these settings. Despite limited *in vitro* activity against HCMV, and lack of efficacy as therapy, oral valaciclovir has been shown to provide significant prophylaxis against HCMV disease in renal transplant recipients, and is licensed for this use.

Passive immunization

CMV hyperimmune globulin is reported to reduce the risk of HCMV disease in renal transplant recipients, but is expensive and little used in practice.

There are reports that HCMV-specific T-cell immunity can be reconstituted in bone marrow transplant recipients by the adoptive transfer of virus-specific T lymphocytes from the immune donor, but this is still the subject of investigational studies.

Active immunization

A live laboratory strain (Towne) of HCMV has been tested as an experimental candidate vaccine in renal transplant recipients, with some evidence of protective immunity, perhaps equivalent to having previous natural HCMV infection. A more recent phase II trial of a recombinant glycoprotein B-based HCMV vaccine in seronegative women showed it has the potential to decrease incident cases of maternal and congenital CMV infection. However, there is currently no available licensed vaccine.

Special problems in pregnant women

Pregnant women who are seronegative should avoid contact with possibly infected children in day-nursery settings, although this may be impractical. Ganciclovir must not be used in pregnancy.

Human herpesvirus 6 and 7

Human herpesvirus 6

Human herpesvirus 6 (HHV-6) was first isolated in 1986 from cultured human lymphocyte lines, and named human B lymphotropic virus, a misnomer since it is trophic principally for T cells, although replication also occurs in macrophages, glial cells, and EBV-transformed B cells. HHV-6 is widely distributed in humans. Primary infection causes roseola infantum (also known as exanthem subitum or sixth disease), an aetiological association first described in Japanese children in 1988.

Aetiology

HHV-6 has typical herpesvirus morphology, and is genetically classified in the beta-herpesvirus subfamily. Two types of isolate, HHV-6A and HHV-6B, are now clearly distinguished by their genetic sequence, and some variation in biological properties. HHV-6B is associated with roseola, whereas HHV-6A has not been associated with disease.

Epidemiology

There is high seroprevalence of HHV-6 in all populations. More than 90% of children are seropositive at 2 years of age. The virus (usually the HHV-6B variant) can be detected in peripheral blood mononuclear cells by PCR-based tests in nearly all healthy people. It is most probably transmitted via maternal saliva, although intrauterine and perinatal transmission could occur. There is also evidence that chromosomally integrated maternal HHV6 can be transmitted in the germline, although the clinical significance is uncertain. The virus is not detectable in breast milk.

Pathogenesis

HHV-6 probably replicates in regional lymphoid tissue in the oropharynx during primary infection, and can be found in circulating lymphocytes. The virus replicates *in vitro* in CD4+ T-cell lines, but during persistent infection in the normal adult, virus can be detected by PCR in both CD4+ T cells and monocytes/macrophages in peripheral blood, which are probably the principal site of carriage during persistent infection. The mechanism of viral latency is uncertain.

Although HHV-6 cannot usually be isolated by culture from the peripheral blood of normal people, specific DNA is easily detected in blood during immunosuppression, indicating reactivation of HHV-6. The mechanism by which HHV6 produces its clinical manifestations remains unclear.

Clinical features

Primary infection with HHV-6 in young children is associated with roseola, and also with a febrile illness without rash.

Roseola infantum (exanthem subitum, sixth disease)

Roseola is an acute illness of infants and young children, typically 3 to 5 days of high fever with upper respiratory tract symptoms, and sometimes cervical lymphadenopathy. As the fever subsides, a rash appears and lasts for 1 to 3 days. The rash is diffuse, macular, or maculopapular, and appears similar to that of rubella. There is mild atypical lymphocytosis and there may be neutropenia. Infections may rarely be complicated by febrile convulsions, meningitis, encephalitis, and hepatitis; the last is usually mild, but occasionally severe.

Roseola has been estimated to occur in only 10 to 20% of children, and primary HHV-6 infection is commonly subclinical.

Febrile Illness

Fever without rash is a more usual manifestation of primary HHV-6 infection than roseola. In a North American study, 10% of 1600 febrile children under the age of 3 years (including 20% of those aged 6–12 months) presenting with acute febrile illness were diagnosed as primary HHV-6 infection, but only 17% of them had clinical roseola.

Febrile convulsions

It is suggested HHV-6 may have a particular association with febrile convulsions in young children. Primary HHV-6 infection was reported to account for one-third of all the febrile seizures in children up to the age of 2 years; however, there were no seizures in 81 children with primary infection in a prospective cohort. HHV-6 DNA can be detected in the cerebrospinal fluid of children with primary infection, and any association may be because HHV-6 specifically infects the nervous system, rather than solely because of high fever.

HHV-6 infection in immunosuppressed patients

A number of studies have shown increases in antibody titres to HHV-6, and increased HHV-6 DNA levels in the peripheral blood of immunosuppressed solid organ and bone marrow transplant recipients. In bone marrow transplant recipients, HHV-6 has been associated with fever, skin rash, graft versus host disease, encephalitis, delayed engraftment, marrow suppression, and pneumonitis. It is not clear whether HHV-6 plays a specific aetiological role in all these syndromes; the evidence is perhaps stronger for a causal role in encephalitis. There is also good evidence that HHV-6 reactivates in patients with advanced HIV infection and AIDS, but again there is less firm evidence that this is associated with disease.

Other disease associations

Studies of chronic fatigue syndrome and multiple sclerosis have not provided convincing evidence of any significant aetiological association with HHV-6.

Differential diagnosis

Primary HHV-6 infection may be confused with many febrile childhood illnesses accompanied by a rash. Roseola may also be misdiagnosed as a sensitivity reaction to recent antibiotic treatment. Other virus infections (EBV, HCMV) may also be associated with atypical lymphocytes and a mononucleosis syndrome.

Pathology

HHV-6 replicates *in vitro* in cells originating from the central nervous system, particularly glial cell lines. HHV-6 DNA can be detected in the brains of apparently normal people, suggesting viral persistence in the central nervous system. No distinctive histopathology has yet been attributed to HHV-6.

Malignancy

HHV-6 DNA has been detected in the blood of patients with several lymphoproliferative disorders, but this probably reflects reactivation rather than any causal association with the tumour. HHV-6 DNA has been reported in some tumour tissues, including the nodular sclerosis variant of Hodgkin's disease, but without a convincing aetiological association between the virus and any tumour.

Laboratory diagnosis

Most assays for HHV-6 antibody do not distinguish between antibody to HHV-6A and HHV-6B, and may crossreact with antibodies to HHV-7. Seroconversion is evidence of primary infection. IgM assays for HHV-6 antibody are not reliable indicators of primary infection, as some HHV-6 carriers may periodically have IgM antibody.

Although HHV-6 can be cultured from peripheral blood mononuclear cells during acute primary infection, few laboratories will undertake this. PCR-based techniques for the detection of HHV-6 DNA in plasma and cerebrospinal fluid are the method of choice for clinical diagnosis, and are becoming more widely available.

Treatment

HHV-6 sensitivity to antiviral drugs corresponds with that of cytomegalovirus. Thus, HHV-6 replication is inhibited *in vitro* by ganciclovir and foscarnet, but not aciclovir; however, there are no controlled clinical trials of these drugs. Their use may be considered for immunosuppressed patients with suspected HHV-6-associated pneumonitis.

Prevention and control

There are no preventative measures for HHV-6 transmission. It seems unlikely that there will be a case for the development of a vaccine because infants may be infected so early in life, while they still have maternal antibody.

Special problems in pregnant women

Nearly all pregnant women will be carriers of HHV-6. There is no evidence that HHV-6 infection harms the fetus or the neonate.

Human herpesvirus 7

Human herpesvirus 7 (HHV-7) was isolated in 1990, and is a beta-herpesvirus similar to, but distinct from, HHV-6. HHV-7 predominantly infects CD4+ T cells and can be reactivated from latency by T-cell activation.

Although there is serological crossreactivity between HHV-6 and HHV-7, data indicate that HHV-7 infects nearly all children, but later than HHV-6, with more than 90% being infected by the age of 5 years. The virus is excreted in saliva.

HHV-7 has been associated with some cases of roseola, which it was reported to cause in Japanese infants with a previous episode of roseola proven to be caused by HHV-6. There is no further evidence of pathogenicity.

The best method of diagnosis is PCR-based testing of serum or cerebrospinal fluid. Laboratory tests for HHV-6 often detect HHV-7 by multiplex PCR. There is no reason to consider any treatment for HHV-7.

Human herpesvirus 8

Human herpesvirus 8 (HHV-8) is the most recently isolated of the human herpesviruses; Chang and colleagues reported the detection of novel DNA sequences with homology to herpesviruses in Kaposi's sarcoma tissue in 1994. Initially named Kaposi's sarcoma-associated herpesvirus, it was subsequently designated HHV-8. It is genetically most closely related to a well characterized simian herpesvirus (herpesvirus saimiri), and less so to EBV; it has consequently been assigned to the rhadinovirus (γ2-herpesvirus) subfamily. Current culture techniques are unreliable, but the virus can be detected by PCR. Serological assays depend on the use of infected cell lines or synthetic antigens from predicted open reading frames. The seroepidemiology, biology, and disease associations of the virus are still being analysed, but HHV-8 is clearly associated with Kaposi's sarcoma, a tumour that has long been suspected of having a viral aetiology; with primary effusion lymphoma; and with multicentric Castleman's disease. Reported associations with multiple myeloma and other cancers are unconfirmed.

Aetiology

HHV-8 has the characteristic morphology of a herpesvirus. The viral genome is composed of a 141 kbp unique segment flanked by multiple 801 bp direct repeats. Sequence analysis suggests that HHV-8, like other herpesviruses, is an ancient human virus; comparative analysis of the variable genes *ORF-K1* and *K15* indicates there are at least four virus subtypes, A to D, reflecting the migrationary divergence of modern human populations. HHV-8 contains genes homologous to mammalian genes encoding cell-cycle regulatory proteins (the cyclins), chemokines, and inhibitors of apoptosis. On the evidence to date, the normal cellular site of latency of HHV-8 almost certainly includes the B cell.

Epidemiology

The emerging epidemiology of HHV-8 suggests it is less ubiquitous than other human herpesviruses. Initial serological assays detected antibodies to a latent nuclear antigen; assays using lytic-cycle antigens gave higher rates of seroprevalence, and newer assays using multiple HHV-8 antigens are currently being applied. Current data suggest a seroprevalence of 90% or more in patients with Kaposi's sarcoma, and 40% in HIV-positive homosexual men without Kaposi's sarcoma. Seroprevalence in normal adults is reported as being more than 50% in African adults in West Africa, 20% in black South African blood donors, and 53% in HIV-positive and -negative adults in Uganda. Seroprevalence is 5% or less in blood donors in the United Kingdom and the United States of America, with intermediate rates in Italy and other Mediterranean countries. HHV-8 can be detected by PCR in nearly all cases of Kaposi's sarcoma, but is less easy to detect in the blood of normal carriers.

The usual route of transmission is probably saliva and sexual contact, but intravenous drug use, blood transfusion, and organ transplantation also transmit the virus. A latent nuclear antigen-based assay detected seroconversion to HHV-8 in HIV-infected homosexual men at a median of 33 months before they subsequently developed Kaposi's sarcoma. HHV-8 infection in children correlates with seropositivity in their mothers, but whether this reflects vertical or horizontal transmission is uncertain.

Pathogenesis

There has been much uncertainty over the cell of origin of Kaposi's sarcoma, but the spindle cells of which the tumour is largely composed are thought to be of lymphatic endothelial origin. In Kaposi's sarcoma tumour tissue, HHV-8 DNA and latent nuclear antigen are present in every spindle cell, suggesting an aetiological role for the virus.

In HIV-associated Castleman's disease, the HHV-8 latent nuclear antigen is present in immunoblasts in the mantle zone of the tumour. HHV-8 is present in the tumour cells of all cases of primary effusion lymphoma so far studied (although so is EBV), and HHV-8 latently infected cell lines derived from these tumours can be induced to release infectious virus. These clear associations of virus DNA with tumour cells suggest a definite oncogenic role for HHV-8. HHV-8 latent transcripts, including latency-associated nuclear antigen (LANA), viral cyclin, viral FLIP, and virus-encoded microRNAs, promote cell proliferation and prevent apoptosis, whereas lytic proteins, such as viral G protein-coupled receptor, K1, and virus-encoded cytokines (viral interleukin-6 and viral chemokines) contribute to the characteristic angioproliferative and inflammatory Kaposi's sarcoma lesions through a mechanism known as paracrine neoplasia.

It has been suggested that HHV-8 may be involved in the pathogenesis of multiple myeloma, but this association is unproven, as is an association with primary pulmonary hypertension. The individual HHV-8 subtypes are not associated with any distinct pathology.

Clinical features

Apart from these malignancies, the only reported clinical syndrome accompanying primary or reactivated HHV-8 infection is fever and bone marrow graft failure in immunosuppressed transplant recipients.

Kaposi's sarcoma

Kaposi's sarcoma appears as purplish-brown macules, papules, or plaques. It is described in four characteristic clinical settings: the classical form in older Mediterranean or Jewish men, the endemic African form (accounting for 10% of cancer in equatorial Africa), in patients with immunodeficiency states, such as transplant recipients, and the AIDS-associated form. In the classical and African forms there are lesions on the extremities; systemic and mucosal involvement is rare, and the disease is indolent. In immunosuppressed patients (other than those with AIDS) the lesions are more widespread and more rapidly progressive, although visceral involvement is still unusual, and lesions may regress if immunosuppressive drugs are stopped. AIDS-associated Kaposi's sarcoma is seen predominantly in homosexual men in western countries, but is commonly associated with heterosexually acquired HIV infection in African countries. The clinical signs are widespread cutaneous lesions, with involvement of the oral mucosa (see Chapter 5.23, Figs. 5.23.12 and 5.23.13), and visceral lesions may occur in the lungs or gastrointestinal tract. Progression can be much more rapid than the other forms. HHV-8 has been isolated from all four types of Kaposi's sarcoma.

Primary effusion lymphomas

Previously known as body-cavity based lymphomas, these are a rare and aggressive type of B-cell lymphoma in patients with AIDS. They present as lymphomatous effusions of the peritoneal, pleural, or pericardial spaces, usually without any identifiable tumour mass. HHV-8 is present in the tumour cells of all cases so far studied, although so also is EBV.

Castleman's disease or angiofollicular lymph node hyperplasia

This can be localized, and is amenable to curative excision. However, a multicentric form is seen particularly in HIV-infected patients, and is more aggressive. HHV-8 is found in a high proportion of these multicentric cases, especially those associated with HIV.

Pathology

No distinctive histopathology has been identified for HHV-8 independent of the pathology of the tumours with which it is associated.

Laboratory diagnosis

HHV-8 can best be detected by PCR-based tests. The antibody assays described above may become commercially available in the near future.

Treatment

In vitro assays in HHV-8-infected lymphoma cell lines indicate that HHV-8 replication is moderately sensitive to foscarnet, ganciclovir, and cidofovir. AIDS patients treated with foscarnet and ganciclovir may be less likely to develop Kaposi's sarcoma. Antiviral drugs are not an established treatment for HHV-8 tumours.

Kaposi's sarcoma confined to the skin can be treated with radiotherapy or intralesional α-interferon. More widespread cutaneous or visceral disease can be treated with single-agent or combination chemotherapy. The treatment of Kaposi's sarcoma in AIDS patients is discussed in Chapters 5.23 and 5.24. Kaposi's sarcoma lesions may regress with antiretroviral treatment, possibly because of improved cellular immunity resulting from the reduction in HIV load.

Prevention and control

Given the uncertainty around the epidemiology and disease associations of HHV-8, prevention and control are not yet possible. No special problems of infection have been identified in pregnant women.

Cercopithecine herpesvirus 1 (herpes B virus)

Cercopithecine herpesvirus 1 is the formal name now given to herpes B virus (replacing the previous term, herpesvirus simiae), the natural hosts of which are members of the *Macaca* genus of Old World monkeys. It produces minimal disease in its natural hosts, but its transmission to humans results in a high incidence of severe disease. Although more than 30 other herpesviruses have been isolated from nonhuman primates, none of these has been unequivocally associated with a disease in humans. The virus was first isolated in 1932 from the brain of Dr W B, who died of encephalitis after a bite from a macaque (hence the name herpes B virus). There have since been about 45 cases of human infection resulting from accidental transmission from captive monkeys.

Aetiology

Herpes B virus is an alpha-herpesvirus closely related to HSV, and appears to behave in an analogous manner to HSV in its natural primate host. Herpes B virus can also infect and produce disease in other nonhuman primates and small mammals.

Epidemiology

Herpes B virus is enzootic in Old World monkeys of the *Macaca* genus, principally rhesus (*M. mulatta*) and cynomolgus (*M. fascicularis*) macaques. The epidemiology in its primate host is similar to that of HSV in humans, with 80% or more of natural and captive adult monkeys being infected. Infected monkeys may develop vesicular oral lesions, and can shed virus intermittently from oral, conjunctival, and genital secretions.

Rhesus and cynomolgus macaques have been quite widely used in medical research, particularly for the development of polio vaccine in the mid 1950s, and in the late 1980s following the AIDS epidemic, for studies of retroviruses. Nearly all the reported human cases resulted from occupational exposure through bites and scratches in workers handling monkeys, but transmission from needlestick injuries and a splash in the eye have also been reported. One case of human-to-human transmission apparently occurred by inoculation onto inflamed skin.

Two clusters of infection have been described in the United States of America (in 1987, involving the case of human-to-human transmission, and 1989). A seroprevalence study of more than 300 monkey handlers showed that none was seropositive, and asymptomatic infection documented by seroconversion appears to be extremely uncommon.

Clinical features

The incubation period, from occupational exposure to the development of symptoms, has usually been 3 to 5 days, but can range from 3 to 30 days. Cutaneous vesicles may occur at or near the site of inoculation, accompanied by regional lymphadenitis. In the first 2 weeks, fever, malaise, headache, and abdominal pain are common, but the dominant and characteristic features are progressive multifocal haemorrhagic myelitis, and encephalitis. Visceral spread of herpes B virus is recorded in fatal cases. The untreated mortality is 80%. The history of monkey bite may lead to a suspicion of rabies (Chapter 5.10).

It is not clear whether herpes B virus in humans can become latent and then be reactivated. Viral shedding has recurred when antiviral treatment was stopped relatively early, so most patients have been maintained on antivirals for long periods.

Laboratory diagnosis

As herpes B virus is a category 4 pathogen, viral culture and isolation are only attempted in a few designated laboratories: in the United Kingdom at the Central Public Health Laboratory, Colindale, London; and in the United States of America at Georgia State University, Atlanta. Monkeys with suspected infection should have serum antibody tests. Serodiagnosis in humans is difficult because of antigenic crossreactivity between herpes B virus and HSV. The inoculation site should ideally be biopsied for culture and analysis.

PCR-based methods are available in specialized centres, and are the standard for definitive diagnosis.

Treatment

Although injuries from macaques carry the risk of herpes B virus infection, most captive macaque colonies are now maintained free of the virus. A suspected contaminated wound should be debrided and cleaned with chlorhexidine or iodine soap. Postexposure prophylaxis may be initiated if the monkey is suspected to be positive for herpes B virus, and there is skin puncture or mucosal exposure. There may be a case for initiating immediate antiviral treatment if infection in the monkey is suspected, or for a deep wound.

Aciclovir and ganciclovir both inhibit herpes B virus replication *in vitro*. For postexposure prophylaxis, valaciclovir 1 g 8 hourly is recommended for at least 2 weeks. If symptomatic disease is suspected or proven, intravenous aciclovir is recommended if CNS symptoms are absent (15 mg/kg 8 hourly), and ganciclovir if CNS symptoms are present (5 mg/kg every 12 h). Treatment has been associated with the limitation of disease, and recovery, in some patients, but prolonged oral therapy with aciclovir or valaciclovir is advised to limit the risk of reactivation.

Prevention and control

Those working with macaques should follow standard procedures to avoid infection. The screening of newly imported monkeys, and the creation of colonies of macaques free of herpes B virus, are now becoming standard practice.

Further reading

Herpes simplex virus infections

Casanova JL, *et al.* (2011). Human TLRs and IL-1Rs in host defense: natural insights from evolutionary, epidemiological, and clinical genetics. *Annu Rev Immunol*, **29**, 447–91. [Review of innate immunity deficiencies associated with HSV encephalitis.]

Corey L, Wald A (2009). Current concepts: maternal and neonatal herpes simplex virus infections. *N Engl J Med*, **361**, 1376–85. [Useful review on this topic.]

Lakeman FD, Whitley RJ (1995). Diagnosis of herpes simplex encephalitis: application of polymerase chain reaction to cerebrospinal fluid from brain-biopsied patients and correlation with disease. NIAID collaborative antiviral study group. *J Infect Dis*, **171**, 857–63. [Study showing the detection of HSV DNA by PCR in 98% of 54 patients with brain biopsy-proven HSV encephalitis.]

Langenberg AGM, *et al.* (1999). A prospective study of new infections with herpes simplex virus type 1 and type 2. *N Engl J Med*, **341**, 1432–8. [Study of incident HSV-1/2 infections, reporting the proportion of symptomatic infections.]

Pellett PE, Roizman B (2007). The Herpesviridae: a brief introduction. In: Knipe DM, *et al.* (eds). *Fields virology*, 5th edition, vol. 2, pp. 2479–99. Lippincott, Williams and Wilkins, Philadelphia.

Roizman B, *et al.* (2007). Herpes simplex viruses. In: Knipe DM, *et al.* (eds). *Fields virology*, 5th edition, vol. 2, pp. 2501–601. Lippincott, Williams and Wilkins, Philadelphia.

Zhang SY, *et al.* (2007). Human toll-like receptor-dependent induction of interferons in protective immunity to viruses. *Immunol Rev*, **220**, 225–36. [Recent work on factors conferring susceptibility to HSV encephalitis.]

Varicella–zoster virus infection

Cohen JI, *et al.* (2007). Varicella–zoster virus. In: Knipe DM, *et al.* (eds). *Fields virology*, 5th edition, vol. 2, pp. 2773–818. Lippincott, Williams and Wilkins, Philadelphia.

Gilden DH, *et al.* (2000). Medical progress: neurologic complications of the reactivation of varicella–zoster virus. *N Engl J Med*, **342**, 635–46. [A good review of the subject, including postherpetic neuralgia.]

Gilden DH, *et al* (2002). The protean manifestations of varicella–zoster virus vasculopathy. *J Neurovirol*, **8** Suppl 2, 75–9. [A less well known aspect of VZV pathogenicity.]

Kimberlin DW, Whitley RJ (2007). Varicella–zoster vaccine for the prevention of herpes zoster. *N Engl J Med*, **356**, 1338–43. [Recent review of current status of the VZV vaccine.]

Wood MJ, *et al.* (1994). A randomised trial of acyclovir for 7 days or 21 days with and without prednisolone for treatment of acute herpes zoster. *N Engl J Med*, **330**, 901–5. [UK study showing that longer courses of aciclovir and prednisolone do not reduce the frequency of postherpetic neuralgia.]

Human cytomegalovirus infection

Boeckh M, Ljungman P (2009). How we treat cytomegalovirus in hematopoietic cell transplant recipients. *Blood*, **113**, 5711–9. [Useful discussion of treatment in this setting.]

Crumpacker CS, Wadhwa S (2005). Cytomegalovirus. In: Mandell GL, Bennett JE, Dolin R, (eds). *Principles and practice of infectious diseases*, pp. 1786–801. Elsevier Churchill Livingstone, Philadelphia.

Hodson EM, *et al.* (2008). Antiviral medications for preventing cytomegalovirus disease in solid organ transplant recipients. *Cochrane Database Syst Rev*, CD003774. [Systematic review of the evidence for the efficacy of primary prevention.]

Mocarski ES, *et al.* (2007). Cytomegaloviruses. In: Knipe DM, *et al.* (eds). *Fields virology*, 5th edition, vol. 2, pp. 2701–72. Lippincott, Williams and Wilkins, Philadelphia.

Pass RF, *et al.* (2009). Vaccine prevention of maternal cytomegalovirus infection. *N Engl J Med*, **360**, 1191–9. [Phase 2 trial of gB based vaccine shows potential for protection.]

Sinclair J, Sissons JGP (2006). Latency and reactivation of human cytomegalovirus. *J Gen Virol*, **87**, 1763–79. [Review of mechanistic basis of latency and reactivation.]

Whitley RJ, *et al.* (1998). Guidelines for the treatment of CMV diseases in patients with AIDS in the era of potent antiretroviral therapy. *Arch Intern Med*, **158**, 957–69. [Recommendations of an international panel on the treatment of CMV disease in AIDS.]

Human herpesvirus 6 and 7

Hall CB, *et al.* (1994). Human herpesvirus-6 infection in children: a prospective study of complications and reactivation. *N Engl J Med*, **331**, 432–8. [A comprehensive study of primary HHV-6 infection in children presenting with febrile illness to a hospital emergency department.]

Yamanishi K, *et al.* (2007). Human herpesvirus-6 and 7. In: Knipe DM, *et al.* (eds). *Fields virology*, 5th edition, vol. 2, pp. 2819–45. Lippincott, Williams and Wilkins, Philadelphia.

Zerr DM, *et al.* (2005). A population-based study of primary human herpesvirus 6 infection. *N Engl J Med*, **352**, 768–76.

Zerr DM, *et al.* (2005). Clinical outcomes of human herpesvirus 6 reactivation after hematopoietic stem cell transplantation. *Clin Infect Dis*, **40**, 932–40.

Human herpesvirus 8

Ganem D (2007). Kaposi's sarcoma-associated herpesvirus. In: Knipe DM, *et al.* (eds). *Fields virology*, 5th edition, vol. 2, pp. 2847–88. Lippincott, Williams and Wilkins, Philadelphia.

Hayward GS (1999). Kaposi's sarcoma HV strains: the origins and global spread of the virus. *Semin Cancer Biol*, **9**, 187–99. [Summarizes the current molecular evidence for the evolution of the virus.]

Martin JN, *et al.* (1998). Sexual transmission and the natural history of human herpesvirus 8 infection. *N Engl J Med*, **338**, 948–54. [Provides evidence for the sexual transmission of HHV-8 and its association with Kaposi's sarcoma in homosexual men.]

Mesri EA, *et al.* (2010). Kaposi's sarcoma and its associated herpesvirus. *Nat Rev Cancer*, **10**, 707–19. [A recent review.]

Cercopithecine herpesvirus 1

Cohen JI, *et al.* (2002). Recommendations for the prevention of and therapy for exposure to B virus. *Clin Infect Dis*, **35**, 1191–203. [Current US recommendations for the management of human herpes B virus infection.]

Sabin AB, Wright AM (1934). Acute ascending myelitis following a monkey bite, with the isolation of a virus capable of reproducing the disease. *J Exp Med*, **59**, 115–36. [The original description of herpes B virus and the case of Dr W B.]

Straus SE (2005). Herpes B virus. In: Mandell GL, Bennett JE, Dolin R, (eds). *Principles and practice of infectious diseases*, pp. 1832–5. Elsevier Churchill Livingstone, Philadelphia.

5.3 Epstein–Barr virus

M.A. Epstein and A.B. Rickinson

Essentials

Epstein–Barr virus (EBV) is a human herpesvirus with a linear double-stranded DNA genome that is carried asymptomatically by most people. Symptomless primary infection is usual in childhood, establishing a lifelong carrier state where the virus persists as a latent infection of circulating B cells. The virus replicates recurrently in oropharyngeal epithelial cells, with consequent shedding of virus in saliva transmitting infection.

Infectious mononucleosis

If delayed beyond childhood, primary infection causes infectious mononucleosis in up to at least 50% of cases. This is typically characterized by sore throat, fever, anorexia, headache, fatigue, malaise (often disproportionately severe), generalized lymphadenopathy, splenomegaly (60%), hepatomegaly (10%), and jaundice (8%). Diagnosis can be confirmed by the Monospot test (which detects heterophil antibodies that are present in 85%) or the presence of IgM antibodies to virus capsid antigen. Treatment is supportive unless there are complications. Most cases resolve within 1 to 2 weeks; chronic or recurrent forms are described but are very rare. Primary infection in boys with the X-linked lymphoproliferative trait, a rare congenital immunodeficiency, gives severe or fatal disease. In other rare cases, most common in Asia, primary infection of immunocompetent people can lead to 'chronic active' EBV syndrome resembling persistent infectious mononucleosis but sometimes fatal.

B-cell tumours

Endemic Burkitt's lymphoma—all cells of this common malignancy of children in areas of Africa and New Guinea carry the EBV genome. A cofactor, hyperendemic malaria, explains the unusual geographical distribution of the high incidence disease. Presentation is with jaw and other tumours, peripheral lymph nodes and spleen are spared, and progression to death is rapid. Cyclophosphamide treatment is remarkably effective.

Other forms of Burkitt's lymphoma—a sporadic type occurs at low incidence worldwide. This is EBV-positive in only a few cases; jaw tumours are rare and lymph nodes are involved; response to treatment is poor—combination therapy is required, and survival after relapse is uncommon. Another form, EBV-positive in 30 to 40% of cases, occurs in AIDS patients.

Other lymphomas—where immune cell control over EBV is impaired in immunosuppressed transplant recipients or long-term AIDS patients, expansions of EBV-transformed B cells can occur as acute polyclonal lymphoproliferative lesions or later monoclonal large cell lymphomas. In transplant patients the first treatment is to reduce immunosuppressive therapy. EBV is also linked to Hodgkin's lymphoma, with the virus genome present in the Reed–Sternberg and mononuclear tumour cells in some 30 to 40% of cases.

Other malignancies and conditions associated with EBV

Undifferentiated nasopharyngeal carcinoma—this epithelial tumour is most common in southern Chinese and Inuit people, and is EBV genome-positive in all cases. Besides virus infection, dietary, genetic, and perhaps herbal remedy cofactors are involved. Radiotherapy is the treatment of choice.

EBV has more tenuous links with salivary gland tumours, some gastric carcinomas, rare smooth muscle tumours of the immunosuppressed, and certain nasal T and NK lymphomas. The nonmalignant lesions of oral hairy leukoplakia in HIV patients are interesting because the squamous epithelial cells forming them are driven by replicating EBV.

Background

The virus

Epstein–Barr virus (EBV) was discovered in 1964 during a sustained search for a viral cause of endemic Burkitt's lymphoma (see 'Endemic ('African') Burkitt's lymphoma' below). EBV is one of the eight human herpesviruses, and consists of an outer envelope, a protein capsid, and an inner double-stranded linear DNA genome. It is a very ancient parasite of humans, and related herpesviruses have been found in both Old World apes and monkeys and in New World monkeys. This indicates that the ancestor of such viruses infected early primates before the evolutionary split between Old World and New World primates occurred (about 35 million years ago based on palaeontology, or 45 million years ago based on DNA sequence analysis).

Viral infectious cycle

Natural infection is limited to humans, and the principal target cells of the virus are circulating B lymphocytes and squamous epithelial cells of the oropharynx. Lytic infection of these cells produces free viral progeny and cell death. The virus also causes latent infection of B cells *in vivo* and can transform normal B lymphocytes *in vitro* into continuously growing, latently infected lymphoblastoid cell lines.

Virus-coded proteins

Different sets of virus-coded proteins are expressed in lytic and latent infection. Lytic-cycle EBV-coded proteins are categorized as immediate early, early, or late antigens, according to when they appear. Many elicit cytotoxic T-cell and serum antibody responses, both of which are important in controlling the infection. Antibodies are used in diagnosis.

Epidemiology

The virus is widespread in all human populations. Primary infection usually occurs in early childhood, when it is almost always clinically silent. This leads to a lifelong carrier state, in which both humoral and cellular immune responses are maintained. The virus becomes latent in a few circulating memory B lymphocytes. There are also subclinical foci of lytically infected epithelial cells (and possibly intraepithelial B cells) in the mouth and pharynx, and perhaps also in the salivary glands and urogenital tract. Virus in the buccal fluid therefore provides the main source for transmission of the infection in the population. In developing countries, 99% of children are infected by the second to the fourth year of life. By contrast, in industrialized countries with higher standards of hygiene, as many as 50% of children, particularly those from high socioeconomic groups, enter adolescence uninfected (Fig. 5.3.1).

Infectious mononucleosis

Up to 50% of those who first acquire the virus in the second or third decade develop some clinical symptoms of infectious mononucleosis. Mononucleosis is therefore mainly a disease of upper socioeconomic groups in Western societies, and is exceptionally rare in developing countries (Fig. 5.3.1). Although most cases occur in adolescents and young adults, children and middle-aged people may sometimes develop the disease, and rarely also older people. Primary infection in adolescence or later is likely to be acquired by kissing a virus-shedding healthy carrier. This explains why case-to-case infection and epidemics are not seen, and why the incubation period, perhaps 30 to 50 days, is difficult to calculate. Symptomatic primary EBV infection may also be acquired through latently infected B lymphocytes present in blood transfusions or organ grafts.

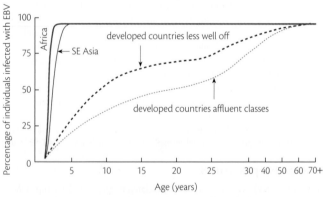

Fig. 5.3.1 Comparison of the ages at which people in different populations become infected with EBV. In developing countries, almost all children have acquired the virus by 2 to 4 years of age, depending on geographical region. In developed countries with high standards of living and hygiene, the time of infection is delayed for many, more markedly among the affluent than the less well off. Among the very rich, as many as 50% may reach adolescence or young adulthood without having encountered the virus, and will undergo delayed primary infection, with a high risk that this will be accompanied by the symptoms of infectious mononucleosis. (Reprinted with permission from Epstein MA (2002). Infectious mononucleosis. In: *Encyclopedia of life sciences*, **10**, 211–16. Nature Publishing Group, London.)

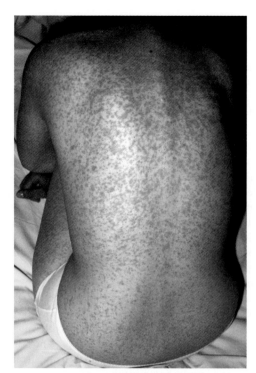

Fig. 5.3.2 Typical maculopapular erythematous rash in a patient with infectious mononucleosis who was treated with ampicillin.
(Copyright D A Warrell.)

Symptoms

Classical infectious mononucleosis may follow days of vague indisposition, or may start abruptly. It presents with sore throat, fever with sweating, anorexia, headache, and fatigue, with malaise quite out of proportion to the other complaints. Dysphagia may be noticed, and also brief orbital oedema. Erythematous and maculopapular rashes occur in a small number of untreated patients, but much more frequently in those that have been taking ampicillin for sore throat before infectious mononucleosis has been diagnosed (Fig. 5.3.2). Tonsillar and pharyngeal oedema can rarely cause pharyngeal obstruction (Fig. 5.3.3).

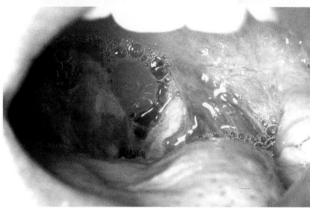

Fig. 5.3.3 Percentage of patients with infectious mononucleosis showing various clinical features during the course of the disease, and the timing and average duration of each.
(Reprinted with permission from Epstein MA (2002). Infectious mononucleosis. In: *Encyclopedia of life sciences*, **10**, 211–16. Nature Publishing Group, London.)

Signs

The fever may rise to 40°C, but swings are not seen. There is redness and oedema of the pharynx, fauces, soft palate, and uvula (Fig. 5.3.4a), and about half the patients develop greyish exudates on the tonsils (Fig. 5.3.4b). Generalized lymphadenopathy is almost always present, and is most marked in the cervical region; the

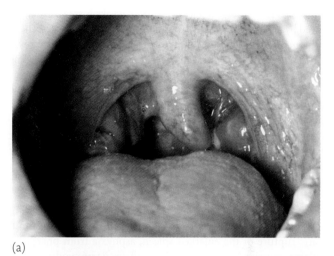

(a)

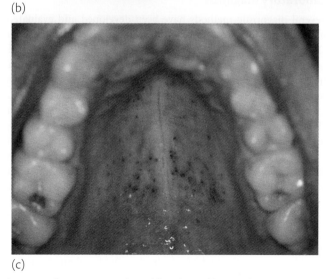

(b)

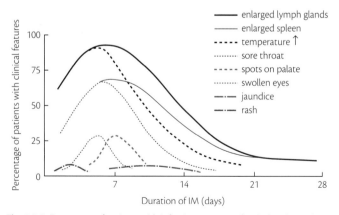

(c)

Fig. 5.3.4 Infectious mononucleosis: (a) Oedema of fauces, soft palate, uvula, and tonsils; (b) tonsillar exudates; and (c) palatal petechiae.
(Courtesy of the late Dr B E Juel-Jensen.)

glands are symmetrical, discrete, and slightly tender. Splenomegaly is seen in about 60% of cases and an enlarged liver in 10%. There is usually a moderate bradycardia. Besides the rash, characteristic palatal enanthematous crops of reddish petechiae (Fig. 5.3.4c) are found in about one-third of patients, and jaundice occurs in about 8%.

Clinical course

Mild cases may resolve in days, but 1 to 4 weeks is more usual, followed by a period of lethargy. The duration of this convalescence is influenced by psychological factors, particularly the speed with which patients are encouraged to resume full activity. About 1 case in 2000 may continue in a truly chronic or recurrent form for several months or years (see 'Chronic active EBV infection' below). Most other cases of so-called chronic infectious mononucleosis are manifestations of chronic fatigue syndrome (Oxford Textbook of Medicine 5e Chapter 26.5.4), but whether this is a true entity rather than a form of depression or a belief disorder is highly controversial. Credible connections with EBV have not been established.

Complications

Minor nonspecific complications may occur. Rare, more serious complications include secondary bacterial throat infections, traumatic rupture of the enlarged spleen, asphyxia from pharyngeal oedema, massive hepatic necrosis, Guillain–Barré syndrome, and autoimmune manifestations such as thrombocytopenia and haemolytic anaemia.

Differential diagnosis

Classical infectious mononucleosis is diagnosed by the clinical features, combined with serological and haematological laboratory investigations (see below). An infectious mononucleosis-like disease can occur in primary cytomegalovirus infection and in toxoplasmosis, but in both conditions the sore throat is much less severe, and with cytomegalovirus the lymphadenopathy may be minimal or absent; an infectious mononucleosis-like syndrome is also sometimes seen during the acute phase of recent HIV infection.

Laboratory diagnosis

Several diagnostic methods have been developed and evaluated, including the Monospot test, detection of EBV viral capsid antigen (VCA) IgM/IgG and EBV nuclear antigen (EBNA) IgM/IgG antibodies using multiplexed bead-based assay (BBA), enzyme immunoassay (EIA), or immunofluorescence assay (IFA) all of which have sensitivities of 80 to 90%, measurement of EBV viral load (EBV-VL) in peripheral blood and real-time polymerase chain reaction (RT-PCR) targeting various EBV genes. The Monospot screening test can be used to detect the presence of heterophile antibodies in the patient's serum. Although these heterophile antibodies are not directed against virally encoded proteins, they are present in up to 85% of acute infectious mononucleosis sera. Cases of Monospot-negative infectious mononucleosis tend to be outside the usual 15- to 25-year age range, and false-positive tests may occur in pregnancy and autoimmune disease. The diagnosis of infectious mononucleosis is confirmed by the presence of serum IgM antibodies to EBV capsid antigen (VCA), which can be detected for about 2 months. RT-PCR is proving useful in the early diagnosis of infectious mononucleosis where EBV IgM immunoassays (multiplexed BBA, EIA, and IFA) proved inconclusive. Targeting the BALF5 gene and

BAHMI-W region of the EBNA1 gene is highly sensitive. Other features include the presence of lymphocytosis up to 15×10^9/litre, composed mainly of activated cytotoxic T cells with an atypical morphology, decreased CD4/CD8 ratio (0.3), and raised C-reactive protein (CRP) concentrations.

Treatment

Bed rest and aspirin or paracetamol for headache and pharyngeal discomfort are the only treatments required. When the fever resolves the patient should be encouraged to get up and resume some activities as fast as is practicable, but violent exercise should be avoided for 3 weeks after an enlarged spleen ceases to be palpable. Only complications need active therapy; splenic rupture requires surgery, bacterial infections call for appropriate antibiotics, airway obstruction must be relieved by tracheostomy, and corticosteroids should be given for life-threatening pharyngeal oedema, and for neurological and haematological complications.

Immunocompetent patients with severe infectious mononucleosis have been treated with a variety of antiviral agents including aciclovir, valciclovir, famciclovir, ganciclovir with or without foscarnet, and vidarabine, together with corticosteroids or intravenous immunoglobulin. Clinical evidence does not support the use of aciclovir alone but more patients receiving a combination of antivirals and immunosuppressives survived compared to those given antiviral therapy alone. Suggested experimental treatments are 5-substituted uracil, azacytosine derivatives aimed at destroying cells expressing EBV thymidine kinase, and peptides inhibiting EBV-mediated membrane fusion.

Pathogenesis

Why children are asymptomatic during primary EBV infection, whereas adolescents and young adults frequently develop infectious mononucleosis, is not fully understood. The higher virus dose likely to be acquired by kissing is one possible factor. In infectious mononucleosis patients, both epithelial and intraepithelial B cells in the oropharynx become productively infected, and infectious virus can easily be found in patients' saliva. The newly replicated virus initiates a latent growth-transforming infection of B cells, causing them to multiply and spread throughout the lymphoid system. These combined lytic and latent infections stimulate an exaggerated cytotoxic T-cell response in the circulation; in lymph nodes, tonsils, and other oropharyngeal lymphoid tissues; and in the spleen and the liver. This exaggerated response, and the cytokine storm that accompanies it, are thought to be responsible for the sore throat, fever, malaise, lymphadenopathy, and hepatosplenomegaly. Thus infectious mononucleosis is an immunopathological disease.

X-linked lymphoproliferative disease (fatal infectious mononucleosis) (OMIM 308 240)

An extremely rare genetically determined susceptibility to EBV occurs in young males of certain kindreds, who develop X-linked lymphoproliferative (XLP) disease following primary infection. This presents initially with acute mononucleosis-like symptoms, but progresses inexorably to haemophagocytosis, which culminates in the necrotic destruction of vital organs, leading to multisystem failure. The mutated X-chromosomal gene (SAP; SH2D1A) responsible for this defect is involved in the normal regulation of T cell and natural killer (NK) cell responses. In patients with XLP, the numbers of cytotoxic T and NK cells are amplified even more dramatically than in classical infectious mononucleosis, and the inflammatory cytokines released from these cells are probably responsible for initiating the haemophagocytosis.

Chronic active EBV infection

There are very rare cases of infectious mononucleosis that fail to resolve, and may continue for years, often developing serious complications leading to death. These cases of chronic active EBV infection can occur in both sexes, are not familially linked, and are more common in people of Asian than European descent.

Symptoms and signs

Persistent fever, lymphadenopathy, and hepatosplenomegaly are frequently accompanied or followed by anaemia, thrombocytopenia, and mononuclear cell haemophagocytosis. The disease can therefore lead to a clinical endpoint not unlike that seen in fatal XLP, but by a different pathogenetic route.

Pathogenesis and treatment

Chronic active EBV infection is unique, in that the virus infects T and/or NK cells, which appear to escape normal immune controls and so proliferate, infiltrating vital organs and releasing the cytokines that are thought to initiate haemophagocytosis. Later on, some of these patients develop monoclonal EBV-positive T- or NK-cell lymphomas.

There is no satisfactory treatment for this disease, but haematopoietic stem cell transplantation is being evaluated.

Endemic ('African') Burkitt's lymphoma

The classical form of this B-cell tumour, first described by Burkitt in 1958, is found in those parts of Africa and Papua New Guinea where the temperature does not fall below 16°C, and the annual rainfall does not fall below 55 cm. Endemic Burkitt's lymphoma is a disease of childhood, is extremely rare over the age of 14 years, and in endemic areas is more common than all other childhood tumours added together.

The association between latent EBV infection and the cells of endemic Burkitt's lymphoma is so close (virtually 100%) that it is generally accepted that the virus is essential, although it requires combination with cofactors in a complicated chain of events to lead to the malignancy. Hyperendemic malaria has been identified as an important cofactor, and its spread by anopheline mosquitoes requiring warmth and moisture explains the climate dependence.

A much rarer, sporadic form of Burkitt's lymphoma occurs worldwide, and there is a remarkably high incidence in AIDS patients (see 'Sporadic Burkitt's lymphoma' below).

Symptoms and signs

The endemic tumour is usually multifocal, and the symptoms depend entirely on the anatomical location. Jaw tumours are present in 70% of patients, are the usual presenting feature, may be multiple in all four quadrants, and are almost always accompanied by tumours elsewhere. The rapidly growing mass causes loosening of teeth, and exophthalmos from orbital spread. Abdominal tumours involve retroperitoneal nodes, liver, ovaries, intestines,

and kidneys. Burkitt's lymphoma sometimes presents in the thyroid, the adolescent female breast, the testicles, and salivary glands; extradural tumours in the spine cause rapid paraplegia, and skeletal tumours also occur. Characteristically Burkitt's lymphoma does not involve the spleen or peripheral lymph nodes. The tumours are firm, very rapidly growing, painless, and cause minimal constitutional disturbance. Their site determines the clinical signs.

Differential diagnosis

In endemic areas, Burkitt's lymphoma can be diagnosed from the clinical picture. Unlike Burkitt's lymphoma, retinoblastoma is intraocular; rhabdomyosarcoma is extraorbital, and does not involve teeth; nephroblastoma is not multifocal; and neuroblastoma and ovarian tumours can be distinguished histologically. Paraplegia of tuberculous origin causes vertebral collapse, and acute transverse myelitis is preceded by pain and fever. The anatomical distribution of other lymphomas is quite different.

Laboratory diagnosis

Histological examination of a biopsy sample is clearly diagnostic. Antibodies to EBV antigens show a unique pattern, and titres rise or fall with disease progression or response to therapy. IgG anti-VCA titres are around 10-fold higher than in controls, and antibodies to EBV-restricted early antigens and membrane antigens are also detectable.

Clinical course and treatment

Tumour growth is relentless, and death ensues within a few months in the absence of treatment.

Surgery and radiotherapy are ineffective, but moderate courses of chemotherapy give excellent results. Cyclophosphamide, the drug of choice, remains effective after relapses.

Pathogenesis

EBV expresses a very limited range of latent gene products in Burkitt's tumour cells. When combined with a key cellular genetic change—a chromosomal translocation that causes hyperexpression of the *MYC* oncogene—these viral gene products appear to complete the malignant conversion of the target cell giving rise to Burkitt's lymphoma. Cofactors such as hyperendemic malaria may contribute, both by chronically stimulating cell—thought to be a germinal centre B cell—turnover in the B-cell system, thereby increasing the chances of rare chromosomal translocations occurring, and also by disturbing the normal virus–host balance, thereby enlarging the pool of EBV-infected cells in the body. It is clear that the virus is a necessary, but not sufficient element in the aetiology of endemic Burkitt's lymphoma.

Sporadic Burkitt's lymphoma

These tumours are seen in children worldwide, but generally at a much lower incidence than endemic Burkitt's lymphoma. The association of these tumours with EBV varies from 15 to 20% in the Western world, where the disease is quite rare, to more than 50% in other areas, where the incidence is intermediate between the two extremes. The role of EBV, when present, is unclear.

Symptoms and signs

Unlike endemic Burkitt's lymphoma, the sporadic form very rarely involves the jaws, and frequently presents in lymph nodes and within the abdomen. The clinical features depend on the location of the tumours.

Diagnosis

The tumour must be distinguished from large-cell and undifferentiated non-Hodgkin's lymphoma by histological examination of biopsies. The *MYC* translocation invariably found in endemic Burkitt's lymphoma is also present in sporadic tumours.

Treatment

The response to chemotherapy is not usually as good as in endemic Burkitt's lymphoma. Cyclophosphamide alone is inadequate; combination therapy is required, and survival after relapse is uncommon.

Lymphoproliferation in immunosuppressed states

T-cell impairment, whether congenital, or caused by immunosuppressive therapy or HIV infection, relaxes host control over persisting EBV infection, leading to increased virus replication in the oral cavity, and increased numbers of circulating virus-carrying B lymphocytes. The higher antigen load induces higher levels of serum antiviral antibodies. This reactivated infection is asymptomatic, but greater degrees of T-cell impairment can lead to the development of EBV-associated lymphoproliferative disease.

In transplant recipients

Transplant recipients who receive lifelong immunosuppressive drugs have up to 100-fold increase in their risk of developing lymphoproliferative disease and lymphoma, compared with normal immunocompetent individuals. Most of these tumours occur within the first year of transplantation, are frequently oligoclonal and consist of EBV-positive B cells expressing the same range of proteins as seen in EBV-transformed lymphoblastoid cell lines in culture. Such lesions arise through a failure of virus-specific immune T cell surveillance and, accordingly, occur with highest incidence in the most heavily immunosuppressed patients, particularly those (most often children) who were uninfected by the virus pretransplant and acquired it in the peritransplant period. The virus therefore appears to be both necessary and sufficient cause of such lymphoproliferative disease. Initial treatment is to reduce immunosuppressive drugs, with or without aciclovir therapy. Experimental treatments with EBV-specific cytotoxic T-cell infusions, or monoclonal antibody (rituximab) to the B-cell surface antigen CD20, have recently shown encouraging results. In addition, it is clear that transplant recipients receiving low but continual immunosuppression also have an increased longer term risk of lymphoma development. Some of these late tumours resemble the above lymphoproliferative lesions, whereas others are monoclonal B cell lymphomas of more varied type only some of which are EBV-positive; the role of the virus in this latter context is unclear.

In HIV/AIDS patients

Two types of lymphoma are seen in patients with HIV infection: large-cell lymphoma and Burkitt's lymphoma, both of which may be associated with EBV.

Large-cell lymphomas similar to those found in transplant recipients (see above) occur in severely immunocompromised patients with AIDS. Their distribution is extranodal, involving many unusual sites, most commonly the central nervous system. At least 50% of these tumours are EBV-positive, and this reaches 100% for cerebral tumours. The progress is rapid, with a mean survival time from diagnosis of 3 to 4 months. Radiotherapy is disappointing because patients with late-stage AIDS are in such poor general health.

Burkitt's lymphoma occurs earlier in the course of HIV disease, while the immune system is still relatively intact, and is therefore more amenable to treatment. Some 30 to 40% of these lymphomas contain EBV DNA.

Hodgkin's lymphoma

There has long been a suspicion that EBV is involved in the induction of Hodgkin's lymphoma, because of the similarity between the age and social class-dependence of this tumour's epidemiology and that of infectious mononucleosis. More recently it has become clear that infectious mononucleosis carries with it an increased risk of developing Hodgkin's lymphoma over the next 10 years. The overall risk is 4-fold but considerably higher within 2–3 years of the original attack of infectious mononucleosis; most of the resulting tumours are the EBV-positive form of Hodgkin's disease. The tumour is derived from post-germinal-centre B cells, and in virus-associated cases, EBV DNA is present and expressed as a monoclonal infection among the entire malignant population of Reed–Sternberg and mononuclear Hodgkin's cells.

In developed countries, up to 50% of Hodgkin's lymphomas are EBV-positive, and show an age-dependent distribution; EBV-positive cases occur relatively rarely in children (mainly boys), but more often in older adults, who characteristically develop the mixed cellularity type of disease. By contrast, nodular sclerosing type tumours, mainly occurring in young adults, are rarely EBV-associated.

In developing countries, the incidence of Hodgkin's lymphoma is high in young boys, and there is also an increased incidence in older people. Overall, 80% of these tumours are EBV positive.

Although the monoclonality of both the tumour cells and, where present, the virus suggest a causal relationship, there is insufficient evidence to be certain, indicating a pressing need for further investigations.

Nasopharyngeal carcinoma

This tumour is restricted to the postnasal space, where it arises from squamous epithelial cells. It is always heavily infiltrated by nonmalignant T cells, and is thus sometimes designated a lymphoepithelioma. The tumour is seen rarely throughout the world, but has a remarkably high incidence among the people of southern China, and the Inuit and related circumpolar peoples. In high-incidence areas, nasopharyngeal carcinoma is the most common cancer of men, and the second most common of women. The disease also occurs with intermediate incidence in Malays, Dyaks, Indonesians, Filipinos, and Vietnamese people, as well as in a belt stretching across North Africa, through Sudan, to the Kenyan highlands.

The tumour usually occurs in middle or old age, but in North Africa it has bimodal age peaks, one involving young people up to 20 years old and a second, much later in life. Irrespective of geographical region, nasopharyngeal carcinoma cells always carry the EBV genome and express viral latent proteins.

Symptoms and signs

Nasopharyngeal carcinoma causes nasal obstruction, discharge, or bleeding; deafness, tinnitus, or earache; and headache and ocular paresis from tumour spread to involve the cranial nerves. Patients may present with a single symptom caused locally by the tumour, or with several symptoms, and about one-third complain only of cervical lymph-node enlargement resulting from metastatic spread from an occult primary tumour.

Direct spread from the primary tumour may involve the soft tissues, bone, parotid gland, buccal cavity, and oropharynx. The neoplasm may extend into the nasal fossae, the paranasal sinuses, or the orbit, and can invade the eustachian tube or the parapharyngeal space, where cranial nerves IX, X, XI, and XII can be involved. Invasion of the skull or cranial foramina may damage cranial nerves II, IV, V, and VI. Lymphatic spread causes enlarged cervical lymph nodes, and subsequently extends to the supraclavicular glands. If bloodborne metastases occur, they are most frequent in the bones, liver, and lungs, but may be in any organ.

Differential diagnosis

Nasopharyngeal carcinoma must be distinguished from other tumours of the nasal cavities, namely adenocarcinomas, sarcomas, malignant lymphomas, and rare malignancies such as chordoma, teratoma, and melanoma.

Laboratory diagnosis

The diagnosis of nasopharyngeal carcinoma is made histologically on a biopsy sample of the primary tumour or an enlarged cervical lymph node. Serum antibody titres to EBV antigens show a characteristic reaction pattern—IgG and IgA antibodies to VCA and diffuse early antigen are raised, with the titre correlating with the tumour burden. Uniquely, IgA antibodies to VCA and early antigen are also found in patients' saliva. These antibody patterns often arise many months before the onset of tumour growth, and have been used in a high-incidence area of China to screen the population.

Treatment

Untreated nasopharyngeal carcinoma progresses inexorably to death, but it responds well to radiotherapy, which is the treatment of choice. In the earliest stages of the disease, radiotherapy gives 5-year survival rates of 50% or more, and of those surviving for 5 years, 70% remain permanently free of relapse. The more advanced stages of nasopharyngeal carcinoma have correspondingly worse prognoses.

Pathogenesis

EBV is now widely accepted as an essential element in the causation of nasopharyngeal carcinoma. Early studies showed that 100% of undifferentiated nasopharyngeal carcinomas are EBV positive, and recent studies have also detected viral DNA in some differentiated tumours. Thus all forms of nasopharyngeal carcinoma, irrespective of whether they originate in high- or low-incidence areas, may be associated with EBV. Both the tumour cells and the EBV genomes within them are clonal, indicating that the malignancy arises from a single malignantly transformed EBV-infected epithelial cell. Evidence from EBV latency genes expressed in nasopharyngeal carcinoma and premalignant lesions shows that viral gene products contribute to the abnormal proliferation.

Nonviral aetiological factors include racial and genetic predispositions; many cases among southern Chinese people show a clear familial link, and certain HLA haplotypes are associated with the disease. Epidemiological studies also suggest that environmental cofactors associated with the Chinese way of life play a role. Two likely candidates are (1) traditional herbal medicines containing tumour-promoting phorbol ester-type substances, taken as snuff, and (2) traditional salted fish, which has been shown to contain carcinogenic nitrosamines.

Salivary gland lymphoepithelioma

These relatively rare tumours resemble nasopharyngeal carcinoma, both histologically and in their prevalence in southern Chinese and circumpolar populations. Although some are in reality nasopharyngeal cancers that have spread to the parotid gland from occult primaries, others are clearly of salivary gland origin. The EBV genome, which is clonal in all the malignant epithelial cells, is not found in any other type of salivary gland tumour. The association with EBV has not been sufficiently explored to assess its significance.

Gastric carcinoma

About 10% of gastric carcinomas worldwide are EBV genome-positive, including all the rare gastric tumours of lymphoepithelioma type, and a minority of common adenocarcinomas. The viral genome is again found in every cell of the EBV-positive tumour, and is monoclonal, providing another example of a tumour arising from a single EBV-infected cell.

Although there is some evidence that EBV gene products contribute to the maintenance of the malignant condition, the role of the virus remains elusive.

Smooth-muscle tumours, T- and NK-cell lymphomas

Surprisingly, certain rare tumours of other cell lineages are consistently EBV positive. These include leiomyomas and leiomyosarcomas, whose incidence is raised in children immunosuppressed by AIDS or after organ transplantation, and those T- and NK-cell lymphomas of the nasal cavity that were previously categorized as lethal midline granulomas. The latter tumours are more common in men than women, and in Asian and South American populations than those of European descent. Presentation is usually in the midline of the face at the nose, or with destructive lesions of the soft palate, or multiple intranasal masses. Other rare forms of T- and NK-cell lymphoma are also associated with chronic active EBV infection (see 'Chronic active EBV infection' above).

Hairy leukoplakia

This nonmalignant lesion occurs in people with HIV, and in other immunosuppressed patients. It usually presents with painless white patches on the tongue or the lateral buccal mucosa. The lesions are usually multiple, up to 3 cm in diameter, slightly raised, poorly demarcated, and have a hairy or corrugated surface.

The differentiated squamous epithelial cells contain large amounts of actively replicating EBV, providing the only example of disease resulting from productive infection by the virus. Such exuberant production of EBV in epithelial cells is also exceptional. Aciclovir treatment arrests virus replication, and the lesions regress, but only for as long as the drug is continued.

Further reading

Bar RS, *et al.* (1974). Fatal infectious mononucleosis in a family. *N Engl J Med*, **290**, 363–7. [The first account of an XLP syndrome family.]

Burkitt D (1958). A sarcoma involving the jaws of African children. *Br J Surg*, **46**, 218–3. [The first description of Burkitt's lymphoma.]

Burkitt D (1963). A lymphoma syndrome in tropical Africa. *Int Rev Exp Pathol*, **2**, 67–138. [An early comprehensive review of Burkitt's lymphoma.]

de Thé, *et al.* (1978). Epidemiological evidence for a causal relationship between Epstein–Barr virus and Burkitt's lymphoma: results of the prospective Ugandan study. *Nature*, **274**, 756–61. [A massive investigation linking EBV to the causation of Burkitt's lymphoma.]

Dharnidkana VR, *et al.* (eds) (2010). Post-transplant lymphoproliferative disorders. Springer-Verlag, Berlin Heidelberg. [An up-to-date survey.

Epstein A (1999). On the discovery of Epstein–Barr virus: a memoir. *Epstein–Barr Virus Report*, **6**, 58–63. [Details of how EBV was discovered.]

Epstein MA, Achong BG, Barr YM (1964). Virus particles in cultured lymphoblasts from Burkitt's lymphoma. *Lancet*, **i**, 702–3. [The first report of the discovery of EBV.]

Gottschalk S, Rooney CM, Heslop HE. Post-transplant lymphoproliferative disorders. *Annu Rev Med* 2005, **56**, 29–44. [A recent review of PTLD and its treatment.]

Greenspan JS, *et al.* (1985). Replication of Epstein–Barr virus within the epithelial cells of oral hairy leukoplakia, an AIDS-associated lesion. *N Engl J Med*, **313**, 1564–71. [The first description of the condition.]

Henle G, Henle W, Diehl V (1968). The relation of Burkitt's lymphoma tumor-associated herpesvirus to infectious mononucleosis. *Proc Natl Acad Sci (USA)*, **59**, 94–101. [The account of the original findings identifying EBV as the cause of infectious mononucleosis.]

Hjalgrim H *et al.* (2003). Characteristics of Hodgkin's lymphoma after infectious mononucleosis. *N Engl J Med*, **349**, 1324–32. [Describes associations between EBV and Hodgkin's lymphoma.]

Hislop AD, *et al.* (2007). Cellular responses to virus infection in humans: lessons from Epstein–Barr virus. *Annu Rev Immunol*, **25**, 587–617. [This review surveys current ideas on T-cell control of EBV infection.]

Hoagland RK (1955). Transmission of infectious mononucleosis. *Am J Med Sci*, **229**, 262–72. [The first recognition of infectious mononucleosis as the 'kissing disease'.]

Kuppers R (2003). B cells under influence: transformation of B cells by Epstein–Barr virus. *Nat Rev Immunol*, **3**, 801–12. [A good account of the pathogenesis of lymphomas.]

Rafailidis PI, *et al.* (2010). Antiviral treatment for severe EBV infections in apparently immunocompetent patients. *J Clin Virol*, **49**, 151–7.

Rickinson AB, Kieff E (2007). Epstein–Barr virus. In: Knipe DM, *et al.* (eds). Fields Virology, 5th edition, vol. 2, pp. 2655–700. Lippincott, Williams and Wilkins, Philadelphia. [A comprehensive review of recent work on EBV.]

Robertson ES (ed) (2005). *The Epstein–Barr virus*. Caister Academic Press, Wymondham. [A multiauthor work covering all aspects of the virus and its associated diseases.]

Schlossberg D (ed) (1989). *Infectious mononucleosis*, 2nd edition. Springer Verlag, Berlin. [A multiauthor work covering many aspects of the disease.]

Sprunt TP, Evans FA (1920). Mononuclear leucocytosis in reaction to acute infections ('infectious mononucleosis'). *Bulletin of the Johns Hopkins Hosp*, **31**, 410–17. [The first description of infectious mononucleosis.]

Torre D, Tambini R (1999). Acyclovir for treatment of infectious mononucleosis: a meta-analysis. *Scand J Infect Dis*, **31**, 543–7.

Vouloumanou EK, *et al.* (2012). Current diagnosis and management of infectious mononucleosis. *Curr Opin Hematol*, **19**, 14–20.

Young LS, Rickinson AB (2004). Epstein–Barr virus: 40 years on. *Nat Rev Cancer*, **4**, 757–68. [A helpful discussion of the biology and oncogenicity of EBV.]

5.4 **Poxviruses**

Geoffrey L. Smith

Essentials

Poxviruses are large, complex DNA viruses that have played several seminal roles in medicine and biological science. Cowpox virus was introduced by Jenner as the first human vaccine in 1796; widespread vaccination with vaccinia virus led to the global eradication of smallpox in 1977, the only human disease to have been eradicated.

Smallpox—caused by variola virus, the most infamous poxvirus. A systemic infection, spread by the respiratory route, with characteristic skin blisters that had a centrifugal distribution on the body and, with variola major, produced mortality rates of 30 to 40% in unvaccinated populations.

Other poxviruses—molluscum contagiosum is the only other poxvirus that infects only humans, causing benign skin tumours that may be single or multiple, typically persisting for months before undergoing spontaneous regression (see Chapter 5.28). Several other poxviruses may cause zoonotic infections in humans, including cowpox virus, vaccinia virus, monkeypox virus, orf virus, psuedocowpox virus, tanapox virus and Yaba monkey tumour virus.

The development of vaccinia virus as an expression vector pioneered the concept of using genetically engineered viruses as live vaccines. Poxviruses remain excellent models for studying virus-host interactions and virus immune evasion strategies.

Introduction

Poxviruses are large DNA viruses that replicate in the cell cytoplasm. The most infamous was variola virus, which caused smallpox, a disease responsible for devastating epidemics with up to 40% mortality and which influenced human history. Smallpox was eradicated (in 1977) by immunoprophylaxis with vaccinia virus, a related orthopoxvirus. Since then, poxvirus infections in humans have been restricted to molluscum contagiosum (Chapter 5.28) and rare zoonoses such as monkeypox, cowpox, orf virus (Chapter 5.27), pseudocowpox, Yaba monkey tumour virus, and tanapox.

Classification

The *Poxviridae* is divided into the *Entomopoxvirinae* and *Chordopoxvirinae* subfamilies whose members infect insects and chordates, respectively. The *Chordopoxvirinae* is subdivided into eight genera (Table 5.4.1), although other genera are likely to be created based on the phylogenetic analysis of genome sequences of eclectic viruses such as deerpox virus and crocodilepox virus (see http://www.poxvirus.org). Viruses within different genera are antigenically distinct, while those within a genus are cross-reactive and cross-protective. Orthopoxviruses have been the most important for humans (Table 5.4.1), and four of the nine poxviruses that infect humans are orthopoxviruses: cowpox, variola, monkeypox, and vaccinia virus. Different orthopoxviruses are distinguishable by their biological properties such as pock type and ceiling

Table 5.4.1 Poxvirus classification

Subfamily	Genus	Species
Entomopoxvirinae		
Chordopoxvirinae	Orthopoxvirus	*Variola virus
		*Vaccinia virus
		*Monkeypox virus
		*Cowpox virus
		Ectromelia virus
		Camelpox virus
		Taterapox virus
	Capripoxvirus	Sheeppox virus
		Goatpox virus
		Lumpy skin disease virus
	Parapoxvirus	*Orf virus
		*Pseudocowpox virus
	Avipoxvirus	Fowlpox virus
		Canarypox virus
	Suipoxvirus	Swinepox virus
	Leporipoxvirus	Myxoma virus
		Shope fibroma virus
	Molluscipoxvirus	*Molluscum contagiosum virus
	Yatapoxvirus	*Yaba monkey tumour virus
		*Tanapox virus

* Viruses that infect humans.

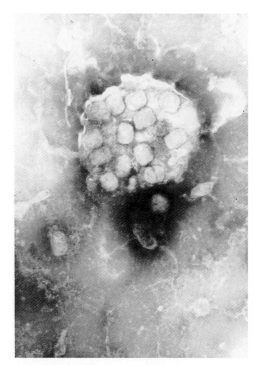

Fig. 5.4.1 Electron micrograph of material from smallpox lesion, viewed by negative contrast, showing a clump of poxvirus particles.
(Courtesy of the late Henry Bedson.)

temperature on the chorioallantoic membrane, or by the restriction pattern of genomic DNA and the genome sequences that have enabled development of species-specific polymerase chain reaction (PCR) detection methods. Vaccinia virus has no known natural animal reservoir and its origin remains a mystery. It caused human disease only as a rare complication after vaccination against smallpox. Cowpox and monkeypox viruses were named after the species from which they were isolated, but the natural reservoir of each virus is rodents. Infections in cows or monkeys, like the occasional transmission to humans, are zoonoses. Human monkeypox virus infections are often caused by handling or consumption of infected 'bush meat'. In 2003, there was an outbreak of monkeypox in the United States of America following the importation of Gambian rodents carrying the virus. Cowpox, monkeypox, and vaccinia viruses have a broad host range, while variola virus infected only humans and the lack of an animal reservoir aided the smallpox eradication campaign.

Poxvirus biology

Poxviruses replicate in the cytoplasm, encode enzymes for transcription and DNA replication, and have large, complex virions (Fig. 5.4.1) and double stranded DNA genomes of 134 to 360 kb. Vaccinia virus is the most intensively studied poxvirus. It encodes about 200 genes (the exact number varying with the strain of virus) of three classes (early, intermediate, and late) that are expressed in a strictly regulated manner. Transcription of each class is dependent upon the prior expression of the previous class.

Virus morphogenesis is complex (Fig. 5.4.2a) and produces two forms of infectious virion: intracellular mature virus (IMV) and extracellular enveloped virus (EEV). IMV remains within the cell until cell lysis and forms most of the progeny, whereas EEV is released by exocytosis (Fig. 5.4.2b) before cell death and represents a small fraction of total infectivity. EEV possesses an additional lipid envelope with which several virus proteins are associated, giving it distinct immunological and biological properties. EEV is necessary for efficient virus dissemination *in vitro* and within the infected host. Immunity to EEV-specific antigens, which are highly conserved among orthopoxviruses, is required for protection against disease and the B5 protein on the EEV surface is the only EEV-specific antigen against which neutralizing Abs are directed.

Pathogenesis

Poxvirus infections cause a local skin lesion or generalized pustular rash. Detailed experimental analysis of human smallpox was impossible, but generalized poxvirus infections have been studied in experimental models, namely monkeypox in monkeys, rabbitpox (a neurovirulent vaccinia virus) in rabbits, ectromelia virus in mice, and myxoma virus in European rabbits. The spread of variola virus in humans was probably similar to that of the ectromelia virus in mice and is characterized by sequential phases of virus infection, replication, and release accompanied by cell necrosis. In the case of vaccinia virus, recent studies of poxvirus entry into cells suggested a two-step process, implicating an unprecedented number of viral proteins and host cellular components involved in signalling and actin rearrangement for initiation of virus–cell membrane fusion.

Virus enters through skin abrasions (ectromelia and cowpox) or inhalation of airborne virus and establishes a respiratory infection (ectromelia, rabbitpox, and variola). In smallpox, the respiratory

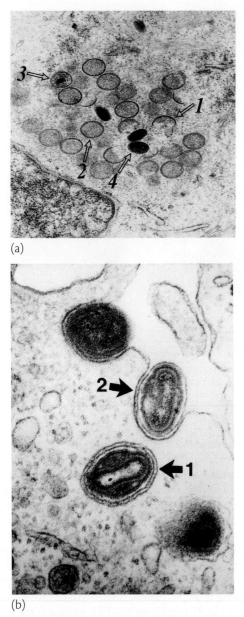

(a)

(b)

Fig. 5.4.2 Electron micrographs showing (a) a cytoplasmic vaccinia virus factory containing maturing virus particles with stages of morphogenesis numbered 1 to 4 and (b) fully enveloped virus particles, one of which is leaving the cell by exocytosis.

distribution (Figs. 5.4.3–5.4.5). Lesions started with a papule that became pustular and then crusted. After 2 to 3 weeks the scab was shed leaving a scar. The incubation period of smallpox was approximately 12 days. Symptoms included headache, fever, malaise, vomiting, and, in severe cases, prostration, toxaemia, and hypotension. Delayed onset of the skin eruptions usually correlated with a grave prognosis. Haemorrhagic or flat confluent-type smallpox had very high mortality rates.

The outcome of infection depended upon the age and physiological and immunological status of the patient and the strain of virus. Variola major was more virulent and produced fatality rates in unvaccinated patients of between 5 and 40%, while the milder variola minor, called alastrim in the Americas, caused only 0.1 to 2% mortality. Morphologically, the viruses were indistinguishable, and vaccination with vaccinia virus was equally effective against both. However, alastrim virus was consistently more thermolabile and had a lower ceiling temperature of 37.5 °C compared to 38.5 °C for variola major, 39 °C for monkeypox, 40 °C for cowpox, and 41 °C for vaccinia virus. The genomes of nearly 50 variola virus strains isolated from different places in the world at different times have been sequenced and compared, allowing the spread and evolution of variola virus in humans to be analysed. Comparisons of variola major and minor virus strains showed the genomes are very closely related, but there are too many minor differences to provide an understanding of why these viruses produced such different mortality rates in humans.

Very young and old patients were most susceptible to smallpox, and those aged 5 to 20 years most resistant. Pregnancy and immunological deficiency, particularly in cell-mediated immunity, increased the severity of infection. Pregnant women were more likely than any other group to develop haemorrhagic-type

route was the most important and sometimes the only possible route of transmission from index cases to contacts; also patients became infectious only after enanthem developed. A respiratory infection was established in the epithelial cells of the alveoli and small bronchioles. Here, alveolar macrophages became infected and transmitted the virus via lymphatics to the local lymph node, where further virus replication occurred. Virus released into the blood (primary viraemia) was mostly cell-associated and spread to other organs of the reticuloendothelial system, notably the liver, spleen, and lymph nodes.

Extensive replication here released larger amounts of virus into the blood (secondary viraemia) enabling the virus to infect other organs such as the kidneys, lungs, and intestines and to reach the skin and produce the skin lesions with the characteristic centrifugal

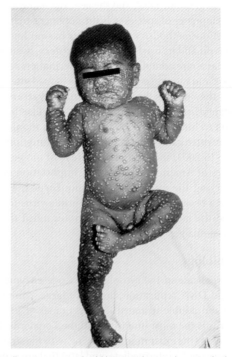

Fig. 5.4.3 Smallpox in a 9-month-old boy in Pakistan, photographed on the eighth day of the rash.
(Courtesy of the World Health Organization.)

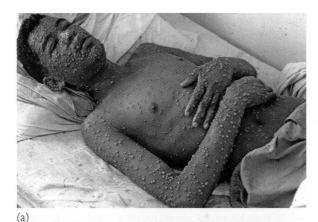

(a)

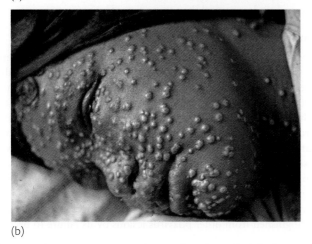

(b)

Fig. 5.4.4 Ethiopian patient, in 1968, showing classical centrifugal distribution of lesions with fewer on trunk (a) than on face (b).
(Copyright D A Warrell.)

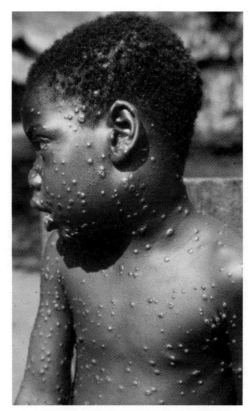

Fig. 5.4.5 Moderately severe monkeypox in a girl of 7 years from Équateur Province, Democratic Republic of the Congo.
(Courtesy of the World Health Organization.)

smallpox, which was usually fatal. The greater importance of cell-mediated immunity rather than antibody in recovery from poxvirus infections was illustrated in several ways. Firstly, in children with severe defects in cell-mediated immunity there was a progressive and uncontrolled virus replication from the vaccination site that was usually fatal. In contrast, defects in antibody production were usually tolerated if the cell-mediated immune response was normal. Secondly, passive administration of antivaccinia virus serum had little effect on mice infected with ectromelia virus, whereas prior infection with vaccinia virus was protective. Thirdly, in mice infected with ectromelia virus, the effective mechanisms that combated infection in the liver and spleen were operative by 4 to 6 days postinfection and coincided with the maximum levels of cytolytic T cells, but preceded the development of systemic antibody.

The eradication of smallpox

Early attempts to control smallpox relied upon variolation or inoculation, in which material isolated from a mild case of smallpox was administered by sniffing or scratching. This was replaced by vaccination in 1798 after Jenner noticed that milkmaids, who often acquired cowpox infections on their hands from the teats of cows, were protected from smallpox. Jenner infected a boy (James Phipps) with poxvirus material (probably cowpox), derived from a cow via a milkmaid (Sarah Nelmes), and challenged him subsequently with smallpox. Protection was achieved and, due to

the efficacy and greater safety of this procedure, it rapidly replaced variolation. Sometime between 1798 and the 20th century vaccinia virus replaced cowpox virus as the smallpox vaccine. In 1959, the World Health Organization (WHO) adopted a recommendation to achieve the global eradication of smallpox. With fresh funding and a plentiful supply of potent freeze-dried vaccine this goal was achieved in 1977. Two years later, the WHO certified that eradication was complete. This triumph of preventive medicine justifies the saying 'prevention is better than cure', but also demonstrates that prevention is best achieved by eradication.

Threat of bioterrorism

Debate continues about what should be done with remaining stocks of variola virus and how the world might prepare itself for bioterrorism employing this agent. Apart from stockpiling vaccine, use of cidofovir, even in an inhaled micronized aerosol as emergency postexposure treatment, is being explored.

Poxvirus genome sequences

The DNA sequence of about 80 orthopoxvirus genomes has been determined (see http://www.poxvirus.org), including 48 strains of variola virus, 14 vaccinia virus strains, nine strains of monkeypox virus, and at least one strain of most orthopoxviruses. The central region (about 100 kb) of these genomes is very highly conserved and 89 of the genes within this region are present in every sequenced chordopoxvirus. These genes probably represent the core genome of an ancestral poxvirus from which the current poxviruses evolved. During their evolution poxviruses acquired additional genes that became located in the more variable terminal regions of the genome and these give each virus its characteristic host range, virulence, and tropism. These genes vary in number and type between poxviruses, and encode nonessential proteins that affect virus virulence, host range, and immune modulation. A surprising feature of some orthopoxviruses is the fragmentation of several genes that are intact in other viruses, indicating that orthopoxvirus evolution has involved both gain and loss of gene function. The retention of these nonfunctional genes by some viruses, such as variola, suggests that they became nonfunctional in the relatively recent evolutionary past, and perhaps that variola virus is a 'recent' human pathogen that never became fully adapted to humans.

Poxvirus expression vectors

Vaccinia virus recombinants expressing foreign genes were developed in 1982 and have become a widely used laboratory tool; they are also being engineered as live vaccines for infectious disease and cancer. Infection with the recombinant virus allows expression and simultaneous delivery of the foreign antigen to the immune system. Moreover, the large capacity of vaccinia virus allows expression of multiple foreign genes from a single virus so creating polyvalent vaccines. Safer vaccinia virus strains that do not cause vaccination complications (eczema vaccinatum, generalized vaccinia, progressive vaccinia, encephalopathy (<2 years), or encephalitis (>2 years)) are being created by genetic engineering. An alternative strategy is to use poxviruses that establish only abortive infections in human cells, such as modified vaccinia Ankara (MVA) or the avipoxviruses fowlpox virus and canarypox virus.

Human monkeypox

Monkeypox was discovered in captive primates in 1958, but in 1970 was isolated in the tropical rainforests of West and Central Africa from humans who had suffered generalized poxvirus rashes visibly very similar to smallpox. The virus is quite distinct from variola in biological properties such as pock morphology, ceiling temperature, and lesion morphology on rabbit skin, and its genome sequence. Moreover, although monkeypox virus produced a very similar disease to smallpox in humans, person-to-person transmission was inefficient. Thus, human monkeypox virus infections are single or multiple sporadic cases restricted to dense tropical rainforests in Central and West Africa. Clinically, human monkeypox closely resembles ordinary, discrete-type smallpox except that there is a pronounced lymph node enlargement (Fig. 5.4.5). Two clades of monkeypox virus have been identified (from Central or West Africa) that differ in their virulence in humans. The Central African strains gave mortality rates in unvaccinated children (<8 years old) between 1970 and 1986 of 11.2%. In contrast, West African strains, such as the one that caused an epidemic in the United States of America in 2003, are milder and no mortalities were reported.

Prevention and treatment

In endemic parts of Africa, or in the face of new epizootics, use of current smallpox vaccine has been discussed, but the prevalence of HIV/AIDS in some areas would restrict widespread, safe use of this approach. Cidofovir cured monkeys infected with monkeypox virus.

Cowpox virus and pseudocowpox virus

Cowpox virus has a broad host range including cattle, humans, large felines, and even elephants, but it is not enzootic in cattle and its natural hosts are rodents. It is distinguishable from vaccinia virus by the pock type, ceiling temperature, genome size and sequence, and the production of cytoplasmic type A inclusion bodies. Pseudocowpox is enzootic in cattle, unlike cowpox. Historically, pseudocowpox virus was important since it was sometimes used mistakenly for vaccination and, being a parapoxvirus, was ineffective in preventing smallpox. Its misuse compromised Jenner's correct assertion that cowpox virus was an effective smallpox vaccine.

In humans, cowpox virus produces an acutely inflamed, local lesion, similar to a primary smallpox vaccination. There is usually fever, enlargement of the local lymph nodes, and pain. Unlike vaccinia virus, which occasionally produced a generalized infection (Fig. 5.4.6), cowpox virus lesions are always local. Human lesions caused by pseudocowpox virus (milker's nodules) are extremely rare and are less painful than those caused by cowpox.

Tanapox virus and Yaba monkey tumour virus

Tanapox virus and Yaba monkey tumour virus are the sole members of the *Yatapoxvirus* genus (another yatapoxvirus called Yaba-like disease virus, is considered a tanapox virus strain). These viruses are characterized by their slow replication rates in cell culture and can cause zoonotic infections in humans. Tanapox virus was isolated in the Tana valley in Kenya (1957–62) from humans suffering from localized skin lesions typical of poxviruses (Fig. 5.4.7). The virus is probably transmitted from infected monkeys by biting insects, particularly during wet weather conditions. It usually produces a solitary lesion that is preceded for a few days by a mild fever. The lesion takes 5 to 6 weeks to clear and is distinguished from other poxvirus lesions by its failure to become

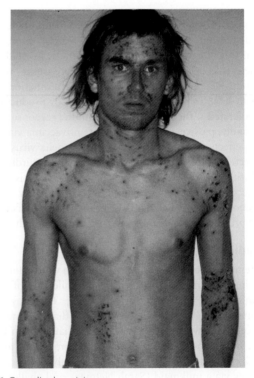

Fig. 5.4.6 Generalized vaccinia.
(Courtesy of the late Dr B E Juel-Jensen.)

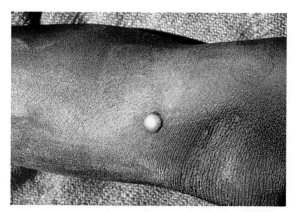

Fig. 5.4.7 Tanapox lesion on the leg of a Kenyan patient.
(Courtesy of the late P E C Manson-Bahr.)

pustular. This virus cannot be cultured on the chorioallantoic
membrane.

Yaba monkey tumour virus was discovered in Yaba, Lagos,
Nigeria in 1957 as a virus causing cutaneous histiocytomas in
rhesus monkeys and can infect humans if injected subcutaneously
or intradermally. The lesions are not neoplastic and are cleared by
the immune response.

Cutaneous poxviruses (orf virus and molluscum contagiosum virus)

See Chapters 5.27 and 5.28.

Further reading

Andrei G, Snoeck R (2010). Cidofovir activity against poxvirus infections.
Viruses, **2**, 2803–30.

Damon IK (2011). Status of human monkeypox clinical disease,
epidemiology and research. *Vaccine*, 2011 Dec 18 [Epub ahead of
print].

Di Giulio DB, Eckburg PB (2004). Human monkeypox: an emerging
zoonosis. *Lancet Infect Dis*, **4**, 15–25.

Fauquet CM, *et al.* (eds) (2005). *Virus taxonomy: Eighth Report of the
International Committee on the Taxonomy of Viruses.*
Elsevier, Amsterdam.

Fenner F, *et al.* (1988). *Smallpox and its eradication.* World Health
Organization, Geneva.

Fenner F, Wittek R, Dumbell KR (1989). *The orthopoxviruses.* Academic
Press Ltd, London.

Hwenda L, Larsen BI (2011). The remaining smallpox stocks: the wrong
debate? *Lancet*, **378**:e7; author reply e7.

Laliberte JP, et al. (2011). The membrane fusion step of vaccinia virus
entry is cooperatively mediated by multiple viral proteins and host cell
components. *PLoS Pathog*, **7**, e1002446.

Mercer AA, Schmidt A, Weber O (2007). *Poxviruses.* Berhäuser-Verlag,
Berlin.

Moss B (2007). Poxviridae: the viruses and their replication.
In: Knipe DM, *et al.* (eds) *Field's virology*, 5th edition, **2**, 2905–2946.
Lippincott Williams & Wilkins, Philadelphia.

Williams G (2010). *Angel of death: the story of smallpox.* Palgrave
Macmillan, Basingstoke.

5.5 Mumps: epidemic parotitis

B.K. Rima

Essentials

Mumps is an acute, systemic, highly infectious, communicable
infection of children and young adults, caused by a paramyxovirus
(with an RNA genome). Transmission is by airborn droplet spread.
After an incubation period of 14 to 18 days, typical presentation
is with fever, pain near the angle of the jaw, and swelling of the
parotid glands. Complications include orchitis, meningitis and
encephalitis. Diagnosis is obvious clinically in cases with a contact
history and parotitis, but serological (mumps-specific IgM and IgA)
and RNA-based (RT-PCR) tests are used when this is not the case,
e.g. the patient presenting with meningitis. Treatment is symptomatic. Prevention is by vaccination, often given as one component
of a trivalent mumps/measles/rubella (MMR) vaccine at 14 to 16
months of age.

Introduction and historical perspective

The primary clinical manifestation in mumps, swelling of the salivary glands, is so characteristic that the disease was recognized very
early as different from other childhood illnesses. Hippocrates
described the disease in the 5th century BCE and also noted swelling of the testes (orchitis) as a common complication of mumps.
In 1790, Hamilton noted the infection in the central nervous system (CNS) and meninges. In 1934, mumps was shown to be a filterable virus by Johnson and Goodpasture, who also fulfilled
Koch's postulates by infecting volunteers with virus propagated in
monkeys. Since 1967, live attenuated vaccines have been licensed
to control and prevent the infection.

Aetiology and genetics

Mumps virus (MuV) can be grown in tissue cultures of chick
embryo, monkey kidney, and most human cells. The virus can also
be cultured in the yolk sac or embryonic cavity of chick embryos.
Cytopathic changes (syncytium formation and cell rounding) may
be seen as early as 24 h postinfection and earlier if immunofluorescence is used. MuV is thermolabile. It can be stored for years at
−70 °C, but infectivity is lost in a few days at room temperature.
Treatment with ether or paraformaldehyde inactivates the virus
rapidly, but does not destroy the antigens responsible for the complement fixation, haemagglutination, or reactivity in the skin test.

MuV is an enveloped RNA virus with a genome of 15 384
nucleotides. Its inner core is a ribonucleoprotein complex (the
nucleocapsid) containing the nonsegmented, negative-strand,
RNA molecule encapsidated by the nucleocapsid protein (N).
The nucleocapsid has the herringbone structure characteristic of
paramyxoviruses (Fig. 5.5.1a). Attached to this are two further proteins involved in transcription and replication of the RNA genome:
the phosphoprotein (P) and the large replicase protein (L). The

nucleocapsid is surrounded by a lipid bilayer (Fig. 5.5.1a, b). On the inner leaflet is a membrane or matrix protein (M) that plays an essential role in virus budding. On the outer surface are two glycoproteins, one carrying the haemagglutinin-neuraminidase activity (HN), the other is the fusion protein (F). A complex between the HN and F proteins is responsible for the fusion of the virion membrane with that of the host cell. The function of a nonstructural, small, hydrophobic protein (SH) is unknown; it is associated with the endoplasmic reticulum in MuV-infected cells. The SH protein sequence is hypervariable and this is used to assign MuV strains to one of 13 currently recognized genotypes. The nonstructural V protein functions in combating the host's innate immune response by targeting STAT 1 and STAT 3 for degradation. The gene order (Fig. 5.5.1c) leads to an expression gradient in which the abundance of mRNAs decreases with increasing distance to the promoter at the 3'-terminal end of the genome, so that the N mRNA is more abundant than the L mRNA.

Epidemiology and pathogenesis

Mumps is highly infectious. Transmission depends on close personal contact with a patient who is excreting virus in the saliva and spreading it in droplets. In the prevaccine era, the peak incidence was in the late winter or early spring, in 3 to 7 year cycles. Most morbidity is associated with meningitis and orchitis. Case fatality is about 2 per 1000. The incubation period lies between 14 and 18 days. In any outbreak, 30 to 40% of those infected have subclinical illness.

MuV causes an infection of the upper respiratory tract that spreads to draining lymph nodes. The subsequent viraemia and infection of lymphocytes and macrophages causes spread to many organs, but because mumps is so rarely lethal, details are scant. Mumps virus can spread to most organs in the body. Lymphocytic infiltration and destruction of periductal cells lead to blockage of the ducts both in salivary glands and in the seminiferous tubules of the testes. The lymphatics in the tissues surrounding and overlying the parotid glands become obstructed, producing a gel-like oedema that may spread down over the chest wall, especially when the swelling of the salivary glands is severe. Rarely, mumps causes hydrocephalus by destruction of the lining of the aqueduct.

Clinical features and diagnosis

Parotitis

A patient with mumps parotitis may have a fever without rigors (40–40.5 °C) as well as pain near the angle of the jaw. The face and neck become distorted with swelling. The skin over the gland is hot and flushed but there is no rash, unlike in the swelling of erysipelas. If the swelling is severe, the mouth cannot be opened for pain and tightness, and is dry because the flow of saliva is blocked. This lasts for 3 or 4 days. Sometimes, as one side clears, the parotid on the other side swells. When there is bilateral parotitis, clinical diagnosis is usually obvious. One condition that must be excluded is bull neck diphtheria (Chapter 6.1), which can look very like mumps.

Rarely, the submaxillary and sublingual salivary glands may also be affected. The symptoms are similar to those in parotitic mumps, but it is difficult or impossible to distinguish the swelling from other forms of submaxillary swellings, especially inflammation of various groups of lymph nodes and Ludwig's angina. In mumps, the neck swelling is ill-defined and the angle of the jaw is impalpable. To determine if cervical lymph nodes are swollen from

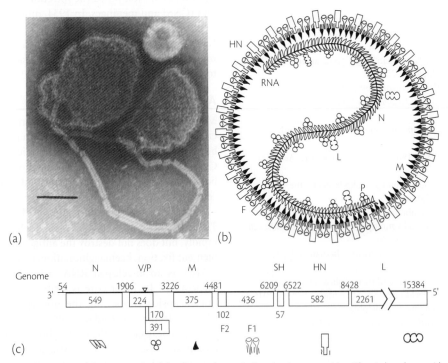

Fig. 5.5.1 Structure and genome organization of the mumps virus: (a) a disrupted, negatively stained, mumps virion. The viral nucleocapsid protrudes from the particle and the fringe of viral spikes is visible (bar = 100 nm); (b) diagram of the localization of the nucleocapsid (N), phospho- (P), large (L), matrix (M), haemagglutinin-neuraminidase (HN), and fusion (F) proteins in the mumps virion; and (c) structure of the genome of mumps virus indicating the localization of the genes, the nucleotide number of their starting and stopping position, and (in boxes) the number of amino acid residues in each of the viral proteins.

some other cause, the pharynx must be examined carefully. The fauces must be examined for signs of tonsilitis that might cause cervical adenitis. The lymph nodes in contact with the submaxillary and sublingual salivary glands drain the corner of the eye, the side of the nose, the cheeks, the lips, and the floor of the mouth, all of which must be explored, before a diagnosis of submaxillary or sublingual mumps can be made. Laboratory tests are needed to confirm the diagnosis.

In infectious mononucleosis, the glands stand out distinctly and the parotid is not affected. In septic parotitis there is more parotid tenderness; there may be fluctuation, and pus exudes from the orifice of Stensen's duct. Calculus causes spasmodic pain and swelling and may be detected radiographically. Recurrent parotitis and Mikulicz's syndrome are unlikely to be confused with mumps except in the earliest stages, nor are uveoparotid fever and tumours of the gland, as they are chronic conditions.

Orchitis

Orchitis may occur 4 or 5 days after the onset of parotitis. Quite often it occurs without preceding parotitis. It is an acute condition, with chills, sweats, headache, and backache, and a swinging temperature as well as severe local testicular pain and tenderness. The scrotum is swollen and oedematous, and the testicles are impalpable. Usually, only one testicle is affected but sometimes both: the second testicle may become affected just as the swelling of the first is subsiding. The illness lasts 3 or 4 days before the swelling begins to subside. Orchitis is unusual before the age of puberty, though it has occurred in young boys and even in infants. In adolescent and young males it develops in 1:5 cases. Some degree of atrophy of the testicle occurs in at least one-third of patients with orchitis. Azoospermia after mumps is rare and only temporary. The fear of sterility after mumps orchitis has been exaggerated and one can reassure the patient. Orchitis when it occurs without parotitis is difficult to distinguish from gonococcal epididymo-orchitis, unless there has been contact with mumps. The rare case of orchitis in infancy may resemble torsion of the testis and perhaps it is safer to operate than risk a serious misdiagnosis.

Meningitis and encephalitis

MuV frequently invades the nervous system: changes in the electroencephalogram and increased levels of protein and lymphocyte levels in the cerebrospinal fluid can be shown in at least half the patients. However, in most cases, neurological symptoms or signs are absent. Mumps virus was one of the most common known causes of lymphocytic meningitis. This may develop a few days after the start of parotitis, but almost as often it occurs in the absence of parotitis. Occasionally, the patient develops transient paralysis of limbs resulting in the occurrence of quadriplegia or single nerve paralysis in some patients. Polyneuritis, neuritis of the trigeminal or facial nerve, and retrobulbar optic neuritis have been described in mumps but all are rare. The meningitis is usually mild and self-limiting.

Mumps encephalitis is a different entity; cerebrospinal fluid is normal and contains no virus. The outlook is different. The patient is confused and may lapse into coma and remain comatose for days, weeks, or months. Almost 2% of the encephalitis cases are fatal. At autopsy there is perivascular demyelination as in other forms of postinfectious encephalitis (Oxford Textbook of Medicine 5e Chapter 24.11.2).

Other complications

Deafness is reported in up to 0.3% of the cases, but it is rarely permanent and often unilateral. Women sometimes complain of ovarian pain during an attack of mumps, but it is rarely as severe as in men with orchitis. There is no evidence that it affects fertility. Mastitis occurs in 15% of the cases, both in men and women, but it is usually mild and fleeting. Mild upper abdominal pain in about 50% of the cases may be related to viral changes in the pancreas. The amount of amylase in duodenal fluid may be less than normal. This is probably caused by a blockage of the ducts in the pancreas. Although there are anecdotal reports of diabetes occurring after an attack of mumps, there is no virological or immunological evidence for a direct link though the virus is known to be able to infect the pancreatic islet B cells.

Mumps in the fetus and infant

Abortion may occur in women with mumps in the first trimester of pregnancy. It is not common and probably not caused by direct viral damage to the fetus. The connection between primary endocardial fibroelastosis and mumps remains vague. The disease's declining incidence has been attributed to mumps vaccination. Some studies using reverse transcription polymerase chain reaction (RT-PCR) indicate that viral RNA can be amplified from myocardial samples in a high percentage of cases. However, the latter technique is open to contamination problems and hence this link remains to be confirmed. Mumps virus has not been isolated from heart tissue at autopsy and these infants have no mumps antibody in their blood. They may show a delayed hypersensitivity response to the skin test. This has not been explained, but may reflect some immune defect in the fetus which could cause myocarditis and fibroelastosis.

In the normal infant, maternal IgG passes to the fetus and seems to protect the infant against mumps during the first year of life. The typical disease of mumps in infants is a rare clinical finding, even in populations with no previous experience of the disease. MuV may be isolated in vague respiratory infections in infants.

Laboratory diagnosis

In patients without parotitis, especially meningitis, and in the absence of contact history, serological tests and RT-PCR are the only means of reaching a firm diagnosis. MuV isolation is an insensitive method and now rarely used. MuV contains several different antigenic components, which provoke distinct antibodies that are useful for laboratory confirmation. Antibody to the N protein rises in the first 2 weeks of infection but then declines rapidly. Antibody to the HN protein appears at the end of the first week, usually in high titre: it may persist for years and indicates past infection. Neutralizing antibodies also develop, but titres are a poor correlate of protection. Nowadays, sensitive enzyme immunoassays allow early diagnosis by detection of mumps-specific IgM and IgA. In recent outbreaks in the United States of America and in the United Kingdom, IgM-negative cases have been identified. IgA can be detected in saliva or mouth washings on about the fourth day after infection, and in the serum early in the disease. Measurement of antibodies in acute and convalescent sera is a reliable method for diagnosis, especially in patients who have no parotitis. RT-PCR methodology targeting the detection of mumps RNA in nose and throat swabs is being developed and slowly replaces serology based techniques in routine laboratory diagnosis and confirmation.

Treatment

There is no specific antiviral treatment. Symptomatic treatment includes simple analgesics, but for the severe pain of orchitis, morphine (15–30 mg) may be required for a day or two. Corticosteroids are worth trying in severe cases of parotitis, more especially in orchitis. An adult dose of 60 mg prednisolone daily for 2 or 3 days sometimes gives dramatic relief from pain, though it may not reduce the swelling.

Prevention and control

The mainstay of prevention is vaccination of susceptible individuals. Isolation is not effective as the patient has been infectious for days before parotitis occurs and inapparent cases are frequent. Attenuated live vaccine gives 95% seroconversion, and protection lasts for at least 15 years. In developed countries, mumps vaccine is currently given between 14 and 16 months of age as one component of a live attenuated trivalent mumps/measles/rubella (MMR) vaccine. A two-dose schedule with follow-up at 4 to 5 years of age is now recommended. This has suppressed the incidence of mumps by more than 98% in United States of America and in the United Kingdom. Nevertheless, both countries have had recent outbreaks of mumps in college age populations in both unvaccinated individuals as well as those with a documented vaccination history. It is not clear whether this is due to primary vaccine failure, or waning immunity in the absence of frequent challenge. The ability of new variant wild-type virus strains to break thought the protective immunity established by older vaccines which are largely based on genotype A strains, appears a less likely cause of the current outbreaks. Mumps vaccination is contraindicated in pregnant women and patients with immunodeficiency due to immunosuppressive therapy or disease. However, HIV seropositive children should be vaccinated with the MMR vaccine.

Further reading

Carbone KM, Rubin S (2006). Mumps virus. In: Fields BN, *et al.* (eds) Fields Virology, 5th edition, pp. 1527–550. Lippincott Williams and Wilkins, Philadelphia.

Christie AB (1980). *Infectious diseases: epidemiology and clinical practice*, 3rd edition. Churchill Livingstone, Edinburgh.

Duprex WP, Rima, BK. (August 2011) *Mumps virus*. In: eLS. 2011, John Wiley & Sons, Ltd: Chichester http://www.els.net/ [DOI: 10.1002/9780470015902.a0000419.pub3]

Feldman HA (1989). Mumps. In: Evans AJ (ed) *Viral infections of humans*, 3rd edition, pp. 471–91. Plenum Medical, New York.

Rima BK, Duprex WP (2008). Mumps virus. In: Mahy BWJ, van Regenmortel MHV (eds) *Encyclopedia of virology*, 3rd edition. Academic Press, London.

Wright KE (2006). Mumps. In: Newton VA, Vallely PJ (eds) *Infection And Hearing Loss*, pp. 109–126. John Wiley and Sons Ltd, Chichester.

5.6 Measles

H.C. Whittle and P. Aaby

Essentials

Measles is a single-stranded RNA virus that is spread by aerosolized droplets and is highly transmissible. It causes a spectrum of disease ranging from mild in the well nourished to severe in the malnourished or immunosuppressed: mortality is 3 to 10% in Africa.

Clinical features—10 to 14 days after infection the viral prodrome typically consists of runny nose and fever, sometimes also diarrhoea or convulsions; signs include mild conjunctivitis, red mucosae, and (on the buccal mucosa) Koplik's spots. After 14 to 18 days a morbilliform rash first appears on the forehead and neck, then spreads to involve the trunk and finally the limbs. Other manifestations include severe conjunctivitis (especially in those who are vitamin-A deficient), pneumonitis and enteritis (which may cause profuse diarrhoea). Early complications include (1) pneumonia—caused by secondary bacterial infection and responsible for most deaths; (2) stomatitis—caused by herpes simplex virus and/or candidal infection; (3) enteritis—due to candidal or bacterial superinfection; (4) eye infection—corneal ulceration may be caused by some combination of measles itself, herpes simplex infection, vitamin A deficiency, and use of traditional eye medicines; more than half of childhood blindness in Africa is related to measles; (5) skin and other infections, e.g. pyoderma; (6) encephalitis—occurs in 0.1 to 0.2% of cases; probably attributable to a neuroallergic process; mortality is 10 to 15%, and 25% of children are left with permanent neurological disability. Late complications include malnutrition, giant cell pneumonia and subacute sclerosing panencephalitis.

Diagnosis and treatment—diagnosis is primarily clinical, but signs may be less clear cut in vaccinated subjects. Detection of measles-specific IgM antibody or detection of measles antigen in saliva or urine may clinch the diagnosis if the rash is mild or atypical. Management is supportive, including administration of vitamin A, and with prompt treatment of secondary infections.

Prevention—(1) Passive immunization—human immunoglobulin is highly effective if given within 2 or 3 days of exposure and should be administered to those in whom vaccination is contraindicated. (2) Active immunization—live vaccine is often given in the developed world as one component of a trivalent mumps/measles/rubella (MMR) vaccine at 14 to 16 months of age. However, this is not appropriate for children in developing countries, who are infected by measles at a much earlier age, where substantial successes in controlling the disease has been obtained with a strategy combining (a) catch-up—a one-time mass campaign covering everybody aged 9 months to 14 years, regardless of previous measles or immunization; (2) keep-up—achieving a high coverage for each birth cohort; (3) follow-up—subsequent mass campaigns covering all children every 3 to 5 years; and (4) mop-up—campaigns that target children who are difficult to reach or during outbreaks. This strategy has eliminated measles from Latin America.

Introduction

Measles is an acute, highly transmissible RNA viral infection of humans that is spread by aerosolized droplets. It causes much death and suffering, especially among poor children in developing countries. Its severity varies according to host and socioeconomic factors, not to antigenic variation or alteration in virulence of the virus. There is no reservoir of infection other than in humans and no evidence of a carrier state and as there is an effective vaccine, global eradication is possible but a dauntingly high vaccine coverage of more than 95% will be needed. The virus causes a generalized infection coupled with severe damage to the immune system due to destruction of T lymphocytes, disturbance of the Th1/Th2 cytokine balance, and impaired antigenic presentation. The chief clinical features result from infection of the skin, mucous membranes, and respiratory tract. Death, which occurs in up to 15% of hospitalized children in Africa, results from secondary infections and immunosuppression. Attack rates in home contacts are very high (of the order of 90%) and long-life immunity follows the disease but not vaccination. Supplemental immunization activities allowing repeated vaccination every 3 to 5 years in endemic countries have lowered measles deaths dramatically. Although the coverage for the first dose of measles vaccine has reached 83% and measles mortality declined to 78% between 2000 and 2008, an estimated 164 000 people still die annually of measles.

Epidemiology

Measles has been the archetypical childhood infection, known and feared by all parents. Nearly everybody contracted this most infectious of childhood diseases. Measles was the single biggest cause of childhood deaths. In the prevaccination era, 6 million children may have died annually of measles. With advances in coverage during the last 25 years, the current estimate (2008) is 164,000 deaths, still the most important of the vaccine-preventable infections (Fig. 5.6.1). The severity and age of infection varies markedly between poor and rich countries. In the West, most children were infected between 3 and 6 years of age, when they attended nursery and primary schools. Mortality was low (<0.05%) and morbidity, although considerable when compared to many other common viral infections, was limited. Most cases occurred in the winter and spring, with a biannual epidemic pattern. Widespread immunization has dramatically reduced both the number of cases and complications in high income countries.

In low income countries, measles is still severe and behaves differently. It kills between 3 and 10% of children in the community and some 10 to 20% of those admitted to hospital. Mortality from measles is considerably higher in Africa (3–10%) than in Asia or South America (1%). West Africa has the highest case fatality rates. There are many reasons for this increase in severity: children are infected at 1 to 2 years of age; severe malnutrition leads to prolonged, severe measles. Overcrowding is another strong determinant, for secondary and tertiary cases in large families are at great risk of death. Exposure to a large dose of the virus when in close contact with the index case may be the critical factor. The severity of measles depends on the severity of disease in the index case. The high mortality found in West Africa is due to this region having the largest polygamous and extended families, which increase the risk of intense exposure. When females stay at home and are constrained in their social contacts, mortality is higher in girls than boys. There is also a high case fatality in children with chronic disease, including kwashiorkor, tuberculosis, and HIV infection. Hospital wards and clinics in developing countries have been important centres of disease transmission.

Though measles may have permanent sequelae, recent research has provided limited support for the previous belief in long-term excess morbidity and mortality after the first 6 weeks of measles infection. Long-term consequences may also depend on intensity of exposure. Index cases apparently have better long-term survival than secondary cases, suggesting a beneficial effect of mild measles infection. Long-term morbidity is most likely to be experienced by young children who have severe measles following intensive exposure.

Measles immunization has dramatically decreased the number of cases (Fig. 5.6.1), but measles deaths through vaccine failures are not infrequent. Immunized cases are characterized by a prolonged incubation period, a short prodrome, mild symptoms, and a favourable outcome. The mild measles of immunized cases leads to less risk of transmission or transmission of less severe disease. Immunization reduces the number of children being susceptible in the same household and hence reduces the risk of intensive exposure (Table 5.6.1).

However, immunization may have negative consequences on herd immunity for an increasing number of unvaccinated children, or children who have responded poorly to the vaccine will reach adulthood without having been exposed to measles. Thus, vaccinated people will have lower antibody levels than naturally infected people, which is particularly important because young immunized mothers will transfer lower antibody levels to their offspring. In West Africa, children of immunized mothers have only half the antibody levels of children of naturally infected mothers and they become susceptible as early as 3 to 5 months of age.

It has been argued that measles vaccines only saved 'weak' children who were likely to die anyway. However, many

Table 5.6.1 Impact of measles immunization on the transmission and severity of measles

Outcome measurements		Bissau 1980–1982	Senegal 1983–1990	Bissau 1991
Case fatality ratio: vaccinated / unvaccinated (95% CI)	Acute mortality within 1 month	0.39 (0.13–1.14)	0.0 (0–0.92)	0.30 (0.13–0.72)
	Delayed mortality from 1 month to 3 years			0.44 (0.22–0.90)
Secondary attack rate ratio according to vaccinated/ unvaccinated index cases		0.28 (0.10–0.79)	0.36 (0.15–0.87)	

Based on data from Aaby P, et al. (1986). Vaccinated children get milder measles infection: a community study from Guinea-Bissau. J Infect Dis, **154**, 858–63, and Samb B, et al. (1997). Decline in measles case fatality ratio after the introduction of measles immunization in rural Senegal. Am J Epidemiol, **145**, 51–7.

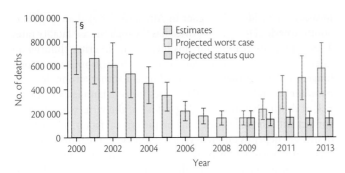

Fig. 5.6.1 Estimated number of measles deaths worldwide, 2000–2008, and worst case/status quo projections of possible resurgence in measles mortality, 2009–2013 (Reproduced from CDC (2009). Global Measles Mortality, 2008–2009. *MMWR*, **58**,1321–6).

epidemiological studies, including small randomized trials, have shown remarkable reductions in all cause mortality after standard measles vaccine. In Bangladesh, measles vaccination was associated with a 49% reduction in all-cause mortality from the age of 9 months, even though acute measles accounted for only 10 to 12% of deaths. This unexpected benefit was not related to prevention of measles. In most studies, this nonspecific benefit is particularly marked for girls. More recent studies have shown that the combination of measles vaccine with other vaccines or vitamin A supplements may influence the nonspecific effects on child survival.

Popular beliefs

In most cultures, measles has a specific local name and is a much feared disease. Popular understanding is centred around the rash, which if it stays within the body will lead to severe disease. This belief has some basis in truth for the prodrome is prolonged in severe cases, and a proportion of deaths reportedly occur before the appearance of the rash during very severe epidemics. Therapeutic practices, such as rubbing the skin with palm oil or kerosene, are aimed at eliciting the rash quickly. In West Africa it is believed that cooling keeps the rash within the body, so the child may be bedded in warm sand or covered with blankets, and is not washed or given cold water to drink.

Popular beliefs can also hamper vaccine uptake, leading to local outbreaks of measles. In the United Kingdom, after the publication of a fallacious medical article in 1998, the myth has arisen that the measles–mumps–rubella (MMR) vaccine can cause autism. Driven by an irresponsible press and the anti-vaccine lobby, measles vaccine coverage fell from 93% to 79% and has yet to fully recover. In Germany some parents believe children benefit from measles and thus shun vaccination. In the Bible Belt of the Netherlands, strong religious beliefs preclude all vaccinations. Marginalized communities like the Roma shun medical and other authorities, and many are unvaccinated. Thus it is difficult to eliminate measles in Europe. In the first half of 2011 there were 6500 cases of measles reported by 33 countries. In northern Nigeria, a predominantly Muslim area, religious and political leaders have warned of the dangers of 'western vaccines': coverage fell, and large outbreaks of polio and measles have ensued.

The virus and its antigens

Measles mainly infects humans, but like the other closely related morbilliviruses (such as rinderpest or canine distemper virus) it is

able to cross species to infect other primates but these outbreaks have not proved to be reservoirs of infection for humans. It contains a single strand of RNA, is highly pleomorphic, and ranges from 100 to 300 nm in diameter. The virus propagates by budding from the cell membrane, from which it acquires an envelope. The membrane of infected cells and the virion envelope contain two surface glycoproteins, the haemagglutinin (H) and fusion (F) proteins, and a nonglycosylated matrix (M) protein, which forms the inner layer. The H protein, which allows attachment of the virus to cells, via the CD46 or CDw150 receptors, is the main target for neutralizing antibodies. The F protein is responsible for fusion and syncytium formation of infected cells. CD46 is a ubiquitous membrane cofactor protein, which together with five other proteins, protects cells from complement activation and lysis. Some wild-type viruses, but not all, bind to the receptor but do not down-regulate it, thus preventing lysis and allowing efficient viral replication. The CDw150 receptor (also known as signalling lymphocyte activation molecule, SLAM) is expressed on immature lymphocytes and on effector memory T cells, and is rapidly induced on T and B cells after activation. The internal components or nucleocapsid consist of RNA, the nucleoprotein (N), which is the major protein, the phosphoprotein (P), and the large protein (L). The F protein is remarkably stable, the H protein shows minor antigenic variation, but the N protein, which contains a variable region in the C-terminal, is highly divergent among different strains of virus. Genetic analysis of Haemagglutinin and Nucleoprotein genes allowed molecular surveillance of the measles virus to track the international spread of the virus. There is also variation in the M protein, which some claim is related to persistent infection. The virus and its antigens are shown in Fig. 5.6.2.

Pathogenesis and the immune response

The course of infection and the immune response to this invasion are shown in Fig. 5.6.3. The measles virus, which is thermolabile and survives best at low humidities, is spread to susceptible contacts in droplets during sneezing and coughing. First, it infects and multiplies in the epithelium of the upper respiratory tract or the conjunctivae. Some 4 to 6 days later, the virus is found in the reticuloendothelial tissue of the liver and the spleen after passage through lymph nodes and spread via the blood. Here it multiplies, causing fusion of cells to form giant cells with many nuclei. Viral antigens, which can be found by immunofluorescent techniques in and on the surface of both these cells and lymphocytes, now induce the immune response. First, natural killer cells and cytotoxic T cells mount a cell-mediated reaction that contains the virus and limits its spread within cells. Later, B cells are primed to produce antibody. Defects in the cellular immune system, as in severe malnutrition, cancer, or primary and secondary immunodeficiencies, allow widespread multiplication of the virus to cause fatal giant cell pneumonia.

Around day 8, the measles virus is carried by the blood, either free or in mononuclear cells, to the target tissues, which are epithelia of the skin, eye, lung, and gut. Again, the agent multiplies to cause a bright erythema of the mucosae and Koplik's spots (see below), which are foci of viral multiplication. At this stage, measles virus may be cultured from nasopharyngeal secretions, and antigen can be detected by immunofluorescent techniques in the characteristic giant cells of the buccal mucosa, in epithelial cells, and in both B and T lymphocytes in the blood.

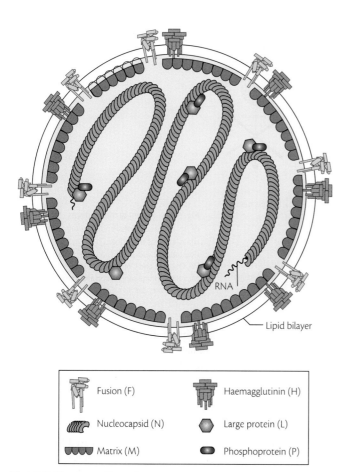

Fig. 5.6.2 The virus and its antigens.
(Reproduced with permission from Moss WJ, and Griffen D E (2006). Global measles elimination. *Nat Rev Microbiol*, **4**, 900–8.)

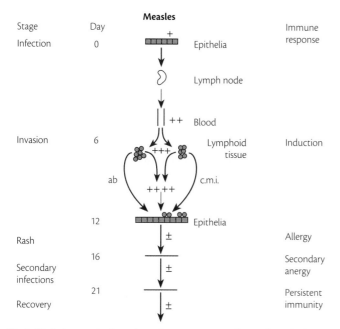

Fig. 5.6.3 Pathogenesis of measles. + Denotes, amount of virus; ab, antibody.
(Reproduced with permission from Parry EHOP (ed) (1984). *Principles of medicine in Africa*, 2nd edition. Oxford University Press, Oxford.)

The rash, appearing around days 14 to 16, is the sign of a strong and complicated allergic reaction to the virus in epithelia. The extent and severity of the rash, which reflects the clinical severity of the disease, is determined by the number of target cells infected. Histological examination shows virus in the disrupted epidermis, in the corium, and in capillary endothelium. These tissues are infiltrated by mononuclear cells together with antibody, immune complexes, and complement. An intact cell-mediated immune response is essential to generate the rash and clear the virus, for if impaired, as in the case of children with leukaemia, or occasionally in severe kwashiorkor, the virus multiplies unchecked and no rash appears. Some 2 or 3 days after the start of the rash, around day 17 or 18, the virus can no longer be cultured from epithelia, for infected cells have been disrupted and the free virus neutralized by antibody. The first antibody to appear is to the nucleoprotein antigens. The second to appear, which is largely responsible for neutralization of the virus, is to the haemagglutinin. Finally, the antibody to the fusion glycoprotein appears in a low titre. This antibody stops cell-to-cell spread of the virus. At this stage the child is markedly immunosuppressed and thus susceptible to secondary infections of the eyes, mouth, gut, and lungs. Latent viruses, such as herpes simplex or cytomegalovirus, may be reactivated and in turn cause further damage to the immune system. The delayed hypersensitivity reaction, as measured by skin tests to old tuberculin or candida antigen, is absent or severely impaired.

By the third week, day 21, as the patient recovers, antibody is in full production. Levels remain elevated for the rest of the patient's life, either because of repeated subclinical infections or because the virus persists in latent form in the spleen and other organs, so stimulating antibody. Occasionally, the virus persists in the brain in a damaging form to cause subacute sclerosing panencephalitis (see below).

Immunosuppression

The mechanisms of immunosuppression are complex (Fig. 5.6.4). The CD4+ and CD8+ cytotoxic T-cell response, which is exuberant, may result in the destruction of infected T cells and dendritic cells thus leading to their depletion, deficient antigen processing, and generalized immunosuppression. Cross-binding of the CD46 cellular receptor down-regulates interleukin 12 (IL-12), a crucial cytokine in the development of Th1 and delayed hypersensitivity responses. Infection of CDw150+ lymphocytes, which are predominantly of the Th0/Th1 type, results in suppression of lymphoproliferation and cell death. Thus, measles ultimately dampens the Th1 response, resulting in a skewing towards a Th2 cytokine response and susceptibility to intracellular and other pathogens. However, this immunosuppression may be in the interest of the host by limiting further autoallergic damage of infected tissues.

Pathogenesis in the underprivileged, in the malnourished, and in the HIV-infected

Measles is severe, prolonged, and carries a high case fatality rate due to secondary infections in children of the developing world, as it was formerly in the underprivileged in Europe. Two explanations are offered. Crowding leads to a high dose of measles virus and also increases the chances of secondary infection. The period of incubation has been found to be short, around 10 to 12 days, in severe and fatal cases, consistent with the concept of infecting dose

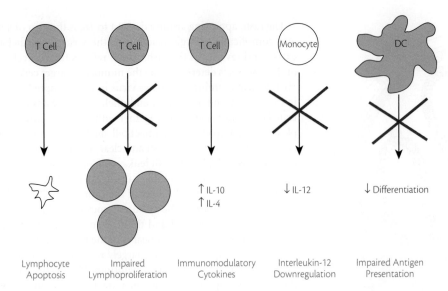

Fig. 5.6.4 Potential mechanisms of immune suppression following measles virus infection.
(Reproduced with permission from Moss WJ, Ota MO, and Griffen DE (2004). Measles: immune suppression and immune responses. *Int J Biochem Cell Biol*, **36**,1380–5.)

as a mechanism of severe disease. Alternatively, or in tandem, malnutrition diminishes the immune response to the virus, allowing great proliferation of virus and subsequent damage to the host. The immune response follows, which generates a severe and widespread rash followed by prolonged immunosuppression. Secondary bacterial infections with, e.g. *Streptococcus pneumoniae*, or latent infections such as herpes simplex or *Mycobacterium tuberculosis* occur in the wake of this intense damage to the immune system, often killing or maiming the child. Virus persists in lymphocytes and epithelial cells for up to 30 days after the start of the rash. Anorexia, increased catabolism, protein loss from the gut, and further malnutrition exaggerate the problem, which is worst in the weanling child (Fig. 5.6.5).

The death rate after measles in hospitalized infants is higher in severely malnourished and HIV-infected children, and prolonged viral shedding occurs in these children. Thus, in regions of high prevalence, HIV-infected children may be unrecognized transmitters of the virus but to date there is no evidence that this has hampered measles control.

Clinical features

There is a spectrum of severity ranging from mild in the privileged and well nourished to severe in the blatantly malnourished or immunosuppressed. However, the rule is not inviolate and other factors such as the age and dose of infection are probably as impor-

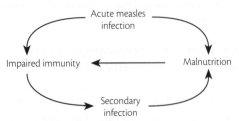

Fig. 5.6.5 The complex interaction between infection, nutrition, and impaired immunity seen in measles.
(Reproduced with permission from Greenwood BM (1996). The host's response to infection. In: Weatherall DJ, Ledingham JGGL, Warrell DA (eds) (1996). *Oxford textbook of medicine*, 3rd edition, p. 282. Oxford University Press, Oxford.)

tant in determining the severity of disease. Measles, often severe, occasionally infects unvaccinated young adults or those who have lived in isolated communities. The clinical features of measles and some complications are shown in Fig. 5.6.6 and discussed below.

Prodrome (days 10–14)

A diagnosis of measles is often missed at this stage, when fever coupled with a runny nose, and sometimes complicated by convulsions, is the main feature. Other signs are mild conjunctivitis, red mucosa, Koplik's spots, and diarrhoea. Koplik's spots are found in the buccal mucosa (Fig. 5.6.7). They are small, irregular, bright-red spots with a minute bluish-white speck in the centre of each of them. The prodrome is prolonged in severe cases, and reduced in individuals with modified measles due to maternal antibodies or the prophylactic use of immunoglobulin.

Rash (days 14–18)

The morbilliform rash first appears on the forehead and neck and then spreads, over a period of 3 to 4 days, to involve the trunk and finally the limbs (Fig. 5.6.8).

In children in Africa and other parts of the developing world the rash is often red, confluent, raised (Fig. 5.6.9), very extensive, and sometimes accompanied by bleeding into the skin and gut. Later, the rash blackens (postmeasles 'staining', see Fig. 5.6.10), then the skin peels causing extensive desquamation (Fig. 5.6.11). Other epithelial surfaces are inflamed, the severity matching that of the rash. Cough may be hoarse and coupled with inspiration difficulty if the larynx and trachea are inflamed. Signs of pneumonitis are apparent, which in severe cases may cause cyanosis or be complicated by mediastinal and subcutaneous emphysema. Conjunctivitis, especially in those who are vitamin A deficient, can be severe. Enteritis may cause profuse diarrhoea with a resulting loss of protein, and malabsorption of food and water. The mouth is painful and red, which adds to the misery of the child, who becomes anorexic and may even refuse to suck the breast. In the uncomplicated case, as is usual in the West, the convalescent period is short, usually lasting less than a week. Complications should be suspected if fever persists while the rash is fading or desquamating.

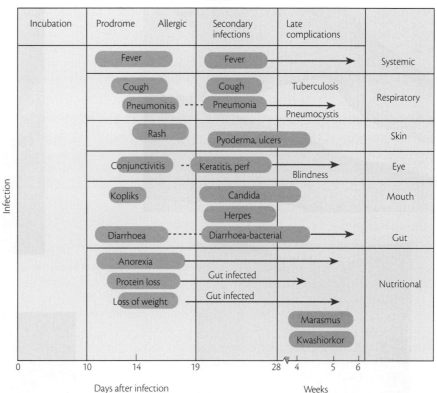

Fig. 5.6.6 Clinical features of measles and some of its complications. (Reproduced with permission from Parry EHOP (ed) (1984). *Principles of medicine in Africa*, 2nd edition, Oxford University Press, Oxford.)

Complications

Early complications (days 18–30)

As a result of the widespread, severe allergic reaction to the measles virus signified by the rash, the patient is left severely immunosuppressed and is susceptible to infection.

Pneumonia

This causes the most deaths (Table 5.6.2) and is heralded by a rise in fever, leucocytosis, and respiratory difficulties. Lobar pneumonia is usually caused by *S. pneumoniae*, but bronchopneumonia, which is more common, results from other bacteria, such as

Staphylococcus aureus, or secondary viral infections with, e.g. herpes simplex or adenovirus. A variety of other organisms such as Gram-negative bacteria, cytomegalovirus, fungi, *M. tuberculosis*, and *Pneumocystis jirovecii* should be considered as potential lung pathogens in the malnourished or immunocompromised child.

Stomatitis and enteritis

Chronic diarrhoea and a sore mouth caused by candidal infection are common complications of measles in children in the developing world. The gut is often superinfected with bacteroides spp., *Escherichia coli*, pseudomonas spp., and *S. aureus*, which results in malabsorption and protein loss. Deep ulcers caused by herpes simplex virus erode the corners of the mouth, gums, and inner surface of the lips causing much misery, illness, and pain (Fig. 5.6.12).

Eye infections

Corneal ulceration leading to impaired vision or blindness is common after measles, especially in malnourished and vitamin A-deficient children (Fig. 5.6.13). Several studies from Africa have shown that more than half of childhood blindness is related to measles. The mechanisms are still under discussion. In northern Nigeria, herpes simplex was found in 47% of active corneal ulcers after measles, and measles virus in 12%: the children often had evidence of oral herpes. In a study in Tanzania, blindness precipitated by measles was associated with vitamin A deficiency (50%), herpes simplex infection (21%), and the use of traditional eye medicine (17%).

Skin and other infections

Pyoderma is common after measles. In the malnourished patient, deep eroding ulcers may bore through the skin even into bone. When originating in the mouth they are known as cancrum oris or noma (Fig. 5.6.14). Otitis media is also common.

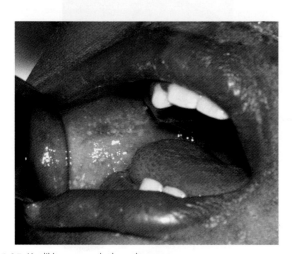

Fig. 5.6.7 Koplik's spots on the buccal mucosa. (Courtesy of the late Dr B.E. Juel-Jensen.)

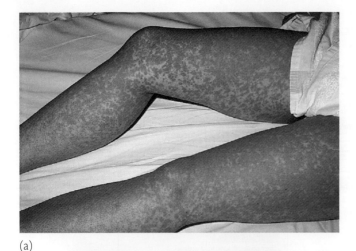

(a)

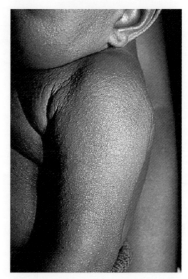

Fig. 5.6.9 Measles rash in an African child.

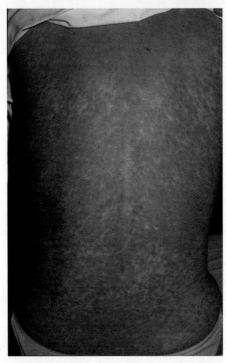

(b)

Fig. 5.6.8 (a, b) The morbilliform rash first appears on the forehead and neck and then spreads, over a period of 3 to 4 days, to involve the trunk and finally the limbs. (Copyright D A Warrell.)

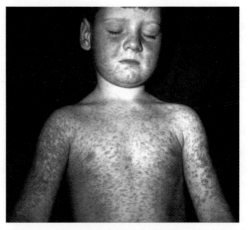

Fig. 5.6.10 Darkening measles rash after several days ('measles staining'). (Courtesy of the late Dr B.E. Juel-Jensen.)

Encephalitis

This is a rare, but much feared, complication found in approximately 1 to 2 per 1000 cases. The onset is usually between 4 and 7 days after the start of the rash, but, rarely, it may occur within 48 h or up to 2 weeks from the onset. In addition to seizures, there is often fever, irritability, headache, and a disturbance in consciousness that may progress to profound coma. The disorder is probably attributable to a neuroallergic process. Lymphocytes from the cerebrospinal fluid have been shown to respond to myelin basic protein, as in experimental allergic encephalomyelitis. The virus cannot be isolated from cerebrospinal fluid, which contains lymphocytes and raised levels of IgG but normal levels of measles antibody. Mortality and morbidity are high: 10 to 15% of patients die and 25% of children are left with permanent brain damage. Treatment is supportive; dexamethasone has no convincing beneficial effect.

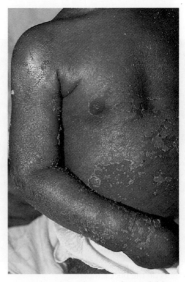

Fig. 5.6.11 Desquamating measles rash in an African child.

Table 5.6.2 Complications and mortality in inpatients with measles, northern Nigeria, July–December 1978

	No.	Died	Percentage dead
Pneumonia	169	32	18.9
Gastroenteritis	65	9	13.8
Marasmic kwashiorkor	25	6	24.0
Laryngotracheobronchitis	21	4	19.0
Encephalitis	10	4	40.0

Reproduced with permission from Parry EHOP (ed) (1984). *Principles of medicine in Africa*, 2nd edition. Oxford University Press, Oxford.

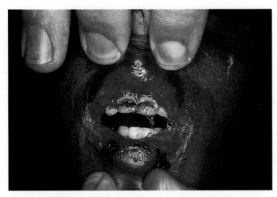

Fig. 5.6.12 Deep ulcers caused by herpes simplex virus. (Copyright D A Warrell.)

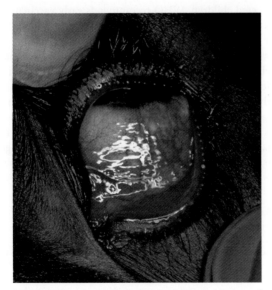

Fig. 5.6.13 Corneal ulceration leading to impaired vision or blindness after measles, especially in malnourished and vitamin A-deficient children. (Copyright D A Warrell.)

Late complications

Malnutrition

This is the most frequent complication, for children of the developing world often lose a lot of weight during measles and may take many weeks to regain it. Those originally underweight, who have had severe measles, are at greatest risk, for anorexia in these

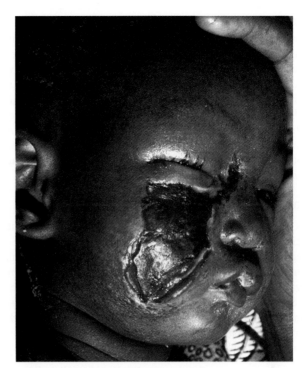

Fig. 5.6.14 Cancrum oris or noma following measles.

children is prolonged, much protein is lost from the gut, and secondary infections, which lead to marasmus or marasmic kwashiorkor, are frequent. Measles has been shown to persist in the epithelia and lymphocytes of the severely malnourished for 30 or more days after the rash.

Persistent infection

Pneumonitis

Giant cell pneumonia is found in patients with defects in cell-mediated immunity. Children with leukaemia or kwashiorkor are particularly vulnerable, as are those with symptomatic HIV infection. The lung disease may develop weeks after measles, and in most cases the rash of measles has been absent and thus the diagnosis may not be suspected. The diagnosis is made by virological and/or histological examination of lung tissue. Most of these children die.

Subacute sclerosing panencephalitis (SSPE)

Persistent measles virus infection in the brain is responsible for this rare, progressive disease of the brain, which is found in 0.1 to 1.4 per million children after measles. The child with SSPE has usually experienced normal measles, albeit at a young age, 5 to 10 years earlier. The first indication is a disturbance in intellect and personality. Behavioural disorders and deterioration in school work are frequently mentioned. There then follows, over a period of weeks and months, myoclonus-like seizures, signs of extrapyramidal and pyramidal disease, and finally a state of decerebrate rigidity followed by death. The electroencephalogram shows a characteristic regular series of high-amplitude, spike-like waves. Very high titres of measles complement-fixing and haemagglutinin-inhibiting antibody are present both in serum and cerebrospinal fluid. Treatments for SSPE have included the use of transfer factor, plasmapheresis, and antiviral drugs, but to no avail.

Multiple sclerosis, autism, Crohn's disease

There is no convincing evidence that measles virus or immune responses to it have a causative role in these diseases. The alleged association between the measles, mumps, and rubella (MMR) vaccine, autism, and Crohn's disease was based on weak science and has now been convincingly refuted by larger and stronger epidemiological studies. Subsequent molecular studies have failed to confirm the original finding of measles virus and genomic RNA in diseased bowel. The false alarm raised by this report caused a substantial reduction in the number of children vaccinated against measles in the United Kingdom.

Diagnosis

This is primarily clinical, although signs may be less clear-cut in vaccinated subjects. Thus, in areas of high vaccine coverage the detection of measles-specific IgM antibody by enzyme-linked immunoassay or, better still, the detection of measles antigen in saliva or urine may clinch the diagnosis if the rash is mild or atypical. Subclinical measles is common in vaccinated children after exposure to measles: the diagnosis is made by detecting a fourfold or greater rise in measles antibody within 2 to 6 weeks of exposure. It is not clear if such cases are infectious.

Treatment of measles and its complications

No effective anti-measles drug exists, yet some children do benefit from treatment in hospital. The following criteria indicate severe measles and a need for hospital admission: a widespread, confluent rash darkening to deep red or purple; signs of laryngeal obstruction; subcutaneous emphysema; marked dehydration; blood in the stool or more than five stools a day; convulsion or loss of consciousness; severe secondary pneumonia; corneal ulceration; severe ulceration of the mouth and skin. These signs should be taken particularly seriously when the child is underweight or frankly malnourished.

Hydrate the child orally or intravenously. Treat lobar pneumonia with benzylpenicillin, and bronchopneumonia with amoxicillin or, if severe, with combined antibiotics such as gentamicin and cloxacillin. Antibiotic eye ointments relieve discomfort and possibly prevent secondary infections of measles conjunctivitis. Antibiotics (topical and systemic) and vitamin A should be given routinely for the treatment of eye ulcers. If herpes simplex virus is the cause, use aciclovir topically or, when severe, systemically. Candida infections of the mouth or gut often respond dramatically to nystatin. Feeding, by tube if necessary, needs careful planning and presentation, for the anorexic infected child will be in severe negative energy balance due to a greatly increased catabolic rate. Case fatality rates are 30 to 50% lower in those children in hospital treated with vitamin A. This should be given orally at the time of diagnosis in a dose of 100 000 IU for children below 12 months of age and in a dose of 200 000 IU for older children. If eye signs of vitamin A deficiency are present, the initial dose should be repeated the next day and again 1 to 4 weeks later.

The prophylactic use of antibiotics such as amoxicillin or co-trimoxazole to prevent secondary infections after measles is a widespread practice based on slender evidence. The only community randomized placebo controlled trial was small: those children who received co-trimoxazole had less pneumonia and conjunctivitis and had a significantly higher weight gain (see Table 5.6.3).

Prevention

Passive immunization with human immunoglobulin is highly effective if given within 2 or 3 days of exposure, in a dose for children of 0.2 ml/kg. Immunoglobulin should be given to those in whom vaccination is contraindicated such as severely immunocompromised children with cancer, AIDS, or congenital immunodeficiencies. For children with severe malnutrition, WHO recommends measles vaccination in the acute phase followed by a second dose on recovery as the immune response is suboptimal. This is widely practised in hospitals in developing countries and in refugee camps where there are practical difficulties in providing immunoglobulin. Although live vaccines are theoretically undesirable in these immunocompromised children, no head-to-head trials of these two preventions have been conducted.

The currently used vaccines are live strains, attenuated by culture in chick fibroblasts. The Edmonston–Zagreb strain, which has been cultured in human diploid cells, is also widely used. It is more effective than other vaccines in the presence of antibody, and should be used in a standard dose if vaccinating infants below 9 months of age, or if a booster dose is required. The complications of vaccination are few and generally mild. Fever of moderate severity is infrequent, and a mild rash with some signs of upper respiratory tract infection occurs rarely. Underweight children respond normally to the vaccine, as do ill children attending the outpatient department and those on the ward. As clinics and hospitals are major sites of transmission of the virus in the developing world, all susceptible children in these places should be vaccinated unless severely immunocompromised. Asymptomatic HIV-infected children are initially protected by measles vaccine but antibody wanes more quickly than in uninfected children. WHO recommends early vaccination at 6 months of age followed by additional vaccinations at 9 months and another later in childhood.

The measles vaccination policy for low income countries has seen major changes in the last 25 years. The optimal age for vaccination in the developed world is between 14 and 16 months, when maternal antibody has disappeared. However, this recommendation could not be applied to children in developing countries, because there measles infects at a much earlier age. In 1980, the World Health Organization recommended vaccination at 9 months of age but, by then, 5 to 15% of children may have had measles. This policy

Table 5.6.3 Prophylactic antibiotic to prevent complications after measles in Guinea-Bissau

Outcome	Co-trimoxazole (n = 46)	Placebo (n = 38)	Adjusted odds ratio (95% CI)
Pneumonia	1 (2%)	6 (16%)	0.14 (0.01–1.50)
Hospitalization	0	3	–
Diarrhoea	3 (7%)	5 (13%)	0.17 (0.01–1.55)
Severe fever	6 (13%)	11 (29%)	0.36 (0.09–1.43)
Stomatitis	4 (9%)	7 (18%)	0.43 (0.08–2.26)
Conjunctivitis	12 (26%)	17 (45%)	0.31 (0.10–1.03)
Weight gain (g/day)	32	15	–

(Adapted and reproduced with permission from Garly M-L, *et al.* (2006). Prophylactic antibiotics to prevent pneumonia and other complications after measles: community based randomised double blind placebo controlled trial in Guinea-Bissau. *BMJ*, **333**, 1245–50.)

was not based on good evidence; it is not known if vaccination at 9 months is better in saving children than vaccination at 7, 8, or 10 months of age, or a two dose regime in infancy.

Through the 1990s it became clear that several doses of measles vaccines were needed to improve measles control. The developed countries have used two-dose strategies with a second dose being given at school entry or to young teenagers. Latin America has obtained major successes with a combination of improved vaccination coverage and regular immunization campaigns providing a second opportunity for measles vaccination. The strategy has the following elements: (1) catch-up—a one-time mass campaign covering everybody between 9 months and 14 years of age regardless of previous measles or immunization; (2) keep-up—achieving a high coverage for each birth cohort; (3) follow-up—subsequent mass campaigns covering all children every 3 to 5 years; and (4) mop-up—campaigns that target children who are difficult to reach or during outbreaks. As a result of this strategy, Latin America has been declared free of internal measles transmission since 2002. Since there is no immediate risk of measles infection, the age of routine vaccination has been raised to 12 months as this is believed to be associated with better antibody responses.

The Latin American model has been transferred to other regions. Rebranded as SIA (supplementary immunization activities), it has assured a spectacular success in reducing measles mortality in Africa. The goal of reducing global measles deaths by 90% by 2010 compared to 2000 has been met. However, these campaigns which are donor driven are expensive and should not be seen as a substitute for an inadequate immunization service. Recently, following the credit crunch, international financial support for this initiative has decreased and many countries have not been able to raise sufficient money for SIAs. Measles cases and deaths have increased: in the worst case scenario WHO predicts an additional 500 000 deaths worldwide in 2013 alone (see Fig. 5.6.1). Unfortunately it is donor policy only to measure vaccination coverage by 12 months of age and therefore some countries are no longer providing routine measles vaccination after 12 months of age. Although it is WHO policy that any unvaccinated child coming to a clinic should receive measles vaccine, there is a drive to reduce wastage and not to open a vial of measles vaccine unless 5 to 7 children are present for vaccination. Such policies make it difficult to achieve high coverage.

Elimination or eradication?

Global measles eradication has yet to be made official policy. However, the Americas have attained elimination (i.e. no internal transmission of the virus), and five other regions are pursuing such a policy. Measles satisfies the criteria for eradication for there is no animal reservoir, it is only transmitted between humans, it is easy to diagnose, and vaccines are available. Measles elimination can be accomplished for prolonged periods in defined geographical regions provided there is sufficient funding and political will. This was obtained for the first time in the Gambia in the mid 1960s as part of the smallpox eradication and measles vaccination campaigns. Rinderpest, a virus closely related to measles that decimated cattle and wild game populations over the centuries, was eradicated in 2010. Now a WHO panel has declared that measles can and should be eradicated by 2020. It stressed that eradication activities should be carried out as part of routine immunization services and estimated it would cost $US 7.8 billion.

However, eradicating measles will be a daunting task. First, it is the most infectious of diseases and will require vaccine coverage of greater than 95%. When there is no risk of infection, it will be increasingly difficult for parents to appreciate the necessity for vaccination especially as risk, although small, is perceived. Secondly, herd immunity will become a problem as with less exposure to the virus vaccine induced immunity will wane more rapidly. Thirdly, Africa will be a stern test for due to political instability, wars, and natural disasters it will be difficult to maintain sufficiently high coverage. Fourthly, with the growing HIV epidemic, there is a risk that the vaccine may be less effective. Fifthly, with the growing fear of bioterrorism, it is unlikely that all immunization can be stopped in the posteradication era. Lastly, but most difficult, will be to assure long-term funding as donors have a tradition of changing priorities.

The international health community is split over whether eradication can be attained with the Latin American strategy using existing vaccines or whether new vaccines and delivery systems such as aerosolization are needed. New vaccines, which can be given in early infancy, or two-dose strategies using the standard Edmonston–Zagreb vaccine at 4 and 9 months of age, might be necessary to contain measles in the developing world. The latter strategy has the advantage that it may confer beneficial nonspecific effects on child survival in countries with high childhood mortality. In Guinea-Bissau, per protocol analysis of a trial of two doses of Edmonston–Zagreb measles vaccine in infancy revealed a mortality rate 30% lower than in the controls who received a single dose of measles vaccine at 9 months of age.

Coverage of at least 95% of all susceptible children, including those between 3 and 9 months of age, with a vaccine that is at least 95% effective is assumed to be necessary if the virus is to be eradicated. Current vaccines do not meet these standards except when two doses have been given in national campaigns. New vaccines such as the modified vaccinia Ankara (MVA) recombinant virus, a nonreplicating mutant of horsepox made to express the F and H proteins, or a DNA vaccine expressing these proteins may possibly fulfill such exacting requirements, for they have been shown to protect macaques from measles. High titre vaccines were used to vaccinate young infants, but were discontinued when an unexplained increase in mortality in girls was found 1 to 3 years after vaccination. Thus, new vaccines need long-term monitoring in order to fully understand the potential nonspecific immunological interactions that may occur between the many vaccines in use and with infections that are common in infants.

Further reading

Aaby P, et al. (1983). Measles mortality, state of nutrition, and family structure. A community study from Guinea-Bissau. *J Infect Dis*, **147**, 693–701. [Groundbreaking paper showing measles mortality depends on family structure and intensity of exposure but not nutrition.]

Aaby P, et al. (1995). Non-specific beneficial effects of measles immunization: analysis of mortality studies from developing countries. *BMJ*, **311**, 481–5.

Aaby P, et al. (2003). Differences in female-male mortality after high-titre measles vaccine and association with subsequent vaccination with diphtheria—tetanus-pertussis and inactivated poliovirus: re-analysis of West African studies. *Lancet*, **361**, 2183–88. [An interesting theory invoking nonspecific effects of vaccines.]

Aaby P, et al. (2010). Non-specific effects of standard measles vaccine at 4.5 and 9 months of age on childhood mortality: randomised controlled trial. *BMJ*, **341**, c6495. [The first trial to demonstate such effects.]

de Quadros CA, *et al.* (1996). Measles elimination in the Americas. Evolving strategies. *JAMA*, **275**, 224–229.

Fenner F (1948). The pathogenesis of the acute exanthems. An interpretation based on experimental investigations with mouse-pox (infectious ectromelia of mice). *Lancet*, **2**, 915–20.

Fowlkes A, *et al.* (2011). Persistence of vaccine-induced measles antibody beyond age of 12 months: a comparison of response to one and two doses of Edmonston–Zagreb measles vaccine among HIV-infected and uninfected children in Malawi. *J Infect Dis*, **204**(Suppl 1), S149–57.

Garly ML, *et al.* (2006). Prophylactic antibiotics to prevent pneumonia and other complications after measles: community based randomized double blind placebo controlled trial in Guinea Bissau. *BMJ*, **333**, 1245–1250. [The only randomized controlled trial of prophylactic antibiotics for measles in Africa.]

Griffen DE (2010). Measles virus-induced suppression of immune responses. *Immunol Rev*, **236**, 176–89. [A scholarly account of this important topic.]

Jaye A, *et al.* (1998). Ex vivo analysis of cytotoxic T lymphocytes to measles antigens during infection and after vaccination in Gambian children. *J Clin Invest*, **102**, 1969–77. [The largest and most complete study of cytotoxic T-cell responses in natural measles.]

Morens DM, *et al.* (2011). Global rinderpest eradication: lessons learned and why humans should celebrate too. *J Infect Dis*, **201**, 502–5.

Morley D (1969). Severe measles in the tropics. *Br Med J*, **1**, 363–5. [Classic clinical studies.]

Moss WJ, Griffen DE (2012) Measles. *Lancet*, **379**, 153–64 [Great review.]

Muscat M (2011). Who gets measles in Europe? *J Infect Dis*, **204** (Suppl 1), S353–5.

Samb B, *et al.* (1997). Decline in measles case fatality ratio after introduction of measles immunization in rural Senegal. *Am J Epidemiol*, **145**, 51–57.

Strebel PM, *et al.* (2011). A world without measles. *J Infect Dis*, **204** (Suppl 1), S1–3. [A commentary on the excellent supplement dealing with measles eradication.]

Whittle HC, *et al.* (1979). Severe ulcerative herpes of mouth and eye following measles. *Trans R Soc Trop Med Hyg*, **73**, 66–9.

Whittle HC, *et al.* (1999). Effect of sub-clinical infection on maintaining immunity against measles in vaccinated children in West Africa. *Lancet*, **353**, 98–101.

5.7 Nipah and Hendra virus encephalitides

C.T. Tan

Essentials

Nipah and Hendra are two related viruses of the Paramyxoviridae family that have their reservoir in large *Pteropus* fruit bats. Human disease manifests most often as acute encephalitis, which may be late-onset or relapsing, or pneumonia, with high mortality. Transmission from bats to human includes direct spread from consumption of food contaminated by infected bats' secretions, and contact with infected animals: human-to-human spread can also occur.

Introduction

Nipah and Hendra viruses are two new zoonotic viruses that have emerged in recent years. Both are paramyxoviridae family sharing many similar characteristics. Because of their homology, a new genus called Henipavirus (Hendra + Nipah) was created for these two viruses.

Hendra virus infection

Hendra virus was first isolated in an outbreak of acute respiratory illness involving horses in Australia in 1994. Horses may become infected by eating hay contaminated by uterine fluids and aborted fetal tissue from fruit bats. All human cases had been in close contact with bodily fluids from sick, moribund, or dead horses. Transmission from bats to humans, humans to horses, or humans to humans has not been documented. A horse trainer and stable hand were also infected, presenting with respiratory illnesses from which the horse trainer died. A second human death occurred in 1995, when a farmer who had been in contact with sick horses about year earlier died from encephalitis. Another two deaths involving a veterinary workers occurred in the Hendra virus outbreaks in July 2008 and July 2009, also in Australia. Thus, up to 2011 there have been 14 outbreaks of Hendra virus infection, all involving horses, 5 of these involving subsequent horse-to-human transmission, with 4 deaths among a total of 7 human cases.

Clinical manifestations

Human patients developed flu-like or feverish illnesses about 2 weeks after exposure to sick horses, but in one case the incubation period was 1 year. Acute or insidious encephalitis then developed after a few days. A survivor suffered persistent residual sensorineural deafness. MRI scans showed hyperintense plaque-like cortical and basal ganglia lesions and perfusion scans suggested widespread cortical vasculitis with infarcts.

The reservoir of Hendra virus is the *Pteropus* genus of fruit bats (see Chapter 5.10, Fig. 5.10.18) which also harbour Nipah, Menangle, Tioman, and Australian bat lyssaviruses.

Nipah virus infection

In late 1998 to early 1999, there was an outbreak of viral encephalitis in several pig-farming villages in peninsular Malaysia which subsequently involved abattoir workers in Singapore. More than 300 patients were affected. Isolation of virus from cerebrospinal fluid specimens of several patients indicated that this was due to previously unknown Nipah virus.

Epidemiology

Human Nipah virus infection was transmitted by close contact with infected pigs. Human-to-human transmission was thought to be rare, although the virus could be readily isolated from patients' respiratory secretions and urine.

Clinical manifestations

During the outbreak, more than half of the patients had affected family members, suggesting a high infection rate. Some of the household members had seroconversion without clinical disease, indicating subclinical infection at a ratio of asymptomatic vs symptomatic infection of 1 to 3. The infection involved all age groups.

The incubation period was less than 2 weeks in most patients. The clinical manifestations were those of an acute encephalitis with fever, headache, vomiting, and reduced level of consciousness. Distinctive clinical features were areflexia, hypotonia, and prominent autonomic changes such as tachycardia and hypertension. Segmental myoclonus found in about one-third of patients was characterized by focal, rhythmic jerking of muscles, commonly involving the diaphragm and anterior muscles of the neck. Respiratory tract involvement with cough was seen at presentation in 14% of patients. There were some patients who had nonencephalitic infection with seroconversion and systemic symptoms but no evidence of encephalitis.

The overall mortality of acute Nipah encephalitis was 40%. Severe brainstem involvement was associated with poor prognosis.

Laboratory investigations

Cerebrospinal fluid examination was abnormal in 75% of patients with elevated protein levels or elevated white cell counts. Glucose levels were within normal limits. These features are nonspecific. IgM and IgG antibody detection in serum and cerebrospinal fluid were critical to the diagnosis of Nipah virus infection. The antibody test utilized an enzyme-linked immunosorbent assay (ELISA) test. The rate of positive IgM was 100% by day 12 of illness. For IgG, it was 100% by 4 weeks of illness.

Brain MRI in acute encephalitis showed multiple, disseminated, small discrete hyperintense lesions best seen in the FLAIR sequence particularly in the subcortical and deep white matter (Fig. 5.7.1). The lesions were likely to correspond to the microinfarctions noted in postmortem tissues. Similar changes were also seen in asymptomatic patients with Nipah virus infection.

Treatment

Treatment is mainly supportive with mechanical ventilatory support for seriously ill patients. Ribavirin, a broad-spectrum antiviral agent, appeared to reduce the mortality rate.

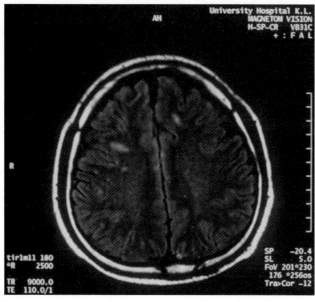

Fig. 5.7.1 Nipah virus encepahalitis: MRI FLAIR showing disseminated, small discrete hyperintense lesions.

Pathology and pathogenesis

Vasculitis of the medium-sized to small blood vessels in brain, causing thrombosis, and vascular occlusion with areas of necrosis and ischaemia, were the major findings (Fig. 5.7.2). There were also viral inclusions indicating direct viral involvement of the neurons. Vasculitis was also seen in lung and kidney.

Relapse and late-onset Nipah encephalitis

Close to 10% of patients suffered a second or even a third neurological episode months or years following recovery from acute encephalitis. About 5% who were either asymptomatic or only had mild nonencephalitic illness initially, also developed similar neurologic episodes (late-onset Nipah encephalitis) for the first time after a delayed period. Clinical, radiologic and pathologic findings indicate that relapse and late-onset Nipah encephalitis was the same disease process,which was distinct from acute Nipah virus encephalitis. The common clinical features were fever, headache, seizures, and focal neurological signs. There was an18% mortality. MRI showed patchy areas of confluent cortical lesions. Necropsy showed focal confluent encephalitis due to a recurrent infection.

The bat as reservoir host

As for Hendra virus, the reservoir of Nipah virus is fruit bats of the *Pteropus* species. Half-eaten fruits dropped by bats near pig farms may have infected an animal that subsequently ingested them. Pigs were the amplifying hosts for the virus. There was pig-to-pig transmission which subsequently spread to human.

Nipah encephalitis in Bangladesh and India

Eleven outbreaks of Nipah encephalitis have been reported in Bangladesh from 2001 to 2011. Two other outbreaks were reported from northeastern India, in Siliguri district in 2001, and Nadia district in 2007.

As in Malaysia, Nipah virus caused a fatal encephalitic illness in humans in Bangladesh and India. However, the Bangladeshi and Indian outbreaks showed prominent human-to-human spread of infection, with physicians who cared for the patients also affected. There was florid pulmonary involvement in some patients. Brain MRI in some patients showed confluent high signal lesions involving both grey and white matter, which is unlike

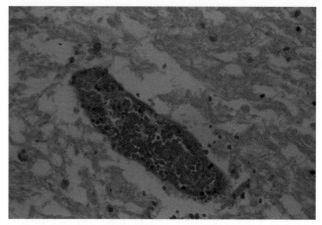

Fig. 5.7.2 Nipah virus encepahalitis: vasculitis of a medium-sized cerebral blood vessel, showing thrombosis and vascular occlusion with areas of necrosis and ischaemia.

the acute Nipah encephalitis in the Malaysian outbreak, suggesting some differences in the pathology from the Malaysian patients. The RNA of Nipah virus in Bangladesh and India was close to but not identical with that causing the outbreak in Malaysia. *Pteropus* bats were also the reservoir of Nipah virus in Bangladesh. There may be a variety of mode of transmission from bats to humans in the Bangladesh and Indian outbreaks. Consumption of raw date-palm juice and half-eaten fruits contaminated by secretions from bats are suggested modes of transmission.

Pteropus bats are widespread in large parts of Asia, Africa, and Australia. Nipah virus has been isolated in urine of *Pteropus* bats in Cambodia, and Nipah viral antigen has been found in saliva of *Pteropus* bats in Thailand. Serological evidence of *Henipavirus* infection has been reported in fruit bats from Papua New Guinea to Ghana, Africa from East to West, and Yunnan, China to Australia from North to South, indicating potential human Nipah virus infection elsewhere.

Menangle and Tioman viruses

These are two other newly identified paramyxoviruses harboured by *Pteropis* fruit bats. Menangle causes disease in pigs but neither has been implicated in human infections.

Further reading

Chadha MS, *et al.* (2006). Nipah virus-associated encephalitis outbreak, Siliguri, India. *Emerg Infect Dis*, **12**, 235–40.
Chong HT, Jahangir Hossain M, Tan CT (2008). Differences in epidemiologic and clinical features of Nipah virus encephalitis between the Malaysian and Bangladesh outbreaks. *Neurol Asia*, **13**, 23–6.
Chua KB, *et al.* (1999). Fatal encephalitis due to Nipah virus among pig-farmers in Malaysia. *Lancet*, **354**, 1257–9.
Goh KJ, *et al.* (2000). Clinical features of Nipah virus encephalitis among pig farmers in Malaysia. *N Engl J Med*, **342**, 1229–35.
Halpin K, *et al.* (2011). Pteropid bats are confirmed as the reservoir hosts of henipaviruses: a comprehensive experimental study of virus transmission. *Am J Trop Med Hyg*, **85**, 946–51.
Hsu VP, *et al.* (2004). Nipah virus encephalitis reemergence, Bangladesh. *Emerg Infect Dis*, **10**, 2082–7.
Nakka P, *et al.* (2011). MRI findings in acute Hendra virus meningoencephalitis. *Clin Radiol* 2011, Nov 29. [Epub ahead of print.]
Tan CT, *et al.* (2002). Relapse and late-onset Nipah encephalitis. *Ann Neurol*, **51**, 703–8.

5.8 Enterovirus infections

Philip Minor and Ulrich Desselberger

Essentials

Enteroviruses are single-stranded RNA viruses comprising poliomyelitis viruses (3 types), Coxsackie A viruses (23 types), Coxsackie B viruses (6 types), and echoviruses (28 types). They have recently been reclassified into 4 human enterovirus species (A–D) on the basis of sequence comparisons. Transmission is by the faeco-oral route, with marked seasonal peaks of infection in areas of temperate climate, but infections occurring all year round in tropical regions with only limited seasonality.

Pathogenesis—following transmission, enteroviruses undergo a first round of replication in cells of the mucosal surfaces of the gastrointestinal tract and in gut-associated lymphoid cells, followed by viraemia, which leads to infection of distant organs (brain, spinal cord, meninges, myocardium, muscle, skin, etc.), where lesions may be produced. Shedding of virus occurs from throat and faeces for many weeks.

Clinical manifestations and diagnosis

Most enterovirus infections are silent or only produce minor illness, but severe major illness can develop in a few of the infected.

Poliomyelitis—infection with poliovirus is normally inapparent, but a few of the infected (1% or less) develop neurological symptoms comprising (1) aseptic meningitis, or (2) paralytic poliomyelitis—5 to 10 days after a mild upper respiratory tract infection presentation is with flaccid paralysis resulting from motor neuron destruction; this may affect the limbs (spinal form) or muscles supplied by the medulla oblongata or bulb (bulbar form), with potentially life-threatening respiratory muscle involvement. Treatment is supportive; mortality is 2 to 5% in children and 15 to 30% in adults, and there is residual paralysis in 90% of survivors.

Other clinical syndromes include: (1) aseptic meningitis, the most frequent clinical presentation of enterovirus infection, caused by Coxsackie viruses and echoviruses; (2) encephalitis, a rare event, possibly following aseptic meningitis; (3) pleurodynia (Bornholm disease), presenting abruptly with fever and chest pain and usually caused by Coxsackie B viruses; (4) myopericarditis; (5) herpangina; (6) exanthema, rubella-like or hand-foot-and-mouth disease; and (7) conjunctivitis.

Diagnosis is by virus isolation in cell culture or by viral genome detection using RT-PCR.

Prevention

Paralytic poliomyelitis has been eradicated in most countries of the world following universal mass vaccination with formaldehyde-inactivated poliovirus (Salk vaccine) and/or live-attenuated viral vaccine (Sabin vaccine). However, it persists in a few countries (e.g. India, Pakistan, Afghanistan, Nigeria) from which it has been exported to otherwise polio-free states. For example, strains from Nigeria have caused disease in other countries of Western Africa, Indian strains have been repeatedly isolated in Angola, there was a major outbreak in Tajikistan caused by strains from Northern India, and in 2011 there were at least 18 cases in China caused by strains from Pakistan. The incident in China was particularly unexpected as the immunization programme has been well executed and was effective for many years. As long as there are pockets of infection, the world remains at risk of re-emergence of the disease.

Introduction

Enteroviruses are a major group of viruses causing systemic infection in humans. They form two genera of the *Picornaviridae* family (the *Enterovirus* and *Parechovirus* genera) and occur in at least

66 serotypes in humans. They infect via the gastrointestinal tract and are mostly clinically inapparent. However, viraemia can be followed by infection of organs distant from the site of entry with often devastating effects in the form of meningitis, encephalitis, paralysis, myopericarditis, and also rashes and conjunctivitis.

The viruses

Viruses of the *Picornaviridae* are nonenveloped icosahedral particles of 27 to 30 nm in diameter and contain single-stranded RNA of positive polarity and 7.2- to 8.4-kb size as their genome. The nucleic acid is polyadenylated at the 3′ end and carries a small protein, VPg, covalently linked at its 5′ end. The enteroviruses and parechoviruses form 2 of the 12 current genera of the *Picornaviridae* family, the others being the genera of *Aphthovirus*, *Avihepatovirus*, *Cardiovirus*, *Erbovirus*, *Hepatovirus*, *Kobuvirus*, *Sapelovirus*, *Senecavirus*, *Teschovirus*, and *Tremovirus*. In turn, the *Picornaviridae* are one of five families of the new order *Picornavirales*. Three serotypes of poliomyelitis virus (poliovirus), 23 types of Coxsackie A virus, 6 types of Coxsackie B virus, and 28 types of enteric cytopathic human orphan (echo) viruses are recognized within the *Enterovirus* genus. The parechoviruses comprise echoviruses 22 and 23 and were established as a separate genus on the basis of highly divergent sequence of their genomes. Other classic features of the enteroviruses, such as their stability at acid pH (in contrast to rhinoviruses or aphthoviruses), their buoyant density in caesium chloride gradients, and the nature of their broad clinical effects and persistence in the environment are also shared by the parechoviruses.

The three-dimensional structure of the poliovirus particle has been elucidated by crystallographic analysis (Fig. 5.8.1). The viral capsid consists of 60 protein subunits, each containing the four unglycosylated viral proteins VP1 to VP4. The capsid proteins are arranged in such a way that VP1 molecules form the apices at the fivefold symmetry axis of the icosahedron, whereas two other proteins VP2 and VP3 are arranged in the centre of the triangular face near the threefold axis of symmetry; VP4 is an internal protein. All proteins interact with each other. The N-terminus of VP4 is myristoylated.

Viruses initiate replication by attaching to their cellular receptors, and some of these have been characterized. The poliovirus receptor (PVR or CD155) is a member of the immunoglobulin superfamily. Transgenic mice expressing the human PVR become susceptible to oral poliovirus infection with a pathology similar to that of infected primates. Tests using these animals have been incorporated into regulatory requirements as supplements and eventual replacements for primates for vaccine testing (see below). Other enterovirus receptors are the decay accelerating factors (DAF; receptor for various echovirus types, Coxsackie B virus types, and coxsackievirus A21), implicated in the complement pathway, and the integrin VLA-2 (receptor for echovirus types 1 and 8). Other cell surface molecules may be involved as coreceptors in the virus–cell receptor interactions of many enteroviruses, as the expression of

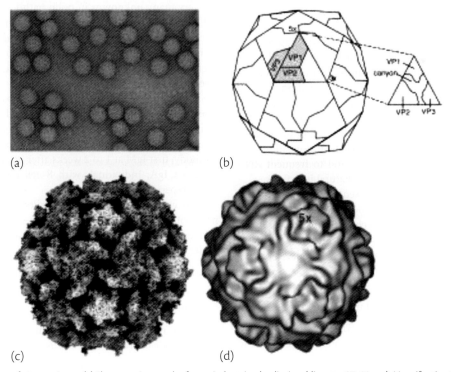

(a)   (b)

(c)   (d)

Fig. 5.8.1 Structural features of picornaviruses. (a) Electron micrograph of negatively stained poliovirus (diameter 27–30 nm). Magnification ×270 000. (b) Diagram of the picornavirus capsid, showing the packing arrangements of VP1, VP2, and VP3, and the interspersed canyon. VP4 is located on the interior of the capsid. The biological protomer (grey) is different from the icosahedral subunit (triangle shown at right). (c) Model of poliovirus type 1, Mahoney, based on X-ray crystallographic structure determined at 2.9 Å. The fivefold axis of symmetry is marked (5×). Surrounding the fivefold axis are canyons, the receptor-binding site. (d) Model of poliovirus type 1, Mahoney, produced by image reconstruction from cryoelectron microscopy data obtained at 20 Å resolution.
From Racaniello VR (2007). Picornaviridae: the viruses and their replication. In: Knipe DM, *et al.* (eds) *Fields virology*, 5th edition, pp. 795–838. Wolters Kluwer Health/Lippincott Williams & Wilkins, Philadelphia. With permission of author and publisher.

a single identified receptor is not always sufficient to make a previously resistant cell line susceptible to productive infection. It is also of interest that some strains of poliovirus, mainly of serotype 2, are able to paralyse mice if injected. The receptor involved in mice has not been identified.

The positive-sense RNA genome acts as a messenger molecule. All enterovirus RNAs have a long 5′ end untranslated region (UTR) of approximately 750 nucleotides in length, which is highly structured and contains an internal ribosomal entry site (IRES). The IRES is important for binding of the RNA to ribosomes and subsequent translation of the RNA into protein. Downstream of the 5′ UTR is a large single open reading frame containing three parts: P1, coding for structural proteins VP1 to VP4; P2, coding for proteins 2A, 2B, and 2C; and P3, coding for proteins 3A to 3D. Proteins 2A and 3C are viral proteases and protein 3D is the RNA-dependent RNA polymerase (RdRp). P2 and P3 proteins (with the exception of VPg = 3B) are only found in infected cells. The P1 to P3 proteins are synthesized as one large precursor from which the individual proteins are produced by complex autocleavage and cleavage cascades. RNA replicates via double-stranded replicative intermediates. The ratio of positive-stranded to negative-stranded RNA molecules in infected cells is approximately 100:1. During replication, RNA recombination does not infrequently occur. Replication of and translation from the same RNA cannot occur at the same time. Poliovirus-infected cells undergo a shut off of cellular mRNA synthesis and cellular protein translation. Naked enterovirus RNA is infectious on transfection (poliovirus was the first RNA virus rescued this way) and can be transcribed and recovered from full-length cDNA clones permitting biochemical manipulation and structure–function studies at the molecular level (reverse genetics).

The extensive antigenic variation of enterovirus capsid proteins allows typing into polioviruses, coxsackieviruses, and echoviruses using type-specific neutralizing antisera, but there is some cross-reactivity. The main antigenic sites are located on all three major virion proteins (VP1–VP3), and some involve sequences from more than one protein. The molecular mechanisms for the high genomic diversity of picornaviruses are thought to be based on misincorporations of nucleotides during chain elongation (due to the high error rate of the viral RdRp) and to frequent RNA recombination events, which also occur in natural infections.

Comparison of complete RNA genome sequences of many enteroviruses shows a very close relationship between some enterovirus and rhinovirus sequences. Within the echoviruses, however, there is great diversity.

A subdivision of human enteroviruses into four species according to genomic relatedness has been proposed:

1 Human enterovirus A: coxsackieviruses A2 to A8, A10, A12, A14, and A16, human enterovirus 71, and human enterovirus 76

2 Human enterovirus B: coxsackieviruses B1 to B6, A9, all echoviruses except types 22 and 23, and human enteroviruses 69, 73 to 75, 77, and 78

3 Human enterovirus C: poliovirus types 1 to 3, coxsackieviruses A1, A11, A13, A17, A19 to A22, and A24

4 Human enterovirus Group D: human enterovirus enteroviruses 68 and 70

(The enterovirus genus also contains three human rhinovirus species and several animal enterovirus species.)

Hepatitis A virus has previously been designated enterovirus 72, but is now in its own genus *Hepatovirus*. Echoviruses types 22 and 23 form the *Parechovirus* genus.

Pathogenesis

The most widely accepted model of the pathogenesis of enterovirus infection is based on that developed by Bodian for poliovirus, in which the virus infects the host via the gastrointestinal tract and undergoes primary replication in lymphoid cells lining the alimentary tract (oropharyngeal, intestinal). A viraemic phase follows, allowing infection of distant target organs: spinal cord and brain, meninges, myocardium, skeletal muscles, skin, and mucous membranes. Other tissues, e.g. lymph nodes and brown fat tissue, can also become infected. Intensive multiplication in the central nervous system (CNS) leads to the destruction of motor neurons and results in paralysis.

A slightly different and more subtle model of poliovirus pathogenesis was proposed by Sabin, in which the virus infects the mucosal surface, thus accounting for the fact that virus can be shed in faeces long after it has become undetectable in lymphoid tissues and when neutralizing antibody is detectable in the blood. The primary replication creates a viraemia which seeds distant, still unknown, sites and virus replication there results in a second viraemia, which may be detected about 1 week postinfection and can lead to systemic infection including CNS involvement. There are very many unknowns in polio pathogenesis. For instance it is still not clear where the virus that is shed in the faeces is produced, nor precisely from which cells. It can be inferred that they are few in number and of limited function because of the level of virus excreted and the fact that infection is almost always silent if confined to the gut.

Shedding of virus occurs from the throat and faeces for many weeks and even months after infection and thus ensures transmission (see below). Virus replication in sites distant from the port of entry normally terminates with the appearance of neutralizing antibody, first IgM at 1 to 2 weeks after infection and then IgG and secretory IgA. Individuals with B-cell immunodeficiencies may develop persistent infections.

Most enterovirus infections are silent or produce a 'minor illness' with the symptoms of a mild upper respiratory tract infection with or without fever. In a minority of infections (1% or less) one of the following systemic 'major diseases' may develop:

- Paralytic poliomyelitis, aseptic meningitis (polioviruses)

- Aseptic meningitis, herpangina, conjunctivitis, hand-foot-and-mouth disease (Coxsackie A viruses)

- Aseptic meningitis, myopericarditis, encephalitis, pleurodynia (Coxsackie B viruses; enterovirus 71)

- Aseptic meningitis, rashes, conjunctivitis (echoviruses)
- Polio-like illness, aseptic meningitis, hand-foot-and-mouth disease, epidemic conjunctivitis (enterovirus types 68–71)

Symptoms of clinical illness caused by enteroviruses are summarized in Table 5.8.1 and are discussed in more detail below.

Table 5.8.1 Clinical symptoms and their possible enteroviral causes

Clinical symptom (phenotype)	Polio 1	Polio 2	Polio 3	CoxA 2	CoxA 4	CoxA 5	CoxA 6	CoxA 7	CoxA 9	CoxA 10	CoxA 16	CoxA 21	CoxA 24	CoxB 1	CoxB 2	CoxB 3	CoxB 4	CoxB 5	Echo 1	Echo 2	Echo 4	Echo 6	Echo 9	Echo 11	Echo 16	Echo 19	Echo 30	Entero 70	Entero 71
Aseptic meningitis (rarely encephalitis)	✓	✓	✓	✓	✓		✓	✓	✓					✓	✓	✓	✓		✓	✓	✓	✓	✓	✓				✓	✓
Paralysis	✓	✓	✓					✓	✓					✓	✓	✓	✓		✓	✓	✓	✓	✓				✓		✓
Severe systemic infection (neonates)														✓	✓	✓	✓	✓	✓	✓	✓	✓							✓
Myo(peri)carditis						✓			✓					✓	✓	✓	✓	✓	✓	✓						✓			
Epidemic pleurodynia								✓						✓	✓	✓	✓	✓	✓	✓									
Exanthemata, enanthema				✓	✓	✓			✓	✓	✓			✓	✓	✓	✓	✓	✓	✓					✓				✓
Conjunctivitis												✓	✓								✓							✓	
Respiratory symptoms (herpangina)							✓		✓	✓	✓	✓		✓	✓	✓							✓	✓	✓				
Diarrhoea																								✓					

Clinical symptoms

Central nervous system infections (Oxford Textbook of Medicine 5e Chapter 24.11.2)

Poliomyelitis

Evidence of poliomyelitis as an ancient human disease is revealed on a funerary stele from Middle Kingdom Egypt, about 1300 bc, but there is little documentation of its occurrence until nearly the end of the 19th century when it appeared in epidemics in children (hence the alternative name 'infantile paralysis'). The appearance of poliomyelitis coincided with the improvement in standards of public hygiene and is explained by the consequent exposure of infants to infection at a later age. Maternal antibody is capable of confining infection to the gut, where the virus can persist until the immune response develops to eliminate it. In contrast, when maternal antibody has declined in older infants, the virus can spread to sites outside the intestine, causing paralysis.

Even under modern conditions of hygiene, infection with all three poliovirus types is normally inapparent, but illness with neurological symptoms results in about 1% of infections or less. This can present as aseptic meningitis with neck stiffness, usually recovering after 10 days (abortive or nonparalytic poliomyelitis). Meningitis is also caused by several other enteroviruses (see below). The more serious presentation is paralytic poliomyelitis, appearing 5 to 10 days after a mild upper respiratory tract infection ('minor illness') and progressing to flaccid paralysis resulting from motor neuron destruction ('major illness'). This may be accompanied by spasms and lack of coordination of nonparalysed muscles. Various forms of the 'major illness' reflect infection of different parts of the CNS. Paralysis of limbs (Fig. 5.8.2) results from destruction of motor neurons in the lower part of the spinal cord ('spinal form'), while the more life threatening bulbar poliomyelitis ('bulbar form') involves infections of the medulla oblongata or bulb. Respiratory functions can be affected in both the spinal and bulbar forms of the disease; encephalitis is rare. In children under 5 years old, paralysis of one leg is most common; in children 5 to 15 years of age, weakness of one limb or paraplegia are frequent; quadriplegia is most common in adults and is often accompanied by urinary bladder

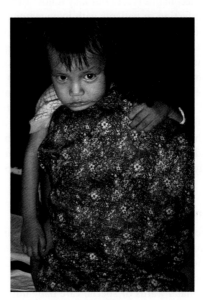

Fig. 5.8.2 Acute monoplegia in a Thai child in 1979 caused by poliomyelitis. Copyright D A Warrell.

and respiratory muscle dysfunction. Muscular function in limbs may return slowly, but there is residual paralysis in 90% of survivors. Of paralytic cases, 10 to 25% have bulbar symptoms with hypertension, shock, and dysphonia. Complications are nosocomial pneumonias (by staphylococci or gram-negative bacteria), urinary tract infections, and emotional problems. The mortality from paralytic polio is 2 to 5% among children and 15 to 30% among adults. Muscle weakness may develop many years after the initial polio disease (postpolio syndrome or postpolio neuromuscular atrophy). A persistent poliovirus infection as cause of this has been assumed, based on the presence of viral RNA in cerebrospinal fluid and neural tissue. However, such RNA has also been found in patients with other neurological and non-neurological diseases and is, therefore, less likely to be related to the postpolio syndrome. The alternative view is that the postpolio syndrome is anatomical in origin, such that the initial attack of polio destroys motor neurons and reduces the backup available as the patient ages.

Aseptic meningitis

Aseptic meningitis is the most frequent clinical presentation of enterovirus infection and can be caused by coxsackieviruses of both groups A and B, and echoviruses, mainly types 4, 6, 11, 14, 16, 25, 30, and 31 (see Table 5.8.1). The disease starts with fever, headache, neck stiffness, and photophobia. Sensory or motor deficits are unusual, but confusion is common. The symptoms may persist for 4 to 7 days. The cerebrospinal fluid usually shows pleocytosis consisting of 10 to 500 leucocytes/µl, mainly lymphocytes. Polymorphonuclear cells may predominate at the onset, but bacterial infection and possibly abscesses should be considered if they persist. The protein concentration in cerebrospinal fluid may be normal or slightly increased; the glucose level is normal. Complete recovery is the usual outcome of aseptic meningitis.

Encephalitis

Enterovirus encephalitis is rare but may follow aseptic meningitis. Enterovirus infection in patients with hypogammaglobulinaemia or agammaglobulinaemia may persist for years with chronic meningitis or encephalitis and a high mortality rate as sequelae.

Enterovirus 71 infection, which is normally associated with hand-foot-and-mouth disease, has been found to cause severe meningoencephalitis (with brain stem involvement), polio-like acute flaccid paralysis, and a high case fatality rate in children during several recent outbreaks in Bulgaria, Taiwan, and Malaysia. In some of the fatal cases there may have been coinfections with a species B adenovirus. Enterovirus 71 occurs in three genotypes and is rapidly evolving; it is most closely related to coxsackievirus A16.

Neonatal infections

Neonatal infection followed by severe generalized disease may be caused by Coxsackie B viruses and echoviruses, mainly of types 6, 7, and 11. These viruses seem to be transmitted late in pregnancy, perinatally, or postnatally by the mother or other virus-infected infants in neonatal wards or special care baby units. The infants develop either heart failure due to a severe myocarditis or a meningoencephalitis; hepatitis and adrenalitis may also occur. The mortality is high. Viruses may be recovered from brain, spinal cord, myocardium, and liver at autopsy.

Bornholm disease (epidemic pleurodynia)

This is usually caused by Coxsackie B viruses but can also be caused by echoviruses of types 1, 6, 9, 16, and 19 and by Coxsackie A viruses of types 4, 6, 9, and 10. The disease can strike families in small outbreaks. It typically starts abruptly with fever and chest pain due to the involvement of the intercostal muscles or abdominal pain resulting from involvement of muscles of the abdomen. There may be severe frontal headache. The symptoms last 3 to 14 days and are followed by complete recovery.

Myopericarditis

Enterovirus-induced myocarditis is mostly due to infection with Coxsackie B viruses in the young. The onset of disease is usually acute, very severe, and may be fatal in neonates; however, in adolescents and adults it is normally mild. The virus may persist after the initial infection and cause dilated cardiomyopathy. In fatal cases (usually neonates 2–11 days after onset of disease) there is cardiac dilatation, myocyte necrosis, and an inflammatory reaction. The diagnosis is often difficult, particularly in older patients, as pericarditis, coronary artery occlusion, or heart failure may have been diagnosed initially. Typical clinical findings are often tachycardia, arrhythmias, murmurs, rubs, and cardiomegaly.

Besides causing acute myocarditis, chronic enterovirus infection may lead to chronic myocarditis and dilated cardiomyopathy, possibly due to immunopathological mechanisms. In chronic disease, neither infectious virus nor viral antigens are normally detected in heart biopsies; however, viral RNA is regularly found in cardiac muscle suggesting that the viral genome persists. The true significance of the presence of the viral genome in such cases is still under discussion.

The disease can be produced with Coxsackie B viruses in mice. In this animal model there is also initial viraemia and replication in myocytes, but this is followed by disappearance of infectious virus and destruction of myocytes, possibly by autoimmune mechanisms.

Herpangina

This is caused by coxsackieviruses of types A1 to A6, A8, A10, and A22. Children and young adults between 2 and 20 years of age are mainly affected. The disease presents with acute onset of fever, sore throat, and pain on swallowing, as well as vomiting and abdominal symptoms. Small vesicular lesions or white papules surrounded by a red halo can be seen on the fauces, pharynx, palate, uvula, and tonsils (Fig. 5.8.3). The disease is mild and self-limiting.

Exanthemas

Rubella-like rashes can be produced by echoviruses of types 4, 9, and 16, but also coxsackieviruses A9, A16, and B5 (Fig. 5.8.4). They usually occur in the summer and may be accompanied by fever, malaise, cervical lymphadenopathy, and aseptic meningitis.

Hand-foot-and-mouth disease

A typical distribution of vesicular lesions in hands, feet, and mouth (but also buttocks and genitalia) is produced by infection with coxsackievirus type A16 and enterovirus 71, and less frequently with coxsackieviruses A4, A5, A9 and A10, B2, and B5 (Fig. 5.8.5a,b).

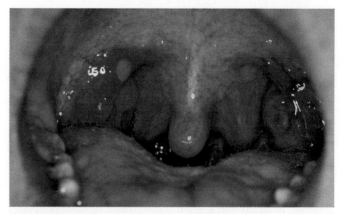

Fig. 5.8.3 Herpangina due to coxsackievirus A6 infection.
Courtesy of the late Dr B E Juel-Jensen.

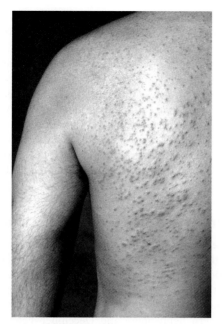

Fig. 5.8.4 Exanthema due to coxsackievirus infection.
Courtesy of the late Dr B E Juel-Jensen.

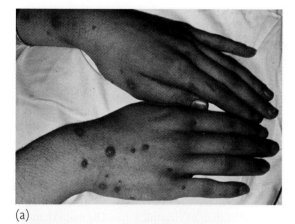

(a)

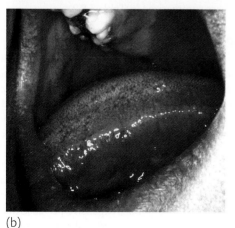

(b)

Fig. 5.8.5 (a, b) Hand-foot-and-mouth disease due to coxsackievirus infection.
Courtesy of the late Dr B E Juel-Jensen.

Enterovirus 71 may produce more severe clinical symptoms (see above).

Foot-and-mouth disease

The aphthovirus causing foot-and-mouth disease in cloven-hoofed animals is endemic in Africa, Asia, and South America. Virus is secreted before blisters on the mouth and feet appear in animals. The zoonosis in humans is very rare, with about 37 recorded cases. Human infection occurs from virus entering through broken skin, drinking unpasteurized milk, or by inhalation of droplets. A 2- to 6-day incubation period is followed by blisters of hands, feet, and mouth, fever, and sore throat; complete recovery ensues. No person-to-person spread is recorded.

Conjunctivitis

Several enterovirus types cause conjunctivitis, often affecting large numbers of people epidemically. Most notable causes are echovirus types 7 and 11, coxsackievirus A24 and B2, and enterovirus 70 that often produces a haemorrhagic conjunctivitis.

Diabetes and pancreatitis

Insulin-dependent diabetes mellitus (IDDM, or type 1 diabetes) is likely to be an autoimmune disorder in which the insulin-secreting pancreatic islet cells (β cells) are destroyed. The human disease has long been thought to be caused by infectious agents, particularly since association between enterovirus infection and the development of IDDM has been shown in animal model studies (infection of mice with Coxsackie B3–B5 viruses). However, there is also a strong genetic component in the development of IDDM.

Chronic fatigue syndrome (Oxford Textbook of Medicine 5e Chapter 26.5.4)

Chronic fatigue syndrome (CFS), also known under the names of myalgic encephalomyelitis (ME), Royal Free disease, Iceland disease, postviral fatigue syndrome, and neuromyasthenia, can occur both sporadically and epidemically. The main clinical feature is excess fatigability of skeletal muscle, accompanied by pain. Other symptoms include headaches, inability to concentrate, paraesthesia, and impairment of short-term memory. A major problem in diagnosis is a clear definition of the clinical entity. Several virus infections have seemed to precede the development of CFS; they are mainly enterovirus infections, chronic Epstein–Barr virus (EBV) infection, and also infections with *Toxoplasma* and *Leptospira* spp. The stringency of the association of chronic enterovirus infection with the appearance of CFS is controversial. A report of a joint working group of the Royal Colleges of Physicians, Psychiatrists, and General Practitioners has concluded that persistence of enteroviruses is unlikely to play a role in the development of CFS. Similar conclusions have been drawn for the possibility of a causal link between chronic EBV infection and CFS (see Chapter 5.3).

Gastroenteritis

Although enteroviruses infect via the gastrointestinal tract and readily replicate there, they very rarely cause diarrhoea. Outbreaks of diarrhoea with echovirus type 11 have been reported. In Japan, an enterovirus termed Aichi virus, which is proposed as the type species of the new genus *Kobuvirus* of the *Picornaviridae* family, has been identified as the cause of multiple outbreaks of gastroenteritis in humans, mostly associated with the consumption of raw oysters. This virus seems to circulate widely in populations of Japan and other south-east Asian countries, with subclinical infections likely to be common (see Chapter 5.9).

Laboratory diagnosis of enterovirus infections

Virus isolation

Virus isolation is an excellent procedure to diagnose enterovirus infections. Virus is shed for weeks, and sometimes months, from the primary infection sites (cells lining the gut, see above). Starting from a few days after infection, virus can be found in concentrations of 10^5 to 10^6 tissue culture infectious doses 50%/g ($TCID_{50}$/g) of faeces. Throat swabs are also a good source for virus, particularly early in infection and when there are respiratory symptoms. In cases of meningitis, enteroviruses can be propagated in cell culture from the cerebrospinal fluid, but the method is much less sensitive than genome detection (see below). Viruses are readily isolated in secondary cultures of monkey kidney cells, or in cultures of permanent cell lines derived from human embryonic kidney, human amnion, or human fetal lung. The cytopathic effect (CPE) produced by enteroviruses is nonspecific. Typing of a cytopathic agent is carried out using antiserum pools (see below) or in multistep procedures. Most Coxsackie A viruses (with the exception of coxsackievirus A9) do not grow well in cell culture but can be readily isolated by intracerebral, intraperitoneal, or subcutaneous infection of mice, causing flaccid paralysis and death. In contrast, Coxsackie B viruses cause spastic paralysis. Polioviruses or echoviruses do not usually grow in mice although polioviruses will replicate in transgenic animals that have appropriate receptors (see above).

Serology

Neutralization assays are the method of choice for typing enteroviruses. Due to the large number of enterovirus types, these tests are labour intensive and not apt for rapid diagnosis. Pools of type-specific antisera (prepared by Drs Lim, Benyesch, Melnick; LMB pools) have greatly helped to establish the epidemiology of enterovirus infections worldwide. Recurrent enterovirus infections during a lifetime often result in elevated serum antibody titres which obscure diagnostic changes. Significant antibody rises are, therefore, rarely observed in paired sera (taken at the onset of and during convalescence from disease).

A Coxsackie B virus-specific IgM test (using an IgM antibody capture technique) has been developed for rapid diagnosis. However, there is cross-reactivity between the IgM responses to different enteroviruses, including different genera of the picornaviruses, and so this test is not very specific. Prolonged presence of enterovirus-specific IgM has also been observed. In summary, the usefulness of serology for the diagnosis of enterovirus infection is limited.

Genome detection

Reverse transcription–polymerase chain reaction (RT-PCR) techniques have been applied to test for the presence of enterovirus genomes. This approach has been very productive, particularly in diagnosing CNS infections from cerebrospinal fluid specimens, and has become the 'gold standard' of diagnosis, surpassing viral culture. Enterovirus RNAs have also been detected in myocardial biopsies from patients with myocarditis and dilated cardiomyopathy, in muscle of people with inflammatory muscle disease and chronic fatigue syndrome, and in brain biopsies. The significance of these findings is not clear, as infectious virus can rarely be isolated and viral antigen cannot be detected. Highly conserved sequences in the 5′ end of enterovirus genomes have allowed the design of PCR primers detecting most enterovirus RNAs. As the echovirus 22 genome is very different from that of the other enteroviruses (see above), tailor-made primers have to be added in a multiplex RT-PCR to include these viruses, which cause infections particularly in neonates and infants. A modified RT-PCR procedure can differentiate between wild-type and vaccine-derived poliovirus infections.

Epidemiology of enterovirus infections

Enteroviruses are mainly transmitted by the faeco-oral route, due to the fact that viruses are shed in faeces for weeks or months after infection. Spread is particularly intense within families, usually starting from the primary infection of young children. In temperate climates, there are seasonal peaks (July–September in the northern hemisphere and December–February in the southern hemisphere), whereas in subtropical and tropical climates enterovirus infections occur all the year round. The vast majority of primary human enterovirus infections occur during the first decade of life. Type-specific surveillance in several geographical regions has shown that coxsackieviruses A9, A16, and B4 and echovirus types 6, 9, 11, 19, 22, and 30 are most frequently found.

Prevention of enterovirus infections

As there are only three poliovirus types and no significant animal reservoir, it has been possible to develop very successful poliovirus vaccines. In 1954, a formalin-inactivated poliovirus vaccine (IPV) was introduced by Dr Jonas Salk in the United States of America, and in 1962 Dr Albert Sabin introduced a vaccine consisting of live attenuated strains of the three poliovirus types which could be given orally (OPV). Protection by the live attenuated vaccine is effected mainly at the site of entry by eliciting locally virus-specific IgAs and IgGs. Inactivated vaccine mainly elicits serum IgGs which prevent infection of the CNS and other sites distant of the port of entry by neutralization of viraemic virus. The main characteristics of IPV and OPV are summarized in Table 5.8.2.

Inactivated poliovirus vaccine

The early IPVs developed by Salk were of relatively low potency. High potency vaccines, based on large-scale cell culture followed by virus purification and concentration but using the same inactivation procedures, were developed in the Netherlands in the 1980s and form the basis of IPVs used today. Much of the developed world including Europe and the United States of America now uses only IPVs, having previously used the live attenuated vaccines. Other countries including Mexico and Russia have changed from using OPV to IPV, and middle income countries such as Argentina and Uruguay are proposing to do so when poliomyelitis is eradicated. IPV is given by injection and is more expensive per dose than the oral vaccine, but has advantages as outlined below, mainly the avoidance of vaccine-associated paralysis. IPV is the vaccine of choice in cases of immunodeficiency.

Table 5.8.2 Characteristics of poliovirus vaccines

Characteristic	Live attenuated poliovirus vaccine (OPV)	Inactivated poliovirus vaccine (IPV)
Virus source	Attenuated virus (Sabin strains)	Virulent virus strains
Primary course	3 doses at monthly intervals starting at age of 2 months (temperate climates; more doses in tropics)	Three doses at 2-month intervals
Administration route	Oral	Parenteral (injection)
Immunity produced—systemic	IgA, IgM, IgG	IgM, IgG, (IgA)
—local	IgA	(IgA, minimal)
Booster doses required	1. at school entry 2. between 15 and 19 years 3. in adult life when exposed (last dose 10 years or more ago)	Yes (every 3–5 years or when exposed)
Efficacy	Good in temperate climates, variable in tropics	Good
Spread to contacts	Yes	No
Vaccine-associated paralysis	0.5–3.4 cases/million first doses in susceptible children	No
Production cost per dose	$0.07	$0.7
Requirement on personnel	Not highly trained	Trained and skilled
Requirement of 'cold chain'	Yes	Less than OPV
Combination with other vaccines	No	Possible
Use in immunodeficient children	No	Possible

Live attenuated poliovirus vaccine

This vaccine has several advantages compared to the inactivated vaccine (Table 5.8.2) as it:

◆ parallels the natural infection;

◆ stimulates both local secretory IgA in the pharynx and alimentary tract, and systemic circulating virus-specific IgG antibody;

◆ is easy to administer as an oral vaccine;

◆ is more cost effective; and

◆ is proven to be capable of interrupting virus circulation and epidemics.

The disadvantage is that in a few cases the attenuated vaccine strains have reverted to virulence in vaccine recipients or their contacts. Since the early 1980s, all cases of polio in the United States of America and Europe were found to be vaccine-related, occurring either in vaccine recipients or their close contacts who became infected by them, or were imported from endemic countries and were not indigenous original wild-type strains. The risk of vaccine-associated poliomyelitis is between 0.5 and 3.4 cases/million of susceptible children immunized. Vaccine-related polio is mostly caused by type 2 or type 3 viruses, probably due to the fact that the number of point mutations in type 1 vaccine virus compared to wild-type virus is much higher than in type 2 and type 3 vaccine viruses. However, as the disease becomes increasingly rare in the countries concerned and the world at large, indigenous cases or importation of virus are increasingly rare, and the risks of oral vaccination begin to outweigh its benefits. The reintroduction of polio by the use of oral vaccine has now been frequently documented in regions where immunization programmes are imperfect and the virus is able to regain the ability to transmit from person to person and cause outbreaks. This poses a risk to the whole eradication programme. These risks are not associated with the use of IPV, which has become the vaccine of choice in many countries.

Polio eradication and surveillance

For many years it was thought that the Sabin oral poliovirus vaccines were ineffective in tropical countries, being unable to control the disease, much less eradicate it. While many reasons were put forward, the lack of impact of polio vaccination programmes was probably due to loss of vaccine potency through failure to maintain storage at cool temperatures ('cold chain'), and also the epidemiology of poliovirus infection. In temperate countries, poliomyelitis is seasonal with infections peaking in the summer months. A strategy of vaccination based on immunization of young children at a set age (usually a few months) is, therefore, able to build up a highly immune population resistant to infection in the winter so that transmission of the wild-type virus becomes more difficult; thus, the virus and the disease are eradicated. In tropical countries, where exposure is year round, it is a matter of chance whether a child will first be naturally infected or immunized, and virus circulation can continue. This was recognized by Sabin in 1960, but not acted upon until some 20 years later when the strategy of National Immunization Days was developed in South America. This approach involves immunizing all children below a certain age in a country within a very short period, so that all susceptible children's intestinal tracts are occupied by vaccine virus and are, therefore, resistant to infection by the wild-type virus. Transmission of wild-type virus is therefore broken, and the virus dies out.

The World Health Organization (WHO) has pronounced the intention of eliminating poliomyelitis due to wild-type virus in 1988, with a target date of 2000 for completion. The Americas have

Polio incidence: 1988

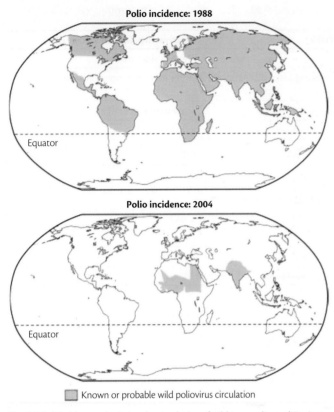

Polio incidence: 2004

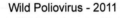

■ Known or probable wild poliovirus circulation

Fig. 5.8.6 World maps depicting the circulation of wild-type poliomyelitis virus for 1988 and 2004, as reported by the World Health Organization.

From Palllansch M, Roos R (2007) Enteroviruses: polioviruses, coxsackieviruses, echoviruses, and newer enteroviruses. In: Knipe DM, *et al.* (eds) *Fields virology*, 5th edition, pp. 839–93. Wolters Kluwer Health/Lippincott Williams & Wilkins, Philadelphia. With permission of author and publisher.

been free of polio since 1992. In 2000, the Western Pacific Region was declared polio-free by WHO, and the European region in 2002. The enormous progress achieved between 1988 and 2004 is shown in Fig. 5.8.6. The scale of the undertaking is colossal, and the progress towards eradication is extraordinary. For example, in 1992 in China, all children aged 5 or less were immunized during a 1-week period. This amounts to one-quarter of the world's children.

However, some regions have proved very difficult. At the time of writing, virus is still known to be endemic in only three countries: Pakistan, Afghanistan, and Nigeria (Fig. 5.8.7), with importation into some of the neighbouring countries. Eradication before long is a real possibility although it is not a trivial matter. It is only in 2011 that India recorded no cases at all and is appearing to be polio-free. The virus has been reintroduced repeatedly into countries where it had been eradicated, particularly into Angola from India and into the Democratic Republic of Congo from Angola. It has also been introduced into Tajikistan (European Region) from India, and most recently into China from Pakistan. In 2004, immunization stopped in Nigeria when it was suggested that the vaccine contained oestrogens to render recipients sterile. The result was the re-emergence and reintroduction of polio into much of Central Africa, where it had been previously considered eradicated, and outbreaks occurred in Yemen and Indonesia; it is surmised that pilgrims returning from Mecca were infected by coreligionists from Nigeria and reintroduced the virus. The situation was only brought under control by massive coordinated immunization activities throughout the region. Lingering on of wild-type polio up until 2010 in India was in part due to vaccine refusals similar to those in Nigeria. Although there have been no cases in India in 2011, in Pakistan the numbers increased by 62% in 2010, due to civilian turmoils, flood catastrophes, and lack of political will to eradicate. So long as pockets of infection persist the world remains at risk of the re-emergence of polio. Thus part of the challenge is to demonstrate that the virus has in fact been eliminated, and this depends on rigorous effective surveillance. One approach is to obtain data on cases of acute flaccid paralysis of whatever

Wild Poliovirus - 2011

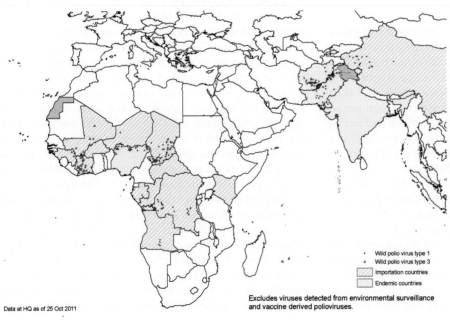

Data at HQ as of 25 Oct 2011

• Wild polio virus type 1
▲ Wild polio virus type 3
▨ Importation countries
▢ Endemic countries

Excludes viruses detected from environmental surveillance and vaccine derived polioviruses.

Fig. 5.8.7 Wild-type poliovirus cases in 2010.
Cases of wild type polio in 2011 from http://www.polioeradication.org. With permission from WHO.

cause, including the Guillain–Barré syndrome. Surveillance of environmental samples for wild-type poliovirus also has a role in global polio eradication, and isolates have been obtained in areas where there are no recorded cases of disease All cases should be investigated to see whether they are due to poliovirus infection or not, and it is considered that the background rate in the absence of poliomyelitis should be one case per 100 000 members of the population, providing a control for the adequacy of the surveillance scheme. Alternative approaches include the investigation of poliovirus isolates to establish whether they are derived from vaccine or represent wild-type strains. There are possible concerns over the adequacy of either approach.

Once wild-type poliovirus has been eradicated, the only sources of the virus will be manufacturers of vaccines, laboratories holding stocks, and recipients of live attenuated vaccine. While manufacturers and laboratory workers can be required to work under high containment level conditions to avoid escape of virulent virus, vaccinees pose a particular problem. The vaccine works by establishing an infection in the recipient, and there are numerous instances of outbreaks caused by vaccine-derived polioviruses that have recovered the ability to circulate (cVDPVs). This has been observed in Haiti, Egypt, the Philippines, and Madagascar among many others, and may be relatively common, particularly where vaccination continues with the live vaccine for a long time with poor coverage so that vaccinated and unvaccinated individuals mix, providing the ideal conditions for the selection of transmissible virus. However, the vaccine virus seems to be poorly transmissible compared to the wild type. In countries such as Cuba where it has been given only in the early part of the year as a matter of policy, virus is not detectable after 6 months. Thus, it might be possible to stop vaccinating with no further precautions, and deal with the re-emergence of polio as cVDPVs on a case-by-case basis.

The solution may be to cease vaccination abruptly, or, as is increasingly the case in developed countries, use IPV which does not pose this risk.

A further concern comes from people with B-cell immunodeficiency who can become chronically infected but be apparently healthy, sometimes for decades. During this time the virus may adapt to an extent that neurotropism is regained, and an unvaccinated population will again be highly susceptible. The numbers and geographical distribution of such long-term excretors are unknown but most exposed individuals do not excrete virus for very long periods, and even those that do usually cease excreting virus spontaneously, albeit after a period of a few years.

The fact that serious consideration has to be given to how to deal with the cessation of vaccination is a tribute to the extraordinary progress which has been made towards polio eradication.

The *de novo* synthesis of infectious particles from poliovirus RNA transcribed from synthetic cDNA in a cell-free HeLa cell extract has created a huge debate on the scientific value of such an experiment, concerns about poliovirus eradication, issues of national security and freedom of virological/biological research. Since then, other viruses (ΦX174, the 1918 H1N1 influenza virus a.o.) have been synthesized *de novo*, allowing the effect of more drastic changes in viral sequence on viral properties to be examined than is possible by established methods of genetic manipulation. The usefulness of the method to carry out broad-based research into questions of viral pathogenesis and attenuation for vaccine production (e.g. by changing codon usage) is becoming appreciated but it has also led to considerable efforts by the scientific community and industry to define and assess possible misuse of this technology.

Further reading

Cello J, Paul AV, Wimmer E. (2002). Chemical synthesis of poliovirus cDNA: generation of infectious virus in the absence of natural template. *Science*, **297**, 1016–18.

Centers for Disease Control and Prevention (CDC) (2011). Progress toward interruption of wild poliovirus transmission worldwide, January 2010-March 2011. *MMWR Morb Mortal Wkly Rep*, **60**, 582–6.

Centers for Disease Control and Prevention (CDC) (2011). Progress toward poliomyelitis eradication—Nigeria, January 2010–June 2011. *MMWR Morb Mortal Wkly Rep*, **60**, 1053–7.

Centers for Disease Control and Prevention (CDC) (2011). Update on vaccine-derived polioviruses—worldwide, July 2009–March 2011. *MMWR Morb Mortal Wkly Rep*, **60**, 846–50.

Hovi T, *et al.* (2011). Role of environmental poliovirus surveillance in global polio eradication and beyond. *Epidemiol Infect*, **140**, 1–13.

Joint Working Group of the Royal Colleges of Physicians, Psychiatrists, and General Practitioners (1997). *Chronic fatigue syndrome*, pp. 58. Royal College of Physicians Publication Unit, London.

Kew OM, *et al.* (2002). Outbreak of poliomyelitis in Hispaniola associated with circulating type 1 vaccine-derived poliovirus. *Science*, **296**, 356–9.

Larson HJ, Ghinai I (2011). Lessons from polio eradication. *Nature*, **47**(7348), 446–7.

Martin J, *et al.* (2000). Evolution of the Sabin strain of type 3 poliovirus in an immunodeficient patient during the entire 637-day period of virus excretion. *J Virol*, **74**, 3001–10.

Melnick JL (1996). Enteroviruses: polioviruses, coxsackieviruses, echoviruses, and newer enteroviruses. In: Fields BN, *et al.* (eds) *Fields virology*, 3rd edition, pp. 655–712. Lippincott-Raven, Philadelphia.

Mendelsohn C, Wimmer R, Racaniello VR (1989). Cellular receptor for poliovirus: molecular cloning, nucleotide sequence and expression of a new member of the immunoglobulin superfamily. *Cell*, **56**, 855–65.

Minor PD (1990). Antigenic structure of picornaviruses. *Curr Top Microbiol Immunol*, **161**, 122–54.

Minor PD (1996). Poliovirus. In: Nathanson N, *et al.* (eds) *Viral pathogenesis*, pp. 555–74. Lippincott-Raven, Philadelphia.

Minor P (2005). Picornaviruses. In: Mahy BW, ter Meulen V (eds) *Topley and Wilson's microbiology and microbial infections. Virology*, 10th edition, pp. 857–87. Hodder Arnold, London.

Nathanson N (2008). The pathogenesis of poliomyelitis: what we don't know. *Adv Virus Res*, **71**, 1–50.

Offit PA (2005). *The Cutter Incident*, pp. 256. Yale University Press, New Haven.

Pallnsch M, Roos R (2007) Enteroviruses: polioviruses, coxsackieviruses, echoviruses, and newer enteroviruses. In: Knipe DM, *et al.* (eds) *Fields virology*, 5th edition, pp. 839–93. Wolters Kluwer Health/Lippincott Williams & Wilkins, Philadelphia.

Racaniello VR (2007). Picornaviridae: the viruses and their replication. In: Knipe DM, *et al.* (eds) *Fields virology*, 5th edition, pp. 795–838. Wolters Kluwer Health/Lippincott Williams & Wilkins, Philadelphia.

Racaniello VR, Baltimore D (1981). Cloned poliovirus complementary DNA is infectious in mammalian cells. *Science*, **214**, 916–19.

Skern T (2010). 100 years poliovirus: from discovery to eradication. A meeting report. *Arch Virol*, **155**, 1371–81.

Stanway G, *et al.* (2005). Picornaviridae. In: Fauquet CM, *et al.* (eds) *Virus taxonomy. Classification and nomenclature of viruses. Eighth Report of the International Committee on Taxonomy of Viruses*, pp. 757–78. Elsevier Academic Press, London.

Wimmer E. (2006). The test-tube synthesis of a chemical called poliovirus. The simple synthesis of a virus has far-reaching societal implications. *EMBO Rep*, **7 Spec No**, S3–S9.

Wimmer E, *et al.* (2009). Synthetic viruses: a new opportunity to understand and prevent viral disease. *Nat Biotechnol*, **27**, 1163–72.

Wimmer E, Paul AV (2011). Synthetic poliovirus and other designer viruses: what have we learned from them? *Annu Rev Microbiol*, **65**, 583–609.

World Health Organization (2008). *Global polio eradication initiative. Annual report 2007. Impact of the intensified eradication effort.* WHO, Geneva. www.polioeradication.org/content/publications/AnnualReport2007_English.pdf

Yamashita T, *et al.* (2000). Application of a reverse transcription-PCR for identification and differentiation of Aichi virus, a new member of the picornavirus family associated with gastroenteritis in humans. *J Clin Microbiol*, **38**, 2955–61.

Websites

http://ictvonline.org/virusTaxonomy.asp?version=2009&bhcp=1

http://www.emro.who.int/polio/ last updated 22 August 2011; accessed 28 Oct 2011

http://www.polioeradication.org/Dataandmonitoring/Poliothisweek.aspx data of 26 Oct 2011; accessed 28 Oct 2011

5.9 Virus infections causing diarrhoea and vomiting

Philip Dormitzer and Ulrich Desselberger

Essentials

Gastroenteritis is frequently caused by rotaviruses, enteric adenoviruses (group F), human caliciviruses (noroviruses, sapoviruses), and astroviruses: these cause much disease worldwide and considerable mortality, mainly in developing countries. Other viruses found in the human gastrointestinal tract are not regularly associated with diarrhoeal disease, except in patients who are immunosuppressed and in whom herpes simplex virus, cytomegalovirus, and picobirnaviruses can cause diarrhoea, as can HIV itself.

Epidemiology—(1) Rotaviruses—the major cause of endemic infantile gastroenteritis worldwide transmission is by the faeco-oral route. There is a strict winter peak of infections in temperate climates, but these occur year round in tropical and subtropical regions. Many animals and birds harbour a large diversity of rotaviruses and may act as a reservoir for human infections. (2) Human caliciviruses—the most important cause of nonbacterial gastroenteritis outbreaks worldwide—frequently spread by contamination of food (oysters, green salads, fresh fruit, cold foods, and sandwiches) and water.

Clinical features and management—following an incubation period of 1 to 2 days, there is sudden onset of watery diarrhoea lasting between 4 and 7 days, vomiting, and varying degrees of dehydration. Other features include abdominal cramps, headache, myalgia and fever. Treatment is supportive, mainly with oral rehydration solutions or—in more severe cases—intravenous rehydration.

Diagnosis—viral infection can be demonstrated by passive particle agglutination tests, by virus-specific enzyme-linked immunosorbent assays, and by viral genome detection using the polymerase chain reaction (PCR) (for adenoviruses) or reverse transcription-PCR (RT-PCR) (for rotaviruses, caliciviruses, and astroviruses).

Prevention and control: two live attenuated oral rotavirus vaccines have recently been licensed in numerous countries, in some of which universal mass vaccination of children as part of childhood vaccination schemes has been accepted. There are no vaccines against other viruses causing gastroenteritis in humans. Outbreak control measures relate mainly to calicivirus-associated gastroenteritis and focus on the interruption of person-to-person transmission and the removal of common sources of infection (food, water, etc).

Introduction

Acute gastroenteritis and vomiting in humans is a well-characterized clinical entity caused by various agents (viruses, bacteria, parasites, etc.). Viral gastroenteritis is a global problem, particularly in infants and young children.

Many viruses are found in the human gut but not all of them produce acute gastroenteritis (Table 5.9.1). Viral infections normally associated with gastroenteritis are caused by rotaviruses, human caliciviruses (noroviruses, sapoviruses), enteric adenoviruses (group F), and astroviruses. Other viruses found in the human gastrointestinal tract (enteroviruses, reoviruses, nongroup F adenoviruses, toroviruses, coronaviruses, parvoviruses) are not regularly associated with diarrhoeal disease. Finally, there are viruses found in the gut of immunosuppressed patients (most commonly those infected with HIV), including herpes simplex virus (HSV),

Table 5.9.1 Virus infections of the human gut

Viruses found as	Genus (Family)
Regular cause of diarrhoea and vomiting	Rotaviruses (*Reoviridae*)[a]
	Human caliciviruses (*Caliciviridae*)[a]
	Group F adenoviruses (*Adenoviridae*)
	Astroviruses (*Astroviridae*)
Occasional cause of diarrhoea and vomiting	Enteroviruses (*Picornaviridae*)[b]
	Reoviruses (*Reoviridae*)
	Adenoviruses other than Group F (*Adenoviridae*)
	Toroviruses (*Coronaviridae*)
	Coronaviruses (*Coronaviridae*)
	Parvoviruses (*Parvoviridae*)
Cause of diarrhoea in immunodeficient patients	Human immunodeficiency virus (*Retroviridae*)
	Herpes simplex virus (*Herpesviridae*)
	Cytomegalovirus (*Herpesviridae*)
	Picobirnaviruses (*Birnaviridae*)

[a] Not all infections cause disease (see text).
[b] Outbreaks of diarrhoea caused by echovirus type 11 infections have been reported (see chapter 5.8).

cytomegalovirus (CMV), and picobirnaviruses. HIV itself can also infect the gut directly.

Only the major virus groups regularly causing gastroenteritis in humans are described here in separate sections. Clinical symptoms, diagnosis, treatment, epidemiology, and vaccine development are reviewed under common headings.

Rotaviruses

Structure

Rotaviruses are the major cause of infantile gastroenteritis worldwide and also of acute diarrhoea in the young of many mammalian species. They are members of the *Reoviridae* family, with a genome of 11 segments of double-stranded RNA encoding six structural viral proteins (VP1–VP4, VP6, VP7) and six nonstructural proteins (NSP1–NSP6). The icosahedral virion has three concentric protein layers and no lipid envelope (Fig. 5.9.1a).

The inner layer (consisting of VP2) encloses the genome segments, the polymerase VP1, and the capping enzyme VP3. The addition of a middle layer consisting of VP6 leads to the formation of a transcriptionally active subviral particle, referred to as the double-layered particle (DLP). VP6 is the most immunogenic rotavirus protein. Infectious virions (triple-layered particles, TLP) have an additional layer, which mediates the translocation of the DLP into the cytoplasm during cell entry. This outermost layer consists of two proteins VP4 and VP7, both of which elicit and are the targets of neutralizing antibodies. VP7 forms a shell, which is shed in the low calcium environment of the cytoplasm. VP4 forms spikes, which are important for attachment and membrane penetration. Electron cryomicroscopy image reconstructions and functional studies have provided evidence that a fold-back rearrangement of the VP4 spike, which is mounted on the VP6 layer and secured by the overlying VP7 shell, is required for membrane penetration during entry. (Fig. 5.9.1b). To achieve maximal infectivity of the virion, the VP4 spike must be cleaved by intestinal trypsin. In electron micrographs of negatively stained specimens, virions have a characteristic appearance as 75-nm wheel-like particles (Fig. 5.9.2), the name of the virus being derived from Latin *rota* = wheel.

Classification

Rotaviruses are classified according to the immunological reactivities and genomic sequences of three of their structural components. Specific epitopes on the inner-shell protein VP6 allow five groups (A–E) to be distinguished, and two more groups (F, G) probably exist. Group A rotaviruses cause the vast majority of human gastroenteritis infections and have been divided into subgroups on the basis of additional determinants on VP6. Group B rotaviruses have caused epidemics of diarrhoea affecting adults and children. Group C rotaviruses generally cause more mild diarrhoeal disease. The remaining groups are only known to infect nonhuman hosts. Recently, all 11 segments of rotaviruses have been classified into genotypes.

Both surface proteins, VP4 and VP7, elicit neutralizing antibodies and thus confer type specificity. A dual-type classification system has been devised for group A rotaviruses, which differentiates glycoprotein (G) types (VP7-specific) and protease-sensitive protein (P) types (VP4-specific). For example, G1P1A[8] is G serotype and genotype 1, P serotype 1A, P genotype 8. At present, rotaviruses carrying a relatively restricted number of G types (G1–G4 and G9) and P types (P[4] and P[8]) cause most human disease in temperate climates. However, at least 11 G types and 11 P types have been

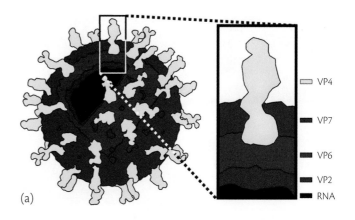

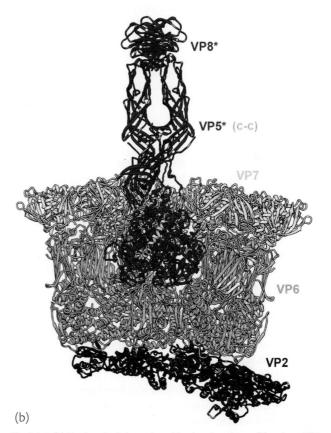

Fig. 5.9.1 (a) The icosahedral rotavirus virion has three layers: (1) an inner VP2 layer that contains the genome, polymerase, and capping enzyme; (2) a middle VP6 layer; and (3) an outer VP7 layer. The VP4 spike is anchored in the VP6 layer and protrudes through the VP7 layer. (b) Interphase of VP4 in the TLP (cutaway view). VP8*, magenta; VP5*, red. The foot of VP5* is anchored at a six-coordinated position in the VP6 layer (green). A VP7 trimer (yellow) caps each VP6 trimer. The VP6 lattice overlays the VP2 shell (dark blue) which surrounds the coiled RNA genome (not shown).

Panel A: based on Dormitzer P, *et al.* (2004). Structural rearrangements in the membrane penetration protein of a non-enveloped virus. *Nature*, **430**, 1053–58; Yeager M, *et al.* (1990). Three-dimensional structure of rhesus rotavirus by cryoelectron microscopy and image reconstruction. *J Cell Biol*, **110**, 2133–44. Panel B: from: Settembre EC, *et al.* (2011). http://www.ncbi.nlm.nih.gov/pubmed/21157433 Atomic model of an infectious rotavirus particle. *EMBO J*, **30**, 408–16. With permission of the authors and the publisher.

found in humans. Zoonotic rotavirus infections of humans are well documented, and previously rare serotypic variants have become established among strains pathogenic to humans (mainly in tropical and subtropical regions). In addition, rotaviruses can exchange

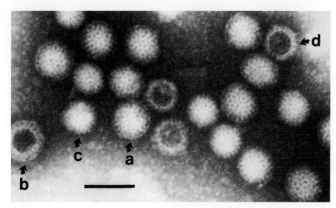

Fig. 5.9.2 Rotavirus particles in the faeces of a child admitted to hospital with acute gastroenteritis. Negative staining with aqueous 2% potassium phosphotungstate, pH 7.0. Scale bar represents 100 nm. Four different morphologies of particles are shown: (a) triple-layered particle containing RNA; (b) triple-layered particle without RNA (empty, core penetrated with stain); (c) double-layered particle containing RNA; and (d) double-layered empty particle. Courtesy of M. Jenkins, Regional Virus Laboratory, East Birmingham Hospital. From Desselberger U (1992). Reoviruses. In: Greenwood D, Slack R, Peutherer J (eds) *Medical microbiology*, 14th edition, p. 620. Churchill Livingstone, Edinburgh, with permission of the publisher.)

genome segments (reassort) during mixed infections, providing an additional mechanism to introduce genetic diversity. Hence, rotavirus epidemiology continues to evolve, and eradication of rotaviruses is not feasible.

Replication

The primary targets of rotavirus infection are the mature epithelial cells at the tips of the villi of the small intestine. Viral entry requires penetration of a membrane to deliver an intact DLP to the cytoplasm. It is not known whether the plasma membrane or an endosomal membrane is the primary site of entry. In the cytoplasm of an infected cell, the DLP extrudes 11 different newly synthesized mRNAs without releasing the genome segments. One viral nonstructural protein, NSP3, binds to the nonpolyadenylated 3′ ends of viral mRNAs, substituting for host poly(A) binding protein in circularizing mRNA, and shutting off host translation by depleting pools of the translation initiation factor eIF4G. New DLPs assemble in the cytoplasmic inclusion bodies, termed viroplasms. Because each infectious unit corresponds to a small number of virus particles, it is likely that one of each of the 11 genome segments is packaged into each new DLP. The mechanism of this specific and highly selective packaging remains a puzzle. Nascent particles bind a virally encoded integral endoplasmic reticulum membrane glycoprotein, NSP4, and bud into the endoplasmic reticulum lumen, acquiring a transient envelope. This envelope is lost as the outermost protein layer is added to complete the virions. Virions are released from infected enterocytes after transport to the cell surface by a vesicular transport pathway that bypasses the Golgi apparatus. Replication in the gut results in very high concentrations of viral particles (up to 10^{11}/ml) in faeces at the peak of the acute diarrhoea. The physical hardiness of the shed particles ensures their efficient transmission to new hosts. In order to carry out rational gene structure–function assignments, reverse genetic systems for rotaviruses have been developed which, however, still require helper virus.

Pathogenesis

The pathogenesis of rotavirus diarrhoea is complex. Viral infection causes direct damage to the enteric epithelium, resulting in the blunting and denudation of villi. The villous damage is repaired by cells emerging and differentiating from the crypts of the gut epithelium, which show a reactive hyperplasia. Loss of functioning absorptive cells leads to a degree of malabsorption and osmotic fluid loss. However, there also appears to be a secretory component to rotavirus diarrhoea. By raising intracellular calcium concentrations in infected cells, NSP4 activates a plasma membrane anion channel causing fluid secretion. There is evidence that a fragment of NSP4 is released from infected cells, acting as a viral enterotoxin to induce a secretory state of uninfected cells. The cellular receptor for the NSP4 fragment has recently been identified. The enteric nervous system also plays a role in pathogenesis. Enteric nervous system inhibitors diminish fluid secretion in the gut of rotavirus-infected animals. Recently, it has been shown that rotaviruses stimulate enterochromaffin cells to release serotonin (5-HT) which activates brain structures involved in nausea and vomiting.

Immune response

A primarily serotype-specific humoral immune response is elicited after neonatal or primary rotavirus infection. However, during the first 2 years of life children are repeatedly infected with rotaviruses leading to multiple serotype-specific and also partially heterotypic protection. The presence of rotavirus-specific secretory IgA coproantibodies seems to correlate best with protection against disease, although the exact correlates remain to be determined. Rotavirus-specific cytotoxic T-cell responses are capable of clearing infections, but appear to be less important than humoral immune responses in protecting against repeated infections. The abundant antibody that is produced against VP6 during infection does not neutralize extracellular virus. However, anti-VP6 IgA, which is transported across enterocytes for secretion into the gut lumen, can inhibit viral replication by binding DLPs in the cytoplasm ('intracellular neutralization'). The role of this phenomenon in protection against human infection is not yet known, but it has become apparent that heterotypic protection (after natural infection and vaccination) plays a considerable role.

Enteric adenoviruses

Structure and classification

Adenoviruses are nonenveloped icosahedral viruses possessing a genome of linear double-stranded DNA approximately 35 000 bp in size. Their capsid is between 70 and 80 nm in diameter and consists of 240 hexons and 12 pentons that stand out as projecting fibres at the apices of the icosahedral virus particle. Human adenoviruses occur in 51 distinct serotypes, ordered in six different subgroups (A–F). Those adenoviruses regularly associated with gastroenteritis are classified as subgroup F, consisting of serotypes 40 and 41. Adenoviruses of different groups (causing respiratory tract infections) are also found frequently in the human gut, but are not regularly associated with diarrhoea.

Replication

Adenoviruses attach to susceptible cells via the fibre proteins, and enter via receptor-mediated endocytosis. Phased early and late gene transcription of the viral DNA in the cellular nucleus is followed by translation and morphogenesis in the cytoplasm, and numerous particles are released after cell death. The virally encoded early proteins E1A and E1B induce host cells to enter the S phase, prevent apoptosis, and inhibit antiviral responses. Late adenovirus gene expression blocks cellular gene expression. Some adenoviruses seem to decrease the expression of major histocompatibility complex class 1 antigens on the surface of infected cells, thus reducing susceptibility to adenovirus-specific cytotoxic T cells. There is a serotype-specific humoral immune response that provides homotypic protection.

Human caliciviruses

Structure and classification

These viruses were first recognized as the cause of gastroenteritis during outbreaks in Norwalk, Ohio, in the late 1960s. Norwalk virus (NV) particles are spherical and measure 27 to 35 nm in diameter. Norwalk virus and Norwalk-like viruses (NLVs) are all members of the *Caliciviridae* family. Their 7.7-kb genome consists of single-stranded RNA of positive polarity. Cup-shaped depressions on the surface of virions have given the name to this viral family (Latin *calix* = goblet, cup) (Fig. 5.9.3c,d). Phylogenetic trees of full-length sequences of caliciviral cDNAs have led to their classification into four genera: viruses of the genera *Norovirus* and *Sapovirus* infect humans, and viruses of the genera *Vesivirus* and *Lagovirus* only infect animals. Until recently, viruses of the *Norovirus* genus were often termed 'small round structured viruses' and those of the *Sapovirus* genus 'classical caliciviruses'. Human noroviruses are genetically very diverse and constantly evolve.

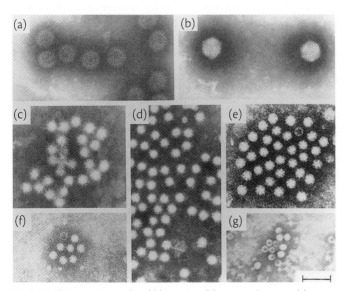

Fig. 5.9.3 Electron micrographs of (a) rotavirus, (b) enteric adenovirus, (c) Norwalk-like virus, (d) sapovirus, (e) astrovirus, (f) enterovirus, and (g) parvovirus. Negative staining with 3% phosphotungstate, pH 6.3; bar represents 100 nm. (Courtesy of Dr J. Kurtz, Oxford Public Health Laboratory (astroviruses) and Dr J Gray, Clinical Microbiology and Public Health Laboratory, Cambridge (all other viruses). Reproduced from Zuckerman A, Banatvala J, Pattison J (eds) (2000). *Principles and practice of clinical virology*, 4th edition, p. 236. Wiley & Sons, Chichester, with permission of the publisher.)

Replication

Details of the replication of human caliciviruses can only be deduced from those of animal caliciviruses, as there is no reproducible *in vitro* cell culture system for the human caliciviruses. The viruses seem to interact with species-specific receptors (various histo-blood group antigens in humans), and a single protein precursor is cotranslationally and post-translationally cleaved in a way similar to that observed in picornaviruses. A reverse genetics system for murine norovirus has recently been developed.

Immune response

Although calicivirus infections elicit humoral and cell-mediated immune responses in humans (with an antibody response mainly directed to the P2 portion of the capsid antigen), they do not seem to give full protection against subsequent infection. Certain histo-blood group antigens act as receptors for noroviruses, and 'secretors' of such antigens have been found to be more susceptible to infection with some norovirus strains than 'nonsecretors', depending, in part, on strain-specific receptor usage. Due to the genetic variability in human susceptibility to some norovirus strains, pre-existing antibody may not necessarily correlate with protection from re-infection. Recently, the level of carbohydrate receptor-blocking antibodies in sera from previously exposed human 'secretors' was shown to be a good correlate of protection from severe disease upon reinfection.

Astroviruses

Structure and classification

Astroviruses are members of the family Astroviridae. They possess a 6.8-kb genome of single-stranded RNA of positive polarity. So far, eight different serotypes have been distinguished and these correlate well with major differences in genome sequences (i.e. genotypes). Astrovirus particles have a characteristic appearance by electron microscopy (Fig. 5.9.3) which has recently been refined by crystallographic characterization of the capsid spike.

Replication

Human astroviruses grow well in particular cell cultures. After viral absorption to unidentified cellular receptors and uncoating in the cytoplasm, full-length and subgenomic RNAs are made. These direct the production of protein precursors, which are post-translationally cleaved. Replication takes place purely in the cytoplasm.

Viral gastroenteritis

Clinical features

The onset of acute viral gastroenteritis follows a short incubation period of 1 to 2 days. It is sudden, with watery diarrhoea lasting between 4 and 7 days, vomiting, and varying degrees of dehydration. Over one-third of children with rotavirus infection have a fever of more than 39°C. Fewer children have a high fever after infection with caliciviruses, and the duration of diarrhoea after infection with caliciviruses is, as a rule, shorter (1–2 days) than after infection with rotaviruses or enteric adenoviruses (4–7 days). Disease due to calicivirus infection may be accompanied by abdominal cramps, headache, and myalgia. In rotavirus infection all degrees of severity are seen. Inapparent infections are not infrequent, particularly in neonates, in whom the infection is caused by so-called nursery strains. It is not known whether the asymptomatic nature of rotavirus infection in neonates is due to infection with particular strains or depends on the presence of maternal antibodies that provide partial protection. Rotavirus infections are frequently accompanied by respiratory symptoms, but there is no strong evidence that rotavirus replicates in the respiratory tract. Viraemia commonly accompanies rotavirus infection; however, the clinical significance of this finding in immunocompetent hosts is not yet established. In immunodeficient children, rotavirus may replicate at extraintestinal sites, and chronic gut infections with rotaviruses, adenoviruses, and astroviruses have been observed, accompanied by virus shedding over weeks and even months.

Diagnosis

The diagnosis of rotavirus, astrovirus, and enteric adenovirus infections is relatively easy as large numbers of particles are shed during the acute phase of the illness. In contrast, human caliciviruses replicate for a shorter period and are shed at lower concentrations. Diagnosis is commonly carried out by passive particle agglutination tests (PPATs), virus-specific enzyme-linked immunosorbent assays (ELISAs), and more recently by viral genome detection using the polymerase chain reaction (PCR) (for adenoviruses) and reverse transcription–PCR (RT-PCR) (for rotaviruses, caliciviruses, and astroviruses). PCRs are extremely sensitive diagnostic tools, allowing both viral detection and typing. Aliquots of PCR amplicons can also be sequenced and the information used to establish phylogenetic trees. Such trees are becoming increasingly important not only for virus classification but also for epidemiological studies and surveillance (see below). Electron microscopy of negatively stained specimen suspensions is a 'catch all' method that can diagnose less common viral enteric pathogens that are not detected by standard assays, such as nongroup A rotaviruses. The morphological appearances of the main viruses pathogenic for humans are shown in Fig. 5.9.3.

Treatment

Treatment is mainly with oral rehydration solutions or, in more severe cases, intravenous rehydration. The enkephalinase inhibitor racecadotril, used as a supplement to oral rehydration, has been shown to significantly decrease the duration and total fluid loss in rotavirus-infected children. In severe rotavirus infections, treatment with oral immunoglobulins can decrease the duration of diarrhoea and virus shedding; however, this is not a routine treatment. Otherwise, treatment is symptomatic, but the use of antimobility drugs (codeine phosphate, diphenoxylate, loperamide) in children is not advised. Specific antiviral agents have been tested in animal models of rotavirus infections but are not used for human treatment.

Epidemiology

Rotaviruses

Rotavirus infections occur endemically worldwide and cause over 600 000 deaths annually in children below the age of 2 years, mainly in developing countries. Therefore, development of vaccine candidates has been a major goal since the early 1980s (see below).

The epidemiology of rotaviruses is complex. Besides children, elderly patients and patients with immunodeficiencies can be affected. There is a strict winter peak of rotavirus infections in temperate climates, but infections occur year round in tropical and subtropical regions. Transmission is by the faeco-oral route. Nosocomial infections on infant hospital wards occur and are difficult to eliminate. Group A rotaviruses of different G and P types are found to cocirculate in various populations within the same geographical location, and the relative incidence of different types changes over time. Various surveys have shown that usually more than 90% of cocirculating strains in temperate climates are types G1 to G4 and occur in combination with different P types as types G1P1A[8], G2P1B[4], G3P1A[8], and G4P1A[8]. Other G types may also be represented, particularly in tropical and subtropical areas but increasingly in temperate climates as well. For instance, G9 strains have recently been found to cause outbreaks of acute gastroenteritis in the United States of America and in many European countries. Most mammalian as well as avian species harbour a large diversity of rotaviruses and may act as a reservoir for human infections. An animal source is suspected for many of the more unusual human group A rotavirus isolates and possibly for group B rotavirus isolates. The latter caused outbreaks in children and adults in China during the 1980s and have also been isolated from patients with diarrhoea in different regions of India and Bangladesh. Group C rotaviruses are associated with small outbreaks in humans.

Human caliciviruses

Age-related seroprevalence studies of human caliciviruses have shown that infection is much more frequent and occurs from younger ages onwards than previously thought. Approximately 50% of children have been infected by the age of 2 years. The rate of inapparent infections is high, particularly in the young. In contrast to rotavirus infections, human caliciviruses cause outbreaks of acute gastroenteritis, mostly due to contamination of food or water, and are now recognized as the most important cause of non-bacterial gastroenteritis outbreaks worldwide. Contaminated oysters, green salads, fresh fruit, cold foods, and sandwiches are often implicated as sources of infection. Outbreaks occur in older children and adults in recreational camps, hospitals, nursing homes, schools, cafeterias, hotels, cruise ships, banquets, etc. Human calicivirus outbreaks occur worldwide throughout the year, in contrast to the regular winter peaks of rotavirus infections in temperate climates. The viruses are highly infectious (i.e. a few virus particles constitute an infectious dose) and spread rapidly. Transmission is by the faeco-oral route and also by projectile vomiting, which scatters viruses into the environment by aerosol. There is cocirculation of different genotypes.

Astroviruses

Endemic infections with astroviruses occur in infants and elderly people, but they can also cause food-borne outbreaks of diarrhoea. There are at least eight genotypes, correlating well with known serotypes, which cocirculate. Serotype 1 is most frequently found, followed by serotypes 2 to 4 at intermediate frequencies and serotypes 5 to 8 at low frequencies. Seroprevalence studies have indicated that infection by more than one serotype is not unusual.

Vaccine development

Vaccines have been confirmed as the best individual and also population-based tools to restrict infection with epidemic viruses. Of the gastroenteritis-inducing viruses, vaccine development has only been intensively directed towards rotaviruses. After many trials with variable success, a live attenuated rhesus rotavirus (RRV)-based human reassortant vaccine eliciting immunity to human rotavirus strains G1 to G4 was found to confer significant protection (70–80%) from severe disease including dehydration. Protection from infection alone was only moderate (40–50%). This vaccine was recommended by the Advisory Committee on Immunization Practices (ACIP) in the United States of America in 1998. However, after 1.5 million doses had been used, the rare complication of gut intussusception was found to be temporally associated with vaccination. In 1999 the ACIP withdrew the recommendation, and the vaccine has been taken off the market by the manufacturer. Studies of the epidemiological findings and possible mechanisms of pathogenesis have not explained the association definitively.

In the search for alternative vaccines, two further live attenuated oral rotavirus vaccines have been developed (Rotarix and Rotateq). The underlying concepts of the vaccines are different. The pentavalent vaccine, containing the human antigens G1 to G4 and P[8] in monoreassortant viruses on a bovine rotavirus (WC3 strain) genetic backbone, is aimed at eliciting type-specific antibodies against all the rotavirus types that are recognized to circulate most frequently. The monovalent vaccine, an attenuated human G1P[8] strain, is based on two clinical observations: (1) cross-protection is accumulated through successive natural infections and rotavirus disease can be prevented by repeated natural infection and (2) vaccination with one rotavirus type can provide protection, even if subsequent infections are by rotaviruses of a different type. Both vaccines have recently been licensed in numerous countries, and in some of them universal mass vaccination of children as part of childhood vaccination schemes has been accepted. The introduction of rotavirus immunization in Australia, the United States of America, and other countries has been associated with substantial reductions in rotavirus disease and some evidence of herd immunity. Although the efficacy of rotavirus vaccination is lower in impoverished settings in sub-Saharan Africa and South East Asia, the Strategic Advisory Group of Experts of WHO have recently recommended worldwide use of the vaccine, since 'vaccine efficacy estimates correlate inversely with disease incidence and child mortality strata'. There is ongoing postmarketing surveillance to estimate the global impact of the vaccines and also to monitor whether or not novel rotavirus strains may emerge. It also remains to be seen to what extent the new vaccines will have an effect in developing countries where they are most needed. Recently, a relatively low risk of intussusception has been recorded in some postmarketing studies, which has led the CDC to recommend that a history of intussusception in an infant should be a contraindication to rotavirus vaccination.

Next generation approaches to immunization against rotavirus infection are under investigation, such as the use of virus-like particles obtained from baculovirus-recombinant coexpressed rotavirus proteins, enhancement of rotavirus immunogenicity by microencapsidation, DNA-based candidate vaccines, and possibly 'edible vaccines'.

No vaccines against other viruses causing gastroenteritis in humans have been developed so far. For human caliciviruses, vaccine development will be challenging because of the extensive genomic and antigenic variation of cocirculating strains, uncertainty about the duration of acquired immunity, and controversy about the true correlates of protection. Nevertheless, virus-like particle norovirus vaccine candidates are now in early clinical development.

Outbreak control

Nosocomial rotavirus outbreaks among paediatric populations (on hospital wards and in day-care centres) are common. There have been numerous reports of outbreaks of diarrhoea and vomiting occurring in adults and children due to infections with caliciviruses acquired from banquets, travel on cruise ships, cafeterias, schools, hotels, fast-food restaurants, etc.

Outbreak control measures should focus on the interruption of person-to-person transmission and the removal of common sources of infection (food, water, etc.) in conjunction with measures to improve environmental hygiene (by food-handlers, etc.).

Further reading

Ball JM, et al. (1996). Age-dependent diarrhoea induced by a rotaviral nonstructural glycoprotein. *Science*, **272**, 101–4.

Carter MJ, Willcocks MM (2005). Human enteric RNA viruses: astroviruses. In: Mahy BWJ, ter Meulen V (eds) *Topley and Wilson's microbiology and microbial infections*, 10th edition, pp. 888–910. Hodder Arnold, London.

Centers for Disease Control and Prevention (CDC) (2009). Reduction in rotavirus after vaccine introduction—United States, 2000–2009. *MMWR Morb Mortal Wkly Rep*, **58**, 1146–9.

Centers for Disease Control and Prevention (CDC) (2011). Addition of history of intussusception as a contraindication for rotavirus vaccination. *MMWR Morb Mortal Wkly Rep*, **60**, 1427.

Clarke IN, Lambden PR (2005). Human enteric RNA viruses: noroviruses and sapoviruses. In: Mahy BWJ, ter Meulen V (eds) *Topley and Wilson's microbiology and microbial infections*, 10th edition, pp. 911–31. Hodder Arnold, London.

Cortese MM, Parashar UD (2009). Prevention of rotavirus gastroenteritis among infants and children. Recommendations of the Advisory Committee on Immunization Practices (ACIP). *Morb Mort Wkly Rec MMWR*, **58**, 1–25.

Desselberger U (2000). Viruses causing gastroenteritis. In: Zuckerman A, Banatvala J, Pattison J (eds) *Principles and practice of clinical virology*, 4th edition, pp. 235–52. Wiley, Chichester.

Desselberger U, Gray J, Estes MK (2005). Rotaviruses. In: Mahy BWJ, ter Meulen V (eds) *Topley and Wilson's microbiology and microbial infections*, 10th edition, pp. 946–58. Hodder Arnold, London.

Desselberger U, Huppertz HI (2011). Immune responses to rotavirus infection and vaccination and associated correlates of protection. *J Infect Dis*, **203**, 188–95.

Donaldson EF, et al. (2010). Viral shape-shifting: norovirus evasion of the human immune system. Nat Rev Microbiol, **8**, 231–41.

Dong J, et al. (2011). Crystal structure of the human astrovirus capsid spike. *Proc Natl Acad Sci U S A*, **108**, 12681–6.

Dormitzer PR (2010). Rotaviruses. In: Mandell GL, Bennett JE, Dolin R (eds) *Principles and practice of infectious diseases*, 7th edition, pp. 2105–15.Churchill Livingston Elsevier, Philadelphia.

Estes MK, Kapikian AZ (2007). Rotaviruses. In: Knipe: DM, Howley PM, et al. (eds) *Fields Virology*, 5th edition, pp. 1917–74. Lippincott Williams & Wilkins, Philadelphia.

Green KY (2007). Caliciviridae: The noroviruses. In: Knipe DM, Howley PM, *et al.* (eds) Fields Virology, 5th edition, pp. 949–80. Lippincott Williams & Wilkins, Philadelphia.

Hagbom M, et al. (2011). Rotavirus stimulates release of serotonin (5-HT) from human enterochromaffin cells and activates brain structures involved in nausea and vomiting. *PLoS Pathog*, 7, e1002115.

Hagbom M, et al. (2011). Rotavirus stimulates release of serotonin (5-HT) from human enterochromaffin cells and activates brain structures involved in nausea and vomiting. *PLoS Pathog*, 7, e1002115.

King CK, *et al.* (2003). Managing acute gastroenteritis among children: oral rehydration, maintenance, and nutritional therapy. *Morb Mort Wkly Rec MMWR*, **52**, 1–16.

Komoto S, *et al.* (2008). Generation of recombinant rotavirus with an antigenic mosaic of cross-reactive neutralization epitopes on VP4. *J Virol*, **82**, 6753–7.

Madhi SA, *et al.* (2010). Effect of human rotavirus vaccine on severe diarrhea in African infants. *N Engl J Med*, **362**, 289–98.

Matthijnssens J, *et al.* (2011). Uniformity of rotavirus strain nomenclature proposed by the Rotavirus Classification Working Group (RCWG). *Arch Virol*, 156, 1397–413.

Mendez E, Arias CF (2007). Astroviruses. In: Knipe DM, Howley PM, *et al.* (eds) *Fields Virology*, 5th edition, pp. 981–1000. Lippincott Williams & Wilkins, Philadelphia.

Nordgren J, *et al.* (2010). Norovirus gastroenteritis outbreak with a secretor-independent susceptibility pattern, *Sweden. Emerg Infect Dis*, **6**, 8–17.

Offit PA (1994). Rotaviruses. Immunological determinants of protection against infection and disease. *Adv Virus Res*, **44**, 161–202.

Patel MM, *et al.* (2011). Intussusception risk and health benefits of rotavirus vaccination in Mexico and Brazil. *N Engl J Med*, **364**, 2283–92.

Pesavento JB, *et al.* (2006). Rotavirus proteins: structure and assembly. *Curr Top Microbiol Immunol*, **309**, 189–219.

Reeck A, *et al.* (2010). Serological correlate of protection against norovirus-induced gastroenteritis. *J Infect Dis*, **202**, 1212–18.

SAGE (2009). Meeting of the Immunization Strategic Advisory Group of Experts, April 2009 – conclusions and recommendations. *Wkly Epidem Rec*, **84**, 220–35.

Settembre EC, *et al.* (2011). Atomic model of an infectious rotavirus particle. *EMBO J*, **30**, 408–16.

Trask SD, *et al.* (2010). Dual selection mechanisms drive efficient single-gene reverse genetics for rotavirus. *Proc Natl Acad Sci U S A*, **107**, 18652–7.

Vesikari T, *et al.* (2008). European Society for Paediatric Infectious Diseases/European Society for Paediatric Gastroenterology, Hepatology, and Nutrition evidence-based recommendations for rotavirus vaccination in Europe. *J Pediatr Gastroenterol Nutr*, **46**, S38–S48.

Wold WSM, Horowitz MS (2007). Adenoviruses. In: Knipe DM, Howley PM *et al.* (eds) *Fields Virology*, 5th edition, pp. 2395–436. Lippincott Williams & Wilkins, Philadelphia.

Yunus MA, *et al.* (2010). Development of an optimized RNA-based murine norovirus reverse genetics system. *J Virol Methods*, **169**, 112–18.

5.10 Rhabdoviruses: rabies and rabies-related lyssaviruses

M.J. Warrell and David A. Warrell

Essentials

The *Rhabdoviridae* are a large family of RNA viruses, two genera of which infect animals: the genus *Lyssavirus* contains rabies and rabies-related viruses that cause at least 55 000 human deaths annually in Asia and Africa.

Transmission and epidemiology

The risks and problems posed by rabies and other lyssaviruses vary across the world. Virus can penetrate broken skin and intact mucosae. Humans are usually infected when virus-laden saliva is inoculated through the skin by the bite of a rabid animal, usually a dog. Although the greatest threat to man is the persistent cycle of infection in stray dogs, several other terrestrial mammal species are reservoirs of infection. In the Americas, bat viruses are also classic genotype 1 rabies and insectivorous bats have become the principal vectors of infection to humans in the United States of America. Elsewhere in the world, there is increasing evidence of widespread rabies-related lyssavirus infection of bats. Unrecognized infection of organ donors has proved fatal to transplant recipients.

Clinical features

After a highly variable incubation period (usually 20 to 90 days), prodromal symptoms include itching at the site of the healed bite wound. These are followed by symptoms of either furious or paralytic rabies, reflecting whether infection of the brain or spinal cord predominates.

Furious rabies—the diagnostic symptom is hydrophobia, a combination of inspiratory muscle spasms, with or without painful laryngopharyngeal spasms, associated with terror, initially provoked by attempts to drink water. Patients may suffer generalized arousal, during which they become wild, hallucinated, fugitive, and rarely aggressive.

Paralytic rabies—flaccid ascending paralysis develops, starting in the bitten limb.

Diagnosis

The diagnosis can be made during life using rapid laboratory methods such as immunofluorescence of brain or punch biopsy specimens of skin taken from a hairy area. The polymerase chain reaction is used increasingly to detect rabies in saliva and skin biopsy material. However, lack of facilities hampers the confirmation of disease in developing countries where the diagnosis usually relies on recognition of hydrophobic spasms and other clinical features of furious rabies. Paralytic disease is rarely identified. Rabies has been misdiagnosed as cerebral malaria, or even drug abuse.

Management and prognosis

The few human survivors of rabies encephalomyelitis had received vaccine and, with one exception were left with severe neurological sequelae. Two unvaccinated patients, at least one of whom was bitten by a bat in North America, have made a good recovery. However, dog rabies virus infection remains universally fatal in man. Patients with furious rabies rarely live more than one week without intensive care but survival can be up to one month with paralytic disease. The mechanism of neuronal dysfunction remains elusive, and no treatment has proved effective experimentally.

Management—intensive care treatment may be appropriate for patients infected by a bat in the Americas if they present early and are already seropositive. Other patients with rabies should be sedated heavily and given adequate analgesia to relieve their pain and terror.

Prevention

Highly effective methods for control and prevention of rabies are available.

Control of rabies in domestic dogs—99% of human rabies deaths could be prevented by controlling the transmission of dog rabies, but education and resources are lacking.

Pre-exposure prophylaxis—a three-dose course of rabies vaccine is recommended for travellers and indigenous people in dog-rabies endemic areas, but the cost is often prohibitive.

Postexposure prophylaxis—at the time of a bite, correct cleaning of the wound and optimum postexposure immunization virtually eliminate the risk of rabies. Effective prophylaxis demands urgent wound cleaning with copious amounts of soap and water, followed by vaccine and rabies immunoglobulin. A new improved economical 4-site intradermal postexposure vaccine regimen could increase the availability of affordable treatment in developing countries.

Epidemiology

Rabies is a zoonosis of mammals that remains endemic in most parts of the world (Fig. 5.10.1). A cycle of infection is maintained in several reservoir species, of which the domestic dog is by far the most important. Many wild mammals including bats are also independent rabies reservoirs (sylvatic infection) with identifiable strains of virus. Any mammalian species is potentially susceptible to rabies and may be a vector, e.g. a cat infected by a dog may then bite and infect a person. However, there is no persistent virus transmission between cats. The vector origin of human disease depends on the likelihood of contact with an infected animal. Hence domestic dog rabies viruses are the source of more than 99% of human cases worldwide, mainly in Africa, Asia, and parts of South America. Rabies control programmes can reduce the risk of rabies in domestic animals to such an extent that wild animals, e.g. insectivorous bats in the United States of America, become the principal vectors of infection to humans. Rabies in wild mammals is usually spread by bites or by ingestion of infected prey.

Rabies and rabies-related viruses

The *Lyssavirus* genus currently includes classic rabies virus, genotype 1, and six rabies-related genotypes that are continent-specific

in Europe, Australasia, and Africa, and are, with one exception, zoonoses of bats (Fig. 5.10.2) (see also 'Rabies-related viruses known to infect humans'). All but Lagos bat virus have caused fatal human disease. New unclassified lyssaviruses are now emerging. No rabies-related viruses have been found in the Americas and only here do bats have genotype 1 rabies. All terrestrial rabies reservoir mammal species (dogs and wildlife) carry genotype 1 rabies, except for the rare Mokola virus in Africa.

Countries currently reported as rabies free include Iceland, Sweden, Norway, (except the Svalbard archipelago), Portugal, Greece, Cyprus and most other Mediterranean islands, Singapore, Sabah, Sarawak, Antarctica, Oceania (including New Guinea and New Zealand), Hong Kong islands (but not the New Territories), Japan, South Korea, Taiwan, and Caribbean islands with the notable exceptions of Cuba, the Dominican Republic, Grenada, Haiti, and Trinidad and Tobago. The British Isles, together with other Western European countries, and Australia have no rabies in terrestrial species, but do harbour rabies-related lyssaviruses in bats (Fig. 5.10.1). Lyssavirus-seropositive bats have been found in every country where surveillance has been carried out, so unusual contact with bats should be considered as a rabies risk anywhere. Inadvertent, usually illegal, importation of infected mammals is a global risk.

Cyclical epizootics of rabies may result from an uncontrolled increase in the population of the key reservoir species, such as the fox epizootic in Europe in the late 20th century. This started in Poland and spread across France, but it has now been eliminated from Western Europe. The AIDS pandemic has increased indirectly the risk of rabies infection in South Africa because many dogs abandoned by people who were sick or dying from AIDS have became feral and rove in packs. Outbreaks in dogs have also followed the movement of refugees.

Although the fox is one of the species most susceptible to rabies, about 3% of animals survive the infection and become immune. Seropositive bats are not uncommon, and rabies antibody has been found in several other species, exceptionally even in dogs. There is no evidence that animals can become chronically infected or be infectious carriers, although an apparently healthy animal may be infectious during the prodromal stage of infection.

Wild mammal reservoir species

Wild mammal reservoir species vary in different areas.

North America

Reservoir species in the central United States of America and California are striped skunks *Mephitis mephitis* and, to a lesser extent, spotted skunks *Spilogale putorius*; in Arizona and Texas grey foxes *Urocyon cinereoargenteus* and red foxes *Vulpes vulpes*; and in Alaska arctic foxes *Alopex lagopus*. However, in the east, rabies is most commonly found in raccoons *Procyon lotor* that transmit it to skunks and foxes. In North America many insectivorous bats are reservoirs of genotype 1 virus, including big brown bats *Eptesicus fuscus*, Mexican free-tailed bats *Tadarida brasiliensis mexicana*, little brown bats *Myotis lucifugus*, and silver-haired bats *Lasionycteris noctivagans* whose virus is a main cause of human rabies infections in the United States of America (see below) where bat infection has been found in every state except Hawaii.

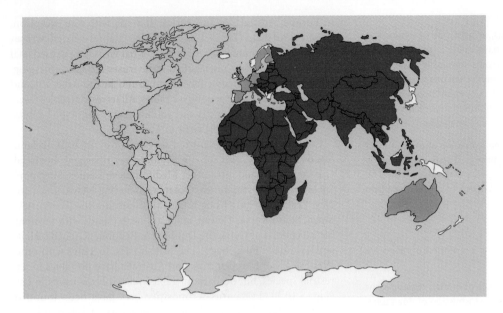

Fig. 5.10.1 Global distribution of rabies and rabies-related lyssaviruses. Red: Rabies in terrestrial mammal species (Lyssavirus Genotype 1) and bat infections by other lyssavirus genotypes. Yellow: Terrestrial and bat rabies are all Genotype 1. Green: Bat lyssaviruses, Genotypes 5, 6 or 7 only. White: No lyssaviruses detected.

Latin America and the Caribbean

Dog rabies persists in some urban areas of South America despite successful control programmes. The three species of true vampire bats *Desmodus rotundus*, *Diaemus youngi*, and *Diphylla ecaudata* (Desmodontinae) occur from sea level to over 3500 m but usually below 1500 m only in Mexico, Central and South America, and some Caribbean Islands (Fig. 5.10.3). The common vampire bat *D. rotundus* (Fig. 5.10.4) is the main reservoir of vampire bat rabies in Trinidad, Mexico, and Central and South America, where humans are occasionally bitten (Fig. 5.10.5). Carnivorous bats of the family Megadermatidae, such as the Indian 'vampire' *Megaderma lyra*, have given rise to the myth that vampires occur elsewhere. In Latin America, thousands of head of cattle are lost each year from vampire bat-transmitted paralytic rabies (derriengue) with locally serious economic consequences. Mongooses *Herpestes auropunctatus* are reservoirs of sylvatic rabies in Central America, Grenada, Puerto Rico, Cuba, Haiti, and the Dominican Republic.

Africa and Asia

Dog rabies predominates but there is sylvatic rabies in Africa in foxes, wolves, jackals, and small carnivores of the families Mustelidae and Viverridae (e.g. the yellow mongoose *Cynictis penicillata* in South Africa), and in Asia in wolves, jackals, ferret-badgers *Melogale moschata* in China, and palm civets *Paradoxurus hermaphroditus* in Indonesia.

Europe

Foxes, wolves, raccoon dogs *Nyctereutes procyonoides*, and insectivorous bats are infected (see also 'Rabies-related viruses known to infect humans').

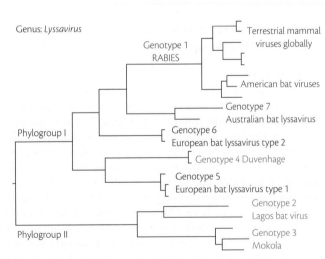

Fig. 5.10.2 Phylogenetic relationships between whole genomes of the lyssaviruses. Viruses in green type are confined to Africa.
(From Delmas O, *et al.* (2008). Genomic diversity and evolution of the lyssaviruses. *PLoS One*, **3**, e2057, with permission.)

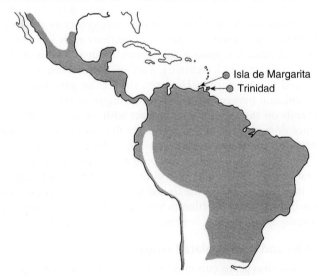

Fig. 5.10.3 Distribution of the three species of true vampire bats (Desmodontinae).

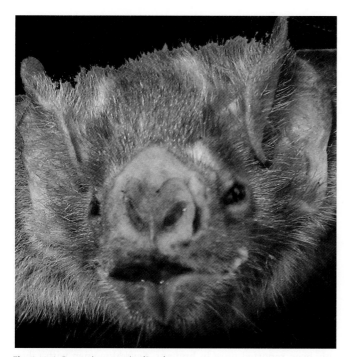

Fig. 5.10.4 *Desmodus rotundus* (Peru).
(Courtesy of Dr Vargas Meneses, Lima, Peru.)

Rodents

There are reports of rabies virus being isolated from wild rodents in many countries but there is no evidence that they are a reservoir species or that rodent bites, which are very common in some places, pose a threat of rabies.

Monkeys

Monkeys are not rabies reservoirs but could occasionally be vectors. Monkey bites are very common in tourists but human deaths have not been reported. However, the risk of rabies should always be considered, especially if an animal is behaving abnormally or the bite is severe.

Incidence of human rabies

The true incidence of human rabies throughout the world is not reflected in official figures; 55 000 deaths annually have been estimated to occur in Asia and Africa, including about 20 000 in India alone. High mortalities also occur in Bangladesh and Pakistan, and recently the incidence has risen in China. Surveillance is minimal, especially in Africa. WHO no longer issues country-specific data. In Latin America, mortality from canine rabies persists in Brazil, El Salvador, Mexico, Bolivia, Colombia, Venezuela, and Haiti. There have been recent outbreaks due to vampire bat rabies in Peru, Ecuador, and Brazil. In the United States of America there are on average two human deaths annually. Among 37 indigenous infections occurring in the last 40 years, 92% were caused by insectivorous bats. Europe reported 45 deaths in 5 years, mainly from the Russian Federation and the Ukraine. Rabies was apparently eliminated from the United Kingdom by 1903, but, since 1980, there have been ten imported cases and one indigenous human European bat lyssavirus infection.

Virology

The Rhabdoviridae are a family of more than 100 bullet-shaped RNA viruses found in vertebrates, insects, and plants (Fig. 5.10.6). Two genera infect animals, *Vesiculovirus* and *Lyssavirus*. Vesicular stomatitis virus is a vesiculovirus of cattle and horses, which occasionally causes an influenza-like illness in farmers or laboratory

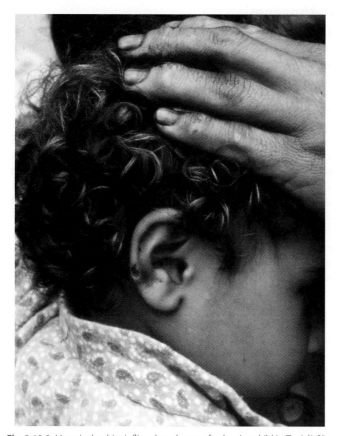

Fig. 5.10.5 Vampire bat bite inflicted on the ear of a sleeping child in Tapiraí, São Paulo, Brazil.
(Courtesy of Dr João Luiz Costa Cardoso, São Paulo, Brazil.)

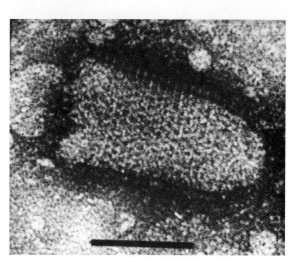

Fig. 5.10.6 Rhabdoviruses. Virion of rabies virus.
(Note the surface projections composed glycoprotein (G). The marker line is 100 nanometres long)

workers. The genus *Lyssavirus* contains rabies and rabies-related viruses.

The rabies virion is approximately 180×75 nm. Its core is a single spiral strand of negative nonsegmented RNA associated with a nucleoprotein, a phosphoprotein, and an RNA polymerase to form a helical ribonucleoprotein (RNP) complex. This is enveloped in a matrix protein, host cell-derived lipid, and a coat of protruding glycoprotein (G) molecules bearing spikes or knobs 10 nm long. The composition of the glycoprotein determines viral virulence.

The virus is readily inactivated by ultraviolet light, drying, boiling, most organic lipid solvents including at least 45% ethanol, soap solution, detergents, hypochlorite, and glutaraldehyde solutions.

Typing by means of monoclonal antibodies or genetic sequencing techniques allows the identification of diverse strains of rabies and rabies-related viruses from different geographical areas and vector species.

Transmission

Virus can penetrate broken skin and intact mucosae. Humans are usually infected when virus-laden saliva is inoculated through the skin by the bite of a rabid dog or other mammal (Fig. 5.10.7). Saliva from a rabid animal can infect if the skin is already broken, e.g. by the animal's claws. In North America, contact with bats leading to rabies has passed unnoticed; only 39% of patients reported a bat bite and 34% had no history of exposure to bats. Animals can be infected through the gastrointestinal tract, but there is no evidence that this happens in humans.

Inhalation of aerosolized virus created by infected nasal secretions of bats may be a method of transmission among cave-dwelling bats. In Texas, two men died of rabies after visiting caves inhabited by millions of Mexican free-tailed bats *Tadarida brasiliensis mexicana*, some of which were rabid; however, fleeting bat contact is more likely to have caused the infection. Two laboratory workers in the United States of America developed rabies after inhaling aerosolized fixed strains of rabies virus during the preparation of

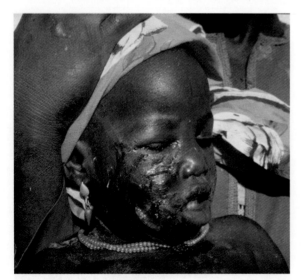

Fig. 5.10.7 Child bitten on the face by a rabid dog. This wound carries a high risk of rabies with a short incubation period.
(Copyright D A Warrell.)

vaccines. The accidental use of vaccine in which the virus was not inactivated has led to fixed virus rabies (rage de laboratoire), e.g. in Fortaleza, Brazil in 1960.

Transmission of rabies between people has been proved in 13 cases of tissue transplantation from donors who had died of undiagnosed neurological diseases. Six recipients of infected corneal grafts developed retro-orbital headache on the side of the graft 22 to 39 days after transplantation and died soon afterwards (other infections spread by corneal grafts include Creutzfeldt–Jakob disease and cryptococcosis). In Texas and Germany, seven recipients of kidney, liver, lung, pancreas, or even just a segment of iliac artery developed rabies encephalitis. Rabies was not suspected in the two young donors despite a history of recent rough travel in India in one and later discovery of a bat bite in the other. Recreational drug abuse was detected in both. One surviving liver transplant patient had had rabies vaccine previously. Postexposure prophylaxis following corneal transplants from infected donors has been successful.

Considering that the saliva, respiratory secretions, and tears of rabies patients contain virus, it is surprising that the disease has not been spread to intimate relatives and nurses.

Transplacental infection has been observed in animals but has only been reported once in humans. Several women with rabies encephalitis have given birth to healthy babies. The transmission of rabies from mother to suckling infant via the breast milk has been suspected in at least one human case and is well known in animals.

Pathogenesis

The mechanism by which the highly neurotropic rabies virus enters the nervous system and travels into the brain and out again to many organs is intriguing. The virus may replicate locally in muscle cells or attach directly to nerve endings. It can bind to many types of receptors including the nicotinic acetylcholine receptors at motor endplates, which may concentrate the virus at this postsynaptic site before entry into the presynaptic axon terminal, possibly via the neural cell adhesion molecule. Several other neuronal binding mechanisms may be involved. Once inside peripheral nerves, virus travels in a strictly retrograde direction within the axoplasm. This progression can be blocked experimentally by local anaesthetics, metabolic inhibitors, and nerve section. The axonal dynein molecular motor is assumed to be the vehicle of transport but the attachment mechanism is elusive. Viral binding might be directly via the naked ribonucleoprotein complex or more likely indirectly within a vesicle containing a whole virion. Rabies virus is experimentally inaccessible to antibodies while concealed in the peripheral nerves.

On reaching the central nervous system, the virus replicates massively within neurons and is transmitted directly from cell to cell across synaptic junctions. Dramatic symptoms can appear before histopathological changes are apparent. Viral virulence is inversely related to neuronal apoptosis. Rabies alters host cell gene expression, but the mechanisms of gross neuronal dysfunction are speculative. Centrifugal spread of virus from the central nervous system, apparently in the axoplasm of somatic and autonomic efferent nerves, deposits virus in many tissues including skeletal and cardiac muscle, adrenal medulla where infection may be clinically significant, and also in kidney, retina, cornea, pancreas, taste buds, respiratory tract, and the skin in nerve twiglets around hair follicles (see below 'Laboratory diagnosis'). At this stage, productive viral replication occurs, with budding from outer cell membranes in the salivary glands and rabies may be transmitted by bites to other mammals. Viraemia has been detected very rarely, only in animals, and is not thought to be involved in pathogenesis or spread.

Immunology

Immunological response to rabies infection in humans

Some patients die without any detectable immune response, because rabies virus evades and suppresses the immune system. Antibody might become detectable in serum 7 days or more after the onset of illness and in cerebrospinal fluid a little later. It may rise to high levels in patients whose lives are prolonged by intensive care. A small amount of rabies-specific IgM is sometimes detectable, but is not useful as a means of diagnosis.

There is little evidence of a lymphocyte-mediated immune response to rabies encephalitis. A pleocytosis appears in only 60% of patients, with a mean leucocyte count of 75×10^3/mm. Peripheral blood lymphocyte transformation is minimal if any. Experimentally, in fatal rabies there is inhibition of innate immunity, particularly interferon activity, and the few immune lymphocytes entering the brain undergo apoptosis, whereas survival of mice is associated with increased permeability of the blood–brain barrier, neutralizing antibody in the brain, expression of rabies glycoprotein, and apoptosis of infected neurons.

In animals, latent infections can be reactivated by corticosteroids and stress. This provides a possible explanation for occasional reports of long incubation periods.

Immunological response to rabies vaccination

The viral glycoprotein induces neutralizing antibody, which is detectable by 2 weeks after the start of primary immunization. In animal studies, the neutralizing antibody titre is the best available measure of protection against death. A titre of 0.5 IU/ml indicates specific seroconversion and is the WHO minimum acceptable level after vaccination. A relatively low response occurs in about 3% of the population, in immunosuppresed patients, and in the elderly. The nucleoprotein antigens also stimulate antibody that is cross-reactive between lyssaviruses, whereas glycoprotein antibody is more strain-specific. Transient low levels of interferon may be induced after the first dose of rabies vaccine. The important anamnestic response after postexposure booster vaccination seems to be initiated by T and NK lymphocytes which stimulate B cell antibody production.

Although neutralizing antibody is undoubtedly protective in the early stages after inoculation of virus, it may be deleterious once central nervous system infection is established. In animals, acceleration of the terminal phase of the encephalitis ('early death phenomenon') is associated with the presence of low titres of rabies antibody in serum.

Rabies in animals

All warm-blooded animals can be infected with rabies but their susceptibility varies. However, only mammals are infected naturally.

In dogs, the incubation period ranges from 5 days to 14 months, but is usually between 3 and 12 weeks. The first symptom, as in many humans, is intense irritation at the site of the infection. Despite the popular idea of the 'mad' rabid dog, probably only a minority develop furious rabies. There is an early and striking change in the dog's behaviour with dysphagia, ptosis, altered bark, paralysis of the jaw, neck, and hind limbs (Fig. 5.10.8), hypersalivation, congested conjunctivae, pruritus, shivering, trembling, snapping at imaginary objects, pica, and extreme restlessness causing the animal to wander miles from home. Dogs with furious rabies attack inanimate objects, often seriously injuring their mouths in the process. Virus has been found in the saliva 3 days before symptoms appear, and the animal usually dies within the next 7 days.

This is the basis for the traditional 10-day observation period for dogs that have bitten humans. Very rare old reports from India, Ethiopia, and Nigeria of persistent or intermittent excretion of virus in the saliva of apparently healthy dogs have not been confirmed by subsequent thorough searches. 'Oulou fato', a clinical variant of canine rabies with reduced virulence, was seen in West Africa 50 years ago. In Tanzania, a rabies virus of apparently low virulence has been identified in hyenas.

Rabid foxes lose their fear of humans and the majority develop paralytic rabies. An extreme degree of furious rabies is seen in 75% of infected cats. Cattle usually develop paralytic symptoms with dysphagia, hypersalivation, groaning, trembling, colic, diarrhoea, tenesmus, and rectal prolapse. Most other domestic ungulates develop paralytic symptoms. Horses often show furious features

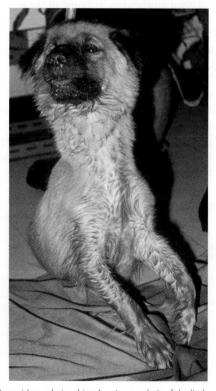

Fig. 5.10.8 Dog with paralytic rabies showing paralysis of the limbs and hypersalivation.
(Copyright D A Warrell.)

with sexual excitement. Most wild animals, like foxes, lose their fear of humans and may appear tame. Rabid skunks, raccoons, badgers, martens, and mongooses may become very aggressive. Dysphagia and inability to drink is common in rabid animals, but they do not exhibit hydrophobia.

Clinical features in humans

The incubation period ranges from 4 days to many years, but it is between 20 and 90 days in three-quarters of cases. It tends to be shorter after bites on the face (average 35 days) than after those on the limbs (average 52 days).

Prodromal symptoms

Often, the first symptom is itching, pain, or paraesthesia at the site of the healed bite wound (Fig. 5.10.9). Nonspecific prodromal symptoms include fever, chills, malaise, weakness, tiredness, headache, photophobia, myalgia, anxiety, depression, irritability, and symptoms of upper respiratory tract and gastrointestinal infections. Subsequently, symptoms of either furious or paralytic rabies will develop, depending on whether the spinal cord or brain are predominantly infected.

Furious rabies

Furious rabies is the more common presentation. Most patients have the diagnostic symptom of hydrophobia, which is a combination of inspiratory muscle spasm, with or without painful laryngopharyngeal spasm, associated with terror (Fig. 5.10.10a–e). Initially provoked by attempts to drink water, this reflex can be excited by a variety of stimuli including a draught of air ('aerophobia'), water splashed on the skin, irritation of the respiratory tract or, ultimately, by the sight, sound, or even mention of water. The inspiratory spasm is violent and jerky. The neck and back are extended, the arms thrown up, and the episode may end with a generalized convulsion complicated by cardiac or respiratory arrest.

Patients experience hyperaesthesia and, at times, generalized arousal during which they become wild, hallucinated, fugitive, and sometimes aggressive (Fig. 5.10.11). This behaviour alternates with periods of mental lucidity during which patients may become distressingly aware of their predicament. Despite these

dramatic symptoms, attributable to brainstem encephalitis, conventional neurological examination may prove surprisingly normal, leading to the false assumption of hysteria. Reported abnormalities include meningism, cranial nerve lesions (especially III, VI, VII, IX–XII), upper motor neuron lesions, fasciculation, and involuntary movements. Disturbances of the hypothalamus or autonomic nervous system are reflected by hypersalivation (Fig. 5.10.12), sweating, lacrimation, hypertension or hypotension, hyperthermia or hypothermia, diabetes insipidus or inappropriate secretion of antidiuretic hormone, and, rarely, priapism with spontaneous orgasms, satyriasis, or nymphomania. Hypersexuality suggests similar aetiology to the Klüver–Bucy syndrome created in rhesus monkeys by bilateral ablation of the hippocampus.

Without supportive treatment, about one-third of the patients will die during a hydrophobic spasm during the first few days. The rest lapse into coma and generalized flaccid paralysis, and rarely survive for more than a week without intensive care.

Paralytic or dumb rabies

This is the clinical pattern in less than one-fifth of human cases except in the case of bat-transmitted rabies, especially vampire bat infection, which is usually paralytic. Patients may become literally dumb ('rage muette') because their laryngeal muscles are paralysed, but symptoms are quieter ('rage tranquille') than in furious rabies. The largest reported outbreak was in Trinidad between 1925 and 1935 when there were 89 human cases, initially misattributed to poliomyelitis or botulism; others have been described from Mexico, Guyana, Brazil, Peru, Ecuador, Bolivia, and Argentina. The paralytic form of rabies was also seen in patients with postvaccinal rabies, in the two patients who inhaled fixed virus, and is said to be more likely to develop in patients who have received antirabies vaccine. After the usual prodromal symptoms, especially fever, headache, and local paraesthesias, flaccid paralysis develops, usually in the bitten limb, and ascends symmetrically or asymmetrically with pain and fasciculation in the affected muscles and mild sensory disturbances. Paraplegia and sphincter involvement then develop, and finally fatal paralysis of deglutitive and respiratory muscles (Fig. 5.10.13). Hydrophobia is unusual, but may be represented by a few pharyngeal spasms in the terminal phase of the illness. Even without intensive care, patients with paralytic rabies have survived for up to 30 days.

Other manifestations and complications

Respiratory system

Asphyxiation and respiratory arrest may complicate the hydrophobic spasms or generalized convulsions of furious rabies and the bulbar and respiratory paralysis of dumb rabies. Bronchopneumonia is a predictable complication if life is prolonged by intensive care, but a primary rabies pneumonitis may occur. Various abnormal patterns of respiration have been described, including cluster and apneustic breathing. There are some similarities to respiratory myoclonus. Pneumothorax may complicate inspiratory spasms.

Cardiovascular system

A variety of dangerous cardiac arrhythmias have been reported, including supraventricular tachycardias, sinus bradycardia, atrioventricular block, and sinus arrest, together with T wave and ST

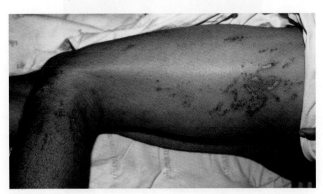

Fig. 5.10.9 This man developed intense itching in the left leg, provoking scratching and excoriation, 6 weeks after being bitten in that limb by a rabid dog. He died with furious rabies a few days later.
(Courtesy of the late Professor Sornchai Looaresuwan.)

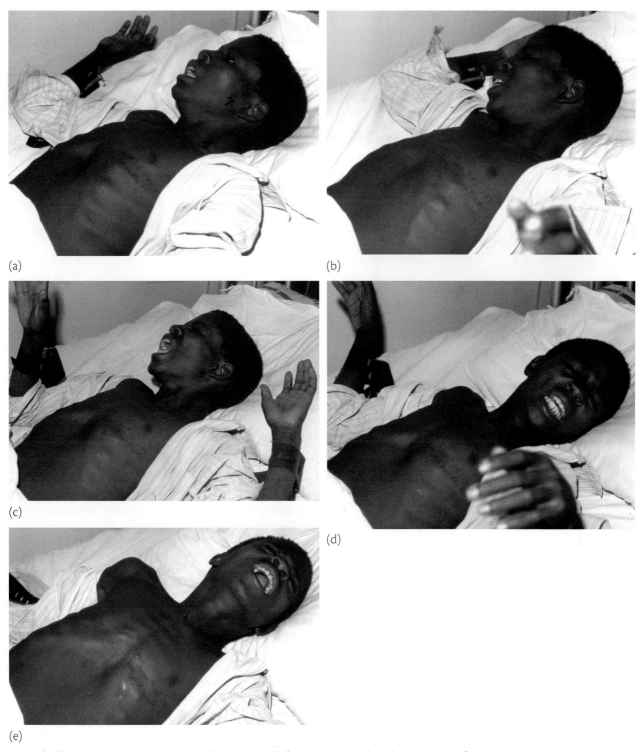

(a)

(b)

(c)

(d)

(e)

Fig. 5.10.10 (a–e) Hydrophobic spasm in a 14-year-old Nigerian boy with furious rabies. Note the violent contraction of inspiratory muscles, sternomastoids and diaphragm, depressing xiphisternum.
(Copyright D A Warrell.)

segment changes (Fig. 5.10.14). Hypotension, pulmonary oedema, and congestive cardiac failure are attributable to myocarditis.

Nervous system

Raised intracranial pressure resulting from cerebral oedema or internal hydrocephalus has been reported in a few cases, but spinal fluid opening pressure is usually normal and papilloedema is rarely seen. There is clinical and electrophysiological evidence of diffuse axonal neuropathy, consistent with histological appearances of degeneration of peripheral nerve ganglia and axons.

Gastrointestinal system

'Stress' ulcers and the Mallory–Weiss syndrome are possible explanations for the haematemesis often reported in rabies.

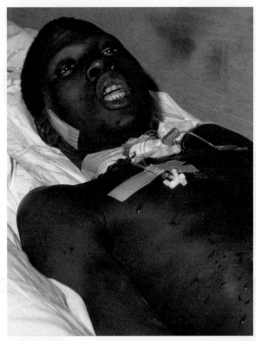

Fig. 5.10.11 Episode of intense arousal in a Nigerian patient with furious rabies. (Copyright D A Warrell.)

Clinical and differential diagnosis

Rabies should be suspected in any patient who develops neurological symptoms after being bitten by a mammal in a rabies endemic area. However, some patients fail to remember that they have been bitten and others may be infected while they are asleep possibly by contact with lip mucosae (North American insectivorous bats) or near-painless bites by vampire bats in parts of Latin America.

Furious rabies

Pathognomonic inspiratory spasms with associated emotional response are provoked by asking the patient to swallow accumulated saliva or by directing a draught of air on to the face.

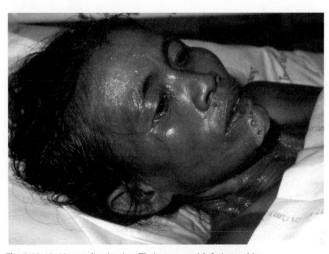

Fig. 5.10.12 Hypersalivation in a Thai woman with furious rabies. (Copyright D A Warrell.)

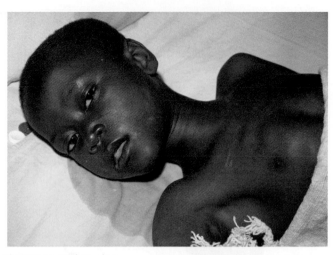

Fig. 5.10.13 Paralytic rabies. (Copyright D A Warrell.)

♦ Psychiatric conditions: Rabies encephalitis has been misdiagnosed as a variety of psychiatric conditions, including hysteria and behavioural disturbances attributed to recreational drugs. Conversely, patients with a morbid fear of rabies (rabies phobia, lyssaphobia, pseudohydrophobia) may simulate the more melodramatic features of the disease but hydrophobia is unlikely to be mimicked accurately, the incubation period after the bite (hours or a few days) is usually much too short for rabies encephalitis, and the prognosis is, of course, excellent.

♦ Otolaryngological conditions: Pharyngeal and upper airway symptoms of hydrophobia may be misinterpreted as pharyngitis or laryngitis so that the patient is referred to an otolaryngologist.

♦ Tetanus: This can also follow an animal bite and is similar to rabies in some respects, especially the pharyngeal form of cephalic tetanus ('hydrophobic tetanus'). It is distinguished by its shorter incubation period (usually less than 15 days in severe tetanus), the presence of trismus, the persistence of muscle rigidity between spasms, the absence of meningoencephalitis (cerebrospinal fluid is universally normal), and the better prognosis.

♦ Other encephalopathies/encephalitides: The typical encephalitic progression from severe headache to continuous coma is unusual in furious rabies. Hydrophobia with intermittent excitation and lucid intervals of full consciousness does not occur in other encephalitides. Among children with suspected cerebral malaria in Malawi, some were proved at biopsy to have died of rabies.

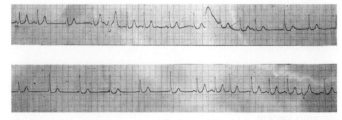

Fig. 5.10.14 Electrocardiogram in a Nigerian patient with furious rabies showing sinus tachycardia, atrial and ventricular premature beats, and a wandering atrial pacemaker. (Copyright D A Warrell.)

◆ Toxic encephalopathies: Delirium tremens, some drugs (pheno-thiazines, amphetamines, modafinil, cocaine, and other recreational drugs), and plant poisonings (e.g. *Datura fastuosa*) can cause excitable and aggressive behaviour that might be confused with rabies.

Paralytic rabies

Other causes of ascending (Landry-type) paralysis may enter the differential diagnosis.

◆ Postvaccinal encephalomyelitis (see below): This usually develops within 2 weeks of the first dose of the now rarely used nervous tissue rabies vaccines.

◆ Poliomyelitis: Objective sensory disturbances are absent and fever rarely persists after paralysis has developed.

◆ Acute inflammatory polyneuropathy (Guillain–Barré syndrome): Cerebrospinal fluid examination will help to distinguish this condition.

◆ *Cercopithecine herpesvirus* (B virus) encephalomyelitis: Bites and other types of contact with Asian macaque monkeys (genus *Macaca*), especially rhesus (*M. mulatta*) and cynomolgus (*M. fascicularis*) transmit this dangerous infection. The incubation period (3–4 days) is usually shorter than in rabies and symptoms develop within 1 month of contact. Vesicles may be found in the monkey's mouth and at the site of the bite, and the diagnosis can be confirmed virologically.

Pathology

The brain, spinal cord, and peripheral nerves show ganglion cell degeneration, perineural and perivascular mononuclear cell infiltration, neuronophagia, and glial nodules. Inflammatory changes are most marked in the midbrain and medulla (Fig. 5.10.15) in furious rabies and in the spinal cord in paralytic rabies.

Negri bodies (Fig. 5.10.16) are eosinophilic intracytoplasmic inclusions, function as viral factories containing rabies RNAs and translated proteins. They can be demonstrated by haematoxylin and eosin stains in histological sections of grey matter in up to 75% of human cases, especially in hippocampal pyramidal cells and cerebellar Purkinje cells.

In view of the appalling prognosis of rabies encephalitis, neuronolysis is often surprisingly mild and patchy, and death can occur without any inflammatory response. Vascular lesions such as thrombosis and haemorrhage have also been described. The brainstem, limbic system, and hypothalamus appear to be most severely affected and, in paralytic disease, the spinal cord and medulla. Outside the nervous system, there is focal degeneration of salivary and lacrimal glands, pancreas, adrenal medulla, and lymph nodes. An interstitial myocarditis with round cell infiltration is found in about 25% of cases.

Laboratory diagnosis

If a mammal suspected of being rabid has bitten, scratched, or otherwise risked infecting a person, it should be killed and its brain examined without delay. The best way to detect rabies antigen in acetone-fixed brain impression smears is by the direct immunofluorescent antibody (IFA) test. Alternatively, if no fluorescent

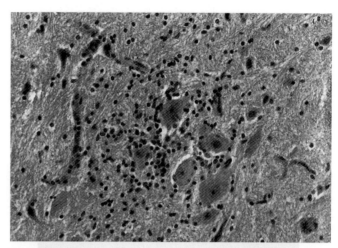

Fig. 5.10.15 Inflammatory cells around neurons in the central medulla (para-ambigualis region) of a patient who died of rabies encephalitis. Magnification×400.
(Courtesy of Dr P Lewis, London.)

microscope is available, rapid enzyme immunodiagnosis can be used. Sellers' stain is insensitive and rarely used. Virus isolation takes up to 3 weeks by intracerebral inoculation of mice, or about 4 days in murine neuroblastoma cell culture.

In humans, rabies can be confirmed early in the illness by demonstration of viral antigen by the direct IFA test in frozen sections of full-thickness skin biopsies taken from a hairy area, usually the nape of the neck. Specific diagnostic staining is seen in nerve twiglets around the base of hair follicles (Fig. 5.10.17). This rapid method is positive in 60 to 100% of cases, and no false-positive results have been reported. Antigen can also be found in brain biopsies, but tests on corneal impression smears are usually falsely negative. The polymerase chain reaction is being used increasingly to detect rabies in saliva, skin biopsy material, and occasionally cerebrospinal fluid.

During the first week of illness, virus may be detected in saliva, brain, cerebrospinal fluid, and very rarely urine. Rabies antibodies are not usually detectable in serum or cerebrospinal fluid before the eighth day of illness in unvaccinated patients. Serum antibody

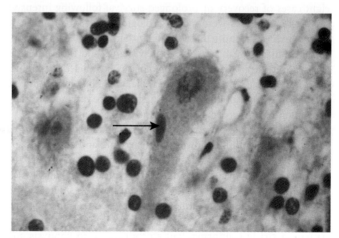

Fig. 5.10.16 Street virus in human cerebellar Purkinje cells as seen with the light microscope. Several Negri bodies can be seen (one is arrowed). Magnification×615.
(Courtesy of Armed Forces Institute of Pathology 73–12 330.)

Fig. 5.10.17 Diagnosis of human rabies during life. Vertical section through a hair follicle and shaft showing fluorescence of nerve cells around the follicle indicating the presence of rabies antigen. Magnification×250.
(Copyright M J Warrell.)

may leak into the cerebrospinal fluid in patients with postvaccinal encephalomyelitis, but a very high titre suggests a diagnosis of rabies. A specific IgM test has not proved useful diagnostically.

Prognosis

There is no specific anti-rabies therapeutic agent. Rabies was formerly regarded as a universally fatal disease, but there are reports of eight cases of recovery or prolonged survival following intensive care. The diagnoses were made serologically except in one case where virus was identified. Two patients had been given postexposure prophylaxis with nervous tissue vaccines and then intensive care. Four further patients, a microbiologist who inhaled fixed rabies virus, two boys in Mexico, a girl in India, and a boy in Brazil were given pre-exposure or postexposure tissue culture vaccines, and survived months or years with profound neurological impairment.

Two unvaccinated patients have to survived rabies and returned to an independent life following intensive care and antiviral therapy. The first, a teenager, was bitten by a bat in Wisconsin in 2004, had no rabies prophylaxis, and developed typical encephalitis without hydrophobia. Rabies neutralizing antibody was detected on the sixth day of illness. Treatment comprised coma induction and antiviral drugs. She made a slow recovery over 5 years. The other patient, a girl in California, had ascending flaccid paralysis and recovered within a few months. The source of her infection is uncertain. Both patients have minor neurological deficits. The antiviral treatments have not proved effective against rabies experimentally;

however, they developed antibody at an early stage of the disease. The treatment possibly maintained vital functions until the spontaneous specific immune response eliminated the virus, probably with loss of infected neurons. In animal experiments, American bat rabies virus infection differs from that of canine virus in that it is slower to evolve and progress, virus replication is not restricted to neurons, and histopathological changes are milder. This suggests that the virus maybe less pathogenic and may also explain the complete recovery of a boy infected by a similar virus in 1970 who had delayed treatment with a nervous tissue vaccine. It is likely that he too had rabies antibody present at an early stage of illness.

The treatment protocol used in Wisconsin has since been used unsuccessfully in >30 other patients with rabies encephalitis who were infected by bats or dogs. Recently, however, a teenager in Texas who had been in bat-infested caves and a girl in California with no known source of rabies infection had relatively mild neurological illnesses and survived. Although unvaccinated, they both had detectable rabies antibody, albeit at a very low level.

Treatment

No treatment has yet proved effective in animal models. Antiserum, antiviral agents, interferon-α, corticosteroid, and other immunosuppressants have proved useless. Human rabies of canine origin remains 100% fatal. Until a new treatment is proved effective experimentally, palliation of the patient and immunization of contacts is recommended. Patients must be sedated heavily and given adequate analgesia to relieve their pain and terror.

Intensive treatment is appropriate for patients infected by an American bat, who present early, and are already seropositive. Intensive care treatment is inappropriate for canine virus infection, especially in developing countries, and the cost is prohibitive. If intensive care is undertaken, the aim is to prevent complications such as cardiac arrhythmias, cardiac and respiratory failure, raised intracranial pressure, convulsions, fluid and electrolyte disturbances including diabetes insipidus and inappropriate secretion of antidiuretic hormone, and hyperpyrexia. A future treatment could be intrathecal live attenuated rabies virus.

Control of rabies in animals

The elimination of dog rabies would reduce the human mortality by over 99% and drastically reduce the need for human vaccination. Rabies control has been achieved most effectively where the principal reservoir is the domestic dog, as in 19th-century United Kingdom, Malaysia, and Japan, and since then in other areas including Western Europe, Taiwan, North America, and parts of urban Latin America.

In countries where rabies is enzootic

The control strategy depends on the local pattern of rabies occurrence in wild and domestic animals. Education and publicity about rabies is always needed. Domestic animals can be protected by regular vaccination. Owned dogs can be muzzled or kept off the streets. People should be discouraged from keeping wild carnivores such as skunks, raccoons, coatis, and mongooses as pets. Unnecessary contact with mammals should be avoided (e.g. stroking stray dogs or apparently friendly wild animals, exploring bat-infested caves). Culling reservoir species has proved an unpopular and ineffective method of long-term control. Impressive reduction of urban rabies in stray dogs has proved possible in India by vaccination, population control, and reducing available food and shelter by removing refuse. Effective oral vaccination of dogs is not yet practicable.

Control of sylvatic rabies has been achieved by vaccination of key wild animal reservoir populations with live oral vaccines distributed in bait. Repeated campaigns distributing attenuated rabies vaccines have eliminated fox rabies in Western Europe, and vaccinia-recombinant vaccine expressing rabies glycoprotein has been used in North American coyotes, foxes, and raccoons. New vaccines are being developed for other species. Vaccination of bats is unlikely to be feasible. Vampire bat rabies is controlled by destroying roosts and poisoning the bats with anticoagulants.

In countries where rabies is not endemic

The inadvertent importation of a mammal incubating rabies is a universal risk. The movement of potential vectors, especially domestic dogs and cats, wild carnivores, and bats, should be strictly controlled. Serological evidence of successful vaccination should be provided for imported mammals, or they should be vaccinated on arrival and quarantined.

Prevention of human infection

Pre-exposure prophylaxis

Pre-exposure vaccination is the most effective form of rabies prevention. No rabies deaths have been reported in anyone who had pre-exposure vaccine followed by postexposure booster doses. It is recommended for people who handle imported animals, workers in zoos and rabies laboratories, and those who are resident in or intend to travel to dog rabies-endemic areas, especially children. Others particularly at risk in certain areas include veterinarians, dog catchers, farm workers, cave explorers, naturalists, and animal collectors. In dog rabies-endemic areas, pre-exposure prophylaxis is advisable but is rarely used. Travellers should be educated to seek immediate local medical help if they are bitten, scratched, or licked by mammals. However, recommendations vary in different areas and local advice may be unreliable. Tissue culture vaccine and especially rabies immune globulin may not be readily available.

Primary pre-exposure vaccine course

A course of three doses of tissue culture rabies vaccine (see below) is given intramuscularly into the deltoid, or the anterolateral thigh in children, on days 0, 7, and 28. The last dose may be advanced towards day 21 if time is short. An effective economical alternative is intradermal injections of 0.1 ml at the same intervals. If the injection is too deep to produce a papule, withdraw the needle and repeat the procedure. Rabies vaccines do not contain preservatives. Strict aseptic precautions are mandatory to avoid contamination. The whole vaccine ampoule should be used within a day or discarded. If chloroquine is being taken for malaria prophylaxis (unlikely today), or in other cases of suspected immunosuppression, the intramuscular route must be used. Many travellers cannot afford three doses of an expensive vaccine, so the economical intradermal route is ideal for family, student, or other groups who can be vaccinated on the same day.

Booster doses

A booster dose 1 to 2 years after the primary course enhances and prolongs the presence of antibody. Although the titre falls more rapidly after intradermal than intramuscular inoculation, the response to a booster dose is still prompt. Confirmation of seroconversion is recommended only if immunosuppression is suspected. Further booster doses may be given intradermally or intramuscularly at intervals of 2 to 10 years depending on the risk of exposure. If the rabies neutralizing antibody level is at least 0.5 IU/ml, boosters are not necessary. Laboratory staff at high risk should have more frequent serology tests. Travellers who will have rapid access to vaccine if exposed need not have further immunization, but, if medical resources will be unreliable, a booster vaccination should be given before departure if 3 to 5 years have elapsed since the previous dose. A personal record of immunization must be kept, and urgent treatment is essential after possible exposure. Lyophilized rabies vaccine is relatively stable even at tropical ambient temperatures. It is sensible to take a dose on expeditions to remote rabies endemic areas. An extra emergency injection can then be given immediately after a risky encounter with an animal. If more than one person is exposed, the ampoule can be shared by giving multiple intradermal doses to each, using the whole dose (see postexposure regimens). This does not replace the normal postexposure treatment, which must still be given as soon as possible.

Postexposure prophylaxis

Despite intensive care, rabies encephalomyelitis of canine origin remains 100% fatal. At the time of the bite, however, correct cleaning of the wound (see below) and optimum postexposure immunization reduce the risk of rabies to nearly zero compared to about 35 to 57% for untreated bites by proven rabid animals. The risk varies with the biting species and the site and severity of the bites. It is highest following bites to the head by proved rabid wolves, which carries a case fatality exceeding 80% in unvaccinated people. The decision to give postexposure treatment depends on an assessment of the risk of infection by asking about the precise geographical location of the exposure; its severity, whether it was a bite or lick on broken skin; the site of the lesion; and the nature, appearance, behaviour, and fate of the biting animal, and, whether it had been recently vaccinated against rabies. The animal's brain must be tested for rabies if possible. If there is any doubt, the patient should be given full postexposure prophylaxis, even if the bite is several months old.

The aim of prophylaxis is to neutralize inoculated virus before it can enter the nervous system. Wound cleaning and active and passive immunization must be implemented as soon as possible.

Wound cleaning

This is effective in killing virus in superficial wounds, but is often neglected. First aid includes vigorous cleaning of the wound with soap or detergent and water under a running tap for at least 5 min. Foreign material should be removed and a viricidal agent such as povidone iodine, or 40 to 70% alcohol, should be applied liberally. Quaternary ammonium compounds such as benzalkonium chloride are inactivated by soap and so are not recommended. Hospital treatment of wounds involves thorough exploration, debridement, and irrigation of deep lesions, if necessary under local or general anaesthetic. Suturing should be avoided or delayed and the wound left without occlusive dressings. Attention should be given to tetanus prophylaxis (Chapter 6.22) and the large range of viral, bacterial, and fungal pathogens particularly associated with mammal bites. These include *Cercopithecine herpesvirus* (B virus) from Asian macaques (Chapter 5.2); *Pasteurella multocida* (Chapter 6.18), *Francisella tularensis* (Chapter 6.19), *Streptobacillus moniliformis*, and *Spirillum minus* (Chapter 6.13) from rodents; and *Pasteurella multocida*, *Capnocytophaga canimorsus*, and *Bartonella henselae* (Chapter 6.42) from dogs and/or cats. Most of the bacteria are sensitive to amoxicillin/clavulanic acid, cefoxitin, or tetracycline.

Active immunization

Rabies vaccines

Three highly immunogenic tissue culture vaccines that meet the World Health Organization (WHO) recommended standards are human diploid cell vaccine (HDCV), purified chick embryo cell (PCEC) vaccine, and purified Vero cell rabies vaccine (PVRV).

Several tissue culture vaccines are produced, mainly for national use, in China, India, Japan, Russia, and other Asian and South American countries.

Obsolete nervous tissue rabies vaccines, no longer sanctioned by the WHO, are still produced in a few countries. Semple vaccine, a sheep or goat brain suspension, or suckling mouse brain (Fuenzalida) vaccine is used in a few countries in Africa and South America. Daily subcutaneous doses for 7 to 21 days, followed by booster doses, are usually given over the abdomen. Neurological reactions including postvaccinal encephalomyelitis still occur.

Postexposure tissue culture vaccine regimens

The standard **intramuscular five-dose (Essen) regimen** is 5 × 1-ml (PVRV 0.5 ml) doses injected into the deltoid (or anterolateral thigh in children) on days 0, 3, 7, 14, and 28. In the United States of America only, the final dose can be omitted providing that rabies immune globulin (RIG) was given and the patient is otherwise healthy.

An alternative **2–1–1 intramuscular regimen** is two full doses (1.0 ml or for PVRV 0.5 ml), injected into the deltoids on day 0, and one dose on days 7 and 21. A total of four full doses are given, but the antibody level may fall more rapidly.

The intramuscular regimens are unaffordable in many countries. However, two economical multisite intradermal methods are available, each requiring only 40% of the vaccine used in the standard intramuscular method. Each of the intradermal injection sites drains to a different group of lymph nodes, intended to stimulate more lymphoid tissue to produce antibody. Aseptic precautions are required as for pre-exposure ID treatment.

The new simplified **four-site intradermal regimen** replaces the eight-site ID regimen. It consists of a whole ampoule of vaccine divided between four intradermal injections over the deltoid and the thigh or suprascapular areas. The volume per site is about 0.1 ml for PVRV and the equivalent dose for vaccines containing 1 ml per ampoule is 0.2 ml. On day 7, two intradermal injections of 0.1/0.2 ml in the deltoid and thigh areas are followed by a single intradermal dose on day 28. If PCECV (1 ml/ampoule) is used, a reduced ID dose of 0.1 ml/ID site was found to be immunogenic. Hence there is a wide safety margin in case of inexperience with ID injection technique or for immunosuppressed patients. If resources are very limited and more than one patient is treated on the same day, ampoules of vaccine could be shared, and an alternative dose is 4 × 0.1 ml ID on day 0, and thereafter 0.1 ml per ID site × 2 on day 7 and one on day 28. The 4-site regimen has several advantages as it requires only three clinic visits on days 0, 7, and 28 and is economical even without sharing any ampoules, using a maximum of 3 doses instead of 5 for the IM regimen. However this involves some vaccine wastage.

The **two-site intradermal regimen** was designed for use with PVRV. A dose of 0.1 ml for PVRV, or 0.2 ml for vaccines formulated in ampoules containing 1 ml, is given ID at two sites in the deltoid area on days 0, 3, 7 and 28. An intradermal dose of 0.1 ml per site is also used with PCEC 1 ml vaccine but higher-potency vaccines are demanded by most countries using this lower dose.

For all other vaccines, the manufacturer's instructions should be followed.

Postexposure vaccine regimen for people who have already received vaccination

If a complete pre-exposure or postexposure course of a potent tissue culture vaccine has been given in the past, or if the neutralizing antibody level has been over 0.5 IU/ml, rabies immune globulin is not required and only two doses of tissue culture vaccine are given IM on days 0 and 3. Alternatively, a new one-day booster regimen is four 0.1 ml ID injections, irrespective of the volume per ampoule. Vaccine should not be wasted, so when using PCECV or HDCV and if immediate sharing is not possible, a whole vial of vaccine is divided between four intradermal sites. Otherwise full postexposure treatment must be given.

Side effects of tissue culture vaccines

Mild and transient local redness, itching (especially after intradermal injection), or pain at the site of injection are not uncommon. Influenza-like symptoms and rashes are infrequent. Type I immediate hypersensitivity occurs rarely during primary courses. Type III immune-complex hypersensitivity was reported in 6% of those receiving booster doses of HDCV in the United States of America. This consisted of urticaria, rash, angio-oedema, and arthralgia 3 to 13 days after injection. No fatal reactions have been reported. Very rarely polyneuritis, Guillain–Barré syndrome has been reported in patients receiving tissue culture vaccines but no more frequently than for other commonly used virus vaccines.

Neurological reactions to nervous tissue vaccines

These occur in up to 1 in 220 courses of Semple vaccine, with a 3% mortality, and are an allergic response to myelin and related neural proteins in the vaccine. Reactions to suckling mouse brain vaccine are rare. The incubation period ranges from 3 to 35 days after the first vaccine injection. Clinical forms include localized neuropathy, transverse myelitis, paralysis with sensory loss or pain (a Landry-type ascending paralysis), meningoencephalitis, and meningoencephalomyelitis. These can be clinically indistinguishable from paralytic rabies, but recovery is usually complete. Permanent neurological sequelae are rare. Corticosteroids are thought to be helpful, and cyclophosphamide therapy has been suggested. Vaccination should be stopped as soon as symptoms appear and the course continued with a tissue culture vaccine.

Passive immunization: rabies immune globulin

Rabies immune globulin (RIG) has proved valuable in providing protection before neutralizing antibody has been actively generated, presumably by neutralizing rabies virus during the first week after initial vaccination. It is recommended as part of primary postexposure treatment, but it is vital following severe bites (on the head, neck, hands, and multiple or deep bites) (see Box 5.10.1).

Box 5.10.1 Specific postexposure prophylaxis for use in a rabies endemic area[a] following contact with a domestic or wild rabies vector species, whether or not the animal is available for observation or diagnostic tests

Minor exposure (including licks of broken skin, scratches, or abrasions without bleeding)

- Start vaccine immediately
- Stop treatment if animal remains healthy for 10 days
- Stop treatment if animal's brain proves negative for rabies by appropriate laboratory tests

Major exposure (including licks of mucosa, minor bites on arms, trunk or legs, or major bites i.e. multiple or on face, head, fingers, or neck)

- Immediate rabies immune globulin and vaccine
- Stop treatment if domestic cat or dog remains healthy for 10 days
- Stop treatment if animal's brain proves negative for rabies by appropriate laboratory tests

[a] This scheme is a simplification of the recommendations of the World Health Organization Expert Consultation on Rabies (2005).

The dose of human RIG is 20 IU/kg body weight and for equine RIG is 40 IU/kg. Reactions to equine and human RIG have been observed in 1.8% and 0.09% of recipients, respectively, and serum sickness in 0.72% and 0.007%, respectively. These are not predicted by a previous intradermal hypersensitivity test and, since RIG must be given even if the test is positive, skin tests are time-wasting and unnecessary. Adrenaline (epinephrine) should always be available in case of reactions.

All the RIG is infiltrated into and around the bite wound if anatomically possible, but any remaining is injected intramuscularly preferably into the thigh, not the buttock, at a site distant from the vaccine. If RIG is given hours or days before the first dose of vaccine, the active immune response will be impaired. RIG is prohibitively expensive and is not available or affordable for 99% of people in developing countries for whom postexposure treatment is indicated.

Failures of postexposure prophylaxis

Deaths from rabies have occurred despite prophylaxis. Failures are attributable to delay in starting vaccination, incomplete vaccine course, use of a substandard (nervous tissue) vaccine, and omission of RIG. Failure to wash the wound or infiltrate RIG around it, injection of vaccine into the buttock, or impaired immune responsiveness of the patient may also contribute. Low vaccine potency has been held responsible only with nervous tissue vaccines. Vaccine protection against rabies-related lyssaviruses may be less efficient than against genotype 1 rabies viruses (see below), but no case of vaccine failure has been attributed to this phenomenon.

A reduced or delayed immune response to vaccine can sometimes be predicted. If treatment is started late (e.g. more than 2 days after exposure), no RIG is available for severe bites, the patient is immunocompromised, or a rabies-related virus infection is suspected, the immune stimulus might be enhanced by dividing the first dose of tissue culture vaccine between four sites intradermally, as for the economical four-site regimen (see above).

Rabies-related virus infections of humans

The genus *Lyssavirus* contains seven genotypes: genotype 1, classic rabies, and six rabies-related genotypes (Fig. 5.10.2). Continent-specific rabies-related viruses occur in Africa, Europe, and Australia, and there is serological evidence of lyssavirus infection across Asia. With the exception of Mokola virus, all are viruses of bats. All are known to be capable of infecting humans except Lagos bat virus. They are occasionally detected in other species, but diagnostic tests are available only in highly specialized laboratories, infection is rarely suspected, and the routine tests for genotype 1 rabies virus may be weakly positive or negative. Their true prevalence is, therefore, unknown. Only 13 human cases of rabies-related virus infections have been reported, and disease is likely to remain unrecognized and misdiagnosed.

African lyssaviruses

- Lagos bat virus (genotype 2) has not been implicated in any human case.
- Mokola virus (genotype 3) has been isolated from shrews (*Crocidura* spp.) and rodents, as well as cats and dogs which are presumably vectors. It was isolated from a child with meningitis who recovered, and from another with fatal encephalitis. Mokola virus also caused mild disease in a rabies-vaccinated laboratory worker.
- Duvenhage virus (genotype 4) has been identified in three people, all of whom had had skin lesions inflicted by bats and had developed a fatal illness with clinical features identical to rabies encephalitis.

European bat lyssaviruses

Infected insectivorous bats have been found in Europe since 1954. The European bat lyssavirus (EBLV) group comprises genotype 5 (also known as EBLV 1) and genotype 6 (EBLV 2), both of which have subgroups a and b. EBLV type 1a is found across Northern and Eastern Europe from the Netherlands to Russia; EBLV type 1b in the Netherlands, France, and Spain; EBLV type 2a in the Netherlands and the United Kingdom; EBLV type 2b very rarely in Switzerland and Finland. Five unvaccinated people with bat bites died of encephalitis indistinguishable from rabies: two in Russia, one each in the Ukraine, Scotland, and Finland. Five new, so far partially classified lyssaviruses have been found in bats in Eastern Europe.

Australian bat lyssavirus

Australian bat lyssavirus (ABL) (genotype 7) has been found in fruit bats (genus *Pteropus*) (Fig. 5.10.18) and insectivorous bats in Eastern Australia since 1996. It caused a fatal rabies-like encephalitis in two women who had handled bats.

The lyssavirus genotypes have been classified into two phylogroups. Mokola and Lagos bat viruses form phylogroup II and the others are phylogroup I. All phylogroup I genotypes have caused fatal rabies-like encephalitis in humans, but experimentally phylogroup II viruses are less pathogenic. This is in keeping with the clinical cases reported. The genetic relationships between the genotypes (Fig. 5.10.2) correlates with the degree of serological

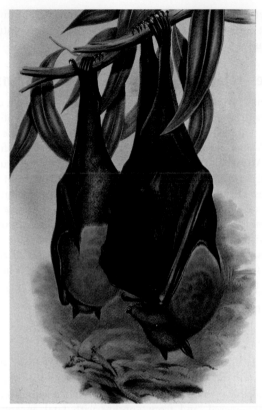

Fig. 5.10.18 Pteropid fruit bat (flying fox) (*Pteropis poliocephalus*), the natural reservoir of Nipah, Hendra, and Menangle paramyxoviruses and of Australian bat lyssavirus.
(From a painting by John Gould.)

cross-protection. Since all rabies vaccines are prepared from genotype 1 rabies virus, protection against ABL, which is closely related to genotype 1, should be undiminished. Protection is less efficient against phylogenetically more distant EBLVs and there is little if any protection against Mokola virus. However, there have been no failures of prophylaxis after exposures to bats, and no other treatment is available. Pre-exposure and postexposure immunization is, therefore, more urgent if exposure to a rabies-related virus infection is suspected.

Further reading

Delmas O, *et al.* (2008). Genomic diversity and evolution of the lyssaviruses. *PLoS One*, **3**, e2057.

Helmick CG, Tauxe RV, Vernon AA (1987). Is there a risk to contacts of patients with rabies? *Rev Infect Dis*, **9**, 511–18.

Hooper D, *et al.* (2011). Therapeutic immune clearance of rabies virus from the CNS. *Future Virol*, **6**, 387–97.

Jackson AC (2007). Pathogenesis. In: Jackson AC, Wunner AH (eds) *Rabies*, 2nd edition, pp. 341–81. Elsevier, Academic Press, London.

Kaplan C, Turner GS, Warrell DA (eds) (1986). *Rabies the facts*, revised edition. Oxford University Press, Oxford. [Detailed review of clinical features with illustrative case histories.]

Manning SE, *et al.* (2008). Human rabies prevention—United States, 2008: recommendations of the Advisory Committee on Immunization Practices. *MMWR Recomm Rep*, **57**(RR-3), 1–28.

Nel LH, Markotter W (2007). Lyssaviruses. *Crit Rev Microbiol*, **33**, 301–24. [A comprehensive compilation of the lyssaviruses from all continents and their distribution.]

Nel LH, Rupprecht CE (2007). Emergence of lyssaviruses in the Old World: the case of Africa. *Curr Top Microbiol Immunol*, **315**, 161–93. [Epidemiological, historical, and genetic details of lyssaviruses in Africa.]

Schnell MJ, *et al.* (2010). The cell biology of rabies virus: using stealth to reach the brain. *Nat Rev Microbiol*, **8**, 51–61.

Warrell DA, *et al.* (1976). Pathophysiologic studies in human rabies. *Am J Med*, **60**, 180–90. [Physiological and histopathological investigations of the mechanism of hydrophobia and brain damage in human rabies encephalitis.]

Warrell MJ (2012). Current rabies vaccines and prophylaxis schedules: preventing rabies before and after exposure. *Travel Med Infect Dis*, **10**, 1–15.

World Health Organization (2007). Rabies vaccines. WHO position paper. *Wkly Epidemiol Rec*, **82**, 425–35. Available from: www.who.int/wer/2007/wer8249_50.pdf

5.11 Colorado tick fever and other arthropod-borne reoviruses

M.J. Warrell and David A. Warrell

Essentials

Human pathogens are found in six genera of *Reoviridae*: *Reovirus*, *Rotavirus*, *Orthoreovirus*, and three arthropod-borne genera—*Coltivirus* (Colorado tick fever, Salmon River virus, and Eyach viruses), *Orbivirus* (Kemerovo, Changuinola, Orungo, and Lebombo) and *Seadornavirus* (Banna virus).

Colorado tick fever—common in parts of north-western North America; acquired from tick (ixodid) bites, most often by hikers and campers, presenting 3 to 6 days later with sudden fever, rigors, generalized aches, myalgia, headache and backache, rashes (12%) and gastrointestinal symptoms (20%). Diagnosis confirmed by detection of viral antigen in erythrocytes or serum, or by serodiagnosis. Management is symptomatic. Illness usually resolves in 10 to 14 days, but convalescence may be prolonged. Prevention is by avoiding, repelling, and rapidly removing ticks; no vaccines are available.

Coltiviruses

Colorado tick fever

The virus responsible for Colorado tick fever or 'mountain fever' is an 80-nm double-shelled particle covered with capsomeres. The icosahedral core contains 12 segments of double-stranded negative-sense RNA. The virus can infect human erythrocytes and this may also occur with the other coltiviruses and orbiviruses.

Colorado tick fever is a zoonosis involving hard (ixodid) ticks (principally *Dermacentor andersoni*, but also *D. occidentalis*, *D. parumapertus*, *D. albipictus*, etc.) and wild mammals, including porcupines, deer, coyotes, squirrels, chipmunks, deer mice, and other rodents. Ticks pass Colorado tick fever virus trans-stadially and transovarially.

Epidemiology

Colorado tick fever is acquired from tick bites in western and north-western parts of the United States of America (including California) and Canada (British Columbia and Alberta). Very rarely, it has been caused by an infected blood transfusion. Several hundred cases are reported each year in the United States of America, but the true incidence is thought to be at least 10 times higher than that. In Montana, Utah, and Wyoming from 1995 to 2003, 91 cases were identified, an overall annual incidence of 2.7 per 1 000 000 population, but there has been a decline in incidence since then. It is the second most commonly diagnosed arboviral infection in the United States of America, after West Nile virus. Hikers and campers are at special risk in rodent- and tick-infested terrain. The prevalence of antibody to Colorado tick fever among shepherds is 32%. The highest incidence is from May to July when ticks are most active. Infection usually confers lasting immunity.

Clinical features

In adults, the infection is nearly always mild, but in children it is occasionally severe but rarely fatal. Three to 6 days after the tick bite (extreme range 1–19 days) there is a sudden fever for about 3 days, with rigors, generalized aches, myalgia, headache, and backache. In one-half of the patients there is a biphasic fever. Rashes then appear in up to 12% of patients, usually a transient peripheral maculopapular rash or petechiae on flexor surfaces of arms or perhaps widespread and it may be hyperaesthetic. Gastrointestinal symptoms occur in 20% of patients. Laboratory findings include leukopenia with relative lymphocytosis, occasional thrombocytopenia, and mild lymphocyte pleocytosis.

The illness usually resolves in about 10 to 14 days, but convalescence may be prolonged. Severe manifestations include meningism and drowsiness, sometimes associated with gastrointestinal symptoms, spontaneous bleeding, thrombocytopenia, and disseminated intravascular coagulation. Late, possibly immunological effects, include myocarditis, pericarditis, pleurisy, arthritis, and epididymitis. Colorado tick fever infection may precipitate abortion, or transplacental infection but the teratogenic effects reported in mice have not been observed in humans.

Diagnosis

Viral antigen may be detected in erythrocytes by immunofluorescence 1 to 120 days after the start of symptoms. Erythrocyte precursors are infected in the marrow, but their survival is apparently not affected. Virus can be isolated from the blood and, if there is central nervous system involvement, the cerebrospinal fluid. Colorado tick fever virus produces a cytopathic effect on several cell lines, but intracerebral injection of ground blood clot or preferably washed erythrocytes into suckling mice is more sensitive for diagnostic isolation. Antigen can be detected in serum during acute infections by polymerase chain reaction (PCR) or Western blot, but enzyme-linked immunosorbent assay (ELISA) techniques have been less sensitive. An indirect fluorescent antibody test can provide early serodiagnosis. Neutralizing antibody and specific IgM enzyme immunoassays become positive after 14 to 21 days and the IgM disappears after 45 days.

Differential diagnosis

Many other tick-borne acute febrile illnesses, some with rashes and nervous system involvement, can be acquired in the area endemic for Colorado tick fever. These include Rocky Mountain spotted fever, tularaemia, Lyme disease, and relapsing fever. Tick paralysis caused by *D. andersoni* and other ixodid ticks presents as a poliomyelitis-like, ascending, flaccid paralysis that is unlikely to be mistaken for the meningitic or encephalitic syndromes of Colorado tick fever.

Treatment

The symptomatic treatment of fever and pain should exclude salicylates in case of thrombocytopenia. Tribavirin (ribavirin) inhibits the replication of Colorado tick fever virus experimentally, but its use in humans has not been reported. Immunity is long lasting.

Salmon River virus

This virus is closely related to Colorado tick fever virus. It was isolated from a patient with similar symptoms in Idaho.

Eyach

This European coltivirus has been found in Germany and France. There is serological evidence of human infection in Czechoslovakia causing meningoencephalitis or neuropathies.

Orbiviruses

Although antibody to the tick-borne Great Island virus and insect-borne Corripata orbiviruses have been found in humans, there is no evidence of their pathogenicity.

Kemerovo

Three serotypes of Kemerovo virus have been isolated from ixodid and hyalomma ticks in Russia and Central Europe. They cause benign febrile illnesses and, occasionally, meningitis or encephalitis in spring and early summer when ticks are active. Rodents and birds are involved in the zoonotic cycle.

Oklahoma tick fever is another Kemerovo virus rarely causing febrile illness in the United States of America.

Changuinola

There is a single report of human febrile illness with the orbivirus Changuinola in Panama. The virus has been isolated from phlebotomine flies and mammals in that area.

Orungo

Orungo virus is found mainly in West Africa but also in Uganda and the Central African Republic. Up to 75% of some human populations are seropositive. The clinical effects are unknown, but fever and diarrhoea occur in some people, perhaps with encephalitis as in experimental mice. There is no rash or jaundice. It is transmitted by anopheles, aedes, and other mosquitoes. Monkeys, sheep, and cattle may be infected.

Lebombo

This orbivirus was isolated from one febrile child in Nigeria. Lebombo is also found in mosquitoes and rodents.

Seadornaviruses

These viruses from south-east Asia and Indonesia include Banna virus (BAV) from China, which has been isolated from patients with encephalitis. In China, 20 new strains of BAVs were identified, widely circulating in areas where Japanese encephalitis virus (JEV) is endemic. These two encephalitis viruses share a common vector, *Culex tritaeniorhynchus*, and they may be clinically confused. BAV cases may be undetected during a JEV outbreak.

Prevention

Tick-borne infections are prevented by avoiding, repelling with diethyl-toluamide, and rapidly removing ticks. No vaccines are available. Long-sleeved, tight-fitting clothing should be worn in the high-risk areas and the body should be checked for ticks at frequent intervals. The nucleoside analogue, 3'-fluoro-3'-deoxyadenosine, inhibits replication *in vitro*.

Further reading

Attoui H, *et al.* (2005). Coltiviruses and seadornaviruses in North America, Europe, and Asia. *Emerg Infect Dis*, **11**, 1673–9.

Brackney MM, *et al.* (2010). Epidemiology of Colorado tick fever in Montana, Utah, and Wyoming, 1995–2003. *Vector Borne Zoonotic Dis*, **10**, 381–5.

Brown SE, Knudson DL (1995). Coltivirus infections. In: Porterfield JS (ed.) *Exotic viral infections*, pp. 329–42. Chapman & Hall, London.

Labuda M, Nuttall PA (2008). Viruses transmitted by ticks. In: Bowman AS, Nuttall PA (eds) *Ticks: biology, disease and control*, pp. 989–92. Cambridge University Press, Cambridge.

Libikova H, *et al.* (1978). Orbiviruses of the Kemerovo complex and neurological diseases. *Med Microbiol Immunol*, **166**, 255–63.

Liu H, *et al.* (2010). Banna virus, China, 1987–2007. *Emerg Infect Dis*, **16**, 514–17.

McGinley-Smith DE, Tsao SS (2003). Dermatoses from ticks. *J Am Acad Dermatol*, **49**, 363–92.

Romero JR, Simonsen KA (2008). Powassan encephalitis and Colorado tick fever. *Infect Dis Clin North Am*, **22**, 545–59.

5.12 Alphaviruses

E.E. Ooi, L.R. Petersen, and D.J. Gubler

Essentials

There are 29 registered alphaviruses belonging to the family Togaviridae, 16 of which are known to cause human infection. They are RNA viruses with global geographical distribution and complex transmission cycles between wild or domestic animals or birds and one or more mosquito species; humans are infected by mosquito bites. They cause a spectrum of clinical manifestations ranging from nonspecific febrile illness to acute encephalitis and death. Diagnosis of infection is made serologically by detection of IgM and IgG antibodies, virus isolation, and polymerase chain reaction , or by immunohistochemistry on tissue samples.

Old World alphaviruses, including Chikungunya, Ross River, Sindbis, Barmah Forest, Mayaro and O'nyong-nyong, generally have mammals as their natural vertebrate host and, cause acute febrile illness characterized by rash and arthritis. Management is symptomatic; prevention and control is by reducing vector mosquito populations and by avoiding mosquito bites. Several efforts to develop vaccines for Chikungunya and Ross River viruses are in progress and are at different stages development.

The New World alphaviruses, including eastern and western equine encephalitides, generally have birds as their natural vertebrate hosts, while the Venezuelan equine encephalitis complex have rodents as their natural hosts. About 2% of adults infected with Eastern Equine Encephalitis virus (less for other types) develop encephalitis, which can be fatal, with permanent neurological sequelae in many survivors; management is symptomatic; prevention and control is by reducing vector mosquito populations and by avoiding mosquito bites. Various vaccines have been used in laboratory workers and others at high risk of exposure. New generation vaccines are in clinical trials.

Introduction

The genus *Alphavirus* of the family Togaviridae comprises 29 registered viruses, 16 of which are known to cause human infection (Table 5.12.1). Alphaviruses are lipid-enveloped virions with a diameter of 60 to 70 nm whose genome is a molecule of single-stranded, positive-sense RNA approximately 12 000 nucleotides in length. Most alphaviruses are maintained in nature in complex transmission cycles between wild or domestic animals and one or more mosquito species. Humans are infected when the infective mosquito takes a blood meal from them. Patients develop high viraemias with some alphaviruses and this may contribute to the transmission cycle by infecting mosquitoes. The epidemiology and geographical distribution of the alphaviruses depend on several factors including the presence of suitable amplifying hosts, the presence and feeding behaviour of a suitable arthropod vector, and the frequency of exposure of nonimmune reservoir hosts and humans to infected vectors. Alphavirus infections are not directly communicable between humans.

Many infections in humans are asymptomatic, but alphaviruses can cause a spectrum of clinical illness ranging from nonspecific febrile illness, often with rash, myalgia, or arthralgia, to frank encephalitis, haemorrhage, and death. They cause two main clinical syndromes: Old World alphaviruses generally cause illness characterized by rash and arthritis while New World alphaviruses are generally associated with neuroinvasive disease. No specific therapy is available. Vaccines for some alphaviruses are used in animals, although none have been licensed for humans.

Laboratory diagnosis

Alphavirus infections are diagnosed serologically by detection of IgM and IgG antibodies. All alphaviruses have common antigenic determinants that result in cross-reactions in immunodiagnostic tests. Neutralization tests may be necessary for serological confirmation in areas where multiple alphaviruses are endemic/enzootic.

Table 5.12.1 Known disease associations of alphaviruses [a]

Virus	Geographical distribution	Disease in humans	Outbreaks	Other features
Aura	South America		No	
Barmah Forest	Australia	SFI, arthropathy	Yes	Clinically similar to Ross River virus infection
Bebaru	Malaysia		No	Laboratory infection only
Cabassou	French Guiana		No	
Chikungunya	Tropical Africa, India, Southeast Asia, Philippines	SFI, arthropathy	Yes	Large outbreaks in urban settings
Eastern equine encephalitis	North and South America on Atlantic and Gulf Coasts, Caribbean	SFI, encephalitis	Yes	Isolated cases or small outbreaks occur mainly in North America
Everglades	Florida	SFI, encephalitis	No	Variant of Venezuelan equine encephalitis
Fort Morgan	Colorado		No	
Getah	Asia	SFI	No	
Highlands J	North America		No	
Mayaro	Trinidad, Brazil, Bolivia, Surinam, French Guiana, Peru, Venezuela	SFI, arthropathy	Yes	
Middleburg	South, West, and Central Africa	Not described	No	
Mosso das Pedras	Brazil		No	Venezuelan equine encephalitis complex
Mucambo	Trinidad, Brazil, Surinam, French Guiana, Colombia, Venezuela	SFI	No	Proposed species in the Venezuelan equine encephalitis antigenic complex
Ndumu	Africa		No	
O'nyong-nyong	East and West Africa, Zimbabwe	SFI, arthropathy	Yes	Igbo-ora virus is a subtype of o'nyong-nyong
Pixuna	Brazil	SFI	No	Laboratory infection only
Rio Negro	Argentina		No	
Ross River	Australia, South Pacific	SFI, arthropathy	Yes	Periodic epidemics in South Pacific
Salmon Pancreas disease	North Atlantic		No	
Semliki Forest	Sub-Saharan Africa	SFI, encephalitis	No	
Sindbis	Africa, East Mediterranean, South and Southeast Asia, Borneo, Philippines, Australia, Sicily, Scandinavia	SFI, arthropathy	Yes	
Babanki	West and Central Africa	SFI, arthropathy	Yes	Subtype of Sindbis
Kyzylagach	Azerbaijan	SFI, arthropathy	Yes	Subtype of Sindbis
Southern elephant seal	Antarctica		No	
Tonate	French Guiana	SFI, encephalitis	No	Venezuelan equine encephalitis complex
Trocara	South America		No	Proposed species in the Venezuelan equine encephalitis antigenic complex; fatal encephalitis in one infant
Una	South America, Trinidad		No	
Venezuelan equine encephalitis	Northern South America, Central America, Mexico	SFI, encephalitis	Yes	Epidemics are caused by epizootic virus strains
Western equine encephalitis	North and South America	SFI, encephalitis	Yes	Human disease rare outside of North America and Brazil
Whataroa	New Zealand, Australia		No	

SFI, systemic febrile illness.
Adapted from Griffin D (2007). Alphaviruses. In: Knipe DM, Howley PM (eds) *Fields virology*, 5th edition, vol. 1, pp. 1023–67. Lippincott Williams & Wilkins, Philadelphia.

Isolation of virus from acute-phase serum is possible with some alphaviruses, but they are seldom recovered from the central nervous system, including cerebrospinal fluid, except from fatal cases. Virological diagnosis may also be made using polymerase chain reaction and immunohistochemistry on tissue samples.

Alphaviruses associated with arthritis and rash

Chikungunya

Aetiology and epidemiology

Chikungunya virus is found in Africa and Asia and is transmitted primarily by day-biting *Aedes* mosquitoes. The primary hosts remain to be conclusively determined, although nonhuman primates such as monkeys and baboons are likely candidates in sylvatic environments in Africa. In urban surroundings in Africa and Asia, the virus is transmitted between humans by *Aedes aegypti* mosquitoes, although *Ae.albopictus* mosquitoes have been implicated in some outbreaks. Explosive urban epidemics occur during the rainy season. Since 2004, a major epidemic has occurred in India (more than 1.3 million cases), adjacent South Asian and South-East Asian countries, Kenya, and Indian Ocean islands (Comoros, Mauritius, Seychelles, Madagascar, Mayotte, and Réunion where 34% of the population was infected), and in 2007 it reached Gabon in Central Africa and Italy. This epidemic was exacerbated by a new variant virus. A single amino acid mutation in the envelope protein increased infectivity to *Ae.albopictus*, a mosquito that has spread throughout the tropics and subtropics and has a wider distribution in urban, semiurban, and rural habitats than *Ae.aegypti*, which favours urban environments. Serological surveys following outbreaks have shown antibody prevalences generally ranging from 30 to 70%. Infections in travellers returning to Europe and the United States of America from areas experiencing outbreaks have been frequently reported. More than 800 cases were imported into France and 100 into the United Kingdom from Réunion and the other islands popular with tourists. In August 2007, local transmission of chikungunya by *Ae.albopictus* mosquitoes was confirmed around Ravenna in Italy, resulting in 205 cases and one death. Neonatal infection has occurred from mothers ill shortly before or at the time of delivery.

Clinical characteristics

'Chikungunya' means 'that which bends up' in Makonde, an East African language, and refers to the crippling arthralgia that characterizes the disease. After an incubation period of 2 to 3 days (range 1–12 days), there is sudden fever and severe arthralgia. In some patients, the fever may remit for 1 to 2 days and then recur ('saddleback' fever). Arthralgias are polyarticular, with the knees, ankles, elbows, and small joints of the hands and feet most commonly affected. They are often associated with low back pain. A useful sign is pain on squeezing the wrists (tenosynovitis). Headache, injected pharynx, gastrointestinal symptoms, and myalgias are frequent during the acute illness. Rashes, typically on the trunk and limbs, occur in about one-half of the patients usually during the second to fifth day of illness. They are variable in appearance: papular or maculopapular erythemas (blanching as in dengue), vesicular, bullous, dyshidrotic, keratolytic, purpuric and hyperpigmented associated with facial oedema, erythema nodosum, and aphthous ulcers. Arthralgia may last several months and is associated with effusions

and bursitis; a few patients may have symptoms 5 years after infection. Haemorrhage, meningoencephalitis, Guillain–Barré polyradiculopathy, myocarditis, and hepatic and renal complications are uncommon but may be fatal. Rheumatological manifestations are less frequent in children. Conjunctival suffusion and cervical or generalized lymphadenopathy are common. Serological surveys suggest that asymptomatic infections may occur.

Diagnosis

Leukopenia and elevation of liver and muscle enzymes are common early in infection. Detection of viral RNA by reverse transcription–polymerase chain reaction (RT-PCR) is useful for diagnosis during the first week of illness. Haemagglutinin inhibition and IgM antibodies will be present in nearly all patients by the seventh day of illness. IgM antibodies detectable in serum by IgM antibody capture enzyme-linked immunosorbent assay (MAC-ELISA) may persist for 6 months after infection. Virus isolation and RT-PCR are confirmatory.

Prevention, control, and treatment

Prevention and control can only be achieved by reducing vector mosquito populations in the large urban centres of the tropics and by avoiding mosquito bites. The American military has an effective vaccine, but it is not licensed for general use. Several new vaccines are all in late stage development. There is no specific treatment. Anti-inflammatory drugs may relieve arthralgia. An uncontrolled study suggested that chloroquine phosphate may be helpful for refractory arthralgias.

Ross River virus

Aetiology and epidemiology

This virus causes 'epidemic polyarthritis' in Australia, south-western Pacific islands, and Fiji. *Aedes vigilax* is an important vector in Australia and *Ae scutellaris* complex mosquitoes in some south Pacific islands, although the virus has been isolated from more than 30 mosquito species. An epidemic in various Pacific islands in 1979 to 1980 affected more than 50 000 people. An average of 4800 cases is reported annually from Australia. Explosive outbreaks and viraemias in humans implicate virus transmission from human to human by certain mosquitoes. Outbreaks tend to be associated with periods of increased rainfall. Camping is a significant risk factor in tropical Australia.

Clinical characteristics

The incubation period ranges from 2 to 21 days (7–9 days on average). The illness begins suddenly with fever and arthralgias predominantly in the ankles, wrists, knees, fingers, and feet. A maculopapular rash occurs in about one-half of patients within 2 days of onset and is most prominent on the trunk and limbs, but can cover the entire body; the rash may progress to small vesicles. Myalgias, headache, anorexia, nausea, and tenosynovitis are common, but the temperature is only slightly elevated. Arthralgia generally resolves within 3 to 6 months. Symptomatic infection is rare in children.

Diagnosis

Isolation of virus from serum is possible for the first few days of illness. IgM antibodies will be detected by MAC-ELISA within 5 to 10 days of onset. Complement fixation, haemagglutinin inhibition, and neutralization tests may be useful, particularly when paired serum samples are available. Virus isolation or PCR is confirmatory.

Prevention, control, and treatment

Avoidance of mosquito bites and peridomestic mosquito control can effectively reduce the risk of infection. No specific treatment is available. Nonsteroidal anti-inflammatory drugs may relieve symptoms. One study suggested that corticosteroids might hasten recovery. Vaccine against this virus is currently in the late stage of development.

Sindbis

Aetiology and epidemiology

Sindbis virus is widely distributed in Africa, India, tropical Asia, Australia, and Europe. However, clinical disease is common only in geographically restricted areas. In Europe, the main vectors to humans are late summer, ornithophilic mosquitoes of the genera *Culex* and *Culiseta*. High antibody prevalences in Africa suggest that human exposure is common. Several outbreaks have been noted.

Clinical characteristics

In northern Europe, symptomatic disease is recognized from Sweden (Ockelbo disease), through Finland (Pogosta disease), to the former Karelian Autonomous Soviet Socialist Republic (Karelian fever). The clinical features include mild fever, rash, arthralgia, myalgia, malaise, headache, and pruritus. The maculopapular rash progresses from trunk to extremities and vesicles can occur on the palms and soles. Ankle, finger, wrist, and knee joints are most commonly affected. Prominent rheumatic symptoms, sometimes persisting for several years, have been noted in Europe and South Africa.

Diagnosis

Haemagglutinin inhibition and IgM antibodies will be present in nearly all patients by the eighth day of illness. IgM antibodies detectable in serum by MAC-ELISA may persist for 6 months after infection. Virus can be infrequently detected by culture or RT-PCR from blood or skin lesions.

Prevention, control, and treatment

Avoidance of mosquito bites can reduce the risk of infection. No specific treatment is available.

Barmah Forest virus

Since its first recognition as a cause of human disease in 1988, the geographical distribution of Barmah Forest virus has expanded recently in Australia. It causes sporadic disease and epidemics, with up to 300 serologically confirmed cases. The disease resembles that of Ross River virus infection, although the rash tends to be more florid and true arthritis is less common. The illness is prolonged in some patients. Little is known about the ecology of Barmah Forest virus, although outbreaks have coincided with Ross River virus outbreaks and the virus has been identified in the same mosquito species.

Mayaro virus

Mayaro virus has been isolated from humans, wild vertebrate reservoir species, and *Haemogogus* mosquitoes, the principal vectors, in Trinidad, Colombia, Brazil, Suriname, Guyana, French Guiana, Peru, Bolivia, and Venezuela. Seroprevalence is high in human populations in many forested areas of South America. The clinical presentation resembles Chikungunya, O'nyong-nyong, Ross River, Barmah Forest, and Sindbis virus infections. In Pará, Brazil, after an incubation period of about a week, fever, chills, headache,

arthralgia, myalgia and lymphadenopathy developed and persisted for 2 to 5 days. Arthralgia was almost universal and could last for months. Small joints in the extremities were principally involved. It was accompanied by joint oedema in 20% of cases, causing severe temporary disability. Maculo- or micropapular rashes appeared on the fifth day and lasted for 3 to 4 days in two-thirds of the cases, more in children (Fig. 5.12.1). All patients had leucopenia and a minority had mild thrombocytopenia and albuminuria. Viraemias as high as as over 5.0 log/1 ml suggested that humans might be amplifying hosts for this virus. In other outbreaks, eye pain, diarrhoea, and vomiting were additional features.

O'nyong-nyong virus

From 1959 to 1962, this virus caused epidemics in Uganda, Kenya, Tanzania, and Malawi involving approximately 2 million people. The virus was isolated in 1978 from *Anopheles funestus* mosquitoes in Kenya after a long period of no apparent o'nyong-nyong virus

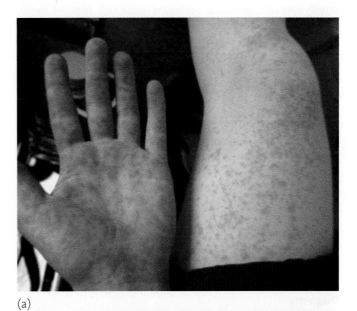

(a)

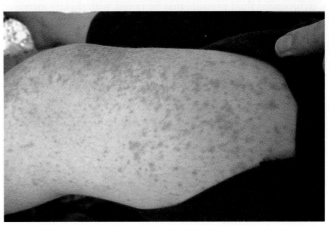

(b)

Fig. 5.12.1 (a and b) Mayaro virus infection acquired in the Peruvian Amazon, showing maculopapular rash that first appeared on the palms of the hands on the fifth day spreading first to arms, knees, and then to entire body and lasting 3 days, accompanied by arthralgia and swelling of the fingers and feet, later affecting the knees. (Courtesy of Dr Celie Manuel) activity. In 1996 to 1997, an outbreak occurred in Uganda. In 2003, an outbreak occurred among refugees in the Côte d'Ivoire and a human infection was confirmed in Chad in 2004. O'nyong-nyong is closely related to chikungunya and produces a similar illness, although fever is less pronounced and lymphadenopathy is more common. *An funestus* and *An gambiae* transmit the virus.

Alphaviruses associated with neuroinvasive disease

Eastern equine encephalitis

Aetiology and epidemiology

The virus is widely distributed throughout North, Central, and South America and the Caribbean. However, little is known about the epidemiology of eastern equine encephalitis outside North America, where it is maintained in a bird–mosquito cycle in hardwood swamps in coastal areas from the Great Lakes to the Gulf Coast. In the United States of America human infections are usually sporadic, and small outbreaks occur each summer mostly along the Atlantic and Gulf Coasts; outbreaks of equine disease are common in Florida. In recent years, 1 to 21 cases have been reported annually. In North America, wild birds and *Culiseta melanura* mosquitoes maintain the virus in hardwood swamps, but a variety of mosquito species act as bridge vectors to humans and domestic animals.

Clinical characteristics

Most infections are inapparent. The incubation period exceeds 1 week and the onset is abrupt with high fever. About 2% of infected adults and 6% of children develop encephalitis. Eastern equine encephalitis is the most severe of the arboviral encephalitides, with a mortality of 35 to 75%. Symptoms and signs include dizziness, decreasing level of consciousness, tremors, seizures, and focal neurological signs. Death can occur within 3 to 5 days of onset. Sequelae are common in nonfatal encephalitis and include convulsions, paralysis, and mental retardation. Illness due to eastern equine encephalitis in South America appears to be less severe.

Diagnosis

Cerebrospinal fluid pressure may be raised, with slightly increased protein, normal sugar, and up to 2000 cells/mm^3. IgM antibodies are readily detected in serum or cerebrospinal fluid by ELISA. Paired serum samples can be tested by haemagglutinin inhibition, ELISA, or neutralization tests. Horse or pheasant deaths and the proximity to swamps provide clues to the diagnosis.

Prevention, control, and treatment

Prevention depends on the avoidance of mosquito bites and mosquito control in suburban areas. Inactivated vaccines have been used successfully in horses, and an inactivated vaccine has been used experimentally in laboratory workers and others at high risk of exposure. No specific treatment is available.

Venezuelan equine encephalitis complex

Aetiology and epidemiology

Six subtypes (I–VI) within the Venezuelan equine encephalitis virus complex have been identified. Five antigenic variants exist within subtype I (IAB, IC, ID, IE, IF). These subtypes and variants are classified as epizootic or enzootic, based on their apparent virulence and epidemiology. Epizootic variants of subtype I (IAB and IC) cause equine epizootics and are associated with more severe human disease. Enzootic strains (ID–F, II (Everglades), III (Mucambo [A,B,D], Tonate [B]), IV (Pixuna), V (Cabassou), VI (Rio Negro)) do not cause epizootics in horses, but may produce sporadic disease in humans. Large epizootics (IAB and IC) have occurred in equines in northern countries of South America and Central America, sometimes reaching the United States of America. In 1969 to 1972, a massive epizootic extending from Ecuador to Texas killed more than 200 000 horses and caused several thousand human infections. In 1995, a large epizootic, which began in Venezuela and spread to Colombia, affected thousands of horses and caused approximately 90 000 human infections. Epizootic strains are carried by a wide variety of mosquitoes including *Aedes*, *Mansonia*, and *Psorophora* spp. Horses are the principal amplifying hosts during epizootics but are not amplifying hosts for enzootic transmission. Enzootic strains are maintained in a cycle involving *Culex* (*Melanoconion*) mosquitoes and rodents.

Clinical characteristics (epizootic virus infections)

After an incubation period of 1 to 6 days, there is a brief febrile illness of sudden onset characterized by malaise, nausea or vomiting, headache, and myalgia. Acute symptoms last 2 to 5 days, and generalized asthenia up to 3 weeks. Clinically, Venezuelan equine encephalitis may be indistinguishable from dengue or other arboviral diseases. Among those with clinical illness, less than 0.5% of adults and less than 4% of children develop encephalitis. Nausea and vomiting, nuchal rigidity, ataxia, convulsions, paralysis, and death may occur. Long-term sequelae following encephalitis are uncommon.

Diagnosis (epizootic virus infections)

A marked leukopenia is universal, often accompanied by neutropenia and thrombocytopenia, with moderate lymphocytosis in the cerebrospinal fluid. Virus can be detected by isolation or by PCR from serum or throat swab is possible within the first few days of illness. Paired sera can be tested by haemagglutinin inhibition and neutralizing tests. Specific IgM can be detected by MAC-ELISA in the second week of illness.

Prevention, control, and treatment

Equine immunization is effective in controlling epizootic disease. Venezuelan equine encephalitis is highly infectious by the aerosol route; many laboratory infections have occurred. Live attenuated and inactivated vaccines have been used in laboratory workers. People in affected areas should avoid mosquito bites. No specific treatment is available.

Western equine encephalitis

Aetiology and epidemiology

This is a complex of closely related viruses found in North and South America, but human disease is rare outside North America and Brazil. Summer outbreaks may be occur with flooding, which increases breeding of *Culex* mosquitoes (particularly *Culex tarsalis* in the western United States of America). Large outbreaks of western equine encephalitis in humans and horses occurred in the western United States of America in the 1950s and 1960s; however, a declining horse population, equine vaccination, and improved vector control have reduced the reported number of human cases to zero in most recent years.

Clinical characteristics

The ratio of apparent to inapparent infection in adults is less than 1 in 1000; however, this ratio increases to 1:1 in infants under 1 year of age. Following an incubation period of about 7 days, headache, vomiting, stiff neck, and backache are typical; restlessness and irritability are seen in children. Weakness and hyporeflexia are common. Convulsions occur in 90% of affected infants and 40% of affected children between 1 and 4 years, but are rare in adults. Recovery in 5 to 10 days is common, but convalescence may be protracted. Although rare in adults and older children, sequelae are common in infants, with one-half of those with encephalitis being left with convulsions and/or severe motor or intellectual deficits. The case fatality rate is 3 to 7%.

Diagnosis

Clinical laboratory findings in western equine encephalitis are often unremarkable. IgM antibodies are readily detected in serum by ELISA. Paired sera can be tested by haemagglutinin inhibition, IgG ELISA, or neutralization tests. Virus can occasionally be isolated from serum or cerebrospinal fluid.

Prevention, control, and treatment

Prevention of western equine encephalitis relies on mosquito control and the avoidance of mosquito bites. Vaccine is available for horses. An inactivated vaccine has been used for laboratory staff and others at high risk of exposure. No specific treatment is available.

Further reading

Aichinger G, et al. (2011). Safety and immunogenicity of an inactivated whole virus Vero cell-derived Ross River vaccine: a randomized trial. Vaccine, 29, 9376–84.

Centers for Disease Control and Prevention (2006). Eastern equine encephalitis: New Hampshire and Massachusetts, August–September 2005 MMWR Morb Mortal Wkly Rep, 55, 697–700.

Griffin D (2007). Alphaviruses. In: Knipe DM, Howley PM (eds) Fields virology, 5th edition, vol. 1, pp. 1023–67. Lippincott Williams & Wilkins, Philadelphia.

Harley D, et al. (2001). Ross River virus transmission, infection, and diseases: a cross-disciplinary review. Clin Microbiol Rev, 14, 909–32.

Kiwanuka N, et al. (1999). O'nyong-nyong fever in South-Central Uganda, 1996–1997: clinical features and validation of a clinical case definition for surveillance purposes. Clin Infect Dis, 29, 1243–50.

Laine M, et al. (2004). Sindbis virus and other alphaviruses as cause of human arthritic disease. J Int Med, 256, 457–71.

Pialoux G, et al. (2007). Chikungunya, an epidemic arbovirosis. Lancet Infect Dis, 7, 319–27.

Pinheiro FP, et al. (1981). An outbreak of Mayaro virus disease in Belterra, Brazil. I. Clinical and virological findings. Am J Trop Med Hyg, 30, 674–81.

Powers AM (2011). Genomic evolution and phenotypic distinctions of Chikungunya viruses causing the Indian Ocean outbreak. Exp Biol Med (Maywood), 236, 909–14.

Schwartz O, Albert ML (2010). Biology and pathogenesis of chikungunya virus. Nat Rev Microbiol, 8, 491–500.

Tesh RB, et al. (1999). Mayaro virus disease: an emerging mosquito-borne zoonosis in tropical South America. Clin Infect Dis, 28, 67–73.

Weaver SC, Frolov IV (2005). Togaviruses. In: Mahy BWJ, ter Meulen V (eds) Topley and Wilson's microbiology and microbial infections, 10th edition, vol. 2, pp. 1010–24. Hodder Arnold, London.

Weaver SC, et al. (2004). Venezuelan equine encephalitis. Annu Rev Entomol, 49, 141–74.

5.13 Rubella

P.A. Tookey and J.M. Best

Essentials

Rubella is caused by an enveloped RNA virus, for which humans are the only known host. Transmission is by airborne droplet spread, with infection seen predominantly in spring and early summer in temperate zones.

Postnatally acquired infection—presents after incubation of 14 to 21 days with rash (maculopapular, usually beginning on the face before spreading to the trunk and extremeties), lymphadenopathy (suboccipital and posterior cervical), and mild fever. Sore throat, coryza, cough, conjunctivitis, and arthralgia may be seen. The illness is usually mild. Management is symptomatic.

Rubella in pregnancy—in the first 10 weeks of gestation this is associated with a 90% risk of congenital fetal abnormalities, most typically comprising sensorineural hearing loss, alone or combined with cataracts and/or cardiac anomalies. Clinical diagnosis is unreliable, hence rapid investigation is essential when a woman develops a rubella-like illness in the first 16 weeks of pregnancy, comprising (1) testing of maternal serum for rubella IgG and IgM antibodies; and sometimes (2) amniotic fluid and/or fetal blood testing; and (3) ultrasonography to detect fetal defects. If a fetus is infected, termination of pregnancy is considered.

Prevention—live attenuated rubella vaccines provide protection to about 95% of vaccinees and are usually given in combination with measles (MR) or measles and mumps (MMR) vaccines. Vaccination of >80% of children is required to prevent circulation of rubella virus. Health care workers and women of childbearing age whose rubella status is unknown (including recent immigrants) should also be targeted for MMR vaccination. Immunization of pregnant women is contraindicated, but women found to be susceptible at antenatal testing should be offered MMR vaccination after delivery.

Introduction

Rubella is a mild exanthematous disease of little clinical significance. However, infection in early pregnancy may result in multiple congenital abnormalities, often referred to as 'congenital rubella syndrome'. As a result of the widespread use of rubella vaccine, congenital rubella syndrome is now rare in many countries.

Aetiology

Rubella is caused by rubella virus, an enveloped RNA virus, which is classified in its own genus Rubivirus within the family Togaviridae. There are no major antigenic differences among rubella virus isolates, although at least seven genotypes have been described.

Epidemiology

Humans are the only known host for rubella virus. In temperate zones the infection is seen predominantly in spring and early summer. Before the introduction of rubella vaccine, rubella was endemic in virtually all countries. Epidemics were superimposed on the endemic infection every 4 to 9 years and pandemics every 10 to 30 years. In most populations, in the absence of a mass immunization programme, 10 to 20% of women are still susceptible to rubella infection when they reach child-bearing age. A review by the World Health Organization in 2000 estimated that more than 100 000 infants were born with congenital rubella syndrome each year in developing countries. In Africa, rubella virus circulates widely but the full impact of congenital rubella syndrome is unclear. In 1996 it was estimated that 22 500 infants with congenital rubella syndrome were born annually in the WHO African Region.

Postnatally acquired infection

The rash usually begins on the face and spreads to the trunk and then the extremities; the pink maculopapular lesions are initially discrete but later tend to coalesce. The suboccipital and posterior cervical lymph nodes are characteristically enlarged. Mild fever, sore throat, coryza, cough, and conjunctivitis may be present; symptoms are usually mild and last 3 to 7 days. There may be a prodrome with malaise and fever, especially in adults. There is no specific treatment.

Transient arthralgia with or without arthritis occurs in up to 70% of postpubertal women, but is less common in men and children. Less common complications include thrombocytopenia with or without purpura, postinfectious encephalitis, transverse myelitis, and rarely the Guillain–Barré syndrome. When rubella is acquired in early pregnancy congenital infection may occur (see below).

Rubella is clinically indistinguishable from several other infections and 20 to 50% of infections are subclinical. Therefore, a history of clinically diagnosed rubella infection is unreliable.

The incubation period is 14 to 21 days. The exact mode of transmission is uncertain but airborne spread by the respiratory route is likely and close contact is usually necessary for transmission. Individuals are most infectious just before the onset of symptoms, and the infectious period lasts from about a week before to a week after the rash appears. Infection usually produces lifelong immunity; however, when rubella is circulating reinfection may occur and is usually asymptomatic.

Congenital infection

Risk to the fetus

The possible consequences of rubella in pregnancy are the birth of an infant with congenital rubella infection with or without congenital defects, the birth of a normal infant, or spontaneous abortion. Infection before conception is not a risk to the fetus. Spontaneous abortion may occur when rubella is acquired early in pregnancy. When maternal infection occurs during the first 10 weeks of pregnancy the rate of fetal infection is about 90%; it then declines until the last few weeks of pregnancy when the rate rises again. Virtually all of those infected during the first 10 weeks of pregnancy are likely to have congenital defects, but the risk declines over the next 6 weeks. After 16 weeks' gestation even sensorineural hearing loss and growth retardation are rare, and no abnormalities have been demonstrated following serologically confirmed maternal infection after 18 weeks' gestation. Most prospective studies of the risk to the fetus have been carried out on women with symptoms, but asymptomatic primary infection is thought to carry a similar risk.

Following maternal reinfection in pregnancy the risk of transmission to the fetus is probably less than 10% and the risk of damage less than 5%, although it may be higher following symptomatic reinfection.

Clinical features

Congenital rubella is typically associated with cataracts, cardiac anomalies, and sensorineural hearing loss, and the term congenital rubella syndrome (CRS) refers to this classic triad of defects. The teratogenic effects may result in a wide range of defects (Box 5.13.1), but sensorineural hearing loss alone or combined with other abnormalities is most common. Severe multiple problems are more likely when infection occurs early in pregnancy.

Some defects, particularly sensorineural hearing loss, may not develop or become apparent until late infancy or childhood. Other reported late-onset problems include diabetes mellitus,

---

Box 5.13.1 Most common defects associated with congenital rubella

Classic triad

◆ Deafness
  • Sensorineural
  • Central auditory
◆ Abnormalities of the cardiovascular system
  • Patent ductus arteriosus
  • Pulmonary stenosis
  • Pulmonary arterial hypoplasia
◆ Abnormalities of the eye
  • Retinopathy
  • Cataracts
  • Microphthalmos
  • Iris hypoplasia

Other defects

◆ Growth retardation
◆ Microcephaly
◆ Mental retardation
◆ Speech defects

Other signs in the neonatal period and infancy

◆ Low birthweight
◆ Hepatosplenomegaly
◆ Jaundice
◆ Meningoencephalitis
◆ Rash
◆ Thrombocytopenia with or without purpura
◆ Adenopathies
◆ Bony radiolucencies
◆ Hypogammaglobulinaemia
◆ Pneumonitis

thyroid dysfunction, autism, and other behavioural and psychiatric disorders. A rare progressive rubella panencephalitis has also been reported.

Laboratory diagnosis

The diagnosis of congenital rubella infection is relatively easy if suspected early, but more difficult to confirm after 3 months of age. The presence of rubella IgM antibody in early infancy is virtually diagnostic of congenital infection because acquired infection is rare at this age. Using sensitive assays, rubella IgM may be detected in 85% of infected infants at 3 to 6 months and about 30% at 6 to 12 months of age. The presence of IgG antibody alone is not diagnostic since it is likely to indicate passively transferred maternal antibody, but persistence of IgG between 6 and 12 months is strongly suggestive of congenital infection. When abnormalities present late, a presumptive diagnosis can be made based on a compatible clinical picture and the presence or persistence of rubella IgG antibodies in a young child who has not yet been vaccinated.

Congenital infection can also be diagnosed by detection of virus during the first months of life when it can be isolated or detected by polymerase chain reaction from a variety of specimens including nasopharyngeal swabs, urine, oral fluid, and conjunctival fluid. Congenitally infected infants shed large amounts of virus from the oropharynx and may be a source of infection for many months; viral shedding occasionally persists for more than a year.

Management of rubella-like illness during pregnancy

Appropriate management of a rash illness in pregnancy will depend on the local epidemiology of rubella. Routine antenatal rubella antibody screening is not designed to identify rubella infection in pregnancy, and specific diagnostic investigations are needed. Pregnant women with a rubella-like rash should be investigated simultaneously for rubella and parvovirus B19, since they are clinically indistinguishable, and even women previously reported to be immune should be investigated in case of laboratory error. Blood should be tested for rubella IgG and IgM antibodies. Rising IgG or detectable IgM antibody indicates recent infection; a positive IgM result alone should be confirmed with a second serum sample. Pregnant women who are susceptible or of unknown rubella antibody status and are in contact with a rubella-like illness should also be investigated as rapidly as possible. The detection of rubella IgM in a woman without a rash or history of contact should be interpreted with caution as rubella IgM may persist for some months or even years after infection or vaccination, or the IgM may be due to cross-reaction with autoantibodies or other viral IgM antibodies. Investigations must be done in consultation with a virologist who should be aware of the date and type of contact, stage of pregnancy, and history of previous immunization and testing. Prenatal diagnosis of congenital infection using amniotic fluid and/or fetal blood may sometimes be indicated. Ultrasound examination may detect such defects as microcephaly, dystrophic calcification, cataracts, microphthalmos, hepatosplenomegaly, and intrauterine growth restriction.

Prevention

Rubella can be prevented by live attenuated rubella vaccines. The RA27/3 strain is commonly used and this produces antibodies in about 95% of recipients; protection is probably lifelong in most vaccinees. Rubella vaccine is usually combined with measles (MR) or measles and mumps (MMR) vaccines.

In children, rubella vaccine causes few side effects. Low-grade fever and rash are occasionally reported, and transient arthralgia has been seen in about 3% of vaccinees; there have also been rare reports of myositis and vasculitis. Joint symptoms are more common in adult women, affecting up to 60% of vaccinees, but are transient and less severe than following naturally acquired rubella.

When rubella vaccines were first licensed in the late 1960s, universal childhood vaccination was implemented in the United States of America with the aim of eliminating rubella. A different strategy was pursued elsewhere, and the selective programmes established in Australia and some European countries targeted prepubertal girls and women of child-bearing age. This provided individual protection while allowing the continued circulation of wild virus and the acquisition of natural immunity by the majority of individuals. When the combined MMR vaccine became available, many countries with high vaccine uptake moved to a universal offer of MMR vaccine for children in the second year of life, usually with a second dose offered preschool or later.

The MMR vaccine was introduced into the United Kingdom schedule in 1988, and uptake by the age of 24 months reached 92% between 1992 and 1996. The schoolgirl programme was discontinued in 1996 and replaced by the offer of a second MMR for four-year-olds. Uptake of MMR subsequently declined to a low point of 80% in 2003, because of unfounded concerns about safety; however, by 2005 there were signs of recovery and uptake increased to over 88% by 2009/10. Antenatal screening continues. Although the circulation of rubella virus has dropped to very low levels since the introduction of MMR, prolonged periods of low vaccine uptake may lead to outbreaks of rubella in the future, putting susceptible pregnant women at risk.

Use of rubella-containing vaccines has led to the elimination of rubella in the United States of America and Scandinavian countries, although outbreaks have occurred in the United States of America due to importations of rubella virus. Similarly, in the United Kingdom there have been dramatic declines in the numbers of susceptible pregnant women, rubella-associated terminations, and children born with congenital rubella syndrome. Fewer than five congenitally infected infants were reported on average each year between 1990 and 1999, compared with about 50 per year in the 1970s. Between 2000 and 2010 fewer than 20 cases were identified, and in over half of these the infant's mother acquired infection abroad. Termination of pregnancy associated with rubella disease or contact is also now a rare occurrence.

The World Health Organization has recommended that all countries undertaking measles elimination should consider the introduction of MR or MMR vaccine in order to eliminate rubella as well. By 2005, rubella vaccine was used by 117 of 214 countries, with particularly good progress seen in the Americas. In 1997 the Pan American Health Organization recommended a regional initiative to eliminate rubella and congenital rubella syndrome, and by 2004 all countries in the region, except Haiti, had incorporated rubella vaccine into their routine vaccination programmes leading to a significant fall in cases of rubella and congenital rubella syndrome. In 2005 the World Health Organization European Region established a goal of reducing congenital rubella syndrome cases to less than 1 per 100 000 births by 2010; however, despite substantial progress by 2010, elimination could not be confirmed throughout the region at that time and the target date was subsequently revised to 2015. The strategy to be adopted in any country seeking to control congenital rubella by vaccination must depend on the projected uptake of vaccination and the long-term prospects for continuing the programme. An important element should be the immunization of susceptible health personnel, particularly those in contact with pregnant women. It is also important to target women who have emigrated from countries without rubella vaccination programmes, as they are more likely to be susceptible than women born in countries with well-established vaccination programmes. In Africa and other developing regions, WHO has recommended that rubella surveillance should be integrated with measles case-based surveillance, congenital rubella syndrome surveillance should be established, the routine immunization programme should be strengthened, and introduction of rubella vaccination should be considered to ensure rubella immunity among women of reproductive age.

Vaccination in pregnancy

There have been persistent concerns that the vaccine virus might be teratogenic if given during pregnancy. Although vaccinees cannot infect other susceptible individuals, the virus can cross the placenta. Data from studies of children born to several hundred women inadvertently vaccinated up to 3 months before conception or during pregnancy show less than 3% with serological evidence of congenital infection, and no reported case of abnormalities attributable to congenital rubella. At least 80 of these infants were born to women vaccinated in the month of conception, probably the period of greatest vulnerability. These data suggest that the likely maximum theoretical risk of rubella-associated abnormalities is less than 5%.

Likely developments

♦ Elimination of rubella by further countries

♦ Introduction of rubella vaccine in additional countries worldwide

♦ Use of mathematical models to guide rubella vaccination strategies in different countries

♦ Use of genotyping to track the source of rubella outbreaks as countries approach elimination of rubella virus

♦ Development of techniques for the diagnosis of congenital rubella syndrome after the age of 3 months

Further reading

Banatvala JE, Brown DWG (2004). Rubella. *Lancet*, **363**, 1127–37.

Banatvala JE, Peckham C (eds) (2007). *Rubella viruses. Perspectives in medical virology*, vol. 15. Elsevier, London.

Best JM, Icenogle JP, Brown DWG (2009). Rubella. In: Zuckerman AJ, (ed) *Principles and practice of clinical virology*, 6th edition, pp. 561–92. John Wiley & Sons, Chichester.

Cooper LZ, Alford CA (2006). Rubella. In: Remington JS, *et al.* (eds) *Infectious diseases of the fetus and newborn infant*, 6th edition, pp. 894–926. Elsevier, Saunders, Philadelphia.

Department of Health (2006). Rubella (chapter updated 2010). In: *Immunisation against Infectious Disease—'The Green Book'*. Available from: http://www.dh.gov.uk/prod_consum_dh/groups/dh_digitalassets/@dh/@en/documents/digitalasset/dh_122641.pdf

Goodson JL, *et al.* (2011). Rubella epidemiology in Africa in the prevaccine era, 2002–2009. *J Infect Dis*, **204**(Suppl 1), S215–25.

HPA Rash Guidance Working Group. *Guidance on viral rash in pregnancy: investigation, diagnosis and management of viral rash illness, or exposure to viral rash illness, in pregnancy*. Available from: http://www.hpa.org.uk/web/HPAwebFile/HPAweb_C/1294740918985

Robertson SE, *et al.* (2003). Rubella and congenital rubella syndrome: global update. *Pan Am J Public Health*, **14**, 306–15.

5.14 Flaviviruses (excluding dengue)

E.E. Ooi, L.R. Petersen, and D.J. Gubler

Essentials

Flaviviruses, family *Flaviviridae*, are enveloped viruses with a single-strand positive-sense RNA genome approximately 11 kb in length. They comprise 53 species (40 of which can cause human infection), divided into three major groups based on epidemiology and phylogenetics. They are maintained in nature in complex transmission cycles involving a variety of animals and hematophagous arthropods, which transmit infection to humans. IgM antibody capture enzyme-linked immunosorbent assay (MAC-ELISA) is widely used for diagnosis, with confirmation requiring a fourfold or greater rise in specific antibodies between acute and convalescent serum samples, virus isolation, detection of specific antigen by immunohistochemistry or of viral RNA by nucleic acid amplification from blood or other a tissue sample.

Mosquito-borne flaviviruses

Dengue and dengue haemorrhagic fever (see Chapter 5.15) is the most important and widespread human disease caused by an arbovirus, causing a broad spectrum of illness ranging from asymptomatic to severe and fatal haemorrhagic disease. It is primarily an urban disease transmitted among humans by the highly domesticated *Aedes aegypti* mosquito.

Japanese encephalitis virus has a widespread distribution throughout Asia; is the most important cause of arboviral encephalitis; is maintained in a cycle involving *Culex* mosquitoes and water birds; about 1/250 infections are symptomatic, with manifestations ranging from a febrile illness with headache, through aseptic meningitis, to encephalitis, and death. Many survivors have residual neurological abnormalities. There is no specific treatment. Vaccination should generally be offered to people spending a month or more in endemic areas, especially if travel includes rural areas.

St Louis encephalitis virus—prevalent throughout the hemisphere from southern Canada to Argentina; maintained in a cycle involving *Culex* mosquitoes and water birds; 1/16 to 1/425 infections are symptomatic, with manifestations ranging from fever with headache, to aseptic meningitis, to encephalitis, and death. There is no specific treatment. No vaccine is available.

West Nile virus—found in Africa, the Middle East, Asia, Australia (Kunjin is a subtype of West Nile virus), parts of Europe and the Americas; maintained in a cycle involving *Culex* mosquitoes and water birds; most infections are asymptomatic, but 20% develop a febrile illness, and 1% neuroinvasive disease including meningitis, encephalitis and acute flaccid paralysis. There is no specific treatment. Several equine vaccines are available, and human vaccines are in clinical trials.

Yellow fever virus—found in tropical America and Africa; forest/jungle transmission cycle involves canopy-dwelling mosquitoes and monkeys, urban cycle involves humans as the vertebrate host and *Aedes aegypti* as the principal vector; 5% of infections present clinically with a viraemic illness, which may be followed after a transient period of remission by relapse with shock, neurological deterioration, jaundice, haemorrhagic manifestations and renal failure. Treatment is symptomatic. A live, attenuated, single-dose vaccine is highly effective.

Other important mosquito-borne flaviviruses include Murray Valley, Rocio and Zika virus.

Tick-transmitted flaviviruses

Tick-borne encephalitis, louping ill, Powassan encephalitis—geographical distribution determined by that of relevant hard tick vectors; rodents are the principal vertebrate hosts, with occupational and vocational pursuits favouring tick exposure as risk factors for human disease; most infections are subclinical, but a nonspecific influenza-like illness may be followed after a few days of apparent recovery by aseptic meningitis or meningoencephalitis that may lead to permanent paralysis in some cases. Treatment is supportive. Effective inactivated vaccines are available.

Tick-borne haemorrhagic fevers—these include Kyasanur Forest disease and Alkhurma (strictly Al Khumra) and Omsk haemorrhagic fevers.

Introduction

The genus *Flavivirus* of the family *Flaviviridae* comprises 53 virus species, 40 of which can cause human infection (Table 5.14.1). Flaviviruses are small (37–50 nm), spherical particles whose genome is a molecule of single-stranded, positive-sense RNA approximately 11 000 nucleotides in length. Based on epidemiological and phylogenetic characteristics, the flaviviruses are classified into three groups: (1) those that are mosquito-borne, (2) those that are tick-borne, and (3) those for which no arthropod vector has been demonstrated. All flaviviruses of human importance belong to the first two groups; the last group contains a few viruses found in vertebrates and mosquitoes.

Most flaviviruses are maintained in nature in complex transmission cycles between wild or domestic animals and one or more haematophagous arthropod vector. Humans become infected from infective arthropod vectors that take a blood meal, but for most of the flaviviruses humans do not usually develop high viraemias and are not thought to contribute to the transmission cycle. However, some flaviviruses such as dengue, yellow fever, and zika viruses do produce high-level viraemias in humans and can be maintained in urban surroundings through a mosquito–human–mosquito transmission cycle.

The epidemiology and geographical distribution of the flaviviruses depend on several factors including the presence of suitable amplifying hosts, the presence and feeding behaviour of a suitable arthropod vector, and the frequency of exposure of nonimmune reservoir hosts and humans to infected vectors. Globalization of

trade and travel, human population growth, urbanization, and neglect of mosquito control programmes have produced conditions conducive to increasing incidence and geographical expansion of the flaviviruses. A recent dramatic example is the introduction and subsequent spread of the West Nile virus in the western hemisphere. Transmission of some flaviviruses directly from one person to another through blood transfusion or organ transplantation has also been documented.

Flavivirus infection in humans can result in asymptomatic infection or a spectrum of clinical illness ranging from nonspecific febrile illness, fever with rash or arthralgia or both, haemorrhagic fever, hepatitis, encephalitis, and death. The same virus can cause a variety of syndromes, and often the majority of those infected have mild nonspecific illness or are asymptomatic. Although no specific therapy is available, prompt supportive treatment and proper management may substantially reduce mortality from some flavivirus infections.

Laboratory diagnosis

All flaviviruses have common group epitopes on the envelope protein that result in extensive cross-reactions in serological tests. The specificity of antibody should, therefore, be confirmed by cross-neutralization tests in areas where multiple flaviviruses are endemic/enzootic.

The IgM antibody capture enzyme-linked immunosorbent assay (MAC-ELISA) is widely used for diagnosis of flaviviruses. IgM antibody is usually detectable 5 to 8 days after onset of symptoms. Because detectable IgM antibody persists for one or more months after infection with most flaviviruses, its presence does not confirm current infection; people with detectable IgM antibody are considered recent or presumptive cases. Confirmatory laboratory diagnosis of most flaviviruses requires isolation of the virus, detection of specific viral RNA by nucleic acid amplification or of specific antigen in autopsy tissues by immunohistochemistry. A fourfold or greater rise in specific neutralizing antibody is also confirmatory.

Important mosquito-borne flavivirus infections

For dengue and dengue haemorrhagic fever, see Chapter 5.15.

Japanese encephalitis

Aetiology and epidemiology

Japanese encephalitis virus is the type species of the Japanese encephalitis antigenic group of flaviviruses that includes several antigenically related viruses, including St Louis encephalitis, West Nile, Kunjin, Koutango, Usutu, Murray Valley encephalitis, Kunjin (a subtype of West Nile), Alfuy, Cacipacore and Yaounde viruses. Sequence analysis of the structural proteins suggests there are several genotypes of Japanese encephalitis in distinct geographical areas.

Japanese encephalitis has a widespread distribution throughout Asia, and its distribution has expanded in recent years with outbreaks in the Pacific, Australia, Nepal, and western India (Fig. 5.14.1). It is the most important cause of arboviral encephalitis and about 50 000 cases are reported annually. The highest incidence of neuroinvasive disease is in temperate and subtropical countries where epidemics may occur. The virus is maintained in a cycle involving *Culex* mosquitoes and water birds and is transmitted to humans by *Culex*

Table 5.14.1 Taxonomy of flaviviruses

Group	Species name[a]	Strain name, synonyms, and tentative species names	Abbreviation
Mosquito-borne viruses			
Aroa virus group	*Aroa virus*	Aroa virus	AROAV
		Bussuquara virus	BSQV
		Iguape virus	IGUV
		Naranjal virus	NJLV
Dengue virus group	***Dengue viruses***	**Dengue virus 1**	**DENV-1**
		Dengue virus 2	**DENV-2**
		Dengue virus 3	**DENV-3**
		Dengue virus 4	**DENV-4**
	Kedougou virus	Kedougou virus	KEDV
Japanese encephalitis virus group	*Cacipacore virus*	Cacipacore virus	CPCV
	Japanese encephalitis virus	**Japanese encephalitis virus**	**JEV**
	Koutango virus	Koutango virus	KOUV
	Murray Valley encephalitis virus	**Alfuy virus**	**ALFV**
		Murray Valley encephalitis virus	**MVEV**
	St Louis encephalitis virus	**St Louis encephalitis virus**	**SLEV**
	Usutu virus	Usutu virus	USUV
	West Nile virus	**Kunjin virus**	**KUNV**
		West Nile virus	**WNV**
	Yaounde virus	Yaounde virus	YAOV
Kokobera virus group	*Kokobera virus*	Kokobera virus	KOKV
		Stratford virus	STRV
Ntaya virus group	*Bagaza virus*	Bagaza virus	BAGV
	Ilheus virus	Ilheus virus	ILHV
		Rocio virus	**ROCV**
	Israel Turkey meningoencephalitis virus	Israel Turkey meningoencephalitis virus	ITV
	Ntaya virus	Ntaya virus	NTAV
	Tembusu virus	Tembusu virus	TMUV
Spondweni virus group	***Zika virus***	**Spondweni virus**	**SPOV**
		Zika virus	**ZIKV**
Yellow fever virus group	*Banzi virus*	Banzi virus	BANV
	Bouboui virus	Bouboui virus	BOUV
	Edge Hill virus	Edge Hill virus	EHV
	Jugra virus	Jugra virus	JUGV
	Saboya virus	Potiskum virus	POTV
		Saboya virus	SABV
	Sepik virus	Sepik virus	SEPV
	Uganda S virus	Uganda S virus	UGSV
	Wesselsbron virus	Wesselsbron virus	WESSV
	Yellow fever virus	**Yellow fever virus**	**YFV**

(Continued)

Table 5.14.1 *(Cont'd)* Taxonomy of flaviviruses

Group	Species name[a]	Strain name, synonyms, and tentative species names	Abbreviation
Tick-borne viruses			
Mammalian tick-borne virus group	*Gadgets Gully virus*	Gadgets Gully virus	GGYV
	Kyasanur Forest disease virus	**Kyasanur Forest disease virus**	**KFDV**
		Alkhumra (Al Khumra) haemorrhagic fever virus	**AKHFV**
	Langat virus	Langat virus	LGTV
	Louping ill virus	**Louping ill virus**	**LIV**
		British subtype	**LIV-Brit**
		Irish subtype	**LIV-Ir**
		Spanish subtype	**LIV-Span**
		Turkish subtype	**LIV-Turk**
	Omsk haemorrhagic fever virus	**Omsk haemorrhagic fever virus**	**OHFV**
	Powassan virus	**Powassan virus**	**POWV**
	Royal Farm virus	Karshi virus	KSIV
		Royal Farm virus	RFV
	Tick-borne encephalitis virus	**Tick-borne encephalitis virus**	**TBEV**
		European subtype	**TBEV-Eu**
		Far Eastern subtype	**TBEV-FE**
		Siberian subtype	**TBEV-Sib**
Seabird tick-borne virus group	*Kadam virus*	Kadam virus	KADV
	Meaban virus	Meaban virus	MEAV
	Saumarez Reef virus	Saumarez Reef virus	SREV
	Tyuleniy virus	Tyuleniy virus	TYUV
Viruses with no known arthropod vector			
Entebbe bat virus group	*Entebbe bat virus*	Entebbe bat virus	ENTV
		Sokoluk virus	SOKV
	Yokose virus	Yokose virus	YOKV
Modoc virus group	*Apoi virus*	Apoi virus	APOIV
	Cowbone Ridge virus	Cowbone Ridge virus	CRV
	Jutiapa virus	Jutiapa virus	JUTV
	Modoc virus	Modoc virus	MODV
	Sal Vieja virus	Sal Vieja virus	SVV
	San Perlita virus	San Perlita virus	SPV
Rio Bravo virus group	*Bukalasa bat virus*	Bukalasa bat virus	BBV
	Carey Island virus	Carey Island virus	CIV
	Dakar bat virus	Dakar bat virus	DBV
	Montana myotis leukoencephalitis virus	Montana myotis leukoencephalitis virus	MMLV
	Phnom Penh bat virus	Batu cave virus	BCV
		Phnom Penh bat virus	PPBV
	Rio Bravo virus	Rio Bravo virus	RBV
Viruses tentatively placed in the genus Flavivirus			
	Cell fusing agent virus		CFAV
	Kamiti River virus	KRV	
	Tamana bat virus		TABV
	Nounané virus	NOUV	
	BYD virus	BYDV	
	New mapoon virus		

[a] Species in bold are discussed in the text.
Adapted with permission from Fauquet C, Fauquet CM, Mayo MA (eds) (2005). *Virus taxonomy: classification and nomenclature of viruses; eighth report of the International Committee on the Taxonomy of Viruses*, pp. 986–8. Academic Press, New York.

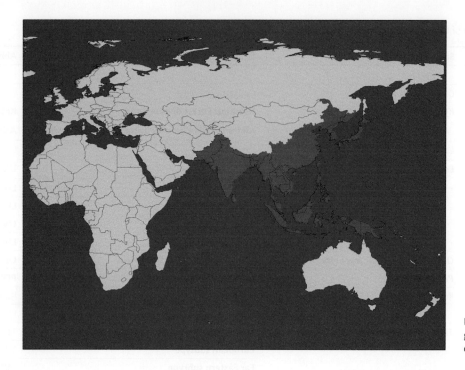

Fig. 5.14.1 Approximate geographical distribution of Japanese encephalitis virus.

mosquitoes, primarily species of the *Culex tritaeniorhynchus* complex which breed in rice fields. Pigs are the primary amplifying host in the peridomestic environment. Epidemics occur in late summer in temperate regions, but transmission occurs throughout the year in some tropical areas of Asia. Children have the highest attack rates because of cumulative herd immunity with age.

Clinical characteristics (see also Oxford Textbook of Medicine 5e Chapter 24.11.2)

Only about 1 in 250 infections results in symptomatic infection, which ranges from a febrile illness with headache, through aseptic meningitis, to encephalitis, and death. After an incubation period of 6 to 16 days, illness usually begins with a prodrome lasting several days followed by abrupt high fever, change in mental status, nausea and vomiting, and headache. Early onset seizures occur in at least one-half of hospitalized children and one-quarter of adults. They are usually generalized tonic–clonic seizures, but may also be partial motor or with more subtle clinical manifestations, such as twitching of a digit or eyebrow, or nystagmus. Patients with subtle seizures are usually in status epilepticus. Extrapyramidal features include dull, expressionless facies, generalized hypertonia, and cogwheel rigidity. Focal motor deficits, including cranial nerve palsies and acute flaccid paralysis resulting from anterior horn cell destruction may also occur. This poliomyelitis-like illness may be the only neurological manifestation of the illness or may proceed or accompany encephalitis. Respiratory dysregulation, coma, abnormal plantar reflexes, and prolonged convulsions are associated with a poor prognosis.

Laboratory examination often reveals a moderate peripheral leukocytosis and mild anaemia. Hyponatraemia, reflecting inappropriate antidiuretic hormone secretion, is common. Cerebrospinal fluid pressure is usually normal, pleocytosis ranges from a few to several hundred cells/mm^3, and cerebrospinal fluid protein is moderately elevated in about one-half the cases.

Five to 40% of cases are fatal; young children are more likely to die, and if they survive are more likely to have residual neurological defects. Overall, up to 70% of survivors have residual neurological abnormalities including parkinsonism, paralysis, behavioural changes, and psychological deficits. Evidence suggests that infection fails to clear in some patients, with clinical relapse several months after resolution of the acute illness. The clinical effects of congenital infection are unknown. Spontaneous abortions of women infected in the first and second trimesters have been reported.

Diagnosis

The differential diagnosis includes other viral encephalitides including arboviruses, herpes, and enteroviral infections, cerebral malaria, and bacterial infections. Epidemiological features such as place of residence or travel, season, and occurrence of other cases in the community provide clues to the diagnosis. Patients with encephalitis are rarely viraemic, although they may be so during the early acute stage of illness. Specific IgM can be detected in cerebrospinal fluid, serum, or both in nearly all patients by the seventh day after onset. Confirmation can be obtained by demonstrating fourfold or greater increase in IgM or neutralizing antibody titre.

Prevention and control

A formalin-inactivated mouse brain vaccine has been used widely in Japan, Korea, Taiwan, Thailand, and other countries in Asia for childhood immunization and is licensed in the United Kingdom, the United States of America, and other developed countries to protect travellers. Hypersensitivity reactions to this vaccine, including generalized urticaria, angio-oedema, and even anaphylaxis, have occurred within minutes to as long as 2 weeks following vaccination at a rate of 1 to 104 per 10 000. An inactivated tissue culture-based vaccine has replaced the mouse brain vaccine in many countries, including for adults in the United States of America. A tissue culture-based live attenuated vaccine (SA 14-14-2) used extensively in China appears to have a remarkably good safety profile and currently is being introduced elsewhere in Asia. The risk to travellers in endemic areas during the transmission season can reach 1 in 5000 per month of exposure. The risk for most short-term travellers may be less than 1 in a million. In general, vaccine should be offered to people spending a month or more in endemic areas during the transmission season, especially if travel includes rural areas. Water and crop management and animal husbandry have been used to decrease human exposure to mosquito bites in the peridomestic environment.

Treatment

No specific therapy is available, but supportive treatment can reduce morbidity and mortality. Interferon-α2a failed to improve clinical outcome in a double-blind placebo-controlled trial. Dexamethasone did not prevent death caused by oedema-induced increases in intracranial pressure in patients with severe encephalitis.

St Louis encephalitis

Aetiology and epidemiology

St Louis encephalitis virus is prevalent throughout the western hemisphere from southern Canada to Argentina. The natural transmission cycle involves wild birds and *Culex* mosquitoes. Although clinical illness has been sporadically reported throughout much of the western hemisphere, the highest incidence occurs in North America during epidemics. Fewer than 100 human cases are generally reported annually; epidemics with hundreds to thousands of cases have occurred in North America every 10 to 20 years.

Clinical characteristics

The ratio of infection to clinical illness is high, ranging from 425:1 in children to 16:1 in elderly persons. Illness ranges from fever with headache, to aseptic meningitis, to encephalitis, and death. Advanced age is the principal risk factor for both symptomatic disease and severity of encephalitis. After an incubation period of 4 to 21 days, the typical presentation of encephalitis is fever, headache, chills, nausea, and dysuria. Within 1 to 4 days, central nervous system signs appear and may include meningism, tremor, abnormal reflexes, ataxia, cranial nerve palsies, convulsions (especially in children), stupor, and coma. Recovery is usually complete, except that 10 to 25% of very young infants have residual mental deficits, personality changes, muscle weakness, and paralysis. Underlying diseases such as hypertension, diabetes, and alcoholism affect the outcome. The case fatality rate is about 7% overall, but is only 1% of those under 5 years of age as the disease is generally milder in children. Short-lived sequelae of nervousness, memory impairment, and headache occur uncommonly in older children and adults.

The peripheral leucocyte count, serum transaminases, and creatine kinase may be elevated. Hyponatraemia due to the syndrome of inappropriate antidiuretic hormone secretion may be noted in up to one-third of patients. The cerebrospinal fluid contains fewer than 500 cells/mm³, principally leucocytes.

Diagnosis

The differential diagnosis includes other viral encephalitides such as West Nile virus and other arboviruses, herpes, and enterovirus, as well as other bacterial and fungal infections of the central nervous system. Epidemiological features (residence, season of the year, and occurrence of other cases in the community) provide diagnostic clues. Because of serological cross-reactivity with other flaviviruses, positive serum samples should be subjected to cross-neutralization tests. From fatal cases, virus may be isolated from brain tissue or demonstrated by immunohistochemistry. Virus has not been isolated from the blood during the acute phase of illness.

Prevention and control

No vaccine is available. Prevention is aimed at personal protection from mosquito bites and mosquito abatement.

Treatment

Treatment is supportive; no specific therapy is available.

West Nile encephalitis (see also Oxford Textbook of Medicine 5e Chapter 24.11.2)

Aetiology and epidemiology

West Nile virus is maintained in a cycle involving *Culex* mosquitoes and wild birds and is enzootic in Africa, the Middle East, western Asia, parts of Europe, and the Americas (Fig. 5.14.2). From the 1950s to the 1970s, sporadic epidemics, rarely associated with severe neurological disease and death, occurred in Israel, France, and Africa. No epidemic activity was then reported until the mid-1990s when epidemics associated with severe neurological disease and death in humans and/or equines and birds were recorded in Algeria, Morocco, Tunisia, Italy, Romania, Israel, southern Russia, and France. The virus was first detected in the New World during an outbreak in New York City in 1999; subsequently, the virus has become enzootic throughout the United States of America (with the exception of Alaska and Hawaii) and southern Canada and has been detected as far south as Argentina. While outbreaks have occurred annually in North America, human or equine cases have been uncommonly reported in the tropical regions of the Caribbean and Latin America despite serological evidence of widespread enzootic transmission. An outbreak of human and equine neuroinvasive disease has recently been reported in Argentina.

In temperate regions, outbreaks typically occur in late summer and early autumn, times when sufficient viral amplification in the bird–mosquito cycle has occurred to produce high mosquito infection rates. Although mosquito transmission accounts for nearly all human infections, infection resulting from receipt of contaminated blood transfusions and transplanted organs, transplacental transmission, needlestick exposure, aerosol exposure in the laboratory, mucous membrane splashes of infected fluids, and possibly ingestion of breast milk from an infected mother have been documented.

Phylogenetic studies indicate five and possibly as many as seven viral lineages: lineage one includes most strains isolated in recent outbreaks in Europe, the Middle East, and North America; lineage two includes many of the strains enzootic in Africa. Kunjin virus (see below) is a variant of West Nile virus and fits within lineage one. The strain introduced into North America was genetically identical to a strain circulating in the Middle East.

Clinical characteristics

Most infections are asymptomatic. Approximately 20% of those infected develop a systemic febrile illness, while less than 1% develop neuroinvasive disease including meningitis, encephalitis, and acute flaccid paralysis. Advanced age is the most important risk factor for developing both encephalitis and death. Immunosuppressed people, such as organ transplant patients, are at extremely high risk of developing neuroinvasive disease after infection. The incubation period is usually 2 to 15 days, but may be longer in the immunosuppressed.

West Nile fever presents as a dengue-like illness with fever, headache, backache, myalgia, muscle weakness, anorexia, nausea, and

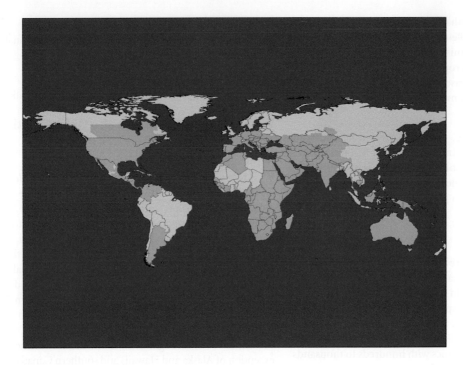

Fig. 5.14.2 Approximate geographical distribution of West Nile virus.

vomiting that lasts 3 to 6 days. Roseola or a maculopapular rash on the trunk and extremities occurs in about one-half of the patients with West Nile fever and generally arises during convalescence. The rash is present in about 20% of patients with neuroinvasive disease. Fatigue lasting longer than a month after acute infection is common.

Among patients with meningitis or encephalitis, fever is present in at least 90%, with weakness, nausea, vomiting, and headache in approximately one-half of patients. Other neurological manifestations include tremor, myoclonus, and parkinsonian features such as rigidity, postural instability, and bradykinesia. West Nile virus infection can cause acute flaccid paralysis following involvement of the anterior horn cell, even without concurrent meningitis or encephalitis. Cranial nerve abnormalities may produce facial paralysis, which has a favourable prognosis. Dysarthria and dysphagia accompanied by acute flaccid paralysis indicate brainstem involvement and thus a high risk of impending respiratory failure. West Nile virus infection infrequently causes other forms of weakness, including brachial plexopathy, radiculopathy, and a predominantly demyelinating peripheral neuropathy similar to Guillain–Barré syndrome. Other neurological complications include seizures, cerebellar ataxia, and optic neuritis.

Numerous other manifestations of West Nile virus infection have been reported. Chorioretinitis and vitritis appear commonly, but are usually of minor clinical significance. Other reported ocular findings include iridocyclitis, occlusive vasculitis, and uveitis. Rhabdomyolysis, myocarditis, hepatitis, pancreatitis, central diabetes insipidus, and haemorrhagic manifestations have been documented.

Recovery from West Nile fever and meningitis is usually complete. Among those with encephalitis, approximately one-half of survivors have residual neurological deficits and initial disease severity may not predict eventual clinical outcome. Case fatality rates among those with encephalitis are approximately 10%. Most patients with acute flaccid paralysis have incomplete recovery of limb strength, often resulting in profound residual deficits. Quadriplegia and respiratory failure are associated with high morbidity and mortality, and recovery is slow and typically incomplete.

Diagnosis

Epidemiological features (residence, season of the year, and occurrence of other cases in the community) provide diagnostic clues. The differential diagnosis includes other causes of acute febrile illness; other viral encephalitides including arboviruses, herpes, and enterovirus, as well as other bacterial and fungal infections of the central nervous system; and other causes of acute flaccid paralysis. West Nile virus should strongly be considered when myoclonic jerking, parkinsonian features, or acute flaccid paralysis occur with encephalitis during peak transmission times. In patients with acute flaccid paralysis, neurological examination should differentiate anterior horn cell dysfunction from Guillain–Barré syndrome.

The cerebrospinal fluid usually contains moderately elevated protein and up to 2000 cells/mm^3, with neutrophils predominating early in infection followed by lymphocytic predominance. IgM ELISA on serum or cerebrospinal fluid samples is positive in nearly all patients by the eighth day after clinical onset, although IgM antibody development may be delayed or even fail in some immunocompromised patients. Nucleic acid amplification testing (NAT) of serum or cerebrospinal fluid may aid in the diagnosis of these patients. In patients with West Nile fever, NAT may increase the yield of testing of early acute-phase samples. In areas endemic for other flaviviruses, serological cross-reactivity may complicate diagnosis and positive samples should be tested by cross-neutralization.

Prevention and control

Several equine vaccines are available. Human vaccines are in clinical trials. Mosquito repellents containing N,N-diethyl-3-methylbenzamide (DEET), picaridin, or oil of lemon eucalyptus are recommended. Community prevention is aimed at surveillance and mosquito abatement. Universal blood donor screening using

NAT has markedly reduced the risk of transfusion-related transmission in the United States of America and Canada.

Treatment

Treatment is supportive; no specific therapy is available. It is imperative that appropriate diagnostic testing including lumbar puncture, electromyography, and nerve conduction studies be obtained before initiating therapies for Guillain–Barré syndrome or other inflammatory neuropathies.

Yellow fever

Aetiology and epidemiology

Yellow fever was first described in the 17th century and was one of the great plagues of humans for over 300 years. In 1900, mosquito transmission and the viral aetiology were proven. The virus was isolated in 1927 and a vaccine developed in 1937. The virus is present in tropical America and Africa, but has not been reported in Asia (Fig. 5.14.3). Epidemics still occur, especially in West Africa. Between 1986 and 1991 a series of outbreaks in Nigeria caused an estimated 100 000 cases (although only about 5000 were officially reported), with attack rates in affected areas of 30/1000 and case fatality rates exceeding 20%. In South America, the disease affects up to 300 people annually, principally young men working in forest areas exposed to haemagogus mosquitoes breeding in tree holes (jungle yellow fever). Disease in unvaccinated travellers has become more common in North America and Europe as ecotourism has increased in recent years; at least six people have died of infection acquired in South America and Africa in recent years. In the past 5 years, yellow fever was reported from the Democratic Republic of the Congo, Côte d'Ivoire, Central African Republic, Liberia, Cameroon, Guinea, Uganda, Peru, Brazil, Argentina, and Paraguay.

Yellow fever virus has two cycles of transmission, jungle (sylvatic) yellow fever and urban yellow fever. The forest or jungle transmission cycle involves canopy-dwelling mosquitoes and monkeys. The urban cycle involves humans as the vertebrate host and *Aedes aegypti* as the principal vector. In the past 30 years, *Ae.aegypti* has reinvaded Central and South America and small outbreaks of urban yellow fever have occurred in Bolivia, Brazil, and Paraguay in recent years. Epidemics in Africa often occur in moist savannah regions, involving forest (sylvatic) or peridomestic *Aedes* mosquitoes and humans as viraemic hosts. In dry areas and urban centres, epidemic transmission occurs where water-storage practices breed domestic *Ae aegypti*. Several hundred thousand people are infected annually and outbreaks are frequent.

Clinical characteristics

Approximately 1 in 20 infections results in clinical disease with jaundice. In its classic form, disease occurs abruptly after an incubation period of 3 to 6 days. The initial phase ('period of infection') is characterized by viraemia, fever, chills, headache, photophobia, lumbosacral pain, myalgia, nausea, and prostration. On examination, the patient may have a relative bradycardia and conjunctival injection. Within several days, the patient may recover transiently ('period of remission') only to relapse ('period of intoxication') with jaundice, albuminuria, oliguria, haemorrhagic manifestations (especially 'black vomit' haematemesis), delirium, stupor, metabolic acidosis, and shock. The prognosis in such cases is poor; 20 to 50% die during the second week of illness.

Clinical laboratory tests reveal leukopenia, thrombocytopenia, hepatic dysfunction, and renal failure. The bleeding diathesis is caused by decreased synthesis of clotting factors and may be complicated by disseminated intravascular coagulation. Pathological findings include midzonal hepatic necrosis and eosinophilic degeneration of hepatocytes (Councilman bodies), possibly representing apoptosis, and acute renal tubular necrosis. Focal myocarditis, brain swelling, and petechial haemorrhages contribute to pathogenesis. There is no postnecrotic hepatic cirrhosis, and recovery is complete.

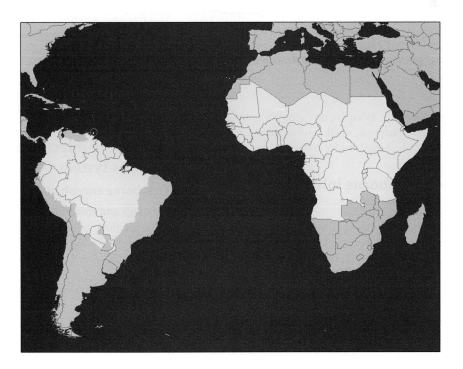

Fig. 5.14.3 Approximate geographical distribution of yellow fever virus.

Diagnosis

Exposure and travel history provide important clues to aetiology. The differential diagnosis includes viral hepatitis, leptospirosis, rickettsial infections, dengue haemorrhagic fever, Rift Valley fever, ebola, Crimean–Congo and other haemorrhagic fevers. Serological cross-reactions with other flaviviruses may complicate serology. Postmortem histopathological examination of the liver may be diagnostic, with or without immunocytochemical staining for viral antigen; severe dengue disease may cause similar liver pathology. Liver biopsy should never be performed on living patients as it may precipitate haemorrhage.

Prevention and control

WHO provides recommendations for the geographical areas where yellow fever vaccination is recommended (see Chapter 7.4). The live attenuated 17D vaccine, delivered as a single 0.5-ml subcutaneous dose, is highly effective and has minimal side effects. Immunity is probably lifelong, but the International Health Regulation published by the WHO recommends revaccination at 10-year intervals. People with documented egg allergy should not be immunized or should be skin tested with the vaccine. The vaccine must not be given to children under 6 months of age, in whom there is a risk of postvaccinal encephalitis, and it is best to delay vaccination until 9 months of age. On theoretical grounds, immunosuppressed patients (including those with clinical AIDS) should not be immunized. The immune response in HIV-infected individuals is impaired. Evidence suggests that vaccine-associated viscerotropic disease is much more common in patients with a history of thymic tumour and thymectomy is contraindicated. No evidence of clinical congenital infection has been found. Immunization during pregnancy is contraindicated, but, if inadvertently performed, recipients should be reassured and followed. The immune response in pregnancy was found to be impaired. Fatal infection following vaccination with the 17D strain has been rarely reported, although postvaccination neurological disease, such as encephalitis and Guillain–Barré syndrome in adults (incidence ranges from 0.8 and 2.3 cases per 100 000 doses of vaccine, respectively) and viscerotropic disease (incidence 0.4 to 2.3 per 100 000 doses) may be increasing. Both of these conditions are more frequent among older vaccinees. Other control measures include reducing the principal urban mosquito vector *Ae.aegypti* in tropical urban centres.

Treatment

Treatment is symptomatic. Intensive care requires prompt awareness and treatment of acidosis, shock, and metabolic imbalance. Patients with renal failure may require dialysis.

Other mosquito-borne infections

Kunjin

Genomic sequencing indicates that Kunjin virus is a variant of West Nile virus. It is found throughout most of tropical Australia and Queensland, although Kunjin-like viruses have been isolated in South-East Asia. It has a similar transmission cycle involving birds and *Culex* mosquitoes. Infection is usually asymptomatic, but occasional cases of encephalitis have been reported. Infections are generally milder than with Murray Valley encephalitis and are not life threatening. Kunjin virus infections that are nonencephalopathic usually present with fever, often with polyarthralgia. Cases

occur sporadically with only 43 reported from 1998 to 2005. Treatment is supportive; there is no vaccine.

Murray Valley encephalitis

Murray Valley encephalitis is enzootic in New Guinea, north Western Australia, and the Northern Territory, and possibly in northern Queensland. The virus has a transmission cycle involving birds and *Culex* mosquitoes and is transmitted to humans by *Culex annulirostris* mosquitoes from the end of March to early June. Only 1 in 1000 to 2000 infections results in clinical illness; of those that have neurological disease, approximately one-third are fatal and one-quarter have residual neurological deficits. Clinical illness resembles Japanese encephalitis. Children and elderly people are at the highest risk. In 1974, the largest recorded epidemic involved 58 cases and 10 deaths; since then, sporadic cases have been identified. Serological diagnosis is complicated by the presence of the closely related Kunjin virus in Australia, which also causes encephalitis. Treatment is supportive; there is no vaccine.

Rocio encephalitis

Rocio virus is a member of the Ntaya virus group and is considered a subtype of Ilheus virus; it is known only in Brazil. Epidemics from 1973 to 1980 caused 1021 cases, principally among young adult male agricultural workers and fisherman. Since then, only sporadic illness has been reported. The virus has been isolated from *Psorophora ferox* mosquitoes and *Aedes scapularis* mosquitoes may be involved in Rocio virus transmission. Wild birds are the likely amplifying hosts. Symptoms include fever, headache, anorexia, nausea, vomiting, myalgia, and malaise followed by confusion, reflex disturbance, motor impairment, and cerebellar dysfunction. The mortality rate is approximately 10%, and 20% of patients have neurological sequelae. Virus is not recoverable from blood, but postmortem diagnosis may be made by virus isolation from brain tissue. Treatment is supportive; there is no vaccine.

Zika virus infection

This flavivirus was first identified in 1947 in rhesus monkey serum in Uganda. It has been responsible for small epidemics in Uganda, Nigeria, Malaysia, Indonesia, and the Pacific. It causes a mild dengue-like illness (fever, conjunctival injection, rash, and arthralgia). A total of 120 confirmed and probable cases occurred in Yap, Micronesia, and possibly Guam, from March to May 2007. Mosquitoes (*Ae. aegypti, Ae.africanus*) are known vectors.

Tick-borne infections of the central nervous system

Tick-borne encephalitis

Aetiology and epidemiology

There are three subtypes of tick-borne encephalitis virus defined phylogenetically, European, Far Eastern, and Siberian, which differ only slightly in viral protein structure. These viruses, along with the louping ill, Powassan, Kyasanur Forest disease, and Omsk haemorrhagic fever viruses, belong to the tick-borne encephalitis antigenic complex. The disease caused by the Far Eastern subtype is also known as Russian spring/summer encephalitis and Russian epidemic encephalitis; the European subtype as also known as FSME (Frühsommer-Meningoenzephalitis), early-summer encephalitis, and Kumlinge's disease. The geographical distribution of disease is determined by that of the hard tick vectors: *Ixodes persulcatus* for the Far Eastern subtype causing human disease principally from the Baltic countries to north-eastern China and northern Japan, and *Ixodes ricinus* for the European subtype which occurs from the Urals in Russia to the Alsace region of France, Scandinavia to the north, and parts of the Mediterranean areas along the Adriatic coast to the south (Fig. 5.14.4). Several other tick species play a role as minor vectors. Switzerland reports more than 100 cases each year, while 3000 clinical cases are reported in Europe. The incidence is increasing in all countries except Austria where an aggressive vaccination policy has proved effective. The Siberian subtype is found in Siberia and the Baltic states. In Russia more than 10 000 cases of tick-borne encephalitis are reported each year.

Infections occur during the period of tick activity from April to November. In Novosibirsk, south-west Siberia, more than 20 000 tick bites are reported annually. Tick-borne encephalitis is largely a rural infection; occupational and vocational pursuits favouring tick exposure are risk factors. Human infection and outbreaks following consumption of raw milk or cheese from asymptomatic goats or, more rarely, sheep or cows have been described. Hundreds to thousands of cases occur annually, with reported attack rates up to 200/100 000 residents in Latvia, the Urals, and western Siberia. Aerosolized virus has caused laboratory infections.

Clinical characteristics

Most human infections are subclinical. The illness produced by each subtype is generally similar but that produced by the Far Eastern subtype carries a worse prognosis. The incubation period is 7 to 14 days (range 2–28 days); incubation periods of 3 to 4 days follow milk-borne exposure. The European subtype typically produces a biphasic illness. The first phase is a nonspecific, influenza-like, febrile illness lasting 2 to 7 days followed by an afebrile and relatively asymptomatic period lasting 2 to 10 days. Flushing, conjunctival haemorrhage, nausea, vomiting, dizziness, and myalgia are common findings. Approximately one-third of patients then develop higher fevers with aseptic meningitis or meningoencephalitis.

The Far Eastern subtype usually progresses without an asymptomatic phase. Signs and symptoms of meningitis, meningoencephalitis, meningoencephalomyelitis, myelitis, or meningoradiculitis include somnolence, coma, asymmetrical paresis of the cranial nerves, tremors of the extremities, nystagmus, severe pain in the extremities, and flaccid paralysis of the neck and upper extremities.

Permanent paralysis develops in 2 to 10% of patients with the European subtype and 10 to 25% with the Far Eastern subtype. Corresponding case fatality rates are 0.5 to 2.0% and 5 to 20% for the European and Far Eastern subtypes, respectively. Severity of illness with the Siberian subtype is intermediate between the European and Far Eastern subtypes, with a case fatality rate of 1 to 3%.

Laboratory findings include neutrophilia, although neutropenia, thrombocytopenia, and elevated liver enzyme levels may occur early. The cerebrospinal fluid white blood cell count is usually below 500 cells/mm^3, primarily of mononuclear cells.

Diagnosis

The differential diagnosis is similar to Japanese encephalitis; the pattern of flaccid paralysis may be confused with poliomyelitis. A history of bite by small ixodid ticks is elicited in less than one-half of patients. Specific diagnosis is made by virus isolation from blood or cerebrospinal fluid during the first week of illness, or by serological tests including IgM enzyme immunoassay and a neutralization test. Virus isolation should be conducted under biosafety level 4 conditions.

Prevention and control

Effective inactivated vaccines are available in Europe in formulations for adults and children. Two doses 4 to 6 weeks apart followed by a booster at 1 year are recommended for those walking and camping in tick-infested coniferous forests of endemic areas, especially during the tick season (May–October). Mass vaccination in Austria produced a dramatic decline in disease incidence. Vaccines appear to produce equal protection against the eastern and western strains. Rapid immunization schedules are available

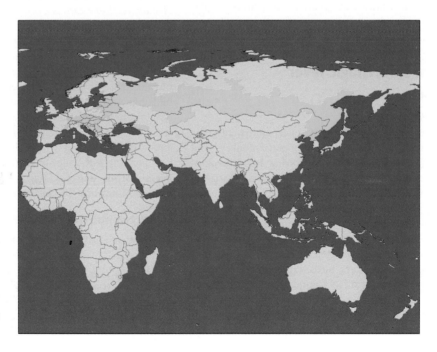

Fig. 5.14.4 Approximate geographical distribution of tick-borne encephalitis virus.

for those with impending travel to endemic areas during the tick season. Tick bites should be prevented by the use of repellents containing DEET and use of permethrin on clothing and camping gear, and attached ticks should be discovered and removed as soon as possible. Unpasteurized goats' milk products should be avoided.

Treatment

Treatment is supportive.

Louping ill

This is a disease of veterinary importance causing neurological illness in sheep and to a lesser extent in cows, horses, farmed deer, sheepdogs, and pigs. The virus, isolated in 1931, is a member of the tick-borne encephalitis complex and is transmitted by *Ix.odes ricinus*. Louping ill occurs in the hill country along the western coast of Scotland and northern England, Ireland, and Norway. Natural infections resulting in human disease have been rare, but laboratory infections are not uncommon. Naturally acquired human infections have mainly occurred in persons with occupational exposure to animals. Some of these cases were attributable to contact with sheep blood. Infection from tick bite is rare. The human disease is typically aseptic meningitis or encephalitis; no fatal infections have occurred. Avoidance of tick bites in enzootic areas is recommended. The licensed tick-borne encephalitis vaccine may be protective.

Powassan encephalitis

The virus was first isolated from the brain of a patient who died in Powassan, Ontario in 1958. Since then, more than 30 human cases have been recognized in eastern Canada and the eastern United States of America, primarily in children, with a case fatality rate of 10% and a high incidence of residual neurological dysfunction. Serological surveys indicate an antibody prevalence of 1 to 4%. The distribution of the virus in North America is considerably wider than indicated by human cases, and the diagnosis should be suspected in any case of summer–autumn encephalitis. The virus is transmitted between *Ix. cookei* (Ix. ricinus complex) ticks and rodents. Cases have also occurred in Russia where the primary vector is *Ix. persulcatus*. The clinical features are those of viral encephalitis, with localizing neurological signs and convulsions. There is no specific treatment or vaccine.

Tick-borne haemorrhagic fever

Kyasanur Forest disease

Aetiology and epidemiology

This virus is a member of the tick-borne encephalitis antigenic complex. The virus has been isolated from humans, monkeys, and ticks since it was first recognized in 1957 during an outbreak of haemorrhagic fever affecting wild monkeys in Karnataka (then Mysore) State, India. Several hundred cases are reported annually, principally among people working in the forest in Karnataka State. In 1983, 1555 cases, including 150 deaths, occurred. The peak seasonal incidence is from January/February to May. The virus is transmitted by *Haemaphysalis spinigera* ticks in a life cycle that involves small mammals, monkeys, birds, cattle, and large mammals at various stages. Humans are incidental hosts and are primarily infected by nymphal ticks. Alkhurma (Al Khumra) virus, a subtype of Kyasanur Forest virus, causes haemorrhagic fever in Saudi Arabia (see below).

Clinical characteristics

After an incubation period of 3 to 8 days, fever starts abruptly with chills, headache, myalgia, abdominal pain, nausea, vomiting, and diarrhoea. Physical signs include bradycardia, lymphadenopathy, and haemorrhagic manifestations. Hypotension is frequently noted during the end of the acute stage. Fatal cases develop shock and pulmonary oedema. A biphasic illness is not uncommon, with resolution of the first phase in 5 to 12 days and return of the fever and signs of meningoencephalitis after an interval of 1 to 3 weeks. Localizing neurological signs are infrequent, and residual defects are rare; convalescence is prolonged. Laboratory abnormalities include leukopenia, thrombocytopenia, and elevated serum transaminases during the acute phase. Fatality rates are 2 to 10%.

Diagnosis

Diagnosis is by virus isolation from blood collected during the first week after onset or by serological tests. Virus isolation should be conducted under biosafety level 4 conditions.

Prevention and control

Tick bites should be avoided in endemic areas. A formalin-inactivated vaccine is available in India.

Treatment

Treatment is supportive; specific therapy is not available.

Alkhurma (Al Khumra) haemorrhagic fever

In 1995, a subtype of Kyasanur Forest disease virus was isolated during an epidemic of dengue from patients from Al-Khumra, south of Jeddah, Saudi Arabia, with clinical symptoms ranging from febrile illness with headache, malaise, myalgia, nausea, and vomiting to fatal haemorrhagic disease. Most of the literature uses the name Alkhurma virus. From 2001 to 2003, 20 cases were identified by national surveillance in Saudi Arabia. Human infections are associated with handling meat or drinking unpasteurized camels' milk. The virus seems to be associated with sheep, goats, and camels, which do not manifest disease themselves, and to be transmitted by ticks. Its natural reservoir is unknown, but the camel tick *Hyalomma dromedarii* is a prime suspect. Fever, headache, malaise, and myalgia are common. About one-half of patients exhibit haemorrhagic manifestations ranging from mild bleeding (epistaxis) to haemorrhagic shock and disseminated intravascular coagulation with thrombocytopenia. Most have elevated serum concentrations of liver transaminases, lactate dehydrogenase, creatine kinase, and bilirubin, and some develop renal failure. About 35% of patients develop encephalitis and the case fatality rate is 25%. Important differential diagnoses include Crimean–Congo haemorrhagic fever and Rift Valley fever which share its epidemiological features. Compared to Rift Valley fever, there is no visual loss, scotomas, or haemolysis in Alkhurma haemorrhagic fever, but haemorrhage is more common and the case fatality rate is higher.

Omsk haemorrhagic fever

This disease was first recognized in 1945 in western Siberia. Cases were frequent between 1945 and 1949, with morbidity rates of 500 to 1400/100 000, but subsequently have been rare, mainly occurring among residents of rural areas working in the fields. Human infections are acquired by *Dermacentor* tick bite or contact with infected muskrats. After an incubation period typically of 3 to 7 days, the disease begins with the abrupt onset of fever, headache, myalgia, facial flushing, conjunctival suffusion, minor haemorrhagic manifestations, and leukopenia. Recovery occurs in the second week, and the case fatality rate is low (0.5–3%). The differential diagnosis includes tularaemia, rickettsial infection, and leptospirosis. Specific diagnosis is made by virus isolation from blood during the acute phase or by serological tests. Only a few laboratories outside Russia with biocontainment level 4 facilities are capable of providing laboratory assistance. Tick-borne encephalitis vaccines may cross-protect against Omsk haemorrhagic fever.

Further reading

Gould EA, *et al.* (2006). Potential arbovirus emergence and implications for the United Kingdom. *Emerg Infect Dis*, **12**, 549–54.

Gritsun TS, Lashkevich VA, Gould EA (2003). Tick-borne encephalitis. *Antiviral Res*, **57**, 129–46.

Gubler DJ, Kuno G, Markoff L (2007). Flaviviruses. In: Knipe DM, Howley PM (eds) *Fields virology*, 5th edition. Lippincott Williams & Wilkins, Philadelphia.

Gubler DJ (2007). The continuing spread of West Nile virus in the western hemisphere. *Clin Infect Dis*, **45**, 1039–46.

Günther G, Haglund M (2005). Tick-borne encephalopathies. Epidemiology, diagnosis, treatment and prevention. *CNS Drugs*, **19**, 1009–32.

Halstead SB, Thomas SJ (2011). New Japanese encephalitis vaccines: alternatives to production in mouse brain. *Expert Rev Vaccines*, **10**, 355–64.

Hayes EB, Gubler DJ (2006). West Nile virus: epidemiology and clinical features of an emerging epidemic in the United States. *Annu Rev Med*, **57**, 181–94.

Hayes EB, *et al.* (2005). Virology, pathology, and clinical manifestations of West Nile virus disease. *Emerg Infect Dis*, **11**, 1174–9.

Kilpatrick AM (2011). Globalization, land use and the invasion of West Nile virus. *Science*, **334**, 323–7.

Mackenzie JS, Gubler DJ, Petersen LR (2004). Emerging flaviviruses: the spread and resurgence of Japanese encephalitis, West Nile and dengue viruses. *Nat Med Suppl*, **10**, S98–109.

Madani TA (2005). Alkhumra (Alkhurma) virus infection, a new viral hemorrhagic fever in Saudi Arabia. *J Infect*, **51**, 91–7.

Marfin AA, *et al.* (2005). Yellow fever and Japanese encephalitis vaccines: indications and complications. *Infect Dis Clin North Am*, **19**, 151–68.

Morales MA, *et al.* (2006). West Nile virus isolation from equines in Argentina, 2006. *Emerg Infect Dis*, **12**, 1559-61.

Pattnaik P (2006). Kyasanur forest disease: an epidemiological view in India. *Rev Med Microbiol*, **16**, 151–65.

Solomon T (2003). Recent advances in Japanese encephalitis. *J Neurovirol*, **9**, 274–83.

5.15 **Dengue**

Bridget Wills and Jeremy Farrar

Essentials

Dengue is caused by a flavivirus and is the most important mosquito-borne viral infection of humans. Some 40 million symptomatic infections are estimated to occur annually. The disease is hyper-endemic in many large Asian cities, and is also a significant problem in the Pacific region and in the Americas. The primary mosquito vector is *Aedes aegypti*. Infection can be caused by any one of four closely related but serologically distinct dengue viral serotypes. Following infection with a single serotype there is life-long immunity to that serotype but the possibility of more severe disease during a subsequent infection with a different serotype.

Clinical features and diagnosis—symptomatic disease ranges from a nonspecific febrile illness through to a syndrome characterized by plasma leakage that may, if severe, result in the development of potentially fatal dengue shock syndrome. Thrombocytopenia and deranged haemostasis also occur, but clinically significant bleeding is unusual except it patients with profound shock. Severe hepatic and neurological complications are also seen in some patients. Diagnosis depends on viral isolation, detection of viral antigen or viral RNA, or serological testing.

Management and prevention—treatment is supportive, with particular emphasis on careful fluid management. Prompt volume resuscitation is essential for patients with shock, with regular monitoring of the pulse rate, blood pressure, and haematocrit to minimize the risk of fluid overload. No vaccine is available as yet but a number of candidates are entering clinical trials. Currently prevention relies on elimination of potential vector breeding sites, biological and chemical vector control strategies, and avoidance of mosquito bites.

Introduction and aetiology

Dengue is the most important mosquito-borne viral infection of humans. 'Dengue' is a West Indian Spanish word derived from Ki Swahili 'ka dinga pepo' ('a kind of cramping plague') that was brought from Africa to the Caribbean. In the British West Indies it was called 'dandy fever' because of the stiff posture of its victims, and in Cuba dengue was later termed 'quebranta huesos' or 'break-bone fever' because of the severe myalgias and arthralgias. Infection can be caused by any one of the four closely related but serologically distinct dengue viral serotypes (DEN-1, -2, -3, and -4) that together constitute one subgroup of the genus *Flavivirus*, family Flaviviridae. Since there is only transient cross-protective immunity between the four serotypes, people living in a dengue-endemic area can be infected up to four times during their lifetime.

Epidemiology

Humans are infected with dengue viruses by the bite of a mosquito. *Aedes aegypti*, the principal vector, is a highly domesticated tropical mosquito that lays its eggs in artificial water containers commonly found in and around homes. The adult mosquitoes rest indoors and prefer to feed on humans during daylight hours, with peak biting activity in the early morning and late afternoon. The adult female mosquitoes are nervous feeders and, if their feeding is interrupted, will return to the same person or different persons to continue feeding. Thus, during a single blood meal several persons may become infected, making *Ae aegypti* a highly efficient epidemic vector. The transmission cycle of most importance is *Ae aegypti*–human–*Ae aegypti* in large urban centres of the tropics.

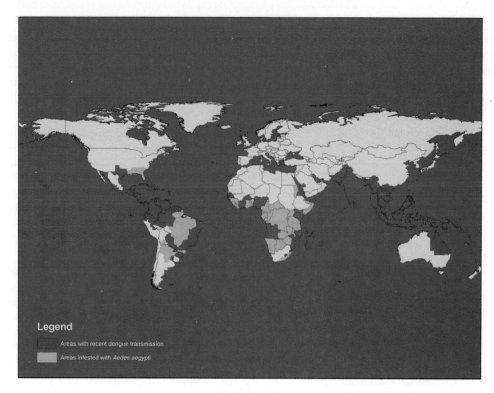

Fig. 5.15.1 Global distribution of dengue.

Multiple virus serotypes often cocirculate within the same city causing periodic epidemics. Epidemics of febrile illness attributed to dengue have been reported at intervals over the last 200 years across Asia, Africa, and North America, likely reflecting progressive expansion in the global distribution of the *Aedes* mosquito vectors. However, from the 1950s onwards a new clinical syndrome, characterized by vascular leakage and bleeding and given the name dengue haemorrhagic fever (DHF), began to emerge in south-east Asia. The first epidemic of DHF in the Americas appeared in 1981 in Cuba, associated with the arrival of a new Asian strain of DEN-2 virus of different genotype from the American strain.

Dengue is now hyperendemic in most Asian cities, with epidemics occurring every 3 to 5 years superimposed on background endemic transmission. Progressive geographical expansion of the disease has also become apparent, attributable to the effects on mosquito ecology of urbanization and climate change. Dengue is now established as a significant problem in the Pacific Region and in the Americas, and outbreaks have also been reported from Africa, the Arabian Peninsula, and even the warmer parts of Europe. More than 3 billion people now live in areas of risk and approximately 40 million symptomatic infections are estimated to occur each year, with some 2 million severe enough to require hospitalization. In parallel with the changing epidemiology and transmission dynamics it is also apparent that different clinical presentations are emerging. Thus in regions with relatively low endemicity, clinical disease tends to be reported among adults rather than children, and the frequency and pattern of complications seen reflects age-related differences in intrinsic physiology as well as the greater likelihood of older patients having underlying comorbidities. Although low mortality rates (0.1–0.2% for severe disease) are usual in experienced hands, much higher rates are still reported from some regions, and among infants and elderly people.

Pathogenesis

All four serotypes can cause disease. Infection with one serotype elicits immunity to that serotype but does not provide long-term cross-protective immunity to the remaining serotypes. Severe disease occurs predominantly in patients experiencing a second or subsequent infection with a dengue serotype different from their first infection, or else in infants with transmitted maternal antibody experiencing their first infection. The generally accepted antibody-dependent enhancement (ADE) hypothesis suggests that residual heterotypic non-neutralizing antibodies bind to the new virus enhancing its infectivity by increasing the efficiency of binding and uptake of virus–antibody complexes through Fc receptors on blood monocyte or tissue macrophage cells, thus amplifying viral replication. The resulting increase in viral load drives an immunopathogenic cascade that alters microvascular function in some way, resulting in capillary leakage and coagulopathy. Rapid mobilization of serotype cross-reactive memory T cells has been suggested as an alternative mechanism to trigger the inflammatory cascade. Other factors considered to influence disease severity include differences in viral virulence, molecular mimicry, and immune complex and/or complement-mediated dysregulation, as well as age and genetic predisposition. However, the pathogenesis of the vascular leakage and coagulopathy associated with severe infections remains poorly understood and, so far, no mechanism has been identified that links the established immunological derangements with a definitive effect on microvascular structure or function.

Clinical manifestations

Dengue virus infection in humans causes a wide variety of illnesses ranging from inapparent infection to mild febrile illness to severe and fatal disease. Most infections are asymptomatic. In the past, symptomatic disease was conventionally separated into two major clinical syndromes, dengue fever (DF) and dengue haemorrhagic fever (DHF), with case definitions and management guidelines for these entities published by the World Health Organization (WHO). The pathognomonic feature of DHF is increased vascular permeability, which may be severe enough to result in hypovolaemic shock; in addition, to qualify for a diagnosis of DHF, a patient must have some evidence of bleeding and a platelet count below 100 x 10^9/litre. Due to practical difficulties in using the old WHO scheme a revised classification system has recently been developed, based on prospective data collected from over 2000 children and adults with dengue from endemic areas around the world, and this has now been adopted in the latest WHO guidelines for dengue published in 2009. The new scheme classifies the disease into dengue and severe dengue, in line with several other complex diseases such as malaria and pneumonia. It is hoped that in the future this will prove to be a simpler system that will be useful for triage, aid clinical management, and improve the quality of surveillance and epidemiological data.

Symptomatic dengue is primarily a disease of older children and adults. After an incubation period of c.4 to 7 days symptoms start suddenly and typically follow three phases—an initial febrile phase, a critical phase around the time of defervescence, and a spontaneous recovery phase.

Febrile phase

There is sudden onset of high fever often accompanied by facial flushing, headache, retro-orbital pain, lumbosacral pain, severe malaise, myalgias, bone pain, anorexia, altered sense of taste, mild sore throat, nausea, and vomiting. Younger children experience high fever, but are generally much less symptomatic. Some patients may have a transient rash or skin mottling in early illness (Fig. 5.15.2a). Other findings associated with infection may include generalized lymphadenopathy, mild haemorrhagic manifestations (e.g. petechiae or easy bruising, Fig. 5.15.3a,b), and palpable hepatomegaly but rarely splenomegaly. Haematuria is uncommon and jaundice is rare. Clinical laboratory findings during the first week include thrombocytopenia and leukopenia, often with moderate elevation of hepatic transaminases.

Critical phase

Most patients recover around the time of defervescence, usually between days 3–7 of illness, but in a small proportion an increase in capillary permeability becomes apparent at this time, marking the onset of the critical phase for complications. A capillary leak syndrome manifests with increasing haemoconcentration, hypoproteinaemia, pleural effusions and ascites, and, if severe, may compromise the circulating plasma volume so that the patient develops the potentially life-threatening dengue shock syndrome (DSS) (Fig. 5.15.4a,b). When the pulse pressure narrows to less than 20 mmHg with a rapid weak pulse and impaired peripheral perfusion, or if hypotension develops, the patient is defined as having DSS. If fluid resuscitation is not instituted promptly the ongoing depletion of plasma becomes critical, the systolic pressure falls rapidly, and irreversible shock and death may follow. However, with judicious fluid management the majority of patients make a full recovery. Warning signs that the patient may be at risk for severe disease include severe vomiting, intense abdominal pain, and increasing tender hepatomegaly.

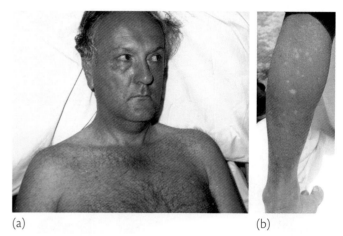

(a)   (b)

Fig. 5.15.2 (a) Early macular rash on the shoulders and conjunctival injection in a European traveller with primary dengue.
(Copyright D A Warrell.)
(b) Convalescent rash in a Vietnamese adult with dengue.
(Copyright OUCRU-VN.)

Haemorrhagic manifestations are common during this period but often limited to the presence of skin petechiae or bruising, or a positive tourniquet test. Mucosal bleeding (e.g. epistaxis, gastrointestinal bleeding, haematuria, menorrhagia) may occur, but is rarely clinically significant in children except in association with profound or prolonged shock. However, adults tend to experience more severe bleeding problems than children (Fig. 5.15.5a,b); gastrointestinal bleeding and menorrhagia may be significant even in patients with little evidence of vascular leakage. Moderate to severe thrombocytopenia is usual, with nadirs below 20×10^9 /litre often observed during the critical period followed by rapid improvement during the recovery phase. An increase in the activated partial thromboplastin time and a reduction in fibrinogen levels are also frequently noted. However, these findings are not indicative of classic disseminated intravascular coagulation and the true nature of the coagulopathy remains unknown. Other laboratory investigations show similar but usually more profound abnormalities to those seen in uncomplicated cases.

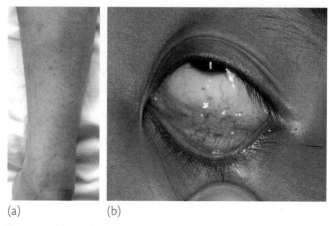

(a)   (b)

Fig. 5.15.3 (a) Petechial rash on the leg of a Vietnamese child with dengue.
(Copyright Dinh The Trung.)
(b) Conjunctival petechiae in a Vietnamese adult with dengue.
(Copyright D A Warrell.)

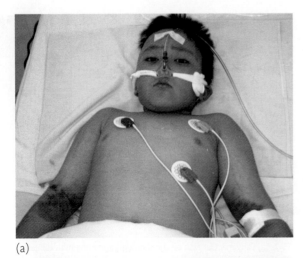

(a)

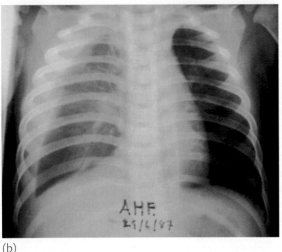

(b)

Fig. 5.15.4 (a) Vietnamese child with severe DSS, pleural effusions, ascites, oedema, and bruising at venepuncture sites. He required crystalloid and colloid infusions, inotropic support, and nasal continuous positive airway pressure (CPAP) but made a good recovery.
(Copyright B A Wills.)
(b) Pleural effusion in a 14-month-old Thai child with DHF and DSS.
(Courtesy of the late Professor Sornchai Looareesuwan.)

Recovery phase

The increase in permeability is transient and reverts to normal after approximately 24–48 h. Fluid is reabsorbed quite rapidly, often with an obvious diuresis, and the patient improves. A second rash, varying in form from scarlatiniform to maculopapular, may appear around day 6 to 7 of illness, typically on the extremities although sometimes involving the trunk and face (Fig. 5.15.2b). The rash blanches on pressure, may be accompanied by intense pruritus, and often resolves with desquamation.

Other syndromes

Unusual manifestations, including acute liver failure and encephalopathy/encephalitis, may be noted, even in the absence of severe plasma leakage or shock. Myocarditis has also been reported in a few cases.

Severe dengue

Under the new scheme, patients who recover without complications are classified as having dengue, while those who experience

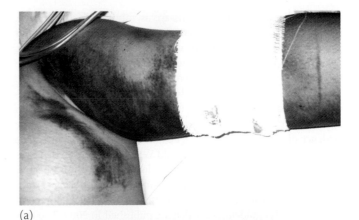

(a)

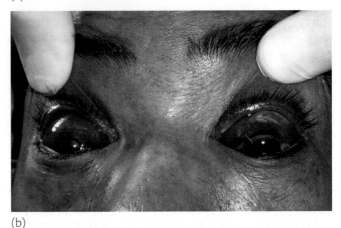

(b)

Fig. 5.15.5 (a) Major bleeding at a venepuncture site in a Vietnamese teenager with severe DSS. (b) Extensive subconjunctival haemorrhages and severe epistaxis requiring nasal packing in a Vietnamese adult with dengue.
(Copyright Dinh The Trung.)

any one of the following problems are classified as having severe dengue: plasma leakage resulting in shock and/or fluid accumulation sufficient to cause respiratory distress; severe bleeding; severe organ impairment, e.g. liver failure, myocarditis etc. However, most deaths from dengue occur in patients with profound shock, particularly if the situation is complicated by fluid overload.

Differential diagnosis

The differential diagnosis during the acute phase of illness includes influenza, Epstein–Barr virus, measles, rubella, typhoid, leptospirosis, rickettsial infection, malaria, other arboviral infections with rash, other viral haemorrhagic fevers, and meningococcaemia.

Laboratory diagnosis

During the early febrile stage (up to about day 5 of illness) laboratory confirmation of dengue infection relies on viral isolation or detection of viral antigen or viral RNA by reverse transcription–polymerase chain reaction (RT-PCR) in blood. After this time IgM antibody capture enzyme-linked immunosorbent assay (MAC-ELISA) is the most widely used serological test for dengue diagnosis; seroconversion or a rising titre of dengue-specific IgM or IgG in paired samples indicates acute infection. Patients with secondary infection (either dengue or another flavivirus infection) often develop high levels of IgG antibodies in the acute phase and the IgM response may be less intense. Serological diagnosis is also complicated by the existence of flavivirus cross-reactivity, making it necessary to perform tests for other locally prevalent flaviviruses in parallel with dengue serology. Because antidengue antibodies persist for several months, diagnosis based on a single positive MAC-ELISA result should be considered provisional. Bedside rapid serological tests are now available but, in common with conventional serological tests, may not become positive until the end of the first week of illness. ELISA tests to detect circulating dengue nonstructural protein 1 (NS1) during the first few days of fever may be a promising tool for early diagnosis.

Management

Good supportive care, with a particular focus on careful fluid management, is critical for a favourable outcome. For patients with mild disease, oral rehydration is usually sufficient. Fever should be controlled with tepid sponging and paracetamol. Aspirin and non-steroidal anti-inflammatory drugs are contraindicated.

Persistent vomiting, severe abdominal pain, mucosal bleeding or severe skin bleeding, a rapidly rising haematocrit, or a marked drop in the platelet count indicate the need for close observation and frequent monitoring of vital signs and haematocrit. Judicious parenteral fluid therapy is indicated for those with a rapidly rising haematocrit. For patients with established DSS, prompt but careful restoration of circulating plasma volume is crucial, followed by maintenance fluids to support the circulation at a level just sufficient to maintain critical organ perfusion until vascular permeability reverts to normal. However, fluid overload with respiratory compromise is a common complication and one of the major contributors to mortality. Thus the volume of parenteral fluid given must be kept to the minimum required to maintain cardiovascular stability and adequate urine output during the phase of active leakage, and as soon as reabsorption begins, usually about 1 to 2 days later, intravenous fluids should be stopped. Isotonic crystalloid solutions should be used initially. Colloid solutions should be reserved for patients presenting with severe DSS and those who fail to improve with crystalloid therapy. Correction of metabolic acidosis, electrolyte imbalance, and hypoglycaemia are also essential. Platelet concentrates are not indicated, even for profound thrombocytopenia unless there is overt bleeding, as the thrombocytopenia improves rapidly during the recovery phase without intervention. However, in the event of significant bleeding transfusion of fresh blood, platelets, and other blood products may be indicated, but should be undertaken with great care because of the risk of fluid overload. No specific drugs are available as yet for the treatment of dengue. Current research is focused on two main therapeutic approaches: first, reduction in viraemia through use of antiviral drugs, and second, immune modulation to suppress the immunopathogenic cascade that is considered to be ultimately responsible for the severe manifestations. Several viral inhibitors are in preclinical trials, and chloroquine, a cheap, safe drug that is known to have modest antiviral effects *in vitro*, was recently assessed in a formal randomized blinded trial in adults with confirmed dengue. However, no effect was seen on the duration of viraemia or NS1 antigenaemia, and use of chloroquine was associated with a higher frequency of adverse events compared to placebo although these were generally mild. Corticosteroid therapy showed no convincing benefit on mortality from shock in

several small clinical trials during the 1980s, but whether deployment before the development of shock influences outcome remains unknown. A recent safety study of early prednisolone use indicated that immune modulation during the viraemic phase did not interfere with viral clearance mechanisms. However, although the study was not powered to assess efficacy, there was no reduction in the incidence of shock or other recognized complications of dengue, suggesting that any protective effect of early steroid use is small.

Outcome

The majority of patients with dengue make a full recovery. Those with DSS and/or significant bleeding usually do well provided they receive appropriate supportive care from experienced health care personnel during the critical phase of the illness. Adults may go on to experience several weeks of extreme tiredness, weakness, skin desquamation, pruritus, and depression during convalescence after infection, but there are no permanent sequelae. In general, children recover more rapidly and do not experience such problems.

Vaccines

The lead dengue vaccine candidate, ChimeriVax-Dengue, is a tetravalent formulation of attenuated yellow fever 17D vaccine strains expressing dengue envelope proteins. Multicentre clinical trials to establish the efficacy of this vaccine are ongoing, but long-term follow-up of vaccinees will be essential to determine if waning vaccine-elicited immunity predisposes recipients to more severe outcomes during any subsequent natural infection. Other candidates in clinical development include live attenuated virus vaccines and recombinant subunit vaccines.

Prevention

Although major efforts are being directed towards development of safe and effective dengue vaccines, it seems unlikely that a suitable candidate will be available for large-scale deployment for some years. Until then prevention of epidemics will continue to rely on elimination of potential vector breeding sites together with biological and chemical vector control strategies. Community control of *Ae aegypti* by eradication of mosquito larvae from stagnant water sources is recommended but has been difficult to achieve in contemporary tropical urban settings. Insecticide-treated bednets have limited use since *Ae aegypti* mosquitoes are primarily daytime feeders. Avoidance of mosquito bites in areas infested with *Ae aegypti* by using repellents containing N,N-diethyl-3-methylbenzamide (DEET) or picaridin and protective clothing are the most effective preventive measures for the traveller.

Further reading

Deen JL, et al. (2006). The WHO dengue classification and case definitions: time for a reassessment. *Lancet*, **368**, 170–3.

Durbin AP, Whitehead SS (2010). Dengue vaccine candidates in development. *Curr Top Microbiol Immunol*, **338**, 129–43.

Halstead SB (1965). Dengue and hemorrhagic fevers of Southeast Asia. *Yale J Biol Med*, **37**, 434–54.

Halstead SB, Nimmannitya S, Cohen SN (1970). Observations related to pathogenesis of dengue hemorrhagic fever. IV. Relation of disease severity to antibody response and virus recovered. *Yale J Biol Med*, **42**, 311–28.

Kay B, Vu SN (2005). New strategy against *Aedes aegypti* in Vietnam. *Lancet*, **365**, 613–7.

Mackenzie JS, Gubler DJ, Petersen LR (2004). Emerging flaviviruses: the spread and resurgence of Japanese encephalitis, West Nile and dengue viruses. *Nat Med*, **10** Suppl, S98–109.

Mongkolsapaya J, *et al.* (2003). Original antigenic sin and apoptosis in the pathogenesis of dengue hemorrhagic fever. *Nat Med*, **9**, 921–7.

Screaton G, Mongkolsapaya J (2006). T cell responses and dengue haemorrhagic fever. *Novartis Found Symp*, **277**, 164–71.

Tricou V, *et al.* (2010). A randomized controlled trial of chloroquine for the treatment of dengue in Vietnamese adults. *PLoS Negl Trop Dis*, **10**, e785.

WHO (1997). *Dengue haemorrhagic fever: diagnosis, treatment, prevention and control.* World Health Organization, Geneva.

WHO (2009). *Dengue: Guidelines for diagnosis, treatment, prevention and control.* World Health Organization, Geneva.

Wilder-Smith A, Schwartz E (2005). Dengue in travelers. *N Engl J Med*, **353**, 924–32.

Wills BA, *et al.* (2005). Comparison of three fluid solutions for resuscitation in dengue shock syndrome. *N Engl J Med*, **353**, 877–89.

5.16 Bunyaviridae

J.W. LeDuc and Summerpal S. Kahlon

Essentials

Viruses of the family Bunyaviridae contain a 3-segmented, single-stranded, negative-sense RNA genome. They are divided into five genera, of which four are known to include human pathogens—*Orthobunyavirus*, *Phlebovirus*, *Hantavirus*, and *Nairovirus*. These viruses are found throughout the world and are transmitted between vertebrate hosts and to humans through the bite of infected arthropod vectors (mosquitoes, ticks, others), or from infectious excreta of rodents and other small mammals, and rarely person to person. Many are transmitted from infected arthropod vector females to the next generation by transovarial transmission, thereby surviving adverse environmental conditions and leading to marked seasonal distribution of disease. There are few vaccines available to protect against infection. Prevention is by avoidance of exposure to potentially infected arthropod and small-mammal vectors.

Clinical features

Bunyaviridae cause a wide range of clinical illnesses, ranging from self-limited febrile disease to severe, life-threatening haemorrhagic fever, acute respiratory distress, or encephalitis. The most important human diseases include those caused by:

La Crosse virus—the commonest cause of 'California encephalitis', most cases of which are relatively mild and with good prognosis; treatment is supportive.

Oropouche fever—causes epidemics of febrile illness, sometimes with meningitis, throughout the Amazon basin; prognosis is good; treatment is supportive.

Haemorrhagic fever with renal syndrome—caused by four distinct viruses (Hantaan, Dobrava, Puumala, Seoul); Hantaan and Dobrava cause the most severe disease, characterized sequentially by (1) febrile phase with features including headache, myalgias,

petechiae and conjunctival haemorrhage, (2) hypotensive phase with shock, (3) oliguric phase, when one-third of cases have severe haemorrhage, (4) diuretic phase, (5) convalescent phase, which may be prolonged; ribavirin is effective if started early in disease. Inactivated vaccines against Hantaviruses are available for use in Asia.

Hantavirus pulmonary syndrome – most commonly reported from the western United States, Canada, Central and South America; symptoms are primarily those of acute unexplained adult respiratory distress syndrome; treatment is supportive; mortality is 20-40%.

Other diseases caused by Bunyaviridae—these include sandfly fever, Rift Valley fever, newly discovered severe fever with thrombocytopenia syndrome (China), and Crimean-Congo haemorrhagic fever. Some viruses of the family, e.g. Rift Valley fever virus and Nairobi sheep disease virus, are important pathogens of domestic animals.

Viral taxonomy and vectors

The family Bunyaviridae currently contains around 300 viruses, and is divided into five genera (Table 5.16.1). The family name, and that of the genus *Orthobunyavirus*, is derived from the type species Bunyamwera virus, which was isolated in Uganda from *Aedes* mosquitoes. The other genera are *Hantavirus* named after Hantaan virus (the cause of Korean haemorrhagic fever), *Nairovirus* after Nairobi sheep disease virus, *Phlebovirus* after phlebotomus or sandfly fever virus, and *Tospovirus* after tomato spotted wilt virus. All members of the family share structural, biochemical, and genetic properties, such as a spherical enveloped virion 80 to 120 nm in diameter (Fig. 5.16.1) and a genome of single-stranded negative-sense RNA divided into three segments (L, M, S). Members of different genera vary substantially in their biological and biochemical properties and in their mechanisms of replication. Orthobunyaviruses, nairoviruses, and phleboviruses, which together make up most of the family, are all arthropod-borne animal viruses (arboviruses). These circulate in a wide variety of different vertebrate hosts and are transmitted between vertebrates, including humans, by the bites of blood-sucking arthropods, principally mosquitoes for orthobunyaviruses, sandflies for phleboviruses, and ticks for nairoviruses. Hantaviruses are zoonotic agents infecting rodents and other small mammals. They may spread to humans who are in close contact with infected excreta. Tospoviruses are arthropod-transmitted plant viruses of no known medical importance.

Viruses within the larger genera are further subdivided into serogroups; orthobunyaviruses have at least 18 serogroups and nairoviruses have 7 (Table 5.16.1). Of over 60 Bunyaviridae that are known to infect humans, the type species and those causing major human diseases are shown in bold type in Table 5.16.1 and are described in more detail. Table 5.16.2 lists the distribution of the remaining viruses that cause minor human infections with their principal arthropod vectors. The habitats of the different viruses and their vectors range from arctic to tropical. The enzootic cycles of arboviruses are poorly understood. Most viruses undergo alternate cycles of replication in vertebrate and invertebrate hosts, but transovarial and trans-stadial transmission within some mosquitoes, ticks, and phlebotomine flies, and venereal transmission from vertically infected male mosquitoes to uninfected females is also known to occur. Most arboviruses have a narrow host range,

Table 5.16.1 The family *Bunyaviridae*: its genera, serogroups, vectors, and viruses infecting humans

Genus	Serogroup	Vector	Viruses infecting humans
Orthobunyavirus (over 150)	Anopheles A (12)	Mosquito	Tacaiuma
	Anopheles B (2)	Mosquito	
	Bakau (5)	Mosquito	
	Bunyamwera (33)	Mosquito	**Bunyamwera**, Calovo, **Garissa**, Germiston, Ilesha, Maguari, Shokwe, Tensaw, Wyeomyia
	Bwamba (2)	Mosquito	**Bwamba**, Pongola
	C group (14)	Mosquito	Apeu, Caraparu, Itaqui, Madrid, Marituba, Murutucu, Nepuyo, Oriboca, Ossa, Restan
	California (14)	Mosquito	**California encephalitis**, Guaroa, **Inkoo, Jamestown Canyon, Keystone La Crosse,** snowshoe hare, **Tahyna,** trivittatus
	Capim (10)	Mosquito	
	Gamboa (8)	Mosquito	
	Guama (12)	Mosquito	Catu, Guama
	Koongol (2)	Mosquito	
	Minatitlan (2)	Mosquito	
	Nyando (2)	Mosquito	Nyando
	Olifantsvlei (5)	Mosquito	
	Patois (7)	Mosquito	
	Simbu (24)	Mosquito	**Oropouche**, Shuni
	Tete (5)	Mosquito	
	Turlock (5)	Mosquito	
	Unassigned (3)	Mosquito	
Hantavirus (8)	Hantaan (39)	None	Amur, **Andes**, Araraquara, Bayou, Bermejo, Black Creek Canal, **Choclo, Dobrava, Hantaan,** Juquitiba, **Laguna Negra,** New York, **Lechiguanas,** Maciel, Monongahela, Oran, Prospect Hill, **Puumala,** Saaremaa, **Seoul, Sin Nombre**
Nairovirus (32)	Crimean–Congo (3)	Tick	**Crimean–Congo haemorrhagic fever**, Hazara
	Dera Ghazi Khan (6)	Tick	
	Hughes (10)	Tick	Soldado
	Nairobi sheep disease (3)	Tick	Dugbe, Ganjam, Nairobi sheep disease
	Qalyub (3)	Tick	
	Sakhalin (7)	Tick	Avalon
	Thiafora (2)	Tick	
Phlebovirus (57)	Phlebotomus (44)	Sandfly[a]	Alenquer, Candiru, **Chagres,** Corfou, **Punta Toro, Rift Valley fever**[a]**, Naples,** sandfly fever, **severe fever with thrombocytopenia syndrome**[a]**, Sicilian, Toscana**
	Uukuniemi (13)	Tick	Uukuniemi, Zaliv-Terpeniya
Tospovirus (1)		Thrips	
Unassigned (53)		Mosquito	Bangui, Kasokero, Tataguine
		Tick	Bhanja, Issyk-kul Keterah, Tamdy, Wanowrie

Numbers in parentheses indicate the approximate number of viruses in the genus or serogroup.
Bold type indicates the type species and viruses causing major disease in humans.
[a] Mosquito vector for Rift Valley fever virus; tick suspected for severe fever with thrombocytopenia virus.

occur within a limited area, and are transmitted by specific vectors to a limited number of vertebrate hosts, but some viruses infect a wider host range, are transmitted by more than one type of vector, and may occur in more than a single continent. Tick transmission predominates in Asia, but is unknown in South or Central America, and although some Bunyaviridae have been isolated in Australia, none is known to infect humans in that continent. Viruses of this family are among the most common apparently emerging diseases. Following viral entry, whether through the skin after the bite of an infected arthropod or by another route, there is replication in draining lymph nodes, which may be enlarged, and then viraemia. Symptoms develop when virus is deposited and replicates in other sites. The viruses are killed by bleach, phenolic disinfectants and detergents, autoclaving, boiling, and γ-irradiation. Enzymes

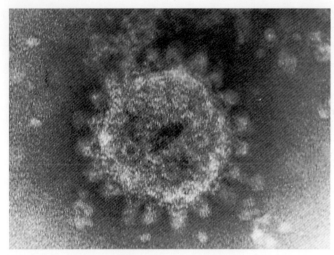

Fig. 5.16.1 Electron micrograph of Crimean–Congo haemorrhagic fever virus. Magnification × 400 000.
(Courtesy of Dr D S Ellis.)

such as nucleases also inactivate these viruses. Biosafety level 3 is recommended for handling most human pathogens with the ability to spread by aerosol (e.g. hantaviruses and Oropouche virus), but level 4 is required for Crimean–Congo haemorrhagic fever virus. Added precautions are necessary when handling hantavirus-infected animals and virus concentrates.

Genus *Orthobunyavirus*

Studies with Bunyamwera and similar viruses show reassortment within the three-segmented genome when two closely related viruses infect the same cell, either in nature or in the laboratory. Such studies have been used to analyse the molecular basis of virulence for vertebrate and invertebrate hosts. Two orthobunyaviruses, Akabane

and Aino viruses in the Simbu serogroup, produce congenital deformities in sheep, goats, and cattle in Japan, Australia, Africa, and the Middle East. However, there is no evidence that any member of the genus or family produces teratogenic effects in humans, but there is concern that Oropouche virus, a Simbu serogroup pathogen of Central and South America, may be a threat to pregnant women.

Bunyamwera virus

Symptoms

A mild febrile illness, usually with headache, joint and back pains, sometimes with a rash, and occasionally with mild involvement of the central nervous system. Serological surveys indicate widespread human infection in sub-Saharan Africa but it is rarely recognized. Laboratory infections have been recorded. Garissa virus, isolated from haemorrhagic fever patients during outbreak investigations in Kenya and Somalia, has genome segments virtually identical to both Bunyamwera and Cache Valley viruses, but neither of these is known to cause haemorrhagic disease in humans.

Treatment and prognosis

No treatment is necessary and the prognosis is excellent.

California encephalitis, Inkoo, Jamestown Canyon, La Crosse, Tahyna, and snowshoe hare viruses

The viruses named above, and perhaps others currently unrecognized, are responsible for the clinical condition known as California encephalitis. The viruses are widely distributed throughout many parts of North America, Europe, and Eurasia. In the United States of America most reported human infections are due to La Crosse virus in Ohio, Wisconsin, West Virginia, and Minnesota, with over 3600 cases reported from 31 states from 1964 to 2010, or approximately 80–100 cases were reported annually. Most occurred in children, usually in boys, although Jamestown Canyon virus is found more often in adults. There is nearly always

Table 5.16.2 *Bunyaviridae* causing only mild or trivial infections in humans, arranged on a geographical basis

Africa	North America	Central America	South America	Europe	Asia
Bangui (M)	Avalon (T)	Fort Sherman	Alenquer (P)	Bhanja (T)	Batai (M)
Bhanja (T)	Keystone (M)	Madrid (M)	Apeu (M)	Calovo (M)	Bhanja (T)
Dugbe (T)	Prospect Hill	Nepuyo	Candiru (P)	Corfou (P)	Issyk-Kul (T)
Germiston (M)	Tensaw (M)	Ossa (M)	Caraparu (M)	Tamdy (T)	Ganjam (T)
Ilesha (M)	Trivittatus (M)	Restan (M)	Catu (M)	Uukuniemi (T)	Hazara (T)
Kasokero (M)		Soldado	Guama (M, P)		Keterah (T)
Nairobi sheep disease		Trivittatus (M)	Guaroa (M)		Wanowrie (T)
Nyando (M)			Itaqui		Zaliv-Terpeniya (M, T)
Pongola (M)			Maguari (M)		
Shokwe (M)			Marituba (M)		
Shuni (M)			Murutucu (M)		
Tataguine (M)			Oriboca		
Thiafora			Restan (M)		
Wanowrie (T)			Tacaiuma (M)		
			Wyeomyia (M)		

M, virus transmitted by mosquitoes; P, virus transmitted by phlebotomine flies; T, virus transmitted by ticks.

a history of outdoor exposure during warmer months in areas where woodland mosquitoes are prevalent. The incubation period is 5 to 10 days. Most cases of La Crosse encephalitis are relatively mild with headache, fever, and vomiting, progressing to lethargy, behavioural changes, and occasional brief seizures, followed by improvement. Severe cases (10–20%) develop sudden fever and headache, disorientation, and seizures during the first 24 h of illness, sometimes progressing to coma and requiring intensive supportive care. Overall, about 50% of symptomatic children have seizures with status epilepticus in 10 to 15%. The case fatality rate approaches 1%. Residual seizures occur in 6 to 13%, persistent hemiparesis in about 1%, and cognitive dysfunction in a few. In appropriate epidemiological settings, the disease should be considered in children presenting with aseptic meningitis or encephalitis.

In Europe, Tahyna virus is widely distributed in Austria, former Czechoslovakia, France, Germany, Italy, Norway, Romania, former Yugoslavia, and the former Soviet Union. Seroprevalence exceeds 95% in parts of former Czechoslovakia, and is about 50% in the Rhone valley in France and the Danube basin near Vienna, but overt disease is seldom recognized. Inkoo virus is prevalent in Finland and also in neighbouring regions of Russia. Most adult Lapps have antibodies. Small children may have signs of central nervous system involvement during acute infection. Antibodies reactive with California serogroup viruses have also been found in human sera collected in Sri Lanka, China, and in the far northern latitudes of Eurasia where several California serogroup viruses have been isolated from mosquitoes, some related to Inkoo and Tahyna viruses, but others to snowshoe hare virus. In another Russian study of c.50 people, mainly 14 to 30 years old, with infections caused by California serogroup viruses, about two-thirds had influenza-like illnesses without central nervous system involvement, while the remaining one-third had aseptic meningitis.

Control, treatment, and prognosis

Measures to limit mosquito breeding, particularly of *Aedes triseriatus*, are useful in endemic regions. No vaccines are available, and there is no specific treatment. Fluid and electrolyte balance must be maintained, and anticonvulsive drugs may be required to control seizures. Intravenous ribavirin has been used to treat severe La Crosse encephalitis.

Oropouche virus

Symptoms

Before 1961, Oropouche virus was known to have caused only a mild fever in a single forest worker in Trinidad, but that year it was responsible for a substantial epidemic in the Belém area of northern Brazil, where c.7000 people were affected. Over the ensuing 50 years, massive epidemics of febrile illness have been recorded throughout the Amazon Basin and beyond, with many thousands infected. Symptoms include headache, generalized pain including back pain, prostration, and fever (40°C). Rash, meningitis, or meningism occasionally accompany infection (Fig. 5.16.2). Illness lasts from 2 to 5 days, occasionally with protracted convalescence. No fatalities have been reported.

Control, treatment, and prognosis

No vaccine is available. Transmission is probably by the biting midge *Culicoides paraensis* and outbreaks appear to be a consequence of agricultural development of the Amazon Basin. Accumulated organic waste from cacao and banana production provides ideal breeding sites for *Culicoides*, leading to massive populations and subsequent epidemic Oropouche disease. Measures to reduce *Culicoides* breeding may be beneficial. Treatment is supportive and the prognosis is good, although convalescence may be protracted.

Genus *Hantavirus*

Haemorrhagic fever with renal syndrome

Hantaan virus of the genus *Hantavirus* is the cause of Korean haemorrhagic fever in Korea. The Hantaan River is near the demilitarized zone between North and South Korea where the virus was first recovered in 1976 from its rodent host *Apodemus agrarius*. The clinical diseases caused by Hantaan and related viruses in the Eurasian continent have long been known by different synonyms: epidemic haemorrhagic fever, Korean haemorrhagic fever, or nephropathia epidemica, but haemorrhagic fever with renal syndrome (HFRS) is preferred. Four distinct viruses are responsible for most recognized cases of HFRS: Hantaan virus, found primarily in Asia; Dobrava virus in an enclave of disease in the Balkan region and sparsely elsewhere in Europe; Puumala virus in Scandinavia, western Russia, and much of Europe; and Seoul virus is probably global wherever uncontrolled populations of *Rattus norvegicus* exist. A few cases of HFRS have been associated with Saaremaa virus in Europe and Amur virus in Asia. Hantaan and Dobrava viruses cause severe life-threatening disease with mortality of about 5%, reaching up to 30% in select populations. Puumala virus infections are less severe, although patients still require admission to hospital, but fewer than 1% of admitted patients die. Seoul virus is thought to be the least severe of the pathogenic strains of Old World hantaviruses, although it has been associated with human deaths.

Each hantavirus is associated with a particular rodent host: Hantaan virus with the striped field mouse *Apodemus agrarius*; Dobrava virus with the yellow-necked mouse *Apodemus flavicollis*; Puumala virus with the bank vole *Myodes*; and Seoul virus with the Norway rat *Rattus norvegicus*. Humans are infected by aerosols of rodent excreta, or rarely by rodent bites. It is seen among adult men in rural environments and may be an occupational disease. Those at greatest risk include farmers, woodcutters, shepherds, and, especially, soldiers in the field. Most hantavirus disease is seasonal, with a peak incidence in late autumn and early winter, although the Balkan form is found most often during summer months in Greece and adjacent countries.

Symptoms

The incubation period for hantaviruses is variable; it is usually 12 to 16 days but it can be up to 2 months. Severe disease, typically associated with Hantaan or Dobrava virus infections in Asia or the Balkans, is characterized by five phases:

1 Febrile: 3- to 7-day duration

2 Hypotensive: lasting from a few hours to 3 days

3 Oliguric: from 3 to 7 days

4 Diuretic: from a few days to weeks

5 Convalescent: prolonged

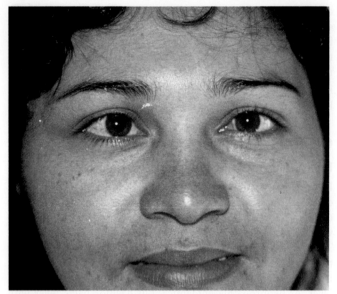

Fig. 5.16.2 Patient convalescent after Oropouche virus encephalitis in Belém, Para, Brazil, showing a left VIIth cranial nerve palsy.
(Courtesy of Dr Pedro Pardal, Hospital Universitário João de Barros Barreto, Brazil.)

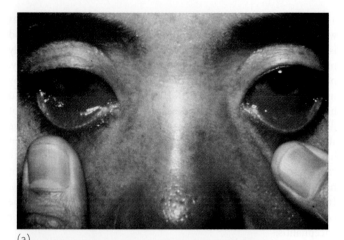

(a)

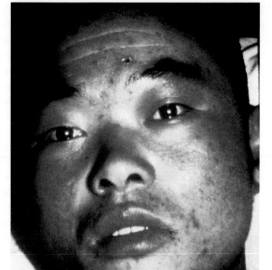

(b)

Fig. 5.16.3 Patient with acute Korean haemorrhagic fever, showing extensive conjunctival haemorrhages (a) and facial swelling (b).
(Courtesy of Professor H W Lee.)

Signs and symptoms of the febrile phase include fever, malaise, headache, myalgia, back pain, abdominal pain, nausea and vomiting, facial flushing, petechiae, and conjunctival haemorrhage (Fig. 5.16.3). In the hypotensive phase, patients have nausea, vomiting, tachycardia, hypotension, blurred vision, haemorrhagic signs, and shock. About one-third of fatalities occur during this phase. In the oliguric phase, nausea and vomiting may persist and blood pressure may rise. Renal failure develops with anuria, and about one-third of cases have severe haemorrhage (epistaxis, gastrointestinal, cutaneous, or bleeding at other sites). Nearly one-half of the deaths occur during the oliguric phase. In the diuretic phase, urine output increases to several litres per day. Convalescence is protracted and it maybe months before full strength and function are regained.

Not all the phases are seen in the less severe forms of the disease. The milder forms of HFRS, such as nephropathia epidemica due to Puumala virus, follow a similar but less severe course, with abrupt onset of fever of 38 to 40°C, headache, malaise, backache, and generalized abdominal pain. Back or loin pain is especially common. Signs of renal failure are usually not as pronounced, and the need for renal dialysis varies. Transient blurred vision occurs in about 10% of cases. Infection due to Seoul virus follows a similar course, but may present with more evidence of liver involvement. There is no evidence of person-to-person transmission.

Treatment and prognosis

Admission to hospital, avoidance of trauma and unnecessary movement, close observation, and careful supportive care are essential for patient survival. Treatment is phase specific, with special attention to fluid balance and volume, and control of hypotension and shock. Renal dialysis may be required. Antiviral therapy using ribavirin has been shown to be effective if started early in disease. Recovery is protracted but usually complete, with the exception of Seoul virus infection which carries the risk of chronic renal disease, hypertension, or stroke.

Hantavirus pulmonary syndrome

Hantavirus pulmonary syndrome, first reported from the United States of America in 1993, also occurs in Canada, Central and South America. The initial cases had a mortality of more than 50%, but rates have declined to 20 to 40% as clinical experience has increased. Most disease was reported from the western United States of America and Canada, and more recently from Argentina, Chile, Brazil, and other Central and South American countries. Sin Nombre virus was first associated with HPS, but many additional hantaviruses have now been recognized as likely causes of this syndrome (Table 5.16.1). As Old World hantaviruses are generally associated with specific microtine rodents (subfamilies Arvicolinae and Microtinae: voles, lemmings, muskrats, rats, and their allies, distributed worldwide), so each American hantavirus appears to be associated with a specific sigmodontine host (Sigmodontinae: cotton rats and their allies found in the western hemisphere). Apparent human-to-human transmission of Andes virus occurred during an outbreak in southern Argentina, including transmission to medical staff. Protective precautions are recommended when treating suspected cases of HPS.

Symptoms

Symptoms are primarily those of acute unexplained adult respiratory distress syndrome and cardiogenic shock, rather than the expected renal disease. Nonspecific prodromal features of fever, myalgia, and malaise may last 4 to 6 days, with nausea, vomiting, and abdominal pain, often accompanied by dizziness. On admission, physical examination of patients with confirmed infection reveals fever (more than 38°C), tachycardia (more than 100 beats/min), tachypnoea (more than 20 breaths/min), and often hypotension (systolic pressure less than 100 mmHg), with audible rales in the chest. Laboratory findings include hypoxia, leukocytosis, haemoconcentration, thrombocytopenia, atypical lymphocytosis, elevated transaminases, and prolonged prothrombin time. Chest radiography shows progression from subtle interstitial findings to bilateral frank pulmonary oedema; pleural effusions are usually present (Fig. 5.16.4). Thrombocytopenia and haemoconcentration are independent statistical predictors of HPS, although not infallible. In a patient with rapidly progressive pulmonary oedema, a blood smear showing four of the following five characteristics is a highly sensitive and specific means of establishing the diagnosis of HPS: (1) thrombocytopenia, (2) haemoconcentration, (3) lack of toxic granulation in neutrophils, (4) more than 10% immunoblasts, and (5) myelocytosis. Disease progresses rapidly once the lungs begin to fill, and death is commonly seen 24 to 48 h after admission, or sooner if there is hypoxia or circulatory failure. The severity of disease correlates with the degree of pulmonary oedema on chest radiography. Hypotension and shock may occur independently in patients whose hypoxaemia is medically controlled.

Treatment and prognosis

Treatment is supportive, ideally in a modern intensive care unit, with careful management of hypoxia, fluid balance, and shock. About two-thirds of patients require intubation and mechanical ventilation. Fluid loss into the lungs leads to haemoconcentration, but infusion of fluids exacerbates pulmonary oedema; therefore fluids should be administered cautiously with careful monitoring. Limited experience suggests that intravenous ribavirin has little effect on the course of HPS, perhaps because of the speed with which the disease progresses.

Control

Prevention involves avoidance of infected rodents either through efficient rodent control programmes in cities, for Seoul virus, or maintenance of clean campsites so that waste food is not allowed to accumulate and attract rodents. Nationally approved inactivated vaccines, reported to be safe and effective against hantaviruses, are available for use in Asia.

Genus *Nairovirus*

The genus *Nairovirus*, named after Nairobi sheep disease, is an acute haemorrhagic gastroenteritis affecting sheep and goats in East Africa, with transmission by the sheep tick *Rhipicephalus appendiculatus*. It has caused laboratory infections, but the genus includes Crimean–Congo haemorrhagic fever virus and several other viruses known to infect humans, e.g. Ganjam virus, almost indistinguishable from Nairobi sheep disease virus but first isolated in India from *Haemaphysalis intermedia* ticks collected from healthy goats; Hazara virus, recovered from *Ixodes redkorzevi* ticks collected from the vole *Alticola roylei* in a subarctic habitat at an altitude of 3660 m in the Kaghan valley of Hazara district, Pakistan; Dugbe virus, isolated in Nigeria from *Amblyomma variegatum* ticks collected from healthy cattle; and Soldado virus, repeatedly isolated from a variety of bird ticks but recently linked to a mild illness in humans.

Crimean–Congo haemorrhagic fever virus

This was first recognized as a cause of an acute febrile haemorrhagic disease affecting humans in the Crimean region of the former Union of Soviet Socialist Republics, transmitted by ticks and carrying a mortality of 5 to 30%. In Africa, Congo virus was first isolated in the then Belgian Congo (now Democratic Republic of the Congo) from the blood of a local 13-year-old boy, and it caused a moderately severe laboratory infection. Related viruses were isolated in Uganda where more laboratory infections occurred, one of which ended fatally after a severe haematemesis. In Asia, a virus indistinguishable from Congo virus was isolated from pools

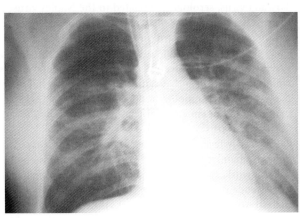
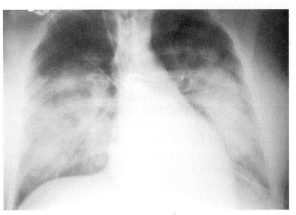

Fig. 5.16.4 Chest radiograph of a patient with early hantavirus pulmonary syndrome (left), and the same patient 24 h later (right) showing development of bilateral perihilar alveolar oedema.
(Courtesy of Dr Loren Ketai.)

of ticks collected from a variety of wild and domestic animals in western Pakistan. Crimean haemorrhagic fever virus was later proved to be serologically indistinguishable from Congo virus, hence the use of the term Crimean–Congo haemorrhagic fever virus. Different strains of this virus have been associated with outbreaks of severe and sometimes fatal disease in the Crimea, Rostov, and Astrakhan regions of Russia, in Albania, Bulgaria, and the Balkans, in East, West, and South Africa, in Iran, Iraq, and western Pakistan, and in China. From 2002 to 2008, ~2500 cases were reported in Turkey, although it was virtually unknown there previously. Most infections are seen among farmers or abattoir workers and acquired by tick bites or exposure to viraemic animal blood, but infections have occurred in both hospitals and laboratories.

Symptoms

The incubation period is 3 to 7 days. Fever usually starts suddenly and is normally continuous, although occasionally it is remittent or biphasic. Other clinical features are headache, nausea, vomiting, joint pains, backache, photophobia, circulatory disorders, thrombocytopenia, and leukopenia. Haemorrhagic manifestations are common. Patients show cutaneous petechiae and extensive ecchymoses, and bleed from nasal, gastric, intestinal, uterine, and urinary tract mucosae (Fig. 5.16.5). Patients may present with acute abdominal pain, mimicking an acute surgical emergency, and operating-theatre staff have become infected and died through exposure to infected blood or secretions at operation. The mortality is about 5 to 30%, but may be up to 40% or higher in hospital or nosocomial outbreaks. Transient hair loss has been reported.

Control, treatment, and prognosis

No vaccine is available. Avoidance of tick bites may reduce the risk of infection. In hospital outbreaks, meticulous attention to the containment of infected secretions is essential and barrier nursing should be used. Overt disseminated intravascular coagulation usually indicates a poor prognosis, and haematemesis, melaena, and somnolence are significantly more common in fatal cases. Supportive therapy is essential, with monitoring of fluid and electrolyte balance. The antiviral ribavirin is recommended for severe cases based on observational studies. Limiting injections and avoidance of aspirin or other drugs affecting coagulation may reduce bleeding. Patients who recover may have residual polyneuritis persisting for months, but eventual recovery is to be expected. Laboratory investigations with live virus require biological safety level 4 containment.

Genus *Phlebovirus*

At least 10 different phleboviruses are known to infect humans (see Table 5.16.1). Pappataci fever, sandfly fever, or phlebotomus fever was recognized as a clinical entity in the Mediterranean area during the 19th century, and the association with *Phlebotomus papatasi* sandflies was demonstrated by showing that filtrates of human blood reproduced the disease in human volunteers. It was thought that humans were the only vertebrate host, but antibody studies indicate that gerbils, cattle, and sheep may also be infected. Naples virus was isolated from human serum collected during an outbreak of sandfly fever in Naples, and the Sicilian virus was isolated from American troops with a similar disease in Palermo, Sicily. The two viruses have many common properties, but are serologically quite distinct. Sandfly

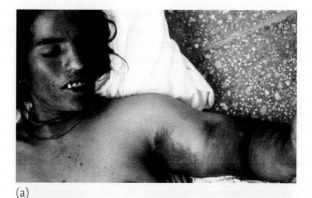
(a)

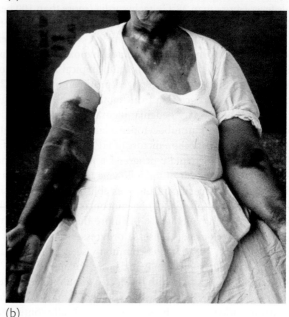
(b)

Fig. 5.16.5 Turkish patients with Crimean–Congo haemorrhagic fever showing petechiae (a) and extensive ecchymoses (a,b) on the arms and thorax. (Courtesy of Professor D I H Simpson.)

fever is widespread throughout the Mediterranean area, and also occurs in Egypt, Greece, Iran, Turkey, the former Yugoslavia, Bangladesh, India, Pakistan, and the southern states of Russia. Toscana virus, serologically related to the Naples virus, is found in countries bordering the Mediterranean; it is notable for its ability to infect the central nervous system, especially in central Italy where it is thought to be responsible for at least 80% of acute summertime infections of the central nervous system in children. The viruses that cause sandfly fever do not occur in the New World, but in South and Central America a similar clinical condition follows infection with Alenquer, Candiru, Chagres, and Punta Toro viruses.

Rift Valley fever has long been known as a disease of domestic animals, mainly sheep, in East Africa, which occasionally spreads to farm workers and others handling infected animals. The infection is endemic, but seldom recognized, in many wild game animals in Africa. Rift Valley fever virus differs from the sandfly fever viruses, Punta Toro virus, and most other members of the genus in being normally transmitted by mosquitoes rather than sandflies. Uukuniemi and Zaliv-Terpeniya viruses are tick-transmitted; the only evidence that Uukuniemi virus can infect humans is the finding of specific antibodies in some human sera collected in Estonia and in former Czechoslovakia. Severe fever with thrombocytopenia syndrome virus is a newly discovered apparently tick-borne phlebovirus found in central and north-east China and affecting farmers living in wooded areas. Zaliv-Terpeniya virus was isolated from bird ticks collected on an island in the Sea of Okhotsk, Sakhalin region, and there is some evidence that it may be pathogenic to humans.

Sandfly fever, Naples, and Sicilian viruses

Symptoms

After an incubation period of 2 to 6 days, fever starts abruptly with chills, nausea and vomiting, epigastric pain, and often severe generalized headache leading to incapacitating prostration. Fever of 38 to 40°C usually resolves after 2 to 3 days, but may be biphasic and persist for a week. There is no rash, but small haemorrhages into the skin and mucous membranes may be seen. Photophobia and eye pain occur, lymphadenopathy is often seen, and the liver may be tender although jaundice is rare. The disease is self-limiting, with complete recovery. No deaths have been attributed to either sandfly fever, Naples, or Sicilian viruses.

Rift Valley fever virus

Following its initial isolation in 1930 as the agent of enzootic hepatitis of domestic animals in Kenya, Rift Valley fever virus was recognized as the cause of sporadic human infections in East, Central, and West Africa, with a particular tendency to infect laboratory workers handling the virus. In East and Central Africa the virus has been isolated from a variety of mosquito species and it is capable of persisting in mosquito eggs during the dry season, emerging when larvae hatch in the rainy season. From 1951 to 1956 there were severe epizootics in lambs in southern Africa, and many human cases occurred. Further human cases with several deaths were seen in South Africa in 1975, and a major outbreak occurred in East Africa following El Niño flooding in 1997 to 1998, apparently seeding a 'virgin soil' outbreak in Saudi Arabia and Yemen in 2000. In 1997–8 and 2006–7 there were epizootics in Kenya, Tanzania, Burundi, and Somalia. In the recent epidemic, 684 cases with 155 deaths were reported in Kenya (case fatality 23%), 264 cases with 109 deaths in Tanzania (case fatality 41%), and 114 cases with 51 deaths in Somalia (case fatality 45%). Heavy rains in East Africa during 2006–7 triggered another outbreak with many human and animal cases.

In the Central African Republic in 1969, a virus isolated from *Mansonia africana* mosquitoes and named Zinga virus was associated with several cases of haemorrhagic fever; Zinga virus was later shown to be a strain of Rift Valley fever virus. In West Africa, Rift Valley fever virus was isolated from mosquitoes in Nigeria and from bats in Guinea, but despite the presence of antibodies in human sera collected in Nigeria and Senegal, human disease was unrecognized until 1987 when a substantial epidemic occurred in Mauritania, with further epidemics in following years. In 1977 the virus spread, apparently for the first time, into Egypt, producing a major epizootic in domestic animals, principally sheep and goats but also cattle, and causing about 600 human deaths within 3 months. The virus has been detected intermittently since then in Egypt. The principal known vector is the mosquito *Culex pipiens*.

Both the Egyptian and the Mauritanian epidemics appeared to be linked to major ecological changes following the construction of the Aswan Dam on the Nile and dams on the Senegal River.

Symptoms

After an incubation period of 3 to 6 days, fever starts abruptly with shivering, nausea and vomiting, epigastric pain, arthralgia, and often severe generalized headache. The fever may be biphasic, with temperatures between 38 and 40°C, and may remain elevated for at least a week. There is no rash, but small haemorrhages appear on mucous membranes. Photophobia and eye pains occur. There may be conjunctival inflammation, and a central serous retinitis leading to central scotoma and sometimes to retinal detachment can occur late in disease. The fundus may show macular exudates that are slow to disappear. There is often a lymphadenopathy and although the liver is frequently involved and may be tender, jaundice is rare. Convalescence may be protracted but is usually uncomplicated.

A few patients develop severe disease with haemorrhage, encephalitis, or eye lesions. Haemorrhagic disease presents as above but progresses with cutaneous and mucous membrane petechiae, ecchymoses (Fig. 5.16.6a), gastrointestinal haemorrhage, and jaundice with severe liver and renal dysfunction often progressing to disseminated intravascular coagulation, hepatorenal syndrome, and death. Patients with encephalitis usually recover from acute febrile disease only to present within a few days to 2 weeks later with headache, meningism, confusion, and fever, often leading to residual defects or ending in death. Ocular complications are characterized by rapid onset of decreased visual acuity with scotomas due to retinal haemorrhage, exudates, and macular oedema (Fig. 5.16.6b). These are also seen after apparent recovery from the initial disease. About one-half of these patients have some degree of permanent visual loss. Death from Rift Valley fever was rarely recognized before the 1977 outbreak in Egypt, but the Mauritanian epidemics with mortality due to jaundice and haemorrhagic manifestations, and the recent East African and Arabian Peninsula outbreaks with several hundred suspect fatalities establish it as a life-threatening infection.

Control, treatment, and prognosis

Veterinary vaccines have been used for some years, and formalin-inactivated vaccines have also had limited use for the prevention of disease in laboratory workers and others exposed to high risk of infection. Improved vaccines based on molecular techniques are under development. Treatment is supportive. Although there are no reports of nosocomial transmission, barrier nursing would be a sensible precaution.

Severe fever with thrombocytopenia syndrome virus

Severe fever with thrombocytopenia syndrome (SFTS) first came to the attention of Chinese health officials in 2009 when cases appeared in rural areas of Henan and Hubei provinces in central China. Adult farmers appear to be at greatest risk, and subsequent studies found evidence of human infection in at least six provinces of central and north-east China. SFTS virus was isolated from ticks (*Haemaphysalis longicornis*), but not from mosquitoes, and molecular characterization of the virus suggests that it is distantly related both to viruses of the sandfly fever complex and to Uukuniemi virus. Of over 150 cases initially reported, the vast majority

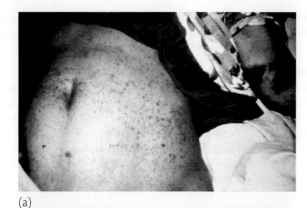

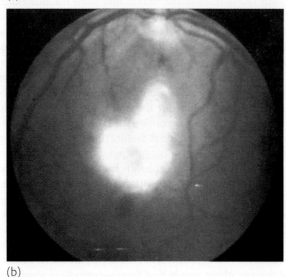

Fig. 5.16.6 Severe Rift Valley fever. (a) Cutaneous petechiae and ecchymosis. (b) Severe central retinal lesion.
(Courtesy of Professor D I H Simpson.)

occurred from May to July, with about 75% of patients over 50 years of age. Transmission by tick bite is suspected; however, recent observations suggest the possibility of person-to-person transmission following contact with bloody secretions or vomited blood of patients.

Symptoms

Symptoms of SFTS include fever, thrombocytopenia and leucopenia, followed by multiorgan failure in severe cases. Patients may present with fever, fatigue, conjunctival congestion, diarrhoea, abdominal pain, proteinuria, and haematuria in addition to thrombocytopenia and leucopenia. Multiorgan failure may develop, rapidly leading to death in 12% or more of hospitalized cases based on limited data now available. Characteristics of less severe disease among nonhospitalized cases have yet to be determined. A robust humoral immune response occurs and neutralizing antibodies persist in surviving patients for at least 1 year. Onset of disease occurred 6 to 13 days after contact with blood of infected persons where person-to-person transmission was suspected.

Control, treatment and prognosis

Assuming transmission from infected ticks, control and prevention should focus on avoidance of tick bite. Barrier nursing and standard precautions against contact with blood and other potentially infectious bodily fluids are prudent precautions. There is no specific treatment and susceptibility to antiviral drugs like ribavirin has yet to be evaluated. Laboratory testing of clinical specimens and experimental manipulation of SFTS virus should be done under appropriate containment.

Unassigned viruses and viruses causing only minor disease in humans

The great majority of the viruses listed in Table 5.16.2 cause only a mild febrile illness, but the following show certain additional features.

Bhanja virus (unassigned)

This virus was first isolated from *Haemaphysalis intermedia* ticks collected from healthy goats in India, but has since been isolated in Sri Lanka, Africa, and Europe. Infection of goats is widespread in Italy and the Balkans where there have been several reported human cases, including some with severe neurological disease and at least two deaths. Laboratory infections have also occurred.

Bwamba virus (*Orthobunyavirus*)

This was first isolated in Uganda in 1941 and is very widespread throughout sub-Saharan Africa. More than 75% of adult human sera collected in Nigeria and over 95% of human sera collected in Uganda and Tanzania have antibodies against Bwamba virus. The original cases showed fever, headache, generalized pain, and conjunctivitis but no rash, although a rash has been described in the Central African Republic. No fatalities have been reported.

Nyando virus (*Orthobunyavirus*)

This virus was first isolated from mosquitoes in Kenya. It has since been isolated from humans in the Central African Republic where it caused fever, myalgia, and encephalitis.

Tataguine virus (unassigned)

This causes fever, rash, and joint pains in at least five African countries (Cameroon, Central African Republic, Ethiopia, Nigeria, and Senegal).

Wanowrie virus (unassigned)

This virus was first isolated in India from *Hyalomma marginatum* ticks collected from sheep. It has also been isolated in Egypt and Iran, and in Sri Lanka where it was recovered from the brain of a 17-year-old girl who died following a 2-day fever with abdominal pain and vomiting.

Further reading

Bartelloni PJ, Tesh RB (1976). Clinical and serologic responses of volunteers infected with phlebotomus fever virus (Sicilian type). *Am J Trop Med Hyg*, **25**, 456–62.

Calisher CH, Thompson WH (eds) (1983). *California serogroup viruses. Progress in clinical and biological research*, vol. 123. Liss, New York.

Ergonul O (2006). Crimean-Congo haemorrhagic fever. *Lancet Infect Dis*, **6**, 203–14.

Jonsson CB, Figueiredo LTM, Vapalahti O (2010). A global perspective on hantavirus ecology, epidemiology and disease. *Clin Microbiol Rev*, **23**, 412–41.

Koster F, *et al.* (2001). Rapid presumptive diagnosis of hantavirus cardiopulmonary syndrome by peripheral blood smear review. *Am J Clin Pathol*, **116**, 665–72.

LeDuc JW (1995). Hantavirus infections. In: Porterfield JS (ed) *Exotic viral infections*, pp. 261–84. Chapman & Hall, London.

LeDuc JW, Pinheiro FP (1989). Oropouche fever. In: Monath TP (ed) *The arboviruses: epidemiology and ecology*, vol. 4, pp. 1–14. CRC Press, Boca Raton.

Lee HW, Calisher C, Schmaljohn CS (1999). *Manual of hemorrhagic fever with renal syndrome and hantavirus pulmonary syndrome.* WHO Collaborating Center for Virus Reference and Research (Hantaviruses), Seoul.

Madani TA, *et al.* (2003). Rift Valley fever epidemic in Saudi Arabia: epidemiology, clinical and laboratory characteristics. *Clin Infect Dis*, **37**, 1084–92.

Monath TP (ed) (1989). *The arboviruses: epidemiology and ecology.* CRC Press, Boca Raton.

Peters CJ (1997). Emergence of Rift Valley fever. In: Saluzzo JF, Dodet B (eds) *Factors in the emergence of arbovirus diseases*, pp. 253–64. Elsevier, Paris.

Peters CJ (1998). Hantavirus pulmonary syndrome in the Americas. *Emerg Infections*, **2**, 17–64.

Peters CJ, LeDuc JW (1991). Bunyaviridae: bunyaviruses, phleboviruses, and related viruses. In: Belshe RB (ed) *Textbook of human virology*, 2nd edition, pp. 571–614. Mosby Year Book, St. Louis.

Peters CJ, Simpson GL, Levy H (1999). Spectrum of hantavirus infection: hemorrhagic fever with renal syndrome and hantavirus pulmonary syndrome. *Annu Rev Med*, **50**, 531–45.

Saluzzo JF, Dodet B (eds) (1999). Factors in the emergence and control of rodent-borne viral disease (hantaviral and arenal diseases). Elsevier, Paris.

Swanepoel R (1995). Nairovirus infections. In: Porterfield JS (ed) *Exotic viral infections*, pp. 285–93. Chapman & Hall, London.

Yu X-J, *et al.* (2011). Fever with thrombocytopenia associated with a novel Bunyavirus in China. *N Engl J Med*, **364**, 1523–32.

5.17 Arenaviruses

J. ter Meulen

Essentials

Arenaviruses are zoonotic RNA viruses that are distributed worldwide and are adapted to various rodent genera. Some are highly pathogenic and cause haemorrhagic fevers that are endemic in restricted regions of a few countries. Humans are thought to become infected mainly through inhalation of aerosolized rodent urine or dust particles to which infectious urine has dried, or by ingestion of contaminated foodstuff: prevention therefore depends on rodent control and avoidance of contact with rodents, their excreta, and nesting materials.

Clinical approach—because arenaviruses cause diseases that start insidiously and therapy is life-saving, they should be considered in all patients with fever of unknown origin and a history of possible exposure in the well-known endemic areas.

Specific infections

Lassa fever—reservoir is a small rodent (*Mastomys natalensis*); occurs regularly in rural areas of Nigeria, Liberia, Sierra Leone and the Republic of Guinea, but may occur also in other West African countries. Clinical picture is highly variable and can be difficult to distinguish from other febrile infections, but may include chest pain, nausea/vomiting/diarrhoea/abdominal pain, facial swelling, pulmonary oedema, and bleeding. Case-fatality is 15 to 30%, but may be reduced by up to 90% through prompt administration of ribavirin. Irreversible sensorineural deafness is a frequent complication. Body fluids of patients are highly infectious and Lassa virus has been transmitted directly from person-to-person, hence strict 'barrier nursing' measures are required and (if possible) patients with severe disease and bleeding should be managed in a negative-pressure room by personnel wearing appropriate protective gear, including respiratory filters; postexposure prophylaxis with ribavirin should be considered. No vaccine is available.

Lymphocytic choriomeningitis virus infection—reservoir is the house mouse. Most commonly causes an influenza-like illness, sometimes with subsequent aseptic meningitis or encephalomyelitis. Intrauterine infection has resulted in nonobstructive hydrocephalus with periventricular calcifications, chorioretinitis, and psychomotor retardation. Use of ribavirin has not been systematically evaluated.

South American haemorrhagic fevers—the reservoir(s) for Argentinian haemorrhagic fever is the vesper mouse, for Bolivian haemorrhagic fever *Calomys callosus*, and for Venezuelan haemorrhagic fever the cotton rat and the cane mouse. These cause an influenza-like illness with marked skin erythema and (in almost half of cases) haemorrhagic manifestations; a late neurological cerebellar syndrome occurs in about 10%. Treatment with convalescent-phase plasma is very effective in Argentinian haemorrhagic fever, and ribavirin may be effective. A live attenuated vaccine for Argentinian haemorrhagic fever is licensed in Argentina.

Introduction

Arenaviruses are pleomorphic enveloped negative-stranded segmented RNA viruses with a characteristic internal granular structure, hence their family name Arenaviridae (Latin *arenosus* = sandy). Several arenaviruses are known to be responsible for severe diseases in humans. Lymphocytic choriomeningitis virus (LCMV) is distributed worldwide and occasionally causes acute central nervous system (CNS) disease and congenital malformations and has been transmitted through solid organ transplantation. Lassa virus in West Africa, and Junin, Machupo, Guanarito, Sabia, and Chapare viruses in South America cause viral haemorrhagic fevers (VHF). Certain rodent species are the principal hosts of arenaviruses and shed them lifelong in high titres in their urine. Humans are thought to become infected mainly through inhalation of aerosolized rodent urine or dust particles to which infectious urine has dried, or by ingestion of contaminated foodstuff. Human-to-human transmission occurs with some of the viruses. In geographically confined endemic rural areas, sporadic infections with these viruses occur regularly and are often linked to seasonal agricultural activities. Novel related viruses are emerging from time to time in previously unaffected areas. In 2000, three patients from California were fatally infected with a novel arenavirus related to Whitewater Arroyo virus, originally isolated from rodents in New Mexico.

Aetiology, genetics, pathogenesis, and pathology

Common to all arenavirus haemorrhagic fevers is disruption of vascular endothelial integrity, originating most likely from the release of endogenous mediators from infected macrophages or endothelial cells, and resulting in extravasations of fluid into extravascular spaces ('capillary leakage syndrome'). Coagulation disorders are subtler than in filovirus infections and disseminated intravascular coagulopathy is not observed. Platelets are dysfunctional despite their adequate or only mildly depressed numbers, and evidence for a soluble protein inhibitor of platelet function, presumably of host origin, has been described in Lassa virus (LASV) and Junin virus (JUNV) infections. Experimentally, LASV-infected nonhuman primates also showed a marked decrease in endothelial prostacyclin production.

Arenaviruses initially infect macrophages and immature dendritic cells, compromising the ability of the latter to mature and stimulate T-cell responses. Infected dendritic cells seem to be eliminated by immunopathological mechanisms, correlating with a decline in the number of lymphocytes and destruction of the architecture of lymphatic organs. In LCMV and LASV infections, this suppression of the innate immune responses is shown by the absence or delayed appearance of a neutralizing antibody response. In contrast, infection with JUNV induces neutralizing antibodies. Hence, immune plasma is used for passive immune therapy.

Arenaviruses replicate in many epithelial cell types with only modest cytopathic effect and there is ominous absence of an inflammatory response in infected organs. Autopsy of LASV-infected nonhuman primates shows pulmonary congestion, pleural effusion, and pericardial oedema and effusion. Major microscopic lesions are necrotizing hepatitis and interstitial pneumonia. The degree of hepatic damage is not sufficient to implicate hepatic failure as the cause of death. In JUNV infection, there are large areas of intra-alveolar or bronchial haemorrhage, petechiae on organ surfaces, and ulcerations of the digestive tract, although bleeding is not massive. Pneumonia with necrotizing bronchitis or pulmonary emboli is observed in one-half of cases. Haemorrhage and a lymphocytic infiltrate have been observed in the pericardium, and splenic haemorrhage is common. Renal damage occurs in about one-half of the fatal cases and consists of severe structural damage in the distal tubular cells and collecting ducts with relative sparing of the glomeruli and proximal tubules.

Neurological involvement during the acute phase of the disease is common in the South American haemorrhagic fevers, but there is no evidence of direct viral infection of the CNS. In Lassa fever, neurological complications, mainly sensorineural deafness, are very common during convalescence and are thought to be due to immunopathology. There is evidence that LASV persists at least for some time because it has been isolated in human urine for up to 60 days.

In one report of a fatal human LCMV infection there was perivascular macrophage infiltration in multiple areas of the brain and antigen was observed in the meninges and cortical cells. LCMV has been recovered from the CNS of newborn children with malformations.

Epidemiology

Lassa fever

Clinical cases of Lassa fever are reported regularly in rural areas of Nigeria, Liberia, Sierra Leone, and the Republic of Guinea, but may occur also in other West African countries. The reservoir of LASV is a small rodent (*Mastomys natalensis*) that lives in and around human dwellings. In West Africa, 300 000 to 500 000 LASV infections are estimated to occur annually, resulting in approximately 150 000 clinical cases, ranging in severity from flu-like illness to haemorrhagic fever, and approximately 5000 deaths. In endemic areas, 75% of all LASV infections are probably asymptomatic, with an overall mortality of 1 to 5%. Lassa fever patients are not infectious during the incubation period and quite close contact with body fluids is required for person-to-person spread of the virus. However, airborne transmission, probably through direct contact with droplets produced during heavy coughing and presumably originating from Lassa pneumonitis, has been reported in a few instances.

Presumed nonpathogenic arenaviruses have been isolated from *Mastomys* spp. and other rodents throughout Africa, and serological evidence of human infection has been detected. Recently, a novel, genetically distinct, and highly pathogenetic arenavirus (named Lujo virus) was isolated from a Zambian patient hospitalized with a fatal Lassa fever-like illness in South Africa, who transmitted the infection to several care givers.

Expatriates working in endemic areas have repeatedly imported Lassa fever into Europe and North America.

Lymphocytic choriomeningitis virus infection

The distribution of LCMV is highly variable within populations of its natural host *Mus musculus*. From infected mouse colonies, LCMV spreads to humans in rural settings or when human habitats are substandard in urban areas. Infected laboratory and pet rodents have also been associated with disease in humans, and aerosol transmission may have occurred. Clinical cases of LCMV infection seem to be rare in the United States of America, even though 9.0% of house mice and 4.7% of residents had measurable antibodies in the Baltimore area in the 1990s. Person-to-person spread has not been demonstrated. Intrauterine LCMV infection has resulted in fetal or neonatal death, as well as hydrocephalus and chorioretinitis in infants, and the virus may be a more frequent cause of CNS disease in newborns than previously recognized. Two clusters of transplantation-associated transmission of LCMV have been reported.

Argentine haemorrhagic fever

The endemic area of Argentine haemorrhagic fever (caused by JUNV) comprises the provinces of Buenos Aires, Córdoba, Santa Fe, and La Pampa. The major rodent hosts of JUNV are the agrarian rodents (vesper mice) *Calomys musculinus* and *C. laucha*. Most human cases are male agricultural workers. About 21 000 cases have been reported since the early 1960s, averaging about 360 a year with wide annual fluctuations. Peak incidence is during summer and early autumn. Overall human antibody prevalence is about 12% and about 30% had no history of typical illness. Occasional hospital or family epidemics have occurred, but cases have not been observed outside of Argentina. Recent introduction of a live attenuated vaccine has reduced the incidence of the disease dramatically.

Bolivian haemorrhagic fever

Bolivian haemorrhagic fever (caused by Machupo virus) is limited to rural areas of Beni department in Bolivia. The only known reservoir is *Calomys callosus*. The largest known epidemic of Bolivian haemorrhagic fever, involving several hundred cases, followed a marked and unusual increase in the *Calomys* population in homes in the town of San Joaquin in 1963 and 1964. This seems to have been a unique event, and there were almost no further cases until 1994, when there was an outbreak in north-eastern Bolivia. Since all ages and both sexes are affected, it can be assumed that most patients were infected in their homes. Person-to-person spread is rarely reported. A novel virus, tentatively designated Chapare virus, was isolated from a fatal haemorrhagic fever case near Cochabamba. The virus is genetically related to Sabia virus from Brazil; its rodent host and geographical distribution are currently unknown.

Venezuelan haemorrhagic fever

Venezuelan haemorrhagic fever (caused by Guanarito virus) is endemic to the southern and south-western parts of Portuguesa state and adjacent regions of Barinas state in Venezuela. From 1989 to 1995, a total of 105 confirmed or probable cases of Venezuelan haemorrhagic fever were reported, of which 34% were fatal. All ages and sexes were infected suggesting that transmission had occurred in and around houses. The incidence peaked each year between November and January, during the period of major agricultural activity. In addition, epidemic activity of the illness appears cyclically every 4 to 5 years. The cotton rat *Sigmodon alstoni* and the cane mouse *Zygodontomys brevicauda* are the rodent reservoirs. Seroprevalence in humans living in the state of Portuguesa is below 2%. Human-to-human transmission has not been reported.

Other arenavirus infections

Sabia virus was isolated in 1990 from a fatal case in São Paulo, Brazil. Its natural distribution and host are still unknown. One patient who acquired the infection in the laboratory treated himself immediately with ribavirin, and made a rapid and full recovery.

Whitewater Arroyo virus was isolated in 1996 from white-throated wood rats or pack rats (*Neotoma albigula* and *Neotoma* spp.) collected in McKinley county, New Mexico. A related virus has caused three fatal human infections in California in 1999 and 2000; they are believed to be rare events because the abundance and habits of wood rats suggest that potential contact with humans is limited. One patient reportedly cleaned rodent droppings in her home during the 2 weeks before illness onset; no history of rodent contact was solicited for the other two patients. Several other arenaviruses isolated from North American rodents have not yet been shown to cause human infections.

Dandenong virus, a new arenavirus related to LCMV, has recently been isolated in Australia from patients who had received organ transplants from a deceased donor who had travelled in eastern Europe.

Prevention

Rodent control

In endemic areas, rodent control is essential and direct contact with rodents, their excreta, and their nesting materials should be avoided.

Management of infected patients

Safe and orderly care of the ill and adequate disinfection procedures should be instituted early (barrier nursing, guidelines from Centres for Disease Control and World Health Organization, see Box 5.17.1), with effective surveillance of high-risk contacts and

---

Box 5.17.1 Principles of barrier nursing in resource-poor settings (World Health Organization)

Protective clothing
- Double gloves
- (Single-use) gown
- Plastic apron
- Mask (P3 protection)
- Goggles
- Disinfect within isolation area or destroy (single-use) material.

Hand washing
- After each patient contact or contact with infected material
- Rinse in disinfectant, then wash with soap and water
- Disinfectant/washing facilities must be located just outside isolation rooms.

Instruments
- Individual thermometer for each patient, keep in receptacle with disinfectant
- Disinfect stethoscope and sleeve of sphygmomanometer between each use
- Place all reusable instruments in disinfecting fluid after use

Bed covering and linen
- Use of plastic sheet to cover and protect entire mattress is essential
- Disinfect after discharge or death of the patient
- Place bedding and linen in plastic bag for sterilization (soak in disinfectant, boil, or autoclave)

Food
- Food should be supplied by hospital, not relatives
- Each patient must have own eating utensils
- Wash and disinfect in isolation area
- Dispose of uneaten food

Charts/records
- Keep outside isolation area

Disinfection methods
- Household bleach—viruses causing viral haemorrhagic fevers are killed by exposure to a 1:10 solution for 1 min, or to a 1:100 solution for 10 min
- Heat sterilization—if autoclave not available, boil at 100°C for 20 min

prompt isolation of further cases. Direct person-to-person transmission occurs in Lassa fever and, although rare, has been documented for some New World viruses. Nosocomial transmission can occur through direct contact with an infected patient's blood, urine, or pharyngeal secretions. If possible, patients with severe disease and bleeding should be placed in a negative-pressure room and all personnel should wear protective gear with P3 filters for respiratory protection. High-risk contacts are associated with percutaneous or mucosal contact with blood or body fluids. Medium-risk contacts (unprotected contact with blood or body fluids) may safely be observed for development of persistent high fever for 3 weeks from the last date of contact by daily temperature measurement and telephone reporting.

Ribavirin postexposure prophylaxis

There are no evidence-based data to support oral ribavirin as postexposure prophylaxis, but, anecdotally, a German physician seroconverted asymptomatically under ribavirin prophylaxis after examining a coughing Lassa fever patient without respiratory protection and gloves (medium-risk contact). Prophylaxis should be given to high-risk contacts of Lassa fever and South American haemorrhagic fever patients, and offered to medium-risk contacts of Lassa fever patients on an individual basis. One recommended dosage is 600 mg orally four times a day for 10 days. Temporary side effects of this regimen were skin rash, tachycardia, myalgia, diarrhoea, and abdominal pain. In one case, there may have been an association between ribavirin and worsening of a pre-existing tachyarrhythmia. Among 16 people there were reversible increases in plasma bilirubin concentrations in 11 and a decrease in haemoglobin concentration in 9. One person stopped prophylaxis after 4 days because of jaundice, and in another the serum lipase concentration increased.

Vaccines

Experimental vaccines based on different viral vector systems have protected against lethal challenge with LASV in animal models, but are far from licensure. A live attenuated vaccine (candid No. 1) against JUNV is licensed in Argentina and produced by the Maiztegui Institute, Pergamino. It was tested in over 200 000 volunteers, showed an estimated effectiveness of 95.5%, and may be cross-protective against Machupo virus only. The Salk Institute, Swiftwater, PA, also produced some quantities of the vaccine, which has an investigational new drug (IND) status from the United States Food and Drug Administration for high-risk populations.

Clinical features

Lassa fever

The clinical picture of Lassa fever is highly variable and may be very difficult to distinguish from other febrile infections. Following an incubation period of 7 to 21 days, Lassa fever begins insidiously with fever, weakness, malaise, severe usually frontal headache, and a painful sore throat. One-half of patients develop joint and lumbar pain and a nonproductive cough. Severe retrosternal chest pain, nausea with vomiting or diarrhoea, and abdominal pain are also common. Respiration rate, pulse rate, and temperature are elevated and blood pressure may be low. There is no characteristic

rash; petechiae and ecchymoses are not seen. About one-third of patients will have conjunctivitis. More than two-thirds of patients have pharyngitis, one-half with exudates; the posterior pharynx and tonsils are diffusely inflamed and swollen, but there are few ulcers or petechiae (Fig. 5.17.1). The abdomen is tender in one-half of the patients. Neurological signs in the early stages are limited to a fine tremor, most marked in the lips and tongue. Thirty per cent of patients progress to a prostrating illness 6 to 8 days after onset of fever, usually with persistent vomiting and diarrhoea. Patients are often dehydrated with elevated haematocrit. Proteinuria occurs in two-thirds of patients, with moderately elevated blood urea nitrogen. About one-half of Lassa fever patients have diffuse abdominal tenderness without localizing signs or loss of bowel sounds. The severe retrosternal or epigastric pain seen in many patients may be due to pleural or pericardial involvement. Facial and conjunctival swelling develop, and severe pulmonary oedema and adult respiratory distress syndrome are common in fatal cases, with gross head and neck oedema, stridor, and hypovolaemic shock (Fig. 5.17.2a,b). Renal and hepatic failure are not seen. Bleeding is seen in only 15 to 20% of patients and is restricted to mucosal surfaces, conjunctiva, and gastrointestinal and/or genital tracts. Over 70% of patients have abnormal electrocardiograms (nonspecific ST-segment and T-wave abnormalities, ST-segment elevation, generalized low voltage complexes, and changes reflecting electrolyte disturbance), but none correlate with disease severity or outcome. There is no clinical evidence of myocarditis. Neurological signs are infrequent but carry a poor prognosis; they progress from confusion to severe encephalopathy with or without general seizures and without focal signs (Fig. 5.17.3). There has been a report of an imported fatal Lassa fever case presenting with only neurological symptoms. Cerebrospinal fluid is usually normal, apart from a few lymphocytes. Pneumonitis and pleural and pericardial rubs develop in early convalescence in about 20% of hospitalized patients, sometimes associated with congestive cardiac failure.

Lassa virus is present in the breast milk of infected mothers, and neonates are therefore at risk of congenital, intrapartum, and

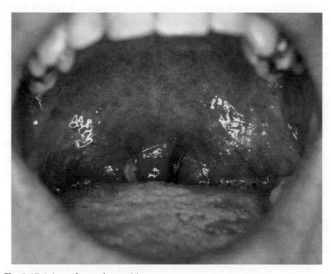

Fig. 5.17.1 Lassa fever: pharyngitis.
(Copyright D A Warrell.)

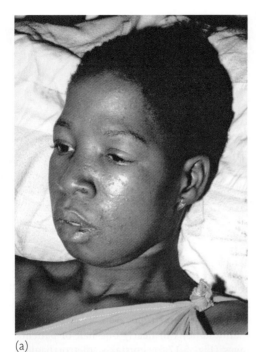

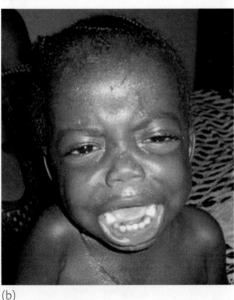

(a)

(b)

Fig. 5.17.2 (a) Lassa fever: facial and generalized oedema and hypovolaemic shock in a pregnant woman in Sierra Leone.
(Copyright D A Warrell.)
(b) Lassa fever: facial oedema in a child.
(Courtesy of Dr S Mardel.)

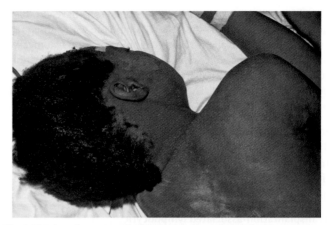

Fig. 5.17.3 Lassa fever: generalized oedema and encephalopathy in a pregnant woman in Sierra Leone.
(Copyright D A Warrell.)

puerperal infection. Lassa fever may be difficult to diagnose in children. In very young babies marked oedema has been reported.

Laboratory findings

A normal mean white blood cell count on admission to hospital (6×10^9/litre) may mask early lymphopenia with later relative or absolute neutrophilia as high as 30×10^9/litre. Thrombocytopenia is moderate, even in severely ill patients, but platelet function is markedly depressed. The ratio of aspartate aminotransferase (AST, SGOT) to alanine aminotransferase (ALT, SGPT) is as high as 11:1. Prothrombin times, glucose, and bilirubin levels are nearly normal, excluding biochemical hepatic failure. Platelet and fibrinogen turnover are normal and there is no indication of disseminated intravascular coagulopathy.

Complications and sequelae

Nearly 30% of patients develop unilateral or bilateral deafness beginning during convalescence. About one-half show a near or complete recovery after 3 to 4 months, but the other one-half remain permanently deaf. Many patients also show transient cerebellar signs during convalescence, particularly tremors and ataxia. Other complications include uveitis, pericarditis, orchitis, pleural effusion, ascites, and acute adrenal insufficiency.

Prognosis

The case fatality rate of hospitalized patients in West Africa is approximately 15%, but it exceeds 50% in patients with haemorrhage. CNS manifestations carry a poor prognosis. Lassa fever is a common cause of maternal mortality in parts of West Africa. Mortality is 20% in the first trimester and 30% in the second trimester of pregnancy, with fetal loss occurring in 87%, apparently not varying with the trimester. Mortality was reduced fourfold in women who spontaneously or were therapeutically aborted.

High viral titre in serum (exceeding 10^4 TCID$_{50}$/ml), AST (SGOT) raised above 150 U/litre, and bleeding, each worsen the prognosis, with the combination of high viral titres and high AST (SGOT) carrying a risk of death of approximately 80%. High neutrophil counts (more than 30×10^9/litre) may be observed in these patients.

In most patients with imported Lassa fever treated in developed countries, diagnosis and ribavirin therapy have often been delayed, and the patients have died despite full supportive care.

Lymphocytic choriomeningitis virus infection

An influenza-like illness is the most common clinical presentation of LCMV. Fever (up to 40°C) with rigors is always present. Frequently noted are malaise, retro-orbital headache, photophobia, lumbar myalgias, anorexia, nausea, bradycardia, and pharyngeal injection without exudate. Mild nontender cervical or axillary lymphadenopathy may occur. Up to 50% of patients have vomiting, sore throat, and dysaesthesias, and one-quarter of patients complain of chest pains and cough, associated with pneumonitis. Arthritis, parotitis, orchitis, myocarditis, rash, and alopecia have also been noted. In some patients, the disease is biphasic with subsequent aseptic meningitis of about 1 week's duration or encephalomyelitis in a smaller number of cases. Other neurological manifestations such as myelitis, Guillain–Barré syndrome, and sensorineural deafness have been reported. The onset of CNS disease may also occur without any prodrome.

Intrauterine infection

This has resulted in nonobstructive hydrocephalus with periventricular calcifications, chorioretinitis, and psychomotor retardation. No cardiac abnormalities were observed. Some mothers had a history of febrile illness during pregnancy.

Transplantation-associated lymphocytic choriomeningitis virus infection

In two clusters of cases, the solid organ transplant recipients had abdominal pain, altered mental status, thrombocytopenia, elevated aminotransferase levels, coagulopathy, graft dysfunction, and either fever or leukocytosis within 3 weeks after transplantation. Diarrhoea, peri-incisional rash, renal failure, and seizures were variably present. Seven of the eight recipients died 9 to 76 days after transplantation.

Prognosis

Patients with aseptic meningitis almost always recover without sequelae, but 25 to 30% of patients with encephalitis have neurological residua.

South American haemorrhagic fevers

In Argentine and Bolivian haemorrhagic fevers, after an incubation period of 7 to 16 days, there is insidious development of malaise, chills, fever, severe myalgia, anorexia, lumbar pain, epigastric pain, abdominal tenderness, conjunctivitis, retro-orbital pain often with photophobia, and constipation. Nausea and vomiting occur frequently after 2 or 3 days of illness. There is no lymphadenopathy, splenomegaly, sore throat, or cough, but there is high fever (up to 40°C), marked erythema of the face, neck, and thorax, and conjunctivitis (Fig. 5.17.4). Respiratory symptoms are uncommon. Petechiae appear by the fourth or fifth day of the illness. There may be

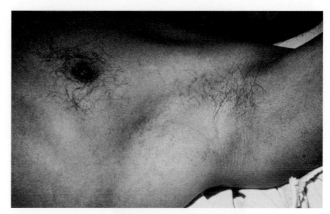

Fig. 5.17.5 Argentine haemorrhagic fever: petechial haemorrhages. (Courtesy of Professor D I H Simpson.)

a pharyngeal enanthema, but pharyngitis is uncommon. The infection either resolves after about 6 days or progresses to severe disease.

South American haemorrhagic fevers are associated with haemorrhagic manifestations in nearly one-half of patients: gingival haemorrhages (Fig. 5.17.5), epistaxis, metrorrhagia, petechiae (Fig. 5.17.6), ecchymoses, purpura, melaena, and haematuria. Severe cases have nausea, vomiting, intense proteinuria, microscopic haematuria, oliguria, and uraemia. Fatal cases develop hypotensive shock, hypothermia, and pulmonary oedema. Renal failure has been reported but glomerular filtration rates, renal plasma flow, and creatinine clearance are usually normal. There is some electrocardiographic evidence of myocarditis. Fifty per cent of patients have neurological symptoms during the second stage of illness, such as tremors of the hands and tongue, progressing in some patients to delirium, oculogyration, and strabismus. Meningeal signs and cerebrospinal fluid abnormalities are rare.

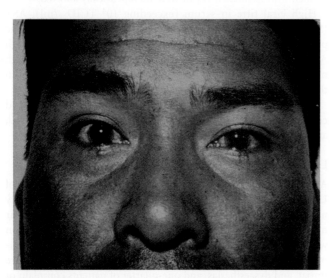

Fig. 5.17.4 Argentine haemorrhagic fever: facial swelling and erythema. (Courtesy of Professor D I H Simpson.)

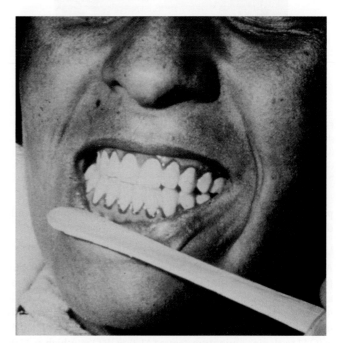

Fig. 5.17.6 Argentine haemorrhagic fever: gingival bleeding. (Courtesy of Professor D I H Simpson.)

The clinical presentation of Venezuelan haemorrhagic fever is similar. Patients are toxic and usually dehydrated, with pharyngitis, conjunctivitis, cervical lymphadenopathy, facial oedema, or petechiae.

Laboratory findings

Thrombocytopenia (below 150×10^9/litre) and neutropenia (range 0.8–6.6×10^9/litre) are almost invariable. Bleeding and clot retraction times are concomitantly prolonged. Although reductions of levels of factors II, V, VII, VIII, and X and of fibrinogen are observed, alterations in clotting functions are usually minor and full-blown disseminated intravascular coagulopathy is not a feature.

Complications and sequelae

A late neurological syndrome in about 10% of cases, consisting mainly of cerebellar signs, is associated with treatment using high titre antiserum. Among survivors of South American haemorrhagic fevers, convalescence typically takes 1 to 3 months, with weight loss, fatigue, autonomic instability, and occasional hair loss. Mild permanent damage to acoustic centres has been detected in a small group of patients.

Prognosis

In endemic areas, the case fatality rate of Argentine haemorrhagic fever is 15 to 30% for untreated hospitalized patients and 1% for patients who received plasma therapy. CNS manifestations carry a poor prognosis. The case fatality rate of Bolivian haemorrhagic fever is higher. In one series of hospitalized patients with Venezuelan haemorrhagic fever, the case fatality rate was reported to be 33% despite vigorous supportive care. Argentine haemorrhagic fever is reported to be severe in pregnancy.

Whitewater Arroyo-like virus

Illnesses were associated with nonspecific febrile symptoms including fever, headache, and myalgias. Within the first week of hospitalization, lymphopenia was observed in all three patients, and thrombocytopenia (30–40×10^9/litre) was seen in two. All three patients had acute respiratory distress syndrome and two developed liver failure and haemorrhagic manifestations. All patients died 1 to 8 weeks after becoming unwell.

Criteria for diagnosis and differential diagnosis

Due to the variable clinical presentation of arenavirus infections, the diseases should be suspected in any patient presenting with a severe febrile illness and evidence of vascular involvement (low blood pressure, postural hypotension, petechiae, haemorrhagic diathesis, flushing of face and chest, nondependent oedema). Sore throat, abdominal symptoms, and CNS symptoms are likewise important. For many regions in the world, the major differential diagnose is malaria.

Lassa fever

Lassa fever should be suspected in a patient living in or coming within the incubation period (7–21 days) from rural areas in Sierra Leone, Liberia, Nigeria, the Republic of Guinea, and adjacent territories, and presenting with otherwise unexplained high fever (above 38.5°C), pharyngitis with dry cough and chest pain or abdominal pain and diarrhoea, facial oedema, mucosal bleeding, or CNS symptoms. In West Africa, fever with pharyngitis, proteinuria, and retrosternal chest pain had a predictive value for Lassa fever of 81% and a specificity of 89%. Due to the variable clinical picture of Lassa fever, there are many differential diagnoses including severe malaria, typhoid fever, rickettsial diseases, relapsing fevers, shigellosis, leptospirosis, meningococcaemia, and gram-negative sepsis. Viral haemorrhagic fevers such as yellow fever, Rift Valley fever, and Marburg and Ebola virus infections are much more likely to cause haemorrhage, disseminated intravascular coagulopathy, and severe liver dysfunction than Lassa fever.

South American haemorrhagic fevers

These should be considered in patients coming from endemic areas of Argentina (particularly male agricultural workers), Bolivia, Venezuela, and Brazil who present with unexplained fever and a bleeding diathesis. Differential diagnoses are similar to those for Lassa fever and, in addition, yellow fever and dengue fever must be considered. Appearance of the blanching maculopapular rash and a shorter duration of fever differentiate dengue from the early stages of arenavirus infections.

The combination of a platelet count of less than 100×10^9/litre and a white blood cell count of less than 2.5×10^9/litre has a sensitivity of 87% and a specificity of 88% for Argentine haemorrhagic fever. These criteria are recommended when screening Argentine haemorrhagic fever patients for treatment with immune plasma or ribavirin in endemic areas.

LCMV infection should be considered in patients presenting in autumn or winter with a biphasic disease characterized by fever and persistent meningeal signs, particularly if there is a history of rodent contact. Other rat bite fevers (Chapter 6.31) enter the differential diagnosis.

Laboratory diagnosis

Laboratory diagnosis of arenavirus infection is by isolation of virus from serum, demonstration of a fourfold rise in antibody titre, or high-titre IgG antibody with virus-specific IgM antibody in association with compatible clinical disease. More recently, detection of viral sequences by reverse transcriptase–polymerase chain reaction (RT-PCR), or by detection of viral proteins using an enzyme-linked immunosorbent assay (ELISA) system have been introduced.

For handling of clinical specimens from suspected cases, see Table 5.17.1.

Treatment

Lassa fever

Ribavirin is effective but must be given as early as possible while laboratory confirmation of the diagnosis is pending. It is administered by intravenous infusion as a 2-g loading dose followed by 1 g every 6 h for 4 days then 0.5 g every 8 h for 6 more days. Another recommended intravenous regimen is an initial dose of 30 mg/kg followed by 15 mg/kg every 6 h for 4 days, followed by 7.5 mg/kg every 8 h for 6 days. Rigors may occur if the drug is infused too rapidly. Oral ribavirin doses are a 2-g loading dose followed by 4 g/day in four divided doses for 4 days followed by 2 g/day for six doses. Oral ribavirin is believed to be only half as effective as intravenous therapy. A five- to tenfold decrease in the case–fatality ratio was demonstrated in patients treated with ribavirin compared to untreated patients when therapy was given within the first 6 days

Table 5.17.1 Inactivation of blood/serum from viral haemorrhagic fever patients for laboratory analysis

Material	Examination	Inactivation
Blood	Thick film	Add formalin to a final concentration of 1% to solution used for lysis of erythrocytes
Blood	Thin film	Methanol fixation
Blood	Leucocyte count	1:100 in 3% acetic acid, 15 min room temperature
Serum/plasma	Serological tests	Heat for 60 min at 60°C[a]
		0.25% β-propiolactone (final concentration), 30 min 37°C
Serum/plasma	Clinical chemistry	Heat for 60 min at 60°C[b]
		0.25% β-propiolactone (final concentration), 30 min 37°C[c]
		0.1% Triton X-100 (final concentration), 60 min room temperature[d]

[a] Loss of reactivity. Heating at 56°C for 1 h preserves antibody reactivity better but leaves sample with residual infectivity. Only recommended if sample can be safely handled in biological safety level 2 cabinet (laminar air flow).

[b] No influence on sodium, potassium, magnesium, urea, creatinine, urate, bilirubin, glucose, C-reactive protein. Reduced levels of bicarbonate, aspartate aminotransferase, calcium, phosphate, albumin, total protein. Measurement not possible for alkaline phosphatase, alanine aminotransferase, γ-glutamyl transpeptidase, creatine kinase.

[c] Liver enzyme values reduced by 20%. pH and bicarbonate not useful.

[d] Influence on clinical chemistry not evaluated.

of illness. Patients with high AST (SGOT) and viraemia, who were treated within the first 6 days of illness, had a 5 to 9% case fatality, and a 26 to 47% fatality when treated after 6 days, compared with 52 to 78% when untreated. Ribavirin is contraindicated in early pregnancy because of potential teratogenicity, but the fetus rarely survives the infection. Fluid, electrolyte, respiratory, and osmotic imbalances should be corrected, and full intensive care support, including mechanical ventilation, offered as required. However, even vigorous support may be insufficient to prevent fatal progression of advanced disease.

Interferon-α has shown efficacy against arenaviruses in animal models but only if given within a couple of days of challenge. A synergistic effect with suboptimal doses of ribavirin was observed.

Lymphocytic choriomeningitis virus infection

Ribavirin treatment has not been evaluated in human CNS disease caused by LCMV. In a cluster of transplantation-associated systemic LCMV infections, one recipient, who received ribavirin and reduced levels of immunosuppressive therapy, survived.

South American haemorrhagic fevers

Convalescent-phase plasma has been shown to be highly successful in Argentine haemorrhagic fever, reducing the mortality from 15 to 30% to 1% in patients treated in the first 8 days of illness. Efficacy is directly related to the concentration of neutralizing antibodies, and delayed treatment is less successful. Availability of appropriately screened plasma may, however, be a problem. Ribavirin is effective against the causative JUNV in experimentally infected primates, but does not prevent CNS involvement. In one small double-blind trial with 18 patients, mortality was 12.5% in those treated compared to 40% in the placebo group. One human case of Bolivian haemorrhagic fever has been successfully treated with ribavirin and Venezuelan haemorrhagic fever is also likely to respond.

Other issues

Lassa fever is a truly neglected re-emerging disease that has a considerable impact on West African health care systems and the economy of affected rural areas. The absence of local diagnostic capacity and the high price of intravenous ribavirin preparations are the main barriers to the introduction of specific therapy to endemic areas.

Areas of uncertainty or controversy

The pathogenic events leading to plasma leakage, bleeding, and shock are not well understood in arenavirus infections, compared to filoviruses. A lack of understanding of the inhibition of neutralizing antibody responses is the main hurdle to the development of a Lassa fever vaccine.

Likely developments in the near future

Candid No. 1 is likely to be licensed in the United States of America. The novel pyrazine derivative favipiravir (T-705, Toyama Chemical Company Ltd), which is currently in phase II trials for the treatment of seasonal influenza, has demonstrated broad-spectrum activity in preclinical investigations against a number of RNA viruses, including several arenaviruses (Junin, Machupo, Guanarito).

Further reading

Bonthius DJ, et al. (2007). Congenital lymphocytic choriomeningitis virus infection: spectrum of disease. Ann Neurol, 62, 347–55.

Fischer SA, et al. (2006). LCMV in transplant recipients. Transmission of lymphocytic choriomeningitis virus by organ transplantation. N Engl J Med, 354, 2235–49.

Geisbert TW, et al. (2005). Development of a new vaccine for the prevention of Lassa fever. PLoS Med, 2, e183.

Günther S, Lenz O (2004). Lassa virus. Crit Rev Clin Lab Sci, 41, 339–90.

McCormick JB, et al. (1986). Lassa fever. Effective therapy with ribavirin. N Engl J Med, 314, 20–6.

McCormick JB, et al. (1987). A case-control study of the clinical diagnosis and course of Lassa fever. J Infect Dis, 155, 445–55.

Mendenhall M, et al. (2011). T-705 (favipiravir) inhibition of arenavirus replication in cell culture. Antimicrob Agents Chemother 55, 782–7.

5.18 Filoviruses

J. ter Meulen

Essentials

Filoviruses are large RNA viruses, of which Ebola virus and Marburg virus cause the most severe forms of viral haemorrhagic fever and have been best-studied because of fear of their misuse as bioterrorism agents. These are zoonotic viruses with reservoirs, most likely fruit-eating bats, in the rainforests of tropical Africa, where they cause sporadic infections and outbreaks among great apes and humans.

Epidemiology—the primary mode of transmission of Ebola virus to humans often involves contact of hunters with dead animals, especially chimpanzees, whose meat is consumed as 'bush meat'; contact with bats has been implicated for Marburg virus. However, the viruses are highly infectious and are transmitted from the index case and subsequently from person to person by all body fluids, including sweat and respiratory droplets.

Clinical features—Ebola haemorrhagic fever is clinically indistinguishable from Marburg haemorrhagic fever. Presentation is with an influenza-like illness, often with gastrointestinal symptoms, followed by development of a maculopapular rash and haemorrhagic manifestations including epistaxis, gum bleeding, haematemesis, melaena, petechiae, and ecchymoses. There is no specific treatment, although recombinant activated protein C (Drotrecogin α) and the investigational anticoagulant rNAPc2 have reduced mortality by 20 to 30% in animal models. Mortality is 50 to 90%.

Diagnosis and prevention—viral haemorrhagic fever is a clinical diagnosis which requires the immediate instalment of the strictest barrier nursing procedures and notification of public health authorities. Care must be taken in both drawing and handling blood specimens, which must be inactivated before performing routine laboratory tests, and samples must be shipped immediately to a reference laboratory for diagnosis by detection of virus by cell culture, viral antigen by ELISA, and viral RNA by PCR. A prophylactic vaccine based on a replication-deficient adenoviral vector is in clinical development.

Introduction

Filoviruses are large, enveloped, negative-stranded, nonsegmented RNA viruses with a characteristic thread-like morphology, hence the family name *Filoviridae* (Latin *filum* = thread). Ebola viruses (EBOV), comprising three genetically distinct species from Côte d'Ivoire, the Democratic Republic of the Congo (DRC, formerly Zaire), and Sudan, and Marburg virus (MARV), cause the most severe forms of viral haemorrhagic fever (VHF). They are now among the best-studied agents of these diseases, mainly because of fear of their misuse as bioterrorism agents (Oxford Textbook of Medicine 5e Chapter 9.5.13). The first appearance of these viruses was in Marburg in 1967, when laboratory, medical, and animal care personnel exposed to tissues and blood from African Green monkeys (*Cercopithecus aethiops*) were infected. In 1976 and 1979, epidemics of a haemorrhagic disease with very high mortality in northern DRC (then Zaire) and in southern Sudan were found to be due to two strains of a related filoviruses, named Ebola virus. Over the next 10 years, rare, sporadic cases of filovirus infections in Africa were the only continuing evidence of the existence of these viruses. Another species of the virus, Ebola virus Reston (EBOv-R), was imported on four occasions between 1989 and 1996 with wild-caught monkeys (*Macaca fascicularis*) from Mindanao, Republic of the Philippines, to animal facilities in the United States of America and Italy. This virus, which is highly lethal for monkeys, has caused asymptomatic infections in animal keepers. Since 1990, both Ebola and Marburg viruses have re-emerged across tropical Africa between latitudes 5° north and 5° south, causing several devastating epidemics.

In total, 18 instances of human Ebola haemorrhagic fever (EHF) have been recorded in Côte d'Ivoire, in the DRC, Gabon, Sudan, and northern Uganda. The outbreaks varied in size from 17 to 425 cases totalling 1880 cases, of which 1302 were fatal. The largest outbreak of Ebola virus disease so far (caused by EBOV Sudan) occurred in 2000 in Gulu, Uganda. There were 425 cases with a case fatality of 53%. Until 2007, Marburg virus cases totalled 567 with 467 fatalities. Outbreaks varied in size from 3 to 374, the largest in Uige, Angola where MARV appeared for the first time in 2005.

Aetiology, genetics, pathogenesis, and pathology

Filovirus infections are characterized by massive, unchecked, and destructive replication of virus in several organs, profound immunosuppression due to infection of immune cells and apoptosis of infected and noninfected cells, and triggering of a cascade of immune-mediated mechanisms resulting in a cytokine storm, endothelial damage, and coagulopathy culminating in shock and organ failure. The immunological and pathological aspects in endstage filoviral disease resemble, in several aspects, those of bacterial sepsis.

Through minute lesions in the skin and mucosa, the pantropic filoviruses infect initially dendritic cells, monocytes, and macrophages. Lymphocytes are spared from the infection. EBOV and MARV infected dendritic cells fail to mature to the antigen-presenting stage and do not produce proinflammatory cytokines required for activation of natural killer cells and T cells. At the molecular level, the expression of viral proteins interferes with the production of interferon-α (IFN-α) and β, and with the ability of these and IFN-γ to induce an antiviral state in cells. Dendritic cells show no increase in costimulatory molecules such as CD40, CD86, and interleukin 12 (IL-12). The early immune response dysfunction originating in dendritic cells is aggravated by continued replication of filoviruses in monocytes and macrophages, accompanied by the secretion of noninhibited proinflammatory cytokines and activation of polymorphonuclear leucocytes. This accumulated release of proinflammatory mediators culminates in a 'cytokine storm', causing thrombocytopenia and endothelial injury, e.g. through the action of tumor necrosis factor-α (TNFα). Fatal human Ebola cases showed a marked elevation of serum levels of IFN-γ, IL-2, and IL-10, whereas elevated IFN-α, TNFα, and IL-6 were associated with fatalities in some, but not all, studies. Increased blood levels of nitric oxide, which has been shown to contribute to hypotension, cardiodepression, and vascular hyporeactivity in sepsis, were also found to be associated with mortality. The likely reason for the variations of cytokine and chemokine release observed *in vivo*, as well as in experimentally infected primary human cells, is currently unknown genetic differences of the host. One study reported that HLA-B*07 and HLA-B*14 alleles were associated with survival, whereas HLA-B*67 and HLA-B*15 were associated with lethality in EBOV-infected patients. Both humans and experimentally infected nonhuman primates show massive apoptotic death of noninfected CD4+, CD8+, and NK cells in the blood and peripheral lymph nodes, a phenomenon which has been termed 'bystander apoptosis'. Lymphocyte apoptosis was thought to be responsible for an elimination of adaptive immune responses; however, studies in transgenic mice have not confirmed it as a major factor in the pathogenesis of disease. In addition, there appears to be also massive apoptotic death of infected macrophages.

The expression of tissue factor is up-regulated in infected monocytes and triggers the extrinsic pathway of coagulation. The procoagulant state amplifies the production of proinflammatory cytokines and the development of vascular leakage, which further provokes activation of coagulopathy. The terminal stage of the disease is therefore characterized by plasma leakage, disseminated intravascular coagulopathy, and bleeding. It is thought that triggering the above outlined cascade of events is more critical to the development of the observed pathology than direct organ damage due to cytopathic virus replication. However, infection of the liver and adrenal glands impairs the synthesis of clotting factors and steroids, thus aggravating hemorrhage and shock. Whether infection of endothelial cells contributes to the overall pathology remains controversial.

At autopsy, both Marburg and Ebola infected humans and primates show widespread haemorrhagic diathesis of skin, membranes, and soft tissue. Extensive necrosis with little infiltration is seen in parenchymal cells of many organs, including liver, spleen, kidneys, and gonads. The most characteristic histopathological features are seen in the liver. Large disseminated deposits of viral antigen can be found in different organs, including the sweat glands and the skin. Virus is also detectable in pneumocytes and as cell-free virions in the alveoli.

Spleen and lymph nodes show various degrees of lymphoid depletion with extensive vascular follicular necrosis. Fatal infection is marked by absence of specific IgG and presence of low levels of specific IgM in only 30% of cases, whereas in human survivors early and increasing levels of Ebola-specific IgM and IgG is followed by activation of cytotoxic T cells. During two outbreaks in Gabon, asymptomatic seroconversion with PCR-proven infection occurred in several people who mounted an early, strong but transient inflammatory response, with high levels of proinflammatory cytokines. This unexpected observation and data from animal models suggest that a tightly controlled, transient early type I IFN and proinflammatory cytokine response is able to induce protective antiviral innate and adaptive immune responses.

The recent successful immunization against EHF in animal models revealed that protection is clearly mediated by cellular immunity, because CD8+ T-cell depletion abrogated vaccine protection in nonhuman primates. Neutralizing antibodies are found neither in natural infection nor after immunization. However, antibodies may contribute to protection by non-neutralizing mechanisms.

Epidemiology

Central African nonhuman primates and monkeys are victims of EBOV, as are other animals such as bushpigs, porcupines, and antelopes living in the tropical rainforest. Data from wildlife surveillance show that epizootics occur more often than previously thought and that EBOV has caused massive die-offs of gorillas and chimpanzees. Phylogenetic analysis of the viruses further suggests that the outbreaks are epidemiologically linked and that EBOV, strain Zaire (EBOV-Z), has spread south-westward since 1976 in a wave-like manner from Yambuku, its site of appearance in the DRC, to the Republic of the Congo and to Gabon at a speed of approximately 50 km per year. This argues against the hypothesis that EBOV-Z was resident, but undetected, in the central African forest block before the mid 1970s. Evidence has now accumulated that fruit-eating bats (*Hypsignathus monstrosus*, *Epomops franqueti*, *Myonycteris torquata* and others) are one, but possibly not the primary, natural reservoir of EBOV, and hunting of bats for human consumption has been linked to an EBOV outbreak in DRC in 2007. Recently, EBOV Reston was detected in domestic swine in the Philippines and a few asymptomatic human infections were reported. The pathogenicity of the virus for these animals and their possible role in a transmission cycle are currently not known.

The primary mode of transmission of EBOV to humans often involves contact of hunters with dead animals, especially chimpanzees, whose meat is consumed as 'bush meat'. In several outbreaks, however, the mode of infection of the index case could not be elucidated. The index cases usually transmit the virus to caring family members, often women, who come into contact with blood and body fluids. These are highly infectious, so that the average rate of secondary cases generated from the index case is around 10 to 20%, but may be considerably higher. Occasionally, the virus has been spread through sexual contact. Nosocomial spread through improperly sterilized reusable syringes or other medical equipment has caused explosive Ebola epidemics in Sudan and the Democratic Republic of the Congo. The mortality among surgical staff operating on EHF patients misdiagnosed as having acute abdominal conditions was also extremely high. Nursing activities and preparing the corpse for burial carry a high risk of infection, as do burial practices which include touching of the corpse and collectively washing hands in a common bowel thereafter. There is no epidemiological evidence that Ebola or Marburg viruses are transmitted as true, small particle aerosols between humans. However, direct mucosal exposure to droplets generated by a patient during coughing poses a considerable risk of infection.

MARV epidemiology is similar to that of EBOV. Evidence of infection has been detected in fruit-eating bats (*Rousettus aegyptiacus*) from Uganda and Kenya, and in insectivorous bats in DRC (*Miniopterus inflatus*, *Rhinolophus elocuens*). However, epizootics have not been observed in mammals. Contact with bats during mining activities was reported for several index cases of Marburg haemorrhagic fever (MHF), in accordance with cave roosting of *R. aegyptiacus*, a habit that is not observed in the bat species implicated in EBOV transmission. Until 2000, the viral origins of cases could be traced to eastern Africa. However, in 2005 the largest outbreak of MHF occurred in Uige, Angola, expanding the known range of the disease to the far western edge of the Congo basin. Continuing population movements in central Africa, destruction of the rainforest, and increased consumption of 'bush meat' increase the likelihood of future filovirus outbreaks. In 2008 a fatal and a nonfatal case of Marburg haemorrhagic fever occurred in the Netherlands and the United States of America, respectively, imported by tourists who had visited a bat-roosting cave in Uganda (Python cave, Queen Elizabeth park). Touching bat excrements or being hit by low-flying bats were identified as possible risk factors for acquisition of the infection. Recently, a genetically distinct filovirus was discovered in Spain in dead insectivorous bats (*Miniopterus schreibersii*) and named Lloviu virus. There is currently no evidence of human infections with this virus.

Prevention

In endemic areas, avoidance of contact with bats and their excrements, with dead and diseased monkeys, and control of monkey sellers are currently the only feasible options for prevention. In case of outbreaks, interruption of person-to-person spread of the virus is essential for control. Early institution of safe and orderly care of the ill, using barrier nursing and disinfection procedures, should be set up with effective surveillance of high-risk contacts and prompt isolation of further cases (barrier nursing, guidelines from the CDC and WHO, see Chapter 5.17, Box 5.17.1). In fully equipped hospitals, patients must be placed in negative-pressure rooms and all personnel must wear protective gear with P3 filters for respiratory protection. Cutaneous or mucosal contact with blood or body fluids from an Ebola patient poses a high risk. Contacts must be followed up for development of persistent high fever for 3 weeks from the last date of contact by daily temperature measurement.

Development of vaccines against filoviruses has recently made astonishing progress, after decades of futile efforts. The first effective vaccine protocol against EBOV in nonhuman primates was based on a prime/boost regimen, expressing the viral nucleoprotein (NP) and glycoprotein (GP) from a plasmid (DNA immunization) and a recombinant, replication-deficient adenovirus, serotype 5 (Ad5). This vector has the advantage of having been tested extensively in humans and found to be safe. Subsequently, a protocol was developed in which a single shot of Ad5-GP given 4 weeks before challenge with 1000 infectious EBOV particles conferred 100% protection in nonhuman primates. This vaccine is currently in clinical trials performed by the National Institutes of Health, United States of America, and may be licensable within a few years. However, Ad5 vectors have the drawback of facing a high level of pre-existing neutralizing antibodies in the general population, which may impede the induction of anti-EBOV immunity. Prime/boost schemes will be required to overcome this problem. The latest amazing finding was that replication-competent vesicular stomatitis virus expressing the EBOV-GP could protect 50% of nonhuman primates when given 30 min after a lethal challenge, making it an ideal postexposure vaccine for health care workers. However, clinical development of this viral vector system faces higher regulatory hurdles, because it has so far not been evaluated in humans. Recently, an experimental preparation of the vaccine was given as a postexposure prophylaxis to a German researcher after a possibly EBOV contaminated needle-stick injury. No severe systemic side effects of the vaccination were reported.

Protection against MARV infection in animal models has been much easier to achieve using a variety of vaccines, including recombinant proteins, than against EBOV. This is probably due to the slightly slower replication of the virus in these models. A vaccine is likely to enter clinical trials soon.

Clinical features

MARV and EBOV cause identical clinical diseases. After an incubation period of 5 to 12 days, the disease starts suddenly with fever, headache, myalgia, and extreme fatigue. Early signs also include conjunctivitis, bradycardia, and sore throat, often associated with severe swelling and dysphagia, but no exudative pharyngitis. Severe nausea,

Fig. 5.18.1 Rash of Ebola haemorrhagic fever acquired through a laboratory accident.
(Courtesy of Professor D I H Simpson.)

vomiting, abdominal pain, and profuse watery diarrhoea are common. Around the fifth day, a perifollicular, nonitching, maculopapular rash frequently appears on the trunk, back, and shoulders, spreading to the face and limbs and becoming confluent (Fig. 5.18.1). It may be difficult to see and has a measles-like appearance on dark skin. The rash fades in 3 to 10 days and is followed by a desquamation in survivors. In about half of the patients, haemorrhagic manifestations occur between the fifth and seventh day, including epistaxis, gum-bleeding, haematemesis (Fig. 5.18.2), melaena, petechiae, ecchymoses (Fig. 5.18.3), haemorrhages from needlesticks and post-mortem evidence of visceral haemorrhagic effusions. Dehydration and prostration are frequent; patients show the ghost-like facial expression typical of the disease. During the first

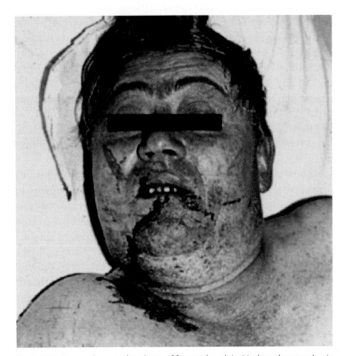

Fig. 5.18.2 Hemorrhage and oedema of face and neck in Marburg haemorrhagic fever.
(Courtesy: Professor S Stille.)

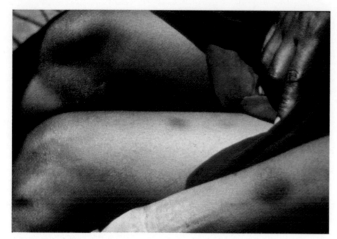

Fig. 5.18.3 Ecchymoses in a patient with Ebola haemorrhagic fever. (Courtesy of Professor D I H Simpson.)

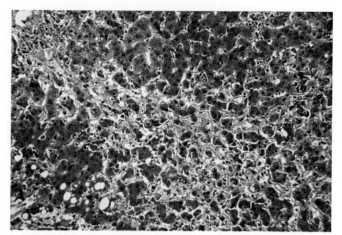

Fig. 5.18.4 Hepatic histology in Ebola haemorrhagic fever. (Courtesy of Professor D I H Simpson.)

week, the temperature remains high around 40°C, falling by lysis during the second week, to rise again between days 12 and 14. Other clinical signs during the second week include hepatosplenomegaly, oedema, orchitis, scrotal or labial reddening, myocarditis, and pancreatitis. Jaundice is not a feature. A poor prognosis is marked by haemorrhagic signs, oliguria or anuria, chest pain, shock, tachypnoea, and neurological symptoms (sudden hearing loss, blindness, painful paresthesia, intractable hiccups). Death in shock usually occurs 6 to 9 days after onset of clinical disease. Infection in pregnancy results in high maternal mortality and virtually 100% fetal death. Central nervous system involvement has led to hemiplegia and disorientation, and sometimes frank psychosis.

The recovery of Marburg and Ebola disease is prolonged with arthralgia or persistent arthritis, ocular disease (ocular pain, photophobia, hyperlacrimation, loss of visual acuity, uveitis), hearing loss and orchitis occurring as late manifestations. Serious but reversible personality changes have been recorded in a few survivors, namely confusion, anxiety, and aggressive behaviour. Blindness has been reported as a sequel.

Marburg virus has been isolated from the anterior chamber of the eye and from seminal fluid 7 weeks after the onset of clinical disease and there has been a documented case of sexual transmission. The shedding of EBOV RNA has been detectable in semen and vaginal fluid by polymerase chain reaction (PCR) for months, but not by virus isolation. Patients should therefore refrain from sexual activities during early reconvalescence.

Haematological studies reveal early leucopenia, thrombocytopenia accompanied by abnormal platelet aggregation, subsequent relative neutrophilia, and the appearance of atypical lymphocytes. Liver enzymes are elevated (AST/SGOT >ALT/SGPT) consistent with histopathological evidence of hepatitis (Fig. 5.18.4), but alkaline phosphatase and bilirubin levels are usually normal or only slightly elevated. Although disseminated intravascular coagulation (DIC) is a prominent manifestation of EBOV infection in primates (prolonged prothrombin (PT) and partial thromboplastin time (PTT), D-dimers, fibrin split products), the presence of DIC in human filoviral infections has been a controversial topic, because logistical problems have hampered systematic studies in the past. However, fibrin deposition has been documented at autopsy, and clinical laboratory data suggest that DIC is likely to be also a prominent feature of human disease. In nonhuman primates, a rapid

decline in plasma protein C levels was observed in EBOV infection, preceding clinical symptoms.

Differential diagnosis and criteria for diagnosis

Clinically, filovirus infections can be confused with nonviral infections such as severe malaria, typhoid fever, shigellosis ('diarrhée rouge' in francophone Africa), leptospirosis, rickettsial diseases, meningococcaemia, Gram-negative sepsis, and other conditions resulting in DIC. There is overlap of clinical presentation with other VHFs. Filovirus HF should be suspected in a patient living in or coming from, within the incubation period, a known endemic area (currently Angola, Côte d'Ivoire, the DRC, Gabon, Sudan, Kenya, and Uganda) and presenting with otherwise unexplained high fever (above 38.5°C) and vascular involvement (subnormal blood pressure, postural hypotension, petechiae, haemorrhagic diathesis, flushing of face and chest, nondependent oedema). Reported contact with another VHF patient or a known VHF vector is obviously a very important risk factor.

Because VHF is a purely clinical diagnosis which requires the immediate instalment of barrier nursing procedures and notification of public health authorities, rapid laboratory confirmation is mandatory. Care must be taken in both drawing and handling blood specimens since virus titre may be extremely high, and the virus is stable for long periods, even at room temperature. During the first week of clinical illness, virus is easily detected by cell culture, viral antigen by enzyme-linked immunoabsorbent assay (ELISA), and viral RNA by PCR, but all methods require specialized equipment. Blood samples have to be handled and shipped to a reference laboratory using special precautions (triple packaging: primary, secondary, and outer container with absorbent material in between) and have to be inactivated for performing routine laboratory tests (Chapter 5.17, Table 5.17.1). In fatal human EBOV cases, antiviral IgM and IgG antibodies were detected in 46% and 30% of patients respectively. ELISA or immunofluorescence can be performed, preferably in paired serum samples. A diagnostic test has been developed based on immunohistochemical detection of abundant filovirus antigen in biopsies. Skin snips taken from the axilla or nape of the neck are fixed with formalin and can be shipped without further safety requirements to reference laboratories.

For handling of clinical specimens from suspected cases, see Chapter 5.17, Table 5.17.1.

Treatment

Conceptually, therapy of EHF and MHF consists of specific antiviral approaches, modulation of the host immune response, and symptomatic treatment. Currently, no specific antiviral therapy is available. The guanosin analogue ribavirin is not effective against filoviruses. Prophylactic treatment of EBOV infection in nonhuman primates with high doses of either polyclonal immune serum, a potent neutralizing human monoclonal antibody (50 mg/kg), or IFN-α2b (2×10^7 IU/kg per day) delayed time to death but did not reduce mortality. However, transfer of convalescent whole blood to EBOV-infected patients protected 8/9 from lethal infection in an uncontrolled study, compared to 20% survival in untreated patients. Experimentally, modulation of the coagulation/inflammation cascade showed some promising results. Treatment with recombinant human activated protein C (continuous perfusion of 48 μg/kg per h drotrecogin-α, on days 0–7) resulted in 18.2% survival and a prolonged time-to-death. Similarly, treatment of nonhuman primates with the recombinant nematode anticoagulant protein c2 (rNAPc2), a potent inhibitor of FVIIa/tissue factor-initiated blood coagulation, by subcutaneous injections of 30 μg/kg bodyweight, administered once daily for up to 14 days after a high-dose lethal injection of Ebola virus, resulted in a 33% survival rate and prolonged survival time.

Fluid, electrolyte, respiratory, and osmotic imbalances should be managed carefully. Patients may require full intensive care support, including mechanical ventilation, along with blood, plasma, or platelet replacement. The maintenance of intravascular volume is a particular challenge, but every effort is justified since the crisis is short lived, and complete recovery can be expected in survivors. Treatment of all concurrent (tropical) infections is important.

Management of an imported EHF or MHF case will therefore require, to a certain degree, experimental therapy, such as the use of investigational drugs for modulation of immune responses and coagulation cascades, which are being evaluated in bacterial sepsis.

Prognosis

The case fatality of filovirus infections is extremely high and possibly dependent on the infecting species, with up to 90% for EBOV Zaire and MARV Angola. Because the lesions in filovirus infections are so widespread and the immune response is so ineffective, it is uncertain whether good supportive care alone has a major effect on the clinical outcome. Despite good clinical care being delivered to the majority of patients during the Ebola outbreak in Uganda in 2000, the overall mortality was not significantly lower than the 50% which would be expected for the Sudan strain of Ebola, which caused the epidemic. Common denominators of survival in filovirus-infected macaques are maintenance of D-dimer levels, maintenance of protein C activity (>50%), maintenance of levels of proinflammatory/procoagulant cytokines, and low viral load.

Areas of uncertainty/controversy

Despite concerted international actions, it has so far neither been possible to implement true standard of care patient treatment during filovirus outbreaks in Africa nor to conduct clinical trials. Therefore, most of the knowledge of the pathogenesis of these diseases and the few available therapeutic data come from experimental infection of nonhuman primates and uncontrolled clinical studies. While the importance of the type I IFN response in controlling filovirus infection is evident, it is unclear what constitutes a protective adaptive immune response either in natural infection or obtained through vaccination. Current data suggest that this may differ between different filoviruses and vaccine platforms.

Likely developments over next 5 to 10 years

The licensing of a recombinant, adenovirus-based EBOV and possibly MARV vaccine is to be expected in the United States of America within 5 years. Combined therapies using antiviral drugs, immune modulators, and anticoagulants will most likely improve survival rates in nonhuman primate models beyond the currently reported 20 to 30%.

Further reading

Bradfute SB, Bavari S. (2011). Correlates of immunity to filovirus infection. *Viruses*, **3**, 982–1000.

Feldmann H, et al. (2007). Effective post-exposure treatment of Ebola infection. *PLoS Pathog*, **3**, e2.

Guenther S, et al. (2011). Management of accidental exposure to Ebola virus in the biosafety level 4 laboratory, Hamburg, Germany. *J Infect Dis*, **204**, S785–90.

Marty AM, Jahrling PB, Geisbert TW. (2006). Viral hemorrhagic fevers. *Clin Lab Med*, **26**, 345–86.

Mohamadzadeh M, Chen L, Schmaljohn AL. (2007). How Ebola and Marburg viruses battle the immune system. *Nat Rev Immunol*, **7**, 556–67.

Rollin PE, et al. (2007). Blood chemistry measurements and D-Dimer levels associated with fatal and nonfatal outcomes in humans infected with Sudan Ebola virus. *J Infect Dis*, **196** Suppl 2, S364–71.

World Health Organization. *Infection control for viral haemorrhagic fevers in the African health care setting* (WHO/EMC/ESR/98.2.). http://www.who.int/csr/resources/publications/ebola/WHO_EMC_ESR_98_2_EN/en/

Zaki SR, et al. (1999). A novel immunohistochemical assay for the detection of Ebola virus in skin: implications for diagnosis, spread, and surveillance of Ebola hemorrhagic fever. *J Infect Dis*, **179** Suppl 1, S36–47.

5.19 Papillomaviruses and polyomaviruses

Raphael P. Viscidi and Keerti V. Shah

Essentials

Papillomaviruses and polyomaviruses are small, nonenveloped, double-stranded DNA viruses.

Human papillomavirus

There are over 100 human papillomavirus (HPV) types that infect epithelia of skin and mucous membranes. They infect only humans, and cause conditions including the following:

Skin warts and verrucas—caused by types 1 and 2; infection initiated when, after e.g. minor skin abrasions, the basal cells of the epithelium come in contact with infectious virus.

Anogenital warts—caused by types 6 and 11; transmitted by direct sexual contact, these are the most common sexually transmitted infection; present clinically as multiple exophytic lesions or as sub-clinical flat lesions. Can be treated topically with podophyllin or imiquimod, or by ablative surgical methods. Recurrences are common. A highly efficacious prophylactic vaccine is available.

Cervical cancer—the second most common tumour in women worldwide; most often caused by types 16 and 18, whose DNA can be recovered from nearly all cases of invasive disease and squamous intraepithelial lesions of the cervix, which precede invasive cancer. Prevention is by cervical screening and vaccination (two highly effective vaccines are available).

Other cancers—HPVs can cause cancers at other lower anogenital tract sites and in the oropharynx. HPV DNA is often detected in nonmelanoma skin cancers, but it is not known whether this is pathogenic.

Respiratory papillomatosis—caused by types 6 and 11; usually involves the vocal cords, leading to presentation with hoarseness or voice change; may rarely cause life-threatening airway obstruction; mainstay of treatment is surgical removal of papillomas, which commonly recur.

Human polyomaviruses

Exposure to polyomaviruses is nearly universal: they cause asymptomatic infection in childhood and then persist as latent infections, primarily in the kidney, producing disease in the context of immunosuppression.

BK virus—can cause (1) nephropathy and renal failure in renal transplant patients; management is by gradual reduction in immunosuppression, but more than 50% of patients lose their allograft; (2) haemorrhagic cystitis in bone marrow transplant patients.

JC virus—causes progressive multifocal leucoencephalopathy, a demyelinating disease of the central nervous system that is usually relentlessly progressive and fatal. Most often seen in patients with HIV/AIDS, but recently reported as a rare complication of treatment with natalizumab in patients with multiple sclerosis or Crohn's disease. Merkel cell polyomavirus has recently been implicated as the aetiological agent of Merkel cell cancer, a rare aggressive skin tumour.

Introduction

Papillomaviruses and polyomaviruses are small, spherical, nonenveloped, doubled-stranded DNA viruses that multiply in the nucleus. The two virus groups are unrelated. Papillomaviruses infect surface epithelia and produce disease at these sites. Polyomaviruses are carried by viraemia, after initial multiplication at the site of entry, to affect internal organs such as the kidney and the brain. Viruses of both families produce experimental tumours in laboratory animals, but only papillomaviruses are related to naturally occurring cancers. Within each family the viruses are immunologically related and share nucleotide similarity.

More than 120 human papillomaviruses have been recognized, about 35 of which infect mucous membranes (genital and respiratory tracts, and the oral cavity) and the remainder infect skin. Human papillomaviruses cause skin warts, genital warts,

respiratory papillomas, and papillomas at other mucosal sites (e.g. mouth, eye). In addition, infection with some genital tract human papillomaviruses causes cervical cancer, one of the most common female malignancies in the world, as well as a proportion of cancers at other genital tract sites and the oropharynx.

JC virus is the aetiological agent of progressive multifocal leukoencephalopathy, a fatal demyelinating disease occurring in immunodeficient people. BK virus is associated with haemorrhagic cystitis in bone marrow transplant recipients, and with nephropathy and renal failure in renal transplant recipients. Merkel cell polyomavirus is implicated as the aetiological agent of Merkel cell cancer, a rare aggressive skin tumour. Trichodysplasia spinulosa-associated polyomavirus is found in the rare skin disease of the same name and may play a role in the development of the disease. Several new human polyomaviruses have been identified recently using molecular techniques, but none of the viruses is known to cause disease.

Human papillomaviruses (HPVs)

Human papillomaviruses cannot be propagated in tissue culture and require nucleic acid hybridization assays for their identification. Their double-stranded circular genome contains about 8000 bp, divided into an early region, necessary for transformation, a late region, encoding for capsid proteins, and a regulatory region, containing control elements (Fig. 5.19.1). Open reading frames of the viral genome are located on one strand: E1 to E8 in the early region and L1 and L2 in the late region. The functions assigned to the different open reading frames are listed in Table 5.19.1.

Human papillomaviruses infect only humans. They show a marked degree of cellular tropism. Mucosal human papillomaviruses do not readily infect cutaneous epithelia and cutaneous human papillomaviruses are rarely present on mucous membranes. Infection is initiated when, after minor trauma (e.g. during sexual intercourse or after minor skin abrasions), the basal cells of the epithelium come in contact with infectious virus. The virus stimulates

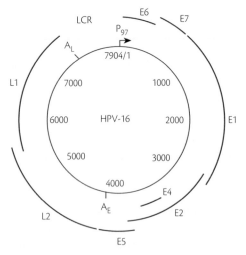

Fig. 5.19.1 Genomic map of HPV-16. On the inner circle, P97 represents the transcriptional promoter and A_E and A_L designate early and late polyadenylation sites. The location of the early region open reading frames (E1–E8), the late region open reading frames (L1, L2), and of the long control or regulatory region (LCR) are shown.
(Reproduced from Shah KV, Howley PM (1996). Papillomaviruses. In: Fields BN, et al. (eds) *Fields Virology*, vol. 2, pp. 2077–109. Lippincott-Raven, Philadelphia., with permission.)

Table 5.19.1 Functions of human papillomavirus open reading frames

Function	ORF
Replication of viral DNA	E1, E2
Regulation of transcription	E2
Coding for late cytoplasmic protein	E4
Cellular proliferation	E5[a]
Transformation	E6, E7
Not known	E3, E8

Abbreviations: ORF, open reading frame.

[a] In bovine papillomavirus, the major transforming activity is in E5.

(Modified from Shah KV, Howley PM (1996). Papillomaviruses. In: Fields BN, *et al.* (eds) *Fields Virology*, vol. 2, pp. 2077–109. Lippincott-Raven, Philadelphia.)

Table 5.19.3 Cancers attributable to HPV infection in 2002

Site	Attributable to HPV (%)	Total cancers	Attributable to HPV	% of all cancers
Cervix	100	492 800	492 800	4.54
Penis	40	26 300	10 500	0.10
Vulva, vagina	40	40 000	16 000	0.15
Anus	90	30 400	27 300	0.25
Oropharynx	50	52 100	26 500	0.
All sites	~5	10 862 500		

(Modified from Parkin DM and Bray F (2006). The burden of HPV-related cancers. *Vaccine* **24**, Suppl 3, S11–S25).

the proliferation of basal cells. The early region open reading frames are expressed in all layers of the infected epithelium, but expression of the late region open reading frames and synthesis of viral particles occur only in the upper differentiating and keratinizing layers.

Important disease associations and characteristics of mucosal HPVs are listed in Table 5.19.2. The burden of human cancers attributable to HPVs is shown in Table 5.19.3. The genital tract is the reservoir for all but a few mucosal human papillomaviruses and genital human papillomavirus infections constitute the most common viral sexually transmitted infections. Genital human papillomaviruses may sometimes infect nonanogenital mucosal sites, e.g. the respiratory tract, the mouth, and the conjunctiva. Transmission of genital tract HPV types 6 and 11 from an infected mother to the baby at birth results in juvenile onset recurrent respiratory papillomatosis. Infection with two types, HPV-13 and HPV-32, appears to be confined to the oral cavity.

Table 5.19.4 lists disease associations of cutaneous HPVs, which are transmitted by direct contact with infected tissue or by contact with a contaminated object.

Anogenital warts

Anogenital warts (condylomas) are the most commonly recognized clinical manifestations of genital HPV infections. More than 90% of condylomas result from infections with HPV-6 and HPV-11. In the United States of America, there are more than a million annual consultations for anogenital warts.

Epidemiology

Genital and anal warts are most common between the ages of 16 and 24 years. They are transmitted by direct sexual contact. Anogenital warts in children can also be due to close but nonsexual contact within a family but, in many cases, sexual abuse by an infected adult is responsible.

Clinical features

The incubation period is between 3 weeks and 8 months (mean=2.8 months). In men, condylomata acuminata (exophytic condylomas) most often appear on areas exposed to coital trauma, the glans penis, coronal sulcus, prepuce, and terminal urethra. The soft fleshy vascular tumours are usually multiple and may coalesce into large masses (Fig. 5.19.2). Sessile or papular warts are more likely to occur on dry areas such as the shaft of the penis (Fig. 5.19.3). The raised pink or grey lesions, 0.5 to 3 mm in diameter, may occur alone or with exophytic condylomas. Subclinical HPV lesions (flat condylomas) are identified by examining the genitalia with magnification after the application of 5% aqueous acetic acid solution. The affected areas are slightly raised and shiny white (acetowhite), with a rough surface. Flat condylomas affect the same areas as exophytic condylomas.

Table 5.19.2 Mucosal human papillomaviruses: chief clinical associations

Clinical association	Viral type(s)
Exophytic condyloma; respiratory papillomas; oral and conjunctival papillomas	HPV-6, -11
Cervical cancer:	
High-risk infections	HPV-16, -18, -31, -45, -33, -35, -39, -51, -52, -56, -58, -59
Low-risk infections	HPV-6, -11, -40, -42, -43, -44, -54, -61, -70, -72, -81
Vulval, vaginal, penile, anal, and oropharyngeal cancers	HPV-16
Focal epithelial hyperplasia of the oral cavity	HPV-13, -32

(Modified from Shah KV, Howley PM (1996). Papillomaviruses. In: Fields BN, *et al.* (eds) *Fields Virology*, vol. 2, pp. 2077–109. Lippincott-Raven, Philadelphia. Includes material from *The Oxford textbook of medicine*, 3rd edition, pp. 3366–9.)

Table 5.19.4 Cutaneous human papillomaviruses: chief clinical associations

Clinical association	Viral type
Deep plantar wart	HPV-1
Common wart	HPV-2, -4
Mosaic wart (superficial spreading wart)	HPV-2
Flat warts	HPV-3, -10, -28, -41
Macular plaques of epidermodysplasia verruciformis	HPV-5, -8, -9, -12, -14, -15, -17, -19, -20, -21, -22, -23, -24, -25, -36, -47, -50
Squamous cell carcinoma	HPV-5, -8, -20, -36, -38

Modified from Shah KV, Howley PM (1996). Papillomaviruses. In: Fields BN, *et al.* (eds) *Fields Virology*, vol. 2, pp. 2077–2109. Lippincott-Raven, Philadelphia.)

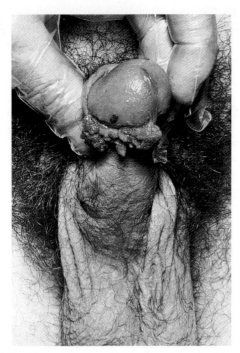

Fig. 5.19.2 Condylomata acuminata (exophytic condylomas) of the penis.

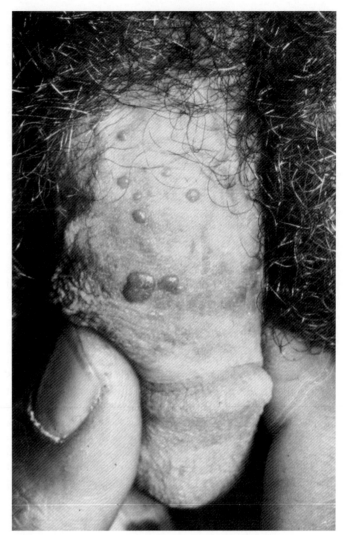

Fig. 5.19.3 Sessile (papular) warts of the penis.

Perianal warts are usually exophytic and in moist conditions around the anus may reach a large size. In 50% of cases, condylomas also appear in the anal canal. Areas of acetowhite epithelium indicative of subclinical HPV infection may be associated with perianal warts or occur alone.

In women, exophytic condylomas (Fig. 5.19.4) appear at the fourchette and adjacent areas, and may spread to the rest of the vulva, the perineum, anus, vagina, and cervix. Multiple sessile warts may affect the labia and perineum. Subclinical HPV infection presents as slightly raised acetowhite lesions: the fissuring of these may cause dyspareunia. About 15% of women with vulval warts have exophytic condylomas on the cervix. Subclinical infection is more common, and consists of acetowhite lesions with punctation due to capillary loops, which can be identified by colposcopy. Large, exophytic vulval condylomas may develop during pregnancy and may become so large that they compromise delivery. Most regress post-partum.

Even with therapy (see below), recurrence of genital warts occurs within 3 months in 25 to 67% of cases. Recurrences are often at sites of previous genital warts and are attributed to persistent infection that then reactivates.

Diagnosis and management

Genital warts must be distinguished from Fordyce's spots, fibroepithelial polyps, molluscum contagiosum, and the papillar lesions of secondary syphilis. Lesions that appear atypical or respond poorly to treatment must be biopsied early.

Associated sexually transmitted diseases must be excluded. Sexual partners should be examined. Intraepithelial neoplasia must be excluded. Cervical cytological examination should always be done on women with vulval warts and on female partners of men with penile warts.

Treatments for genital warts can be classified as topical, immunomodulatory, or surgical. Podophyllin and podophyllotoxin, which are derived from the root of the mayapple plant, are antimitotic agents that disrupt viral activity by inducing local tissue necrosis. Patient-applied topical podophyllotoxin, 0.5%, has a clinical cure rate of 56%; however, recurrence rates range from 23 to 65%. Disadvantages of podophyllin compounds include local adverse reactions, risk of systemic absorption, and teratogenicity. Imiquimod, a topical treatment for genital warts, induces macrophages to secrete cytokines, principally interferon-α, and is thought to work by stimulation of a cell-mediated immune response against HPV. Imiquimod is as effective as podophyllin for initial clearance of genital warts and results in a lower recurrence rate. The side effect profile of imiquimod is benign. Warts may be destroyed by cryotherapy with liquid nitrogen, electrocautery, electrodessication, scissor excision, or carbon dioxide laser therapy. Although these ablative therapies are successful in initially removing genital warts, recurrences are common. In a comparative trial, imiquimod 5% cream alone or in combination with ablative treatments was superior to ablation alone in reducing the recurrence rate of successfully treated anogenital warts. A prophylactic vaccine that prevents 100% of genital warts due to HPV-6 and HPV-11, if administered prior to exposure to HPV, is now commercially available in many countries (see below).

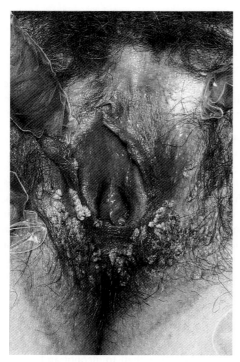

Fig. 5.19.4 Condylomata acuminata of the vulva.

Respiratory papillomatosis

This rare disease may have onset in childhood or in adult life. It is most common in children under the age of 5 years. It may become life-threatening if it obstructs the airways. Papillomatosis usually involves the vocal cords and the patient presents with hoarseness or voice change. Papillomas may recur after surgical removal.

HPV-6 and HPV-11, genital tract HPVs that are responsible for most of the exophytic genital warts, also cause respiratory papillomatosis. Patients with juvenile-onset disease are infected at birth during passage through an infected birth canal. In adult-onset disease, transmission may occur by sexual contact. Respiratory papillomas rarely progress to invasive cancer. Irradiation of papillomas with X-rays (a practice now discontinued) increases the risk of malignancy.

Caesarean delivery for mothers who are found to have genital warts or are infected with HPV-6 or HPV-11 would reduce the risk of juvenile-onset respiratory papillomatosis, but it is not generally recommended because of the small risk of disease following perinatal infection. The mainstay of treatment is surgical removal of papillomas; however, recurrence of lesions is common. Various adjunct therapies have been tried, including interferon-α, indole-3-carbinol, cidofovir, and photodynamic treatment. These therapies have had only modest success in reducing the need for surgery. It is anticipated that a child born to a mother who has received the HPV Gardasil vaccine, will have a markedly reduced risk of developing respiratory papillomatosis.

Cervical cancer (Oxford Textbook of Medicine 5e Chapter 6.1)

Human papillomavirus DNA is recovered from nearly 100% of cases of invasive cervical cancer and squamous intraepithelial lesions of the cervix, which precede invasive cancer. The viral genome is present in the tumour cells of primary as well as metastatic cervical cancer. The progression from low grade squamous

intraepithelial lesions to invasive cancer may take more than 10 years; human papillomaviruses are found throughout this disease process. The viruses are recovered much less frequently from cytologically normal women of comparable age. In prospective studies of women with normal cervical cytology, the presence of HPV is a strong risk factor for the subsequent development of squamous intraepithelial lesions.

Certain HPV types are preferentially associated with invasive cancers. From their distribution in normal individuals and in preinvasive and invasive cervical disease, genital tract HPVs have been categorized as high-risk, or low-risk types (Fig. 5.19.5; Table 5.19.2). HPV-16 and HPV-18 are the predominant viruses in invasive cancers and account for 40 to 60% and 5 to 20%, respectively, of HPV-positive cancers in different studies. About a dozen additional types of HPV are found in small proportions of invasive cancers. The low-risk HPVs are almost never detected in invasive cervical cancers.

Comparisons of different HPV types for their ability to transform human keratinocytes *in vitro* show that HPV-16 and HPV-18, types most clearly associated with naturally occurring cervical cancers, also have the greatest oncogenic potential in laboratory studies. The transforming functions of HPVs are localized to open reading frames E6 and E7; these are the viral genes consistently expressed in naturally occurring HPV-positive cancers. The viral genome is integrated into the cellular DNA in most cervical cancers. The break in the circular viral genome that is required for integration occurs most frequently in the E1/E2 region and results in an enhanced expression of the transforming E6 and E7 open reading frames. The transforming HPV proteins E6 and E7 interact with cellular tumour suppressor proteins p53 and Rb, respectively. The oncogenic effect of HPVs is mediated largely by their ability to inactivate the tumour suppressor proteins which normally regulate the cell cycle.

Epidemiology

Human papillomavirus infections of the genital tract are extremely common in sexually active populations. In young sexually active

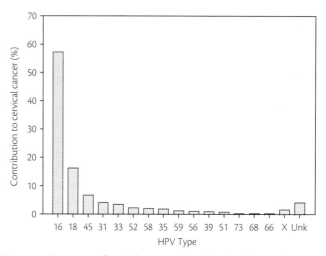

Fig. 5.19.5 Percentages of cervical cancer cases attributed to the most frequent HPV types in all world regions combined. X includes the rare types 40, 42, 53, 54, 55, 83, and 84. 'Unk' includes specimens that were positive for HPV DNA but could not be genotyped by current methods.
(Data from Munoz N, *et al.* (2004). Against which human papillomavirus types shall we vaccinate and screen? The international perspective. *Int J Cancer*, **111**, 278–85.)

women, point prevalence (single sampling) of HPV infection as measured by the detection of HPV DNA in genital tract specimens by the sensitive polymerase chain reaction (PCR) may be as high as 40%, and the cumulative prevalence (multiple sampling of women over time) may be as high as 80 to 90%. The prevalence decreases with increasing age. Most of these infections are found in women with normal cervical cytology and undoubtedly resolve without leaving a trace. Only a small proportion of infections persists and progresses to squamous intraepithelial lesions and then to invasive cancer. The cofactors that might be associated with progression to cancer include smoking, use of oral contraceptives, parity, and presence of other sexually transmitted diseases. Human immunodeficiency virus (HIV) infection and associated immunosuppression, leads to a much higher prevalence, and longer persistence, of HPV infections and to greater incidence of squamous intraepithelial lesions.

Prevention and control

Screening for cervical cytological abnormalities by cervical smear and treatment of preinvasive and invasive cancers identified by screening, have been credited with the decrease in incidence of cervical cancer and mortality due to the disease that has been observed in many developed countries over the last 40 to 50 years. Women who have cytological abnormalities which are low grade or of uncertain significance may benefit from an HPV diagnosis. The presence of cancer-associated HPVs would indicate a need for closer monitoring and colposcopy; HPV-negative women would be monitored routinely. Tests for the presence of high risk HPVs may replace cervical smears as cervical cancer screening strategy.

Prophylactic vaccines

The discovery that the L1 coat protein of papillomaviruses could assemble into a virus-like particle (VLP), when expressed as a recombinant protein, and the demonstration that immunization of rabbits, cattle, and dogs with VLPs of their respective papillomaviruses protected against papillomavirus-induced disease, stimulated the development of vaccines for human papillomaviruses. L1 VLPs appear to induce very limited cross-neutralization against other genotypes necessitating a multicomponent vaccine to provide coverage against disease caused by more than one type. Two HPV L1 VLP vaccines have been developed commercially; Cervarix is a bivalent HPV-16/18 L1 VLP vaccine and Gardasil is a quadrivalent HPV16/18/6/11 L1 VLP vaccine. Both vaccines are generally safe and well tolerated and are highly immunogenic. Both vaccines have demonstrated truly remarkable efficacy, preventing nearly 100% of incident infections and preinvasive cervical cancers due to the HPV types in the vaccines. Gardasil is also 100% effective in preventing genital warts associated with HPV 6/11. Since genital HPV infection is sexually transmitted, the vaccines ideally should target prepubertal and young adolescent girls. The vaccines are also recommended for young women 13 to 26 years of age, because many of them may not yet have been exposed to the HPV types in the vaccines. If HPV vaccines are proven to be safe and efficacious in males, future recommendations will likely include immunization of boys and young men in order to reduce the risk of genital warts, protect against penile and oropharyngeal cancer, and provide herd immunity. The durability of the immune response engendered by HPV vaccines and thus the possible need for a booster in vaccinated individuals is unknown. Because protection may wane over time and because vaccination does not protect against the HPV types not included in the vaccines, screening programmes will need to be maintained, but the strategy may change with longer intervals between screening and a greater emphasis on HPV DNA testing as a screening method.

Therapeutic vaccines

Human papillomavirus-associated cancers express HPV E6 and E7 proteins in their tumour cells. Candidate therapeutic vaccines targeted to these proteins are being developed for the treatment of high grade squamous intraepithelial lesions and invasive cancer.

Cancers at other lower anogenital tract sites

Human papillomavirus infections are very common on the vulva, vagina, penis, perineum, and anus. Synchronous neoplasia at multiple sites in the female lower genital tract is almost always associated with HPVs, especially HPV-16. Carcinoma of the vulva is aetiologically heterogeneous. Vulval cancers occurring in younger women are associated with HPVs, but the typical squamous cell carcinoma of the vulva in older women is not. Neoplasia of the anal canal, seen frequently in HIV-seropositive homosexual men, is strongly associated with HPVs.

Cancer of the oropharynx

A subset of oropharyngeal cancers, especially tonsillar cancers, is aetiologically linked to high-risk HPVs, most often HPV-16. Patients with HPV-associated cancers have risk factors related to their sexual history rather than to alcohol and tobacco use. As compared to HPV-negative cancers, the HPV-positive cancers are characterized by more frequent basaloid pathology, less frequent p53 and Rb mutations, and better prognosis. Demonstration of HPV genome in tumour cells, presence of HPV transcripts, and immunostaining for cellular p16 characterize HPV-caused cancers, which are increasing in incidence in North America and Europe. It is estimated that the number of HPV-caused oropharyngeal cancers in men and women will exceed the number of cervical cancers in the United States of America by 2020.

Skin warts (Oxford Textbook of Medicine 5e Chapter 23.10)

Skin warts and verrucas may occur anywhere on the skin and are morphologically diverse. They are most common in older children and young adults. Except in the rare condition known as epidermodysplasia verruciformis (see below), they almost never become malignant. Most regress within 2 years. Specific HPV types are strongly associated with specific types of warts (Table 5.19.4).

Epidermodysplasia verruciformis

This is a rare, lifelong disease in which a patient has extensive warty involvement of the skin that cannot be resolved. It generally begins in infancy or childhood with multiple, disseminated polymorphic wart-like lesions on the face, trunk, and extremities that tend to become confluent. The warts are either flat or reddish-brown macular plaques that resemble pityriasis versicolor. In about a third of the cases, foci of malignant transformation occur in macular plaques in areas of the skin exposed to sunlight. The tumours are slow growing and rarely metastasize.

Epidermodysplasia verruciformis (EV) is often a familial disease. Patients sometimes have a history of parental consanguinity. A susceptibility locus has been mapped to chromosome 17q25 and truncating mutations in either of two novel adjacent genes, *TMC6* and *TMC8*, are associated with the disease in different pedigrees. The function of the gene products of TMC6 and TMC8 and how they confer increased risk for EV are unknown. A second putative susceptibility locus is located on chromosome 2p21-p24. The flat warts yield the same HPV types as those of normal individuals, but a very large number of HPVs that are seldom encountered in normal individuals are recovered from the macular plaques (Table 5.19.3). It is unclear how patients with epidermodysplasia verruciformis become infected with these particular papillomaviruses. The factors that contribute to the occurrence of carcinoma in these patients therefore include a genetic defect, infection with specific HPVs, e.g. HPV-5 and HPV-8, and exposure of the affected area to sunlight.

Nonmelanoma skin cancers

HPV DNA has been detected in 30 to 50% of nonmelanoma skin cancers (NMSC) in immunocompetent populations and in up to 90% of NMSC from immunocompromised populations, in particular organ transplant recipients. The HPV prevalence is generally higher in squamous cell carcinoma than in basal cell carcinoma. The sequences represent cutaneous HPV types, EV-associated HPVs, and many novel HPV sequences. No single HPV type predominates and there is no evidence of high-risk types analogous to those seen in cervical cancer. The amount of HPV DNA in skin tumours is very low, indicating that not every tumour cell harbours an HPV genome. Because HPV DNA is frequently detected in normal skin samples, it is not clear to what extent HPVs contribute to the development of NMSC. Ultraviolet (UV) light is considered the most significant risk factor for NMSCs. Cutaneous HPVs through the antiapoptotic activity of their E6 gene may act as cocarcinogens by preventing elimination of cells with UV-induced DNA damage.

Human polyomaviruses

In 1971, BK virus was isolated from the urine of a renal transplant recipient and JC virus was recovered from the brain of a patient with progressive multifocal leukoencephalopathy. Recently, two new human polyomaviruses, KI virus and WU virus, were detected in respiratory tract secretions of children by using molecular techniques. The viruses were detected in upper respiratory tract specimens in the presence of other recognized respiratory tract pathogens and thus their role in disease is unclear. In 2008, another new human polyomavirus, Merkel cell virus, was identified in tumour cells from patients with Merkel cell carcinoma, a rare aggressive skin cancer.

Trichodysplasia spinulosa (TS) is a rare skin disease primarily affecting immunosuppressed patients and presenting as follicular-based papules and keratin spicules widespread on the face, along with variable degrees of alopecia and dysmorphism. In 2010, a new human polyomavirus, designated TS-associated polyomavirus, was identified in the TS lesions of a heart transplant recipient. Two new human polyomaviruses, designated type 6 and 7, were detected in the skin of healthy persons. Another new human polyomavirus, type 9, was identified in the blood and urine of a renal transplant patient. Subsequently the virus was independently identified in the skin of a Merkel cancer patient. No diseases have been associated with polyomavirus types 6, 7, and 9. All the new polyomaviruses were detected by using a variety of molecular techniques that do not rely on prior knowledge of the DNA sequence of the virus. Polyomaviruses have a double-stranded DNA genome of about 5000 bp, which is divided into an early region encoding viral T proteins, a late region encoding viral capsid proteins, and a noncoding regulatory region. The T proteins regulate viral transcription, initiate viral DNA replication, and mediate inactivation of host cell tumour suppressor proteins, which contribute to the oncogenic potential of polyomaviruses. The viral regulatory region contains elements for viral DNA replication and promoters for transcription of early and late genes, as well as binding sites for cellular transcription factors, which determine the host and tissue tropism of polyomaviruses.

The early and late regions are transcribed from different strands of the viral DNA. Although BK and JC viruses are homologous for 75% of their nucleotide sequence, the infections are readily distinguishable by conventional tests.

Infection occurs in childhood and is largely subclinical. Most children acquire antibodies to BK virus by the age of 10; infection with JC virus occurs at a later age. Infection occurs by the respiratory route and possibly by ingestion. Both viruses establish latent, often lifelong, infection in the kidney and are often shed in the urine of normal people. Reactivation in immunodeficient people is responsible for most associated illnesses. The viruses are reactivated in pregnancy, but without any apparent harm to the mother or the newborn.

Polyomavirus-associated illnesses

Nephropathy in renal transplant recipients

This condition is associated most often with BK virus and rarely with JC virus. It occurs in 3 to 10% of renal transplant recipients and results in a loss of the allograft in 50 to 80% of the affected patients. The recent increase in the incidence of this complication is related to the introduction of new and intensive immunosuppressive therapies. Pathologically, the disease is characterized by inclusion-bearing enlarged nuclei in renal tubular and glomerular epithelial cells which are readily detected by microscopy (Fig. 5.19.6). Monitoring of the patients for BK virus viraemia has predictive value for the incidence of the disease.

Haemorrhagic cystitis in bone marrow transplant recipients

Late-onset haemorrhagic cystitis in bone marrow transplant recipients is associated with BK virus infection. Large amounts of BK virus are shed in urine during the haemorrhagic episodes.

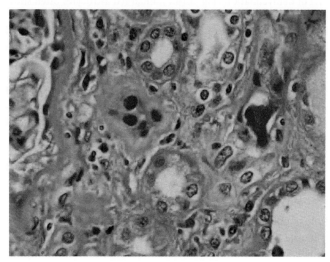

Fig. 5.19.6 BK virus infected cells (dark and hyperchromatic) in renal parenchyma, with some cells shed in the tubular lumen.

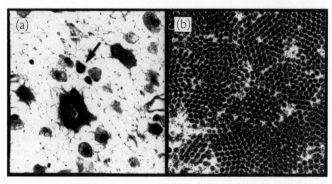

Fig. 5.19.7 A lesion of progressive multifocal leukoencephalopathy showing oligodendrocytes with enlarged, deeply staining nuclei (arrow) and giant astrocytes (left), and a crystalloid array of JC virus particles in an infected oligodendrocyte nucleus (right).
(Reproduced, with permission, from Shah KV (1992). Polyomavirus, infection and immunity. In: Roitt IM (ed) *Encyclopedia of Immunology*, pp. 1256–8. Academic Press, New York.)

Progressive multifocal leucoencephalopathy (PML) (Chapters 5.23 and Oxford Textbook of Medicine 5e 24.11.2)

JC virus causes progressive multifocal leucoencephalopathy, a sub-acute demyelinating disease of the central nervous system occurring in individuals with impaired cell-mediated immunity. Until the advent of AIDS, it was a rare disease found mainly in older patients with lymphoproliferative disorders or chronic diseases. Because PML is a complication in 1 to 2% of AIDS cases, it is a more common disease and is seen much more frequently in younger patients. It has also been recognized in children who have inherited immunodeficiency diseases or have AIDS. Recently, PML has been recognized as a complication in patients with Crohn's disease or multiple sclerosis participating in clinical trials of natalizumab monoclonal antibody, which inhibits migration of cells across the blood–brain barrier.

The key pathogenetic event in PML is the cytocidal JC virus infection of oligodendrocytes, which are responsible for the production and maintenance of myelin. This leads to foci of demyelination that tend to coalesce and eventually involve large areas of the brain. Infected oligodendrocytes, containing large inclusion-bearing nuclei filled with abundant virus particles, surround the foci of demyelination (Fig. 5.19.7). Enlarged astrocytes often show bizarre nuclear changes but are mostly virus negative. They are found within the foci of demyelination. JC virus is disseminated haematogenously to the central nervous system, probably through virus-infected B lymphocytes.

PML starts insidiously. Early signs and symptoms indicate the presence of multifocal asymmetrical lesions in the brain and involve impairment of vision and speech, and mental deterioration. The disease is usually relentlessly progressive and fatal within 3 to 6 months, but rarely it can become stabilized with survival for many years. CT and MRI have been successfully used for diagnosis (Fig. 5.19.8). Treatment with cytosine arabinoside and the presence of an inflammatory response in the brain have been associated with the few relatively successful outcomes.

Role of polyomaviruses in human tumours

The role of polyomaviruses in human tumours is the subject of debate. JC virus and BK virus are oncogenic for laboratory animals and they transform cultured cells. There are reports of finding JC virus DNA in brain and colon tumours and BK virus DNA in

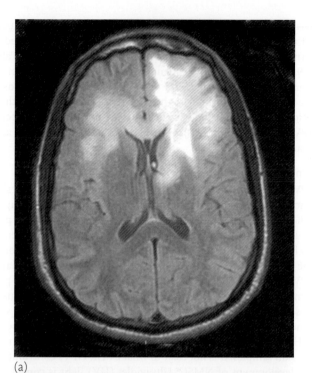

(a)

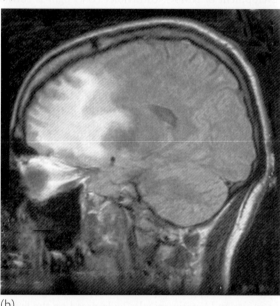

(b)

Fig. 5.19.8 Brain fluid attenuation inversion recovery (FLAIR) MRIs in axial (a) and sagittal (b) planes of a 36-year-old man with AIDS and progressive multifocal leukoencephalopathy proven by detection of JC virus DNA in cerebrospinal fluid by PCR.

prostate, bladder, and brain tumours, as well as neuroblastomas and insulinomas. However, a reproducible and consistent aetiological association of either virus with any human tumour has not been demonstrated. The Merkel cell virus provides a more convincing example of a polyomavirus-induced human tumour, since the viral genome was found to be integrated into tumour cell DNA, a key event in experimental polyomavirus-induced animal tumours. Further supporting the carcinogenic potential of the virus is the observation that survival of virus-positive Merkel cancer cell lines is dependent on expression of the viral oncoprotein. The virus has been detected in approximately 80% of Merkel cell cancers worldwide. Serological studies have revealed that exposure to Merkel cell polyomavirus is very high in human populations. Thus the precise role of the virus and modifying cofactors in the aetiology of Merkel cell carcinoma remains to be established.

Further reading

Berger JR, *et al.* (1998). Progressive multifocal leukoencephalopathy in patients with HIV infection. *J Neurovirol*, **4**, 59–68.

Bosch FX, *et al.* (2002). The causal relation between human papillomavirus and cervical cancer. *J Clin Pathol*, **55**, 244–265.

Chatuevedi AK, *et al.* (2011) Human papillomavirus and rising oropharyngeal cancer incidence in the United States. *J Clin Oncol*, **29**, 4294–301.

D'Souza G, *et al.* (2007). Epidemiological evidence that human papillomavirus is a cause of oropharyngeal squamous cell carcinomas. *N Engl J Med*, **356**, 1944–56.

Koutsky LA, *et al.* (2002). A controlled trial of a human papillomavirus type 16 vaccine. *N Engl J Med*, **347**, 1645–51.

Munoz N, *et al.* (2004). Against which human papillomavirus types shall we vaccinate and screen? The international perspective. *Int J Cancer*, **111**, 278–85.

Randhawa P, Brennan DC. (2006). BK virus infection in transplant recipients: an overview and update. *Am J Transplant*, **6**, 2000–5.

Shah KV. (1992). Polyomavirus, infection and immunity. In: Roitt IM (ed) *Encyclopedia of immunology*, pp. 1256–8. Academic Press, New York.

Shah KV, Howley PM. (1996). Papillomaviruses. In: Fields BN, *et al.* (eds) *Fields virology*, vol. 2, pp. 2077–109. Lippincott-Raven, Philadelphia.

Yousry TA, *et al.* (2006). Evaluation of patients treated with natalizumab for progressive multifocal leukoencephalopathy. *N Engl J Med*, **354**, 924–33.

5.20 **Parvovirus B19**

Kevin E. Brown

Essentials

Parvovirus B19 (B19V) is a small DNA virus that replicates in erythroid progenitor cells, with virus-induced cytotoxicity stopping red cell production. It only infects humans, is endemic in most places, and is transmitted predominantly by the respiratory route. In healthy people it causes erythema infectiosum, also known as 'fifth disease' or 'slapped cheek disease', associated with minimal drop in haemoglobin, but in patients with increased red cell turnover, e.g. haemolytic anaemia or haemoglobinopathy, it causes transient aplastic crisis; in immunocompromised patients it causes chronic anaemia; and following maternal infection it leads to hydrops fetalis or fetal loss. Treatment is supportive in most instances, but reduction in iatrogenic immunosuppression and/or intravenous immunoglobulin may be appropriate in some cases. No vaccine is available.

Introduction

Parvovirus B19 (B19V) is a member of the Parvoviridae, small (*c.*22 nm), nonenveloped, icosahedral-shaped viruses (Fig. 5.20.1), with a linear single-stranded DNA genome of about 5000 nucleotides. At least four types of parvovirus infect humans: B19V; adeno-associated viruses (AAVs); the recently described Parv4/5, and human bocavirus. To date, only B19V has definitively been shown to be a human pathogen.

Aetiology, pathogenesis, and pathology

Based on viral sequence, B19V can be divided into three distinct genotypes (1, 2, and 3). Genotypes 2 and 3 are infrequently detected in Europe or the United States of America. No differences in pathogenicity are observed between the different genotypes, and they are all a single B19V serotype.

B19V replication occurs primarily in erythroid progenitors, with the specificity in part due to the limited tissue distribution of the B19V receptor, blood group P antigen (globoside). Infection leads to high titre viraemia (>10^{12} virus particles/ml or IV/ml) (Fig. 5.20.2), and the virus-induced cytotoxicity stops red cell production. In immunocompetent people, viraemia and arrest of erythropoiesis is transient, and resolves as the antibody response is mounted. In those with normal erythropoiesis the drop in haemoglobin is minimal, but in patients with increased red cell turnover, infection induces a transient crisis with severe anaemia (Fig. 5.20.2b). Similarly, in the fetus or anyone who does not mount a neutralizing antibody response which halts the lytic infection, erythroid production is compromised and patients develop chronic anaemia (Fig. 5.20.2c).

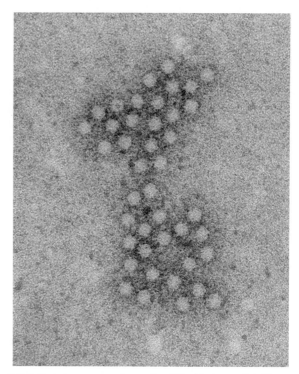

Fig. 5.20.1 Typical appearance of parvovirus B19, with characteristic 22 nm icosahedral particles.

(Courtesy of Dr Hazel Appleton, Virus Reference Department, Health Protection Agency.)

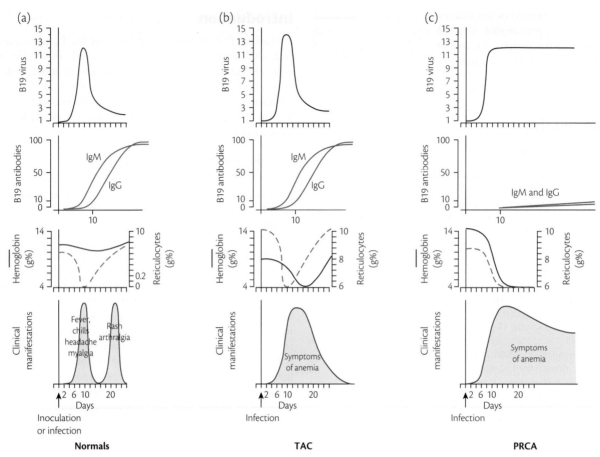

Fig. 5.20.2 Schematic of the time course of B19 infection in (a) erythema infectiosum (EI), (b) transient aplastic crisis (TAC), and (c) pure red cell aplasia (PRCA) or chronic anaemia. The B19 virus titres are given in log 10 IU/ml.
(From Young NS, Brown KE (2004). Parvovirus B19. *N Engl J Med*, **350**, 586–97.)

The immune-mediated phase of illness begins 2 to 3 weeks postinfection as the IgM response peaks, and the rash of fifth disease, arthralgia, and/or frank arthritis appear.

The B19 receptor is found on other cell types, including megakaryocytes, endothelial cells, placenta, myocardium, and liver. B19 infection at these sites may be responsible for some of the more unusual presentations. Rare people who lack P antigen are naturally resistant to B19V.

Epidemiology

B19V exclusively infects humans, and the virus is endemic in virtually all parts of the world. Transmission is predominantly via the respiratory route, prior to the onset of the rash or arthralgia. About 50% of 15-year-old children have detectable IgG, increasing to more than 90% of older people. In pregnant women there is an estimated annual seroconversion rate of approximately 1%. The secondary infection rate within households approaches 50%.

Prevention

High titre B19V is not unusual in blood, and transmission occurs via transfusion, particularly of pooled components. B19V is resistant to heat and solvent/detergent inactivation. Plasma pools are currently screened by nucleic acid testing (NAT) and high titre pools are discarded.

Clinical features

The clinical manifestation of B19V infection varies widely, depending on the host (Table 5.20.1). The majority of infections are asymptomatic. In healthy, immunocompetent people, B19 infections causes erythema infectiosum (EI), also known as 'fifth disease' or 'slapped cheek disease' due to the characteristic facial rash which appears several days after a minor febrile prodrome. The rash may spread and develop a lacy reticular appearance, but the intensity and distribution of the rash varies and is difficult to distinguish from other viral exanthems. Rarely the rash can present as papular-purpuric gloves and socks syndrome (PPGSS) (Fig 5.20.3). In adults, the 'slapped cheek' may not be apparent. Although uncommon in children, a symmetrical polyarthropathy, affecting the small joints of the hands and occasionally the ankles, knees, and wrists occurs in *c*.50% of adults, more often in women than men. Resolution usually occurs within a few weeks, but recurring symptoms can continue for months.

Patients with increased erythropoiesis (i.e. those with haemolytic anaemia or haemoglobinopathy) develop transient aplastic crisis (TAC), with symptoms of acute anaemia. Bone marrow examination reveals an absence of erythroid precursors and the presence of characteristic giant pronormoblasts.

In the immunocompromised (i.e. patients with AIDS, leukaemia, and following transplantation), B19 infection may lead to chronic anaemia or pure red cell aplasia. Patients have persistent anaemia

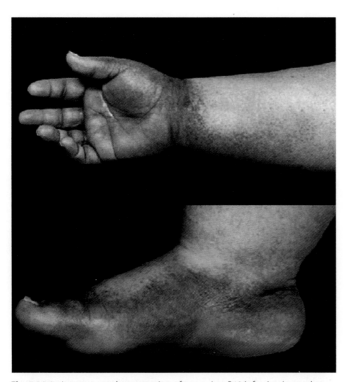

Fig. 5.20.3 A very unusual presentation of parvovirus B19 infection is papular-purpuric gloves and socks syndrome.
(From Gutermuth J, *et al.* (2011), *Lancet*, **378**, 198, *with permission from Elsevier.*)

B19V infection is rarely associated with hepatitis, vasculitis, myocarditis, glomerulosclerosis, and CNS disease.

Diagnosis

In immunocompetent people, B19V infection is usually diagnosed by the detection of B19 IgM antibodies (Table 5.20.1). IgM can be found at the time of rash in EI and by the third day of TAC in patients with haematological disorders. IgM remains detectable for about 3 months. B19 IgG appears by the seventh day of illness and remains for life. Detection of B19 DNA should be used for the diagnosis of early TAC or chronic anaemia. Although levels fall rapidly with the development of the immune response, low levels of DNA can be detectable by polymerase chain reaction (PCR) for months and even years after infection, even in healthy people, so a quantitative PCR should be used for diagnosis. At the height of viraemia, more than 10^{12} B19 DNA IU/ml of serum can be detected, but titres fall rapidly within 2 days. Patients with aplastic crisis or B19-induced chronic anaemia generally have more than 10^5 IU/ml B19 DNA.

Treatment

No antiviral drug is available, and treatment is often only symptomatic. B19-induced TAC may require blood transfusions, and intrauterine blood transfusion can prevent fetal loss in some cases of fetal hydrops. In patients on chemotherapy, stopping treatment temporarily may result in an immune response and resolution, but if unsuccessful or inapplicable, intravenous human normal immunoglobulin (HNIG) may cure or improve persistent B19 infection. These patients and those with TAC should be considered infectious. Administration of immunoglobulin is not beneficial for EI or B19-associated polyarthropathy.

Table 5.20.1 Diseases associated with parvovirus B19 infection and methods of diagnosis

Disease	Host(s)	Pathogenesis	IgM	IgG	Quantitative PCR
Fifth disease	Healthy children	Immune-mediated	Positive	Positive	(Low positive)
Polyarthropathy syndrome	Healthy adults (especially women)	Immune-mediated	Positive within 3 months of onset	Positive	(Low positive)
Transient aplastic crisis (TAC)	Patients with increased erythropoiesis	Erythroid cytotoxicity			Often >10^{12} IU/ml, but rapidly decreases
Persistent anaemia/ pure red cell aplasia	Immunocompromised patients	Impaired neutralizing antibody	Negative/weak positive	Negative/ weak positive	Often >10^{12} IU/ml, but should be >10^6 IU/ml in the absence of treatment
Hydrops fetalis	Fetus	Erythroid cytotoxicity and impaired neutralizing antibody			Positive amniotic fluid or tissue

with reticulocytopenia, absent or low levels of B19 IgG, high levels of B19 DNA in serum, and often scattered giant pronormoblasts in the bone marrow. Transient neutropenia, lymphopenia, and thrombocytopenia, may be seen and B19V occasionally causes a haemophagocytic syndrome.

Infection with B19V during pregnancy can lead to hydrops fetalis and fetal loss. The risk of transplacental fetal infection is about 30%, and the risk of fetal loss, predominantly in the second trimester, 9%. The risk of congenital infection is less than 1%. Although B19V does not appear to be teratogenic, there are anecdotal reports of eye damage and CNS abnormalities. Cases of congenital anaemia have also been described. B19V probably causes 10 to 20% of all cases of nonimmune hydrops.

Prevention in the future

No vaccine is currently approved for parvovirus B19. A vaccine based on viral-like particles expressed in insect cells is under development and results of phase 1 trials were promising.

Further reading

Brown KE, Young NS (2006). Parvovirus B19. In: Young NS, Gerson SL, High KA (eds) *Clinical Hematology*, pp. 981–991. Mosby Elsevier, Philadelphia.

Brown KE, *et al.* (1994). Resistance to parvovirus B19 infection due to lack of virus receptor (erythrocyte P antigen). *N Engl J Med*, **330**, 1192–96.

Gutermuth J, *et al.* (2011). Papular-purpuric gloves and socks syndrome. *Lancet*, **378**, 198.

Kerr JR, *et al.* (eds) (2006). *Parvoviruses*. Hodder Arnold, London.

Kurtzman GJ, *et al.* (1987). Chronic bone marrow failure due to persistent B19 parvovirus infection. *N Engl J Med*, **317**, 287–94.

Young NS, Brown KE (2004). Parvovirus B19. *N Engl J Med*, **350**, 586–97.

5.21 Hepatitis viruses (excluding hepatitis C virus)

N.V. Naoumov

Essentials

The group of hepatitis viruses includes five unrelated human viruses (A to E), which differ in their genome organization, biology, and epidemiology, while being united by their hepatotropism. About 10 to 15% of cases of viral hepatitis are considered as non-A to E hepatitis, whose aetiology is still unknown, but the search for which has led to the identification of several new viruses (e.g. HGV or GB virus-C, TT, and SEN viruses) of uncertain pathogenic significance.

Clinical aspects of viral hepatitis are discussed in the Oxford Textbook of Medicine 5e Chapter 15.21.1.

Hepatitis A virus (HAV)

A single-stranded RNA virus with four genotypes in humans. HAV replicates primarily in hepatocytes and is excreted via the biliary system into the faeces, where it can be found in high concentrations prior to clinical symptoms. HAV causes acute hepatitis with significant morbidity and occasional mortality. Anti-HAV IgG remains detectable after acute infection and provides protective immunity.

Hepatitis B virus (HBV)

HBV is the smallest human DNA virus. Eight genotypes, designated A to H, have been determined, each having a distinct geographical distribution. The virus is noncytopathic, with virus-specific cellular immunity being the main determinant for the outcome of infection. Eradication of HBV is rare, but in cases with resolution of HBV infection an effective immune response controls HBV replication and there is no liver disease. The natural evolution of chronic infection includes four consecutive phases: (1) early 'immunotolerant' phase—high levels of virus replication and minimal liver inflammation; (2) immune reactive phase—significant hepatic inflammation and elevated serum aminotransferases; with some patients progressing to (3) 'non-replicative' phase—seroconversion to anti-HBe; undetectable or low level of viraemia (below 2000 IU/ml by polymerase chain reaction-based assays); resolution of hepatic inflammation; and (4) HBeAg-negative chronic hepatitis B—due to the emergence of viral mutations; characterized by fluctuating serum HBV DNA and serum ALT levels, and progressive liver disease.

Hepatitis C virus (HCV)

See Chapter 5.22.

Hepatitis delta virus (HDV)

A defective virus with a single-stranded circular RNA genome. Eight genotypes have been determined in humans; genotype 1 is most common in the Western world and genotype 2 is predominant in East Asia. HDV infection is always associated with HBV infection and occurs as a consequence of coinfection or superinfection. Clinical manifestations vary from acute to fulminant hepatitis and from an asymptomatic carrier state to progressive chronic liver disease. Diagnosis is based on the detection of serum HDag and serum HDV RNA. The optimal treatment of HDV is uncertain. Prevention is by vaccination against HBV.

Hepatitis E virus (HEV)

A single-stranded RNA virus. HEV is widely distributed and transmitted by the faeco-oral route and may be zoonotic, with evidence of infection in pigs, cattle and sheep in endemic regions. It causes acute viral hepatitis which may be fulminant in those who are pregnant, malnourished or have existing liver disease. Chronic infection has been reported in transplant recipients. Immunity can be transient and may wane if acquired in childhood. An effective vaccine has been developed but is not yet commercially available.

Introduction

Viral hepatitis (Fig. 5.21.1) is an ancient disease which remains a major health problem worldwide. Five viruses have been identified as aetiological agents and named A, B, C, D, and E (Table 5.21.1). These unrelated human viruses differ in their genome organization, biology, and epidemiology, while being united by their hepatotropism. Approximately 10 to 15% of cases with viral hepatitis are considered as non-A to E hepatitis and the aetiology is still unknown. The search for additional hepatitis agents led to the identification of several new viruses, named hepatitis G virus (HGV or GB virus-C), TT, and SEN viruses. These viruses have been detected in high proportions of the general population and their pathogenic role, if any, remains uncertain. Thus, the search for new hepatitis agents responsible for the small proportion of cases with cryptogenic hepatitis continues. Clinical aspects of viral hepatitis are discussed in the Oxford Textbook of Medicine 5e Chapter 15.21.1.

Hepatitis A virus (HAV)

HAV particles were first discovered by immune electron microscopy in 1973 in stool samples of patients with hepatitis A. The virus is classified in the genus *Heparnavirus* of the family Picornaviridae. The genome of HAV is a single-stranded, linear RNA of 7474 nucleotides (Table 5.21.1). This includes a 5′ untranslated region (5′ UTR) of 742 nucleotides, followed by a single, long, open reading frame (ORF, 6681 nucleotides), which encodes a polyprotein of 2227 amino acids, and a short 3′ noncoding region (63 nucleotides). After translation, HAV polyprotein undergoes multiple cleavages by a virally-encoded enzyme, 3C protease. The polyprotein contains three functionally separate domains. At the N-terminal end is domain P1 which includes the major structural polypeptides of HAV in the following sequence—VP2, VP3, and VP1. A fourth very small polypeptide, VP4, which is presumed to be involved in HAV capsid formation, is located at the extreme N-terminal end of the polyprotein. These four structural polypeptides assemble into a viral capsid containing 60 copies of each. It is not known how the viral RNA is incorporated into the virion, but both empty and

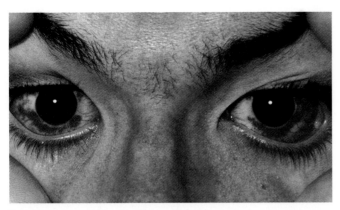

Fig. 5.21.1 Acute viral hepatitis (HBV) with jaundice and subconjunctival haemorrhages.
(Copyright D A Warrell.)

RNA-containing capsids have been observed in most virus preparations. The other P2 and P3 domains of the viral polyprotein include at least six separate proteins which are involved in viral replication. These include 2B and 2C helicase, 3A and 3B proteins, 3C (the viral protease), and 3D (an RNA-dependent RNA polymerase).

Hepatocytes are the predominant site of HAV replication *in vivo*. Recent data indicate that HAV may also replicate within the epithelial cells of the gastrointestinal tract. However, the mechanism by which HAV reaches the liver remains unknown. The maximal HAV replication in hepatocytes occurs before serum aminotransferases rise. The virus is excreted via the biliary system into the faeces where it can be found in high concentrations around 1 to 2 weeks prior to the onset of clinical symptoms. Viraemia is present from the earliest phase of infection and is due to HAV replication within hepatocytes. HAV differs from other picornaviruses because of its noncytolytic replication. Liver injury is immune mediated by natural killer cells, virus-specific CD8+ cytotoxic T cells, and nonspecific inflammatory cells recruited to the liver. At the onset of clinical symptoms there is a humoral immune response and antibodies to structural HAV proteins (anti-HAV) are detectable in patients' serum. Initially, these are mainly IgM antibodies (IgM anti-HAV) which usually persist for approximately 6 months. During convalescence, anti-HAV IgG become predominant and remain detectable indefinitely, representing protective immunity to HAV.

Hepatitis B virus (HBV)

Two discoveries related to HBV mark the beginning of the understanding of hepatitis viruses. In 1965, Baruch Blumberg identified the hepatitis B surface antigen (HBsAg) of HBV, initially termed 'Australia antigen', and in 1970 the complete virion (a 42 nm particle) was identified by Dane and colleagues using electron microscopy. HBV belongs to a virus family named Hepadnaviridae, which includes similar hepatotropic DNA viruses specific for woodchucks, ground squirrels, and Pekin ducks.

Genome organization

The HBV genome contains only 3200 nucleotides and is the smallest DNA virus (Table 5.21.1). One of the DNA strands, known as the 'minus' strand, is almost a complete circle and contains four overlapping ORFs encoding enveloped (pre-S/S), core (precore/core), polymerase, and X proteins (Fig. 5.21.2). The other ('plus') strand is shorter and varies in length.

The envelope ORF contains 3 start codons which separate the pre-S1, pre-S2, and S regions, encoding the large (L), middle (M), and small (S) envelope proteins respectively. The surface gene encodes the major envelope protein (HBsAg), which has 226 amino acids. The translation product of the pre-S2 and S gene is the middle envelope protein and the product of pre-S1, pre-S2, and S gene is the large envelope protein. In addition to the complete virion, a much greater amount of noninfectious, 22 nm in diameter, spherical, and filamentous subviral particles are produced in infected hepatocytes. HBsAg and the middle envelope protein are present in all viral and subviral particles, while the large protein is present in the virions and in some subviral filaments. The domain which binds to a specific HBV receptor (still not defined) on the plasma membrane of hepatocytes resides within the pre-S1 region.

The precore/core ORF has two start codons which encode two closely related proteins. Translation from the preC start codon produces a precursor molecule, designated precore protein. In the endoplasmic reticulum this protein undergoes two proteolytic steps at the N- and at the C-terminal ends, and the resultant polypeptide is secreted from hepatocytes as hepatitis B e-antigen (HBeAg). This is a nonstructural protein, which is not essential for viral replication. Translation from the C start codon results in the nucleocapsid protein (HBcAg), which has 183 amino acids. In the cytoplasm of hepatocytes HBcAg assembles spontaneously into nucleocapsid particles. HBeAg and HBcAg share about 90% of the amino acids but differ substantially in their conformation.

The polymerase ORF encodes the HBV polymerase protein with 832 amino acids. It has three functional domains—terminal protein, reverse transcriptase, and RNAse H activity. The X ORF encodes a protein with 154 amino acids. Its role is not fully understood, but it functions as a transactivator of cellular and other viral genes. The X protein is not essential for the replication of hepadnaviruses, but is believed to contribute to HBV-related hepatocarcinogenesis.

Eight genotypes of HBV (designated with the letters A to H) have been determined. The variations involve approximately 10% of the genome. Data on the geographical distribution indicate that genotype A is predominant in central and northern Europe, genotypes B and C in Asia, genotype D in the Mediterranean basin, and genotype E in Africa.

Viral replication

Following HBV entry into hepatocytes, the nucleocapsid is transported to the nucleus (Fig. 5.21.3). Cellular enzymes repair the open circular HBV DNA into covalently closed circular DNA (cccDNA), which serves as a template for the synthesis of pregenomic and messenger RNAs. Viral DNA does not integrate into the host genome as part of the normal replication cycle. The pregenomic RNA is transported to the cytoplasm and serves as mRNA for translation of new core and polymerase proteins. When these three components (pregenomic RNA, core, and polymerase proteins) reach sufficient quantities, they assemble into nucleocapsid particles, with the polymerase protein being directly involved in the pregenomic RNA encapsidation. Inside the particles the pregenomic RNA is reverse transcribed into DNA 'minus' strand, while the RNA template is simultaneously degraded by RNAse H. Finally, the 'plus' strand is produced which completes a new, partially double-stranded, HBV DNA. Some of the newly synthesized nucleocapsids with HBV DNA are transported back to the nucleus, which maintains a stable pool of cccDNA.

Table 5.21.1 Main characteristics of hepatitis viruses

Virus	Family	Morphology	Genome	Proteins	Antibodies	Pathogenesis	Specific features
HAV	*Picornaviridae*	27–28 nm nonenveloped, spherical particles	Single-stranded linear RNA, 7474 nt	Four capsid proteins, viral polymerase, and proteases	Anti-HAV	Noncytopathic virus Immune-mediated acute hepatitis	No chronic infection Effective vaccines available
HBV	*Hepadnaviridae*	42 nm particle with nucleocapsid (core) and outer envelope (surface)	Partially double-stranded, circularDNA, 3200 nt	*Envelope* Major protein (HBsAg) Middle protein (PreS2+S) Large protein (PreS1+S2+S) *Nucleocapsid* (HBcAg) HBeAg nonstructural, soluble protein	Anti-HBs Anti-HBc Anti-HBe	Noncytopathic virus Immune-mediated acute and chronic hepatitis Weak T-cell reactivity—a dominant cause for persistent viral replication	In chronic infection spontaneous evolution from HBeAg(+) to anti-HBe(+) phase Mutant strains (surface, precore, polymerase) evolve under selection pressure DNA integration into host genome Transactivation of cellular genes Effective vaccines available
		22 nm spherical and filamentous subviral particles		Envelope proteins only	Anti-HBs		
HCV	*Flaviviridae*	50–60 nm enveloped spherical particles	Single-stranded linear RNA, approx. 9500 nt	*Structural* Envelope 1 (E1) Envelope 2 (E2) Nucleocapsid (core)	Anti-E1 Anti-E2 Anti-core	Usually noncytopathic virus Neutralizing antibodies (?)	High degree of virus heterogeneity (genotypes and quasi species) High propensity to chronic infection No integration in host genome
			Six major genotypes	*Nonstructural* NS2 NS3 NS4 NS5	Anti-NS3 Anti-NS4 Anti-NS5	T-cell reactivity—major role for resolution of acute infection	
HDV	Resembles viroids and plant viruses	35–37 nm enveloped particles	Single-stranded circular RNA, 1700 nt	HD-Ag (nucleocapsid) HBsAg (envelope)	Anti-HD Anti-HBs	Direct cytopathic and/or immune-mediated liver injury	Defective RNA virus Requires help from HBV for providing the envelope HBsAg
HEV	*Caliciviridae*	32–34 nm nonenveloped spherical particles	Single-stranded linear RNA, 7500 nt	ORF1—nonstructural proteins ORF2—structural proteins ORF3—unknown function	Anti-HEV	Probably immune mediated (?)	Enterically transmitted hepatitis mainly in Asia, Middle East, and Central America No chronic infection
HGV/GBV-C	*Flaviviridae*	?	Single-stranded linear RNA, 9400 nt	Conserved E2 No core protein	Anti-E2	Primary site of replication unknown Does not cause hepatitis	Can establish chronic infection No clear pathogenic role
TTV	*Circinoviridae* (?)	?	Single-stranded, circular DNA, approx. 3850 nt	?	?	Does not cause hepatitis	Can establish chronic infection High degree of virus heterogeneity No clear pathogenic role

NS, nonstructural; nt, nucleotides; ORF, open reading frame.

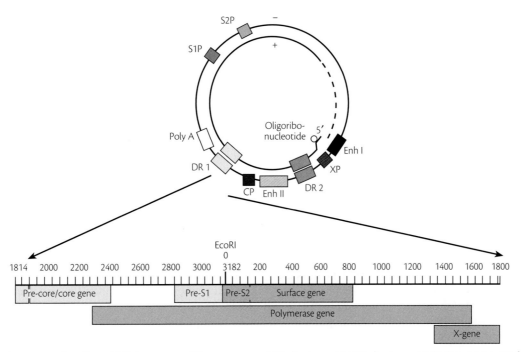

Fig. 5.21.2 Schematic representation of hepatitis B virus genome. CP, core promoter; DR1, direct repeat 1; DR2, direct repeat 2; EcoRI, restriction site for EcoRI enzyme used as a starting point for numbering; EnhI, enhancer I; EnhII, enhancer II; S1P, pre-S1 promoter; S2P, pre-S2 promoter; XP, X gene promoter.

Others are enveloped and leave the cell as new virions. The replication strategy used by hepadnaviruses differs from that of retroviruses in two main aspects: 1) integration into the host genome is not obligatory during replication; 2) functional mRNAs are produced from several internal promoters of the circular DNA genome.

Host immune response and pathogenesis

HBV is a noncytopathic virus. The virus-specific cellular immune response mainly determines the outcome of infection. Both HLA class I and class II-restricted T-cell responses are strong and directed to multiple viral antigens in patients with acute self-limited

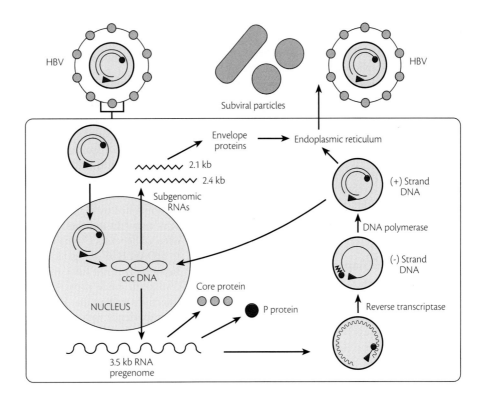

Fig. 5.21.3 Replicative cycle of hepatitis B virus.

hepatitis B. Despite clearance of serum HBsAg, HBV DNA remains detectable by polymerase chain reaction (PCR) in most cases, and HBV-specific CD4+ and CD8+ T-cell reactivity has been demonstrated 10 to 20 years after the time of acute infection. Cytokines released from these cells, especially interferon-γ, have been shown to exert a noncytolytic inhibition on HBV replication without causing cell death. Thus, eradication of HBV may be rare, but an effective immune response controls HBV DNA expression and there is no liver disease. Patients with chronic HBV infection (defined by detection of HBsAg in serum for longer than 6 months) show weak virus-specific T-cell reactivity, which is the dominant cause for HBV persistence. This ineffective response, together with antigen nonspecific inflammatory cells recruited at the site of inflammation, is responsible for the progression of liver damage.

The humoral immune response involves antibodies directed at different HBV antigens (Table 5.21.1). The clinical significance is based on several aspects: 1) diagnosis—the antibody profile in the serum, together with the result of HBsAg and HBeAg, is used to define different phases of HBV infection; 2) prophylaxis—the development and the level of the protective antibody (anti-HBs) is used to monitor the response to vaccination; 3) pathogenesis—the humoral immune response contributes to viral elimination from the circulation by forming immune complexes. In some cases, the tissue deposition of antigen-antibody complexes is responsible for extrahepatic pathology such as glomerulonephritis, polyarteritis nodosa, arthritis, and skin changes.

Evolution of chronic HBV infection

HBV–host interactions change over time, typically in four consecutive phases, which are characterized by different levels of HBV replication and associated liver disease. The early 'immunotolerant' phase is associated with high levels of virus replication. HBeAg and HBV DNA are readily detectable in serum, while there is minimal liver inflammation. Over the years this is followed by a phase with enhanced immune reactivity to the virus, as reflected by significant hepatic inflammation and elevated serum aminotransferases. Serum HBeAg is still positive and serum HBV DNA level is usually lower. Some patients will progress spontaneously to the next 'nonreplicative' or low-replicative phase, manifested by seroconversion to anti-HBe, undetectable or less than 2000 IU/ml viraemia (by polymerase chain reaction-based assays), and resolution of hepatic inflammation. In a proportion of patients, HBeAg loss may be due to the emergence of mutations in the core promoter and/or in the precore region (usually the $G_{1896}A$ stop codon), which prevent the translation of HBeAg. These HBe-minus mutants are replication competent and when viraemia levels are high, they cause HBe-negative chronic hepatitis B. The latter is characterized by fluctuating serum HBV DNA levels, mirrored by serum alanine aminotransferase (ALT) fluctuations, and progressive liver disease.

Hepatitis C virus (HCV) (Chapter 5.22)

Hepatitis D virus (HDV)

HDV is a defective virus that causes acute and chronic liver disease only in association with hepatitis B virus. This unique pathogen was discovered in 1977 by Mario Rizzetto in liver biopsies from patients with hepatitis B. HDV particles contain the viral RNA nucleocapsid, which is hepatitis delta antigen (HDAg), and an outer envelope (HBsAg), which is provided by the helper virus HBV. The HDV genome is a single-stranded, circular RNA (Table 5.21.1), and is the smallest known animal virus genome. Because of a high degree of internal complementarity, 70% of the nucleotides are base-paired. This gives an unusual, rod-like structure of the HDV genome. HDV RNA replicates via RNA-directed RNA synthesis by transcription of genomic RNA to a complementary antigenomic delta RNA. The latter serves as a template for subsequent genomic RNA synthesis. HDV produces a single protein, hepatitis delta antigen (HDAg), which is encoded by the antigenomic RNA. RNA editing of the antigenomic RNA allows the virus to make two forms of HDAg—small (HDAg-S, 195 amino acids) and large (HDAg-L, 214 amino acids). Both forms are present in the virions and have different functions in the HDV replicative cycle. HDAg-S facilitates HDV RNA replication, while HDAg-L inhibits replication and is required for assembly of the virion. Although the formation of delta virions requires the helper function of HBV, the replication of HDV RNA within the cell can occur without HBV.

Eight phylogenetically distinct HDV genotypes have been identified. The most widespread is genotype 1, identified in Africa, Asia, Europe, and North America, which is associated with a broad spectrum of chronic liver disease. Genotype 2 is found only in East Asia and seems to cause mild hepatitis delta. Genotype 3 is found exclusively in northern parts of South America and is associated with particularly severe hepatitis. At least five additional HDV genotypes have been described; their clinical features are less well characterized than genotypes 1 to 3.

Clinical manifestations vary from acute to fulminant hepatitis and from an asymptomatic carrier state to progressive chronic liver disease. Clinical outcome may be related to different HDV genotypes. Persistent HDV replication is associated with annual rates of development of cirrhosis and hepatocellular carcinoma of 4% and 2.8% respectively. Diagnosis is based on the detection of serum HDAg (detectable in acute infection), serum HDV RNA, and anti-HDV antibodies. The optimal treatment of HDV is uncertain. Interferon alpha is the only licensed treatment but responses have been poor. Pegylated interferon may be better but data are limited and the addition of nucleoside analogues does not appear to be beneficial. Prevention of HDV is by vaccination against HBV.

Host immune response and pathogenesis

HDV can infect a person either simultaneously with HBV (coinfection) or as superinfection of a person with chronic HBV infection. Because HDV requires the helper function of HBV, the duration of delta infection is determined by the duration of HBsAg positivity. Analogous to the antibodies to HBV nucleocapsid (anti-HBc), antibodies to HDAg are not protective. Chronic HDV infection is accompanied by high titres of IgG anti-HD. A high serum level of IgM anti-HD indicates acute delta infection or exacerbation of chronic hepatitis D. The relative role of cellular immune reactions to HDAg, HBV antigens, or both in the immunopathogenesis of hepatitis D is not fully understood. The lack of liver pathology in transgenic mice expressing HDV and data from experimental infections suggest that HDV is not cytopathic. This is supported by the experience with patients undergoing liver transplantation for HDV cirrhosis. Although HDV recurs universally in the graft, necroinflammation is absent unless HBV recurs as well. The presence of microvesicular steatosis in severe hepatitis D indicates a possible direct cytopathic effect in some circumstances.

Hepatitis E virus (HEV)

HEV was first identified in 1983 by immune electron microscopy in the faeces of patients and classified in the genus *Hepevirus*, family Hepeviridiae. HEV is an icosahedral, nonenveloped single-stranded RNA virus that is 27 to 34 nm in diameter. The HEV genome is a single-stranded, polyadenylated RNA of approximately 7500 nucleotides and contains three ORFs (Table 5.21.1). ORF1 encodes nonstructural proteins involved in virus replication—helicase and RNA-dependent RNA polymerase. ORF2, comprising approximately 2000 nucleotides, codes for the major structural proteins. ORF3 has 328 nucleotides and also appears to code for a structural protein. The genomic organization of HEV is different from HAV and HCV because the structural and nonstructural proteins are coded by discontinuous, partially overlapping ORFs. HEV is widely distributed with the highest incidence of infection in Asia, Africa, the Middle East, and Central America. It is spread by the faeco-oral route in endemic areas. Person-to-person transmission is uncommon. HEV may be transmitted by blood transfusion, particularly in endemic areas. Unlike HAV, HEV infection may be zoonotic. HEV RNA has been found in the faeces of wild pigs and serological evidence of infection was found in pigs, cattle, and sheep in endemic regions. Transmission has been reported in the context of consumption of undercooked meat.

Four genotypes of HEV have been identified, which show 25% nucleotide variability. Geographically, genotype 1 has been isolated from tropical countries in Asia and Africa; genotype 2 was found in Mexico, whereas genotype 3 has worldwide distribution, including America, Asia, and Europe. Genotype 4 in contrast has been found only in Asia. Non-travel-associated hepatitis E has been diagnosed in indigenous patients in England and Wales. In the majority of cases it was caused by HEV genotype 3. For vaccine development, it is important that all HEV strains share at least one major, serogically cross-reactive, epitope.

HEV usually causes an acute self-limited infection, although fulminant infection may occur. Fulminant infection is more common in pregnancy, malnutrition, and in those with pre-existing liver disease. Chronic HEV infection has been reported in transplant recipients and in immunosuppressed individuals, e.g. patients with non-Hodgkin's lymphoma treated with rituximab, and HIV patients. Treatment is supportive; case reports have suggested a benefit from ribavirin.

The primary site of HEV replication is not fully understood. Following intravenous HEV inoculation in experimental models, serum aminotransferases levels rise after 24 to 38 days. Expression of HEV antigens has been detected in the cytoplasm of hepatocytes as early as 7 to 10 days after inoculation. Experimental data indicate that during an initial phase with high HEV replication the virus may be released from hepatocytes into bile, which occurs before the elevation of liver enzymes and morphological changes in the liver. The virus shedding appears to end with the normalization of serum aminotransferases. HEV RNA is detectable in the stool 1 week before the onset of illness and persists for 2 weeks thereafter. HEV RNA is detectable in the serum by real-time polymerase chain reaction (PCR) in the serum of virtually all patients within 2 weeks after the onset of hepatitis. Prolonged periods of viraemia, between 4 to 16 weeks, have also been reported. The detection of anti-HEV by enzyme immunoassays, involving recombinant HEV antigens or synthetic peptides, is the most frequently used method for diagnostic purposes and for epidemiological studies.

During acute infection, the humoral immune response gradually develops in parallel with the ALT rise. The serum level of anti-HEV IgM reaches a maximal titre around the time of peak ALT levels and is detectable for 5 to 6 months. Although the IgG anti-HEV response persists for several years after the acute phase, the natural history of protective immunity to HEV is not fully established. In contrast to HAV, hepatitis E shows an unusually high attack rate amongst adults, suggesting that immunity to HEV, if acquired in childhood, may wane.

Vaccines against HEV are being developed and two large randomized controlled trials have shown 96% preventive efficacy in endemic settings. There is no evidence for the efficacy of pre- or postexposure prophylaxis with immune globulin for the prevention of HEV.

New hepatitis-associated viruses

GB virus C (GBV-C) or hepatitis G virus (HGV)

The genome of GBV-C was identified in 1995 by molecular hybridization techniques in the serum of a patient with the initials GB. In parallel, another group of investigators identified the genome of a new RNA virus, named hepatitis G virus. The comparison of HGV and GBV-C genomes revealed very high homology, both at nucleotide (86%) and amino acid level (100%). It is now accepted that they represent two isolates of the same virus. GBV-C/HGV is an RNA virus with a single ORF encoding a polyprotein of approximately 3000 amino acids (Table 5.21.1). Together with another two RNA viruses, GBV-A and GBV-B, it belongs to the Flaviviridae and these three viruses show various similarities with HCV. Specific features of the GBV-C/HGV genome include absence of core gene (nucleocapsid); long 5′ and 3′ NTR and lack of poly A tail. Unlike HCV, this virus has a very conserved E2 region. GBV-C has a global distribution with a high prevalence in the North American blood donor population. Longitudinal studies have shown that GBV-C/HGV can establish chronic infection with RNA persistence in serum for up to 15 years. A proportion of patients clear the virus spontaneously and develop anti-E2 reactivity, which is used as a marker of past infection. Anti-E2 also seems to confer protective immunity. A large body of evidence suggests that GBV-C/HGV does not cause liver disease. Evidence suggests a protective effect of GBV-C in patients coinfected with HIV. The protective effect may be related to maintenance of an intact T-helper 1 cytokine profile, induction of HIV-1 inhibitory cytokines and interference with HIV-1 replication; the therapeutic implications of these findings remain unclear.

TT virus (TTV)

TTV was identified in 1997 by investigators in Japan. By applying the methodology used for the identification of GBV-C, they detected the genome of a new DNA virus in the serum of a patient with cryptogenic post-transfusion hepatitis. The patient's initials (TT) prompted the name of this new virus and a causative role for acute and chronic hepatitis was suggested. TTV and its smaller variant are now spelt as Torque teno virus (TTV) and Torque teno minivirus (TTMV), after the Latin for 'thin necklace'.

The TTV genome is circular, single-stranded DNA of approximately 3850 nucleotides (Table 5.21.1). Three partially open reading frames have been predicted, but TTV proteins have not been expressed, so far. It is suggested that TTV belongs to the genus *Anellovirus* in the Circinoviridae family. TTV DNA has been detected in nonhuman primates and in farm animals. The primary site of TTV replication and the biological nature of TTV are still unknown.

Unlike other DNA viruses, TTV shows remarkable genomic variability. Phylogenetic analyses of TTV isolates have identified at least 20 genotypes, which differ between each other by more than 40% of the DNA sequences. As recombinant viral proteins are not available, the diagnosis of TTV infection is based on the detection of TTV DNA by PCR. TT virus population is very heterogeneous, and frequently a mixed infection with 3 to 5 TTV genotypes is present in one patient.

TTV infection is ubiquitous in more than 90% of adults worldwide. The virus was initially thought to have mainly a parenteral route of transmission, although the high prevalence of TTV infection in the general population indicates the importance of non-parenteral routes as well. The prevalence of TTV infection was shown to increase with age in paediatric and adult groups.

The pathogenic role of TTV, if any, is unknown. Analysis of liver histology in patients with TTV infection, longitudinal studies, as well as experimental TTV inoculation in chimpanzees all demonstrate that this virus does not cause hepatitis. Possible associations with other diseases, such as severe idiopathic inflammatory myopathies, systemic lupus erythematosus, pancreatic cancer, diabetes mellitus, laryngeal cancer, and periodontal disease have been reported. TTV may replicate in the respiratory tract of children and has been implicated in acute respiratory diseases in infants and exacerbations of asthma and bronchiectasis. However, TTV remains an example of a human virus with no clear disease association.

SEN virus (SEN-V)

SEN-V is a recently discovered single-stranded DNA virus, distantly related to TTV, with a worldwide distribution. Eight genotypes of SEN-V, designated A to H, have been identified. SEN-V is transmitted via transfusion of blood products and parenteral contact. Interest in SEN-V was triggered by the initial reports that two SEN-V genotypes, SEN-V-D and H, were associated with post-transfusion non-A, non-E hepatitis. No causative agent and no evidence of hepatitis due to SEN-V infection have yet been established.

Further reading

Hino S, Miyata H (2007). Torque teno virus (TTV): current status. *Rev Med Virol*, **17**, 45–57.

Hoofnagle JH, *et al.* (2007). Management of hepatitis B: summary of a clinical research workshop. *Hepatology*, **45**, 1056–75.

Hughes SA, Wedemeyer H, Harrison PM (2011). Hepatitis delta virus. *Lancet*, **378**(9785), 73–85. [Review.]

Naoumov NV (2006). Hepatitis A and E. *Medicine*, **35**, 35–38.

Rehermann B, Nascimbeni M (2005). Immunology of hepatitis B virus and hepatitis C virus infection. *Nat Rev Immunol*, **5**, 215–29.

Taylor JM (2006). Structure and replication of hepatitis delta virus RNA. *Curr Top Microbiol Immunol*, **307**, 1–23.

Tellinghuisen TL, *et al.* (2007). Studying hepatitis C virus: making the best of a bad virus. *J Virol*, **81**, 8853–67.

Teshale EH, Hu DJ, Holmberg SD (2010). The two faces of hepatitis E virus. *Clin Infect Dis*, **51**, 328–34. [Review.]

5.22 Hepatitis C

Paul Klenerman, K.J.M. Jeffery, and J. Collier

Essentials

Hepatitis C virus (HCV) is an RNA virus that has evolved into multiple genotypes (1–6) and subtypes. Humans are the only known natural host. HCV replication is highly error-prone, hence within any one person the virus exists as a swarm of closely related variants, known as 'quasispecies'.

Epidemiology—HCV is a major cause of liver disease worldwide, with 170 million people probably infected. Spread is parenteral and usually associated with needle use, most commonly by injection drug users in the West; mother-to-child infection does occur but is infrequent, as is sexual spread. Before the screening of blood products was introduced, blood transfusion recipients and patients with haemophilia were also at risk, and outbreaks in some countries (e.g. Egypt) have been associated with mass vaccination and parenteral therapy programmes.

Clinical aspects—these are discussed in detail in the Oxford Textbook of Medicine 5e Chapter 15.21.1, but HCV tends to become persistent in most of those infected, although around 25% clear the virus as a result of effective innate and adaptive immune responses at the time of acute infection. The clinical course is variable in those with persistent infection: most develop some degree of hepatic inflammation and fibrotic liver disease, with a fraction going on to develop cirrhosis, with an increased risk of hepatocellular carcinoma. Cofactors which predispose to progression include simultaneous HIV infection and drinking alcohol.

Treatment: now and in the future—treatment is currently a combination of pegylated interferon-α and ribavirin with or without a protease inhibitor, with outcome dependent on viral genotype. Future therapies will include other compounds directed against specific viral gene products (direct acting antiviral compounds, DAA) such as polymerase inhibitors may be useful, but the capacity of the virus to mutate and thus evade both drug therapy and immune responses may be a major barrier to universal virus eradication. .

Introduction

Hepatitis C virus (HCV) is a major global pathogen. Humans are the only known natural hosts, although chimpanzees have been infected experimentally. The origin of the virus in humans is not well established, but the huge genetic diversity and global distribution, together with analyses of the viral molecular clock, suggest that it has coevolved with human populations for centuries. In the 1990s, spread through changes in medical practice and injection drug use was recognized to have created an emerging problem. The capacity of the virus to persist despite host innate and adaptive immune responses makes it extremely challenging to develop vaccines. Although there have been major improvements in the efficacy of treatment regimens, they are still expensive, hard to deliver, and associated with serious side effects. Therefore, it is important to identify those who are most likely to benefit from the available therapies, based on the observed progression and likely response to treatment. Improved understanding of the viral replication cycle and the most effective immune responses is leading to more selective drugs and vaccines.

Historical perspective

Previously known as non-A, non-B hepatitis, HCV was recognized for many years before its discovery by Kuo and Houghton in 1988. It was soon identified as a major infectious agent and the development of antibody-based assays revealed its prevalence, and allowed the development of screening tools for blood products. The majority of chronic viral carriers were identified by detection of viral RNA in blood, while sequencing and bioinformatics approaches led to the description of diverse viral genotypes. Inability to culture the virus proved a major obstacle, but the development of a replicon system by Bartenschlager in 1999 was a major breakthrough, allowing a dissection of viral replication *in vitro*. However, no infectious virus system was available until 2005, when several groups used an unusual Japanese strain (JFH-1) to develop cell culture infectious systems.

Aetiology, genetics, pathogenesis, and pathology

HCV is a positive-sense single-stranded RNA virus. It is classed individually as an hepacivirus and is genetically closely related to flaviviruses, such as dengue virus. The viral RNA genome is approximately 10 kb in length and comprises a long, single open reading frame. The genome is typically divided into structural and nonstructural proteins. The structural proteins, contained within virions, comprise core and envelope (E1 and E2). The latter are glycosylated, form a heterodimer, and are important targets for antibodies. They are also highly variable and contain hypervariable regions (HVR1 and HVR2), which evolve rapidly under antibody selection pressure. The nonstructural proteins include enzymes with defined protease and helicase activity, and a viral polymerase.

Viral replication is initiated using an internal ribosomal entry site (IRES) in the 5′ untranslated region (5′ UTR). The latter is highly conserved, varying only slightly between genotypes and so is an important target for molecular diagnosis. The polymerase replicates the virus through a double-stranded intermediate, which is a substantial trigger for host innate responses. However, the virus can disable triggering of one of these pathways (RIG-I; retinoic acid inducible gene I) through the action of the protease, which cleaves a cellular target (Cardif; CARD adapter inducing interferon (IFN)-β). Another important feature is that replication is highly error-prone. Thus, within any one person, the virus exists as a swarm of closely related variants, known as 'quasispecies'.

HCV usually replicates in hepatocytes. Virus has been observed in other cell types, including lymphocytes and dendritic cells, and within the central nervous system, but it is uncertain how this contributes to disease pathogenesis. A number of cellular receptors for HCV have been described including: CD81 (a member of the tetraspanin family with signalling properties on lymphocytes); the LDL (low-density lipoprotein) receptor; DC-SIGN (dendritic cell-specific ICAM3-grabbing nonintegrin); a macrophage scavenger receptor class B1 (SR B1); and Claudin-1and Occludin, both components of tight junctions. None of these fully explains the hepatotropism of the virus.

After natural or experimental infection, virus may be detectable for weeks or months without any apparent clinical, biochemical, or immunological disturbance. During this time, virus may replicate to high levels in blood and within the liver, indicating the minimal direct cytopathic effects of the virus in the absence of host immune responses. This silent phase is followed by the onset of acute hepatitis, which is not always clinically apparent. Detailed intrahepatic studies in animal models (not possible in man) reveal that the first responses at this stage of infection are production of innate immune mediators (IFNs, NK cells), followed by an influx of T cells (both CD4+ and CD8+). In human studies of acute hepatitis C, the emergence of highly activated, virus-specific CD8+ T cells correlates quantitatively and temporally with the peak of the alanine aminotransferase (ALT), suggesting that tissue damage at this stage is a result largely of the host T-cell response.

The subsequent events vary substantially between different patients, but three clinical patterns are observed: clearance of virus below the level of detection in blood; persistence of virus without host control; or an intermediate state, where the virus is transiently controlled, but relapses. The immunological differences determining these outcomes are not clear, but include both innate and adaptive components. Polymorphisms linked to the *IL28B* gene indicate a major role for interferon-lambda in acute outcome (see below). Similarly, the association of specific HLA genes, both class II (such as *HLA DR11/DQ3*) and class I (such as *HLA B27* and *B57*), with spontaneous resolution point to the importance of T-cell responses. The broader and more sustained in number and function the responses are, the more likely they are to be successful in viral control. B-cell responses are also likely to be involved. However, the rapid emergence of viral escape mutants in the hypervariable envelope regions may limit the efficacy of neutralizing antibody responses in containing viral replication. Viral mutation within T-cell epitopes is also a major cause of persistence despite T-cell responses, although other phenomena such as T-cell exhaustion and the emergence of regulatory T-cell subsets also contribute to T-cell failure.

In the 25% in whom virus is cleared below the level of detection long term, antibody and T-cell responses may be detected for many years. In most people, virus persists after the acute hepatitis, despite the presence of antibody. T-cell responses in blood at this stage are weak, but infiltrates of T cells may be found within the liver.

Liver histopathology due to HCV infection can vary greatly, and there is no diagnostic staining pattern. Portal tract infiltrates of T and B cells are typical, sometimes with the emergence of lymphoid follicles within liver tissue. Histological scores (Ishak's, Metavir) have been developed to quantify the degree of liver damage. These assess the degree of hepatic inflammation (typically portal tract infiltration, 'interface' hepatitis, lobular infiltration and necrosis), and the degree of hepatic fibrosis.

The viral genotype is not thought to have a major effect on pathogenesis, although genotype 3 has been associated with the development of hepatic steatosis, which might contribute to increased inflammation and fibrosis.

Epidemiology

HCV is estimated to infect around 170 million people worldwide. Spread is parenteral, and usually associated with needle use (intravenous drug users, patients in parenteral therapy programmes, nosocomial spread) and exposure to infected blood products (recipients of unscreened blood or plasma fractions, haemophiliacs). Mother-to-child infection does occur, but at relatively low rates (around 3–5%), and sexual spread is also infrequent.

In the West, injection drug users have particularly high rates of acquisition and now represent the main focus of the infection. In some countries, notably Egypt, medical programmes have resulted in the spread of HCV in specific groups, and the 20 to 30% prevalence of HCV in some communities in Egypt is the highest worldwide.

HCV has evolved into multiple genotypes (1–6) and subtypes. Molecular typing techniques can trace the spread of individual strains within populations (including those from a single source). The Egyptian outbreak is genotype 4a, the older circulating Western strains were typically genotype 1a and 1b, and the more recent strains acquired by Western drug users are 3a. Genotype 3 viruses were originally found in Asia, where genotype 6 is still prevalent. Genotypes 2 and 5 have remained mainly localized to West and South Africa respectively, but all strains are tending to spread worldwide.

Prevention

Primary prevention

There are no licensed HCV vaccines. Primary prevention of HCV worldwide depends on ensuring a safe blood supply and sterile injection devices for all health care applications. Provision of sterile equipment to injection drug users has been shown to reduce the prevalence of HCV. Infection is not transmitted by normal household exposure, but household contacts of HCV-positive people should avoid sharing razors and toothbrushes. Sexual transmission of HCV is inefficient and studies show a low prevalence (average 1.5%) of HCV infection in long-term partners of patients with chronic HCV infection who had no other risk factors. Multiple published studies have demonstrated that the prevalence of HCV infection among men who have sex with men (MSM) who were not injecting drugs, was similar to that in heterosexuals. However, a high incidence of acute hepatitis C in HIV-positive MSM has recently been recognized.

No intervention has been shown clearly to decrease the risk of mother-to-child transmission of HCV, and breastfeeding is not discouraged. The risk of mother-to-child transmission is increased two-to threefold if there is HIV/HCV coinfection. Medical workers should ensure aseptic techniques and appropriate equipment and facilities to reduce the risk of percutaneous injury.

Postexposure prophylaxis

Immune globulin is not effective in preventing HCV infection following exposure. Anyone exposed to the virus, e.g. following needle-stick injury or perinatally, should be offered follow-up testing for HCV. The average risk of infection following a percutaneous injury is 1.8% (range 0–7%) and those who become infected should be offered early antiviral therapy.

Clinical features

Acute hepatitis C

Acute HCV infection is usually asymptomatic, but is otherwise clinically indistinguishable from other causes of acute viral hepatitis. There is prodromal fever, myalgia, and malaise. Compared with hepatitis A or B, classical symptoms of jaundice, pruritus, pale stools, and dark urine are unusual. Serum transaminase levels can be markedly elevated, although values of up to 10 times the upper limit of normal would be more usual. Fulminant hepatic failure is rare in acute HCV infection. There is evidence that patients with symptomatic acute HCV infection have a higher rate of spontaneous viral clearance than those with asymptomatic infection. Overall, approximately one in four patients will clear the virus spontaneously. In those with persistent virus, serum transaminases may return to normal, but they usually remain elevated at about twice the upper limit of normal (Fig. 5.22.1).

Polymorphisms in the region of the *IL28B* gene are important predictors of spontaneous clearance. In a single-source outbreak amongst Irish women, those with a favourable polymorphism had an odds ratio for spontaneous clearance of nearly fourfold. However, the mechanism underlying this substantial effect remains unclear.

Chronic infection

Chronic infection with HCV is defined as the persistence of HCV RNA in blood for more than 6 months. Most patients with chronic HCV are unaware of their diagnosis, and many will have been tested following an incidental finding of abnormal liver function tests or on routine screening, e.g. for blood donation, or having given a history of potential HCV exposure, such as injection drug use. Such patients may be asymptomatic or have nonspecific symptoms such as fatigue. Clinical features of liver disease are unlikely to be present unless cirrhosis has developed. Laboratory abnormalities such as hypoalbuminaemia, thrombocytopenia, and coagulopathy suggest cirrhosis, although this can only be confirmed histologically by liver biopsy.

HCV is associated with several extrahepatic manifestations, the best documented of which are HCV-related lymphoproliferative disorders, characteristically with mixed cryoglobulinaemia. Although studies suggest a high prevalence of serum cryoglobulins in HCV-positive patients, they are generally present at low levels with few, if any, symptoms. Occasionally, patients will present with neuropathies, arthralgias, and purpura. In more severe cases, there may be renal involvement (e.g. glomerulonephritis). In some studies, B-cell non-Hodgkin's lymphomas, porphyria cutanea tarda, Sjögren's syndrome, lichen planus, autoimmune thyroiditis, and type 2 diabetes mellitus have been found more frequently in association with HCV infection than in control groups.

Prognosis

The rate of progression of HCV is highly variable. Risk factors for progression include: older age at acquisition of infection; male gender; immunosuppression including HIV coinfection; and concurrent heavy alcohol consumption. It is estimated that 7 to 20% will develop cirrhosis within 20 years of infection. Progression rates are highest in those with transfusion-associated hepatitis.

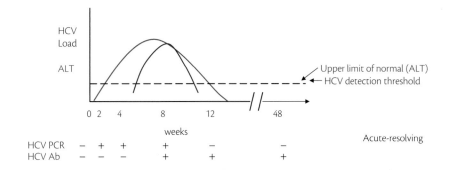

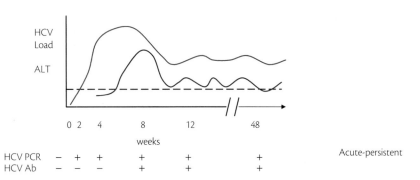

Fig. 5.22.1 Typical virological and biochemical test results following infection with hepatitis C in (a) patients who clear the virus (acute resolving) and (b) those that go on to get persistent infection (acute persistent). The time lines vary between patients and these are approximations based on human and chimpanzee model infections. Some patients, such as those with HIV, may never develop an antibody response. ALT, alanine aminotransferase.

However, some groups, such as a cohort of Irish women infected in 1977 through contaminated blood products, show very low rates, with only 3% developing cirrhosis within 20 years of infection.

Once cirrhosis has developed, 80% will have complications such as ascites and variceal bleeding within 10 years. Fifty per cent of these patients will develop liver failure within a further 5 years. Hepatocellular carcinoma occurs only in the presence of cirrhosis, with an incidence of 1 to 5% per year. HIV coinfected patients progress more rapidly to liver failure once complications of cirrhosis have occurred.

Liver transplantation is indicated for decompensated HCV cirrhosis and for cirrhotics who develop a small hepatocellular carcinoma despite good liver function. The infection always recurs in the transplanted liver and progression to cirrhosis occurs in about 10% of transplant recipients within 5 years. Only about 20% of patients with recurrent HCV post-transplantation can be cured with pegylated IFN and ribavirin, which is often poorly tolerated.

Diagnosis

Serology

Initial diagnosis of HCV infection is usually made by detecting HCV antibody to recombinant HCV proteins in sensitive screening immunoassays. In low prevalence populations, the probability of a false positive antibody result is high, and supplementary confirmatory tests should be performed, such as immunoassays using different antigens. Alternatively, highly specific line or strip immunoblots (which have individual synthetic or recombinant antigens applied as separate lines to a solid phase) can distinguish different antigens to which the serum is reacting, and confirm the presence of HCV antibody.

Recent developments include assays which combine tests for antibody and HCV core antigen. These are more useful for the diagnosis of acute infection (Fig. 5.22.1) as the HCV core antigen can be used to detect HCV infection during the window phase of infection. These assays are likely to be particularly useful for screening programmes (e.g. blood donation services and renal dialysis units). HCV core antigen may also have a role in informing response-guided therapy with treatment regimens which include protease inhibitors. The appearance of HCV antibody after infection can take up to 2 months in immunocompetent people, and may be delayed or even absent in immunocompromised patients, such as those with HIV infection or those who are on haemodialysis. By 6 months, 97% of those infected will have developed an antibody response. It is good practice to confirm the presence of HCV antibody with a second sample.

HCV RNA testing

Nucleic acid tests are essential for the diagnosis of acute and chronic HCV infection, and should be used as supplementary tests for confirmation of HCV antibody tests. HCV RNA can be detected by polymerase chain reaction (PCR) as early as 2 weeks after infection, before the appearance of antibody. Several amplification techniques, including reverse transcriptase PCR (RT-PCR), transcription-mediated amplification (TMA), and branched DNA (bDNA) are available. Most commercial assays now produce quantitative results with increasingly sensitive limits of detection. Although quantitative tests (i.e. a measure of viral load, which may vary across several logs between individuals) may be important to predict the response to interferon (IFN) therapy (see below), in contrast to HIV infection they are not useful in predicting disease severity or long-term progression. Some countries have successfully introduced nucleic acid screening of pools of samples for blood donation. Dried blood spot testing for both hepatitis C antibody and RNA is now widely available, and can be used to facilitate screening in certain groups, e.g. injection drug users engaging in needle-exchange programmes.

Pretreatment evaluation

HCV virus genotyping is essential before treatment as it determines the duration of treatment and the response (see below). Most genotyping methods are based on viral sequencing and subsequent phylogenetic analysis, or on the detection of nucleic acid mutations specific for individual genotypes. A pretreatment liver biopsy is frequently, but not always, performed to assess the degree of fibrosis. Noninvasive methods of assessing the degree of liver fibrosis using serum markers, and assessment of liver stiffness using an ultrasound probe (e.g. Fibroscan, FibroSure/FibroTest) are an alternative to liver biopsy as they can differentiate mild fibrosis from cirrhosis.

Genotyping of the patient for *IL28B* polymorphisms can also contribute to pretreatment evaluation. In genome-wide association studies (GWAS) of interferon/ribavirin therapy for genotype 1, a major impact of those *IL28B* polymorphisms which favour spontaneous clearance has been shown for treatment response. Together with other clinical markers this information can now be used to provide an indication of the likelihood of a successful response to conventional therapy.

Treatment

The aim of HCV therapy is to eradicate HCV RNA from serum. Although loss of viraemia is associated with improvement in liver histology, the risk of hepatocellular carcinoma by ultrasound remains if cirrhosis is present. Tumours have been detected up to 5 years after successful treatment with antiviral therapy. Screening of cirrhotic patients for hepatocellular carcinoma should therefore be continued.

HCV viraemia may re-emerge within 6 months of stopping treatment (relapse), but those who remain HCV RNA negative for 6 months are considered to be cured (sustained virus response, (SVR)) and viraemia will not recur.

Chronic hepatitis C

Interferon-α and ribavirin underpin current treatments for chronic HCV infection. Interferon-α (IFN–α) induces the expression of multiple genes with antiviral and antiproliferative actions, including those encoding RNAses, 2′,5′-oligoadenylate synthetase, and protein kinase R. It is given as pegylated IFN once weekly in combination with ribavirin. The two types of pegylated IFN-α, 2a and 2b, are IFN-α molecules with modified side chains that prolong their half-lives. Ribavirin is a guanosine analogue which does not reduce HCV RNA levels when used alone but sustains virological suppression when combined with IFN-α.

Treatment success (SVR) is dependent on virus genotype. Following combination treatment with ribavirin (800–1000 mg/day orally) and pegylated IFN-α(180 μg/kg subcutaneously weekly for IFN-α2a, or 1.5 μg/kg subcutaneously weekly for IFN-α2b) the SVR in genotype 2 and 3 infection is 76 to 82%. For genotype 1 patients, 12 months of combination therapy only achieves an SVR in 42 to 46%. Predictors of an SVR include younger age, absence of cirrhosis, low HCV viral load (<400 000 IU/ml) and in genotype 1 patients, the presence of a favourable *IL28B* genotype. Response rates in genotype 4 are slightly better than for genotype 1 following 12 months of therapy. The poor response in genotype 1 patients has led to the development of first-generation directly acting antiviral (DAA) compounds with the licensing of two protease inhibitors, to be used in combination with pegylated interferon and ribavirin.

In trials, both boceprevir and telaprevir increased the SVR in treatment-naive patients to around 70%, and may allow the duration of therapy to be reduced from 48 to 24 weeks. In previously treated patients who relapsed following therapy within 6 months, retreatment with interferon and ribavirin with the addition of teleprevir or boceprevir resulted in SVR in up to 88% of subjects, with up to 59% SVR rate in partial responders and 33% in previous nonresponders. The absence of a one-log drop in HCV viral load at 4 weeks is a useful predictor of nonresponse. The next generation of protease inhibitors and other DAAs are likely to have efficacy against other genotypes.

Coinfection with HIV is not a contraindication to therapy, although the efficacy of treatment is reduced. Twelve months of ribavirin and pegylated IFN-α results in a sustained viral response in 29% of genotype 1 HCV/HIV coinfected patients and 62% in those with genotype 2 or 3. Data are awaited on the efficacy of newer agents in HCV/HIV coinfected patients.

Side effects of treatment are common and the quality of life is universally affected, although many patients are able to continue work during therapy. Treatment with IFN-α is associated with fatigue, depression, and mood swings. Other adverse effects include rashes and thyroid abnormalities. Influenza-like symptoms are frequent within 6 h of the first dose, but often improve over the first few weeks. Bone marrow suppression is common and may warrant dose reductions, a particular problem in cirrhotic patients who are pancytopenic before starting treatment. IFN-α is contraindicated in renal and cardiac transplant recipients for fear of inducing acute cellular rejection. Ribavirin causes haemolysis and frequently leads to a 2 to 3 g/dl drop in haemoglobin during treatment. As it is excreted by the kidney, it is contraindicated in renal failure. Complications of the protease inhibitors include severe rash (telaprevir) and anaemia (boceprevir).

Acute hepatitis C

The results of treating acute HCV infection are much better than in chronic infection. Up to 50% of patients with acute symptomatic HCV infection may clear the virus spontaneously within the first 3 months. Treatment should be started between 12 and 24 weeks of infection, allowing time to assess whether spontaneous resolution has occurred, without losing the clinical benefit of early treatment. Genotype does not substantially affect response and cure rates of 80 to 95% can be achieved.

The optimal regimen for treatment of acute hepatitis C remains to be determined but guidelines suggest that pegylated IFN should be used in equivalent doses to those in chronic infection, and that ribavirin may be added (800 mg daily), although success may be achieved with monotherapy. At least 24 weeks of therapy is recommended. In HCV HIV coinfected patients, cohort studies support the addition of ribavirin to pegylated interferon.

Areas of uncertainty or controversy

The significance of finding residual viral RNA in lymphocytes and liver tissue after successful treatment with HCV or spontaneous resolution of acute infection is unclear. The mechanism of action of ribavirin, including its effect on the immune response, is not understood. The role of adaptive immunity in the pathogenesis of HCV and the response to treatment in acute and chronic infection is debated. The functional impact of the polymorphisms in and around *IL28B* require further dissection and the specific protective role of IFN lambdas remain to be defined.

Likely future developments

There are more than 50 new DAAs targeting specific HCV enzymes in development: in addition to further protease inhibitors, these include drugs which interfere with NS5B RNA-dependent RNA polymerase, essential for virus replication. Nucleoside inhibitors of the HCV NS5B polymerase have been shown to have antiviral activity against several HCV genotypes, although the non-nucleoside polymerase inhibitors are primarily active against genotype 1. Phase 2 studies have demonstrated potent antiviral effects with polymerase inhibitors in combination with IFN and ribavirin, but drug toxicity has caused some agents to be withdrawn. Resistance to these agents can arise readily, resulting in reduced drug susceptibility. There is some evidence that resistance to the nucleoside inhibitors (which act as chain terminators) may arise less readily than resistance to the non-nucleoside (allosteric) inhibitors.

Other DAAs in development include the cyclophilin inhibitors. Cyclophilins are ubiquitously expressed proteins and have a role in the folding and isomerization of other proteins including those necessary for virus replication. Preliminary clinical studies have shown that in combination with IFN and ribavirin, cyclophilin inhibitors can boost SVR rates in treatment-naive genotype 1 patients, including those with unfavourable *IL28B* genotypes. Studies are under way in genotype 2 and 3 patients. Potential advantages may include a high barrier to resistance and a lack of cross-resistance with other DAAs.

It is hoped in future that combinations of DAAs acting at different points of the virus life-cycle will provide well tolerated, successful, oral, IFN-free regimens for both treatment-naive and treatment-experienced patients. The combination should be optimized to cross-resistance and prevent virological breakthrough. Proof-of-concept studies of protease and polymerase inhibitor combinations in human subjects achieved profound viral suppression and were well tolerated. In contrast to HIV, eradication of HCV infection should be achievable with short-course combination DAA.

Accessibility of current and newer HCV treatments on a global scale is essential if cirrhosis and hepatocellular carcinoma are to be prevented in most of the world's HCV-infected population.

Further reading

Bacon BR, *et al.*; HCV RESPOND-2 Investigators. (2011). Boceprevir for previously treated chronic HCV genotype 1 infection. *N Engl J Med*, **364**, 1207–17.

Benvegnu L, *et al.* (2004). Natural history of compensated viral cirrhosis: a prospective study on the incidence and hierarchy of major complications. *Gut*, **53**, 744–49. [Important study showing the risk of complications of cirrhosis occurring over a 10 year period of follow-up.]

Dienstag JL, McHutchison JG (2006). American Gastroenterological Association technical review on the management of hepatitis C. *Gastroenterology*, **130**, 231–64. [Comprehensive review of the management of HCV.]

di Iulio J, *et al.*; Swiss HIV Cohort Study (2011). Estimating the net contribution of interleukin-28B variation to spontaneous hepatitis C virus clearance. *Hepatology*, **53**, 1446–54. [Study identifying IL28B haplotypes highly predictive of spontaneous hepatitis C clearance.]

Feld JJ, Hoofnagle JH (2005). Mechanism of action of interferon and ribavirin in treatment of hepatitis C. *Nature*, **436**, 967–72.

[A review of how interferon and ribavirin act to eliminate HCV, with data on viral kinetics during treatment.]

Ge D, *et al* (2009). Genetic variation in IL28B predicts hepatitis C treatment-induced viral clearance. *Nature*, **461**, 399–401. [Study showing that a genetic polymorphism near the IL28B gene, encoding interferon-lambda-3, is associated with an approximately twofold change in response to treatment.]

Gee I, Alexander G (2005). Liver transplantation for hepatitis C virus related liver disease. *Postgrad Med J*, **81**, 765–71. [Comprehensive review of management of recurrent HCV following liver transplantation and natural history.]

Hadziyannis SJ, *et al.* (2004). Peginterferon –alpha 2a and ribavirin combination therapy in chronic hepatitis C: a randomized study of treatment duration ribavirin dose. *Ann Intern Med*, **140**, 346–55. [A study showing that it is possible to treat genotypes 2 and 3 HCV with lower doses of ribavirin and shorter courses of pegylated interferon-α.]

Jacobson IM, *et al.*; ADVANCE Study Team (2011). Telaprevir for previously untreated chronic hepatitis C virus infection. *N Engl J Med*, **364**, 2405–16.

Johnson RJ, *et al.* (1993). Membranoproliferative glomerulonephritis associated with hepatitis C virus infection. *N Engl J Med*, **328**, 465–70. [One of the earliest papers to make a clear association between hepatitis C infection and an extrahepatic disorder.]

Levine RA, *et al.* (2006). Assessment of fibrosis progression in untreated Irish women with chronic hepatitis C contracted from immunoglobulin anti-D. *Clin-Gastroenterol Hepatol*, **4**, 1271–7. [Study of young women infected with hepatitis C showing that the risk of progression to cirrhosis 20 years following infection is much lower than 20% in some cohorts.]

Maheshwari A, Ray S, Thuluvath PJ (2008). Acute hepatitis C. *Lancet*, **372**, 321–32. [A comprehensive review of the presentation and treatment of acute hepatitis C.]

Manns MP, *et al.* (2001). Peginterferon alfa -2b plus ribavirin compared with interferon alfa-2b plus ribavirin for initial treatment of chronic HCV: a randomised trial. *Lancet*, **358**, 958–65. [One of two large studies showing the improved efficacy of pegylated interferon in combination with ribavirin over standard interferon-α.]

McHutchison JG, *et al.* (2009). Telaprevir with peginterferon and ribavirin for chronic HCV genotype 1 infection. *N Engl J Med*, **360**, 1827–38. [Shows the added benefit of a novel targeted protease inhibitor in improved SVR and reduced treatment times for genotype 1.]

Micallef JM, Kaldor JM, Dore GJ (2006). Spontaneous viral clearance following acute hepatitis C infection: a systematic review of longitudinal studies. *J Viral Hepat*, **13**, 34–41. [Although clearance rates in the 19 studies (682 individuals) reviewed in this paper range from 0–80%, the overall clearance rate was 26%, with the largest study (67 individuals) having a clearance rate close to this. Women appeared to have a higher clearance rate than men.]

Pépin J, Labbé AC (2008). Noble goals, unforeseen consequences: control of tropical diseases in colonial Central Africa and the iatrogenic transmission of blood-borne viruses. *Trop Med Int Health*, **13**, 744–53.

Poynard T, Bedossa P, Opolon P (1997). Natural history of liver fibrosis progression in patients with chronic hepatitis C. The OBSVIRC, METAVIR, CLINIVIR, and DOSVIRC groups. *Lancet*, **349**, 825–32. [The first large retrospective cross-sectional study showing the wide variation in progression of hepatitis C fibrosis with cirrhosis occurring in around 20% within 20 years of infection.]

Poordad F, *et al.*; SPRINT-2 Investigators (2011). Boceprevir for untreated chronic HCV genotype 1 infection. *N Engl J Med*, **364**, 1195–206.

Thursz M, *et al.* (1999). Influence of MHC class II genotype on outcome of infection with hepatitis C virus. The HENCORE group. Hepatitis C European Network for Cooperative Research. *Lancet*, **354**, 2119–24. [A host genetics study confirming the importance of specific HLA Class II genes (and CD4+ T cells) in determining the outcome of HCV.]

Walker C, Bowen, D (2005). Adaptive immune responses in acute and chronic hepatitis C virus infection. *Nature*, **436**, 946–52. [A comprehensive account of the immunological responses against hepatitis C virus in human and model studies, including a discussion of the importance of immune escape through mutation.]

Wakita T, *et al.* (2005). Production of infectious hepatitis C virus in tissue culture from a cloned viral genome. *Nat Med*, **11**, 791–6. [A description of tissue culture replication competent virus—one of the studies opening the way to address fundamental aspects of HCV biology *in vitro*.]

Zeuzem S, *et al.*; REALIZE Study Team. (2011). Telaprevir for retreatment of HCV infection. *N Engl J Med*, **364**, 2417–28 [Four randomised phase III studies demonstrating improved sustained virus response rates with the addition of protease inhibitor agents to interferon-α and ribavirin.]

Zignego AL, *et al.* (2006). Extrahepatic manifestations of Hepatitis C Virus infection: A general overview and guidelines for a clinical approach. *Dig Liver Dis*, **39**, 2–17. [A review outlining recent evidence for extrahepatic disorders possibly associated with hepatitis C.]

5.23 HIV/AIDS

Graz A. Luzzi, T.E.A. Peto, P. Goulder, and C.P. Conlon

Essentials

Since its discovery in 1983, the human immunodeficiency virus (HIV) has been associated with a global pandemic that has affected more than 60 million people and caused more than 30 million deaths. The highest prevalence rates are in sub-Saharan Africa and other parts of the developing world. The impact of HIV in some African countries has been sufficient to reverse population growth and reduce life expectancy into the mid thirties, although HIV incidence has recently declined in some of these high-prevalence countries. However, there are large-scale epidemics of HIV elsewhere, e.g. India, the Russian Federation, and eastern Europe.

Transmission

Worldwide, the principal mode of transmission is heterosexual intercourse. Other risk factors for acquisition of HIV include unprotected sex between men, injecting drug use, transfusion of contaminated blood products and mother-to-child transmission.

Cellular biology

HIV-1 (derived from a simian immunodeficiency virus in the chimpanzee) and HIV-2 (animal reservoir the sooty mangabey monkey) belong to the lentivirus subfamily of retroviruses. The viral genes in infectious particles are carried as RNA, but upon infection of the host cell, reverse transcriptase catalyses the synthesis of a double-stranded DNA viral genome that is inserted into the chromosomal DNA of the infected cell by viral integrase.

Genomic structure—HIV has only nine genes: (1) *gag*—encoding the core proteins p17, p24, and p15; (2) *pol*—encoding the enzymes protease, reverse transcriptase, and integrase; (3) *env*—encoding envelope glycoproteins (gp120 and gp41); (4) two major regulatory genes—*tat* and *rev*—encoding proteins that are not assembled into

the virus but are essential for replication in the cell; (5) four accessory genes, whose functions are not clearly understood.

HIV receptors and cellular tropism—CD4 is the cell surface receptor for HIV, which binds to it via gp120; gp41 is then thought to effect membrane fusion. However, another cellular component or coreceptor is required, and different substrains of HIV (even those isolated from the same patient) exhibit specific tropisms for different cell types in culture, dependent on the ability of each particular substrain to bind to particular chemokine receptor family coreceptors.

Knowledge of the cell biology of HIV has facilitated the development of pharmacological agents that have transformed the disease from a uniformly fatal illness to a chronic condition in those countries able to provide antiretroviral treatment.

Diagnostic tests and screening

Reliable tests that detect HIV antibodies and antigen are used for diagnosis and screening. In all countries, many HIV-infected people are unaware of their infection, increasing the risk of sexual and perinatal transmission and requiring the development of targeted screening programmes.

Clinical features

Primary HIV infection—a few weeks after acquisition of HIV, many people develop a nonspecific influenza-like illness (seroconversion illness/acute retroviral syndrome), with a transient macular or maculopapular rash affecting the upper body. Rarely, there are neurological complications and severe immunodeficiency with secondary opportunistic infections. Most do not seek medical help, and whether treatment of primary HIV infection with antiretroviral drugs would improve long term prognosis is not known.

Clinical latency—following primary infection (symptomatic or asymptomatic) a period of clinical latency follows, typically lasting 8 to 10 years before development of further illness. The infected person is asymptomatic, but some have persistent generalized lymphadenopathy, and they may develop minor opportunistic conditions affecting the skin and mucous membranes, e.g. viral warts, oropharyngeal candidiasis, oral hairy leucoplakia.

Progression to symptomatic HIV disease (AIDS)—the value of making a distinction between AIDS and HIV infection at other stages is questionable, especially in industrialized countries: it is more useful to consider progressive HIV disease as a continuous spectrum. Complications of late-stage HIV disease include (1) opportunistic infections—e.g. *Pneumocystis* pneumonia, oesophageal candidiasis, cerebral toxoplasmosis, and cytomegalovirus retinitis; (2) opportunistic tumours—e.g. Kaposi's sarcoma and non-Hodgkin's lymphoma; and (3) direct HIV effects—e.g. HIV encephalopathy/dementia.

Clinical management and prognosis

CD4+ T-lymphocyte count (CD4 count) and plasma HIV-1 viral load are the two laboratory markers with the best prognostic value. (1) CD4 count—this is an indicator of HIV-related immune impairment, with decline to below 200/mm^3 associated with the risk of life-threatening opportunistic infection; antiretroviral treatment is currently considered when it has fallen to around 350/mm^3.

(2) Viral load—quantitative estimation of HIV RNA in the blood plasma adds additional prognostic information before starting antiretroviral treatment, and is useful in monitoring the effectiveness of therapy, which aims to maintain suppression of viral RNA at undetectable levels (<40 copies/ml). The choice of initial antiretroviral regimen should take into account the results of baseline genotypic resistance testing.

Prognosis—the outlook for people with HIV infection in well-resourced countries was transformed in the late 1990s by the advent of highly active antiretroviral therapy (HAART), but access to antiretroviral drugs continues to be difficult in less-developed countries (see Chapter 5.24).

Drug regimen—more than 20 agents are now available: a minimum of 3, drawn from at least 2 drug classes, is required for effective treatment. Initial regimens usually include (1) a backbone of two nucleoside/nucleotide analogues (inhibitors of HIV reverse transcriptase), e.g. tenofovir and emtricitabine or abacavir and lamivudine with either (2) a non-nucleoside reverse transcriptase inhibitor (NNRTI), e.g. efavirenz or nevirapine, or (3) a boosted protease inhibitor, e.g. lopinavir and ritonavir or atazanavir and ritonavir. Factors considered when selecting the initial antiretroviral combination include potential drug interactions with other medications, presence of renal or hepatic dysfunction, likelihood of pregnancy, and the presence of cardiovascular risk factors. An important development has been the availability of simplified regimens involving small numbers of coformulated tablets taken once or twice daily. Adherence to treatment and avoidance of suboptimal therapy (such as regimens involving fewer than three active agents, or use of agents in the presence of HIV mutations conferring resistance) are important in avoiding treatment failure.

Other drugs for HIV—(1) New agents in established drug classes—these have activity against HIV despite mutations conferring resistance to other drugs in the class, e.g. etravirine (a NNRTI), and tipranavir and darunavir (protease inhibitors); (2) fusion entry inhibitors; (3) CCR5 receptor antagonists (e.g. maraviroc); and (4) integrase inhibitors (e.g. raltegravir). The role of these newer agents in HIV therapy is being determined in clinical trials.

Adverse reactions to antiretroviral drugs—these are relatively common and include. (1) Short-term reactions—gastrointestinal disturbances, rashes, and neuropsychiatric reactions may require early adjustments to the treatment regimen. (2) Longer-term reactions—metabolic complications include (a) mitochondrial toxicity; (b) disturbances of lipid and glucose metabolism associated with a risk of cardiovascular disease including myocardial infarction—the absolute risk is small but requires consideration in patients with pre-existing cardiovascular risk factors; (c) renal impairment, e.g. with tenofovir; (d) metabolic bone disease. (3) Paradoxical reactions—called immune reconstitution syndromes, these occur in up to 20% of patients starting treatment and include new or worsening inflammatory symptoms, especially in patients who have opportunistic infections such as tuberculosis, *Mycobacterium avium* infection, cryptococcal meningitis, and cytomegalovirus retinitis.

Coinfections involving HIV and tuberculosis, hepatitis B or hepatitis C are common and require specialized treatment.

Prevention

Strategies to raise awareness and provide education, and promote risk reduction, underpin HIV control programmes worldwide. Control of coexistent sexually transmitted genital ulcers and other genital infections reduces HIV transmission. Mother-to-child transmission can be reduced to below 1% if antiretroviral treatment is administered to the mother during pregnancy, delivery is by planned caesarean section (vaginal delivery may be an option if HIV viral load is below the detection threshold), and breastfeeding is avoided. Despite decades of research, an effective HIV vaccine is not available.

Introduction

Acquired immunodeficiency syndrome (AIDS) was first recognized in 1981 in the United States of America, when outbreaks of *Pneumocystis* pneumonia and Kaposi's sarcoma were reported in men who have sex with men (MSM) in New York and California. The variety of unusual infections and other conditions declared a new form of cellular immunodeficiency and was described as the acquired immune deficiency syndrome (AIDS). In 1983, the causative retrovirus was isolated and subsequently named human immunodeficiency virus (HIV). At the time of its discovery, HIV was already widespread, the earliest infections probably having occurred before the 1950s.

In 1986, a second retrovirus causing AIDS, HIV-2, was identified in West Africa. It remains largely confined to this region, while HIV-1 is the cause of the world pandemic of AIDS. HIV infection may be regarded as a zoonosis: HIV-1 is derived from a simian immunodeficiency virus in the chimpanzee (*Pan troglodytes troglodytes*), and the animal reservoir for HIV-2 is the sooty mangabey monkey (*Cercocebus atys*).

Epidemiology

The global HIV-1 pandemic has had the greatest impact in developing countries (see Chapter 5.24). The World Health Organization (WHO) estimated that in 2006, 33.3 million people were living with HIV worldwide, of whom 22.5 million were in sub-Saharan Africa (Fig. 5.23.1). Worldwide, the WHO estimated there were over 2.6 million new HIV infections in 2010, 2009, of which 1.8 million were in sub-Saharan Africa. Globally, AIDS caused 1.8 million deaths of which 1.3 million were in sub-Saharan Africa.

In North America, western Europe, and Australasia the epidemic began among MSM and injecting drug users. However, in these regions the proportion attributable to heterosexual transmission subsequently increased. In 2010, over 80 000 people were living with HIV in the United Kingdom, nearly a third of whom were unaware of their diagnosis. The proportion of newly diagnosed cases in the United Kingdom attributed to heterosexual transmission rose steadily from 1999 onwards, largely due to increased numbers arriving from countries with high prevalence, and increased HIV detection through routine antenatal testing. However, injecting drug use, unprotected sex between men, and unprotected paid sex remain important modes of transmission in Europe, as well as in Asia and Latin America.

In contrast, HIV transmission in regions with the highest prevalence rates, such as sub-Saharan Africa, is predominantly

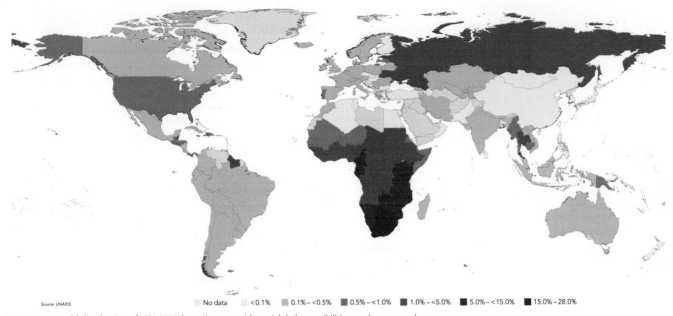

Fig. 5.23.1 World distribution of HIV, 2009. http://www.unaids.org/globalreport/HIV_prevalence_map.htm
(Reproduced with permission from: UNAIDS. *2010 Report on the global AIDS epidemic*, http://www.unaids.org/en/media/unaids/contentassets/documents/unaidspublication/2010/20101123_
globalreport_en.pdf.)

heterosexual and perinatal. The estimated overall adult prevalence there is 6%, rising to between 20 and 30% in some countries such as Botswana and Zimbabwe, where AIDS has curtailed population growth and life expectancy has fallen into the mid thirties. Swaziland (population 1 million) is the country with the highest adult seroprevalence, of 33%. The country with more infected people than any other is believed to be South Africa (5.5 million adults living with HIV, adult seroprevalence 20%), although in India, where prevalence data are less easily accessible, the overall numbers may be similar (despite adult seroprevalence below 1%).

The overall prevalence of HIV has risen worldwide in recent years because new transmissions exceed AIDS-related deaths, and because antiretroviral treatment has reduced mortality. However, there have been notable declines in some high-prevalence countries such as Kenya, Zimbabwe, and parts of India, and a levelling off in other parts of sub-Saharan Africa, attributable to prevention efforts. Uganda is seen as one of the best examples of a country where prevalence has declined significantly, believed to be, at least in part, due to the timely government campaign of public education.

The global distribution of HIV is currently characterized by very variable rates of prevalence and scattered areas of very high transmission in epidemics. Consequently, the risk of acquisition of HIV is also highly variable from region to region. In some countries, such as Russia and Ukraine, HIV has caused large scale epidemics and transmission rates remain high. The risk of onward transmission is especially high soon after sexual acquisition of HIV, when plasma viral load is high, and the virus is present in genital secretions in sexually active people. Therefore, it is particularly important to detect primary HIV infection in population screening programmes. HIV transmission continues at a high level in many countries because of poverty, low condom usage, high rates of other sexually transmitted infections, and higher risk behaviour such as unprotected paid sex and use of nonsterile injecting drug equipment.

HIV-2 is endemic in parts of West Africa and is also prevalent in Angola, Mozambique, France, and Portugal. In other parts of the world, the prevalence is very low, although it is present in India. The clinical features of HIV-2 are similar to those of HIV-1, but some patients with HIV-2 appear to progress much more slowly than those with HIV-1 for unknown reasons.

Variation of HIV-1 RNA sequences has been identified, leading to a classification of 11 sequence subtypes (or clades), A to K, of the main group M, and N (new) and O (outlier) as two quite distinct groups in west central Africa. The subtypes have varying geographical distributions. For instance, subtypes A and D are found in central Africa, B in North America and Europe, and E in Thailand. More people are infected with clade C virus than any other, being the predominant clade of virus in southern Africa as well as India. A new group, P, was designated after the discovery of a novel HIV strain in a female from Cameroon in France in 2009, which was closely related to the simian immunodeficiency virus found in gorillas. Study of the genetic and geographical divergence of subtypes has shed light on the emergence and global spread of HIV.

Cellular biology of HIV

The viral replication cycle

HIV-1 (Fig. 5.23.2) and HIV-2 belong to the lentivirus subfamily of retroviruses. Retrovirus implies a 'backwards' step in biological information during viral replication attributable to its enzyme, reverse transcriptase. As with all retroviruses, the viral genes in infectious particles are carried as RNA, but upon infection of the host cell, reverse transcriptase catalyses the synthesis of a double-stranded DNA viral genome (Fig. 5.23.3). Insertion of the DNA genome into the chromosomal DNA of the infected cell is effected by viral integrase. The integrated provirus may remain latent, particularly in resting lymphocytes. In actively infected cells, however, RNA transcripts and proteins are synthesized, leading to the formation of new virus particles.

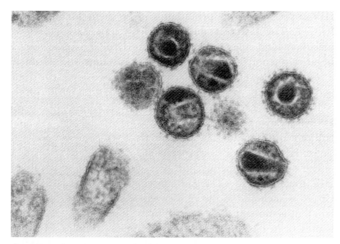

Fig. 5.23.2 Electron micrograph of HIV-1.
(Reproduced by courtesy of H Gelderblom.)

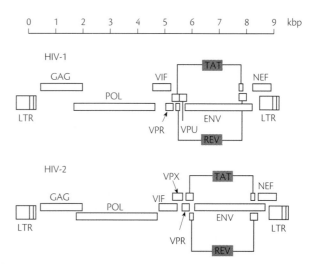

Fig. 5.23.4 HIV genome map.

The core proteins derived from the *gag* and *pol* genes are made as large polypeptides that are then cleaved into smaller components representing the enzymes and building blocks of the virus. This cleavage is achieved by the viral protease. The unique reverse transcriptase and protease are targets of antiretroviral therapy (see below). Reverse transcriptase inhibitors such as zidovudine and lamivudine affect an early step in HIV replication, whereas the protease inhibitors, such as lopinavir, block a late stage of virus assembly (Fig. 5.23.3). Compounds that inhibit any stage of HIV replication, without being too toxic to the infected person, are potential antiviral drugs. Agents have recently been developed to block viral entry (e.g. fusion entry inhibitors and CCR5 receptor antagonists) and integration into the host cell DNA (integrase inhibitors).

Although regarded as a complex retrovirus, HIV has only nine genes (Fig. 5.23.4). The three structural genes are *gag*, *pol*, and *env*, encoding the core proteins p17, p24, and p15, the enzymes (protease, reverse transcriptase, and integrase), and the envelope glycoproteins (gp120 and gp41), respectively. The major regulatory genes *tat* and *rev* encode proteins that are not assembled into the virus but are essential for replication in the cell. The Tat

protein acts in positive feedback to enhance transcription of viral RNA from the DNA provirus, while the Rev protein helps the efficient transport of viral RNA from the nucleus to the cytoplasm. Either of these proteins could be a suitable target for antiviral therapy, particularly Tat, because the synthesis of all the other viral proteins depends on its activity.

The functions of the four accessory genes of HIV are less well understood. *Vif* encodes a protein assembled in virus particles that appears necessary for the infectivity ('viral infectivity factor') at a stage soon after entry. Vif binds and hastens the degradation of the cellular protein APOBEC which, in the absence of Vif, hypermutates HIV, thereby disabling it. *Nef* also affects an early postentry function; it is not needed by laboratory-adapted HIV strains or if virus enters via endosomal vesicles rather than fusing with the outer cell membrane. It also down-regulates surface expression of the primary cell-surface receptor for HIV, the CD4 antigen, by drawing CD4 into clathrin-coated pits. *Vpu* similarly interacts with CD4, promoting its degradation by directing it to the ubiquitin–proteasome pathway. *Vpr* has dual functions; first, it directs the preintegration complex of the virus, containing the newly synthesized DNA, into the nucleus so that it can integrate into chromosomal DNA; second, it blocks cell proliferation in the G2 phase of the cell cycle, thereby enhancing the amount of viral progeny released per cell.

Unlike HIV-1, HIV-2 and the simian immunodeficiency viruses (SIV) lack *vpu*, but have an alternative gene, *vpx*. HIV-2 Vpr leads the viral genome into the cell nucleus, but does not arrest the cell cycle. These proteins presumably recognize cellular proteins and some of these interactions are species-specific. Thus the Vpr and Vif proteins in SIV of African green monkeys do not function in human cells, while the equivalent proteins of SIV from sooty mangabey monkeys work well in human cells. This could explain why sooty mangabey SIV was able to infect humans and become HIV-2, whereas the more widespread African green monkey SIV has not led to a zoonosis. Another difference is that HIV-1 incorporates the cellular protein cyclophilin A (the target of the drug ciclosporin A) into virus particles, where it may cooperate with Vif and is required for steps early in the infection. In contrast, HIV-2 does not contain cyclophylin A and replicates well without it.

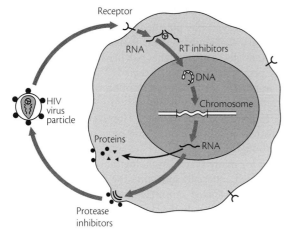

Fig. 5.23.3 Replicative cycle of HIV.

HIV receptors and cellular tropism

CD4 is the cell-surface receptor for HIV; it is expressed on T-helper lymphocytes, the cells that become depleted in AIDS. CD4 is also expressed (to a lesser extent but sufficient to permit infection) on macrophages, Langerhans dendritic cells in mucous membranes, and brain microglial cells. These are the other target cells for HIV infection. CD4 is necessary to initiate HIV infection but is not sufficient to allow the virus to fuse with host-cell membranes: another cellular component or coreceptor is required.

Different substrains of HIV, even those isolated from the same patient, exhibit specific tropisms for different cell types in culture. All isolates can infect primary CD4 lymphocytes, but only some infect macrophages while others can infect cell lines established from CD4+ leukaemic cells. Macrophage-tropic strains predominate early in the course of HIV infection, and may be more transmissible from person to person. They do not cause CD4 lymphocytes to fuse together in culture and hence are referred to as non-syncytium-inducing (NSI) strains. In contrast, many HIV isolates established from late-stage infection rapidly adapt in culture to infect T-cell lines and are syncytium-inducing (SI). Approximately 50% of patients with AIDS develop SI strains in addition to NSI strains. The differences in cellular tropism and SI/NSI phenotype occur in all HIV subtypes or clades, which appear to reflect geographical variation of HIV rather than specific biological properties of the virus.

The complex cellular tropism of HIV has been explained by the discovery that different members of the chemokine receptor family act as coreceptors to CD4 for HIV entry into cells. Chemokines are chemoattractant, locally acting hormones or cytokines that bind to one or more receptors which are structurally related to olfactory and neurotransmitter receptors. Following binding to the CD4 receptor, primary NSI strains use CCR5, the chemokine receptor for macrophage-inhibitory proteins (MIP-1α, MIP-1β) and RANTES. In contrast, the SI strains of HIV use the CXCR4 coreceptor, the receptor for another chemokine, stromal-derived factor-1 (SDF-1). Other receptors such as CCR3 (the receptor of eotaxin) can be used by some NSI strains.

High levels of MIP-1α or -β in the blood correlate with relative resistance to HIV infection. Some exposed yet uninfected individuals are homozygous for an inherited defect of the CCR5 receptor involving a 32 bp deletion in the *CCR5* gene. This mutation is present in approximately 20% of white people (approximately 1% of white people are homozygous), but is not found in African and Asian populations. Individuals who are homozygous for the deletion are healthy, indicating that the CCR5 receptor is not essential for the development of immune competence, probably because MIP-1 and RANTES can also bind to alternative receptors. However, homozygotes are genetically resistant to infection by NSI strains of HIV, and the few homozygotes with Δ32 deletions who are HIV-positive appear to have been infected with SI strains that utilize CXCR4 instead. Other, more subtle, mutations in the promoter region of the *CCR5* gene allowing only low levels of coreceptor expression may confer relative resistance to HIV infection and also, if infection occurs, slower the progression to AIDS.

Recently, a blood group antigen on red blood cells, the Duffy antigen receptor for chemokines (DARC), was shown to be another non-HLA genetic factor influencing HIV transmission and disease progression. In addition to forming a receptor for certain HIV-suppressive and proinflammatory chemokines such as RANTES, DARC serves as the red cell receptor for *Plasmodium vivax* malaria and consequently nonexpression of DARC on red cells (Duffy negative phenotype) confers complete resistance to *P. vivax*. As a result of selection pressure from malaria, most West Africans and two-thirds of African Americans do not express DARC on red cells (although expression is preserved on endothelial cells). The DARC-negative red cell phenotype is associated with an increased risk of acquisition of HIV-1; however, it is also associated with slower HIV-related disease progression.

The outer envelope glycoprotein, gp120, is the molecule on HIV that binds to CD4 and subsequently to the coreceptor. Gp120 is anchored to the viral envelope via gp41, the viral protein that is thought to effect membrane fusion. The gp120–gp41 is present in the viral envelope as a trimeric complex. SI strains have a gp120–gp41 structure that is less stable than NSI strains, readily undergoing conformational change on binding to CD4. This property makes SI strains more sensitive to neutralization by gp120 antibodies and also to inactivation by soluble forms of recombinant CD4, which were once seen as promising therapeutic agents. NSI strains, however, are more resistant. Mutations in the V3 loop of gp120 can convert NSI strains to SI strains. These mutations arise naturally during progression to AIDS and may allow HIV to switch to infect different cell types via new coreceptors.

The natural chemokines act as competitive inhibitors of HIV entry; certain chemically modified chemokines and chemical analogues act as strong HIV inhibitors without triggering the downstream signalling of the receptor. This has led to a new class of anti-HIV drugs, called CCR5 receptor antagonists.

Diagnosis of HIV infection

Following seroconversion, antibody to envelope protein persists indefinitely in the serum and forms a highly specific test for HIV infection. Most laboratories use one or more sensitive enzyme immunoassay tests that detect HIV-1 and HIV-2 antibodies and p24 antigen as the initial screening test. Positive screening tests are usually referred to a specialist laboratory for additional tests to confirm the presence of HIV antibodies. Most seroconversions occur within 3 months of infection, and very rarely up to 6 months. Routine diagnostic tests, if negative, should be repeated 3 months after the last possible exposure. If primary infection is suspected, or after high risk exposure, additional tests may be indicated (see Primary HIV infection, below). Near patient testing for HIV, e.g. using saliva, is available, but the place for such testing is not well defined. Easy availability of near patient testing or home testing could potentially increase higher risk behaviour.

Many people are unaware of their HIV infection. Detection of HIV is important for timely intervention with antiretroviral treatment, reduction of risk of perinatal transmission, and behavioural change to protect sexual partners. However, early diagnosis may cause distress and disruption of domestic, social, and professional lives, although the infected person may not need antiretroviral treatment for many years. Psychological support and counselling may be needed, especially soon after the diagnosis.

Many industrialized countries are developing strategies to increase HIV detection. In the United Kingdom, it is standard practice that all patients attending sexual health clinics for screening or treatment for sexual infections are offered HIV testing, and it is recommended that HIV testing should be considered in all general medical admissions to hospital and all adults registering in general practice if the HIV prevalence in the local population exceeds 2 in 1000 (typically larger cities). In the United States of America, where more than 25% of those infected are unaware of their HIV infection, the Centers for Disease Control and Prevention (CDC) has recommended that HIV testing should be routinely offered in all health care settings. In patients with unexplained symptoms that could be caused by HIV, testing is essential for diagnosis so that appropriate treatment can be provided. If the patient is too ill to give consent, testing is justified on these grounds as being in the patient's best interest. As there is still stigma associated with HIV, confidentiality must be maintained; disclosure of HIV-positive status is acceptable only in the medical interests of the patient and in general with their knowledge and consent. Patients unwilling to inform their sexual partners should be advised of the possible legal implications of nondisclosure if transmission occurs. In the United Kingdom, there have been successful prosecutions of individuals knowingly exposing their partners to HIV.

Clinical presentation and features

Primary HIV infection

Between 2 and 6 weeks after exposure to HIV, 50 to 70% of those infected develop a transient, often mild, nonspecific illness (sometimes called seroconversion illness or acute retroviral syndrome) similar to infectious mononucleosis, with fever, malaise, myalgia, lymphadenopathy, and pharyngitis. However, unlike infectious mononucleosis, over 50% of people develop a rash, typically erythematous, maculopapular, and affecting the face and trunk. Other rashes and patterns of distribution, and oral and genital ulcers have also been reported. The illness begins abruptly and usually lasts for 1 to 2 weeks, but may be more protracted. Most cases are so mild that patients do not seek medical help. In addition, neurological complications can occur and include acute encephalitis, lymphocytic meningitis, and peripheral neuropathy. Severe or long-lasting illness and neurological involvement are associated with accelerated progression to AIDS and a bad prognosis, which may be influenced by early antiretroviral therapy. A transient decrease in CD4 lymphocytes is usual during primary illness. Occasionally, this may be substantial and associated with opportunistic infections such as oral or oesophageal candidiasis, and rarely pneumocystis pneumonia (PCP).

Diagnosis requires a high index of suspicion. Primary HIV infection is a time of high viraemia (typically 10^5–10^6 viral particles/ml) during which antibodies to HIV may initially be absent (Fig. 5.23.5). However, new fourth-generation tests can detect p24 antigen as well as HIV antibodies and may be positive early in primary infection. Serum antibodies to the core and surface proteins of the virus usually appear within 2 to 6 weeks. However, if primary infection is suspected and the initial test is negative, additional tests may be required; rapid diagnosis may be provided by detecting HIV viraemia using tests for HIV RNA or proviral cDNA (by polymerase chain reaction, PCR), which may confirm HIV infection before antibodies become detectable.

Aggressive therapy of primary HIV infection with antiretroviral drugs does not eradicate the infection but, on theoretical grounds, might alter the natural history. After primary infection, the viral load becomes relatively stable after 6 to 9 months at an average level of 30 000 HIV RNA copies/ml plasma (Fig. 5.23.5). The

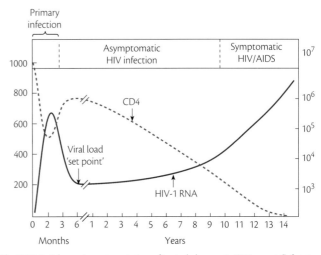

Fig. 5.23.5 Schematic representation of typical changes in CD4 count (left axis, per mm³) and plasma HIV-1 RNA (right axis, copies/ml) with time, during the natural history of HIV infection.

plasma HIV RNA level at this virological steady state or 'set point' is of prognostic importance; therefore, treatment of the initial viraemic illness could theoretically lower the risk of progression if viral set point off therapy is lowered. A placebo-controlled trial of zidovudine monotherapy during primary HIV infection showed a short-term benefit, but a recent trial currently underway (Short Pulse Anti Retroviral Therapy at HIV Seroconversion, SPARTAC) which compared early treatment for a limited period (12 weeks or 48 weeks) with early treatment that is continued indefinitely, or no treatment for primary infection, showed no significant difference in mortality rate or progression to AIDS for the three groups after an average of 4.2 years' follow-up. Forty-eight weeks of antiretroviral treatment delayed disease progression, but not significantly longer than the time already spent on treatment.

Early HIV infection

Following the primary illness or subclinical seroconversion, there usually follows an asymptomatic period lasting an average of 10 years without antiretroviral therapy. Although a time of clinical latency, there is intense viral turnover: 10^9 to 10^{10} viral particles are replaced daily and the half-life of circulating CD4 lymphocytes is substantially reduced.

During the asymptomatic period, physical examination may be normal, but about one-third of patients have persistent generalized lymphadenopathy. The enlarged nodes, caused by a reactive follicular hyperplasia, are usually symmetrical, mobile, and nontender. The cervical and axillary nodes are most commonly affected. Nodes that are markedly asymmetrical, painful, or rapidly enlarging should be biopsied to exclude tumours such as lymphoma and opportunistic infections such as tuberculosis.

Symptoms of progressive HIV infection can be prevented by antiretroviral treatment. In the absence of treatment, patients often develop minor opportunistic conditions affecting the skin and mucous membranes. These are also common throughout the later stages of HIV disease. They include a range of infections: fungal (e.g. tinea, pityrosporum), viral (e.g. warts, molluscum contagiosum, herpes simplex, herpes zoster), and bacterial (e.g. folliculitis, impetigo); and also eczema, seborrhoeic dermatitis, and psoriasis.

Oral hairy leucoplakia usually appears as corrugated greyish-white lesions on the lateral borders of the tongue in homosexual men. The condition is symptomless and nonprogressive, but may be a clue to HIV seropositivity. Epstein–Barr virus DNA has been demonstrated in these lesions.

One of the characteristic clinical presentations of HIV disease is a sore mouth and throat due to oropharyngeal candidiasis (oral thrush) (Fig. 5.23.6). This is a sign of worsening immunodeficiency and may be recurrent. *Candida albicans* is usually responsible, but other species (e.g. *Candida glabrata*) may be implicated.

There is an increased incidence of periodontal disease in those with untreated HIV, including inflammation of the gums (gingivitis) and the more serious and extensive periodontitis that can lead to loss of teeth. Two distinctive forms are associated with HIV: a linear gingival erythema that causes a typical red band along the gum line, and in advanced immunosuppression, necrotizing ulcerative periodontitis which may require extensive debridement and antimicrobials. Recurrent oropharyngeal aphthous ulceration is common and may be painful. Recurrent ulcers may occur in the oesophagus and other parts of the gastrointestinal tract. They usually respond to local or systemic corticosteroid therapy. Resistant cases may respond to thalidomide. The availability of antiretroviral therapy has reduced the need for specific treatment.

Later in the course of untreated HIV infection, intermittent or persistent nonspecific constitutional symptoms may develop, which include lethargy, anorexia, diarrhoea, weight loss, fever, and night sweats. These symptoms may presage severe opportunistic infections or tumours.

Progression to symptomatic HIV disease (AIDS)

Various staging systems for HIV infection and case definitions of AIDS were developed and modified as understanding of the pathogenesis and natural history increased (Fig. 5.23.7). The CDC in the United States of America listed a range of specific diseases and other criteria, such as a CD4 lymphocyte count of less than 200/mm^3 (0.2×10^9/litre), as indicative of AIDS. AIDS-defining illnesses were essential for surveillance when HIV status was frequently unknown, the natural history of HIV infection was poorly understood (the proportion developing opportunistic complications was uncertain), and disease-modifying drugs were not available.

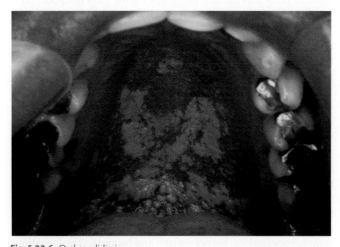

Fig. 5.23.6 Oral candidiasis.
(By courtesy of the late Dr B E Juel-Jensen)

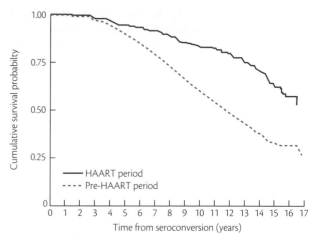

Fig. 5.23.7 Natural history of HIV. Estimated proportions of individuals surviving from HIV-1 seroconversion in the pre-HAART era. HAART, highly active antiretroviral therapy.
(From CASCADE collaboration (2000). Survival after introduction of HAART in people with known duration of HIV-1 infection. The CASCADE Collaboration. Concerted Action on SeroConversion to AIDS and Death in Europe. *Lancet*, **355**, 1158–9.)

Effective prevention of many of the opportunistic infections has led to an increase in the proportion of symptomatic patients who do not fulfil the criteria for AIDS. Antiretroviral therapy usually improves the clinical condition and survival, even when started after progression to AIDS. These factors have undermined the epidemiological value and prognostic importance of a strict AIDS case definition. Therefore, the current value of making a distinction between AIDS and HIV infection at other stages is questionable, especially in industrialized countries. It is more useful to consider progressive HIV disease as a continuous spectrum.

However, clinical criteria to identify symptomatic HIV disease and AIDS were needed in resource-poor countries, if laboratory confirmation of HIV was not possible. The WHO therefore adopted clinical case definitions for AIDS surveillance in resource-limited countries, based on clinical manifestations with or without laboratory confirmation of HIV infection. This approach has been superseded by the WHO clinical staging system, which assumes that an HIV test has been done. Rapid HIV tests can now be done even in field conditions. For surveillance, it is suggested that HIV case reporting should supersede AIDS case reporting, though that may not yet be possible everywhere (Chapter 5.24).

Nonprogression

While the average time between infection with HIV and the development of AIDS is about 10 years, approximately 20% of patients progress rapidly to AIDS within 5 years and 10 to 15% remain clinically well for 15 to 20 years. Age is an independent risk factor for progression; acquisition of HIV in later life is associated with a less favourable prognosis. Long-term healthy survivors are often called nonprogressors, and this subgroup generally represents the tail end of a normal distribution of progression rates. Cohort studies have demonstrated that most apparent nonprogressors are actually slow progressors, in whom a gradual decline in the CD4 lymphocyte count and increments in HIV viral load can be demonstrated. Although several investigators have reported virological, genetic, and cellular and humoral immunological factors that may be associated with nonprogression, limitations in study design have made it difficult to identify what is responsible.

In white cohorts of antiretroviral treatment-naive, HIV-infected persons who show unusually successful control of HIV to levels of below 50 copies/ml plasma, more than 50 to 90% express one or both of the HLA class I alleles HLA-B*5701 and HLA-B*2705. The protective value of these HLA class I alleles is related to the importance of the CD8+ T-cell response in successful immune control of HIV, and in particular where the CD8+ T-cell response includes broad targeting of epitopes in the conserved internal Gag protein. Infected persons expressing the HLA class I alleles HLA-B*3502 or B*5802 tend not to make Gag-specific CD8+ T-cell responses, and progress to AIDS significantly more rapidly. In addition to defining the nature of the CD8+ T-cell response, the particular HLA alleles expressed have important influences on the natural killer cell response against HIV, also affecting rates of progression to HIV disease. Non-HLA genes that affect rates of progression include the macrophage chemokine receptor CCR5 gene mutation (see Cellular biology of HIV, above) associated with nonprogression in the heterozygous state.

Late complications and their management
Pneumocystis jirovecii pneumonia (Chapter 7.6)

P. jirovecii (previously *Pneumocystis carinii*) pneumonia, one of the hallmarks of AIDS, is now less common because of primary prophylaxis and antiretroviral therapy. Some 85% of cases occur in patients with CD4 counts below 200/mm³, and mostly at counts below 100/mm³. Symptoms typically include increasing shortness of breath, dry cough, and fever, usually developing subacutely over a few weeks. Malaise, fatigue, weight loss, and chest pains or tightness may occur. Chest signs are usually minor (crackles) or absent. The characteristic chest radiograph shows bilateral mid zone interstitial shadowing (Fig. 5.23.8), but can be normal. Other appearances include localized infiltrates or consolidation, upper lobe shadows resembling tuberculosis, nodular lesions, and pneumothorax; effusions are very rare. The arterial oxygen saturation is usually less than 95% at rest or falls after exercise.

Infection with *P. jirovecii* is associated with an interstitial inflammatory infiltrate and progressive impairment of lung function. The diagnosis can sometimes be confirmed by microscopy of sputum, which is induced by nebulized saline in properly ventilated isolation rooms to reduce the risk of tuberculosis transmission (see Multidrug-resistant tuberculosis, below). *P. jirovecii* cysts and trophozoites are visualized by the use of special stains. If the result is negative, fibreoptic bronchoscopy with bronchial lavage is indicated (Fig. 5.23.9); other causes of lung disease or coexistent infection may also be diagnosed by this technique, including tuberculosis, fungal infections, and Kaposi's sarcoma. Immunofluorescence using monoclonal antibodies, or DNA amplification by PCR, may improve diagnostic sensitivity when compared with conventional staining techniques, but these methods are not yet used routinely. In a minority of patients with *P. jirovecii* pneumonia the diagnosis is not confirmed but treatment is given empirically.

High-dose co-trimoxazole (120 mg/kg daily in divided doses) for 3 weeks is the first-line treatment for pneumocystis pneumonia. Oral therapy is often adequate, but in moderate and severe cases the drug should be given intravenously. The drug can be given orally if fever, symptoms, and oxygenation have improved after 10 days. Adverse reactions to co-trimoxazole—especially neutropenia, anaemia, rash, and fever—occur in up to 40% of patients, usually after 6 to 14 days. Intravenous pentamidine (4 mg/kg per day) is the second-line choice for patients who do not tolerate co-trimoxazole.

Patients intolerant of co-trimoxazole and pentamidine may be treated with clindamycin plus primaquine or dapsone plus trimethoprim. These regimens have only been evaluated in patients with mild to moderate pneumocystis pneumonia, as has atovaquone, an antiprotozoal drug that is active against *P. jirovecii*. Although slightly less effective than co-trimoxazole, atovaquone causes fewer adverse effects.

In patients with moderate or severe pneumocystis pneumonia, high-dose corticosteroids reduce morbidity and mortality. If the arterial partial pressure of oxygen (Pao_2) is less than 9.3 kPa or the alveolar–arterial oxygen gradient is greater than 4.7 kPa, oxygen and intravenous methylprednisolone or oral prednisolone should be given for 5 to 10 days. Patients who develop respiratory failure may require ventilatory support. After treatment for pneumocystis pneumonia has been completed, secondary prophylaxis should be given to prevent recurrence. This can be discontinued if there is a

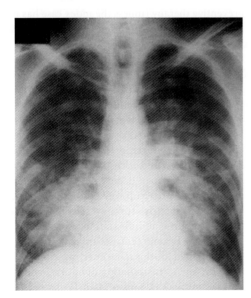

Fig. 5.23.8 Chest radiograph: *Pneumocystis jirovecii* pneumonia.

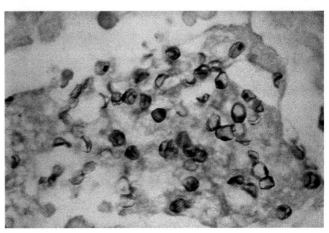

Fig. 5.23.9 *Pneumocystis jirovecii* cysts in bronchoalveolar lavage aspirate.

good response to antiretroviral treatment, with a rise in the CD4 count sustained above 200/mm^3.

Bacterial pneumonia

The risk of bacterial pneumonia is increased in HIV, especially if the CD4 count is below 200/mm^3. The most common cause is *Streptococcus pneumoniae*, although *Haemophilus influenzae* and *Moraxella catarrhalis* are also relatively common, and *Staphylococcus aureus*, *Klebsiella*, and other Gram-negative rods are important causes in advanced HIV disease. Rare causes include *Nocardia* and *Rhodococcus equi*. The presentation may be atypical, and radiological appearances frequently include diffuse infiltrates that resemble pneumocystis pneumonia, as well as more typical segmental or lobar patterns. Cavitation with abscess formation, pleural effusion, and empyema may occur. HIV predisposes to recurrent invasive pneumococcal infections with bacteraemia; recurrent bacterial pneumonia in a 12-month period is an AIDS-defining condition. Chronic lung damage with bronchiectasis and colonization by *Pseudomonas aeruginosa* have been reported.

Other pulmonary complications

Disseminated fungal infections, including *Cryptococcus*, may involve the lungs (Chapter 2.4, Section 7). In endemic areas, histoplasmosis, coccidioidomycosis, and disseminated *Penicillium marneffei* infection need to be considered (see below). Invasive *Aspergillus fumigatus* infections may occur in patients with advanced HIV disease who have additional risk factors such as severe neutropenia. Patients usually have severe systemic illness. The radiographic appearances in all these fungal infections are usually nonspecific. Bronchoalveolar lavage may be needed for diagnosis. HIV-associated lymphocytic interstitial pneumonitis causes diffuse abnormalities, usually in children but occasionally in adults. Cryptogenic organizing pneumonia is a steroid-responsive cause of lung infiltrates, probably a tissue response to various underlying conditions, which has also been reported in HIV and may be confused with pneumocystis pneumonia.

Tuberculosis (Chapter 6.25)

The interaction between HIV and tuberculosis (TB) was recognized early in the HIV epidemic. Studies in central Africa in the mid 1980s showed that more than 60% of newly diagnosed tuberculosis patients were HIV-positive at a time when the background seroprevalence of HIV in the population was much lower. Injecting drug users were shown to have an increased risk of developing active tuberculosis if they were HIV-positive. After decades of progressive decline in the incidence of tuberculosis in the United States of America, notifications increased during the mid-1980s, soon after the emergence of the HIV epidemic. A similar trend was subsequently observed in western Europe. Globally, tuberculosis remains the most frequent life-threatening opportunistic infection in AIDS.

Most cases of tuberculosis in HIV-positive individuals represent reactivation of dormant bacilli. However, molecular typing of isolates of *Mycobacterium tuberculosis* by restriction fragment length polymorphism (RFLP) analysis suggests that up to 40% are new infections. The WHO estimates that one-third of the world's HIV-positive population is coinfected with tuberculosis. In communities where *M. tuberculosis* is endemic those who are immunosuppressed by HIV have an increased risk of relapsing or contracting new infections. Where the background prevalence of tuberculosis is low, the disease is uncommon in HIV-positive patients unless they become exposed, e.g. through travel. Testing for HIV should be done in all patients presenting with active tuberculosis, and tuberculosis should be considered as a cause of unexplained symptoms in patients with HIV.

Active tuberculosis may occur at any time during the course of HIV infection. In early-stage HIV, it is more likely to present with the typical clinical features: subacute history of cough, fever, and weight loss, upper lobe cavitary disease and/or pleural disease on chest radiographs, and a positive skin test to tuberculin. In late-stage HIV, infected patients are more likely to present atypically with unusual chest findings, extrapulmonary involvement, and cutaneous anergy. The chest radiograph may be normal in up to 40% of cases and, when abnormal, upper lobe involvement is less common. Sputum smears should be examined for acid-fast bacilli, but are less likely to be positive in HIV. Blood cultures may be positive for *M. tuberculosis*.

Patients with HIV and TB are more likely to relapse after completion of therapy and to die prematurely if their HIV disease is not treated. Patients with advanced HIV infection are more likely to develop extrapulmonary tuberculosis involving lymph nodes, pericardium, liver, bone marrow, or meninges. Diagnosis can be difficult and frequently relies on invasive procedures to obtain appropriate specimens. The role of interferon-γ release assays (IGRA) in the diagnosis of HIV-associated TB is uncertain.

The standard 6-month regimen of three or four antituberculosis drugs (isoniazid, rifampicin, pyrazinamide, and ethambutol) is generally effective in patients with HIV, unless there is resistance to one or more of these first-line drugs. The drug regimen may need to be adjusted when *in vitro* sensitivity results are known. For fully sensitive organisms, after 2 months on three or four drugs, isoniazid and rifampicin should be continued for a further 4 months. It should be noted that rifampicin interacts with many of the antiretroviral drugs, particularly protease inhibitors, and these interactions need to be considered in deciding on drug regimens. Patients with pulmonary tuberculosis should be isolated initially. Contact tracing is important; HIV-positive contacts of a smear-positive TB case are at particular risk and should be offered isoniazid preventive therapy (unless the index case has multidrug-resistant TB). The tuberculin skin test may be negative, especially if the CD4 count is low.

Up to 20% of patients with HIV experience adverse reactions to antituberculosis drugs. In HIV-positive patients with tuberculosis in Africa, the sulpha-based drug thiacetazone has been associated with serious skin reactions, including toxic epidermal necrolysis and fatal cases of Stevens–Johnson syndrome. Whereas response rates for conventional short-course tuberculosis treatment in industrialized countries are similar to those achieved in HIV-negative patients, in resource-limited countries and where compliance is less easily achieved, cure rates are lower and there is a risk that resistance will develop. Several countries have adopted a 'directly observed therapy' strategy (DOTS) to address this problem. Supervised drug administration is a component of this strategy but political commitment, secure drug supply, and good organization are needed for this to be effective.

The optimal timing of the initiation of antiretroviral treatment in patients presenting with HIV-associated TB has been controversial. Early initiation of HAART increases the pill burden and risks IRIS reactions, whereas starting too late risks HIV disease progression. However, three recent studies have clarified this area and have shown that in patients with TB and HIV whose initial CD4 count is less than 50/mm^3, HAART and TB therapy should be started together. Although the incidence of IRIS reactions is increased, this does not increase mortality. For patients with CD4 counts greater than 200/mm3, antiretroviral therapy can be deferred for 8 to 12 weeks. HIV therapy should not be delayed beyond 12 weeks, however. It should be noted that these studies were mainly carried out in patients with pulmonary TB and a study in TB meningitis showed no benefit with immediate HAART and an increased frequency of severe adverse effects.

Multidrug-resistant tuberculosis

Over 15 outbreaks of multidrug-resistant tuberculosis (MDR-TB) have been reported since the late 1980s. MDR-TB isolates are resistant to at least two first-line antituberculosis drugs, most commonly isoniazid and rifampicin, and are often resistant to several agents. Most have occurred in HIV units in hospitals, but there have been outbreaks in prisons, drug treatment centres, and nursing homes. Most documented outbreaks have been in the United States of America. Elsewhere, over 200 people were involved in Buenos Aires, Argentina, and another outbreak affected over 100 people in Lisbon, Portugal. In MDR-TB outbreaks, health care workers may become infected. Initially, the mortality among HIV-positive patients was very high (up to 93%), but the outcome has subsequently improved because of more rapid diagnosis and treatment with at least four drugs to which the *M. tuberculosis* isolate is sensitive *in vitro*. More recently, extensively drug-resistant TB (XDR TB) in HIV infected patients in South Africa has caused outbreaks, with 100% mortality.

To prevent outbreaks of MDR-TB, special precautions are required when HIV-positive patients with possible tuberculosis are admitted to hospitals. Diagnosis must not be delayed, appropriate treatment must be started as soon as possible, and drug resistance identified although this can be difficult in resource-limited settings. Precautions include the isolation of patients in negative-pressure rooms, use of respiratory protection for staff, and special care during certain procedures such as bronchoscopy or nebulized pentamidine administration. With effective treatment, patients rapidly become noninfectious, but precautions need to be continued until the sputum is repeatedly culture-negative.

Mycobacterium avium complex

In the absence of antiretroviral treatment, patients with advanced HIV infection and CD4 counts below 50/mm^3 are at high risk of disseminated *Mycobacterium avium* complex (MAC) infection, particularly in industrialized countries where historically it was reported to develop in up to 40% of patients with AIDS. *M. avium* is a ubiquitous environmental organism of low pathogenicity that can be isolated from domestic water supplies. Infection is likely to be through the gastrointestinal tract. MAC infection becomes widely disseminated in those with advanced HIV and causes fever, night sweats, weight loss, diarrhoea, abdominal pain, anaemia, disturbed liver function, and reduced overall survival. The organism can usually be cultured from blood or bone marrow, or may be recognized as acid-fast bacilli in tissue biopsies (e.g.

from lymph node, small bowel, or liver). It is unclear why the diagnosis is uncommon in low-income countries; high mortality from other opportunistic infections at earlier stages of immunosuppression may be partly responsible.

MAC infection is intrinsically resistant to most first-line antituberculosis drugs. Comparative trials suggest that initial therapy should be with two or three drugs: clarithromycin or azithromycin and ethambutol should be used, and additional rifabutin or a quinolone (e.g. ciprofloxacin) considered. In severely ill patients, intravenous amikacin may be useful as the third agent. In the absence of antiretroviral treatment, lifelong treatment may be required to prevent relapse; but if immunity is restored by highly active antiretroviral therapy, such maintenance therapy can be discontinued.

Other nontuberculous mycobacteria

Other mycobacteria, notably *Mycobacterium kansasii*, *Mycobacterium genavense*, and *Mycobacterium celatum*, may cause opportunistic infections in those with HIV. *M. genavense*, which colonizes pet birds, was discovered in European patients with HIV and causes fever, diarrhoea, and severe weight loss. HIV does not seem to affect the incidence or natural history of leprosy (*Mycobacterium leprae*).

Gastrointestinal disease

Oesophageal candidiasis

Oesophagitis presents with retrosternal pain on swallowing, and in patients with HIV is most commonly caused by *C. albicans*. Oesophageal candidiasis indicates advanced immunosuppression and is an AIDS-defining condition. The diagnosis should be suspected in a patient with oral candida and dysphagia, and may be supported by barium swallow or confirmed by endoscopy and biopsy. Treatment is with oral azole antifungal agents such as fluconazole. It may recur and in patients with severe immunosuppression, and in the absence of antiretroviral treatment, *Candida* may become resistant to prolonged azole treatment. Resistance tends to develop gradually and can be monitored by *in vitro* testing. Such patients require treatment or continuous suppression with high doses of fluconazole (which is better tolerated than high doses of ketoconazole or itraconazole). Azole-resistant oro-oesophageal candidiasis has become rare since the advent of highly active antiretroviral therapy. Echinocandins may be an option in this case.

The differential diagnosis of oesophageal candidiasis includes oesophagitis caused by cytomegalovirus (CMV) or herpes simplex virus (HSV), which require specific antiviral therapy, and aphthous ulceration, which may respond to oral prednisolone or thalidomide.

Intestinal infections

Some infections are much more common in HIV disease than in other settings. *Cryptosporidium parvum* can lead to cholera-like diarrhoea. An ascending cholangitis may occur with fever, pain, and jaundice and have the imaging appearance of sclerosing cholangitis. Other protozoan parasites, such as *Isospora belli* and *Cyclospora cayetanensis* may also cause diarrhoea, as can microsporidia. Cytomegalovirus can cause an acute colitis with pain and bloody diarrhoea. Sigmoidoscopy shows ulceration and biopsies show characteristic CMV inclusions. Tuberculosis may also present as intestinal disease.

HIV enteropathy

Many patients with HIV, especially in the tropics, present with diarrhoea and malnutrition leading to wasting in the absence of detectable gastrointestinal opportunist infections. Biopsies often show villous blunting and increased inflammatory cells in the lamina propria of the small bowel and functional tests suggest increased bowel permeability. The pathogenesis of this enteropathy is poorly understood, but may involve cytokine activation secondary to HIV infection.

HIV and the nervous system (Oxford Textbook of Medicine 5e Chapter 24.11.4)

The nervous system is a major site of involvement for direct and indirect complications of HIV at all stages of infection. All parts of the nervous system may be affected. In advanced HIV, opportunistic infections and tumours (lymphoma), and tissue damage caused by HIV replication in the brain and spinal cord, are important and relatively common during progressive HIV disease.

Cerebral toxoplasmosis (Chapter 8.4)

Cerebral infection with the intracellular protozoan *Toxoplasma gondii* is the most frequent infection of the central nervous system in AIDS, occurring when the CD4 count is below 200/mm^3. It usually results from reactivation of *Toxoplasma* cysts in the brain, leading to the formation of focal lesions that are typically multiple but may be single. Symptoms develop subacutely and include focal neurological disturbance, headache, confusion, fever, and convulsions. On CT scan the lesions appear as ring-enhancing masses with surrounding oedema (Fig. 5.23.10). MRI is more sensitive and frequently detects lesions not visible on CT. Serum antibodies to *Toxoplasma* spp. are usually detectable; their absence makes the diagnosis unlikely but does not exclude it. Detection of *Toxoplasma* DNA in cerebrospinal fluid by PCR is being evaluated as a diagnostic test. The principal differential diagnosis is primary cerebral lymphoma; other causes of focal brain lesions in AIDS include cryptococcoma, cerebral abscess (including infection with *Nocardia* spp.), tuberculoma, progressive multifocal leukoencephalopathy, and neurosyphilis. Brain biopsy is required for a definitive diagnosis, but is rarely performed. As toxoplasmosis is by far the most common treatable cause of focal cerebral lesions in HIV, it is standard

practice to treat for this and only consider biopsy if there is no clinical improvement in 7 to 10 days.

The condition responds well if treatment is started early; a combination of sulfadiazine at 4 to 6 g/day and pyrimethamine at 50 to 75 mg/day is the treatment of choice. More than 40% of patients experience adverse effects, especially rash and nephrotoxicity caused by sulfadiazine. The haematological toxicity of pyrimethamine may be reduced by adding folinic acid (10 mg/day). If sulpha drugs are not tolerated, clindamycin with pyrimethamine is an effective alternative. Corticosteroids can be used to reduce cerebral oedema in patients with large lesions and serious mass effects, but this is controversial.

Treatment is usually given for 3 to 6 weeks, and in the absence of effective antiretroviral treatment relapse is common after stopping. In these circumstances, lifelong maintenance treatment is usually required using pyrimethamine (25–50 mg/day) with a sulpha drug or clindamycin. However, these can be discontinued if antiretroviral treatment leads to sustained immunological recovery. The use of primary prophylaxis against *Pneumocystis jirovecii* also reduces the risk of toxoplasmosis.

Cryptococcal meningitis (Chapter 7.2)

Although infection of the central nervous system with *Cryptococcus neoformans* can occur in the absence of immunodeficiency, it most commonly arises in association with HIV infection. Before the widespread use of azole antifungals for mucosal candidiasis, it accounted for 5 to 10% of opportunistic infections in patients with AIDS. The presentation is usually subacute and may be subtle and nonspecific with headache, vomiting, and mild fever, and few neurological signs. Less frequently, psychiatric disturbance, convulsions, cranial nerve palsies, truncal ataxia, or focal intracerebral lesions may occur. Neck stiffness is unusual. The diagnosis is made by detecting cryptococci in the cerebrospinal fluid by India ink staining, detection of cryptococcal antigen in the cerebrospinal fluid (uniformly positive), and culture. Cryptococcal antigen is also usually detectable in serum. *C. neoformans* in patients with AIDS causes minimal inflammation, so the white cell count of the cerebrospinal fluid is often only mildly raised and the protein and glucose levels of the cerebrospinal fluid may be normal.

A randomized, controlled trial showed that the combination of amphotericin B and flucytosine was superior to amphotericin B alone or fluconazole alone for the treatment of cryptococcal meningitis. Amphotericin B and flucytosine together lead to more rapid sterilization of the cerebrospinal fluid, but are not as well tolerated as fluconazole. Resistance of cryptococci to fluconazole is very rare. Adverse reactions to amphotericin are frequent, especially fever, myalgia, renal impairment, and electrolyte disturbances. Close monitoring is required. Lipid formulations of amphotericin are increasingly used and likely to become the standard of care; otherwise they are used for patients intolerant of the conventional formulation. Raised intracranial pressure is associated with clinical deterioration and the risk of blindness: repeated lumbar punctures and, sometimes, ventricular shunting are needed in these circumstances.

Without secondary prophylaxis, cryptococcal meningitis relapses in 50 to 80% of patients with HIV in the absence of antiretroviral treatment. Oral fluconazole (200 mg/day) is effective for maintenance, and can be discontinued if antiretroviral treatment leads to sustained immunological recovery. A recent trial has found that

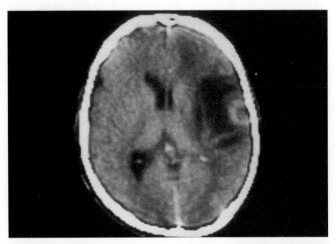

Fig. 5.23.10 Cerebral toxoplasmosis: ring enhancement and surrounding cerebral oedema (CT with contrast).

oral fluconazole is safe and effective as primary prophylaxis against cryptococcal disease in patients awaiting or starting antiretroviral therapy in Uganda.

Progressive multifocal leukoencephalopathy

Progressive multifocal leukoencephalopathy is a progressive demyelinating condition of advanced HIV disease caused by JC virus, a polyomavirus cytopathic for oligodendroglia. It presents with focal neurological deficits, personality changes, or ataxia; headache and mass effects are absent. Brain MRI, the investigation of choice, usually shows multiple white matter lesions. JC virus is detectable in cerebrospinal fluid by PCR, but this is not usually necessary for diagnosis. There is no specific treatment. Survival of less than 6 months is usual, but progression may sometimes be halted or reversed by highly active antiretroviral therapy. Cidofovir is active against JC virus and is being evaluated. The other human polyomavirus, BK virus, is a very rare cause of encephalitis and interstitial nephropathy in AIDS.

Primary cerebral lymphoma

These are B-cell non-Hodgkin's lymphomas that are associated with EBV, which is usually detectable in the cerebrospinal fluid by PCR. Lymphoma of the central nervous system may present in a manner similar to toxoplasmosis, with focal signs or seizures. CT or MRI of the brain often reveals a single space-occupying lesion but the disease is typically multifocal. Without treatment the prognosis is only a few weeks. Treatment with radiotherapy and steroids, with or without chemotherapy, and HAART, prolongs the median survival to several months, but longer-term survival is exceptional.

HIV-associated dementia (HAD)

HIV can infect the nervous system directly, leading to a variety of clinical problems. Most patients dying of AIDS show histological evidence of brain involvement including neuronal loss. Patients with brain involvement may be asymptomatic or develop minor functional impairment (mild neurocognitive disorder). A smaller number (up to 10%) develop the cognitive, behavioural, and motor abnormalities of dementia. In the early stages, there is impairment of concentration and memory and mood changes mimicking depression; gradual progression leads to intellectual incapacity and motor disability so that patients cannot care for themselves. Neurological signs include slow movement, incoordination, motor weakness, hyperreflexia, and extensor plantar responses; brain imaging shows reduced grey matter volume in the cortex and basal ganglia. Ultimately, a nearly vegetative condition develops with virtual mutism, inability to walk, and incontinence. These patients die within 2 years. Antiretroviral treatment prevents, and in the earlier stages reverses, HIV-related dementia.

Other psychological/psychiatric problems include anxiety, panic attacks, and depression. Psychotherapy may be helpful. Antidepressants may be needed in severe cases. Acute psychosis is rare. Dystonic reactions to various drugs, such as metoclopramide, are more common in patients with HIV.

In the late stages of HIV disease, the differential diagnosis of HIV dementia includes cytomegalovirus (CMV) encephalitis. This usually presents with rapidly progressive confusion and dementia, impaired consciousness, fever, cranial nerve lesions, and convulsions. MRI shows necrotizing periventriculitis; protein levels in cerebrospinal fluid may be elevated and CMV DNA is detectable in the cerebrospinal fluid by PCR. Ganciclovir and other anti-CMV agents may reduce progression.

Peripheral neuropathy and myelopathy

Peripheral neuropathy can occur at any stage of HIV infection, even at seroconversion, but is most common in advanced disease, when 10 to 15% of patients have a distal symmetrical sensorimotor neuropathy of axonal type causing pain and paraesthesias that may limit walking and, less often, distal weakness and atrophy. Mononeuritis multiplex and acute inflammatory demyelinating polyneuropathy resembling the Guillain–Barré syndrome are also described, generally at an earlier stage. Drugs used in patients with HIV, including stavudine, didanosine, and vincristine, may cause or exacerbate peripheral neuropathy. HIV-related autonomic neuropathy may cause postural hypotension, diarrhoea, impotence, impaired sweating, and bladder symptoms. CMV infection in patients with AIDS presents with a lumbosacral polyradiculopathy causing sacral paraesthesiae and numbness, lower limb weakness, and urinary retention that may progress to flaccid paraparesis if untreated.

HIV may involve the spinal cord directly, causing a vacuolar myelopathy. This usually presents with bilateral leg weakness and sensory symptoms, usually paraesthesias, and may progress to spastic paraparesis, ataxia, and incontinence. Rarely, a myopathy can occur.

Ocular disease

Cytomegalovirus retinitis

Without antiretroviral therapy, up to 30% of patients with AIDS (and a CD4 lymphocyte count below 50/mm^3) develop reactivation of CMV in the form of a destructive and blinding retinitis. This is rare in other types of immunosuppression. It usually presents with blurring of vision, scotomas, floaters, or flashing lights. The characteristic retinal changes are patches of irregular retinal pallor, caused by oedema and necrosis, and haemorrhages in a perivascular distribution (Fig. 5.23.11). The retinitis usually starts peripherally and progresses rapidly to involve the macula and whole retina, leading to blindness. Complications include retinal detachment, branch retinal artery occlusion, persistent iritis, and cataract. CMV retinitis should not be confused with cotton wool spots (HIV retinopathy)—small, pale retinal lesions without haemorrhages that commonly occur in patients with HIV. These are benign and often come and go.

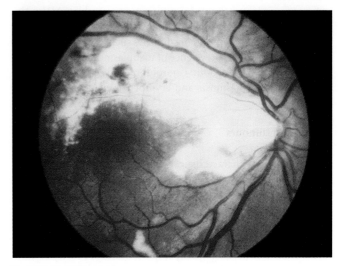

Fig. 5.23.11 CMV retinitis.

The diagnosis of CMV retinitis is clinical, based on the characteristic retinal appearance (see Oxford Textbook of Medicine 5e Chapter 25.1). CMV viraemia may be detectable by PCR, and high or rising CMV viral load is associated with an increased risk of developing retinitis and other CMV disease. Anti-CMV drugs (ganciclovir, foscarnet, cidofovir) are virustatic; before the availability of highly active antiretroviral drug combinations, the aim of treatment was to stop progression rather than to cure disease. First-line treatment is with intravitreal ganciclovir injection or implant; oral valganciclovir is often given in conjunction with intravitreal ganciclovir as patients treated without systemic therapy may develop contralateral or extraocular CMV disease. Oral valganciclovir alone may be used as an alternative in patients without sight-threatening disease. Other effective treatments include intravenous ganciclovir, foscarnet, or cidofovir.

Intravenous ganciclovir and forscarnet require administration via a central vein, whereas foscarnet may be given via a peripheral vein, The main adverse effects of ganciclovir are bone marrow suppression, in particular neutropenia, central nervous system symptoms, abnormal liver function tests, fever, and rash. Foscarnet is associated with decreased renal function, electrolyte abnormalities, and infusion-related nausea.

With the advent of highly active antiretroviral therapy, CMV retinitis is much less common in developed countries. Sustained suppression of HIV viral load and improvement in immune status can allow discontinuation of maintenance treatment. New manifestations of ocular CMV, such as vitritis, have been reported in patients treated with highly active antiretroviral therapy (see Immune reconstitution syndromes, below).

Other ocular syndromes

Acute retinal necrosis is a rare condition originally reported in reactivation of varicella zoster virus in otherwise healthy adults. In patients with advanced HIV infection, it is usually preceded by dermatomal herpes zoster and typically presents with blurring of vision and pain in the affected eye. Progressive necrotizing retinitis leads to visual deterioration that may be associated with uveitis. An outer retinal necrosis syndrome with little ocular inflammation also occurs in patients with AIDS. There is a high risk of visual loss and retinal detachment. Both eyes may be affected. Suspected acute retinal necrosis should be treated with intravenous aciclovir.

Acute toxoplasma choroidoretinitis may resemble CMV retinitis, but the retinal scarring that follows treatment is distinctive. The disease is more common in countries such as Brazil and France where the background prevalence of toxoplasmosis is much higher than in the United Kingdom. Choroidoretinitis is also a rare complication of histoplasmosis and cryptococcosis, and uveitis may occur in syphilis.

HIV-related tumours

Kaposi's sarcoma

Kaposi's sarcoma characteristically presents as multiple, purplish, nodular skin lesions (Fig. 5.23.12). Lesions start as small, pink, deep purple, or brown macules, and develop into nodules or plaques that may ulcerate. They also occur on mucosal surfaces, most commonly on the hard palate. Local or regional oedema and lymph node enlargement may occur. Mucocutaneous lesions are cosmetically and psychologically important but are rarely of clinical importance (Fig. 5.23.13). However, visceral disease, which most commonly affects the lungs and gastrointestinal tract, is an important cause of morbidity and even mortality. Lung lesions cause dyspnoea, cough, or haemoptysis, and gut involvement may cause abdominal pain, bleeding, or a rare protein-losing enteropathy. Extensive visceral involvement can cause constitutional symptoms such as fevers, night sweats, and weight loss. Kaposi's sarcoma rarely affects the central nervous system.

In industrialized countries, Kaposi's sarcoma is over 2000 times more common in HIV-infected individuals than in the general population. Classic Kaposi's sarcoma in HIV-negative individuals occurs in middle-aged and older men of Eastern European or Mediterranean origin. Endemic Kaposi's sarcoma in Africa has been known for decades. It is predominantly a disease of older men that has a fairly indolent course. HIV-related Kaposi's sarcoma, on the other hand, is a more aggressive disease and occurs mostly in those people who have acquired HIV via a sexual route, namely homosexual and bisexual men and in younger African men and women. The epidemic of Kaposi's sarcoma in central and East Africa exactly mirrors the HIV epidemic in these regions. Kaposi's sarcoma is rare in intravenous drug users and very rare in recipients of blood products, including those with haemophilia. These epidemiological features suggested a sexually transmissible aetiological agent.

In 1994, a new herpesvirus, human herpesvirus 8 (HHV-8), was found in HIV-related Kaposi's sarcoma and was soon detected in the lesions of all forms of Kaposi's sarcoma. Seroepidemiological studies show that HHV-8 is common only in certain geographical regions, corresponding to where Kaposi's sarcoma was endemic before the era of HIV. HHV-8 is detectable in saliva but less often in semen. This may explain why both sexual and other routes of transmission occur. In Africa, where HHV-8 infection is common, it is transmitted perinatally from mother to child.

Kaposi's sarcoma lesions are characterized by proliferating spindle cells of lymphatic and blood vascular endothelial origin, thin-walled slit-like vascular spaces, infiltration by lymphocytes and plasma cells, and extravasated red cells. Multiple lesions appear synchronously in widely dispersed areas. The clonality of Kaposi's sarcoma lesions has not been fully resolved. Although some studies have suggested a monoclonal origin, others have shown a mixed picture and the lesions may be reactive proliferative rather than truly cancerous. HHV-8 is detectable in spindle cells and flat endothelial cells lining the vascular spaces of Kaposi's sarcoma lesions. It is likely that the virus triggers the release of cellular and virus-encoded cytokines that promote the proliferation of spindle cells.

Highly active antiretroviral therapy has led to a dramatic reduction in the frequency and mortality of Kaposi's sarcoma in developed countries. In early Kaposi's sarcoma, the progression is often halted or reversed by starting antiretroviral treatment alone. Otherwise, cutaneous lesions may be left untreated or treated with local radiotherapy, cryotherapy, or intralesional vinblastine. Widespread skin or visceral disease is usually treated by systemic chemotherapy, usually with a liposomal anthracycline such as daunorubicin or doxorubicin, which are more effective than the previously used combination of vincristine and bleomycin. Paclitaxel, a taxane, is potentially more toxic than liposomal anthracyclines, but may be useful as a second line agent after treatment failure. Treatment of disseminated Kaposi's sarcoma has not been considered to be curative, but remissions may be induced by a combination of highly active antiretroviral treatment and systemic chemotherapy.

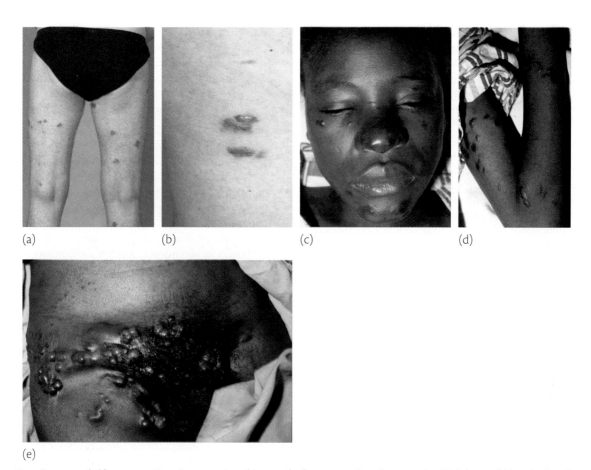

Fig. 5.23.12 Kaposi's sarcoma. (a, b) cutaneous Kaposi's sarcoma in a white man; (c, d), cutaneous Kaposi's sarcoma in a Zimbabwean; (e) invasive Kaposi's sarcoma in a Kenyan.
(Copyright D A Warrell)

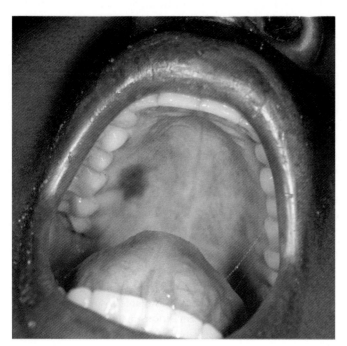

Fig. 5.23.13 Palatal Kaposi's sarcoma.
(Copyright D A Warrell.)

Non-Hodgkin's lymphoma

Non-Hodgkin's lymphoma develops in 3 to 10% of HIV-positive patients, an incidence 60 to 100 times higher than in the general population. Most tumours are extranodal and, histologically, 60% are large cell B-cell lymphomas; 30% are Burkitt's type and the rest are of T-cell or non-B-, non-T-cell origin. Some 50% are associated with Epstein–Barr virus (EBV) infection and are more aggressive with a shorter survival. A minority of HIV-related lymphomas are associated with HHV-8. They present as body cavity lymphomas, causing pleural or peritoneal effusions (primary effusion lymphoma). Patients on highly active antiretroviral therapy have a reduced risk of developing non-Hodgkin's lymphoma, and consequently the incidence of HIV-related lymphomas in developed countries has declined in recent years.

HIV-associated lymphoma outside the central nervous system may respond well to standard lymphoma chemotherapy regimens, in addition to highly active antiretroviral treatment. Response is better in those who are less immunosuppressed (CD4 above 200/mm^3 and no previous AIDS diagnosis). Opportunistic infections cause many deaths during chemotherapy. Lower dose or less toxic chemotherapy protocols are sometimes advocated for patients with more advanced HIV disease.

Non-AIDS defining cancers

It is now apparent that HIV increases the frequency of several cancers other than those that have been categorized as AIDS-defining (i.e. Kaposi's sarcoma, non-Hodgkin's lymphoma, and cervical carcinoma), and non-AIDS-defining cancers cause a high proportion of deaths in HIV patients in industrialized countries (50% in a recent study from France). These include Hodgkin's disease, particularly of the mixed cellularity type and associated with EBV. Disseminated disease with a poor prognosis seems to be more frequent than for HIV-negative Hodgkin's disease.

Other cancers that arise with higher frequency than in HIV-negative individuals include hepatocellular carcinoma (caused by hepatitis C and probably hepatitis B); lung carcinoma; skin tumours (basal cell carcinoma, squamous cell carcinoma, and malignant melanoma); and cancers of the head and neck, probably associated with human papillomavirus (HPV), especially type 16. There is an increased incidence of squamous cell carcinoma of the conjunctiva in patients with HIV infection, especially in Africa. HPV is also associated with a higher incidence of cervical intraepithelial neoplasia (CIN) and predisposition to cervical carcinoma in HIV-infected women, and the higher incidence of vulvar intraepithelial neoplasia (VIN) in women; and also anal carcinoma and its precursor anal intraepithelial neoplasia (AIN), which occurs at a greatly increased frequency in HIV-positive homosexual men.

Other cancers that may arise with greater frequency, but where this is less clear cut, include colorectal cancer, testicular cancer, myeloma, and acute myeloid leukaemia. Cancers that do not arise with greater frequency include prostate, bladder, and breast.

Miscellaneous conditions
Castleman's disease
Castleman's disease (angiofollicular lymph node hyperplasia) is a lymphoproliferative condition that can be HHV-8 related and, in the multicentric form, is associated with HIV. It can sometimes be difficult to distinguish from Kaposi's sarcoma.

Bacillary angiomatosis
Disseminated infection with *Bartonella henselae*, the principal agent of cat-scratch disease, is the cause of bacillary angiomatosis, an HIV-associated condition that typically causes multiple subcutaneous vascular lesions, fever, liver lesions (bacillary peliosis hepatis), and osteolytic bone lesions. The skin lesions are usually purplish nodules that may be mistaken for Kaposi's sarcoma, but the histology is distinct—acute neutrophilic inflammation and capillary proliferation, and clusters of bacilli revealed by modified silver staining. The organism may be cultured from blood. A similar syndrome in HIV-positive patients can be caused by the agent of trench fever, *Bartonella quintana*. Bacillary angiomatosis usually responds to treatment with a macrolide antibiotic. Cats and cat fleas form a reservoir for *B. henselae*, and patients who develop bacillary angiomatosis frequently have a history of contact with cats.

Disseminated fungal infections
In regions where invasive fungal infections are endemic (such as *Histoplasma capsulatum* in the Mississippi river region, *Coccidioides immitis* in the southern United States of America, and *Penicillium marneffei* in South East Asia) or where there is a relevant travel history, disseminated fungal infection should be considered in HIV-positive patients presenting with fever, weight loss, anaemia, pulmonary infiltrates, lymphadenopathy, and hepatosplenomegaly. Papular skin lesions may be seen in disseminated histoplasmosis and *P. marneffei* infection. Similar lesions resembling giant molluscum (see below) may occur with disseminated cryptococcosis.

Blood or bone marrow cultures or direct identification by the use of special stains on tissue obtained from skin lesions, bone marrow, or liver are required for diagnosis. Initial therapy is generally with intravenous amphotericin; itraconazole (for histoplasmosis and *P. marneffei*) or fluconazole (for coccidioidomycosis) may be adequate for subsequent maintenance treatment.

Leishmaniasis
HIV-associated disseminated leishmaniasis is mostly reported from the Mediterranean littoral, South America, and Africa. It is caused by dissemination of leishmania spp., protozoan parasites transmitted by sandflies. A high index of clinical suspicion is required, because although the classic features are fever, weight loss, anaemia, and hepatosplenomegaly, a high proportion of patients have fever alone. The disease may present months or years after exposure in an endemic country. Leishmania may be transmitted by shared needles in injecting drug users. Most cases can be diagnosed by bone marrow examination or splenic aspirate; serology may be helpful. Treatment is with lipid formulations of amphotericin B.

Haematological conditions
Thrombocytopenia is relatively common (5–15%) in HIV infection and may be how the disease first presents. It is associated with antiplatelet antibodies. Symptomatic thrombocytopenia is uncommon but more likely in the later stages of HIV infection. Life-threatening bleeding is rare. Thrombocytopenia is not a marker for HIV progression and spontaneous remissions are frequent. Antiretroviral treatment is first-line when the CD4 count is low; zidovudine is known to increase platelet production. When specific treatment for thrombocytopenia is required, the principles and response are similar to those that apply in the treatment of HIV-negative immune thrombocytopenia, and include the use of prednisolone, intravenous immunoglobulin, and splenectomy.

Anaemia is common in patients with advanced HIV infection, and is frequently related to medications (such as zidovudine). Human (B19) parvovirus infection is a reversible cause of chronic anaemia in HIV infection. Bone marrow biopsy typically shows an absence of erythroid development with occasional giant pronormoblasts, and B19 parvovirus is detected by PCR. The anaemia may respond to treatment with intravenous immunoglobulin.

Mild neutropenia is common in HIV-positive patients at all stages of infection, and may be partly responsible for the increased risk of pyogenic bacterial infections; however, profound neutropenia (below 0.5×10^9/litre) is rare. Antineutrophil antibodies may be present. Drugs (such as co-trimoxazole, ganciclovir, and antiretrovirals) may increase the incidence and severity of neutropenia. In selected HIV-positive patients with refractory or life-threatening bacterial or fungal infection and severe neutropenia, the addition of recombinant human granulocyte colony-stimulating factor to the treatment regimen may improve the outcome.

Skin conditions in advanced HIV
In the later stages of HIV infection, a number of infections have atypical cutaneous manifestations. All have become rare in settings where antiretroviral treatment is available to prevent advanced immunosuppression. These conditions include giant molluscum contagiosum, characterized by large, flesh-coloured, nontender umbilicated lesions often affecting the face in homosexual men. In advanced HIV disease, genital herpes simplex infection may cause

painful chronic genital or anal ulcers that can become resistant to aciclovir and related compounds; intravenous foscarnet or cidofovir are effective. Aciclovir-resistant varicella zoster virus also occurs in AIDS; and reactivation of varicella zoster virus can take an unusual form, with a subacute course and dissemination causing scattered vesicular lesions in the absence of dermatomal zoster. CMV is a cause of chronic perianal ulceration that can be treated with ganciclovir. Atypical cutaneous presentations of syphilis may occur at any stage of HIV infection. In Asia, the varied skin manifestations of *P. marneffei* infection are familiar.

HIV-associated nephropathy (HIVAN)

HIV can directly infect glomerular and tubular epithelial cells and renal disease is relatively common in HIV-infected patients, most commonly caused by a collapsing focal segmental glomerulosclerosis (FSGS) also known as HIV-associated nephropathy (HIVAN). This typically presents as a nephritic syndrome, but with minimal oedema. It appears to be more common in Africans and African Americans than in the white population. Renal function usually improves with the use of antiretroviral medication, but some patients progress to chronic renal failure and require renal replacement therapy or transplantation. Other renal diseases are described in HIV including membranoproliferative glomerulonephritis associated with hepatitis C, immune complex glomerulonephritis with IgA deposits, and membranous nephropathy. Drug toxicity is an important cause of renal impairment in HIV patients, including drugs used to treat opportunistic infections (e.g. cidofovir, amphotericin B, pentamidine). Antiretroviral treatment (e.g. tenofovir) may cause Fanconi's syndrome due to tubular damage; atazanavir and indinavir may induce renal calculi and a nephropathy). Renal impairment caused by concurrent conditions such as diabetes or hypertension may also arise in patients with HIV infection.

HIV and hepatitis virus coinfections

Because of common risk factors for blood-borne virus infections, there are increasing numbers of individuals with HIV who are coinfected with either hepatitis C (HCV) or hepatitis B (HBV) virus, or both. Over the past few years, new data have become available on the size of this problem and some management strategies have emerged.

HIV/HCV coinfection

HCV coinfection occurs in up to a third of those with HIV. The group with the highest prevalence is the haemophiliac population, but the group most at risk now is injecting drug users (IDU). Anywhere between 50 and 75% of IDU with HIV are coinfected. More recently, there is an awareness that growing numbers of men who have sex with men (MSM) are acquiring HCV sexually.

HCV/HIV coinfection increases the risk of liver disease progression compared to HCV infection by itself. In addition, the treatment of HIV with antiretrovirals may carry an increased risk of hepatotoxicity in those with coinfection. There is little evidence to suggest that HCV worsens HIV disease.

Treatment aimed at clearing HCV in those with coinfection can be successful, but is less likely to lead to a sustained virological response compared to HCV infection alone. Trials in HIV coinfected patients show that pegylated interferon-α 2a with ribavirin is the treatment of choice and, as in those without coinfection, HCV genotypes 2 and 3 respond better than genotypes 1 and 4. Treatment in those with coinfection is more likely to lead to anaemia and may cause transient drops in CD4 count. The new HCV

protease inhibitors, boceprevir and telaprevir, show promise for HCV genotype 1 infections in non-HIV-infected patients and trials are under way in patients with dual infection.

HIV/HBV coinfection

The scale of the HIV epidemic in Africa and, now, in Asia means that up to 90% of those with HIV will have evidence of past or current HBV infection. Estimates vary, but up to 10% of those with HIV may be HBV carriers.

Unlike with HCV, there is no evidence that liver disease due to HBV is worse in HIV coinfected individuals. Although HBV DNA levels are higher in HIV coinfection, there is evidence that there is less liver injury. New HBV infections in HIV positive individuals are less likely to cause acute hepatitis and jaundice, but are more likely to result in chronic HBV carriage. HBV infection does not seem to affect the progression of HIV disease.

Treatment of HBV coinfection is less well defined than treatment of HCV coinfection. Although pegylated interferon may be useful, there are no large trials of its efficacy in HIV. Lamivudine monotherapy is more likely to lead to resistant HBV with the 'YMDD' mutant in the presence of HIV. Drugs currently used to treat HBV in the absence of HIV coinfection also have anti-HIV activity, particularly lamivudine, emtricitabine, and tenofovir. Caution must be used in treating HBV with these agents in coinfected patients as monotherapy with these drugs will lead to resistant HIV. A recently introduced drug to treat HBV, entecavir, was thought not to have activity against HIV but had now been shown to have an anti-HIV effect and this can also lead to HIV resistance. By contrast, if HBV coinfected patients require antiretroviral therapy, a combination of lamivudine and tenofovir, or emtricitabine and tenofovir, is recommended as part of the antiretroviral regimen to decrease HBV replication.

Management of HIV infection and prognosis

The advent of highly active antiretroviral therapy (HAART) in the mid 1990s led to marked reductions in morbidity and mortality attributable to HIV and its complications—although not in resource-limited countries, where the epidemic is concentrated and access to antiretroviral treatment remains limited. A decline in the incidence of opportunistic infections, notably pneumocystis pneumonia, disseminated *M. avium* complex (MAC) infection, CMV retinitis, cerebral toxoplasmosis and cryptococcal meningitis, and associated mortality was reported from the United States of America and Europe after the introduction of treatment based on a minimum of three antiretroviral drugs. HIV infection in adults in resource-rich countries is now almost exclusively managed on an outpatient basis. Antiretroviral treatment has transformed HIV/AIDS from a uniformly fatal disease to a long-term condition. Although the prognosis is variable and influenced by adherence to HAART, a large-scale study of mortality in HIV-infected adults in Europe has shown that in patients who are stable on treatment the standardized mortality ratio (SMR) approaches normal (1.05) and nearly half of patients have SMR less than 2, which is lower than for type 1 diabetes.

In industrialized countries, HAART has also influenced the proportion of deaths from non-AIDS causes, which now exceed AIDS-related deaths and typically include non-AIDS-defining cancers, cardiovascular disease, and liver disease.

There is no evidence that HAART can ever achieve eradication or 'cure' of HIV. Although HIV may be undetectable in plasma for many months, a long-lived reservoir of infectious virus can be recovered from latently infected (resting) memory CD4 lymphocytes. The half-life of this cell population is long, about 6 months, and it is not known whether HIV can ever be eradicated from this infected cell line. Other compartments exist that are relatively inaccessible to drugs—e.g. in the central nervous system, retina, and testes—and unless viral replication can be successfully prevented at such sites there is also the risk of reinfection of compartments previously cleared by therapy.

Initial assessment and management

Ideally, HIV infection should be identified at the asymptomatic stage. At the time of diagnosis, patients should undergo a baseline assessment that includes taking a detailed history, including a sexual history, and determination of risk factors for HIV infection. An assessment of cardiovascular risk factors should be made, including smoking and family history. A detailed physical examination should be performed with attention to the skin and mucous membranes, blood pressure, and body mass index (BMI), fundoscopy, and should include a search for lymphadenopathy and signs of liver disease. Initial investigations include full blood count, biochemical screen including liver profile, bone profile and estimated GFR, lipids, chest radiography, and serological screening for infections that may require additional treatment (hepatitis B and C, syphilis) or which can reactivate during immunosuppression (CMV and toxoplasma). Baseline investigations include CD4 lymphocyte (T-helper cell) count (lymphocyte subsets profile), quantitative estimation of HIV RNA in the blood plasma (viral load), and HIV genotypic resistance testing; and should include tissue typing for HLA-B*5701, a marker for abacavir hypersensitivity. In women, cervical cytology screening is indicated at annual intervals.

Following initial assessment, hepatitis B immunization can be provided to susceptible individuals, and pneumococcal vaccine can be offered. Psychological support and counselling are often needed. There should be a discussion on who should be informed about their HIV status, including the primary care physician, and family members and friends for support. The issue of disclosure to sexual partners should also be raised, with advice on reducing risk of transmission (including the importance of barrier methods such as condoms). Antiretroviral treatment of the HIV-infected partner might be offered earlier than usually indicated to reduce risk of transmission to their HIV-negative sexual partner, although safe sex counselling should still be provided.

The CD4 lymphocyte count and HIV viral load are the two laboratory markers that have the best prognostic value. The CD4 count is a reliable indicator of HIV-related immune impairment. CD4 counts, normal at or above 600/mm^3, vary considerably, even in the absence of HIV infection. A fall in the CD4 lymphocyte count to below 200/mm^3 is associated with a risk of opportunistic infections of about 80% over 3 years without antiretroviral treatment. However, progression is variable and a minority remain well for several years with stable low CD4 counts. This variability is explained partly by differences in HIV viral load. The level of CD4 lymphopenia generally determines the spectrum of potential infections (Table 5.23.1). For instance, whereas oral and oesophageal candidiasis and pneumocystis pneumonia can occur at CD4 counts of 100 to 200/mm^3, disseminated MAC infection and CMV retinitis are rarely seen until the CD4 count is below 50/mm^3.

The prognostic value of measuring HIV RNA in plasma was reported from the United States of America in 1996. In HIV-positive men, in a subgroup of the Multicenter AIDS Cohort Study, only 8% with less than 5000 copies of HIV RNA/ml progressed to AIDS over 5 years, whereas 62% with viral loads above 35 000 developed AIDS. For a given level of CD4 lymphocytes, variations in viral load broadly predict the risk of progression. The most useful prognostic information is therefore derived from the CD4 count and viral load taken together (Fig. 5.23.14).

In industrialized countries, HIV viral load measurements are widely available. Techniques include reverse transcription followed by amplification by the polymerase chain reaction (RT-PCR), branched DNA (bDNA) signal amplification, and nucleic acid sequence-based amplification (NASBA). Highly sensitive tests with very low detection limits (40 copies/ml) are generally used.

Antiretroviral therapy

Nucleoside/nucleotide analogues

Knowledge of the viral lifecycle (Fig. 5.23.3) led to the development of a number of antiretroviral compounds with clinically useful activity against HIV (Table 5.23.2). The forerunner of these was zidovudine (AZT or ZDV), first shown to be active against HIV *in vitro* in 1985. Zidovudine, a nucleoside analogue that inhibits HIV reverse transcriptase, slowed down the rate of disease progression over a 12-month period in patients with AIDS and improved short-term survival, well-being, body weight, and neurological features. However, clinical progression associated with viral resistance to the drug was observed after a year or two of therapy. When early treatment with zidovudine was compared to deferred zidovudine, there was no difference in survival or disease progression after 3 years.

The clinical failure of monotherapy prompted combination therapy in an attempt to reduce the development of drug resistance. Double nucleoside combinations proved superior to zidovudine monotherapy, especially in patients without prior exposure to zidovudine. Treatment with at least three drugs is more effective and has become the standard of care. In general, two nucleoside drugs are used with either a non-nucleoside reverse transcriptase inhibitor or a protease inhibitor. A combination of three nucleoside analogues (zidovudine, lamivudine, and abacavir) can also be used in a single tablet taken twice daily, but is less effective than other combinations and is not routinely recommended (Table 5.23.3). A nucleotide agent, tenofovir, has similar properties and is usually grouped in the same category as the nucleoside analogues.

Non-nucleoside reverse transcriptase inhibitors

The prototype of the class is nevirapine, a potent and selective inhibitor of HIV reverse transcriptase. When nevirapine is given alone, resistance develops rapidly; this drug is of limited effectiveness in double therapy or when added to failing regimens. However, in antiretroviral-naive patients without AIDS (CD4 200–600/mm^3), over 50% of patients treated with nevirapine plus two nucleosides (zidovudine and didanosine) had undetectable plasma HIV RNA after 1 year of therapy, compared with 12% for zidovudine/didanosine only. Efavirenz and delavirdine (which is not licensed for use in the United Kingdom) are other non-nucleoside reverse transcriptase inhibitors (NNRTIs) with similar properties to nevirapine. More recently, a new NNRTI, etravirine, has been licensed and has activity against viral isolates resistant to the older NNRTIs. The most recently licensed NNRTI, rilpivirine, has been shown to

Table 5.23.1 Principal complications of untreated HIV infection

Infections	Neoplasms	Direct HIV effects
Early/intermediate HIV infection (CD4 >200/mm³)		
Herpes zoster	Non-Hodgkin's lymphoma[a]	Persistent generalized lymphadenopathy
Oral hairy leucoplakia	Cervical intraepithelial neoplasia	Atopy; eczema
Oral candidiasis; candidal vaginitis	Anal intraepithelial neoplasia	Recurrent aphthous ulcers (oral and gastrointestinal tract)
Pulmonary tuberculosis[a]		Immune thrombocytopenia
Bacterial pneumonia, especially pneumococcal		Neutropenia
Bacteraemia, especially pneumococcal and salmonella		Neuropathy (mononeuritis multiplex; Guillian–Barré syndrome)
Bacillary angiomatosis		HIV-associated nephropathy (HIVAN)
		Lymphocytic interstitial pneumonitis (LIP)
Late HIV infection (CD4 <200/mm³)		
Pneumocystis pneumonia[a]	Kaposi's sarcoma[a]	HIV enteropathy
Candidal oesophagitis[a]	Primary cerebral lymphoma[a]	Peripheral neuropathy (distal, axonal)
Cerebral toxoplasmosis[a]	Hodgkin's lymphoma	Autonomic neuropathy
Cryptococcal meningitis[a]	Conjunctival carcinoma	Myelopathy
Chronic cryptosporidial diarrhoea[a]	? Cervical carcinoma[a]	HIV dementia[a]
Chronic isosporiasis[a], microsporidiosis	? Anal carcinoma	Wasting syndrome[a]
Chronic HSV[a] ulceration		Cardiomyopathy
Extrapulmonary tuberculosis[a]		
Disseminated *M. avium* complex (MAC)[a]		
CMV (retinitis and disseminated)[a]		
Progressive multifocal leucoencephalopathy[a]		
Recurrent bacterial pneumonia[a]		
Recurrent bacteraemia, especially salmonella[a]		
Disseminated histoplasmosis[a], and *P. marneffei*		

[a] AIDS-defining conditions; incomplete list.

? Signifies suspected but unproven association. Many of the early/intermediate manifestations also occur in late-stage HIV disease; non-Hodgkin's lymphoma is more common during the later stages.

be as effective as efavirenz in treatment-naive patients who have HIV viral loads of less than 100 000 copies/ml but was not noninferior at higher viral loads. NNRTIs are not active against HIV-2.

Protease inhibitors

The HIV-encoded protease (or proteinase) is required for the production of mature infectious viral particles. This enzyme cleaves a number of structural proteins and enzymes from the polyprotein precursors produced by translation of the *gag* and *gag–pol* genes. Inhibitors of HIV protease act synergistically with nucleoside drugs and are potent inhibitors of HIV replication.

In early studies, indinavir, in combination with two nucleoside analogues (zidovudine/lamivudine or stavudine/lamivudine) produced good results in a large controlled trial with clinical endpoints (ACTG 320 clinical trial). Similar results were subsequently reported for combination therapy with other protease inhibitors (PIs). The PIs in current use are generally 'ritonavir-boosted', i.e. they are used in combination with low dose ritonavir to improve pharmacokinetics (via cytochrome P450 interactions) of the principal PIs (especially saquinavir, lopinavir, atazanvir, and fosamprenavir).

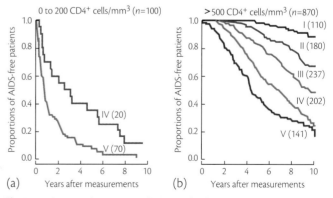

Fig. 5.23.14 Curves showing AIDS-free survival with time among groups with different baseline CD4 lymphocyte counts, according to HIV-1 RNA category. The five categories were (copies/ml): I, 500 or less; II, 501–3000; III, 3001–10 000; IV, 10 001–30 000; and V, above 30 000. (Sample sizes are shown in brackets.)

244 CHAPTER 5 VIRUSES

Table 5.23.2 Principal antiretroviral agents

Nucleoside reverse transcriptase inhibitors	Non-nucleoside reverse transcriptase inhibitors	Protease inhibitors	Entry inhibitors
Zidovudine (AZT/ZDV)	Nevirapine	Lopinavir[a]	*Fusion inhibitor*
Lamivudine (3TC)	Efavirenz	Ritonavir	Enfuvirtide
Emtricitabine (FTC)	Etravirine	Atazanavir[a]	
Abacavir (ABC)	Rilpivirine	Saquinavir[a]	*CCR5 antagonists*[b]
Didanosine (ddI)	Lersivirine[b]	Fosamprenavir[a]	Maraviroc
Stavudine (d4T)		Indinavir[a]	Vicriviroc[c]
		Nelfinavir	Cenicriviroc[b]
Nucleotide reverse transcriptase inhibitor		Tipranavir[a]	*Integrase inhibitors*
Tenofovir (TDF)		Darunavir[a]	Raltegravir
			Elvitegravir[b]
			Dolutegravir[b]

Other compounds (not shown) are at earlier phases of development and evaluation.

[a] Given with low-dose ritonavir for pharmacokinetic enhancement.

[b] Experimental, in advanced clinical trials.

[c] Development discontinued due to poor results in recent clinical trials

PIs have a higher threshold for development of resistance mutations compared to NNRTIs, so that when resistance does occur it is more likely to be due to poor absorption and suboptimal blood levels. Nevertheless, PI mutations do occur and can be a problem in drug-experienced patients. Newer PIs, such as tipranavir and darunavir, are active against some of the PI-resistant isolates and have an increasing role in salvage therapy.

Table 5.23.3 Initial antiretroviral regimens

Regimen	Examples	Comment
2 NRTIs + NNRTI	3TC/ABC + efavirenz OR nevirapine	Preferred initial regimens[a]; avoid efavirenz if risk of pregnancy
	TDF/FTC + efavirenz OR nevirapine	
	AZT/3TC + efavirenz OR nevirapine	Alternative regimen; avoid efavirenz if risk of pregnancy
2 NRTI + 2PIs[b]	AZT/3TC + ritonavir/other PI[b]	Alternative initial regimen; caution about drug interactions with ritonavir
	3TC/ABC + ritonavir/other PI[b]	
	TDF/FTC + ritonavir/other PI[b]	

3TC, lamivudine; ABC, abacavir; AZT, zidovudine; FTC, emtricitabine; NNRTI, non-nucleoside reverse transcriptase inhibitor; NRTI, nucleoside reverse transcriptase inhibitor; PI, protease inhibitor; TDF, tenofovir.

[a] If HLA-B*5701 -ve

[b] Low-dose ritonavir (to improve pharmacokinetics) plus usually lopinavir, atazanavir or fosamprenavir.

Entry inhibitors

HIV entry inhibitors are a new class of antiretroviral drugs that target viral entry into cells. This class contains two subgroups, fusion inhibitors and coreceptor antagonists. The fusion inhibitor enfuvirtide (T-20) stops the HIV glycoprotein gp41 from effecting fusion of the viral and cellular membranes, and thereby prevents HIV entry into host cells. This drug is licensed for use in treatment-experienced patients in combination with other drugs. It must be given by subcutaneous injection and is associated with a high rate of injection site reactions.

Coreceptor antagonists act as functional antagonists of the chemokine receptor CCR5 and are active against the R5-tropic subgroup of HIV-1 viruses. Maraviroc is the first to be licensed from this subgroup, but others, such as cenicriviroc are in clinical trials. These drugs are not effective against strains of virus using CXCR4 (more common in late disease), so tropism assays to determine the type of coreceptor usage of a patient's virus are needed before these drugs are used. The place of these agents in HIV therapy is yet to be determined.

Integrase inhibitors

This new class of drugs inhibits an essential enzyme that catalyses the integration of HIV proviral DNA into the host cell genome. The enzyme, integrase, is also involved in viral assembly and is not a feature of host cells. The first drug to be licensed in this group, raltegravir, is a potent inhibitor of HIV replication which currently should only be used in combination with other active antiretrovirals in patients with high exposure to all three major drug classes. Another drug in this class, elvitegravir, is at an advanced stage of development.

Other drugs

There is a need for new drug classes for use after development of drug resistance, allowing additional options for switching after treatment failure or drug intolerance, and also to provide compounds that avoid the long-term toxicities associated with current antiretrovirals. Immunotherapy with interleukin-2 (IL-2), which raises CD4 lymphocyte counts and is given by subcutaneous injection, has been shown to be clinically ineffective in recent studies.

When to start antiretroviral treatment

The optimum time to start antiretroviral therapy is not known, and no trials have adequately addressed this question; large scale, long-term clinical trials are needed. Data from several clinical cohorts suggest that patients who start treatment when the CD4 count is below 350/mm^3 (and definitely <200/mm^3) have an increased mortality or progression to AIDS when compared with those starting at higher CD4 levels, therefore, current guidelines recommend that treatment should be considered when the CD4 count falls to around 350/mm^3 or if symptoms related to HIV develop. A major trial (Strategic Timing of Anti-Retroviral Treatment, START) is investigating whether treatment should be started early, immediately at presentation regardless of CD4 count, or deferred until the CD4 count declines to less than 350/mm3 or AIDS develops. It is expected to report in 2015. The decision to start treatment should take into account other factors of prognostic importance, including the rate of CD4 decline, the viral load, age, and presence of coinfection with hepatitis B or C. Patients who are clinically well and have high CD4 counts at presentation should be seen for follow-up at intervals of 3 to 6 months for CD4 and viral load measurements.

What to start with

Highly active antiretroviral therapy consists of at least three drugs from two different drug classes, usually a backbone of two nucleosides with either a non-nucleoside reverse transcriptase inhibitor or a protease inhibitor (see Table 5.23.3). For improved pharmacokinetics, the protease inhibitor is usually combined ('boosted') with a second protease inhibitor, i.e. low-dose ritonavir. A triple nucleoside regimen is also available, but is not suitable for initial therapy because of lower potency. A number of initial regimens have equivalent efficacy.

The most important cause of treatment failure is inadequate treatment, which may relate to failure to take the drugs regularly, i.e. nonadherence, lack of availability of drugs, or poor absorption. Before starting treatment it is therefore important to discuss the patient's views about taking medication regularly. Simplified regimens have helped with adherence (see below). A number of other factors also influence the selection of the initial regimen, including potential drug interactions (e.g. with antituberculosis treatment), toxicity (e.g. avoidance of stavudine if possible), ease of administration (didanosine is taken on an empty stomach), presence of renal or hepatic dysfunction, female gender (avoidance of efavirenz in women who may be at risk of pregnancy). HIV viral load and CD4 count should be checked within 2 months. The aim of initial treatment is to achieve a sustained reduction in viral load to undetectable levels (<40 copies/ml) within 2 to 3 months of starting treatment.

Patient adherence

A substantial proportion of HIV patients do not follow treatment recommendations. Reasons for nonadherence include poor communication, the complexity of drug regimens and number of tablets, disruption of life (including timing and food restrictions), side effects, concerns about long-term effects, and lack of confidence in noncurative treatments of indefinite duration. Adherence to treatment requires a high level of understanding and motivation in the patient. This is of particular concern in HIV therapy because of the risk of developing drug resistance mutations during suboptimal therapy. The recent development of simplified regimens (one or two tablets taken once or twice daily) has helped. Patients may be helped to be adherent by skilled support from trained professionals such as counsellors or pharmacists.

Changing therapy

The principal reasons for changing antiretroviral treatment are treatment failure, toxicity, and poor adherence. There is no agreed definition for treatment failure. Patients whose viral load is not suppressed to less than 40 copies/ml within 3 months, or was initially suppressed and subsequently rises, should be considered for changing to a completely new regimen of at least three drugs. This should be guided by a resistance test (see below). Continuing viral replication in the presence of antiretroviral treatment should be avoided because of progressive accumulation of resistance mutations which can compromise future treatment options. If adherence is poor or likely to be the cause of treatment failure, changing to a combination that is simpler to take should be considered, e.g. based on once or twice daily dosage and low pill burden.

Poor absorption of protease inhibitors may sometimes cause treatment failure related to low blood levels, without development of resistance; measurement of blood levels may be useful in this context. If treatment needs to be changed because of drug toxicity (e.g. a severe rash), a single drug substitution can be made if the responsible agent is identified.

'Salvage' therapy

Salvage therapy is generally defined as treatment following exposure to multiple antiretroviral drugs. In this situation, numerous drug resistance mutations are usually present and the likelihood of achieving sustained viral suppression below the detection level is much lower than for patients who have limited or no previous antiretroviral exposure. This is especially true if drugs from all three major classes have previously been used. Studies using clinical endpoints suggest that declines in viral load correlate with improvements in clinical outcome, even if suppression to below the detection limit is not achieved. Several factors may be considered when selecting a treatment regimen in these circumstances, including the history of drug classes to which the patient has not been exposed and the results of tests for viral resistance. It may be possible to recycle some drugs with less likelihood of resistance, or to include new drugs active against resistant isolates (e.g. darunavir) or new classes of drugs (e.g. raltegravir). When initiating salvage therapy it is important to use at least two new drugs to which the patient has not been exposed in order to reduce the risk of further resistance developing.

Drug resistance

Viral resistance is a major factor in treatment failure. Resistant mutants can arise spontaneously even in the absence of antiretroviral therapy; however, the selection of drug-resistance mutants occurs rapidly when HIV replicates in the presence of subtherapeutic levels of antiretroviral drugs, and is eliminated when HIV replication is completely suppressed by a potent drug combination.

Extensive genotypic variation of HIV occurs because of very high viral turnover and transcription errors by the reverse transcriptase enzyme, so that all possible single point mutations are likely to occur over time. Although mutations causing resistance to single agents may arise before antiretroviral treatment is started, on statistical grounds it is unlikely that specific combinations of multiple mutations will be present. Control of viral replication with a highly potent treatment regimen limits the appearance of resistant HIV mutants.

Genotypic and phenotypic assays have been developed to test for drug resistance in HIV isolates. Genotypic assays that identify codon mutations correlating with *in vivo* resistance to antiretrovirals are relatively easy to perform, inexpensive, and most widely used. Phenotypic assays that measure the ability of the virus to grow in increasing concentrations of drugs are time-consuming and expensive, but provide more direct evidence of resistance to a particular drug. Resistance assays are widely used in the selection of drug regimens and investigation of treatment failure. Interpretation of resistance patterns is increasingly difficult as the number of drugs and mutations involved increases.

Resistance mutations to antiretroviral agents in newly acquired HIV, indicating transmitted drug resistance, are identified in approximately 10% of recent seroconverters in Europe. However, the presence of a mutation does not necessarily denote clinical resistance. In the absence of therapy, wild-type virus predominates and resistance mutations may be undetectable though present in small copy numbers. This can lead to treatment failures with the resistant mutants increasing as wild-type virus is eradicated by drugs. For this reason, baseline resistance testing at diagnosis is now advocated in an attempt to identify resistance mutations at the outset.

Drug toxicity and interactions

Adverse reactions to antiretroviral agents are relatively common and may lead to the patient stopping their therapy (Table 5.23.4). Minor gastrointestinal disturbances (nausea, vomiting, and diarrhoea), rashes, and headache are common, but some adverse reactions are serious. Drug interactions must be considered when prescribing antiretroviral drugs, especially in advanced HIV disease. Antiretroviral agents may interact with each other and with other drugs. For example, phenytoin drastically reduces plasma levels of efavirenz. Ritonavir, a potent inhibitor of cytochrome P450, is especially prone to raising blood levels of other drugs and should not be given with most antiarrhythmics, anxiolytics, and antihistamines. Caution is required with several analgesics, anticonvulsants, and other categories of medication.

Metabolic complications, especially mitochondrial toxicity and disturbances of lipid and glucose metabolism, have emerged as important adverse effects of antiretroviral therapy. Mitochondrial toxicity is associated with nucleoside drugs (especially didanosine and stavudine, which are now much less often prescribed) and may result in neuropathy, myopathy, pancreatitis, hepatic steatosis, hyperlactataemia, and lactic acidosis. Lactic acidosis causes nonspecific symptoms, including malaise, gastrointestinal disturbance, and liver function abnormalities, and can progress to death, particularly if antiretrovirals are not stopped. There is no evidence that routine monitoring of lactate levels is helpful. Nucleoside drugs are thought to cause mitochondrial dysfunction by inhibiting mitochondrial DNA polymerase-γ.

A syndrome of lipodystrophy (progressive loss of fat from face and limbs) and hyperlipidaemia is associated with thymidine analogue nucleoside drugs, especially stavudine, and to a lesser extent zidovudine. Truncal fat accumulation, hyperlipidaemia, and insulin resistance have been associated with protease inhibitors.

After the introduction of antiretroviral treatment, early reports suggested a possible increase in cardiovascular disease. Several variables potentially affect the risk of myocardial infarction and other cardiovascular events in patients with HIV. Uncontrolled viraemia may cause endovascular inflammation. The Data Collection on Adverse Events of Anti-HIV Drugs (DAD) study group has shown an association with antiretrovirals and cardiovascular events. The relative risk of myocardial infarction may be increased by about 10% when other factors, such as lipid levels, are taken into account. The INITIO trial has showed an increased incidence of the metabolic syndrome with antiretroviral treatment, with an associated increased risk of cardiovascular disease. The absolute risk is very small when compared to the risks associated with smoking and diabetes mellitus. Nevertheless, increasing attention is being paid to modifying cardiovascular risk factors in those on HIV therapy, such as smoking cessation programmes, treatment of hypertension, and managing hyperlipidaemia.

Recent attention has also focused on changes in bone metabolism. HIV-infected patients have an increased risk of osteoporosis and bone fractures, which are often multifactorial. Antiretroviral therapy seems to be a factor, but other contributing causes include smoking, vitamin D deficiency, elevated cytokines and systemic inflammation, low testosterone levels in males, low oestrogen

Table 5.23.4 Principal toxicities of antiretroviral drugs

Nucleoside reverse transcriptase inhibitors (NRTI)	
Class effects	GI disturbances, raised liver enzymes, hepatic steatosis, lactic acidosis
AZT	Headache, nausea (usually resolve within 2–4 weeks)
	Anaemia (avoid if anaemic at baseline)
	Macrocytosis (benign)
	Nail pigmentation
	Myopathy (rare on lower dosages 500–600 mg/day)
	Lipodystrophy with facial wasting (long-term effect, unknown incidence)
ABC	Hypersensitivity 5%; may be fatal if rechallenged (closely associated with HLA B*5701)
ddI	Pancreatitis, peripheral neuropathy
d4T	Lipodystrophy with facial wasting; peripheral neuropathy
3TC, FTC	No major toxicities
Nucleotide RTI	
Tenofovir	Renal failure (case reports, rare, incidence unknown)
Non-nucleoside RTI (NNRTI)	
Efavirenz	Neuropsychiatric disturbances (8%) – vivid dreams, impaired concentration, mood changes (usually transient, <4 weeks duration); rash
Nevirapine	Rash (20%, severe 6%); rarely Stevens–Johnson syndrome; hepatitis (esp. in women with CD4 >250/mm^3 or men with CD4 >400 / mm^3—avoid)
Protease inhibitors (PI)	
Class effects	GI disturbances; hyperlipidaemia, truncal fat accumulation, diabetes, bleeding in haemophiliacs, raised liver enzymes
Lopinavir	Diarrhoea
Ritonavir	Circumoral and peripheral parasthesiae (unusual in low dosage)
Saquinavir	Rash, peripheral neuropathy
Nelfinavir	Diarrhoea
Indinavir	Renal calculi, haemolysis
Atazanavir	Hyperbilirubinaemia, jaundice
Tipranavir	Rash (caution in sulphonamide allergy), liver dysfunction
Darunavir	Diarrhoea, rash (caution in sulphonamide allergy)
Entry inhibitors	
Fusion inhibitors	
Enfuvirtide	Injection site reactions (painful, erythematous nodules); headache, dizziness, nausea, eosinophilia
CCR5 antagonists	
Maraviroc	Cough, muscle and joint pain, diarrhoea, sleep disturbance, raised liver enzymes (and possibly hepatitis)
Integrase inhibitors	
Raltegravir	Nausea, diarrhoea, headache; raised CPK in some patients

levels in postmenopausal women, and increasing age. Patients on HIV therapy also have an increased incidence of avascular necrosis of the femoral head, which may be a consequence of vascular disease, but the mechanism involved in the development of osteoporosis is not clear.

Treatment interruptions

In general, once treatment is started it is continued indefinitely. There has been recent interest in whether interrupting treatment (in supervised or structured treatment interruptions) can be beneficial. In theory, such interruptions might enhance immune responses, reduce long-term toxicity, or reduce resistant virus by allowing repopulation with wild-type virus. A large trial (SMART) was stopped early because of a paradoxical result. The study randomized patients with stable disease on therapy to continuing therapy or to stopping (and restarting if the CD4 count fell below 250). Not only were there more HIV complications in the stopping group, but this group, surprisingly, also had a higher incidence of cardiovascular disease. It is postulated that the increased cardiovascular risk is related to endothelial inflammation secondary to uncontrolled viraemia. It is thus unlikely that treatment interruption will be a sensible management strategy and patients should be counselled about the need for long-term treatment.

Immune reconstitution inflammatory syndrome (IRIS)

Since the introduction of highly active antiretroviral therapy (HAART), there have been reports of unusual symptoms and signs appearing in patients some time after starting therapy. Because these clinical problems arise in the face of increasing CD4 counts, the syndrome has been called the immune reconstitution inflammatory syndrome (IRIS) or immune reconstitution disease (IRD). In the absence of HIV, paradoxical clinical responses have been described in tuberculosis and in leprosy. In the setting of HIV, IRIS often takes the form of an exacerbation of a previously treated opportunistic infection or an unusual clinical presentation of an opportunistic infection that was subclinical at the time HAART was started.

The incidence of IRIS is difficult to determine, particularly as there is no currently agreed definition, but it may occur in up to 20% of patients starting HAART. Usually, IRIS starts within a few months of starting HAART and is temporally related to a rise in CD4 count. A proposed definition includes (1) new or worsening symptoms of an infection or inflammation after starting antiretrovirals, (2) symptoms not explained by a new infection or the expected course of an infection previously diagnosed, and (3) a decrease in viral load by at least 1 $\log_{10}$. The pathogenesis of IRIS is poorly understood, but many patients have been found to have raised IL-6 levels, possibly related to a brisk Th-1 lymphocyte response.

The most common opportunistic infections complicated by IRIS are tuberculosis, *M. avium* (MAC) infections, pneumocystis pneumonia, cryptococcal meningitis, and cytomegalovirus. IRIS complicating tuberculosis is probably the most common problem. Patients may develop fever or lymphadenopathy or may present with pleural effusions. Bone and joint involvement also occurs. IRIS is possibly more common in those presenting with extrapulmonary tuberculosis and can be fatal in tuberculous meningitis.

IRIS may occur in those receiving treatment for MAC and in one series complicated 30% of cases. The usual problem is lymph node enlargement, which may be massive and can mimic lymphoma. Some cases are complicated by hypercalcaemia.

Cryptococcal meningitis, when complicated by IRIS, may present as an apparent relapse with fever, headache, and signs of meningeal irritation. Rapidly expanding cerebral cryptococcomas may lead to fatal increases in intracranial pressure. Cytomegalovirus infections may also be complicated by IRIS with a worsening of signs of retinitis or a more benign vitritis. Rarely, patients have presented with a uveitis some years after starting HAART.

Some of the common features in the above conditions are that affected patients often started HAART at very low CD4 counts and with very high HIV viral loads. There is no consensus on the best management of IRIS, but there is no rationale for stopping HAART and most cases are self-limiting. Steroids and nonsteroidal anti-inflammatory drugs are frequently used, but there are no trial data to provide guidance.

Children and HIV

Most paediatric infections result from the mother-to-child transmission (MTCT) of HIV, although some children may be infected by blood products or sexual abuse. The risk of MTCT is increased during advanced maternal HIV disease, by vaginal delivery, and by breastfeeding (see Mother-to-child transmission, below). Diagnosis is important during the first year of life because about 20% of HIV-infected children progress rapidly to AIDS during that time; however, a special diagnostic approach is needed before 18 months of age, because over this period uninfected children may have maternal HIV antibody. Techniques for virus detection (e.g. HIV DNA by PCR) allow confirmation of HIV infection in 95% of nonbreast-fed perinatally infected infants by 1 month of age.

The natural history is very different in resource-rich versus resource-limited countries. In the latter, HIV-infected children without antiretroviral therapy have a mortality rate of 45 to 59% at 2 years. In Europe and the United States of America, about 20% of untreated children would develop AIDS or die in infancy; by 5 years, 40% of children would have developed AIDS and 25% would have died. The most common AIDS diagnosis in infancy is pneumocystis pneumonia, typically presenting at 10 to 14 weeks of age. HIV encephalopathy is also common in untreated HIV-infected infants, with severe developmental delay occurring in about 10% and more subtle delays in an additional 40%.

In older children, clinical conditions suggestive of HIV infection include persistent oral candida, parotid swelling, and recurrent or frequent serious bacterial infections including pneumonia, meningitis, and sepsis. Failure to thrive, diarrhoea, fever, lymphadenopathy, and hepatosplenomegaly are more common in HIV-infected infants but are nonspecific and less predictive. HIV dementia and other neurological and developmental problems are associated with a poor prognosis. HIV-related lymphocytic interstitial pneumonitis (LIP) typically occurs in children and is characterized by progressive, widespread, reticulonodular shadowing on chest radiography. LIP develops insidiously and may initially be asymptomatic; chronic lung disease develops with cough, breathlessness, hypoxia, clubbing, and secondary bacterial infections, and bronchiectasis occurring in severe cases. LIP is often associated with other lymphoproliferative manifestations (such as parotitis) and relatively well-preserved immune function, and may be treated with oral prednisolone.

HIV-infected children should be managed by paediatricians with experience in HIV care, usually in specialized units. The absolute CD4 lymphocyte count is less valuable for monitoring than in adults, particularly in very young children; consequently, prophylaxis against pneumocystis is usually given regardless of the CD4 count during the first year. In older children, the principles of monitoring are similar to those in adults, using clinical status, CD4 counts, and viral load estimation by plasma HIV-1 RNA measurement. The CD4 percentage (percentage of total lymphocytes) varies less with age and is more useful than absolute CD4 counts in children under the age of 5 years.

Principles of antiretroviral treatment are similar in children and adults. Particular challenges to the effective use of HAART that are specific to children include the need to adjust drug dose as the child grows (to avoid underdosing and drug resistance), the lack of paediatric formulations suitable for infants, fewer drug choices, limited paediatric toxicity data and nonspecific presentation of drug toxicity in children, reliance of children on caregivers who themselves may have HIV and be ill, and, in adolescents, problems of adherence and coming to terms with an HIV diagnosis. An additional problem in the use of HAART in infants, where infected mothers have received single-dose nevirapine (or other antiretroviral therapy during pregnancy to reduce MTCT), is that the transmitted virus in such a setting is usually nevirapine resistant. Clinical trials are used to determine optimal antiretroviral combinations, when to start treatment, and the tolerability of the newer drugs in all the major categories. Triple and even quadruple therapy regimens are well tolerated in infants and older children and may produce sustained elevations in CD4 lymphocyte counts, but adherence is particularly difficult. As HIV-infected children grow older, the number of adolescents with perinatally acquired HIV is increasing, raising the need for advice on reducing the risk of sexual transmission.

Prevention of opportunistic infections (see Table 5.23.5)

The risk of developing an opportunistic infection rises greatly once the peripheral CD4 lymphocyte count falls consistently below 200/mm^3. It is standard practice to introduce low-dose co-trimoxazole prophylaxis for pneumocystis pneumonia at this stage. This also reduces the risk of cerebral toxoplasmosis and may prevent bacterial pneumonia. Studies in Africa, in both children and adults, have shown that co-trimoxazole prophylaxis is associated with decreased mortality.

The risk of developing active tuberculosis in HIV-positive American intravenous drug users with positive tuberculin skin tests has been shown to be about 8% per year and can be reduced by taking isoniazid for a year. In developing countries, in particular, the risk of active tuberculosis in HIV-positive individuals is high and isoniazid alone or in combination with rifampicin can reduce the risk, but there is a challenge in implementation, which includes addressing the need to exclude active TB. BCG vaccination does not appear to be protective in HIV.

Primary prophylaxis may prevent other conditions, such as CMV retinitis, cryptococcal meningitis, and histoplasmosis, but because of the relatively low incidence and lack of predictors of risk for these conditions, it is not cost-effective. Before the advent of highly active antiretroviral therapy, after treatment of an opportunistic infection the predisposition to the infection usually remained. Thus, in early studies, following an episode of pneumocystis pneumonia, patients had a 50% chance of a further episode within a year. Secondary prophylaxis with co-trimoxazole proved effective. Secondary prophylaxis for pneumocystis and other opportunistic infections, including MAC and CMV, is discontinued if there is a good response to antiretroviral treatment, with CD4 counts sustained above 200/mm^3 and low plasma levels of HIV RNA.

Simple measures, other than drugs, may reduce the risk of some infections. Avoiding undercooked eggs and poultry may reduce the risk of disseminated salmonella infection and adequate boiling of drinking water can prevent cryptosporidiosis. Stopping cigarette smoking reduces the risk of bacterial chest infections.

Prevention of HIV transmission

Sexual transmission

Sexual transmission accounts for most new cases of HIV infection. Education to alter behaviour and reduce the risk of HIV infection is a key component of HIV control programmes. Condom promotion in Thailand has made an impact on HIV transmission rates. The presence of other sexually transmitted infections, especially those causing genital ulcers, facilitates HIV transmission. Accordingly, studies in Tanzania and elsewhere have demonstrated that programmes to prevent and treat sexually transmitted infections reduce the incidence of new HIV infections. Herpes simplex virus type 2 (HSV-2) is of particular importance in facilitating HIV-1 transmission, because of its high prevalence worldwide, including developing countries. Aciclovir suppression of HSV-2 infection has been shown to reduce genital shedding of HIV-1 and plasma HIV viral load, but field studies have not demonstrated a consequent reduction in risk of HIV acquisition.

The risk of HIV transmission is related to the HIV viral load, and is reduced dramatically by antiretroviral treatment. A systematic review in 2009 showed no transmissions in over 5000 serodiscordant heterosexual couples when the index patient's viral load was less than 400 copies/ml. HIV may be detected in the semen of patients with undetectable viral load and so it should not be assumed that the risk of transmission is zero. These findings have led to a debate on the potential value of large-scale antiretroviral treatment as a strategy for controlling HIV transmission in populations with high prevalences of HIV.

The foreskin in males, rich in Langerhans cells, is an important portal of entry for HIV infection. Randomized trials in Africa have confirmed that the risk of acquiring HIV is reduced by half in circumcised men compared to uncircumcised men. Adult male circumcision, although not fully protective, may therefore be a valuable addition to HIV prevention programmes in resource-limited countries.

Large studies to assess the efficacy of vaginal microbicides in the prevention of sexually transmitted infections (STIs) and HIV have been disappointing. However, a controlled study to assess the feasibility of using antiretroviral drugs for pre-exposure prophylaxis (PrEP) of sexually acquired HIV yielded promising results using tenofovir and emtricitabine in a daily single tablet. The cost-effectiveness and appropriate use of PrEP remain to be determined.

Mother-to-child transmission

As the number of women infected with HIV increases, the problem of mother-to-child transmission (MTCT) of the virus assumes

Table 5.23.5 Prophylaxis of major opportunistic infections in HIV

Infection	Indications	Regimens		Comments
		First line	**Alternatives**	
Pneumococcal pneumonia	All HIV-positive patients	Pneumococcal vaccine	None	Clinical effectiveness unproved; antibody response greater if CD4 >350/mm^3
P. jirovecii pneumonia	CD4 <200/mm^3; or symptomatic HIV; or following PCP	Co-trimoxazole 480–960 mg daily (or 960 mg, 3 times per week)	Dapsone; dapsone with pyrimethamine; monthly nebulized pentamidine; atovaquone	May be stopped if CD4 is sustained >200/mm^3 on anti-HIV treatment
Cerebral toxoplasmosis	CD4 <100/mm^3 plus toxoplasma IgG-positive following treatment of cerebral toxoplasmosis	As above	Dapsone with pyrimethamine	Primary prophylaxis usually incidental to that for PCP prophylaxis; pentamidine not protective
		Sulfadiazine 0.5–1 g, 4 times daily with pyrimethamine 25–75 mg/day, and folinic acid; protects against *P. jirovecii* as well	Clindamycin with pyrimethamine, and folinic acid;	May be stopped if CD4 is sustained >200/mm^3 on anti-HIV treatment
Tuberculosis[a]	Tuberculin reaction >5 mm induration with no previous BCG; or high-risk exposure to tuberculosis[a]	Isoniazid 300 mg/day with pyridoxine 50 mg/day for 6–12 months	Rifampicin with isoniazid for 3 months	Rifampicin should not be given with protease inhibitors or nevirapine
M. avium complex (MAC)	CD4 <50/mm^3 following treatment of disseminated MAC	Clarithromycin 500 mg, twice daily, or azithromycin 1200 mg/week	Rifabutin; rifabutin with azithromycin	Primary prophylaxis not recommended
		Clarithromycin 500 mg, twice daily, with ethambutol 15 mg/kg per day with or without rifabutin 300 mg/day	Azithromycin with ethambutol, with or without rifabutin	May be stopped if CD4 is sustained >200/mm^3 on anti-HIV treatment
Cytomegalovirus (CMV)	CD4 <50/mm^3 and CMV antibody-positive	Valganciclovir 900 mg daily	None	Primary prophylaxis not recommended
	Following CMV retinitis or other CMV disease	Valganciclovir 900 mg daily; or ganciclovir 5–6 mg/kg IV on 5–7 days/week	Foscarnet IV; cidofovir IV; ganciclovir intraocular implant	May be stopped if CD4 is sustained >200/mm^3 on anti-HIV treatment
Cryptococcal meningitis	CD4 <50/mm^3 following treatment of cryptococcal meningitis	Fluconazole 100–200 mg/day orally	Itraconazole orally	Primary prophylaxis recommended in endemic settings
		Fluconazole 200 mg/day orally	Itraconazole orally; amphotericin B IV weekly or 3 times/week; itraconazole orally	Fluconazole superior to itraconazole for secondary prophylaxis. May be stopped if CD4 is sustained >200/mm^3 on anti-HIV treatment

IV, intravenous; PCP, pneumocystis pneumonia.

[a] In circumstances of contact with MDR-TB, specialist advice about prophylaxis should be sought.

greater importance. Currently, an estimated 1500 infants are infected by MTCT daily worldwide. In developed countries, the risk of MTCT without interventions is 15 to 30%, but 25 to 40% in sub-Saharan Africa because of population differences and breast-feeding. Without interventions, approximately one-third of peripartum MTCT occurs in late pregnancy, the remaining two-thirds during labour. Post-partum transmission through breastfeeding can double the risk of MTCT. However, in resource-limited settings where the vast majority of infected mothers live, breastfeeding for 6 months is still recommended because of the substantial nutritional and immunological benefits that accrue, and these outweigh even the increased risk of HIV infection in the infants. In resource-rich settings, the risk of MTCT is below 1% as a result of HAART administered to the mother during pregnancy and delivery by elective Caesarean section. Vaginal delivery is a safe option if the viral load is fully suppressed by HAART. Simpler, cheaper regimens have been employed widely in resource-limited settings, such as single-dose nevirapine given to the mother during labour and to the infant within the first 72 h of life. These have also been shown to be effective (50% reduction in MTCT); but not as effective as highly active antiretroviral treatment. The routine offer of HIV testing is incorporated into antenatal care in developed countries where antiretroviral treatment is available.

Blood products

Screening of blood products began as soon as testing for HIV became available, and heat treatment for factor VIII concentrate was also introduced. These measures dramatically reduced the risk of virus transmission by blood and blood products in industrialized countries. However, there may still be a problem in resource-limited countries where screening is not efficient, or where the background seroprevalence of potential donors is so high that HIV-infected blood may be screened as negative when donated by an individual in the 'window period' immediately after initial infection (see Diagnosis of HIV infection, above).

Injecting drug use

Needle exchange programmes and the prescription of controlled drugs to registered addicts may reduce the incidence of new HIV infections in injecting drug users. Major problems still exist in countries such as India and Russia, where injecting drug use is more common and education about the risk and the availability of clean needles is very limited.

Occupational exposure and postexposure prophylaxis

Based on data from more than 3000 occupational exposures to HIV, the average risk of HIV infection after needlestick injury or other percutaneous exposure was calculated to be 0.3% (about 1 in 325). The risk following mucous membrane exposure has been estimated to be around 0.1%. The risk of transmission is greatest for deep injuries; if there is visible blood on the device; during procedures involving direct cannulation of blood vessels; or if the source patient has advanced HIV disease. A small retrospective case-control study demonstrated an 80% reduction in the likelihood of seroconversion in health care workers who took zidovudine soon after percutaneous exposure to HIV. In view of the greater activity of antiretroviral drug combinations but without direct evidence, it is currently recommended that high-risk occupational exposures to HIV are treated as soon as possible with two nucleoside inhibitors and a protease inhibitor (such as zidovudine, lamivudine, and lopinavir/ritonavir) for 1 month. Nevirapine is not currently recommended in postexposure prophylaxis regimens because of a relatively high rate of adverse reactions. A careful risk assessment should be done, and if a significant risk of HIV transmission is identified antiretroviral therapy should be offered and started promptly to maximize the chance of success.

Following possible sexual exposure to HIV, antiretroviral therapy may reduce the risk of seroconversion, but there are no randomized studies to confirm this. A comparative study in men who have sex with men in Brazil reported that individuals who took antiretroviral therapy after sexual intercourse were less likely to acquire HIV infection (0.6% vs 4.2%). Unprotected receptive anal intercourse (including sexual assault) is associated with the greatest risk (estimated up to 3%). After possible sexual exposure to HIV, a risk assessment is recommended and antiretroviral therapy should be offered if a significant risk is identified. Treatment should be started as soon as possible and is unlikely to be effective if started more than 72 h after exposure.

Vaccine development

The high degree of viral variation and immune escape present difficulties for the development of an effective preventive HIV vaccine. Nonetheless, group-specific neutralizing antibodies have been identified. In particular, there is evidence that broad CD8+ T-cell responses directed against the relatively invariant, internal p24 Gag 'capsid' protein can be successful in achieving durable immune control of HIV at very low or undetectable (below 50 HIV RNA copies/ml plasma) levels. Current vaccine efforts are therefore focused principally on inducing broad CD4+ and CD8+ T-cell responses against HIV. These responses, however, would be expected to control rather than eliminate the virus altogether, and may lead to disease modification rather than complete prevention. Although a vaccine capable of inducing broadly neutralizing antibodies against the range of HIV variants would eliminate the virus, no antigen capable of doing so has been identified to date.

So far, noninfectious killed whole virus or recombinant subunit vaccines have not been successful in protecting chimpanzees from HIV infection, or macaques from SIV infection and disease. Certain live attenuated strains of SIV, with deletion mutations in *nef* and other regulatory genes, initially appeared to protect adult monkeys from challenge with virulent SIV strains, but subsequently were reported to cause AIDS in neonatal macaques.

Human testing of candidate HIV vaccines, including a vaccine made from tiny recombinant fragments of gp120, the surface glycoprotein of HIV that binds to host cell CD4 receptors, has so far not been successful. Large phase III trials in Thailand and the United States of America involving over 5000 uninfected high risk volunteers showed no protection by a vaccine using recombinant gp120 (VaxGen) that had produced good neutralizing antibodies in pilot studies.

Several new approaches are being examined, which may prove more effective in inducing protective humoral and killer T-cell-mediated immunity. These include DNA vaccines, consisting of pieces of HIV DNA incorporated into harmless plasmid DNA from bacteria, and the use of live vectors (e.g. poxviruses such as canarypox and modified vaccinia) to deliver portions of the HIV envelope. A common approach now is to use a 'prime-boost' strategy whereby a DNA vaccine dose is given, followed by a boosting with the DNA incorporated in a vector, such as modified vaccinia. One of the most potent vaccines uses a replication-incompetent adenovirus type 5 as the vector. However, a phase IIb efficacy trial (STEP/HVTN 502) using the adenovirus type 5 vector with *gag*, *pol*, and *nef* genes was stopped prematurely. Not only was no efficacy shown, but there was evidence that those already immune to human adenovirus from natural infection were more likely to become infected by HIV. The reasons for this are not clear, but the National Institutes of Health (NIH) has stopped or paused other trials using adenovirus vectors as a result. Trials with canarypox and other vectors continue.

This approach, using DNA vaccines to stimulate CD8+ responses, is also being evaluated for therapeutic vaccination in HIV-positive patients with suppressed viraemia who are being treated with antiretroviral agents, to determine if vaccination will allow interruption of treatment without loss of virological control. Effective vaccination is likely to hold the greatest promise for controlling HIV infection in the future, but experience to date would indicate that researchers face a formidable challenge.

Further reading

Abdool Karim SS, Naidoo K, Grobler A, *et al.* (2010). Timing of initiation of antiretroviral drugs during tuberculosis therapy. *N Engl J Med*, **362**, 697–706.

Altfeld M, Goulder P (2007). 'Unleashed' natural killers hinder HIV. *Nat Genet*, **39**, 708–10.

Bartlett JG, Gallant JE (2006). *Medical Management of HIV infection*. Johns Hopkins Medicine, Health Publishing Business Group, Baltimore.

Fisher M, *et al.* (2006). UK guideline for the use of post-exposure prophylaxis for HIV following sexual exposure. *Int J STD AIDS*, **17**, 81–92.

Friis-Møller N, *et al.* (2003). Cardiovascular disease risk factors for HIV patients—association with antiretroviral therapy. Results from the Data Collection on Adverse Events of Anti-HIV Drugs (DAD) study. *AIDS*, **17**, 1179–93.

Goulder P, Watkins D (2004). HIV and SIV CTL escape: implications for vaccine design. *Nat Rev Immunol*, **4**, 630–40.

He W, *et al.* (2008). Duffy antigen receptor for chemokines mediates trans-infection of HIV-1 from red blood cells to target cells and affects HIV-AIDS susceptibility. *Cell Host Microbe*, **4**, 52–62.

Johnston MI, Fauci AS (2008). An HIV vaccine—challenges and prospects. *N Eng J Med*, **359**, 888–890.

McMichael AJ (2006). HIV vaccines. *Ann Rev Immunol*, **24**, 227–255.

Prendergast A, *et al.* (2007). International perspectives, progress, and future challenges of paediatric HIV infection. *Lancet*, **370**, 68–80.

Robertson J, *et al.* (2006). Immune reconstitution syndrome in HIV: validating a case definition and identifying clinical predictors in persons initiating antiretroviral therapy. *Clin Infect Dis*, **42**, 1639–46.

The Strategies for Management of Antiretroviral Therapy (SMART) Study Group. (2006). CD4+ count–guided interruption of antiretroviral treatment. *N Eng J Med*, **355**, 2283–96.

Online resources

Joint United Nations Programme on HIV/AIDS. *2008 Report on the Global AIDS Epidemic.* http://www.unaids.org/en/KnowledgeCentre/HIVData/GlobalReport/2008/2008_Global_Report.asp

Joint United Nations Programme on HIV/AIDS. *UNAIDS, Uniting the world against AIDS.* http://www.unaids.org

NAM. *Aidsmap.* http://www.aidsmap.com [UK national guidelines (British HIV Association, regularly updated).]

University of California (San Francisco). *HIV InSite Gateway.* http://hivinsite.ucsf.edu/ [University of California Center for HIV Information.]

US Department of Health and Human Services (DHHS). *AIDSinfo.* http://www.hivatis.org [United States of America HIV Treatment Guidelines Library; regularly updated.]

graphically-restricted opportunistic pathogens, e.g. *Leishmania* and *Penicillium marneffei.*

Diagnosis and management—diagnosis of HIV-related disease may be difficult where there is limited access to laboratory diagnostics, and presumptive therapy based on the most likely aetiologies is often necessary. Antiretroviral therapy (ART) is increasingly available using clinical eligibility criteria, standardized drug regimens, and simpler monitoring.

Prognosis—the underlying natural history of HIV infection in the developing world is little different from that in industrialized nations, but survival with advanced HIV disease is short if there is no access to ART or interventions to prevent and treat HIV-related infections.

Prevention—this requires political commitment to create an environment that supports education about HIV, and prevents stigma and discrimination. Some countries have implemented successful control programmes and have seen declining HIV prevalence, but the goal of preventing HIV transmission remains elusive in many settings. Trial results showing high efficacy of ART in preventing transmission between discordant couples has led to renewed optimism; work is ongoing to explore how these results should be translated into policy and practice. Prevention interventions for general populations should include information and education; promotion of partner reduction and of condoms, which are highly protective against sexual transmission if used correctly and consistently; and encouragement of universal knowledge of HIV serostatus. Targeted interventions should be focused on groups and situations in which HIV transmission is most intense, guided by local epidemiology. Male circumcision has a protective efficacy of almost 60% against heterosexual acquisition of HIV infection in men, but other methods of prevention must still be promoted among circumcised men. No vaccine is available.

5.24 HIV in the developing world

Alison D. Grant and Kevin M. De Cock

Essentials

The developing world is disproportionately affected by the HIV pandemic. In many countries in sub-Saharan Africa, HIV infection is established in the general population: in southern Africa, which is particularly severely affected, HIV prevalence among pregnant women reached around 40% by 2003 in some areas. Local epidemiology depends on the relative contribution of the three major routes of HIV transmission: sexual contact (heterosexual and homosexual); mother to child; and exposure to blood or blood products. The main route of transmission is sex between men and women.

Clinical features—these vary by geographical region, reflecting increased exposure in developing countries to common pathogens such as tuberculosis, nontyphoid salmonellae, and *Streptococcus pneumoniae* throughout the course of HIV infection. People with advanced immunosuppression are also at risk of disease due to geo-

Epidemiology

At the end of 2010, the Joint United Nations Programme on HIV/AIDS (UNAIDS) and the World Health Organization (WHO) estimated that 34 million people were living with HIV infection worldwide (Chapter 5.23). This global pandemic comprises a mosaic of local epidemics, each with its own characteristics. Variation, both between regions and between groups of individuals affected within one region, is one of the pandemic's striking features. Broadly, there are two patterns: generalized epidemics, established in the general population in most countries in sub-Saharan Africa; and concentrated epidemics, in specific populations in most other regions.

Local epidemiology depends on the relative contribution of the three major routes of HIV transmission: sexual contact (heterosexual and homosexual); mother-to-child; and exposure to blood or blood products. Within sub-Saharan Africa, there have been substantial regional differences in the evolution of the epidemic. The main route of transmission is sex between men and women, although recent studies have shown that in some cities, sex between men is more important than previously realized. In West Africa, where the HIV epidemic was recognized from the mid 1980s, the highest prevalence among women attending antenatal clinics was in Abidjan, Côte d'Ivoire, peaking at around 14% in 1999 and subsequently falling to around 10% in 2002. By contrast, in southern Africa, where HIV prevalence was very low until the 1990s, HIV prevalence among pregnant women in some areas reached around 40% by 2003.

The reasons for these regional differences are not clearly understood. In a study comparing countries with high (Zambia and Kenya) and lower (Benin and Cameroon) prevalences, the main behavioural differences in cities with high prevalence were young age of sexual debut in women, young age at first marriage, and a large age difference between spouses. The main biological risk factors were herpes simplex virus type 2 (HSV-2) infection, trichomoniasis in women, and lack of male circumcision.

Global HIV incidence probably peaked in the late 1990s, and in 2010 was estimated at 2.7 million new cases (1.9 million in sub-Saharan Africa). The reduction in HIV incidence, in some countries, is attributed to a range of reasons including maturation of the epidemic, successful prevention campaigns, and behaviour change. HIV prevalence among young people has fallen in many, but not all, high-prevalence countries, reflecting this reduction in HIV incidence. In South Africa, the country with the highest number of HIV-infected people, the national prevalence of HIV infection among women aged 20 to 24 in 2008 was 21.1% compared with 5.1% among men of the same age, implying very high HIV incidence among young women. Since the turn of the 21st century, the global prevalence of HIV has stabilized, in many places, reflecting high incidence balanced by high mortality. In 2010, global deaths due to HIV were estimated at 1.8 million, and in sub-Saharan Africa at about 1.2 million; these have fallen since 2006, as ART coverage has increased. As ART becomes more widely used, the prevalence of HIV infection will rise as treatment prolongs survival. Prevention of new infections remains the key to controlling the epidemic. Understanding the local epidemiology is essential to guide prevention and control efforts.

Prevention

Prevention of HIV infection requires political commitment to creating an environment that supports education about HIV, and prevents stigma and discrimination. Everyone should know about prevention, but efforts must be focused on groups and situations in which HIV transmission is most intense, guided by local epidemiology. Involvement of civil society and those living with HIV is especially important, as is emphasis on 'positive prevention' to ensure that people with HIV benefit from interventions and support to prevent transmission to others.

Sexual transmission

A traditional approach has been that of 'ABC', standing for Abstinence, Being faithful, and using Condoms if neither abstinent nor monogamous. While abstinence is an appropriate strategy for the youngest age group, there is no evidence that promoting abstinence is effective as a broader strategy. Reduction in the number of sexual partners, and avoidance of concordant different partnerships and intergenerational sex are important. Correct and consistent use of condoms is highly protective against acquiring HIV infection, but is difficult to sustain in long-term relationships. HIV-infected people who are aware of their HIV status tend to alter their behaviour to prevent transmission to others. A randomized trial of imme-

diate ART for the HIV-infected partner in discordant couples, where the HIV-infected partner had a CD4 count of 350 to 550/mm³ (thus not fulfilling usual criteria for ART), found a 96% reduction in HIV transmission to the HIV-negative partner. Studies are in progress to explore the feasibility of earlier ART initiation as a prevention strategy at population level. Tenofovir-based ART prevented HIV acquisition among HIV-negative men having sex with men, in discordant couples and young heterosexuals, but not in early results from two studies among African women; adherence seems an important determinant of efficacy. A tenofovir-based vaginal microbicide provided 39% protection from HIV acquisition in one study using a pericoital dosing schedule, but another study of tenofovir vaginal gel, with daily dosing, was stopped early for lack of efficacy. Further studies, including other antiretroviral agents and sustained-release delivery systems, are in progress. Clinical trials of herpes suppressive therapy have failed to show reductions in HIV acquisition or transmission.

Male circumcision has a protective efficacy of almost 60% against heterosexual acquisition of HIV infection in men, but it affords only partial protection and other methods of prevention must still be promoted among circumcised men. Male circumcision could have considerable public health impact in southern Africa and, to a lesser extent, in East Africa, but cultural difficulties, logistical challenges, and health system weaknesses pose practical obstacles to its implementation.

For commercial sex workers and their clients, correct and consistent condom use and prompt diagnosis and treatment of other sexually transmitted infections must be promoted. Important interventions for men who have sex with men include voluntary HIV counselling and testing, correct and consistent condom use, and addressing drug use that may lead to unsafe behaviour. The quest continues for an effective HIV vaccine.

Transmission by injecting drug use

The public health approach emphasizes harm reduction. Essentials include information and education, access to HIV testing and counselling, sterile needle and syringe programmes, interventions to assure safe disposal of contaminated injection equipment, treatment for drug dependence including opioid substitution, and interventions to prevent sexual transmission of HIV.

Blood transfusion and nosocomial transmission

Although eliminated in the industrialized world, transmission of HIV by blood transfusion remains a possibility in many countries. Basic measures to prevent transfusion-transmitted HIV include appropriate management of conditions predisposing to the need for transfusion (such as childbirth and malaria), and avoidance of all but essential transfusions. Family and paid donors should be avoided in favour of regular, low risk donors. All blood destined for transfusion should be screened for HIV, and, as far as possible, obtained from centralized services that can assure safe blood.

Preventive measures against nosocomial transmission include universal precautions, which treat all body fluids as potentially infectious, not to be handled without gloves. Infection-prone procedures may require other protection such as masks, gowns, and goggles. Injection safety requires absolute avoidance of re-use of needles and syringes, and assurance of their safe use and disposal. Health care institutions require policies and availability of postexposure antiretroviral prophylaxis following occupational exposure.

Mother to child transmission

In industrialized countries, combination ART for pregnant women, elective caesarean section, and avoidance of breastfeeding have rendered perinatal HIV transmission rare. An integrated approach in developing countries requires primary prevention of HIV infection in girls and young women, prevention of unintended pregnancy in HIV-infected women, interventions to prevent transmission of HIV from infected women to their offspring, and diagnosis and care of infants and their mothers.

Health care workers should recommend HIV testing and counselling to all pregnant women. Pregnant women requiring ART for their own health should receive standard therapy, but avoid starting efavirenz during the first trimester because of possible teratogenicity. WHO recommendations for pregnant women in low and middle income countries are shown in Table 5.24.1.

All women should receive information and support about infant feeding. National programmes in low and middle income countries should decide whether to advise mothers to breastfeed in combination with antiretroviral interventions, or to advise replacement feeding, aiming to maximize HIV-free survival among infants. Where breastfeeding is advised, this should be exclusive breastfeeding for the first 6 months, with introduction of complementary food thereafter; breastfeeding should continue to 12 months, with gradual weaning over 1 month.

Clinical features

Acute HIV disease

Symptoms associated with seroconversion, which is rarely specifically diagnosed, are described in Chapter 5.23. In a study of women in Kenya, the most common symptoms reported by seroconverters were fever, headache, fatigue, and arthralgia, whereas the clinical features most strongly associated with seroconversion were lymphadenopathy, vomiting, diarrhoea, fever, and myalgia.

Progression from HIV infection to symptomatic disease

Contrary to early assumptions, data from representative cohorts with well-defined dates of seroconversion show that the progression of HIV disease from seroconversion to the stage of advanced immunosuppression in developing countries is little different from that observed in the pre-ART era in industrialized countries. Once people reach the stage of advanced immunosuppression, survival is likely to be shorter than in industrialized countries if they do not have access to ART and interventions to prevent and treat opportunistic infections.

People with early HIV disease in developing countries frequently experience symptoms suggestive of more advanced immunosuppression such as weight loss, chronic fever or diarrhoea, and severe bacterial infections, which may give the impression of rapid HIV disease progression. However, such symptoms are also common among individuals without HIV infection, and thus are more likely to be explained by a high background morbidity in the community.

Symptomatic HIV disease

HIV-infected people suffer much higher incidence of diseases caused by pathogens common in developing countries, such as tuberculosis, pneumococcal disease, and nontyphoid salmonella,

Table 5.24.1 WHO recommendations for antiretroviral therapy for pregnant women

Women needing antiretroviral treatment for their own health	
Mother	
Preferred	Zidovudine plus lamivudine plus nevirapine or efavirenz[a]
Alternative	Tenofovir plus lamivudine (or emtricitabine) plus nevirapine or efavirenz[a]
Infant	
Irrespective of mode of infant feeding	Nevirapine (daily) or zidovudine (twice daily) until 4 to 6 weeks of age
Women who do not yet require antiretroviral therapy for their own health **Option A: maternal AZT**	
Mother	
Antepartum	Zidovudine daily starting from as early as 14 weeks of gestation and continued during pregnancy
Onset of labour	Single-dose nevirapine; initiation of zidovudine plus lamivudine[b]
During labour and delivery	Zidovudine plus lamivudine[b]
Postpartum	Zidovudine/lamivudine × 7 days[b]
Infant	
Breastfeeding	Nevirapine daily for minimum 4 to 6 weeks, and until 1 week after all exposure to breast milk has ended
Nonbreastfeeding	Nevirapine (daily), or single-dose nevirapine plus zidovudine (twice daily), from birth until 4 to 6 weeks of age
Option B: maternal triple antiretroviral therapy prophylaxis	
Mother	From 14 weeks gestation until one week after all exposure to breast milk has ended: ◆ Zidovudine plus lamivudine plus lopinavir/ritonavir OR ◆ Zidovudine plus lamivudine plus abacavir OR ◆ Zidovudine plus lamivudine plus efavirenz[a] OR ◆ Tenofovir plus lamivudine (or emtricitabine) plus efavirenz[a]
Infant	
Irrespective of mode of infant feeding	Nevirapine (daily) or zidovudine (twice daily) from birth until 4 to 6 weeks of age
Nonbreastfeeding	Zidovudine or nevirapine for 6 weeks

[a] Avoid starting efavirenz in the first trimester of pregnancy: use nevirapine.
[b] Single-dose nevirapine and zidovudine/lamivudine intrapartum and postpartum may be omitted if mother receives more than 4 weeks of zidovudine during pregnancy.

than those uninfected with HIV. Tuberculosis is often the first manifestation of HIV disease, although by the time they present with tuberculosis about half the patients will already have a CD4 count below 200/mm^3. Other early presenting symptoms of HIV disease are skin conditions such as generalized pruriginous dermatitis and herpes zoster, both of which have a high positive predictive value for underlying HIV infection among populations with high HIV prevalence.

Advanced HIV disease

When HIV-infected people reach the stage of advanced immuno-suppression, the spectrum of disease varies by geographical region. Tuberculosis, bacterial infections due to pathogens such as *Streptococcus pneumoniae* and nontyphoid salmonella sp., and cryptococcal disease are common worldwide, whereas the risk of some other opportunistic infections depends on the risk of exposure, which differs by geographical region. Penicilliosis, caused by *Penicillium marneffei*, is largely confined to South-East Asia and southern China (Chapter 7.7). Pneumocystis pneumonia is relatively common in Asia and South Africa, but in many countries in sub-Saharan Africa, it is less common as a cause of severe respiratory symptoms than bacterial infections and tuberculosis. Diseases characteristic of very advanced immunosuppression such as those due to cytomegalovirus and *Mycobacterium avium intracellulare* have been rare in many developing countries, probably because survival with advanced disease in the absence of ART is short. This could change with increasing ART coverage, particularly if ART prevents death but does not fully restore immunocompetence.

Tuberculosis (Chapter 6.25)

Tuberculosis is the most important cause of HIV-related severe morbidity and mortality in developing countries. It results both from reactivation of latent infection as well as rapid progression following new or re-infection. Molecular epidemiological studies show that new infections are an important mechanism of recurrence, which is common in HIV-infected people.

The diagnosis of tuberculosis is more challenging in developing countries. The changing clinical presentation of tuberculosis with advancing immunosuppression is described in Chapter 5.23. HIV-infected people are more likely to have atypical clinical presentations and to have smear-negative tuberculosis, making the diagnosis harder to confirm, particularly where the main diagnostic test is sputum microscopy. This is a particular problem for those with advanced immunosuppression, among whom a delay in initiating tuberculosis treatment may be fatal. Sputum culture has higher sensitivity than microscopy, particularly if liquid culture media are used, but in many developing countries facilities for mycobacterial culture are very limited. Current initiatives are improving microscopy-based tuberculosis diagnosis and are making culture-based diagnosis more widely available. An automated, nucleic acid amplification-based assay (Xpert MTB/RIF) holds promise for rapid diagnosis both of tuberculosis and of rifampicin resistance, with potential as a near-patient assay. It is recommended by WHO for people with suspected HIV-associated tuberculosis, but logistical barriers and cost currently limit its use in resource-constrained settings (see Chapter 6.25).

A particular challenge is posed by drug-resistant tuberculosis. Extensively drug-resistant tuberculosis (XDR-TB) (defined as resistance to at least rifampicin, isoniazid, any quinolone, and one of the injectable agents amikacin, capreomycin, or kanamycin) has been identified in every world region. The susceptibility of HIV-infected people to drug-resistant tuberculosis was highlighted by a survey in rural South Africa in 2005 to 2006. All those with XDR-TB who were tested had HIV infection, and almost all died rapidly after diagnosis. Those with XDR-TB included health care workers, raising concerns about nosocomial transmission. This problem is made worse by the paucity of facilities for drug susceptibility testing in most countries that carry the highest burden of tuberculosis, making interruption of transmission or rapid appropriate treatment challenging. This emphasizes the urgent need for stronger tuberculosis programmes, better diagnostic tests for drug resistance, improved detection and treatment of people with resistant tuberculosis, and better infection control in health facilities to prevent nosocomial transmission to both patients and staff.

Everyone with newly diagnosed HIV infection should be screened for tuberculosis. Those who do not have active tuberculosis may benefit from isoniazid preventive therapy (see Chapter 6.25). ART reduces the risk of a new tuberculosis episode, although the risk remains high, particularly among those with low CD4 counts. Those with newly diagnosed tuberculosis should be recommended testing for HIV infection because in some places more than 70% will also have HIV infection. Patients with HIV-associated tuberculosis should receive co-trimoxazole prophylaxis. For patients whose HIV infection is diagnosed at the time of a tuberculosis episode, WHO guidelines recommend that tuberculosis treatment should be started first, followed by ART as soon as possible afterwards, regardless of the CD4 count. Randomized controlled trials suggest that people with newly diagnosed HIV-associated tuberculosis and CD4 less than 50 cells/mm^3 are most likely to benefit from early initiation of ART, shortly after initiation of tuberculosis treatment. Among individuals with tuberculous meningitis, data from one trial showed no survival benefit from immediate vs deferred ART, and further data are needed to determine the optimum timing of ART initiation for these patients.

Interaction between HIV infection and 'tropical' diseases

Malaria (Chapter 8.2)

In areas of year-round (stable or holoendemic) malarial transmission, studies from Uganda and Malawi suggest that HIV infection impairs acquired immunity to falciparum malaria, resulting in increased frequency of malarial parasitaemia and clinical malaria among adults and older children proportional to the degree of immunosuppression, but no increase in severe or complicated malaria. However, HIV-infected infants in a holoendemic area of Kenya were at increased risk of severe anaemia and hospitalization for malaria. In studies from South Africa of nonimmune adults and older children resident in areas of intermittent (low or unstable) malaria transmission, HIV was associated with an increased risk of severe and fatal falciparum malaria, inversely proportional to their CD4 counts. In HIV-infected pregnant women, the beneficial effects of parity on severity of malaria are attenuated, and their peripheral and placental parasitaemia, and risk of suffering an episode of malaria or anaemia during pregnancy are increased. Malaria-HIV coinfection is associated with an increased risk of low birth weight, preterm birth, intrauterine growth retardation, and postnatal infant mortality. Malaria transiently increases peripheral blood and placental HIV viral load, but whether this affects the risk of vertical transmission of HIV infection or accelerates HIV disease progression is unknown. ART and co-trimoxazole reduce the risk of febrile malarial episodes; HIV-infected patients in malaria endemic areas should sleep under insecticide-treated bed nets; and nonimmune people travelling to malarial areas should use bednets and antimalarial chemoprophylaxis. Pregnant women who are not taking continuous co-trimoxazole should receive at least three doses of intermittent preventive therapy. In malaria-endemic areas, those on co-trimoxazole prophylaxis who develop fever should be investigated for causes other than malaria rather than being treated presumptively for malaria. They should not be given pyrimethamine with sulfadoxine as malaria treatment. ART may interact with antimalarial drugs (see http://www.hiv-druginteractions.org).

Leishmaniasis (Chapter 8.12)

The HIV epidemic has led to localized increases in visceral leishmaniasis, predominantly in people with CD4 counts below 200/mm^3, particularly among injecting drug users around the Mediterranean; in the north-east of Africa (Ethiopia and Sudan); Brazil; and India. In those with HIV infection, visceral leishmaniasis most often presents classically with fever, hepatosplenomegaly, and pancytopenia, although presentations range from asymptomatic to multiorgan involvement. The treatment of choice is liposomal amphotericin B. Amphotericin B deoxycholate or sodium stibogluconate are less satisfactory. Without secondary prophylaxis, relapse after treatment is almost inevitable until the CD4 count has risen on ART.

Cutaneous leishmaniasis may present with atypical skin lesions, which may be disseminated and may recur after treatment.

Trypanosomiasis (Chapters 8.10–8.11)

Asymptomatic infection with Chagas' disease (*Trypanosoma cruzi*) may be reactivated by HIV-related immunosuppression, most often resulting in meningoencephalitis or cerebral mass lesions. Myocarditis is common at autopsy, although rarely apparent clinically. There is no evidence of an interaction between human African trypanosomiasis and HIV infection, although reports suggest high mortality among HIV-infected patients treated for central nervous system disease.

Helminths

There is little evidence of interaction between intestinal nematodes and HIV infection; the expected association with *Strongyloides stercoralis* hyperinfection has not been observed, although it is common with another retroviral infection, human T-lymphotropic virus (HTLV-1) (Chapter 9.4). HIV infection does not affect the management of onchocerciasis, although skin disease may be more severe. Higher prevalence of *Wuchereria bancrofti* infection in HIV-infected than uninfected people has been reported. Schistosomiasis does not appear to be more common or more severe in HIV-infected people, although genital schistosomiasis in women is associated with HIV infection and could be a risk factor for HIV transmission. Atypical forms of neurocysticercosis, such as giant brain cyst and spinal epidural lesions, are reported.

Fungi

Penicilliosis (Chapter 7.7) is a common opportunistic infection among those with advanced immunosuppression in South East Asia and China. Paracoccidioidomycosis (*Paracoccidioides brasiliensis* infection—Chapter 7.4) is the most common invasive fungal infection in South America, but reports of coinfection with HIV are uncommon.

There is no evidence of important interactions between HIV infection and typhoid fever, melioidosis, amoebiasis, or giardiasis. Leprosy may be unmasked by ART as an immune reconstitution phenomenon.

Clinical staging of HIV disease

Given limited laboratory facilities in many developing countries, HIV viral load estimation and CD4 counts are often not available. A system designed to estimate HIV disease stage based on clinical symptoms, modified by CD4 count if available, was published by WHO in 1990 and revised in 2006 (Table 5.24.2). This is widely used in developing country settings to guide when to start interventions such as preventive therapy with co-trimoxazole and ART.

Diagnosis and testing

Serological tests for HIV infection first became available in 1985, the driving force for their development being concern to assure the safety of blood for transfusion. From early on, because of concerns about discrimination, there was a strong commitment to ensure HIV testing was only conducted with informed consent after pre- and post-test counselling and with assured confidentiality (voluntary counselling and testing, VCT), unlike the approach to diagnostic testing for other communicable diseases. Compulsory testing was not thought to bring public health benefit and was strongly discouraged. VCT emphasized discussion with a counsellor about the desirability of being tested, the implications of positive or negative results, advice about disclosure, etc. An important incentive for VCT was to avoid people at risk donating blood primarily to discover their HIV serostatus. As HIV treatment has improved, VCT has become more popular and services, especially in Africa, have increased substantially, facilitated by the advent of simple rapid tests. If the initial test is positive, confirmatory testing using a test based on a different antigen and/or platform is important to minimize false positive results.

As HIV treatment programmes began to be introduced, VCT was recognized to be poorly adapted to the needs of clinical medicine, and patients were going undiagnosed. WHO and UNAIDS introduced the concept of provider-initiated HIV testing and counselling, where health care providers recommend HIV testing to patients. Pretest information is provided and patients have the right to decline, ensuring that the test is voluntary. Results must be returned with post-test counselling, and patients must be linked

Table 5.24.2 WHO clinical staging system

WHO clinical stage	HIV-associated symptoms	Examples of defining conditions
1	Asymptomatic	Asymptomatic Persistent generalized lymphadenopathy
2	Mild symptoms	Recurrent respiratory tract infections Herpes zoster Seborrhoeic dermatitis
3	Advanced symptoms	Unexplained severe (>10%) weight loss Persistent oral candidiasis Pulmonary tuberculosis Severe bacterial infections
4	Severe symptoms	HIV wasting syndrome Extrapulmonary tuberculosis Recurrent severe bacterial pneumonia Kaposi's sarcoma

to appropriate services. To distinguish it from provider-initiated testing, VCT is now also referred to as client-initiated HIV testing and counselling. Table 5.24.3 shows the indications for provider-initiated HIV testing and counselling according to different epidemic situations.

HIV testing is also conducted for surveillance. In low and middle income countries, blood collected for syphilis testing from pregnant women attending antenatal services is most often used. To ensure completeness of testing, identifiers from the specimens are removed and the blood is tested for HIV anonymously (unlinked anonymous testing).

Treatment, care, and prevention of HIV-related disease

Prior to 2000, ART was considered too expensive and too complex to be made widely available in developing countries. Supported by unprecedented funding from initiatives such as the Global Fund to Fight AIDS, Tuberculosis and Malaria, and the United States President's Emergency Plan for AIDS Relief, the number of people receiving ART in low and middle income countries has increased from around 240 000 in 2001 to 6.6 million by the end of 2010. Despite this success, more needs to be done to make ART available to all of the estimated 14.2 million people in need of it.

The approach to ART delivery in developing countries takes a public health rather than an individualized approach. The aim is to maximize the survival of all HIV-infected people in the population by using ART regimens which are standardized rather than tailored to the individual; by simplifying management so that HIV care can be undertaken by health care workers where there are few doctors; and using clinical and basic laboratory monitoring so that ART can be delivered even if CD4 counts and HIV viral load measurements cannot be done. The current WHO guidelines for adults and adolescents (2010) for starting ART are summarized in Table 5.24.4; additionally, ART is recommended for all people (irrespective of CD4 count) with HIV and active tuberculosis or hepatitis B requiring treatment.

The recommended first line regimen for HIV-1 infections comprises two nucleoside reverse transcriptase inhibitors (NRTIs) and one non-nucleoside reverse transcriptase inhibitor (NNRTI). For

Table 5.24.3 WHO recommendations for provider-initiated counselling and testing

Type of HIV epidemic	HIV testing and counselling recommended to:
All	All patients with signs, symptoms, or conditions which could indicate HIV infection, including tuberculosis Children born to HIV-infected women Men seeking male circumcision for HIV prevention
Generalized	All patients presenting to health facilities, regardless of the reason for presentation. Priorities may include: medical wards and outpatient facilities, antenatal, childbirth, and postpartum health services, sexually transmitted infection services
Low level or concentrated	Prioritize symptomatic and perinatally-exposed people, as above. Consider for: Sexually transmitted infection services Most-at-risk populations Maternal health services

Table 5.24.4 WHO guidelines on when to start antiretroviral therapy in adults and adolescents

WHO clinical stage	Action
1 or 2	Treat if CD4 350/mm³ or below
3 or 4	Treat irrespective of CD4 count

HIV-2 infections, NNRTIs are ineffective, and a boosted protease inhibitor-based regimen would be the preferred first line regimen. Second line therapy is based on a boosted protease inhibitor in combination with two previously unused NRTIs.

Immune reconstitution inflammatory syndrome (IRIS; see also Chapter 5.23), either paradoxical worsening of an existing HIV-associated disease, or unmasking of a previously undiagnosed disease after the start of ART, occurs in about 16% patients, and is associated with a low baseline CD4 count, and (for paradoxical IRIS) with earlier ART initiation. Case fatality for patients with IRIS is relatively low (4.5% overall) but appears higher (around 21%) in patients with cryptococcal meningitis, and in these patients ART initiation should be deferred until there is evidence of a response to antifungal therapy (usually 2 to 6 weeks, depending on the antifungal regimen used (see Chapter 5.23).

In addition to the provision of ART, much can be done to prevent illness among HIV-infected people. Co-trimoxazole prophylaxis reduces morbidity and mortality among HIV-infected children and symptomatic adults. WHO guidelines recommend, in the absence of CD4 counts, starting co-trimoxazole prophylaxis for those with symptomatic HIV disease (WHO stage 2, 3, or 4), or, if CD4 counts are available, at any WHO stage if the CD4 count is below 350/mm³, or for WHO stage 3 or 4, irrespective of the CD4 count. Where health infrastructure is limited, co-trimoxazole may be offered to everyone with HIV infection, regardless of their CD4 count or clinical disease stage. People with HIV should be screened for symptoms of active tuberculosis (cough, fever, weight loss, night sweats) at each clinical encounter, and those who do not have active tuberculosis should be offered a course of isoniazid preventive therapy. Where cryptococcal disease is common, screening for cryptococcal antigen followed by pre-emptive antifungal treatment if cryptococcal antigen positive may be considered prior to ART for people with CD4 less than 100/mm³. Interventions to prevent malaria should be offered. Appropriate vaccines may include those against hepatitis B, pneumococcal disease, and influenza. Nutritional support should be provided for the malnourished. To reduce infective diarrhoea, household-based water treatment methods are recommended, along with proper disposal of faeces and hand washing with soap.

The WHO document 'Priority interventions: HIV/AIDS prevention, treatment and care in the health sector' brings together recommendations relevant to HIV care in resource limited settings and is available on the WHO website (details in the reading list).

Further reading

Corbett EL, *et al.* (2006). Tuberculosis in sub-Saharan Africa: opportunities, challenges, and change in the era of antiretroviral treatment. *Lancet*, **367**, 926–37.

Friedland G, Churchyard GJ, Nardell E (2007). Tuberculosis and HIV infection: current state of knowledge and research priorities. *J Infect Dis*, **196** Suppl 1, S1–S3.

Joint United Nations Programme on HIV/AIDS. *UNAIDS epidemic update.* http://data.unaids.org/pub/Report/2009/JC1700_Epi_Update_2009_en.pdf

Karp LC, Auwaerter PG (2007). Coinfection with HIV and tropical infectious diseases. I. Protozoal pathogens. *Clin Infect Dis*, **45**, 1208–13.

Karp CL, Auwaerter PG. (2007). Coinfection with HIV and tropical infectious diseases. II. Helminthic, fungal, bacterial, and viral pathogens. *Clin Infect Dis*, **45**, 1214–20.

Mermin J, *et al.* (2005). Developing an evidence-based, preventive care package for persons with HIV in Africa. *Trop Med Int Health*, **10**, 961–970.

Muller M, *et al.* (2010). Immune reconstitution inflammatory syndrome in patients starting antiretroviral therapy for HIV infection: a systematic review and meta-analysis. *Lancet Infect Dis*, **10**, 251–61.

Sanders EJ, *et al.* (2007). HIV-1 infection in high risk men who have sex with men in Mombasa, Kenya. *AIDS*, **21**, 2513–20.

Slutsker L, Marston BJ (2007). HIV and malaria: interactions and implications. *Curr Opin Infect Dis*, **20**, 3–10.

Todd J, *et al.* (2007). Time from HIV seroconversion to death: a collaborative analysis of eight studies in six low and middle-income countries before highly active antiretroviral therapy. *AIDS*, **21** Suppl 6, S55–S63.

World Health Organization. (2008) *Essential prevention and care interventions for adults and adolescents living with HIV in resource-limited settings.* http://www.who.int/hiv/pub/prev_care/OMS_EPP_AFF_en.pdf

World Health Organization. (2009) *Priority interventions: HIV/AIDS prevention, treatment and care in the health sector.* http://www.who.int/hiv/pub/priority_interventions_web.pdf

World Health Organization (2010). *Antiretroviral therapy for HIV infection in adults and adolescents. Recommendations for a public health approach. 2010 revision.* http://whqlibdoc.who.int/publications/2010/9789241599764_eng.pdf

World Health Organization (2011). *Guidelines for intensified tuberculosis case-finding and isoniazid preventive therapy for people living with HIV in resource-constrained settings.* http://whqlibdoc.who.int/publications/2011/9789241500708_eng.pdf.

5.25 HTLV-1, HTLV-2, and associated diseases

Kristien Verdonck and Eduardo Gotuzzo

Essentials

Human T-lymphotropic virus (HTLV)-1 and HTLV-2 belong to the genus *Deltaretrovirus* of the family *Retroviridae*. They only infect humans, produce a lifelong infection, and can be transmitted from mother to child, through sexual intercourse, and via cellular blood components. Both viruses are present in all continents. The highest HTLV-1 prevalence in the general population (10%) has been found in southern Japan. There are endemic foci of HTLV-2 among native Amerindians and Central African pygmy tribes. HTLV-2 is also frequent among injecting drug users. It is unclear why some infected people develop associated diseases while others remain asymptomatic.

Clinical features—(1) HTLV-1—up to 10% of carriers develop clinical manifestations, including adult T-cell leukaemia/lymphoma, HTLV-associated myelopathy/tropical spastic paraparesis, and infectious diseases such as strongyloidiasis, scabies, and tuberculosis. (2) HTLV-2—causes a milder form of HTLV-associated myelopathy/tropical spastic paraparesis and pulmonary disorders, arthritis, bronchitis, and pneumonia.

Diagnosis and prevention—HTLV enzyme immunosorbent assays and particle agglutination tests are used for screening, followed by confirmatory testing of positive results. Mother-to-child transmission of HTLV-1 can be reduced by avoiding breastfeeding; condom use protects against sexually transmitted infection; screening of blood donors is performed in many countries. No vaccine is available and there are no effective antiviral drugs.

Historical perspective

In 1979, human T-lymphotropic virus 1 (HTLV-1) was isolated from a patient with a T-cell malignancy. In the years that followed, several syndromes, previously considered idiopathic, were linked to this virus: adult T-cell leukaemia/lymphoma (ATL), tropical spastic paraparesis, uveitis, and infective dermatitis. Originally, tropical spastic paraparesis had been attributed to malaria by Strachan in Jamaica in 1897, but was named Jamaican neuropathy by Cruickshank in the 1950s. HTLV-2 was discovered in 1982, and HTLV-3 and HTLV-4 in 2005. It is not yet known whether HTLV-3 and -4 cause human disease.

Pathogenesis

The genomes of HTLV-1 and HTLV-2 consist of RNA, which, during infection, is transcribed to DNA and inserted into the DNA of human lymphocytes. HTLV-1 shows tropism for CD4 and HTLV-2 for CD8 lymphocytes. Three molecules (glucose transporter 1, neuropilin-1, and heparan sulfate proteoglycans) are involved in HTLV-1 binding and entry. HTLV-1 can spread between T cells via a tight and organized cell-cell contact (virological synapse). During chronic infection, HTLV-1 mainly propagates via mitosis of infected lymphocytes (clonal expansion).

A viral protein, Tax, regulates the expression of viral genes and interferes with host cell gene expression, resulting in spontaneous proliferation of infected lymphocytes among other phenomena. The effects of Tax on cells include potent nuclear factor-kappa B (NF-κB) activation, cell cycle perturbation, and cell transformation. In HTLV-1 infection, the effects of Tax can lead to ATL. It is now thought that another viral regulatory protein, the antisense coded HTLV-1 basic leucine zipper (HBZ), also plays a crucial role in leukemogenesis by HTLV-1.

The proviral load (the proportion of peripheral blood mononuclear cells carrying integrated HTLV provirus) remains relatively stable in any given subject, but varies between subjects. A high HTLV-1 proviral load is related to the risk of human T-lymphotropic virus associated myelopathy (HAM)/tropical spastic paraparesis (TSP), and perhaps also of ATL.

HTLV infection is a necessary but insufficient condition for the development of associated diseases. Other viral, host genetic and environmental factors contribute to the risk of disease. The risk of

HAM/TSP in HTLV-1 carriers is influenced by the viral subgroup, the rate of HTLV-1 expression, and the efficiency of the cytotoxic lymphocyte response (CTL) against the virus. FoxP3+CD4+ T cells are abnormally frequent in HTLV-1 infection. These cells reduce the CTL lysis of HTLV-1-infected cells and could codetermine the outcome of HTLV-1 infection. There are no vaccines and no effective antiviral drugs against HTLV-1 and HTLV-2.

Epidemiology

The origin of HTLV is in Africa. Several HTLV-1 and HTLV-2 subtypes have spread to the rest of the world, in ancient and more recent times. It has been estimated that 20 million people are infected with HTLV-1 worldwide and that the number of HTLV-2-infected people also amounts to several millions. However, the prevalence estimates are usually based on serological screening of blood donors, pregnant women, and other selected population groups and should be interpreted with caution. New studies of the general population are needed to re-evaluate the global burden of HTLV infection.

The highest HTLV-1 prevalence (>10% of the general population) is found in southern Japan. Countries with a moderate prevalence (1–10%) include Papua New Guinea and the Solomon Islands in Oceania; Guinea-Bissau, Togo, Gabon, and Cameroon in Central Africa; Jamaica, Haiti, and Martinique in the Caribbean; and Guyana, French Guyana, and Peru in South America. In Brazil, Mozambique, Iran, Romania, and Taiwan, the prevalence is 0.1 to 1%. The infection is uncommon in Western Europe and the United States of America.

For HTLV-2, there are two endemic foci: among native Americans (prevalence 1–58%) and Central African pygmy tribes (prevalence up to 14%). The virus is also frequent among injecting drug users (IDU) in all continents (prevalence up to 20%).

In endemic populations, the prevalence of HTLV-1 and HTLV-2 tends to increase with age and is higher in women than in men. Other risk factors include prolonged breastfeeding, unsafe sexual practice, blood transfusion, and drug abuse.

There are six molecular subtypes of HTLV-1 and four of HTLV-2 connected with specific populations and geographical locations, but they have little or no influence on disease outcome.

Diagnosis of infection

HTLV enzyme immunosorbent assays are available for screening. In samples with a positive result, confirmatory testing with western blot, line immunoassay, immunofluorescence, and/or polymerase chain reaction (PCR) is recommended to eliminate false-positive reactions and to discriminate between HTLV-1 and HTLV-2.

Prevention

HTLV-1 mother-to-child transmission can be reduced from 15 to 25% to less than 5% by avoiding breastfeeding.

The incidence of sexual transmission among stable partners is about 1 per 100 person-years for HTLV-1 and -2. Condom use protects against infection.

Transfusion of HTLV-1-contaminated cellular blood components leads to infection in more than 40% of recipients. In many countries, candidate blood donors are screened for HTLV.

HTLV-1 disease outcomes

The lifetime risk for HTLV-1 carriers to develop ATL is 1 to 5% (see Table 5.25.1). HAM/TSP occurs in 0.3 to 4%, and for HTLV-1-associated diseases in general, the risk is estimated in 10%.

Adult T-cell leukaemia/lymphoma (ATL)

ATL is an aggressive malignancy of HTLV-1-infected CD4 lymphocytes. Clinical features include lymphadenopathy, hepatosplenomegaly, skin lesions, and opportunistic infections. Hypercalcaemia and lytic bone lesions are found in up to 70% of

Table 5.25.1 HTLV-1 and HTLV-2 disease outcomes and main clinical features

HTLV-1	
Malignant disease	
ATL	Lymphadenopathy, hepatosplenomegaly, skin lesions, opportunistic infections, hypercalcaemia. Poor prognosis. Affects more men than women, mostly adults
Inflammatory syndromes	
HAM/TSP	Weakness of the legs with signs of pyramidal tract involvement (hyperreflexia, clonus, spasticity, Babinski's sign), loss of vibration sense, pain, urinary problems, constipation, and sexual disorders. Progressive disease. Affects more women than men; mostly adults
Uveitis	Blurred vision with floaters, iritis, vitreous opacities, retinal vasculitis, uni- or bilateral. Intermediate uveitis in >50% of cases. Sometimes preceded by an episode of thyroiditis. Resolves spontaneously, but more rapidly with corticosteroids. Relapse is frequent. Affects more women than men; mostly adults, sometimes children
Arthritis	Resembles rheumatoid arthritis
Infectious complications	
Strongyloidiasis	Disseminated, life-threatening strongyloidiasis can develop. Relapse after treatment is common
Infective dermatitis	Generalized papular rash, with exudates and crusting on scalp, ear, eyelid margins, paranasal skin, neck, axilla, and groin. Watery nasal discharge, lymphadenopathy. Chronic syndrome; good response to antibiotics but frequent relapse. The syndrome has an inflammatory as well as an infectious component. Affects usually young children
Scabies	Severe forms can occur, with extensive, crusted lesions, located mainly in pressure areas
Tuberculosis	Increased risk of active tuberculosis. Specific clinical features remain to be clarified
Bronchiectasis	Reported among indigenous people in Central Australia. High mortality. Linked to recurrent respiratory tract infections
HTLV-2	
HAM/TSP	Similar symptoms as in HTLV-1, but milder and more slowly progressive disease
Acute bronchitis and pneumonia	Specific clinical features remain to be clarified
Arthritis	

ATL, adult T-cell leukaemia/lymphoma; HAM/TSP, HTLV-associated myelopathy/tropical spastic paraparesis.

patients. Peripheral blood smears may show lymphoid cells with basophilic cytoplasm and convoluted nuclei ('flower cells').

HTLV-1-induced ATL is classified as acute, lymphoma-type, chronic, and smouldering, based on total lymphocyte count, presence of abnormal lymphocytes in peripheral blood, calcium and lactate dehydrogenase levels, and lymphadenopathy.

The median survival time after diagnosis of acute ATL is 6 months. Chronic and smouldering forms have a better prognosis, but can evolve to acute ATL.

Allogenic haematopoietic stem cell transplantation, intensive chemotherapy, and antiviral therapy (combination of interferon-α with zidovudine) have been evaluated for the treatment of ATL. In most reports, the median survival remained less than 1 year despite treatment.

HTLV-associated myelopathy/tropical spastic paraparesis (HAM/TSP)

HAM/TSP is a chronic, debilitating condition characterized clinically by spastic weakness of the legs (Fig. 5.25.1), back pain, bladder problems, sensory signs and symptoms, constipation, and/or sexual dysfunction. The main pathological feature is an inflammation of the white and grey matter of the spinal cord. Cerebrospinal fluid examination may show mild lymphocytosis and protein increase.

The diagnosis of HAM/TSP requires demonstration of HTLV-1 and exclusion of other causes of myelopathy, such as spinal cord compression, vitamin B_{12} and folate deficiency, multiple sclerosis, amyotrophic lateral sclerosis, and lathyrism.

Several treatment strategies have been proposed, including corticosteroids, interferon-α, interferon-β-1a, reverse transcriptase inhibitors (e.g. zidovudine, lamivudine, and tenofovir), histone deacetylase inhibiton (valproate), NF-κB inhibition, fucoidan, ciclosporin, and monoclonal antibodies to CD25 or interleukin-15. There are reports of good response to zidovudine and lamivudine in combination with corticosteroids in patients with rapidly progressive disease. However, only two of these treatment strategies (interferon-α and zidovudine and lamivudine) have been tested in randomized controlled studies. They showed no satisfactory effect on symptoms or proviral load.

Infective dermatitis

Infective dermatitis is a chronic, relapsing disease that affects mostly children. Clinical characteristics include a papular rash, with exudates and crusting, mainly on the scalp, but also on the ears, eyelid margins, paranasal skin, neck, axilla, and groin (Figs. 5.25.2, 5.25.3). Watery nasal discharge and crusting of the nostrils are frequent. Clinical and histopathological images may resemble atopic dermatitis. The response to corticosteroids and antibiotics is generally good, but relapses are frequent after withdrawal of treatment. Case reports suggest that HTLV-1-infected children with infective dermatitis have an increased risk to develop HAM/TSP and ATL.

Other diseases

An increasing body of evidence shows that symptoms and signs suggestive of neurological disease are frequent among HTLV-1-infected people, also among those who do not have a formal diagnosis of HAM/TSP. Arthropathy, uveitis, dry eye syndrome,

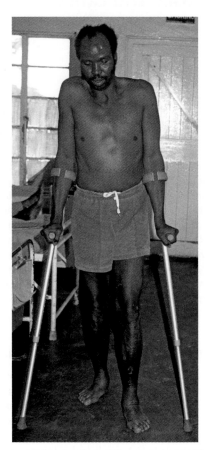

Fig. 5.25.1 Spastic paraplegia in a South African patient with HTLV-1 infection. (Copyright D A Warrell.)

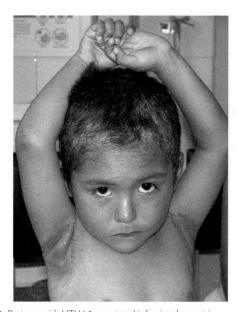

Fig. 5.25.2 Patients with HTLV-1-associated infective dermatitis.
The child has a papular rash on the forehead, crusting on the scalp, and lesions in the armpits.
(Courtesy of Dr Francisco Bravo, Institute of Tropical Medicine Alexander von Humboldt, Lima, Peru.)

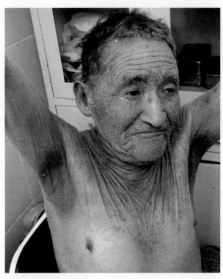

Fig. 5.25.3 Patient with HTLV-1-associated infective dermatitis. This disease can affect adults, although it mostly occurs in children. Typical characteristics are crusting on the scalp and lesions on the eyelid margins, in the neck and in the armpits. (Courtesy of Dr Francisco Bravo, Institute of Tropical Medicine Alexander von Humboldt, Lima, Peru.)

thyroiditis polymyositis, and alveolitis are other inflammatory conditions linked to HTLV-1. Carriers of HTLV-1 are also at increased risk of infectious complications, notably invasive strongyloidiasis (superinfection) (Chapter 9.4), scabies, tuberculosis, and perhaps also leprosy, onychomycosis, paracoccidioidomycosis, periodontal disease, and bronchiectasis. These infectious complications of HTLV-1 appear to be associated with far more morbidity and mortality than was previously appreciated. When HTLV-1 carriers live in an overcrowded and contaminated environment with inadequate sanitation, they are more likely to suffer severe infectious outcomes. This has been reported among Aboriginal people of central Australia and is likely to occur in other HTLV-1-endemic areas as well.

HTLV-2 disease outcomes (see Table 5.25.1)

HTLV-2 is less pathogenic than HTLV-1, but has been linked with HAM/TSP, arthritis, pneumonia, and bronchitis. A prospective study of HTLV-2-infected candidate blood donors in the United States of America found a twofold increase in mortality compared to uninfected control subjects.

Likely future developments

Developments in the near future will probably include the following:

- Treatment trials for HAM/TSP and ATL
- Clearer picture of HTLV-1, -2, -3, and -4 epidemiology and disease outcomes
- Better understanding of pathogenesis of associated diseases (role of viral, genetic, and environmental factors)
- Availability of surrogate markers in addition to proviral load

- Better understanding of interaction with HIV
- Research into vaccines and antiretroviral therapy

Further reading

Bangham CR, *et al.* (2009). The immune control of HTLV-1 infection: selection forces and dynamics. *Front Biosci*, **14**, 2889–903.

Biswas HH, *et al.*; HTLV Outcomes Study (2010). Increased all-cause and cancer mortality in HTLV-II infection. *J Acquir Immune Defic Syndr*, **54**, 290–6.

De Castro-Costa CM, *et al.* (2006). Proposal for diagnostic criteria of tropical spastic paraparesis/HTLV-I-associated myelopathy (TSP/HAM). *AIDS Res Hum Retroviruses*, **22**, 931–5.

Hlela C, *et al.* (2009). The prevalence of human T-cell lymphotropic virus type 1 in the general population is unknown. *AIDS Rev*, **11**, 205–14.

Martin F, Taylor GP. Prospects for the management of human T-cell lymphotropic virus type 1-associated myelopathy (2011). *AIDS Rev*, **13**, 161–70.

Roucoux DF, Murphy EL (2004). The epidemiology and disease outcomes of human T-lymphotropic virus type II. *AIDS Rev*, **6**, 144–54.

Tsukasaki K, *et al.* (2009). Definition, prognostic factors, treatment, and response criteria of adult T-cell leukemia-lymphoma: a proposal from an international consensus meeting. *J Clin Oncol*, **27**, 453–9.

Verdonck K, *et al.* (2007). Human T-lymphotropic virus 1: recent knowledge about an ancient infection. *Lancet Infect Dis*, **7**, 266–81.

5.26 Viruses and cancer

R.A. Weiss

Essentials

Viruses are important in cancer for three main reasons: (1) As a cause of cancer—about 15% of the worldwide cancer burden is due to viruses: retroviruses can activate cellular oncogenes (2) In understanding of the biology of cancer—through the discovery and characterization of oncogenes and tumour-suppressor genes. (3) In the treatment of cancer—some viruses selectively replicate in and destroy proliferating cells; viruses as foreign antigens may aid the recognition of cancer cells by the host's immune system ('xenogenization'), and viruses can also be used as vectors for immunization and for gene therapy. Viral cancers are prevented by early screening for tumours, screening for the virus in order to prevent transmission, and immunization as in the cases of hepatitis B virus (HBV) and human papilloma virus (HPV).

Viruses as aetiological agents of cancer

Oncogenic viruses establish persistent infections, which usually occur decades before malignancy. Table 5.26.1 lists the viruses implicated in human cancer. In most but not all cases, the viral genome is present in the malignant cells; the exceptions appear to be those that promote cancer indirectly, such as HIV and hepatitis C virus (HCV). Table 5.26.1 also lists the diseases associated with oncogenic viruses that are not malignancies.

Table 5.26.1 Viruses implicated in human cancer

Virus	Malignancy	Nonmalignant disease
DNA viruses		
HPV-16, 18	Cervical cancer	
HPV-5, -8	Skin cancer	Warts
HBV	Primary liver cancer	Hepatitis
MCPyV	Merkel cell skin cancer	
	Burkitt's lymphoma	
	Immunoblastic lymphoma	
	Hodgkin's disease	
	Leiomyosarcoma	
EBV	Nasopharyngeal carcinoma	Infectious mononucleosis
KSHV	Kaposi's sarcoma	
	Primary effusion lymphoma	
	Castleman's disease	
Retroviruses		
HTLV-1	Adult T-cell leukaemia	Tropical spastic paraparesis
HIV-1	Non-Hodgkin's lymphoma	AIDS
	Kaposi's sarcoma	
RNA virus		
HCV	Primary liver cancer	Hepatitis

EBV, Epstein–Barr virus; HBV, hepatitis B virus; HCV, hepatitis C virus; HPV, human papillomavirus; HTLV, human T-lymphotropic virus; MCPyV, Merkel cell polyomavirus

Cancer is usually a rare outcome of virus infection, and other cofactors play a part in viral carcinogenesis. For example, Epstein–Barr virus (EBV) is a ubiquitous infection, yet childhood Burkitt's lymphoma occurs only in areas of holoendemic malarial infection, whereas undifferentiated nasopharyngeal carcinoma occurs mainly in southern Chinese populations. Aflatoxin acts synergistically with hepatitis B virus (HBV) to induce liver cancer, and in hereditary epidermodysplasia verruciformis the ultraviolet radiation acts with human papilloma virus strains (HPV-5 and HPV-8) to cause skin cancer. The underlying cause of all forms of Kaposi's sarcoma (KS) is human herpes virus 8 (HHV-8 or KSHV), which also causes primary effusion lymphoma and plasmablastic multicentric Castleman's disease. KS occurs much more frequently in immunodeficient patients. Its relative risk in recipients of organ transplants is about 400, and in persons with AIDS about 20 000.

Oncogenic viruses belong to many virus families with different routes of transmission. HBV is frequently acquired perinatally or through subsequent exposure to blood. Human T-cell lymphotropic virus type 1 (HTLV-1) is transmitted vertically through infected cells in breast milk. Sexual transmission is common to HIV, HTLV-1 (with a male to female bias), HBV, and HPV. Oncogenic viruses do not appear to be transmitted by the respiratory route or via arthropod vectors, except for some veterinary cases, e.g. bovine leucosis virus. Whereas EBV (transmitted through saliva) occurs worldwide, HBV, HTLV-1, and HHV-8 have a higher prevalence in those population groups in which the associated cancers occur.

Certain common human viruses are highly oncogenic in experimental animals but are not linked epidemiologically to human cancer, namely the polyomaviruses BK and JC, and the adenoviruses types 2 and 12. There are claims that a simian relative of BK virus, simian vacuolating virus 40 (SV40), is linked with mesothelioma, osteosarcoma, and ependymoma in humans, but these findings remain controversial. In 2008, a novel human polyomavirus, MCPyV, was linked to Merkel skin cell cancer. In 1996 a retrovirus related to murine leukaemia virus (XMRV), was detected in the certain human prostate cancers, but there is also a large literature on 'false alarms' of human retroviruses and this turned out to be one of them.

Mechanisms of viral carcinogenesis

Physical and chemical carcinogens are usually mutagens. They cause DNA mutations in specific genes that contribute to the eventual malignant phenotype of the cancer. Oncogenes were first discovered in animal retroviruses, such as the Rous sarcoma virus of chickens, and are now known to originate from cellular genes. Most retroviruses do not carry oncogenes, but the DNA provirus integrates into chromosomal DNA and can activate adjacent cellular oncogenes. Oncogene activation by retroviruses is comparable to activation by chromosomal translocation.

The mechanism of cell transformation by HTLV-1 is different from that of the majority of animal retroviruses. HTLV-1 encodes a viral protein, Tax, which is essential to promote full viral gene transcription. Tax acts as a transcriptional activator, by associating with host nuclear proteins which activate expression of the viral genome. However, Tax also up-regulates certain cellular genes such as the interleukin-2 receptor. HTLV-1 'immortalizes' CD4+ T lymphocytes in culture, rather as EBV 'immortalizes' B lymphocytes, but this is only one step in the pathway to malignancy.

Cell transformation by DNA viruses is best understood for polyomaviruses and adenoviruses. The transforming genes of these viruses are expressed early in the infection cycle and prevent tumour suppressor protein function. Adenovirus proteins E1A and E1B and BK virus T antigen bind to p53 and retinoblastoma (Rb) proteins and block their normal interaction in the cell cycle. Thus, instead of mutating these cellular tumour suppressor genes, DNA tumour viruses block the normal function of their proteins, which similarly results in unregulated cell proliferation. The KSHV genome carries several oncogenes, including a homologue of *cyclin D2* (*CCND2*), which inactivates Rb by a different mechanism, phosphorylation.

Most oncogenic viruses persist in the tumour cells, often by integrating into chromosomal DNA. Oncogenic herpesviruses do not integrate but are maintained episomally. Epstein–Barr virus-associated nuclear antigen 1 (EBNA-1) is required for episomal replication of EBV (and latency-associated nuclear antigen (LANA) for KSHV), while other nuclear and latent membrane proteins are responsible for the transformed cell phenotype. With HBV, integrated copies are found in many liver carcinoma lines, but a requirement for integration has not been unequivocally shown. HBV expresses transactivating functions from the *X* gene, so its transformation may resemble that of HTLV-1.

Indirect carcinogenic effects are those in which damage to tissues by viruses may allow clones of premalignant cells to proliferate that would not otherwise do so. HCV and possibly HBV do this by destroying normal liver cells, resulting in a much greater rate of liver cell regeneration. HIV promotes tumour development by destroying helper T-cell immunity to other oncogenic viruses.

The cancers which occur more frequently in AIDS are also seen in immunosuppressed transplant patients, e.g. non-Hodgkin's lymphoma and Kaposi's sarcoma, and have a viral aetiology.

Treatment and prevention

Oncogenesis is multifactorial, requiring several sequential events before a patient presents with a fully malignant tumour. Yet, if a virus plays a crucial role in oncogenesis, its elimination should prevent that type of cancer. Currently, there is no special approach to the treatment of cancers that have a viral aetiology. Among the lymphoid malignancies, some respond well to radiotherapy or chemotherapy, such as Hodgkin's disease, whereas others seldom show remission, such as adult T-cell leukaemia (ATL). Cancers that express viral antigens should be responsive to immunotherapy. For tumours in which viral proteins are required for the maintenance of the malignant state, those proteins are potential molecular targets, as drugs that block them might spare normal cellular functions.

Prevention is preferable to cure, and offers the greatest promise of reducing cancer mortality due to viruses. Prevention can be accomplished by three strategies: (1) early screening for tumours, (2) screening for the virus with prevention of transmission, and (3) immunization. Early screening is exemplified by cervical smears. Screening to prevent iatrogenic transmission via blood and blood products is routinely employed in many countries for potentially oncogenic viruses such as HBV, HCV, HIV, and HTLV-1. In Kyushu, Japan, where infection was endemic, HTLV-1 is being steadily eradicated through a policy of antenatal screening to prevent transmission via mothers' milk.

Prevention of cancer by immunization against infection by oncogenic viruses is likely to have a major impact on world cancer mortality in the 21st century. The HBV vaccine is based on surface antigen and two HPV vaccines protective against cervical cancer were licensed in 2006. Intensive research is also being undertaken on vaccines for HIV and HCV, but there are immense obstacles to successful immunization against HIV as the virus is extraordinarily variable. Nevertheless, immunization against oncogenic viruses is becoming a most effective cancer prevention strategy.

Viruses as therapeutic agents

Viruses may be put to use in the fight against cancer. First, some cytopathic viruses preferentially replicate in proliferating cells and destroy them, such as parvoviruses and mutant adenoviruses. Second, viruses as foreign antigens may aid the recognition of cancer cells by the host's immune system. Although the mechanism is ill understood, 'xenogenization' of tumour cells by virus infection can, in some cases, enhance immune attack against noninfected cells in the same tumour. Third, viruses are used as vectors for immunization and for gene therapy, by restoring tumour suppressor functions, by enhancing immune responses through the expression of antigens or cytokines, and by locally delivering genes for enzymes that convert inert prodrugs into active, chemotherapeutic agents.

Further reading

Astbury K, Turner MJ (2009). Human papillomavirus vaccination in the prevention of cervical neoplasia. *Int J Gynecol Cancer*, **19**, 1610–13.

Boshoff CH, Weiss RA (2002). AIDS-related malignancies. *Nature Cancer Rev*, **2**, 373–82.

Feng H, *et al.* (2008). Clonal integration of a polyomavirus in human Merkel cell carcinoma. *Science*, **319**, 1096–100.

Plymoth A, Viviani S, Hainaut P (2009). Control of hepatocellular carcinoma through hepatitis B vaccination in areas of high endemicity: perspectives for global liver cancer prevention. *Cancer Letters*, **286**, 15–21.

Voisset C, Weiss RA, Griffiths D (2008). Human RNA rumor viruses: the search for novel human retroviruses in chronic disease. *Microbiol Mol Biol Rev*, **72**, 157–96.

Weiss RA, Vogt PK (2011). 100 years of Rous sarcoma virus. *J Exp Med*, **208**, 2351–5.

Zur Hausen H (2009). Papillomaviruses in the causation of human cancers. *Virology*, **384**, 260–65.

5.27 Orf

David A. Warrell

Essentials

Orf ('ecthyma contagiosum') is caused by an epitheliotropic parapox DNA virus of sheep and goats that is able to subdue the host's immune response. It is an occupational zoonosis of people working with these animals. A painful papule/pustule develops, usually on a finger, the site of contact with lesions on the animal's muzzle. Systemic effects are unusual, but include local lymphadenopathy, fever, erythema multiforme, and other generalized rashes. Spontaneous resolution within 6 weeks is usual. Multiple, giant lesions may develop in the immunosuppressed. Topical cidofovir is effective in severe cases.

Aetiology

Orf virus, a member of the *Parapox* genus of the Chordopoxvirinae subfamily, causes 'scabby mouth' (ecthyma contagiosum, contagious pustular dermatitis), a debilitating disease of sheep and goats. Orf virions are ovoid (approximately 260×160 nm), with a characteristic basketweave pattern visible by negatively stained and transmission electron microscopy. Other parapoxviruses infect cattle (pseudocowpox; bovine papular stomatitis virus, BPSV), camels, seals, and reindeer. Full genome sequences of orf and BPSV have been published. The orf virus genome is double-stranded DNA of 135 kbp, encoding a polypeptide homologous to interleukin 10 (IL-10), inhibitors of interferon, interleukin 2 (IL-2), and granulocyte-macrophage colony-stimulating factor (GM-CSF), and a vascular endothelial growth factor. These contribute to the dermal lesions characterized by capillary proliferation and dilatation.

Epidemiology

Orf has been recognized for more than 200 years as a disease of mainly young lambs and kids, which contract the infection from one another, or possibly from persistence of the virus in the pastures where the virus can remain viable for long periods in dried scabs from lesions. Human disease is an occupational zoonosis, following contact with infected sheep. Since orf is familiar to veterinarians, shepherds, farmers, abattoir workers, and butchers and is generally self-limiting, it often goes unreported. In the United Kingdom it is known to be prevalent in sheep farming communities in Wales. Outbreaks are associated with the end of the lambing season and with Islamic religious festivals associated with animal sacrifice. Transmission is by direct contact with the animals' lesions and possibly with fomites. Human to human spread has not been recorded. Infection confers only partial immunity, so that repeated milder attacks are possible.

Immunopathology

Orf virus infects skin keratinocytes and excites a brisk immune response locally and in lymphoid tissue, involving CD4+ and CD8+ cells, interferon, and antibody. However, orf virus genome encodes a variety of virulence and immunomodulatory factors that subvert or suppress the host's immune response, allowing viral replication. These include viral IL-10, interferon resistance protein, chemokine binding protein, GM-CSF, vascular endothelial growth factor, and heparin binding protein. In vaccinology, orf is proving a promising viral vector for delivering pathogen antigens to the immune system, and inactivated virus is immunoenhancing.

Clinical features

In sheep and goats, papules and vesicles appear on the muzzle or nostrils (Fig. 5.27.1) and gradually heal without scarring over 4 to 8 weeks, although more persistent infections may occur. In humans, after an incubation period of 2 to 6 days, a painful, small, red, firm papule enlarges to form a flat-topped haemorrhagic pustule or bulla with prominent margin and an eroded, crusted centre, sometimes surrounded by pustular satellite lesions (Fig. 5.27.2). The lesion is usually 1 to 3 cm in diameter, but may be as large as 5 cm. They are usually solitary or few in number and commonly occur on the extensor surface of a finger or hand, but also on the palm, forearm, and occasionally the face or scalp. The surrounding skin may be reddened, sometimes diffusely, and erysipelas-like lesions have been described. Lymphangitis or regional lymphadenopathy is not uncommon. Giant, multiple, fungating granulomatous or tumour-like lesions have been reported, usually in immunocompromised patients with haematological malignancies or undergoing transplan-

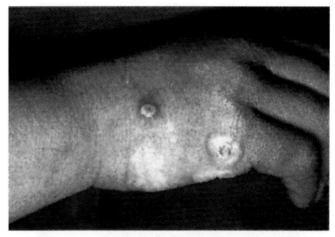

Fig. 5.27.2 Typical lesions of orf on a farmer's hand.

tation. Patients with atopic eczema may develop widespread eruptions. Slight fever and malaise can occur. Complications include secondary infection, generalized vesicular rashes, usually classified as erythema multiforme, in as many as one-third of cases (Fig. 5.27.3), which develop typically 10 to 14 days after the initial lesion,

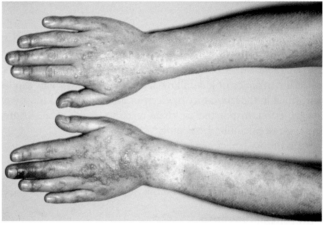

(a)

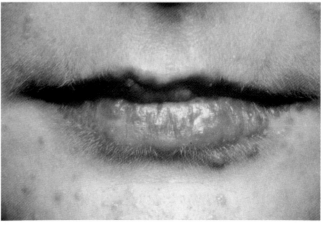

(b)

Fig. 5.27.3 Generalized vesicular eruption 'erythema multiforme' complicating orf of the left middle finger in a veterinary student: (a) arms, (b) mouth.

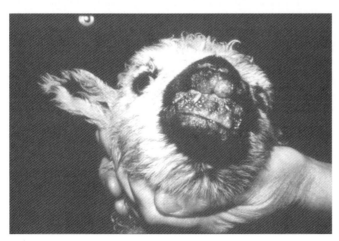

Fig. 5.27.1 Contagious pustular dermatitis ('orf') in a lamb.

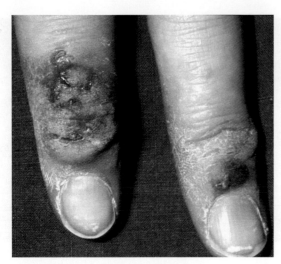

Fig. 5.27.4 Herpetic whitlows on adjacent fingers.
(Courtesy of the late Dr B E Juel-Jensen.)

and other generalized rashes. An autoimmune bullous disease, previously designated as bullous pemphigoid, has been reported. A lesion on the precanthal skin resulted in follicular conjunctivitis. Spontaneous recovery without residual scarring is usually complete within 6 weeks.

Diagnosis

The characteristic lesion in someone exposed to sheep or goats, especially to lambs or kids, allows a clinical diagnosis. This can be confirmed in the laboratory by electron microscopy of a biopsy of the orf lesion, by polymerase chain reaction (PCR), viral culture, and fluorescent antibody staining.

Skin biopsy specimens show distinctive histopathological changes. There is hyperkeratosis with cellular swelling, balloon degeneration and vacuolation in the upper epidermis, and the presence of eosinophilic B type intracytoplasmic inclusion bodies.

Differential diagnosis

In those at occupational risk of orf, differential diagnoses include milkers' nodules, caused by another parapox virus, and cowpox (Chapter 5.4), an orthopoxvirus. Whitlows (felons), including herpetic whitlow (Fig. 5.27.4), impetigo, pyogenic granuloma, cutaneous anthrax, and tumours might also cause confusion.

Treatment

Secondary infection should be treated if it occurs. Large lesions can be removed surgically, but recurrence can occur in the immunocompromised. Cidofovir (topically or intravenously) and imiquimod (topically) have been used successfully to treat giant or persistent lesions, especially in immunosuppressed patients.

Prevention

Live attenuated virus vaccines have been used to protect sheep and goats from orf. Farmers should avoid handling animals with obvious lesions.

Further reading

Al-Salam S, *et al.* (2008). Ecthyma contagiosum (orf)—report of a human case from the United Arab Emirates and review of the literature. *J Cutan Pathol*, **35**, 603–7.

Gill MJ, *et al.* (1990). Human orf. *Arch Dermatol*, **126**, 356–8.

Groves RW, Wilson-Jones E, MacDonald DM (1991). Human orf and milkers' nodule: a clinicopathologic study. *J Am Acad Dermatol*, **25**, 706–11.

Haig DM (2006). Orf virus infection and host immunity. *Curr Opin Infect Dis*, **19**, 127–31.

Torfason EG, Gunadóttir S (2002). Polymerase chain reaction for laboratory diagnosis of orf virus infections. *J Clin Virol*, **24**, 79–84.

5.28 Molluscum contagiosum

David A. Warrell

Essentials

Molluscum contagiosum is caused by a Molluscipox DNA virus which infects keratinocytes of the epidermal stratum spinosum, producing distinctive small umbilicated papules on the skin. Its genome encodes a variety of proteins that suppress the host's immune response. In children it is spread by skin contact, producing few or many lesions, while in sexually active adults it causes anogenital lesions. Molluscum is self-limiting within a few years in the immunocompetent, but those with preexisting atopic eczema and immunosuppression, notably AIDS, commonly develop persistent diffuse eruptions with larger papules. Lesions can be removed mechanically or chemically. More severe infections can be treated with imiquimod or cidofovir.

Aetiology

Molluscum contagiosum (MCV), first described clinically in the early 19th century, is caused by a virus of the genus Molluscipox. This enormous (200–300 nm long), brick-shaped, double-stranded DNA virus, is a member of the Chordopoxvirinae subfamily of the Poxviridae. It multiplies in the cytoplasm of keratinocytes of the deep epidermal stratum spinosum. MCV shares unique genomic features with parapoxviruses such as orf (Chapter 5.27), including a GC-rich nucleotide composition, three orthologous genes, and a paucity of nucleotide metabolism genes. Restriction endonuclease analysis of the genome has identified four types, MCV-1, MCV-1a, MCV-2, and MCV-3. MCV-1 causes most childhood infections while MCV-2 is transmitted sexually in older people. Like orf virus, MCV encodes several proteins that suppress host immunity. MC54L is a human (IL-18) binding protein homologue. MC148 antagonizes CC chemokine receptor 8. MC013L promotes viral replication by inhibiting the differentiation of infected keratinocytes. MC159L causes abnormal proliferation of epithelium by inhibiting tumour necrosis factor (TNF) and apoptosis-inducing factors. MC80R, an MHC class I homologue, interferes with the presentation of MCV peptides. Glutathione peroxidase protects infected cells from oxidative damage by peroxides.

MCV has not been transmitted to laboratory animals and no *in vitro* cultivation system is available. It has been grown in human prepuce grafted to athymic mice.

Epidemiology

Molluscum contagiosum has a worldwide incidence of 2 to 8%. It also affects animals: chimpanzees, kangaroos, dogs, horses, and birds. In tropical climates, it is more common in younger children (1–4 years), and in temperate climates, in older school-age children (10–12 years). The prevalence in American children is less than 5%. It is highly contagious by skin-to-skin contact, especially in humid and unhygienic conditions. Fomites such as shared towels, the use of communal bathtubs and swimming pools, contact sports such as wrestling, and tattooing all promote infection. Lesions are spread over the body by autoinoculation. Sexual transmission accounts for a second peak of incidence in young adults. The risk and extent of infection is increased in those with generalized skin diseases such as atopic eczema and in those with congenital or acquired immunodeficiency, caused by HIV, lymphomas, sarcoidosis, organ transplantation, and immunosuppressive therapy. In HIV seropositive people, the prevalence of molluscum contagiosum is 5 to 20%, but in those with CD4 cell counts below 100/ml it increases to 30%.

Clinical features

The incubation period varies from 7 days (in newborns) to 50 days or even up to 6 months. The classic lesion is a painless, discrete, shiny, pearly, hemispherical, firm papule with a central umbilication (depression).

In immunocompetent children, lesions can occur singly but are commonly multiple, fewer than 30 to several hundred (Figs. 5.28.1, 5.28.2). They grow gradually to a diameter of 5 to 10 mm over 6 to 12 weeks. Occasionally, a single lesion may grow to 1.5 cm in diameter, or a plaque of very small lesions develops (agminate form). New lesions may continue to appear for 6 to 8 months,

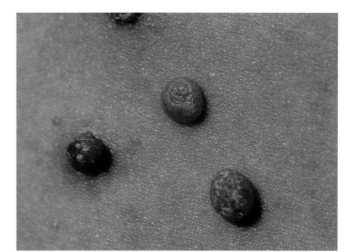

Fig. 5.28.2 Molluscum contagiosum: characteristic papules with central punctum.
(Courtesy of Dr Susan M Burge.)

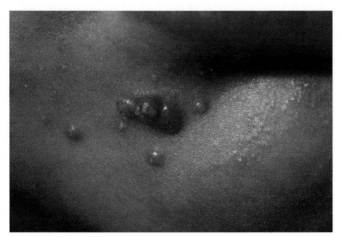

Fig. 5.28.1 Molluscum contagiosum: cluster of lesions in an immunocompetent child.
(Courtesy of Dr Susan M Burge.)

but spontaneous clearance is complete without scarring within 2 to 4 years. In about 10% of cases, especially where there is a history of atopy, a patchy erythema or dermatitis develops around the lesions, causing itching which encourages scratching and autoinoculation. Lesions are most commonly seen on the axilla and other flexures, trunk, neck, or face, but any part of the skin can be affected. Conjunctival inoculation may result in unilateral conjunctivitis or corneal or conjunctival nodules. Lesions are rare on the palms, soles, and buccal mucous membrane. In immunocompetent sexually active teenagers and adults, infections usually result in anogenital lesions.

In patients with HIV and other types of immunosuppression or with atopic eczema, molluscum can be widespread, but particularly involves the face (eyelids), neck, trunk, and around and inside the mouth in homosexual men. Lesions often lack the classic umbilication and may become so large, atypical, and even necrotic that they are mistaken for basal cell carcinomas or other skin tumours. The disease persists and spreads, especially when HIV is advanced.

Diagnosis

The diagnosis is usually clinical, but histological and electron microscopic examination of a curetted papule establishes the diagnosis. The demarcated lesion shows lobules of epidermis, depleted of Langerhans cells, penetrating down to the dermis with a central crater opening onto the surface through a narrow pore (Fig. 5.28.3). It contains keratinocyte debris with numerous Henderson–Paterson molluscum bodies. These are 35 μm in diameter, ovoid, eosinophilic, intracytoplasmic inclusion bodies within keratinocytes (Fig. 5.28.4). They stain purple with Tzanck reagent in scrapings from the lesions. In HIV patients, histological appearances may different.

Differential diagnosis

The differential diagnosis includes lepromatous leprosy, Darier's disease (keratosis follicularis), epithelial naevi, and skin tumours such as basal cell epithelioma or trichoepithelioma. Giant lesions

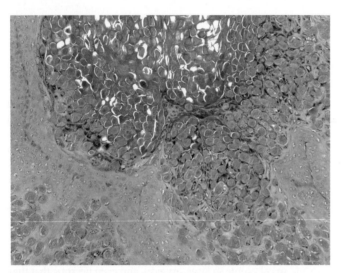

Fig. 5.28.3 Molluscum contagiosum showing the characteristic demarcated lesion.
(Courtesy of K Hollowood.)

Fig. 5.28.4 Molluscum contagiosum showing keratinocyte debris with Henderson–Paterson molluscum bodies.
(Courtesy of K Hollowood.)

might be confused with keratoacanthoma, common warts, or warty dyskeratoma. In the genital area, genital warts (condylomata acuminata) may look similar. In immunosuppressed people, cutaneous lesions of disseminated *Penicillium marneffei* infection, histoplasmosis, paracoccidioidomycosis, or cryptococcosis may appear identical to molluscum.

Treatment (see also Oxford Textbook of Medicine 5e Section 23)

Treatment may not be necessary, depending on the site and number of lesions and the age of the patient. An enormous number of local treatments are claimed to be effective, but evidence is lacking. Mechanical methods include picking out lesions on the tip of a needle or with adhesive tape, curettage, cryotherapy with liquid nitrogen, and diathermy. Topical chemicals include tretinoin, podofilox, cantharidin, acetic acid, phenol, salicylic acid, silver nitrate, trichloroacetic acid, lactic acid, and benzoin. Agents can be delivered to the inside of the lesion using the sharpened end of a

wooden applicator stick. In children, local anaesthetic cream should be applied beforehand.

In patients with HIV, molluscum usually responds dramatically to highly active antiretroviral therapy (HAART). In severe cases, 5% imiquimod cream or cidofovir (intravenously or topically) have proved effective.

Prevention

In schoolchildren, spread can be prevented by avoiding swimming pools, contact sports, and shared towels, until the lesions have resolved.

Further reading

Brown J, *et al.* (2006). Childhood molluscum contagiosum. *Int J Dermatol*, **45**, 93–9.

De Clercq E (2003). Clinical potential of the acyclic nucleoside phosphonates cidofovir, adefovir, and tenofovir in treatment of DNA virus and retrovirus infections. *Clin Microbiol Rev*, **16**, 569–96.

Lee R, Schwartz RA (2010). Pediatric molluscum contagiosum: reflections on the last challenging poxvirus infection, Part 1. *Cutis*, **86**, 230–6, 287–92.

Schwartz JJ, Myskowski PL (1992). Molluscum contagiosum in patients with human immunodeficiency virus infection. A review of twenty-seven patients. *J Am Acad Dermatol*, **27**, 583–8.

Smith KJ, Skelton H (2002). Molluscum contagiosum: recent advances in pathogenic mechanisms, and new therapies. *Am J Clin Dermatol*, **3**, 535–45.

Smith KJ, Yeager J, Skelton H (1999). Molluscum contagiosum: its clinical, histopathologic, and immunohistochemical spectrum. *Int J Dermatol*, **38**, 664–72.

van der Wouden JC, *et al.* (2006). Interventions for cutaneous molluscum contagiosum. *Cochrane Database Syst Rev*, **2**, CD004767.

5.29 Newly discovered viruses

H.C. Hughes

Essentials

Although humans are affected by an enormous range of micro-organisms, almost all newly discovered emerging pathogens are viruses that are often zoonotic or vector-borne. These emerging viruses often have high baseline mutation rates, allowing them to adapt relatively easily to new hosts and enabling them to take advantage of new epidemiological opportunities provided by the changing environment. A range of apparently new human viral pathogens has been reported increasingly in international outbreak information over the last few years. How they will influence global public health remains to be seen.

Emerging viruses that may be of particular public health importance include (1) respiratory SARS-like coronaviruses; (2) Garissa and Ngari viruses, Alkhurma virus and Lujo virus—discovered during investigations of haemorrhagic fever; (3) KI and WU human polyomaviruses, new human coronaviruses, human bocavirus, human parechovirus, and mimivirus—causing predominantly respiratory disease; (4) Toscana and, Usutu, viruses—causing viral meningitis and encephalitis; (5) Merkel cell polyomavirus—with oncogenic potential. The human pathogenicity of other emerging viruses, e.g. Vesivirus, Ljungan virus, Aichi virus, Titi Monkey adenovirus, gamma-retrovirus and Saffold virus is less certain.

SARS-like coronaviruses (Chapter 5.1)

Coronaviruses (CoV) are single-stranded RNA viruses commonly associated with respiratory illness and less often with gastrointestinal and neurological disease in a wide variety of mammals and birds. The severe acute respiratory syndrome (SARS) outbreak of a new human coronavirus, SARS-associated coronavirus (SARS-CoV), between November 2002 and July 2003 spread across 5 continents and caused over 700 human deaths. This pandemic triggered renewed interest in this area, leading to increased understanding of the origin of SARS-CoV, as well as the discovery of two previously unknown human coronaviruses.

In the early phase of the outbreak, the infecting SARS viruses showed closer similarities to animal viruses than later on in the pandemic. Virological studies suggest that the animal viruses crossed over to humans on more than one separate occasion, so repeated similar events should be expected in the future. Bats are increasingly recognized as reservoirs of emerging viruses. The discovery of species-specific, SARS-like coronaviruses in horseshoe bats with the same genome organization as human SARS coronaviruses indicates that a human SARS virus originated in one or more bat species. It is likely that an intermediate animal host is also required to allow modification of the mutating progenitor virus before transmission to humans is possible. Understanding this reservoir might help to prevent future human outbreaks of SARS-CoV.

New human coronaviruses

Two new human coronaviruses have been discovered since the SARS epidemic: HCoV-NL63 and HCoV-HK. HCoV-NL63 was first identified in a child with bronchiolitis in the Netherlands. Studies published in 2004 and 2005 found 8 to 9% of children aged under 5 years old with known respiratory illness were positive for HCoV-NL63 by polymerase chain reaction (PCR), while tests for common respiratory viruses were negative. Longitudinal studies showed that seroconversion usually occurred by the age of 3.5 years. Significant sequence heterogeneity exists and it is likely therefore that there are two closely related genotypic subgroups.

In 2005, another human coronavirus was discovered, HCoV-HKU1. It was first described in Hong Kong in a 71-year-old man with pneumonia who had recently returned from China. It has since been reported in patients in Australia and the United States of America. Common clinical findings in young children included rhinorrhoea, cough, fever, and abnormal breath sounds on auscultation. The possibility of central nervous system infection and hepatitis (in a liver transplant recipient) were suggested in two separate patients in one study. Genomic and phylogenetic analysis suggests that this virus is most closely related to the mouse hepatitis virus, a coronavirus studied since the 1930s.

New human polyomaviruses: KI, WU, and Merkel cell polyomavirus

The double-stranded DNA human polyomaviruses, JC virus and BK virus, are ubiquitous worldwide and are pathogenic in immunocompromised hosts. In 2007, two new human polyomaviruses were described, KI virus and WU virus. They share a phylogenetic relationship and together may form a new subclass. They have been isolated primarily from respiratory secretions. KI was discovered after molecular screening of respiratory samples. WU was first detected by high-throughput sequencing of respiratory secretions from a patient with an acute respiratory disease of unknown aetiology. Analysis of two more cohorts in different continents revealed that the majority of patients positive for WU were aged under 3 years, and that all infected adults were immunocompromised. The clinical spectrum of the disease included upper and lower respiratory tract infection, bronchiolitis, croup, and, rarely, gastroenteritis. However, the role of these viruses as respiratory pathogens has since been questioned after further studies detected them both in asymptomatic children and those concurrently infected with other respiratory viruses. Studies to establish the role of WU and KI in immunocompromised adults have been inconclusive. The relatively high seroprevalence of these viruses in healthy blood donors suggest that a benign primary infection with these viruses occurs in childhood, followed by a period of latency and subsequent reactivation in the context of immunosuppression.

In 2008, another novel polyomavirus termed 'Merkel Cell polyomavirus' was found to be integrated within the cellular genome of cells of the rare skin cancer Merkel cell carcinoma which primarily occurs in elderly and immunosuppressed people. This is consistent with the oncogenic potential of other polyomaviruses. Merkel cell polyomavirus has also been isolated in respiratory samples from symptomatic adult and paediatric patients though its precise role as a pathogen in this context is yet to be confirmed.

Human bocavirus

Human bocavirus (HBoV) is a nonenveloped, single-stranded DNA virus in the family Parvoviridae, first described in September 2005 following isolation by random PCR in pooled respiratory samples from hospitalized children in Sweden. HBoV is closely related to canine minute virus and bovine parvovirus. The only other parvovirus known to be pathogenic in humans is parvovirus B19, the cause of fifth disease in children (Chapter 5.20).

Although Koch's postulates have not yet been fulfilled, supportive molecular evidence demonstrated this virus in respiratory samples from children with lower respiratory tract disease who tested negative for common respiratory viruses. It has been found most commonly in children aged under 3 years old, particularly in preterm infants with mild to severe respiratory symptoms. Although a study conducted in the Netherlands showed no difference between the detection of HBoV in children with or without LRTI in paediatric intensive care, higher levels of HBoV were seen in the symptomatic patients compared to asymptomatic controls. This may reflect differences in viral load of acute infection versus asymptomatic shedding. A more recent study of patients hospitalized with acute LRTI in Argentina in 2010 found a bimodal age distribution of HBoV (<1 year and >30 years) with a significantly higher rate of coinfection (predominantly with RSV) found in children compared to adults.

Related viruses HBoV2, HBoV3, and HBoV4 and a recombinant HBoV-1/-2 have more recently been identified in faecal samples of children in several countries including the United Kingdom, Pakistan, and Thailand. An association with acute gastroenteritis has been described: in one study, HBoV2 was the third most prevalent virus seen in children with AGE after rotavirus and astrovirus. Absence of HBoV2 in more than 6500 paediatric respiratory samples in one study suggests a very different tissue tropism to HBoV despite its close phylogenetic lineage. HBoV-3 has also been described though a clinical association is yet to be shown.

Further quantitative studies are needed before the precise role of these viruses in human disease is reliably established.

Vesivirus

Single-stranded RNA vesiviruses of the Calciviridae family are common marine microorganisms, but are also known to infect land mammals. They cause a broad spectrum of disease in animals including vesicular rash, encephalitis, haemorrhagic disease, spontaneous abortion, and hepatitis. Their effect on humans is not well established, but a recent seroprevalence study has shown that 12% of tested successful blood donors had evidence of past exposure to vesivirus. This was significantly higher (29%) in patients with hepatitis of unknown but suspected infectious cause, and even higher (47%) in patients with hepatitis of unknown cause associated with blood transfusion or dialysis. Vesivirus viraemia was also shown to be present in some of those tested.

Picornaviridae

New parechoviruses: Human parechovirus and Ljungan virus

Human parechovirus and Ljungan virus are the two species of the genus parechovirus of the family *Picornaviridae*. Human parechoviruses are single-stranded RNA viruses which differ from other family members in having only three, rather than four, capsid proteins, and in exerting atypical cytopathic effects. HPeV-1 and HPeV-2 were previously designated Enterovirus 22 and 23 but were reclassified in 1999. By the end of 2011, 16 human parechoviruses genotypes had been described.

HPeV infections are common with at least 95% of the adult population positive for HPeV-specific antibodies. Most infections are thought to predominantly affect neonates and young children and, although the clinical spectrum of disease differs between the viruses, it has been compared to infection with enterovirus. Earlier studies of HPeV-1 suggested infection resulted in more gastrointestinal and respiratory illness which was often severe, and was occasionally found as a copathogen with other respiratory viruses such as respiratory syncytial virus (RSV). The role of HPeV-1 as a respiratory pathogen has since been challenged. HPeV-2 and HPeV-3 have been shown to present as sepsis-like syndromes, predominantly affecting neonates. Children with HPeV-3 positive CSF specimens in the United States of America showed a predominance of male infants presenting with sepsis-like syndromes in a late summer/autumn distribution. This seasonal distribution was not reflected in a similar survey in the United Kingdom, in which patients presented in the spring in even-numbered years, and were almost always infants less than 3 months of age. The combination of prominent abdominal distension with erythematous rash has been described in four of eight infants with confirmed HPeV infection; such symptoms are postulated to be important clues to the diagnosis in the absence of a raised CRP or lymphocyte count.

More recently described HPeV-8 (Brazil, 2009) and HPeV-10 (Sri Lanka, 2010) were both found in stool specimens of children with acute gastroenteritis. It is also likely that further novel human parechoviruses will be discovered and their contribution as human pathogens investigated.

Another parechovirus, Ljungan virus (LV) has recently been postulated as a major aetiological agent in sudden infant death syndrome (SIDS). LV mainly affects rodents and is known to be associated with perinatal rodent death both in the wild and in laboratory mice. Interestingly, a strong epidemiological link between small rodent numbers and human intrauterine fetal death has been described in Sweden. In addition, LV has been detected in brain, heart and lung tissue in cases of SIDS. Whether true causation can be proven is yet to be established.

Aichi virus

Aichi virus is a novel human picornavirus which was initially described in 1991 and linked epidemiologically with food- and water-associated diarrhoea, aqlthough its role in the aetiology of acute gastroenteritis is yet to be established. A recently published study overcame previous technical difficulties in using specific molecular detection methods to look at stool samples from patients in Germany with acute gastroenteritis over a 1 year period. Viral shedding with Aichi virus appeared unrelated to the severity of symptoms, and no food association was found despite investigation. A detection rate of 2% was seen across all age groups, comparable to similar studies elsewhere in Europe and Asia. However, there was a distinct geographical and temporal association more in keeping with faeco-oral transmission than a point-source outbreak.

Human cardiovirus: Saffold virus

Investigation of an 8 month old girl with pyrexia of unknown origin, led to the discovery in 2007 of a novel cardiovirus of the family *Picornaviradae*, named Saffold virus (SAFV). Several strains of SAFV have since been described and have been detected in faecal and respiratory specimens of children worldwide, from a patient with aseptic meningitis and from children with nonpolio acute flaccid paralysis, though causality has not yet been proven. Interestingly, SAFV is grouped with Theiler's murine encephalomyelitis virus (TMEV) which is known to cause a multiple sclerosis-like syndrome in mice. Although this may be the first human cardiovirus, a specific clinical association is yet to be found.

Usutu virus

Usutu virus, named after a river in Swaziland, was first isolated from mosquitoes in South Africa in 1959. It is a mosquito-borne flavivirus of the Japanese encephalitis group and was isolated once from a man with fever and rash. Although a virus of tropical or subtropical Africa, the epidemiology might be changing, following its isolation from several bird species during a die-off in Austria in 2001. This reflects the pattern of the emergence of West Nile virus in the United States of America in 1999, which first affected birds and subsequently humans. Neuroinvasive infection secondary to Usutu virus was reported for the first time worldwide in 2009 when USUV was detected by RT-PCR in CSF and serum samples in two immunocompromised patients in Italy who had both received blood transfusions. Clinical symptoms in both patients included fever (>39.5°C), headache, and neurological disease. The extent of the human pathogenic potential of USUV remains to be seen, but there is concern that it may follow a recurrent theme of flavivirus emergence in previously cooler climates following climate change. Surveillance systems already in place in areas of endemic West Nile virus could be adapted to detect more cases of Usutu virus if surveillance in wild birds and vectors indicated a need.

Garissa and Ngari virus

Genetic reassortment of segmented RNA viruses such as influenza is well known to have an important role in the emergence of viruses with new disease potential and host range. There is less genetic information on bunyaviruses, but there is increasing evidence that this mechanism could account for their evolution and increase their potential to cause disease in humans.

The first association of Ngari virus with human haemorrhagic fever (HF) was discovered during an extensive investigation of a large outbreak in Kenya, Tanzania, and Somalia in 1997 to 1998. A previously unidentified member of the orthobunyavirus genus (family Bunyaviridae) was found in two cases. The virus was initially named Garissa virus, but subsequent genetic analysis showed that it was not a separate orthobunyavirus but had arisen by genetic segment reassortment between two known orthobunyaviruses, Bunyamwera virus and Ngari virus. Further sequence analysis of multiple orthobunyaviruses revealed that Ngari virus is a reassortment Bunyamwera virus.

Alkurma virus

Alkhurma virus, a re-emerging tick-borne flavivirus, is related to Kysanur Forest disease and shares clinical features with Dengue Fever. It was first described in a butcher in Saudi Arabia in the 1990s, and over the next 10 years, had a case fatality rate of around 25%. In 2009, 4 further sporadic cases were described in Jeddah in the post Hajj period and all may be linked to the slaughtering/processing of sheep. The cases have highlighted the need to further understand the epidemiology of this re-emerging disease.

Lujo virus

Lujo virus is a novel, genetically distinct, highly pathogenic arena virus associated with haemorrhagic fever with an exceptionally high case fatality rate of 80%. It was first isolated in South Africa in 2008 during a nosocomial outbreak of 5 cases following the transfer of the index case from Zambia. The technique of unbiased pyrosequencing used during the investigation of this outbreak may well be useful in identifying other novel pathogens in the future.

Toscana virus

Toscana virus (TOSV) is an arthropod-borne bunyavirus transmitted by sandflies. Two genotypes have been described (TOSV A and B) with different geographical distributions. Though TOSV

was first identified in Italy in 1971, epidemiological studies and clinical research over the last three decades has shown that it is an increasingly important cause of seasonal aseptic meningitis and encephalitis across the Mediterranean. It is the most common cause of this disease in Italy from May to October and has also been associated with human infection in France. Lethal infections and long-term sequelae have been reported. The RNA of TOSV has been isolated in a different species of sandfly in France from that in Italy, although there is no confirmation that human disease is arthropod-borne.

Mimivirus

With a diameter of 600 nm and with a dsDNA genome of 1.2 Mb, mimivirus is the largest virus so far discovered. It was initially thought to be a Gram-positive coccoid bacterium and is visible with the light microscope.

The virus species *Acanthamoeba polyphaga mimivirus* is within a family of its own, the Mimiviridae. Phylogenetic analysis has shown its relationship to other large DNA viruses including the Iridoviridae and Poxviridae, though its precise position in the phylogenetic tree remains under debate. Discovered during the investigation of respiratory pathogens using an amoeba coculture system, it may have originated in marine environments. Although it replicates within amoebae, it is yet to be shown to multiply effectively in mammalian cells. Mimivirus may have a role in respiratory disease. A pneumonic illness can be produced in mice and a laboratory technician occupationally exposed to high concentrations of mimivirus antigens developed a subacute, spontaneously resolving pneumonia with seroconversion to Mimivirus. The prevalence of antibodies to mimivirus was 9.66% in 376 Canadian patients with community acquired pneumonia compared to 2.3% of healthy controls. Two studies of pneumonia in intensive care units have shown seroconversion to the virus in more patients with ventilator-associated pneumonia than in controls. Seropositivity to mimivirus in ventilated patients in a prospective matched cohort study was associated with longer duration of ventilation and longer ICU stay. There was no mortality difference between seropositive patients and matched seronegative controls. Mimivirus antibodies have been found to be more prevalent in populations admitted from nursing homes and in those rehospitalized after discharge. These seroprevalence studies must be interpreted cautiously because of possible cross-reactivity with other pathogens. More recent studies using real-time PCR have also been inconclusive. Although mimivirus DNA was recovered from a bronchoalveolar lavage of a patient with relapsing pneumonia in the absence of other causative pathogens, a prevalence study in 69 ventilated patients in an intensive care setting found no evidence of mimivirus infection using real-time PCR. A study of paired serological and DNA detection in lower respiratory samples may be useful in investigating the role of mimivirus in respiratory disease.

Gamma-retrovirus: xenotropic murine leukaemia virus-related virus

A novel retrovirus termed xenotropic murine leukaemia virus-related virus (XMRV) was linked previously to prostate cancer in the United States of America but not in Europe. In 2009, it was reported that 68 of 101 patients with chronic fatigue syndrome in the United States of America were infected with the virus though this finding has not been replicated in a similar United Kingdom cohort. It may be that these findings reflect differences in the prevalence of this virus in North America and Europe rather than a specific association with CFS per se.

Titi Monkey adenovirus

An outbreak of fulminant pneumonia affected 34% of New World monkeys housed in a closed colony in the United States of America. The Virochip microarray was used to identify the causative agent, a novel adenovirus—the Titi Monkey adenovirus (TMAdV). An exposed worker subsequently developed an acute respiratory tract infection lasting 4 weeks and seroconverted to TMAdV. A critically ill family member of this person also developed symptoms and tested positive serologically, suggesting potential for primate–human and human–human transmission of this novel agent.

Further reading

Abed Y, *et al.* (2006). Human parechovirus types 1, 2 and 3 infections in Canada. *Emerg Infect Dis*, **12**, 969–75.

Allander T, *et al.* (2005). Cloning of a human parvovirus by molecular screening of respiratory tract samples. *Proc Natl Acad Sci U S A*, **102**, 12891–96.

Allander T, *et al.* (2007). Identification of a third human polyomavirus. *J Virol*, **81**, 4130–36.

Arthur JL, *et al.* (2009). A novel bocavirus associated with acute gastroenteritis in Australian children. *PLoS Pathog*, **5**, e1000391.

Babakir-Mina M, *et al.* (2011) The novel KI, WU, MC polyomaviruses: possible human pathogens? *New Microbiol*, **34**, 1–8.

Charrel RN, *et al.* (2005). Emergence of Toscana virus in Europe. *Emerg Infect Dis*, **11**, 1657–63.

Charrel RN, *et al.* (2005). Low diversity of Alkhurma hemorrhagic fever virus, Saudi Arabia, 1994–1999. *Emerg Infect Dis*, **11**, 683–88.

Chen EC (2011). Cross-species transmission of a novel adenovirus associated with a fulminant pneumonia outbreak in a New World monkey colony. *PLoS Pathog*, **7**, e1002155.

Drexler JF, *et al.* (2009). Novel human parechovirus from Brazil. *Emerg Infect Dis*, **15**, 310–13.

Drexler JF, *et al.* (2011). Aichi virus shedding in high concentrations in patients with acute diarrhea. *Emerg Infect Dis*, **17**, 1544–8.

Erlwein O, *et al.* (2010). Failure to detect the novel retrovirus XMRV in chronic fatigue syndrome. *PLoS One*, **5**, e8519.

Esper F, *et al.* (2006). Coronavirus HKU1 infection in the United States. *Emerg Infect Dis*, **12**, 775–79.

Gaynor AM, *et al.* (2007). Identification of a novel polyomavirus from patients with acute respiratory tract infections. *PLoS Pathog*, **3**, e64.

Gerrard SR, *et al.* (2004). Ngari virus is a Bunyamwera virus reassortant that can be associated with large outbreaks of hemorrhagic fever in Africa. *J Virol*, **78**, 8922–26.

Ghietto LM, *et al.* (2011). High frequency of human bocavirus 1 DNA in infants and adults with lower acute respiratory infection. *J Med Microbiol*. Epub ahead of print Nov 24 2011.

Harvala H, *et al.* (2008). Epidemiology and clinical associations of human parechovirus respiratory infections. J Clin Microbiol, **46**, 3446–53.

Harvala H, *et al.* (2011). Comparison of human parechovirus and enterovirus detection frequencies in cerebrospinal fluid samples collected over a 5-year period in Edinburgh: HPeV type 3 identified as the most common picornavirus type. *J Med Virol*, **83**, 889–96.

Kim Pham NT, *et al.* (2010). Novel human parechovirus, Sri Lanka. *Emerg Infect Dis*, **16**, 130–32.

Nguyen NL, *et al.* (2009). Serologic evidence of frequent human infection with WU and KI polyomaviruses. *Emerg Infect Dis*, **15**, 1199–1205.

Pyrc, K *et al.* (2007). The novel human coronaviruses NL63 and HKU1. *J Virol*, **81**, 3051–57.

Raoult D, *et al.* (2007). The discovery and characterization of Mimivirus, the largest known virus and putative pneumonia agent. *Clin Infect Dis*, **45**, 95–102.

Ren, L *et al.* (2009). Saffold cardiovirus in children with acute gastroenteritis, Beijing, China. *Emerg Infect Dis*, **15**, 1509–11.

Smith AW, *et al.* (2006). Vesivirus viremia and seroprevalence in humans. *J Med Virol*, **78**, 693–701.

Vabret A, *et al.* (2005). Human coronavirus NL63, France. *Emerg Infect Dis*, **11**, 1225–29.

van de Pol AC, *et al.* (2009). Human bocavirus and KI/WU polyomaviruses in pediatric intensive care patients. *Emerg Infect Dis*, **15**, 454–57.

Vincent A, *et al.* (2009). Clinical significance of a positive serology for mimivirus in patients presenting a suspicion of ventilator-associated pneumonia. *Crit Care Med*, **37**, 111–8.

Wang LF, *et al.* (2006). Review of bats and SARS. *Emerg Infect Dis*, **12**, 1834–40.

Wattier RL, *et al.* (2008). Role of human polyomaviruses in respiratory tract disease in young children. *Emerg Infect Dis*, **14**, 1766–68.

Weissenbock H, *et al.* (2002). Emergence of Usutu virus, an African mosquito-borne flavivirus of the Japanese encephalitis virus group, central Europe. *Emerg Infect Dis*, **8**, 652–56.

6 Bacteria

Contents

6.1 Diphtheria

Delia B. Bethell and Tran Tinh Hien

Essentials

Diphtheria is a potentially lethal infection caused by toxin-producing strains of *Corynebacterium diphtheria*, a Gram-positive bacillus. Humans are the only known reservoir, with spread via respiratory droplets or direct contact with skin lesions. Although now rare in developed countries, this vaccine-preventable disease remains an important problem in countries with poor or failing health systems, and is estimated to cause about 5000 deaths per year worldwide, most in children under 5 years of age.

Pathogenesis—diphtheria develops when toxigenic bacteria lodge in the upper airway or on the skin of a susceptible individual. An intense inflammatory reaction develops, leading to a characteristic greyish-coloured pseudomembrane that is adherent to underlying tissues. Systemic effects are caused by release of diphtheria toxin, carried by a lysogenic corynebacteriophage, a single molecule of factor A of which can kill a eukaryotic cell.

Clinical features—after an incubation period of 2 to 6 days the disease presents acutely in a number of ways, classified by the location of the pseudomembrane: (1) anterior nasal—usually relatively mild; (2) tonsillar (faucial)—the commonest form, with malaise, fever, sore throat, painful dysphagia and tender cervical lymphadenopathy; (3) tracheolaryngeal—with particular risk of airway obstruction; (4) malignant—with rapid onset, circulatory shock, cyanosis, gross cervical lymphadenopathy ('bull neck'), and very poor prognosis; (5) cutaneous—usually mild but chronic; morphological features can be extremely variable. Later complications include (1) myocarditis—seen in 10% of cases; and (2) segmental demyelinative neuropathy—most often palatal paralysis, and more sinister paralyses of pharyngeal, laryngeal, respiratory and limb muscles.

Diagnosis—infection may be confirmed by bacterial culture, with detection of toxin production by one of several laboratory techniques, or of the toxin-producing gene by PCR.

Treatment and prognosis—aside from supportive care, this involves (1) antitoxin—20000 to 100000 units, depending on disease severity; preferably given within 48 h of the onset of symptoms; (2) antibiotics—benzylpenicillin (or penicillin V), or erythromycin in those allergic to penicillin; (3) maintaining the airway—life-saving procedures such as tracheostomy may be required. Recovery is usually complete if the patient survives.

Prevention—diphtheria is completely preventable by vaccination, but immunity is not life-long and may wane in adult life if booster doses are not given regularly. Similarly, infection does not necessarily confer complete protection and the disease may recur in previously infected individuals.

Introduction

Diphtheria is an acute and potentially highly lethal infection of the upper respiratory tract caused by toxigenic strains of *Corynebacterium diphtheriae* and *C. ulcerans*. Today diphtheria has been virtually eliminated from most developed countries by mass immunization, yet it remains a threat in countries with poor vaccine coverage. During the 1990s there was a huge epidemic in parts of the former Soviet Union. Smaller outbreaks have been reported in several other countries.

Historical perspective

Since ancient times diphtheria has been one of the most feared childhood diseases, characterized by devastating outbreaks. Diphtheria was recognized as an infectious disease by Brentonneau in 1819. The causative bacillus was described by Löffler in 1884 and a soluble toxin was identified by Roux and Yersin in 1889. In 1890, Fränkel developed an attenuated vaccine and von Behring produced an antitoxin, the first therapeutic antiserum that was first used clinically by Roux in 1894. Before the introduction of antitoxin, mortality in some epidemics had exceeded 50%. In 1913, von Behring produced a successful vaccine and the Schick (skin) test was used to detect immunity. In the United Kingdom there was an average of 50 000 cases and 4000 deaths each year from 1915 to 1942 and it was the leading cause of death among children aged 4 to 10 years. During the Second World War, more than a million cases were reported, including 50 000 deaths. In the United States of America, W. Barry Woods Jr declared in 1961 that: "Were it possible merely to apply what is now known about diphtheria to every part of the world, this devastating malady could be wiped from the face of the earth". However, even in that country, epidemic outbreaks continued in major cities, e.g. the 1970 San Antonio epidemic involving 201 cases with 3 deaths mainly in the unimmunized poor nonwhite population aged less than 15 years. In the United Kingdom, mass vaccination had reduced diphtheria to approximately 8 to 10 notified cases each year. In 2002 there were still an estimated 5000 deaths from diphtheria worldwide, of which 4000 were in children under 5 years of age.

Pathogenesis

C. diphtheriae are slender pleomorphic Gram-positive rods or clubs. There are four biotypes: *gravis*, *intermedius*, *belfanti*, and *mitis*, any of which can cause diphtheria if they produce exotoxin. Early manifestations of diphtheria, including pseudomembrane formation, result from an inflammatory reaction to the multiplying toxigenic *C. diphtheriae*. Fluid and leucocytes move from dilated blood vessels to surround necrotic epithelial cells. The fluid clots to enmesh dead cells, leucocytes, diphtheria bacilli, cellular debris, and occasionally small blood vessels. The resulting pseudomembrane is therefore adherent to underlying tissues and bleeds when pulled away.

C. diphtheriae does not usually pass beyond the pseudomembrane site; it is the toxin that causes the later complications of diphtheria. Diphtheria toxin is a 535-amino acid residue 62-kDa exotoxin consisting of three domains, A (enzymatic), B (binding), and T (translocation). Domain B binds on the cell surface to heparin-binding epidermal growth factor (EGF)-like growth factor precursor and CD9 complex, allowing the lethal factor A to pass through the endosome membrane into the cytosol where it catalyses the NAD$^+$-dependent ADP-ribosylation of eukaryotic elongation factor 2 preventing protein synthesis leading to cell death, facilitated by apoptosis. Delivery of a single molecule of factor A to the cytosol of a eukaryotic cell will kill it. Employing this mechanism, recombinant diphtheria toxin with its B domain truncated and fused with the human interleukin (IL)-2 receptor is marketed as denileukin diftitox (DT388-IL2) for the treatment of cutaneous T-cell lymphoma, chronic lymphocytic leukaemia, and non-Hodgkin's lymphoma.

The structural gene of the toxin (*TOX*) is carried by a lysogenic corynebacteriophage. However, *TOX* gene expression is regulated by the bacterial chromosome and requires low extracellular iron concentrations. Locally the toxin causes tissue necrosis and, when absorbed into the bloodstream, systemic complications. In addition to bacterial exotoxin, cell wall components such as the O- and K-antigens are important in disease pathogenesis.

Pathological changes may be seen in all human cells, but the most profound changes are seen in the myocardium, peripheral nerves, and kidneys. Common cardiac changes include fatty degeneration of cardiac muscle (myocarditis) and infiltration of the interstitium with leucocytes, which may involve the conduction fibres. Although the heart can recover completely from these effects, severe fibrosis and scarring may lead to death in late convalescence. Mural endocarditis may cause embolism leading to cerebral infarction and hemiplegia. Valvular endocarditis is extremely uncommon. Neuritic changes may be seen in the nerves to the heart during the late paralytic stage of the disease. Diphtheria toxin also causes demyelination and degeneration of both sensory and motor nerves. It affects the nerves to the eye, palate, pharynx, larynx, heart, and limb muscles. It is unclear whether the toxin crosses the blood–brain barrier to cause central lesions.

Epidemiology

Humans are the only known reservoir for *C. diphtheriae*. In most cases transmission to susceptible individuals results in transient pharyngeal carriage rather than disease. Spread is via respiratory droplets or direct contact with skin lesions. Cutaneous diphtheria is more contagious than respiratory diphtheria and chronic skin infections are the main reservoir in environments of poverty and overcrowding. Patients may become carriers of the infection and continue to harbour the organism for weeks or months. The organism can survive for up to 5 weeks in dust or on fomites.

Today diphtheria remains an important health problem in countries with poor vaccine coverage. In these areas, children generally meet *C. diphtheriae* early, sometimes becoming a carrier, and young children may have severe or fatal attacks of diphtheria. *C. diphtheriae* tends to die out in highly immunized populations, and children may grow to adult life without encountering the bacillus. Recent serological studies in several countries indicate that up to 50% of adults are susceptible to diphtheria, and their immunity decreases significantly with increasing age. This potential risk is becoming increasingly important with the growth in international travel.

Immunity to systemic disease depends on the presence of IgG antitoxin antibodies. Type-specific protection against carriage and mild forms of local disease is induced by antibodies to the variable K antigens of the bacterial cell wall. Infection does not always confer protective immunity and outbreaks of mild disease have been reported even in highly vaccinated populations. In endemic countries protective immunity is boosted naturally through circulating strains of toxigenic *C. diphtheriae*.

Diphtheria is a devastating but preventable disease. Experience suggests that declining immunity in adults poses the risk of outbreaks, but is probably not sufficient in itself to sustain a large diphtheria epidemic unless there are large numbers of susceptible children and adolescents. In the newly independent states of the former Soviet Union (NIS), economic hardship, large urban migration, and low vaccination coverage due to failing health systems probably contributed to the massive outbreak of the 1990s. This started in Russia but spread to all the NIS, leading to more than 150 000 cases and 5000 deaths between 1990 and 1998 and more than 2700 cases subsequently. Widespread immunization campaigns have largely controlled the epidemic but the risk of diphtheria remains in all countries of the former Soviet Union (e.g. there were outbreaks in Western Siberia in 2003 and the southern Urals in 2004) and rare cases of diphtheria continue to be reported in tourists and travellers to the NIS.

Since 2002 *C. ulcerans* infections have been more commonly reported than *C. diphtheria* in the United Kingdom and France. The patients usually contracted the infection from raw milk or animals or close contact with companion animals and pets (cow, goat, cat, and dog). The increasing incidence of the diseases has resulted in the expansion of the notification criteria of the E-CDC and US-CDC for diphtheria to include infection caused by *C. diphtheria* and *C. ulcerans*. This increase in the number of clinical cases of diphtheria also emphasized the need to maintain vaccination coverage in the population above the 95% as recommended by the World Health Organization.

In May 2010, a diphtheria outbreak was reported from Cite Soleil district, Port-au-Prince, Haiti, in one of the settlements housing people displaced by the January 2010 earthquake. Another diphtheria outbreak causing 11 cases and 5 deaths over a 4-week period was also reported in Haiti in October 2009.

Clinical features

Early features

Diphtheria has an incubation period of 2 to 6 days and presents acutely in a variety of forms, classified according to the location of the pseudomembrane:

Anterior nasal

This is usually unilateral and relatively mild unless it coexists with other forms. It is relatively common in infancy. There is a nasal discharge, initially watery, then purulent and blood-stained. The nostril may be sore or crusted and a thin pseudomembrane can sometimes be seen within the nostril itself.

Tonsillar (faucial)

This is the commonest form of diphtheria. Malaise, sore throat, and moderate fever develop gradually. At the onset of symptoms only a small, yellow-grey spot of pseudomembrane may be present on one or both tonsils and is easily mistaken for other types of tonsillitis; it is associated with marked fetor. The surrounding areas are dull and inflamed. Over the next few days the pseudomembrane enlarges and may extend to cover the uvula, soft palate, oropharynx, nasopharynx, or larynx (Fig. 6.1.1). There is tender cervical lymphadenopathy, nausea, vomiting, and painful dysphagia. The pseudomembrane becomes greenish-black and eventually sloughs off.

Tracheolaryngeal

Some 85% of tracheolaryngeal presentations are secondary to faucial diphtheria, but occasionally there may be no pharyngeal pseudomembrane. Initial symptoms include moderate fever, hoarseness, and a nonproductive cough. Over the next day or two, as the pseudomembrane and associated oedema spread, the patient becomes increasingly dyspnoeic with severe chest recession, cyanosis, and eventual asphyxiation unless the obstruction is relieved. Tracheostomy brings instant relief if the obstruction is confined to the larynx and upper trachea. In a minority of cases the pseudomembrane also involves the bronchi and bronchioles and tracheostomy has little effect.

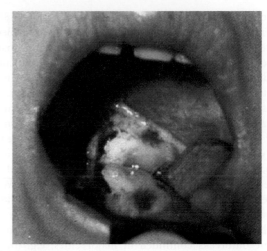

Fig. 6.1.1 Severe diphtheria in Vietnamese children. Typical faucial pharyngeal pseudomembrane.
(Copyright Bridget Wills.)

Malignant

The onset is rapid, with high fever, tachycardia, hypotension, and cyanosis. Pseudomembrane spreads from the tonsils to cover much of the nasopharynx. It has a thick edge and as this advances the earlier parts become necrotic and foul-smelling. There is gross cervical lymphadenopathy. Individual lymph nodes are difficult to feel because of surrounding oedema; this is the characteristic 'bull neck' of malignant diphtheria (Fig. 6.1.2). The patient may bleed from the mouth, nose, or skin (Figs. 6.1.3, 6.1.4). Cardiac involvement with heart block occurs within a few days. Acute renal failure may ensue. Survival is unlikely.

Cutaneous diphtheria

In contrast to respiratory forms, cutaneous diphtheria is usually chronic but mild. The morphological features of individual lesions can be extremely variable as *C. diphtheriae* can colonize any pre-existing skin lesion (such as impetigo, scabies, surgical

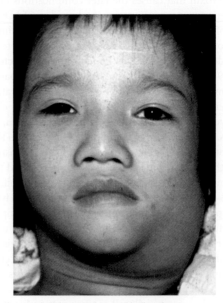

Fig. 6.1.2 Malignant diphtheria with typical bull neck.
(Copyright Rachel Kneen.)

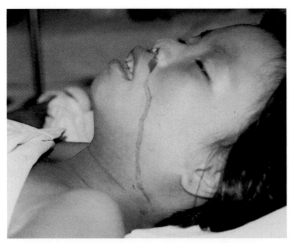

Fig. 6.1.3 Malignant diphtheria with serosanguinous nasal discharge.
(Copyright Rachel Kneen.)

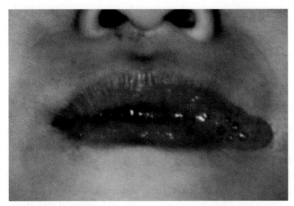

Fig. 6.1.4 Malignant diphtheria with serosanguinous oral discharge.
(Copyright Tran Tinh Hien.)

wounds, or insect bites) without altering their picture. However, the ulcerative form is the most frequent and typical (Fig. 6.1.5). Initially vesicular or pustular, and filled with straw-coloured fluid, it soon breaks down to leave a punched-out ulcer several millimetres to a few centimetres across. Common sites are the lower legs, feet, and hands. During the first 1 to 2 weeks it is painful and may be covered with a dark pseudomembrane which separates,

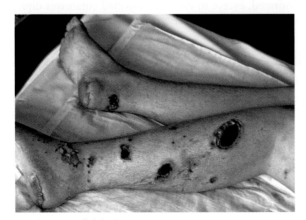

Fig. 6.1.5 Cutaneous diphtheria.
(Courtesy of the late Dr B E Juel-Jensen.)

revealing a haemorrhagic base, sometimes with a serous or serosanguinous exudate. The surrounding tissue is oedematous and pink or purple in colour. Spontaneous healing to leave a depressed scar usually takes 2 to 3 months, and sometimes much longer. Systemic complications such as myocarditis are rare. Occasionally, the affected limb becomes paralysed.

Other sites

A mild conjunctivitis may accompany faucial diphtheria. Occasionally, pseudomembrane forms in the lower conjunctiva and spreads over the cornea causing considerable damage. Dysphagia may indicate that pseudomembrane has spread from the tonsils to the oesophagus. Other parts of the gastrointestinal tract are not usually affected, but melaena with colicky abdominal pain is described. Diphtheria may spread by fingers from the throat to vulva or penis causing localized sores. *C. diphtheriae* occasionally invades the vagina and cervix, allowing the absorption of toxin. Endocarditis is rare, but at least one reported case recovered following antimicrobial treatment.

Diphtheria caused by other corynebacteria

C. ulcerans produces two toxins, one of which seems to be the same as diphtheria toxin. It may cause membranous tonsillitis but toxic manifestations are rare. *C. ulcerans* has been spread to humans in cows' milk.

C. pseudodiphtheriticum is commonly present in the flora of the upper respiratory tract. It is nontoxigenic, but can cause exudative pharyngitis with a pseudomembrane identical to that produced by *C. diphtheriae*. More commonly it causes endocarditis in patients with anatomical abnormalities or infections of the lungs, trachea, or bronchi in immunosuppressed patients or those with pre-existing respiratory disease.

Later complications

Patients surviving acute diphtheria may develop one or more later complications. These result from delayed effects of the toxin following haematogenous spread. The risk and severity of complications correlates directly with the extent of the pseudomembrane and the delay in administration of antitoxin.

Cardiovascular

Approximately 10% of patients with diphtheria will develop myocarditis, usually those with clinically severe infection. There is a much greater frequency of cardiac involvement in laryngeal and malignant diphtheria than in faucial diphtheria, and where antitoxin administration was delayed more than 48 h after onset of symptoms.

Cardiac toxicity usually appears after the first week of illness, but in malignant diphtheria can occur after just a few days. Patients complain of upper abdominal pain and may vomit. They become very lethargic and tired. Examination reveals a rapid, thready pulse with hypotension. At this stage profound shock may lead to death. In less severe cases, congestive cardiac failure may develop with a displaced apex beat, gallop rhythm, and murmurs audible over all areas of the heart. Profound bradycardia may result from heart block. There is hepatomegaly and oliguria.

Electrocardiography (ECG) is the best way to demonstrate cardiac involvement (Fig. 6.1.6). The most common abnormalities are T-wave inversion with ST-segment changes in one or more chest leads and prolonged QTc and PR intervals. There may be right or left axis deviation, bundle branch block, or heart block.

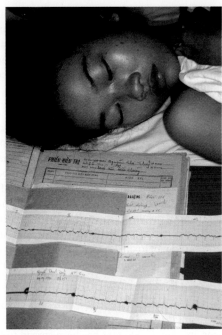

Fig. 6.1.6 Fifteen-year-old girl with cardiac and neurological complications (paralysis of muscles innervated by cranial nerves IX, X, and XII). (Copyright D A Warrell.)

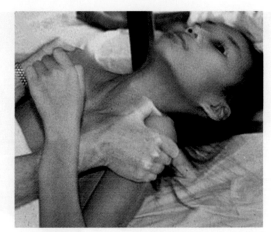

Fig. 6.1.7 Generalized muscle weakness. (Copyright Rachel Kneen.)

Very occasionally, atrial fibrillation or tachyarrhythmias are seen. Many more bursts of arrhythmias can be demonstrated if 24-h ECG monitoring is performed. Numerous ectopic beats have been recorded in patients who lacked other manifestations of cardiac involvement. Although most patients surviving myocarditis recover completely, the presence of left bundle branch block at discharge is associated with poor long-term outcome.

Neurological

Diphtheria toxin causes a segmental demyelinative neuropathy. Neurological complications usually appear weeks after the onset of the disease, when the patient appears to be recovering, and may show a temporal progression. Palatal paralysis is relatively common and may be seen from the third week onwards. The patient develops a nasal voice and regurgitates fluids through the nose. This usually resolves within a week or so. From the third to the fifth week there may be blurred vision from paralysis of accommodation, or a transient squint from external rectus paralysis. About the sixth or seventh week more sinister paralyses may develop involving pharyngeal, laryngeal, respiratory, and limb muscles (Fig. 6.1.7). The nerves to the heart may be affected causing tachycardia and dysrhythmias. In severe cases patients may become profoundly hypotonic over a few hours and can die from respiratory arrest. However, if intensive care facilities and skilled staff are available, complete recovery over the following weeks or months should ensue.

Differential diagnosis

Clinical diagnosis is difficult where diphtheria is rare. The differential diagnosis includes infectious mononucleosis, streptococcal or viral tonsillitis, peritonsillar abscess, Vincent's angina, oral thrush, anthrax (Chapter 6.20, Fig. 6.20.2), Lassa fever (Chapter 5.17),

and leukaemia and other blood dyscrasias. The bull neck of malignant diphtheria may be mistaken for mumps. In adults, secondary syphilis can sometimes cause a glairy (resembling egg white) exudate on the tonsils, and may be accompanied by rash and laryngitis.

Clinical investigation

Bacterial culture of *C. diphtheriae* is the mainstay of investigation. Material for culture should be obtained preferably from the edges of the mucosal lesions and inoculated onto appropriate selective media. Suspected colonies may be tested for toxin production by gel precipitation (Elek's test), guinea pig inoculation, or enzyme immunoassay. Direct smears of infected areas of the throat are often used for diagnostic purposes, but are only of value in experienced hands. More reliably the diphtheria toxin gene may be detected directly in clinical specimens using polymerase chain reaction techniques.

Criteria for diagnosis

In areas where diphtheria is relatively common and during outbreaks, the disease should be suspected in any patient with exudate in the throat. Treatment must not be delayed until the disease is confirmed, except in cases of suspected cutaneous diphtheria without associated respiratory symptoms.

Other corynebacterial skin infections

C. diphtheriae and some other corynebacteria are associated with cutaneous 'desert sores'. Erythrasma is caused by *C. minutissimum* and, in HIV-immunosuppressed patients, *C. striatum* can cause exuberant ulceration (Fig. 6.1.8).

Treatment

Antitoxin is the mainstay of treatment, but to be maximally effective it must be given before the toxin has reached tissues such as the heart and kidneys, preferably within 48 h of the onset of symptoms, implying that it must be given empirically before

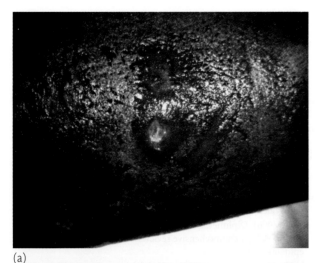

(a)

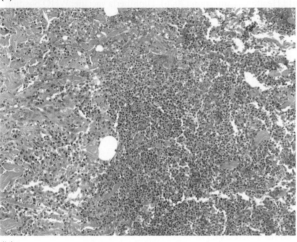

(b)

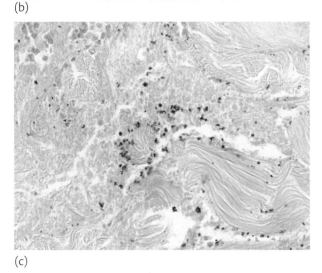

(c)

Fig. 6.1.8 *Corynebacterium striatum* infection on the thigh of an African patient with HIV-immunosuppression (a) clinical appearance of exuberant ulcerative lesion, (b) and (c) histopathological appearances of a biopsy of the lesion showing Corynebacteria (Gram-positive short rods, banded forms that look like diplococci and clubbed forms).
(a) (Courtesy of Dr C P Conlon, Oxford.) (b) and (c) (Courtesy of Kevin Hollowood, Oxford.)

bacteriological confirmation. Dosage depends on the site of primary infection, the extent of pseudomembrane, and the delay between the onset of symptoms and antitoxin administration. Between 20 000 and 40 000 units are given for faucial diphtheria of less than 48 h duration or for cutaneous infection, 40 000 to 80 000 units for faucial diphtheria in excess of 48 h duration or for laryngeal infection, and 80 000 to 100 000 units for malignant diphtheria. For doses over 40 000 units a portion is given intramuscularly followed by the bulk of the dose intravenously after an interval of 30 min to 2 h. Anaphylaxis can occur following antitoxin administration, and adrenaline (epinephrine) should always be available.

Antibiotics are given to eradicate the organism and prevent further toxin production. Benzylpenicillin 150 000 to 250 000 units/kg per day (90–150 mg/kg per day) is given intravenously in four to six divided doses in children aged 1 month to 12 years. In adults the dosage is 12 million to 20 million units/day (7.2–12 g/day) in four to six divided doses. Oral penicillin V is substituted when the patient is able to swallow. Erythromycin may be used for penicillin-sensitive individuals, but it may not be as effective in eradicating carriage. Antibiotic therapy should continue for 10 to 14 days.

Facilities for urgent tracheostomy should always be available in case of respiratory obstruction. Indications include increasingly laboured breathing and agitation. This procedure will be lifesaving in many cases. Most tracheostomies can be closed after just a few days. Steroids may be used in conjunction with tracheostomy to reduce airway swelling, but there have been no controlled trials to support their use. Steroids are of no benefit in preventing myocarditis or neuritis.

Patients with signs or symptoms of cardiac involvement need to be managed in intensive care units. Oxygen should be given. Temporary cardiac pacing is useful in patients with heart block, but is of doubtful value in cases of malignant diphtheria. An isoprenaline infusion may buy valuable time while the patient is transferred to a centre with facilities for pacing. Digoxin has been used in congestive cardiac failure. It has been suggested that carnitine may prevent some cases of myocarditis.

There is no specific treatment for neuritis. The severest cases will need mechanical ventilation and intragastric or intravenous feeding. With skilled nursing care full recovery can be expected. Patients recovering from clinical disease should complete active immunization during convalescence.

Prevention

Diphtheria toxoid is highly effective in conferring protection against clinical disease. Circulating antitoxin levels of less than 0.01 IU/ml are considered nonprotective, while levels of 0.01 IU/ml may confer some protection. Levels of 0.1 IU/ml or more are considered fully protective, and levels above 1.0 IU/ml are associated with long-term protective immunity. The potency of diphtheria vaccine is reduced in children aged 7 years and older so that reactogenicity is minimized.

The recommended schedule for vaccination against diphtheria varies between countries. In the United Kingdom three primary doses of adsorbed diphtheria–tetanus–pertussis–haemophilus influenzae type b vaccine (DTP-Hib) are given at 2, 3, and 4 months; a first booster dose with DTP at age 3 to 5 years, and a second booster dose with DT at school leaving. The primary course does not need to be repeated if boosters are delayed. People living in low-endemic or nonendemic countries should receive booster doses of DT approximately every 10 years. It is now recommended by the World Health Organization that DT rather than T (tetanus toxoid alone) should be used when tetanus prophylaxis is needed following injury. Tetanus-diphtheria vaccine is recommended for all travellers who have not received the vaccine within the last 10 years.

Where diphtheria is endemic the primary course alone should be sufficient to prevent an epidemic of diphtheria, as natural mechanisms such as frequent skin infections caused by *C. diphtheriae* probably contribute to maintaining immunity. One or two DT or DTP booster doses may need to be added to the routine schedule in areas at increased risk of diphtheria. Adults in developing countries do not require routine immunization.

Aggressive action is needed in the event of a diphtheria outbreak. Groups at risk should be immunized, there should be prompt diagnosis and management of cases, and identification of close contacts should be made so that the spread of infection can be halted. A single dose of DTP should be used for children under 3 years of age, and DT for children aged over 3 years and adults. Additional doses of vaccine will be needed in nonimmunized (Schick test positive) people.

Susceptibility to diphtheria may be assessed using the Schick test: 0.1 ml of toxin is injected into the skin of one forearm (test site) and the same quantity of a heat-inactivated toxin injected into the other forearm (control site). A positive reaction occurs in individuals without toxin-neutralizing antibodies and consists of an area of redness appearing after 24 to 36 h at the test site only and persisting for 4 to 5 days. If no toxin-neutralizing antibodies are present there will be either no reaction at either site (negative test) or a pseudoreaction at either site due to antibodies to substances other than diphtheria toxin in the test materials. This test is no longer commonly performed due to limited availability of the test materials.

Further reading

Celik T, *et al.* (2006). Prognostic significance of electrocardiographic abnormalities in diphtheritic myocarditis after hospital discharge: a long-term follow-up study. *Ann Noninvasive Electrocardiol*, **11**, 28–33. [Thirty-two patients surviving diphtheritic myocarditis were followed after discharge. All seven with left bundle branch block at discharge eventually died.]

Christie AB (ed) (1987). Diphtheria. In: *Infectious diseases: epidemiology and clinical practice*, 4th edition, pp. 898–928. Churchill Livingstone, New York. [Still the best clinical account.]

Crowcroft NS, *et al.* (2006). Screening and toxigenic corynebacteria spread. *Emerg Infect Dis*, **12**, 520–1. [A brief discussion of the factors influencing diphtheria surveillance in the United Kingdom.]

European Centre for Disease Prevention and Control (2009). http://ecdc.europa.eu/en/healthtopics/diphtheria

Health Protection Agency (n.d.). *Diphtheria*. http://www.hpa.org.uk/HPA/Topics/InfectiousDiseases/InfectionsAZ/1191942152928 [Includes information on United Kingdom notifications and vaccine uptake.]

Hofler W (1991). Cutaneous diphtheria. *Int J Dermatol*, **30**, 845–7. [A useful review of cutaneous diphtheria.]

Jayashree M, Shruthi N, Singi S (2006). Predictors of outcome in patients with diphtheria receiving intensive care. *Indian Pediatr*, **43**, 155–60. [Myocarditis was found to be the only independent predictor of death in 48 children admitted to a paediatric intensive care unit.]

Mikhailovich VM, *et al.* (1995). Application of PCR for detection of toxigenic *C. diphtheriae* strains isolated during the Russian diphtheria epidemic, 1990 through 1994. *J Clin Microbiol*, **33**, 3061–3. [A comparison of PCR with Elek's plate method.]

ProMed-mail (2009). http://www.promedmail.org/ 30 Oct 2009 Diphtheria—Haiti: RFI 20091030.3755

ProMed-mail (2010). http://www.promedmail.org/ 19 May 2010 Diphtheria—Haiti: (Port-au-Prince) 20100519.1644

Rakhmanova G, *et al.* (1996). Diphtheria outbreak in St. Petersburg: clinical characteristics of 1,860 adult patients. *Scand J Infect Dis*, **28**, 37–40.

Statutory notifications of infectious diseases 1994–2008—England and Wales.

Vitek CR (2006). Diphtheria. *Curr Top Microbiol Immunol*, **304**, 71–94. [A comprehensive review of the disease and its epidemiology.]

World Health Organization (2006). Diphtheria vaccine: WHO position paper. *Weekly Epidemiol Rec*, **81**, 24–32. [A detailed yet concise summary of the disease and its prevention.]

World Health Organization (2009). *Diphtheria*. www.who.int/topics/diphtheria/en [Up-to-date information on global and regional figures for diphtheria.]

Wren MW, Shetty N (2005). Infections with *Corynebacterium diphtheriae*: six years' experience at an inner London teaching hospital. *Br J Biomed Sci*, **62**, 1–4. [Suggests C. diphtheriae infections are underdiagnosed in the United Kingdom.]

6.2 **Streptococci and enterococci**

Dennis L. Stevens

Essentials

The streptococci are a diverse group of Gram-positive pathogenic cocci that cause clinical disease in humans and domestic animals. They are traditionally classified on the basis of serological reactions, particularly Lancefield grouping based on cell-wall carbohydrates, and haemolytic activity on blood agar. Six groups can be defined by genetic analysis: pyogenic streptococci, milleri or anginosus group, mitis group, salivarius group, mutans group, and bovis group.

Group A streptococci (*S. pyogenes*)

Group A streptococci are carried, usually in the nose or throat, by 5 to 20% of children and 0.5% of adults. More than any other human pathogen, group A streptococci cause a wide variety of infections ranging from pharyngitis, erysipelas, cellulitis, and necrotizing fasciitis to the postinfectious sequelae; rheumatic fever and poststreptococcal glomerulonephritis. These microbes continue to evolve, as evidenced by over 150 different genetic types and the emergence of novel infections such as streptococcal toxic shock syndrome.

Acknowledgement: The author of the present chapter and the editors acknowledge the inclusion of much material from the chapter in the previous edition by Professor S K Eykyn.

Group A streptococci are easy to culture in the laboratory from appropriate samples; diagnosis can also be made by detection of the group A antigen or confirmed serologically. All strains remain sensitive to penicillin, which is the antibiotic of choice, with erythromycin usually given to those who are penicillin allergic, although epidemics of pharyngitis caused by erythromycin-resistant strains have been widely reported. Genetic differences and the presence of multiple virulence factors have frustrated efforts to develop effective vaccines.

Group B streptococci (*S. agalactiae*)

Group B streptococci are carried in the throat by 5 to 10% of adults, as well as in the urethra, vagina, perineum, and anorectum. They cause a variety of infections: (1) neonatal infection—including bacteraemia and meningitis; screening for vaginal carriage during the third trimester of pregnancy and intrapartum treatment with intravenous penicillin has reduced the incidence of early onset neonatal disease; (2) postpartum infection—puerperal infection usually manifests as endometritis with fever and uterine tenderness, occurring within 24 to 48 h of delivery or abortion; also (3) skin and soft tissue infections, urinary tract infections, and bacteraemias (especially in patients with diabetes mellitus, malignancy, HIV infection, and chronic renal or liver disease).

Group B streptococci are readily isolated from any clinical specimen in the laboratory, and detection of group B antigen in body fluids by latex particle agglutination enables rapid diagnosis. They are sensitive to penicillin (the antibiotic of choice), erythromycin and cephalosporins. The polysaccharide capsule of group B streptococcus is a major virulence factor, with at least six different serotypes identified: experimental immunization using the polysaccharide provides type specific protection, but no such vaccine has yet been developed for human use.

Other groups of streptococci

Groups C and G—produce infections that are similar to those caused by group A streptococci, but tend to be less virulent. They are important causes of cellulitis, particularly recurrent cellulitis associated with saphenous vein donor site infections in patients with coronary artery by-pass surgery.

Streptococcus milleri or *Streptococcus anginosus* group—includes *S. constellatus*, *S. intermedius*, and *S. anginosus*. These are found in the normal flora of the upper respiratory tract, gastrointestinal tract and genital tract; commonly isolated from a range of pyogenic infections (e.g. dental or other abscesses), sometimes in pure culture, but often with other organisms, particularly anaerobes.

Streptococcus mitis, *Streptococcus salivarius*, and *Streptococcus mutans* groups of streptococci (oral/viridans streptococci)—these include *S. pneumoniae* (see Chapter 6.3) and those oral streptococci that are the commonest causes of infective endocarditis of oral or dental origin. Occasionally cause bacteraemia in neutropenic patients, particularly those who have received prophylaxis with fluoquinolones such as ciprofloxacin.

Streptococcus bovis group—a gastrointestinal commensal; most patients with *S. bovis* bacteraemia will have endocarditis in association with colonic pathology or cirrhosis of the liver.

Streptococcus suis—an occupational cause of septicaemia, meningitis, septic arthritis, pneumonia, and endophthalmitis among those working with pigs and pork in South-East Asia.

Enterococci

Part of the normal gut flora of humans and animals, these are an increasingly important cause of nosocomial infection and colonization, possibly the result of the large-scale use of antibiotics such as cephalosporins and quinolones to which they are inherently resistant. *Enterococcus faecium* and *E. faecalis* have also become vancomycin resistant, a characteristic dramatically increasing treatment failures, although they remain sensitive (at the time of writing) to linezolid, an oxazolidinone antimicrobial.

Introduction

The term streptococcus was first used by Billroth in 1874 to describe chain-forming cocci found in infected wounds. In 1879, Pasteur also found them in the blood of women with puerperal sepsis. In 1884, Rosenbach defined these streptococci as *Streptococcus pyogenes*. This organism remains one of the most important human pathogens. The genus *Streptococcus* contains many other species of varying degrees of pathogenicity for humans and animals. *S. faecalis* and *S. faecium* were split from the genus *Streptococcus* in 1984 and became *Enterococcus* spp. and numerous other species have since been included in this genus. The nutritionally variant streptococci *S. adjacens* and *S. defectivus* have also been assigned to a new genus *Abiotrophia* to which the newly described species *A. elegans* has been added.

Classification

Traditionally, classification of streptococci has relied on serological reactions, particularly the Lancefield grouping based on cell wall carbohydrates, and haemolytic activity on blood agar, which has led to rather unsatisfactory streptococcal taxonomy. Genetic analysis has now enabled the subdivision of the species of *Streptococcus* into six clusters or groups as follows: pyogenic streptococci, milleri or anginosus group, mitis group, salivarius group, mutans group, and bovis group. Since the medically important members of the mitis, salivarius, and mutans groups are all oral streptococci and are of clinical relevance predominantly in endocarditis, they will be considered together.

Pyogenic streptococci

The pyogenic streptococci include the major human pathogen *S. pyogenes* (Lancefield group A), group B streptococci (*S. agalactiae*), and groups C and G streptococci. These organisms are β-haemolytic on blood agar.

S. pyogenes (β-haemolytic group A)

The prevalence and severity of streptococcal pharyngitis has remained constant over the centuries of recorded history, although the incidence of complications such as peritonsillar abscess and mastoiditis have declined with the advent of antibiotics. Since the beginning of the 20th century, and long before the introduction of antibiotics, the prevalence and severity of scarlet fever and rheumatic fever following infections with *S. pyogenes* declined until the 1980s. In the mid-1980s, highly virulent streptococci appeared causing very severe infections such as streptococcal toxic shock syndrome and necrotizing fasciitis, often in otherwise healthy people. Such cases occurred not only in the United Kingdom but also in most of the developed world. *S. pyogenes* infection is usually community-acquired but may be acquired in hospital where the most serious infections are postoperative.

Carriage

Although *S. pyogenes* is an invasive organism, it survives on epithelial surfaces (asymptomatic carriage) usually in the nose and throat. Carriage can also be anal, vaginal, and on the scalp. Pharyngeal carriage rates are usually much higher in children (5–20%) than in adults (0.5%) and also vary with season, year, and geographical location. They are higher in crowded living conditions. *S. pyogenes* can persist for months after acute pharyngitis, though in decreased numbers. Survival in the environment is poor and *S. pyogenes* can only survive on skin and inanimate objects for a limited period of time.

Pathogenicity, virulence, and typing

S. pyogenes is an extracellular pathogen and produces virulence factors that enable it to avoid host defences and spread in tissues. An important virulence factor is the M protein and streptococci rich in M protein resist phagocytosis by granulocytes. Immunity to *S. pyogenes* infection is associated with the development of opsonic antibodies to antiphagocytic epitopes of M protein; the immunity is usually type specific and lasts for many years. M protein was first described in the 1920s by Rebecca Lancefield; over 100 M types have now been differentiated. Lancefield also developed the supplementary T typing system which distinguishes 26 serotypes of a trypsin-resistant surface protein (T antigen), most of which can be expressed by several different M types. Certain M types also produce a serum opacity factor (OF+). These typing systems are still widely used in epidemiological studies to distinguish between strains of *S. pyogenes*. However, more modern methods utilize procedures to sequence the M protein gene. Recent studies have shown considerable genetic diversity in *S. pyogenes*, and horizontal transfer and recombination of virulent genes have played a major role. This finding is likely relevant to the emergence of new unusually virulent clones of the organism.

In addition to M protein, lipoteichoic acid, important in the host–bacterial interaction, is expressed on the surface of the organism and is the adhesin that binds the organism to fibronectin on the surface of the oral epithelial cell membranes and initiates the colonization that precedes infection. *S. pyogenes* has a hyaluronate capsule which, like M protein, is also antiphagocytic, and is an additional virulence factor. The extent of encapsulation varies, and colonies with prominent capsules are very mucoid on blood agar. Strains of *S. pyogenes* that are both rich in M protein and heavily encapsulated are readily transmitted from person to person and have been associated with epidemics of acute rheumatic fever.

S. pyogenes produces many extracellular substances, several of which are important in the pathogenesis of infection. The most familiar are streptolysin O, deoxyribonuclease (DNase) B, and hyaluronidase, as serum antibodies to these provide retrospective confirmation of recent streptococcal infection. Other extracellular products include DNases A, C, and D, streptolysin S, proteinase, streptokinase, and the substances previously known as erythrogenic toxins. These toxins have now been designated streptococcal pyrogenic exotoxins (SPE)-A, -B, -C, and more recently several others. SPE-A and SPE-C are coded by a phage gene and readily transmitted to susceptible strains. These toxins, known as superantigens,

have diverse effects on the host. In addition to the rash of scarlet fever, they cause fever and induce lethal shock in animals. They have profound effects on the immune system including increasing susceptibility to endotoxic shock, induction of cytokine production, and cause clonal proliferation of T lymphocytes.

Recently, nicotine adenine dinucleotidase (NADase) has been found in 100% of strains of group A streptococci (GAS) associated with invasive GAS infections such as toxic shock syndrome and necrotizing fasciitis. There is evidence that the gene for NADase is found in all strains of GAS but only produced extracellularly in these invasive strains. In addition, production of NADase by M1 strains, the most common strain associated with invasive types of infections, began around 1985, just before the recognition of severe invasive GAS infections.

S. pyogenes may penetrate the upper respiratory tract mucosa or a break in the skin causing local infection or may spread along tissue planes or lymphatics. The M protein is not toxic in itself but protects the streptococcus from phagocytosis, and antibodies to the M protein are opsonic. In about two-thirds of patients with serious invasive disease, who may present with fever, shock, and renal impairment, the portal of entry is the skin and infection of soft tissue is apparent, but in others the site of infection may be deep in the fascia or muscle.

Infections caused by S. pyogenes

S. pyogenes causes a variety of illnesses ranging from very common infections such as pharyngitis, impetigo, and cellulitis to less common more severe infections such as puerperal sepsis, necrotizing fasciitis, bacteraemia, and toxic shock. *S. pyogenes* is also associated with the nonsuppurative sequelae of acute rheumatic fever and acute glomerulonephritis.

Streptococcal pharyngitis

Streptococcal pharyngitis or tonsillitis is one of the commonest bacterial infections in children from 5 to 15 years, but all ages are susceptible. The incubation period, at least in outbreaks, is short (1–3 days) and the onset of the infection is marked by the abrupt onset of sore throat and pain on swallowing with malaise, fever, and headache. The signs are redness and oedema of the pharynx, enlarged red tonsils (Fig. 6.2.1) with spots of white exudate, fever, and

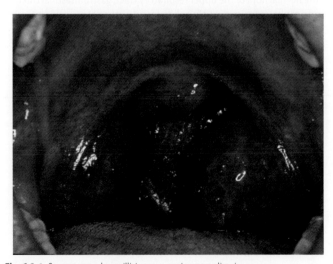

Fig. 6.2.1 Streptococcal tonsillitis: suppurative complications. (Copyright D A Warrell.)

enlarged tender anterior cervical lymph glands. Nausea, vomiting, and abdominal pain are common in children, and in infants and preschool children there may be few definite signs of pharyngitis but fever, nasal discharge, enlarged cervical lymph glands, and otitis media occur.

Direct extension of streptococcal pharyngitis can give rise to acute sinusitis or otitis media, and other suppurative complications include peritonsillar abscess (quinsy), mastoiditis, retropharyngeal abscess, and suppurative cervical lymphadenitis.

Scarlet fever

Scarlet fever results from infection with a strain of *S. pyogenes* that produces SPE (erythrogenic toxin). It is usually associated with streptococcal pharyngitis but may follow streptococcal infections at other sites including surgical site infections. Scarlet fever rarely follows streptococcal pyoderma. Most cases occur in school-age children and the rash must be distinguished from viral exanthems, Kawasaki's disease, and staphylococcal toxic shock syndrome. The rash, which generally appears on the second day of clinical illness, is usually a diffuse erythema, symmetrical, and blanches on pressure. It is seen most often on the neck, chest, folds of the axilla, and groin. Occlusion of sweat glands gives the skin a 'sandpaper' texture, a useful sign in dark-skinned patients. The face appears flushed with circumoral pallor. There are small red haemorrhagic spots on the palate, and the tongue is initially covered with a white fur through which red papillae appear ('strawberry tongue'); after the rash develops, the white fur peels off leaving a raw red papillate surface ('raspberry tongue'). The rash persists for several days and later (up to 3 weeks) peeling (desquamation) may occur, usually on the tips of the fingers, toes, or ears and less often over the trunk and limbs. A similar rash may develop as a reaction to streptokinase thrombolytic therapy.

Streptococcal perianal infection (cellulitis)

This is a superficial well-demarcated rash spreading out from the anus in young children, usually boys, associated with itching, rectal pain on defaecation, and blood-stained stools. *S. pyogenes* is isolated from perianal cultures and usually also from pretreatment throat swabs.

Streptococcal vulvovaginitis

Vulvovaginitis in prepubertal girls is often caused by *S. pyogenes* and presents with serosanguinous discharge and erythema of the labia and vaginal orifice. As with perianal infections, *S. pyogenes* is usually also found in the throat. In both streptococcal perianal infection and vulvovaginitis, more than one child in the family may be affected and nasopharyngeal carriage is likely in both infected and uninfected children.

Streptococcal skin and soft tissue infections

Pyoderma/impetigo Almost any purulent lesion of the skin can yield *S. pyogenes*, sometimes with *Staphylococcus aureus*. Such lesions include impetigo, infected cuts and lacerations, insect bites, scabies, intertrigo, and ecthyma. *S. pyogenes* often causes secondary infection in varicella, occasionally with resultant bacteraemia. The term pyoderma is used synonymously with impetigo for discrete purulent apparently primary infections of the skin that are prevalent in many parts of the world, especially in children. These lesions are initially papules, then vesicular with surrounding erythema, and finally pustules with crusting exudate; they may be localized to one part of the body or generalized. Outbreaks of impetigo can occur

among adults subject to skin trauma, such as rugby football players (scrumpox), and streptococcal infection of cuts on the hands and forearms are an occupational hazard for workers in the meat trade. Epidemics of impetigo can occur in day care centres, prisons, and schools. Ecthyma is an ulcerated form of impetigo in which ulceration extends into the dermis. In recent times, approximately 50% of cases of impetigo are caused by *Staphylococcus aureus*.

Invasive streptococcal infections of skin and soft tissues

Erysipelas This is an acute inflammation of the skin with lymphatic involvement. The streptococci are localized in the dermis and hypodermis. It usually affects the face, particularly in elderly people, but may occur elsewhere. It may be bilateral (Fig. 6.2.2) and is sometimes recurrent. There is generally a history of sore throat, but the mode of spread to the skin is unknown. It is usually accompanied by fever, rigors, and toxicity. The cutaneous lesion begins as a localized area of brilliant erythema and swelling and then spreads with rapidly advancing raised red margins that are well demarcated from adjacent normal tissue. Facial erysipelas begins over the bridge of the nose and spreads over the cheeks. Vesicles and bullae appear, which become crusted when they rupture. There is marked oedema and the eyes are often closed. When the infection resolves it is often followed by desquamation. Intense local allergic reactions to topical agents, such as cosmetics, may cause confusion.

Cellulitis Cellulitis (Fig. 6.2.3) is commonly caused by streptococci and *Staphylococcus aureus*. This is an acute spreading inflammation of the skin and subcutaneous tissues with local pain swelling and erythema. Fever, rigors, and malaise may precede by a few hours the appearance of the skin lesion and associated lymphangitis and tender lymphadenopathy. Streptococcal cellulitis differs from erysipelas in that the lesion is not raised and the demarcation between affected and unaffected skin is indistinct. It may result from infection of burns, mild trauma, or surgical wounds. When this involves the leg, fungal infection of the feet is often present and predisposes to streptococcal invasion. After the first episode, there

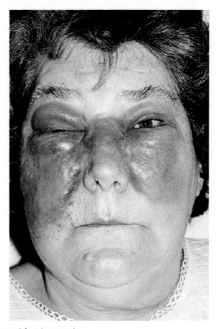

Fig. 6.2.2 Bilateral facial erysipelas.
(Copyright S J Eykyn.)

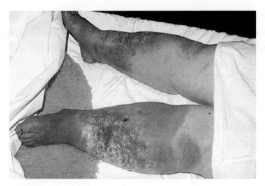

Fig. 6.2.3 Cellulitis.
(Copyright S J Eykyn.)

is a tendency for recurrence in the same area. Recurrences are more common in patients with chronic venous insufficiency, lymphatic obstruction, and at the saphenous vein donor site in patients following coronary bypass surgery. These latter infections are most commonly caused by group C or G streptococci. Intravenous drug users are also at risk of streptococcal cellulitis associated with skin and tissue infection and septic thrombophlebitis.

(Type II) necrotizing fasciitis (streptococcal gangrene) This infection, described by Meleney in 1924, involves the deep subcutaneous tissues and fascia (and occasionally muscle as well) with extensive necrosis and gangrene of the skin and underlying structures. It is generally community-acquired, usually involving the arm or leg, but may also occur after surgery, which can sometimes be quite minor. Some people with this infection are diabetic, but the majority are previously healthy. Risk factors providing a portal of entry include surgery, trauma, childbirth, intravenous drug abuse, and chickenpox. Blunt trauma and muscle strain and the use of nonsteroidal anti-inflammatory agents are also risk factors. The infection begins at the site of trivial or even inapparent trauma with redness, swelling, fever, and rapidly escalating focal pain followed by purple discoloration and the development of bullae, which are often haemorrhagic. In patients who develop infection deeply in traumatized tissue such as muscle, fever and severe pain may be the only initial signs and symptoms of infection. Bacteraemia is often present and within days skin necrosis occurs followed by extensive sloughing. The patient is profoundly ill and the disease has a high case fatality rate of 30 to 70%. Features of streptococcal toxic shock syndrome are associated in many cases. The United Kingdom media memorably dubbed *S. pyogenes* the 'flesh-eater' in reports of a cluster of cases of necrotizing fasciitis in 1994. Treatment involves early intravenous antibiotics. The organisms are sensitive to penicillin but, paradoxically, the drug may not be effective in high concentrations (the 'Eagle effect'). Clindamycin has advantages over penicillin, based on animal studies and one retrospective study in humans. The efficacy of clindamycin is likely due to its ability rapidly to inhibit toxin production by Gram-positive pathogens. Urgent surgical debridement of necrotic tissue and intensive care to support failing organs and systems (e.g. cardiovascular and renal) are extremely important. Benefits of immunoglobulin are suggestive but inconclusive.

Streptococcal toxic shock syndrome

This syndrome was described in 1989 in patients with severe *S. pyogenes* infection and clinical features remarkably similar to those of the staphylococcal toxic shock syndrome described a decade earlier. Streptococcal toxic shock syndrome is defined as any acute *S. pyogenes* infection associated with the sudden onset of shock and multiorgan failure. Streptococcal toxic shock syndrome may be associated with necrotizing fasciitis, myositis, pneumonia, peritonitis, or postpartum sepsis. It can occur at all ages and many of those affected are young and previously healthy. Most cases have been community-acquired, though it can be acquired in hospital. M1 has been the predominant serotype in many countries, though others, especially 3, 4, 6, 11, 12, and 28, have also been implicated. Most strains produce SPE-A. Interestingly there is an amino acid homology of 50% and immunological cross-reactivity between SPE-A and staphylococcal enterotoxins B and C, which together with staphylococcal toxic shock syndrome toxin-1 are relevant in nonmenstrual staphylococcal toxic shock syndrome. Diffuse scarlatina type rash is present in only 5 to 10% of cases (Fig. 6.2.4).

Streptococcal bacteraemia

In parallel with the increase in serious *S. pyogenes* infections, there has been an increase in bacteraemic infections, both community- and hospital-acquired (usually postoperative) (Fig. 6.2.5). While many patients have an underlying disease, generally malignancy, immunosuppression, or diabetes, others are previously healthy adults between 20 and 50 years old. The portal of entry is usually the skin. The mortality is higher in patients with underlying disease, those with necrotizing fasciitis, myositis, pneumonia, or postpartum sepsis, and the very young or old.

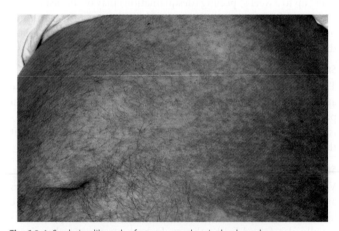

Fig. 6.2.4 Scarlatina-like rash of streptococcal toxic shock syndrome.
(Copyright D A Warrell.)

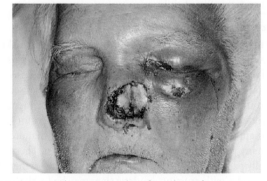

Fig. 6.2.5 *S. pyogenes* bacteraemia 3 days after a skin graft.
(Copyright S J Eykyn.)

Puerperal and neonatal infection

Historically *S. pyogenes* has always been an important cause of puerperal sepsis ('childbed fever'). However, in the postantibiotic era, it was rarely encountered in obstetric practice until the 1980s when sporadic cases occurred, some with streptococcal toxic shock syndrome, and some women have died. These infections follow abortion or delivery when streptococci (usually colonizing the patient herself) invade the endometrium, lymphatics, and bloodstream. They can be devastatingly severe and present with nonspecific signs such as restlessness and gastrointestinal upset that may not immediately suggest sepsis. Fever may be absent resulting in further diagnostic confusion. The streptococcal infection involves the uterus and adnexa and sometimes distant sites such as joints as well. It can also affect the baby, causing serious neonatal infection including meningitis. Instrumentation in the presence of asymptomatic vaginal or anorectal carriage of *S. pyogenes* can result in severe infection. Small epidemics of puerperal sepsis have been reported where a health care provider has been a carrier that caused infection.

Other infections

S. pyogenes can cause pneumonia (usually associated with viral infection or pulmonary disease), osteomyelitis, septic arthritis, meningitis, pericarditis (Fig. 6.2.6), endophthalmitis, and endocarditis.

Laboratory diagnosis of *S. pyogenes* infection

S. pyogenes is easy to culture in the laboratory and usually grows on blood agar in 24 h in atmospheres containing 10% CO_2. Throat swabs must be taken before antibiotics are given or the chance of recovery is greatly reduced. Kits for the detection of the group A antigen directly from throat swabs are available and give few false-positive reactions; they are seldom used in the United Kingdom but are commonly used in the United States of America. Ideally, two swabs are obtained. One is used for the rapid test and, if negative, the other is cultured appropriately. Even trivial

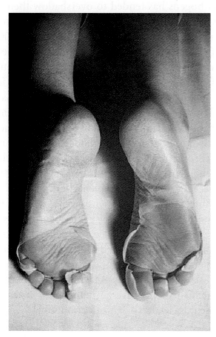

Fig. 6.2.6 Peeling of the skin of the soles of the feet in a patient with *S. pyogenes* pericarditis.
(Copyright S J Eykyn.)

skin lesions such as impetigo or surgical site infection are worth swabbing (if necessary with a moistened swab). Swabs from the surface of cellulitis and erysipelas rarely yield streptococci, although they may be recovered from specimens obtained by aspiration approximately 20% of the time, although this is seldom carried out. Blood cultures should be done in any patient who is ill whether febrile or not. Serological confirmation of infection with *S. pyogenes* when the organism has not been isolated can be obtained by the detection of raised antibodies to its extracellular products. Most laboratories tend to use two or more tests. Interpretation requires knowledge of the level of titres in the community for those without a history of recent streptococcal infection. In the United Kingdom the upper limit of titres in teenagers and young adults without such a history is antistreptolysin O (ASO) 200, antideoxyribonuclease B (ADB) 240, and antihyaluronidase (AHT) 128.

Management and antibiotic treatment of *S. pyogenes* infection

Remarkably, *S. pyogenes* remains exquisitely sensitive to penicillin and this is the antibiotic of choice for treatment, parenterally for severe infections and orally otherwise. Conventionally, 10 days treatment is recommended for pharyngeal infections to eradicate the organism and prevent acute rheumatic fever. In practice, compliance with this regimen is poor as once the symptoms abate there is a natural reluctance to continue the antibiotic. Treatment of patients allergic to penicillin is usually with erythromycin or the newer macrolides (azithromycin and clarithromycin), but some 3 to 5% of strains are erythromycin resistant in most of the Western world. Epidemics caused by erythromycin-resistant strains have been described in Japan, Finland, Sweden, and the United States of America. *S. pyogenes* is also sensitive to cephalosporins. Topical agents such as mupirocin and fusidic acid are useful in addition to systemic antibiotic treatment in impetigo and other skin lesions. Patients with streptococcal toxic shock syndrome require intensive care and many require inotropic support, ventilation, and haemodialysis. Urgent surgical intervention is needed for necrotizing fasciitis and myositis. Clindamycin (in addition to penicillin) has been recommended for patients with established invasive streptococcal infections since this drug stops the metabolic activity of the streptococci and thus halts further production of toxin. This is especially relevant in type II necrotizing fasciitis/myositis and streptococcal toxic shock syndrome. Intravenous immunoglobulin has also been used in an attempt to neutralize the streptococcal toxins, but reports of its effects are inconclusive. Prevention of recurrent cellulitis of the lower legs involves meticulous foot hygiene with treatment of tinea pedis (if present) and reduction in skin carriage using topical mupirocin. Oedematous limbs can benefit from elastic stockings. Antibiotic prophylaxis may be required in cases of frequent recurrence refractory to these measures. Lastly it should be remembered that *S. pyogenes* is readily transmitted from person to person and thus appropriate infection control precautions should be taken until swabs show that the organism has been eradicated.

β-Haemolytic group B streptococci (*S. agalactiae*)

The group B streptococcus has been known for over a century as a cause of bovine mastitis, and in the 1930s it was recognized as a vaginal commensal, an occasional cause of puerperal fever, and an uncommon cause of invasive disease in adults. Not until the 1960s was it realized that the group B streptococcus was an important neonatal pathogen, and some 20 years later it had replaced *Escherichia coli* as the predominant neonatal pathogen. Group B streptococcus can also cause a broad range of infections in nonpregnant adults including skin and soft tissue infections, bacteraemia, urinary tract infections, bone and joint infections, endocarditis, and meningitis.

Carriage

Group B streptococci can be recovered from various sites in healthy adults but vaginal carriage has been most extensively investigated. Swabs from the lower vagina are more often positive than cervical swabs and carriage rates of 3% to over 40% have been reported. Higher rates have been obtained with selective media and enrichment techniques. Carriage also increases with sexual activity and is highest in women attending genitourinary clinics. The urethra, vagina, perineum, and anorectal region have all been suggested as the prime site of carriage. Approximately 5 to 10% of healthy adults carry group B streptococci in the throat, independent of urogenital and anorectal carriage.

Pathogenicity, virulence, and typing

The chief determinant of virulence appears to be the capsular polysaccharide, and most human strains carry one of six sialic acid-containing polysaccharides that surround the cell wall. In addition, a protein antigen (c, X, or R) may be carried. Certain combinations are common; serotypes III or III/R form one-quarter of all isolates from superficial sites on women, but three-quarters of all group B streptococci causing meningitis in infants. They are also the commonest serotypes found in adult (nonpregnant) infections. The type polysaccharide, like the M protein of *S. pyogenes*, inhibits phagocytosis. Colonization of the mucous membranes of the neonate results from vertical transmission of the organism from the mother either *in utero* by the ascending route or at delivery. The rate of vertical transmission in neonates born to mothers colonized with group B streptococci is about 50%, but the incidence of symptomatic infection in neonates born to colonized mothers is only about 1 to 2%. It is much higher in preterm infants. Nosocomial colonization of neonates can also occur. In most cases of adult infections (other than in pregnant women) the source of the infection is unknown.

Infections caused by group B streptococci

These are commonly neonatal or puerperal infections, but group B streptococci also cause infection in nonpregnant adults.

Neonatal infection

The frequency of neonatal infection (bacteraemia, meningitis, or both) has been variously quoted as between 0.3 and 5.4 cases/1000 live births, but these figures have wide confidence limits. Two fairly distinct clinical patterns of disease predominate, but the spectrum is wide and includes impetigo neonatorum, septic arthritis, osteomyelitis, pneumonitis, peritonitis, pyelonephritis, facial cellulitis, conjunctivitis, and endophthalmitis.

Early-onset disease Symptoms of group B streptococcus (GBS) disease develop within the first 6 days of life with a mean of 20 h, although they can present at birth suggesting an intrauterine onset of infection. Early-onset disease usually presents with bacteraemia with no identifiable focus of infection, but can also be pneumonia or, infrequently, meningitis. The presenting signs include lethargy, poor feeding, jaundice, grunting respirations, pallor, and hypotension and they are common to all types of disease. Respiratory symptoms are nearly always present. The only reliable way of

detecting meningitis is by lumbar puncture. Mortality rates are high in low birth weight babies. In addition to positive blood cultures, the infecting strain can be found in the mother's vagina and cultured from 'screening' sites on the baby; these include ear, throat, and nasogastric aspirate.

Late-onset disease Late-onset GBS disease usually presents between 7 days and 3 months after birth, often in previously healthy babies born after a normal labour who are admitted unwell from home. The pathogenesis is less clear than in cases of early-onset disease and only about one-half of these cases are associated with mucosal colonization during delivery. Most babies have meningitis and concomitant bacteraemia and present with nonspecific symptoms such as lethargy, poor feeding, irritability, and fever. Neurological sequelae are common among survivors.

Late, late-onset disease This is also called very-late-onset or GBS beyond early infancy. It occurs in infants more than 3 months of age and is more common in babies born before 28 weeks' gestation or in those with underlying immunodeficiency.

Puerperal infection

Puerperal infection with group B streptococci usually occurs within 24 to 48 h of delivery or abortion. The source of the organism is always the vagina and infection is more likely when there has been premature rupture of the membranes and chorioamnionitis. Most infections are endometritis with fever and uterine tenderness sometimes associated with retained products of conception, but group B streptococci can also cause wound infection after caesarean section. Bacteraemia is common. Other bacteria, both aerobes and anaerobes, are sometimes isolated from the genital tract and wounds in addition to the group B streptococcus. Very rarely the streptococcus may spread to other sites in puerperal women.

Infection in nonpregnant adults

The prominence given to group B streptococci as neonatal and puerperal pathogens has tended to overshadow their importance in men and nonpregnant women in whom they cause significant morbidity and mortality. The incidence is 4 to 7 per 100 000 population although rates as high as 26 per 100 000 have been reported in those aged over 65 years. In view of the reductions in GBS infection seen in pregnant women and infants, infection in nonpregnant adults now account for three-quarters of invasive disease. Most infections are community-acquired, occur in middle-aged and elderly people, and are as common in men as women. Risk factors for invasive infection include diabetes mellitus, malignancy, alcoholism, chronic renal or liver disease, cardiovascular disease, collagen vascular diseases, and trauma. Skin and soft tissue infections are especially common in patients with diabetes. Occasional urinary tract infections occur, in men as well as women. Bacteraemic infections serve to emphasize the virulence of group B streptococci, and they have increased in incidence, or perhaps have been increasingly recognized, since the early 1990s. Other clinical manifestations include endocarditis, vertebral osteomyelitis, septic arthritis, endophthalmitis, and meningitis. As with staphylococcal infections, some bacteraemic patients have more than one metastatic focus of infection, which can lead to diagnostic confusion.

Laboratory diagnosis of group B streptococcal infection

Group B streptococci are readily isolated from any clinical specimen in the laboratory and easily identified by Lancefield grouping.

The group B antigen is not shared by any other streptococcus. Importantly the antigen can be reliably detected in fluids such as blood, urine, or cerebrospinal fluid by latex particle agglutination enabling a rapid diagnosis.

Treatment of group B streptococcal infection

Group B streptococci are sensitive to penicillin and this is the antibiotic of choice for treatment. They are rather less sensitive to penicillin than *S. pyogenes* with minimum inhibitory concentrations some fourfold to tenfold higher. For this reason penicillin is sometimes combined with gentamicin for meningitis and other serious infections, though this is not of proven benefit. Certainly, the maximum recommended dose of parenteral penicillin should be given whether combined with gentamicin or not. Penicillin allergy is not likely to be an issue in neonates; adults with meningitis can be treated with chloramphenicol. Most group B streptococci are sensitive to erythromycin and they are sensitive to cephalosporins.

Prevention of neonatal infection with group B streptococci
Intrapartum antibiotic prophylaxis

Risk factors for early-onset GBS disease include: delivery at less than 37 weeks' gestation; premature rupture of membranes; prolonger rupture of membranes (>18 h before delivery); chorioamionitis; GBS bacteriuria during pregnancy; temperature >38°C during labour); sustained intrapartum fetal tachycardia; previous infant with GBS disease. These factors have been used to develop guidelines for the prevention of early-onset GBS disease. The United States Centers for Disease Control recommends screening of pregnant women by culture at 35 to 37 weeks' gestation and intrapartum antibiotic prophylaxis for women found to be colonized with GBS. This has resulted in a dramatic decline in the incidence of early-onset GBS disease from 1.8 to 0.28 cases per 1000 live births between 1990 and 2008. In contrast the United Kingdom Royal College of Gynaecologists advocates a risk-factor based approach, as there are no clinical trial data to support routine antibiotic prophylaxis and concerns related to antibiotic use. Recent analyses, however, suggest that culture-based screening may be more cost effective than the current risk factor based strategy.

Vaccination

The capsular polysaccharide antigens (Ia, Ib, II, III, IV, V, VI, and VIII) and C surface proteins of GBS have long been recognized to generate protective antibody responses. Analysis of genome sequences from GBS strains has identified a number of antigens and proteins that could potentially be used as vaccine candidates and some of these are in clinical trials.

β-Haemolytic groups C and G streptococci

These streptococci are sometimes referred to as 'large colony-forming group C and G streptococci' to distinguish them from the small colony-forming strains of streptococci with the same Lancefield antigens that belong to the anginosus or milleri group (see below). Groups C and G streptococci are closely related genetically. They are most conveniently regarded as 'pyogenes-like' as the infections they cause are similar to those caused by *S. pyogenes* though these streptococci tend to be less virulent than *S. pyogenes*. Infections with these streptococci are less common than *S. pyogenes* infections. Although poststreptococcal glomerulonephritis has been associated with pharyngitis caused by both groups C and G streptococci, acute rheumatic fever has not.

Group C streptococci are less frequently encountered in human infections than group G and most group C infections are caused by *Streptococcus dysgalactiae* subsp. *equisilmilis*. Those caused by *Streptococcus dysgalactiae* subsp. *zooepidemicus* have an animal source. Animal infections include mastitis in cows and 'strangles' in horses. Risk factors for infection with group C and G streptococci include: advanced age; underlying medical condition (e.g. diabetes mellitus, cardiovascular disease, cirrhosis, alcoholism, bone and joint disease, skin conditions); immunocompromise (e.g. malignancy, immunosuppressive drugs, HIV infection); surgical procedures; animal exposure. Clinical manifestations include pharyngitis, cellulitis, septic arthritis, bacteraemia, endocarditis, and a wide range of other infections.

Streptococci of the anginosus or milleri group

This group of streptococci has been a source of considerable taxonomic confusion, partly as a result of a lack of international consensus on nomenclature but also because of a lack of reliable phenotypic differences between taxa within the group. Most clinicians are familiar with the organism they know as 'Streptococcus milleri'. There are three species of milleri streptococci, *S. anginosus*, *S. constellatus*, and *S. intermedius*, but despite increasing awareness of the clinical significance of the milleri group little is known about the association between individual species and specific sites of isolation and diseases. These streptococci are found in large numbers in the normal flora of the upper respiratory tract, gastrointestinal tract, and genital tract, and are commonly isolated from a range of pyogenic infections, sometimes in pure culture but often with other organisms, particularly anaerobes. These infections include dental abscesses, intra-abdominal abscesses (especially of the liver), subphrenic abscesses, lung abscesses and empyema, and brain abscesses. Such is the propensity of these organisms to cause deep-seated abscesses that isolation of a milleri streptococcus from a blood culture should prompt investigations to detect such a focus. Milleri streptococci are also commonly isolated from inflamed appendices and postappendicectomy wound infection. Unlike other viridans and nonhaemolytic streptococci, milleri streptococci seldom cause endocarditis. They form minute colonies on blood agar and are preferentially anaerobic on primary isolation. They may be α-, β-, or non-haemolytic. Some have the Lancefield antigens A, C, G, or F. All group F streptococci are milleri group whereas not all milleri streptococci are group F. Another useful clue to their identity in the laboratory is the distinct caramel smell of many strains on blood agar, the result of the diacetyl metabolite. Most strains are very sensitive to penicillin.

Streptococci of the mitis, salivarius, and mutans groups (oral/viridans streptococci)

This group of usually α-haemolytic (viridans) streptococci includes *S. pneumoniae* and those oral streptococci (*S. mitis*, *S. oralis*, *S. sanguis*, *S. gordonii*, and, rarely, *S. salivarius*) that are the commonest cause of infective endocarditis of oral or dental origin. These streptococci occasionally cause bacteraemia in neutropenic patients, who sometimes have detectable mouth lesions, and neonatal infection, as they are found as part of the normal vaginal flora. These infections should be suspected in neutropenic patients who have received prophylaxis with fluoroquinolones such as ciprofloxacin.

Streptococci of the bovis group

Although this group comprises at least three species, *S. bovis* is the main species of medical importance. *S. bovis* is similar to the enterococci in that it bears the Lancefield group D antigen and is a gastrointestinal commensal, but, unlike the enterococci, it is sensitive to penicillin. It can be misidentified in the laboratory either as an oral streptococcus or as an enterococcus. Most patients with *S. bovis* bacteraemia will have endocarditis and it is seldom isolated from other sites. It is important to recognize *S. bovis* in a blood culture as the organism is associated with colonic pathology or liver cirrhosis, and patients should be specifically investigated for these.

Nutritionally variant organisms previously classified as streptococci, now *Abiotrophia* spp.

These organisms, which occasionally cause endocarditis, require pyridoxal or thiol group supplementation for growth in the laboratory and tend to form satellite colonies surrounding colonies of *Staphylococcus aureus*. Although most blood culture media will support their growth, successful subculture requires supplementation or cross-streaking of the plates with *Staphylococcus aureus* to provide the necessary growth factors. The *Abiotrophia* include three species, *S. adjacens*, *S. defectivus*, and the recently described *A. elegans*. They are less susceptible to penicillin than other streptococci.

Streptococcus suis

This streptococcus, which can be misidentified in the laboratory as *S. bovis* or an enterococcus as it reacts with group D antiserum, is an important pathogen of young pigs causing meningitis, septicaemia, arthritis, pneumonia, and endocarditis and is also carried in the pharynx of healthy pigs. *S. suis* type II (also referred to as group R streptococci) is not only the most invasive type in pigs, it can cause serious infection—mainly septicaemia and meningitis, but also septic arthritis, pneumonia, and endophthalmitis—in humans, in whom it is an occupational disease of pig farmers, abattoir workers, and factory workers handling pig meat (Fig. 6.2.7) (see Oxford Textbook of Medicine 5e Chapter 24.11.1). The streptococcus probably enters the bloodstream via skin abrasions that are common in the above occupations. *S. suis* type II meningitis results in deafness in about one-half of those affected.

Enterococci

Enterococci are Lancefield group D, Gram-positive cocci that can grow and survive in extreme cultural conditions, and are also more resistant to antibiotics than streptococci. They form part of the normal gut flora of humans and animals. Overall, the commonest clinical isolates of enterococci are *Enterococcus faecalis*, but the

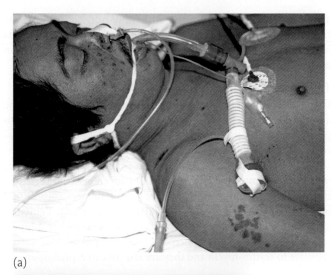

(a)

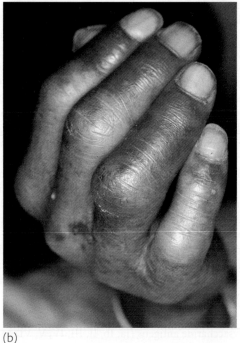

(b)

Fig. 6.2.7 (a) *S. suis* septicaemia with meningitis in a Vietnamese pig farmer. (b) *S. suis* pyogenic arthritis in a Thai abattoir worker. (a) (Copyright D A Warrell.) (b) (Courtesy of the late Professor Prida Phuapradit.)

more antibiotic-resistant species *E. faecium* is increasingly encountered in hospitals. Nosocomial isolates of enterococci have dramatically increased in the 1990s. Other species, including *E. casseliflavus*, *E. durans*, and *E. avium*, are occasionally isolated. In most cases it is unnecessary to determine the species of enterococci in a clinical laboratory but sometimes differentiation between *E. faecalis* and *E. faecium* is helpful, e.g. in epidemiological studies and in endocarditis because of their different antibiotic susceptibilities.

Infections caused by enterococci

Enterococci are an increasingly important cause of nosocomial infection and colonization, possibly as a result of the large-scale use of antibiotics such as cephalosporins and quinolones to which they are inherently resistant. They occasionally cause community-acquired urinary tract infections but the most important community-acquired infection is endocarditis, which is increasing in incidence. This infection is almost always caused by *E. faecalis*. Any patient admitted from the community with *E. faecalis* in blood cultures should be assumed to have endocarditis until proved otherwise. Enterococci are predominantly hospital pathogens and cause urinary infection, particularly after instrumentation, intra-abdominal infections, wound infections (usually with other organisms), infections associated with intravascular devices and dialysis, and occasionally endocarditis.

Antibiotic sensitivity and treatment

Enterococci are not only intrinsically resistant to many antibiotics, they show a remarkable ability to acquire new mechanisms of resistance. This allows them to survive in environments in which large quantities of antibiotics are used and also has important therapeutic consequences, particularly for the treatment of endocarditis and other serious infections. Fortunately many patients from whom enterococci are isolated do not require antibiotic treatment. Sensitive enterococci cannot be killed by ampicillin/amoxicillin alone, although combination with an aminoglycoside is bactericidal (synergy); but many strains now exhibit high-level gentamicin resistance and for them the combination is not bactericidal. *E. faecium* is almost always resistant to ampicillin/amoxicillin and *E. faecalis* is occasionally. The first published report of vancomycin-resistant enterococci (VRE) was in 1988 from a London hospital outbreak, though such strains had been recognized a year before in Paris. Most strains of VRE in the London outbreak were *E. faecium* and overall most VRE are *E. faecium*. There are four recognized phenotypes of vancomycin resistance; the first isolates of VRE were highly resistant to vancomycin and teicoplanin and exhibit what is known as the VanA resistance phenotype. Since then, levels of resistance to teicoplanin in this phenotype have been more varied. Most VanA enterococci are *E. faecium*, but this phenotype also occurs in *E. faecalis* and occasionally in other species. The VanB phenotype is associated with low-level vancomycin resistance and sensitivity to teicoplanin and is found in both *E. faecalis* and *E. faecium*. Both VanA and VanB are acquired traits. The VanC phenotype is an intrinsic property of *E. casseliflavus* and *E. gallinarum* and these species have low-level resistance to vancomycin but are sensitive to teicoplanin. A fourth phenotype, VanD, has been described in a single strain of *E. faecium*. Vancomycin-resistant *E. faecium*, though not vancomycin-resistant *E. faecalis*, is sensitive to quinupristin/dalfopristin and all VRE are sensitive to the oxazolidinone linezolid.

The antibiotic susceptibilities of the enterococci outlined above serve to emphasize that these bacteria are the most antibiotic-resistant Gram-positive bacteria now encountered in hospital practice. Fortunately many, perhaps most, of the patients from whom they are isolated do not require antibiotic treatment at all, but for those who do, the effective treatment of serious infection caused by enterococci and particularly antibiotic-resistant strains requires microbiological expertise.

Further reading

Bisno AL, Stevens DL (2000). *Streptococcus pyogenes* (including streptococcal toxic shock syndrome and necrotizing fasciitis). In: Mandell GL, Bennett JE, Dolin R (eds) *Principles and practice of infectious diseases*, pp. 2101–17. Churchill Livingstone, New York.

Bisno AL, Brito MO, Collins CM (2003). Molecular basis of group A streptococcal virulence. *Lancet*, **3**, 191–200.

Colman G, et al. (1993). The serotypes of *Streptococcus pyogenes* present in Britain during 1980 to 1990 and their association with disease. *J Med Microbiol*, **39**, 165–78.

Edwards MS, Baker CJ (2000). *Streptococcus agalactiae* (group B streptococcus). In: Mandell GL, Bennett JE, Dolin R (eds) *Principles and practice of infectious diseases*, pp. 2156–67. Churchill Livingstone, New York.

Jacobs JA (1997). The 'streptococcus milleri' group: *Streptococcus anginosus*, *Streptococcus constellatus* and *Streptococcus intermedius*. *Rev Med Microbiol*, **8**, 73–80.

Katz AR, Morens D (1992). Severe streptococcal infections in historical perspective. *Clin Infect Dis*, **14**, 298–307.

Murray BE (1990). The life and times of the *Enterococcus*. *Clin Microbiol Rev*, **3**, 46–65.

Royal College of Obstetricians and Gynaecologists (2003). *Green Top Guideline 36. Prevention of early onset neonatal group B streptococcal diseases*. http://www.rcog.org.uk/files/rcog-corp/uploaded-files/GT36GroupBStrep2003.pdf Accessed 1 January 2012.

Stevens DL (1992). Invasive group A streptococcus infections. *Clin Infect Dis*, **14**, 2–13.

Stevens DL (1995). Streptococcal toxic shock syndrome: spectrum of disease, pathogenesis and new concepts of treatment. *Emerg Infect Dis*, **1**, 69–78.

Stevens DL (2004). Streptococcal infections. In: Goldman L, Ausiello D (eds) *Cecil textbook of medicine*, 22nd edition, pp. 1782–7. Saunders, Philadelphia.

Stevens DL, et al. (2000). Molecular epidemiology of *nga* and NAD glucohydrolase/ADP-ribosyltransferase activity among *Streptococcus pyogenes* causing streptococcal toxic shock syndrome. *J Infect Dis*, **182**, 1117–28.

Stevens DL, et al. (2005). Practice guidelines for the diagnosis and management of skin and soft-tissue infections. *Clin Infect Dis*, **41**, 1373–1406.

Verani JR, McGee L, Schrag SJ; Division of Bacterial Diseases, National Center for Immunization and Respiratory Diseases, Centers for Disease Control and Prevention (CDC) (2010). Prevention of perinatal group B streptococcal disease—revised guidelines from CDC. *MMWR Recomm Rep*, 59(RR-10), 1–36.

Woodford N (1998). Glycopeptide-resistant enterococci: a decade of experience. *J Med Microbiol*, **47**, 849–62.

6.3 Pneumococcal infections

Anthony Scott

Essentials

Streptococcus pneumoniae is an encapsulated Gram-positive bacterium that lives almost exclusively in the human nasopharynx. Each pneumococcus expresses one or more than 90 immunologically distinguishable capsular polysaccharides that are the principal target of systemic human immunity and define its serotype.

Epidemiology

Pneumococci are transmitted through contact with infected nasal secretions or by airborne dissemination, and most preschool children carry them in their nasopharynx. The risk of acquisition is increased by contact with other children, crowded environments, and cold weather. The incidence of pneumococcal disease is highest in young children and elderly people, and also increased in males, certain indigenous populations, smokers, alcoholics, and patients with chronic medical illnesses or immune susceptibility, including HIV infection, sickle cell disease, and splenectomy.

Clinical features

Pneumonia—pneumococci are the commonest cause of severe community-acquired pneumonia at all ages in the developed and developing world. Typical presentation of pneumococcal lobar pneumonia is with abrupt onset of fever, followed by cough, difficulty breathing, pleuritic chest pain, haemoptysis, and purulent sputum. Physical signs include high pyrexia, raised respiratory rate, cyanosis, and chest features of lobar consolidation, namely reduced chest movement, dullness on percussion, fine crepitations, and bronchial breathing over the affected area. The chest radiograph shows a lobar opacity, often with a pleural effusion.

Other diseases—pneumococci cause significant morbidity in adults and children through meningitis and septicaemia, and they can also cause bronchopneumonia and multiple disease syndromes simultaneously (e.g. meningitis and pneumonia). In children, the most common pneumococcal disease is otitis media. Other less common presentations include sinusitis, pleural empyema, pericarditis, endocarditis, septic arthritis, osteomyelitis, peritonitis, and conjunctivitis.

Diagnosis

S. pneumoniae is a fastidious organism that grows successfully on blood agar, producing α-haemolysis. Blood culture is the principal aetiological tool to diagnose pneumococcal pneumonia, but cultures are positive in only 15 to 30% of cases. The capsular serotype is identified by a positive Quellung reaction with specific rabbit antisera. In addition: (1) pneumococci can be observed on microscopy as Gram-positive diplococci in sputum or, in cases of meningitis, in cerebrospinal fluid, and can be cultured from both specimens; (2) a urinary antigen test for the common pneumococcal constituent C-polysaccharide is sensitive and specific for pneumococcal pneumonia in adults, but not in children; (3) PCR is useful in cerebrospinal fluid, especially when the patient is partially treated and cultures are sterile.

Treatment and prognosis

Most pneumococci are sensitive to β-lactam antibiotics, but some are resistant. (1) Pneumonia—when caused by sensitive or intermediately resistant pneumococci, this should be treated with high-dose oral amoxicillin or intravenous cefotaxime, the latter being effective against pneumococci with cephalosporin MICs up to 1 to 2 μg/ml. Macrolides and newer fluoroquinolones may be used to treat infections that are fully resistant to β-lactam antibiotics. (2) Meningitis—when caused by susceptible pneumococci, ceftriaxone is effective; vancomycin should be added as empirical meningitis therapy in areas with penicillin-resistant pneumococci; dexamethasone

is an effective adjunctive treatment for pneumococcal meningitis where HIV prevalence is low.

The case fatality of pneumococcal pneumonia is 5%, but in bacteraemic pneumonia and pneumococcal meningitis it is 30%.

Prevention

A single dose of 23-valent capsular polysaccharide vaccine prevents invasive pneumococcal disease in elderly or high-risk populations. In infants and young children, 10- or 13-valent pneumococcal conjugate vaccine is highly effective in preventing invasive pneumococcal disease as well as pneumococcal pneumonia, meningitis and otitis media. It is given routinely as two or three doses in infancy, with a booster dose at 12 to 15 months of age. Immunization of children reduces pneumococcal transmission and prevents pneumococcal disease in older family members.

Introduction

Streptococcus pneumoniae (the pneumococcus) is an ubiquitous yet potentially fatal human pathogen. Its only viable habitat is the human nasopharynx. Throughout the world, most children and a significant minority of adults carry it at any one time. Most people are exposed to the pneumococcus several times a year but only rarely does this result in illness. When it invades it causes a diverse range of disease syndromes of which pneumonia, meningitis, and septicaemia have high case fatalities, and yet its most common disease manifestation, otitis media, is relatively benign. In old age it affects the healthy, but throughout life it is a burden to those with chronic medical illnesses. Pneumococcal disease is common in temperate and tropical climates; however, because the pneumococcus is fastidious in culture, it is rarely identified and the disease burden is frequently underestimated. Its differentiation into more than 90 serotypes indicates the complexity of its immunological interaction with humans and its need for adaptability in this long-enduring host–pathogen relationship. Microbiologists and physicians have regarded the pneumococcus as a formidable opponent for over 125 years. They have fought it with antibiotics and, more recently, with efficacious vaccines, each of which renders its nasopharyngeal niche a hostile home. Yet, through its capacity to combine DNA from other bacteria into its own chromosome, it has evolved and survived. It has all the fascination of the esoteric, yet a busy doctor will not pass a week in practice without seeing a case.

Historical perspective

S. pneumoniae is a Gram-positive bacterium described historically as *Diplococcus pneumoniae* because of its tendency to appear microscopically in pairs. It was first isolated in 1881 by Sternberg in the United States of America and, simultaneously, by Pasteur in France through experiments inoculating the saliva of a patient dying of rabies into rabbits. Serotypes of pneumococcus are defined by the rabbit immune response to its variable capsular polysaccharide. In 1910, Neufeld and Händel described two serotypes; by 2010, more than 90 serotypes had been defined.

Convalescent sera from surviving pneumonia patients were shown to be protective against pneumococcal disease in rabbit models in 1891. The protective substance was identified as homologous anticapsular antibody and this underpinned the development of serum therapy in the early years of the 20th century. Although successful, serum therapy required knowledge of the serotype of the infecting pneumococcus, usually determined from sputum or lung aspirate cultures, leading to a delay in treatment. With the introduction of sulphonamide antibiotics in 1938, serum therapy was abandoned.

Antibiotic chemotherapy has been the mainstay of management of pneumococcal disease ever since, but the rapid evolution of resistant strains in the 1990s reactivated interest in vaccine development. A polyvalent capsular polysaccharide vaccine had been shown to protect South African miners from putative pneumococcal pneumonia in 1976. It was poorly immunogenic in infants, among whom most episodes of pneumococcal disease occur, but conjugation of the polysaccharide to immunogenic proteins overcame this limitation and a pneumococcal conjugate vaccine (PCV) against seven serotypes was introduced into the childhood immunization programme in the United States of America in 2000.

In 1928, Griffith inoculated rabbits with a suspension of live avirulent unencapsulated pneumococci and heat-killed serotype 3 pneumococci. The rabbits subsequently succumbed to serotype 3 septicaemia. The avirulent isolate was derived from a serotype 2 strain suggesting that it acquired the type 3 capsule, and virulence, from the heat-killed organisms. In 1944, Avery isolated and purified the 'active principle' that brought about this transformation and characterized it chemically as DNA. The sequence of the pneumococcal genome was first described in 2000 and numerous strains have now been fully annotated. These sequences have been used to identify conserved surface-expressed proteins that may serve as antigens in noncapsular vaccines. Comparison of the genome sequences of 240 strains from a multidrug-resistant lineage spanning 1984–2008 revealed 700 recombinations. This has illustrated the dominance of recombination in determining the survival of the pathogen in a period of significant pressure from antibiotics and capsule-specific vaccines.

Epidemiology

Incidence

Throughout the world, the risk of pneumococcal disease is highest in infancy and declines throughout the first 5 years of life. The lowest risk is in older children and young adults and from the age of 50 years onwards disease risk rises progressively (Fig. 6.3.1).

Among children older than 5 years, the incidence of culture-proven pneumococcal disease was 70 to 100 per 100 000 population in the United States of America before vaccine introduction; in Africa it is 110 to 430 per 100 000 population. In developed countries, the incidence is 15 to 20 per 100 000 population among adults of all ages and at least 50 per 100 000 population among adults aged 65 or over. There are no measurements from developing countries, although some estimate can be extrapolated from studies of indigenous peoples living in developed countries. Native Australians and Alaskans and White Mountain Apaches have incidence rates of 200 to 1000 per 100 000 population among children, 50 to 180 per 100 000 population among adults 18 to 59 years old, and 120 to 170 per 100 000 population among older adults.

The epidemiology of pneumococcal disease is markedly different in the meningitis belt of West Africa. Here, infants and working-age adults are at highest risk, the disease is strongly associated with the dry season, and the case-fatality rate is greater than 60% among adults aged 40 years or more. Serotype 1 accounts for more than half of all infections and the burden of meningitis caused by pneumococcus, with an incidence of 8 to 12 per 100 000 population, rivals that caused by *Neisseria menigitidis*.

The total burden of pneumococcal disease is frequently underestimated because it is difficult to detect. Studies of 'invasive pneumococcal disease', which rely on cultures of *S. pneumoniae* from specimens of blood, cerebrospinal fluid, and pleural fluid, fail to identify the majority of cases of pneumococcal pneumonia that are not bacteraemic. Lung aspirates obtained by percutaneous fine needle puncture significantly increase the yield of pneumococci from pneumonia cases at all ages but are rarely undertaken. The World Health Organization (WHO) has modelled the incidence of pneumococcal pneumonia, meningitis, and other serious manifestations using global data to derive country-based estimates of

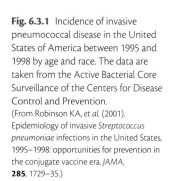

Fig. 6.3.1 Incidence of invasive pneumococcal disease in the United States of America between 1995 and 1998 by age and race. The data are taken from the Active Bacterial Core Surveillance of the Centers for Disease Control and Prevention.
(From Robinson KA, *et al.* (2001). Epidemiology of invasive *Streptococcus pneumoniae* infections in the United States, 1995–1998: opportunities for prevention in the conjugate vaccine era. *JAMA*, **285**, 1729–35.)

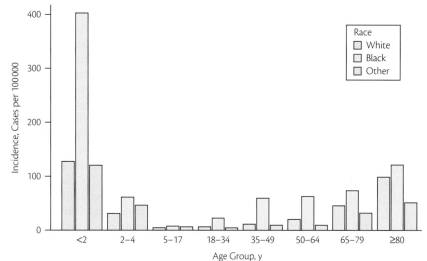

disease burden in children aged less than 5 years. In this estimate, there are more than 14.5 million cases of pneumococcal disease worldwide leading to approximately 26 000 deaths per year. The majority of these deaths take place in Africa and Asia. The global burden of disease in adults is not known.

Carriage, transmission, and serotypes

Viable *S. pneumoniae* have been described in collections of dust and in epizootics of some mammals, but the principal habitat and critical ecological niche of the pneumococcus is the human nasopharynx. Infants can acquire infection within hours of birth and most infants in developing countries become infected in the first 3 months of life. In The Gambia more than 90% of children aged less than 5 years old are colonized by the pneumococcus at any one time. In the United Kingdom, carriage prevalence among children is approximately 50%. Adults also carry *S. pneumoniae* in the nasopharynx but at lower prevalence.

Although the pneumococcus has evolved more than 90 capsular serotypes, 58 to 66% of disease in children is caused by just seven (serotypes 1, 5, 6A, 6B, 14, 19F, and 23F), depending on region. The likelihood that a serotype will cause disease is a function of the prevalence of that type in the nasopharynx and the likelihood of invasion once colonization is established. The ratio of the incidence of invasive disease to the incidence of nasopharyngeal acquisition provides an index of the invasiveness of pneumococcal serotypes and can be used to group them. Serotypes 1, 5, 12F, and 46 are found among series of invasive isolates but are rarely isolated in the nasopharynx. These are labelled 'adult' types because they are associated with disease in adults. Other serotypes, including 10A, 11A, 15B, 15C, 16F, and 33F, are found among series of colonizing isolates but are uncommon causes of disease. A third group, which includes serotypes 6A, 6B, 14, 19A, 19F, and 23F, are found very commonly in the nasopharynx but also cause invasive disease. These are labelled 'paediatric' types because they cause the majority of invasive disease episodes among young children. Serotypes that are highly prevalent in the nasopharynx tend to be less invasive than others but when they do cause disease the case-fatality ratios are higher. Success in colonization is a function of evading the host defences (neutrophil-mediated killing) and outcompeting other serotypes for the ecological niche of the nasopharynx. The capsules of the most successful colonizing serotypes are less biochemically costly, with fewer carbon repeats.

The duration of carriage can be as short as 3 h or as long as 3 years; in most instances it is between 1 and 6 months. It declines with the age of the host, probably as a result of CD4+ T-cell acquired immunity mediated by IL-17A. For some serotypes, circulating anticapsular IgG appears to reduce the acquisition of carriage and vaccine induced anticapsular antibodies are also highly effective in reducing carriage prevalence.

The pneumococcus is transmitted by carriers, particularly preschool children, through direct contact with nasal secretions or by infected fomites. The rapid spread of pneumococcal pneumonia in outbreaks in adults suggests that airborne dissemination, facilitated by cough, is another mechanism of spread.

Risk factors

Risk of pneumococcal disease is a function of exposure to the bacterium, leading to colonization, and of host resistance to invasion. Exposure is increased in crowded environments at home and in institutions (e.g. military barracks, homeless shelters, jails, miners' compounds) and by contact with preschool children. In temperate climates pneumococcal disease follows a consistent seasonal variation with winter peaks and summer troughs. Risk is especially high at New Year when families gather and generations intermingle (Fig. 6.3.2).

Throughout life, males have an incidence of pneumococcal disease 1.2 to 1.5 times greater than females. Chronic medical conditions predispose to pneumococcal invasion (see Box 6.3.1). Alcoholism is consistently associated with pneumococcal disease and may act directly on macrophage function or, like seizure disorders, by compromising laryngeal defences leading to aspiration. HIV infection increases the risk of invasive pneumococcal disease by approximately 50-fold. Where HIV prevalence is greater than 2%, as in much of Africa, most cases of pneumococcal disease occur among HIV-positive patients. Recurrent pneumococcal disease is especially common in this group.

Respiratory viral infections, especially influenza, increase the risk of invasive pneumococcal disease. Influenza enhances the acquisition of pneumococci in the nasopharynx, in animal models, and increases the density of colonization in children. The virus facilitates pneumococcal binding by damaging respiratory epithelial cells and synergy between the two pathogens enhances the action of their separate neuraminidases and stimulates type 1 interferons, impairing macrophage function.

Antibiotic resistance

Epidemiology

Laboratory isolates of penicillin-resistant pneumococci were first reported in 1967 and by the early 1970s they were being isolated in clinical specimens in Australia and Papua New Guinea. During the 1990s, penicillin resistance spread widely throughout the world reaching a prevalence of 35% in several countries (e.g. France, South Africa, Japan, Hong Kong). Pneumococci are classified as either intermediately resistant (minimum inhibitory concentration (MIC) between 0.12 and 1.0 μg/ml) or fully resistant to penicillin (MIC 2 μg/ml and above). In developed countries resistance is dominated by fully resistant isolates whereas the reverse is found in developing countries. Resistance to other antibiotic classes, including macrolides, also increased during the 1990s. The use of long-acting macrolides appears to be responsible for the observed increase in resistance to erythromycin.

Multidrug-resistant pneumococci were first observed in South Africa in 1978. Their presence indicates that the use of one antibiotic can select for resistance against another. Penicillin-resistant strains are transmitted more successfully than penicillin-susceptible strains but multiresistant strains spread most successfully within populations. Much of this spread is driven by the expansion of a small number of clones. In the United States of America, 78% of all resistant isolates are represented by just 12 clonal groups.

In the United Kingdom, antimicrobial prescriptions have fallen since 1995 and at the same time there has been a reduction in both penicillin-resistant and macrolide-resistant pneumococci. Use of 7-valent PCV in the United States of America has resulted in a decrease in penicillin-resistant and multiresistant strains, although continued surveillance has revealed disease caused by new strains of pneumococcus some of which are also resistant. Pneumococcal resistance to fluoroquinolones has increased in prevalence but remains less than 5%.

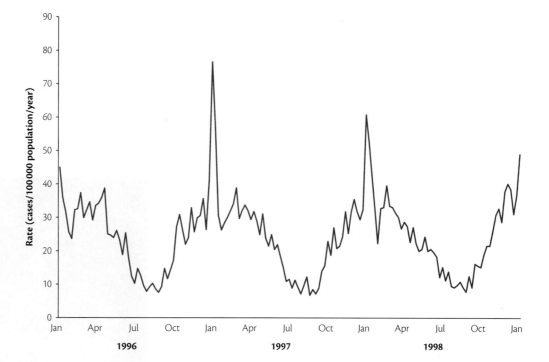

Fig. 6.3.2 Annualized weekly incidence of pneumococcal disease among adults in the United States of America between 1996 and 1998 showing a consistent increase in incidence in the winter and a sharp increase in incidence during the Christmas/New Year holiday season. (From Dowell SF, *et al.* (2003). Seasonal patterns of invasive pneumococcal disease. *Emerg Infect Dis*, **9**, 573–9.)

Box 6.3.1   Risk factors for pneumococcal disease

Social and demographic

- Older age
- Male sex
- Black race
- Indigenous populations
- Lower level of education
- Unemployment
- Excess alcohol use

Exposure to pneumococci

- Contact with preschool children
- Day care attendance[a]
- Crowding in the home
- Crowded adult environments (homeless shelters, military or occupational barracks)
- Institutionalized care
- Winter season
- Hospital admission

Respiratory tract damage

- Currently smoking
- Passive smoking
- Indoor air pollution

- Chronic obstructive pulmonary disease
- Recent viral respiratory tract infection

Preexisting medical conditions

- Chronic renal failure
- Congestive heart failure
- Cirrhosis
- Cerebrovascular disease
- Dementia
- Seizure disorder
- Asthma
- Diabetes
- Malignancies of the lung

Immune susceptibility

- HIV
- Hypogammaglobulinaemia
- Sickle cell disease
- Asplenia/splenectomy
- Pregnancy
- Not breastfeeding[a]
- Previous pneumococcal disease

[a] These apply only to infants or children.

Resistance mechanisms

Pneumococcal resistance to penicillin is entirely due to the accumulation of genetic variations among the six penicillin binding proteins (PBPs) that normally catalyse cross-linkage of the bacterial cell wall. By binding to PBPs, β-lactam antibiotics inhibit cell wall synthesis and promote cell lysis. Resistance to penicillin occurs when a PBP variant arises which has low binding affinity for β-lactams. Sensitive pneumococci have MICs for benzylpenicillin and cefotaxime which are approximately 0.02 µg/ml. Mutations in PBP 2b or 2x genes lead to a 2- to 30-fold increase in MIC. However, isolates that are fully resistant to penicillin usually contain alterations at three PBP genes, 2b, 2x, and 1a. High-level resistance to cefotaxime may be observed with a combination of changes in only two (PBP 2x and 1a).

Resistant strains come about through horizontal transfer and recombination into chromosomal DNA of large sequence blocks of mosaic genes acquired from other streptococci. This transfer may include capsular and resistance genes simultaneously. Pneumococci colonizing the nasopharynx are then exposed to antibiotics, which are commonly prescribed for community-acquired respiratory tract infections, and this selects resistant strains.

Pneumococcal genes *cat*, *erm*(B), and *tet*(M), which confer resistance to chloramphenicol, macrolides, and tetracyclines, respectively, have been found together on DNA elements (conjugative transposons) which spread between pneumococci without involving recombination thus facilitating multidrug resistance. Resistance to fluoroquinolones and trimethoprim/sulfamethoxazole is acquired by point mutations in topoisomerase genes and folate synthesis genes, respectively. Exposure to low levels of antibiotic selects single gene mutants which then acquire higher resistance through additional mutations.

Pathogenesis

Pneumococci exist in two morphologically distinct phenotypes; in the opaque phase they have abundant capsular expression and in the transparent phase they have little. In the nasopharynx, transparent-phase pneumococci predominate as abundant capsule prevents attachment of pneumococcal cell wall structures to epithelial cells. This attachment is mediated by binding of pneumococcal phosphorylcholine and choline binding protein A (CbpA) to human platelet activating factor receptors and polymeric immunoglobulin receptors. Once attached, pneumococci can cause disease by local spread to the middle ear or sinuses, by aerosol inhalation to the lung, or by blood stream invasion to the meninges, joint spaces, or heart valves. Blood stream invasion begins with endocytosis across the mucosal barrier although the components of this pathway are not well understood. In the blood stream pneumococci are found in the opaque phase since capsule is effective in evading opsonophagocytosis.

Pneumococci colonizing the nasopharynx cannot bind to the ciliated epithelium of the bronchi and therefore make their way to the lung in aerosols. However, if the ciliated epithelium is damaged, by antecedent viral infection or by cigarette smoke, it reveals a basement membrane to which pneumococci can adhere easily. Pneumolysin released from pneumococci causes further epithelial damage by direct cytotoxicity and encourages inflammation of the larger bronchioles, which leads to bronchopneumonia.

In the alveoli, pneumococci multiply in serous fluid and spread from one alveolus to another through the pores of Kohn. They adhere to the alveolar type 2 cells, through expression of

CbpA, and stimulate production of the inflammatory mediators tumour necrosis factor-α, nitric oxide, and interleukins IL-1, IL-6, and IL-10, which initiates oedema. This creates the first pathological phase of pulmonary consolidation—engorgement.

In the second phase—red hepatization—erythrocytes leak into the alveolar spaces, reducing the compliance of the lung and leading to a liver-like appearance of the gross lung specimen (Fig. 6.3.3). Fibrin deposition creates a mesh of erythrocytes, leucocytes, and damaged epithelial cells and the lymphatics become dilated with

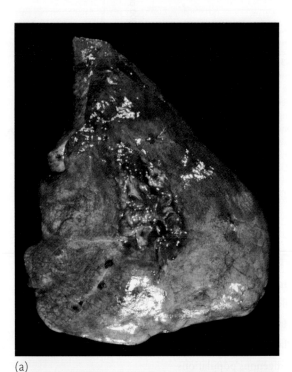

(a)

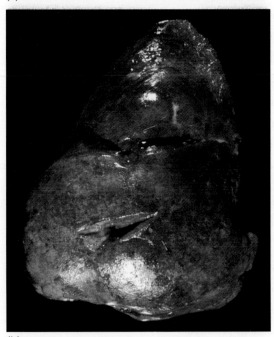

(b)

Fig. 6.3.3 Red hepatization in fatal pneumococcal pneumonia. (Copyright D A Warrell.)

cells and fibrin. Without ventilation, perfusion declines and the lung becomes maximally consolidated.

CbpA binding stimulates epithelial cells to release chemokines that attract leucocytes to the lung which initiates the third phase of consolidation—grey hepatization. Neutrophils trap pneumococci against the alveolar wall and engulf them by surface phagocytosis. C-reactive protein enhances this process by binding to choline residues on pneumococcal surfaces. The chemokines activate complement that, together with anticapsular antibody, facilitates opsonophagocytosis. Thereafter, lung inflammation begins to decline simultaneously with neutrophil apoptosis, fever declines, and macrophages are recruited to the lung to absorb the debris. Over a period of weeks this leads to complete resolution of the pathology.

Immunity to pneumococcal disease

Historically, the role of anticapsular antibody in recovery from pneumonia and the efficacy of serotype-specific serum therapy suggested that anticapsular IgG was the primary mechanism of immunity to pneumococcal disease. The age groups at highest risk of pneumococcal disease, infants and elderly people, have little anticapsular antibody or have antibody that lacks avidity. The genetic diversity of capsular expression into more than 90 variants suggests the antigen is under considerable immune selection and the success of polysaccharide antigens as vaccines further reinforces the importance of anticapsular immunity.

Capsular polysaccharides are complex molecules with repeating epitopes that create cross-linkage of antigen receptors on B lymphocytes and which produce antibodies of the IgM and IgG2 isotypes. Antibody production can occur in the absence of T lymphocytes (T-independent) but it does not induce memory responses and can lead to antigen tolerance following repeated stimulation. Pneumococcal capsular and cell wall components both activate the human complement system leading to deposition of C3b and C3d on capsular polysaccharide. In the presence of both anticapsular antibody and complement, encapsulated pneumococci are opsonized and taken up by phagocytes expressing the receptor Fcγ-RIIa (CD32).

In contrast to natural immunity, conjugates of polysaccharides and highly immunogenic proteins (e.g. diphtheria toxoid) induce T-cell-dependent immunity with a predominance of IgG1 antibody and a memory response. These responses are inducible even in very young infants. Anticapsular antibody responses are measured by IgG enzyme-linked immunosorbent assay (ELISA) and a serum concentration of 0.35 μg/ml correlates with vaccine-induced protection in infancy.

In addition to adaptive immunity, innate mechanisms (e.g. lipoteichoic acid stimulation of Toll-like receptor (TLR) 2, or pneumolysin stimulation of TLR4) appear to be important in shaping the inflammatory response to pneumococcal disease and in determining host survival. Furthermore, several lines of evidence suggest that CD4+ T cells play an important role in nasopharyngeal immunity that could be exploited by vaccines consisting of pneumococcal proteins or even whole cell killed pneumococci.

Prevention

Pneumococcal polysaccharide vaccine

In 1976, Austrian reported a trial of a 13-valent vaccine among South African gold miners in which the efficacy against putative pneumococcal pneumonia was 78%. This led to the commercialization of a pneumococcal polysaccharide vaccine (PPV), initially with 14 serotypes and later extended to 23 serotypes. Trials of PPV in the older people or in high-risk populations do not provide consistent evidence of protection against pneumococcal pneumonia. Observational studies using case-control designs or the indirect cohort method have more consistently indicated protection against bacteraemic pneumococcal disease. The evidence of effect is greater for older people than for those with chronic disease. On the basis of meta-analyses of the observational studies, PPV is recommended in the United Kingdom for all adults aged 65 years or more and for all persons aged 5 or more years who belong to an at-risk group (e.g. with asplenia, splenectomy, chronic respiratory disease, chronic heart, liver or renal disease, diabetes, or immunosuppression, including HIV infection at all stages). Revaccination of elderly people is recommended at 5-year intervals. Among patients having planned splenectomy, vaccination should take place well before the operation. Although PPV is recommended for United Kingdom patients with HIV this remains controversial. In a study of PPV in HIV-positive individuals from Uganda, the vaccinated group had an elevated risk of pneumonia. PPV is not recommended for HIV-positive populations in the developing world.

Pneumococcal conjugate vaccine

A 7-valent PCV, consisting of separate protein–polysaccharide conjugates for serotypes 4, 6B, 9V, 14, 18C, 19F, and 23F, was licensed in the United States of America in 2000 following successful trials in Californian infants and Native American children. The seven serotypes in the vaccine accounted for 83% of invasive disease in American children less than 2 years old. The efficacy against invasive pneumococcal disease caused by these serotypes was 97% after a four-dose schedule given at 2, 4, 6, and 15 months of age. The vaccine was also shown to protect against pneumococcal meningitis, bacteraemia, pneumonia, and otitis media.

PCV reduces nasopharyngeal colonization by pneumococci of the serotypes included in the vaccine and increases colonization by other serotypes commensurately. In routine immunization, this has produced two effects. First, the transmission of vaccine-serotype pneumococci has declined providing 'herd protection' for older children and adults whose pneumococcal disease rates have fallen substantially. Second, the incidence of disease caused by serotypes not included in the vaccine has increased slightly. So far this 'serotype replacement disease' has been much smaller in magnitude than the substantial reductions in vaccine-serotype disease. However, to mitigate the effects of serotype replacement disease new vaccines with 10 serotypes (including 1, 5 and 7F) or 13 serotypes (also including 3, 6A and 19A) have been introduced in childhood immunization programmes in developed countries.

Vaccine trials in children in South Africa and The Gambia have shown that 9-valent PCV, which includes two additional serotypes (1 and 5), can protect against invasive pneumococcal disease among HIV-infected children and can reduce childhood mortality and admissions to hospital with pneumonia among young children. In 2007, WHO recommended introduction of PCV into childhood immunization programmes in developing countries and, by 2011, 16 developing countries had introduced PCV with financial support from the GAVI Alliance; 40 more developing countries will introduce the vaccine in the next 4 years.

Among HIV-infected Malawian adults, with a previous history of invasive pneumococcal disease, 7-valent PCV reduced recurrent invasive pneumococcal disease by 74%. Pneumococcal disease is a significant problem among African adults, including both HIV seropositive adults in Southern Africa and otherwise healthy adults in the meningitis belt of West Africa. However, arguments in favour of adult vaccination have not yet been translated into health policy.

In the United Kingdom, the recommended immunization schedule for infants is two doses of 13-valent PCV given at 2 and 4 months of age followed by a booster dose at 13 months of age. For children 2 to 5 years of age who belong to an at-risk group, the recommendation is for a single dose of PCV followed 2 months later by a single dose of PPV.

Other forms of prevention

For children who are at high risk of invasive pneumococcal disease, including those with sickle cell disease or nephrotic syndrome, or following splenectomy, daily prophylaxis with oral penicillin reduces risk by over 80%. It should be continued until at least 5 years of age.

In developing countries, simple measures such as reducing indoor smoke from cooking stoves and improving nutrition are likely to be effective in prevention. Zinc supplementation can reduce the incidence of pneumonia in children by 40%. In Pakistan, a community intervention to promote hand washing reduced pneumonia incidence in children by one-half.

Diagnosis

Culture of S. pneumoniae

Pneumococcal disease is most convincingly diagnosed by culture of *S. pneumoniae* from a normally sterile site in a patient with a compatible illness. Pneumococci are fastidious organisms but they grow readily on 5% blood agar incubated in 5% CO_2. Colonies are small and grey with a draughtsman like central indentation and are surrounded by a greenish zone of α-haemolysis. Species identity is confirmed by sensitivity to optochin (ethylhydroxycupreine), bile solubility, and serotyping. The capsular type of *S. pneumoniae* is differentiated by a change in the refractive index around the cell seen on microscopy in the presence of specific rabbit antisera, the (Neufeld) Quellung reaction (Fig. 6.3.4).

In pneumococcal meningitis, cerebrospinal fluid frequently yields a positive culture. Pneumococci are also cultured from pleural and joint fluid in thoracic empyema and septic arthritis, respectively. Diagnosis of pneumococcal pneumonia by culture is, however, highly insensitive. Blood culture is a poor diagnostic test for several reasons; infection can be confined to the lungs; episodes of bacteraemia are only intermittent; the density of bacteraemia is too low, especially in children; or the patient can have taken antibiotics that inhibit growth. Sputum culture lacks specificity, since the pharynx is colonized by pneumococci even in healthy individuals, and also has relatively poor sensitivity. Most cases of pneumococcal pneumonia are, therefore, not formally diagnosed. A measure of this insensitivity is obtained from the Gambian trial of PCV where 15 cases of radiographic pneumonia were prevented by vaccination for every two cases of detectable bacteraemic disease prevented.

Antigen detection

Patients with pneumococcal pneumonia excrete pneumococcal breakdown products including C-polysaccharide, a universal

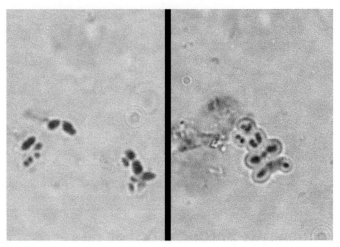

Fig. 6.3.4 The (Neufeld) Quellung reaction. Pneumococci show an apparent increase in the thickness of capsule when mixed with homologous anticapsular antibodies. The negative control is shown on the left and the positive reaction on the right.
(From Werno AM, Murdoch DR (2008). Medical microbiology: laboratory diagnosis of invasive pneumococcal disease. *Clin Infect Dis*, **46**, 926–32.)

component of pneumococcal cell walls, and capsular polysaccharides. Detection of C-polysaccharide in urine has been commercialized in a rapid immunochromatographic test that has a sensitivity of approximately 80% for bacteraemic pneumococcal pneumonia in adults and is highly specific. In children it lacks specificity as positive results may be obtained from healthy individuals who are merely colonized with pneumococci. Antigen detection is a useful adjunct to the testing of cerebrospinal fluid in cases of suspected meningitis.

Polymerase chain reaction

Primers targeting genes encoding the pneumococcal proteins pneumolysin, autolysin, pneumococcal surface adhesin A, and PBPs have been used for polymerase chain reaction (PCR) diagnosis. These assays have the same limitations as culture-based detection. PCR of respiratory specimens does not distinguish colonization from lung infection, and PCR of blood has poor sensitivity for pneumococcal pneumonia. Conversely, PCR of cerebrospinal fluid is sensitive and specific and has proven useful in the investigation of epidemic meningitis. In contrast to PCR using gel-based amplicon detection, quantitative real-time PCR for the autolysin gene, *lytA*, has shown high specificity and good sensitivity in validation studies and may become a useful diagnostic, particularly in epidemiological studies.

Clinical features

S. pneumoniae causes pneumonia, meningitis, septicaemia, otitis media, endocarditis, peritonitis, sinusitis, conjunctivitis, and purulent infections of the pleura, joints, and bone. These conditions do not necessarily occur in isolation; pneumococcal meningitis is quite frequently accompanied by pneumonia.

Pneumococcal pneumonia

Symptoms

Typically, the illness starts suddenly although there may be an antecedent upper respiratory tract infection. Fever is usually the first symptom and it is frequently accompanied by rigors. The patient feels weak and anorexic and may have severe headache and myalgia. Cough develops within 24 to 72 h and becomes a prominent symptom. At first the cough is nonproductive but it becomes productive of blood-tinged ('rusty') sputum and later of purulent sputum.

Pleuritic chest pain also develops during the course of the illness. The pain is sharp and stabbing and is aggravated by deep inspiration or coughing. The patient may try to obtain relief by splinting the affected side of the chest or lying on the affected side. Involvement of the diaphragmatic pleura leads to misleading abdominal pain or referred pain in the shoulder.

Among young children, a history of cough and difficulty breathing should raise suspicion of pneumonia. Elderly and immunocompromised patients may present with general malaise and confusion and have few respiratory symptoms and no fever. Prior antibiotic treatment also modifies the classic presentation.

Physical signs

On general examination, adults have tachycardia and pyrexia, with a rectal temperature as high as 40°C. With early presentation the respiratory system may appear normal, but pneumonia patients go on to develop rapid and difficult breathing (of which flaring of the alae nasi is a subtle early sign), cyanosis, and signs of lobar consolidation including reduced chest movement, dullness on percussion, fine crepitations, and, occasionally, bronchial breathing over the affected area. A pleural rub is sometimes audible.

Abdominal distension, upper abdominal tenderness, and guarding suggest involvement of the diaphragmatic pleura. Mild jaundice occurs in a minority. Concomitant herpes labialis ('cold sores') is common. Confusion is a sign of severity and is frequently observed in elderly patients.

In infants, the signs of pneumonia are nonspecific; most will have a raised respiratory rate and nasal flaring but only a minority will have crepitations. In developing countries, most cases of pneumonia are diagnosed and treated by nonmedical health workers. To facilitate diagnosis and promote early treatment, the WHO has designed a simple diagnostic algorithm as part of its Integrated Management of Childhood Illness (IMCI), which defines pneumonia on the respiratory rate (Fig. 6.3.5). Severe pneumonia, requiring admission to hospital, is indicated by lower chest wall indrawing; very severe pneumonia, requiring oxygen treatment, is indicated by hypoxia or mental changes (Fig. 6.3.6).

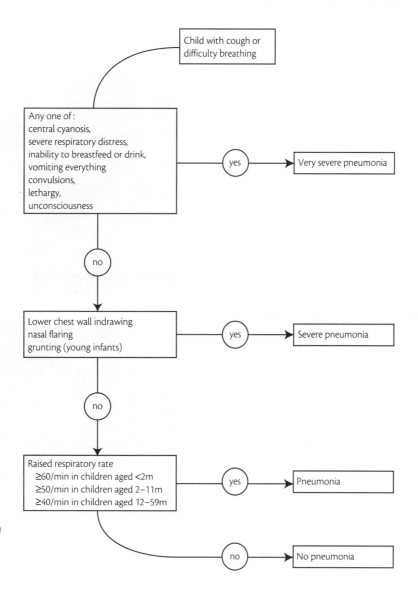

Fig. 6.3.5 The WHO classification of pneumonia in developing countries. (Adapted from World Health Organization (2004). *Serious childhood problems in countries with limited resources. Background book on management of the child with a serious infection or severe malnutrition.* World Health Organization, Geneva.)

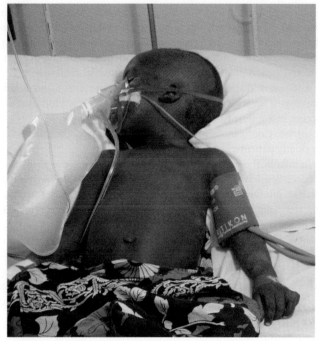

Fig. 6.3.6 Kenyan child with very severe pneumonia, as defined by the WHO, receiving high-flow oxygen therapy.
(Taken in the clinical service of Kilifi District Hospital; supplied by Dr Mike English. The patient's parents gave written consent for the taking of this photograph and for its use for educational purposes.)

Investigations

The pathological process of pneumonia is confirmed by the chest radiograph. This typically shows a homogenous area of opacification confined within the lobar structure (Fig. 6.3.7). The lower lobes are affected more frequently than the upper lobes. The area of pathology may be localized to a single lobule or extend over several lobes; early in the presentation there may be no abnormality at all. In children, widespread patchy opacification (bronchopneumonia) is common. Lateral radiographs add to the sensitivity of posteroanterior projections particularly for lower lobe disease hidden beneath the dome of the diaphragm.

In adults, pneumococcal aetiology is defined most sensitively by the C-polysaccharide antigen test in urine. Many patients are severely dehydrated on admission and cannot readily produce a urine specimen. Blood culture is positive for *S. pneumoniae* in about 10 to 30% of adults and about 15% of children. Genuine sputum samples should be differentiated from upper respiratory tract secretions by a high ratio of pus cells to epithelial cells on microscopy. The appearance of large numbers of Gram-positive diplococci on microscopy together with culture of *S. pneumoniae* is diagnostic. However, because prior antibiotic use is common, sputum microscopy is positive in only about one-quarter of patients and sputum culture is positive in only one-half. Young children cannot normally produce a sputum specimen.

Other laboratory investigations determine the prognosis. A Pao_2 less than 8 kPa marks out severe pneumonia but $Paco_2$ is usually unaffected unless terminal ventilatory failure occurs. A plasma urea exceeding 7 mmol/litre is a mark of severity (Fig. 6.3.8).

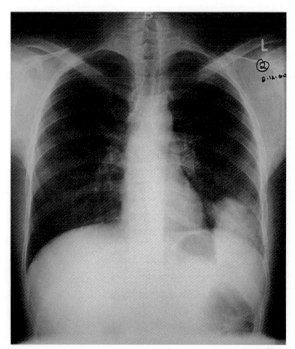

Fig. 6.3.7 Chest radiograph of an adult with clinical signs of left lower lobe pneumonia illustrating a well-demarcated area of alveolar consolidation.

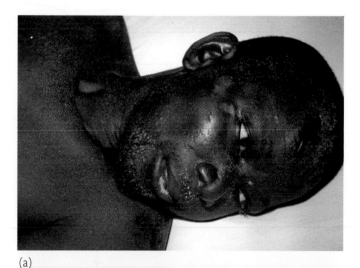
(a)

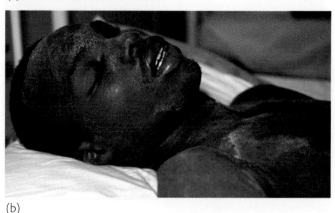
(b)

Fig. 6.3.8 Urea frost in two patients with uraemia complicating pneumococcal pneumonia.
(Copyright D A Warrell.)

The peripheral white blood cell count is elevated in most cases and may be as high as 40×10^9/litre. A low white cell count is a poor prognostic sign.

Differential diagnosis

The abrupt onset of symptoms often leads the patient to seek care before focal signs become established and it is not possible to differentiate pneumonia from other causes of acute febrile illness. In tropical countries, malaria is the main differential at this stage. When localizing symptoms and signs are established, pneumonia must be distinguished from pulmonary infarction. Both conditions lead to chest pain and haemoptysis and are accompanied by tachycardia. Pyrexia and rigors favour a diagnosis of pneumonia, while a very sudden history of chest pain and frank haemoptysis favour pulmonary embolism. Pulmonary oedema (secondary to heart failure), pulmonary atelectasis, pleurisy, lung abscess, tuberculosis, and acute bronchitis should also be considered in the differential diagnosis. Outside the chest, subdiaphragmatic lesions such as cholecystitis, a subphrenic abscess, or an amoebic liver abscess can mimic the clinical picture of lower lobe pneumonia.

Bacterial pneumonia is differentiated from viral or mycoplasma pneumonia by its abrupt onset, severity of symptoms and systemic illness, raised peripheral white blood cell count, and C-reactive protein level exceeding 125 mg/litre in serum. Confusion, signs of multiorgan involvement, lymphopenia, or a low serum sodium should raise the possibility of legionnaires' disease. Tuberculosis occasionally presents with an acute pneumonia in adults. In HIV-infected patients, the differential diagnosis also includes infection by *Pneumocystis jirovecii*, mycobacteria, and cytomegalovirus.

Treatment

Management of pneumonia first requires an assessment of severity to determine whether the patient should be treated at home, admitted to hospital, or admitted to the intensive care unit. The British Thoracic Society (BTS) recommendations define pneumonia as severe if there are three or more CURB-65 features: **C**onfusion, **U**rea exceeding 7 mmol/litre, **R**espiratory rate equal to or exceeding 30 breaths/min, abnormal **B**lood pressure, either systolic (<90 mmHg) or diastolic (≤60 mmHg) hypotension, and age equal to or exceeding **65** years. Additional features that may influence this assessment include the presence of coexisting disease, hypoxaemia (Pao_2 less than 8 kPa or Sao_2 less than 92%), and bilateral or multilobe involvement on the chest radiograph. Bacteraemia is itself an indicator of severity and increased risk of death. Supportive care includes analgesia for chest pain, ample hydration and nutrition, advice to stop smoking, and oxygen for inpatients with hypoxaemia.

Empirical guidelines for pneumonia treatment focus on treatment of pneumococcal pneumonia. High-dose penicillin or amoxicillin therapy will provide serum concentrations sufficiently high to treat pneumonia that is caused by pneumococci with MICs up to 4 μg/ml. Based on efficacy, cost, and acceptability, the optimum antibiotic is amoxicillin. The BTS recommends oral amoxicillin 500 to 1000 mg three times daily for 7 days for nonsevere cases of community-acquired pneumonia treated at home. Erythromycin 500 mg four times daily and clarithromycin 500 mg twice daily are acceptable alternatives. A fluoroquinolone with enhanced pneumococcal activity (e.g. levofloxacin, moxifloxacin) may be considered in outbreaks of resistant pneumococcal disease or in patients unresponsive to first-line antibiotics.

Severe cases of pneumonia requiring admission to hospital should be treated empirically with a broad-spectrum intravenous antibiotic such as co-amoxiclav (1.2 g three times daily), cefuroxime (1.5 g three times daily), cefotaxime (1 g three times daily), or ceftriaxone (2 g once daily) for 10 days. Cefotaxime or ceftriaxone are most active against pneumococci and should be effective against pneumonia caused by pneumococci with high cephalosporin MICs of 1 to 2 μg/ml. Empiric therapy with either erythromycin (500 mg four times daily) or clarithromycin (500 mg twice daily) should also be given to cover other causes of pneumonia. After 3 days of intravenous antibiotics, clinically stable patients may be safely switched to oral therapy.

Course and prognosis

Historically, untreated patients who survived long enough to make specific anticapsular polysaccharide antibody recovered spontaneously by crisis, or by a more gradual lysis, 7 to 10 days after the onset of illness. The significance of the observation, dating from Hippocrates and perpetuated by Osler, that crisis was most likely on uneven days (the 5th and especially the 7th) after the start of fever, remains obscure. However, mortality from pneumococcal pneumonia in the preantibiotic era was 20 to 40%. With antibiotic treatment, mortality is about 5% overall but is 30% among the subset of patients with bacteraemia. Mortality is highest among elderly and very young patients, and among those with an underlying illness such as cirrhosis, alcoholism, or heart disease. Most deaths occur within the first few days of admission to hospital. The causes of death are difficult to establish but include shock, cardiac arrhythmias, and respiratory failure.

Pneumococcal pleural effusion and empyema

A large pleural effusion or an empyema develops during treatment in 2 to 5% of patients with established pneumococcal pneumonia. In children these complications have increased in incidence over recent years and are frequently caused by serotype 1.

Symptoms

Some patients with pneumococcal empyema give a history of recent lung infection but others develop the disease without any previous illness. Hectic fever, rigors, sweats, malaise, anorexia, and marked weight loss are characteristic symptoms, often going back several weeks. Patients with a large pleural collection are breathless and may complain of dull pain on the affected side. A productive cough is unusual unless a bronchopleural fistula has developed.

Physical signs

General examination reveals pyrexia, tachycardia, and evidence of recent weight loss. Examination of the chest usually shows the characteristic signs of a pleural effusion: diminished chest movement, stony dullness on percussion, and diminished breath sounds over the accumulated fluid. The chest wall overlying an empyema may be tender.

Investigations

The effusion will usually be visible on the chest radiograph but loculated effusions may require localization by ultrasonography. On aspiration, turbid fluid or thick pus is obtained which contains pneumococci and degenerate white cells. If antibiotics have been given it may not be possible to culture pneumococci, but the fluid contains detectable pneumococcal antigens. The peripheral white blood cell count is raised predominantly with neutrophils.

Differential diagnosis

The principal differential diagnosis is pulmonary tuberculosis, and pleural biopsy may be required if the pleural fluid is sterile. The absence of copious, purulent sputum differentiates pleural empyema from a lung abscess.

Treatment

Successful treatment requires both intravenous antibiotics and pleural drainage. Appropriate antibiotic treatment for pneumococcal empyema follows the recommendations for pneumococcal pneumonia, with intravenous amoxicillin or a cephalosporin. Because of the frequent coexistence of penicillin-resistant aerobes and anaerobes, a β-lactamase inhibitor or metronidazole should also be given. Antibiotics should be continued for 4 to 6 weeks.

Course and prognosis

If untreated, an empyema may rupture through the chest wall (empyema necessitatis) or into a bronchus causing a bronchopleural fistula. Even when pus is aspirated and healing achieved, subsequent fibrosis and calcification may seriously restrict expansion of the underlying lung.

Pneumococcal meningitis

Pneumococci colonizing the nasopharynx can gain access to the subarachnoid space either by direct spread (from paranasal sinusitis or otitis media), following damage to the base of the skull, or, more commonly, via the bloodstream where they cross the blood–brain barrier at the choroid plexus and cerebral capillaries.

Symptoms

Adults with pneumococcal meningitis usually have fever, headache, neck stiffness, and impaired consciousness. At presentation, one-half of all patients have been ill for less than 24 h. Nausea and photophobia are common and seizures occur before diagnosis in 5 to 10% of patients. Among elderly patients, confusion may be the only symptom. Deterioration in the psychological or neurological state of an elderly patient with community-acquired pneumonia should be investigated with lumbar puncture. The presentation of meningitis in infants may be subtle, beginning with inability to feed and followed by irritability or lethargy.

Physical signs

Patients with pneumococcal meningitis are pyrexial and toxaemic. Classic signs such as nuchal rigidity, Kernig's sign, and Brudzinski's sign are absent in many patients with pyogenic meningitis. Bulging of the anterior fontanelle may be present in infants. Consciousness is often impaired, varying from drowsiness and confusion to deep coma. Raised intracranial pressure due to cerebral oedema or a cerebral abscess may be indicated by bradycardia and hypertension, but papilloedema is rarely seen. A cranial CT or MRI is mandatory before lumbar puncture in the presence of signs of cerebral or cranial nerve damage including a dilated pupil, ocular palsies, hemiparesis, history of focal seizures, decreased or rapidly falling level of consciousness, irregular respiration, tonic seizures, and decerebrate or decorticate posturing.

An associated pneumococcal lesion, such as otitis media or pneumonia, may be detected.

Investigations

Lumbar puncture should be undertaken whenever meningitis is suspected. In pneumococcal meningitis the cerebrospinal fluid is usually turbid and the leucocyte count is equal to or exceeds 1000×10^6/litre. Most of the leucocytes are neutrophils. A few patients have a low leucocyte count ($<100 \times 10^6$/litre) and in patients who present very early the leucocyte count may be normal; a repeat lumbar puncture several hours later will confirm the diagnosis. In pneumococcal meningitis, the concentration of protein in cerebrospinal fluid is increased and the ratio of glucose concentrations in cerebrospinal fluid and plasma is usually less than one-third. In untreated cases, culture of cerebrospinal fluid is usually positive and pneumococci are visible following Gram's staining. In patients who have received less than 48 h of antibiotic therapy the leucocyte count remains high and pneumococcal antigen may be detectable in cerebrospinal fluid. In developing countries, particularly in Asia, the use of immunochromatographic tests for C-polysaccharide antigen in cerebrospinal fluid has increased the number of cases of pneumococcal meningitis diagnosed. Culture of blood also frequently reveals the pneumococcus. The peripheral white cell count is usually elevated.

Differential diagnosis

Pneumococcal meningitis cannot be differentiated clinically from other forms of meningitis and the aetiology must be defined by investigation of the cerebrospinal fluid. An associated ear infection or pneumonia, or a history of head trauma favours pneumococcal infection. Conversely, rashes are rarely found in pneumococcal meningitis and petechiae or purpura on skin or mucosae strongly suggest meningococcal disease.

Treatment

Standard empirical therapy for meningitis in adults is cefotaxime (300 mg/kg per day divided into three or four doses) or ceftriaxone (100 mg/kg per day divided into two doses) for 10 to 14 days. In parts of the world where strains with intermediate or full resistance to cefotaxime or ceftriaxone have emerged, vancomycin (60 mg/kg per day divided into four doses) should be added to the empiric therapy. Meropenem is a useful alternative to cefotaxime and is active against pneumococci of intermediate but not full cefotaxime resistance. Imipenem increases susceptibility to seizures. Penicillin or ampicillin are effective therapy for culture-proven pneumococcal meningitis caused by penicillin-sensitive strains, but intermediately resistant strains are not adequately treated by these drugs.

In children in developing countries, for several decades the recommended therapy for acute pyogenic meningitis has been chloramphenicol with penicillin. The spread of intermediate penicillin resistance among pneumococci and the expiry of the patent for ceftriaxone have recently led to a change in this policy. In nonepidemic situations, the WHO now recommends treatment with ceftriaxone 100 mg/kg once daily for 5 to 7 days with a maximum daily dose of 2 g. A multicountry trial of 5 days versus 10 days of ceftriaxone therapy in children has provided empiric support for short-course therapy for 5 days, provided there is good clinical evidence of response.

Treatment with antibiotics should be started as soon as a clinical diagnosis of bacterial meningitis is made. Delay in treatment until after hospitalization is associated with increased mortality. Other supportive therapies include adequate oxygenation, maintenance of normal blood pressure, prevention of hypoglycaemia and hyponatraemia, and control of seizures (which may be covert and unsuspected in an unconscious patient) with anticonvulsants.

The use of dexamethasone in bacterial meningitis in adults has been controversial for many years. In a Cochrane review of five randomized controlled trials, the summary mortality reduction attributable to dexamethasone adjunctive treatment was 43%; the effect was greatest in meningitis caused by *S. pneumoniae*. The summary findings were influenced to a large extent by a single study of European patients. In a more recent study of HIV-infected adults in Africa, among whom case fatality rates were very high, dexamethasone was not beneficial, suggesting that dexamethasone may only be useful in populations with low HIV prevalence who are less sick at presentation. The recommended dose is 10 mg every 6 h for 4 days. Meningeal inflammation facilitates diffusion of vancomycin into the cerebrospinal fluid and the anti-inflammatory action of dexamethasone may lead to suboptimal antibiotic concentrations. Patients on treatment for cephalosporin-resistant pneumococcal meningitis should therefore be monitored both clinically and by repeat lumbar puncture. In children, dexamethasone is highly protective against hearing loss in *H. influenzae* meningitis but also provides some protection in pneumococcal meningitis if given with or before administration of antibiotics. For children in developing countries, however, the evidence suggests there is no benefit to adjunctive dexamethasone.

Course and prognosis

The prognosis of patients with pneumococcal meningitis is poor. Most patients develop complications of which the most important are seizures, brain infarction, brain swelling, hydrocephalus, and cranial nerve palsies. Subdural collections are commonly seen on brain imaging and may require needle puncture to exclude subdural empyema, especially if there is persistence of fever, irritability, neck stiffness, or continued cerebrospinal fluid leucocytosis detected by repeat lumbar puncture.

Over one-third of patients also develop systemic complications such as shock, cardiorespiratory failure, and disseminated intravascular coagulation, and these are frequently the final cause of death among older patients. Among children, supportive therapy to sustain adequate blood pressure is important to maintain cerebral blood flow against the resistance of raised intracranial pressure.

The mortality from pneumococcal meningitis in industrialized countries varies between 10 and 40%, being lower in children than in adults. In developing countries, the mortality range is higher (30–60%). Features on admission that are associated with a poor outcome include advanced age, seizures, cranial nerve palsies, deep coma, low cerebrospinal fluid leucocyte count (below 1000×10^6/litre), low glucose concentration in cerebrospinal fluid, and associated pneumonia. Death is almost inevitable in patients who are in deep coma at the time they are admitted to hospital. Survivors are frequently affected by neurological sequelae: hearing loss occurs in one in five; cerebral damage is common leading to hemiparesis, ataxia, and aphasia; and cranial nerve palsies, particularly of the oculomotor nerve, occur in a small percentage. Among those who appear to make a good recovery from pneumococcal meningitis, one-quarter have residual cognitive slowness.

Otitis media

In young children aged below 2 years, otitis media is one of the commonest reasons for seeking medical advice. The pneumococcus causes a significant fraction of all cases. Following conjugate pneumococcal vaccine introduction in the United States of America, the incidence of all otitis media has fallen by one-fifth. Beyond childhood, otitis media is uncommon.

Symptoms

Acute otitis media starts suddenly, although there may be a history of a recent upper respiratory tract infection. Fever, crying, and extreme irritability are the usual features in young children, in whom febrile convulsions may also occur. Fever and severe pain in the ear are the usual presenting complaints in older children and adults, and patients may also complain of deafness and tinnitus.

Physical signs

On otoscopic examination of the affected ear, the tympanic membrane is red and swollen and lacks the normal light reflection. It may bulge outwards into the external ear and there may be an air–fluid level indicating a middle ear effusion. Pus or blood in the external auditory canal suggests a perforation that is confirmed by observing a ragged hole in the tympanic membrane. The affected ear is usually partially deaf. In children, meningism may be present; if so, meningitis must be excluded by lumbar puncture.

Investigations

Fine needle puncture of the tympanic membrane (tympanocentesis) and aspiration of middle ear fluid is used with variable frequency in different countries but is of most value where antibiotic resistance is prevalent. In complicated cases or in those not responding to initial antibiotics, culture of middle ear fluid may guide therapy. A tympanogram can identify increased middle ear pressure and accumulation of fluid.

Treatment

Most episodes of otitis media are diagnosed clinically without microbiological confirmation. Randomized controlled trials show that otitis media resolves in the majority of otherwise healthy children whether or not they take antibiotics. This evidence underpins a policy of observation without treatment. Immediate antibiotics are indicated in young infants (<6 months) and in older children (>2 years) with a clear bacteriological diagnosis of otitis media or symptoms of severity. The antibiotic of choice for pneumococcal otitis media is oral amoxicillin (90 mg/kg per day) for 5 days. For penicillin-resistant pneumococcal infection the appropriate antibiotic is intravenous ceftriaxone for 3 days.

Course and prognosis

Pneumococcal otitis media normally resolves rapidly and completely. However, rupture of the drum can lead to partial conductive deafness and pneumococcal otitis media can give rise to a chronic discharging ear requiring prolonged or complicated treatment. The infection can spread to cause acute mastoiditis, meningitis, or a cerebral abscess.

Other clinical syndromes

The pneumococcus is an important cause of bacterial sinusitis resulting from direct spread from the nasopharynx. Sinusitis that does not resolve within 5 to 7 days may require treatment with an antibiotic effective against pneumococcus. A mild form of pneumococcal bacteraemia, variously labelled as 'occult bacteraemia' or 'walk-in bacteraemia', is encountered relatively commonly in children. The child presents with fever or febrile convulsions but without any obvious focus of pneumococcal infection. Although there is a small risk of dissemination to the meninges, the patient is usually successfully treated as an outpatient with oral antibiotics before the culture results are known. Significant bloodstream infection is less common but may lead to septicaemia or purulent localization in meninges, vertebrae, joints, orbits, or testes. Pneumococcal conjunctivitis has been observed in outbreaks among college students and has two unusual features: (1) the causative strain is unencapsulated and (2) the attack rates are high, suggesting little pre-existing immunity.

Septicaemia

Acute septicaemia is a less common form of pneumococcal infection and is encountered most frequently in immunocompromised patients or those without a spleen. Sudden fever, peripheral circulatory collapse, and bleeding (purpura fulminans) are the usual presenting features of this condition, which is indistinguishable from other forms of overwhelming bacterial septicaemia. Leucopenia is usually found. Bleeding is due to disseminated intravascular coagulation. The mortality from septicaemia is very high, even when treatment is started promptly. The pneumococcus has been rarely associated with toxic shock syndrome and with haemolytic uraemic syndrome.

Endocarditis and pericarditis

Cardiac manifestations of pneumococcal infection are well described but where there is good access to antibiotics they are now rare, occurring in less than 1% of all pneumococcal infections. Acute endocarditis may complicate pneumococcal septicaemia to affect healthy heart valves, especially the aortic valve, which may rupture and cause severe aortic incompetence. Emboli derived from cardiac vegetations may reach the brain and other organs. Progressions of the cardiac lesions may be very rapid and the prognosis of this condition is poor. Valve replacement may be necessary for patients who survive the initial episode.

Pneumococci may spread directly from the lower lobes of the lung to produce pericarditis which is clinically silent in some patients or may be manifest only as a transient pericardial rub or an abnormal electrocardiogram. Patients with a pericardial empyema usually complain of dull or pleuritic central chest pain and give a history of persistent fever, malaise, anorexia, and weight loss over several days or weeks. Many patients with a pneumococcal pericardial empyema are critically ill by the time they reach hospital and have pericardial tamponade: a rapid small-volume pulse, pulsus paradoxus, a low blood pressure, elevation of the jugular venous pressure with a further increase during inspiration, peripheral oedema, and ascites. The heart sounds are usually faint and a chest radiograph may show globular enlargement of the heart together with evidence of an associated lung infection. An ultrasonographic examination may help to define the best sites for diagnostic and therapeutic drainage. The electrocardiogram shows low-voltage potentials and ST elevation or depression may be present. Pneumococcal aetiology can be confirmed by culture or antigen detection of drained pus. Mortality is high, and among patients who survive the initial episode constrictive pericarditis may develop within weeks or months of their acute illness.

Peritonitis

Pneumococcal peritonitis is an uncommon condition that is encountered among three risk groups: (1) patients with cirrhosis of the liver or nephrotic syndrome; (2) patients with gastrointestinal disease (e.g. appendicitis), intra-abdominal surgery, or peritoneal dialysis; and (3) otherwise healthy young girls, possibly as a complication of pelvic infection. The condition is characterized by sudden fever and abdominal pain and tenderness. The ascitic fluid is turbid and contains neutrophils and pneumococci. The prognosis of pneumococcal peritonitis is determined principally by the severity of the underlying illness.

Future developments

Of great concern for future treatment of pneumococcal disease is the global spread of multidrug-resistant isolates of *S. pneumoniae*. Resistance to new agents such as fluoroquinolones is established in adult disease and is now reported among paediatric cases in South Africa. Judicious use of antibiotics has curbed the rise in resistance in developed countries but resistant strains still have a competitive advantage in many developing countries where antibiotic use is relatively unregulated. The clinical relevance of *in vitro* resistance to antibiotics, especially intermediate β-lactam resistance in the treatment of pneumonia, remains an area requiring further investigation.

The significance of pneumococcal disease will be shaped to a large extent during the next decade by the global introduction of new vaccines and by the evolutionary response of the pathogen to these interventions. New conjugate vaccines are being introduced that cover 10 and 13 serotypes each. These protect against more cases of pneumococcal disease in developing countries where serotypes 1 and 5, which are not included in the 7-valent PCV, predominate. The potential of PCV to reduce the incidence of childhood pneumonia and reduce childhood deaths is enormous; however, the success of the vaccine will be determined by its population effects, particularly serotype replacement disease. Third-generation vaccines which use surface expressed pneumococcal proteins and virulence factors to stimulate immunity are not restricted to a subset of serotypes and avoid this limitation. These are now beginning to enter clinical trials.

Genome sequencing and phylogenetic analysis of specific lineages of *S. pneumoniae* may help to reveal the selection pressures which both antibiotics and vaccines impose on the species and the nature of the pathogen's response. Such studies will guide the introduction of new drugs and vaccines to minimize horizontal transfer of both antibiotic resistance genes and serotype capsular genes leading to vaccine-serotype escape strains.

Further reading

Austrian R, Gold J (1964). Pneumococcal bacteremia with especial reference to bacteremic pneumococcal pneumonia. *Ann Intern Med*, **60**, 759–76. [Classic description of the effect of antibiotics on pneumonia mortality.]

Austrian R, *et al.* (1976). Prevention of pneumococcal pneumonia by vaccination. *Trans Assoc Am Physicians*, **89**, 184–94. [Vaccine trial of 13-valent polysaccharide vaccine in South African miners.]

Bentley SD, *et al.* (2006). Genetic analysis of the capsular biosynthetic locus from all 90 pneumococcal serotypes. *PLoS Genet*, **2**, e31, 1–8.

Berkley JA, *et al.* (2005). Bacteremia among children admitted to a rural hospital in Kenya. *N Engl J Med*, **352**, 39–47. [A conservative estimate of invasive pneumococcal disease incidence from Africa.]

Black S, *et al.* (2000). Efficacy, safety and immunogenicity of heptavalent pneumococcal conjugate vaccine in children. Northern California Kaiser Permanente Vaccine Study Center Group. *Pediatr Infect Dis J*, **19**, 187–95.

Briles DE, *et al.* (2000). Immunization of humans with recombinant pneumococcal surface protein A (rPspA) elicits antibodies that passively protect mice from fatal infection with *Streptococcus pneumoniae* bearing heterologous PspA. *J Infect Dis*, **182**, 1694–701. [First study to show human antibodies against pneumococcal proteins are protective.]

British Thoracic Society (2001). BTS guidelines for the management of community acquired pneumonia in adults. *Thorax*, **56** Suppl 4, 1–64.

[United Kingdom professional guidelines on management of pneumonia, last updated in 2004 and available at www.brit-thoracic.org.uk/]

Croucher NJ, *et al.* (2011). Rapid pneumococcal evolution in response to clinical interventions. *Science*, **331**, 430–4.

Cutts FT, *et al.* (2005). Efficacy of nine-valent pneumococcal conjugate vaccine against pneumonia and invasive pneumococcal disease in The Gambia: randomised, double-blind, placebo-controlled trial. *Lancet*, **365**, 1139–46.

Dowell SF, *et al.* (2003). Seasonal patterns of invasive pneumococcal disease. *Emerg Infect Dis*, **9**, 573–9.

Dowson CG, *et al.* (1989). Horizontal transfer of penicillin-binding protein genes in penicillin-resistant clinical isolates of *Streptococcus pneumoniae*. *Proc Natl Acad Sci U S A*, **86**, 8842–6. [Early description of the genetic basis of penicillin resistance in pneumococcus.]

Fedson DS, Scott JA (1999). The burden of pneumococcal disease among adults in developed and developing countries: what is and is not known. *Vaccine*, **17** Suppl 1, 11–18.

French N, *et al.* (2010). A trial of a 7-valent pneumococcal conjugate vaccine in HIV-infected adults. *N Engl J Med*, **362**, 812–22.

Gessner BD, *et al.* (2010). African meningitis belt pneumococcal disease epidemiology indicates a need for an effective serotype 1 containing vaccine, including for older children and adults. *BMC Infect Dis*, **10**, 22.

Giefing C, *et al.* (2008). Discovery of a novel class of highly conserved vaccine antigens using genomic scale antigenic fingerprinting of pneumococcus with human antibodies. *J Exp Med*, **205**, 117–31. [Use of pneumococcal genomics to discover antigenic common pneumococcal proteins.]

Gilks CF, *et al.* (1996). Invasive pneumococcal disease in a cohort of predominantly HIV-1 infected female sex-workers in Nairobi, Kenya. *Lancet*, **347**, 718–23. [Epidemiology and clinical presentation of pneumococcal disease in HIV-positive adults.]

Gordon SB, *et al.* (2000). Bacterial meningitis in Malawian adults: pneumococcal disease is common, severe, and seasonal. *Clin Infect Dis*, **31**, 53–7. [In a setting with high HIV prevalence, pneumococcus caused 18% of bacterial meningitis cases and 32% of bacterial meningitis deaths.]

Greenwood B (1999). The epidemiology of pneumococcal infection in children in the developing world. *Philos Trans R Soc Lond B Biol Sci*, **354**, 777–85.

Heffron R (1939). *Pneumonia with special reference to pneumococcus lobar pneumonia*. The Commonwealth Fund, New York. (Second printing 1979, Harvard University Press, Cambridge, Mass.) [Classic book summarizing the first 60 years of research on pneumococcal pneumonia.]

Hill PC, *et al.* (2006). Nasopharyngeal carriage of *Streptococcus pneumoniae* in Gambian villagers. *Clin Infect Dis*, **43**, 673–9. [Reveals the enormous exposure to pneumococci in a developing world setting.]

Johnson HL, *et al.* (2010). Systematic evaluation of serotypes causing invasive pneumococcal disease among children under five: the pneumococcal global serotype project. *PLoS Med*, **7**, e1000348.

Kadioglu A, *et al.* (2008). The role of *Streptococcus pneumoniae* virulence factors in host respiratory colonization and disease. *Nat Rev Microbiol*, **6**, 288–301.

Klugman KP, *et al.* (2003). A trial of a 9-valent pneumococcal conjugate vaccine in children with and those without HIV infection. *N Engl J Med*, **349**, 1341–8.

Malley R, *et al.* (2001). Intranasal immunization with killed unencapsulated whole cells prevents colonization and invasive disease by capsulated pneumococci. *Infect Immun*, **69**, 4870–3.

Mangtani P, Cutts F, Hall AJ (2003). Efficacy of polysaccharide pneumococcal vaccine in adults in more developed countries: the state of the evidence. *Lancet Infect Dis*, **3**, 71–8.

Musher DM (1992). Infections caused by *Streptococcus pneumoniae*: clinical spectrum, pathogenesis, immunity, and treatment. *Clin Infect Dis*, **14**, 801–7.

O'Brien KL, *et al.* (2009). Burden of disease caused by *Streptococcus pneumoniae* in children younger than 5 years: global estimates. *Lancet*, **374**, 893–902.

Ogunniyi AD, *et al.* (2007). Development of a vaccine against invasive pneumococcal disease based on combinations of virulence proteins of *Streptococcus pneumoniae*. *Infect Immun*, **75**, 350–7. [Illustrates the state of common protein vaccine development and especially the role of vaccines consisting of combinations of different proteins.]

Pallares R, *et al.* (1995). Resistance to penicillin and cephalosporin and mortality from severe pneumococcal pneumonia in Barcelona, Spain. *N Engl J Med*, **333**, 474–80. [Large retrospective study fails to find an increase in mortality from pneumococcal pneumonia caused by penicillin-resistant strains when it was treated with penicillin.]

Prymula R, *et al.* (2006). Pneumococcal capsular polysaccharides conjugated to protein D for prevention of acute otitis media caused by both *Streptococcus pneumoniae* and non-typable *Haemophilus influenzae*: a randomised double-blind efficacy study. *Lancet*, **367**, 740–8.

Reingold A, *et al.* (2005). Direct and indirect effects of routine vaccination of children with 7-valent pneumococcal conjugate vaccine on incidence of invasive pneumococcal disease: United States, 1998–2003. *MMWR Morb Mortal Wkly Rep*, **54**, 893–7. [Illustration of the herd protection provided to older children and adults by pneumococcal conjugate vaccine when children are routinely immunized.]

Scott JA, *et al.* (2000). Aetiology, outcome, and risk factors for mortality among adults with acute pneumonia in Kenya. *Lancet*, **355**, 1225–30.

Siber GR, Klugman, KP, Mäkelä PH (eds) (2008). *Pneumococcal vaccines: the impact of conjugate vaccines*. ASM Press, Washington, DC.

Sleeman KL, *et al.* (2006). Capsular serotype-specific attack rates and duration of carriage of *Streptococcus pneumoniae* in a population of children. *J Infect Dis*, **194**, 682–8. [Provides an estimate of invasiveness of each pneumococcal serotype based on acquisition rates and incidence of invasive disease.]

Tettelin H, *et al.* (2001). Complete genome sequence of a virulent isolate of *Streptococcus pneumoniae*. *Science*, **293**, 498–506.

Trzcinski K, Thompson CM, Lipsitch M (2004). Single-step capsular transformation and acquisition of penicillin resistance in *Streptococcus pneumoniae*. *J Bacteriol*, **186**, 3447–52. [Demonstrates in vitro the capacity of pneumococcus to exchange DNA coding for capsular serotype and penicillin resistance in a single genetic step.]

Tuomanen EI, *et al.* (eds) (2004). *The pneumococcus*. ASM Press, Washington, DC. [Modern summaries of research into genomics, pathogenesis, immunity, virulence, colonization, epidemiology, and treatment of invasive pneumococcal disease as well as antibiotic resistance and vaccines.]

van de Beek D, *et al.* (2004). Clinical features and prognostic factors in adults with bacterial meningitis. *N Engl J Med*, **351**, 1849–59.

van der Poll T, Opal SM (2009). Pathogenesis, treatment, and prevention of pneumococcal pneumonia. *Lancet*, **374**, 1543–56.

Watera C, *et al.* (2004). 23-Valent pneumococcal polysaccharide vaccine in HIV-infected Ugandan adults: 6-year follow-up of a clinical trial cohort. *AIDS*, **18**, 1210–3. [In a randomized controlled trial among HIV-infected adults, risk of all causes of pneumonia was, surprisingly, 1.6 times greater in recipients of polysaccharide vaccine.]

Watson DA, *et al.* (1993). A brief history of the pneumococcus in biomedical research: a panoply of scientific discovery. *Clin Infect Dis*, **17**, 913–24.

Weiser JN, *et al.* (1994). Phase variation in pneumococcal opacity: relationship between colonial morphology and nasopharyngeal colonization. *Infect Immun*, **62**, 2582–9.

Weisfelt M, *et al.* (2006). Pneumococcal meningitis in adults: new approaches to management and prevention. *Lancet Neurol*, **5**, 332–42.

Werno AM, Murdoch DR (2008). Laboratory diagnosis of invasive pneumococcal disease. *Clin Inf Dis*, **46**, 926–32. [Up-to-date review of laboratory diagnosis of pneumococcal disease.]

White B (1938). *The biology of pneumococcus*. The Commonwealth Fund, New York. (Second printing 1979, Harvard University Press, Cambridge, Mass.) [Classic book describing the first 70 years of research on the pneumococcus.]

Whitney CG, *et al.* (2003). Decline in invasive pneumococcal disease after the introduction of protein-polysaccharide conjugate vaccine. *N Engl J Med*, **348**, 1737–46. [Surveillance study documenting the large impact of pneumococcal conjugate vaccine on invasive pneumococcal disease among children following routine use in the United States of America.]

World Health Organization (2009) *Integrated management of childhood illness*. http://www.who.int/child_adolescent_health/topics/prevention_care/child/imci/en/index.html

6.4 Staphylococci

Bala Hota , Kyle J. Popovich, and
Robert A. Weinstein

Essentials

Staphylococci are Gram-positive cocci that form clusters, but can occur singly, in pairs, chains, or tetrads. They are classically distinguished from other Gram-positive cocci by presence of catalase, an enzyme that degrades hydrogen peroxide (H_2O_2). *S. aureus* is distinguished from other coagulase-negative staphylococci, which are generally less virulent, by the presence of coagulase, an enzyme that coagulates plasma. Many toxins and regulatory elements enhance virulence in staphylococci.

Epidemiology

Colonization—staphylococci are skin commensals. About 20% of adults are persistently colonized by *S. aureus*, 60% are intermittently colonized, and 20% are never colonized. High-risk groups for *S. aureus* colonization include infants, insulin-dependent diabetics, intravenous drug users, HIV-infected patients, and renal dialysis patients.

Methicillin-resistant *S. aureus* (MRSA)—risk factors for MRSA colonization and infection among hospitalized patients include antibiotic exposure, surgery, nursing-home residence, or high MRSA 'colonization pressure', i.e. frequent exposure to colonized or infected patients. However, MRSA is no longer only a hospital-related infection, with community-associated MRSA affecting individuals without health care exposures.

Clinical features

S. aureus infection—clinical syndromes can be divided into three groups: (1) Illness due to release of toxins, leading to disease at sites often remote from infection—including (a) staphylococcal scalded skin syndrome—release of epidermolytic toxins leads to bullae and desquamation; (b) food-borne illness due to preformed toxin—a heat-stable superantigen toxin produces sudden vomiting and diarrhoea; (c) toxic shock syndrome—superantigen toxins cause multisystem organ dysfunction; may be menstrual (e.g. tampon-associated) or nonmenstrual. (2) Illness due to local tissue destruction and abscess formation—including (a) impetigo, folliculitis, and cellulitis; (b) furuncles and carbuncles; (c) mastitis; (d) pyomyositis; (e) septic bursitis; (f) septic arthritis; (g) osteomyelitis; (h) epidural abscess; (i) pneumonia; (j) urinary tract infection. (3) Hematogenous infection—including bacteraemia and endocarditis.

Coagulase-negative staphylococci—most infections with these skin commensals are the consequence of medical interventions leading to foreign bodies, e.g. prosthetic joints or heart valves, indwelling intravascular catheters or grafts, or peritoneal catheters. Conditions include endocarditis (5–8% of native valve infections, c.40% of prosthetic valve infections), intravascular catheter infections (6–27% of vascular-catheter infections), prosthetic joint infections (up to 38% of arthroplasty infections), peritoneal dialysis, catheter infections, and postoperative ocular infections.

Diagnosis

Diagnosis relies on characteristic clinical and epidemiological features, supported by positive cultures from the relevant clinical site, with identification (when appropriate) of exotoxin-positive strains. Outbreak and epidemiological investigations use molecular fingerprinting techniques to assess relatedness of staphylococci.

Treatment

Aside from supportive care, the mainstays of therapy are (1) prompt drainage of infected foci; and (2) antimicrobials— (a) coagulase-negative staphylococci—vancomycin is the mainstay of therapy because of the high rates of methicillin resistance; (b) *S. aureus*—antimicrobial choice should be based on the local prevalence of MRSA and the clinical severity of illness; a bactericidal agent, preferably a β-lactam, is used whenever possible; oral agents active against MRSA include clindamycin, trimethoprim/sulfamethozaxole, doxycycline, minocycline, linezolid; glycopeptides (i.e. vancomycin or teicoplainin) have been the usual therapy of severe infections due to MRSA, but vancomycin resistance is emerging.

Prevention

Prevention of illness due to *S. aureus*, particularly MRSA, relies on proactive infection control measures, including (1) surveillance for MRSA colonization; (2) imposed grouping (cohorting) of infected and colonized patients; (3) barrier precautions—e.g. gowning and gloving by health care staff; (4) improved hand hygiene; (5) cleaning patients—e.g. with chlorhexidine; (6) improved environmental cleaning; (7) antimicrobial stewardship.

Better strategies for treatment and salvage of infected catheters or methods for treatment of biofilm may improve treatment of coagulase-negative staphylococcal infections. No vaccines are available.

Introduction and historical perspective

Staphylococci are named for their microscopic appearance, the name coming from Greek words meaning 'bunch of grapes' and 'berry'. First described in 1880 by Ogston as an important cause of abscesses in humans, staphylococci are among the most common causes of bacterial colonization and infection in the community and in hospitals.

Staphylococcus aureus, the pre-eminent human staphylococcus, has adapted efficiently to improvements in therapeutics. In the 1940s, shortly after the introduction of penicillin, penicillin-resistant *S. aureus* was noted in the United Kingdom and the United States of America, and by the end of the decade 50% of isolates were resistant. From 1940 to 1960, a particularly invasive clone of penicillin-resistant *S. aureus*, 'phage type 80/81', caused pandemic hospital infections. Following the introduction of methicillin, that strain faded from concern only to be replaced in subsequent decades with endemic health care-associated methicillin-resistant *S. aureus* (MRSA) that frequently was resistant to multiple antimicrobial classes. Most recently, reminiscent of the 1940 to 1960 experience, invasive strains of community-associated MRSA (CA-MRSA) have emerged rapidly in some communities among otherwise healthy individuals. Coagulase-negative staphylococci infections, in contrast, are infecting implanted devices and occurring in association with health care, thereby filling a niche created by medical success.

Microbiology and molecular genetics

Staphylococci stain purple ('positive') with Gram's stain and form grape-like clusters, but can occur singly, in pairs, in chains, or in tetrads. Of 32 staphylococcal species, 16 colonize or infect humans. Classically, staphylococci are distinguished from other Gram-positive cocci by the presence of catalase, an enzyme that degrades hydrogen peroxide. *S. aureus* is distinguished from other staphylococci by the presence of coagulase, an enzyme that coagulates plasma. Most laboratories use latex agglutination tests to detect coagulase; other assays include the tube coagulase and free coagulase tests.

Outbreak and epidemiological investigations use molecular 'fingerprinting' techniques to assess relatedness of staphylococci, i.e. bacteriophage typing, pulsed-field gel electrophoresis (PFGE), multilocus sequence typing (MLST), or more recently, whole bacterial genome sequencing.

Pathogenesis

The infectiveness of staphylococci depends in part on bacterial factors that promote growth, colonization, invasiveness (i.e. regulation and virulence determinants), and antibiotic resistance and in part on host susceptibility (e.g. presence of diabetes mellitus).

Regulation and virulence determinants

Regulation determinants 'autoregulate' staphylococci based on environmental conditions or host factors. The major *S. aureus* regulatory gene is the accessory gene regulator (*agr*) that facilitates intercell communication. This and other systems may have roles in tissue destruction (through exoprotein production) and endocarditis (through adhesin regulation).

Virulence determinants, e.g. peptidoglycan, lipoteichoic acids, protein toxins, and biofilm, enhance bacterial pathogenicity but can also activate patient protective mechanisms. Peptidoglycan, an important component of Gram-positive bacterial walls, and lipoteichoic acids, bound to the plasma membrane, are implicated in triggering the inflammatory response in humans that can enhance bacterial killing. Exoproteins and 'superantigens' (i.e. antigens that lead to nonspecific immune activation) can be released by *S. aureus* to cause a severe immune response or disease remote from infection, while local toxins, e.g. Panton–Valentine leucocidin (PVL), may increase bacterial invasiveness. Biofilm, an extracellular complex of polysaccharides, enhances binding to foreign objects (e.g. intravascular catheters) and serves as a bacterial sanctuary from host defences and antimicrobials.

Antimicrobial resistance

S. aureus resistance to β-lactams is mediated by β-lactamases (penicillin resistance) or, more commonly, by altered enzymes responsible for cell wall formation (methicillin resistance). Penicillinases propagate by plasmids or phage transfer; methicillin resistance results from spread of a genomic island of DNA called the staphylococcal chromosomal cassette (SCC). The SCC carries the *mecA* gene (termed SCCmec). The product of *mecA* is penicillin-binding protein 2a (PBP2a), which has low affinity for methicillin and enables cell wall synthesis in spite of active antibiotics. SCCmec type IV primarily is associated with CA-MRSA, while types I, II, and III are associated primarily with hospital strains.

Glycopeptides (i.e. vancomycin or teicoplanin) have been the usual therapy of severe infections due to MRSA. However, vancomycin resistance is emerging among MRSA. Two resistance patterns exist: (1) vancomycin- (or glycopeptide-) intermediate *S. aureus* (VISA or GISA) and (2) vancomycin-resistant *S. aureus* (VRSA). The VISA phenotype has vancomycin minimum inhibitory concentrations (MICs) of 4 to 8 µg/ml, and is thought to arise from thickening of the cell wall, changes in *agr* function, and changes in cell metabolism that arise from subinhibitory exposure to vancomycin. VRSA have higher MICs (≥16 µg/ml) due to a gene (*vanA*) that has been passed from vancomycin-resistant *Enterococcus faecalis* to *S. aureus*. Clinical isolates of VRSA (12 so far) have been reported in the United States of America; VRSA has also been isolated in Hyderabad, India. Although new agents (linezolid and daptomycin) exist for therapy of MRSA and could be used for VISA/VRSA, fledgling resistance has been reported.

Outbreaks of linezolid-resistant MRSA have been identified, with the *cfr* gene believed to mediate resistance. One outbreak was felt to be associated with high usage of linezolid; the outbreak was controlled with antibiotic stewardship and enhanced infection control measures.

Resistance to antimicrobials in the macrolide–lincosamide–streptogramin (MLS) group is not predictably concordant. Clindamycin resistance can be inducible, producing misleading susceptibility phenotypes in automated testing that are erythromycin resistant and, seemingly but erroneously, clindamycin susceptible, or constitutive (readily detected resistance to erythromycin *and* clindamycin). The double-disc diffusion test, or D test, will detect inducible clindamycin resistance. Clindamycin therapy is unreliable in organisms with either inducible or constitutive resistance.

Among the coagulase-negative staphylococci, 80% of isolates are resistant to methicillin due to the action of *mecA*. Laboratory testing of coagulase-negative staphylococci is complicated by heterotypic expression of methicillin resistance, which may lead to deceptively low methicillin MICs. PCR testing for *mecA* or slide agglutination testing for PBP2a will reveal resistance; methicillin or oxacillin will not effectively treat such strains.

Epidemiology: *S. aureus*
Colonization

Among staphylococci, as a general rule, colonization precedes infection. *S. aureus* colonizes multiple sites but predominately the anterior nares. Some CA-MRSA may share the ability of coagulase-negative staphylococci to colonize intact skin. Among adults, 20% are persistently colonized by *S. aureus*, 60% are intermittently colonized, and 20% are never colonized. Meticillin-susceptible *S. aureus* (MSSA) colonization prevalence rates are about 30% in the community. High-risk groups for *S. aureus* colonization include infants, insulin-dependent diabetics, intravenous drug users, HIV-positive patients, and patients undergoing either haemodialysis or peritoneal dialysis. Host factors promoting colonization may be antibiotic treatment and polymorphisms in host genes.

Health care-associated MRSA

Health care-associated MRSA infection causes significant morbidity and mortality, and has been associated with 29% longer stays and 36% greater hospital charges for patients with MRSA compared to MSSA bacteraemia. Among hospitalized patients, risk factors for MRSA colonization and infection include antibiotic exposure, surgery, nursing home residence, or high MRSA 'colonization pressure', i.e. frequent exposure to colonized or infected patients.

There is a large 'resistance iceberg' for MRSA; the ratio of infected-to-colonized patients may reach 1:3, which complicates control measures. The hands of health care workers probably represent a major vector for MRSA cross-transmission. Another mechanism of staphylococcal transmission is bacterial shedding from nares of colonized patients or staff, which can be enhanced by rhinitis. Spread via contaminated environmental surfaces may account for an additional 10 to 15% of MRSA transmissions in health care settings.

Community-acquired MRSA (CA-MRSA)

MRSA are no longer exclusively nosocomial pathogens. They have been affecting people without exposure to health care. Although CA-MRSA colonization rates have lagged behind those of MSSA, infection rates for those colonized with CA-MRSA are up to 10 times higher than rates for those colonized with MSSA.

Worldwide, CA-MRSA infections have been mainly due to only a few PFGE types, e.g. USA300 strain. Rates of infection with USA300 CA-MRSA are rising and in some locations have exceeded MSSA infection rates. Risk factors for infection or colonization with CA-MRSA include African American race, HIV infection, drug use, tattooing, and situations and environments associated with increased person-to-person contact such as military service, jails, homosexual contacts, sports activity, and children's day care.

Potential reservoirs and sources for CA-MRSA may include animals (e.g. pigs, cattle, horses, chickens, and companion animals). One study found that a novel strain of MRSA in the Netherlands was associated with pig or cattle farmers. Another MRSA strain with an altered *mecA* gene has been identified in Europe among humans and dairy cows. The extent of transmission occurring between humans and animals, and how this contributes to spread of MRSA in the community among humans, is unclear.

Secular trends and morbidity

Overall trends in hospitalizations for *S. aureus* infections suggest an increasing burden of illness. Trends fostering increases include aging of populations in western societies with increased comorbidities and use of prosthetic devices such as joint replacements; the emergence of CA-MRSA, which is occurring in addition to, not in place of, community-associated MSSA; and use of broad-spectrum antibiotics. In the United States of America, it has been estimated that about 9 of every 1000 hospitalizations may be due to *S. aureus*, and about 43% of *S. aureus* admissions are due to MRSA. Mortality rates among patients infected with *S. aureus* are 15 to 34% in various studies. Clinical factors enhancing the likelihood of death include pneumonia, older age, diabetes, inadequate therapy, and failure to drain infected foci. With spread of CA-MRSA into hospitals, the epidemiology and control of nosocomial MRSA may change.

CA-MRSA strains are now a common cause of skin and soft tissue infections (SSTIs) in ambulatory clinics and emergency rooms in the United States of America. In addition, CA-MRSA strains now account for a significant proportion of healthcare-associated and nosocomial bacteraemias in several United States hospitals.

In addition, *S. aureus* has been increasingly recognized as a bacterial pathogen that can complicate influenza. CA-MRSA strains have been linked to severe pneumonia among young healthy patients following influenza.

Prevention: *S. aureus*

General interventions

Prevention of illness due to *S. aureus*, particularly MRSA, relies on proactive infection control measures. These may include surveillance for MRSA colonization to detect the resistance iceberg, barrier precautions (use of gowning and gloving) for care of infected and colonized patients, imposed grouping (cohorting) of infected and colonized patients, isolation wards, improved hand hygiene, antimicrobial stewardship, cleaning patients with chlorhexidine, improved environmental cleaning, and use of intensive care unit 'monitors' to promote adherence to infection control measures.

MRSA

Studies of MRSA control suggest that multiple simultaneous interventions can reduce colonization and infection rates. Highly promoted among packages or bundles of interventions are hospital admission surveillance nasal cultures for MRSA colonization. These are recommended in high-risk units (although results of recent randomized trials question the effectiveness of surveillance for MRSA colonization in intensive care unit patients) or when other control measures fail to reduce MRSA infection rates. The role of decolonization of patients colonized by MRSA detected by surveillance is currently being studied. The strongest support for decolonization comes from outbreak investigations, particularly in neonatal units. The evaluation of risks/benefits of decolonization programmes, and of the impact on overall nosocomial infection rates, awaits the findings from ongoing studies.

CA-MRSA

Control of CA-MRSA presents distinct challenges. The feasibility of contact precautions or isolation of infected persons in the community may be limited. Additionally, the role of fomites in transmission of CA-MRSA is unknown, and community environmental decontamination may be difficult. Current guidelines for people with CA-MRSA infections and their community contacts include proper dressings for infected areas, hand hygiene, washing clothes contaminated with infected secretions, and avoiding contact sports while lesions exist. If infection is recurrent or spreading in specific settings, such as families, search for and decolonization of carriers may be useful.

Agents useful for decolonization

Potential agents used for staphylococcal decolonization include topical agents (mupirocin, chlorhexidine, tea tree oil) or short courses of systemic antimicrobials. Mupirocin 2% is effective for decolonization but has not been shown to reduce nosocomial infection rates and is of limited use when mupirocin resistance occurs. Tea tree oil, from the Ti (or Tea) tree (*Melaleuca alternifolia*, Myrtaceae), has been effective for some colonized patients. Chlorhexidine gluconate has potent antibacterial effects for decolonizing skin or as a nasal gel. Failure to control spread of specific clones of MRSA due to efflux of chlorhexidine from resistant bacteria has been reported, but, resistant strains have been very rare in systematic studies. Baths containing dilute bleach solutions have been advocated by paediatricians for interrupting cycles of MRSA skin infection in infants, and assiduous application of approved detergents/disinfectants or bleach can decontaminate the environment.

Clinical features: *S. aureus*

Risk factors for infection

Groups commonly at risk of colonization and infection include AIDS patients, intravenous drug users, and patients with diabetes mellitus. Multiple risk factors for *S. aureus* infection often coexist. For example, haemodialysis and peritoneal dialysis patients are at increased colonization risk and have high-risk foreign bodies. Conditions that predispose specifically to tissue invasion include skin trauma, haematomas, burns, or chronic diseases (e.g. dermatitis or psoriasis); surgical wounds; indwelling vascular catheters; and postviral sequelae such as influenza-related mucosal damage. Rarer conditions associated with increased risks of staphylococcal infection include Chédiak–Higashi syndrome and Job's syndrome (Oxford Textbook of Medicine 5e Chapter 5.2).

Clinical syndromes

S. aureus infection syndromes can be divided into three groups: (1) illness due to release of toxins, leading to disease at sites often remote from infection; (2) illness due to local tissue destruction and abscess formation; and (3) haematogenous infection. Therapy for these syndromes is based on the use of active drugs at appropriate dosages with appropriate concern for common side effects and toxicities.

Toxin-related syndromes
Staphylococcal scalded skin syndrome

In 1878, staphylococcal scalded skin syndrome (SSSS), or Ritter's disease, was described in 297 children by the German physician Ritter von Rittershain. After release of epidermolytic toxins by *S. aureus*, patients develop bullae and desquamation. Though clinically impressive (Fig. 6.4.1a), this superficial desquamation can be distinguished clinically and histologically from deeper exfoliative illnesses such as toxic epidermal necrolysis (TEN). In SSSS, skin separation occurs within the epidermis, at the stratum granulosum, while in TEN, separation occurs deeper, at the dermal–epidermal junction, leading to more severe skin loss. The absence of mucosal disease in SSSS also distinguishes these syndromes.

SSSS occurs more commonly in children (Fig. 6.4.1b). Disease may be generalized or localized (i.e. bullous impetigo), and the burden of *S. aureus* may be low. Nasal or mucosal colonization may cause disease. When cases occur in epidemics, such as in neonatal units, patients and health care workers should be screened for carriage. Diagnosis relies on the characteristic clinical and epidemiological features and is supported by identification of exotoxin-positive strains colonizing or infecting clinical sites. Treatment involves topical or systemic antibiotics for infected sites and supportive care for areas of skin/soft tissue destruction.

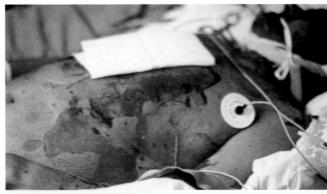

(a)

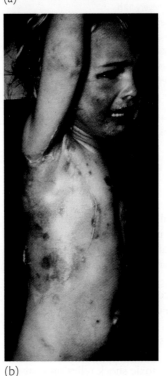

(b)

Fig. 6.4.1 Staphylococcal scalded skin syndrome: (a) in an adult; (b) in a child. (a, copyright Professor S J Eykyn; b, copyright Professor W C Noble.)

Food-borne illness due to preformed toxin

S. aureus can produce a heat-stable superantigen toxin that can persist even after cooking has eradicated the organism. Ingestion of toxin in contaminated, often unrefrigerated, food can result in epidemic gastrointestinal disease. There is a short incubation of only 2 to 6 h, followed by sudden vomiting (82%), diarrhoea (68%), and occasionally fever (16%). The differential diagnosis includes other short-incubation toxin-mediated gastrointestinal pathogens such as *Bacillus cereus* and toxins (Oxford Textbook of Medicine 5e Chapter 9.2). Treatment involves supportive care, particularly rehydration. The illness is typically self-limited, lasting less than 12 h.

Toxic shock syndrome

Staphylococcal toxic shock syndrome is caused by superantigen toxins released by *S. aureus*, resulting in multisystem organ dysfunction. Staphylococcal toxic shock is clinically similar to streptococcal toxic shock (high fever, mental confusion, erythroderma,

Table 6.4.1 Therapy of toxic shock due to *S. aureus*

Drug	Dosage	Duration/comment
For penicillin-susceptible *S. aureus*:		Duration based on focus of infection
Penicillin[a]	2–4 MU IV every 4 h	Adequate drainage is critical
Ampicillin	1–2 g IV every 4–6 h	
Ampicillin + sulbactam	1.5–3 g IV every 6 h	Data to support adjunctive use of immunoglobulin and/or clindamycin are needed
For methicillin-susceptible *S. aureus*:		
Oxacillin/flucloxacillin[a]	1–2 g IV every 4–6 h	
Cefazolin	1–2 g IV every 8 h	
For methicillin-resistant *S. aureus* (or β-lactam allergy):		
Vancomycin[a]	15 mg/kg IV every 12 h	
Clindamycin[b]	600 mg IV every 8 h	
Daptomycin	6 mg/kg IV every 24 h	
Teicoplanin	At least 400 mg IV BID	
Linezolid[b]	600 mg IV every 12 h	
Quinupristin/dalfopristin	7.5 mg/kg every 12 h	
Intravenous immunoglobulin	Dosage not standardized	

BID, twice daily; IV, intravenously. Note: dosing recommendations assume normal renal and hepatic function.
[a] First-line agent.
[b] These agents may be useful for reduction of protein synthesis and toxin production, but require further study.

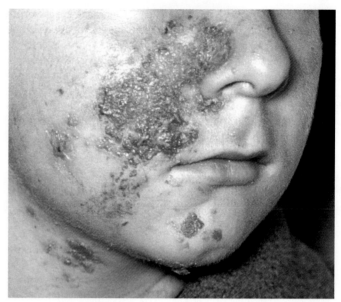

Fig. 6.4.2 Staphylococcal impetigo.
(Copyright Dr Renwick Vickers.)

diarrhoea, hypotension, and renal failure), but streptococcal toxic shock is typically associated with invasive infection such as necrotizing fasciitis while staphylococcal toxic shock may be precipitated by clinically minor infections that are overshadowed by the systemic effects of the toxin.

Staphylococcal toxic shock occurs in two major forms, menstrual (e.g. tampon-associated) and nonmenstrual. In women with vaginal colonization by *S. aureus*, it is presumably the favourable microenvironment during menses that leads to increased production of toxin (TSST-1).

Management of staphylococcal toxic shock relies on systemic antimicrobial therapy (Table 6.4.1), supportive care, and prompt drainage of infected/colonized foci. Common adjunctive therapies such as intravenous immunoglobulin to bind free toxin and antibacterials (especially clindamycin) with activity at the ribosome, which decreases bacterial protein (toxin) synthesis, have a theoretical rationale and some support from animal models; however, clinical data are limited.

Illness due to local tissue invasion/destruction

S. aureus and β-haemolytic streptococci cause approximately 80% of soft tissue infections. *S. aureus* is the aetiological agent of 37 to 65% of native monoarticular joint infections in healthy adults and of 75% of joint infections in rheumatoid arthritis. Osteomyelitis, either of haematogenous or contiguous origin, is caused by *S. aureus* or coagulase-negative staphylococci in more than 50% of cases. Any local infection can lead to secondary bacteraemia and haematogenous seeding of distant sites.

Impetigo, folliculitis, and cellulitis

The most superficial *S. aureus* infections are impetigo, folliculitis, and cellulitis. Impetigo is limited to the epidermis, folliculitis to the hair follicles, and cellulitis to the dermis and/or the subcutaneous fat.

Impetigo can appear as small round honey-crusted lesions on the skin, primarily on exposed areas (Fig. 6.4.2). Impetigo typically is caused by streptococci; in the United Kingdom, *S. aureus* is an infrequent cause. However, bullous impetigo is a clinical variant (caused by *S. aureus* phage type 71), reported in up to 10% of impetigo cases. Initially, the lesions can be vesicles that enlarge into bullae containing clear or yellow fluid.

Cellulitis is typically due to streptococci, but when associated with penetrating trauma, furuncles, or carbuncles *S. aureus* should be considered. Diagnosis depends on the clinical appearance and the presence of purulence that can be cultured. However, aspirates of cellulitic areas are positive in fewer than one-third of cases and bacteraemia is rare.

Treatment of impetigo (Table 6.4.2) should reflect local antibiotic resistance patterns. Topical therapy may be effective for limited disease, though EMRSA-16, one of two predominant MRSA types in the United Kingdom, often shows high-level mupirocin resistance. Systemic therapy should be used in patients with impetigo who have many lesions or who fail topical therapy. In areas where CA-MRSA prevalence exceeds 10%, initial therapy should be directed by local susceptibility patterns.

Suspicion of more invasive infection, such as necrotizing fasciitis, should be high in cases of soft tissue infections with disproportionate pain, bullae, haemorrhagic or necrotic lesions, cutaneous anaesthesia, rapid progression of lesions, gas in the tissues, presence of risk factors, and when laboratory tests show elevated creatine kinase, acidosis, leucocytosis, or C-reactive protein exceeding 13 mg/litre. Necrotizing infections should prompt inpatient antibiotic therapy assuming MRSA and urgent surgical consultation.

Furuncles and carbuncles

Furuncles and carbuncles are deep suppurative infections that occur in the dermis and originate at hair follicles. Infection can be limited to small lesions that appear as painful nodules, sometimes with necrotic centres (Fig. 6.4.3a). Confluence leads to the formation of carbuncles (Fig. 6.4.3b). Several members of a family may

Table 6.4.2 Therapy of impetigo and mild soft tissue lesions caused by *S. aureus*

Therapy	Drug	Dosage	Duration
Topical	Mupirocin	2% ointment TID	14 days
	Fusidic acid	2% cream TID	
Oral	**For methicillin-susceptible *S. aureus*:**		
	Dicloxacillin[a]	250 mg PO QID	
	Cefalexin	500 mg PO QID	
	For methicillin-resistant *S. aureus* (or β-lactam allergy):		
	Clindamycin (Ery[s], Clin[s], or D-test negative)	300–450 mg PO QID	7 days
	Trimethoprim/ sulfamethoxazole	1–2 double-strength[b] tablets PO BID	7 days
	Doxycycline	100 mg PO BID	
	Minocycline	100 mg PO BID	
	Linezolid	600 mg po BID	

BID, twice daily; Clin[s], clindamycin-sensitive; D, double-disc diffusion; Ery[s], erythromycin-sensitive; PO, by mouth; QID, four times daily; TID, three times daily.

[a] First-line agent.

[b] 160 mg trimethoprim and 800 mg sulfamethoxazole in a double-strength tablet.

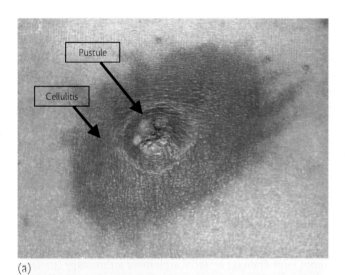

(a)

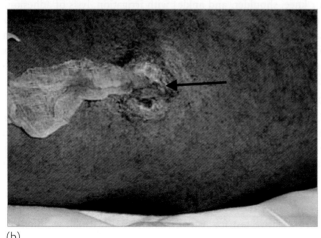

(b)

Fig. 6.4.3 (a) Pustule/early furuncle with surrounding cellulitis due to *S. aureus*. (b) Coalescent furuncles, i.e. carbuncle, that required incision and drainage.

be affected. Mild lesions cause limited systemic complaints, whereas fever, malaise, or symptoms and signs of sepsis can occur with extensive disease.

Furunculosis is caused increasingly by the emerging pathogen CA-MRSA and has been attributed to the presence of PVL toxin, although the causal role requires validation. Additionally, toxin-containing *S. aureus* has been associated with more fulminant courses in which skin lesions, pneumonia, a sepsis-like picture, or even Waterhouse–Friderichsen syndrome occur. PVL occurs in about 2% of MSSA and most CA-MRSA.

Drainage, spontaneously or surgically, is the mainstay of therapy. Early furuncles may be treated by application of moist heat to stimulate drainage. Lesions on the face, lesions with cellulitis (especially exceeding 5 cm in diameter), or the presence of systemic symptoms and/or signs (fever, chills, or haemodynamic changes) should lead to use of antistaphylococcal antibiotics (Table 6.4.3) in addition to drainage. Oral agents are sufficient in most cases, but in severe infections or for bacteraemia parenteral agents should be used.

Mastitis

Mastitis is most commonly caused by *S. aureus*, occurs in 1 to 3% of nursing mothers typically within 3 weeks of birth, and may lead to breast abscesses. Infection can appear as a painful nodule or a draining abscess. Therapy (Table 6.4.3) should include topical moist heat, oral antimicrobials with efficacy against *S. aureus* (and MRSA in endemic areas), and abscess incision and drainage.

Pyomyositis

Pyomyositis, or primary bacterial abscess of skeletal muscle, is most common in the tropics where 'tropical pyomyositis' can account for 1 to 4% of hospital admissions (Oxford Textbook of Medicine 5e Chapter 24.24.6). In nontropical areas the syndrome is uncommon. *S. aureus* is the cause in about 95% of tropical cases and about 70% of other cases. Associations are with muscle trauma (20–50% of cases), HIV infection, and possibly *Toxocara canis* infection.

Symptoms develop subacutely over 2 to 3 weeks with variable degrees of fever, muscle pain, swelling, and induration. Large lower extremity and trunk muscles are most commonly affected. Regional lymphadenopathy is typically absent. Diagnosis relies on clinical suspicion, helpful radiographic findings (i.e. gas or soft tissue swelling on plain radiographs, abscess or muscle enlargement on ultrasound examination, inflammation, oedema, or focal abscess in muscles on MRI or CT, and the results of aspirating the lesion. Antibacterial therapy for *S. aureus* (Table 6.4.3) and open or radiographically assisted percutaneous drainage of abscesses are essential parts of therapy.

Septic bursitis

Infection can occur in any of the approximately 160 bursae found in humans, but septic bursitis usually affects prepatellar or olecranon bursae, usually is a result of trauma. It is due to *S. aureus* in more than 80% of cases but is accompanied by bacteraemia in 8% or less. Diagnosis relies on clinical recognition of the characteristic findings of fever and pain, swelling, redness, and warmth in the area of an affected bursa. Leucocytes and *S. aureus* are found if there is enough bursal fluid to aspirate.

Treatment of septic bursitis includes appropriate antimicrobials (Table 6.4.4) and, if possible, drainage. Treatment failures have been described when erythromycin is used as the sole agent. Localized infection with no systemic signs may be treated with

Table 6.4.3 Therapy of cellulitis, abscess, mastitis, furunculosis, and pyomyositis caused by *S. aureus*

Therapy	Drug	Dosage	Duration/comment
Oral	**For methicillin-susceptible *S. aureus*:**		5 days for cellulitis
			For deeper infection duration depends on proper drainage when necessary and clinical response
	Flucloxacillin or dicloxacillin[a]	500 mg PO QID	With incision and drainage, lesions with <5 cm of cellulitis in immunocompetent patients may be cured
	Cefalexin	500 mg PO QID	without systemic antibiotics
	For methicillin-resistant *S. aureus* (or β-lactam allergy):		For deeper infection duration depends on proper drainage when necessary and clinical response
	Clindamycin (Ery[S], Clin[S], or D-test negative)	300–450 mg PO QID	Early change to oral therapy may be employed in stabilizing, nonbacteraemic patients
	Trimethoprim/sulfamethoxazole	1–2 double-strength[b] tablets PO BID	May have a future role
	Doxycycline	100 mg PO BID	
	Minocycline	100 mg PO BID	
	Linezolid	600 mg PO BID	
	Erythromycin[c]	250 mg PO every 6 h or 500 mg PO every 12 h	
Parenteral	**For methicillin-susceptible *S. aureus*:**		
	Oxacillin/flucloxacillin[a]	1–2 g IV every 4–6 h	
	Cefazolin	1–2 g IV every 8 h	
	For methicillin-resistant *S. aureus* (or β-lactam allergy):		
	Vancomycin[a]	15 mg/kg IV every 12 h	
	Erythromycin[c]	250 mg IV every 6 h or 500 mg IV every 12 h	
	Clindamycin (Ery[S], Clin[S], or D-test negative)	600 mg IV every 8 h	
	Linezolid	600 mg IV every 12 h	
	Daptomycin	4 mg/kg IV every 24 h	
	Quinupristin/dalfopristin	7.5 mg/kg every 12 h	
	Tigecycline	100 mg initially, then 50 mg IV every 12 h	
	Dalbavancin, oritavancin, telavancin		

BID, twice daily; Clin[S], clindamycin-sensitive; D, double-disc diffusion; Ery[S], erythromycin-sensitive; PO, by mouth; QID, four times daily; TID three times daily; IV, intravenously.
[a] First-line agent.
[b] 160 mg trimethoprim and 800 mg sulfamethoxazole in a double-strength tablet. Note: dosing recommendations assume normal renal and hepatic function.
[c] In many areas high rates of resistance should prevent empiric use of erythromycin.

oral therapy, since high antimicrobials levels are achieved in bursal fluid. Adequate drainage is important. Patients with systemic signs or symptoms or who are immunocompromised should receive parenteral therapy.

Patients who present within 7 days of developing symptoms may be treated successfully with antibiotics and aspiration every 1 to 3 days. In this situation, bursal fluid may become sterile within 4 days and therapy should be continued for an additional 5 days. Surgical intervention is needed only for patients whose fluid remains infected or cannot be aspirated because the bursa is deep, who have foreign or necrotic material in the bursal space, or who need exploration or removal of the bursa because of recurrences.

Septic arthritis

S. aureus is the most common cause of nonprosthetic monoarticular septic arthritis. The typical pathogenesis is haematogenous seeding, but traumatic direct inoculation can occur. Important differential diagnoses include gonococcal infection in adolescents and adults and urosepsis pathogens and crystal-induced arthropathies in older patients. Because joint destruction is rapid, prompt diagnosis through joint aspiration is essential.

The mainstays of therapy are antimicrobials (Table 6.4.4) and prompt joint drainage by serial aspiration; arthroscopy (preferred for knee, shoulder, and ankle) with irrigation, lysis of adhesions, and removal of purulent material; or open drainage (useful for hip or shoulder infections to protect blood supply to femoral or humeral heads, and in instances where repeated aspirates or arthroscopy fail). *S. aureus* can be a cause of infected prosthetic joints, which may have a more indolent atypical presentation.

Osteomyelitis

S. aureus osteomyelitis results from bacteraemia or contiguous spread from a soft tissue focus or chronic ulcer. Risk groups are patients with diabetes mellitus, those with vascular disease or at risk for haematogenous infection (i.e. haemodialysis), children, and elderly people.

Diagnosis usually depends on radiographic studies. Plain radiographs may show evidence of periosteal reaction. However, the most sensitive test for osteomyelitis is MRI, which will demonstrate changes within bone and bone marrow. The most specific test is CT, which will reveal the presence of periosteal reaction or other bony changes not evident on plain radiographs. 'Probing

Table 6.4.4 Therapy of septic bursitis and septic arthritis caused by *S. aureus*

Therapy	Drug	Dosage	Duration/comment
Oral	**For methicillin-susceptible *S. aureus*:**		
	Flucloxacillin or dicloxacillin[a]	500 mg PO QID	
	Cefalexin	500 mg PO QID	
	For methicillin-resistant *S. aureus* (or β-lactam allergy):		
	Clindamycin (Ery[s], Clin[s], or D-test negative)	300–450 mg PO QID	
	Trimethoprim/sulfamethoxazole	1–2 double-strength[b] tablets PO BID	
	Doxycycline	100 mg PO BID	
	Minocycline	100 mg PO BID	
	Ciprofloxacin or levofloxacin	500 mg PO BID or 500 mg PO once daily	
	With		
	Rifampin	300 mg PO every 12 h	
	Linezolid	600 mg PO BID	
	Erythromycin[c]	250 mg PO every 6 h or 500 mg PO every 12 h	
Parenteral	**For methicillin-susceptible *S. aureus*:**		
	Oxacillin/flucloxacillin[a]	1–2 g IV every 4–6 h	
	Cefazolin	1–2 g IV every 8 h	
	For methicillin-resistant *S. aureus* (or β-lactam allergy):		
	Vancomycin[a]	15 mg/kg IV every 12 h	
	Linezolid	600 mg IV every 12 h	

BID, twice daily; Clin[s], clindamycin-sensitive; D, double-disc diffusion; Ery[s], erythromycin-sensitive; PO, by mouth; QID, four times daily; TID three times daily; IV, intravenously.
[a] First-line agent.
[b] 160 mg trimethoprim and 800 mg sulfamethoxazole in a double-strength tablet. Note: dosing recommendations assume normal renal and hepatic function.
[c] In many areas high rates of resistance should prevent empiric use of erythromycin.

to bone' in the case of a chronic ulcer is highly sensitive for a diagnosis of osteomyelitis. The microbiological diagnosis of osteomyelitis relies on positive blood or bone cultures; superficial wound or sinus track culture results are not reliable and may be misleading.

Therapy for osteomyelitis includes drainage of pus (acute osteomyelitis) or debridement of areas of avascular or 'dead' bone (sequestra in chronic osteomyelitis) and antibacterials with activity against the culture-proven pathogen(s). The duration of therapy sufficient to eradicate the organism and prevent relapse is based on common experience and usually is 4 to 6 weeks. Children with acute haematogenous *S. aureus* osteomyelitis may be treated with surgical drainage of purulent collections and short-course intravenous therapy (e.g. 1 week) followed by oral therapy for 4 to 6 weeks as outpatients. Initial choice for therapy is based on the presence of MSSA or MRSA (Table 6.4.5); copathogens may require broader therapy. An open-label study showed that for diabetic foot infections, linezolid performed as well as ampicillin–sulbactam for infected ulcers or osteomyelitis.

Epidural abscess
Epidural abscesses occur adjacent to vertebral osteomyelitis and are medical/surgical emergencies (Fig. 6.4.4). Enlarging epidural sites can compress the spinal cord or reduce vascular supply through thrombophlebitis. About 50% of cases follow haematogenous spread from known or occult trauma or from parenteral use of illicit drugs, while about 30% result from contiguous spread. *S. aureus* accounts for more than 60% of cases. Risks for MRSA infection include recent health care exposure or rising CA-MRSA rates.

Symptoms and physical findings progress at variable rates, sometimes rapidly, through four stages: (1) back pain at the infected level, (2) pain radiating in the distribution of affected nerve roots, (3) motor weakness (including bladder and bowel dysfunction) and sensory deficit at the appropriate level, and (4) paralysis. The triad of back pain, fever, and neurological findings is highly suggestive of epidural abscess.

MRI or CT scanning is most useful for evaluating epidural abscesses (Fig. 6.4.4). For diagnosis and therapy, a space-occupying lesion in the epidural space requires surgical evaluation and emergency laminectomy/decompression or drainage by interventional radiography.

Table 6.4.5 Therapy of osteomyelitis caused by *S. aureus*

Therapy	Drug	Dosage	Duration
Parenteral	**For methicillin-susceptible *S. aureus*[b]:**		4–6 weeks IV
	Oxacillin/flucloxacillin[a]	1–2 g IV every 4–6 h	
	Cefazolin	1–2 g IV every 8 h	
	For methicillin-resistant *S. aureus* (or β-lactam allergy):		
	Vancomycin[a]	15 mg/kg IV every 12 h	
	Linezolid	600 mg IV every 12 h	

IV, intravenously. Note: dosing recommendations assume normal renal and hepatic function.
[a] First-line agent.
[b] In 2011, the Infectious Disease Society of American came out with first guidelines for treatment of MRSA. Although the optimal duration of treatment of osteomyelitis due to MRSA has not been established, the guidelines suggest at least 8 weeks of therapy.

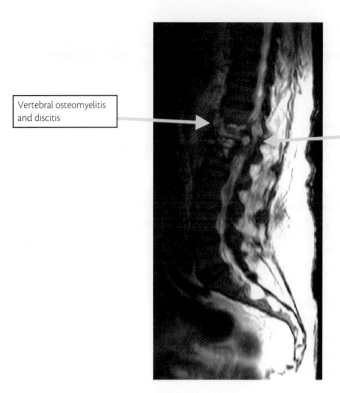

Fig. 6.4.4 Epidural abscess and vertebral osteomyelitis due to *S. aureus*.

Preoperative neurological status predicts outcome. Broad empirical antimicrobial therapy should include coverage for MRSA (Table 6.4.6) and Gram-negative bacilli. If MSSA infection is diagnosed, β-lactams are preferred over glycopeptides.

Pneumonia

S. aureus pneumonia can result from haematogenous spread or direct inoculation following mucosal damage. *S. aureus* causes less than 10% of cases of community-acquired pneumonia but causes approximately 20 to 30% of cases of nosocomial pneumonia. Case fatality of *S. aureus* pneumonia ranges from 8% to more than 30%. Risks for a more severe course include MRSA, acute respiratory distress syndrome (ARDS), comorbidities, and renal dysfunction.

S. aureus is a cause of postviral, particularly postinfluenza, pneumonia. Patients may report a biphasic illness. CA-MRSA may cause a necrotizing pneumonia with more severe course.

Additionally, *S. aureus* pneumonia may be associated with complications such as empyema, lung abscesses, and bronchopleural fistulae. Lung abscess must be differentiated radiographically from pneumatocele, a common and relatively benign complication of staphylococcal pneumonia.

Diagnostic studies for patients with pneumonia in the presence of staphylococcal bacteraemia or embolic-appearing lesions on chest imaging (Fig. 6.4.5) should seek an intravascular source (e.g. endocarditis or infectious thrombophlebitis). Therapy (Table 6.4.7) should include use of an active drug for at least 8 days in less complicated cases or longer if pulmonary involvement is secondary to an intravascular infection, presence of MRSA, or

Table 6.4.6 Therapy of epidural abscess caused by *S. aureus*

Therapy	Drug	Dosage	Duration
Parenteral	**For methicillin-susceptible *S. aureus*:**		≥6 weeks IV
	Oxacillin/ flucloxacillin[a]	1–2 g IV every 4–6 h	
	Cefazolin	1–2 g IV every 8 h	
	For methicillin-resistant *S. aureus* (or β-lactam allergy):		
	Vancomycin[a]	15 mg/kg IV every 12 h	
	Linezolid	600 mg IV every 12 h	
	Daptomycin	6 mg/kg IV every 24 h	

IV, intravenously. Note: dosing recommendations assume normal renal and hepatic function.

[a] First-line agent.

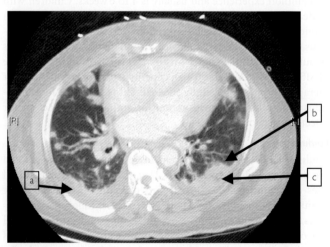

Fig. 6.4.5 Pneumonia due to *S. aureus*, from septic pulmonary emboli. Note presence of (a) empyema, (b) nodular (including pleural-based) infiltrate, and (c) early cavitation of abscess.

Table 6.4.7 Therapy of pneumonia due to *S. aureus*

Drug	Dosage	Duration/comment
For methicillin-susceptible *S. aureus*:		7–14 days for uncomplicated infection
Oxacillin/flucloxacillin[a]	1–2 g IV every 4 h	
Cefazolin	1–2 g IV every 8 h	
For methicillin-resistant *S. aureus* (or β-lactam allergy):		Requires longer courses if empyema, lung abscess, or bacteraemia present
Vancomycin[a]	15 mg/kg IV every 12 h	
Linezolid	600 mg IV every 12 h	

IV, intravenously. Note: dosing recommendations assume normal renal and hepatic function..
[a] First-line agent.

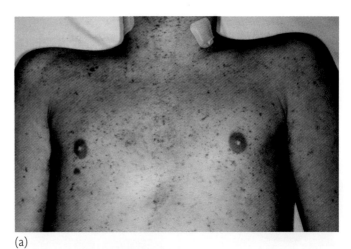

(a)

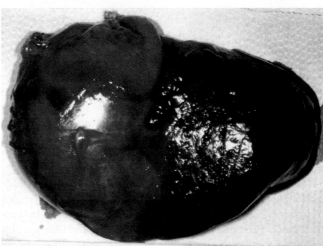

(b)

Fig. 6.4.6 *S. aureus* bacteraemia and infective endocarditis. (a) Meningococcal-like rash in a patient with *S. aureus* endocarditis of a bicuspid aortic valve and aortic root abscess. (b) Splenic abscess complicating *S. aureus* endocarditis. (Copyright Professor S J Eykyn.)

complications such as emboli or empyema. Surgical drainage is indicated for empyema. Daptomycin should be avoided because of its poorer activity in pulmonary infections. Linezolid may emerge as a drug of choice for MRSA pneumonia based on its greater penetration due to smaller molecule size and putative clinical benefit.

Urinary tract infections

S. aureus urinary tract infections (UTIs) result from ascending infection in catheterized patients or haematogenous seeding, which may lead to renal carbuncles (abscesses). Staphylococcal UTIs should prompt consideration of sources of bacteraemia such as endovascular infection. Clinically, patients with renal abscesses have fever and flank pain, but urinary complaints may be absent and urinalyses and urine cultures may be negative. Renal ultrasonography or CT may show a range of findings from 'lobar nephronia' (renal phlegmon) to large multilocular abscesses. Treatment may require percutaneous or open drainage; antimicrobial therapy (Table 6.4.8) should reflect results of cultures.

Haematogenous infections

Bacteraemia

S. aureus is among the commonest causes of bacteraemia in hospitals and the community. It causes 18 to 27% of endocarditis cases (Fig. 6.4.6), is responsible for 13% of nosocomial bloodstream infections, and causes up to 78% of cases of intravascular catheter-related thrombophlebitis. Rates of community-associated *S. aureus* bacteraemia in the United States of America are estimated at 17/100 000 people, similar to rates of invasive *Streptococcus*

Table 6.4.8 Therapy of urinary tract infection due to *S. aureus*

Drug	Dosage	Duration/comment
For methicillin-susceptible *S. aureus*:		7 days for ascending infection
Oxacillin/flucloxacillin[a]	1–2 g IV every 4 h	
Cefazolin	1–2 g IV every 8 h	≥ 14 days for renal abscess, bacteraemia, or complicated infection (duration is based on resolution of infected foci and/or use of drainage)
For methicillin-resistant *S. aureus* (or β-lactam allergy):		
Vancomycin[a]	15 mg/kg IV every 12 h	
Linezolid	600 mg IV every 12 h	

IV, intravenously. Note: dosing recommendations assume normal renal and hepatic function.
[a] First-line agent.

pneumoniae infection, with mortality of 10 to 20%, depending on underlying illnesses. In Oxfordshire, England, the incidence of nosocomial MRSA bacteraemia increased from 50/100 000 admissions in 1997 to 300/100 000 admissions in 2004, increasing the overall burden of *S. aureus* disease.

S. aureus in blood should always be considered a true pathogen. Bacteraemia has traditionally been categorized as 'health care-associated' (i.e. onset more than 2 days after admission) and 'community-associated' (i.e. onset within 2 days of admission). Complications of bacteraemia include endocarditis (itself a major cause of bacteraemia) and 'metastatic' seeding of distant sites, especially joints, bone, kidney, and skin (Fig. 6.4.7). An estimated 13% of nosocomial bacteraemias with *S. aureus* include endocarditis.

If MSSA is isolated from cultures, a penicillinase-resistant penicillin (oxacillin or nafcillin) should be used instead of vancomycin as these agents have better activity against MSSA. A cephalosporin, cefazolin, has also been widely used to treat MSSA infections because of its convenient dosing. There are limited data comparing these

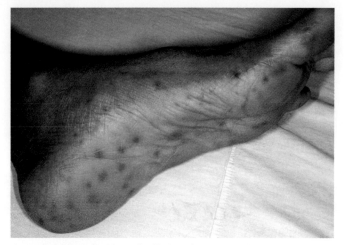

Fig. 6.4.7 Seeding of MRSA to the skin in a Vietnamese patient. (Copyright D A Warrell.)

agents for treatment of MSSA infections. Recently, a retrospective case–control study comparing cefazolin to nafcillin for the treatment of MSSA bacteraemia observed that they had similar treatment failure rates with cefazolin having fewer adverse drug effects. However, a limitation of this study is that there were few endocarditis cases and no meningitis cases, limiting the generalizability of these findings.

The principles of therapy for *S. aureus* bacteraemia include evaluation for endocarditis; use of a parenteral agent; removal of infected foci (i.e. catheters or abscesses); and use of a bactericidal agent, preferably a β-lactam, whenever possible. Occasionally, uncomplicated bacteraemia with drainage of infected foci and no embolic sites may respond to only 14 days of therapy (Table 6.4.9); however, more often, prolonged bacteraemia, residual disease, undrained foci of infection, infected clots, or endocarditis all warrant longer therapy (at least 4 weeks).

Endocarditis (Oxford Textbook of Medicine 5e Chapter 16.9.2)

Many features of endocarditis are nonspecific (fever, tachycardia, arthralgias and myalgias, wasting, and back pain). Finding a new cardiac (especially diastolic) murmur or septic emboli provides strong supportive evidence. Other suggestive findings include petechiae, Janeway's lesions, mycotic aneurysms of arterial vessels (with resultant pain, vascular leak, or adjacent deep venous thrombosis), discitis or osteomyelitis (particularly vertebral disease), and neurological complications such as septic infarcts or mycotic cerebrovascular aneurysms. Conduction abnormalities, e.g. AV delay, may be noted in the presence of myocardial abscess. In the setting of right-sided endocarditis, septic pulmonary emboli are common.

The presence of multiple positive blood cultures is a necessary criterion for diagnosis of endocarditis in the untreated patient. Diagnosis is aided by specific criteria (e.g. modified Duke's criteria). Transthoracic echocardiography is indicated as a noninvasive method to evaluate the presence of cardiac vegetations in those with low pretest probability of disease; individuals with nondiagnostic studies or worsening clinical course should undergo transoesophageal echocardiogram. Patients with high clinical risk, despite nondiagnostic transoesophageal studies, should be restudied after 7 to 10 days.

Table 6.4.9 Therapy of bacteraemia, without endocarditis, due to *S. aureus*

Drug	Dosage	Duration/comment
For methicillin-susceptible *S. aureus*:		14 days with removable focus of infection
Oxacillin/flucloxacillin[a]	1–2 g IV every 4–6 h	
Cefazolin	1–2 g IV every 8 h	
For methicillin-resistant *S. aureus* (or β-lactam allergy):		Longer course of therapy for complicated infection
Vancomycin[a]	15 mg/kg IV every 12 h	
Daptomycin[a]	6 mg/kg IV every 24 h	
Teicoplanin	At least 400 mg IV BID	
Linezolid	600 mg IV every 12 h	
Quinupristin/dalfopristin	7.5 mg/kg every 12 h	
Sodium fusidate	500 mg IV every 8 h	
Dalbavancin, oritavancin, telavancin	May have future role	

BID, twice daily; IV, intravenously. Note: dosing recommendations assume normal renal and hepatic function.
[a] First-line agent.

Therapy for staphylococcal endocarditis requires a bactericidal antibiotic (Tables 6.4.10–6.4.12). In general, therapy should last for 4 (in uncomplicated disease) to 6 or more (in the setting of metastatic infection, perivalvular abscess, or other complications) weeks. Combination therapies (agents given with either vancomycin or β-lactams) have not been demonstrated to improve outcomes in native valve endocarditis but are commonly used.

Table 6.4.10 Therapy of native valve left-sided endocarditis due to *S. aureus*

Drug	Dosage	Duration/comment
For methicillin-susceptible *S. aureus*:		4–6 weeks after negative cultures
Oxacillin/flucloxacillin[a]	2 g IV every 4 h	
Cefazolin	1–2 g IV every 8 h	
For methicillin-resistant *S. aureus* (or β-lactam allergy):		
Vancomycin[a]	15 mg/kg IV every 12 h	
Teicoplanin[a]	At least 400 mg IV BID	
Linezolid	600 mg IV every 12 h	
Quinupristin/dalfopristin	7.5 mg/kg every 12 h	
Daptomycin	6 mg/kg IV every 24 h	
Sodium fusidate	500 mg IV every 8 h	
Trimethoprim/sulfamethoxazole	320 mg/1600 mg IV every 12 h	
Above therapies can be used with:		
Gentamicin[b] (3–5 days at start of therapy)	1 mg/kg IV every 8 h	

BID, twice daily; IV, intravenously. Note: dosing recommendations assume normal renal and hepatic function.
[a] First-line agent.
[b] Gentamicin therapy is optional, and has not been demonstrated to change clinical outcomes.

Table 6.4.11 Therapy of native valve right-sided endocarditis due to *S. aureus*

Drug	Dosage	Duration/comment
β-Lactams	As for left-sided disease (Table 6.4.10)	4–6 weeks after negative cultures
Vancomycin[a]	As for left-sided disease (Table 6.4.10)	
Daptomycin[a]	6 mg/kg IV every 24 h	
Above therapies can be used with:		
Gentamicin[b]	1 mg/kg IV every 8 h	3–5 days at start of therapy, or combined therapy with β-lactam for MSSA infection
Ciprofloxacin/ rifampicin[b]	750 mg/300 mg PO BID	For use in patients with tricuspid valve endocarditis who cannot/will not be admitted for intravenous therapy

BID, twice daily; IV, intravenously; PO, by mouth. Note: dosing recommendations assume normal renal and hepatic function.
[a] First-line agent.
[b] Use is indicated in only limited circumstances. Gentamicin therapy is optional and has not been shown to improve clinical outcomes.

Table 6.4.12 Therapy of prosthetic valve endocarditis due to *S. aureus*

Drug	Dosage	Duration/comment
For methicillin-susceptible *S. aureus*:		
Oxacillin/flucloxacillin[a] With	2 g IV every 4 h	≥6 weeks
Rifampicin And	300 mg PO/IV every 8 h	≥6 weeks
Gentamicin	1 mg/kg IV every 8 h	3–5 days at start of therapy
Cefazolin (second choice for MSSA)	1–2 g IV every 8 h	
For methicillin-resistant *S. aureus* (or β-lactam allergy):		
Vancomycin[a] With	15 mg/kg IV every 12 h	
Rifampicin And	300 mg PO/IV every 8 h	≥6 weeks
Gentamicin	1 mg/kg IV every 8 h	3–5 days at start of therapy

IV, intravenously; PO, by mouth. Note: dosing recommendations assume normal renal and hepatic function.
[a] First-line agent.

For example, the addition of gentamicin for 3 to 5 days shortens the duration of bacteraemia by about 1 day but does not influence outcome. Addition of rifampicin for bacteraemic patients with putative failure of therapy (e.g. bacteraemia or fever persisting for more than 4–5 days) is a common strategy. Rifampicin is recommended as part of the standard treatment of prosthetic valve endocarditis.

The average time to clearance of *S. aureus* from the bloodstream is 5 days of β-lactam or 1 week of vancomycin therapy. Prolonged bacteraemia should prompt a closer evaluation of antibiotic MICs (especially for vancomycin), a search for sequestered sites of infection or undrained foci, or a myocardial or valvular abscess.

The 2011 Infectious Disease Society of America guidelines for the treatment of MRSA suggest a vancomycin trough concentration of 15–20 μg/ml for serious infections (e.g. bacteraemia, infective endocarditis, osteomyelitis, meningitis, pneumonia, and severe SSTI such as necrotizing fasciitis). Part of the impetus for higher trough levels comes from studies that have suggested that there is an increased chance of treatment failure with vancomycin as the MIC for vancomycin increases to the upper limit of the susceptible range. However, in a study of an Australian cohort of patients with *S. aureus* bacteraemia, elevated vancomycin MIC was associated with increased 30 day mortality but meticillin resistance and specific antibiotic selection were not, suggesting that vancomycin itself may be a marker for more difficult-to-treat strains but not the driver per se of worse outcomes in these patients.

Increasing vancomycin dosing has not been demonstrated clearly to improve outcomes, although consensus supports increased trough levels of 15 to 20 μg/ml (requiring close monitoring of renal function) for serious infections. Although close monitoring of renal function is recommended, the data establishing the causal link between serum vancomycin concentration and nephrotoxicity are limited since concomitant nephrotoxic agents may play a role in toxicity. Indications for surgical valve replacement include new congestive heart failure (associated with higher mortality), failure to clear the bloodstream, recurrent emboli, and myocardial or valvular abscess. As daptomycin has concentration-dependent bactericidal activity against Gram-positive organisms, some have suggested higher doses (e.g. 8 mg/kg per day or greater) may be effective for treatment of complicated Gram-positive infections. However, further evaluation of this is needed, in particular the safety and tolerability of higher doses.

Clinical syndromes: coagulase-negative staphylococci

Coagulase-negative staphylococci are generally less virulent than *S. aureus*. Most infections with these organisms are the consequence of medical progress, related to foreign bodies (e.g. prosthetic joints or heart valves, indwelling intravascular catheters or grafts, or peritoneal catheters), and occur in association with health care. Syndromes caused by coagulase-negative staphylococci include endocarditis (5–8% of native valve infections, c.40% of prosthetic valve infections), intravascular catheter infections (6–27% of vascular catheter infections), prosthetic joint infections (up to 38% of arthroplasty infections), peritoneal dialysis catheter infections, and postoperative ocular infections. Production of biofilm by coagulase-negative staphylococci aids infection of both intravascular and peritoneal catheters. Therapy for infections with coagulase-negative staphylococci and side effects and toxicities are outlined in Tables 6.4.13 and 6.4.14.

Bacteraemia and infected vascular catheters
Clinical features and diagnosis
Coagulase-negative staphylococci are the most commonly reported bacteria in positive blood cultures; however, unlike *S. aureus*,

Table 6.4.13 Therapy for coagulase-negative staphylococcal infections

Indication	Drug	Dosage	Duration
Bacteraemia (with prompt catheter removal)	Vancomycin[a] Oxacillin/flucloxacillin (methicillin-susceptible *S. epidermidis*)	15 mg/kg IV every 12 h 1–2 g IV every 4 h	10–14 days
Bacteraemia (with attempted catheter salvage)	Vancomycin catheter lock (for catheter salvage)	1–5 mg/ml vancomycin, mixed with 50–100 U heparin or normal saline, to fill catheter lumen (total 2–5 ml of solution) when catheter not in use	14 days
	Vancomycin[a] Oxacillin/flucloxacillin (methicillin-susceptible *S. epidermidis*)	15 mg/kg IV every 12 h 1–2 g IV every 4 h	10–14 days

Prosthetic valve endocarditis	Vancomycin[a]
	with
	    Rifampicin[a]
	and
	    Gentamicin
	Oxacillin/flucloxacillin (methicillin-susceptible *S. epidermidis*)
		15 mg/kg IV every 12 h
		
		300 mg PO/IV every 8 h
		
		1 mg/kg IV every 8 h
		1–2 g IV every 4 h
			≥6 weeks

Peritoneal dialysis-associated peritonitis	Vancomycin[a] Or Vancomycin	30–50 mg vancomycin per litre of dialysate given intraperitoneally 1 g IV once, then based on levels (keep trough >10–15 mcg/ml)	10–21 days 10–21 days

IV, intravenously; PO, by mouth. Note: dosing recommendations assume normal renal and hepatic function.
[a] First-line agent.

coagulase-negative staphylococci are frequently blood culture contaminants. Typical rates of blood culture contamination by skin flora are approximately 2 to 3%; higher rates may be a sign of poor phlebotomy technique.

Infected intravascular catheters are common sources of coagulase-negative staphylococcal bloodstream infections. However, given the association of *S. epidermidis* and contaminated blood cultures, a careful physical examination for signs of catheter infection is critical to determine whether a single positive blood culture represents true infection and/or an infected catheter. Suggestive findings include fever, erythema at or purulence expressible from the site of catheter insertion, or tenderness.

Methods to enhance the identification of true bloodstream infection as opposed to contamination include proper skin preparation and obtaining at least two sets of blood cultures from sites separated by location and time. The use of quantitative catheter tip cultures (more than 15 colonies) or differential time to positivity (more than 2 h) for peripheral compared to catheter-drawn blood cultures helps assess whether a catheter is infected.

Management of bacteraemia and catheter infection

An approach for management of presumed infected catheters is to remove the catheter when the index of suspicion is high and/or the patient is unstable, with insertion of a new catheter at an uninvolved site. When likelihood of infection is unclear and the patient is stable, the catheter can be changed over a guidewire and the tip cultured. Positive tip cultures should prompt removal of the replacement catheter and new catheter insertion at a different site. A negative culture may allow the replacement catheter to remain in place, although its risk of subsequent infection is increased by the exchange process.

Parenteral vancomycin is the mainstay of therapy for vascular catheters infected by methicillin-resistant coagulase-negative staphylococci, and should be continued for 7 to 14 days unless there is metastatic seeding requiring longer treatment. Antibiotic lock therapy (Table 6.4.13) may be useful in carefully selected patients for 'line salvage'. The presence of tenderness along the course of a tunnelled catheter is highly predictive of failure of medical management and should lead to catheter removal.

Endocarditis

Multiple positive blood cultures with coagulase-negative staphylococci may indicate the presence of infective endocarditis. More than 80% of patients with prosthetic valve infection have persistent fever, deep valve involvement (e.g. infection of the sewing ring or valve dysfunction, dehiscence, or abscess), and/or cardiac conduction abnormalities. Infections within the first 6 to 12 months following surgery typically reflect acquisition of the organism in the perioperative period and may have a higher likelihood of complicated infection.

Diagnosis of prosthetic valve infection should be sought aggressively when multiple positive cultures with coagulase-negative staphylococci have been obtained in the postcardiac operative period. Physical examination usually shows fever and a new or worsening murmur or valve dysfunction. Evaluation includes serial blood cultures to document degree and persistence of bacteraemia, electrocardiography to search for conduction delay,

Table 6.4.14 Information on indications and toxicity for selected drugs

Drug class	Indications/use	Side effects/toxicities
Semisynthetic penicillins		
Flucloxacillin Oxacillin	Drugs of choice in penicillin-resistant MSSA infection	Interstitial nephritis (which limits methicillin use in adults)
Nafcillin	Not effective in MRSA infection	Neutropenia (nafcillin)
Dicloxacillin	CA-MRSA may equal or exceed 50% prevalence in some areas Range of prevalence of nosocomial MRSA is 2–70% Adequate incision and drainage of infected foci is critical	Elevated transaminases (oxacillin, nafcillin)
First-generation cephalosporins		
Cefazolin Cefalexin	Alternative agents for penicillin-resistant, MSSA infection Not effective in MRSA infection CA-MRSA may equal or exceed 50% prevalence in some areas Range of prevalence of nosocomial MRSA is 2–70% Adequate incision and drainage of infected foci is critical	15% cross-reaction for penicillin-allergic patients Hypersensitivity Eosinophilia
Penicillins and aminopenicillins		
Penicillin Ampicillin Amoxicillin Ampicillin + sulbactam Amoxicillin + clavulanate	Penicillin is the drug of choice in known penicillin-sensitive *S. aureus* infection Duration of therapy and indications similar to those of oxacillin	Hypersensitivity
Glycopeptides		
Vancomycin Teicoplanin Dalbavancin Oritavancin Telavancin	Indicated for MRSA infections or MSSA infections in penicillin-allergic patients	3–11% of patients given vancomycin may develop anaphylactoid reaction (i.e. 'red man' or 'red-neck' syndrome) due to overly rapid infusion
	Indicated for coagulase-negative staphylococcal infections	Nephrotoxicity with vancomycin (0–7% alone, 14–20+% in conjunction with aminoglycoside) and teicoplanin (5%)
	MRSA that are vancomycin susceptible but have increased MIC may require higher doses	Neutropenia with vancomycin (1–2%)
	Vancomycin trough levels should be 10–15 mg/litre and monitored closely in the setting of renal dysfunction; ≥15 if vancomycin MIC >1 mcg/ml	Erythematous rash with teicoplanin (7%)
	Teicoplanin levels should be >10 mg/litre in bacteraemia and >20 mg/litre in endocarditis	
Lincosamide		
Clindamycin	Indicated for nonsevere MRSA infections that are erythromycin and clindamycin susceptible or that are erythromycin resistant and double-disc diffusion (D) test is negative	20% of patients develop diarrhoea
	An option for nonsevere MSSA infections in penicillin-allergic patients	Increased risk of *Clostridium difficile*-associated diarrhoea (10%)
Tetracyclines		
Doxycycline Minocycline Tigecycline	Not recommended in children aged <8 years	Photosensitivity
	Bacteriostatic, not recommended for bacteraemia or severe infections	Eosinophilia
	Recent review in osteomyelitis demonstrated success rate in over 80%; retained foreign body in osteomyelitis may lead to failure	SLE-like reaction with minocycline
	Likely need additional agent for treatment of long duration (i.e. rifampicin or fluoroquinolone) to prevent emergence of resistance	Pseudotumour cerebri or vestibular toxicity
	Potency/activity of drugs: tigecycline > minocycline > doxycycline > tetracycline	Antianabolic

Table 6.4.14 (*Cont'd*) Information on indications and toxicity for selected drugs

Drug class	Indications/use	Side effects/toxicities
Dihydrofolate reductase inhibitors		
Trimethoprim/ sulfamethoxazole	Higher failure rate as compared with vancomycin in MSSA endocarditis seen in one study MRSA endocarditis success equivalent to vancomycin TMP/SMX resistance may be common among nosocomial MRSA (up to 50%) but is generally uncommon among CA-MRSA (<10%)	Hypersensitivity, may progress to erythema multiforme and/or Stevens–Johnson syndrome Macrocytic anaemia Photosensitivity Methaemoglobinaemia (rare)
Fluoroquinolones		
Ciprofloxacin Levofloxacin Moxifloxacin Ofloxacin	Should not be used as monotherapy due to rapid emergence of resistance May possibly be used with other agents (e.g. TMP/SMX, rifampicin) Ciprofloxacin or levofloxacin in combination with rifampicin may be an option for patients with uncomplicated tricuspid valve endocarditis who cannot/will not be admitted; or those with skin/soft tissue infection with CA-MRSA	Neurological (0.9–11% delirium and/or seizures) Arthropathy, tendinitis, tendon rupture Hypoglycaemia
Rifamycins		
Rifampicin	Part of combination treatment of prosthetic valve endocarditis, or in setting of endovascular infection with a foreign body Should be used with another agent given rapid acquisition of resistance	Gastrointestinal complaints Hepatitis Myeloid suppression Acute tubular necrosis or acute interstitial nephritis SLE-like syndrome
Macrolides		
Erythromycin Clarithromycin Azithromycin	May be used in penicillin-allergic patients for skin/soft tissue infections Should be used with caution based on local susceptibility to erythromycin in *S. aureus* and emergence of resistance	Gastrointestinal complaints (prokinetic) QT prolongation in conjunction with other medications
Oxazolidinones		
Linezolid	Comparable indications to vancomycin; of use in therapy for MRSA or VISA/VRSA Data suggest better efficacy than vancomycin for pneumonia and skin/soft tissue infections with MRSA Has been used for bacteraemia in small open label trials Bacteriostatic Limited clinical experience	Myelosuppression Serotonin syndrome Peripheral neuropathy Lactic acidosis (due to mitochondrial toxicity)
Lipopeptides		
Daptomycin	Bactericidal May have use in VISA/VRSA Resistance has been noted to develop on therapy Not indicated for treatment of pneumonia 'Noninferior' to vancomycin for right-sided endocarditis and uncomplicated bacteraemia with *S. aureus* and possibly better for MRSA	Myopathy, especially with higher doses or in the setting of renal insufficiency Cases of eosinophilic pneumonia reported
Streptogramins		
Quinupristin/dalfopristin	May have use in soft tissue infections, bacteraemia, or osteomyelitis in settings where other agents are not available/ useful May have use in MRSA or VISA/VRSA infections Presence of inducible or constitutive clindamycin resistance (i.e. MLS resistance) may indicate elevated MICs for quinupristin/ dalfopristin	Phlebitis (30%)—limits general usefulness Arthralgias (9.1%) Myalgias (6.6%)

(Continued)

Table 6.4.14 (*Cont'd*) Information on indications and toxicity for selected drugs

Drug class	Indications/use	Side effects/toxicities
Sodium fusidate	Topical therapy for impetigo	Thrombophlebitis (parenteral use)
	May be used parenterally in therapy of MRSA bacteraemia or endocarditis, depending on susceptibility	Reversible jaundice (parenteral use)
	Should not be used in newborns	Thrombocytopenia (parenteral use)

CA, community-acquired; MIC, minimum inhibitory concentration; MLS, macrolide–lincosamide–streptogramin, MRSA, methicillin-resistant *S. aureus*; MSSA, methicillin-susceptible *S. aureus*; SLE, systemic lupus erythematosus; TMP/SMX, trimethoprim/sulfamethoxazole, VISA/VRSA, vancomycin-intermediate/vancomycin-resistant *S. aureus*.

and echocardiography or angiography for documentation of valve function. Therapy for prosthetic valve endocarditis should include parenteral vancomycin (for methicillin-resistant strains), gentamicin, and/or rifampicin (Table 6.4.13).

Peritoneal dialysis-associated peritonitis

Peritoneal dialysis catheter infection is characterized by abdominal pain, cloudy exchange fluid, and peritoneal fluid containing predominantly polymorphonuclear leucocytes (>100 leucocytes/mm³). To improve diagnostic yield of peritoneal dialysate fluid cultures, 2 to 3 ml of fluid can be inoculated into thioglycolate broth or blood culture bottles.

Therapy for catheter-associated *S. epidermidis* peritonitis depends on susceptibility results. For susceptible organisms, β-lactams, trimethoprim/sulfamethoxazole, and vancomycin have all been effective, and both parenteral and oral antibiotics have been used. However, if methicillin-resistant *S. epidermidis* is suspected, vancomycin therapy (Table 6.4.13) with monitoring of serum levels may be indicated. Therapy can consist of either systemic or intraperitoneal antimicrobial administration. Intraperitoneal therapy is advantageous because it allows continued ambulatory care and therapy directly to the site of infection. Catheter salvage is frequently possible, but relapses may lead to catheter removal.

Other organisms

S. saprophyticus is a common cause of UTIs (20% of UTIs in women 16–35 years old). *S. lugdunensis* has been reported as a cause of endocarditis, including native valves, and bloodstream infection; its true incidence is not clear given the lack of speciation of most coagulase-negative staphylococci in many laboratories. *S. lugdunensis* infections have been characterized by a clinical course more like that of *S. aureus*, with valve destruction a prominent part of the illness.

Likely developments in the near future

Future directions in the management of *S. aureus* infections include vaccine development, new antimicrobials, enhanced understanding of epidemiology and control of nosocomial-associated and CA-MRSA, and evaluation and control of the emergence of VISA/VRSA. A bivalent vaccine containing *S. aureus* polysaccharides 5 and 8 briefly reduced risk of bacteraemia in haemodialysis recipients in a prospective study published in 2002. Further testing of booster doses of the vaccine to demonstrate increased efficacy is in progress. An additional target for vaccine synthesis is the PVL toxin, which may provide protection against CA-MRSA. Another preventive measure may be screening for nasal or skin colonization

with MRSA, with subsequent decolonization of colonized persons. However, populations that require screening (i.e. universal or targeted screening), actions to pursue among the colonized, and efficacy and costs of such a programme are all variables that require further clarification. The promise of such a strategy may be control of MRSA and reduction of the costs and morbidity associated with MRSA infection.

New glycopeptides (telavancin, oritavancin, and dalbavancin), new cephalosporins with activity against MRSA (ceftobiprole and ceftaroline), and existing agents with evolving indications (daptomycin, linezolid) may improve treatment options for MRSA and VISA/VRSA. Better strategies for treatment and salvage of infected catheters with catheter coating (e.g. with chlorhexidine) or methods for treatment of biofilm may improve treatment of coagulase-negative staphylococci.

Further reading

Baddour LM, *et al.* (2005). Infective endocarditis: diagnosis, antimicrobial therapy, and management of complications: a statement for healthcare professionals from the Committee on Rheumatic Fever, Endocarditis, and Kawasaki Disease, Council on Cardiovascular Disease in the Young, and the Councils on Clinical Cardiology, Stroke, and Cardiovascular Surgery and Anesthesia, American Heart Association: endorsed by the Infectious Diseases Society of America. *Circulation*, **111**, e394–434. [Guidelines in the United States of America for the treatment of infective endocarditis, including staphylococcal endocarditis.]

Darouiche RO (2006). Spinal epidural abscess. *N Engl J Med*, **355**, 2012–20. [Review of clinical features and therapy of epidural abscess.]

Drees M, Boucher H (2006). New agents for *Staphylococcus aureus* endocarditis. *Curr Opin Infect Dis*, **19**, 544–50. [A review of new and soon to arrive therapy for *S. aureus*.]

Elliott TS, *et al.* (2004). Guidelines for the antibiotic treatment of endocarditis in adults: report of the Working Party of the British Society for Antimicrobial Chemotherapy. *J Antimicrob Chemother*, **54**, 971–81. [Guidelines in the United Kingdom for the treatment of infective endocarditis, including staphylococcal endocarditis.]

Fowler VG Jr, *et al.* (2005). *Staphylococcus aureus* endocarditis: a consequence of medical progress. *JAMA*, **293**, 3012–21. [Interesting data regarding the epidemiology of *S. aureus* endocarditis.]

Gemmell CG, *et al.* (2006). Guidelines for the prophylaxis and treatment of methicillin-resistant *Staphylococcus aureus* (MRSA) infections in the UK. *J Antimicrob Chemother*, **57**, 589–608. [United Kingdom review of the evidence for practices in control and treatment of MRSA infection.]

Grundmann H, *et al.* (2006). Emergence and resurgence of meticillin-resistant *Staphylococcus aureus* as a public-health threat. *Lancet*, **368**, 874–85. [A recent review of the emergence of community-associated MRSA infections.]

Heldman AW, *et al.* (1996). Oral antibiotic treatment of right-sided staphylococcal endocarditis in injection drug users: prospective randomized comparison with parenteral therapy. *Am J Med*, **101**, 68–76. [A comparison of oral ciprofloxacin with rifampin vs parenteral agents in the treatment of right-sided endocarditis.]

Holland TL, Fowler VG, Jr. (2011). Vancomycin minimum inhibitory concentration and outcome in patients with *Staphylococcus aureus* bacteremia: pearl or pellet? *J Infect Dis*, **204**, 329–31. [A review of the literature on the relationship between vancomycin MIC and outcome.]

Holmes NE, *et al.* (2011). Antibiotic choice may not explain poorer outcomes in patients with *Staphylococcus aureus* bacteremia and high vancomycin minimum inhibitory concentrations. *J Infect Dis*, **204**, 340–7.

Huang SS, Datta R, Platt R (2006). Risk of acquiring antibiotic-resistant bacteria from prior room occupants. *Arch Int Med.* **166**, 1945–51. [Evidence to support the risk of nosocomial and environmental spread of MRSA.]

Klevens RM, *et al.* (2006). Changes in the epidemiology of methicillin-resistant *Staphylococcus aureus* in intensive care units in US hospitals, 1992–2003. *Clin Infect Dis*, **42**, 389–91.

Lal Y, Assimacopoulos AP (2011). Two cases of daptomycin-induced eosinophilic pneumonia and chronic pneumonitis. *Clin Infect Dis*, **50**, 737–40.

Lee S, *et al.* (2011). Is cefazolin inferior to nafcillin for treatment of methicillin-susceptible *Staphylococcus aureus* bacteremia? *Antimicrob Agents Chemother*, **55**, 5122–6.

Lipsky BA, Itani K, Norden C (2004). Treating foot infections in diabetic patients: a randomized, multicenter, open-label trial of linezolid versus ampicillin-sulbactam/amoxicillin-clavulanate. *Clin Inf Dis*, **38**, 17–24. [A trial examining linezolid in the treatment of diabetic foot infections.]

Liu C, *et al.* (2011). Clinical practice guidelines by the infectious diseases society of america for the treatment of methicillin-resistant Staphylococcus aureus infections in adults and children. *Clin Infect Dis*, **52**, e18–55. [First guidelines issued by the Infectious Disease Society of America for the treatment of MRSA.]

Markowitz N, Quinn EL, Saravolatz LD (1992). Trimethoprim-sulfamethoxazole compared with vancomycin for the treatment of *Staphylococcus aureus* infection. *Ann Int Med*, **117**, 390–8. [Parenteral trimethoprim/sulfamethoxazole is compared with vancomycin in this double-blind randomized trial.]

Mermel LA, *et al.* (2001). Guidelines for the management of intravascular catheter-related infections. *Clin Inf Dis*, **32**, 1249–72. [Guidelines for the treatment of catheter-related bloodstream infections; includes information about antibiotic lock in coagulase-negative staphylococcal infections.]

Mulligan ME, *et al.* (1993). Methicillin-resistant *Staphylococcus aureus*: a consensus review of the microbiology, pathogenesis, and epidemiology with implications for prevention and management. *Am J Med*, **94**, 313–28. [A review of nosocomial MRSA colonization and infection. Reviews strategies for decolonization of carriers.]

Ruhe JJ, *et al.* (2005). Use of long-acting tetracyclines for methicillin-resistant *Staphylococcus aureus* infections: case series and review of the literature. *Clin Inf Dis*, **40**, 1429–34. [A review of tetracyclines in treatment of MRSA infections.]

Safdar N, Fine JP, Maki DG (2005). Meta-analysis: methods for diagnosing intravascular device-related bloodstream infection. *Ann Int Med*, **142**, 451–66. [Summary of studies and most effective methods for diagnosis of catheter-related bloodstream infections.]

Shorr AF, Kunkel MJ, Kollef M (2005). Linezolid versus vancomycin for *Staphylococcus aureus* bacteraemia: pooled analysis of randomized studies. *J Antimicrob Chemother*, **56**, 923–9. [Pooled data from two randomized trials show efficacy of linezolid.]

Stevens DL, *et al.* (2005). Practice guidelines for the diagnosis and management of skin and soft-tissue infections. *Clin Inf Dis*, **41**, 1373–406. [Guidelines for the treatment of soft tissue infections.]

Van Loo I, *et al.* (2007). Emergence of methicillin-resistant Staphylococcus aureus of animal origin in humans. *Emerg Infect Dis*, **13**, 1834–9.

Wertheim HF, *et al.* (2004). Risk and outcome of nosocomial *Staphylococcus aureus* bacteraemia in nasal carriers versus non-carriers. *Lancet*, **364**, 703–5.

Wertheim HF, *et al.* (2004). Mupirocin prophylaxis against nosocomial *Staphylococcus aureus* infections in nonsurgical patients: a randomized study. *Ann Int Med*, **140**, 419–25. [Two studies that evaluate the impact of nasal colonization, and decolonization, in infection rates of hospitalized patients.]

Wyllic DH, Crook DW, Peto TE (2006). Mortality after *Staphylococcus aureus* bacteraemia in two hospitals in Oxfordshire, 1997–2003: cohort study. *BMJ*, **333**, 281. [Epidemiology of *S. aureus* bacteraemia in the United Kingdom is reviewed in this cohort study.]

Zimmermann B 3rd, Mikolich DJ, Ho G Jr (1995). Septic bursitis. *Semin Arthritis Rheum*, **24**, 391–410. [Review of the treatment of septic bursitis.]

6.5 Meningococcal infections

Petter Brandtzaeg

Essentials

Neisseria meningitidis is an obligate human Gram-negative diplococcus. It is carried in the nasopharynx by about 10% of people, with most strains being harmless and inducing immunity. Pathogenic strains usually belong to specific clones that are encapsulated, express pili and the major porin, PorA. Serogroups A, B, and C usually account for more than 90% of all invasive isolates.

Epidemiology

Young asymptomatic adults are the main reservoir. Meningococci are transmitted by droplets and susceptible people usually develop the first symptoms within 2 to 4 days. The incidence of disease is highest during the first 4 years of life, with a secondary lower peak in adolescents. Pathogenic strains tend to cause single cases or small clusters in industrialized countries, whereas they cause large outbreaks in developing countries, particularly in the meningitis belt of Africa. Host factors predisposing to invasive disease include (1) lack of protective antibodies, (2) defects in the complement system or mannose-binding lectin, (3) polymorphisms of complement factor H and related proteins as well as tumour necrosis factor α.

Clinical features and prognosis

Initially, *N. meningitidis* induces bacteraemia, with growth velocity in the circulation a major determinant of the clinical presentation and outcome. The two major clinical presentations are meningitis and septic shock.

Meningitis—the commonest presentation; preceded by low grade meningococcaemia ($<10^3$/ml); characterized by fever, subsequently a petechial rash (30–80% of cases) and increasing symptoms of meningitis. If adequately treated with antibiotics, case fatality is <5% in industrialized countries, but higher in developing countries. Brain oedema leading to herniation of the cerebellum is the main cause of death. Neurosensory hearing loss is the major complication.

Septic shock—symptoms develop very rapidly; within 6 to 12 h of initial symptoms the patient may have persistent circulatory failure and severe coagulopathy leading to thrombosis and extensive haemorrhage of the skin, thrombosis and gangrene of the extremities, and impaired renal, adrenal, and pulmonary function. Mortality is high (29–53%).

Mild meningococcaemia—in industrialized countries, 20 to 30% of cases present with fever and petechial or macular rash, but without marked signs of meningitis or shock. Occasional complications include pericarditis, arthritis, ocular infection or chronic meningococcaemia. Prognosis is good (with appropriate antibiotic treatment).

Diagnosis

Intra- and extracellular diplococci can be observed in the cerebrospinal fluid, peripheral blood buffy coat (fulminant septicaemia), and biopsies of haemorrhagic skin lesions using Gram or acridine orange stains. *N. meningitidis* can be grown from blood culture and swabs from the nasopharynx/tonsils. Polymerase chain reaction (PCR) methods are increasingly used to detect and classify *N. meningitidis* in blood, cerebrospinal fluid, and other bodily fluids.

Treatment

Aside from supportive care, appropriate antibiotic treatment should be started immediately in suspected cases of meningococcal infection: this should not be delayed while the patient is transferred to hospital, or for the results of investigations to become available. Benzylpenicillin (intravenously or intramuscularly) remains the drug of choice in most countries; third-generation cefalosporins and chloramphenicol are also effective.

Prevention

Vaccination—conjugate vaccines comprising serogroup A, C, Y, and W135 polysaccharide are effective. A vaccine covering serogroup B strains is in the final stage of evaluation. The outer membrane vesicle vaccines used during a serogroup B outbreak in Norway and New Zealand, containing the porin A (PorA) of the epidemic strain, induced 57 to 73% protection.

Secondary prophylaxis—health authorities in most countries advise that close contacts of cases of meningococcal disease have eradication treatment, e.g. with a single dose of ciprofloxacin 500 mg or ofloxacin 400 mg.

Introduction

Neisseria meningitidis infection remains a major public health problem worldwide by causing clusters or epidemics of meningitis and acute lethal sepsis. Case fatality has gradually declined from 70 to 90% to approximately 10% but has remained at this level since the introduction of antimicrobial chemotherapy in 1937.

The bacterium

N. meningitidis is an obligate human Gram-negative diplococcus classified as a β-proteobacterium and is a member of the family Neisseriaceae. Meningococci are normally located in the mucous membrane of the nasopharynx and tonsils. Invasive isolates from blood and cerebrospinal fluid or as detected in tissue biopsies are encapsulated and express pili and the major porin PorA. Capsule polysaccharides that inhibit phagocytosis and bacterial adhesion are divided into at least 13 different serogroups (A, B, C, D, E, H, I, K, L, W135, X, Y, and Z). Serogroups A, B, and C usually account for more than 90% of all invasive isolates. Less than 10% of clinical isolates are from serogroups X, Y, and W135.

The cell wall of meningococci consists of an outer lipid bilayer, containing lipopolysaccharides (LPS, endotoxin), lipids, and outer membrane proteins, and an inner thin peptidoglycan layer. LPS is the major inflammatory (toxic) component of *N. meningitidis* (Fig. 6.5.1). Lipoproteins and fragments of peptidoglycan are weaker inflammatory molecules. They activate the innate immune system via CD14 and the Toll-like receptors 4 (LPS) and 2 (lipoproteins, peptidoglycan) located on monocytes, macrophages, and to a lesser extent neutrophils (Fig. 6.5.2). During growth, meningococci release a large number of outer membrane vesicles containing LPS and other outer membrane molecules that trigger the innate immune system in a dose-dependent manner.

Outer membrane proteins are classified according to electrophoretic mobility into five major classes. PorA (class 1 protein) and PorB (class 2 or 3 proteins) are cation-selective and anion-selective porins, respectively. PorB and PorA define serotype and serosubtype, respectively. Loops 1 and 4 in PorA are surface exposed major epitopes inducing bactericidal and opsonophagocytic antibodies when exposed to the human immune system.

Meningococci are fastidious bacteria that readily autolyse. They grow well on blood agar, supplemented chocolate agar, trypticase soy agar, Mueller–Hinton agar, and selective GC medium. Optimal growth occurs at 35 to 37°C in a humid atmosphere with 5 to 10% carbon dioxide. The convex colonies (diameter 1–4 mm) are transparent, nonpigmented, and nonhaemolytic. They produce cytochrome oxidase and ferment glucose and maltose, but not lactose and sucrose, to acid without gas formation.

Practical handling of clinical specimens

Blood culture (10 ml for adults, 2–4 ml for infants/children) and swabs from the nasopharynx and the tonsils are collected immediately. Media for blood culture and transportation of swabs should be optimal for recovery of meningococci. Cerebrospinal fluid is best cultured by direct plating of 0.1 ml on supplemented chocolate agar or a similar medium. If direct plating is impossible or delayed, the sample should be stored at +4°C to +20°C but preferably at refrigerator temperature. Recovery of live meningococci may increase if some drops of the cerebrospinal fluid are stored on a sterile swab in transport medium or injected into blood culture medium and incubated at 35 to 37°C.

Direct visualization of *N. meningitidis* in clinical specimens

Intracellular and extracellular diplococci can be observed in the cerebrospinal fluid, peripheral blood buffy coat (fulminant

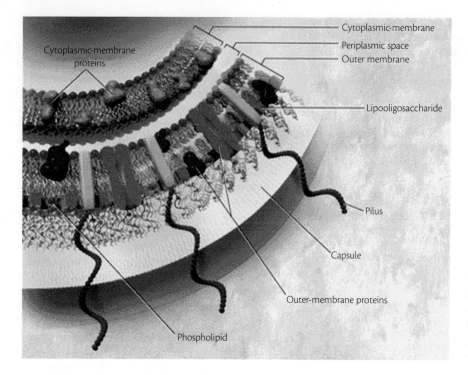

Fig. 6.5.1 Cross-sectional view of *N. meningitidis*. (Reproduced with permission from Rosenstein NE, Bradley BA, Stephens DS, Popovic T, Hughes JM (2001). Meningococcal disease. *N Engl J Med*, **334**, 1378–88.)

septicaemia), and biopsies of haemorrhagic skin lesions using Gram's or acridine orange stains.

Polymerase chain reaction

Polymerase chain reaction (PCR) is increasingly used to detect and classify *N. meningitidis* in blood, cerebrospinal fluid, joint fluid, and pericardial fluid. Real-time PCR has made it possible to quantify the total number of meningococci, i.e. live plus dead bacteria, in plasma and cerebrospinal fluid. In shock plasma, nonviable meningococci outnumber those that can be cultured by a factor 1000:1. The number of *N. meningitidis* DNA copies is closely correlated to the LPS levels, clinical presentation, disease severity, and outcome. Blood anticoagulated with EDTA is optimal for the PCR reaction but other anticoagulants (heparin, citrate) or even serum have been used.

Epidemiology

Industrialized countries

Infection presents as single cases or in small clusters. The incidence is usually 1 to 3 per 100 000 inhabitants per year. Strains belonging to specific clonal complexes may cause a hyperendemic situation characterized by a much higher incidence than usually observed (4 to 30 per 100 000 per year). This epidemiological situation may last for more than a decade in defined geographical areas before slowly declining. Serogroup A has disappeared as a cause of significant epidemics. Outbreaks in Finland in the 1970s and in New Zealand in the 1980s were exceptions. In Europe 70% of the cases are presently caused by serogroup B. Immunization of infants with serogroup C conjugate vaccine in various countries has reduced the incidence significantly. Serogroup Y strains belonging to several clonal complexes are gradually increasing. In the United States of America serogroups B, C, and Y accounted for approximately one-third of the cases each (Fig. 6.5.3).

Developing countries

Large-scale epidemics are confined to developing countries, primarily in sub-Saharan Africa where the incidence approaches 10 to 25 per 100 000 inhabitants per year. During epidemic peaks in Africa, as many as 500 to 1000 per 100 000 inhabitants may contract meningococcal infections. Serogroup A and to lesser extent serogroups W135 and C dominate the isolates of large epidemics (Fig. 6.5.3).

Meningitis belt in sub-Saharan Africa

The area stretches from the Gambia in the west to Ethiopia in the east and includes Senegal, Guinea, Mali, Burkina Faso, Ghana, Togo, Benin, Nigeria, Niger, Chad, Cameroon, the Central African

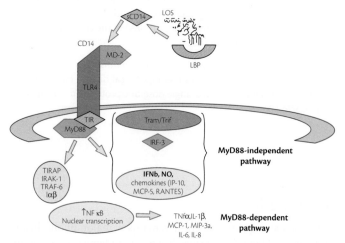

Fig. 6.5.2 Activation of Toll-like receptor 4 by endotoxin (lipopolysaccharides or lipooligosaccharides, LOS). (Reproduced with permission from Stephens DS, Greenwood B, Brandtzaeg P (2007). Epidemic meningitis, meningococcaemia, and Neisseria meningitidis, *Lancet.*, **369**, 2196–210.)

Republic, and Sudan (Fig. 6.5.3). Mainly serogroup A strains belonging to a few clonal complexes cause the increased attack rate. In some of these countries large-scale epidemics occur every 8 to 12 years. Since the 1990s serogroup W135 has caused epidemics in West Africa.

Season

In temperate climates most cases occur during the winter and early spring. In the sub-Saharan African meningitis belt the incidence increases from the middle of the dry season and reaches its maximum at the end of that season (harmattan). New cases decline rapidly after the start of the rainy season.

Preceding infections

Influenza A predisposes to invasive meningococcal infections. Mycoplasma infections and rubella have been associated with outbreaks.

Age distribution

Cases are seen in all age groups; however, most occur from 0 to 4 years with a smaller peak from 13 to 20 years. During epidemics the median age appears to increase. Complement-deficient patients may contract the infection at an older age than average.

Genetic diversity

N. meningitidis can exchange and incorporate DNA from other Neisseria species or closely related bacteria. Meningococci are genetically more diverse than most other human pathogens. However, strains from certain clonal complexes may persist for many decades over wide areas, retaining their pathogenicity. Strains from seven clonal complexes have predominated since the late 1960s.

Nasopharyngeal colonization

Upper respiratory tract mucosa is the natural habitat of N. meningitidis. It is spread from person to person by droplets and direct mucosal contact. Most colonizing meningococci are nonpathogenic and are genetically and phenotypically different from virulent invasive strains. Only a minority of those colonized with virulent strains will develop invasive disease. Colonization is asymptomatic; it induces local and systemic immune responses within 1 to 2 weeks.

Carriage

Cross-sectional studies in England and Norway in the 1980s and 1990s indicated that approximately 10% of the population harboured meningococci in the upper respiratory tract. However, only 1% of the healthy normal population carried strains from typical virulent clones prevalent at the time. The acquisition rate leading to carriage appears to be independent of season.

The carriage rate in England is low (2–3%) in the first 4 years of life, rises in children aged 10 to 14 years (9–10%), reaches a maximum among young adults of 15 to 19 years (20–25%), and then gradually declines to less than 15% in persons above 25 years. It increases in closed or semiclosed communities and is particularly high in military camps where strains change frequently. In university communities with bar and catering facilities the carriage rate is high. Smoking increases the carriage rate.

Reservoir of virulent meningococci

Healthy adults carrying virulent strains of N. meningitidis are the main reservoir. Household members and kissing contacts of a patient harbour virulent strains more often than the average population. In industrialized countries, infants and children are

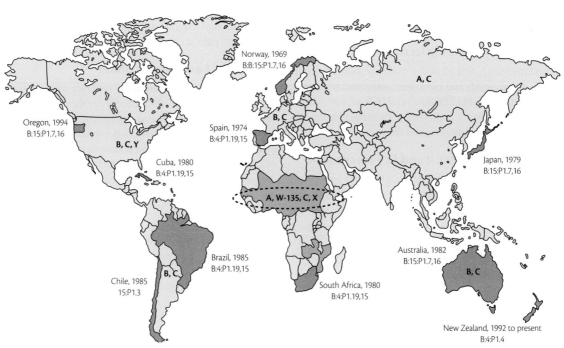

Fig. 6.5.3 Outbreaks of different serogroups of N. meningitidis since the 1960s. Purple areas indicate countries with serogroup B epidemics.
(Reproduced with permission from Stephens DS, Greenwood B, Brandtzaeg P (2007). Epidemic meningitis, meningococcaemia, and Neisseria meningitidis, Lancet, **369**, 2196–210 and Caugant D A (1998). Population genetics and molecular epidemiology of Neisseria meningitides. APMIS, **106**, 505–10.)

usually infected by a local adult carrier. Spread from patients to medical staff is very uncommon. In Africa, children may more commonly infect each other with serogroup A strains.

Predisposing factors for invasive disease

These are summarized in Box 6.5.1.

Lack of protective antibodies

Antibodies against serogroups A, C, W135, and Y capsule polysaccharides are bactericidal and confer protection at concentrations of 1 to 2 μg/ml of serum. Serogroup B polysaccharide induces a weak transient IgM but no protective IgG response. Bactericidal and opsonophagocytic antibodies recognizing surface-exposed epitopes of the outer membrane protein, in particular PorA, are important for protection. Antibodies to newly discovered outer membrane proteins including factor H binding protein, neisserial adhesion A, neisserial heparin binding antigen (components in a serogroup B vaccine to be licensed soon) are bactericidal and may hopefully confer protection. Antilipopolysaccharide antibodies, recognizing commonly shared epitopes among virulent and non-pathogenic neisseria and closely related species, presumably play a role in protection.

Defects in the complement system

Reduced function of the complement system caused by defects in the alternative or terminal pathways increases the susceptibility up to 6000 times. Defects in the classic pathway appear not to not predispose to meningococcal infection. Complement defects are rare; they play a minor role in the development of invasive serogroup A, B, and C infections in Europe. Complement defects were over-represented in patients with the less common and presumably less virulent serogroups W135, X, Y, and Z in studies from the Netherlands. High serum levels of factor H appear to increase the risk of invasive meningococcal infections in England.

Defects in the mannose-binding lectin

Mutations in codons 54, 57, and 52 of the mannose-binding lectin gene result in low serum levels and have been associated with one-third of all meningococcal cases in England and Ireland. Low serum levels of mannose-binding lectin combined with properdin defects increase the risk of invasive meningococcal disease.

Polymorphism of Fcγ-receptor II and Fcγ-receptor III

Polymorphisms of Fcγ receptor II (Fcγ-RIIa, CD32) and Fcγ receptor III (Fcγ-RIIIb, CD16) on phagocytic cells are associated with reduced binding of antibodies. They are over-represented in patients with defects in the late complement components (C5–C9) and in children with fulminant meningococcal sepsis. Fcγ-RIIa receptors where arginine has replaced histidine at position 131 are associated with reduced binding of IgG2 subclass (antipolysaccharide) antibodies. The influence of these polymorphisms in adults is uncertain.

Other genetic predisposition for invasive infection and outcome

In a European genome-wide association study, genetic variants in the complement factor H region were associated with susceptibility to meningococcal disease. Polymorphism in TNF-α gene appears to be associated with invasive meningococcal infection. Genes coding for mannose-binding lectin, Fcγ receptors (CD16, CD32), and Toll-like receptor (TLR)-4 have previously been implicated in increased susceptibility and outcome. TLRs play an important role in protecting the host from intruding microorganisms. Studies from the United Kingdom and Gambia suggest that the most common polymorphism in the *TLR4* gene (Asp299Gly) is not over-represented among cases. Polymorphism in genes coding for plasminogen activator inhibitor 1 (PAI-1), interleukin-1 receptor antagonist (IL-1RA) and interleukin-1 (IL-1) are associated with increased disease severity.

Invasive infection

Most patients appear to develop invasive disease 2 to 4 days after acquiring the virulent strain in the upper respiratory tract, but some are carriers for up to 7 weeks before invasive infection develops. *N. meningitidis* adheres to specific molecules on nonciliated epithelial cells in the nasopharynx and on the tonsils (Fig. 6.5.4).

During a period of adaptation and proliferation, meningococci presumably alter various surface structures (lipopolysaccharides, pili, outer membrane proteins) by phase variation before starting transepithelial migration. They reach submucosal tissue and, via capillaries, gain access to the circulation (Fig. 6.5.5).

The initial bacteraemic phase

Bacteraemia is a prerequisite for systemic meningococcal infection. Meningococci may be eliminated from the blood by lysis induced by bactericidal antibodies and complement and by phagocytosis of opsonized bacteria. Persistent bacteraemia allows meningeal invasion.

Bacterial proliferation and accompanying inflammatory response may occur predominantly in either the subarachnoid space, causing meningitis, or in the circulation, causing meningococcaemia with or without shock.

The rash

Haemorrhagic skin lesions are the hallmark of systemic meningococcal disease, occurring in 70 to 80% of all cases in industrialized countries. They appear as red or bluish petechiae. These lesions are larger and more irregular in size than the petechiae of thrombocytopenic purpura. Each lesion represents a local nidus of meningococci within the endothelial cells, thrombus formation, and extravasation of erythrocytes. The petechial rash indicates meningococcaemia, not necessarily severe sepsis. However, in fulminant meningococcal septicaemia the haemorrhagic lesions are larger (ecchymoses) with a propensity to locate on extremities (Fig. 6.5.6).

Box 6.5.1 Factors predisposing for meningococcal infections

- Lack of bactericidal and/or opsonizing antibodies
- Lack of alternative pathway or late complement components, polymorphism of factor H
- Low levels of mannan-binding lectin
- Polymorphism of complement factor H and closely related proteins and tumour necrosis factor-α

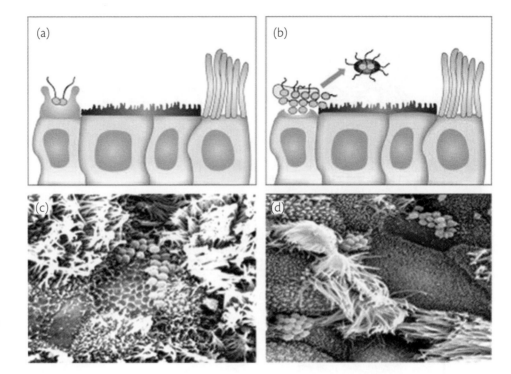

Fig. 6.5.4 Attachment to and proliferation of meningococci on nonciliated epithelial cells in nasopharynx.
(Reproduced with permission from Stephens DS, Greenwood B, Brandtzaeg P (2007). Epidemic meningitis, meningococcaemia, and *Neisseria meningitidis*, *Lancet*, **369**, 2196–210.)

Some patients develop relatively large nonspecific maculopapular lesions, with or without haemorrhagic lesions, at an early stage (Figs. 6.5.7, 6.5.8). The petechial lesions are difficult to discover on dark skin but may be observed in the conjunctivae (Fig. 6.5.9).

Clinical presentations

The initial symptoms of systemic meningococcal infection are attributable to meningococcaemia. This may persist as a low-grade bacteraemia or develop into septic shock in a few hours. Most commonly, the patient develops meningococcaemia without circulatory impairment which gradually evolves to meningitis within 12 to 72 h. Occasionally, patients develop distinct meningitis and persistent shock simultaneously. Based on easily recognizable clinical symptoms, meningococcal infections can be classified as: (1) meningitis without shock, (2) shock without meningitis, (3) meningitis and shock, and (4) meningococcaemia without shock or meningitis. Each clinical presentation is associated with a distinct pathophysiological background and prognosis (Table 6.5.1).

Distinct meningitis without persistent shock

Meningism dominates the clinical presentation and the onset is often insidious. The patients, particularly children, may complain of general malaise, nausea, and headache. They vomit and become febrile. The temperature may fluctuate and can be normal at times. Many patients are initially diagnosed as 'gastric flu', gastroenteritis, or upper respiratory tract infection. Gradually, the symptoms of meningitis dominate the clinical picture. The patient complains of headache, vomits, and develops nuchal and back rigidity, photophobia, and in more advanced cases altered consciousness; Kernig's and Brudzinski's signs become positive. Many patients are lethargic and some are agitated. The blood pressure is normal or slightly elevated by stress. Occasionally it is low but can be restored to normal by infusion of a limited volume of fluid. In untreated cases brain oedema develops, the intracranial pressure rises,

and the central circulation is increasingly compromised. Finally, herniation of the cerebellum occurs with arrest of the brain circulation. The case fatality rate is usually less than 5% in industrialized countries.

Meningococcal meningitis without persistent shock accounts for more than 50% of all cases of systemic meningococcal infections in industrialized countries and an even higher proportion of cases reaching hospitals in developing countries. The combination of multiple petechiae and symptoms of meningitis supports a diagnosis of meningococcal meningitis.

Pathophysiological background

N. meningitidis multiply in a compartmentalized manner with the main proliferation occurring in the subarachnoid space. Quantitative PCR indicates that the real number of meningococci is usually less than 10^3/ml in plasma and may increase to 10^9/ml in the cerebrospinal fluid (Fig. 6.5.10). This distribution is reflected in the levels of endotoxin and various cytokines which are low in plasma and 100 to 1000 times higher in the cerebrospinal fluid. Meningococci can be cultivated from both compartments in untreated patients. Plasma proteins, mainly albumin, leak into the cerebrospinal fluid, and the influx of mainly neutrophils causes the pleocytosis. The glucose level of the cerebrospinal fluid is reduced mainly as a result of increased central glucose consumption rather than the pleocytosis.

Laboratory findings

The erythrocyte sedimentation rate, C-reactive protein, and leucocyte count in the peripheral blood are markedly elevated with increased numbers of band forms. Sodium, potassium, calcium, and magnesium ions, pH, renal, hepatic, and coagulation parameters are usually within normal range. Cerebrospinal fluid shows a marked pleocytosis (more than 100×10^6 leucocytes/litre), with increased levels of protein and decreased levels of glucose.

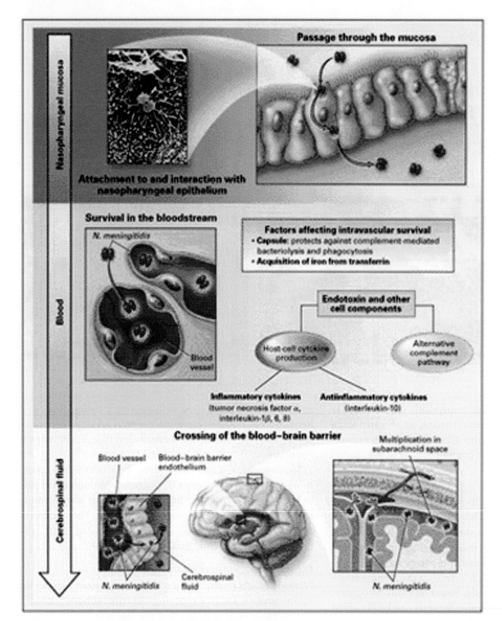

Fig. 6.5.5 Events leading to the different clinical presentations of meningococcal infections. Reproduced with permission from Rosenstein NE, Bradley BA, Stephens DS, Popovic T, Hughes JM (2001).Meningococcal disease. *N Engl J Med,* **334**, 1378–88.

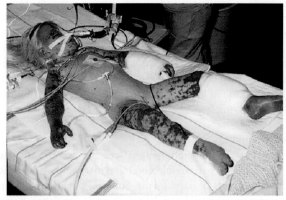

Fig. 6.5.6 Massive skin haemorrhage on the extremities of a 4-year-old girl with fulminant meningococcal septicaemia. The infection was caused by *Neisseria meningitidis* group B. The left leg had to be amputated below the knee. She needed extensive skin transplantation and several fingers had to be amputated.

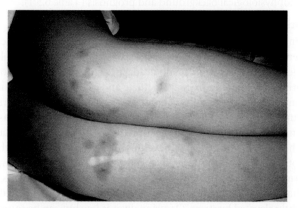

Fig. 6.5.7 Macular lesions on the legs, some with a central haemorrhagic spot in a 17-year-old girl with mild meningococcaemia caused by *Neisseria meningitidis* group C. She recovered completely after 5 days treatment with benzylpenicillin.

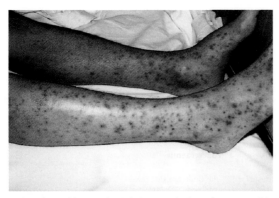

Fig. 6.5.8 Macular and haemorrhagic lesions on the legs of a 21-year-old man with mild meningococcaemia caused by *Neisseria meningitidis* group B. He recovered completely after 5 days of penicillin treatment.

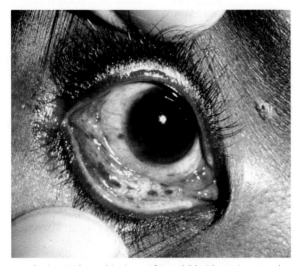

Fig. 6.5.9 Conjunctival petechiae in an African child with meningococcal group A meningitis.
(Copyright D A Warrell.)

Table 6.5.1 Levels of *N. meningitidis* DNA, lipopolysaccharides, and inflammatory mediators related to the clinical presentation

	No shock	Shock[a]	Shock	No shock
	Meningitis[b]	No meningitis	Meningitis	No meningitis
Circulation	(+)	++++	++	(+)
Subarachnoid space	+++++	(+)	+++	(+)

[a] Shock denotes persistent hypotension requiring treatment with volume and pressor for 24 h.
[b] Meningitis denotes 100×10^6/litre or more leucocytes in the cerebrospinal fluid or clinically distinct signs of meningism.

Intracellular and extracellular Gram-negative diplococci can be detected by direct microscopy.

Persistent septic shock without distinct meningitis

Fulminant meningococcal septicaemia (Waterhouse–Friderichsen syndrome) is characterized by persistent circulatory failure and severe coagulopathy leading to thrombosis and extensive haemorrhage of the skin, thrombosis and gangrene of the extremities, and impaired renal, adrenal, and pulmonary function.

Symptoms develop very rapidly. Six to 12 h after recognizing their first symptoms the patients are often desperately ill. Initially, they complain of 'flu-like' symptoms such as fever, aching muscle, prostration, abdominal pain, and nausea. The temperature rises rapidly, commonly to between 39.0 and 41.5°C, but occasionally lower. Diarrhoea may occur during the first few hours. The patient appears worryingly sick to relatives. The parents usually recognize cold extremities indicating impaired circulation before the skin haemorrhagic lesions appear but misinterpret the acute symptoms as influenza or acute gastroenteritis.

The haemorrhagic skin lesions are first seen as bluish petechiae, which rapidly increase in size and number. They are distributed all over the body but are often more pronounced and detected earliest on the extremities. Occasionally they are seen on the conjunctivae and other mucous membranes.

The circulation is severely impaired. The extremities are often cold and cyanotic with a capillary refill time of more than 3 s. The blood pressure is low despite tachycardia. The tissue perfusion remains inadequate despite extensive fluid and pressor therapy. Initially, the circulation is hyperdynamic, but gradually becomes hypodynamic from persistent vasodilatation and gradually reduced myocardial performance. The heart becomes dilated with a reduced ejection fraction, as observed by serial ultrasound examinations.

Patients usually lack nuchal and back rigidity, and Kernig's sign is negative. Despite impaired circulation, many patients remain awake and alert on hospital admission, being able to communicate their complaints. They hyperventilate to compensate for the pronounced metabolic acidosis. Urine output gradually dwindles. They may develop acute respiratory distress syndrome (ARDS), i.e. pulmonary oedema after fluid volume repletion of more than 40 ml/kg.

Circulatory collapse dominates the clinical picture during the first 48 to 96 h. Fifty per cent of the nonsurvivors die within 12 h of hospital admission. Few patients die after 48 h. Later, ARDS, renal failure, and the consequences of the diffuse thrombosis of the extremities and the skin dominate the picture. The case fatality rate ranges from 16 to 53%.

Rapidly evolving symptoms with fever, circulatory shock, and extensive skin haemorrhages in a person without a history of splenectomy makes the diagnosis of fulminant meningococcal septicaemia likely. The same clinical picture is, however, observed in cases of overwhelming infections caused by *Streptococcus pneumoniae*, *Haemophilus influenzae*, *Streptococcus pyogenes*, and *Capnocytophaga canimorsus* (after animal bite) and with viral haemorrhagic fevers (Fig. 6.5.11).

Pathophysiological background

The pathophysiological changes are explained by the very rapid proliferation of *N. meningitidis* in the circulation. On admission 5×10^5 to 5×10^8 meningococci/ml plasma are detectable by quantitative PCR (Fig. 6.5.10). This massive bacterial growth generates very high levels of endotoxin and other bacterial molecules in the blood.

Few meningococci have yet penetrated into the subarachnoid space, which is explained by the short duration of symptoms. The levels of lipopolysaccharides in the plasma are closely associated with the copy number of meningococcal DNA and predict the development

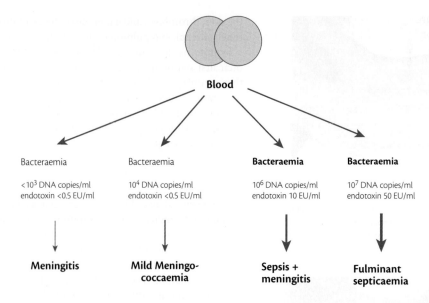

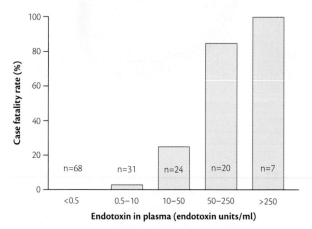

Fig. 6.5.10 Median number of *N. meningitidis* (number of DNA copies) as determined by real-time PCR and median level of endotoxin in plasma in the different clinical presentations of systemic meningococcal disease.

of persistent septic shock, multiple organ failure, and death. Plasma levels of lipopolysaccharides below 10 endotoxin units/ml were associated with 1% mortality due to circulatory impairment whereas levels above 250 endotoxin units/ml, i.e. 1.4 log higher, were associated with 100% mortality among 150 Norwegian patients (Fig. 6.5.12).

Coagulopathy

Coagulation is activated primarily via the extrinsic (tissue factor, FVIIa) pathway. In patients with fulminant meningococcal septicaemia there are increased levels of tissue factor in monocytes and on microparticles released from monocytes. The platelets disappear rapidly and remain at a low level for many days due to extensive consumption at the altered endothelial surface. Thrombopoietin increases in plasma without detectable increase of circulating platelets. The activation of the coagulation system, as measured by formation of fibrin, gradually reduces after antibiotic and fluid therapy is initiated (Table 6.5.2).

Inhibited fibrinolysis

Concurrently with activation of coagulation, fibrinolysis is inhibited by high levels of plasminogen activator inhibitor 1 (PAI-1) released from activated endothelial cells and platelets. High levels of PAI-1 are associated with development of persistent septic shock

and a fatal outcome. Allelic variations in the promoter region of the PAI-1 gene enhance production and are associated with an increased risk of dying.

Thrombus formation

Thrombosis occurs particularly in the vessels of the skin, adrenals, kidneys, muscles, choroid plexus, peripheral extremities, and to

Fig. 6.5.12 Relationship between the levels of endotoxin (lipopolysaccharides) in plasma and case fatality rate related to the development of septic shock and multiple organ failure in 150 Norwegian patients with systemic meningococcal disease.

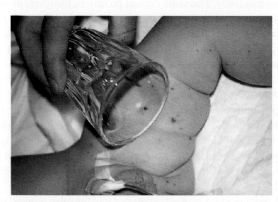

Fig. 6.5.11 The 'tumbler test' used to differentiate haemorrhagic skin lesions from viral or drug rash in an infant with meningococcal meningitis caused by *Neisseria meningitidis* group B. There was complete recovery after 5 days treatment with benzylpenicillin.

Table 6.5.2 Factors contributing to the coagulopathy in fulminant meningococcal septicaemia

Procoagulant factor	Tissue factor in monocytes ↑
Anticoagulant factors	Antithrombin ↓
	Protein C ↓↓
	Tissue factor pathway inhibitor ↑
Profibrinolytic factor	Tissue plasminogen activator ↑↓
Antifibrinolytic factor	Plasminogen activator inhibitor 1 ↑↑

some extent in the lungs. The thrombomodulin–thrombin complex on the endothelial cells converting protein C to activated protein C, and the protein C endothelial cell receptor enhancing this activity, are down-regulated. Glycosaminoglycans including heparan sulphate, molecules with an antithrombotic effect, are released from the endothelial surface. Both processes may facilitate formation of thrombi. Concomitantly natural coagulation inhibitors are consumed. Protein C is reduced to 20% and antithrombin to median 50% of normal functional plasma levels (>70%). Tissue factor pathway inhibitor increases.

Proinflammatory and anti-inflammatory mediators

A multitude of bioactive proinflammatory and anti-inflammatory mediators are released into the plasma. The complement and the kallikrein–kinin systems generate anaphylatoxins (C3a, C4a, C5a) and bradykinin, which are potent vasodilators. Proinflammatory cytokines, notably TNF-α, interleukin (IL)-1β, IL-6, and various chemokines are massively up-regulated. Concomitantly, high levels of soluble receptors of the same cytokines are released. The anti-inflammatory cytokines IL-10 and IL-1 RA are present at high levels and suppress the cell-activating effect of the bacterial lipopolysaccharides and the many proinflammatory cytokines. Nitric oxide production is increased in meningococcal septic shock and is thought to contribute to the vasodilation.

The subarachnoid space

The number of meningococci is very low, if present at all. They can be cultured from cerebrospinal fluid in up to 50% of untreated cases. The inflammatory response is very limited with a leucocyte count usually in the range of 10 to 100×10^6/litre and normal contents of protein and glucose.

Laboratory findings

The erythrocyte sedimentation rate and C-reactive protein are only moderately elevated on admission, rising to high levels within 48 h. The leucocyte count is usually low with a marked shift to young band forms of neutrophils. There is evidence of a partly compensated metabolic acidosis with decreased levels of pH and $P\text{CO}_2$. Creatinine and urea are elevated, serum glucose is variable (high, normal, or low), and potassium, calcium, and magnesium are low. Potassium rises with the renal failure. Serum aspartate aminotransferase and alanine aminotransferase are slightly elevated, whereas γ-glutamyl transferase remains normal. Creatine kinase rises within 1 to 3 days, indicating rhabdomyolysis. Prothrombin, activated partial thromboplastin, and thrombin times are prolonged. The levels of platelets, fibrinogen, coagulation factors VII, X, and V, and prothrombin are low. Antithrombin and protein C are low, whereas tissue factor pathway inhibitor is elevated. Fibrin(ogen) degradation products, thrombin–antithrombin complexes, PAI-1, and plasmin-α2-antiplasmin complexes are elevated. Lumbar puncture should be avoided since the procedure may deteriorate the general condition of the patient, particularly the unstable circulation.

Distinct meningitis and persistent shock

There are meningeal and circulatory symptoms. Usually the symptoms from the inflamed meninges dominate the picture. On admission there are classic signs and symptoms of meningitis such as headache and nausea, nuchal and back rigidity, and a positive Kernig's sign. The blood pressure remains low despite fluid volume repletion.

Circulating levels of endotoxin and inflammatory mediators are lower than in patients with fulminant septicaemia, and case fatality is lower (Fig. 6.5.12). However, it is higher than in patients with meningitis without compromised circulation.

Meningococcaemia without distinct meningitis and persistent shock

Twenty to 30% of patients with invasive meningococcal disease are hospitalized because of fever and petechial or uncharacteristic rash. They lack distinct signs of meningitis although slight pleocytosis (less than 100×10^6 leucocytes/ml) may be present. The circulation is not severely compromised. They represent a composite group of patients. Many are admitted to hospital early, 12 to 24 h after their first symptoms. Left untreated they might have developed symptoms of meningitis or fulminant shock. The endotoxin level in plasma is less than 7 endotoxin units/ml and the number of *N. meningitidis* DNA copies less than 10^4/ml (Fig. 6.5.10). The case fatality rate is close to zero.

Transient benign meningococcaemia

These patients develop fever and often an uncharacteristic rash, but no meningism. They are diagnosed as most likely having a viral infection and receive no antibiotic. When the blood culture results are known, the symptoms have disappeared spontaneously, usually within 1 to 3 days. This syndrome may occur in all age groups.

Subacute meningococcaemia

A few patients develop fever, an uncharacteristic maculopapular rash, general malaise, and arthralgia but no signs of meningitis or shock. They feel uncomfortable but are not severely ill. Meningococci are isolated from blood cultures. Untreated the symptoms may last for days to several weeks but disappear within 1 to 2 days after penicillin therapy is initiated.

Chronic meningococcaemia

The patient develops undulating fever, arthralgia, and maculopapular rash (Fig. 6.5.13). The symptoms may last for months, but at times they may disappear completely. Blood cultures are sometimes repeatedly negative. Patients are often treated with corticosteroids because an underlying autoimmune disease is suspected. The fever disappears temporarily before reappearing and at this stage meningococci may well be isolated from blood cultures. Antibiotic treatment clears the symptoms within a few days. Meningococci with an abnormal lipopolysaccharide (endotoxin) containing five and not six fatty acids in the lipid A moiety have been isolated in many of such patients.

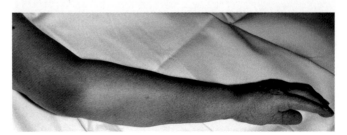

Fig. 6.5.13 Maculopapular rash and peri-articular swellings in an adult patient with chronic meningococcaemia.
(Copyright D A Warrell.)

Other organ manifestations

Pericarditis

The pericardium is seeded during a transient meningococcaemia. Subsequent inflammation and exudate may lead to cardiac tamponade if left untreated. The patient is febrile, nauseated, and may complain of epigastric pain. The condition is often misdiagnosed as an acute abdominal condition. Blood cultures may be negative. *N. meningitidis* can be cultured, detected by PCR, and seen in aspirated pus by direct microscopy. Treatment consists of evacuating the pus and administering antibiotics. The condition should be followed daily by ultrasound examination. Serogroup C organisms have been particularly implicated in these cases.

Arthritis

Acute meningococcal arthritis is an uncommon clinical manifestation of a preceding, often low-grade, meningococcaemia. It is usually located to one, or more rarely, several large joints. If the characteristic petechial rash is absent, detection of meningococci in blood or joint fluid is necessary for a correct diagnosis. Arthritis caused by *Neisseria gonorrhoeae* is considerably more common than primary meningococcal arthritis. The symptoms disappear rapidly after penicillin treatment and there are no long-term complications.

Arthritis induced by immune complexes

This is more common than the meningococcal arthritis. One or several large joints become swollen and painful. The symptoms usually develop at the end of the first week of treatment. Blood and joint cultures are negative. The temperature and inflammatory markers may rise after an initial decline. The symptoms disappear gradually after some days of treatment with nonsteroidal anti-inflammatory drugs. Extended antibiotic therapy is not necessary.

Cutaneous vasculitis and episcleritis

This appears simultaneously with the immune complex arthritis and is commonly observed in sub-Saharan Africa (Figs. 6.5.14, 6.5.15). The vasculitis causes multiple blisters that readily rupture leading to multiple superficial skin ulcers.

Ocular infections

Conjunctivitis or panophthalmitis may precede other symptoms of invasive meningococcal infection. They are primarily observed in infants and children. The patient develops a red eye which in the case of panophthalmitis becomes painful with impaired vision. Formation of microthrombi and haemorrhage in retina and corpus vitreum, leading to blindness, may complicate the infection.

Pneumonia

Strains belonging to serogroups Y and W135 or more rarely other serogroups may cause pneumonia in adults and children. The diagnosis depends on detecting meningococci in a representative specimen from the low respiratory tract or blood culture. It cannot be differentiated from pneumonia caused by other agents on the clinical symptoms alone.

Treatment

Prehospital antibiotic treatment

Since as many as 30% of the patients in industrialized countries infected with *N. meningitidis* develop septic shock characterized by rapidly increasing levels of meningococci and lipopolysaccharides (endotoxin) in the blood. Early antibiotic treatment to stop further growth is regarded as vital. Consequently, health authorities in many countries advise general practitioners to start prehospital antibiotic treatment (i.e. benzylpenicillin) in suspected cases of meningococcal infection. The doses in Table 6.5.3 rapidly lead to bactericidal concentrations in plasma.

The penicillin is injected intravenously or intramuscularly in one or both thighs. The patients most likely to benefit from this strategy, if applied early enough, are those who are distant from the hospital and have rapidly evolving symptoms leading to a compromised circulation and extensive haemorrhagic skin lesions.

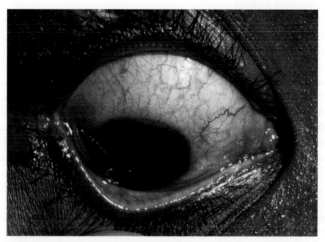

Fig. 6.5.15 Episcleritis in an African child with meningococcal group A meningitis.
(Copyright D A Warrell.)

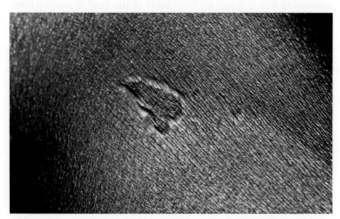

Fig. 6.5.14 Vasculitic lesion in an African child with meningococcal group A meningitis.
(Copyright D A Warrell.)

Table 6.5.3 Doses of prehospital antibiotic to be administered in suspected cases of meningococcal infection

Age (years)	Dose
<2	300 mg (0.5×10^6 IU) benzylpenicillin intramuscularly
2–7	600 mg (1×10^6 IU) benzylpenicillin intramuscularly
>7	1.2 g (2×10^6 IU) benzylpenicillin intravenously or intramuscularly

Initial evaluation in hospital

The patients should be regarded as emergency cases. The main clinical presentation and severity should be evaluated immediately. A variety of prognostic scores have been developed. The Glasgow Meningococcal Septicaemia Prognostic Score is the one most commonly used. Scores can be used to select patients for intensive care treatment. They should never be used to justify withholding treatment as they may overestimate case fatality.

Antibiotic treatment

Adequate doses of benzylpenicillin, cefotaxime, ceftriaxone, or chloramphenicol effectively stop further proliferation of *N. meningitidis* in the circulation, cerebrospinal fluid, and other extravascular sites. Induction of an explosive release of bacterial lipopolysaccharides leading to a Jarisch–Herxheimer reaction has never been documented in patients receiving antibiotics for meningococcal infection. Plasma levels of lipopolysaccharides and the levels of important inflammatory mediators decline immediately after treatment with antibiotics is initiated in these patients (Table 6.5.4).

Benzylpenicillin, chloramphenicol, cefotaxime, ceftriaxone, and meropenem are bactericidal to *N. meningitidis*. Benzylpenicillin remains the drug of choice in most countries. It is effective, cheap, and nontoxic in high doses as long as renal function is normal. High doses are necessary since it penetrates the cerebrospinal fluid relatively poorly. In patients with fulminant septicaemia and severe renal dysfunction the doses should be reduced after 24 to 48 h.

Strains whose sensitivity to penicillin is reduced because of altered penicillin-binding protein 2 are an increasing problem. In most industrialized countries they account for less than 5% of all meningococcal isolates, but the frequency is higher in Mediterranean countries, particularly Spain. Patients infected with these strains have been adequately treated with benzylpenicillin as long as dosage is adequate. A recent study from the United Kingdom indicated the same outcome among patients infected with fully sensitive strains as compared with strains with reduced sensitivity to penicillin. Penicillinase-producing meningococci remain extremely rare.

Chloramphenicol is a good alternative in patients hypersensitive to β-lactam antibiotics. In developing countries it is the best and cheapest alternative to benzylpenicillin. Meningococcal strains resistant to chloramphenicol occur in certain areas. In many industrialized countries cefotaxime or ceftriaxone is combined with vancomycin as empirical treatment of bacterial meningitis until the aetiological agent has been identified. Cefotaxime and ceftriaxone are highly effective antibiotics that penetrate the blood–brain barrier better than benzylpenicillin. Nonsusceptible strains have emerged in India. Meropenem is a carbapenem highly active against *N. meningitidis*, *H. influenzae*,

and *S. pneumoniae*. It does not induce seizures as observed with the imipenem–cilastatin combination.

In each country the health authorities and microbiological laboratories should recommend the optimal and affordable drug regimen.

Antibiotic treatment should be initiated promptly. Therapy should start immediately after the first clinical evaluation and collection of the necessary samples for microbiological diagnosis. If there are contraindications to lumbar puncture or if it is delayed until after brain imaging, antibiotic treatment should be started immediately. Three to 4 days of treatment is adequate to eradicate sensitive meningococci.

Supportive treatment

Patients with persistent shock should be given extensive volume replacement, whereas patients with meningitis should receive a moderate amount of fluid. All patients should be monitored closely to detect early signs of a deteriorating circulation, renal and pulmonary failure, or increasing intracranial pressure.

Volume treatment

Patients in industrialized countries with persistent hypotension and signs of inadequate peripheral circulation have routinely been treated with massive fluid volume repletion. The extensive capillary leak syndrome increases the volume required. Children and adults may require an infused volume that is one to several times their circulating blood volume in the first 24 h. Sodium chloride 0.9% solution is recommended as basic treatment, later supplemented with Ringer's solution. However, in a recently conducted clinical controlled trial in several African countries evaluating children with severe febrile illness and impaired circulation, the results showed unexpectedly that an initial bolus infusion with 20 to 40 ml/kg of 5% albumin or NaCl 0.9% increased the mortality significantly. Whether these results also apply to meningococcal shock in Africa is unknown since the pathophysiology with capillary leakage, cardiac dysfunction, and DIC differs from malaria. In many countries the use of fresh frozen plasma is no longer recommended because of the risk of transmitting pathogens, especially HIV.

Patients presenting with distinct signs of meningitis without shock should receive the basic daily requirement of fluid supplemented with extra volume for dehydration and loss due to vomiting and fever to ensure a normal dieresis (≥1 ml/kg per hour for children). Excessive hydration should be avoided since it may precipitate irreversible brain oedema and cerebellar herniation. In patients with persistent shock and meningitis, treatment of shock is the priority.

Inotropic support

If initial volume repletion fails to improve the circulation, inotropic support should be added. Dopamine, dobutamine, noradrenaline, and adrenaline are used. Most physicians start with dopamine at 3 to 10 µg/kg per min which at an early stage is combined with noradrenalin at 0.03 to 3.0 µg/kg per min or dobutamine at 1 to 10 µg/kg per min. Ideally, patients should be infused through a central line.

Corticosteroid therapy for shock

In adults with septic shock and reduced adrenal function, low doses of cortisol increased survival in one study but was not confirmed in a larger follow up study. Similar studies do not exist for children.

Table 6.5.4 Antibiotics in meningococcal meningitis or sepsis

Antibiotic	Dose/24 h		Dose interval (h)
	Adult (g)	Child (mg/kg)	
Benzylpenicillin	14.4 (24×10^6 IU)	200 (300 000 IU/kg)	4–6
Cefotaxime	9	200	6–8
Ceftriaxone	4	100	12–24
Chloramphenicol	3	100	6

Adrenal haemorrhage is common in patients with fulminant meningococcal septicaemia. Serum cortisol is lower and ACTH higher in nonsurviving than surviving children with meningococcal shock; a relative adrenal insufficiency may therefore exist. Recently many clinicians have treated meningococcal shock with low doses of cortisol in an attempt to reduce inotropic support.

Corticosteroid therapy for meningitis

The United Kingdom National Institute for Health and Clinical Excellence (NICE) guidelines advocate the use of dexamethasone 0.15 mg/kg × 4/24 h (maximum dose 10 mg × 4/24 h) for 4 days for bacterial meningitis. Dexamethasone should ideally be given 15 min before or at least within 4 h after antibiotic treatment is initiated. However, the benefit of dexamethasone in meningococcal meningitis is controversial and has not been documented in randomized clinical controlled trials in Europe and North America. Dexamethasone did not improve the outcome in any type of bacterial meningitis in two large double-blind randomized clinical controlled trials (children and adults) in Malawi, one (adults) in Vietnam and one (children) in Chile. Corticosteroids reduce the penetration of antibiotics over the blood-brain barrier. In developing countries corticosteroids are presently not recommended as adjunct treatment for meningitis. The American Academy of Pediatrics does not advise any adjunct therapy, given the lack of evidence.

Ventilatory support

Patients receiving volume treatment for profound shock are in danger of developing ARDS. Hyperventilation, increasing oxygen demand, decreased pulmonary compliance, and the appearance of diffuse infiltrates on chest radiograph indicate the development of ARDS. At a partial oxygen pressure in arterial blood (Pao_2) of less than 8 kPa with the fraction of inspired oxygen (Fio_2) above 0.6 (60% O_2 in the inspiration air), the patient usually requires intubation and artificial ventilation. Infants and children often require mechanical ventilation if the resuscitation fluid volume exceeds 40 ml/kg per 24 h to combat the septic shock, even if the oxygenation is normal.

Renal support

Patients with persistent septic shock and coagulopathy develop renal dysfunction from acute proximal tubular necrosis. Thrombosis in the small peritubular vessels and in glomeruli, and myoglobinaemia may contribute to renal dysfunction. Serum creatinine and urea are elevated on admission and continue to increase for many days without adequate treatment. Hyperkalaemia, which may develop during the first 24 to 48 h, is an immediate threat. Haemodialysis or peritoneal dialysis and continuous haemofiltration are used to treat the renal failure and remove oedema. The renal failure is usually reversible but may last for weeks. Complete kidney failure is uncommon in survivors.

Treatment of disseminated intravascular coagulation

The first priority is to stop further bacterial proliferation with antibiotics. This reduces the thrombin activity by 50% within 2 to 6 h. In the 1970s heparin was extensively used. Two small controlled trials did not document any survival benefit in patients receiving heparin. Infusion of a continuous low-dose unfractionated heparin (10–15 IU/kg per h) has been advocated as supplement to treatment with concentrated protein C. The antithrombin levels should be kept above 35 to 40 IU/ml. Antithrombin does not reduce the fatality rate in other types of severe sepsis.

Infusion of the natural anticoagulant protein C (loading dose 100 IU/kg, followed by 15 IU/kg per h for 4 days to keep the plasma concentration between 0.8 and 1.2 IU/ml) may possibly limit thrombus formation, skin necrosis, and the need for amputation. If used it should be started early. In the few uncontrolled studies that have been published, several patients treated with protein C concentrate still needed amputation. Randomized controlled trials are lacking.

Recombinant human activated protein C (Xigris) did not improve the outcome in patients with septic shock in a recently conducted randomized clinical controlled trial. The drug was withdrawn from the market (November 2011). Routine transfusion of platelets is controversial. In patients with life-threatening bleeding, massive platelet transfusion can be lifesaving; however, it may also aggravate thrombus formation.

Fibrinolysis

To overcome inhibition by PAI-1, recombinant human tissue plasminogen activator (0.25–0.5 mg/kg in 1.5–4 h) has been infused to enhance fibrinolysis. Retrospective studies suggest that it increases the rate of cerebral haemorrhages. It is not recommended for routine use in severe meningococcaemia.

Plasmapheresis and blood exchange

Plasmapheresis and exchange blood transfusion have been tried to remove pathologically activated plasma and leucocytes; 50 ml plasma/kg body weight has been exchanged with fresh plasma. These techniques do not increase the clearance of bacterial lipopolysaccharide (endotoxin) substantially. Results suggest improved survival but adequate control groups are lacking. Even desperately ill patients have tolerated the procedures.

Extracorporeal membrane oxygenation

A limited number of children have been treated with extracorporeal membrane oxygenation in a few centres with apparently good results. However, equally good results have been achieved in another paediatric intensive care unit without using the procedure, suggesting that the experience of the intensive care unit is more important than the procedure *per se*.

Neutralization of bacterial lipopolysaccharides

Three different antiendotoxin principles, the anti-J5 serum, the human monoclonal IgM (HA-1A) antibody, and the recombinant bactericidal/permeability increasing protein (BPI_{21}) have been evaluated in randomized double-blind controlled clinical trials. None increased survival significantly; however, fewer patients treated with BPI_{21} required multiple severe amputations and more patients had a functional outcome similar to that before illness 60 days after treatment. None of the principles are presently commercially available.

Antimediator therapy

Strategies to neutralize TNF-α, IL-1β, bradykinin, platelet-activating factor, and prostaglandins in patients with septic shock have not increased the 28-day survival rate. They have not been specifically evaluated in meningococcal septic shock.

Sequelae

Meningitis

Sensorineural hearing loss or impaired vestibular function occurs in 4 to 19% of patients. It develops at an early stage, is usually irreversible, and is more common in adults than children. Epilepsy, hydrocephalus, and diffuse brain damage are at present rare complications in industrialized countries.

Persistent headache, altered sleep pattern, concentration difficulties, irritability, and neurasthenia may persist in 5 to 8% of all patients.

Shock and coagulopathy

Most long-term complications are related to development of gangrene of the extremities requiring amputation and necrotic skin lesions requiring extensive grafting. The renal failure is usually reversible although reduced function may persist. Permanent adrenal insufficiency, i.e. Addison's disease, develops very rarely in survivors. ARDS may lead to permanent pulmonary fibrosis and reduced function.

Prevention

Vaccination

Conjugate protein capsule polysaccharide vaccines (A, C, Y, and W)

Serogroup C conjugate vaccines are immunogenic from 2 months of age. They are very effective and induce immunological memory. Booster doses are required for those vaccinated in the first year of life. Combined conjugate vaccines containing serogroups A, C, Y, and W135 have been licensed in many countries for children and adults from 2 to 55 years of age. Evaluation is ongoing for infants and toddlers.

Mass vaccination of African children with a newly developed serogroup A conjugate vaccine appears to be very effective as indicated by preliminary results from Burkina Faso (October 2011). It induces bactericidal anti-capsule antibodies and reduces carriage resulting in heard immunity. Serogroup A, combined A–C, and other combinations of conjugate vaccines are under development and will be licensed in the near future for use in infants.

Capsule polysaccharide vaccine (A, C, Y, and W)

The protective effect of these vaccines in infants below 2 years of age is uncertain. When vaccination is required to prevent serogroup A infection, infants of less than 24 months should receive two doses with at least a 1-month interval, whereas those above 2 years should receive one dose. For serogroup C infection, one dose should be given from 18 months. Revaccination with serogroup C polysaccharide may reduce the antibody level. Malaria reduces the immune response. They do not induce immunological memory. An antibody level of 1 to 2 µg/ml appears to be necessary for protection which lasts for 3 to 5 years. The vaccines are cheap and have for many years been used successfully to contain outbreaks for those above 2 years of age.

Outer membrane vesicle vaccine (B)

Since the capsule polysaccharide of serogroup B strains induces a short-lived IgM but no lasting IgG response, several countries (Cuba, Norway, New Zealand) have developed and used an outer membrane vesicle vaccine protecting against outbreaks of one virulent clone. The protection rate in adolescents after two doses is lower (57–80%) than for the non-B polysaccharide and conjugate vaccines and is relatively strain specific. The immunodominant epitope is the outer membrane protein PorA. Three doses given 6 weeks apart and a fourth dose 8 months later induce a significantly better immune response than two doses. Studies in New Zealand with a strain-specific vaccine has resulted in 73% protection.

The duration of the protection is not known. The Norwegian and New Zealand vaccines are presently not on the market.

New serogroup B vaccines are in phase 2 and 3 immunogenicity trials and will presumably soon be licensed. The method known as 'reverse vaccinology' has identified genes in the *N. meningitidis* DNA coding for previously unknown surface exposed outer membrane proteins present in most of the invasive strains. The genes are cloned, the proteins produced in *E. coli*, purified, and, in one vaccine, combined with outer membrane vesicles from the New Zealand strain. The vaccine induces bactericidal antibodies in infants. The effectiveness in the different age groups remains to be determined.

Indications for vaccination

Routine immunization with the A, C, Y, and W vaccine is advocated for people with documented deficiencies in the alternative pathway and late complement components.

Nonoutbreak situation

Indications for vaccination with A or C vaccine are close contacts of an index case, travellers to high-risk areas, military recruits, persons with asplenia, and alcoholics.

Outbreak situation

Vaccination has been recommended if two or more persons are attacked by the same strain in a school class or day care centre, the attack rate exceeds 10 cases/100 000 population per 3 months, or the attack exceeds 1/1000 with 3 or more cases in a closed group setting.

Epidemic situation

An advocated threshold for mass vaccination is 15 cases/100 000 population per week for 2 consecutive weeks caused by the same strain. A steadily increasing number of cases and an increase in the median age of the patients indicate an epidemic.

Secondary prophylaxis

Antibiotic prophylaxis

Household contacts of an index case have a 100 to 1000 times increased relative risk for developing meningococcal infections. Usually the second case occurs within 2 weeks of the index case if no eradication treatment is given. However, there is doubt about the effectiveness of eradication treatment when the causative strain belongs to serogroup B.

Health authorities in most countries advise that close contacts have eradication treatment. Presently, adults receive 500 mg ciprofloxacin or 400 mg ofloxacin as a single dose. Pregnant women and children of less than 12 years should receive 250 mg and 125 mg ceftriaxone, respectively, as one intramuscular injection. Alternatively children are treated with rifampicin 10 mg/kg, maximum dose 600 mg, every 12 h for 48 h.

Further reading

American Academy of Pediatrics (2009). *Meningococcal infections. Red Book*, pp. 455–63. Elk Grove Village, IL.

Brandtzaeg P, van Deuren M (2005). Meningococcal infections at the start of 21st century. *Adv Pediatr*, **52**, 129–62.

Brower MC, Read RC, van de Beek (2010). Host genetics and outcome in meningococcal disease: a systematic review and metaanalysis. *Lancet Infect Dis*, **10**, 262–74.

Davila S, *et al.* (2010) Genome-wide association study identifies variants in the CFH region associated with host susceptibility to meningococcal disease. *Nat Genet*, **42**, 772–6.

Frosch M, Maiden M (eds) (2006). *Handbook of meningococcal disease.* Wiley, Weinheim.

Gardner P (2006). Prevention of meningococcal disease. *N Engl J Med*, **355**, 1466–73.

NICE (2010). Guidelines for bacterial meningitis and meningococcal septicaemia. www.nice.org.uk/guidance/CG102

Pace D, Pollard AJ, Messonier NE (2009). Quadrivalent meningococcal conjugate vaccines. *Vaccine*, **27S**, B30–41.

Rosenstein NE, *et al.* (2001). Meningococcal disease. *N Engl J Med*, **344**, 1378–88.

Stephens DS, Greenwood B, Brandtzaeg P (2007). Epidemic meningitis, meningococcemia and *Neisseria meningitidis*. *Lancet*, **369**, 2196–3210.

Tan LKK, Carlone GM, Borrow R (2010). Advances in the development of vaccines against Neisseria meningitidis. *N Engl J Med*, **362**, 1511–20.

Van Deuren M, Brandtzaeg P, van der Meer JWM (2000). Update on meningococcal disease, with special emphasis on pathogenesis and clinical management. *Clin Microbiol Rev*, **13**, 144–66.

Welch SB, Nadel S (2003). Treatment of meningococcal infection. *Arch Dis Child*, **88**, 608–14.

6.6 *Neisseria gonorrhoeae*

D. Barlow, Jackie Sherrard, and C. Ison

Essentials

Neisseria gonorrhoeae is a Gram-negative, intracellular (within the cytoplasm of a leucocyte), diplococcus that primarily colonizes the columnar epithelium of lower genital tract, only occasionally progressing to the upper genital tract or causing systemic disease. It is almost exclusively transmitted by sexual activity.

Clinical features—(1) Oropharyngeal and rectal infections usually produce no symptoms; (2) men—dysuria (50%) and urethral discharge (98%) develop after a median of more than 5 days; complications, e.g. epididymitis, orchitis, are rare; (3) women—there are no specific symptoms in the absent of complications, e.g. salpingitis, bartholinitis; (4) disseminated gonococcal infection—a comparatively benign bacteraemia affecting joints (particularly shoulder and knee) and skin; more common in women than men.

Diagnosis—microscopy of a Gram-stained smear from a genital site (urethral or cervical) will give a presumptive diagnosis of gonorrhoea; nucleic acid amplification tests (NAATs) are now the most sensitive test for the confirmation of gonorrhoea but a single result from an extragenital site or from samples from low-prevalence populations should be confirmed using a second test with a different nucleic acid target; culture is the most specific test and provides a viable organism for susceptibility testing but can lack sensitivity.

Treatment—the gonococcus has adapted rapidly to prevalent antimicrobial usage, leading to reduced susceptibility to many antibiotics, notably penicillins, fluoroquinolones, macrolides , tetracycline,

and oral cephalosporins. First-line treatment of uncomplicated infection in adults should be ceftriaxone 500 mg intramuscularly as a single dose plus azithromycin 1 g orally as a single dose. Spectinomycin 2 g by intramuscular injection is suitable for those with penicillin allergy.

Introduction

Gonorrhoea is an ancient disease. Galen coined its name in the 2nd century AD (from Greek works meaning 'semen' and 'flow'), but there are older references including most of Chapter 15 of Leviticus in the Old Testament. The name of the causative bacterium, *Neisseria gonorrhoeae*, credits Albert Neisser with its discovery in 1879 although Hallier had described its characteristic microscopic appearance 7 years earlier.

In the era of HIV/AIDS, this treatable disease plays an important role as an indicator of risky sexual activity.

Epidemiology

In the United Kingdom since the Second World War, the peak incidence in 1946 resulted from a combination of returning infected soldiers and ascertainment bias (Fig. 6.6.1). Changing incidence thereafter seemed independent of the availability of effective antibiotics. The rising numbers of infections since the late 1950s, peaking in 1974, coincided with the introduction of the oral contraceptive pill and greater sexual promiscuity, and an increasing availability of different classes of effective antibiotics and was independent of resistance, first to penicillin and then to tetracyclines, macrolides, and quinolones. The rapid fall in incidence in the late 1980s coincided with a self-imposed regime of safer sex in the gay community.

Differences in the incidence of gonorrhoea between ethnic groups are not explained by genetic susceptibility.

Changes in gonococcal infection

Probably as a result of the availability of effective antibiotics, there have been changes in clinical manifestations of gonococcal infection. In men, the incubation period increased during the last century, from 2 to 3 days before the First World War to more than 8 days in recent years. In the 1990s, the median incubation period of 5.5 days lies outside the often quoted '2 to 5 days'. In women, the incubation period cannot be reliably estimated.

The time from symptoms to presentation for treatment (the infectious period) increased from under 2 days in 1932 to over 6 days in 1991, possibly because symptoms are less severe. The severe burning dysuria of previous times has been replaced by mild 'stinging' and, in 50% of men with gonococcal urethritis in one large study, no dysuria at all.

The complication rate has declined in parts of the world where management and treatment of sexually transmitted infections (STIs) is readily available. However, the availability of effective antimicrobial agents for gonorrhoea is declining worldwide as resistance rapidly emerges to current agents.

Changes in the gonococcus have been driven until now by antibiotic pressures. An intriguing and worrying problem, with the

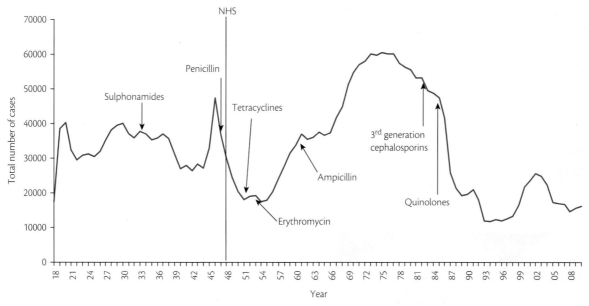

Fig. 6.6.1 Reported cases of gonorrhoea in England between 1918 and 2010 (Health Protection Agency).

increasing use of NAATs for diagnosis, is the evolution of strains that become 'invisible' to the test as a result of loss of the chosen target sequence; this has already happened with tests for *C. trachomatis* in Sweden in 2006.

Pathogenesis

N. gonorrhoeae has evolved mechanisms of evading host defences and causing repeated infection. Major outer membrane antigens exposed to the immune response are pili, lipo-oligosaccharide (LOS), and three major outer membrane proteins Por, Opa, and Rmp. *N. gonorrhoeae* primarily colonizes the columnar epithelium of the lower genital tract, only occasionally spreading to the upper genital tract or causing systemic disease. To colonize successfully, the organism must attach to and invade the epithelial layer to avoid being swept away by cervical secretions in women or urine in men. Iron is essential to multiplication; *N. gonorrhoeae* expresses transferrin or lactoferrin receptors on its surface. *In vivo*, gonococci resist the bactericidal activity of serum by sialylation of LOS. *In vitro*, most strains become serum sensitive. Pili, Opa, and LOS antigens can alter the part of the molecule exposed to the immune response. This antigenic variation occurs at a frequency higher than the normal mutation rate. On each encounter between the organism and the host, the gonococcus presents a range of immunologically distinct proteins that are not recognized by the host. Host cell receptors are complex carbohydrates, glycosamines, lipoproteins, and glycoproteins.

Gonorrhoea in women

Signs and symptoms

Initially, there are no specific symptoms. Uncomplicated gonorrhoea in women affects the cervix (90%), urethra (75%), rectum (40%), or oropharynx (5–15%). Gonococcal cervicitis may result in an increased purulent or mucopurulent exudate from the os, which can present as an increased vaginal discharge (50%). This vaginal discharge has no specific characteristic. Dysuria (12%),

without frequency, is not found consistently enough to make it a diagnostically helpful symptom. The occasional urethral discharge is not profuse enough to cause symptoms. Rectal infection may occur without anal intercourse and rarely produces slight dampness or discharge; throat infection is asymptomatic in both sexes. Abdominal pain signifies spread to the pelvic organs.

Complications

Spread to the endometrium, fallopian tubes, and pelvic adnexae is the most common complication (5%). It occurs at or soon after the menstrual period, probably resulting from retrograde flow of menses. Pelvic pain may be unilateral causing confusion with acute appendicitis. Coincidental infection with *Chlamydia trachomatis* is sufficiently common to justify treatment of both organisms. Infection of Bartholin's, Skene's, or periurethral glands is rare in the United Kingdom.

Perihepatitis (Fitz-Hugh–Curtis syndrome) occurs more frequently with *C. trachomatis* than *N. gonorrhoeae*. Right hypochondrial pain, referred to the shoulder, occasionally with pleural effusion and rub, may lead to referral to a surgical or general medical clinician rather than a genitourinary physician.

Disseminated gonococcal infection (DGI) is rare but more common in women than men, reflecting the lack of genital symptoms in women. It is almost always caused by penicillin-sensitive organisms and is a comparatively benign bacteraemia affecting joints and skin. The shoulder and knee are most commonly affected, followed by wrist, elbow, and small joints of the hands and feet, often with an associated tenosynovitis. The pathognomonic painless usually 4 to 10 skin lesions evolve through vesicular, pustular, and haemorrhagic stages before healing (Figs. 6.6.2, 6.6.3). Erythema nodosum-like lesions have been described. Systemic symptoms are minimal. White cell count and erythrocyte sedimentation rate are not greatly raised. The response to antibiotic treatment is rapid, but joints may need to be aspirated. Blood or joint fluid culture may yield gonococci, but the quickest diagnosis comes from anogenital and throat culture.

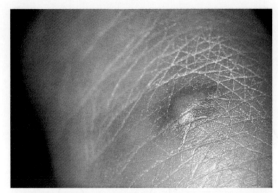

Fig. 6.6.2 Disseminated gonococcal infection, haemorrhagic vesiculopustule.

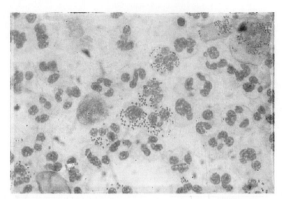

Fig. 6.6.4 Gram-stained urethral discharge showing Gram-negative intracellular diplococci.

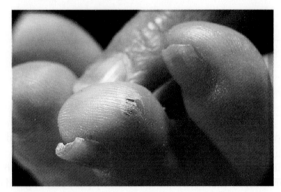

Fig. 6.6.3 Disseminated gonococcal infection: healing lesions with desquamation and deposition of haemosiderin.

Gonorrhoea in men

Signs and symptoms

Classically, urethral gonorrhoea causes discharge and dysuria although the severity and frequency of the dysuria has diminished in recent years. The diagnostic thick, profuse, purulent, white or off-white exudate is preceded by a mucopurulent or scanty mucoid discharge. Even if untreated, the discharge may, after some weeks, diminish to a simple clear mucus; asymptomatic patients (less than 10%) thus include presymptomatic, postsymptomatic, and unobservant men. Urethral gonorrhoea acquired by fellatio is increasingly seen in gay men practising 'safe' sex. It may be transmitted to a regular partner resulting in rectal gonorrhoea. Rectal and oropharyngeal infections are asymptomatic in almost all cases. Sore throat after oral sex does not indicate any particular STI.

Complications

Complications are rare in the developed world. Spread to the epididymis and testis is more often due to *C. trachomatis*. Tysonitis, (infection of the Tyson's or preputial glands), prostatitis, periurethral abscess, and infection of the median raphe are rare in the United Kingdom.

Diagnosis

Microscopy

Diagnosis is easier in men than in women. Microscopy of a suitably stained specimen is the first line in diagnosis. The organism is a

Gram-negative intracellular (within the cytoplasm of a leucocyte) diplococcus (GNID) (Fig. 6.6.4). In samples from the male urethra, microscopy is sensitive (identifying up to 98% of positives in symptomatic men and rather fewer in those without symptoms) and highly specific (<1% will be found on culture to be *Neisseria meningitidis* or other species).

Microscopy of stained samples from the cervix is much less sensitive (55% or less of true positives), but when positive enables immediate treatment. In known contacts of gonorrhoea, microscopy of urethral samples is indicated. Because of the preponderance of other neisseria species in the oropharynx, microscopy of samples from this site is not helpful. Microscopy of anorectal swabs is not recommended because of the large number of other Gram-negative cocci present in faecal flora. However, microscopy of samples of a rectal discharge taken through a protoscope can be helpful.

Laboratory detection of *N. gonorrhoeae*

Isolation of *N. gonorrhoeae* has been the diagnostic gold standard because of its high sensitivity and 100% specificity, but can be hampered by inadequacies in sample taking, transport to the laboratory, and isolation media. NAATs have now been shown to be more sensitive than culture for gonococcal infection because they are more tolerant to delays before testing and can be used on a wide range of samples including urine and self-collected vaginal swabs. NAATs are demonstrably more sensitive than culture in samples from the oropharynx and rectum, although they are not currently licensed for use at these sites, but cross-reacting commensal neisseria species can reduce specificity and require confirmation using second test with a different nucleic acid target. Because NAATs are now the standard test methodology for *C. trachomatis* infection, commercial kits offering testing for both organisms have become the norm. Care is needed in their use in low-prevalence populations; false-positives may be unacceptably common. Culture is recommended following a positive NAAT test, to allow susceptibility testing of the organism.

Isolation and identification of *N. gonorrhoeae*

N. gonorrhoeae requires an enriched medium, such as Thayer–Martin or modified New York City which consist of gonococcal (GC) agar base supplemented with a source of iron (lysed horse blood) and essential amino acids and glucose, and incubation in moist conditions with 5 to 7% carbon dioxide at 37°C. Good specimen collection and efficient transport to the laboratory are crucial for successful isolation.

Specimens are taken from appropriate sites using disposable loops or swabs for inoculation in the clinic or transfer to the laboratory in transport medium. Isolation is enhanced by adding antibiotics to the medium to suppress other organisms that colonize the anogenital tract. Vancomycin inhibits Gram-positive organisms, colistin and trimethoprim inhibit other Gram-negative organisms, and amphotericin or nystatin inhibit yeasts.

Gram-negative cocci on primary isolation that are oxidase positive (presence of cytochrome *c* oxidase) are considered to be *Neisseria* spp. In the industrialized world confirmation of identity as *N. gonorrhoeae* is considered normal practice. This is achieved using carbohydrate utilization tests, either alone or in combination with iminopeptidases in commercial kits; *N. gonorrhoeae* differs from other species in that it produces acid from glucose alone. An alternative approach is to use immunological reagents such as those that contain antibodies raised to epitopes on the two types of the major outer membrane protein, Por or PI, linked to staphylococcal protein A (Phadebact Monoclonal GC OMNI test). These sensitive and specific reagents can identify colonies direct from the primary isolation medium and a result can be obtained on the same day as the organism is isolated. Correct identification of *N. gonorrhoeae* is always desirable but is most important in cases of sexual or child abuse when more than one identification test should be used to confirm an isolate as *N. gonorrhoeae*.

Molecular detection of *N. gonorrhoeae*

NAATS (see above) have historically not been used as extensively for *N. gonorrhoeae* as for *C. trachomatis*, with which it commonly coexists, because they failed to offer much advantage over Gram staining and culture and they do not provide an organism for susceptibility testing. However, the increasing pressure to screen more patients attending for sexual health care, or asymptomatic individuals in other healthcare settings, together with the evolution of improved commercial kits, has escalated their use recently. The sensitivity and specificity of NAATs is high, they are less affected by suboptimal handling or transport, and can be used with noninvasive specimens as urine or self-taken swabs. No molecular tests are available for determining antibiotic susceptibility and so a representative sample of viable organisms will be required for surveillance purposes to guide antimicrobial therapy.

Typing

This has been used to study reinfection, treatment failure, antimicrobial susceptibility patterns, sexual networks, and for forensic purposes. Molecular typing has largely replaced phenotypic methods (auxotyping, determination of nutritional requirement, serotyping, reactivity with a panel of monoclonal antibodies) because it is more robust and discriminating. However, *N. gonorrhoeae* is nonclonal and highly competent for genetic exchange and therefore exhibits marked genetic diversity. For this reason, genotyping is more appropriate for short-term studies such as analysis of sexual networks, rather than temporal studies or comparisons at different geographical locations. Techniques based on diversity in the *por* gene and sequence-based methods, such as *N. gonorrhoeae* multiantigen sequence typing (NG-MAST) which examines diversity in two genes *por* and *tbp*B1, have proved useful. The combination of a highly discriminatory typing method and detailed epidemiological and behavioural data can provide information on the epidemiology that can be used for public health purposes.

Antimicrobial resistance

N. gonorrhoeae is inherently sensitive to most antimicrobial agents but with increased usage both chromosomally mediated and plasmid-mediated resistance has developed. Resistance is most prevalent in the developing world where the incidence of gonorrhoea is high and appropriate antibiotics are often unavailable or misused. However, in the industrialized world these strains are often imported and then spread by the indigenous population. Penicillin was used as first-line therapy for gonorrhoea for many years, until in 1989 the World Health Organization issued new guidelines for the treatment of gonorrhoea following increasing levels of resistance worldwide. Alternative treatments were recommended: ciprofloxacin (a quinolone), ceftriaxone (a third-generation cephalosporin), or spectinomycin (a macrolide), with penicillin recommended only if the gonococcal population was known to be sensitive. Ciprofloxacin was the treatment of choice in the United Kingdom because it is administered orally and was highly effective and inexpensive, whereas in the United States of America ceftriaxone was more widely used. In 2002 resistance to ciprofloxacin reached levels over 5% in England and Wales resulting in a change in guidelines for first-line therapy to a third-generation cephalosporin, ceftriaxone or cefixime. Emerging reports of treatment failure to the oral cephalosporins such as cefixime and surveillance data indicating increasing prevalence of decreased susceptibility are worrying and national guidelines are being changed to recommend the injectable agent ceftriaxone, sometimes at the increased dose of 500 mg. The lack of new alternative treatments after ceftriaxone is a concern and raises the possibility of gonorrhoea as a potentially untreatable infection.

Chromosomally mediated resistance

Decreased susceptibility to penicillin was detected as early as 1958 but this could be overcome by increasing the dose of penicillin and by adding probenecid. It was not until the 1970s that strains began to appear with minimum inhibitory concentrations (MIC) to penicillin of more than 1.0 mg/litre and posed a therapeutic problem. Chromosomal resistance to penicillin in *N. gonorrhoeae* (CMRNG) is the result of the additive effects of mutations at multiple loci *penA, mtr penB, ponA,* and *penC,* the products of which reduce the permeability of the cell wall to penicillin.

Resistance to ciprofloxacin emerged initially in gonococcal strains primarily originating from the Western Pacific with mutations in the DNA gyrase gene *gyrA* and the topoisomerase IV gene *parC*. The level of resistance may be enhanced by additional mutations in the *gyrB* gene or in changes in cell wall permeability possibly due to efflux mechanisms. Ciprofloxacin-resistant gonorrhoea is now endemic in most countries and in many instances is highest among infections in men who have sex with men (MSM).

Therapeutic failure to the oral cephalosporins such as cefixime and ceftibuten is now emerging and is thought to be mediated by a penA mosaic, at least in part. With the increasing use of these highly active agents it is likely that resistance will emerge over time. Spectinomycin may be an alternative choice as resistance, which is high-level and due to a mutation on the chromosome that affects ribosomal binding, has only been reported sporadically.

Azithromycin, primarily used for chlamydial infection, is being used for gonorrhoea but resistance has emerged possibly under selective pressure of the lower 1 g dose recommended for chlamydial infection compared to the 2 g dose for gonorrhoea.

Plasmid-mediated resistance

N. gonorrhoeae exhibiting plasmid-mediated resistance to penicillin was first described in 1976. Simultaneous reports appeared of two strains, one from Africa carrying a plasmid of 3.2 MDa and the second from the Far East carrying a plasmid of 4.4 MDa. Both plasmids encode for the TEM-1 type β-lactamase (penicillinase). The smaller 3.2-MDa plasmid has a deletion from the 4.4-MDa plasmid in a nonfunctional region. Penicillinase-producing *N. gonorrhoeae* (PPNG) carrying the 3.2-MDa and 4.4-MDa plasmids have now disseminated worldwide although their prevalence is greatest in countries of the developing world. PPNG carrying plasmids of differing size (2.9, 3.0, and 4.8 MDa) have been described but have not spread in the same manner.

In 1985, plasmid-mediated resistance to tetracycline was first detected. It is high-level (MIC ≥16 mg/litre) and is due to the acquisition of the *tetM* determinant by the conjugative plasmid of *N. gonorrhoeae* resulting in a plasmid of 25.2 MDa. Strains carrying this plasmid are known as tetracycline-resistant *N. gonorrhoeae* (TRNG). Tetracycline is not the treatment of choice for gonorrhoea but was commonly used, particularly in African countries until the emergence of TRNG, because it was inexpensive and available.

Susceptibility testing

The primary aim of susceptibility testing of *N. gonorrhoeae* is to predict therapeutic failure. However, it is also important to monitor drifts in susceptibility and to detect the emergence of resistant strains to the main first-line therapies. There is much controversy over the correct method for achieving this for gonococci. Determination of zones of inhibition around antibiotic-containing discs has been the method chosen by most clinical laboratories. Gonococci are fastidious organisms that vary in their growth patterns and therefore this method can be difficult to control and interpret. Determination of the full MIC is not necessary for most laboratories and is best performed by reference centres. Etests, which are strips that contain a gradation of concentrations of antibiotics and give a MIC using a similar methodology to disc testing, are very useful for laboratories testing small numbers of strains, albeit still an expensive choice. E-tests are particularly useful for testing susceptibility to cefixime and ceftriaxone and are preferable to disc testing.

Plasmid-mediated resistance to penicillin can be easily detected using the chromogenic cephalosporin (nitrocefin) test. Penicillinase-producing strains change the yellow reagent to a pink/red colour within a few seconds and this can be performed direct from the primary isolation plate. Plasmid-mediated resistance to tetracycline can be detected using either the absence of a zone of inhibition around a 10-μg tetracycline disc or presence of growth on GC agar containing 10 mg/litre tetracycline. Both these screening tests are known to be good predictors of the presence of the 25.2-MDa plasmid and the *tetM* determinant. In a similar manner high-level resistance to ciprofloxacin can be detected by screening for isolates that can grow on agar containing 1 mg/litre ciprofloxacin.

Treatment of gonococcal infection

Ideally, the choice of treatment will depend on the antibiotic susceptibilities of the prevalent gonococci. In the absence of such information, the fluoroquinolones recommended previously , like penicillin, can be used only if the organism is known to be susceptible. The same holds for oral cefixime.

Since the spectrum of antibiotic resistance is continually changing, up-to-date advice should be sought, for example from the websites of the Health Protection Agency (HPA) and the British Association of Sexual Health and HIV (BASHH).

First-line treatment of uncomplicated infection in adults, including oropharyngeal infection, is ceftriaxone 500 mg intramuscularly with azithromycin 1 g orally as a single dose. Spectinomycin 2 g intramuscularly, also with 1g azithromycin, is an alternative and is suitable for those with penicillin allergy. Both regimens can be used to treat infection in pregnant or breastfeeding women. Azithromycin should not be used on its own for gonorrhoea because of the presence of high-level resistance (shared with other macrolides).

Pelvic infection and epididymo-orchitis may be due to the gonococcus *C. trachomatis*, or any number of organisms, and treatment regimens reflect this. British guidelines suggest that gonococcal pelvic infection and perihepatitis should be treated with parenteral antibiotics. Ceftriaxone 1 g intramuscularly or intravenously once daily with doxycycline 100 mg and metronidazole 400 mg, both twice daily intravenously or orally, are recommended. For gonococcal epididymo-orchitis, the treatment is ceftriaxone 500 mg intramuscularly plus doxycycline 100 mg twice daily for 2 weeks.

Infected individuals should be screened for other sexually transmitted infections and their partners identified and, ideally, tested for infection before treatment.

For disseminated gonococcal infection, British guidelines suggest ceftriaxone 1 g intramuscularly or intravenously daily; or cefotaxime 1 g intravenously every 8 h; or spectinomycin 2 g intramuscularly every 12 h continuing for 7 days. This may be switched 24 to 48 h after symptoms improve to an oral regimen such as cefixime 400 mg twice daily or, if quinolone resistance is excluded, ciprofloxacin 500 mg twice daily. Laboratory testing should provide full sensitivities of the causative organism and, unless disseminated gonococcal infection is caused by a resistant strain (an extremely rare occurrence at the time of writing), treatment can be switched to oral amoxicillin 500 mg and probenecid 500 mg, both four times daily.

We now recommend a test of cure following treatment particularly if symptoms persist and in cases of pharyngeal infection. Studies from the pre-NAATS era demonstrated a small but significant failure rate in samples from the rectum even when a fully sensitive organism had originally been isolated.

Further reading

Alexander S, Tosswill J, Ison CI (2010). Laboratory diagnosis of STIs. *Medicine*, **38**, 242–4.

Barlow D, Phillips I (1978). Gonorrhoea in women: diagnostic, clinical and laboratory aspects. *Lancet*, **i**, 761–4.

Bignell CJ , Fitzgerald M (2011). UK *National guideline for the management of gonorrhoea in adults 2011*. www.bashh.org/guidelines

British Association of Sexual Health and HIV (2010). *2010 HPA guidance on gonorrhoea testing in England & Wales*. www.bashh.org/guidelines

Health Protection Agency (2011). http://www.hpa.org.uk/web/
    HPAweb&HPAwebStandard/HPAweb_C/1316016753645 and
    gonorrhoea: therapeutic choice, resistance and susceptibility testing.
    Genitourin Med, **72**, 253–7.

Ison CA (1998). Gonorrhoea. In: Woodford N, Johnson AP (eds)
    Methods in molecular medicine, vol. 15. *Molecular bacteriology:
    protocols and clinical applications*, pp. 293–308. Humana Press,
    Totawa, New Jersey.

Nassif X, *et al.* (1999). Interactions of pathogenic neisseria with host cells.
    Is it possible to assemble the puzzle? *Mol Biol*, **32**, 1124–32.

Ohnishi M, *et al.* (2011). Is Neisseria gonorrhoeae initiating a future era of
    untreatable gonorrhea?: detailed characterization of the first strain with
    high-level resistance to ceftriaxone. *Antimicrob Agents Chemother*, **55**,
    3538–45.

Sherrard J, Barlow D (1996). Gonorrhoea in men: clinical and diagnostic
    aspects. *Genitourin Med*, **72**, 422–6.

Tabrizi SN, *et al.* (2011). Evaluation of six commercial nucleic acid
    amplification tests for the detection of Neisseria gonorrhoeae and other
    Neisseria species. *J Clin Microbiol*, **49**, 3610–16.

Whiley DM, *et al.* (2008). Exploring 'best practice' for nucleic acid detection
    of *Neisseria gonorrhoeae*. *Sex Health*, **5**, 17–23.

6.7 Enterobacteria

Contents

6.7.1 Enterobacteria and bacterial food poisoning

Hugh Pennington

Essentials

The worldwide impact of food poisoning is very great. Such infections kill many children in the developing world, where diarrhoeal diseases stunt their physical and cognitive development. The number of illnesses is also large elsewhere: in the United Kingdom the commonest cause of food poisoning, *Campylobacter*, accounts for about 500 000 cases every year.

The commonest bacterial pathogens are *Campylobacter* and various members of the Enterobacteriaceae, a large family of Gram-negative organisms, of which *Escherichia coli*, *Shigella*, and *Salmonella* are considered in this chapter.

Escherichia coli

Pathogenic *E. coli* include the following:

Enteropathogenic (EPEC)—virulence-positive EPEC are now rare in industrialized countries; food- and water-borne and person-to-person

spread occur, resulting in diarrhoeal illness; fewer than 500 cases are recorded annually in the United Kingdom.

Enteroaggregative (EaggEC)—first isolated from malnourished children in Chile suffering from chronic diarrhoea; not routinely tested for in industrialized countries but probably common.

Enterotoxigenic (ETEC)—an important cause of mortality in children under 5 years of age in developing countries, and causes travellers' diarrhoea; adheres to the mucosal surface of epithelial cells of the proximal small bowel, a process mediated by at least 12 different kinds of pili encoded by transferable plasmids, and produce enterotoxins.

Enteroinvasive (EIEC)—like *Shigella*, for all practical purposes.

Enterohaemorrhagic (EHEC)—the most important EHEC is *E. coli* O157:H7, which produces a toxin virtually identical to that of *Shigella dysenteriae*. *E. coli* O157 is a normal nonpathogenic inhabitant of the gastrointestinal tract of cattle and sheep; most human infections are contracted either by the consumption of foods contaminated with animal manure or by its direct ingestion, probably from hands that have touched contaminated surfaces. Clinical presentation is with diarrhoea (becoming bloody in 90% of cases) and abdominal pain, with a few cases (15% of children <10) going on to develop haemolytic uraemic syndrome (HUS). Diagnosis is by culture. Management is supportive.

EHEC/EaggEC hybrid—caused the serious *E. coli* O104:H4 outbreak in Germany in May to July 2011; attributed to an organic farm producing fenugreek seed sprouts.

Shigella

Infections are exclusively human, spread by the faecal–oral route from person to person, and with a very low infectious dose. Shigellosis is endemic in developing countries in tropical areas, and it probably kills about 600 000 annually, mostly young children. Presentation is with watery diarrhoea, fever and malaise, with severe infections (most often caused by *S. dysenteriae*) progressing to diarrhoea comprising mucus, blood, and pus, along with severe abdominal cramps and tenesmus. Management of mild cases is supportive; severe cases are given antibiotics (ampicillin, co-trimoxazole, tetracycline, ciprofloxacin, others) as guided by local antimicrobial susceptibility data.

Salmonella

There are over 2000 *Salmonella* serotypes, all belonging to the single species *Salmonella enterica*. Those that cause food poisoning infect both animals and humans, and most infections are food-borne, most often by poultry, with *S. enteritidis* (strictly a serotype rather than a species) the paradigmatic organism. Clinical presentation is typically with headache, vomiting (not usually a prominent feature), diarrhoea, abdominal pain, and fever. Metastatic infection sometimes occurs, particularly osteomyelitis and in atherosclerotic vessels, abnormal heart valves, and joint prostheses. Management of mild cases is supportive; severe cases are given antibiotics, usually ciprofloxacin.

Campylobacter

This is by far the commonest cause of bacterial gastroenteritis in the industrialized world, with an annual incidence of infection perhaps as high as 1 per 100 in the United Kingdom. The organisms are very common in the intestines of wild birds, poultry, cattle, and sheep, but the source of infection in most human cases is unknown. A prodrome of fever and general aching sometimes precedes abdominal pain (sometimes severe) and diarrhoea (frequently bloody). Complications include reactive arthritis (1% of cases) and Guillain–Barré syndrome. Most infections are self-limiting, but aside from supportive care, antibiotics (often erythromycin or ciprofloxacin) are given to severe cases.

Prevention

Prevention of food poisoning depends on Hazard Analysis and Critical Control Points (HACCP), which identifies hazards, identifies the points in a process where they may occur, and decides which points are critical to control to ensure consumer safety, e.g. in milk pasteurization the critical control points are the temperatures reached during heating, its duration, and the measures taken to prevent subsequent contamination.

Introduction

Food poisoning denotes gastrointestinal diseases caused by microbes transmitted in food or by microbial toxins preformed there. Food spoilage by microbes also has important consequences for human health because of its impact on food supply. Each year 10 to 20% of the world's annual cereal crop of approximately 2×10^9 tonnes is lost through spoilage by moulds. Much of this loss occurs in the humid tropics and contributes there to the nutritional deficiencies caused by other factors.

The terms food poisoning and food-borne disease overlap but are not synonymous. Thus variant Creutzfeldt-Jacob disease (vCJD), contracted by eating meat products from cows with bovine spongiform encephalopathy, only fits under the food-borne rubric because of its very long incubation period despite the absence of gastrointestinal symptomatology. It is the same for bovine tuberculosis transmitted by milk.

The worldwide impact of food poisoning is very great, as recognized by the World Health Organization Global Strategy for Food Safety (2002), and is the cause of death of many children in the developing world. Diarrhoeal diseases stunt the growth of children and impair their physical and cognitive development. Mortality rates are much lower in developed countries, but the number of illnesses is still large. Quantitation is difficult because of underreporting. A large national study of the number and causes of cases of infectious intestinal disease (IID) in the United Kingdom estimated that in 2009 there were 16.9 million cases and over 1 million GP consultations due to IID every year. Routes of transmission were not established in this study but aetiologies indicate that food-borne transmission occurred in a significant minority; for example, campylobacter was responsible for 500 000 cases. In the United States of America, it has been estimated that each year 3.645 million people contract bacterial food-borne disease with 35 796 being hospitalized and 865 deaths.

The human intestine is home to 10^{13} to 10^{14} microorganisms. Their collective genome contains at least 100 times as many genes as the human one. They metabolize glycans and amino acids, detoxify xenobiotics, and synthesize isoprenoids and vitamins. A prominent member of the distal gut and faecal flora is the methane synthesizer, *Methanobrevibacter smithii*. However, the taxonomic identity and precise properties of most gut microbes is unknown because they cannot be grown in the laboratory. Cultivable ones that cause disease comprise a small minority, even when those opportunistic pathogens which occur primarily as commensals are included, such as members of the Enterobacteriaceae. This family contains several important causes of disease. *Salmonella* Typhi and *S. Paratyphi*, the causes of typhoid and paratyphoid fevers, are members of the Enterobacteriaceae. They cause systemic disease and are described in detail in Chapter 6.8.

Gastroenteritis caused by non-Enterobacteriaceae, i.e. the Gram-negative organisms *Aeromonas*, *Plesiomonas*, *Vibrio parahaemolyticus* and other noncholera vibrios, and, most important quantitatively by incidence, *Campylobacter*, are included here, together with accounts of food poisoning caused by *Bacillus* spp. For descriptions of diseases caused by *Clostridium botulinum* and *C. perfringens* see Chapter 6.24, *C. difficile* see Chapter 6.23, and *Staphylococcus aureus* see Chapter 6.4. An overview of infections of the intestinal tract is given in the Oxford textbook of Medicine 5e Chapter 15.18.

Enterobacteriaceae

The Enterobacteriaceae is a large family of Gram-negative bacteria. Many species are free-living, some are associated with plants and can be plant pathogens, and others live in the intestines of animals and humans. The pathogens considered in detail in this chapter belong to the genera *Escherichia*, *Shigella*, and *Salmonella*.

The formal bacteriological definition of the family is that its members are nonsporing Gram-negative rods that are often motile, usually by peritrichous flagella. They are easily cultivable on ordinary laboratory media. They may or may not have capsules. All are aerobes, although many grow anaerobically as well. All ferment glucose with the formation of acid and sometimes gas, and most reduce nitrate to nitrite. They are oxidase negative and, with the exception of one type of *Shigella dysenteriae*, are catalase positive.

For a century, species in the family have been identified by carbohydrate fermentation patterns and by testing the reactivity of the bacteria to antisera prepared against their surface structures.

Salmonella and *Shigella* do not ferment lactose. With the exception of proteus, providencia, and morganella, all other Enterobacteriaceae ferment this sugar freely with acid production. After cultivation on agar medium containing lactose and a pH indicator, nonlactose-fermenting colonies stand out because of their colour difference, making the initial detection of salmonella or shigella a fairly straightforward task. A similar approach is used to detect the most frequently occurring enterohaemorrhagic *Escherichia coli* serotype, *E. coli* O157:H7, most isolates of which do not ferment sorbitol. Antigenic epitopes key in identification schemes reside in the thick outer bacterial layer (the O antigens) and in flagella (the H antigens). The outer layer is a complex of lipopolysaccharide (LPS) protein and lipid. The LPS has a hydrophobic lipid A component (responsible for the pathological effects of endotoxin) and a hydrophilic polysaccharide made up of an O-specific polysaccharide and a core oligosaccharide. K-antigen epitopes reside on a capsular polysaccharide which when present covers the O antigens. It can be removed by boiling.

Enterobacteriaceae have a clonal population structure. Each individual pathogen has a common ancestor and the incidence of the disease it causes correlates with the population size of the clone that has grown from it. The task of the diagnostic laboratory is to detect and identify these clones as quickly and as cheaply as possible. In general, the traditional tests described above satisfy these requirements. Enterobacteriaceae clones evolve in real time, however, so markers can often be found to distinguish strains, even those with a recent common clonal origin. Tests that determine the susceptibility of isolates to a range of bacterial viruses, bacteriophage typing, have been widely used for this purpose, particularly in the United Kingdom. Molecular methods that detect DNA sequence differences are widely used internationally and have universal applicability and high discriminatory power.

The Enterobacteriaceae considered here live in the intestines of animals and humans. This environment facilitates gene exchange between individual bacteria. It has been known for many years that plasmids, bacteriophages, and transposons are mobile genetic elements. Studies on *E. coli* virulence factors in the 1990s led to the discovery of pathogenicity islands, large genomic regions that are present in pathogenic strains but not in related nonpathogens. They carry genes associated with virulence, are often associated with tRNA genes, and are frequently flanked by repeat sequences. Their G+C content is different from the rest of the bacterial chromosome. DNA sequencing studies have shown more recently that similar islands also occur in nonpathogenic strains. The functions they encode contribute to increased adaptability, fitness, and competitiveness. Genomic islands have been acquired from other bacteria, not necessarily closely related ones. With the other mobile genetic elements they form part of a flexible gene pool which confers beneficial traits supplementing the essential functions encoded by the conserved core genome.

Promiscuous plasmid exchange coupled with the spread of clones has been responsible for the emergence and spread of Enterobacteriaceae that produce New Delhi metallo-β-lactamase-1 (NDM-1). This inactivates all β-lactam antibiotics except aztreonam. The bla_{NDM-1} gene responsible usually occurs in isolates already resistant to most antibiotics; they only remain sensitive to colistin, fosfomycin, and, less consistently, to tigecycline. The first NDM-1 infection was identified in 2008. Since then they have been identified worldwide, mostly in *E. coli* and *Klebsiella pneumoniae* and usually in patients who have been treated in hospitals in the Indian subcontinent. In New Delhi the bla_{NDM-1} gene has been found in Enterobacteriaceae (including shigella), aeromonads, and *Vibrio cholerae*, and in tap water and environmental water.

Molecular genetics has shown that *Shigella* spp. and *E. coli* are so closely related that formally they belong to a single genus. *Escherichia* has priority; however, *Shigella* is a useful name and is likely to continue in use for the foreseeable future. Likewise, the enthusiasm of those who gave hundreds of specific names to *Salmonella* strains distinguished by serotyping was misplaced. The strains are so closely related they are now referred to as serovars of the single species, *Salmonella enterica*.

Escherichia coli

Theodor Escherich was the first to grow *E. coli* in pure culture. He employed the 'Plattenmethode' described by Robert Koch in 1881 in his investigation in Munich in 1885 of the intestinal bacterial flora of newborns. It was the first detailed study of human commensal

bacteria; appropriately so, because an overwhelming majority of the hundred billion billion *E. coli* bacteria that live in the world at any time are normal inhabitants of the intestines of healthy humans and animals. The perception in the 1940s by molecular biologists of its harmless nature coupled with its nonfastidious cultural requirements and rapid growth (2–3 generations/h in the laboratory) led to its choice as a model organism. The strain most often studied is K12, isolated from the faeces of an American convalescent diphtheria patient in 1922. More Nobel prizes have been won by researchers on *E. coli* than any other species (with the exception of *Homo sapiens*).

The identification of *E. coli* using traditional bacteriological methods is straightforward. It is a nonsporing Gram-negative rod, usually motile with peritrichous flagella, facultatively anaerobic, and a gas producer from fermentable carbohydrates. The methyl red reaction is positive and the Voges–Proskauer reaction negative. Many strains have a polysaccharide capsule or microcapsule and most rapidly ferment lactose. Finding such an organism in a normally sterile site such as cerebrospinal fluid or in larger numbers in urine than can be accounted for by contamination is sufficient to indicate an aetiological role. Different approaches have to be used to detect enterovirulent *E. coli* in stools. Selective indicator media have been developed for *E. coli* O157. Other kinds are not looked for routinely; the best methods for detection use DNA probes or polymerase chain reaction (PCR) amplification procedures that are only available in reference laboratories. Few studies have been done on the carriage of commensal *E. coli* by healthy individuals but it is known that some carry a single clone for long periods, whereas others carry several simultaneously, acquiring and losing different clones rapidly. Some clones have a worldwide distribution; others seem to be only local. The genome sequence of strain K12 was published in 1997 and since then the genomes of representative pathogenic clones have been sequenced. A general principle has emerged that within the species there is an enormous amount of genetic diversity. Comparison of K12, a uropathogenic isolate, and an *E. coli* O157 showed that only 39.2% of the combined set of proteins was common to all. The genomes of the pathogens were as different from each other as each pathogen was from the commensal strain. Another *E. coli* characteristic is that different clones share a common genomic backbone of vertically evolved genes which is punctuated by many islands that have been acquired by different horizontal transfer events in each strain.

All pathogenic *E. coli* are sticky, in that they produce structures on their surfaces that act as organelles of attachment. The proteins that make them sticky are adhesins, which recognize host cell structures—receptors—with stereochemical specificity. This fit is an important determinant of host specificity and tissue tropism. Adhesins are often assembled into hair-like fibres, pili. Some take the form of a fuzzy mass on the bacterial surface, curli. Others form no particular oligomeric structures.

The genomes of uropathogenic strains are also rich in genes coding for autotransporters, phase-switch recombinases, and iron-sequestration systems.

Enteropathogenic *E. coli* (EPEC)

The isolation of antigenically identical *E. coli* strains during the investigation of outbreaks of diarrhoea in young babies in the 1940s in London, Aberdeen, and Liverpool provided the first clear evidence that *E. coli* could be an intestinal pathogen.

Subsequent serotyping showed the isolates to be O111 and O55. The disease they caused had a mortality of about 50% and mostly occurred in babies aged 6 months or less. Although volunteer studies in Liverpool showed that isolates from babies caused gastroenteritis in adults, a dose of 2×10^9 organisms only led to a mild short illness.

Typical EPEC cause illness in infants and children under 2 years old; the hospital outbreaks that occurred in the 1940s are no longer seen. Intestinal colonization by typical EPEC involves virulence plasmid-encoded type IV bundle-forming pili which mediate bacterium to bacterium adherence and the formation of compact microcolonies on the surface of host cells, a pattern called localized adherence. EPEC fall into two related groups. Each contains several clones, some of which have been circulating for many years and have been found on several continents. O type does not always correlate with clonal type; thus type O142 marked two clones, one responsible for a high mortality outbreak in a Mexico City hospital in 1965 and the other for much less lethal infections of infants in Indonesia in 1960, hospital outbreaks in England, Scotland, and Ireland from 1969 to 1972, and sporadic cases in Canada in 1972 and Arizona in 1975.

Virulence-positive EPEC are now rare in industrialized countries. Surveys in Brazil showed that they were common there in the 1980s and 1990s. In Europe and North America, EPEC lacking the virulence plasmid are now much more frequent causes of diarrhoea. These atypical EPEC are now becoming proportionally commoner in Brazil as well.

A mechanism central to EPEC pathogenesis is the attaching and effacing (A/E) lesion. At the sites of adhesion in the colon, intestinal cell microvilli disappear. Actin accumulates beneath the bacteria, which become seated on pedestal-like structures. The bacterial genes for the production of attaching and effacing lesions are located on the locus of enterocyte effacement (LEE) pathogenicity island. It codes for intimin, an outer membrane protein responsible for adherence of the bacteria to enterocytes, Esp molecules, which are involved in the machinery that translocates bacterial proteins into enterocytes, and tir, which is translocated and inserts into the enterocyte cell membrane to act as the receptor for intimin.

The incubation period of the diarrhoeal illness caused by EPEC ranges from 12 to 72 h, and the illness can last for several days. Food-borne, water-borne, and person-to-person spread occur. Less than 500 cases are recorded annually in the United Kingdom.

Enteroaggregative E. coli (EAggEC)

These adhere to cell cultures in a 'stacked brick' pattern, a property often encoded on a 60-MDa plasmid. EAEC were first isolated from malnourished children in Chile who had chronic diarrhoea and have been found since in Brazil, Mexico, India, and Zaire. They are not routinely tested for in industrialized countries but are probably common. They have diverse O and H types. Little is known about their virulence factors or their precise pathogenic potential.

Enterotoxigenic E. coli (ETEC)

ETEC are an important cause of mortality in children under 5 years old in developing countries, and a significant cause of travellers' diarrhoea; 31 to 75% of Peace Corps volunteers in Africa with diarrhoea have been found to have ETEC in their stools. An incubation period of 12 to 72 h is followed by diarrhoea and vomiting lasting 3 to 5 days. ETEC adhere to the mucosal surface of epithelial cells of the proximal small bowel, a process mediated in different strains by at least 12 different kinds of pili encoded by transferable

plasmids. There they produce enterotoxins, either a heat-labile (LT) or a heat-stable (ST) one, or both. LTs resembles cholera toxin in structure, mode of entry into cells, and toxic effects therein (see Chapter 6.11). There are different forms but are all made up of one A subunit and five B subunits. There are two kinds of the low molecular weight ST; ST-1 increases intestinal secretion through a route that involves the activation of cyclic guanosine monophosphate. ETEC enterotoxins are often plasmid encoded.

Many E. coli O serotypes have ETEC virulence factors; different clones vary in pilus type and in the enterotoxins they express.

Enteroinvasive E. coli (EIEC)

For all practical purposes EIEC are like shigella (see below); they have the same virulence factors and cause watery diarrhoea.

Enterohaemorrhagic E. coli (EHEC)

The most important EHEC is E. coli O157:H7. Because it produces a toxin which is lethal to cultured African green monkey (Vero) cells and is virtually identical to that of Shigella dysenteriae serotype 1 it is often called VTEC or STEC.

Epidemiology

E. coli O157 is a new pathogen. It came to notice abruptly and dramatically in the United States of America in 1982 where it infected consumers of beef burgers at a well-known chain of fast food restaurants. The first outbreak in England was in 1983. There is a rough correlation between closeness to the north and south poles and the national incidence of infection, which is higher in Scotland than England, in Canada than the United States of America, and in Argentina than Brazil. Accurate figures on its incidence in tropical countries are not available; it is probably uncommon. E. coli O157 is a normal nonpathogenic inhabitant of the gastrointestinal tract of cattle and sheep.

A significant minority of animals, up to 9%, carry it at any one time. The majority of tissue-associated E. coli O157 in them adhere to mucosal epithelium in a region extending up to 5 cm proximal to the rectoanal junction characterized by a high density of lymphoid follicles. Transmission of infection in humans is by the faecal–oral route. Person-to-person spread between young children occurs, and most infections are contracted either by the consumption of foods contaminated with animal manure or by its direct ingestion, probably from hands that have touched contaminated surfaces. Prevention of the contamination of carcasses in slaughter houses is difficult, which explains why transmission by meat occurs. Transmission by burgers has been significant in the United States of America because they are often consumed rare; maintaining 60°C for 2 min in their centre makes them safe. Many ready-to-eat foods have been vectors, e.g. lettuce. Poorly pasteurized milk, unpasteurized apple juice, and untreated drinking water have been important vehicles of transmission. Contamination of meats after cooking was important in the big Scottish outbreak in 1996, in which about 500 people were infected and 17 died.

About 80% of infections are sporadic. In North America and Europe they are commoner in people who live in or who have visited rural areas; in a majority of infections a food vehicle cannot be identified and direct transmission probably occurs.

Pathogenesis

E. coli O157 has the locus of enterocyte effacement pathogenicity island and adheres to enterocytes with the production of attaching and effacing lesions. In this respect it resembles EPEC; it may be that the latter was its progenitor. It also produces Shiga toxins (Stx1, Stx2). They are made of a single A subunit and a B pentamer. Stx1 is almost identical to the toxin produced by *Shigella dysenteriae* type 1; there are several allelic variants of Stx2 which are 50% homologous to Stx1 in amino acid sequence. The B subunit binds to the glycosphingolipid globotriaosylceramide on the surface of host cells; the A subunit enters and turns off protein synthesis by disrupting the large ribosomal subunit in a ricin-like fashion. Shiga toxins induce apoptosis in human renal cells as well. Most pathogenic *E. coli* O157 are Stx2 gene positive; about two-thirds are positive for Stx1.

Clinical features

After an incubation period ranging from 2 to 12 days, most commonly 3 days, diarrhoea starts. In up to 90% of cases it becomes bloody after another 1 to 3 days. Asymptomatic infections are not rare. Most symptomatic cases are afebrile; abdominal pain is more severe than in other forms of bacterial gastroenteritis and abdominal tenderness is common. After between 5 and 13 days of diarrhoeal onset, a minority of cases develop haemolytic uraemic syndrome (HUS). The risk is much greater at the extremes of age; about 15% of children under 10 years develop HUS. Other risk factors are antibiotic administration and the use of antimotility agents. Thrombocytopenia is the first abnormality to develop. There is increased activity of plasminogen activator inhibitor 1 and the concentration of fibrin D-dimers and thrombin fragments 1 and 2 becomes high. In full HUS (some cases never progress beyond thrombocytopenia) the kidneys fail. Neurological complications—thrombotic or haemorrhagic strokes, seizures, and coma—occur in 10% of HUS cases and cardiac dysfunctions occur in about the same proportion; they are important determinants of mortality. No treatment has been shown to prevent the development of HUS or specifically affect its course; the vascular damage that causes it is almost certainly well under way when patients present with diarrhoea. There is no bacteraemia and at this time the Shiga toxin has probably already reached its target organs via the blood stream. Management is supportive rather than specific. Antibiotics, antimotility agents, and nonsteroidal anti-inflammatory drugs should not be given. Fluid balance should be monitored and treated carefully to avoid cardiac overload. Platelet monitoring will indicate whether the HUS risk period has passed. Anaemia sometimes requires transfusion. Renal failure requires specialist management, and renal function returns in a majority. The sequelae of *E. coli* O157 HUS mostly relate to renal function; risk factors for long-term problems are the severity of the HUS itself and the need for dialysis. In most cases of HUS, long-term problems have not been described.

Laboratory diagnosis

The diagnosis of *E. coli* O157 infection is by culture. Growth on selective media containing sorbitol leads to the formation of colourless colonies that are provisionally identified using O157 antiserum. For the detection of small numbers or organisms in, e.g. food suspected to be a vehicle of transmission, enrichment cultures followed by a specific concentration step using magnetic beads covered with O157 antiserum is carried out. Direct tests for Shiga toxin have been developed. Subtyping by phage typing and by pulsed-field gel electrophoresis (for high resolution and in countries where phage typing is not available) is an essential tool in outbreak investigation.

E. coli O157 is the commonest EHEC and cause of HUS. Other serotypes fall into these categories, and O26:H11, O103:H2, O111:H−, and O113:H21 have caused outbreaks in Australia and in continental Europe. Some pathogenic strains of *E. coli* O157 ferment sorbitol. Routinely used selective media detect none of these.

Control

The inability to influence the outcome of EHEC infections once established means that prevention is paramount. The development and implementation of preventive policies has been driven by the impact of big dramatic outbreaks, particularly those associated with burger chains in the United States of America in the 1990s and a butcher's shop in Scotland in 1996. In the United States of America, the Food and Drug Administration classifies *E. coli* O157 as a food adulterant; in consequence its detection has very bad commercial effects. In the United Kingdom and in Europe as a whole, the implementation of Hazard Analysis and Critical Control Points (HACCP)—the evidence-based food safety system—has probably been driven more rapidly than it otherwise would have been. With occasional exceptions these measures have worked well. For example, in Scotland rural/environmental risk factors for infection now far outweigh food ones. Further reductions in the number of cases will be difficult to achieve. No effective measures for reducing *E. coli* O157 in ruminants have been devised, and ruminants shed large numbers into the environment. In north-east Scotland (human population 5×10^5) it has been estimated that cattle and sheep drop about 3×10^{13} live *E. coli* O157 on the ground every day; the infectious dose of *E. coli* O157 for humans is very small, less than 100. Fortunately, the chain of events that leads to transmission from manure to mouth only occurs infrequently. In most years since the mid-1990s the annual incidence of infection in Scotland by *E. coli* O157 has been the highest in the world, but it is usually about 4 per 100 000, so infections are uncommon.

EHEC/EAggEC hybrid

Between May and July 2011 more than 3500 cases of gastroenteritis caused by *E. coli* O104:H4 occurred in Germany. A small outbreak in France at the same time caused by the same organism assisted epidemiological investigations which showed a very clear association with the consumption of fenugreek seed sprouts. Big differences with *E. coli* O157 were that many (c.25% of those with gastroenteritis) went on to develop HUS and that most of these were adults. The incubation period (median 8 days) was longer but the interval between the onset of diarrhoea (median 5 days) was shorter. The causative organism had EHEC characteristics (the *Stx2* gene, a high pathogenicity island encoding an iron uptake system, and adhesin genes) as well as those characteristic of EAggEC (the virulence plasmid pAA, the *aggA* (coding for the pilin subunit of aggregative adherence fimbriae), *aggR* (a transcriptional regulator), *plc* (coding for an intestinal colonisation protein) and *set1* (coding for *Shigella* enterotoxin) genes. The fenugreek was contaminated with faeces during growth, or harvesting, or processing. The source—animal or human—is not known.

Shigella

Bacteriologists working in Japan, Germany, and the Philippines in the early 20th century demonstrated the bacterial aetiology of many cases of dysentery, and that the causative organisms belonged to a group of related but different nonmotile noncapsulate Gram-negative bacilli closely resembling *E. coli* but differentiated from it by their inability to ferment lactose on overnight incubation. The names of the genus, *Shigella*, and three of the four species, *S. flexneri*, *S. boydii*, and *S. sonnei*, commemorate them. The pioneer was Kiyoshi Shiga, who discovered *S. dysenteriae* in Tokyo in 1898.

Epidemiology

As countries become more affluent there is a fall in the number of shigella types circulating as common causes of disease. There is also a relative shift towards types that cause milder disease. *S. dysenteriae* type 1 causes the most severe disease. In the United Kingdom it had disappeared by the mid-1920s, when several *S. flexneri* types and *S. sonnei* were endemic. In England and Wales after 1950, 95 to 98% of infections were caused by *S. sonnei*, although *S. flexneri* was still commoner in Scotland. In the United States of America *S. flexneri* became less common than *S. sonnei* in 1968; currently in Thailand *S. sonnei* is becoming commoner than *S. flexneri*. However, the propensity of shigella to cause epidemics has meant that the change in incidence of infection has not been one of unremitting reduction. Thus in England and Wales after a postwar peak of 49 000 notifications of *S. sonnei* dysentery in 1956, the incidence declined steadily to an annual average of 3000 notifications between 1970 and 1990. However, they rose sharply in 1991 and again in 1992, peaking at 17 000 cases and then falling again. *S. dysenteriae* type 1 became commoner in Mexico and Central America in 1968, in the Indian subcontinent in 1975, and Central Africa during 1985.

Shigella infections are exclusively human (monkeys are susceptible but very probably catch their infections from humans) and are spread by the faecal–oral route. Volunteer studies and information from outbreaks caused by the faecal contamination of water and food on cruise liners have shown that the infectious dose is very low; dysentery can follow the ingestion of 10 viable organisms. Most spread is person-to-person and infection is greatly facilitated by bringing people close together in institutions and circumstances where unsanitary defaecation and inadequate hand washing is common; well-described examples are prisons in England in the early 19th century, mental hospitals in the United Kingdom, Germany, Denmark, and the United States of America later in the 19th century and in the early 20th century, British soldiers in Greece and Mesopotamia (now Iraq) in the First World War, and children in nursery and primary (elementary) schools in the United Kingdom in the early 1990s. It is considered that those with diarrhoea are by far the most effective transmitters of infection. After recovery many individuals continue to excrete organisms for a few weeks; temporary carriers of this kind are not thought to be important sources of infection, even if they are food handlers. Large and dramatic water-borne outbreaks have occurred occasionally in industrialized countries; milk and ice cream have also been vectors. Vegetables contaminated with human faeces during growth, harvesting, or preparation have also caused outbreaks. Molecular typing has revealed the international nature of some; e.g. more than 100 cases in the United Kingdom, Denmark, Norway, and Sweden in 1994 were shown in this way to be due to lettuce contaminated with an identical strain of *S. sonnei*. Shigellosis is endemic in developing countries in tropical areas; a long-standing estimate is that it kills about 600 000 people—mostly young children—annually.

Pathogenesis

Central to the pathogenesis of shigellosis (including that of enteroinvasive *E. coli*, which can be regarded as a variant of *S. sonnei*) is invasion of the colonic mucosa. Organisms gain access to the basolateral pole of enterocytes through M cells, components of intestinal lymphoid follicles (Peyer's patches). Bacteria infect macrophages in these structures and kill them by apoptosis. Their release allows direct invasion and is associated with a cytokine-induced inflammatory response that facilitates bacterial invasion by disrupting the epithelial architecture. The entry of shigella into intestinal cells is actin-microfilament dependent. Shortly after entry the bacterium lyses its phagocytic vacuole and grows in the cytoplasm at a rate of about 40 min/generation; most of the bacterial proteins responsible are plasmid-encoded. Bacteria then spread from cell to cell. Infected cells die and bacterial spread continues deep into the lamina propria. There is an acute inflammatory response dominated by polymorphonuclear leucocytes. Rectocolitis with epithelial desquamation and purulent necrosis with ulcers leads to the production of bloody mucus. Spread of bacteria from the intestines to other parts of the body is rare.

Shiga toxin is only produced by *S. dysenteriae* type 1 (see above). As with EHEC, infections with *S. dysenteriae* type 1 lead, in a minority of cases, to HUS. The increased severity of *S. dysenteriae* type 1 rectocolitis compared with that caused by other *Shigella* spp. is probably due to the local effects of Shiga toxin on the colonic vasculature.

Clinical features

After an incubation period ranging from 12 h to 7 days, but most commonly 2 to 3 days, symptoms usually start suddenly, often with abdominal colic. Watery diarrhoea follows, usually with fever and malaise. The symptomatology of most *S. sonnei* infections progresses no further and, commonly, the number of watery stools is small. The most severe infections are caused by *S. dysenteriae*. After 1 to 3 days the diarrhoea becomes bloody and very frequent, being composed of mucus, blood, and pus. Abdominal cramps and tenesmus are severe. Serious complications, sometimes lethal, are hyponatraemia, hypoglycaemia, septic shock, and HUS. Recovery in complicated cases is slow. More straightforward but severe illnesses such as those not infrequently caused by *S. flexneri* and *S. boydii* usually last about 4 days but may continue for 10 days or more.

Laboratory diagnosis

Diagnosis is by culture and traditional bacteriological methods work well; faeces are the best samples. *Shigella* dies rapidly when swabs dry and such samples should be transported to the laboratory quickly. Inoculation of enrichment cultures from broths or direct inoculation onto special media gives colonies recognizable as shigella by morphology. Further identification is by biochemical tests and type-specific antisera. DNA probes for plasmids are available and Shiga toxin can be looked for.

Treatment

S. sonnei infections in healthy individuals other than those at the extremes of age do not benefit from antibiotic treatment. Agents reducing gut motility should be avoided. Antibiotic treatment of severe infections must be guided by antimicrobial susceptibility data; antibiotic-resistant strains are common in areas where these infections have a high incidence. Ampicillin, co-trimoxazole, tetracycline, or ciprofloxacin have worked well; ceftriaxone and pivmecillinam have been successfully used to treat infections in children caused by antibiotic-resistant strains.

Control

The occurrence of urban epidemic shigellosis in countries like the United Kingdom long after the universal provision of treated town water shows that, while the provision of safe water in parts of the world where serious shigella infections are common is a necessary general public health measure, it will not be sufficient. Interrupting faecal–oral spread needs the provision of toilets and wash hand basins in homes—more a concomitant of economic development than of public health programmes.

Salmonella

The number of different *Salmonella* clones is very large, but they all belong to the single species *Salmonella enterica*. Traditional bacteriological methods—serotyping using O and H antigens and simple biochemical tests—have been used to identify different kinds of *Salmonella* since the 1930s and they are good markers of clonal identity. The custom of referring to the entities they define as though they were species, e.g. *Salmonella enteritidis* is taxonomically incorrect (they are serotypes) but operationally useful. A minority of *Salmonella* serotypes has a host range limited to a single species, e.g. for humans *Salmonella* Typhi (see Chapter 6.8), and these serotypes not considered further here. The serotypes that cause food poisoning infect both animals and humans, and well over 2000 have been described.

Epidemiology

Person-to-person spread is uncommon and the infected/carrier food handler is not an important source; faecal–oral spread after contact with carrier animals such as terrapins and other reptiles occurs from time to time, but most infections are food-borne. In the United Kingdom a big increase in microbiologically confirmed *Salmonella* infection rates and the number of serotypes causing infections occurred in the late 1940s and early 1950s. A common pattern, which continues, is that a serotype appears, persists, and then declines. Their source for humans is food animals. Cattle, sheep, and pigs are far less important than poultry, although *S.* Typhimurium of bovine origin has remained quite common for many years. However, poultry dominate and the paradigmatic organism is *S.* Enteritidis. It caused a panzootic in broiler and layer chicken flocks in Europe and the United States of America starting in the 1980s and concomitantly a human pandemic. In England and Wales it peaked in 1993, when 17 257 infections accounted for 56% of all *Salmonella* isolates. In chickens, *S.* Enteritidis not only grows in the intestines but also invades the reproductive tract leading to egg contamination. Since the early 1990s, control in flocks by slaughter, vaccination, and heightened biosecurity in hen houses has markedly reduced carriage levels in poultry, accounting for the decline in the number of human cases; in England and Wales in 2004 there were 2201 infections. The propensity of certain *Salmonella* serotypes to expand their population size has been enormously facilitated by the scale and nature of the poultry industry. The increase in the number of human infections since the 1940s has followed the expansion of broiler production. In 1950, United States broiler production was 631 million heads and *per capita* consumption was 8.7 pounds ready to cook; in 1990, it was 5864 million and 61.0 pounds, respectively.

Cross-contamination, where organisms from chicken carcasses have been transferred to ready-to-eat foods in the kitchen, has caused large outbreaks. Undercooked egg products are important vectors of *S.* Enteritidis. Many other foods have been vehicles of transmission: unpasteurized milk, dried milk, desiccated coconut, alfalfa sprouts, lettuce, mung bean sprouts, and chocolate. Multicontinental outbreaks occur because of international trade, e.g. 4000 cases of *S.* Agona infection were caused by a contaminated kosher snack in the United Kingdom, Israel, the United States of America, and Canada in 1996.

Pathogenesis

Volunteer studies give an infectious dose ranging from 125 000 to 50 million organisms. For some foods, particularly those with much fat, e.g. cheese, potato chips, peanut butter, and chocolate, it is much less and ranges from fewer than 10 to 100. Organisms attack the distal small intestine and large intestine. At points of contact there is a transient denaturation of brush border microvilli, bacteria are internalized, and they remain in membrane-bound compartments. Replication is necessary for virulence; their presence triggers a transepithelial migration of neutrophils. These processes need the action of many bacterial genes, some of which are in pathogenicity islands.

Clinical features

The incubation period ranges from 4 to 48 h but most commonly it is between 8 and 24 h. Onset is often sudden, with headache, vomiting (not usually a prominent feature), diarrhoea, and abdominal pain; fever is common. The clinical course is usually short, up to 2 to 3 days; in a minority it is severe and prostrating with dehydration. Mortality rates are low but are higher in infants (meningitis sometimes occurs) and elderly people with preexisting pathologies. Some serotypes, e.g. *S.* Dublin are more virulent; bacteraemia with any serotype is usually transient but sometimes leads to metastatic infection, particularly in atherosclerotic vessels, abnormal heart valves, and joint prostheses. Osteomyelitis most frequently occurs in long bones, costochondral junctions, and the spine. Sickle cell anaemia is an important predisposing condition. Arthritis may be septic or reactive; the latter follows more than 1% of infections. It is commonest in those with the HLA-B27 haplotype. Faecal excretion of organisms continues for 4 to 8 weeks and is longer for infants; the number of organisms excreted is usually low. Carriage for longer than 6 months is rare.

Laboratory diagnosis

Diagnosis is by culture. Direct plating of faeces onto selective media and testing of suspicious colonies by slide agglutination for O antigens can give a presumptive diagnosis in 24 h. Enrichment broth cultures increase test sensitivity and are used to search for small numbers of bacteria in faeces or food. Phage typing schemes, available for *S. enteritidis*, *S. typhimurium*, and *S. virchow*, and pulsed-field gel electrophoresis have high resolution and are used to type isolates from patients and other sources in outbreaks.

Treatment

Fluid and electrolyte replacement is the management mainstay. Drugs that reduce gut motility are contraindicated. In uncomplicated cases antibiotics have no place and they may prolong the excretion of organisms. In patients with a high risk of bacteraemia and invasive disease (infants under 3 months, immunosuppressed patients, patients with cancer, and those with haemoglobinopathies) they should be considered. Ciprofloxacin is usually the agent of choice but antibiotic-resistant strains have emerged and therapy must be guided by susceptibility testing. Cefotaxime and ceftriaxone have been of value in treating meningitis in infants.

Prevention

Preventing the infection of food animals is central and it has been successful in poultry in Northern Europe and North America. HACCP has been adopted worldwide; refrigeration and adequate cooking are very important critical control points.

Campylobacter

Campylobacter was discovered as a pathogen of sheep at the beginning of the 20th century, but 70 years elapsed before it was recognized as a common cause of human gastroenteritis. Its high optimum growth temperature (42°C), need for a microaerobic atmosphere, and requirement for help from selective medium to inhibit other competing gut bacteria hindered its detection. *Campylobacter* shares about 50% of its genes with helicobacter; both have a spiral shape and flagella. Most human infections are caused by *Campylobacter jejuni* and some by *C. coli*. Occasional infections are caused by *C. fetus*, an important pathogen of cattle and sheep, and sometimes in patients with immune deficiency.

Epidemiology

Campylobacter is by far the commonest cause of bacterial gastroenteritis in the industrialized world. In England and Wales in 2010, 62 684 laboratory isolates were recorded, 7.3 times more than for nontyphoidal salmonellae In the United Kingdom it is estimated that for every case reported to national surveillance there are 9.3 cases in the community.

Campylobacteriosis is a zoonosis. The organisms are very common inhabitants of the intestines of wild birds, poultry, cattle, and sheep. Mechanized processes in chicken abattoirs mean that the majority of carcasses leave with surface contamination. However, the source of infection in most human cases is unknown; outbreaks, an invaluable epidemiological investigative tool, are rare, and the very great genotypic and phenotypic diversity of the *C. jejuni* genome caused by frequent horizontal gene exchange seriously impedes the development of epidemiologically useful typing systems. Multilocus sequence typing allows the identification of genetically related clonal complexes. The commonest, ST-21, has been isolated from human cases and healthy cattle, broiler chickens, wild birds, and sheep.

Unlike *Salmonella*, the organisms do not grow on contaminated food, so outbreaks are uncommon. They have been associated with failures in milk pasteurization and water chlorination. The incidence of sporadic human cases in the United Kingdom rises sharply in weeks 21 to 24 (May and June); the reason for this is unknown.

Pathogenesis

The infectious dose is low, less than 1000 viable organisms. The jejunum and ileum are colonized first, with extension distally, often to the colon and rectum. Infection is invasive; the mesenteric lymph glands enlarge and become inflamed and neutrophil polymorphonuclear leucocytes accumulate in the intestinal mucosa. A cytolethal distending toxin, phospholipase A, and flagellar structural proteins as well as other bacterial proteins with unknown functions are produced by all pathogenic isolates.

Clinical features

The incubation period ranges from 1 to 7 days and averages 3 days. A prodrome of fever and general aching sometimes precedes abdominal pain and diarrhoea; vomiting is not a prominent feature. Abdominal pain may be severe and acute appendicitis is a frequent differential diagnosis. The diarrhoea contains leucocytes, is frequently bloody, and seldom lasts more than 2 to 3 days. Most patients have culture-negative stools after 5 weeks. Ten to 15% of patients have a recurrence of symptoms.

About 1% of patients develop reactive arthritis 1 to 3 weeks after the onset of illness. It is indistinguishable from that which follows *Salmonella* infections. *Campylobacter* gastroenteritis is the commonest event that leads to the development of the Guillain–Barré syndrome (Oxford Textbook of Medicine 5e Chapter 24.16); 26 to 41% of cases have a history of its occurring 1 to 3 weeks after the onset of diarrhoea.

Laboratory diagnosis

Laboratory diagnosis is by culture. Stools are plated onto selective media and incubated for 48 h at 42 to 43°C in 5 to 15% oxygen and 1 to 10% CO_2. Infectivity is labile; if delays in transport to the laboratory are expected, faeces should be refrigerated or placed in transport medium. Diagnosis of recent infections is by serology.

Treatment

Most *Campylobacter* infections are self-limiting. Fluid and electrolyte replacement may be needed. Most strains are sensitive to erythromycin; ciprofloxacin and other fluoroquinolones are also effective in more severe infections, but resistant strains are becoming commoner.

Miscellaneous food poisoning bacteria

Listeria monocytogenes

See Chapter 10.34.

Vibrio parahaemolyticus

Vibrio parahaemolyticus is the commonest bacterial cause of diarrhoea (usually watery, sometimes explosive) in Japan. Infection follows the consumption of seafood, particularly those prepared raw in the Japanese style. The incubation period is commonly 10 to 20 h (range 4–9 h) and the illness lasts 1 to 2 days. Pathogenic strains produce a heat-stable toxin and are Kanagawa positive (produce haemolysis on Wagatsuma's agar). Other vibrios that cause seafood-associated gastroenteritis are *V. fluvialis*, *V. hollisae*, *V. mimicus*, and *V. vulnificus*.

Aeromonas hydrophila

This Gram-negative rod is frequently isolated from diarrhoea. Virulence factors remain unidentified.

Exotoxin producers

See Chapters 6.23 and 6.24 for *Clostridium difficile*, *C. botulinum*, and *C. perfringens*, and Chapter 6.4 for *Staphylococcus aureus*.

Bacillus cereus

This Gram-positive saprophyte produces heat-resistant spores. It is common in raw foods, especially rice, and causes two kinds of food poisoning, emetic and diarrhoeic. Vomiting occurs 6 h or less after eating food containing preformed toxin, usually lightly cooked rice that has then been stored at room temperature and reheated, conditions which stimulate the bacterium to produce the low molecular weight heat-, acid-, and protein-resistant peptide toxin. Diarrhoea occurs 8 to 24 h after eating contaminated food. A heat-labile enterotoxin is produced in the intestine. Both kinds of illness are short lived. Other *Bacillus* species, *B. licheniformis*, *B. pumilis*, and *B. subtilis*, have caused *B. cereus*-like illnesses.

Prevention of food poisoning

The production of safe food rests on evidence-based practical technologies and management systems; HACCP is central to their delivery. The system was developed by the National Aeronautics and Space Administration (NASA) and others in the 1960s to prevent food poisoning in space; the notion of diarrhoea and vomiting in zero gravity was too awful to contemplate. HACCP is now used worldwide and in many countries for some food businesses it is a legal requirement. It identifies hazards, identifies the points in a process where they may occur, and decides which points are critical to control to ensure consumer safety. A good example is milk pasteurization; critical control points are the temperatures reached during heating, its duration, and the measures taken to prevent subsequent contamination.

As a written scheme testable by food law enforcers, HACCP stops at the farm gate and the dwelling door. However, its principles apply on the farm and in the home, and their promulgation there currently exercises all promoters of food safety. Ignorance of them is not restricted to these environments; large food poisoning outbreaks have followed failures of food processors to follow them. Milk pasteurization is again a good example. Political resistance to its implementation in England meant that 65 000 died there from milk-borne bovine tuberculosis between 1912 and 1937. Thirty-nine milk-borne salmonella outbreaks with deaths in Scotland between 1970 and 1981 drove legislation preventing the sale of unpasteurized milk there, and now nearly all United Kingdom milk is pasteurized. However, pasteurization failures or postpasteurization contamination still lead to campylobacter and *E. coli* O157 outbreaks.

Further reading

Advisory Committee on the Microbial Safety of Food (2005). *Second report on campylobacter.* Food Standards Agency, London.

Cheasty T, Smith HR (2005). Escherichia. In: Borriello SP, Murray PR, Funke G (eds) *Topley and Wilson's microbiology and microbial infections (bacteriology)*, pp. 1360–75. Hodder Arnold, London.

Granum PE, Lund T (1997). *Bacillus cereus* and its food poisoning toxins. *FEMS Microbiol Lett*, **157**, 223–82.

Maskell D, Mastroeni P (eds) (2006). *Salmonella infections: clinical, immunological and molecular aspects. (Advances in molecular and cellular microbiology)*. Cambridge University Press, Cambridge, UK.

Nair GB, *et al.* (2007). Global dissemination of *Vibrio parahaemolyticus* serotype 03;K6 and its serovariants. *Clin Microbiol Rev*, **20**, 39–48.

Nordmann P,Naas T, Poirel L (2011). Global spread of carbapenemase-producing Enterobacteriaceae. *Emerg Infect Dis*, **17**, 1791–8.

Pennington TH (2010). Review. Escherichia coli O157. *Lancet*, **376**, 1428–35.

Schroeder GN, Hilbi H (2008). Molecular pathogenesis of shigella species: controlling host cell signaling, invasion and death by type III secretion. *Clin Microbiol Rev*, **21**, 134–56.

Tarr PI, Gordon CA, Chandler WI (2005). Shiga-toxin-producing *Escherichia coli* and haemolytic uraemic syndrome. *Lancet*, **365**, 1073–86.

The Public Inquiry into the September 2005 outbreak of E. coli O157 in South Wales 2009. www.ecoliinquirywales.org

Threlfall EJ (2005). Salmonella. In: Borriello SP, Murray PR, Funke G (eds) *Topley and Wilson's microbiology and microbial infections (bacteriology)*, pp. 1398–434. Hodder Arnold, London.

Young KT, Davis LM, Dirita VJ (2007). *Campylobacter jejuni*: molecular biology and pathogenesis. *Nat Rev Microbiol*, **5**, 665–79.

6.7.2 *Pseudomonas aeruginosa*

G.C.K.W. Koh and S.J. Peacock

Essentials

Pseudomonas aeruginosa is a highly versatile environmental Gram-negative bacterium that can be isolated from a wide range of habitats, including soil, marshes, and the ocean, as well as from plants and animal tissues. It is resistant to many disinfectants and antibiotics, giving it a selective advantage in hospitals. It rarely causes infection in the healthy host but is a major opportunistic pathogen.

Clinical features—(1) In hospitals—causes a range of infections, including bacteraemia (often in association with neutropenia), ventilator-associated pneumonia, urinary tract infection, skin and soft-tissue infections, and bacteraemia associated with burns. (2) In the community—the largest group of people affected by *P. aeruginosa* are those with cystic fibrosis, who develop long-term colonization of the airways punctuated by episodes of clinical infection.

Diagnosis—this is usually straightforward when the organism is cultured from samples collected from normally sterile sites, but is often challenging when infection is suspected in sites such as a catheterized urinary tract, burns, or ulcers. Serology is of no value.

Treatment—*P. aeruginosa* is intrinsically resistant to a broad range of antimicrobial drugs. Appropriate and effective prescribing for high-risk patients requires (1) clinical awareness of risk factors for *P. aeruginosa*, combined with knowledge of the spectrum of diseases caused by this organism; (2) carefully considered empirical regimens based on local antimicrobial susceptibility data—these will typically include a β-lactam (e.g. ceftazidime, meropenem, or piperacillin) plus a second agent (e.g. a fluoroquinolone or aminoglycoside) for serious infections, although single agents may be used for uncomplicated infections; and (3) attention to susceptibility profiles once the causative strain has been isolated and tested.

Genetics and pathogenesis

The *Pseudomonas aeruginosa* genome is composed of a single chromosome of 6.3 Mbp containing around 5700 predicted open reading frames. This is markedly larger than most other sequenced bacterial genomes, and approaches the size of the simple eukaryote *Saccharomyces cerevisiae*, the genome of which encodes around 6200 proteins. The *P. aeruginosa* genome contains a high proportion of regulatory genes and a large number of genes involved in catabolism, transport, and efflux of organic chemicals. The size and complexity of the genome underpins its ability to thrive in diverse environments. *P. aeruginosa* produces a single polar flagellum and numerous fimbriae or pili which allow it to adhere to the respiratory epithelium. More than one-half of all clinical isolates produce pyocyanin (a blue pigment) and pyoverdin (a green pigment), which are responsible for the characteristic blue-green colour of *P. aeruginosa* colonies growing on solid media. Pyocyanin is an exotoxin that has immunomodulatory effects on respiratory epithelial cells, is toxic to neutrophils, and is involved in iron acquisition. Alginate mediates adherence to epithelial surfaces and protects the organism from phagocytosis. The production of alginate exopolysaccharide by mucoid strains of *P. aeruginosa* has been shown to be involved in the colonization of the lungs of patients with cystic fibrosis, and is an adverse prognostic factor.

P. aeruginosa in the environment

P. aeruginosa is ubiquitous in the environment. In homes, it is often found in the aerators and traps of sinks, shower heads, water coolers, contact lens solutions, and cosmetics, as well as in swimming pools, whirlpool baths, and jacuzzis. It may also be cultured from a wide variety of raw fruit and vegetables. It is difficult to eradicate from the hospital environment, where it has been found in soap dishes, dialysis fluid, irrigation fluids, eye drops, disinfectants, ointments, and mechanical ventilators. *P. aeruginosa* is resistant to several commonly used disinfectants: ammonium acetate-buffered benzalkonium chloride solution will support the growth and division of *P. aeruginosa*, and the organism readily develops resistance to chlorhexidine. *P. aeruginosa* is killed by povidone-iodine, glutaraldehyde, bleach, and alcohol, but may be relatively resistant to these when present in a biofilm or embedded within proteinaceous material.

Human colonization and disease

Colonization

P. aeruginosa is probably consumed regularly and is capable of colonizing the human gastrointestinal tract. It is rarely present on the intact skin or mucous membranes of healthy individuals but often colonizes severely ill patients, particularly those on broad-spectrum antibiotics. *P. aeruginosa* often colonizes areas of broken skin, such as ulcers, and medical devices in contact with the environment, such as long-term urinary catheters. The organism may cause a broad range of infections, most commonly in patients with one or more risk factors.

Bacteraemia

Bacteraemia occurs primarily in immunocompromised patients, particularly those with haematological malignancies, neutropenia, or severe burns. *P. aeruginosa* accounts for approximately one-quarter of all hospital-acquired bacteraemias, and has a mortality of 18%. In 2007, there were 3823 reported cases of *Pseudomonas* bacteraemia in the United Kingdom (6.9 per 10 000 population), a 20% increase compared to 2003. Clinical features of sepsis associated with *P. aeruginosa* infection do not differ from those associated with other bacterial infections, and empirical antimicrobial prescribing for high-risk patients should include cover for *P. aeruginosa*. A primary source of infection (e.g. a chronic ulcer in a diabetic patient, a urinary catheter, etc.) should be sought and removed wherever possible. In rare cases of *P. aeruginosa* infection, patients may develop a skin lesion called ecthyma gangrenosum (Fig. 6.7.2.1) which, although not pathognomonic for *P. aeruginosa*, is rarely a feature of infection by any other organism. This presents as a painful, well-circumscribed, erythematous lesion anywhere on the body that progresses to necrosis within hours or days. Ecthyma rarely appears in a non-neutropenic host, and its appearance marks the failure of the host immune response to control the infection. In these patients, *P. aeruginosa* may often be cultured both from blood and from the lesion, but not every patient with ecthyma is detectably bacteraemic.

Pulmonary infection

P. aeruginosa consistently ranks either first or second in frequency as a cause of ventilator-associated pneumonia in United States of America surveys (National Healthcare Safety Network). Diagnosis is complicated by the fact that severely ill patients commonly become colonized by *P. aeruginosa*, and appropriate sampling of patients with suspected ventilator-associated pneumonia requires the use of bronchoalveolar lavage or protected-specimen brush sampling of the distal airways. Tracheal aspirates are easier to obtain but less helpful (positive cultures are suggestive but not diagnostic). The diagnosis and treatment of ventilator-associated pneumonia is described in Oxford Textbook of Medicine 5e Section 18 and Chapter 18.4.3. *P. aeruginosa* commonly colonizes the respiratory tract of people with cystic fibrosis and is the leading cause of respiratory infection in this group. Asymptomatic *P. aeruginosa* colonization is associated with a more rapid decline in lung function and increased mortality from respiratory failure. It is difficult to obtain adequate sputum samples from children, and so in the context of cystic fibrosis, bronchoscopy is sometimes the only available diagnostic technique. Some clinicians have attempted to avoid invasive sampling by using serological tests, but the results are unreliable. Current evidence is that early treatment with nebulized tobramycin is capable of eradicating of *P. aeruginosa* from cystic fibrosis patients. Cystic fibrosis is discussed in Oxford Textbook of

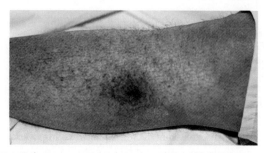

Fig. 6.7.2.1 Ecthyma gangrenosum lesion in a patient with Pseudomonas aeruginosa septicaemia.
(Courtesy of the late Dr BE Juel-Jensen).

Medicine 5e Chapter 18.10. *P. aeruginosa* may cause a fulminant necrotizing pneumonia in neutropenic patients as part of a syndrome of disseminated infection.

Skin and soft tissue infection

P. aeruginosa rarely invades healthy skin and a breach of the integument (e.g. skin maceration from chronic immersion in water, a burn, a cut or nick from a razor blade or rose thorn, a surgical wound, or an ulcer) is usually required for infection to become established. 'Hot tub' dermatitis is a self-limiting skin infection in healthy people caused by exposure to water contaminated with *P. aeruginosa* and manifests as folliculitis or vesicular lesions. Outbreaks have been associated with jacuzzis, spas, and swimming pools. *P. aeruginosa* is a cause of surgical wound infections (4.6–11% according to annual National Nosocomial Infections Surveillance System surveys), but is far less common than *Staphylococcus aureus*. *P. aeruginosa* colonization of chronic leg ulcers is common, but it is rarely the only organism found from superficial swabs taken from this type of lesion and is usually a colonizer rather than an invader. Superficial swabs of ulcers are best avoided in the absence of clinical signs of active infection. When infection is present (e.g. cellulitis, associated osteomyelitis, bacteraemia), cultures from deep tissue that does not communicate with the ulcer or wound surface should be obtained. Ecthyma gangrenosum is described under the section on bacteraemia (see above). *P. aeruginosa* is an important cause of infection in patients with burns, the other important pathogen being *S. aureus*.

Urinary tract

The initiating event in *P. aeruginosa* urinary tract infection is usually urinary catheterization or instrumentation of the urinary tract, although infection may occasionally occur by haematogenous spread to the kidneys. Patients with long-term indwelling urinary catheters are at particular risk, a combined effect of the presence of prosthetic material that provides a nidus for infection and because frequent antimicrobial therapy for recurrent urinary infection selects for resistant organisms such as *P. aeruginosa*. No specific clinical features distinguish *P. aeruginosa* urinary infections from infection caused by other pathogens. The diagnosis is made on urine culture in the presence of appropriate clinical features, predominant of which is fever. *P. aeruginosa* infection in this patient group is rarely cured without removal/replacement of the urinary catheter on which organisms persist within a biofilm. Catheter change should be performed towards the end of therapy once the burden of planktonic bacteria (bacteria free in urine) is much reduced. Routine urine culture of patients with long-term urinary catheters provides no useful information in the absence of clinical features of active infection. Renal imaging may be useful to exclude renal abscesses or calculi if the reason for the infection is not obvious.

Ear infection

P. aeruginosa is a leading cause of otitis externa, an infection of the external auditory canal that causes inflammation, pain (which is exacerbated by traction on the pinna), and, if severe, a purulent discharge. It is common to find lymphadenopathy just anterior to the tragus. The disease is usually seen in children and the source of infection includes underchlorinated swimming pools or fresh water (lakes or rivers). The diagnosis is based on signs and symptoms, and empiric treatment with eardrops is usually effective. Malignant otitis externa is rare but much more serious. It is not a neoplastic process, but is so called because of the risk of localized destructive spread to the central nervous system. It most commonly occurs in elderly patients with diabetes and people with HIV infection, and is essentially an osteomyelitis of the mastoid and petrous temporal bone. Affected patients present with an erythematous oedematous inflamed external auditory canal, and the tympanic membrane is often hidden by oedema. Otoscopy is necessary to make the diagnosis, but is often poorly tolerated because of pain. Lymphadenopathy of the ipsilateral cervical lymph nodes may be present; facial nerve involvement produces an ipsilateral lower motor neuron seventh nerve palsy. Spread to the temporomandibular joint causes pain on mastication, and spread to the apex of the petrous temporal nerve produces Gradenigo's syndrome (trigeminal and trochlear nerve palsies). Features of malignant otitis externa should prompt immediate referral to an ear, nose, and throat surgeon for assessment and debridement of the ear canal and adjacent bone. The diagnosis is made by demonstrating osteomyelitis of the skull base on a technetium-99 bone scintigram or on MRI, along with *P. aeruginosa* cultured from the discharge or from a bone biopsy.

Eye infection

The most common manifestation of *P. aeruginosa* eye infection is keratitis, which occurs following direct inoculation from trauma (e.g. contact sports, industrial accidents) or minor abrasions (e.g. contact lens use). Contact lens keratitis has been associated with contaminated contact lens disinfectant solutions. *P. aeruginosa* keratitis requires prompt ophthalmological referral and treatment since infection may be rapidly progressive and can result in corneal opacification and even perforation within 48 h. Pseudomonal endophthalmitis most commonly occurs as a consequence of penetrating injury or surgery, but there is also a rare syndrome of neonatal endophthalmitis that may be bilateral, the main risk factor for which is prematurity. Clinical features include severe pain, chemosis, loss of the red reflex, hypopyon, and corneal clouding. Neonatal pseudomonal endophthalmitis most commonly arises from haematogenous spread, frequently in association with a syndrome of disseminated disease that includes meningitis and pneumonia, and is commonly fatal. Endophthalmitis is diagnosed by culture of a vitreous humour biopsy.

Endocarditis

P. aeruginosa endocarditis is a disease confined almost exclusively to injecting drug users, in whom it is usually right-sided. Extended intravenous combination therapy with a β-lactam and an aminoglycoside is required, and valve replacement is often necessary. In the case of left-sided endocarditis, antibiotic therapy alone is rarely sufficient and valve replacement is mandatory.

Bone and joint infection

Patients with diabetes may develop osteomyelitis of the foot following penetrating injury or local extension of an untreated chronic ulcer. Results from superficial swabs are of minimal clinical relevance, and diagnosis should be based on the results of bone biopsy which should be processed for culture and histopathology. Parenteral antimicrobials are not always successful and radical debridement or amputation may be necessary to clear the infection. Intravenous drug users are susceptible to *P. aeruginosa* septic arthritis and osteomyelitis of the axial skeleton.

HIV infection

Patients with HIV infection are more susceptible to *P. aeruginosa* infection, usually when the CD4 count is below 100 cells/µl. The incidence has fallen since the advent of highly active antiretroviral therapy (HAART). The presentation of *P. aeruginosa* infection in HIV patients is more indolent than that in neutropenic patients, but mortality is 22 to 34%. The fever is frequently low grade and ecthyma gangrenosum is rare. It is most commonly intravenous device related. Pneumonia is the most common community-acquired presentation, followed by sinusitis, and infections of the urinary tract, all of which may be associated with bacteraemia.

Antimicrobial therapy

P. aeruginosa elaborates a range of β-lactamases (penicillinases and cephalosporinases) and has a relatively impermeable outer membrane, which makes it intrinsically resistant to a wide variety of antimicrobials, including all first-generation and second-generation cephalosporins, most penicillins, and all macrolides. The antipseudomonal cephalosporins ceftazidime and cefepime are effective; of the carbapenems, imipenem and meropenem are effective. The antipseudomonal penicillins are piperacillin and ticarcillin (commonly available in combined preparations with tazobactam or clavulanate). The β-lactams are bactericidal and there is good clinical evidence for their efficacy and safety, except that cefepime monotherapy is associated with a higher all-cause mortality and cannot therefore be recommended. There is evidence from animal studies that continuous infusions of β-lactam are superior to intermittent dosing. The monobactam, aztreonam, has not found widespread use because isolates that are resistant to ceftazidime or piperacillin are generally also resistant to aztreonam. However, there are rare metallo-β-lactamase-producing strains of *P. aeruginosa* that may be resistant to carbapenems but sensitive to aztreonam. The aminoglycosides (gentamicin, amikacin, kanamycin, tobramycin, etc.) are effective *in vitro* and may be used in combination with β-lactams in empiric regimens for febrile neutropenic patients and for *P. aeruginosa* ventilator-associated pneumonia. Concerns that aminoglycosides are not efficacious in neutropenia has led to the use of other empirical combinations (e.g. β-lactam plus fluoroquinolone). The aminoglycosides also have poor tissue penetration and are renal/ototoxic. Depending on the site of infection, inhaled or topical aminoglycosides may be preferable, e.g. inhaled tobramycin for cystic fibrosis patients, or topical gentamicin for otitis externa and superficial eye infections. The fluoroquinolone ciprofloxacin is active when administered orally, an attribute that makes it almost unique among the therapeutic options available for *P. aeruginosa* treatment.

Acquired drug resistance is a problem in patients who are antibiotic experienced (an important example being patients with cystic fibrosis), but resistance to commonly used antibiotics is a problem even outside this patient group. The United Kingdom Health Protection Agency reported that of the *P. aeruginosa* strains isolated from blood in 2009, 11% were not susceptible to ciprofloxacin, 8% to ceftazidime, 8% to piperacillin/tazobactam, 14% to imipenem, and 11% meropenem, with a rise in the proportion of isolates resistant to carbapenems. It is not uncommon for resistance to develop during the course of treatment, an event that is associated with excess mortality. Gentamicin-resistant strains may remain susceptible to kanamycin or neomycin, but cross-resistance to tobramycin is common. Strains that colonize patients with cystic fibrosis frequently become multiply resistant; older antimicrobial agents such as colistin and polymyxin B may then be used.

The antimicrobial treatment and management of *P. aeruginosa* infection is complex because the infections are often system or patient-group specific and so a single guideline is not appropriate. For patients with serious suspected *P. aeruginosa* infection, increasing resistance rates mean first line therapy should include a β-lactam (e.g. piperacillin-tazobactam or meropenem) in combination with a second agent in order to achieve adequate coverage. Therapy should be reviewed when culture and susceptibility results are known. There is good *in vitro* evidence that monotherapy is associated with a slower rate of bacterial killing and the emergence of resistance; however, for uncomplicated infections, therapy with a single agent is probably adequate. Decisions on empirical antimicrobial therapy should be taken in the light of local information on patterns of resistance. The reader is encouraged to study this section in conjunction with other relevant chapters on the management of conditions including neutropenic sepsis, ventilator-associated pneumonia, cystic fibrosis, and urinary tract, ear, and eye infections.

Prevention

Groups of patients (e.g. neutropenic patients, or patients with severe burns) who are particularly susceptible to invasive pseudomonal infection may be housed in clean units. Such units are equipped with filtered air supplies, and incoming water is chlorinated and continuously heated to 60°C. Attention is paid to the regular maintenance of air conditioning, hydrotherapy units, and water coolers. Visitors and staff are required to wear protective gowns and gloves, and to remove their shoes to avoid contaminating the hospital environment with bacteria brought in from outside the hospital. Fresh flowers and fruit are prohibited for the same reasons, and a rigorous regimen of hand washing is instituted for all visitors and staff. The emergence over the last decade of highly transmissible strains of multidrug-resistant *P. aeruginosa* in people with cystic fibrosis has necessitated the institution of measures to segregate affected patients. A number of vaccine candidates have entered II and III trials (e.g. IC43), but none are currently licensed for clinical use.

Further reading

Flume *et al.* (2009). Cystic fibrosis pulmonary guidelines: treatment of pulmonary exacerbations. *Am J Respir Crit Care Med*, **180**, 802–8.

Fujitani S, *et al.* (2011). Pneumonia due to Pseudomonas aeruginosa: part I: epidemiology, clinical diagnosis, and source. *Chest*, **139**, 909–19.

Kaushik V, Malik T, Saeed SR (2010). Interventions for acute otitis externa. *Cochrane Database Syst Rev*, **1**, CD004740.

Langton Hewer SC, Smyth AR (2009). Antibiotic strategies for eradicating Pseudomonas aeruginosa in people with cystic fibrosis. *Cochrane Database Syst Rev*, **4**, CD004197.

Louie A, *et al.* (2010). The combination of meropenem and levofloxacin is synergistic with respect to both Pseudomonas aeruginosa kill rate and resistance suppression. *Antimicrob Agents Chemother*, **54**, 2646–54.

Paul M, *et al.* (2010). Anti-pseudomonal beta-lactams for the initial, empirical, treatment febrile neutropenia: comparison of beta-lactams. *Cochrane Database Syst Rev*, **11**, CD005197.

Shuman EK, Chenoweth CE (2010). Recognition and prevention of healthcare-associated urinary tract infections in the intensive care unit. *Crit Care Med*, **38**, S373–9.

Wu DC, *et al.* (2011). Pseudomonas skin infection: clinical features, epidemiology, and management. *Am J Clin Dermatol*, **12**, 157–69.

6.8 Typhoid and paratyphoid fevers

C.M. Parry and Buddha Basnyat

Essentials

Typhoid and paratyphoid fever (the enteric fevers) are caused by specific serovars of the Gram-negative bacillus, *Salmonella enterica*. Sources of typhoid transmission are excreting chronic or convalescent carriers and the acutely infected, with transmission occuring through contamination by carriers of food or water by effluents containing infected urine or faeces. There are an estimated 27 million cases of enteric fever in the world each year, almost all in the developing world, with about 200 000 deaths.

Clinical features—the main symptom is fever (39–40° C); headache and malaise are common; constipation is a frequent early symptom, but most patients will experience diarrhoea; abdominal pain is usually diffuse and poorly localized. Physical examination is often unremarkable, apart from fever, but rose spots and relative bradycardia may be observed. In developing countries, patients may progress in the second to fourth week, with life-threatening manifestations including gastrointestinal bleeding, intestinal perforation, and the syndrome of mental confusion.

Diagnosis—the principal method for confirming the diagnosis is by isolating *Salmonella* Typhi or *Salmonella* Paratyphi from blood or bone marrow. The organisms may also be isolated from stool, urine, and bile aspirates, but such demonstration should be interpreted with caution in areas with many chronic carriers as the acute illness may be due to another cause.

Treatment—aside from supportive care, antibiotic therapy reduces mortality and complications and shortens the illness. Antibiotic resistance is a common and increasing problem, hence the choice of antibiotic should be informed by knowledge of likely local susceptibility. Fluoroquinolones are often given as first-line treatment, although low-level resistance to these agents (marked by nalidixic acid resistance) is widespread in Asia, with extended-spectrum cephalosporins and azithromycin as alternatives.

Acknowledgement: The authors acknowledge the contribution of Dr John Richens to previous editions of this chapter.

Prevention—typhoid has been eliminated from industrialized countries by (1) the provision of safe drinking water and safe disposal of sewage; (2) legal enforcement of high standards of food hygiene, and programmes to detect, monitor, and treat chronic carriers; and (3) prompt investigation and intervention when these safeguards are breached. Measures for individual protection are to (1) kill the organism in water by heating to 57° C, iodination, or chlorination; (2) take care with uncooked or reheated food; and (3) immunization—two typhoid vaccines are available and widely used in travellers, but their role as a public health tool in endemic areas is undefined; there is no paratyphoid vaccine.

Introduction

The organisms classically responsible for enteric fever are *Salmonella* Typhi and *Salmonella* Paratyphi A, B, and C. They commonly present as a prolonged febrile illness with a paucity of physical signs. The spectrum of disease varies from a mild self-limiting febrile illness to severe disease associated with gastrointestinal bleeding, intestinal perforation, or mental confusion with shock. In the 19th century typhoid fever was a leading cause of death in Europe and America. The disease today is predominantly found in developing countries.

Aetiology

The Gram-negative bacilli *Salmonella enterica* subspecies *enterica* serovar Typhi (*S.* Typhi) and *S.* Paratyphi A are the principal causative agents of enteric fever. Three antigens are important for identification: in Typhi the somatic oligosaccharide O antigen (9 and 12), the protein flagellar H-d antigen, and the polysaccharide envelope Vi antigen; in Paratyphi A the relevant O antigens are 1,2,12 and H antigens a:[1,5]. Antibiotic resistance is conferred by R plasmids, usually of the incompatibility group IncH-1 (chloramphenicol, amoxicillin, co-trimoxazole), and by mutations in the chromosomal *gyrA* gene (fluoroquinolones). The sequencing of isolates of *S.* Typhi and *S.* Paratyphi A is shedding light on the pathogenicity of these organisms. It is apparent that the genome of *S.* Typhi has a remarkable plasticity compared to other bacteria, with recombination of homologous rRNA operons as well as insertion of nonhomologous DNA.

Transmission

Sources of typhoid transmission are excreting chronic or convalescent carriers and the acutely infected. Transmission occurs through contamination by carriers of food or water by effluents containing infected urine or faeces. 'Typhoid Mary' was a faecal carrier and cook who infected 53 people early last century, while the Aberdeen outbreak in 1964 was traced to a leaking corned beef tin which had been cooled with faecally contaminated river water. Transmission of typhoid has also been attributed to flies, laboratory mishaps, unsterile instruments, and anal intercourse. Hornick demonstrated that 10^7 organisms of Quailes strain of *S.* Typhi given orally infected 50% of experimental subjects. Susceptibility is increased by medicines which decrease the gastric acidic environment or vagotomy. Infection may lead to acute disease, transient symptoms, or a symptomless carrier state.

Multiplication and dissemination

Bacteria are thought to pass from the gut through the cytoplasm of enterocytes and M cells overlying lymphoid tissue (Peyer's patches) of the small intestine to reach the lamina propria from which they are conveyed to the mesenteric nodes before reaching the blood stream via the thoracic duct. During a transient primary bacteraemia the organism is seeded to reticuloendothelial sites where intracellular multiplication occurs during a 7- to 14-day incubation period. A second bacteraemia follows, accompanied by symptoms as the infection spreads throughout liver, gallbladder, spleen, Peyer's patches, and bone marrow. Multiplication occurs mainly in macrophages. Concentrated sites of infection in reticuloendothelial tissues, known as typhoid nodules, are characterized by infiltrates of lymphocytes and macrophages. At postmortem examination, hypertrophy of lymphoid tissue is often visible within liver, spleen, mesenteric nodes, and Peyer's patches. Ulceration of Peyer's patches is seen where the inflammatory process has resulted in ischaemia and necrosis.

Endotoxin plays a central role in stimulating the release of cytokines, such as tumour necrosis factor and interleukin-6, from macrophages and neutrophils by activating the complement cascade and upregulating the adhesive capacity of neutrophils and endothelial cells. Unlike in meningitis and malaria, no clear correlation between levels of tumour necrosis factor and clinical outcome has been demonstrated in typhoid. The capacity of whole blood to produce proinflammatory cytokines following stimulation is reduced in patients with severe typhoid.

Immune response

There is a cell-mediated immune response lasting about 16 weeks, a mucosal immune response lasting for up to 48 weeks, and persistent circulating anti-O and anti-H agglutinins for up to 2 years. The predominance of clinical typhoid among children and young adults in endemic areas suggests a degree of acquired immunity. Only 25% of volunteers given a standard inoculum of *S.* Typhi 20 months after an initial infection developed clinical illness. Prolonged elevation of Vi antibody occurs in typhoid carriers. Immunodeficiency reduces the ability to clear salmonella infections.

Epidemiology

Worldwide, an estimated 27 million cases of enteric fever occur each year with about 200 000 deaths. In affluent countries, enteric fever is seen in returned travellers visiting friends and relatives abroad in areas of endemicity or when food or water safety measures fail. With appropriate antibiotic treatment, death is rare. In the Indian subcontinent, Central and South-East Asia, Indonesia, and sub-Saharan Africa, high rates of transmission are seen and annual incidence rates of 100 to 1600 cases per 100 000 population have been recorded. In these countries, transmission has been exacerbated by antibiotic resistance. Peaks of transmission occur in dry weather or at the onset of rains. Case fatality rates have exceeded 10% in some reports of hospitalized patients in Indonesia and Papua New Guinea. *S.* Paratyphi was previously thought to cause less severe disease that *S.* Typhi; a recent study of 609 cases of bacteraemic enteric fever in Nepal (409 with *S.* Typhi and 200 with *S.* Paratyphi) found that the clinical syndromes were indistinguishable and of similar severity.

Prevention

The elimination of typhoid from industrialized countries can be attributed to the provision of safe drinking water, safe disposal of sewage, legal enforcement of high standards of food hygiene, programmes to detect, monitor, and treat chronic carriers, and prompt investigation and intervention when these safeguards are breached. Outbreaks can be investigated using phage typing of isolates, pulsed-field gel electrophoresis and other molecular typing methods, registers of known carriers, and sewer swabs used to trace isolates back to their source.

Measures for individual protection are to kill the organism in water by heating to 57°C, iodination, or chlorination, care with uncooked or reheated food, and immunization. Patients and convalescents with typhoid should be advised to wash their hands after using the toilet and before preparing food and to use separate towels. Western travellers visiting friends and relatives in areas of endemicity are vulnerable to acquiring enteric fever; therefore counselling needs to be targeted on this group. The approach of travel medicine, which has evolved around the tourist industry, will miss this susceptible group.

Clinical features

Enteric fever is predominantly an infection of infants, children, and young adults, affecting both sexes equally. The incubation period ranges from 3 to 60 days, but most infections occur 7 to 14 days after exposure. The main focus of typhoid is in the small bowel, but systemic symptoms often overshadow abdominal symptoms. The predominant symptom is the fever which rises gradually to a high plateau of 39 to 40°C, and shows little diurnal variation. Rigors are uncommon, except in late or complicated typhoid or in patients treated with antipyretics. Patients usually complain of headache and malaise, and constipation is a frequent early symptom. Most patients will experience diarrhoea, and typhoid can present as an acute gastroenteritis and occasionally bloody diarrhoea. Severe diarrhoea or colitis has been reported in HIV-infected patients. The abdominal pain is usually diffuse and poorly localized but occasionally sufficiently intense in the right iliac fossa to suggest appendicitis. Nausea and vomiting are infrequent in uncomplicated typhoid but are seen with abdominal distension in severe cases. Other early symptoms include cough, sore throat, and epistaxes. In developing countries, patients with typhoid in its second to fourth week present with accelerating weight loss, weakness, altered mental state, intestinal haemorrhage and perforation, refractory hypotension, pneumonia, nephritis, and acute psychosis. Those infected with multidrug-resistant infections may have more severe disease.

Physical examination is often unremarkable apart from fever. A coated tongue is often observed. Rose spots appear at the end of the first week and form a sparse collection of maculopapular lesions on the abdominal skin, which blanch with pressure and fade after 2 or 3 days (Fig. 6.8.1). Osler found them in 90% of white-skinned patients and 20% of patients with black skin. The rash may extend on to the trunk and arms. Melanesian typhoid patients develop purpuric macules that do not blanch (Fig. 6.8.2). Petechiae are sometimes visible on the conjunctivae (Fig. 6.8.3) Tachycardia is common although temperature–pulse dissociation (relative bradycardia) is considered characteristic. Hypotension has

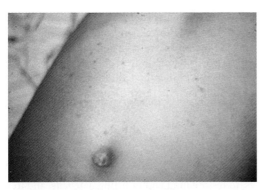

Fig. 6.8.1 Rose spots on the abdomen in typhoid fever.

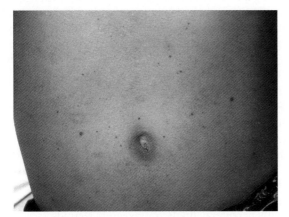

Fig. 6.8.2 Typhoid rash in a Melanesian child: sparse purpuric (nonblanching) macules.
(Copyright D A Warrell.)

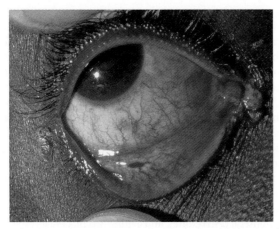

Fig. 6.8.3 Conjunctival petechial haemorrhage in an African child with typhoid.
(Copyright D A Warrell.)

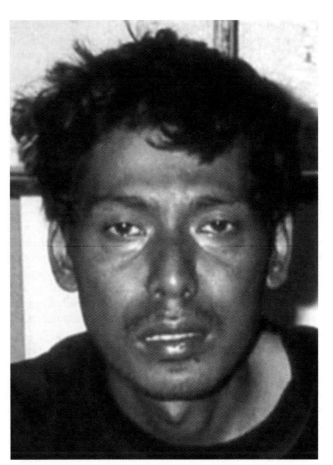

Fig. 6.8.4 Typhoid facies: a man with the apathetic expression seen in severe typhoid.

important implications (see below 'Severe typhoid'). Adventitious lung sounds, especially scattered wheezes, are common and may suggest pneumonia. These findings with a normal chest radiograph and high fever should prompt consideration of typhoid. Abdominal examination may reveal the typhoid rash, distension, or a diffuse tenderness, occasionally localized to the area of the terminal ileum. Intra-abdominal inflammation sometimes provokes retention of urine. A moderate soft tender hepatosplenomegaly eventually develops in most patients but it less likely to be found early.

Patients with advanced illness may display the 'typhoid' facies (Fig. 6.8.4), a thin flushed face with a staring apathetic expression. Mental apathy may progress to an agitated delirium, frequently accompanied by tremor of the hands, tremulous speech, and ataxic gait. If the patient's condition deteriorates further the features described in the writings of Louis and Osler make their appearance—muttering delirium, twitchings of the fingers and wrists (subsultus tendinum), agitated plucking at the bedclothes (carphology/carphologia), and a staring unrousable stupor (coma vigil).

Typhoid in children

Community-based studies in highly endemic areas have shown that enteric fever is more common in children less than 5 years old than was once appreciated. The main differences, compared to adults, are a greater frequency of diarrhoea and vomiting, jaundice, febrile convulsions, nephritis, or typhoid meningitis. Relative bradycardia is of greater diagnostic significance for typhoid in febrile children. In some reports case fatality rates are high in the under-fives. The disease can also take a milder course in very young children, behaving like a mild respiratory illness that is not clinically recognized as enteric fever. Typhoid may also occasionally develop in neonates born to infected mothers.

Differential diagnosis

Many viral, bacterial, and protozoal infections as well as noninfectious conditions characterized by fever, including lymphoproliferative disorders and vasculitides, resemble enteric fever. Typhoid should always be considered when suspected malaria has not been confirmed or has not responded to antimalarial therapy. In areas of endemicity, typhus, leptospirosis, and dengue should be considered in the differential diagnosis.

Diagnosis

Culture

The definitive diagnosis of enteric fever rests on the isolation of *S*. Typhi or *S*. Paratyphi from blood, bone marrow, cerebrospinal fluid, and rose spots. In mild typhoid, the number of bacteria in blood may be as low as 1 colony-forming unit/ml. The median number of bacteria in the blood of children is higher than adults and declines with increasing duration of illness. Successful culture from blood can be achieved in up to 80% of patients but depends on taking a generous volume of blood and using the correct volume of blood to broth (1:10). Bone marrow gives the highest yield, including those exposed to antibiotics, but yields only marginally more than blood. Rose spots, when present, can give a positive culture in 70% of patients.

The organisms may also be isolated from stool, urine, and bile aspirates. The number of organisms recoverable from faeces increases through the illness. The results should be interpreted with caution in areas with many carriers, as the acute illness may be due to another cause in chronic carriers. Isolation from urine is more common in areas endemic for schistosomiasis. Culture of bile obtained from an overnight duodenal string capsule gives a similar yield to blood and offers additional means to isolate *S*. Typhi and *S*. Paratyphi from children or from carriers.

Serology

The use of a tube or slide agglutination test (the Widal test) to diagnose typhoid is cheaper and simpler than culture but fraught with pitfalls. The demonstration of a fourfold rise in titre of antibodies to *S*. Typhi or *S*. Paratyphi antigens suggests enteric fever but is too delayed to help clinical decision-making and is not observed in all patients. Single measurements of antibody titres have been found useful in populations where accurate up-to-date information about the predictive value of the test at specific cut-off points is available. False-positive serological tests are obtained from persons with previous infection, infection with cross-reacting organisms, or following vaccination.

Other tests for typhoid

Many other tests for the detection of antibodies, antigens, and salmonella DNA in body fluids have been described. Few have so far been adopted for routine use. Newer serological assays using enzyme-linked immunosorbent assay (ELISA) and lateral flow (dipstick) devices perform somewhat better, but sensitivity and specificity are not adequate for routine diagnostic use. An ELISA for antibodies to the Vi antigen is useful for detecting carriers.

Other laboratory findings in typhoid

A mild normochromic anaemia, mild thrombocytopenia, and an increased erythrocyte sedimentation rate are common. Most patients have a total white cell count within the normal range. Leucocytosis suggests either perforation or another diagnosis.

Laboratory evidence of mild disseminated intravascular coagulation is common but rarely of clinical significance. Common biochemical findings include hyponatraemia, hypokalaemia, and elevation of liver enzymes, which may mimic acute viral hepatitis. The urine often contains some protein and white cells. Examination of the cerebrospinal fluid may be normal or show a mild pleocytosis (<35 cells/mm^3) in patients with central nervous system symptoms.

Treatment

The aims of management are to eliminate the infection swiftly with antibiotics, to restore fluid and nutritional deficits, and to monitor the patient for dangerous complications. In many parts of the world antibiotic treatment for typhoid fever is started empirically based on the syndrome of fever of 3 or 4 days and constitutional symptoms with no known source of infection and a negative malaria smear. Because there are no reliable clinical predictors, in areas of endemicity concurrent treatment with doxycycline to cover for typhus and leptospirosis may be considered.

Supportive care

Cooling is preferred to antipyretics for relief of fever, and simple analgesics may be used to relieve headache. Most patients can eat and drink normally; special diets do not protect the bowel from perforation. Daily assessment of the patient's mental and circulatory status is required plus examination of the abdomen for signs of impending perforation. Severely ill patients require intensive care with parenteral fluids, intravenous steroids (see below), inotropic support, and sedation.

Antibiotics

Effective antibiotic therapy in typhoid reduces mortality and complications and shortens the illness (see Table 6.8.1 for doses). Chloramphenicol was the first antibiotic found to be effective and the standard against which subsequent antibiotics have been measured. Symptom resolution occurs over a period of 4 to 6 days although the antimicrobial should be given for at least 2 weeks to prevent relapse. Ampicillin, amoxicillin, and co-trimoxazole have been shown to have comparable efficacy to chloramphenicol while having less toxicity; they must also be given for at least 2 weeks. In many areas these drugs are no longer used because of the spread of multidrug-resistant (MDR) strains of *S*. Typhi and *S*. Paratyphi A. Alternative antibiotics active against MDR infections include the fluoroquinolones, although resistance has in turn emerged to these agents, the extended-spectrum cephalosporins (e.g. parenteral ceftriaxone), and azithromycin.

In recent years many physicians have given a fluoroquinolone, ciprofloxacin or ofloxacin, as first-line therapy. Treatment can be completed in a week or less with minimal toxicity. In controlled trials in endemic areas, infections with fully susceptible isolates have resulted in a rapid resolution of symptoms with high cure rates and low relapse and faecal carriage rates. Response rates in endemic areas may be better than those of nonimmune travellers. There have been questions about the safety of fluoroquinolones in children and during pregnancy. Careful follow-up studies of children in Asia following fluoroquinolone therapy have shown no toxicity and there has been a growing consensus that the advantages of therapy outweigh the potential dangers.

Table 6.8.1 Guidelines for the antibiotic treatment of enteric fever

Antibiotic	Daily dose	Route[a]	Doses/day	Duration in nonsevere enteric fever (days)	Duration in severe enteric fever[b]
Acute infection					
Chloramphenicol[c]	50–100 mg/kg	O/IM/IV[d]	4	14	14–21
Co-trimoxazole[e]	Trimethoprim 6.5–10 mg/kg	O/IM/IV	2–3	14	14
	Sulfamethoxazole 40 mg/kg				
Amoxicillin	75–100 mg/kg	O/IM/IV	3	14	14
Ceftriaxone	50–60 mg/kg	IM/IV	2	7–14	14
Cefixime	20 mg/kg	O	2	7–14	
Ciprofloxacin[f]	20–25 mg/kg	O/IV	2	7–14	14
Ofloxacin[f]	15–20 mg/kg	O/IV	2	7–14	
Pefloxacin[f]	800 mg	O/IV	2	7–14	
Fleroxacin[f]	400 mg	O/IV	1	7–14	
Gatifloxacin	10 mg/kg	O	1	7	
Azithromycin	10–20 mg/kg	O	1	7	
Treatment of carriers					
Ampicillin or amoxicillin with probenecid	100 mg/kg	O	3–4	90[g]	
	30 mg/kg				
Co-trimoxazole	6.5–10 mg trimethoprim	O	2	90	
Ciprofloxacin	1500 mg	O	2	28	

O, oral; IM, intramuscular; IV, intravenous.

[a] Oral therapy is satisfactory for most patients. Parenteral therapy is generally reserved for severely ill patients.

[b] In intestinal perforation, the antibiotic therapy should also cover other aerobic and anaerobic gastrointestinal bacteria contaminating the peritoneum. In severe typhoid (characterized by delirium, obtundation, coma, or shock) dexamethasone is beneficial (see text).

[c] May cause bone marrow suppression.

[d] The oral route is preferred; there are reports of lower blood levels of chloramphenicol in patients given parenteral therapy.

[e] May cause allergic reactions and nephrotoxicity. Not suitable for children younger than 2 years or during pregnancy.

[f] Infection with isolates that have low-level fluoroquinolone resistance (nalidixic acid resistance) may not respond.

[g] The duration of treatment can be shortened if parenteral therapy is given, e.g. 8-hourly intravenous ampicillin for 2 weeks.

Unfortunately strains of *S.* Typhi and *S.* Paratyphi A with low-level resistance to the commonly used fluoroquinolones (ciprofloxacin and ofloxacin) have become common in Asia and have sporadically been reported in sub-Saharan Africa. These strains are not detected by current ciprofloxacin disc susceptibility breakpoints but are usually nalidixic acid resistant and this has proved to be a useful, although not a completely sensitive, laboratory marker. Where possible fluoroquinolones should be avoided in patients infected with these strains. They should be treated with extended-spectrum cephalosporins (ceftriaxone) or, in nonsevere cases, with azithromycin. If fluoroquinolones are the only available option they should be used at the maximum dose. Recent data from Vietnam and Nepal suggest that the new fluoroquinolone gatifloxacin is effective in these infections. Cefixime, an oral third-generation cephalosporin, is another alternative although there have been concerns about its efficacy in some studies. Some areas in the Indian subcontinent now report fully fluoroquinolone-resistant isolates but also an increase in isolates that have regained susceptibility to the old first-line drugs, chloramphenicol, ampicillin, and co-trimoxazole, and in such circumstances these older drugs are appropriate. Some antibiotics such as gentamicin appear sensitive *in vitro* but are ineffective *in vivo* and should not be used in enteric fever.

Ampicillin, amoxicillin, or ceftriaxone are considered safe in pregnancy with enteric fever. There are limited data on the management of immunocompromised patients with enteric fever, but data from patients with nontyphoidal salmonella infections suggest that they may need extended treatment to prevent relapse.

Complications

Box 6.8.1 lists the complications of typhoid. Most are rare and only likely to be encountered in patients who present with untreated disease lasting 2 weeks or more. Occasionally, a complication dominates the clinical picture and deflects attention from the underlying diagnosis of typhoid.

Severe typhoid

Studies from Indonesia and Papua New Guinea have revealed an important subgroup of patients with mental confusion or shock (defined as a systolic blood pressure of less than 90 mmHg in adults or less than 80 mmHg in children), with evidence of decreased skin, cerebral, or renal perfusion, who have a 50% fatality rate and account for most typhoid deaths. In one study in Jakarta, high doses of dexamethasone substantially reduced the mortality of such severe cases. The criteria for severe typhoid were marked mental confusion or shock. In adults treated with chloramphenicol, 3 mg/kg dexamethasone infused intravenously over 30 min, followed by eight doses of 1 mg/kg every 6 h, resulted in a 10% case fatality rate compared to 55.6% in controls. It has proved almost impossible to duplicate this study because the number of severe

Box 6.8.1 Complications of typhoid

Abdominal

- Intestinal perforation
- Intestinal haemorrhage
- Hepatitis
- Cholecystitis (usually subclinical)
- Spontaneous splenic rupture
- Rupture and haemorrhage from mesenteric nodes
- Pancreatitis

Genitourinary

- Retention of urine
- Glomerulonephritis
- Pyelonephritis
- Cystitis
- Orchitis

Cardiovascular

- Asymptomatic ECG changes
- Myocarditis
- Pericarditis
- Endocarditis
- Phlebitis and arteritis
- Deep venous thrombosis
- Gangrene
- Shock
- Sudden death

Respiratory

- Bronchitis
- Laryngeal ulceration
- Glottal oedema
- Pneumonia (*S.* Typhi, *Streptococcus pneumoniae*)

Neuropsychiatric

- Delirium

- Psychotic states
- Depression
- Deafness
- Meningitis
- Encephalomyelitis
- Transverse myelitis
- Signs of upper motor neuron lesions
- Signs of extrapyramidal disorder
- Impairment of coordination
- Optic neuritis
- Peripheral and cranial neuropathy
- Guillain–Barré syndrome
- Pseudotumour cerebri

Haematological

- Disseminated intravascular coagulation (usually subclinical)
- Anaemia
- Haemolysis
- Haemolytic uraemic syndrome

Focal infections

- Abscesses of brain, liver, spleen, breast, thyroid, muscles, lymph nodes
- Parotitis
- Pharyngitis
- Osteitis, especially tibia, ribs, spine
- Arthritis

Other

- Myopathy
- Hypercalcaemia
- Decubitus ulceration
- Abortion
- Relapse

typhoid patients has decreased, probably because of the ready availability of over-the-counter antibiotics.

Intestinal haemorrhage and perforation

Perforation of ileal ulcers occurs in less than 5% of typhoid patients (Fig. 6.8.5). The development of acute abdominal signs is often gradual, making diagnosis difficult. Severely ill patients display only restlessness, hypotension, and tachycardia. A chest radiograph may show free gas under the diaphragm. Ultrasonography is useful for demonstrating and aspirating faeculent fluid in the peritoneal cavity. Management includes nasogastric suction, administration of fluids to correct hypotension, and prompt surgery. Simple closure of perforations is adequate but experienced surgeons use procedures to bypass the worst-affected sections of the ileum in order to reduce postoperative morbidity. Closure of perforations should be accompanied by vigorous peritoneal toilet. Metronidazole or clindamycin should be added to the therapy of ceftriaxone or fluoroquinolone-treated patients. Metronidazole and aminoglycosides are recommended for patients receiving chloramphenicol, ampicillin, or co-trimoxazole. The survival of

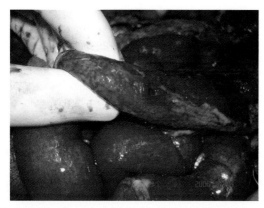

Fig. 6.8.5 Typhoid perforation of the distal ileum at operation.

patients undergoing surgery for perforation is generally 70 to 75%, but reaches 97% in the best series. This compares with survival rates of around 30% in conservatively managed patients.

Evidence for silent gastrointestinal bleeding may be sudden collapse of a patient or a steadily falling haematocrit. Most bleeding episodes are self-limiting. Severe bleeding is sometimes seen in advanced typhoid but is rarely fatal. A few require transfusion. In exceptional circumstances surgery or intra-arterial vasopressin have been used to halt haemorrhage.

Relapse

Relapse in typhoid is a second episode of fever, usually milder than the first, occurring a week or two after recovery from the first episode. Isolates from relapsing patients usually have identical antibiotic susceptibility to those identified during the first episode. Relapse rates of 10% have been described in untreated typhoid and chloramphenicol-treated patients. Relapse is managed with a similar or abbreviated course of the same therapy used in the initial episode. Reinfection may also occur but can only be distinguished by differences in the sensitivity pattern or molecular typing of isolates.

Carriers

Many patients excrete S. Typhi or S. Paratyphi in their stools or urine for some days after starting antibiotic treatment. Convalescent carriers excrete for periods of up to 3 months. Patients still excreting at 3 months are unlikely to cease and at 1 year meet the formal definition of 'chronic carrier'. Among carriers detected by screening, 25% give no history of acute typhoid. Faecal carriage is more frequent in individuals with gallbladder disease and is most common in women over 40; in the Far East there is an association with opisthorchiasis. Urinary carriage is associated with schistosomiasis and nephrolithiasis. Acute typhoid in carriers has been reported. There is an increased risk of carcinoma of the gallbladder.

Patients discharged after treatment for typhoid with six negative stool and three negative urine specimens and negative Vi serology are considered free of infection. Most patients with positive stools at the completion of treatment excrete temporarily and can be safely followed up. Antibiotic eradication of carriage is advised in those still excreting at 3 months, or earlier in those at particular risk of communicating infection to others. The patient with a persistently elevated or rising Vi antibody titre is likely to be a carrier. Repeated checks of urine and faeces should be made and consideration given to obtaining bile cultures if these are negative.

Eradication of carriage requires prolonged, high-dose antibiotics (Table 6.8.1). Ampicillin, amoxicillin, and co-trimoxazole have been used with some success. More recently, good results have been reported with fluoroquinolones. Cholecystectomy and nephrectomy, once used to eliminate carriage (and not without operative mortality), are hard to justify on public health grounds alone, but can be considered if antibiotic methods fail and there are additional indications for operation. The success rates of surgery are increased by giving antibiotics as well.

Vaccines

The greatest need for typhoid vaccination is among infants, children, and young adults in endemic areas, especially where antibiotic resistance is increasing, and among laboratory workers handling the organisms. In practice, vaccines are given mostly to travellers to endemic areas. The most currently available vaccines are the parenteral Vi vaccine, given as a single injection, and the live attenuated Ty21a vaccine, given as three or four oral doses. The Ty21a vaccine should not be given to immunosuppressed persons or those taking mefloquine or antibiotics. Current typhoid vaccines do not protect against paratyphoid infection and the protection afforded by vaccination can be overcome by large inocula of bacteria. Efficacy figures derive largely from trials conducted in partly immune populations and overestimate the benefit in persons without prior exposure.

The risks of typhoid among travellers are low (3 to 30 cases per 100 000) and the precise efficacy of currently recommended doses in previously unexposed adults remains unknown. However, circumstantial evidence indicates typhoid vaccine affords protection to travellers visiting endemic areas. Travellers without the vaccine seem more susceptible to the disease, and this is true for even short-term (less than 1 week) travellers to endemic areas. Several new vaccines are currently being developed or evaluated, notably a Vi conjugate vaccine and single-dose oral vaccines.

Paratyphoid fever

Paratyphoid A occurs chiefly in Asia and Africa, Paratyphoid B worldwide, and paratyphoid C in Asia and the Middle East. Paratyphoid A has recently been increasing in South Asia, including drug-resistant disease. Outbreaks of paratyphoid are more often food-borne than water-borne, probably because larger inocula are needed to establish infection. Paratyphoid has a shorter incubation period (4–5 days). Recent reports suggest that the clinical syndromes caused by Typhi and Paratyphi A are indistinguishable, in particular that Paratyphi A may be as severe as Typhi. The management of paratyphoid is the same as that of typhoid.

Areas of uncertainty and controversy

The recommendation for first-line antibiotic therapy in endemic areas has been debated. Many practitioners have used fluoroquinolones for first-line therapy where multidrug resistance is common. The emergence of low-level resistance to fluoroquinolones has bought that approach into question. The laboratory detection of such isolates has proved problematic. Although nalidixic acid resistance is a useful laboratory marker of low-level resistance, it is not completely reliable and new fluoroquinolone breakpoints are needed.

The optimum treatment for such infections is also undefined. The extended-spectrum cephalosporins, such as ceftriaxone, and azithromycin are available options and new fluoroquinolones, such as gatifloxacin, may be effective. In some areas isolates have regained sensitivity to first-line agents and chloramphenicol is being used. Whether isolates with full fluoroquinolone and extended-spectrum cephalosporin resistance become common in the next decade remains to be seen.

A second area of controversy is the use of vaccination as a public health tool in endemic areas. The emergence of multidrug resistance may swing the cost–benefit ratio in favour of vaccination. Several Vi vaccine demonstration trials are in progress to evaluate the cost-effectiveness of vaccination and these projects should provide an evidence base to inform policy. The realization that typhoid is common in children under 5 years has also focused attention on the development of vaccines appropriate for this age group. A Vi conjugate vaccine and single-dose oral vaccine are likely to become available in the near future.

Further reading

Basnyat B, *et al.* (2005). Enteric fever (typhoid) fever in travellers. *Clin Infect Dis*, **41**, 1467–72. [A recent review of issues relating to travellers.]

Bhan MK, Bahl R, Bhatnager S (2005). Typhoid and paratyphoid fever. *Lancet*, **366**, 749–62. [A useful, recent, and general review.]

Butler T, *et al.* (1985). Typhoid fever complicated by intestinal perforation: a persisting fatal disease requiring surgical management. *Rev Infect Dis*, **7**, 244–56.

Christie AB (1987). Typhoid and paratyphoid fevers. In: Christie AB (ed) *Infectious diseases: epidemiology and clinical practice*, 4th edition, vol. 1, pp. 100–64. Churchill Livingstone, Edinburgh. [An outstanding, detailed, and generously referenced monograph on typhoid.]

Forsyth JRL (1998). Typhoid and paratyphoid. In: Smith GR, Easmon CSF (eds) *Topley and Wilson's principles of bacteriology, virology and immunity*, 9th edition, vol. 3, pp. 459–78. Arnold, London. [A useful chapter covering microbiological aspects of typhoid in depth.]

Hoffman SL, *et al.* (1984). Reduction of mortality in chloramphenicol-treated severe typhoid fever by high-dose dexamethasone. *N Engl J Med*, **310**, 82–8.

Sanger Institute. *Bacterial genomes*. www.sanger.uk/Projects/Microbes [Information concerning the S. enterica ser. Typhi genome sequence.]

6.9 Intracellular klebsiella infections (donovanosis and rhinoscleroma)

J. Richens

Essentials

Two rare intracellular species of *Klebsiella*, a Gram-negative bacillus, cause granulomatous disease in humans that is found in small endemic foci in warm climates, linked to poverty and poor hygiene.

Donovanosis—caused by *Klebsiella granulomatis* (until recently named *Calymmatobacterium granulomatis*); presumed to be sexually transmitted; presents with genital ulcers or growths, often accompanied by an inguinal 'pseudobubo' (granuloma inguinale). Diagnosed by demonstrating Donovan bodies (vacuoles containing capsulated coccoid bacteria) lying within histiocytes in material taken from a typical lesion. Treatment is with azithromycin; surgery may be needed for complications.

Rhinoscleroma—caused by *Klebsiella rhinoscleromatis*; transmission believed to occur from person to person; following a period of rhinitis most typically manifests with bulky growths in the upper respiratory tract. Diagnosed by demonstrating intracellular organisms in typical lesions, combined with culture. Treatment is with ciprofloxacin; surgical debulking of lesions and/or reconstruction may be required.

Donovanosis

Introduction

Donovanosis was first described in Calcutta by Donovan in 1905. It is a sexually transmitted infection best known in Papua New Guinea, India, southern Africa, and Brazil. An important focus among Australian aborigines has recently been eliminated. Donovanosis seems to be retreating, raising hopes of eventual eradication. Dark-skinned people appear to have greater susceptibility. The predilection of lesions for the anogenital region of sexually active adults and the frequent association with other sexually transmitted infections point strongly to sexual transmission. In the past, epidemics of donovanosis in New Guinea were linked to ritual homosexual and heterosexual practices. Perinatal transmission has been observed in a few cases.

Aetiology

An unusual Gram-negative bacillus can be isolated in HEp-2 cells or human peripheral blood mononuclear cells from patients with the characteristic lesions of donovanosis. This organism will not grow on conventional solid media. Previously named *Donovania* and subsequently *Calymmatobacterium* by Aragão and Vianna in 1913, it has now been classed as *Klebsiella granulomatis* on the basis of close DNA homology with other *Klebsiella* species. *K. granulomatis* shows morphological identity with Donovan bodies observed within clinical lesions of donovanosis and patients with characteristic lesions have high levels of antibody that react equally with Donovan bodies and with *K. granulomatis*. *K. granulomatis* is pathogenic only to humans. Experimental transmission has been reported with lesion material, but to date not with a pure culture of this organism. Donovanosis shows a close macroscopic and microscopic similarity to rhinoscleroma which produces granulomatous lesions of the upper airways. These lesions contain intracellular clusters of the closely related organism *Klebsiella rhinoscleromatis*.

Pathogenesis

The organism has a special tropism for dermal macrophages. The response to infection is characterized by vigorous granulomatous inflammation that damages the skin and subcutaneous tissues. Extension of the infection is a local process of spreading ulceration.

The inguinal lesions are probably seeded by lymphatic spread. Haematogenous dissemination and spread to the upper genital tract of women are exceptional. Lesions in women tend to be more extensive and may progress rapidly during pregnancy.

Clinical features

After an incubation period of 3 to 40 days, the disease usually starts with a small genital lesion. A nonspecific papule evolves into a painless ulcer displaying a deep red colour, contact bleeding, and a rolled edge. Hypertrophic lesions that pout outwards from the surrounding skin are frequent. Local lymphoedema is seen commonly in women. Chronic lesions tend to expand gradually along skin folds forming a large continuous area of ulceration with a characteristic serpiginous outline (Fig. 6.9.1). Inguinal lesions are common (Fig. 6.9.2). They start as a firm, subcutaneous swellings and often ulcerate. The term 'pseudobubo' tends to be applied to any inguinal lesion in donovanosis although it was originally coined to describe a subcutaneous inguinal abscess, which is a rare event. Such lesions have even given rise to suspicion of bubonic plague when Donovan bodies in the aspirate were misinterpreted. Primary lesions of the cervix simulate carcinoma of the cervix. Upper genital tract involvement in women may simulate pelvic inflammatory disease or malignancy and hydronephrosis may ensue. Anal lesions in have been described in homosexual men. Involvement of the rectum seldom occurs.

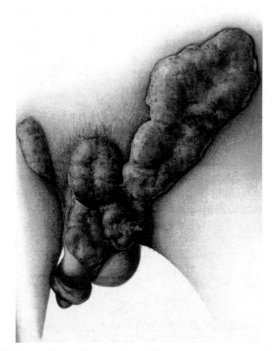

Fig. 6.9.2 Inguinal lesion: from Aragão and Vianna's paper on the value of trivalent antimony in treating donovanosis.
(From Aragão H, Vianna G (1913). Resquizas sobre o *Granuloma venereo. Mem Inst Oswaldo Cruz*, **5**, 211–38.)

Oral lesions of donovanosis with extension to cervical nodes have been described. Haematogenous dissemination is associated with pregnancy and causes lesions of bone, liver, and spleen. Lesions in infants tend to involve the ears and nearby lymph nodes.

Complications of donovanosis include extensive scar formation, lymphoedema of the genitalia, penile autoamputation, and the development of squamous carcinoma in active or healed lesions. Secondary infection with fusospirochaetal organisms can cause rapid, extensive, and sometimes fatal tissue destruction.

Diagnosis

Klebsiella granulomatis is difficult to culture and the diagnosis is made by demonstrating Donovan bodies lying within histiocytes in material taken from a typical lesion. Donovan bodies show well with Giemsa's, Leishman's, and Wright's stains but poorly with haematoxylin and eosin. Histology typically shows a heavy plasma cell infiltrate and epithelial hyperplasia in addition to histiocytes containing Donovan bodies (Fig. 6.9.3). Common misdiagnoses are squamous carcinoma of cervix, vulva, or penis, secondary syphilis, and conditions that produce genital lymphoedema such as filariasis and lymphogranuloma venereum. Molecular diagnostic tests for the detection of *K. granulomatis* DNA have been developed but are not validated or approved for diagnostic use by the United States Food and Drug Authority (FDA).

Treatment

In 1913, Aragão and Vianna described the value of trivalent antimony in treating donovanosis (Fig. 6.9.2). The European guidelines (2010) recommend treatment with azithromycin 1 g weekly until complete healing of lesions. The United States CDC (2010) guidelines recommend doxycycline 100 mg twice daily for at least

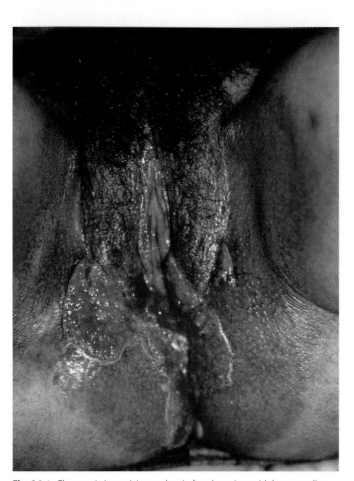

Fig. 6.9.1 Characteristic serpiginous ulcer in female patient with long-standing donovanosis.

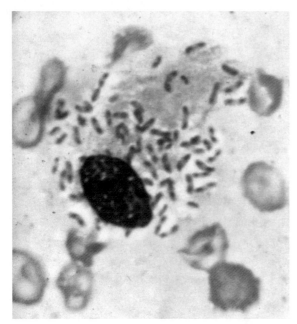

Fig. 6.9.3 Donovan bodies: Giemsa-stained smear from donovanosis lesion demonstrating the characteristic 'closed safety pin' appearance of encapsulated organisms within a large histiocyte.

3 weeks or until lesions have healed. Alternative regimens include azithromycin (1 g weekly) or ciprofloxacin (750 mg twice daily) or erythromycin (500 mg four times daily) or co-trimoxazole (960 mg twice daily). The addition of an aminoglycoside (e.g. gentamicin 1 mg/kg) may be considered if there is no improvement within a few days of treatment. Erythromycin is safe and gives good results in pregnant women. Women in labour found to have untreated lesions of the cervix should be delivered by caesarean section to reduce known risks of haematogenous dissemination and transmission to the neonate. A week of prophylactic treatment may be offered to healthy contacts to abort incubating infections. Patients with genital deformity may benefit from plastic surgical procedures.

Rhinoscleroma

Introduction and aetiology

Rhinoscleroma or scleroma is characterized by inflammatory growths of the upper airways. Endemic foci have been described in Africa (especially Egypt and Uganda), Siberia, Turkestan, the Middle East, the Indian subcontinent, China, the Philippines, Indonesia, and Papua New Guinea. There are many foci in South and Central America where it has been identified in terracotta Maya heads of AD 300 to 600. The disease has retreated in Eastern and Central Europe where it was first described by Hebra and Kaposi in 1870. The histological features were first described by Johann von Mickulich in 1877 and the causative organism was identified by von Frisch in 1882. The term 'scleroma respiratorium' was proposed by Belinov in 1832.

Klebsiella rhinoscleromatis can be isolated from about 60% of patients.

Pathogenesis

Transmission is believed to occur from person to person in endemic areas. Initially patients infected with this organism may complain

of an exudative rhinitis. An atrophic rhinitis may follow. The most characteristic phase of the disease is the nodular stage during which a granulomatous reaction to the organisms within macrophages leads to the development of bulky masses within any part of the respiratory tract from nares to tracheal bifurcation. The process can extend into and destroy neighbouring soft tissues, cartilage, bone, and skin. Fibrosis and strictures are seen in the final stage. Patients with rhinoscelroma appear to have impaired cellular immunity with a decrease in the CD4+ T-lymphocyte count. A Mexican study has shown that the HLA DQA1*03011-DQB1*0301 haplotype is associated with the development of rhinoscleroma.

Clinical features

Rhinoscleroma runs a slow fluctuating course over several years, progressing through exudative, atrophic, nodular, and fibrotic stages. Systemic symptoms are not seen. The usual presentations are with nasal obstruction and bleeding and nasal deformity (splaying of the lower nose, often with a visible growth extending down to the upper lip, known as Hebra nose) (Fig. 6.9.4). Some patients present with ozaena, which is an atrophic rhinitis accompanied by

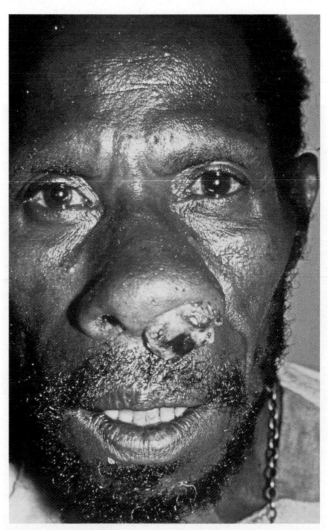

Fig. 6.9.4 Rhinoscleroma with characteristic nasal splaying (Hebra nose) and obstruction of the left nostril in a 30-year-old man from Papua New Guinea.
(From Cooke R (1987). *Colour atlas of anatomical pathology*, p. 31. Churchill Livingstone, Edinburgh, with permission.)

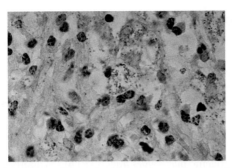

Fig. 6.9.5 Rhinoscleroma. Silver-stained preparation showing bacteria. (Copyright J Richens.)

a foul smell and formation of crusts within the nose. Patients with tracheal involvement may present with stridor. With the help of sinus endoscopy and newer imaging techniques it is not unusual to find evidence of spread into the sinuses, orbits, cranial cavity, middle ear, and regional lymph nodes.

Diagnosis

Histology shows a dense infiltrate of plasma cells among which are seen large foamy histiocytes (Mikulicz cells) containing Gram-negative bacteria and Russell bodies which are thought to be effete plasma cells (Fig. 6.9.5). The diagnosis is usually made by demonstrating intracellular organisms in Giemsa-stained or silver-stained sections taken from typical lesions, combined with culture for *K. rhinoscleromatis*. Culture is only positive in 50 to 60% of cases. CT scanning and endoscopic techniques provide useful ways to define the extent of the disease.

Treatment

Treatment with ciprofloxacin 250 mg twice daily for 4 weeks appears to be substantially superior to previously used antibiotic regimens (rifampicin, streptomycin, tetracyclines, ampicillin, and co-trimoxazole). Debulking operations may be needed for obstructing nasal and tracheal disease, and tracheostomy may be required as a temporary measure. Reconstructive surgery may be needed to deal with late fibrotic stenosis.

Further reading

Borgstein J, Sada E, Cortes R (1993). Ciprofloxacin for rhinoscleroma and ozena. *Lancet*, **342**, 122.

Bowden FJ, *et al.* (1996). Pilot study of azithromycin in the treatment of genital donovanosis. *Genitourin Med*, **72**, 17–19.

Canalis RF, Zamboni L (2001). An interpretation of the structural changes responsible for the chronicity of rhinoscleroma. *Laryngoscope*, **111**, 1020–6.

Carter JS, *et al.* (1999). Phylogenetic evidence for reclassification of *Calymmatobacterium granulomatis* as *Klebsiella granulomatis* comb. nov. *Int J Syst Bacteriol*, **49**, 1695–1700.

Centers for Disease Control and Prevention (2010). Sexually transmitted diseases treatment guidelines. *MMWR*, **59** (No. RR-12), 1–109.

Mackay IM, *et al.* (2006). Detection and discrimination of herpes simplex viruses, *Haemophilus ducreyi*, *Treponema pallidum*, and *Calymmabacterium (Klebsiella)* granulomatosis from genital ulcers. *Clin Infect Dis*, **42**, 1431–8.

O'Farrell N (2002). Donovanosis. *Sex Trans Infect*, **78**, 452–7.

O'Farrell N, Moi H; IUSTI/WHO European STD guidelines Editorial Board. (2010). European guideline for the management of donovanosis, 2010. *Int J STD AIDS*, **21**, 609–10.

Richens J (1991). The diagnosis and treatment of donovanosis (granuloma inguinale). *Sex Transm Infect*, **67**, 441–52.

Velho PE, Souza EM, Belda Jr W (2008). Donovanosis. *Braz J Infect Dis*, **12**, 521–5.

6.10 Anaerobic bacteria

Anilrudh A. Venugopal and David W. Hecht

Essentials

Anaerobic bacteria will not grow when incubated with 10% CO_2 in room air, but vary in their tolerance of different levels of oxygen. They are important commensal flora of the skin and oral, intestinal, and pelvic mucosae, and are classified according to their Gram staining characteristics and ability to produce spores: (1) Gram positive—cocci, non-spore-forming bacilli, and spore-forming bacilli (notably clostridium); (2) Gram negative—cocci and bacilli. Many anaerobic bacteria possess virulence factors that facilitate their pathogenicity, e.g. histiolytic enzymes and various toxins.

Clinical features—anaerobes typically cause clinically significant infections when there is tissue compromise, ischaemia or mucosal injury. These infections are often polymicrobial in nature and include (1) bacteraemia; (2) central nervous system infection—intracranial abscesses by contiguous spread, e.g. from chronic otitis media, or haematogenous spread, e.g. from tooth abscess; (3) head and neck infections—periodontal and pharyngeal infections from spread of gingival disease; (4) pleuropulmonary infections—e.g. lung abscess from aspirated oropharyngeal flora; (5) intra-abdominal infections—often caused by mixed colonic flora that have been displaced by bowel injury; (6) gastrointestinal infections; (7) genitourinary infections; (8) skin and soft-tissue infections—ranging from cellulitis to necrotizing fasciitis; should be considered in cases of infected animal and human bites, and in intravenous drug users; diabetic foot ulcers often have polymicrobial infections that include anaerobes.

Diagnosis—a putrid odour of the affected tissue or discharge is very suggestive of anaerobic infection, as is the presence of gas in tissues. Care must be taken when collecting specimens for anaerobic cultures because many of the organisms are very sensitive to oxygen, and some cannot tolerate more than a few minutes at ambient oxygen levels. However, anaerobic spores are aerotolerant, can survive in harsh oxygen-laden environments, and will germinate under appropriate conditions.

Treatment and prevention—aside from supportive care, treatment requires (1) drainage of abscesses and resection of devitalized tissue; and (2) antibiotics—agents that are active against anaerobes include clindamycin, metronidazole, vancomycin, β-lactam/β-lactamase combinations, carbapenems, moxifloxacin, and tigecycline but resistance patterns are changing and the choice of empirical therapy is best guided by knowledge of local susceptibility testing. Prophylaxis against anaerobic bacteria significantly reduces postoperative infection rates following intra-abdominal surgery.

History

In 1690 Antonie van Leeuwenhoek first described anaerobic bacteria as 'animalcules' that could survive in the absence of air. This observation was overlooked until nearly 200 years later. In 1861 Louis Pasteur had observed that the bacteria near the surface of a droplet of water had stopped moving while the organisms at the centre of the droplet continued to move about. He hypothesized that oxygen in the air had caused the death of the surface bacteria. Pasteur's early experiments with bacterial fermentation led to the development of anaerobic bacteriology.

Initially there was uncertainty about the importance of these organisms, but the invention of the anaerobic jar by James McIntosh and Paul Fildes in 1916 allowed the repeated culture and study of anaerobes. This led to the discovery of many anaerobic bacteria responsible for various human diseases.

Definition

Anaerobic bacteria are organisms that cannot grow in the presence of various levels of oxygen. Room air is approximately 20% oxygen and when cultured in this environment, anaerobes will not grow on solid media. Reduced oxygen tensions are required for their growth. Anaerobes are described as strict, moderate, or facultative anaerobes, according to their tolerance of oxygen.

Strict anaerobes may grow only at oxygen levels of less than 0.5%. They are usually catalase negative and lack superoxide dismutase rendering them susceptible to toxic oxygen radicals, although this is not always the case. Moderate anaerobes also grow poorly in air and prefer media that have oxygen levels of 2 to 8%. Facultative anaerobic bacteria are organisms that can grow in various levels of oxygen including normal oxygen tensions.

Taxonomy of important anaerobic organisms

Table 6.10.1 lists the species of anaerobes that colonize human mucosal surfaces and skin or produce clinically significant disease. They are classified according to their Gram-staining characteristics and ability to produce spores.

Epidemiology

Limited data about the incidences of anaerobic infections are available. A few well-known anaerobic infections occur frequently enough to deserve mention here.

Clostridium difficile (see Chapter 6.23) is the most frequently isolated bacterial agent in diarrhoeal illnesses when a causative agent is established. It is a common cause of hospital-acquired diarrhoea and can present in different ways that are discussed later in this chapter.

Enterotoxigenic *Bacteroides fragilis* (ETBF) is another emerging enteric pathogen causing diarrhoeal illness in humans. It has been known to cause epidemics of diarrhoeal illness in industrialized and developing nations.

Human commensal flora

Commensal bacteria are organisms that live on both mucosal surfaces and skin of humans but under normal circumstances do not cause disease. They play an important role in normal host physiology by colonizing and helping to prevent infections by pathogenic organisms. By producing toxic metabolites, lowering the local pH, and depleting the area of nutrients they make the surrounding area uninhabitable to other pathogenic organisms. Anaerobes make up a large part of this commensal flora in humans, as outlined below.

Skin

The commensal flora of the skin consists predominantly of aerobes, anaerobes, and yeasts. The principal anaerobes present are Gram-positive bacilli of the genus *Propionibacterium*. The three main species are *P. acnes*, *P. granulosum*, and *P. avidum*. They occur mainly in hair follicles and sebaceous glands. *P. acnes* produce free fatty acids from triglycerides, but, while this may control the growth of pathogenic bacteria on the surface of skin, it has also been associated with the development of acne.

Upper respiratory tract and oral cavity

The nasal cavity mucosa tends to be colonized with organisms that are similar to the organisms found on skin surfaces and the sebaceous glands. Oropharyngeal flora typically includes *Peptostreptococci*, *Tannerella forsythensis*, and *Fusobacterium*. In the oral cavity, areas such as the tonsillar crypts, gingival crevices, and the clefts on the

Table 6.10.1 Taxonomy of important anaerobic bacteria

Gram-positive anaerobes			Gram-negative anaerobes	
Cocci	Bacilli		Cocci	Bacilli
	Nonspore-forming	Spore-forming		
	Actinomyces spp.	*Clostridium* spp.	*Veillonella* spp.	*Bacteroides fragilis* group
Peptostreptococcus spp.	*Bifidobacterium* spp.			Other *Bacteroides* spp.
Streptococcus spp.	*Eubacterium* spp.			*Bilophila wadsworthia*
Finegoldia magna	*Eggerthella* spp.			
	Lactobacillus spp.			*Fusobacterium* spp.
	Mobiluncus spp.			*Porphyromonas* spp.
	Propionibacterium spp.			*Prevotella* spp.

tongue have a more favourable atmosphere for anaerobes. Their lower oxygen levels promote colonization with *Prevotella*, *Peptostreptococci*, *Fusobacterium*, and other anaerobic Gram-positive bacilli.

Gastrointestinal tract

The upper gastrointestinal tract from oesophagus to jejunum is relatively free of microorganisms but can become transiently colonized with bacteria following meals or from the swallowed secretions of the upper airway. The terminal ileum tends to have a flora more closely resembling that of the large intestines where anaerobes can outnumber the aerobes 100 to 1000:1. Among a diverse group of anaerobes, the *Bacteroides fragilis* group predominates. *B. vulgatus* and *B. thetaiotaomicron* are more common than *B. fragilis*. Another group of colonizing anaerobes found in the stool are *Clostridium* spp., including *C. perfringens* and *C. novyi*. Infants have been found to be colonized with *C. difficile* but without symptoms. Infantile intestinal mucosal cells in rabbits lack the receptors to bind the disease-producing *C. difficile* toxin, but they acquire the receptors with increasing age.

Genitourinary tract

The kidneys, ureters, urinary bladder, and proximal part of the urethra are normally free of organisms as they are constantly flushed with urine if the anatomy of the urinary tract is normal. The distal portion of both male and female urethras have a scanty flora including aerobic skin colonizers and some anaerobic organisms including *Bacteroides*, *Fusobacterium*, *Peptostreptococcus*, and *Clostridium* spp. The vaginal flora can include both aerobes and anaerobes but, by adulthood, anaerobes such as *Lactobacillus*, *Prevotella*, *Fusobacterium*, and *Peptostreptococci* predominate (Fig. 6.10.1)

Pathogenesis

Several factors predispose to the pathogenesis of anaerobic infections, including tissue injury and destruction, impaired blood supply, or any breakdown in the integrity of mucosa or skin.

Many anaerobic bacteria possess one or more characteristics that enhance their pathogenic virulence. Histolytic enzymes such as collagenase, fibrinolysin, lipases, and other enzymes are produced by bacteroides and *Prevotella*. These enzymes cause tissue destruction, whereas the α-toxin found in *C. perfringens* can also cause haemolysis. Enterotoxigenic *B. fragilis* is known to produce a metalloproteinase toxin that causes cell proliferation and protein shedding resulting in a diarrhoeal illness. Various organisms including *C. perfringens* and *C. difficile* have also been found to have enterotoxins that alter intestinal cell function and cause cell death leading to diarrhoea. Certain species of clostridium including *C. botulinum* and *C. tetani* produce neurotoxins that block neuromuscular transmissions leading to paralysis or spasms plus rigidity, respectively. Gram-negative anaerobes, like their aerobic

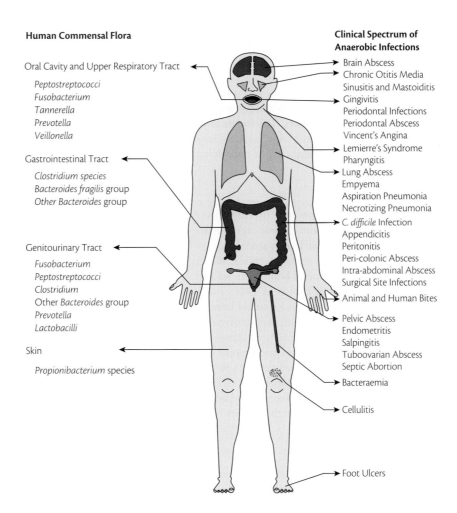

Fig. 6.10.1 Human anaerobic commensal flora (left) and clinical spectrum of anaerobic infections (right).

counterparts, have a lipopolysaccharide layer in their outer membrane that can act as an endotoxin. Endotoxins can cause macrophage and complement activation leading to fever, hypotension, and oedema from the release of cytokines. However, the endotoxin of the *B. fragilis* group is defective and weak when compared to those of other facultative anaerobic bacteria. *Porphyromonas gingivalis*, *Bacteroides* spp., and *Fusobacterium* produce heparinases that can promote coagulation leading to tissue ischaemia. The capsular polysaccharides associated with the *B. fragilis* group, *Prevotella melaninogenica*, and *Peptostreptococcus*, are associated with impaired phagocytosis by host cells and can lead to abscess formation. *Porphyromonas gingivalis*, *B. fragilis*, and *Fusobacterium nucleatum* produce catalase and superoxide dismutase which are believed to help the organisms tolerate higher levels of oxygen. Spore-producing organisms like the clostridial species can survive in harsh oxygen-laden environments by developing spores that will later germinate when environmental conditions become favourable again. Finally, several organisms produce surface ligands and charges that help to improve mucosal adherence and bacterial aggregation, while others produce metabolites that inhibit the growth of normal flora.

Clinical spectrum

Anaerobic bacteraemia

Anaerobes account for 1 to 17% of all positive blood cultures. The predisposing factors for anaerobic bacteraemia in newborns include prematurity, prolonged labour, chorioamnionitis, and necrotizing enterocolitis. Underlying risk factors for anaerobic bacteraemia in children and adults include malignancies, immunosuppression, hepatic failure, and diabetes mellitus. The organism isolated depends on the underlying infectious condition. In cases of gastrointestinal or necrotic skin infections it is usually a member of the *B. fragilis* group. *Peptostreptococcus* and *Clostridium* spp. are other commonly found blood isolates. The isolation of *Clostridium septicum* or the facultative anaerobe *Streptococcus bovis* in bacteraemic patients should raise the suspicion of underlying cancer, especially of colonic origin.

Central nervous system infections

Intracranial infections with anaerobes can arise by contiguous spread from surrounding structures, e.g. with chronic otitis media, mastoiditis, or sphenoidal sinusitis. This can lead to abscess formation, septic thrombophlebitis, or venous sinus infections. When frontal sinusitis spreads to involve the frontal bone it can lead to osteomyelitis and subperiosteal abscess known as Pott's puffy tumour. Intracranial abscesses may also arise as a result of haematogenous seeding of the brain parenchyma from suppurative distant foci such as dental abscesses and alveolar infections. Abscesses that arise may be single or multiple in number and involve any portion of the brain, although the site involved depends on the mode of infection. Anaerobic organisms commonly associated with infections of the central nervous system include *Prevotella*, *Peptostreptococci*, and *Fusobacterium* spp., although these are often polymicrobial infections involving aerobes.

Head and neck infections

The origin of oral, head, and neck infections is often the anaerobic flora of the oral cavity. Lower oxygen tension in the gingival crevices promotes colonization with anaerobes. When dental hygiene is poor, dental plaque develops leading to gingivitis, periodontal infections, and abscesses. Periodontal infections result from spread of gingival disease to the surrounding tissue. As infection spreads from more superficial gingival disease to deeper infections there is a shift in the pathogenic organisms from Gram-positive cocci and bacilli to Gram-negative bacilli. Anaerobic pharyngeal infections may arise in relation to gingivitis. Complications may arise by contiguous spread of these infections along medial, lateral, or submaxillary spaces. Ludwig's angina is described as a brawny induration of the submaxillary and sublingual spaces with cellulitis usually arising from spread of lower molar dental infections. Severe infections threaten the airway and may extend to the mediastinum. Vincent's angina is an acute necrotizing ulcerative gingivitis manifested by inflamed gingivae, interdental ulcerations, and halitosis. Otitis media and sinusitis occasionally involve anaerobes, although they are more common in chronic infections of these spaces. *Fusobacterium necrophorum* may be a cause of pharyngitis in up to 10% of cases. Lemierre's syndrome frequently occurs in young previously healthy patients as the result of spread of an oropharyngeal infection leading to septic thrombophlebitis of the internal jugular vein. Clinical features helpful in diagnosing this condition are recent oropharyngeal infection, clinical evidence of thrombophlebitis including ipsilateral neck tenderness with fevers and chills, as well as isolation of the anaerobic pathogen. Most commonly, the organism isolated is *Fusobacterium necrophorum*, although other organisms have been identified. Early diagnosis is required to reduce morbidity associated with distant septic emboli and mortality.

Pleuropulmonary infections

The spectrum of anaerobic lung infections extends to include lung abscesses, empyema, aspiration pneumonitis, and necrotizing pneumonias. The origins of these anaerobes are usually from aspirated oropharyngeal flora. *Peptostreptococcus*, *Fusobacterium*, pigmented *Prevotella*, *Porphyromonas*, and *Bacteroides* spp. are most commonly isolated, often in combination with aerobes and other microaerophilic anaerobes such as *Streptococcus* spp. Patients with an anaerobic lung abscess will often complain of fevers, weight loss, and foul-smelling or foul-tasting sputum. This odour is frequently detectable on entering the patient's room.

Intra-abdominal infections

The presence of an intra-abdominal infection can usually be diagnosed clinically from a thorough history and physical examination. If the patient is not being taken for an immediate laparotomy then patients with suspected intra-abdominal infection should undergo CT scanning to evaluate the abdomen. Intra-abdominal infections are often caused by mixed colonic flora that have been displaced by surgery, penetrating trauma, intestinal malignancy, inflammatory bowel disease, or perforation of colonic diverticula. Intra-abdominal abscesses, pericolonic abscesses, and peritonitis may develop. Isolates are most commonly mixed facultative and strict anaerobes, notably the facultative anaerobe *Escherichia coli* and the anaerobe *B. fragilis* group. Other commonly occurring anaerobes include *Peptostreptococcus* spp., *Fusobacterium* spp., and *Clostridium* spp.

Gastrointestinal infections

C. difficile-associated disease (CDAD) is discussed in Chapter 6.23. Risk factors include recent or current antibacterial therapy (especially clindamycin, cephalosporins, and fluoroquinolones), advanced age, recent hospitalization or long-term care residence, and recent gastrointestinal surgery or procedures. Severity of CDAD ranges from diarrhoea to ileus, pseudomembranous colitis, toxic megacolon, and death. Clinical symptoms often include abdominal pain and distension, fevers, and profuse foul-smelling watery diarrhoea. Laboratory findings include leucocytosis (leukaemoid reactions) and hypoalbuminaemia. PCR assays of stool samples that target the presence of the toxin B gene have sensitivities ranging from 85 to 95% and specificities of 95 to 99%, which are improved compared to the toxin immunoassays. Recommendations about the use of oral metronidazole and vancomycin are discussed in detail in the adult clinical practice guidelines (see Further reading) and also in Chapter 6.23. Fidaxomicin is a newer treatment option that offers the advantage of lower recurrence rates compared to oral vancomycin. It is important to perform strict contact isolation measures for patients suspected of *C. difficile* disease to prevent nosocomial transmission and encourage proper hand hygiene with soap and water.

Enterotoxigenic *Bacteroides fragilis* has been associated with a diarrhoeal illness in humans. The ETBF organism produces a metalloprotease *Bacteroides fragilis* toxin that is proinflammatory and causes disruption of the colonic epithelial cells. Patients often present with tenesmus, abdominal pain and an inflammatory diarrhoea. In the mouse model, chronic colonization with ETBF has shown to have oncogenic potential, but the effects in humans are not yet known.

Genitourinary infections

Like the oral cavity and colon, the female genital tract has an increased colonization ratio of anaerobes to aerobes of nearly 10:1. Disruption of the integrity of the tissues of the female genital tract increases the risk of anaerobic infections such as periurethral and labial pyogenic infections, pelvic abscesses, postpartum endometritis, salpingitis, tubo-ovarian abscess, and septic abortions. *B. fragilis* group, *Prevotella* spp. including *P. bivia*, *P. disiens*, and *P. melaninogenica*, *Peptostreptococci*, and *Clostridium* spp. are commonly isolated. Actinomyces have been associated with intrauterine device-related infections. Bacterial vaginosis (see Oxford Textbook of Medicine 5e Chapter 14.15) is an infection characterized by malodorous vaginal discharge caused by a polymicrobial infection often including *Prevotella*, *Peptostreptococci*, *Mobiluncus*, and the facultative anaerobe *Gardnerella vaginalis*. *Clostridium sordellii* is a toxin-producing Gram-positive anaerobe that has been known to cause pelvic infections. This usually presents with vague symptoms causing deep infections following childbirth, medically induced abortions, or trauma. There is rapid clinical deterioration with profound hypotension, an intense leukaemoid reaction, and it is associated with a high mortality rate.

Skin and soft tissue infections

These usually arise after the integrity of the skin has been lost from injury, ischaemia, or surgery and there is contamination by either faecal or oral secretions. These are usually polymicrobial infections with aerobic and anaerobic bacteria. The spectrum of disease ranges from cellulitis to necrotizing fasciitis. Anaerobic skin infections should also be considered in cases of infected animal and human bites and decubitus ulcers, and also with intravenous drug users. Often intravenous drug users will clean their needles with saliva and they may present with cellulitis at a recent injection site.

Diabetic foot ulcers often have polymicrobial infections that include anaerobes. Common isolates from soft tissue infections include *B. fragilis* group, *Peptostreptococci*, and *Clostridium* spp.

Bone and joint infections

Osteomyelitis and septic arthritis from anaerobes are rare but can result when infection spreads from surrounding soft tissue, as in the case of diabetic foot ulcers. Diagnosis is made by the careful collection of fluids in anaerobic containers or by bone biopsy cultures. *Fusobacterium* spp. and other *Bacteroides* spp. have been isolated from joint infections on a few occasions.

Diagnosis

Clinical clues

A putrid odour of the affected tissue or discharge is very suggestive of anaerobic infections. Underlying illnesses such as diabetes mellitus, abscess formation, tissue ischaemia, and necrotic tissue are predisposing factors. Another important clue is the location of the infection in relation to mucosal surfaces that are normally colonized by anaerobes such as intra-abdominal and oral infections. Gas in tissues suggests anaerobic infection. It can often be detected on radiographs in cases of skin and soft tissue infections or with CT or MRI in deeper infections. However, gas formation in tissues is not specific to anaerobes and can be found in many aerobic infections as well. Some characteristic anaerobic infections such as actinomycosis may be identified on smears or tissue biopsy by the presence of filamentous Gram-positive bacilli and 'sulphur granules', although these may be easily missed.

Collection of specimens

The greatest barrier to the diagnosis of anaerobic infections (aside from not considering anaerobes) is faulty collection and transport of specimens. Aspirated pus or excised infected tissue should be despatched to the microbiology laboratory under anaerobic conditions as soon as possible. The use of swabs is discouraged because of the low yield of organisms collected with these specimens. Gram's stains and plating of the specimens should be done promptly with minimal exposure to air to minimize the loss of obligate anaerobes during handling. Immediately after inoculation, the media should be kept under anaerobic conditions in either anaerobic jars or chambers at 35 to 37°C. Most microbiology laboratories will not set up anaerobic cultures if the specimens have been collected improperly or were not transported in anaerobic transport media. Another potential method to culture anaerobic bacteria is to inoculate from 1 to 10 ml of the suspected infected fluid specimen in to an anaerobic blood culture bottle with proper labelling of the specimen source.

Anaerobic blood cultures

The collection of anaerobic blood cultures for the routine surveillance of bacteraemia has been debated for several years. Recent studies have confirmed their importance in detecting both anaerobic and early facultative anaerobic bacteraemia. Paired cultures should be drawn, including both aerobic and anaerobic bottles, and these should be collected from peripheral sources. This is important as positive cultures for anaerobes often occur when not suspected.

Treatment

Susceptibility and resistance

Anaerobic susceptibility patterns have consistently demonstrated resistance by members of the *B. fragilis* group since the late 1970s. Antibiotics vary in their *in vitro* activity against anaerobes. One of the most active agents is metronidazole which is the preferred agent for the treatment of *B. fragilis* and *C. tetani* and demonstrates activity against most species of *Clostridium*. It is effective in the treatment of *C. difficile* infections and is often used as initial therapy in patients with mild to moderate disease. Oral vancomycin must be recognized as the agent of choice for severe cases of *C. difficile* disease. Among 110 isolates of toxigenic *C. difficile*, no resistance to vancomycin and metronidazole was demonstrated.

β-lactam/β-lactamase combinations such as ampicillin/sulbactam, piperacillin/tazobactam, and ticarcillin/clavulanate demonstrate a high degree of *in vitro* activity against anaerobes including members of the *B. fragilis* group. Tigecycline has activity against many Gram-positive and Gram-negative anaerobic bacteria including the *Bacteroides fragilis* group, *C. perfringens*, and *Peptostreptococcus* spp. Carbapenems such as imipenem/cilastatin, meropenem, ertapenem, and doripenem also demonstrate excellent *in vitro* activity against nearly all anaerobes, while chloramphenicol has continued to maintain good *in vitro* activity against most anaerobic isolates due to its limited use.

Moderate anti-anaerobic *in vitro* activity is seen with cephamycins such as cefoxitin and cefotetan. Among fluoroquinolones, moxifloxacin has demonstrated moderate to good *in vitro* activity against most anaerobes. Over recent years, the *B. fragilis* group has shown the most significant increase in resistance to clindamycin.

Resistance patterns of the *B. fragilis* group members from isolates tested in both the United States of America and Europe are shown in Table 6.10.2. Updated data on anaerobic resistance in the United States will be available in the CLSI M100-S22 document in 2012. Anaerobes from the non-*Bacteroides* group are generally more susceptible to antianaerobic antibiotics. Exceptions to this rule include the resistance of *Prevotella* spp.

(clindamycin and moxifloxacin resistance at 38% and 29%, respectively), other *Clostridium* spp. (non-*C. perfringens* show cefoxitin, clindamycin, and moxifloxacin resistance at 30%, 10%, and 20%, respectively), and *P. acnes* (metronidazole resistance 100%). *Peptostreptococcus* spp. demonstrate clindamycin and moxifloxacin resistance of 14% and 17%, respectively, and penicillin resistance in the range of 4 to 8% among tested isolates (personal communication D.W. Hecht, 2007). Antibiotic resistance among anaerobes is less predictable than with aerobic and facultative anaerobes. Institutions should perform susceptibility testing at least annually to establish patterns of resistance to be reported with the hospital's antibiogram. Susceptibility of individual isolates should be performed if they were cultured from otherwise sterile sites and in cases of severe infections or those requiring long-term antibiotics.

Surgery

Often, antimicrobial therapy alone is not sufficient to cure anaerobic infections. Since many infections are associated with abscess formation or occur in areas with tissue ischaemia, surgical intervention frequently becomes imperative with drainage of abscesses and resection of devitalized tissue.

Complicated intra-abdominal infections

Patients with advanced age, malnutrition, or malignancy; those who have a delay in antibiotics; or those who have inadequate source control are at higher risk for treatment failure and also a higher severity of illness. Empiric initiation of antibiotics is recommended based on the severity of illness and whether it is associated with community or health-care onset. For mild to moderate community-onset infections, some possible empiric choices could be cefoxitin, ertapenem, tigecycline, or a cephalosporin with metronidazole. For severe community-onset disease, broader empirical treatment should be used until it can be narrowed down based on cultures. Some potential empirical choices include the use of imipenem/cilastatin, doripenem or piperacillin/tazobactam. Ampicillin/sulbactam is no longer recommended as an initial

Table 6.10.2 *In vitro* resistance of six species of the *B. fragilis* group from the United States of America and Europe to selected agents[a] (given in percentages)

Isolate	Cefoxitin		Clindamycin		Imipenem/cilastatin		Piperacillin/tazobactam		Metronidazole		Moxifloxacin		Tigecycline	
	USA[b]	Europe[c]	USA	Europe	USA	Europe	USA	Europe	USA	Europe	USA	Europe	USA	Europe
B. fragilis	3.5–9.4	13.7	29.4–30.2	28.5	0–2.7	1.2	0.8–2.7	1.7	<0.001	0.2	30.0–43.4	14.0	3.0–6.5	1.8
B. thetaiotaomicron	8.8–23.0	27.1	36.3–47.1	42.2	0	0	0–1.2	12.0	0	1.2	29.2–67.1	14.5	1.5–9.6	0
B. vulgatus	3.7–8.0	14.3	34.1–60.0	47.6	0	0	0	4.8	0	2	44.4–77.3	21.4	0–4.5	4.8
B. ovatus	0–17.9	24.5	30.0–43.8	44.9	0	0	0	0	0	0	36.4–72.0	8.2	0–7.7	2.0
B. disatonis[d]	5.3–25.9	35.7	19.2–50.0	28.6	0	0	0	14.3	0	0	31.8–43.8	0	0–3.8	0
B. uniformis	7.1–17.6	20.0	36.4–47.1	60.0	0	0	0	10.0	0	0	40.9–64.3	0	0–9.5	10.0

[a] Testing of the isolates was performed using the reference agar dilution method recommended by the Clinical and Laboratory Standards Institute.

[b] Percentage of resistance of seven species of the *B. fragilis* group members against six antibiotics, 2006 to 2009, from eight medical centres in the United States of America.
(Snydman DR, *et al.* (2011). Update on resistance of *Bacteroides fragilis* group and related species with special attention to carbapenems 2006–2009. *Anaerobe*, **17**, 147–51.)

[c] Percentage of resistance of seven species of the *B. fragilis* group members against six antibiotics, 2008 to 2009, from 13 European medical centres.
(Nagy E, *et al.* (2011). Antimicrobial susceptibility of Bacteroides fragilis isolates in Europe: 20 years of experience. *Clin Microbiol Infect*, **17**, 371–9.)

[d] *Bacteroides distasonis* was reclassified as *Parabacteroides distasonis* in 2006.

empiric agent because of growing resistance among enteric organisms. The choice for empiric treatment in health-care associated onset intra-abdominal infections should be chosen based on the local rates of resistant organisms including *Pseudomonas*, extended-spectrum-lactamases producing Enterobacteriaceae, multidrug-resistant Gram negatives, and meticillin-resistant *Staphylococcus aureus*. Surgical drainage or drainage by interventional radiology should be performed when a drainable focus is present and the patient is not improving with antibiotics alone.

Surgical antimicrobial prophylaxis

In cases where contamination of surgical wounds by the local flora could result in infection, it has become common practice for surgeons to use antimicrobial prophylaxis in the intraoperative and postoperative periods. In intra-abdominal procedures, prophylaxis against anaerobic bacteria significantly reduces postoperative infection rates. The regimens may cover both aerobes and anaerobes. The choice and duration of therapy depends on the nature of the surgery and whether it is an elective or emergency procedure. These decisions are based on timing, type of clinical presentation, and intraoperative findings. The antimicrobials used include cephamycins such as cefoxitin and cefotetan or other more specific antianaerobic agents such as metronidazole. Ertapenem has proved an effective alternative to cefotetan in prophylaxis of infections for elective colorectal surgery.

Further reading

Aldape MJ, Bryant AE, Stevens DL (2006). *Clostridium sordellii* infection: epidemiology, clinical findings and current perspectives on diagnosis and treatment. *Clin Infect Dis*, **43**, 1436–46.

Bartlett JG (2006). Narrative review: the new epidemic of *Clostridium difficile*-associated enteric disease. *Ann Int Med*, **145**, 758–64.

Brook I (2010). The role of anaerobic bacteria in bacteremia. *Anaerobe*, **16**, 183–9.

Centor RM (2009). Expand the pharyngitis paradigm for adolescents and young adults. *Ann Intern Med*, **151**, 812–15.

Chow AW (2006). Anaerobic infections. In: Dale DC, *et al.* (eds) *ACP medicine*, pp. 1604–20. Web MD, New York.

CLSI (2012). *Performance standards for antimicrobial susceptibility testing; twenty-second informational supplement*. CLSI document M100-S22. Clinical and Laboratory Standards Institute, Wayne, Pennsylvania.

Cohen SH, *et al.* (2010). Clinical practice guidelines for *Clostridium difficile* infection in adults: 2010 update by the society for healthcare epidemiology of America (SHEA) and the infectious diseases society of America (IDSA). *Infect Control Hosp Epidemiol*, **31**, 431–55.

Cohen-Poradosu R, Kasper DL (2009). Anaerobic infections: general concepts. In: Mandell GL, Bennett JE, Dolin R (eds) *Principles and Practices of Infectious Diseases*, pp. 3083–9. Churchill Livingstone, Philadelphia, Pennsylvania.

Finegold SM, George WL (eds) (1989). *Anaerobic infections in humans*. Academic Press, New York.

Hagelskjaer L, Prag J (2000). Human necrobacillosis, with emphasis on Lemierre's syndrome. *Clin Infect Dis*, **31**, 524–32.

Hecht DW (2004). Prevalence of antibiotic resistance in anaerobic bacteria: worrisome developments. *Clin Infect Dis*, **39**, 92–7.

Hecht DW, *et al.* (2007). In vitro activities of 15 antimicrobial agents against 110 toxigenic Clostridium difficile clinical isolates collected from 1983 to 2004. *Antimicrob Agents Chemother*, **51**, 2716–19.

Itani KMF, *et al.* (2006). Ertapenem versus cefotetan prophylaxis in elective colorectal surgery. *N Engl J Med*, **355**, 2640–51.

Jenkins SG (2001). Infections due to anaerobic bacteria and the role of antimicrobial susceptibility testing of anaerobes. *Rev Med Microbiol*, **12**, 1–12.

Lassmann B, *et al.* (2007). Reemergence of anaerobic bacteremias. *Clin Infect Dis*, **44**, 895–900.

Nagy E, *et al.* (2011). Antimicrobial susceptibility of Bacteroides fragilis group isolates in Europe: 20 years' experience. *Clin Microbiol Infect*, **17**, 371–9.

Snydman DR, *et al.* (2011). Update on resistance of Bacteroides fragilis group and related species with special attention to carbapenems 2006–2009. *Anaerobe*, **17**, 147–51.

Solomkin JS, *et al.* (2010). Diagnosis and management of complicated intra-abdominal infection in adults and children: guidelines by the Surgical Infection Society and the Infectious Diseases Society of America. *Clin Infect Dis*, **50**, 133–64.

Wick EC, Sears CL (2010). Bacteroides spp. and diarrhea. *Curr Opin Infect Dis*, **23**, 470–4.

6.11 Cholera

Aldo A.M. Lima and Richard L. Guerrant

Essentials

Vibrio cholerae is a Gram-negative organism that can be subdivided into over 200 serogroups based on the somatic O antigen, with only serogroups O1 and O139 causing epidemic and pandemic disease. Historically it has killed millions from dehydrating diarrhoea, encouraged the birth of modern epidemiology, the sanitary revolution, and oral rehydration therapy; it persists today as a glaring reminder of poverty and inadequate water/sanitation. Contaminated food (especially undercooked seafood) is the usual route of transmission in developed countries; contaminated water and street food vendors are more common vehicles in less developed countries.

Clinical features and diagnosis—typical presentation is with sudden onset of voluminous, painless, watery diarrhoea, which can exceed 500 to 1000 ml/h, leading to severe dehydration in a couple hours and risk of death. Definitive diagnosis is by isolating *V. cholerae* from stool or rectal swab samples.

Treatment—oral rehydration therapy with sugar or starch, water, and salts must be provided in the community and at field stations, clinics, and hospitals where most patients present: this reduces the case fatality of untreated severe cholera from about 50% to 1% or less. Antibiotics can shorten the illness and decrease diarrhoeal purging: tetracycline, cotrimoxazole, ciprofloxacin, or azithromycin have been effective, but there is increasing resistance.

Prevention—effective preventive measures include (1) ensuring a safe water supply; (2) improving sanitation; (3) making food safe for consumption by thorough cooking of high-risk foods, especially seafood; and (4) health education through mass media. Newer-generation killed oral cholera vaccines have been licensed and proved to be well tolerated, protective, cost-beneficial, and a potential tool to control cholera together with the other preventive recommendations.

Introduction and historical perspective

Cholera, the dreaded scourge causing death from dehydrating diarrhoea, existed for centuries in South Asia until, in 1817, it broke out along trade routes; since then there have been seven pandemics across all six inhabited continents. Recent outbreaks in Zimbabwe (2008 to 2009) and Haiti (2010) indicate that this seventh pandemic is still ongoing across the continents. The whole-genome sequences of globally and temporally representative *V. cholerae* isolates have shown that since the 1950s these isolates have spread from the Bay of Bengal in three independent waves with a common ancestor. Cholera was largely responsible for encouraging the birth of modern epidemiology and for driving the sanitary revolution in Western Europe and North America in the 19th century. In the last one-third of the 20th century, it helped drive scientific discoveries of cell signalling, intestinal ion transport, and oral rehydration therapy (ORT), which have brought global diarrhoea mortality down from over 5 million/year to below 2 million/year. Yet cholera persists today as a disease of poverty, along with other faecally transmitted pathogens, a sign of inadequate water and sanitation among the desperately poor and displaced around the world.

Aetiology, genetics, and pathophysiology

Thirty years before the causative agent *Vibrio cholerae* was discovered during the fifth pandemic in 1884 in Kolkata, India, by Robert Koch, John Snow's classic epidemiological study of cholera in London in 1854 suggested that it was transmitted by contaminated drinking water. Snow even postulated that a toxin might cause the dramatic fluid loss. *V. cholerae* is a halophilic flagellated curved Gram-negative organism classified by biochemical tests and further subdivided into serogroups based on the somatic O antigen. Among over 200 serogroups, only O1 and O139 cause epidemic and pandemic disease. The other strains are classified as non-O1 and non-O139 *V. cholerae*. Serogroup O1 is further subdivided into three serotypes (Inaba, Ogawa, and Hikojima) and into two phenotypically different biogroups (Classical and El Tor). The latter is named for the Egyptian village quarantine station where it was first isolated in 1905 from Indonesian pilgrims travelling to Mecca. This strain then became the cause of the seventh pandemic that continues around the world today. The O139 serogroup, first seen in 1992, appears to have emerged from horizontal gene transfer of a fragment of DNA that encodes O-antigen biosynthesis from another serogroup (perhaps O22) into the seventh pandemic *V. cholerae* O1 El Tor strain. O139 and O1 (both Classical and El Tor biotypes) now coexist and continue to cause large outbreaks in India and Bangladesh. *V. cholerae* O1 (biotype El Tor) has two circular chromosomes and the entire genome sequence was recently described. The large chromosome has most of the genes required for growth and pathogenicity and the small chromosome encodes components of several essential metabolic and regulatory pathways. Critical to the pathogenicity of *V. cholerae* (and distinct from environmental isolates) is the acquisition of two distinct phages. The first contains a 'pathogenicity island' (VPI) encoding the 'toxin coregulated pilus' (TCP). Remarkably, TCP serves as both a major intestinal colonization factor and as the receptor for the second phage, CTXφ, that encodes for cholera toxin and accessory proteins (including ACE and Zot) as well as containing genes required for phage replication, integration, and regulation in the RS2 region.

Genes encoding colonization factors or toxin are regulated in response to environmental conditions. The 32-kDa transmembrane protein ToxR binds upstream of *ctxAB* to increase transcription and synthesis of cholera toxin. ToxR also regulates the expression of other genes in the ToxR regulon; hence, the expression of ToxR is controlled by environmental factors. Recent characterization of *V. cholera* O1 El Tor biotype variant clinical isolates from Bangladesh and Haiti showed that all strains produced increased cholera toxin (2- to 10-fold) compared to the wild type El Tor strains and also produced more TCP and ToxT. These essential virulence factors are regulated primarily by ToxT via the ToxR virulence regulon.

Vibrios are acquired from contaminated water or food and they must pass though the acidic stomach before they are able to colonize the upper small intestine. Colonization occurs with filamentous protein fimbriae, called toxin coregulated pili, which extend from the vibrio wall and attach to receptors on the mucosa. *V. cholerae* adhere to the M cells without causing tissue damage and rapidly multiply to 10^7 to 10^8 cells/g of tissue. Attached vibrios efficiently deliver cholera toxin directly to the epithelial cells (Fig. 6.11.1). The A subunit consists of two peptides linked by a disulphide bond. The larger, A1, containing the toxic activity, is endocytosed following toxin binding via its B subunit to GM1 ganglioside. A1 subunit catalyses the covalent bonding of adenosine diphosphoribose from nicotinamide adenosine dinucleotide to the α-subunit of Gs, the heterotrimeric adenylyl cyclase-stimulating G protein, thus activating adenylate cyclase to form cAMP. cAMP then acts to open the cystic fibrosis transmembrane conductance regulator (CFTR) chloride channel causing increased chloride secretion by the intestinal crypt cells and a blockade of neutral sodium and chloride absorption by villous cells. This leads to voluminous fluid efflux into the small intestinal lumen which exceeds the absorptive capacity of the bowel and results in watery diarrhoea. The diarrhoeal fluid contains large amounts of sodium, chloride, bicarbonate, and potassium, but little protein or blood cells. The loss of electrolyte-rich isotonic fluid leads to blood volume depletion with attendant low blood pressure and shock. Loss of bicarbonate and potassium leads to metabolic acidosis and potassium deficiency.

Epidemiology

Ever since Snow's seminal epidemiological treatise, cholera has been described as the classic water-borne disease. However, it is also transmitted by contaminated food, especially undercooked seafood or food mixed with contaminated water. Contaminated food (especially undercooked seafood) is the usual vehicle for transmission in developed countries, and contaminated water and street food vendors are more common vehicles in less developed countries. *V. cholerae* is found in brackish surface water and in shellfish, and survives and multiplies in association with zooplankton and phytoplankton independently of infected human beings. There is no known other animal reservoir for *V. cholerae*. *V. cholerae* is endemic in the Indian subcontinent and the re-emergence of cholera in other continents is highly dependent on environmental factors. The association of the bacteria with plankton has led to the suggestion that ship ballast is a cause of its global spread. *V. cholerae* has evolved to survive in the aquatic environment and then in the host. In water, *V. cholerae* vibrios are free swimming or attached to plants, green algae, copepods, crustaceans, or insects.

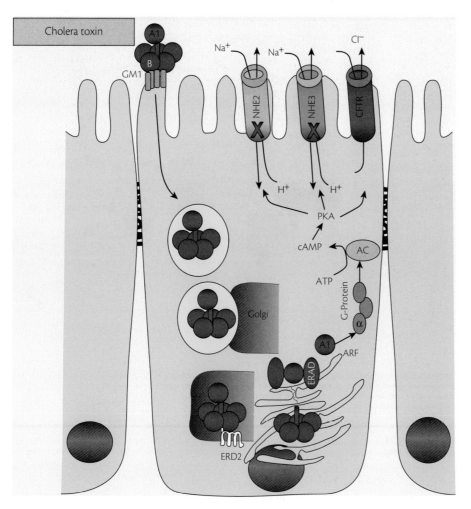

Fig. 6.11.1 Pathophysiology of cholera. *V. cholerae* produces a major virulence factor, cholera toxin, an 84-kDa protein consisting of a dimeric A subunit and five identical B subunits. Cholera toxin binds to a monosialoganglioside GM1 receptor at the host mucosal surface and triggers endocytosis of the holotoxin. The A1 domain of the A subunit is transported through the Golgi and endoplasmic reticulum to activate the Gsα subunit of G-protein. This A1 domain interacts with ADP-ribosylating factors (ARFs) to ADP-ribosylate this the Gsα subunit leading to activated G-protein and consequent activation of adenylyl cyclase (AC). The AC cleaves ATP to cAMP which subsequently activates protein kinase A which inhibits NaCl absorption (NHE transporters) and increases chloride secretion through the cystic fibrosis transmembrane regulator (CFTR).

In humans, the intestinal milieu fosters the acquisition of genetic elements from the TCP bacteriophage, lacking in most environmental strains. TCP phage encodes type IV fimbria which serves as colonization factor and receptor for the CTX phage that carries genes encoding cholera toxin. Thus both bacteriophages integrate into the bacterial genome and form episomal replication intermediates. The production of cholera toxin and the biogenesis of CTX phage both depend on a type II secretion apparatus, encoded within the bacterial genome. In Bangladesh and Peru, where the disease has been endemic and epidemic, cholera tends to occur in the warm seasons albeit before and after the monsoon rains in Bangladesh.

Most *V. cholerae* infections are asymptomatic (case:infection = 1:3 to 1:100) or associated with mild nonspecific diarrhoea. Since a high inoculum dose is required for infection, person-to-person infection is rare without intervening water or food contamination. Infection and its severity also depend on the gastric acid barrier, local intestinal immunity, and blood group. Those with blood group O are at higher risk of severe El Tor cholera than are those with other blood groups. This susceptibility may explain the lower prevalence of blood group O in the Ganges delta area. A recent study showed that Lewis blood group antigen type Le(a+b−) are more susceptible and Le(a−b+) are less susceptible to *V. cholerae* O1 associated symptomatic disease. This may be important in evaluating population risk factors for cholera and in vaccine efficacy studies. In cholera-endemic areas, the highest attack rates are in children aged 2 to 4 years. In newly invaded areas, attack rates are similar for all ages. First illnesses are often seen in adult men, presumably because of greater exposure to contaminated food and water.

The current seventh pandemic began in 1961, in Sulawesi (Celebes), Indonesia. By 1966 the disease had spread to other countries in eastern Asia including Bangladesh, India, the former Union of Soviet Socialist Republics, Iran, and Iraq. Cholera reached West Africa in 1970, and in 1991 it appeared in Latin America for the first time in more than a century. Until 1992 only serogroup O1 had been implicated in epidemics while other serogroups had caused only sporadic cases of diarrhoea. However, in late 1992 cholera broke out in India and Bangladesh caused by a previously unrecognized serogroup of *V. cholerae*, designated O139. It is unclear whether this new serogroup from Southeast Asia will spread to other regions of the world. It is estimated that 120 000 people die from cholera worldwide each year (Fig. 6.11.2).

All cases of suspected cholera should be reported to local and national health authorities, since cholera outbreaks can become massive epidemics. These cases should be confirmed by laboratory investigation. If a patient older than 5 years develops severe dehydration or dies from acute watery diarrhoea, or if there is a sudden increase in the daily number of patients with acute watery diarrhoea, a cholera outbreak should be suspected.

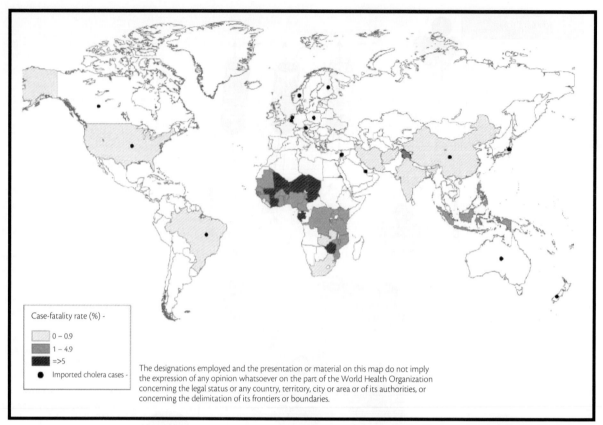

Fig. 6.11.2 Countries and areas reporting cholera cases in 2005.
(From Cholera. *Weekly Epidemiological Record* (2006), **81**(31), 297–307.)

Prevention and vaccines

Since contaminated water and food are the main vehicles of transmission, effective preventive measures include ensuring a safe water supply (especially for municipal water systems), improving sanitation, making food safe for consumption by thorough cooking of high risk foods (especially seafood), and providing health education through mass media (Box 6.11.1).

Two safe and well-tolerated oral cholera vaccines that provide significant protection have been licensed for commercial use:

1 Killed whole cell *V. cholerae* plus recombinant B subunit of cholera toxin vaccine given as two doses 1 to 6 weeks apart (rCTB-WC; Dukoral). In Dukoral the A subunit of cholera toxin is deleted.

2 Live attenuated *V. cholerae* O1 strain, CVD 103-HgR vaccine given as a single dose (Orochol; known as Mutachol in Canada). In Orochol, the gene for encoding the A subunit of cholera toxin has been largely deleted.

Neither vaccine is licensed in the United States of America.

Twenty-five trials of oral cholera vaccines were reviewed to assess the effect of cholera vaccines in preventing cases of cholera and preventing deaths. Eighteen efficacy trials of relatively good quality, testing parenteral and oral killed whole cell vaccines and involving over 2.6 million adults, children, and infants were included. Eleven safety trials were conducted using killed whole cell vaccines and involving 9342 people. The efficacy of the killed whole cell vaccines compared to placebo to prevent cholera at 12 months was 49%.

Both parenteral and oral administrations were effective, although killed whole cell vaccines had a significant protection extended in older children and adults. Parenteral killed whole cell vaccines were associated with increased systemic and local adverse effects compared to placebo. Oral killed whole cell vaccines were not associated with adverse events compared to placebo. In conclusion, killed whole cell cholera vaccines are relatively effective and safe. Because vaccine efficacy is overcome by larger infectious doses, vaccine should be seen as synergistic with improvements in water and sanitation that reduce the numbers of vibrios ingested.

A newer generation of oral cholera vaccines have been tested and licensed which provide direct protection and vaccine herd immunity. The current killed oral cholera vaccines (Shanechol and mORCVAX) are highly cost-effective and attractive for use in

---

Box 6.11.1 Prevention of cholera

- ◆ Ensure a safe water supply.
- ◆ Wash hands after defecation and before food preparation.
- ◆ Improve sanitation, making water and food safe for consumption.
- ◆ Provide health education through mass media.
- ◆ Vaccination and improvements in sanitation work synergistically.

developing countries. They do not require qualified medical personnel for administration. The two-dose regimen of these killed oral cholera vaccines in children 1 year of age or less gave a protective efficacy of 66% during 3 years of follow-up. This study is still in progress and continued follow-up will be important to evaluate the vaccine's duration of protection as well as a single-dose regimen which has shown similar protective efficacy in one study.

Clinical features

The incubation period of cholera usually ranges from 18 h to 5 days. There is a sudden onset of voluminous watery diarrhoea with occasional vomiting. Diarrhoea is severe in 5 to 10% of those infected. Its most distinctive feature is the painless purging of voluminous stools resembling rice-water with a fishy odour. The vomitus is generally a watery and alkaline fluid. Severe diarrhoea can exceed 500 to 1000 ml/h, leading to severe dehydration in 2 h and risk of death. Dehydration can be classified based on the presence and severity of clinical findings (Table 6.11.1). Signs of severe dehydration include absent or low-volume peripheral pulse, undetectable blood pressure, poor skin turgor, sunken eyes, and wrinkled hands and feet. Metabolic acidosis can develop and lead to gasping (Kussmaul) breathing. Urine output is diminished or absent until dehydration is corrected.

Complications generally result from inadequate fluid replacement, acute renal failure due to protracted hypotension, hypoglycaemia, hypokalaemia, and cramps due to electrolyte imbalance.

Differential diagnosis

Most cases are indistinguishable from other cases of diarrhoeal diseases, but since the treatment of any dehydrating diarrhoea is the same—fluid replacement—identification of the pathogen is not essential for patient management. However, if an adult patient becomes severely dehydrated and is in the right epidemiological setting or with a history of travelling, the clinician and public health authorities should be alert to the possibility of cholera.

Table 6.11.1 Assessment of patients with diarrhoea for dehydration

Feature	No dehydration	Some dehydration[a]	Severe dehydration[a, b]
General appearance	Well, alert	Restless, irritable	Lethargy or unconscious; floppy
Eyes	Normal	Sunken*	Very sunken and dry*
Tears	Present	Absent*	Absent*
Mouth and tongue	Moist	Dry*	Very dry*
Thirst	Drinks normally, not thirsty	Thirsty, drinks eagerly	Drinks poorly or not able to drink
Skin pinch[c]	Goes back quickly	Goes back slowly	Goes back very slowly

[a] Two or more of these signs including one indicated by *.
[b] Absence of radial pulse and low blood pressure are also signs of severe dehydration in adults and children older than 5 years.
[c] The skin pinch is less useful in patients with marasmus (severe wasting), kwashiorkor (severe malnutrition with oedema), or in obese patients.
(From Azurin JC, et al. (1967). A long-term carrier of cholera: cholera Dolores. *Bull World Health Organ*, **37**, 745–9.)

Criteria for diagnosis

Definitive diagnosis is by isolating *V. cholerae* from stool or rectal swab samples on selective media. *V. cholerae* survives in faecal specimens if kept moist. Cary–Blair transport medium should be used for transport to the laboratory for plating onto thiosulphate citrate bile salts sucrose (TCBS) agar that inhibits most other normal faecal flora but supports the growth of the vibrios. Specimens should also be inoculated into alkaline peptone water, an enrichment broth that preferentially supports the growth of vibrios. After 6 to 12 h of incubation, a second TCBS plate is inoculated. These plates are incubated for 18 to 24 h, and *V. cholerae* colonies appear as smooth yellow colonies with slightly raised centres. *V. cholerae* is a Gram-negative, polar monotrichous oxidase-positive asporogenous curved rod that ferments glucose, sucrose, and mannitol and is positive in the lysine and ornithine decarboxylase tests. The organism is classified by biochemical tests and is further subdivided into serogroups based on the somatic O antigen. Presumptive identification of *V. cholerae* O1 or O139 can be made on the basis of typical colonies, which are oxidase-positive and agglutinate with O1 or O139 antiserum.

Rapid tests include dark-field microscopy and rapid immunoassays which can be useful for monitoring epidemiological patterns in remote areas where cultures are not readily available. New outbreaks must be confirmed by cultures. Polymerase chain reaction (PCR) and DNA probes are available but are not practicable in many areas where cholera is common.

Treatment

Treatment must be provided at the community and field stations, clinics, and hospitals where most of the patients present. ORT was a major therapeutic breakthrough that has drastically decreased mortality from cholera and other dehydrating diarrhoeal diseases. The case fatality rate of untreated severe cholera approaches 50%, but with ORT it is decreased to 1% or less. The physiological basis for ORT is Na^+-coupled transport with glucose; transport from the enterocyte to the lateral intercellular space creates a local osmotic gradient that initiates water flow (Fig. 6.11.3). The oral rehydration salts (ORS) formulation approved by the World Health Organization (WHO) is based on the electrolyte composition lost in stool in patients with cholera. Table 6.11.2 summarizes the electrolyte concentrations from cholera stool and several oral rehydration formulations, including that approved and recommended by the WHO.

Table 6.11.1 summarizes the clinical assessment and management of patients with mild, moderate, or severe dehydration. In all cases the key is to rapidly replace fluid deficits, correct metabolic acidosis and potassium losses, and to continue replacing ongoing fluid losses. Because cholera toxin has prolonged effects, it is imperative to continue replacing fluid losses, for which a 'cholera cot' with a central hole, plastic sheet, and bucket to monitor purging can be tremendously helpful to both the patient and medical attendants.

Five to 7.5% of the bodyweight should be given as ORS with additional ORS to compensate for other losses. In patients who are severely dehydrated, having lost at least 10% (5 litres for a 50-kg patient) of their bodyweight, volume replacement must be rapid. Lactated Ringer's solution is an excellent commercially available

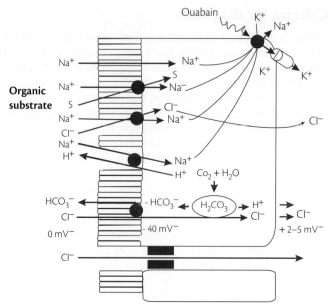

Fig. 6.11.3 The pharmacological principle and basis for oral rehydration therapy. Na^+ coupling permits the organic substrate to be transported 'uphill', i.e. from low luminal to higher concentration, a gradient opposite to that for Na^+. The Na^+ gradient is the driving force for sugar and amino acids. As these organic solutes are absorbed, salt is absorbed with them, and water follows osmotically—transport from enterocytes to lateral intercellular space creates a local osmotic gradient that initiates water flow. This coupled transport of Na^+ and organic substrate is the theoretical basis for oral rehydration therapy in cholera and other diarrheal diseases.

intravenous fluid. Other polyelectrolyte solutions with added potassium can also be used. Since ORS is the best polyelectrolyte solution to compensate for the acidosis and potassium deficiency, they should be given as soon as possible after initial intravenous fluid resuscitation.

A formulation of ORS that uses rice rather than glucose is better for cholera patients because it reduces the purging rate by providing polymeric glucose with lower osmolarity. ORS have been modified to prevent hypernatraemia (more common with other diarrhoeas) by having a reduced concentration of sodium (75 mmol/litre). This hypo-osmolar solution is also acceptable for cholera. ORS are easily prepared by adding the following simple ingredients to 1 litre water: 2.6 g sodium chloride, 2.9 g trisodium citrate, 1.5 g potassium chloride, and 13.5 g glucose (or 50 g boiled and cooled rice powder).

Adults and children are encouraged to eat, and breastfeeding can continue as there is no scientific basis for resting the gut.

Antibiotics can shorten the illness and decrease diarrhoeal purging. One- to 3-day courses of tetracycline, co-trimoxazole, or ciprofloxacin have been effective but there is increasing resistance. Azithromycin has been used more recently, but growing macrolide resistance may limit its use as well. Antibiotic sensitivity testing is therefore recommended during outbreaks. Antibiotics are not indicated for asymptomatic contacts. Prophylactic use of antibiotics increases the risk of the development of resistance and it is not indicated to prevent cholera.

Prognosis

Case fatality should be 1% or less if adequate ORT is used early in the illness, even at the community level. Adequate fluid and electrolyte replacement reverses or prevents complications such as acute renal failure or hypoglycaemia even in moderate or severe cholera. Cholera may well persist in its brackish marine reservoir, but improved water and sanitation and increasingly available vaccines promise to control this dreaded disease.

Other issues (health economics, areas of uncertainty or controversy, and likely developments ahead)

Areas of uncertainty or controversy include the mechanisms and importance of natural reservoirs of cultivable and even noncultivable vibrios and marine organisms from plankton to shellfish in the

Table 6.11.2 Composition of cholera stools and electrolyte rehydration solutions used to replace stool losses

Fluid	Sodium (mmol/litre)	Chloride (mmol/litre)	Potassium (mmol/litre)	Bicarbonate (mmol/litre)	Carbohydrate (g/litre)	Osmolality (mmol/litre)
Cholera stool						
Adults	130	100	20	44	–	–
Children	100	90	33	30	–	–
Oral rehydration salts						
Glucose	75	65	20	10[a]	13.5[b]	245
Rice	75	65	20	10[a]	30–50[c]	About 180
Intravenous fluids						
Lactated Ringer's	130	109	4	28[d]	–	271
Dhaka solution	133	154	13	48[e]	–	292
Normal saline	154	154	0	0	–	308

[a] Trisodium citrate (10 mmol/litre) is generally used, rather than bicarbonate.

[b] Glucose 13.5 g/litre (75 mmol/litre).

[c] Depending on degree of hydrolysis, 30–50 g rice contains about 30 mmol/litre glucose.

[d] Base is lactate.

[e] Base is acetate.

(From Sack DA, *et al.* (2004). Cholera. *Lancet*, **363**, 223–33.)

ecology of cholera. Despite the remarkable advances in understanding the pharmacological mechanisms of cholera toxin action, reliable, effective, and inexpensive means of blocking the effects of the toxin remain elusive.

With molecular genetic understanding of virulence and protective immunity, likely developments in the near future include the promise of new and better vaccines, toxin-blocking or absorption-enhancing drugs, and continued improvements in ORT, perhaps with nutrients, micronutrients, or probiotics that compete with vibrio colonization or deliver proabsorptive drugs or nutrients.

Further reading

Arifuzzaman M, *et al.* (2011). Individuals with Le(a+b−) blood group have increased susceptibility to symptomatic Vibrio cholerae O1 infection. *PLoS Negl Trop Dis*, **5**, e1413.

Chin CS, *et al.* (2011). The origin of the Haitian cholera outbreak strain. *N Engl J Med*, **364**, 33–42.

Clements J, *et al.* (2011). New-generation vaccines against cholera. *Nat Rev Gastroenterol Hepatol*, **8**, 701–10.

Desai SN, Clements JD (2011). An overview of cholera vaccines and their public health implications. *Curr Opin Pediatr*, **24**, 85–91.

Faruque SM, *et al.* (2003). Reemergence of epidemic *Vibrio cholerae* O139, Bangladesh. *Emerg Infect Dis*, **9**, 1116–22.

Field M (2003). Intestinal ion transport and the pathophysiology of diarrhea. *J Clin Invest*, **111**, 931–43.

Guerrant RL (2006). Cholera: still teaching hard lessons. *N Engl J Med*, **354**, 2500–2.

Mutreja A *et al.* (2011). Evidence for several waves of global transmission in the seventh cholera pandemic. *Nature* **477**, 462–5.

Sack DA, *et al.* (2004). Cholera. *Lancet*, **363**, 223–33.

Saha DS, *et al.* (2006). Single-dose azithromycin for the treatment of cholera in adults. *N Engl J Med*, **354**, 2452–62.

Salim A, *et al.* (2005). *Vibrio cholerae* pathogenic clones. *Emerg Infect Dis*, **11**, 1758–60.

Son MS, *et al.* (2011). Characterization of Vibrio cholera O1 El Tor biotype variant clinical isolates from Bangladesh and Haiti, including a molecular genetic analysis of virulence genes. *J Clin Microbiol*, **49**, 3739–49.

Sur D, *et al.* (2009).Efficacy and safety of a modified killed-whole-cell oral cholera vaccine in India: an interim analysis of a cluster-randomized, double-blind, placebo-controlled trial. *Lancet*, **374**, 1694–702.

Sur D, *et al.* (2011). Efficacy of a low-cost, inactivated whole-cell oral cholera vaccine: results from 3 years of follow-up of a randomized, controlled trial. *PLoS Negl Trop Dis*, **5**, e1289.

World Health Organization (2006). Cholera 2005. *Weekly Epidemiol Rec*, **81**, 297–308.

6.12 *Haemophilus influenzae*

Derrick W. Crook

Essentials

Haemophilus influenzae is a Gram-negative bacillus that is an exclusively human pathogen. There are six capsular serotypes (a–f), of which type b (Hib) is a major cause of childhood infectious disease.

Transmission occurs by close bodily contact, the main source being other children, and is usually followed by nasopharyngeal carriage, following which susceptible people may develop disease.

Clinical features—in infants Hib causes symptoms ranging from a mild nonspecific febrile illness (occult bacteraemia) to fully blown sepsis with meningitis, epiglottitis, pneumonia, septic arthritis, and cellulitis. Nontypeable *H. influenzae* (NTHi) are common nasopharyngeal commensals and may cause otitis media and conjunctivitis in children, and exacerbations of chronic bronchitis, sinusitis, and pneumonia in adults. *H. parainfluenzae, H. aphrophilus, H. paraphrophilus,* and *H. segnis* are rare causes of infective endocarditis and other sepsis.

Diagnosis and treatment—Gram staining of cerebrospinal, synovial, or pleural fluid is a key investigation, but definitive diagnosis requires culture or detection of *H. influenzae* DNA by polymerase chain reaction (PCR) methods. Aside from supportive care, treatment requires (1) appropriate antibiotics—resistance is an increasing problem: the agent of choice for invasive Hib disease is a third-generation cephalosporin with good cerebrospinal fluid penetration (e.g. ceftriaxone or cefotaxime); chloramphenicol with or without ampicillin remains effective in some developing countries. (2) corticosteroids—except in children in low-income countries, these reduce mortality, severe hearing loss, and neurological sequelae of Hib meningitis. Antibiotic treatment of noncapsulate *H. Influenzae* otitis media, sinusitis, and chronic bronchitis is widely practised but largely unsupported by evidence.

Prevention—conjugate Hib vaccines are given as part of the routine infant immunization schedule and have virtually eliminated invasive Hib disease from North America, Europe and some other countries.

Introduction

Haemophilus influenzae is a human-adapted pathogen with no other reservoir. Typically, it inhabits the nasopharynx but may also be recovered from other mucosal surfaces including genital and intestinal tracts. Despite being a fastidious organism that is relatively difficult to grow, it was first isolated as early as 1890 by Pfeiffer who mistakenly thought it was the cause of a current influenza pandemic.

Description of the organism

The genus *Haemophilus* includes *H. influenzae, H. ducreyi,* which causes chancroid, the sexually transmitted infection (Chapter 6.13), and other human-adapted species all of which are commensals: *H. parainfluenzae* (the most abundantly colonizing species), *H. aegyptius, H. aphrophilus, H. haemolyticus, H. paraphrophilus,* and *H. segnis.*

H. influenzae is a small (0.2–0.3 × 0.5–0.8 µm) Gram-negative nonmotile coccobacillus that grows well on rich media (e.g. chocolate agar which is the preferred medium) incubated in 5% CO_2. It is fastidious with the following specific growth requirements: it does not grow on nutrient agar, such as Columbia, without growth supplements X factor (haemin) and V factor (NAD). *H. influenzae* produces 2- to 3-mm-diameter grey translucent colonies after 18 to 25 h incubation. Precise speciation requires bacterial genome sequence analysis, e.g. 16s ribosomal DNA.

H. influenzae are phenotypically and genetically diverse. A minority have polysaccharide capsules and can be serologically classified in six serotypes (a to f). These strains are relatively nondiverse, consisting of few lineages, suggesting that the genes encoding the capsule were acquired relatively recently. The type b capsule is essential for the pathogenesis of bacteraemia and meningitis, a feature recognized in the early 1930s. The majority of strains are nonencapsulated and are nontypeable; these strains genetically heterogeneous.

Pathogenicity

H. influenzae expresses several cell surface features essential for colonization of the nasopharynx. These are virulence factors of which the capsule is the most important. Of the six antigenically distinct structures (types a–f), type b accounts for virtually all the invasiveness of *H. influenzae* in children. The serotype b capsule consists of a negatively charged phosphodiester-linked linear polymer of disaccharide units of polyribosylribitol phosphate (PRP) which resists phagocytosis by interfering with binding of serum complement. The capsule also resists desiccation, perhaps promoting host-to-host transmission. Serum antibody directed against serotype b capsular polysaccharide is protective. This simple observation stimulated the development of the highly successful *H. influenzae* type b (Hib) vaccine, now used routinely in national childhood immunization programmes. Modern vaccines contain PRP covalently conjugated to a protein carrier such as tetanus toxoid.

Other cell surface structures involved in pathogenesis, particularly in those strains lacking a capsule (nontypeable *H. influenzae*), include lipopolysaccharide, pili, and other adhesion proteins.

Epidemiology

Haemophilus influenzae type b

Hib is a major cause of childhood infectious disease. Acquisition occurs by close bodily contact, the main source being other children, and is usually followed by carriage. The organism dwells harmlessly for months in the nasopharynx. However, in a few susceptible individuals, acquisition immediately precedes invasive disease. Carriage rates increase from birth until 4 years and are

Table 6.12.1 Clinical manifestations of *H. influenzae* type b disease

Disease	Percentage
Meningitis	52
Pneumonia	12
Epiglottitis	10
Septicaemia	8
Cellulitis	5
Osteoarticular	4
Multifocal	6
Other	3

higher in developing countries especially where there is crowding, day care attendance, and contact with siblings. Hib immunization virtually eliminates carriage and produces a marked herd effect, protecting against disease. In 2000, it was estimated that as many as 60% of the world's children were unimmunized, but Hib vaccine is now being introduced to most parts of the world. In some parts of Asia, particularly China, Hib is far less prevalent and so the health benefits of mass vaccination may be insufficient to justify a national vaccination programme.

The main diseases caused by Hib are meningitis, bacteraemia, pneumonia, epiglottitis, and arthritis (Table 6.12.1). Before the introduction of immunization, Hib was the most important cause of childhood meningitis in the United States of America, accounting for 80% of cases (Fig. 6.12.1), and in the United Kingdom accounting for approximately 50% of cases. In contrast, it was a much less prominent cause of meningitis than *Neisseria meningitidis* in the 'meningitis' belt of Africa. In Western countries, the case fatality of Hib meningitis was about 5% and long-term morbidity (deafness and neurological and learning deficits) occurred in at least 10% of cases.

The incidence of Hib infections varies with age. Neonates are protected, after which disease peaks by 9 months of age and declines to very low levels by 4 years. Age-specific disease incidence is inversely related to serum antibodies to Hib. Risk factors for *H. influenzae* infection include complement deficiency, hypogammaglobulinaemia, hyposplenism, sickle cell anaemia, malignancy, and HIV

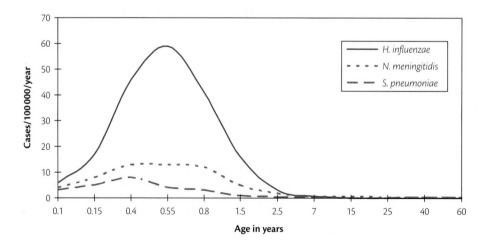

Fig. 6.12.1 Incidence of meningitis in the United States of America caused by *H. influenzae*, *N. meningitides*, and *S. pneumoniae* before the implementation of the Hib conjugate vaccine.
(Data derived from various sources.)

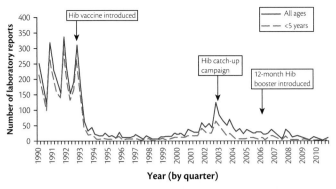

Fig. 6.12.2 Number of cases of Hib reported in England and Wales 2000–2010. (Source: Health Protection Agency http://www.hpa.org.uk/Topics/InfectiousDiseases/InfectionsAZ/HaemophilusInfluenzaeTypeB/EpidemiologicalData/HibGraph/ accessed 1 January 2012.)

infection. Ethnicity is also important, with higher rates of invasive disease observed in Native American and Aboriginal populations.

Since the implementation of Hib conjugate vaccination, the disease has virtually disappeared from North America and Europe and there has been a similar dramatic decline in The Gambia and Kenya. A striking but temporary re-emergence of Hib disease in the United Kingdom (Fig. 6.12.2) was attributed to the introduction, in 2000, of a combined Hib-acellular pertussis vaccine that induced lower Hib antibody levels.

Nontypeable *H. influenzae* (NTHi)

Nontypeable *H. influenzae* is acquired soon after birth: 20% of children are colonized in the first year of life and over 50% by 5 years. Colonization persists throughout adulthood. NTHi causes noninvasive infections in children and older adults. It is an important cause of otitis media, sinusitis, bronchitis, and post-traumatic meningitis. NTHi can cause community-acquired pneumonia in adults, which can be severe. Bacteraemia is uncommon apart from in neonates or the immunocompromised host.

Antibiotic resistance

Resistance of *H. influenzae* to antibiotics was first reported in the early 1970s. Since then, the prevalence of ampicillin-resistant β-lactamase-producing strains has risen rapidly in most parts of the world and strains resistant to tetracycline, chloramphenicol, and trimethoprim or multiresistant to these antibiotics have emerged. In recent years, β-lactamase resistance rates have remained reasonably constant in Europe at 10 to 20%. β-Lactamase-negative (BLNAR) *H. influenzae* is an emerging pathogen and high rates have been reported in certain countries, e.g. Japan (*c*.34%) and Spain (*c*.56%) although prevalence elsewhere remains low. Possible explanations for this include low vaccine coverage, under-dosing of oral ampicillin, or frequent use of cephalosporins. These strains appear to remain susceptible to ceftriaxone.

Clinical features

Hib invasive disease

In infants, clinical features vary from a mild nonspecific febrile illness, reflecting so-called occult bacteraemia, to fully blown sepsis with meningitis. Infants may present with fever and irritability alone

but severe cases show typical features of meningitis including altered mental status, stiff neck, and sepsis. In some cases there is disseminated intravascular coagulation with purpuric rash and septicaemic shock, reminiscent of meningococcaemia. Diagnosis is by examination of cerebrospinal fluid and blood culture. In older children, lumbar puncture should not be performed until cerebral oedema can be excluded by CT, but antibiotic treatment must not be delayed.

Epiglottitis is an acutely life-threatening medical emergency. Against a background of sepsis (fever, tachycardia, and tachypnoea), pronounced local signs and symptoms evolve rapidly, including sore throat, drooling, dysphagia, hoarseness, barking 'brassy' cough, and stridor. The epiglottis is inflamed and swollen, looking like a red cherry, but attempts to examine the throat may precipitate acute airway obstruction. Pneumonia is an important but relatively unrecognized feature of Hib disease. The main features are fever with signs of respiratory distress including tachypnoea, nasal flaring, and intercostal indrawing. Chest examination and radiography are diagnostic.

The child with septic arthritis shows features of sepsis, is unwilling to use the affected limb, and resists movement of the painful joint. Examination and culture of joint fluid are diagnostic. Cellulitis is rare in children and cellulitis of the neck is unusual in adults. These presentations have been increasingly associated with *H. influenzae* type f infection, especially since the introduction of Hib conjugate vaccine.

Nontypeable *H. influenzae*

Otitis media is the main clinical presentation of NTHi. This common childhood illness presents with irritability and, on otoscopy, an inflamed tympanic membrane is visible and may perforate discharging pus. Although not used routinely, tympanocentesis is the most reliable means of aetiological diagnosis. A high proportion of cases of conjunctivitis in children are caused by NTHi. Historically, *H. aegyptius* has also been associated with conjunctivitis. Culture of conjunctival swabs is the main test for making a diagnosis. Brazilian purpuric fever, a fulminant septicaemic illness with high case fatality, is also caused by *H. aegyptius*.

NTHi sinusitis presents with local pain, a sense of pressure in the head, local facial oedema, and visible pus draining from the ostia of the sinuses. Diagnosis is by skull radiography, with special (Towne's and Water's) views, or CT scan, which reveals sinus opacification and a fluid level. Sinus aspiration provides an aetiological diagnosis.

In adults, exacerbations of chronic bronchitis are commonly associated with NTHi. *H. influenzae* and *S. pneumonia* are cultured from sputum of up to 50% of cases although their precise aetiological role is uncertain.

NTHi can cause severe invasive disease such as neonatal sepsis, resembling group B streptococcal neonatal sepsis, and pneumonia in adults, particularly older people. It has also been implicated in meningitis associated with head trauma, particularly skull fracture.

Laboratory diagnosis

Culture or detection of specific DNA is essential for aetiological diagnosis. Direct examination of cerebrospinal, pleural, or synovial fluids by Gram's stain may reveal organisms with the morphological features of *H. influenzae*. This is very helpful in indicating bacterial infection but is nonspecific. Blood culture using most commercial systems yields excellent growth in both anaerobic and aerobic bottles. However, growth on agar and differentiation of *Haemophilus* spp. requires special conditions (see above).

Antibiotic susceptibility testing using antibiotic discs requires supplemented media to support the growth of *Haemophilus* spp. but this may be inaccurate and should be supplemented by measurement of β-lactamase activity. Chloramphenicol disc susceptibility is frequently inaccurate and should be supplemented by an assay for chloramphenicol acetyltransferase activity.

Capsular type b antigen can be rapidly detected in cerebrospinal fluid, sterile site fluid, or urine but is seldom used since the implementation of Hib vaccination. Polymerase chain reaction (PCR) of cerebrospinal fluid has been developed for diagnosing *Haemophilus* spp. meningitis. Capsular typing of *H. influenzae* can be achieved serologically but a PCR-based method has proved more reliable.

Treatment

Antibiotics

A third-generation cephalosporin with good cerebrospinal fluid penetration is the first-line antibiotic treatment for invasive Hib disease. High-dose ceftriaxone or cefotaxime are effective for treating *H. influenzae* meningitis and septicaemia, but cefuroxime must not be used. In developing countries, chloramphenicol alone (depending on the prevalence of chloramphenicol resistance) or in combination with ampicillin is effective therapy.

Antibiotics are commonly prescribed for otitis media, sinusitis, and chronic bronchitis, but large meta-analyses have failed to demonstrate convincing efficacy although some subgroups are benefited. Oral amoxicillin is the first-line drug. Amoxicillin/clavulanate, trimethoprim, tetracycline (adults only), and quinolones (adults only) can also be used. BLNAR *H. influenzae* appear to have *in vitro* sensitivity to ceftriaxone, which is the drug of choice, depending on local antimicrobial susceptibility patterns.

Corticosteroid treatment

Corticosteroids significantly reduce mortality, severe hearing loss, and neurological sequelae. In adults with community-acquired bacterial meningitis, corticosteroid therapy should be started with the first antibiotic dose. In children, data support the use of adjunctive corticosteroids in children only in high-income countries.

Prevention and control

PRP-conjugate vaccines are the best preventive measure for controlling Hib disease. Highly effective vaccines contain capsular antigen PRP conjugated to tetanus toxoid (PRP-T), outer membrane protein (PRP-OMP), or mutant diphtheria toxoid (PRP-CRM, HbOC). Three doses are given at intervals between the ages of 2 and 6 months. In many countries, a booster dose is given at age 1 to 2 years.

Rifampicin, 20 mg/kg orally once a day for 4 days, eradicates carriage and is believed to prevent secondary cases among close contacts. This is appropriate only where they have not received Hib vaccine.

Other nasopharyngeal *Haemophilus* spp.

H. parainfluenzae

H. parainfluenzae is a well-adapted commensal that colonizes virtually everyone soon after birth but is rarely associated with disease. It has been isolated in cases of infective endocarditis, neurosurgical meningitis, prosthetic device infection, and brain and liver abscesses. It is treated in the same way as *H. influenzae*.

Rare species

H. aphrophilus, *H. paraphrophilus*, and *H. segnis* are implicated in fewer than 2% of all cases of infective endocarditis and in brain or lung abscesses and empyema fluid. Since they are slow growing, they may be missed if blood cultures are not incubated for prolonged periods. Antibiotic treatment is the same as for *H. influenzae*.

Further reading

Adegbola RA, *et al.* (2005). Elimination of *Haemophilus influenzae* type b (Hib) disease from The Gambia after the introduction of routine immunisation with a Hib conjugate vaccine: a prospective study. *Lancet*, **366**, 144–50.

Barbour ML, *et al.* (1995). The impact of conjugate vaccine on carriage of *Haemophilus influenzae* type b. *J Infect Dis*, **171**, 93–8.

Frazer DW (1982). *Haemophilus influenzae* in the community and the home. In: Sell SH, Wright PF (eds) *Haemophilus influenzae*: epidemiology, immunology and prevention of disease. Elsevier Science, New York.

Kim KS (2010). Acute bacterial meningitis in infants and children. *Lancet Infect Dis*, **10**, 32–42.

Morris SK, Moss WJ, Halsey N (2008). *Haemophilus influenzae* type b conjugate vaccine use and effectiveness. *Lancet Infect Dis*, **8**, 435–43.

Murphy TF (2003). Respiratory infections caused by non-typeable *Haemophilus influenzae*. *Curr Opin Infect Dis*, **16**, 129–34.

Peltola H (2000). Worldwide *Haemophilus influenzae* type b disease at the beginning of the 21st century: global analysis of the disease burden 25 years after the use of the polysaccharide vaccine and a decade after the advent of conjugates. *Clin Microbiol Rev*, **13**, 302–17.

Prasad K, Karlupia N, Kumar A (2009). Treatment of bacterial meningitis: an overview of Cochrane systematic reviews. *Respir Med*, **103**, 945–50.

Schaad UB, *et al.* (1990). A comparison of ceftriaxone and cefuroxime for the treatment of bacterial meningitis in children. *N Engl J Med*, **322**, 141–7.

Ulanova M, Tsang RS (2009). Invasive *Haemophilus influenzae* disease: changing epidemiology and host-parasite interactions in the 21st century. *Infect Genet Evol*, **9**, 94–605.

Watt JP, Wolfson LJ, O'Brien KL, *et al.* (2009). Burden of disease caused by *Haemophilus influenzae* type b in children younger than 5 years: global estimates. *Lancet*, **374**, 903–11.

Zwahlen A, *et al.* (1989). The molecular basis of pathogenicity in *Haemophilus influenzae*: comparative virulence of genetically-related capsular transformants and correlation with changes at the capsulation locus cap. *Microb Pathog*, **7**, 225–35.

6.13 *Haemophilus ducreyi* and chancroid

Nigel O'Farrell

Essentials

Haemophilus ducreyi, which should on phylogenetic grounds be reclassified as an *Actinobacillus* is a Gram-negative, facultative anaerobic bacillus that is the cause of chancroid, which is endemic in sub-Saharan Africa and the Caribbean, although the overall global incidence of the condition has decreased dramatically since the mid 1990s.

Clinical features—after an incubation period of 4 to 7 days, presentation is with a tender genital papule that develops into a pustule and then an ulcer with a ragged undermined edge and a yellow base that bleeds readily. The usual sites of infection in men are the prepuce and coronal sulcus, and in women the labia minora and fourchette. Inguinal lymphadenopathy is found in about half the male cases. Chancroid is an important risk factor for the transmission of HIV infection. HIV infection may result in atypical manifestations if chancroid.

Diagnosis and treatment—nucleic acid amplification tests are the optimal method of diagnosing *H. ducreyi*. Treatment is with ciprofloxacin, erythromycin, azithromycin, or ceftriaxone.

Introduction

The causative organism is *Haemophilus ducreyi*, a Gram-negative facultative anaerobic bacillus. Chancroid has also been known as soft sore (*ulcus molle*) and was first differentiated from syphilis by Ricord in 1838 in France. In 1889 in Naples, Ducrey inoculated the forearms of patients with material from their own genital ulcers and maintained serial ulcers through multiple generations. The first successful culture was undertaken by Lenglet in 1898. The Ito–Reenstierna test was developed subsequently using a commercial antigen for intradermal testing and proved positive in 90% of true cases.

Aetiology

Recent phylogenetic studies suggest that the causative organism should be reclassified as an *Actinobacillus* of the Pasteurellaceae. The organism is small, nonmotile, and nonspore-forming Gram-negative rod that requires enriched media for growth. Colonies can be seen after 48 h incubation in 5% CO_2 and are greyish in colour. These colonies are cohesive and can be pushed across culture media with a thin wire. Microscopic examination using Gram's stain shows streptobacillary chaining.

Epidemiology

Chancroid is endemic in eastern and southern Africa and the Caribbean. In Asia, cases in India and Thailand used to be fairly common but have decreased recently and are now only sporadic.

Overall, the global incidence of chancroid has decreased dramatically since the mid-1990s when it accounted for 30 to 50% of genital ulcers in southern Africa. This may reflect changes in sexual behaviour, the increased use of and adherence to syndromic management for genital ulcers that included effective antibiotic cover for chancroid, or some other unknown factors.

Sporadic outbreaks have been reported in the West. These have usually been associated with sex work and have been brought under control using intensive partner notification schemes.

The male to female ratio is about 5 to 1. Chancroid is more common in uncircumcised than circumcised men. This may reflect inferior standards of genital hygiene and a tendency for small microabrasions to develop in the subpreputial space that might provide a portal of entry for infection. Asymptomatic carriage has been identified in women but is uncommon.

Pathology and pathogenesis

The pathogenesis of chancroid is incompletely understood. Bacterial adherence to susceptible cells appears to involve interaction between a protein mediator and liopoligosaccharide with fibronectin contained in the extracellular matrix, followed by the elaboration of a heat shock protein (GroEL). A cytotoxin, similar to cytolethal distending toxin, appears to play an important role in epithelial injury and ulcer formation.

The histological features include a superficial purulent exudate in the epidermis and a perivascular and interstitial mononuclear cell infiltrate, containing CD4+ T-lymphocytes, in the dermis. This may partly explain the increased risk of HIV transmission among people with chancroid.

Clinical features

The usual incubation period is 4 to 10 days (range 1–5 days) and there are no prodromal symptoms. Lesions start as a tender papule that develops into a pustule and then an ulcer. Classically, ulcers have a ragged undermined edge with a grey or yellow base that bleeds when touched. Lesions may be single or multiple.

The usual sites of infection are the prepuce, coronal sulcus, frenulum, and glans in men, and the labia minora and fourchette in women. Ulcers of the vaginal wall and cervix are uncommon. Extragenital lesions are rare but have been reported on the fingers, breasts, and inner thighs. *H. ducreyi* does not disseminate systemically.

Clinical variants can occur. These include giant phagedenic ulcers, dwarf chancroid similar to herpes, follicular chancroid similar to pyogenic infection, and single painless ulcers not unlike syphilis.

Painful inguinal lymphadenopathy is found in about one-half the male cases but less so in women. These lymph glands may develop into buboes that should be managed by aspiration rather than incision and drainage. Fluctuant buboes may rupture spontaneously causing delayed healing.

The differential diagnosis includes syphilis, genital herpes, lymphogranuloma venereum, and donovanosis. Mixed infections with other causes of genital ulceration should always be considered as coinfection with syphilis has been documented.

The presence of HIV infection may result in atypical manifestations, for example numerous lesions, extragenital involvement, or slow resolution after treatment.

Laboratory diagnosis

Nucleic acid amplification tests (NAATs) are now the optimal method of diagnosing *H. ducreyi* but their availability remains limited in areas where chancroid is found. Primers have been developed to amplify sequences from the *H. ducreyi* 16S ribosomal RNA gene, the *rrs* (16S) to *rrl* (23S) ribosomal intergenic spacer region, and the *groEL* gene. Multiplex polymerase chain reaction tests have been developed that can identify infection with *H. ducreyi*, *Treponema pallidum*, and *Herpes simplex* virus types 1 and 2 from genital ulcers.

Antigen detection using fluorescence techniques may be useful but is expensive. Serological tests are unable to differentiate between old and new infections and have limited application.

Culture was the usual method of diagnosis of chancroid until relatively recently but has now been overtaken by NAATs. Culture media must be fresh and may need fine adjustment depending on the characteristics of local strains of *H. ducreyi*. Two culture media are required to achieve a reasonable sensitivity of 50 to 80%. Media used include gonococcal agar base and Mueller–Hinton with various additives and supplements. Vancomycin may be used to inhibit Gram-positive bacteria. Cultures should be incubated at 33°C with 5% carbon dioxide in a humid atmosphere. Thioglycolate haemin-based transport medium may allow storage of viable organisms at 4°C for 24 h or possibly longer. Most strains are β-lactamase producers. *H. ducreyi* reduces nitrate to nitrite and all strains are oxidase positive and catalase negative. Gram-stained smears of material from ulcers may show characteristic Gram-negative coccobacilli in a 'school of fish' or 'railroad track' appearance.

Histology shows superficial necrosis with large numbers of neutrophils, endothelial proliferation, and infiltration with plasma cells, lymphocytes, and fibroblasts.

Treatment

Current treatment of chancroid comprises one of the following regimens: ciprofloxacin (500 mg twice daily for 3 days), erythromycin (500 mg three times daily for 7 days; can be used in pregnant women), azithromycin (a single oral dose of 1 g), or ceftriaxone (a single dose of 250 mg intramuscularly). Trimethoprim/sulphamethoxazole is no longer recommended. Healing of ulcers is usually achieved after 7 to 14 days. Longer courses of treatment are sometimes required in HIV-positive patients who should be followed up until healing is complete. Single-dose treatment should probably not be given to HIV-positive patients.

In the preantibiotic era, circumcision, saline soaks, and improved hygiene were recommended. Initially organisms were sensitive to penicillin but resistance emerged fairly rapidly. Trimethoprim/sulphamethoxazole then became the mainstay of treatment but resistance to this antibiotic emerged in the early 1990s.

Chancroid and HIV

Chancroid has been identified as an important risk factor for the bidirectional transmission of HIV, particularly in eastern and southern Africa. In some high-risk groups it was undoubtedly an important factor in driving the initial spread of HIV. At the biological level, the mechanism for this is likely to be that chancroid ulcers allow a route of entry and exit for HIV and are likely to bleed when subject to trauma. In addition, subpreputial lesions in men that subsequently heal might result in partial phimosis with thinning of the superficial mucosa. This mucosa would then be more susceptible to trauma during sexual intercourse thereby increasing the potential risk of HIV transmission through microulcerations. There are some reports that HIV-positive men have increased numbers of ulcers that heal slowly, although this may be related to low CD4 counts.

Prevention and control

In developed countries intensive partner notification and epidemiological treatment of sexual contacts have formed the basis for managing outbreaks.

The World Health Organization has recently renewed interest in the elimination of chancroid as an additional HIV prevention strategy. In most developing countries genital ulcers have been managed by the syndromic approach. This involves treating for the most likely causes of ulceration that in the past have been syphilis and chancroid. However, the prevalence of chancroid in previously endemic countries has reduced considerably leaving genital herpes as the most frequent cause of genital ulceration. With this emergence of genital herpes, the case for treating empirically for chancroid has weakened and it may be that new epidemics of chancroid will emerge as treatment regimens change.

Further reading

Bong CT, Bauer M, Spinola SM (2002). *Haemophilus ducreyi*: clinical features, epidemiology, and prospects for disease control. *Microbes Infect*, **4**, 1141–8.

Spinola S (2008). Chancroid. In: Holmes KK, *et al.* (eds) *Sexually transmitted diseases*. McGraw-Hill, New York.

Spinola SM, Bauer ME, Munson RS (2002). Immunopathogenesis of *Haemophilus ducreyi* infection (chancroid). *Infect Immun*, **70**, 1667–76.

Trees DL, Morse SA (1995). Chancroid and *Haemophilus ducreyi*: an update. *Clin Microbiol Rev*, **8**, 357–75.

6.14 Bordetella infection

Cameron Grant

Essentials

Bordetella are small Gram-negative coccobacilli, of which *Bordetella pertussis* is the most important human pathogen. It is the cause of whooping cough, which is one of the 10 leading causes of childhood death worldwide. Transmission of this highly infectious organism is primarily by aerosolized droplets, and the condition is very infectious.

Clinical features—presentation varies with age, immunization and previous infection: (1) infants—apnoea, cyanosis, and paroxysmal cough; (2) nonimmunized children—cough, increasing in severity with distressing, repeated, forceful expirations followed by a gasping inhalation (the 'whoop'); (3) children immunized in infancy—whooping, vomiting, sputum production; (4) adults—cough, post-tussive vomiting. Atypical mild illness is common.

Complications include pneumonia, pulmonary hypertension, seizures and encephalopathy. Most deaths occur in those less than 2 months old.

Diagnosis and treatment—culture lacks sensitivity; the preferred diagnostic methods are polymerase chain reaction (PCR) detection from nasopharyngeal samples and serology (IgG antibodies to pertussis toxin). Macrolide antibiotics (usually erythromycin) are recommended if started within 4 weeks of illness onset.

Prevention—Pertussis vaccines protect against disease more than infection. Preventing severe disease in young children remains the primary goal, hence schedules consist of a three-dose infant series and subsequent booster doses. Acellular vaccines enable immunization schedules to include adolescents and adults. Antibiotic prophylaxis is given when there is an infant at risk of exposure.

Introduction

Seven *Bordetella* species cause human infections. *Bordetella pertussis*, as the principal cause of whooping cough (pertussis), is the most important. Pertussis is one of the 10 leading causes of childhood death.

The epidemiology of *B. pertussis* infection and pertussis disease differ. Immunization has caused a large reduction in pertussis disease but minimal change in the circulation of *B. pertussis*. Eradication of the disease is not currently possible.

Historical perspective

Before the introduction of immunization, pertussis was a predominant child killer. In the 1930s in the United States of America pertussis caused more infant deaths than measles, diphtheria, poliomyelitis, and scarlet fever combined. With mass immunization, disease incidence has decreased dramatically.

Aetiology, genetics, pathogenesis, and pathology

Two of the seven *Bordetella* species that infect humans, *B. pertussis* and human-adapted *B. parapertussis*, are strictly human pathogens. They evolved independently from a common *B. bronchiseptica* ancestor. The *B. pertussis* population is continuously evolving. As a result antigenic variation occurs between *B. pertussis* in circulation and the *B. pertussis* vaccine strains.

In immunocompromised hosts *B. bronchiseptica* and *B. hinzii* causes respiratory illnesses and *B. holmesii* causes respiratory illnesses, bacteraemia, and endocarditis. *B. trematum* is occasionally isolated from ear and skin infections and *B. petrii* from patients with cystic fibrosis.

B. pertussis is highly infectious and each primary case produces approximately 15 secondary cases. Transmission is primarily by aerosolized droplets. There is an average of 2 weeks between successive cases. In immunized populations the household secondary attack rate remains greater than 80%, although many such infections are asymptomatic.

Pathogenesis is incompletely understood. *Bordetella* spp. have numerous virulence factors including filamentous haemagglutinin, fimbriae, pertactin, pertussis toxin (PT), adenylate cyclase, and lipopolysaccharides. Several affect immune regulation. Filamentous haemagglutinin interacts with macrophages, altering cytokine production and inhibiting T-cell proliferation. Pertactin and fimbriae are implicated in attachment to host epithelial cells, and fimbriae interact with monocytes/macrophages. Adenylate cyclase has anti-inflammatory and antiphagocytic functions. Pertussis is characterized by an inadequate immunological response. Impairment of the immune response by *B. pertussis* virulence factors is a potential mechanism that contributes to disease severity.

B. pertussis organisms multiply on the ciliated respiratory epithelium. Necrosis occurs within the bronchial epithelium. A necrotizing bronchitis and bronchopneumonia is present in most fatal cases. Coinfection with other respiratory pathogens is frequent in fatal cases.

Epidemiology

Underestimation and how this varies with age and surveillance intensity is central to understanding pertussis epidemiology. Pertussis affects all ages; however, incidence has always been highest in infants and children. Since the 1990s there has been an increase in reported pertussis in many countries. This re-emergence of pertussis is due to several factors including suboptimal immunization coverage and timeliness plus greater awareness and improved laboratory diagnosis of a disease for which neither natural infection nor immunization induces lifelong protection. There is also evidence of pathogen adaptation with clonal expansion of strains in recent epidemics in Europe.

Mortality

The propensity for pertussis to kill young infants is unique among vaccine-preventable diseases, with the exception of tetanus.

Pertussis causes approximately 2% of deaths globally of children younger than 5 years old. Estimates are complicated by the relationship between pertussis and malnutrition. Malnutrition contributes to more than one-half of the deaths in this age group. A prolonged period of weight loss frequently complicates pertussis in the developing world.

In the developed world it is estimated that there are three times more deaths from pertussis than are reported. Pertussis deaths occur despite intensive care. Treatment of infants with critical pertussis illness remains challenging.

Morbidity

Most pertussis incidence estimates are based on passive notification which identifies only 6 to 25% of cases. The proportion of cases notified decreases with increasing age and decreasing severity.

Countries with consistently low pertussis hospitalization rates have, in common, high immunization coverage rates sustained over decades. Higher disease rates are due primarily to lower coverage, but also sometimes to lower vaccine efficacy or suboptimal immunization schedules.

Prevention

Neither disease nor immunization confer lifelong immunity. Pertussis vaccines protect against disease more than infection. Schedules consist of a three-dose infant series and subsequent booster doses. Pertussis remains endemic in adolescents and adults. Without boosters it is also endemic in school children.

Whole cell and acellular pertussis vaccines are combined with other antigens. Acellular vaccines contain between one and five *B. pertussis* antigens. The most efficacious whole cell and acellular vaccines induce protection against clinical disease in approximately 85% of recipients.

In order to minimize the pertussis risk to infants the primary series must be completed without delay. However, without booster doses, timely completion of the primary series is insufficient to prevent disease in infants.

Immunity induced by whole-cell and acellular pertussis vaccines persists for 5 to 10 years after completion of a primary series. T-cell responses to whole-cell and acellular vaccines differ. Protection following both disease and immunization is superior to either alone; hence those who have had pertussis should be immunized.

With the recognition that adolescents and adults spread pertussis to infants, the timing of booster doses has been reconsidered. Randomized trials have confirmed the efficacy and safety of acellular vaccines in adolescents and adults. Several counties have scheduled adolescent booster doses. The targeted immunization of adults in close contact with infants, for example child healthcare workers, is also recommended in some countries.

Clinical features

Presentation varies with age, immunization, and previous infection. Atypical mild illness is common.

In infants apnoea, cyanosis, and paroxysmal cough are key symptoms. These can occur sufficiently early in the illness that clinical differentiation from other infections is impossible. Thus pertussis must be considered in infants presenting with an acute life-threatening event or apnoea.

Pertussis in the nonimmunized child is a coughing illness increasing in severity over several weeks with distressing repeated forceful expirations followed by a gasping inhalation. Between paroxysms symptoms can be minimal. The contrast between parental descriptions of the previous night's events and the normal appearance the following morning is deceiving. Following pertussis, viral respiratory tract infections can cause the coughing paroxysms to recur.

In school-aged children immunized in infancy, clinical symptoms which distinguish pertussis are whooping, vomiting, sputum production, and the absence of wheezing.

Most *B. pertussis* infections in adults are asymptomatic or are atypical with few symptoms. Persistent cough, not infrequently for more than a month, is the cardinal feature of clinical pertussis in adults. Cough is worse at night and often paroxysmal. Adults describe being woken by a choking sensation. Post-tussive vomiting and whoop are frequent.

Differential diagnosis

Not considering pertussis in someone with prolonged cough is a more important cause of a missed diagnosis than is an atypical presentation. In infants, coinfection with respiratory viruses occurs not infrequently, causing more severe disease and diagnostic confusion.

A careful history of coughing illnesses in other household members is critical. Successive household members of varying ages are symptomatic over weeks to months rather than having almost concurrent respiratory illnesses.

Infections with *Mycoplasma pneumoniae*, *Chlamydia pneumoniae*, *C. trachomatis*, adenoviruses, and other respiratory viruses can cause illnesses which overlap clinically with pertussis. Particularly because it is also worse at night, cough from sinusitis can be confused with pertussis.

B. pertussis infection causes approximately 20% of prolonged coughing illnesses in adolescents and adults. Presentation is often delayed until symptoms have persisted for several weeks. Other causes of chronic cough such as asthma, gastro-oesophageal reflux, tuberculosis, and malignancy need to be considered.

Table 6.14.1 Antibiotics for the treatment or prevention of pertussis

Drug	Dosage	Regimen	Side effects	Contraindications
Erythromycin	Children, 40–50 mg/kg per day Adults, 1–2 g/day	Four divided doses for 14 days[a]	Gastrointestinal irritation, abdominal cramps, nausea, vomiting; hypertrophic pyloric stenosis has been reported in infants	Known sensitivity to any macrolide antibiotic; use with caution in neonates
Azithromycin[b]	10 mg/kg (maximum 500 mg) as a single dose on day 1; 5 mg/kg (maximum 250 mg) thereafter	Lower dose once daily for an additional 4 days	Allergic reactions and hepatic toxicity	Known sensitivity to any macrolide antibiotic
Clarithromycin	20 mg/kg per day (maximum 1 g/day)	Two divided doses daily for 7 days	Allergic reactions and hepatic toxicity	Known sensitivity to any macrolide antibiotic
Trimethoprim/ sulfamethoxazole	Trimethoprim, 8 mg/kg per day (maximum 320 mg/day); sulfamethoxazole, 40 mg/kg per day (maximum 1600 mg/day)	Two divided doses daily for 7 days	Rash, kernicterus in newborns	Known allergy to sulphonamides or trimethoprim; should not be given to pregnant women shortly before delivery, breastfeeding mothers, or infants< 2 months old because of the risk of kernicterus

[a] A 7-day regime of erythromycin estolate has similar efficacy to a 14-day regimen.
[b] Azithromycin is the preferred antibiotic for infants < 1 month old because of risk of idiopathic hypertrophic pyloric stenosis associated with erythromycin.
(From Hewlett EL, Edwards KM (2005). Clinical practice. Pertussis—not just for kids. *N Engl J Med*, **352**, 1215–22.)

Clinical investigation

Laboratory diagnosis of pertussis has improved with the development of polymerase chain reaction (PCR) and serological assays.

B. pertussis is a small Gram-negative coccobacillus. It is strictly aerobic and fastidious; special media such as charcoal blood agar are important. Culture lacks sensitivity. Careful collection and rapid transport of the nasopharyngeal sample to the laboratory is required. Immunization and antibiotic treatment both reduce the yield. The organism is most abundant before the onset of paroxysmal cough and is rarely recovered once cough has been present for 3 weeks.

PCR is more sensitive and rapid than culture. Sensitivity decreases with illness duration and less so with antibiotic treatment. Real-time PCR assays enable laboratory confirmation within 24 hours of specimen collection.

Antibodies to pertussis toxin are specific to *B. pertussis* with measurement of only IgG antibodies recommended. In the absence of immunization in the previous 2 years a single antibody titre of 100 IU/ml has been shown to be sensitive and specific for recent *B. pertussis* infection. A sensitive and specific oral fluid assay that measures IgG to pertussis toxin has been developed.

The preferred laboratory test varies with age and cough duration. PCR is particularly useful in infants. In older children, adolescents, and adults the sensitivity of culture and PCR is lower, and, particularly with later presentation, serology is more useful.

Criteria for diagnosis

The World Health Organization surveillance case definition is a case diagnosed as pertussis by a physician, or a person with cough for 2 weeks with at least one of paroxysms of coughing, inspiratory whoop, or post-tussive vomiting without other apparent cause. Laboratory confirmation is by isolation of *B. pertussis*; or detection of genomic sequences by PCR, or positive paired serology. Pertussis should be considered in anyone with paroxysmal cough of any duration, or cough with inspiratory whoop, or cough ending in apnoea, vomiting, or gagging.

Treatment

Antibiotic treatment reduces infectivity. *B. pertussis* cannot be isolated from most patients after 5 days of antibiotics. If started within 2 weeks of symptom onset, antibiotic treatment may decrease symptom severity.

Antibiotics are always recommended if started within 4 weeks of illness onset. To minimize transmission to young infants, treatment is recommended for 6 to 8 weeks after illness onset for pregnant women in the third trimester and healthcare workers.

Erythromycin or the newer macrolides are first-line treatment. Azithromycin is now the preferred macrolide for infants less than 1 month old. Azithromycin is as efficacious, better tolerated and requires a shorter treatment course than erythromycin. Compliance is also better with azithromycin. Antibiotic resistance is uncommon.

Prophylaxis is most important when there is an infant at risk of exposure. Interruption of household transmission is only possible if treatment is started within 3 weeks of symptom onset in the primary case and before any symptomatic secondary cases.

There are no proven efficacious agents for the treatment of pertussis-induced cough; salbutamol, diphenhydramine, and pertussis immunoglobulin are no more efficacious than placebo.

Prognosis

Pertussis in young infants is unpredictable with the potential for rapid deterioration. Complications include pneumonia, pulmonary hypertension, seizures, and encephalopathy.

Pneumonia, seizures, and encephalopathy also complicate pertussis in adults. Complications include cough-induced urinary incontinence and syncope, herniated intervertebral disc, inguinal hernia, hearing loss, angina, carotid artery dissection, and death.

Areas of uncertainty or controversy

Alternatives to the current immunization schedule of acellular vaccines that could improve protection of young infants are being considered. Potential strategies include maternal immunization during pregnancy or the postpartum period and infant immunization at birth.

The role that transplacentally acquired antibodies could play in preventing infant pertussis is not known. They appear to reduce severity of infant pertussis.

Vaccine adverse events

Many adverse events have been attributed to the whole cell pertussis vaccine. Febrile convulsions (risk 1 in 1750 to 1 in 13 400 doses), persistent crying (6 in 100 to 1 in 1000 doses), hypotonic hyporesponsive episodes (1 in 350 to 1 in 28 500 doses), and anaphylaxis (1 in 50 000 doses) are recognized associations. There is no causal relationship between pertussis vaccine and infantile spasms, cot death, brain damage, or death. Although acellular pertussis vaccines are less reactogenic (Table 6.14.2), the potential exists for causal relationships to be proposed for temporal associations between vaccine administration and otherwise unrelated events.

The frequency of local injection-site reactions increases in children receiving a fourth or fifth dose of acellular pertussis vaccine and with pain only for a sixth dose given during adolescence.

Table 6.14.2 Frequency of reactions after any doses during immunization with three doses of one of 13 acellular or one whole cell pertussis vaccine

Reaction	Acellular pertussis vaccine (n = 1818) (%)	Lederle whole cell pertussis vaccine (n = 371) (%)
Local reactions		
Redness	35	73
Swelling	24	61
Pain	7	40
Systemic reactions		
Fever ≥ 38°C	16	38
Fussiness	17	42
Drowsiness	43	62
Vomiting	13	14
Anorexia	22	35

(From Decker MD, *et al.* (1995). Comparison of 13 acellular pertussis vaccines: adverse reactions. *Pediatrics*, **96**, 557–66.)

Future research

Much remains to be learnt about the pathogenesis. What causes the prolonged cough remains unknown. Vaccines containing antigens with greater efficacy against *B. pertussis* infection would potentially decrease endemic disease. Improved surveillance is required in both developed and developing countries.

Likely developments in the near future

The need to extend the duration of immunization-induced protection will lead to further refinement of immunization schedules.

Further reading

Black RE, *et al.* (2010). Global, regional, and national causes of child mortality in 2008: a systematic analysis. *Lancet*, **375**, 1969–87. [Contribution of pertussis to global child mortality.]

Cherry JD. (2005). The epidemiology of pertussis: a comparison of the epidemiology of the disease pertussis with the epidemiology of *Bordetella pertussis* infection. *Pediatrics*, **115**, 1422–7. [Review of pertussis epidemiology.]

Centers for Disease Control (2011). Updated recommendations for use of tetanus toxoid, reduced diphtheria toxoid and acellular pertussis vaccine (Tdap) in pregnant women and persons who have or anticipate having close contact with an infant aged <12 months—Advisory Committee on Immunization Practices (ACIP). *MMWR Recomm Rep*, **60**, 1424–6. [Safety of pertussis immunization during pregnancy.].

Crowcroft NS, Pebody RG. (2006). Recent developments in pertussis. *Lancet*, **367**, 1926–36. [Comprehensive review of pertussis.]

Crowcroft NS, *et al.* (2003). How best to estimate the global burden of pertussis? *Lancet Infect Dis*, **3**, 413–18. [This manuscript defines the global pertussis burden.]

Fry NK, *et al.* (2004). Laboratory diagnosis of pertussis infections: the role of PCR and serology. *J Med Microbiol*, **53**, 519–25. [Review of laboratory diagnosis of pertussis.]

Halperin SA (2007). The control of pertussis—2007 and beyond. *N Engl J Med*, **356**, 110–13. [Recent changes in pertussis epidemiology.]

He Q, Mertsola J (2008). Factors contributing to pertussis resurgence. *Future Microbiol*, **3**, 329–39. [Adaptation of B. pertussis to immunization.]

Hewlett EL, Edwards KM. (2005). Clinical practice. Pertussis—not just for kids. *N Engl J Med*, **352**, 1215–22. [Comprehensive clinical review of pertussis.]

Langley JM, *et al.* (2004). Azithromycin is as effective as and better tolerated than erythromycin estolate for the treatment of pertussis. *Pediatrics*, **114**, e96–101. [Trial demonstrating that azithromycin was as effective and better tolerated than erythromycin for the treatment of pertussis.]

Litt DJ, et al. (2006). Detection of anti-pertussis toxin IgG in oral fluids for use in diagnosis and surveillance of Bordetella pertussis infection in children and young adults. *J Med Microbiol*, **55**, 1223–8. [Oral fluid assay for diagnosis of pertusiss].

Mattoo S, Cherry JD. (2005). Molecular pathogenesis, epidemiology, and clinical manifestations of respiratory infections due to *Bordetella pertussis* and other *Bordetella* subspecies. *Clin Microbiol Rev*, **18**, 326–82. [Comprehensive review of bordetella infections.]

Sawal M, *et al.* (2009). Fulminant pertussis: a multi-center study with new insights into the clinico-pathological mechanisms. *Pediatr Pulmonol*, **44**, 970–80. [Review of pathophysiology of fatal pertussis.]

Ward JI, *et al.* (2005). Efficacy of an acellular pertussis vaccine among adolescents and adults. *N Engl J Med*, **353**, 1555–63. [Important trial demonstrating efficacy of an acellular pertussis vaccine in adults.]

Wood N, McIntyre P (2008). Pertussis: review of epidemiology, diagnosis, management and prevention. *Paediatr Respir Rev*, **9**, 201–11. [Review of treatment of pertussis.]

6.15 Melioidosis and glanders

S.J. Peacock

Essentials

Melioidosis is a serious infection caused by the soil-dwelling Gram-negative bacillus *Burkholderia pseudomallei*. It is most commonly reported in north-east Thailand and northern Australia, but is increasingly recognized around the world. Infection is predominantly acquired through bacterial inoculation, often related to occupation, and mostly affects adults between the fourth and sixth decade who have risk factors such as diabetes mellitus and renal impairment.

Clinical features—these are very varied, ranging from a septicaemic illness (the commonest presentation), often associated with concomitant pneumonia (50%) and other features including hepatic and splenic abscesses, to a chronic illness characterized by fever, weight loss, and wasting. Case fatality is 43% in north-east Thailand (20 to 30% in children) and 14% in Australia.

Diagnosis and treatment—diagnosis requires culture of *B. pseudomallei* (a hazard group 3 biological agent) from any specimen. Serological tests should be with used in caution in those with suspected melioidosis who are culture-negative. Aside from supportive care and drainage of collections of pus, prolonged antimicrobial therapy is required, with a parenteral phase of 10 to 14 days (ceftazidime or a carbapenem) followed by oral therapy for 12 to 20 weeks (trimethoprim-sulfamethoxazole). *B. pseudomallei* is difficult to eradicate and recurrence occurs in 6% of cases within the first year.

Glanders—this resembles melioidosis and is caused by *Burkholderia mallei*, which appears to have evolved from a single clone of *B. pseudomallei*.

Genetics and pathogenesis

The *Burkholderia pseudomallei* K96243 genome is composed of two chromosomes of 4.07 Mbp and 3.17 Mbp which show functional partitioning of genes. The large chromosome encodes many of the core functions associated with metabolism and growth, while the smaller chromosome carries more accessory functions associated with adaptation and survival in different environments. At least 6% of the genome is made up of putative genomic islands that have probably been acquired via horizontal gene transfer. Findings from multilocus sequence typing (MLST) of *B. pseudomallei* are indicative of a high rate of genetic recombination, and comparison by MLST of isolates from Thailand and northern Australia has demonstrated intercontinental geographical segregation between the two groups.

Experimental studies indicate a role in virulence for lipopolysaccharide, capsular polysaccharide, flagella, a type IV secretion system and a type III secretion system (TTSS3) that shares homology with the *inv/spa/prg* TTSS of *Salmonella typhimurium* and the *ipa/mxi/spa* TTSS of *Shigella flexneri*. Other candidate virulence factors include a siderophore for iron acquisition, and secreted proteins such as haemolysin, lipases, and proteases. Data from *in vitro* models and postmortem studies indicate that *B. pseudomallei* is equipped for intracellular survival. The organism survives and replicates within neutrophils and monocytes, and employs multiple mechanisms to escape macrophage killing and evade host immunity.

Epidemiology, aetiology, and prevention

The first reported case of melioidosis occurred in a 40-year-old morphine addict in Rangoon (Yangon), Myanmar in 1911. The incidence of recognized cases is highest in north-east Thailand and northern Australia, but melioidosis is also known to occur in numerous countries across south and east Asia, in Central America, Ecuador, and Brazil, and in several countries in Africa. The route of infection is most commonly via skin inoculation or bacterial contamination of wounds, but other routes include ingestion, inhalation, and aspiration including near drowning. Factors associated with disease acquisition include adverse weather conditions especially heavy rain, and integrity of the host immune system. Melioidosis incidence peaks between the fourth and sixth decades; children represent one-sixth of infected individuals in north-east Thailand. Diabetes mellitus, excess alcohol consumption, chronic renal failure, and chronic lung disease are independent risk factors. One or more risk factors are present in approximately 80% of affected adults but only 30% of children (most commonly penetrating injury). The majority of cases in Thailand occur in rice farmers who work without protective footwear. Avoidance of contact with the environment in which *B. pseudomallei* exists is likely to prove an effective preventive measure, but such strategies are not in place across rural Asia.

Clinical features, differential diagnosis, and criteria for diagnosis

The period between *B. pseudomallei* exposure and onset of clinical manifestations is difficult to define since most patients do not report a specific inoculation event. An incubation period of 1 to 21 days (mean 9 days) was determined for 25% of cases in Australia with a specific inoculation event, but this may not be representative for cases overall. The longest recorded incubation period is 62 years. Time from onset of disease to clinical presentation is also variable; in north-east Thailand, approximately one-third of patients have symptoms for less than 7 days, one-half for 7 to 28 days, and the remainder have symptoms for more than 28 days.

Manifestations range from a fulminant sepsis and rapid death to a chronic illness characterized by fever, weight loss, and wasting. The most frequent clinical picture is a septicaemic illness, often associated with bacterial dissemination to distant sites such that concomitant pneumonia (Fig. 6.15.1) and hepatic and splenic abscesses are common. Pneumonia occurs in around 50% of patients. Infection may also occur in bone, joints, skin (superficial pustules and cutaneous abscesses, Fig. 6.15.2), soft tissue (pyomyositis), and prostate. A specific syndrome of meningoencephalitis with brain stem involvement and risk of respiratory arrest, flaccid paraparesis, or peripheral motor weakness occurs in 4% of cases in northern Australia. Central nervous system infections occur in around 1.5% of melioidosis patients in Thailand (Fig. 6.15.3), although meningoencephalitis is not recognized in this setting. Involvement of the vascular tree is recognized but unusual. Acute parotitis accounts for one-third of

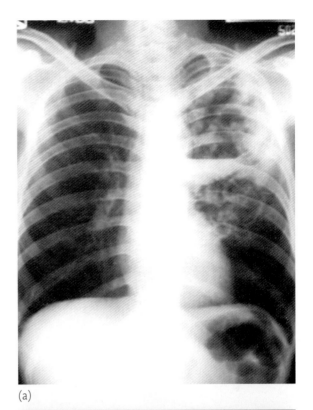

(a)

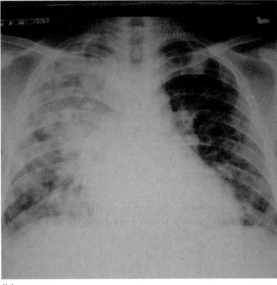

(b)

Fig. 6.15.1 Chest radiographs of two patients with melioidosis. (a) Left upper lobe involvement with abscess formation. (b) Diffuse pulmonary involvement with marked radiological changes in the right lung field.

childhood cases in Thailand but is unusual in adulthood. The number of sites involved is variable and possible combinations include positive blood cultures but no other focus, positive blood cultures and one or more distant foci, and negative blood cultures with one or more foci. Classification of patients into different categories based on these observations has been suggested, but it may be more accurate to consider disease as a continuum.

A high index of suspicion is required in order to diagnose melioidosis in the nonendemic setting. Clinicians should consider

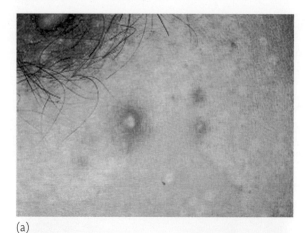

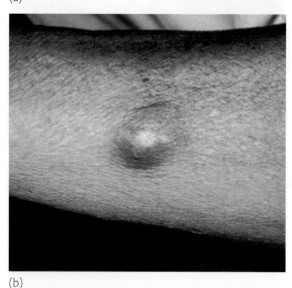

(a)

(b)

Fig. 6.15.2 Skin and soft tissue involvement in two patients with melioidosis. Skin pustules (a) and subcutaneous abscess (b) occurring as secondary foci of infection associated with disseminated infection.

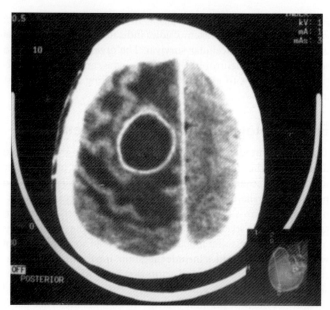

Fig. 6.15.3 CT brain scan of a patient presenting with fever, headache, confusion, and hemiparesis. The image shows a ring-enhancing lesion with surrounding oedema in the right frontoparietal lobe, pus from which grew *B. pseudomallei*.

In addition, *B. pseudomallei* is classified as a hazard group 3 biological agent and safe handling requires use of a containment level 3 laboratory. Samples of blood, urine, throat swab, and respiratory secretions should be obtained for culture from all patients, together with pus and wound swabs where relevant. All sample types should be taken where possible since site of culture positivity may not necessarily relate to clinical foci of infection (as an extreme example, it is possible for a throat swab to be positive in a patient with a splenic abscess in the absence of features of respiratory infection). *B. pseudomallei* colonization is extremely rare and isolation of even a single colony from a low quality sample can clinch the diagnosis. Bacterial detection and identification using the polymerase chain reaction is described but is not available in routine microbiology laboratories, and is reported to be less sensitive than culture.

Negative microbiological cultures do not rule out melioidosis since patients who have been commenced on effective antimicrobial agents may be culture-negative. Serodiagnostic tests should be considered for the investigation of persons with suspected melioidosis who are culture-negative, but should be interpreted with caution. A rising antibody titre to *B. pseudomallei* in paired serum samples taken 2 weeks or more apart in an individual who does not normally reside in an area where melioidosis is endemic is highly supportive of the diagnosis of melioidosis in the presence of clinical features of disease. This ideal is often difficult to achieve since the potential exposure event may have occurred months or years before presentation and may not be remembered. In this case, a single high antibody titre at presentation is indicative of exposure. Serodiagnostic tests in people who have resided in areas where melioidosis is endemic have very limited value since background seropositivity in the healthy population is high and the detection of antibodies to *B. pseudomallei* has a low

the possibility in patients with a fever who have one or more of the following: (1) residency at any time in an endemic region or a relevant travel history; (2) an occupation or other pursuits that may have resulted in contact with soil or water containing *B. pseudomallei* (including military personnel who are on exercise or active service); and (3) the presence of risk factors such as diabetes mellitus or renal disease. The variability in clinical features is such that it is often impossible on clinical grounds to differentiate between melioidosis and other acute and chronic bacterial infections, including tuberculosis. Confirmation of the diagnosis relies on good practices for specimen collection, laboratory culture, and isolation of *B. pseudomallei*.

Clinical investigation and confirmation of diagnosis

Early discussion with the clinical microbiology laboratory is important during investigation of suspected cases. This will raise awareness for the presence of a significant pathogen in a mixed culture.

diagnostic accuracy for active melioidosis. A small number of patients with culture-proven melioidosis do not mount a detectable antibody response, and a negative serological result does not rule out exposure or active infection. The most commonly used serodiagnostic method is the indirect haemagglutination assay (IHA). Cut-off points ranging from an IHA titre of 1:10 to 1:40 have been used to indicate exposure.

In patients with melioidosis, laboratory tests should be employed to detect acute renal failure, abnormal liver function tests, and anaemia, all of which are well recognized during severe melioidosis. Arterial blood gases should be taken in patients with lung involvement and/or any evidence of respiratory impairment. Serum C-reactive protein levels do not give an accurate reflection of disease severity. Chest radiographs should be taken in all patients. Features are highly variable and include focal, multifocal, or lobar consolidation, localized patchy alveolar infiltrate, diffuse interstitial shadowing (consistent with blood-borne spread of infection), pleural effusion, and upper lobe involvement which may include cavitation. The radiographic pattern may be indistinguishable from tuberculosis. The development of empyema and/or lung abscess(es) is well recognized, and repeat chest radiographs are indicated for patients with respiratory involvement. Abdominal ultrasound examination or CT scan should be performed to exclude the presence of abscesses in liver and spleen. Clinical evidence of prostatic involvement requires appropriate imaging (transrectal ultrasonography or CT scan). The need for other imaging should be guided by clinical features and organ involvement.

Management, prognosis, and outcome

Appropriate antimicrobial agents should be started immediately on suspicion of the diagnosis of melioidosis. Recommendations are given in Box 6.15.1. Treatment is divided into intravenous and oral phases. Initial parenteral therapy is given for 10 to 14 days or until clinical response is seen (which ever is the longer). Ceftazidime or a carbapenem antibiotic is the treatment of choice. Ceftazidime is used as first-line therapy in Thailand, with a switch to a carbapenem antibiotic in the event of treatment failure on ceftazidime. Parenteral treatment at the Royal Darwin Hospital, Australia, consists of ceftazidime or meropenem plus granulocyte colony stimulating factor (G-CSF) if the patient has septic shock. The routine addition of trimethoprim/sulfamethoxazole (TMP-SMX) to ceftazidime or meropenem during the initial intensive therapy phase has been discontinued, although this drug is still used in some centres for patients with neurological or prostatic melioidosis in view of its excellent penetration. Intravenous amoxicillin/clavulanate is second-line therapy but is associated with higher rates of treatment failure and there are few indications for this agent if first-line agents are available. Oral treatment is given for 12 to 20 weeks or longer if clinically indicated, and consists of TMP-SMX. The routine addition of doxycycline to oral regimens has ceased following the outcome of a randomized controlled trial conducted in Thailand, which found equivalence between TMP-SMX alone and TMP-SMX plus doxycycline. First-line oral treatment for pregnant women and children is amoxicillin/clavulanate; this is also an alternative for adults who cannot tolerate TMP-SMX.

> **Box 6.15.1** Antimicrobial therapy for melioidosis
>
> **Initial parenteral therapy**
> - Ceftazidime 50 mg/kg per dose (up to 2 g) every 6–8 h, or meropenem 25 mg/kg per dose (up to 1 g) every 8 h.
> - Intravenous amoxicillin/clavulanate can be used as a second-line agent and is associated with equivalent mortality but a higher rate of treatment failure compared with ceftazidime. Dosage 20/5 mg/kg every 4 h.
> - Duration of parenteral therapy: a minimum of 10 days or until clear clinical improvement (which ever is the longer). Extend therapy to 4–8 weeks for deep-seated infection.
>
> **Oral eradication therapy**
> *Adults*
> - Trimethoprim/sulfamethoxazole using a weight-based dosing schedule: 2 × 160/800 mg (960 mg) tablets if more than 60 kg, 3 × 80/400 (480 mg) tablets if 40–60 kg, and 1 × 160/800 mg (960 mg) OR 2 × 80/400 (480 mg) tablets if less than 40 kg
>
> *Children ≤8 years and pregnant women*
> - Amoxicillin/clavulanate 20/5 mg/kg orally every 8 h.
> - For adult patients <60 kg, a dose of 1000/250 mg three times daily is suggested. In regions where amoxicillin/clavulanate is only available in fixed 2:1 combinations, use 500/250 mg three times daily with additional amoxicillin (500 mg three times daily). For patients >60 kg, use a maximum dose of 1500/375 mg three times daily.
> - Duration of oral therapy: 12–20 weeks.

Collections of pus should be drained wherever feasible. Patients with severe melioidosis associated with septic shock, respiratory failure, acute renal failure, and other manifestations of a severe septic illness require intensive care management, although many cases occur in geographical regions where such resources are scarce. Fever clearance is often slow (median fever clearance time of around 9 days), and without evidence of clinical deterioration is not normally sufficient to indicate a change in therapy. Sputum and draining abscess cultures may remain positive for several weeks in a patient who is otherwise responding to treatment. The benefit of other interventions for critically ill septic patients such as goal-directed therapy and intensive glycaemic control have not been evaluated in patients with melioidosis. A randomized placebo-controlled trial of G-CSF for severe melioidosis conducted in Thailand failed to show an outcome benefit.

Several features can be used to predict risk of death. The Acute Physiology and Chronic Health Evaluation II (APACHE II) score is an independent predictor of death from melioidosis. Time to blood culture positivity has prognostic significance, with a mortality rate of 74% for those with a positive culture within 24 h compared with 41% in those with a positive culture after 24 h. In patients who have a positive blood culture, counts of <1 colony-forming unit (CFU)/ml blood have been reported to be associated with a mortality of 42%, compared with a mortality of 96% in those with counts of >100 CFU/ml. *B. pseudomallei* count in urine is also associated with mortality. Patients with melioidosis whose urine culture was negative for *B. pseudomallei* had the lowest death rate (39%). Mortality was 58% in those with positive spun urine pellet only, 61% in those with between 10^3 CFU/ml and 10^5 CFU/ml *B. pseudomallei* in neat urine, and 71% in those with $\geq 10^5$ CFU/ml *B. pseudomallei* in neat urine. Sputum culture positive for *B. pseudomallei* in patients with culture-confirmed melioidosis is associated with a higher mortality (72%) compared with that for melioidosis patients with sputum culture negative for *B. pseudomallei* (42%).

Recurrent melioidosis is not uncommon (6% in the first year and 13% over 10 years). Three-quarters of recurrent cases are due to relapse caused by a strain that has persisted within the host following the primary episode, and the remainder represent reinfection by a different strain. One-quarter of patients with recurrence die as a direct result.

The risk of nosocomial infection between patients or transmission to family or other contacts has not been the subject of specific study. Several case reports have been published. Melioidosis in two infants in northern Australia was related to breastfeeding by mothers with mastitis caused by *B. pseudomallei*, and the wife of a Vietnam veteran with chronic prostatitis caused by *B. pseudomallei* developed an antibody response to the organism in the absence of clinical manifestations of melioidosis. Person-to-person transmission occurred between two siblings with cystic fibrosis and may have occurred between a diabetic brother and sister living in northeast Thailand, and a case of nosocomial infection from a suspected environmental source has been reported from an endemic area.

Likely developments in the near future

The overall incidence of melioidosis is likely to rise among wealthier nations within Asia as the number of susceptible elderly people increases. The number of reported cases worldwide is also likely to increase alongside the dissemination of diagnostic laboratories. Probably the most important strategy required to reduce mortality from melioidosis in rural Asia is early recognition and timely administration of antimicrobial drugs together with adequate fluid resuscitation. Further studies are required to define safe and affordable interventions that improve outcome where intensive care facilities are unavailable, such as protocols to optimize fluid management and glycaemic control in a general ward setting.

Overview of glanders

Burkholderia mallei, the cause of glanders, appears to have evolved through genomic downsizing from a single clone of *B. pseudomallei*. Historically, this pathogen was an important cause of morbidity and mortality in horses worldwide and was occasionally transmitted to humans or other animals. In horses, donkeys, and mules it causes nodules and ulcerations in the upper respiratory tract and lungs. The cutaneous form is known as 'farcy'. The mallein skin test is a sensitive and specific clinical test for equine glanders.

No naturally acquired case has been reported in the United States of America or the United Kingdom since 1938, but it is thought to still occur in the Middle East, Africa, and Asia. Outbreaks of equine glanders reported in Bahrain since 2010 and in Lebanon since 2011 may be linked to importation of horses from elsewhere in the region, including Syria. Clinical manifestations of glanders in humans resemble those of melioidosis. The untreated case fatality rate is 95% in 3 weeks. The approach to investigation, diagnosis, and management is as for melioidosis. The organism requires handling in a containment level 3 laboratory; important differentiating bacterial features between *B. mallei* and *B. pseudomallei* are that the former is nonmotile and susceptible to gentamicin. *In vitro* susceptibility is otherwise similar to that for *B. pseudomallei*, and glanders should respond to the regimens used to treat melioidosis.

Further reading

Cheng AC, *et al.* (2005). Melioidosis: epidemiology, pathophysiology, and management. *Clin Microbiol Rev*, **18**, 383–416.

Cheng AC, *et al.* (2008). Consensus guidelines for dosing of amoxicillin-clavulanate in melioidosis. *Am J Trop Med Hyg*, **78**, 208–9.

Chierakul W, *et al.* (2005). Two randomized controlled trials of ceftazidime alone versus ceftazidime in combination with trimethoprim-sulfamethoxazole for the treatment of severe melioidosis. *Clin Infect Dis*, **41**, 1105–13.

Currie BJ, *et al.* (2010). The epidemiology and clinical spectrum of melioidosis: 540 cases from the 20-year Darwin prospective study. *PLoS Negl Trop Dis*, **4**, e900.

6.16 **Plague: *Yersinia pestis***

Michael B. Prentice

Essentials

Bubonic plague is a flea-borne zoonosis caused by the Gram-negative bacterium *Yersinia pestis*, which mainly affects small burrowing mammals including domestic rats. Human disease occurs in endemic countries—currently mainly in Africa (including Madagascar)—following bites from fleas recently hosted by a bacteraemic animal. Historical use of *Y. pestis* as a biological warfare agent has raised fears of its future use in bioterrorism.

Clinical features—the commonest presentation is acute painful lymphadenitis (80–95% of suspected cases), with sudden onset of fever, chills, weakness, headache and development of an intensely painful swollen lymph node (bubo). Spread to the lungs occurs in less than 10% of cases, resulting in pneumonia which can result in onward respiratory transmission by droplet infection. Overall mortality without treatment is 50 to 90%.

Diagnosis and treatment—diagnosis is usually by culture from appropriate specimens (blood culture, bubo aspirate, sputum, cerebrospinal fluid), but rapid confirmation can be provided by detection of *Y. pestis* F1 antigen by immunofluorescence in clinical material. Aside from supportive care, early antimicrobial therapy (usually with streptomycin, gentamicin, or doxycycline) greatly improves survival.

Prevention—is by reducing the likelihood of people being bitten by infected fleas, or being exposed to infected droplets from humans or animals with plague pneumonia. Postexposure chemoprophylaxis may be advised for those who have been in unprotected close contact with a person with pneumonic plague. There is no current vaccine.

Acknowledgement: The author gratefully acknowledges the substantial contribution to this chapter made by Dr Tom Butler based on previous editions.

Introduction and historical perspective

Alexandre Yersin isolated the bacterium now known as *Yersinia pestis* in 1894 from a patient with bubonic plague in Hong Kong, during a plague pandemic when disease spread to ports all over the world from a focus in China. Most mortality in this pandemic was seen in India and China in the late 19th and early 20th century when millions died. Experimental work in India in the early years of the 20th century confirmed the flea–rat cycle of transmission, allowing rational control measures to be developed. This pandemic is called the third plague pandemic because of a retrospective association of bubonic plague with two historical disease pandemics. The second pandemic was the Black Death, which killed one-third of the European population between 1347 and 1352. The first plague pandemic refers to an outbreak which began in the reign of the Roman Emperor Justinian in the 6th century AD.

Aetiology, genetics, pathogenesis, and pathology

Y. pestis strains form a clonal group within *Y. pseudotuberculosis*, an enteric pathogen of mammals spread by the faeco-oral route (this has implications for laboratory identification, see below; see also Chapter 6.17). These are Gram-negative bacteria within the family Enterobacteriaceae. The change to a two-stage life style alternately parasitizing an arthropod and a mammalian host was very recent in evolutionary terms, and linked to the acquisition of two plasmids, pFra and pPst, with adaptation of preexisting properties of *Y. pseudotuberculosis*.

In the arthropod-parasitizing portion of its life cycle, *Y. pestis* multiplies and forms biofilm-embedded aggregates in the flea midgut after ingestion of a blood meal containing bacteria. Blocked fleas die, but make persistent efforts to feed, regurgitating oesophageal contents and inoculating *Y. pestis* into each bite site. Recent work suggests some fleas may be long-lived successful vectors without blockage. The ability to colonize and multiply in the flea requires a factor encoded by the pFra plasmid. *Y. pestis* dissemination from the fleabite and bubo formation requires plasminogen activator, encoded by the small pPst plasmid.

Y. pestis travels inside macrophages to the regional lymph nodes from the site of inoculation, before switching to extracellular replication in growing necrotic foci which form in infected tissues. Extracellular survival requires expression of a type III secretion system (injectisome) encoded by the yersinia virulence plasmid pCD/pYV to inject virulence effectors (Yop proteins) into mammalian host immune effector cells. This forestalls the usual immune response, preventing phagocytosis. The injectisome component LcrV (V antigen) also has an extracellular anti-inflammatory activity, preventing recruitment of inflammatory cells and granuloma formation which would normally terminate an infection. An antiphagocytic polypeptide capsule (fraction 1 or F1 antigen) is specified by pFra plasmid.

Maintenance of flea transmission requires extreme virulence in the mammalian host. Because of the small volume of blood in a flea meal and a large minimum infectious dose for the flea, a very high level of bacteraemia (10^8/ml) is required in the mammalian host to infect fleas. Few bacteria are transmitted by a flea bite and the organism has a low minimum infectious dose for mammals.

Epidemiology

Between 1989 and 2003, 25 countries reported a total of 38 310 cases and 2845 deaths to the World Health Organization. The 10 countries reporting most cases between 1987 and 2001 (accounting for over 92% of the total) were, in descending order: Madagascar, Tanzania, Democratic Republic of the Congo, Vietnam, Mozambique, Namibia, Peru, Zambia, India (all cases from an outbreak in 1994), and Myanmar. Notably, the very large enzootic focus covering the western United States of America contributed only 125 human cases (12 fatalities) over this period. The plague is seasonal in most endemic countries, with a well-defined geographical distribution correlated with that of the predominant flea vectors and rodent reservoirs and their ecology. Most cases in the United States of America occur from May to October, when people are outdoors in contact with rodents and their fleas. Countries reporting several recent outbreaks include the Democratic Republic of the Congo, Uganda, and China (northern and north western provinces).

Plague is a zoonosis with humans figuring as an incidental host. It is transmitted among animal reservoirs by flea bites and ingestion of animal tissues. The fleas of many major animal reservoirs such as burrowing rodents, including ground squirrels and prairie dogs in the United States of America and tarbagans in Asia, can only contact humans in rural areas. Human infection is more frequent when disease occurs in small mammals in closer contact with humans, particularly urban and domestic rats. The oriental rat flea *Xenopsylla cheopis* is the most efficient vector. Risk factors for acquiring plague include contact with rodents or carnivores in endemic areas and presence of refuges or food sources for wild rodents near homes. Human-to-human transmission of pneumonic plague is limited to rare outbreaks in endemic areas. Although there are no reports of the use of *Y. pestis* as a biological weapon since the Second World War, the possibility of bioterrorism would nowadays be investigated if any cases of plague, particularly pneumonic plague, were diagnosed in a nonendemic area (e.g. Europe, eastern United States of America).

Prevention

Plague prevention measures seek to reduce the likelihood of people being bitten by infected fleas or exposed to infected droplets from humans or animals with plague pneumonia. In plague-endemic areas, monitoring and control of the local plague hosts is important, as well as rat-proofing and insecticide treatment of houses and wearing shoes and garments to cover the legs. Because removing the flea food supply by poisoning their normal hosts can increase human contact with starving fleas, flea control by application of insecticides before vector control in plague outbreak areas is required. Infection control measures for patients with suspected pneumonic plague centre on respiratory isolation with droplet precautions (wearing of disposable masks by medical attendants to reduce the risk from large respiratory droplets) until they have received antibiotic treatment for 48 h. Postexposure chemoprophylaxis is advised for persons who have been in unprotected close contact (defined as coming within 2 m) with a person with known or suspected pneumonic plague who has not received antibiotic treatment for at least 48 h. Doxycycline is used for adults and trimethoprim-sulfamethoxazole for children or pregnant women. Standard isolation precautions are recommended for non-pneumonic plague patients. There is no currently available plague vaccine, but a variety of different prospective subunit vaccines are in development and clinical trials, mostly based on combinations of immunogenic plasmid-specified protein antigens LcrV and fraction 1, which in animal models protect against pneumonic challenge.

Clinical features

Three clinical syndromes are associated with plague: bubonic plague, septicaemic plague, and pneumonic plague. The most common presentation is acute painful lymphadenitis (80–95% of suspected cases). There is sudden onset of fever, chills, weakness, and headache. At the same time, or shortly afterwards, patients notice the bubo, which is signalled by intense pain in one anatomical region of lymph nodes, usually the groin, axilla, or neck (Fig. 6.16.1). The swelling is so tender that patients avoid any motion that might provoke discomfort. If the bubo is in the femoral area, the patient will flex, abduct, and externally rotate the hip to relieve pressure on that area, and will walk with a limp. With an axillary bubo, the patient will abduct the shoulder or hold the arm in a splint. When the bubo is in the neck, patients will tilt their neck to the opposite side.

Buboes are oval swellings varying from 1 to 10 cm in length and elevate the overlying skin, which may appear stretched or erythematous. They may consist of a single smooth uniform mass or an irregular cluster of several nodes with intervening and surrounding oedema. The overlying skin is warm with an underlying tender firm nonfluctuant mass. Patients are typically prostrate and lethargic, but can show restlessness or agitation. Occasionally they are delirious with fever, and seizures are common in children. Fever of 38.5 to 40°C is usual, with a pulse of 110 to 140/min. Blood pressure is characteristically low, 100/60 mmHg, and may be unobtainable if systemic sepsis syndrome occurs as a consequence of the host response to large amounts of circulating bacterial endotoxin. As part of this response, disseminated intravascular coagulopathy (DIC) may occur involving arteriolar thrombosis, skin and serosal haemorrhage, acral cyanosis, and tissue necrosis, as well as multiple organ failure and adult respiratory distress syndrome.

A minority of patients (10–20%) develop systemic *Y. pestis* sepsis with no bubo (primary septicaemic plague) and less than 10% develop secondary pneumonic plague or meningitis as a consequence of bacteraemia.

Differential diagnosis

Other infections producing acute lymphadenitis (streptococcal lymphadenitis, cat-scratch fever, etc.) do not generally share the same suddenness of onset leading to death 2 to 4 days after the onset of symptoms. The plague bubo is also distinctive in the usual absence of a detectable skin lesion or ascending lymphangitis. A minority of patients show various skin lesions (pustules, eschars, or papules) presumably representing the site of flea bite in the skin area draining to the bubo (Fig. 6.16.2).

Clinical investigation

The diagnosis should be suspected in febrile patients exposed to rodents or other mammals in endemic areas. *Y. pestis* is on a short list of pathogens to be excluded in any unexplained outbreak of severe respiratory disease which could follow an aerosol release by bioterrorists.

Appropriate diagnostic specimens include blood culture (positive in 27 to 96% of patients with bubonic plague), bubo aspirate, sputum, and cerebrospinal fluid, depending on clinical presentation and, if necessary, taken at postmortem examination. A bubo aspirate is obtained by inserting a 10-ml syringe with a 21-gauge

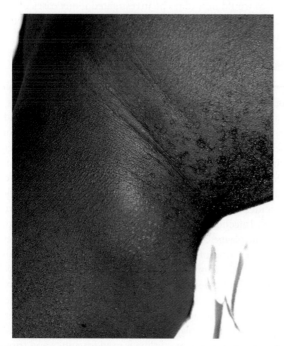

Fig. 6.16.1 A right femoral bubo consists of an enlarged tender lymph node with surrounding oedema in a Kenyan patient.
(Copyright D A Warrell.)

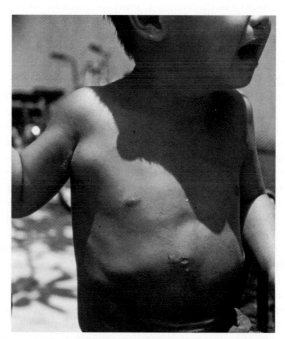

Fig. 6.16.2 Right axillary bubo was accompanied by a purulent ulcer on the abdomen, which was the presumed site of the fleabite.
(Copyright Tom Butler.)

needle containing 1 ml sterile saline through the skin into the bubo. The saline is injected and reaspirated until blood-tinged fluid appears in the syringe. *Y. pestis* grows on standard laboratory media but should be processed in containment level 3 laboratory conditions.

The organism is characterized as a slow-growing non-lactose-fermenting nonmotile Gram-negative rod, first seen at 24 h on standard laboratory media. Biochemically, *Y. pestis* is oxidase negative, catalase positive, urease negative, and indole negative. It may be misidentified as *Y. pseudotuberculosis* or another Enterobacteriaceae species by routine biochemical identification systems and it is important to notify the laboratory if the diagnosis is clinically suspected. In the United States of America *Y. pestis* is a 'select agent' under bioterrorism legislation and diagnostic cultures are strictly notified and controlled.

Gram's stain of smears of sputum, bubo aspirate, or cerebrospinal fluid may show small Gram-negative rods or coccobacilli; bipolar staining may be seen with Wayson's or Giemsa's stains (Figs. 6.16.3, 6.16.4). Rapid diagnosis is provided by detection of *Y. pestis* F1 antigen by immunofluorescence in clinical material.

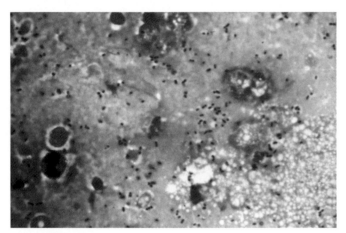

Fig. 6.16.3 Bubo aspirate shows bipolar bacilli stained with methylene blue (Wayson's stain).
(Copyright Tom Butler.)

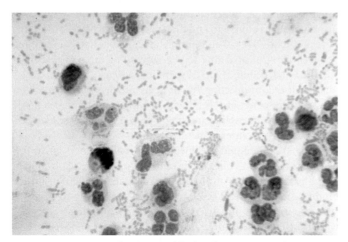

Fig. 6.16.4 Gram's stain of cerebrospinal fluid in plague meningitis shows numerous Gram-negative bacilli.
(Copyright Tom Butler.)

A dipstick containing F1 antibody has been shown to be a sensitive and specific assay in field conditions in Madagascar on a variety of clinical specimens (sputum, bubo aspirate, cerebrospinal fluid). Current trials of this dipstick in Africa are ongoing. Polymerase chain reaction (PCR) assays for various targets and an enzyme-linked immunosorbent assay (ELISA) for *Y. pestis* LcrV antigen have also been developed but are not in widespread clinical use, although one real time PCR kit is now licensed by the United States Food and Drug Administration for *in vitro* diagnosis.

Criteria for diagnosis

Diagnosis is by culture of the organism, F1 antigen detection, a fourfold rise in antibody titre to *Y. pestis* F1 antigen using the passive haemagglutination testing of paired serum specimens (PHA test) or a single titre greater than 1:16. Specificity of the PHA test requires confirmation with the F1 antigen haemagglutination inhibition test. Seroconversion can occur 5 days after onset of symptoms, but is more usual between 1 and 2 weeks after onset.

Treatment

Streptomycin is traditionally regarded as the most effective treatment for plague at a dose of 1 g IM twice daily (30 mg/kg per day) for 10 days, and was the first antimicrobial shown to be effective against pneumonic plague. The more readily available aminoglycoside gentamicin is as effective as streptomycin in the treatment of human plague when given at standard doses for severe sepsis. Trial data in Africa shows seven-day courses of intramuscular gentamicin 2.5 mg/kg 12 hourly or oral doxycycline therapy 100 mg (adults) and 2.2 mg/kg (children) orally every 12 h are highly effective in adults and children with bubonic, septicaemic, or pneumonic plague (tetracyclines are contraindicated in pregnancy, breastfeeding, and children younger than 7 years because of tooth discoloration). In a mouse septicaemia model, third-generation cephalosporins and quinolones were as effective as streptomycin and tetracycline. In a mouse model of pneumonic plague, β-lactam antibiotics were less effective than aminoglycosides and quinolones. Oral chloramphenicol is recommended for plague meningitis at a loading dose of 25 mg/kg followed by 60 mg/kg per day in four divided doses, reducing to 30 mg/kg per day orally on clinical improvement to complete a total course of 10 days. Trimethoprim-sulfamethoxazole has been used to treat bubonic plague but response may be delayed or incomplete. Fluoroquinolones are active against *Y. pestis in vitro* and in animal models although clinical data are limited.

General therapeutic measures for systemic bacterial sepsis including intravenous fluids are appropriate, but no available trial data for the use of these in plague are available. A consensus view of treatment for pneumonic plague resulting from biological weapon attack suggests streptomycin, gentamicin, tetracycline, or fluoroquinolones may be effective.

Although still very rare, natural antimicrobial resistance has been detected. A wild-type *Y. pestis* strain resistant to multiple antimicrobials was first reported from Madagascar in 1997, and subsequently a different strain resistant to the first-line antibiotic streptomycin was also identified. Worryingly, both plasmids responsible for these resistance patterns were self-transferrable to other bacteria. Fortunately, no other *Y. pestis* strains with multiple antimicrobial resistance have subsequently been isolated in Madagascar.

Prognosis

Untreated bubonic plague has a mortality of 50 to 90% and untreated meningitis, pneumonia, or septicaemia is fatal in most cases. Diagnosis and appropriate therapy reduce bubonic plague and septicaemia mortality to 10 to 20%, but delay in diagnosis and therapy can be fatal. Primary pneumonic plague mortality approaches 100% untreated and is still over 50% with antimicrobial therapy.

Areas of uncertainty or controversy

A long-standing controversy about the aetiology of the 14th-century Black Death pandemic has recently been resolved. Two independent ancient DNA sequencing studies have confirmed that the Black Death was caused by *Y. pestis* strains ancestral to current pandemic clades. The minor genetic differences found between ancient and current *Y. pestis* strains over the whole genome suggests the enhanced dissemination of the Black Death compared with contemporary plague was not due to specific bacterial virulence factors. This reduces the likelihood that a hypervirulent *Y. pestis* strain could re-emerge to cause a new Black Death pandemic.

Likely future developments

Novel subunit vaccines now in clinical trials will come into clinical use. Knowledge of plague evolution and pathogenesis will improve with the completion of numerous genome sequences and intensive genome resequencing of strain collections.

Further reading

Achtman M, *et al.* (1999). *Yersinia pestis*, the cause of plague, is a recently emerged clone of *Yersinia pseudotuberculosis*. *Proc Natl Acad Sci U S A*, **96**, 14043–8.

Bos, KI, *et al.* (2011) A draft genome of *Yersinia pestis* from victims of the Black Death. *Nature*, **478**, 506–10.

Dennis DT, *et al.* (1999). Plague manual: epidemiology, distribution, surveillance and control. World Health Organization, Geneva. www.who.int/csr/resources/publications/plague/WHO_CDS_CSR_EDC_99_2_EN/en/ [Accessed 31/10/2011].

Eisen RJ, *et al.*(2012). Transmission of flea-borne zoonotic agents. *Annu Rev Entomol*, **57**, 61–82.

Haensch, S, *et al.* (2010). Distinct clones of Yersinia pestis caused the Black Death. *PLoS Pathog*, **6**, e1001134.

Kool JL (2005). Risk of person-to-person transmission of pneumonic plague. *Clin Infect Dis*, **40**, 1166–72.

Mwengee W, *et al.* (2006). Treatment of plague with gentamicin or doxycycline in a randomized clinical trial in Tanzania. *Clin Infect Dis*, **42**, 614–21.

Parkhill J, *et al.* (2001). Genome sequence of *Yersinia pestis*, the causative agent of plague. *Nature*, **413**, 523–7.

Prentice MB, Rahalison L (2007). Plague. *Lancet*, **369**, 1196–207.

Sebbane F, *et al.* (2006). Role of the *Yersinia pestis* plasminogen activator in the incidence of distinct septicemic and bubonic forms of flea-borne plague. *Proc Natl Acad Sci U S A*, **103**, 5526–30.

Sharp S, Saubolle MA (2010). Sentinel level clinical microbiology laboratory guidelines for suspected agents of bioterrorism and emerging infectious diseases: *Yersinia pestis* American Society for Microbiology, Washington, DC. http://asm.org/images/pdf/Clinical/Protocols/ypestis06-11-10.pdf [Accessed 31/10/2011].

6.17 Other *Yersinia* infections: yersiniosis

Michael B. Prentice

Essentials

Yersiniosis is caused by the enteropathogenic Gram-negative organisms *Yersinia enterocolitica* and *Yersinia pseudotuberculosis*, which are worldwide zoonotic pathogens. Disease is acquired by consumption of contaminated food or water and is commonest in childhood, and in colder climates. Presentation is with diarrhoea, fever and abdominal pain, which may mimic appendicitis. Late complications include reactive arthritis, erythema nodosum, and erythema multiforme. Systemic infection is more likely with *Y. pseudotuberculosis* and a subgroup of *Y. enterocolitica*, and also in patients with diabetes or iron overload. Diagnosis is by culture of the organism or convalescent serology. Most cases of enteritis are self limiting and antimicrobials are not indicated, but septicaemia or focal infection outside the gastrointestinal tract requires antimicrobials (usually cefotaxime, ceftriaxone, or ciprofloxacin). Prevention is by standard food hygiene precautions.

Introduction and historical perspective

Yersinia pseudotuberculosis was first identified in 1883 and *Y. enterocolitica* in 1939. Water-borne outbreaks of *Y. pseudotuberculosis* were recognized in Japan and Korea from the 1920s onwards. *Y. enterocolitica* was rarely reported before the 1960s and the first large-scale outbreak of human disease was reported in 1976.

Aetiology, genetics, pathogenesis, and pathology

The genus *Yersinia* includes 17 species, 3 of which cause human disease: *Y. pestis* (Chapter 6.16) causes plague; *Y. enterocolitica* and *Y. pseudotuberculosis* cause diarrhoeal diseases. Enteropathogenic *Yersinia* are Gram-negative organisms of the order Enterobacteriaceae. Ingested enteropathogenic *Yersinia* expressing invasin proteins adhere to and then pass through M cells overlying Peyer's patches. They then multiply in lymphoid tissue, remaining extracellularly located due to the activity of the pYV plasmid-specified injectisome (type III secretion system). This inactivates phagocytic cells by injecting Yop proteins into them. *Y. enterocolitica* classically causes terminal ileitis with or without adjacent mesenteric adenitis (microabscesses inside lymph nodes), while *Y. pseudotuberculosis* causes mesenteric adenitis without terminal ileitis. Some strains of *Y. enterocolitica* (biovar 1B, so-called American strains which are rarely found in Europe) and *Y. pseudotuberculosis* contain a high pathogenicity island (HPI) and produce an additional iron-binding siderophore. These strains are more likely to produce systemic infection and bacteraemia. Correspondingly, patients with iron overload (polytransfused, haemochromatosis) are at risk of serious or fatal consequences if infected by enteropathogenic *Yersinia*, especially when using iron chelators. Recent evidence from mice suggest *Y. enterocolitica* and *Y. pseudotuberculosis* strains penetrating from the gut to the liver and spleen may not be entering via Peyer's patches. Some strains of *Y. pseudotuberculosis* produce a superantigenic toxin, *Y. pseudotuberculosis*-derived mitogen (YPM). *Y. enterocolitica* strains produce a heat-stable enterotoxin. Genome sequences of *Y. enterocolitica* shows the presence of several metabolic operons found in salmonella not present in *Y. pseudotuberculosis*, which may account for epidemiological differences.

Epidemiology

Both enteropathogenic yersiniae are zoonotic pathogens distributed worldwide but are more common in temperate and cold countries. *Y. enterocolitica* commonly colonizes and infects domestic animals, particularly pigs. *Y. pseudotuberculosis* is associated with wild mammals such as rodents, rabbits, and deer, and birds and human infection is more rarely diagnosed. *Y. enterocolitica* infection is commonest in children under the age of 5 years. In Germany 40% of blood donors have anti-*Yersinia* Yop antibodies thought to relate to *Y. enterocolitica* infection, and it is the third commonest cause of bacterial diarrhoea in Scandinavian countries and New Zealand. Seroepidemiology and culture studies suggests human disease is at least 10-fold rarer in the United Kingdom, although United Kingdom animals frequently carry the organism. In the United States of America, high virulence 'American' strains of *Y. enterocolitica* have been displaced by European strains of lower virulence in recent years. Recent outbreaks of yersiniosis involving *Y. enterocolitica* have been mainly pork meat related, for example children in New Zealand consuming cocktail sausages, although large raw and pasteurized milk-related outbreaks have been reported from the USA, Japan and Canada in the past. Recent outbreaks of *Y. pseudotuberculosis* have followed consumption of lettuce and raw carrot (Finland), various raw vegetables (Russia), well water (Korea and Japan) and homogenized milk (Canada). In rare cases *Y. enterocolitica* septicaemia has been reported after transfusion of packed red cells.

Prevention

Standard food hygiene precautions are effective including avoiding consumption of undercooked or raw meat (e.g. pork chitterlings), especially by children, and pasteurization of milk. Chlorination of water supplies is important for *Y. pseudotuberculosis* control. *Yersinia* grow (slowly) at refrigerator temperature, and prolonged cold storage of contaminated food or blood products may greatly increase their contamination.

Clinical features

Following an incubation period of 1 to 11 days (usually 4–6 days), enteric *Yersinia* infection usually presents with diarrhoea, fever, and abdominal pain. Abdominal pain in older children and adults is often central or right sided, simulating appendicitis (pseudoappendicitis). Diarrhoea can be minimal or absent. *Y. enterocolitica* diarrhoea contains blood in 25 to 50% of cases. Infection is usually self-limiting, but bacteraemia and systemic spread can occur.

Gastrointestinal complications of acute yersiniosis are rare and include diffuse ulcerating ileitis and colitis, intestinal perforation, peritonitis, toxic megacolon, intussusception, mesenteric vein thrombosis, and intestinal ischaemia. Extraintestinal complications

are also rare and include septicaemia, intra-abdominal abscesses, pharyngeal abscess, endocarditis, mycotic aneurysm, meningitis, osteomyelitis, septic arthritis, lung abscess, empyema, ophthalmitis, suppurative lymphadenitis, and skin infections. The majority of patients experiencing systemic enteropathogenic *Yersinia* sepsis have diabetes, iron overload, or immunosuppression.

Contamination of blood for transfusion with *Y. enterocolitica*, presumably introduced at the time of donation and multiplying on storage, is a rare but usually fatal cause of blood transfusion reactions and systemic sepsis.

The most common postinfectious sequelae of yersiniosis are reactive arthritis and erythema nodosum. Immunological complications of enteric infection are common in northern Europe where HLA-B27 is frequent. Reactive arthritis follows several weeks after diarrhoea with other complications such as erythema nodosum, erythema multiforme, vasculitis and glomerulonephritis. A specific *Yersinia*-associated variant of erythema multiforme has been reported from Germany with localization of eruption to the neck, shoulders and arms, accompanied by erythema nodosum, conjunctivitis and arthralgia.

Y. pseudotuberculosis strains producing superantigenic toxin YPM are associated with Far Eastern scarlet-like fever (FESLF) in eastern Russia, a childhood illness with desquamating rash, arthralgia, and polyarthritis also seen in Japan (Izumi fever) and Korea. There is epidemiological overlap between populations exposed to *Y. pseudotuberculosis* and the incidence of Kawasaki disease, an idiopathic acute systemic vasculitis of childhood.

Differential diagnosis

Differential diagnosis includes appendicitis, other causes of terminal ileitis, mesenteric adenitis (Crohn's disease, tuberculosis), and fever with abdominal pain. Other causes of community-acquired septicaemia should be considered for the rarer systemic infection presentation.

Clinical investigation

Culture of material from normally sterile sites (blood culture, lymph nodes) is carried out on standard media. Selective cefsulodin-irgasan-novobiocin (CIN) agar is used for faeces and other contaminated specimens. Standard biochemical identification to species level is possible in most laboratories, but some *Y. enterocolitica* strains isolated from faeces lack the virulence plasmid and their pathogenicity is uncertain. Reference laboratories separate *Y. enterocolitica* into distinct biotypes and serotypes of more or less established virulence, serotype *Y. pseudotuberculosis*, and provide convalescent serology. A new multilocus sequence typing (MLST) scheme for *Y. pseudotuberculosis* has recently shown that the same serotypes are present in different lineages and serotype is poorly predictive of genetic relatedness or pathogenicity for humans.

Criteria for diagnosis

Diagnosis is by culture of the organism from a sterile site, bioserotyping of faecal isolates of *Y. enterocolitica* into a pathogenic group, convalescent serology by agglutinating antibodies, enzyme-linked immunosorbent assay (ELISA), or Western blot. *Y. pseudotuberculosis* is rarely isolated from faeces and serology is the usual diagnostic method.

Treatment

Most cases of enteritis are self-limiting and antimicrobials are not indicated. Septicaemia or focal infection or scarlet-like fever (FESLF) outside the gastrointestinal tract require antibiotics. *Y. enterocolitica* strains possess two different β-lactamases and, in the absence of controlled trial data, therapy with cefotaxime, ceftriaxone, or ciprofloxacin are most commonly recommended for acute sepsis. Gentamicin is sometimes given in addition to β-lactams. *Y. pseudotuberculosis* sepsis can be treated by the same agents, although this organism does not produce β-lactamase and is generally ampicillin sensitive.

Prognosis

Acute enteritis is usually self-limiting. Reported mortality is low, ranging between 0.5% in a Norwegian study and 1.2% in the United States of America. Septicaemic illness has a high mortality (up to 50%), probably associated with predisposing illnesses. In northern European countries with high HLA-B27 prevalence, *Yersinia* postinfectious complications including reactive arthritis can result in chronic illness which responds poorly to antimicrobials.

Areas of uncertainty or controversy

Virulence plasmid-negative biovar 1A *Y. enterocolitica* strains may have some role in diarrhoea. A Cochrane review is in progress evaluating the evidence of efficacy of antimicrobial treatment of reactive arthritis, including cases caused by *Yersinia*.

Likely future developments

Because chronic oropharyngeal colonization with *Y. enterocolitica* is frequent in apparently healthy domestic animals such as pigs, breaking the transmission chain requires selective breeding of specific pathogen-free herds. This is under way in Norway. Sequencing of more strains of *Y. enterocolitica* (including *Y. enterocolitica* biovar 1A strains) and *Y. pseudotuberculosis* will shed more light on pathogenic mechanisms and organism evolution.

Further reading

Bottone EJ (1997). *Yersinia enterocolitica*: the charisma continues. *Clin Microbiol Rev*, **10**, 257–76.

Carniel E, *et al.* (2006). *Y. enterocolitica* and *Y. pseudotuberculosis*. In: Dworkin M, *et al.* (eds) *The prokaryotes*, vol. 6, *Proteobacteria: Gamma subclass*, pp. 270–398. Springer, New York.

Chain PS, *et al.* (2004). Insights into the evolution of *Yersinia pestis* through whole-genome comparison with *Yersinia pseudotuberculosis*. *Proc Natl Acad Sci U S A*, **101**, 13826–31.

Laukkanen-Ninios R, *et al.* (2011). Population structure of the *Yersinia pseudotuberculosis* complex according to multilocus sequence typing. *Environ Microbiol*, **13**, 3114–27.

Rimhanen-Finne R, *et al.* (2009). *Yersinia pseudotuberculosis* causing a large outbreak associated with carrots in Finland, 2006. *Epidemiology and Infection*, **137** (Special Issue 03), 342–47.

Sato K, Ouchi K, Taki M (1983). *Yersinia pseudotuberculosis* infection in children, resembling Izumi fever and Kawasaki syndrome. *Pediatr Infect Dis*, **2**, 123–6.

Tennant SM, *et al.* (2005). Homologues of insecticidal toxin complex genes in *Yersinia enterocolitica* biotype 1A and their contribution to virulence. *Infect. Immun.* **73**, 6860–867.

Thomson N, *et al.* (2006). The complete genome sequence and comparative genome analysis of the high pathogenicity *Yersinia enterocolitica* strain 8081. *PLoS Genet*, **2**, 1–13.

Vincent P, *et al.* (2007). Similarities of Kawasaki disease and *Yersinia pseudotuberculosis* infection epidemiology', *Pediatr Infect Dis J*, **26** (7), 629–31.

Wang, X, *et al.* (2011). Complete genome sequence of a *Yersinia enterocolitica* "Old World" (3/O:9) strain and comparison with the "New World" (1B/O:8) strain. *J Clin Microbiol*, **49**, 1251–9.

6.18 **Pasteurella**

Marina S. Morgan

Essentials

Pasteurella multocida is an important human Gram-negative pathogen residing primarily in the oropharynx of mammals and transmitted through bites and scratches. Presentation is typically within 12 h of the injury with rapidly spreading cellulitis or sepsis, leading to serious morbidity and mortality (up to 40%) if untreated. Diagnosis is clinical: fresh bite wound cultures are unhelpful, but the organism may be cultured in cases with established infection. Treatment requires thorough wound debridement, with delayed closure if possible, along with antimicrobials to provide empirical cover against pasteurellae and other expected pathogens, e.g. amoxicillin-clavulanate plus ciprofloxacin, or imipenem plus clindamycin. Prevention is by avoidance of animal bites or scratches and prompt hygienic management of wounds: antibiotic prophylaxis (amoxicillin-clavulanate) should be reserved for high-risk bites (e.g. cat bites) or high-risk wounds that are difficult to debride adequately.

Introduction

Pasteurella multocida (literally 'killer of many species') is a major human pathogen and causes severe morbidity. Pasteurella septicaemia is associated with a mortality of 40% and a propensity for metastatic infection.

Infection usually follows close animal contact or bites. The organism is part of the colonizing oral flora in virtually every species from birds to elephants and water buffalo, but especially in domestic cats.

Historical perspective

The genus *Pasteurella* was named in honour of Pasteur who, in 1880, discovered *P. multocida* to be the cause of fowl cholera. *Pasteurella* spp. cause haemorrhagic septicaemia, 'shipping fever' in cattle, and respiratory infections in goats, sheep, and rabbits.

Aetiology, genetics, pathogenesis, and pathology

Nearly all infected patients have a history of animal exposure. *Pasteurella* spp. such as *P. dagmatis*, *P. pneumotropica*, *P. bettyae*, *P. haemolytica*, and *P. caballi* rarely cause human infection.

Pasteurella spp. are small Gram-negative coccobacilli, often with bipolar staining. Unusually for a Gram-negative rod, *P. multocida* is sensitive to penicillin and fails to grow on MacConkey's agar. Potential virulence factors include capsule lipopolysaccharide, a cytotoxin, iron acquisition proteins, and other surface structures including homologues of the *Bordatella pertussis* filamentous haemagglutinin. One complete genome sequence of *P. multocida* has been determined.

An aggressive and opportunistic pathogen, *P. multocida* infection can colonize the oropharynx in those working with animals, and cause invasive infection in those with underlying pathology such as liver cirrhosis or bronchiectasis. *P. multocida* is particularly associated with infection following animal bites. Cat-related trauma is particularly likely to result in pasteurella infection, especially septic arthritis and osteomyelitis following hand bites. Small, sharp cat teeth leave a septic focus in deeper tissues, under an apparently innocuous puncture wound. Necrotizing soft-tissue infections such as tenosynovitis, septicaemia, and liver and brain abscesses are the commoner manifestations, with very rare reports of epiglottitis, chorioamnionitis, and neonatal sepsis.

Epidemiology

Infection may be occupationally related, e.g. in veterinary surgeons, farmers, and postmen, but more commonly follows bites from companion animals, accounting for roughly 2% of attendances at Emergency Departments in the United Kingdom. Nearly 60% of cat bites are infected with. *P. multocida*, together with anaerobes.

Prevention

Avoidance of animal bites or scratches and prompt hygienic management of wounds are key to preventing infection.

Antibiotic prophylaxis should be reserved for high-risk bites (e.g. cat bites) or high-risk wounds that are difficult to debride adequately. Oral co-amoxiclav, 625 mg three times daily for 3 to 5 days will cover *Pasteurella* spp. as well as the other 172 other possible oral commensals present.

Patients who have undergone mastectomy and those with diabetes, immunosuppression, cirrhosis, steroid therapy, splenectomy, or prosthetic joints are 'high-risk patients' for whom prophylaxis should be seriously considered. 'High-risk wounds' include puncture wounds, particularly to the hand or wrist, and crush wounds with devitalized tissue.

Erythromycin, clindamycin, and flucloxacillin are ineffective against *Pasteurella* spp. and should not be used for prophylaxis or treatment in the absence of sensitivity information. Numerous reports of breakthrough *P. multocida* septicaemia and meningitis have occurred during erythromycin therapy. Alternative prophylaxis for penicillin-allergic patients includes cefoxitin, tetracycline, or combination therapy (clindamycin and ciprofloxacin or ciprofloxacin and linezolid).

Clinical features of pasteurella infection

The most common presentation of pasteurella infection is soft tissue infection but septic arthritis, osteomyelitis, osteomyelitis, septicaemia, and meningitis may occur, particularly in infants and immunocompromised individuals. Soft tissue infections are usually cat or dog bites or cat scratches but may occur if an animal licks

broken skin. Since *Pasteurella* spp. are extremely pyogenic, bite-related or scratch-related infections usually present 8 to 12 h after the incident and rapidly spreading cellulitis is typical (Fig. 6.18.1) lymphadenopathy in 10%.

P. multocida can cause bone and joint infections such as septic arthritis (usually monoarticular and involving the knee joint) or osteomyelitis. Most cases of septic arthritis occur after an animal bite distal to the joint. Osteomyelitis results either from extension of soft tissue infection or via direct inoculation of bacteria into the periosteum by the animal bite; osteomyelitis is more frequently associated with cat bites than dog bites, presumably because of cats' small, sharp teeth.

Respiratory tract *Pasteurella* spp. may be commensals or cause infections such as glossitis, pharyngitis, sinusitis, otitis media, epiglottitis, bronchitis, pneumonia, and empyema. In one study of 108 patients with pleuropulmonary *P. multocida* infections an underlying disease was found in 90% and mortality was 29%.

P. multocida may also cause a number of other serious invasive infections such as meningitis, bacteraemia, endocarditis, and peritonitis. Intra-abdominal infections include peritonitis and appendicitis. Chorioamnionitis is associated with neonatal sepsis.

Differential diagnosis

Of the hundreds of species contaminating animal bites, other major pathogens to consider include streptococci, staphylococci, and especially anaerobes, the latter more common in deep penetrating wounds.

Clinical investigation

A history of animal bite or scratch preceding any presentation of sepsis should alert the clinician to the possibility of pasteurella infection. Fresh bite wound cultures are unhelpful. Established infections necessitate the taking of blood cultures and culture of any discharge. The microbiology laboratory should be alerted to the possibility of *Pasteurella* so that specimens can be cultured appropriately. Unlike most Gram-negative rods it does not grow on MacConkey's agar

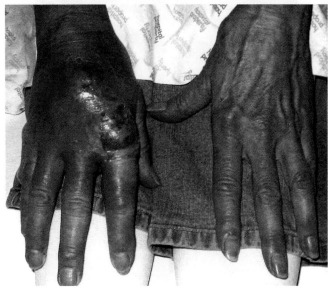

Fig. 6.18.1 *Pasteurella multocida* hand infection, preoperative.

and is susceptible to penicillin. Selective media containing vancomycin, clindamycin and amikacin have been used to isolate pasteurella. Most strains are catalase, oxidase, indole, sucrose, and decarboxylate ornithine positive.

Antibiotic susceptibility testing is warranted for isolates cultured from normally sterile sites and respiratory specimens, particularly in the immunocompromised. *Pasteurella* is usually susceptible to penicillin, amoxicillin-clavulanate, piperacillin-tazobactam, doxycycline, fluoroquinolones, extended spectrum cephalosporins (e.g. ceftriaxone, cefpodoxime, and cefixime), and carbapenems (imipenem, meropenem, and doripenem).

Typing of *P. multocida* has traditionally been done serologically. There are five capsular serogroups and 16 somatic serotypes; most human infections are caused by serotypes A, D, and F. New typing methods rely on molecular methods. Subspecies of *P. multocida* can be identified by polymerase chain reaction (PCR) fingerprinting. Human infections have been reported with *P. multocida* subsp. *multocida*, *P. multocida* subsp. *septica*, *P. multocida* subsp. *gallicida*, *P. canis*, *P. dagmatis*, and *P. stomatis*.

Treatment

Indications for hospital admission after animal bites include systemic sepsis, involvement of joint or tendon, immunocompromise, bites requiring reconstructive surgery, severe cellulitis, and infection refractory to oral therapy. Hands are especially prone to infection because of the numerous small compartments and lack of soft tissues separating the skin from bone and joint.

Inadequate debridement and incorrect antibiotic prophylaxis are major contributors to the excessive morbidity of *P. multocida* infection. Where adequate debridement of deep wounds, especially cat bites, is not possible, irrigation with 250 ml saline, using a 19- or 20-gauge needle or plastic intravenous catheter on a 30-ml syringe, followed by prophylactic antibiotics may be effective (Fig. 6.18.2).

Thorough irrigation and debridement of the wound, and, where possible, delayed closure of limb bites maximizes salvage. Limbs

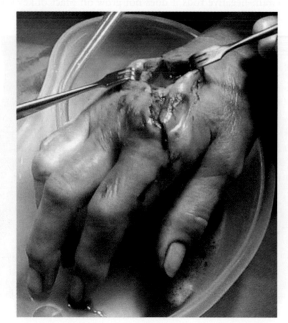

Fig. 6.18.2 The same patient: infected area being incised and drained.

should be elevated and immobilized. Tenosynovitis may be so advanced on presentation that amputation is the only option.

Pus must be drained and affected joints washed out, and the wound left open where possible. Facial bites can be closed primarily since bleeding is profuse and wounds are easily cleaned.

Broad-spectrum empiric antimicrobial therapy should be directed at polymicrobial infection that occurs after bite infections and a combination of a penicillin and a β-lactamase inhibitor (e.g. amoxicillin-clavulanate or piperacillin-tazobactam) is recommended in patients without penicillin allergy. Definitive treatment is based on the result of wound cultures and should be continued for 7 to 10 days.

Alternative agents for patients allergic to penicillins or infected with β-lactamase producing strains include oral levofloxacin, moxifloxacin or doxycycline. In patients without immediate hypersensitivity to penicillins can be treated with ceftriaxone, cefixime, or cefpodoxime. Aztreonam may be an acceptable alternative in patients with immediate type hypersensitivity to penicillins.

For established soft-tissue infection, 10 days therapy is usual, compared with 3 weeks for tenosynovitis, 4 weeks for septic arthritis, and 6 weeks for osteomyelitis. In practice, intravenous therapy until the C-reactive protein (CRP) falls to less than 50 mg/litre is a useful objective guideline for switching to oral therapy.

Prognosis

The prognosis of *P. multocida* infections depends on the site of infection and the existence of underlying medical conditions. Soft tissue infections usually resolve with wound drainage and oral antibiotics. Established bite-related hand infection often results in permanent impairment of function, justifying aggressive management and thorough documentation. Factors associated with poor outcome include inadequate initial antimicrobials and inadequate debridement. Pasteurella septicaemia may result from inappropriate therapy with erythromycin or flucloxacillin. *P. multocida* prosthetic joint infection, usually associated with rheumatoid arthritis and female gender, results in loss of the prosthesis in 70% of patients, even with early appropriate antibiotic therapy. The mortality of systemic pasteurella infections is high; 25% in meningitis, 30% in bacteraemia and endocarditis.

Areas of controversy

The role of antimicrobial prophylaxis following animal bites, in the absence of any other risk factor for infection, is debatable. One meta-analysis of eight randomized trials concluded that the relative risk for infection in patients given antibiotics compared with controls was 0.56 (95% confidence interval, 0.38–0.82), whereas another meta-analysis included trials with few cat bites, resulting in no evidence for the benefit of prophylaxis.

Further reading

Adlam C, Rutter JM (1989). *Pasteurella and pasteurellosis*. Academic Press, London.

Antuna SA, *et al.* (1997). Late infection after total knee arthroplasty caused by *Pasteurella multocida*. *Acta Orthop Belg*, **63**, 310–12.

Cummings P (1993). Antibiotics to prevent infection in patients with dog-bite wounds: a meta-analysis of randomised trials. *Ann Emerg Med*, **23**, 535–40.

Medeiros I, Saconato H (2001). Antibiotic prophylaxis for mammalian bites. *Cochrane Database Syst Rev*, **2**, CD001738.

Morgan MS (2005). The hospital management of animal bites. *J Infect*, **61**, 1–10.

Talan DA, *et al.* (1999). Bacteriologic analysis of infected dog and cat bites. *N Engl J Med*, **340**, 85–92.

Weber DJ, *et al.* (1984). *Pasteurella multocida* infections: report of 34 cases and review of the literature. *Medicine*, **63**, 133–54.

6.19 *Francisella tularensis* infection

Petra C.F. Oyston

Essentials

Fransicella tularensis is a small Gram-negative coccobacillus that circulates in small rodents, rabbits and hares, most frequently in Scandinavia, northern North America, Japan, and Russia. Clinical presentation depends on the route of infection. Most commonly this follows the bite of an infected arthropod vector, resulting in ulceroglandular tularaemia. The most acute and life-threatening disease, respiratory or pneumonic tularaemia, arises following inhalation of infectious aerosols or dusts. The organism is highly fastidious, requiring rich media for isolation and specialized reagents for positive identification; most cases are diagnosed serologically. Treatment is with supportive care and antibiotics (usually ciprofloxacin, doxycycline or gentamicin). There is no vaccine.

Historical perspective

Francisella tularensis was first isolated during an outbreak of a plague-like disease in rodents in California in 1911. Since then it has been recognized as a zoonotic infection of humans capable of causing significant morbidity or death. Human infection occurs following contact with infected animals or invertebrate vectors. It is also called Francis' disease, deer fly fever, rabbit fever, water-rat trappers' disease, wild hare disease (yato-byo), and Ohara's disease. It is highly infectious by the aerosol route and, as such, has been of concern as a biological threat agent.

Aetiology, genetics, pathogenesis, and pathology

The genus *Francisella* includes two species, *Francisella tularensis* and *Francisella philomiragia*. *F. tularensis* is a small (0.2–0.5 μm × 0.7–1.0 μm) Gram-negative coccobacillus that is nonmotile and an obligate aerobe. The four subspecies of *F. tularensis* are: *F. tularensis* subsp. *tularensis* (also called *F. tularensis* type A or *F. neoarctica*); *F. tularensis* subsp. *holarctica* (also called *F. tularensis* type B); *F. tularensis* subsp. *novicida* and *F. tularensis* subsp. *mediastica*. Molecular typing methods have identified distinct genotypes of *F. tularensis* subsp. *tularensis* that differ in their grographic location

and virulence. The majority of human and animal infections are caused by *F. tularensis* subsp. *tularensis* and *F. tularensis* subsp. *holoarctica*. Human disease has also been reported with *F. tularensis* subsp. *novicida* and and *F. philomiragia*.

F. tularensis is able to infect a wide range of hosts including humans to cause tularaemia. An intracellular pathogen, it is one of the most highly infectious bacteria known with an infectious dose in humans as low as 10 bacteria by the inhalational route. It multiplies to high levels within macrophages, and mutants unable to multiply in macrophages are avirulent. *F. tularensis* susbp. *tularensis* causes more severe infections than *F. tularensis* susbp. *holoarctica*. *F. tularensis* susbp. *tularensis* genotype A1b are more likely to be associated with invasive disease and higher mortality than type A1a, A2, or B.

F. tularensis multiplies at the site of inoculation and spreads to the regional lymph nodes and then systemically. An acute inflammatory reaction with neutrophils, macrophages, and lymphocytes is seen at the site of inoculation, resulting in tissue necrosis and, sometimes granuloma formation. *F. tularensis* is an intracellular pathogen that replicates primarily on host macrophages. Macrophage uptake occurs by an unusual process called 'looping phagoyctosis' that involves symmetric and spacious pseudopod loops. Once ingested, phagosome maturation and phagosome -lysosome fusion are impaired resulting in organism escape and multiplication in the cytosol. Similar events occur in neutrophils where the organism suppresses oxidative burst and escapes into the cytoplasm. Within the macrophage cytosol the organisms activate a multimolecular complex, the inflammasone, which leads to the release of proinflammatory cytokines and trigger caspase-1 dependent cell death. The virulence of *F. tularensis* has been correlated with several phenotypic characteristics including capsule formation, lipopolysaccharide, pili, production of acid phosphatases, and a siderophore. Genomic studies have identified genes in the *Francisella* pathogenicity island (FPI) which are involved in intracellular survival and animal virulence.

Epidemiology

F. tularensis is mainly isolated in the northern hemisphere, most frequently in Scandinavia, northern America, Japan, and Russia (100–400 cases/year), but has never been isolated in the United Kingdom. *F. tularensis* subsp. *tularensis* accounts for 90% of infections in North America whereas *F. tularensis* subsp. *holarctica* infections are more common in the rest of the world. The organism infects more than 100 species of wild and domestic vertebrates, such as small rodents, rabbits, hares, squirrels, hamsters, mice, and voles. Outbreaks in human populations frequently mirror outbreaks of disease occurring in wild animals. A wide range of arthropod vectors have been implicated in the transmission of the disease within wild animal populations and to humans. Rural populations and especially those individuals who spend periods of time in endemic areas such as farmers, hunters, walkers, and forest workers are most at risk of contracting tularaemia.

Transmission to humans occurs from contact with an infected animal or biting insect. Contaminated meat and water are important environmental sources of the infection and outbreaks have also been associated with contaminated water supplies and can involve large numbers of cases. Transmission can also occur from airborne spread of contaminated materials such as dust, hay, and water. Airborne transmission was the suspected source of an outbreak of pneumonic tularaemia in the United States of America and was associated with lawn mowing or brush cutting. Recent reports of tularaemia have been from Russia (following a sable bite), northern Spain (possibly associated with aerosolized contaminated water), and the United States of America (Utah).

Prevention

No licensed vaccine is available for prevention of tularaemia. Avoidance of contact with infected animals and vectors reduces the risk of infection. Hunters in particular should wear gloves when skinning dead animals, and meat should be thoroughly cooked before eating. Reducing the risk of inhalation of infectious dusts, e.g. during farming activities in endemic areas, by wearing respiratory protection should be considered.

Clinical features

Tularaemia in humans can occur in several forms depending on the route of infection. Although tularaemia can be a severely debilitating and even fatal disease, especially when caused by virulent strains, many cases of disease caused by lower virulence strains go undiagnosed owing to the nonspecific nature of the symptoms. The incubation period is normally 3 to 5 days (range 1–21 days), and patients develop influenza-like symptoms which may be protracted and relapsing if untreated.

Infection through skin or mucous membranes

Infection through the skin results in ulceroglandular tularaemia (Figs. 6.19.1, 6.19.2); where no ulcer is reported, this is termed glandular tularaemia. These forms of tularaemia are the most common presentations of the disease and can arise following the bite of an infected vector or through direct contact with the flesh of infected animal. A lesion develops at the site of infection, often a single papule which develops into an ulcer surrounded by a zone of inflammation. The ulcer is relatively painless and heals within a week. Within 3 to 5 days following infection, the patient

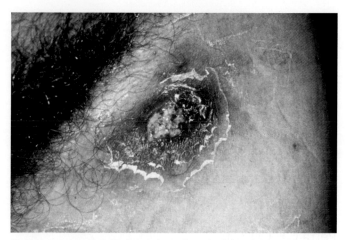

Fig. 6.19.2 Inguinal lymphadenopathy in ulceroglandular tularaemia. (Courtesy of A Berglund, Fallund, Sweden.)

develops fever, chills, malaise, headaches, and a sore throat. The local draining lymph nodes become enlarged and painful, like a bubo. Lymphadenopathy can take a significant period to resolve even with treatment, and without treatment suppuration occurs in approximately 30% of patients. Symmetrical rashes have been attributed to hypersensitivity (Fig. 6.19.3).

Less commonly, infection can occur through the conjunctiva. This is termed oculoglandular tularaemia and arises following direct contamination of the eye, e.g. through rubbing the eyes after skinning an infected rabbit. The patient develops conjunctivitis in the infected eye, swollen eyelids, and a purulent secretion.

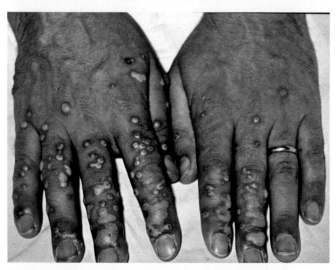

Fig. 6.19.1 Hands in a case of ulcero-(cutano-)glandular tularaemia. (Courtesy of A Berglund, Fallund, Sweden.)

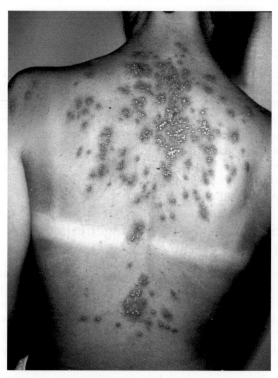

Fig. 6.19.3 Hypersensitivity reaction in infection with *Francisella tularensis* (Courtesy of A Berglund, Fallund, Sweden.)

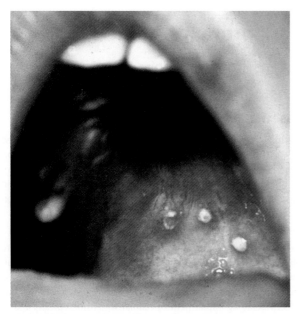

Fig. 6.19.4 Oral tularaemia in a case from northern Sweden. (Courtesy of A Berglund, Fallund, Sweden.)

Table 6.19.1 Differential diagnosis of tularaemia

Tularaemia	Differential diagnosis
Ulceroglandular	Pyogenic bacterial infection, orf, pasteurella infections, syphilis, chancroid, lymphogranuloma venereum, scrub typhus, streptococcal and staphylococcal cellulitis, mycobacterial infections (including tuberculosis), sporotrichosis, herpes simplex virus, anthrax
Glandular	Pyogenic bacterial infection, cat-scratch disease, toxoplasmosis, mycobacterial infections, sporotrichosis, streptococcal and staphylococcal adenitis, syphilis, plague
Oropharyngeal	Streptococcal pharyngitis, infectious mononucleosis, adenoviral infection, diphtheria
Oculoglandular	Pyogenic bacterial infection, cat-scratch disease, herpes simplex virus, syphilis, adenovirus
Typhoidal	Enteric fever, brucellosis, leptospirosis, malaria, Q fever, rickettsial infection, toxic shock syndrome, endocarditis
Gastrointestinal	Enterohaemorrhagic *E. coli*, GI anthrax, *Clostridium perfringens*, listeriosis
Respiratory	Q fever, other atypical bacterial pneumonias (mycoplasma, *Chlamydia pneumoniae*, Legionnaire's disease, psittacosis), viral pneumonia (influenza, hantavirus, respiratory syncytial virus, cytomegalovirus), tuberculosis, pneumonic plague

Untreated, the infection can spread to the local lymph nodes, in a similar way to ulceroglandular tularaemia.

Ingestion of infected meat can result in oropharyngeal (Fig. 6.19.4) or gastrointestinal tularaemia. Ulcers, pharyngitis, and swollen cervical lymph nodes develop, and a yellow-white pseudomembrane may be seen in oropharyngeal tularaemia. Gastrointestinal tularaemia can range from a mild but persistent diarrhoea to an acute fatal disease with extensive ulceration of the bowel, depending on the size of the infecting dose.

Any of the above infections may disseminate and progress to systemic disease without the appearance of swollen lymph nodes or ulcers. This is termed typhoidal tularaemia. Severe complications may also occur, such as septic shock.

Infection through inhalation

Inhalation of *F. tularensis* results in respiratory or pneumonic tularaemia. Pneumonia can also arise following haematogenous spread in other forms of tularaemia. Symptoms can be variable and depend on the virulence of the strain involved. Infection with the most highly virulent strains can have a case fatality rate of up to 30% if untreated, but antibiotic therapy reduces this to approximately 2%. Presentation can range from a mild pneumonia to an acute infection with high fever, malaise, chills, cough, delirium, and pulse–temperature dissociation. Radiological examination may reveal parenchymal infiltrates, most commonly in one lobe, and hilar lymphadenopathy may be present.

Differential diagnosis

Diagnosis of tularaemia is difficult due to the nonspecific nature of most of the symptoms, particularly if the ulcer has already healed. A high index of clinical suspicion is therefore required. Other diseases which must be rapidly excluded in patients presenting with acute respiratory distress and fever or influenza-like disease include plague and Q fever (Table 6.19.1). Oculoglandular tularaemia may be confused with severe infection caused by a range of viral and bacterial conjunctival pathogens.

Criteria for diagnosis

Most cases of tularaemia are diagnosed on the basis of epidemiological and clinical picture. The diagnosis is confirmed serologically and a range of serological tests for the detection of antibodies against *F. tularensis* is commercially available. The antibody response peaks at 4 to 6 weeks, but can be detected from 2 weeks. Routine cultures of specimens such as blood, sputum, pleural fluid, skin lesions, and lymph nodes are frequently negative as the organism is fastidious and requires enriched media and prolonged culture. The microbiology laboratory should be alerted to the possibility of *F. tularensis* as it is a biohazard group 3 pathogen and should be processed in a containment level 3 laboratory. Most strains require cystine or cysteine for growth and more than 2 days' incubation at 35°C to produce colonies. Some strains grow on conventional media such as chocolate agar, modified Thayer–Martin medium, or buffered charcoal yeast agar. The organisms are tiny, poorly staining Gram-negative coccobacilli on Gram stain and oxidase negative, weakly catalase positive, β-lactamase positive, urease negative, and satellite or XV test negative. Polymerase chain reaction (PCR) and enzyme-linked immunosorbent assay (ELISA) can be used to positively identify the bacteria, both following isolation and in specimens. Such direct detection of the pathogen is useful in patients who are serologically negative, e.g. in the early days of infection.

Treatment

Antimicrobial therapy should be administered to patients in whom tularaemia is suspected or confirmed. There are no randomized controlled trials comparing the efficacy of different drug regimens. Historically, aminoglycosides have been the drugs of choice for the treatment of tularaemia. Although it is clinically effective, streptomycin is rarely used now; gentamicin is a suitable alternative and is usually given for 7 to 14 days.

For patients with milder disease, oral therapy with tetracyclines or fluoroquinolones has been recommended. Doxycycline is effective in treatment of tularaemia and can also be used in children and pregnant women.

Ciprofloxacin has been shown to be highly effective and can be considered the current drug of choice for uncomplicated tularaemia. It has been shown to be effective in treating tularaemia in children and may be suitable for use in pregnant women. Both tetracyclines and fluorquinolones have been associated with relapse after cessation of treatment.

Meningitis should be treated with an aminoglycoside in combination with chloramphenicol.

Supportive care should be provided as appropriate; some patients may require intensive care with respiratory support should sepsis develop. Suppurating nodes should be drained.

Prognosis

Tularaemia responds well to antibiotic therapy, especially if started early in infection. The mortality rate of the more acute forms of the disease is reduced from 30% to 2% if the patient receives suitable antibiotics. Most deaths are associated with pneumonic or typhoidal forms. Relapse may occur when antibiotic therapy is withdrawn (even with aminoglycosides or fluoroquinolones).

Other issues

Patients are not considered an infection risk and do not require isolation. Tularaemia is notifiable in some countries, although not in the United Kingdom.

Autopsies should only be performed by personnel wearing respirators if death from tularaemia is suspected. Bodies should not be embalmed before burial.

Likely future developments

Work is under way to identify a vaccine against tularaemia that will be suitable for licensing. It is highly likely that progress will be made in this area in the next few years, although it can take many years to obtain approval.

Further reading

Centers for Disease Control and Prevention. *Emergency preparedness and response: tularaemia.* www.bt.cdc.gov/agent/tularemia/index.asp

Dennis DT, *et al.* (2001). Tularemia as a biological weapon: medical and public health management. *JAMA*, **285**, 2763–73.

Health Protection Agency (2007) *Tularaemia.* www.hpa.org.uk/infections/topics_az/tularemia/menu.htm

Jacobs RF, Condrey YM, Yamauchi T (1985). Tularemia in adults and children: a changing presentation. *Pediatrics*, **75**, 818–22.

© Crown copyright Dstl 2010.

6.20 Anthrax

Arthur E. Brown and Thira Sirisanthana

Essentials

Anthrax is primarily a disease of herbivorous mammals, caused by the Gram-positive rod *Bacillus anthracis*, which causes human infection when its spores enter the body, most commonly from handling infected animals or animal products. The disease occurs in most countries of the world, but not in those where the condition is controlled in livestock by vaccination programmes. Anthrax is a leading agent of biological warfare.

Pathophysiology—after entry into the body, anthrax spores are phagocytosed by macrophages and carried to regional lymph nodes, where they germinate to produce vegetative bacilli that enter the blood stream. These produce anthrax toxin, which has effects including impairment of cellular water homeostasis and of many intracellular signalling pathways.

Clinical features—anthrax occurs in three clinical forms based on the route of exposure. (1) Cutaneous—lesions are usually found on exposed areas of skin; a small papule develops at the site of infection, enlarges and ulcerates, with the painless ulcer becoming covered with a black leathery eschar surrounded by nonpitting oedema before healing in 2 to 6 weeks; associated systemic symptoms are usually mild. (2) Gastrointestinal—acquired by eating contaminated food and comprising (a) oropharyngeal anthrax, presenting with fever, neck swelling, sore throat, oropharyngeal ulcer, and dysphagia, or (b) terminal ileal/caecal anthrax, presenting with fever, nausea, vomiting, and abdominal pain, followed by rapidly developing ascites and bloody diarrhoea. (3) Inhalation—aerosol exposure leads to a nonspecific viral-type prodrome which progresses to a fulminant stage of severe respiratory distress, cyanosis, stridor, and profuse sweating; up to half of patients develop anthrax meningitis; shock and death typically follow in hours or days.

Diagnosis—may be very difficult in the absence of a known outbreak, particularly for inhalation anthrax, where a clinical clue is widening of the mediastinum caused by lymphadenopathy. Confirmation is by laboratory identification of *B. anthracis*. Serological testing can be used for retrospective diagnosis.

Treatment—this is with supportive care and antibiotics, which are effective against the multiplying (vegetative) form of *B. anthracis*, but not against the spore form. Mild cases of cutaneous anthrax are usually treated with oral penicillin. For gastrointestinal, inhalational and meningeal anthrax, at least two antibiotics should be given intravenously, e.g. ciprofloxacin or doxycycline along with another antimicrobial expected to be effective (e.g. penicillin, ampicillin, rifampin, vancomycin, chloramphenicol, imipenem, clindamycin, and clarithromycin).

Prognosis—the mortality of untreated cutaneous anthrax is 10 to 20%, but fatalities are rare with appropriate antibiotic treatment. Almost all cases of inhalation anthrax and anthrax meningitis are

---

The views expressed in this chapter are those of A E Brown and do not represent the positions of the United States Department of Defense or Army.

fatal; initiation of treatment after the start of fulminant disease is rarely effective.

Prevention—routine immunization of livestock should be instituted in endemic areas with continuing cases of animal anthrax. Carcasses of animals suspected of dying from anthrax must be disposed of appropriately. Anthrax vaccines should be offered to members of high-risk groups, e.g. those at occupational risk, laboratory workers and some military groups. Postexposure prophylaxis should be given following suspected exposure to aerosolized anthrax spores (e.g. ciprofloxacin for 60 days).

Introduction

Anthrax is a zoonotic disease, primarily of herbivorous mammals, caused by *Bacillus anthracis*. Herbivores are particularly susceptible to anthrax, acquiring the infection via contact with soil-borne spores through oral or gastrointestinal mucosa. The bacteria multiply rapidly to high concentrations and these animals are the common source of exposure to humans. Human infections occur when spores of *B. anthracis* enter the body, most commonly from handling infected animals or animal products. The disease occurs in three clinical forms based on the route of exposure: cutaneous, gastrointestinal, and inhalation. Septicaemia and meningitis may occur from any primary focus. Other names for anthrax include malignant pustule, Siberian ulcer, charbon, malignant oedema, *Milzbrand*, and woolsorters' disease.

Anthrax is present in most countries of the world but has practically disappeared from North America, Western Europe, and Australia since the control of disease in livestock by extensive vaccination programmes. However, it is still prevalent in less developed countries of Asia, Africa, and the Middle East where control programmes are weak or compromised by social disruptions.

Anthrax has gained further importance due to its use as a biological weapon (Oxford Textbook of Medicine 5e Chapter 9.5.13). Evidence exists that at least 13 countries have offensive biological weapons programmes and anthrax is one of the most threatening potential agents. Nonstate groups may attempt to use anthrax as a tool of bioterrorism. Recognition of these threats has led to an increase in resources for development of improved methods of diagnosis, therapy, and prevention.

Historical perspective

Anthrax in agricultural settings has been recognized for more than 2400 years. With the industrial revolution, workers processing animal hides and wool became another risk group. Use as a weapon of biowarfare or bioterrorism is now perceived as the major public health threat posed by anthrax. This was made clear by its accidental release from a Soviet military facility in 1979 and its distribution by letter in the United States of America in 2001.

Industrial exposure to anthrax spores carried by animal hides and wool led to cases of cutaneous and inhalation ('woolsorters' disease') anthrax in industrializing countries at the end of the 19th century. In Liverpool, a disinfection station was established where imported wool and other animal fibres were bathed in formaldehyde. This public health measure led to a marked decrease in industrial anthrax in the United Kingdom.

Anthrax played a central role in the birth of medical microbiology. In the 1870s, Robert Koch and Louis Pasteur carried out complementary studies that proved the causal relation between *B. anthracis* and the disease anthrax. Koch cultured the organism on artificial media, described the vegetative and spore phases of its life cycle, and demonstrated disease causality by fulfilling 'Koch's Postulates'. Pasteur added extensively to the anthrax-based evidence for the germ theory of disease. In the early 1880s, Pasteur in France and Greenfield in England each demonstrated that heat-attenuated strains of *B. anthracis* protected sheep, goats, and cows from anthrax. This disease of livestock had enormous economic importance and by the mid-1890s millions of sheep and cattle had been given this first animal vaccine. In the 1930s, Sterne developed nonencapsulated strains of *B. anthracis* that induce protection within weeks after a single injection. This live attenuated vaccine became the main vaccine in the world for domesticated animals and is still used.

Aetiology, genetics, pathogenesis, and pathology

Anthrax is caused by *B. anthracis*, combining a dormant spore phase in the environment with a rapidly multiplying vegetative phase in animals which resists phagocytosis and produces a lethal toxin-mediated disease. The organism is a large nonmotile Gram-positive rod; in clinical specimens it has a large capsule and occurs singly or in short chains that appear as 'jointed bamboo' rods. Key to the pathogen's life cycle and epidemiology is the property of spore formation outside living animals, related to nutrient depletion in its microenvironment. These spores are resistant to heat, desiccation, ultraviolet light, gamma irradiation, and some disinfectants.

Genetically, *B. anthracis* consists of a 5.2-Mbp chromosome and two plasmids, pXO1 (182 kbp) and pXO2 (96 kbp), which contain hundreds of predicted protein-coding sequences. The nucleotide sequences are highly conserved, with interisolate identity is believed to be greater than 99.99%. This genetic homogeneity complicates the strain typing needed for molecular epidemiology. Based on genome sequencing, tandem repeat markers and single-nucleotide polymorphisms, three major lineages (A, B, and C) have been identified which can be subdivided into 12 subgroups. Since spores long dormant in the environment will cause new disease outbreaks, further revision of this typing system is expected. Genetic typing of isolates from bioterrorist events has special forensic importance.

Transmission of anthrax to humans is via spores entering the skin or gastrointestinal or respiratory tracts. In the skin, entry is enhanced by abrasion and germination may occur in extracellular tissue fluid. In the respiratory tract, airborne spores reach the alveoli where they are phagocytosed by macrophages and potentially dendritic cells, and are carried to regional lymph nodes. Intracellular spores germinate, producing vegetative bacilli that multiply and activate genes carried on plasmids pXO1 and pXO2 which are the basis of its virulence. pXO1 expresses anthrax toxin, which is made up of three proteins, protective antigen (PA), lethal factor (LF), and oedema factor (EF), expressed from the genes *pag*, *lef*, and *cya*, respectively. pXO2 expresses poly-D-glutamic acid that forms a capsule resistant to phagocytosis. LF and EF impair leucocyte function, and contribute to tissue necrosis, oedema, and relative absence of leucocytes. Multiplying bacteria enter the blood stream, reaching bacteraemias of 10^7 to 10^8 bacilli/ml.

Anthrax toxin causes the massive oedema, organ failure, and immune compromise seen in severe anthrax. Transfer of sterile plasma containing anthrax toxin was shown in the 1950s to be lethal in a guinea pig model. The toxicology of the binding (PA) and active (LF and EF) proteins is complex. PA (83 kDa) binds to cell surface receptors, is cleaved by a furin protease which releases a 20-kDa segment, and oligomerizes into heptamers on cell surface lipid rafts. The final step in forming the toxin–receptor complex is the additional binding of three EF and/or LF proteins. The surface-bound structures are internalized by endocytosis; PA is degraded and EF/LF protected while transported to, and released into, the cytoplasm. EF, a calmodulin-dependent adenylate cyclase, increases intracellular cAMP levels and interferes with water homeostasis. LF, a zinc metalloprotease, cleaves key protein kinases on pathways linking surface receptors to transcription of specific nuclear genes resulting in cellular dysfunction. These toxins also interfere with immune responses, including production of inflammatory cytokines and phagocyte function.

When spores of *B. anthracis* are introduced cutaneously they germinate and multiply, protected by the antiphagocytic capsule. EF and LF impair leucocyte function and contribute to tissue necrosis, oedema, and the paucity of leucocytes in the skin lesion. Spread to draining lymph nodes results in haemorrhagic, oedematous, and necrotic lymphadenitis. Gastrointestinal anthrax follows ingestion of food contaminated with *B. anthracis*. Localization and multiplication of bacilli in the oropharynx and the draining lymph nodes causes oropharyngeal ulcers localized oedema, neck swelling. Localization and multiplication in the stomach, duodenum, ileum, or caecum cause mucosal inflammation, ulcers, and ascites. Bacteria drain to mesenteric lymph nodes causing haemorrhagic adenitis. Inhalation anthrax follows deposition of spores in alveoli, phagocytosis and transport to tracheobronchial and mediastinal lymph nodes, and intracellular germination. Production of toxins leads to haemorrhagic, oedematous, and necrotic lymphadenitis in the mediastinum.

All primary forms of anthrax can be complicated by septicaemia and, at times, haemorrhagic meningitis. This is especially common with inhalation anthrax; autopsies of untreated cases reveal numerous bacteria in blood vessels, lymph nodes, and multiple organs.

Epidemiology

The natural life cycle of anthrax involves vegetative multiplication in susceptible animals and dormancy of spore forms in soil. Anthrax in animals is usually acquired by exposure of mucous membranes of the mouth and gastrointestinal tract to soil contaminated with spores of *B. anthracis*. Once internalized, the spores germinate to yield vegetative cells which multiply and produce either localized or systemic infection. Animal species vary in susceptibility to infection and disease severity. Herbivores such as horses, sheep, goats, and cattle are most susceptible, dying with overwhelming bacteraemias. They often bleed from the nose, mouth, and bowel, and thereby contaminate soil with vegetative *B. anthracis* which sporulate and can persist for decades. Carcasses of infected animals are additional sources of contamination. *B. anthracis* spores in soil may undergo bursts of vegetative multiplication that increase the local concentration of organisms in the soil of 'hot' zones. The factors controlling this *ex vivo* multiplication of anthrax are poorly understood, but seem associated with major shifts in soil microenvironment when water and nutrients become available after periods of drought.

Human anthrax may occur in agricultural or industrial settings, or by the intentional use of anthrax spores as biological weapons. Agricultural cases (usually cutaneous form) result from direct contact with infected animals, generally by herders, butchers, and slaughterhouse workers. Industrial cases (often inhalation form) involve workers in contact (direct or via aerosol) with contaminated animal products such as hides, wool, goat's hair, or bone. No human-to-human transmission of anthrax has been reported. Cutaneous anthrax typically follows skin exposure to infected animals or animal products. Gastrointestinal anthrax follows ingestion of *B. anthracis*-contaminated food, usually meat, and may be more common than appreciated in endemic regions of Asia and Africa. Inhalation anthrax is a result of the spores, which are 1 to 2 μm in diameter. Historically, woolsorters and those working with herbivore hides in industrial mills were at risk, but naturally occurring inhalation anthrax is now rare.

The worldwide incidence of human anthrax is not known, but is estimated to be 2000 to 20 000 cases annually, of which some 95% are cutaneous. Based on reporting of anthrax outbreaks in animals, the World Health Organization (WHO) characterizes several countries in Africa, the Middle East, and Asia as hyperendemic/epidemic. Many other countries in these regions, as well as in southern Europe and the Americas, have an endemic level of anthrax, while most remaining countries have at least sporadic cases. The largest reported outbreak of agricultural anthrax occurred in Zimbabwe in the late 1970s during the civil war. Most of the estimated 10 000 human cases were cutaneous, while a small number were gastrointestinal. Disruption of veterinary health services, especially anthrax vaccination, led to epizootic anthrax in cattle and the associated epidemic in humans.

An outbreak of the oropharyngeal form of anthrax occurred in Thailand in 1982 when 24 people developed anthrax after eating poorly cooked meat from infected cattle and water buffalo. In Switzerland in 1991, 25 workers in one textile factory contracted anthrax, 24 had cutaneous disease and one had inhalation disease. The factory had imported contaminated goat hair from Pakistan. An unnatural outbreak of inhalation anthrax occurred among residents of Sverdlovsk in the former Soviet Union in 1979. Spores accidentally released into the atmosphere from a military laboratory were carried downwind and caused at least 79 cases of inhalation anthrax and 68 deaths. In the United Kingdom and Europe in 2000 and again in 2009–10, there were infections and deaths among parenteral drug users due to anthrax-contaminated heroin. Thirty-one confirmed cases, including 11 deaths, have been reported from Scotland, England, and Germany. Patients reported snorting, smoking, and/or injecting heroin. Clinical presentations were atypical for anthrax and varied greatly.

State-sponsored biological weapons programmes have often selected anthrax as an ideal organism for tactical use (Oxford Textbook of Medicine 5e Chapter 9.5.13). It is easily obtained and cultured, and spores are very stable and small enough to reach alveoli when aerosolized; inhalation infections are usually fatal. In the early 1970s, more than 140 countries signed or ratified the Biological Weapons Convention, agreeing to terminate offensive weapons programmes and destroy existing weapons stockpiles. Monitoring compliance of this convention remains problematic.

Anthrax has also been used by terrorist groups. In the early 1990s, members of the Aum Shinrikyo cult dispersed aerosols of *B. anthracis* (Sterne strain) spores over a Japanese city but caused no disease. In 2001, at least five letters containing anthrax spores (Ames strain) were mailed in the United States of America to several government and news offices, leading to 11 cases of inhalation anthrax with five deaths, and another 11 cases of suspected or confirmed cutaneous anthrax. Thus, in industrialized countries, the threat of human infection due to agricultural and industrial anthrax has lessened while that due to biological warfare has increased.

Prevention

Control of anthrax in animals limits human exposure. Routine immunization of livestock should be instituted in endemic areas with continuing cases of animal anthrax. The most widely used animal vaccine is a live nonencapsulated strain of *B. anthracis* developed in the United States of America by Sterne in the 1930s. Cases of animal and human anthrax should be reported to the appropriate authorities. Carcasses of animals, domestic or wild, suspected of dying from anthrax should be incinerated in a manner that also sterilizes the underlying soil, or buried intact to a depth of six feet and covered with lime to avoid sporulation. Gastrointestinal anthrax can be prevented by proper cooking of meat and avoidance when contamination is suspected. Anthrax vaccines should be offered to members of high-risk groups, such as those at occupational risk, laboratory workers, and some military groups.

Current anthrax vaccines for humans are all produced from attenuated strains of *B. anthracis* that are nonencapsulating. In the United Kingdom and the United States of America vaccines made from cell-free culture supernatants are used to induce antitoxin immunity, PA being the main immunizing antigen. In Russia and China, live spore vaccines have been developed. The licensed vaccine in the United States of America is anthrax vaccine adsorbed (AVA); it is given intramuscularly at 0, 1, 6, 12, and 18 months, with yearly boosters. More than 95% of vaccinees are seropositive after the first three doses. The licensed vaccine in the United Kingdom is anthrax vaccine precipitated (AVP); it is given intramuscularly at 0, 3, 6, and 26 weeks, with yearly boosters. The Russian anthrax vaccine is a suspension of live spores (strain STI-1) in use since 1953; it is given by scarification through a drop of vaccine containing 10^8 spores or subcutaneously at 0 and 3 weeks, with yearly boosters. The Chinese anthrax vaccine is a live spore (strain A16R) product in use since the 1960s; it is given by scarification with a dose of 10^8 colony-forming units and boosted at 6 to 12 months.

Drawbacks of the current cell-free vaccines are the incomplete characterization of the vaccine and the complex immunization regimens. These, along with the increased risk of *B. anthracis* use as a biological weapon, have stimulated renewed efforts to develop improved vaccines. A recombinant PA vaccine is in clinical development. Additional approaches under investigation include antigen and adjuvant modification, live vaccines, and DNA and vectored constructs.

Postexposure prophylaxis is given following suspected exposure to aerosolized anthrax spores. Ciprofloxacin has been approved for this indication in the United States of America (500 mg twice daily). A 60-day course is recommended because antibiotics are not effective against the spore form that may be dormant in alveoli for many weeks. Antibiotics protect against multiplying organisms, but prevent development of protective immune responses. Therefore, disease may occur if the strain is drug resistant, after cessation of antibiotics, or when compliance is poor. For these reasons, concurrent vaccination has been recommended by the Advisory Committee on Immunization Practices in the United States, although this indication is not approved by the Food and Drug Authority (FDA).

Clinical features

Cutaneous anthrax

Anthrax acquired its name from the Hippocratic description of the skin lesion's characteristic eschar as being the colour of coal (Greek *anthrakos* = coal). These cutaneous lesions are usually found on exposed areas of skin, such as the face, neck, arms, or hands, and may be single or multiple depending on the type of exposure. The incubation period ranges from 1 to 12 days, usually 2 to 7 days. Initially a small papule develops at the site of infection, and it then enlarges and ulcerates. The depressed ulcer becomes covered with a black leathery eschar surrounded by nonpitting oedema (Fig. 6.20.1) that is occasionally massive ('malignant oedema'). Established lesions are characteristically painless and may be hypaesthetic. Small satellite vesicles, containing many organisms and few white cells, may surround the original lesion; regional lymphadenitis is common. Associated systemic symptoms are usually mild; lesions heal without scarring, although slowly (2–6 weeks), after eschar separation. In 10 to 20% of untreated patients the disease becomes systemic, with bacteraemia and toxaemia. Cutaneous anthrax should be considered in patients with painless ulcers associated with oedema and vesicles, and who have had prior contact with animals or animal products. Differential diagnosis includes staphylococcal or streptococcal skin infections, ulceroglandular tularaemia, bubonic plague, bites of brown recluse spiders, orf, rickettsial pox, and scrub typhus.

Gastrointestinal anthrax

Gastrointestinal anthrax is acquired by eating contaminated and inadequately cooked food, and thus may occur in familial clusters. The disease has an incubation period of 2 to 5 days and occurs in two forms. Oropharyngeal anthrax follows deposition of bacteria in the oropharynx. Patients present with fever, neck swelling, sore throat, and dysphagia. The neck swelling is caused by enlargement of the jugular lymph nodes together with subcutaneous oedema as in diphtheria. The lesion in the oral cavity or oropharynx starts as inflamed mucosa, progressing through necrosis and ulceration to formation of a pseudomembrane (no eschar) covering the ulcer (Fig. 6.20.2). In severe cases, subcutaneous oedema extends to the anterior chest wall and axilla, with the overlying skin showing signs of inflammation. Death may result from systemic toxaemia or local airway obstruction. Oropharyngeal anthrax should be considered in patients who present with fever, neck swelling, sore throat, and oropharyngeal ulcer, and who give a history of eating raw or undercooked meat. The differential diagnosis includes diphtheria and peritonsillar abscess.

In the other form of gastrointestinal anthrax, organisms are deposited in the terminal ileum or caecum, and occasionally in more proximal parts of the gastrointestinal tract. Disease onset

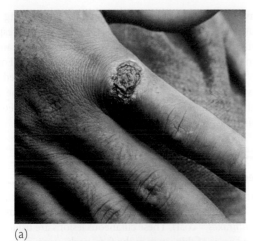

(a)

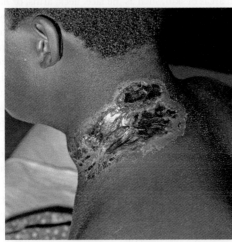

(b)

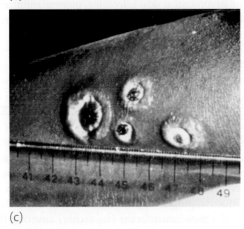

(c)

Fig. 6.20.1 Cutaneous anthrax. (a) Early lesion. (b) Large eschar in a Nigerian patient who carried an infected carcass on his shoulder. (c) Ulcer with satellite lesions in a Thai patient.
(a) (Copyright Dr S Eykin.) (b) (Copyright D A Warrell.) (c) (Copyright the late Sornchai Looareesuwan.)

is nonspecific with fever, nausea, vomiting, and abdominal pain, followed by rapidly developing ascites and bloody diarrhoea. Haematemesis, melaena, haematochezia, and/or profuse watery diarrhoea may occur. In severe cases, toxaemia, shock, and death follow. Early diagnosis is difficult, except in an epidemic setting, and the disease is likely under reported.

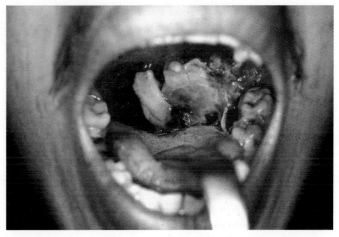

Fig. 6.20.2 Oropharyngeal anthrax in a Thai man showing extensive lesion in posterior pharynx.
(From Sirisanthana T, *et al.* (1984). Outbreak of oral-pharyngeal anthrax: an unusual manifestation of human infection with *Bacillus anthracis. Am J Trop Med Hyg,* **33**, 144–50.)

Inhalation anthrax

Inhalation anthrax has an incubation period of 1 to 43 days, which modelling suggests is dose dependent. A prodrome consists of malaise, myalgia, fever, and nonproductive cough, nonspecific symptoms similar to those of viral respiratory diseases. In some patients there is transient improvement after 2 to 4 days. A fulminant stage follows which begins with severe respiratory distress, cyanosis, stridor, and profuse sweating. Subcutaneous oedema of the chest and neck may develop. A characteristic radiographic finding is mediastinal widening usually with pleural effusion. By CT, nearly all patients have mediastinal enlargement secondary to lymphadenopathy, as well as pleural effusions (Fig. 6.20.3). Blood cultures collected before the start of antibiotics will grow *B. anthracis.* Up to one-half of patients develop anthrax meningitis. Shock and death typically follow in less than 24 h. During the prodrome, and

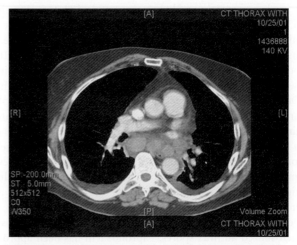

Fig. 6.20.3 CT image of an American adult with inhalation anthrax showing mediastinal enlargement secondary to lymphadenopathy. Note small bilateral pleural effusions and nearly clear lung fields.
(From Jernigan JA, *et al.* (2001). Bioterrorism-related inhalational anthrax: the first 10 cases reported in the United States. *Emerg Infect Dis,* **7**, 933–44.)

in the absence of a known outbreak, the disease is very difficult to diagnose. Advanced disease may be suspected in the presence of a characteristically widened mediastinum despite otherwise normal chest radiographic findings. Inhalation anthrax must be distinguished from pneumonic plague.

Meningeal anthrax

Anthrax meningitis, associated with overwhelming *B. anthracis* bacteraemia, may complicate any primary form of anthrax. Rarely, a case of anthrax meningitis has been reported in which the primary site was not identified. Within a few days of the primary lesion the patient suddenly develops confusion, loss of consciousness, and focal neurological signs. The cerebrospinal fluid may be haemorrhagic, but of note is the high concentration of organisms. The disease is almost always fatal.

Criteria for diagnosis

The diagnosis of anthrax may be suspected on clinical and epidemiological grounds, and is confirmed by laboratory identification of *B. anthracis*. Clinical signs and symptoms are discussed above. Clinical specimens containing large Gram-positive rods, singly and in short chains of 2 to 4 cells, should be interpreted as possible *Bacillus* spp. Demonstration of encapsulation of these bacilli by India ink, Giemsa's, or polychrome methylene blue stain leads to a presumptive identification of *B. anthracis*. Culture isolates are identified by classic morphological and biochemical characteristics: Gram-positive broad spore-forming rods, the spores do not swell the vegetative cell and are oval shaped; nonmotile; colonies have a ground-glass appearance and are (nearly always) nonhaemolytic on sheep blood agar. Standard confirmatory tests include lysis by gamma phage and direct immunofluorescent assays for cell wall or capsular antigens on the vegetative cells.

Serological testing is not helpful for diagnosis at the onset of symptoms but can be used for retrospective diagnosis. Specific IgG antibodies are detectable by enzyme-linked immunosorbent assay (ELISA), with testing of paired samples preferred. In 2004, the United States Food and Drug Administration approved a rapid blood test for diagnosis of anthrax based on antibodies to anthrax protective antigen. Delayed-type hypersensitivity is assessed by antigen skin test (Anthraxin) in the former Soviet Union for diagnosis of former infection or response to vaccination. Other technologies include immunohistochemistry, polymerase chain reaction (PCR), and genetic sequencing.

Treatment

Antibiotics are effective against the multiplying (vegetative) form of *B. anthracis*, but not against the spore form. They should be used in combination for all severe anthrax disease. Most strains of *B. anthracis* are susceptible to penicillin, and mild cases of cutaneous anthrax may be treated with oral penicillin at the dosage of 250 mg 6-hourly for 5 to 7 days. For extensive lesions, parenteral penicillin G, 2 million units every 6 h, should be given for a total treatment period of 7 to 10 days. Ciprofloxacin, erythromycin, doxycycline, or chloramphenicol can be used in penicillin-sensitive patients. Antibiotics decrease the likelihood of systemic disease and thus mortality, but the time to resolution of skin lesions is unchanged. The skin lesion should be covered with a sterile dressing and used dressings should be decontaminated.

In gastrointestinal, inhalational, and meningeal anthrax, at least two antibiotics should be given intravenously. If naturally acquired, penicillin G (4 million units every 4 h) has been the drug of choice; ciprofloxacin (400 mg every 12 h) or doxycycline (100 mg every 12 h) are currently recommended in the United States of America. Of note, doxycycline should not be used for meningitis which should be assumed in the management of inhalation anthrax. Many patients will require intensive supportive care.

Anthrax caused by a biological weapon will generally be acquired by inhalation. In this setting, drug resistance due to genetic modification is of concern and drug sensitivity testing is imperative. Treatment should begin intravenously with ciprofloxacin (400 mg every 12 h) or doxycycline (100 mg every 12 h), along with one or two other antimicrobials expected to be effective (penicillin, ampicillin, rifampicin, vancomycin, chloramphenicol, imipenem, clindamycin, and clarithromycin are candidates). Factors associated with lower mortality are initiation of treatment during the prodrome phase, drainage of pleural fluid, and use of multidrug regimens. Initiation of treatment after the start of fulminant disease is rarely effective.

Prognosis

The mortality of untreated cutaneous anthrax is 10 to 20%. With appropriate antibiotic treatment, fatalities are rare. Almost all cases of inhalation anthrax and anthrax meningitis are fatal. An exception to this is suggested by the recent experience in the United States of America where initiation of multidrug treatment during the prodromal stage, along with drainage of pleural effusions and extensive supportive measures, resulted in a reduction of mortality to about 50%. Mortality of oropharyngeal anthrax is about 15% in treated patients; mortality of the other form of gastrointestinal anthrax is uncertain, but high if disease becomes systemic.

Other issues

The WHO has estimated that 50 kg of *B. anthracis* spores released over a city of 5 million people would infect 250 000 people, killing 40% of them. Numbers would be influenced by the quality of the aerosol, dispersal method, and ambient weather conditions. Cases would be largely inhalation and intensive medical care would be required. Most cities would not have the required medical surge capacity. Antibiotics and vaccine would be needed in great quantities for postexposure prophylaxis. These realities are among the challenges to preparedness planning.

Areas of uncertainty

Specificity of environmental assays will remain challenging, since true-positives will be rare and false-positives disruptive and expensive. The increasing capacity to genetically modify anthrax strains may lead to biological weapons that are resistant to antibiotics or have altered vaccine target sites.

Likely future developments

Methods for detection of spores in the atmosphere will improve. The mechanisms by which anthrax toxins compromise immune responses and cause rapid death will become clear and result in improved therapies. New vaccines with simpler immunizing regimens will become available.

Further reading

Abrami L, Reig N, Gisou van der Goot F (2005). Anthrax toxin: the long and winding road that leads to the kill. *Trends Microbiol*, **13**, 72–8. [Good review of anthrax toxicology.]

Beatty ME, *et al.* (2003). Gastrointestinal anthrax: review of the literature. *Arch Intern Med*, **163**, 2527–31. [Review of gastrointestinal anthrax, clinical, microbiological, and epidemiological aspects.]

Booth MG, *et al.* (2010). Anthrax infection in drug users. *Lancet*, **375**, 1345–6. [Lethal, but atypical, cases of anthrax in heroin users in Scotland, England and Germany.]

Brachman PS, Friedlander AM, Grabenstein JD (2008). Anthrax vaccine. In: Plotkin SL, Orenstein WA, Offit PA (eds) *Vaccines*, pp. 111–126. Saunders, Philadelphia. [Comprehensive and expert review of anthrax vaccines.]

Brachman PS, *et al.* (1962). Field evaluation of a human anthrax vaccine. *Am J Public Health*, **52**, 632–45. [Report of controlled human efficacy study of vaccine against anthrax.]

Brittingham KC, *et al.* (2005). Dendritic cells endocytose *Bacillus anthracis* spores: implications for anthrax pathogenesis. *J Immunol*, **174**, 5545–52. [Evidence for potential role of dendritic cells in pathogenesis.]

Centers for Disease Control and Prevention (2006). Inhalation anthrax associated with dried animal hides: Pennsylvania and New York City, 2006. *MMWR Morb Mortal Wkly Rep*, **55**, 280–2. [Report of first case of naturally acquired inhalation anthrax in the United States of America in 30 years.]

Centers for Disease Control and Prevention (2010). Use of anthrax vaccine in the United States. *MMWR Morb Mortal Wkly Rep*, **59**, 1–30. [2009 recommendations of the Advisory Committee on Immunization Practices on use of anthrax vaccine.]

Davies JCA (1982). A major epidemic of anthrax in Zimbabwe, part 1. *Cent Afr J Med*, **28**, 291–8. [First of three articles describing the largest known anthrax outbreak.]

Holty J-EC, *et al.* (2006). Systematic review: a century of inhalational anthrax cases from 1900 to 2005. *Ann Intern Med*, **144**, 270–80. [Retrospective case review of inhalation anthrax showing factors associated with survival.]

Inglesby TV, *et al.* (2002). Anthrax as a biological weapon, 2002: updated recommendations for management. *JAMA*, **287**, 2236–52. [Comprehensive review of bioweapons-related concerns.]

Maguina C, *et al.* (2005). Cutaneous anthrax in Lima, Peru: retrospective analysis of 71 cases, including four with a meningoencephalic complication. *Rev Inst Med Trop Sao Paulo*, **47**, 25–30. [Large retrospective review of cutaneous cases.]

Marano N, *et al.* (2008). Effects of reduced dose schedule and intramuscular administration of anthrax vaccine absorbed on immunogenicity and safety at 7 months. *JAMA*, **300**, 1532–43. [Basis for shift to IM administration of vaccine and drop of dose at 2 weeks.]

Meselson M, *et al.* (1994). The Sverdlovsk anthrax outbreak of 1979. *Science*, **266**, 1202–8. [Description of the bioweapons-related outbreak in the former Soviet Union.]

Perl DP, Dooley JR (1976). Anthrax. In: Binford CH, Connor DH (eds) *Pathology of tropical and extraordinary diseases*, vol. 1, pp. 118–23. Armed Forces Institute of Pathology, Washington. [Description and illustrations of gross and microscopic human pathology.]

Plotkin SA, *et al.* (1960). An epidemic of inhalation anthrax, the first in the twentieth century: I. Clinical features. *Am J Med*, **29**, 992–1001. [Landmark description of industrial anthrax.]

Rasko DA, *et al.* (2011). *Bacillus anthracis* comparative genome analysis in support of the Amerithrax. *Proc Natl Acad Sci USA*, **108**, 5027–32. [Shows forensic value of genetic typing of isolates, spurred on by the 2001 outbreak in the United States of America.]

Sirisanthana T, *et al.* (1984). Outbreak of oral-pharyngeal anthrax: an unusual manifestation of human infection with *Bacillus anthracis*. *Am J Trop Med Hyg*, **39**, 144–50. [Largest reported outbreak of an unusual variant of gastrointestinal anthrax.]

Van Ert ML, *et al.* (2007). Global genetic population structure of Bacillus anthracis. *PLoS ONE*, **2**(5), e461. [Description of genetic groupings of B. anthracis, geographic distribution and global spread.]

Vietri NJ, *et al.* (2006). Short-course post-exposure antibiotic prophylaxis combined with vaccination protects against experimental inhalational anthrax. *Proc Natl Acad Sci*, **103**, 7813–6. [Evidence from primates showing benefit of postexposure vaccination with antibiotics.]

6.21 Brucellosis

M. Monir Madkour[†]

Essentials

There are four species of the Gram-negative, aerobic brucella bacillus, each comprising several biovars: *Brucella melitensis* ('Malta fever', most commonly associated with goats, sheep, and camels), *B. abortus* (cattle), *B. suis* (pigs), and *B. canis* (dogs). The disease that they cause—brucellosis—occurs worldwide, but is especially prevalent in the Mediterranean region, the Indian subcontinent, Mexico, and Central and South America. Transmission is commonly by ingestion of untreated dairy products or other contaminated foods, but can also be by inhalation or inoculation.

Clinical features—symptoms are highly variable, simulating other febrile illnesses, hence travel to endemic areas (with details of drinking and eating behaviour) and occupation are crucial elements in the history. Joint pains, back pain and headache are common (each found in >80% of cases). Signs include spinal tenderness (48%), arthritis (40%), lymphadenopathy (32%), splenomegaly (25%), hepatomegaly (20%), and epididymo-orchitis (21% of men).

Diagnosis and treatment—definite diagnosis requires the isolation of the organism from the blood, body fluids, or tissues. Treatment is with supportive care and antibiotics: regimens containing doxycycline in combination with streptomycin/gentamicin/netilmicin are most effective, incurring fewer therapeutic failures and relapses.

Prevention—human brucellosis can be prevented by eradicating the disease in animals by vaccination. Other preventive measures include avoiding keeping farm animals in close proximity to houses, drinking raw milk and its products, and consumption of raw liver, meat, and bone marrow. There is no effective vaccine for human use.

Aetiological agent

There are four species of *Brucella*, each comprising several biovars: *B. melitensis* ('Malta fever', most commonly associated with goats, sheep, and camels), *B. abortus* (cattle), *B. suis* (pigs), and *B. canis* (dogs). They are small nonencapsulated nonmotile nonsporulating Gram-negative aerobic bacilli. Genomes of *B. abortus*, *B. melitensis*, and *B. suis* have been fully sequenced. They may survive in unpasteurized soft white goat cheese for up to 8 weeks but

---

[†] It is with regret that we report the death of Professor M. Monir Madkour during the preparation of this edition of the textbook.

die within 60 to 90 days in cheese that has undergone lactic acid fermentation. Freezing dairy products or meat does not destroy the organisms but pasteurization or boiling are effective. Organisms shed in animal urine, stool, and products of conception remain viable in soil for 40 days or more.

Epidemiology

The global incidence of human brucellosis is difficult to determine as it is not a notifiable disease in many countries. However, more than 500 000 new cases are reported to the World Health Organization (WHO) each year. In the United States of America, only 4 to 10% of cases are recognized. Illegal importation of unpasteurized dairy products is responsible. Brucellosis is distributed worldwide but is especially prevalent in the Mediterranean region, Indian subcontinent, Mexico, and Central and South America. *B. melitensis* is the commonest cause of brucellosis worldwide. The incidence of human and animal brucellosis is increasing and animal disease has been eradicated in only 17 countries because of the recent expansion of animal industries and lack of scientific and modern methods of animal husbandry. Other factors contribute including traditional eating habits, poor standards of personal and environmental hygiene, methods of processing milk and its products, and the rapid movement of animals both locally and internationally. Control and eradication programmes in animals are expensive and difficult to implement. The ease of modern travel exposes travellers to the disease while visiting endemic countries. In endemic areas, brucellosis affects predominantly young men. Traditionally, farm animals considered as pets are kept in close contact to humans. Childhood disease indicates endemicity in the community. Where animal brucellosis is controlled, human brucellosis is mostly an occupational disease.

Mode of transmission

Ingestion of untreated dairy products, raw meat, liver, or bone marrow are common sources of infection through the gastrointestinal tract. Inhalation is the most frequent occupational hazard in herdsmen, dairy farm workers, meat processors, and laboratory workers. Abattoir workers are commonly infected by pieces of bone penetrating their skin. Veterinary surgeons are vulnerable to accidental autoinoculation or conjunctival contamination by live brucella vaccine while vaccinating animals. Transmission transplacentally or by breastfeeding, blood transfusion, marrow or organ transplantation, or sexual intercourse is rare.

Pathogenesis

How brucella survives and replicates inside host macrophages is uncertain. Immunity involves antigen-specific T-cell and humoral responses. Brucella lacks classic virulence factors and typical lipopolysaccharide pathogenicity. However, genes that modify phagocytosis, phagolysosome fusion, cytokine secretion, and apoptosis have been identified. Brucella virulence factor consists of a type IV secretion system responsible for injecting toxins into the cytoplasm of infected cells, resembling the VirB system.

Soon after brucella penetrates the mucosa, there is a polymorphonuclear leucocytosis and migration of activated macrophages to the site of invasion. The initial response is neither antigen nor organism specific (innate immunity), involving γδ T-cell (Vγ9Vδ2), natural killer (NK), and CD4 and CD8 T-cell activation. Lipopolysaccharide

on the surface of brucella is recognized by these cells, which activate macrophages and facilitate phagocytosis. Activated γδ T cells may provide the initial γ-interferon (INFγ), tumour necrosis factor-α (TNFα), and other cytokine secretions which become cytotoxic for brucella-infected monocytes and the bacteria, impairing their intracellular survival. Most brucella are rapidly eliminated by phagolysosome fusion. Killing inside macrophages is initiated by cytokines secreted by T-helper cells. Macrophages activate TNFα secretion, initiating a complex cascade of host defence mechanisms, resulting in hydrolytic enzymes and the peroxide–halide system ('oxidativeburst' or 'oxygen-based killing'). Some brucella survive in compartments which are rapidly acidified. Brucella resists being killed by oxidative-burst using the myeloperoxide–hydrogen peroxide–halide system. Bacteria enter the macrophages through lipid rafts or lipid microdomains. Brucella requires smooth lipopolysaccharide to avoid the bactericidal arsenal of the macrophages.

Impaired Th1 immunity, T-cell proliferation, NK-cell cytotoxic activity, and IFNγ production allow invasion. Brucella resists lysosome-mediated killing and phagosome acidification. The mechanism of trafficking of the brucella-containing phagosome within macrophages and the lack of fusion with the lysosome is not understood. Brucella multiplies in the macrophage endoplasmic reticulum without affecting host-cell integrity. The organisms are released by cell lysis and necrosis. Brucella protects infected cells from apoptosis by using IFNγ or TNFα. In the early stage of infection, brucella activates the cAMP/PKA pathway which regulates a variety of mechanisms favouring infection. Brucella later passes through lymphatics to regional lymph nodes, then via the blood stream to all organs of the body particularly those rich in reticuloendothelial tissue. Organ localization is associated with inflammatory cellular infiltrates with or without granuloma formation, caseation, necrosis, or even abscess formation. In the first week of infection, antilipopolysaccharide IgM appears in the serum, followed 1 week later by IgG and IgA which peak during the fourth week. Antilipopolysaccharide antibodies have a limited role in host protection, but are important for diagnosis.

Clinical features

The incubation period ranges from 1 to 3 weeks (maximum several months). Symptoms are highly variable and simulate other febrile illnesses. Travel to endemic areas and occupation are important details in the history. Symptoms may start suddenly (1–2 days) or gradually (1 week or more). Brucellosis is a febrile illness, with or without organ localization. Infection is classified usefully according to whether it is active (i.e. history, clinical features, and significantly raised brucella agglutinins with or without positive blood cultures) and whether it is localized to a particular organ. This determines the treatment regimen and its duration. Classification as acute, subacute, chronic, serological, bacteraemic, or mixed types is not helpful for diagnosis or management. The most frequent symptoms noted in 500 patients with *B. melitensis* who attended the author's clinic are given in Table 6.21.1. The fever pattern is neither distinctive nor diagnostic. The patient's temperature is usually normal in the morning and high in the afternoon and evening. Chills or rigors with profuse sweating may simulate malaria. Patients with brucellosis usually look deceptively well. Less frequently, they may look acutely ill. Physical signs may be lacking despite the multiplicity of symptoms. The frequency of

Table 6.21.1 History and symptoms in 500 patients with *B. melitensis* who attended the author's clinic

History/symptoms	Number	Percentage
Animal contact	368	73.6
Raw milk/cheese ingestion	350	70
Raw liver ingestion	147	29.4
Family history	188	37.6
Fever	464	92.8
Chills	410	82.0
Sweating	437	87.4
Body aches	457	91.4
Lack of energy	473	94.6
Joint pain	431	86.2
Back pain	431	86.2
Headaches	403	80.6
Loss of appetite	388	77.6
Weight loss	326	65.2
Constipation	234	46.9
Abdominal pain	225	45.0
Diarrhoea	34	6.8
Cough	122	24.4
Testicular pain (of 290 males)	62	21.3
Rash	72	14.4
Sleep disturbances	185	37.0

Table 6.21.2 Signs in 500 patients with *B. melitensis* who attended the author's clinic

Signs	Number	Percentage
Ill looking	127	25.4
Pallor	110	22.0
Lymphadenopathy	160	32.0
Splenomegaly	125	25.0
Hepatomegaly	97	19.4
Arthritis	202	40.4
Spinal tenderness	241	48.0
Epididymo-orchitis (of 290 males)	62	21.3
Skin rash	72	14.4
Jaundice	6	1.2
Central nervous system abnormalities	20	4.0
Cardiac murmur	17	3.4
Pneumonia	7	1.4

aneurysms, thrombophlebitis, and pulmonary embolism. Patients from endemic areas with 'culture-negative infective endocarditis' should have their blood culture extended for a period of up to 6 weeks. Respiratory symptoms are common but may be missed because they are usually mild. An influenza-like illness with sore throat and mild dry cough is common. Hilar and paratracheal lymphadenopathy, pneumonia (solitary or multiple nodular lung shadows or abscess formation), soft tissue miliary shadowing, pleural effusion, empyema, or mediastinitis are rare.

Gastrointestinal infections are usually mild and are rarely a presenting feature of the disease. They include tonsillitis and

physical signs seen in the same group of patients is shown in Table 6.21.2.

Localizations

Septic monoarthritis may result from haematogenous spread to the synovium or via direct extension from neighbouring brucella osteomyelitis (Fig. 6.21.1). Knee (Fig. 6.21.1), shoulder (Fig. 6.21.2a,b), sternoclavicular (Fig. 6.21.3), sacroiliac (Fig. 6.21.4), and hip (Fig. 6.21.5) joints are commonly affected. Joint destruction with loss of function may occur if diagnosis and treatment are delayed. In the spine, infection starts at the superior endplate anteriorly, an area of rich blood supply (Fig. 6.21.6). The infection may either regress and heal or progress to involve the entire vertebra, intervertebral disc, and adjacent vertebrae (Fig. 6.21.7a,b). Brucella spondylitis may involve single or, less frequently, multiple sites. The lumbar spine, particularly L4, is the most frequent site (Fig. 6.21.7a). Extraspinal brucella osteomyelitis is rare but may affect femur, tibia, humerus, or the manubrium sterni (Fig. 6.21.8). Bursitis, tenosynovitis, and subcutaneous nodules are rare. The peripheral white cell count is normal in brucella septic arthritis and spondylitis. The total white cell count in the synovial fluid ranges from 400 to 40 000/mm^3 with 60% polymorphonuclear cells. Glucose may be reduced and culture is positive in about 50% of cases.

Cardiovascular infections include endocarditis (Fig. 6.21.9), myocarditis, pericarditis, aortic root abscess (Fig. 6.21.10), mycotic

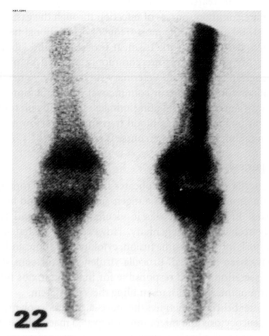

22

Fig. 6.21.1 Brucellar arthritis and osteomyelitis. Scintigram showing increased uptake in the osseous components of the left knee and the distal half of the left femur.

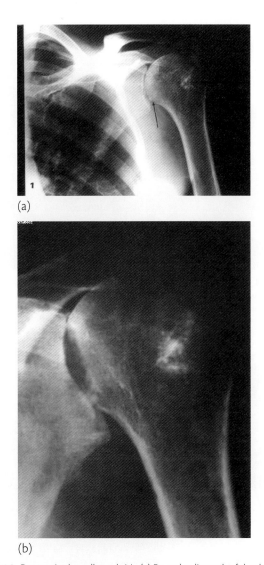

(a)

(b)

Fig. 6.21.2 Destructive brucellar arthritis. (a) Frontal radiograph of the shoulder joint showing diffuse cartilage loss in the glenohumeral joint (arrowed). (b) Radiograph taken 6 months after (a).

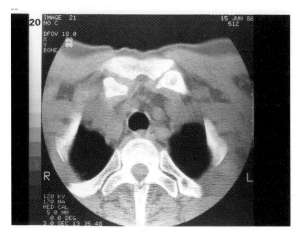

Fig. 6.21.3 Destructive brucellar arthritis. High-resolution CT scan showing marked cartilage loss and sternoclavicular erosions in the left sternoclavicular joint.

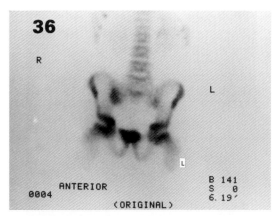

Fig. 6.21.4 Brucella sacroiliitis. There is increased uptake in the right sacroiliac joint which can be noted on the anterior view of the scintigram.

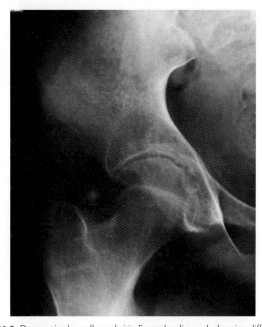

Fig. 6.21.5 Destructive brucellar arthritis. Frontal radiograph showing diffuse osteopenia and diffuse cartilage loss in the right hip.

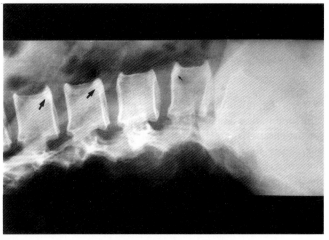

Fig. 6.21.6 Early brucellar spondylitis. There is sclerosis at the anterior aspect of the superior endplate of L4 (small arrow). Similar areas are seen in the inferior endplates of L1 and L2 (larger arrows). Note the normal disc spaces.

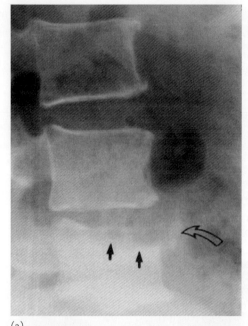

(a)

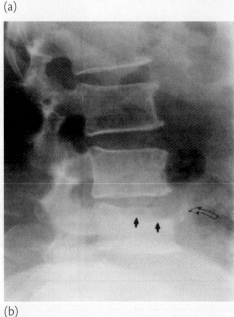

(b)

Fig. 6.21.7 (a,b) Progression of brucellar spondylitis to advanced disease. Lateral radiographs show anterior erosions (black arrows), reduction of the L3/L4 disc space and lateral osteophytes (outlined arrow).

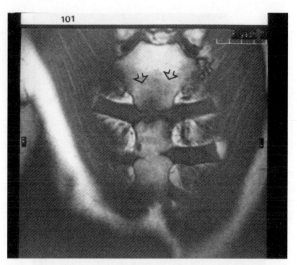

Fig. 6.21.8 Brucellar osteomyelitis. MRI of the sternum, coronal cut T1-weighted image, showing an area of patchy decreased signal intensity in the lower half of the manubrium (arrows).

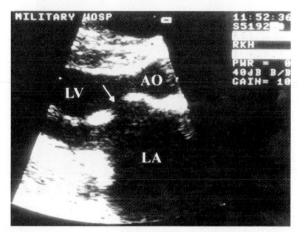

Fig. 6.21.9 Brucellar endocarditis. Two-dimensional transthoracic echocardiography showing perforation of the anterior mitral valve leaflet (arrow) due to brucellar endocarditis. AO, aorta; LA, left atrium; LV, left ventricle.

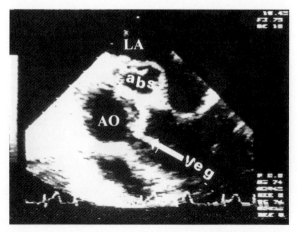

Fig. 6.21.10 Horizontal transoesophageal endocardiograph showing brucellar aortic root abscess (abs) and aortic valve vegetation (veg) (arrow). AO, aorta; LA, left atrium.

hepatitis with mild jaundice (either nonspecific or granulomatous with suppuration and abscess formation); frank cirrhosis is rare. Splenic abscess is rarely reported. Mesenteric lymphadenopathy with abscess formation, cholecystitis, peritonitis, pancreatitis, and ulcerative colitis are described. The liver transaminases, alkaline phosphatase, and serum bilirubin may be mildly raised.

Genitourinary involvement may be the presenting feature of brucellosis: unilateral or bilateral epididymo-orchitis prostatitis or seminal vesiculitis in males; dysmenorrhoea, amenorrhoea, tubo-ovarian abscesses, chronic salpingitis, and cervicitis in female. Acute nephritis or acute pyelonephritis-like features, renal calcifications, and calyceal deformities may occur. Renal granulomatous lesions with abscess formation, caseation, and necrosis may occur, as may cystitis and proximal urethritis.

Urine culture may be positive in about 50% of patients with brucellosis. Brucella has been isolated from human semen during investigation of possible sexual transmission.

Neurobrucellosis is uncommon but serious and can include meningoencephalitis, multiple cerebral or cerebellar abscesses, ruptured mycotic aneurysm, cranial nerve lesions, transient ischaemic attacks, hemiplegia, myelitis, radiculoneuropathy and neuritis, Guillain–Barré syndrome, a multiple sclerosis-like picture, paraplegia, sciatica, granulomatous myositis, and rhabdomyolysis. Psychiatric features are no more frequent than in other infections. Neurobrucellosis may result from direct blood-borne invasion, pressure from destructive spinal lesions, vasculitis, or an immune-related process. In meningoencephalitis the cerebrospinal fluid pressure is usually elevated and the fluid may look clear, turbid, or rarely, haemorrhagic. Protein concentration and cells (predominantly lymphocytes) are raised, while glucose may be reduced or normal. Brucella may be cultured from cerebrospinal fluid. Brucella agglutinins in cerebrospinal fluid are usually raised but are sometimes undetectable.

In endemic areas, pregnant women may experience abortion, intrauterine fetal death, premature delivery, and retention of the placenta and other products of conception. They may transmit infection by breastfeeding.

The uncommon skin manifestations include maculopapular eruptions, contact dermatitis (particularly among veterinary surgeons and farmers assisting animal parturition), erythema nodosum, purpura, petechiae, chronic ulcerations, multiple cutaneous and subcutaneous abscesses, vasculitis, superficial thrombophlebitis, discharging sinuses, and, rarely, pemphigus.

Splashing live brucella vaccine into the eyes may cause conjunctivitis. Keratitis, corneal ulcers, uveitis, retinopathies, subconjunctival and retinal haemorrhages, retinal detachment, and endogenous endophthalmitis with positive vitreous cultures are well documented.

Diagnosis

Definite diagnosis of brucellosis requires the isolation of the organism from the blood, body fluids, or tissues. Positive blood culture yield ranges between 40 and 70%. Extended culture for up to 6 weeks using biphasic culture media (solid and liquid) or with the Castaneda bottle (incubated at 37°C with and without an atmosphere of carbon dioxide) is commonly used. Automated culture systems are more sensitive and rapid. Bone marrow culture may rarely be required. Brucella species and biotypes are differentiated by their carbon dioxide requirements; ability to use glutamic acid, ornithine, lysine, and ribose; hydrogen sulphide production; growth in the presence of thionine or basic fuchsin dyes; agglutination by antisera directed against certain lipopolysaccharide epitopes; and susceptibility to lysis by bacteriophage. Molecular diagnosis is achieved by polymerase chain reaction (PCR) and 16S rRNA-based fluorescence in situ hybridization assay. Many varieties of PCR have been developed, including restriction fragment length polymorphism (PCR-RFLP), nested PCR, real-time PCR, and PCR–enzyme-linked immunosorbent assay (ELISA). They have superior specificity and sensitivity. Identification of specific antibodies against bacterial lipopolysaccharide and other antigens can be detected by the standard agglutination test (SAT), rose Bengal, 2-mercaptoethanol (2-ME), antihuman globulin

(Coombs' test), and indirect ELISA. The SAT is the most commonly used serological test in endemic areas. An agglutination titre of 1:160 or higher is considered significant in nonendemic areas and 1:320 or higher in endemic areas.

Since the O-polysaccharide of brucella is similar to that of various other Gram-negative bacteria (e.g. *Francisella tularensis*, *Escherichia coli*, *Salmonella urbana*, *Yersinia enterocolitica*, *Vibrio cholera*, *Xanthomonas maltophilia*), cross-reactions of IgM may occur. The inability to diagnose *B. canis* by SAT due to lack of cross-reaction is another drawback. False-negative SATs may be caused by the presence of blocking antibodies (the prozone phenomenon) in the α_2-globulin (IgA) and in the α-globulin (IgG) fractions. New dipstick assays, based on the binding of brucella IgM antibodies, have proved simple, accurate, and rapid.

ELISAs typically use cytoplasmic proteins as antigens. They detect IgM, IgG, and IgA without some of the shortcomings of the SAT. PCR is fast and specific.

In other laboratory investigations, the peripheral white cell count is normal or occasionally reduced with relative lymphocytosis. Blood biochemistry is commonly normal.

Treatment

Two classic regimens, doxycycline plus streptomycin (DS) or doxycycline plus rifampicin (DR), are recommended by the WHO and have been used all over the world for outpatient management; they have remained effective for many years. Doxycycline (preferred to other tetracyclines) is the most effective agent for the treatment of brucellosis. Its activity is enhanced by the acidic environment of the macrophage phagolysosomes. Regimens containing doxycycline are associated with fewer therapeutic failures and relapses than other regimens. The streptomycin-containing regimen is slightly more efficacious in preventing relapses as rifampicin reduces doxycycline levels in the serum. Doxycycline is given by mouth, 100 mg 12-hourly for 6 weeks; streptomycin is given intramuscularly, 15 mg/kg daily for 2 to 3 weeks; and rifampicin is given by mouth, 600 to 900 mg daily for 6 weeks. Patients with spondylitis, endocarditis, neurobrucellosis, and abscesses may require hospitalization for surgery (urgent valve replacement or drainage of abscesses) and triple antibiotics (doxycycline, aminoglycoside, and rifampicin) for a period of up to 6 months. The overall therapeutic failure rate ranges from 3 to 10%. Parenteral administration of aminoglycoside and the risk of nephrotoxicity and ototoxicity require monitoring. Monotherapy has been abandoned because of unacceptably high rates of therapeutic failure and relapse.

Since 1990, an alternative regimen has been used. Gentamicin or netilmicin are administered intramuscularly or intravenously as a single daily dose of 5 mg/kg for 7 days with doxycycline 100 mg 12-hourly for 45 days. This proved as effective as the DS regimen. In my experience, longer duration of gentamicin plus doxycycline (GD) or netilmicin plus doxycycline (ND) for 14 to 28 days, followed by doxycycline alone for a further 30 to 60 days was associated with no therapeutic failures and only 3% relapse/reinfection rate. Co-trimoxazole by mouth, two tablets (480 mg each) twice daily for 2 months plus doxycycline (CD) or plus rifampicin (CR) have been used; CD proved to be better than CR. In endemic areas, tuberculosis may also be common and the use of rifampicin may be restricted to avoid the emergence of resistance.

Quinolones (ciprofloxacin and ofloxacin) have been used in a limited number of clinical studies in patients without localizations. The activity of quinolones is decreased in the acidic environment of macrophage phagolysosomes but quinolones may have some role in replacing doxycycline or rifampicin when toxicity occurs. Quinolones may be used as second-line regimen in patients who fail to respond or develop relapse after using other regimens. Ofloxacin is given by mouth, 400 mg 12-hourly plus doxycycline or rifampicin combination for 6 weeks. Ciprofloxacin is given by mouth, 500 mg 12-hourly, in combination with doxycycline or rifampicin for 6 weeks. The expense of quinolones is a major draw back. The macrolide azithromycin is rapidly distributed into tissue and cells, particularly phagocytes. However, the acidic macrophage phagolysosomal environment reduces its activity and there were high rates of therapeutic failure and relapses when used against *B. melitensis*.

Children younger than 8 years with brucellosis are treated with the CR regimen. Rifampicin can be given orally or intravenously as a single dose of 10 to 20 mg/kg per day. Co-trimoxazole is given by intravenous infusion, 36 to 54 mg/kg per day in two divided doses. A paediatric suspension is given by mouth, 240 mg/ml 12-hourly.

Oral minocycline 2.5 mg/kg in combination with intravenous rifampicin 10 mg/kg (both given 12-hourly) for 3 weeks proved effective in infants and children in Italy. No dental defects were observed. Pregnant women with brucellosis are treated with the CR regimen. In patients with renal impairment, blood urea, creatinine, and aminoglycoside levels should be carefully monitored or else DR should be used.

Therapeutic response is assessed by improvement of symptoms (within 14 days) and signs (within 2–4 weeks) after starting antibiotics. Lack of clinical improvement 14 days after starting antibiotics until the end of therapy indicates therapeutic failure. Serological tests are not ideal for monitoring response. Titres may not decline and, if the patient develops a Jarisch–Herxheimer reaction with initial worsening of symptoms a few days after starting treatment, the titre may increase. In the first 3 months after completion of treatment, SAT titres decline to less than 1:320 in only 8.3% of patients and in 71.4% after 2 years or more. Of cured patients, 28.6% continue to have a titre of 1:320 or higher, 2 years after completion of clinically successful treatment. Patients receiving doxycycline in the treatment regimen are more likely to achieve serological cure than those who did not. Relapse is indicated by recurrence of clinical features and rise in agglutination titre, with or without positive blood culture, usually in the first 3 to 6 months but may be up to 1 year after completion of treatment. In endemic areas, reinfection may be difficult to differentiate from relapse.

Prevention

Human brucellosis can be prevented by eradicating the disease in animals by vaccination. There are five effective and marketed animal vaccines: *B. abortus* 4-5/20, *B. melitensis* Rev. 1, *B. suis* strain 2, *B. abortus* strain 19, and *B. abortus* RB51. These vaccines offer an animal protection rate of between 65% and 90%. Other preventive measures include changing the habits and traditions of keeping farm animals in close proximity to houses, drinking raw milk and its products, and consuming raw liver, meat, and bone marrow. Currently there is no effective vaccine for human use.

Further reading

Al Dahouk S, et al. (2005). Identification of brucella species and biotypes using polymerase chain reaction fragment length polymorphism (PCR-RFLP). *Clin Rev Microbiol*, **31**, 191–6.

Cascio A, et al. (2004). No findings of dental defects in children treated with minocycline. *Antimicrob Agents Chemother*, **48**, 2739–41.

Celli J, Gorvel J (2004). Organelle robbery: brucella interactions with the endoplasmic reticulum. *Curr Opin Microbiol*, **7**, 93–7.

Clavijo E, et al. (2003). Comparison of a dipstick assay for detection of brucella-specific immunoglobulin M antibodies with other tests for serodiagnosis of human brucellosis. *Clin Diagn Lab Immunol*, **10**, 612–15.

Falagas ME, Bliziotis IA (2006). Quinolones for treatment of human brucellosis: critical review of the evidence from microbiological and clinical studies. *Antimicrob Agents Chemother*, **50**, 22–33.

Ficht TA, et al. (2009). Brucellosis: the case for live, attenuated vaccines. *Vaccine*, **27**, Suppl 4, D40–3.

Franco MP, et al. (2007). Human brucellosis. *Lancet Infect Dis*, **7**, 775–86.

Ismail TF, et al. (2002). Evaluation of dipstick serologic tests for diagnosis of brucellosis and typhoid fever in Egypt. *J Clin Microbiol*, **40**, 3509–11.

Madkour MM (ed) (2001). *Madkour's brucellosis*, 2nd edition. Springer, Berlin.

Mantur BG, Amarnath SK. Brucellosis in India - a review. *J Biosci*, **33**, 539–47.

Maria-Pilar JB, et al. (2005). Cellular bioterrorism: how brucella corrupts macrophage physiology to promote invasion and proliferation. *Clin Immunol*, **114**, 227–38.

Morata P, et al. (2003). Development and evaluation of a PCR–enzyme-linked immunosorbent assay for diagnosis of human brucellosis. *J Clin Microbiol*, **41**, 144–8.

Oliveira SC, et al. (2008). The role of innate immune receptors in the control of *Brucella abortus* infection: toll-like receptors and beyond. *Microbes Infet*, **10**, 1005–9.

Pappas G, et al. (2006). The new global map of human brucellosis. *Lancet Infect Dis*, **6**, 91–9.

Roop RM 2nd, et al. (2009). Survival of the fittest: how Brucella strains adapt to their intracellular niche in the host. *Med Microbiol Immunol*, **198**, 221–38.

Skalsky K, et al. (2008). Treatment of human brucellosis: systematic review and meta-analysis of randomised controlled trials. *BMJ*, **336**, 701–4.

Wellinghausen N, et al. (2006). Rapid detection of *Brucellosis* spp. in blood cultures by fluorescence in situ hybridization. *J Clin Microbiol*, **44**, 1828–30.

Whatmore AM (2009). Current understanding of the genetic diversity of Brucella, an expanding genus of zoonotic pathogens. *Infect Genet Evol*, **9**, 1168–84.

Yingst S, Hoover DH (2003). T cell immunity to brucellosis. *Crit Rev Microbiol*, **29**, 313–31.

6.22 **Tetanus**

C.L. Thwaites and Lam Minh Yen

Essentials

Clostridium tetani is a Gram-positive, spore-forming anaerobic bacterium that is ubiquitous, being found throughout the world in human and animal faeces, soil, and street dust. In children and adults, superficial skin wounds are the common entry sites, although in 20% no portal of entry can be found.

Pathophysiology—under favourable anaerobic conditions, clostridial spores germinate and bacteria grow and multiply, producing a pathogenic toxin which—either locally or after circulation in the bloodstream—enters motor nerves, with the eventual effect of preventing discharge of γ-aminobutyric acid (GABA) inhibitory interneurons, resulting in unrestricted motor nerve activity, increased muscle tone, and spasms characteristic of tetanus.

Clinical features—after an incubation period of 7 to 14 days the disease presents with symptoms including trismus ('lockjaw', 98%), muscle stiffness (95%), back pain (94%), dysphagia (83%), muscle spasms (46%, with 'risus sardonicus' due to facial muscle spasm), and difficulty breathing (7%). Life-threatening complications include laryngeal muscle spasms and spasm and hypertonus of the respiratory muscles, and in severe cases there are violent autonomic disturbances. Tetanus continues to be a common cause of death in developing countries.

Diagnosis and treatment—tetanus is a clinical diagnosis: the presence of generalized muscle rigidity with trismus being characteristic, and risus sardonicus virtually pathognomonic. Key elements of treatment are (1) wound toilet and antibiotics, usually metronidazole; (2) antitoxin—most commonly human tetanus immune globulin 100 to 300 IU/kg intramuscularly; (3) spasm control—benzodiazepines are the first-line agents, with chlorpromazine, phenbarbitone, and propofol as alternatives; (4) control of any autonomic disturbance. Many patients require intensive care management and nursing.

Prevention—tetanus has largely been eliminated in countries with good immunization programmes and standards of hygiene. The World Health Organization recommendation is for a primary immunization course of three doses in infancy, followed by boosters aged 4 to 7 years and 12 to 15 years, with a further dose given in adult life. All patients with tetanus require a full course of active immunization as the disease itself does not confer long-lasting immunity.

Historical perspective

Tychon the soldier [was hit by] an arrow in his back ... [He] sounded like someone gnashing his teeth in a fury of rage… He was arched back in opisthotonos, his jaws locked together against his will. A friend forced some wine between his teeth, but Tychon could not swallow, and the liquid was expelled in spurts from his nostrils.

Hippocrates (*c.*425 BC)

Tetanus has been known since ancient times, with the earliest descriptions included in the Edwin Smith papyrus of ancient Egypt (1000 BC). It has been a well-recognized complication of battle injuries (Fig. 6.22.1). In 1880, Nicolaier demonstrated that soil contamination of wounds resulted in tetanus and discovered the bacterium responsible when he isolated *Clostridium tetani* bacilli from wounds. Ten years later Faber discovered tetanus toxin, and von Behring and Kitasato produced the first antitoxin. Ramon detoxified tetanus toxin and in 1926 performed the first successful vaccination of humans. Tetanus vaccination was introduced to British armed

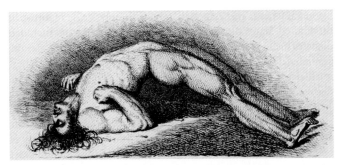

Fig. 6.22.1 Opisthotonus in a soldier wounded at the battle of Corunna (1809) and illustrated by Sir Charles Bell in his *The Anatomy and Philosophy of Human Expression* (1832).

forces in 1938, and during the 1950s was gradually incorporated into infant immunization programmes throughout the United Kingdom, finally becoming part of the national schedule in 1961.

Aetiology, genetics, pathogenesis, and pathology

Tetanus results from wound inoculation. In neonates the umbilical stump is the usual portal of entry. The bacteria are ubiquitous and have been found throughout the world in human and animal faeces, soil, street dust, and even the air of operating theatres. *C. tetani* is a Gram-positive spore-forming anaerobic bacterium. Under favourable anaerobic conditions the spores will germinate and the bacteria grow and multiply producing the pathogenic toxin. Tetanus toxin (tetanospasmin) is a 150-kDa protein consisting of one heavy and one light chain linked by a disulphide bond. The amino acid sequence is similar to that of the botulinum toxins and the toxins act in similar ways, but as botulinum toxins are not transported into the central nervous system they produce a different clinical picture.

The heavy chain of the tetanus toxin mediates toxin entry into the motor nerves, either locally or after circulation in the bloodstream. Its motor specificity is due to binding to specific domains within the motor nerve membrane. The heavy chain is also necessary for the subsequent retrograde axonal transport of the toxin and its passage across the synaptic cleft, where it preferentially enters γ-aminobutyric acid (GABA) inhibitory interneurons. The light chain of the toxin is a zinc-dependent endopeptidase that cleaves vesicle-associated membrane protein II (VAMP II or synaptobrevin) at a single peptide bond. This molecule is essential for synaptic release of neurotransmitters and cleavage disrupts synaptic transmission. By preventing inhibitory discharge, unrestricted motor nerve activity occurs, resulting in the increased muscle tone and spasms characteristic of tetanus. In severe forms of tetanus the autonomic nervous system is also affected giving rise to marked cardiovascular instability.

Epidemiology

In developed countries with good immunization programmes and standards of hygiene the incidence of tetanus has declined steadily since the 1940s. In the United States, for example, 233 cases of tetanus were reported between 2001 and 2008. The annual incidence rate was 0.1 cases per million in the general population and 0.23 cases per million in those over 65 years of age. The case-fatality rate was 13.2% overall and 31.3% in patients over 65 years of age.

Neonatal tetanus was extremely rare, with only 1 case reported in the United States during the same period. Risk factors included diabetes mellitus and injection drug use. In England and Wales the annual incidence was 0.2 cases/million population with the highest incidence in those aged 65 years or older. In Italy the incidence rate declined from 0.5 to 0.2 cases per 100 000 population between the 1970s and the 1990s.

By contrast, in developing countries tetanus remains endemic and is common cause of morbidity and mortality, particularly of neonates but also of children and young adults. One million cases of tetanus are estimated to occur worldwide each year. In 1988, an estimated 787 000 neonatal deaths occurred, prompting the World Health Assembly to call for the elimination of tetanus by 1995. Slow progress resulted in this goal being postponed until 2000 and then 2005 (when maternal tetanus was added).

In 2008 neonatal tetanus accounted for approximately 59 000 deaths, representing a 92% decrease in mortality compared with 1988. Nevertheless, as of 2010, 39 countries had still not achieved the target elimination (defined as <1 case of neonatal tetanus per 1000 live births in every district).

Neonatal tetanus is usually acquired through contamination of the umbilical stump and is associated with delivery on unclean surfaces or traditional midwifery practices such as cutting the umbilical cord with bamboo or applying soil to the umbilical stump. Mortality rates are high, often greater than 90% in areas with few resources, and even in those with good facilities mortality remains approximately 40 to 50%.

In children and adults, superficial skin wounds are the common entry sites, although in 20% no portal of entry can be found. Mortality is higher with deep entry sites such as postoperative infections, intramuscular injections, or postpartum. Injecting drug users (especially those using the skin 'popping' method of administration) are prone to develop a particularly severe form of tetanus.

Prevention

Tetanus is preventable by immunization and good hygiene. Tetanus vaccines are made from tetanus toxoid adsorbed onto aluminium to increase immunogenicity. They are available as single-dose tetanus toxoid (TT) or combined with diphtheria toxoid. There are two preparations of the latter: (1) DT or high dose for use in children under 7 years and (2) dT or low dose for use in older people. Further combinations of DT or dT are available with whole cell or acellular pertussis (DTwP, DtaP, dTwP, or dTaP). In addition, preparations are now available containing *Haemophilus influenzae* B, hepatitis B, or polio. Tetanus toxoid or standard combinations are safe and effective and adverse events are mild and infrequent. They can be used during pregnancy or in immunodeficient people, including those with HIV, but responses may be diminished. Adequate tetanus vaccination requires a primary course (three doses), boosters (two or three), and further boosters after tetanus-prone wounds.

The World Health Organization (WHO) recommend that five doses of vaccine should be given during childhood: a primary immunization course of three doses in infancy followed by boosters between the ages of 4 and 7 years and 12 and 15 years. They differ from current United Kingdom guidelines by recommending a further booster in adult life, e.g. during a woman's first pregnancy. In the United Kingdom, a total of five doses is recommended. Further doses are deemed necessary only after tetanus-prone wounds (see below).

In nonimmunized adolescents and adults, a three-dose primary course is recommended. The first two doses should be given at least 4 weeks apart and the third at least 6 months after the second. In these people, a total of five doses is expected to confer lifelong protection. This schedule is also recommended for pregnant women with incomplete or unknown vaccination histories who should be given at least two doses (usually dT) at least 4 weeks apart during the pregnancy, a third 6 months later, and two boosters at yearly intervals. If they have had a primary course in infancy, two further doses (at least 4 weeks apart) are recommended. This can be reduced to one dose if they also had a childhood booster. A final (sixth) booster at least 1 year later should confer lifelong immunity.

Booster doses of tetanus toxoid should also be given after certain tetanus-prone wounds (Table 6.22.1). In very high-risk situations, additional passive immunization should be given using human or equine tetanus immune globulin.

Table 6.22.1 Management of tetanus-prone wounds

Wound type		Active immunization	Passive immunization
Clean wound		Only if vaccination history incomplete (i.e. give booster if not up to date or initiate primary course as described in text)	No
Low risk tetanus-prone	**1** Wounds or burns: Requiring surgical intervention or when treatment delayed >6 h With significant degree of devitalized tissue Containing foreign bodies Individuals with systemic sepsis **2** Puncture-type injury, particularly in contact with soil and/or manure **3** Open fractures	Only if vaccination history incomplete (i.e. give booster if not up to date or initiate primary course as described in text)	If vaccination history incomplete, one dose human immune globulin (in different site to vaccination)
High risk tetanus-prone	As above but with heavy contamination with material likely to contain tetanus spores and/or extensive devitalized tissue	Only if vaccination history incomplete (i.e. give booster if not up to date or initiate primary course as described in text)	All one dose human immune globulin (in different site to vaccination, if given)

Clinical features

Symptoms evolve gradually over a period of days and weeks or, in very severe cases, hours, and the time course is divided into specific periods. The incubation period is the period from inoculation to the first symptom (therefore may be unknown if no entry site is found) and is usually around 7 to 14 days. The period of onset is the period from the first symptoms to the first spasm and is usually 2 to 5 days. Both these periods can be shorter in severe disease which tends to progress more rapidly. The initial symptoms complained of on admission by 2422 patients (excluding neonates) admitted to the Hospital for Tropical diseases, Ho Chi Minh City, are shown in Table 6.22.2.

As tetanus develops, muscle tone gradually increases until spasms occur. In the face trismus ('lockjaw') commonly occurs (Fig. 6.22.2) and the characteristic risus sardonicus is seen due to facial muscle spasm. Involvement of the erector spinae group of muscles results in opisthotonus (Fig. 6.22.3). Sometimes, tetanus

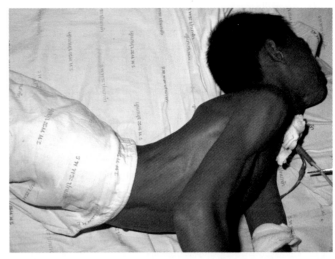

Fig. 6.22.3 Opisthotonus.
(Copyright D A Warrell.)

Table 6.22.2 Presenting clinical features of tetanus

Symptom	Percentage of admissions
Trismus	98
Dysphagia	83
Back pain	94
Muscle stiffness	95
Muscle spasms	46
Difficulty breathing	7
Fever	8

is confined to a local group of muscles producing only local muscle spasm. If this occurs in the head, it is termed 'cephalic tetanus' (Fig. 6.22.4). Unlike local tetanus elsewhere, this form is potentially dangerous if laryngeal muscle spasms cause airway obstruction leading to asphyxiation. This occurs commonly in generalized tetanus and is a life-threatening emergency. Respiratory tract secretions are increased in tetanus, due perhaps to a combination of autonomic nervous system stimulation and pharyngeal and laryngeal muscle spasms that prevent swallowing. Spasm and hypertonus of the respiratory muscles is a serious occurrence that, without artificial respiratory support, is a common cause of death in tetanus.

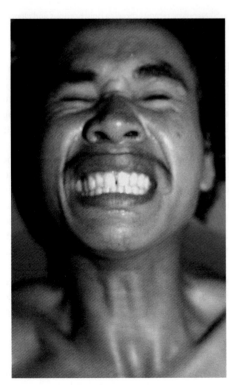

Fig. 6.22.2 Risus sardonicus resulting from trismus.
(Courtesy of the late Professor Sornchai Looareesuwan.)

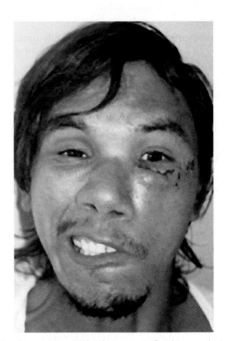

Fig. 6.22.4 Brazilian patient with local tetanus confined to muscles innervated by the left VIIth cranial nerve and with trismus, showing the wound causing the infection.
(Courtesy of Dr Pedro Pardal, Belém, Brazil.)

Table 6.22.3 Ablett score

Grade	Clinical features
I	Mild to moderate trismus (little or no dysphagia) General spasticity No respiratory embarrassment No spasms
II	Moderate trismus Well-marked rigidity Mild to moderate but short spasms Moderate respiratory embarrassment with an increased respiratory rate greater than 30 breaths/min Mild dysphagia
III	Severe trismus Generalized spasticity Reflex prolonged spasms Increased respiratory rate greater than 40 breaths/min Apnoeic spells Severe dysphagia Tachycardia greater than 120 beats/min
IV	Grade III and violent autonomic disturbances involving the cardiovascular system Severe hypertension and tachycardia alternating with relative hypotension and bradycardia, either of which may be persistent

In centres having facilities to control muscle spasm and provide mechanical ventilation, autonomic system effects are responsible for a second group of major complications. The syndrome of autonomic instability usually takes the form of labile hypertension and tachycardia which is difficult to control. However, it may manifest as more sustained hypertension and tachycardia or, less commonly but more seriously, with periods of hypotension and bradyarrhythmias. It is associated with acute renal failure (nonoliguric or oliguric) and adult respiratory distress syndrome (ARDS).

The clinical severity of tetanus is commonly described using a modified version of the score described by Ablett (Table 6.22.3).

Neonatal tetanus has a similar clinical picture (Fig. 6.22.5). Abnormalities of muscle tone usually present as difficulty in feeding and crying and is followed by frank spasms. The WHO define neonatal tetanus as 'an illness occurring in a child who has the normal ability to suck and cry in the first 2 days of life but who loses this ability between days 3 and 28 of life and becomes rigid and has spasms'. Fluctuations in blood pressure and heart rate are common, as are secondary infections and septicaemia.

Severity of illness can be predicted on admission from clinical measures. Previously the Dakar (described 1975) and Phillips (described 1967) scores have been used, but the recent tetanus severity score shows superior predictive value. This score (Table 6.22.4) is simple to use, is calculated using only baseline observation data and features of the history, and is, therefore, suitable for use in most clinical settings.

Differential diagnosis

Tetanus is a clinical diagnosis. Presence of generalized muscle rigidity with trismus are characteristic, and the risus sardonicus virtually pathognomonic. Wound cultures commonly do not yield *C. tetani*. The differential diagnosis includes local causes of trismus and

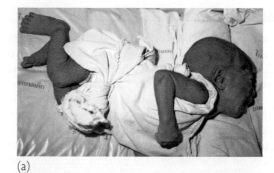
(a)

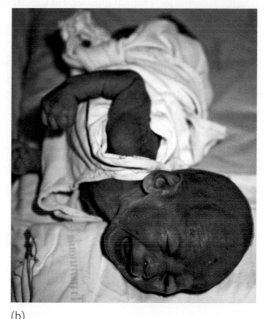
(b)

Fig. 6.22.5 (a, b) Neonatal tetanus showing opisthotonus and clenched fist. (Copyright D A Warrell.)

pharyngeal muscle spasm such as oropharyngeal infection or temporomandibular joint pathology.

Rabies, like tetanus, may result from an infected animal bite, but its incubation period is usually much longer (Chapter 5.10). Hydrophobic spasms may resemble tetanic spasms, particularly in the case of cephalic tetanus.

Strychnine is a competitive antagonist of the inhibitory neurotransmitter glycine that causes hyperreflexia and severe muscle spasms leading to convulsions. It may be very hard to distinguish this from tetanus. The diagnosis may be suggested by a history of ingestion and confirmed by toxicological tests of urine, serum, or gastric contents. Clinically the continuous muscle rigidity characteristic of tetanus is not present, although this may be difficult to detect with frequent convulsions.

Other causes of muscle tone abnormality are dystonic reactions to antidopaminergic drugs such as metoclopramide or phenothiazines. These may be associated with torticollis or eye and tongue movements which are not features of tetanus. The administration of anticholinergics and withdrawal of the precipitating drug can eliminate these.

In children, hypocalcaemic tetany and meningoencephalitis may present with some of the features of tetanus, but more careful clinical examination and investigation will differentiate these.

Table 6.22.4 Tetanus severity score (TSS), calculated from the total of individual section scores

		Score
Age (years)	≤70	0
	71–80	5
	>80	10
Time from first symptom to admission (days)	≤2	0
	3–5	−5
	>5	−6
Difficulty breathing on admission	No	0
	Yes	4
Coexisting medical conditions[a]	Fit and well	0
	Minor illness or injury	3
	Moderately severe illness	5
	Severe illness not immediately life-threatening	5
	Immediately life-threatening illness	9
Entry site[b]	Internal or injection	7
	Other (including unknown)	0
Highest systolic blood pressure recorded during first day in hospital (mmHg)	≤130	0
	131–140	2
	>140	4
Highest heart rate recorded during first day in hospital (beats/min)	≤100	0
	101–110	1
	111–120	2
	>120	4
Lowest heart rate recorded during first day in hospital (beats/min)	≤110	0
	>110	−2
Highest temperature recorded during first day in hospital (°C)	≤38.5	0
	38.6–39	4
	39.1–40	6
	>40	8[c]

[a] Defined according to the American Society of Anesthesiologists' physical status scale.

[b] 'Internal' site includes postoperative / postpartum or open fractures; 'injection' includes intramuscular, subcutaneous, or intravenous injections.

[c] Scores ≥ 8 are associated with worse prognosis.

Management

The principal areas of management are wound management, antimicrobial therapy, neutralization of unbound tetanus toxin, control of muscle spasms, management of autonomic dysfunction, and supportive management. Wounds should be cleaned and debrided to remove necrotic tissue and spores.

Antibiotics probably play a relatively minor role but are generally given to prevent further bacterial multiplication. Metronidazole is the preferred agent, although benzylpenicillin is a safe and effective alternative. Two randomized controlled trials have found no difference in mortality between penicillin and metronidazole but, in one study, patients receiving metronidazole required fewer sedatives and muscle relaxants. This may be potentially be explained by the neuroexcitatory effects of penicillins.

Antitoxin is given to neutralize any unbound toxin and, if given early enough, may limit the severity of tetanus. Debate has centred on whether an intrathecal route would be more effective. An existing meta-analysis failed to show any benefit, but a recent randomized controlled trial showed that patients given intrathecal human tetanus immune globulin (HTIG) had less severe tetanus and a shorter duration of mechanical ventilation and hospital stay. Preparations containing thimerosal must never be given intrathecally. If given by conventional methods, HTIG is given at a dose of 100 to 300 IU/kg intramuscularly. If this is unavailable or too expensive, as is the case in countries where most tetanus occurs, equine antitoxin (500–1000 IU/kg intramuscularly) is an alternative. However, its use is associated with an increased risk of anaphylactic reactions.

Spasms are treated with benzodiazepines as first-line agents. Diazepam is the commonest choice due to its low cost and widespread availability, but other preparations such as midazolam are more suited to long-term administration. High-dose regimes are commonly used, such as diazepam 100 mg/h intravenously. Other agents that may be used include phenobarbitone or chlorpromazine. Chlorpromazine has the potential advantage of α-adrenergic antagonistic activity and has been used alone or as an adjunct. In 1966, Hendrickse reported one of the few randomized trials comparing diazepam, chlorpromazine, and phenobarbitone with chlorpromazine and phenobarbitone alone in 104 neonates and 45 older children. Mortality in the neonates was identical but in the older children the death rate was almost halved in those treated with diazepam, although numbers were too small to reach statistical significance. More modern sedatives such as propofol can also be used, although there are limited data to provide efficacy and safety profiles.

Autonomic disturbance of severe tetanus is difficult to treat. Heavy sedation is used as a means of improving cardiovascular stability. Intravenous morphine is commonly used as it inhibits central sympathetic discharge resulting in peripheral arteriolar vasodilatation. Other authors report the use of calcium antagonists or other vasodilators to reduce blood pressure in hypertension. More recently, several trials have been published using magnesium sulphate to treat tetanus. Initially its use was intended to reduce the autonomic instability of severe tetanus, but it also has muscle relaxant properties that may be beneficial in all patients with tetanus. Results of a randomized controlled trial have shown that intravenous magnesium sulphate (with infusions titrated to produce serum concentrations between 2 and 4 mmol/litre) improves cardiovascular stability and reduces the requirements for sedatives and muscle relaxants. However, those with severe tetanus still required neuromuscular blocking agents and mechanical ventilation. In those with low cardiac output, inotropes such as adrenaline, noradrenaline, or dobutamine may be needed. If bradyarrhythmias occur, cardiac pacing may be necessary. Labetatol has frequently been administered because of its dual α- and β-blocking properties; β-blockade alone should be avoided because of reports of sudden death. Other treatments that have been reported to be useful for autonomic dysfunction include atropine, clonidine, and bupivacaine.

Patients with severe tetanus are critically ill and require intensive care management and nursing. In patients with respiratory muscle involvement, endotracheal intubation and ventilation is life-saving.

Early tracheostomy is frequently indicated because of the likelihood of prolonged mechanical ventilation. Fluid balance must be carefully monitored as insensible fluid losses are particularly high in tetanus. Care must be taken to ensure adequate fluid replacement. Patients require regular turning to prevent pressure sores, which can be especially difficult in those with many spasms or high muscle tone. Frequent suctioning is required to maintain airway patency due to the copious secretions, but it provokes spasms. Some authors report high incidence of venous thrombosis in tetanus patients and recommend routine anticoagulant prophylaxis. Almost all units report a high incidence of nosocomial infections, particularly ventilator-associated pneumonia and line-related sepsis. Optimal management of these involves bacterial cultures, appropriate antibiotics, and infection-control procedures and has been associated with improved outcome.

All patients with tetanus require a full course of active immunization as the disease itself does not confer long-lasting immunity.

Prognosis

Case-fatality rates in developing countries range from 8 to 50% for non-neonatal tetanus and 10 to 60% for neonatal tetanus. Patients with shorter incubation periods (<7 days) have more severe disease and higher mortality. Death is uncommon in developed countries with intensive care support.

Further reading

Attygalle D, Rodrigo N (2002). Magnesium as first line therapy in the management of tetanus: a prospective study of 40 patients. *Anaesthesia*, **57**, 811–17.

Attygalle D, Rodrigo N (2004). New trends in the management of tetanus. *Expert Rev Anti Infect Ther*, **2**, 73–84.

Beeching NJ, Crowcroft NS (2005). Tetanus in injecting drug users. *BMJ*, **330**, 208–9.

Blasi J, *et al.* (1993). Botulinum neurotoxin A selectively cleaves the synaptic protein SNAP-25. *Nature*, **365**, 160–3.

Brauner JS, Vieira SR, Bleck TP (2002). Changes in severe accidental tetanus mortality in the ICU during two decades in Brazil. *Intensive Care Med*, **28**, 930–5.

Cook TM, Protheroe RT, Handel JM (2001). Tetanus: a review of the literature. *Br J Anaesth*, **87**, 477–87.

Humeau Y, *et al.* (2000). How botulinum and tetanus neurotoxins block neurotransmitter release. *Biochimie*, **82**, 427–46.

Lipman J, *et al.* (1987). Autonomic dysfunction in severe tetanus: magnesium sulfate as an adjunct to deep sedation. *Crit Care Med*, **15**, 987–8.

Miranda-Filho Dde B, *et al.* (2004). Randomised controlled trial of tetanus treatment with antitetanus immunoglobulin by the intrathecal or intramuscular route. *BMJ*, **328**, 615.

Okoromah CN, Lesi FE (2004). Diazepam for treating tetanus. *Cochrane Database Syst Rev*, **1**, CD003954.

Salisbury DM, Begg NT (2006). Tetanus. In: *Immunisation against infectious diseases (the green book)*. www.doh.gov.uk/greenbook/greenbookpdf-chapter-30-layout.pdf

Thwaites CL, *et al.* (2006). Predicting the clinical outcome of tetanus: the tetanus severity score. *Trop Med Int Health*, **11**, 279–87.

Thwaites CL, *et al.* (2006). Magnesium sulphate for treatment of severe tetanus: a randomized controlled trial. *Lancet*, **368**, 1436–43.

World Health Organization (2006). Tetanus vaccine. *Wkly Epidemiol Rec*, **81**, 198–208.

6.23 *Clostridium difficile*

John G. Bartlett

Essentials

Clostridium difficile is a Gram-positive spore-forming anaerobic bacillus found in the environment. Its spores are part of the colonic flora in about 2 to 3% of healthy adults, with colonization rates increasing during hospitalization to 20 to 40%. Disease occurs when the organism shifts to its replicating vegetative form with toxin (A and B) production, this typically happening when there is inhibition of the competing colonic flora by antibiotics. *C. difficile* infection is now recognized as the most important bacterial enteric pathogen in wealthier countries, with a new NAP-1 epidemic strain appearing to produce more toxin than many others.

Clinical features—these range from trivial diarrhoea that subsides rapidly when antibiotics are stopped to fulminant pseudomembranous colitis, which may progress to toxic megacolon; most cases have watery and voluminous diarrhoea, accompanied by evidence of colonic inflammation.

Diagnosis and treatment—the condition should be suspected in any patient who has diarrhoea in association with antibiotic use. Diagnosis is established by demonstrating *C. difficile* toxin in stool by enzyme immunoassay or cytotoxin assay. Treatment is by stopping the implicated antibiotic, supportive care, avoiding antiperistaltic agents, and giving oral metronidazole or vancomycin.

Prevention—the most important issues are avoidance of the major antibiotic causes of *C. difficile*, and infection control in acute and chronic care facilities, including patient isolation and barrier precautions.

Historical perspective

The history of *Clostridium difficile* has three elements: the bacterium, the animal model of the disease, and the clinical features of antibiotic-associated colitis. *C. difficile* was originally described as a component of the normal flora of newborn infants by Hall and O'Toole in 1935. At that time, the organism was known to produce an exotoxin that was highly lethal when injected intraperitoneally in mice. However, the clinical implications of this were unclear. Review of the relatively rare cases of *C. difficile* infection (CDI) at various anatomical sites showed no unusual clinical features suggesting a histotoxic clostridial syndrome. Work with animal models began during the Second World War, with attempts to determine the efficacy of penicillin for the treatment of gas gangrene in guinea pigs. However, penicillin proved more lethal to rodents than *Clostridium perfringens*. When antibiotics became available in clinical practice, a potentially important complication was staphylococcal enterocolitis, also known as antibiotic-associated colitis. In 1974, a prospective study at Barnes Hospital, St. Louis, by Tedesco *et al.* showed that 10% of patients receiving clindamycin developed pseudomembranous colitis (PMC). In retrospect, this was one of the first outbreaks of *C. difficile* colitis. Unexpectedly, *Staphylococcus aureus* could not be cultivated from the stool despite the ease of recovering this pathogen. This observation stimulated studies to determine the cause of antibiotic-pseudomembranous colitis which had also become known as clindamycin colitis. In 1977–78, *C. difficile* was identified as the agent of antibiotic-associated colitis, presumably involving Hall and O'Toole's *C. difficile* toxin that had been responsible for antibiotic-induced disease in rodents. Retrospectively, stool samples from Tedesco *et al.*'s study of PMC were found to contain *C. difficile* toxin. During the period 1970–80, work from many clinical groups defined the epidemiology, clinical features, methods of diagnosis, and treatment of *C. difficile*. During the 1980s and 1990s, it was recognized as a relatively frequent and important cause of antibiotic-associated diarrhoea. It was readily diagnosed by detecting *C. difficile* toxin in stool and was effectively treated with oral metronidazole or vancomycin. However, occasionally patients had fulminant disease and about 20% relapsed after treatment. Since 2000, the NAP1 strain of *C. difficile* (also known as ribotype 027 or toxinotoxin III), which appears to be a relatively new, has been increasingly recognized in Canada, the United States of America, and much of Europe. NAP1 seems particularly important because it produces large amounts of toxin *in vitro* and, unlike previous strains, is resistant to fluoroquinolones which are now implicated in many cases of antibiotic-associated diarrhoea.

Aetiology, pathogenesis, and pathology

Like all enteric pathogens, *C. difficile* causes a range of clinical and pathological expressions, ranging from asymptomatic carriage that may be accompanied by positive toxin assays to a fulminant and life-threatening PMC. The organism forms part of the colonic flora in about 2 to 3% of healthy adults, but colonization rates increase during hospitalization to 20 to 40%. Under ordinary circumstances, the organism exists as a spore in the colon and presumably shifts to the replicating vegetative form with toxin production when there is inhibition of the competing colonic flora by antibiotics. The organism produces two toxins, designated toxin A and toxin B. Initial studies using intestinal loop assays indicated that toxin A was a cause of a severe inflammatory disease and toxin B was a particularly potent cytopathic toxin, readily detected with tissue culture assays. However, more recent studies with human colonic tissue indicated that both toxin A and toxin B are important causes of colitis in humans. The pathological findings with endoscopy or histopathology show a range of changes from a completely normal colonic mucosa with minimal histological evidence of inflammation to the other end of the spectrum which is PMC. The pseudomembranes are almost always restricted to the colon, and small bowel involvement is rare. This is in contrast to *S. aureus* enterocolitis which generally involves the small bowel as well as the colon.

Epidemiology

Most at risk of *C. difficile* infection (CDI) are older people and those hospitalized in acute or chronic care facilities and exposed to antibiotic treatment. The association with care facilities is presumably due to clustering of large numbers of elderly patients with high rates of antibiotic exposure where there is widespread environmental contamination by spores of *C. difficile*. Almost any drug with antibacterial activity has been implicated, but the most frequently implicated are broad-spectrum β-lactams (third- and fourth-generation cephalosporins, β-lactam–β-lactamase inhibitors,

amoxicillin and carbapenems, clindamycin, and fluoroquinolones). Despite these strong associations, some of the more recent studies have defined cases of CDI in substantial numbers of children and adults receiving proton pump inhibitor treatment without any recent history of antibiotic exposure.

Prevention

The most important facets of prevention are avoidance of the major antibiotic causes of CDI and infection control in acute and chronic care facilities. Antibiotic selection is not usually altered by concern for CDI except in institutional epidemics, elderly patients, and patients who have had previous bouts of this complication, especially those who had severe or relapsing disease. Control of implicated antibiotics during institutional epidemics has proven effective. Recommendations for infection control from the Society for Healthcare Epidemiology of America include patient isolation in a single room preferably with a bathroom, barrier precautions, room cleaning with a 1 in 10 solution of bleach, avoidance of rectal thermometers, and the use of soap and water for hand washing.

Clinical features

Clinical symptoms of CDI range from trivial diarrhoea that subsides rapidly when antibiotics are stopped to fulminant PMC, sometimes complicated by toxic megacolon, sepsis syndrome, renal failure, shock, and death. Cardinal features of the disease that apply to most cases are diarrhoea that is frequently watery and voluminous, accompanied by evidence of colonic inflammation, reflected by cramps, fever, leucocytosis, and typical features of colonic inflammation on endoscopy or CT. The small bowel is rarely involved. Three important observations suggest CDI specifically in some cases: hypoalbuminaemia, leukaemoid reactions, and ileus or toxic megacolon, all following recent antibiotic exposure.

Differential diagnosis

The main differential is antibiotic-associated diarrhoea, a common complication of antibiotics that generally resolves with reduction in dose or simply stopping the drug. However, only about 10 to 15% of specimens submitted to laboratories for detection of *C. difficile* toxin are positive. Assuming that most of these are to investigate suspected CDI in patients with diarrhoea following recent antibiotic exposure, the conclusion is that CDI accounts for a relatively small proportion of antibiotic-associated diarrhoea cases. Distinctive features of CDI are evidence of inflammation as summarized above and severity of disease. Diarrhoea is often caused by medications other than antibiotics including many drugs commonly used in hospitals. In patients with inflammatory diarrhoea, other potential causes include enteric pathogens (salmonella, shigella, *Campylobacter jejuni*, etc.), ischaemic colitis, and idiopathic inflammatory bowel disease. Rare cases of antibiotic-associated colitis may be due to *S. aureus*, *Klebsiella oxytoca*, *C. perfringens*, salmonella and candida.

Diagnosis

CDI should be suspected in any patient who has diarrhoea that occurs in association with antibiotic use. The probability of this diagnosis increases substantially with clinical evidence of inflammation and exposure to the agents that are most frequently implicated. The diagnosis is established by demonstrating *in vivo* production of *C. difficile* toxin. This is detected in stool using enzyme immunoassay (EIA) or cytotoxin assay. Advantages of EIA are that it is rapid (results are available in 1–2 h), the reagents are commercially available, it is technically quite easy to perform, and the specificity is good. The disadvantage is lack of sensitivity. The cytotoxin assay is frequently considered the gold standard and has good sensitivity and specificity, but it is technically demanding and gives results only after 24 to 48 h. Perhaps the most sensitive test is the culture–toxin test in which *C. difficile* carriage is demonstrated either by culture or by detection of common antigen. Subsequently, the strain can be tested for toxogenicity either by *in vitro* toxin production or by detecting toxin in stool using the cytotoxin assay. Although detecting *C. difficile* is highly sensitive, the disadvantage is the relatively high carriage rate of this organism without clinical disease in 20 to 40% of hospitalized patients.

Polymerase chain reaction (PCR) assays that detect the gene for toxin B have been developed. An evaluation of a real-time PCR assay showed that PCR was more sensitive than EIA and equally rapid. Three PCR assays have been licensed by the United States Food and Drug Administration in 2009 and one has been further developed to detect the epidemic 027/NAP1/BI strain as well as the toxin B gene.

Organism detection assays include common antigen testing and anaerobic culture. Common antigen tests detect the GDH antigen, an enzyme produced by all *C. difficile* isolates. Some laboratories use this as a screening method prior to confirmation with a cytotoxin assay.

Stool culture is rarely performed for the diagnosis of *C. difficile*. Although culture is highly sensitive it relatively slow and does not distinguish toxin-producing from non-toxin-producing strains.

Treatment

CDI should be managed by stopping the implicated antibiotic, supportive care, and avoiding antiperistaltic agents such as loperamide and narcotics. Up to one-third of patients will respond to simply stopping the implicated antibiotic. However, in the era of severe disease with hypervirulent NAP1 strain there is often reluctance simply to observe patients without initiating antibiotic treatment that appears effective in the vast majority of patients. However, the drugs for therapy also appear to cause the disease. This may account for one of the major complications of treatment which is relapses. Only two antibiotics have been used frequently, vancomycin and metronidazole. Both are active against virtually all strains of *C. difficile* so that resistance is not an issue. Their pharmacology is very different. Vancomycin given orally is not absorbed but provides levels that are about 100 to 1000 times the minimum inhibitory concentration in the colon where *C. difficile* resides. In contrast, oral metronidazole is almost completely absorbed and so colonic levels are erratic and often undetectable. Comparative trials of metronidazole versus vancomycin have generally shown equivalent responses, but more recently, vancomycin was shown to be superior, especially in patients with severe disease. There is concern about the high cost of oral vancomycin therapy and the fear that its excessive use might lead to vancomycin resistance, not by

C. difficile but by other organisms such as enterococci. As a result, many authorities now recommend metronidazole (500 mg orally three times a day for 7–10 days) for mild-moderate CDI and oral vancomycin (125 mg orally four times a day for 7–10 days) for those with more serious disease. Patients with fulminant CDI are a special challenge, often because it is so difficult to get antibiotics to the site of infection due to ileus. Recommendations in these cases include oral vancomycin in doses of 500 mg orally or via nasogastric tube four times a day combined with intravenous metronidazole. Many of these patients and especially those with ileus or toxic megacolon may require colostomy.

Another complication of antibiotic treatment of CDI is relapse, which occurs in approximately 20% of patients with their first course of treatment, about 40% treated for a single relapse, and 60% for those treated for two relapses. Several different therapeutic strategies have been recommended for relapses but none is uniformly effective. The most frequently recommended strategy is oral vancomycin in standard dose for 7 to 10 days to control the relapse episode, followed by vancomycin tapered over 2 weeks, followed by a prolonged course of 'pulse vancomycin' (125 mg orally every other day) for a total of 2 to 6 weeks. The presumed mechanism for pulse therapy is to give sufficient vancomycin to maintain the pathogen in spore state, but insufficient to inhibit recolonization by the normal flora which will ultimately control replication and toxin production of *C. difficile*. Other strategies include intravenous immune globulin, probiotics, other antibiotics such as rifamycins, and several experimental agents. Data are inadequate for use of these strategies at present.

Small case series have suggested that sequential therapy with vanomcyin followed by rifaximin may be effective for the treatment of recurrent CDI.

Fidaxomicin is a macrocylic antibiotic that is bactericidal against *C. difficile* and has been shown to have similar efficacy to but lower relapse rates that vancomycin in randomized controlled trial.

Other strategies include probiotics, anion binding resins, intravenous immunoglobulin, and faecal bacteriotherapy. Studies of probiotics and anion binding resins have proven inconclusive. A retrospective review of the use of intravenous immunoglobulin showed no benefit. Faecal bacteriotherapy has been reported to be efficacious in case reports and uncontrolled case series of patients with chronic recurrent CDI. An optimal standardized regimen has not been developed and treatment is administered either via an enema or colonoscope or via a nasogastric, nasojejunal or nasoduodenal tube. Reported cure rates are high but concerns remain about potential transmission of infectious agents to the recipient.

Areas of controversy

Diagnostic testing

A range of tests are now used to detect *C. difficile*. Choice is based on speed of results, cost, sensitivity, specificity, and availability of reagents. In the United States of America, 95% of hospital laboratories use EIA as the only diagnostic test. In Europe and Australia, there is much more frequent use of culture–toxin assays based on better sensitivity, but there is an increase in the cost and a delay in receiving results.

Treatment

Most groups have traditionally recommended metronidazole as the drug of choice for CDI, including Centers for Disease Control, Society of Health Care Epidemiology of America, and Infectious Diseases Society of America. However, the use of oral vancomycin is increasingly advocated, especially for patients who are seriously ill, but controversy continues about its cost and the consequences of its excessive use.

Infection control

The recommendation is for a private room and private bathroom to prevent nosocomial spread, but many older hospitals and most chronic care facilities cannot provide these. Another controversy concerns the use of soap and water hand washing, which is favoured because the standard alcohol-based hand cleaning does not eradicate clostridial spores. The problem is lack of easy access to soap and water in many facilities and concern that this is a largely theoretical issue with no demonstrated clinical benefit, while alcohol-based cleaning prevents many other important pathogens.

Antibiotic selection

The most important causative agents have been identified and some workers in the field have felt that their use should be discouraged more aggressively especially during epidemics in which a specific agent has been implicated. Controversy surrounds the definition of an epidemic, clarity in implicating a single agent, and methods of discouraging use while still providing optimal therapy.

Strain identification

The NAP1 strain is implicated as a cause of a particularly severe disease, but most physicians do not know if it is the responsible strain in a particular patient as this would require stool culture with referral to a reference source for *C. difficile* strain typing. This is possibly important in epidemics, but is not important in individual cases since management strategies are based on severity of disease and infection control to prevent spread of the epidemic strain regardless of strain type.

Likely developments in the near future

C. difficile poses many challenges. In recent years there has been progress in diagnosis, treatment, and prevention of CDI. However, recent events have called attention to many deficits in current practice and many now feel that much more attention to diagnosis, treatment, and infection control is needed. For detection, the challenge is to find a test that is fast, cheap, sensitive, and specific. Some current research favours the use of a sensitive method to detect *C. difficile*, such as common antigen detection by EIA or PCR to detect toxigenic strains accompanied by EIA for detection of toxin A and toxin B, with the more sensitive cytotoxin assay to detect those that are *C. difficile* positive and EIA negative for toxin A. For treatment, a drug superior to oral vancomycin for the treatment of acute disease, especially severe acute disease, is unlikely to emerge. The challenge is getting the drug to the site of infection. Future research may define better the role of ancillary methods such as probiotics, indications for colectomy, and the role of intravenous immune globulin. For relapses, the most promising results will be use of nonantibiotic treatment, since the drugs currently in use have the paradox that they cause as well as cure *C. difficile*. Most promising in this category will be antibiotics that selectively inhibit *C. difficile* without altering the colonic flora or the use of nonantibiotics such as anion exchange resins. For infection control, perhaps the biggest challenge is antibiotic stewardship to eliminate abuse of these drugs which is a well-recognized problem, but very difficult to control in terms of physician understanding and patient acceptance.

Further reading

Al-Nassir WN, *et al.* (2008). Comparison of clinical and microbiological response to treatment of *Clostridium difficile*-associated disease with metronidazole and vancomycin. *Clin Infect Dis*, **47**, 56–62.

Aslam S, Hamill RJ, Musher DM (2005). Treatment of *Clostridium difficile*-associated disease: old therapies and new strategies. *Lancet Infect Dis*, **5**, 549–57.

Bartlett JG (2006). Narrative review: the new epidemic of *Clostridium difficile*-associated enteric disease. *Ann Intern Med*, **145**, 758–64.

Blossom DB, McDonald LC (2007). The challenges posed by reemerging *Clostridium difficile* infection. *Clin Infect Dis*, **45**, 222–7.

Dial S, *et al.* (2005). Use of gastric acid-suppressive agents and the risk of community-acquired *Clostridium difficile*-associated disease. *JAMA*, **294**, 2989–95.

Gerding DN, *et al.* (1995). *Clostridium difficile*-associated diarrhea and colitis. *Infect Control Hosp Epidemiol*, **16**, 459–77.

Hall IC, O'Toole E (1935). Intestinal flora in newborn infants with a description of a new pathogenic anaerobe, *Bacillus difficilis*. *Am J Dis Child*, **49**, 390–402.

Hambre LDS, *et al.* (1943). The toxicity of penicillin as prepared for clinical use. *Am J Med Sci*, **206**, 642–52.

Johnson S, *et al.* (1999). Epidemics of diarrhea caused by a clindamycin-resistant strain of *Clostridium difficile* in four hospitals. *N Engl J Med*, **341**, 1645–51.

Lamontagne F, *et al.* (2007). Impact of emergency colectomy on survival of patients with fulminant *Clostridium difficile* colitis during an epidemic caused by a hypervirulent strain. *Ann Surg*, **245**, 267–72.

Louie TJ, *et al.* OPT-80-003 Clinical Study Group. (2011). Fidaxomicin versus vancomycin for Clostridium difficile infection. *N Engl J Med*, **364**, 422–31.

McFarland LV, *et al.* (1989). Nosocomial acquisition of *Clostridium difficile* infection. *N Engl J Med*, **320**, 204–10.

Monaghan T, Boswell T, Mahida YR (2008). Recent advances in *Clostridium difficile*-associated disease. *Gut*, **57**, 850–60.

Pépin J, *et al.* (2004). *Clostridium difficile*-associated diarrhea in a region of Quebec from 1991 to 2003: a changing pattern of disease severity. *Can Med Assoc J*, **171**, 466–72.

Peterson LR, *et al.* (2007). Detection of toxigenic Clostridium difficile in stool samples by real-time polymerase chain reaction for the diagnosis of C. difficile-associated diarrhea. *Clin Infect Dis*, **45**, 1152–60.

Riegler M, *et al.* (1995). *Clostridium difficile* toxin B is more potent than toxin A in damaging human colonic epithelium in vitro. *J Clin Invest*, **95**, 2004–11.

Tedesco FJ, Barton RW, Alpers DH (1974). Clindamycin-associated colitis. A prospective study. *Ann Intern Med*, **81**, 429–33.

Ticehurst JR, *et al.* (2006). Effective detection of toxigenic *Clostridium difficile* by a two-step algorithm including tests for antigen and cytotoxin. *J Clin Microbiol*, **44**, 1145–9.

Warny M, *et al.* (2005). Toxin production by an emerging strain of *Clostridium difficile* associated with outbreaks of severe disease in North America and Europe. *Lancet*, **366**, 1079–84.

Zar FA, *et al.* (2007). A comparison of vancomycin and metronidazole for the treatment of *Clostridium difficile*-associated diarrhea, stratified by disease severity. *Clin Infect Dis*, **45**, 302–7.

6.24 Botulism, gas gangrene, and clostridial gastrointestinal infections

Dennis L. Stevens, Michael J. Aldape, and Amy E. Bryant

Essentials

Botulism

Human botulism is caused by seven serological types of *C. botulinum*, which is ubiquitously distributed in the soil. Poisoning usually results from ingestion of preformed toxin in food, although this is rapidly inactivated at ordinary cooking temperatures, but it can also result from contaminated wounds. *C. botulinum* toxin binds irreversibly to the neuromuscular junction and is the most lethal known microbial toxin.

Clinical features, diagnosis, and treatment— there are five forms of clinical botulism: (1) foodborne botulism—ingestion of food contaminated by preformed toxin; (2) wound botulism—infection of a wound with *Cl. botulinum* and *in vivo* toxin production (3) infant botulism—ingestion of clostridial spores that colonize the gastrointestinal tract and release toxin; (4) adult enteric infectious botulism—similar to infant botulism; (5) inhalational botulism—considered a potential agent of bioterrorism. Clinical presentation is with symptoms suggesting gastrointestinal tract illness, followed by neurological symptoms including diplopia, blurred vision, dizziness, and difficulty with speech or swallowing, leading on to generalized flaccid paralysis. The diagnosis can be confirmed by testing for botulinum toxin in the patient's serum, urine, or stomach contents, or in the suspect food. Treatment requires (1) supportive care—this, including mechanical ventilation, may be needed for many months until new synapses have developed; (2) antitoxin—this reduces case fatality and shortens the illness.

Gas gangrene

Gas gangrene is caused by *C. perfringens* (most commonly), *C. histolyticum*, *C. novyii*, *C. sordellii*, and *C. septicum*, which occur naturally in soil and in the gastrointestinal tracts of humans and animals. Common causes of the condition are severe trauma that interrupts the blood supply to the soft tissues (gunshot wounds, penetrating or crushing injuries) with contamination by dirt, vegetation, or clothing containing vegetative forms of clostridia or spores. Skin popping of black tar heroin is another recently recognized cause. The clostridia responsible elaborate a wide range of toxins with varying effects: the principle toxin of *C. perfringens* is α-toxin, a phospholipase C that cleaves phosphatidylcholine in eukaryotic cell membranes and activates neutrophils, platelets, and endothelial cells, causing obstruction of local blood flow.

Acknowledgement: The authors acknowledge inclusion of material from the chapter in the previous edition by Dr H E Larson.

Clinical features—severe and sudden pain is the most characteristic symptom. Infection progresses rapidly with local ecchymosis, blistering, massive swelling, and crepitus indicating gas in the tissue as progressive necrotizing soft-tissue infection destroys muscle, fascia, fat, and skin. Without rapid and appropriate treatment, bacteraemia, hypotension, and multiple organ failure ensue.

Diagnosis and treatment—diagnosis must be made on clinical grounds, although Gram stain of the wound discharge or tissue sample may be helpful. Treatment requires (1) early recognition and aggressive surgical debridement of devitalized tissue; (2) antimicrobials—most commonly penicillin and clindamycin (which suppresses α-toxin production); (3) anti-α-toxin serum. The benefit of hyperbaric oxygen (HBO) has not been proven in controlled trials. In an experimental model of gas gangrene, HBO did not improve the efficacy of clindamycin or penicillin.

Prevention—prophylactic antibiotic treatment reduces the risk, but this depends upon factors including the time interval between the injury and surgical debridement.

Particular forms of gas gangrene—(1) *C. septicum* can grow at ambient oxygen tensions, causing 'spontaneous gas gangrene' in normal tissues, most commonly when bacteria spread from a colonic adenocarcinoma to uninjured muscle. (2) *C. sordellii* causes haemoconcentration, leukaemoid reaction without fever, and gradually progressive shock that is fatal in 75 to 80% of patients. Women infected during parturition, after medical abortion, or following gynaecological surgery almost always die.

C. perfringens gastrointestinal infections

Food poisoning—if foods such as meat and heavy gravy infected with type A strains of *C. perfringens* are allowed to sit at room temperature, bacilli can multiply greatly. If the food is then inadequately heated before consumption, preformed heat labile enterotoxin, combined with toxin produced in the gut, causes self-limiting abdominal pain and diarrhoea, usually without fever or vomiting.

Necrotizing enterocolitis—*C. perfringens* type C β-toxin causes fulminating enterocolitis that destroys intestinal mucosa. Epidemic outbreaks occurred in postwar Germany (Darmbrand) and New Guinea (enteritis necroticans, 'pig bel') following ingestion of contaminated food, or dramatic change from vegetarian to meat diets. Treatment consists of supportive care and antibiotics (usually benzylpenicillin). Complications, e.g. intestinal perforation, may require surgery, in which case mortality is high. A toxoid vaccine is protective and should be considered in areas of Papua New Guinea where the disease still occurs.

Botulism

Definition

Botulism is an acute symmetrical descending paralysis caused by a neurotoxin produced by *Clostridium botulinum*. Food contaminated by *C. botulinum* spores and elaborated toxin produces illness when ingested. Wound infections with *C. botulinum* or intestinal tract colonization in infants and adults occasionally cause botulism. Although the illness is most commonly described in humans, botulism can occur in wild ducks feeding off the bottoms of alkaline lakes in the western United States of America. The illness is called 'limber neck'.

Occurrence

C. botulinum is ubiquitously distributed in the soil. The surfaces of potatoes, vegetables, and other foods are easily contaminated with spores, which survive brief heating at 100°C. Autoclaving or use of pressure cookers that are appropriately adjusted are very effective at killing spores. In the 1920s in the United States of America, pressure cookers calibrated at sea level which were then used at several thousand feet above sea level in the western states were the cause of outbreaks of botulism among families that home-canned food. The anaerobic conditions created by canning, smoking, or fermentation facilitate clostridial growth and toxin release. Canned food with neutral pH, such as canned corn, is particularly prone to promoting the growth of clostridia. Spores germinate in sausage or cheese kept for extended periods at room temperature. An 18th-century report associated paralytic illness with eating sausages, hence *botulus*, a Latin word for 'sausage'. Cases have been associated with fermented milk in Africa, cheese sauce on baked potatoes in North America, fermented stew in Japan, and imported fish in the United Kingdom.

Although past outbreaks typically involved small groups of people, home-canned peppers served in a restaurant caused two large outbreaks in the United States of America. Outbreaks caused by commercially processed foods are infrequent, but contamination of hazelnut purée added to commercially produced yoghurt caused 27 cases of botulism in Wales and north-west England in 1989, the largest recorded outbreak in the United Kingdom. Most of the contaminated cartons could not be accounted for, suggesting that the attack rate varied or that mild symptoms were not diagnosed as botulism. Commercially prepared chopped garlic in soybean oil caused 36 cases dispersed over 8 provinces and states in North America.

Some outbreaks involved only single contaminated items, such as in the Loch Maree episode in 1922 where eight people died after eating duck paste, the 1978 outbreak in Birmingham involving four people who ate tinned Alaskan salmon, and one case in 1989 following a meal on a commercial airliner. Uneviscerated fresh fish have been associated with botulism, usually where there have been deficiencies in refrigeration.

Purified botulinum toxin has recently come into therapeutic use. Toxin injections produce temporary muscle weakness and are effective in the treatment of strabismus, blepharospasm, and torticollis, and are also used for cosmetic purposes. Treatment doses are considered too small to elicit systemic symptoms. Under experimental conditions, aerosolized botulinum toxin causes illness in monkeys, and the toxin has been utilized as an agent for biological warfare or terrorist activity. For example, botulinum toxin was loaded into Scud missile warheads by Iraq during the first Gulf War and stockpiled by the Aum Shinrikyo cult in Japan.

The toxin

There are seven serological types of botulinum toxin (A–G). Types A, B, and E account for nearly all human cases. Serotypes implicated in outbreaks of botulism parallel the geographical distribution of soil spores. Type E is nearly always associated with fish, but outbreaks caused by fish products can also involve types A and B.

C. botulinum toxin is heat labile and rapidly inactivated at ordinary cooking temperatures. It is a protein neurotoxin, and a dose as small as 0.1 μg is sufficient to cause death in humans. The 150-kDa molecule is composed of two peptide chains connected by disulphide bonds. One chain binds to and penetrates the neuron, and the other cleaves a protein essential for neurotransmitter release, reducing acetylcholine availability for impulse transmission. Toxin types A, C, and E hydrolyse a protein in the presynaptic membrane while types B, D, F, and G hydrolyse a protein in the synaptic vesicle.

Pathogenesis

Botulinum toxin is absorbed directly across mucous membranes. Locally acting toxin may produce some symptoms but cranial nerve paralysis results from blood stream distribution. Cranial nerves are preferentially affected because botulinum toxin binds more rapidly to sites where the cycles of depolarization and repolarization are frequent. Binding is irreversible and the toxin cannot thereafter be neutralized by antitoxin. Recovery occurs when nerve terminals sprout from the axon to form new motor endplates.

Botulinum toxin blocks impulse transmission mediated by acetylcholine at neuromuscular junctions, at autonomic ganglia, and at parasympathetic nerve terminals. Nerve stimulus transmission is blocked because the toxin prevents release of acetylcholine from the presynaptic membrane. Impulse conduction within peripheral nerves and muscle contraction are not affected. The synthesis of acetylcholine and impulse transmission within terminal nerve fibrils remain intact. On the other hand, the miniature endplate potentials spontaneously generated by release of acetylcholine in a resting nerve decrease and eventually disappear in the presence of toxin. If a poisoned nerve is stimulated repetitively, temporary summation of acetylcholine release occurs producing an augmented response.

History

The symptoms of botulism vary from mild fatigue to severe weakness and collapse leading to death within a day. Initially, nausea, vomiting, abdominal bloating, and dryness in the mouth and throat may suggest gastrointestinal tract illness. Diplopia, blurred vision, dizziness, unsteadiness on standing, and difficulty with speech or swallowing are common early neurological symptoms. Subsequently, there is progression to weakness or paralysis in the limbs, and generalized weakness and lassitude. The dryness of the mouth and throat may become so severe as to cause pain. Eventually there may be difficulty holding up the head, constipation, urinary hesitancy, and problems in breathing. The incubation period is between 12 and 72 h. Patients with short incubation periods are likely to have ingested large amounts of toxin. However, individuals are known to have ingested large amounts of contaminated food without developing symptoms.

Physical examination

Negative findings in botulism are pertinent. Higher mental functions are preserved, although sometimes patients are drowsy. Sensation is intact. Fever is unusual. The mouth is dry and the tongue is furrowed. Lateral rectus weakness in the eyes produces internal strabismus. Failure of accommodation is common and the pupils may be fixed in mid position or dilated and unresponsive to light. Ptosis, weakness of other extraocular muscles, and inability to protrude the tongue or to raise the shoulders are other early findings. Weakness in the limbs is of the flaccid, lower motor neuron type and deep tendon reflexes are initially preserved. Facial muscles may be spared; gag and corneal reflexes are not lost.

Weakness of the respiratory muscles develops early in relation to other findings and deterioration can be rapid. Paralysis descends symmetrically from cranial nerves to upper extremities to respiratory muscles to the lower extremities in a proximal to distal pattern. Hypotension without compensatory tachycardia, intestinal ileus, and urinary retention are evidence of the widespread autonomic paralysis. Symptoms and signs can be confined to the autonomic nervous system.

Diagnosis

The diagnosis in the first case of an outbreak can be missed because cranial nerve symptoms and signs are ignored in what is apparently a gastrointestinal disturbance. The differential diagnosis usually lies between botulism and the descending form of acute inflammatory polyneuropathy or Guillain–Barré syndrome. There can be similarities in the clinical presentation and progression of symptoms in the two diseases. Patients with botulism have normal cerebrospinal fluid findings and respiratory weakness and failure develop early, before the presence of severe limb weakness. Patients with the Guillain–Barré syndrome have marked limb weakness before the development of respiratory failure. Sensation and mental status are preserved in botulism.

Other diagnoses that may be considered include diphtheria, intoxication with atropine or organophosphorus compounds, myasthenia gravis, cerebrovascular disease involving the brainstem and producing bulbar palsy, paralytic rabies, tick paralysis, and neurotoxic snake bite. Botulism is distinguished from polymyositis and periodic paralysis by its rapid progression and cranial nerve abnormalities. Sometimes patients with other types of poisoning are thought to have botulism, most often with an outbreak of staphylococcal food poisoning. Individuals with carbon monoxide poisoning have been mistakenly been thought to be poisoned by food, but they invariably have headaches and altered consciousness. Poisoning from chemicals or fish produces rapid onset of symptoms. Mushroom poisoning is characterized by severe abdominal pain.

The diagnosis of botulism can be confirmed by testing for botulinum toxin in the patient's serum, urine, stomach contents, or in the suspect food. Ten millilitres of serum should be taken before antotoxin treatment. Mice are inoculated intraperitoneally with 0.5 ml of sample, with and without mixing with polyvalent botulinum antitoxin, and observed for signs of botulism. Appropriate samples for microbiological investigation should also be collected: suspected food sample; faeces, rectal washout, vomitus, and gastric contents in suspected foodborne or infant botulism; pus or tissue in wound botulism. These should be inoculated into a cooked meat broth or other anaerobic medium.

Electromyography can be helpful in confirming a diagnosis of botulism. Single or low-frequency stimuli evoke muscle action potentials that are reduced in amplitude; tetanic or rapid stimuli produce an enhanced response. Nerve conduction velocities are normal. This result readily differentiates botulism from the Guillain–Barré syndrome. Patients with myasthenia gravis usually have muscle action potentials of normal or minimally decreased amplitude.

Treatment

The priorities in management are assessment of respiratory function followed by administration of antitoxin. Respiration should be monitored closely with a view to elective intubation since deterioration can occur rapidly. Prolonged respiratory support may be required. Profound hypotension can be secondary to hypoxaemia, acidosis, and accumulated fluid deficits or can be a feature of the autonomic paralysis. Treat autonomic paralysis by expanding the intravascular volume using whole blood, protein, and/or saline while monitoring central venous pressure or by infusing a low dose of dopamine.

Trivalent (types A, B, and E) antitoxin reduces case fatality and shortens the course of the illness. To be useful it must be given early, before free circulating toxin has bound to its peripheral targets and before the diagnosis can be confirmed by animal tests. Heptavalent equine antitoxin is available from the Health Protection Agency in the United Kingdom and through the State Departments of Health in the United States of America; one-half of the dose is given intramuscularly and one-half intravenously. An intradermal 0.1-ml test dose is given, but most serum reactions are not predicted by this test. As the antitoxin is derived from horse serum, serum sickness and anaphylaxis may occur. A pentavalent ovine antitoxin is available for military use only. One study of 132 patients with type A foodborne botulism reported reduced mortality in those treated with antitoxin compared with those who were not. Earlier administration appears to reduce the duration of symptoms and duration of mechanical ventilation.

Human-derived botulinum immunoglobulin (called BIG-IV or BabyBIG) is available for use in infants less than 1 year of age who are diagnosed with infant botulism. BIG-IV should be administered as early as possible in the illness.

Many years ago it was shown that patients dying of botulism carried bacilli in their intestine. The discovery that clinical disease can result from toxin formed within the gastrointestinal tract of infants and adults makes antimicrobial treatment theoretically appealing. Gastric lavage, repeated high enemas, and cathartics have been utilized in an attempt to remove unabsorbed toxin. Drugs capable of reversing neuromuscular blockade have been used to treat patients with botulism, but without any noticeable effect on respiratory muscle weakness or tidal volume.

The mortality from botulism in the early part of the 20th century was 60 to 70%, but this improved to 23% for cases reported between 1960 and 1970 since the use of respiratory support. In a single large outbreak in 1977 there were no deaths among 59 cases. Recovery from botulism depends on the formation of new neuromuscular junctions; clinical improvement thus takes weeks to months. One severe case required respiratory support for 173 days with eventual recovery. Very prolonged fatigue and dyspnoea on exertion can be due to factors other than the neuromuscular blockade.

Wound botulism

Symptoms and signs of botulism can develop in people with injuries. Recognition may be complicated by the presence of fever from wound infection or gas gangrene, or by the absence of gastrointestinal symptoms. The diagnosis is confirmed by electromyography; botulinum toxin is detected in serum in only about one-half of the reported cases. The incubation period averages 7 days with a range of 4 to 17 days. Clinical findings and management are the same as for patients with food-borne botulism. Since 1991, wound botulism has increasingly become a complication of injection drug abuse; small abscesses at injection sites yield *C. botulinum*. An epidemic of wound botulism in the United States of America has been associated with the injection of black tar heroin. *C. botulinum* can be recovered from wounds in the absence of clinical botulism.

Infant botulism

Sporadically, cases of botulism are recognized in infants less than 6 months of age. Previously healthy babies develop constipation, which progresses over 3 to 10 days to poor feeding, irritability, a hoarse cry, and weakness in head control. Examination shows a generally weak, hypotonic, afebrile infant. Abnormalities in eye movements and pupillary reactions are sometimes present and deep tendon reflexes are reduced or absent. There is considerable range in severity; respiratory failure can develop but most recover completely.

The diagnosis can be confirmed by finding *C. botulinum* and toxin in the faeces, and by electromyography. Botulinum toxin is not present in the serum. The disease is thought to follow ingestion of *C. botulinum* spores, which multiply in the infant's gastrointestinal tract and produce toxin. Excretion of *C. botulinum* and toxin may continue for as long as 3 months. Honey has been a source of spores in some cases. Other than supportive measures, no consistent pattern in treatment using antitoxin, antibiotics, cathartics, or enemas has been established.

Gas gangrene

Definition

Gas gangrene is a rapidly developing and spreading infection of muscle caused by toxin-producing clostridial species. Gas gangrene is accompanied by bacteraemia, hypotension, and multiorgan failure and is invariably fatal if untreated.

Aetiology

Clostridia are mainly saprophytes, occurring naturally in soil and in the gastrointestinal tracts of humans and animals. Most cases of gas gangrene are caused by *Clostridium perfringens* type A, but some are due to *C. novyi* and a few to *C. septicum*, *C. histolyticum*, *C. sordellii*, and *C. fallax*; not uncommonly more that one species is isolated. Oxygen inhibits growth of most, although *C. septicum* is quite aerotolerant.

Gas gangrene has been a major cause of wound infection on the battlefield, although recently civilian and iatrogenic traumas have become more common. Disease development requires an anaerobic environment and contamination of the wound with spores or vegetative organisms usually through soil contact. However, proximity to faecal sources of bacteria is also a risk factor for cases occurring after hip surgery, adrenaline injections into the buttock, or amputation of the leg for ischaemic vascular disease. Wound contamination with dirt, shrapnel, or bits of clothing reduces local oxygen concentrations. Traumatic gas gangrene develops in deep wounds involving large muscle masses in the shoulder, hip, thigh, and calf and particularly in those situations where damage to major arteries has occurred. Thus, gunshot wounds, crush injuries, and open fractures account for most of the cases. High-velocity bullets of large calibre are commonly used in contemporary times in civilian and military firearms and these produce extensive tissue damage. Necrotic tissue, foreign bodies, and ischaemia in a wound reduce the locally available oxygen and favour outgrowth of vegetative cells and spores.

The incidence of gas gangrene after trauma reflects the speed at which injured people can be evacuated and receive appropriate treatment. During the Vietnam and Falklands conflicts there were very few cases of gas gangrene among American and British wounded cared for by highly organized surgical teams. This reduction was likely due to more timely cleansing of wounds, maintaining blood flow by vascular surgery, and the use of antibiotics. In comparison, when a jet airliner crashed in the Florida everglades, eight of the 77 injured survivors developed the disease.

Nontraumatic or 'spontaneous gas gangrene' occurs without a preceding injury. Classically, it presents as a primary infection of the perineum or scrotum or in a limb secondary to seeding from clostridial colonization of a colonic neoplasm. These cases are most commonly caused by the more aerotolerant *C. septicum* where production of superoxide dismutase permits the organisms to survive in the presence of small amounts of oxygen.

Recently, *C. novyi*, *C. sordellii*, and *C. perfringens* have been associated with necrotizing soft tissue infections at injection sites in drug addicts. Outbreaks of these infections were reported in Scotland, Ireland, England, and the United States of America in 2000 and were characterized by extensive soft tissue necrosis, hypotension, severe constitutional toxicity, and a high case fatality rate.

C. sordellii infections have been described in women following natural childbirth or therapeutic abortion, and in men, women, and children following a variety of traumatic and surgical procedures. The infections are perhaps the most aggressive of all clostridial infections, in part because of a unique syndrome of absence of fever, profound hypotension, diffuse capillary leak, haemoconcentration, and leukaemoid reaction resulting in 70% mortality within 2 to 4 days of hospital admission. The toxins responsible for this remarkable infection have not been fully elucidated.

Toxins

The clinical and histological manifestations of gas gangrene are attributable to the production of potent bacterial exotoxins. The clostridia responsible for gas gangrene elaborate a wide range of toxins. More than 12 have been described for *C. septicum*, *C. novyi*, and *C. perfringens*. The principal toxin of *C. perfringens* is α-toxin, a phospholipase C. This toxin cleaves phosphatidylcholine found in cell membrane of eukaryotic cells, releasing diacylglycerol and phosphorylcholine. In small doses, this toxin can hyperactivate a variety of cells including neutrophils, platelets, endothelial cells, and macrophages; in high doses it is cytotoxic. Interestingly, this toxin can cause the rapid and irreversible cessation of blood flow to normal tissue. This perfusion deficit is the consequence of toxin-induced platelet/neutrophil aggregates that irreversibly occlude small to medium-sized vessels. Experimentally, active or passive immunization against α-toxin is protective against active infection. A second toxin, θ-toxin, is a cholesterol-dependent thiol-activated cytolysin that lyses red blood cells and other cells by its ability to form pores in cell membranes. Electron microscopy of θ-toxin-treated cells shows arc and ring structures of 7.5 to 18 nm appearing in the plasma membrane as early as 1 h postexposure. These plasma membrane defects increase with time and can be visualized adjacent to toxin molecules that have been labelled with ferritin. α-Toxin and θ-toxin are not readily detected in the tissues or serum of patients with gas gangrene, possibly because the toxin binds rapidly and irreversibly to lipid moieties in the cytoplasmic membranes.

History

The incubation period of gas gangrene is usually less than 4 days, often less than 24 h, and occasionally as short as 1 to 6 h. Pain is the most characteristic symptom. Patients describe this as severe or excruciating and sudden in onset. Evolution of symptoms and signs can be very rapid. Toxicity may prevent the patient from giving an adequate history.

Physical examination

Early on, it may be difficult to account for the patient's pain by objective physical findings. Swelling, bluish discoloration, or darkening of the skin occurs at the affected site. The traumatic or surgical wounds become oedematous and a thin, serous discharge emerges from the site. Pain steadily increases in severity; the overlying skin becomes stretched and develops a brown or 'bronzed' discoloration. Haemorrhagic vesicles and finally areas of frank necrosis appear. A sweet odour from the wound has been described. Gas is not invariably present early in the course, but radiographs may detect gas earlier than can physical examination. Later, crepitus and exquisite tenderness are present in the wound.

Profound constitutional changes occur. Patients become sweaty and febrile, and though alert and oriented, are very distressed. The pulse is elevated out of proportion to the fever. Death may occur within 48 h. At operation, infected muscle appears dark red with purple discoloration; frank gangrene and liquefaction may be seen. Involved muscle does not bleed when cut or contract when directly stimulated.

Rapidly progressing necrotizing infections of the soft tissue may be monomicrobic, caused by clostridia, *Streptococcus pyogenes*, *Staphylococcus aureus*, *Vibrio vulnificus*, or *Aeromonas hydrophila*. Alternatively, necrotizing infections may be polymicrobic and caused by mixed aerobic and anaerobic microbes. Clostridia and polymicrobial infections are usually associated with gas in the tissue, whereas the others are not. Polymicrobial necrotizing infections occur most commonly following gastrointestinal surgery, penetrating injury to the abdomen, surgical incisions in the vaginal mucosa (episiotomy), or in diabetic patients with peripheral vascular disease. All of these necrotizing infections may destroy fascia, but frequently also destroy muscle, subcutaneous tissue, and skin.

Diagnosis

The diagnosis of gas gangrene must be made on clinical grounds and prompt recognition and treatment improve the prognosis. Sudden deterioration in a postoperative patient or following trauma requires examination of the wound and surrounding tissue. Cases of primary gas gangrene and cases following elective surgery may have a higher fatality because recognition is delayed. Gram's staining of the wound discharge, of an aspirate, or of a needle biopsy may aid diagnosis. In gas gangrene there are many large plump Gram-positive bacilli, usually without spores. Few, if any, polymorphonuclear leucocytes are present in the tissues or exudates, likely due to toxin-induced inhibition of cellular extravasation.

CT scanning can detect gas deep in muscle, but the absence of gas does not exclude the diagnosis. Culture of clostridia does not confirm a diagnosis of gas gangrene as simple colonization without clinical disease occurs in up to 30% of traumatic wounds.

Treatment

Surgical removal of all affected muscle is essential to eliminate the conditions that allow the organism to grow. High-velocity missiles distribute energy radially from their path, producing more extensive tissue damage than missiles at low speeds or with a small mass. Thus, wounds should be excised widely by resection back to healthy, viable muscle and skin. Closure should be delayed for 5 to 6 days until it is certain that the wound is free of infection.

Administration of appropriate antimicrobial agents is also required. Penicillin has been the drug of choice based on *in vitro* susceptibility testing, but experimental evidence has demonstrated that clindamycin or tetracycline is superior to penicillin. This improved efficacy is most likely because these two protein synthesis inhibitors prevent the production of toxins. This has led to the use of penicillin and clindamycin as combination therapy. Ceftriaxone or erythromycin are alternative choices for severely penicillin-allergic patients.

Hyperbaric oxygen therapy (typically 100% oxygen at 303 kPa for 60–120 min, 2–3 times daily) has been used to treat gas gangrene; however, an effect on mortality has never been shown by controlled trials and comparable survival rates have been achieved without using it. Experimental studies have demonstrated that hyperbaric oxygen alone was neither effective in an animal model of *C. perfringens* gas gangrene nor did it improve the efficacy of clindamycin or penicillin.

Therapeutic administration of gas gangrene antitoxin made from horse serum is controversial. Use during the Second World War reduced mortality, but serum sickness and other allergic reactions occurred. It is no longer produced in the United States of America. In recent studies, active immunization of animals with a truncated, nontoxic form (C-domain) of the α-toxin was 100% protective against active muscle infection with *C. perfringens*.

Prevention

Prophylactic antibiotic treatment reduces the risk of gas gangrene but this depends on the time interval between the injury and surgical debridement, the associated vascular deficit, the presence of foreign body, the presence of a compound or open fracture, and the duration of antibiotic administration. Patients have clearly developed gas gangrene after prophylactic administration of β-lactam antibiotics. Gas gangrene can develop from wounds contaminated with either vegetative organisms or spores. Antibiotics may be more effective in the former case since spores, until they germinate, are not affected by antibiotics. Metronidazole or clindamycin may be useful in patients who are hypersensitive to β-lactam antibiotics. Experimentally, active immunization against the α-toxin provides impressive protection against *C. perfringens* gas gangrene, but no active or passive vaccine is currently available.

Clostridial infections of the gastrointestinal tract

Necrotizing enterocolitis

Definition

Necrotizing enterocolitis is a fulminating clinical illness characterized by extensive necrosis of the intestinal mucosa and wall. Terms such as *darmbrand* (Germany), enteritis necroticans, pig bel (Papua

New Guinea), or gas gangrene of the bowel describe geographic variants. Cases occur sporadically in adults or as epidemics in all ages. Necrotizing enterocolitis occurs in infants, and some of these cases have demonstrated clostridia in the wall of the intestine.

Aetiology

Gram's staining of the necrotic mucosa and the bowel wall shows many Gram-positive bacilli that are typically identified as *C. perfringens* (*C. welchii*). Sporadic cases usually yield *C. perfringens* type A. However, in the German and especially in the Papua New Guinea outbreaks, there is substantial evidence implicating *C. perfringens* type C. Type C produces large amounts of β-toxin, which has lethal and necrotizing effects. Papua New Guinea highlanders have a high prevalence of antibodies to β-toxin; antibodies are rare in people who live where the disease is uncommon. Patients with pig bel have rising levels of antibodies to β-toxin, and specific passive or active immunization prevents disease. It is not clear whether exogenous human infection with these organisms occurs or whether the lesions are produced by the overgrowth of endogenous clostridia. Sweet potato, a local dietary staple, contains an inhibitor of trypsin. Combined with a low-protein diet this may impair the ability of the intestine to inactivate endogenously produced β-toxin. However, the methods used for roasting the pigs offer many opportunities for clostridial contamination.

History and physical examination

Sporadic cases in patients over 50 years of age or among those recovering from gastric surgery are regularly reported from Scandinavia, Europe, the United States of America, Australia, and the Middle East. Alternatively, epidemic outbreaks as described in postwar Germany and among the highlanders of Papua New Guinea follow ingestion of contaminated food or a dramatic change in eating habits. Severe intermittent abdominal pain is the first symptom and pain rapidly becomes continuous. Bloody diarrhoea and vomiting are common. Patients quickly develop tachycardia, followed by hypotension and evidence of multiorgan failure. On examination there is fever with abdominal distension, localized or diffuse tenderness, and reduced bowel sounds. A tender mass may be palpated. Following resolution of infection, malabsorption and partial small bowel obstruction may develop because of intestinal scarring.

Treatment and prevention

Patients with suspected pig bel should be treated with nasogastric suction and intravenous fluids. Pyrantel is given by mouth and the bowel rested by fasting. Benzylpenicillin, 1 MU, is given intravenously every 4 h and the patient observed for complications requiring surgery. Mild cases recover without surgical intervention, but if surgical indications are present the mortality ranges from 35 to 100%, in part due to perforation of the intestine. As pig bel continues to be a common disease in Papua New Guinea, consideration should be given to the use of a *C. perfringens* type C toxoid vaccine in local areas. Two doses spaced 3 to 4 months apart are preventive.

Clostridium perfringens food poisoning

Occurrence and clinical findings

In the United Kingdom and the United States of America, food poisoning caused by *C. perfringens* is the third most common type of food-borne illness. Meat and poultry are responsible for at least 90% of the outbreaks, which occur where food is prepared in large quantities. Two-thirds of the reported outbreaks are in schools, hospitals, factories, restaurants, or catering establishments, and in a typical outbreak 35 to 40 people are affected. An estimated 12 000 cases were associated with a single outbreak in 1969.

The circumstances surrounding an outbreak repeat themselves with monotonous regularity. A meat dish is prepared by stewing, braising, boiling, or steaming and this is allowed to stand at ambient temperatures for a period of 4 to 24 h. The food is served cold or after rewarming. Six to 12 h after eating the meal, people complain of cramping abdominal pain and then diarrhoea. Vomiting is unusual and fever inconsequential. Twelve to 24 h later the diarrhoea and pain have subsided. Fatal cases occur rarely; at autopsy they show severe enterocolitis.

Undoubtedly many cases of *C. perfringens* food poisoning occur at home but are not reported. Antibodies to the toxin mediating the symptoms are very common and it is likely that nearly everyone has experienced this disease once or more in their lifetime.

Aetiology

C. perfringens is an ubiquitous sporulating anaerobe with an unparalleled virtuosity for production of biologically significant toxins. The clinical effects of infection with any particular strain may depend largely on its toxin-producing capacity. Strains associated with food poisoning have several special characteristics. They are type A, although their production of α-toxin is variable; the organisms are often heat resistant to 100°C. Eighty-six per cent of food-poisoning strains produce a specific heat-labile enterotoxin. Toxin production *in vitro* is closely associated with sporulation rather than with the multiplication of vegetative cells. *In vivo*, toxin probably acts by damaging enterocyte membranes. Free enterotoxin has been detected in diarrhoeal stool after *C. perfringens* food poisoning. Antibody to enterotoxin increases after such episodes, and ingestion of 8 to 12 mg enterotoxin by volunteers produces abdominal pain and diarrhoea.

C. perfringens is a normal human faecal organism, is regularly found in the intestinal tract of domestic animals, often contaminates raw meat, and can be carried by flies. The distribution of enterotoxin-producing strains may be more restricted. However, surface contamination of meat with *C. perfringens* is common and subsequent rolling or grinding distributes these organisms throughout. Spores germinate and multiply to 10^6 to 10^7 cells/g in the anaerobic environment created when meat or meat gravy cools slowly or stands at ambient temperature. Reheating may not kill these cells and, when ingested, they multiply still further, sporulate, and release their toxin.

Enterotoxin-producing strains of *C. perfringens* may sometimes cause diarrhoea by means of overgrowth in the gut. Patients, usually elderly, can experience diarrhoea without known contact with contaminated food. The diarrhoea may be short lived or persist intermittently for several months. Colony counts of 10^8 to 10^{10}/g of faeces are associated with the presence of high titres of free toxin. Previous antimicrobial treatment may encourage the overgrowth and the same strain has been found to cross-infect patients.

Further reading

Botulism

Arnon SS, *et al*. (2006). Human botulism immune globulin for the treatment of infant botulism. *N Engl J Med*, **354**, 462–71.

Cherington M (2004). Botulism: update and review. *Semin Neurol*, **24**, 155–63.

Chertow DS, *et al.* (2006). Botulism in 4 adults following cosmetic injections with an unlicensed, highly concentrated botulinum preparation. *JAMA*, **296**, 2476–79.

Fox CK, Keet CA, Strober JB (2005). Recent advances in infant botulism. *Pediatr Neurol*, **32**, 149–54.

Lalli G, *et al.* (2003). The journey of tetanus and botulinum neurotoxins in neurons. *Trends Microbiol*, **11**, 431–7.

Sobel J (2009). Diagnosis and treatment of botulism: a century later, clinical suspicion remains the cornerstone. *Clin Infect Dis*, **48**, 1674–5.

Gas gangrene

Aldape MJ, Bryant AE, Stevens DL (2006). *Clostridium sordellii* infection: epidemiology, clinical findings and current perspectives on diagnosis and treatment. *Clin Infect Dis*, **43**, 1436–46.

Bryant AE, Stevens DL (1996). Phospholipase C and perfringolysin O from *Clostridium perfringens* upregulate ELAM-1 and ICAM-1 expression, and induce IL-8 synthesis in cultured human umbilical vein endothelial cells. *Infect Immun*, **64**, 358–62.

Bryant AE, *et al.* (1993). *Clostridium perfringens* invasiveness is enhanced by effects of theta toxin upon PMNL structure and function. *FEMS Immunol Med Microbiol*, **7**, 321–36.

Bryant AE, *et al.* (2000). Clostridial gas gangrene I: cellular and molecular mechanisms of microvascular dysfunction. *J Infect Dis*, **182**, 799–807.

Bryant AE, *et al.* (2000). Clostridial gas gangrene II: phospholipase C-induced activation of platelet gpIIbIIIa mediates vascular occlusion and myonecrosis in *C. perfringens* gas gangrene. *J Infect Dis*, **182**, 808–15.

Bryant AE, *et al.* (2006). *Clostridium perfringens* phospholipase C-induced platelet/leukocyte interactions impede neutrophils diapedesis. *J Med Microbiol*, **55**, 495–504.

Centers for Disease Control (2000). Update: *Clostridium novyi* and unexplained illness among injecting-drug users. *MMWR Morb Mortal Wkly Rep*, **49**, 543–5.

Cohen AL, *et al.* (2007). Toxic shock associated with *Clostridium sordellii* and *Clostridium perfringens* after medical and spontaneous abortion. *Obstet. Gynecol*, **110**, 1027–33.

Darke SG, King AM, Slack WK (1977). Gas gangrene and related infection: classification, clinical features and aetiology, management and mortality. A report of 88 cases. *Br J Surg*, **64**, 104–12.

Maclennan JD (1962). The histotoxic clostridial infections of man. *Bacteriol Rev*, **26**, 177–276.

Shouler PJ (1983). The management of missile injuries. *J R Nav Med Serv*, **69**, 80–4.

Stevens DL, Bryant AE (2005). Clostridial gas gangrene: clinical correlations, microbial virulence factors, and molecular mechanisms of pathogenesis. In: Proft T (ed) *Microbial toxins: molecular and cellular biology*, pp. 313–35. Horizon Bioscience, Norfolk, UK.

Stevens DL, *et al.* (1993). Evaluation of therapy with hyperbaric oxygen for experimental infection with *Clostridium perfringens*. *Clin Infect Dis*, **17**, 231–7.

Stevens DL, *et al.* (2004). Immunization with the C-domain of alpha-toxin prevents lethal infection, localizes tissue injury, and promotes host response to challenge with *Clostridium perfringens*. *J Infect Dis*, **190**, 767–73.

Gastrointestinal infections

Abrahao C, *et al.* (2001). Similar frequency of detection of *Clostridium perfringens* enterotoxin and *Clostridium difficile* toxins in patients with antibiotic-associated diarrhea. *Eur J Clin Microbiol Infect Dis*, **20**, 676–7.

Alfa MJ, *et al.* (2002). An outbreak of necrotizing enterocolitis associated with a novel clostridium species in a neonatal intensive care unit. *Clin Infect Dis*, **35**, S101–S105.

Bos J, *et al.* (2005). Fatal necrotizing colitis following a foodborne outbreak of enterotoxigenic *Clostridium perfringens* type A infection. *Clin Infect Dis*, **40**, e78–e83.

Fisher DJ, *et al.* (2005). Association of beta2 toxin production with *Clostridium perfringens* type A human gastrointestinal disease isolates carrying a plasmid enterotoxin gene. *Mol Microbiol*, **56**, 747–62.

Lawrence GW, *et al.* (1990). Impact of active immunisation against enteritis necroticans in Papua New Guinea. *Lancet*, **336**, 1165–7.

Li DY, *et al.* (2004). Enteritis necroticans with recurrent enterocutaneous fistulae caused by *Clostridium perfringens* in a child with cyclic neutropenia. *J Pediatr Gastroenterol Nutr*, **38**, 213–15.

Obladen M (2009). Necrotizing Enterocolitis—150 Years of Fruitless Search for the Cause. *Neonatology*, **96**, 203–10.

Sobel J, *et al.* (2005). Necrotizing enterocolitis associated with *Clostridium perfringens* type A in previously healthy north American adults. *J Am Coll Surg*, **201**, 48–56.

6.25 Tuberculosis

Richard E. Chaisson and Jean B. Nachega

Essentials

Tuberculosis is caused by organisms of the *Mycobacterium tuberculosis* complex, including *M. tuberculosis* (the most important), *M. bovis*, and *M. africanum*. It has been present since antiquity and is the second leading infectious cause of death after HIV infection. An estimated 2 billion people worldwide carry latent infection, when *M. tuberculosis* persists within cells and granulomas, with the potential to reactivate to cause disease decades later.

Tubercle bacilli are transmitted between people by aerosols generated when an infectious person coughs. Proximity to an infectious person determines the risk of infection. Host immunity and factors affecting it—most importantly HIV infection but also diabetes, cigarette smoking, and alcohol and drug abuse—determine the risk of active disease following infection.

Clinical presentation of active tuberculosis is highly variable, depending on the site and extent of disease and the immune status of the host. Disease is generally classified as pulmonary or extrapulmonary, with considerable clinical heterogeneity within each group.

Clinical features—pulmonary tuberculosis

Following deposition of tubercle bacilli in the alveoli of the lungs, they are ingested by alveolar macrophages, multiply intracellularly and eventually cause cell lysis with release of organisms. Over a period of weeks, infection spreads to regional lymph nodes, elsewhere in the lungs and systemically. Infected people who successfully contain viable bacilli in granulomas retain a latent infection, with lifetime risk of reactivation of about 10%.

Active pulmonary tuberculosis—this is usually a subacute respiratory illness, the most frequent symptoms of which are cough, fever, night sweats and malaise. The cough is initially nonproductive, but often progresses to sputum production and occasionally haemoptysis. Loss of appetite and excessive weight loss are common.

Clinical features—extrapulmonary tuberculosis

This may be generalized or confined to a single organ, and is found in 15 to 20% of all cases of tuberculosis in otherwise immunocompetent adults, more than 25% of cases under 15 years of age, and in more than 50% of HIV-related cases. Children under 2 years of age have high rates of miliary or disseminated tuberculosis and meningeal disease.

Infection spreads from the lungs by lymphatic and haematogenous routes. The tissues and organs most likely to be affected are the pleura, lymph nodes, kidneys and other genitourinary organs, bone, and central nervous system. Tuberculosis bacteraemia is unusual, but seen most often in patients with HIV infection and low CD4 lymphocyte counts.

Pleural tuberculosis—this is usually the result of relatively small numbers of tubercle bacilli invading the pleura from adjacent lung tissue, in which case the duration of symptoms is generally brief, with patients complaining of symptoms including fever, chest pain, and nonproductive cough. Pleural tuberculosis involving larger numbers of bacilli produces frank empyema and is commoner in older patients.

Lymphatic tuberculosis—classic scrofula of the cervical or supraclavicular lymph node chains is the most common presentation, but multiple lymph node groups can be involved in HIV-infected patients.

Genitourinary tuberculosis—the most common manifestation is renal tuberculosis, resulting from haematogenous seeding of the renal cortex during primary infection; this is frequently asymptomatic, but may be evident as sterile pyuria.

Bone and joint tuberculosis—the most common form is vertebral tuberculosis (Pott's disease), resulting from haematogenous seeding of the anterior portion of vertebral bodies during primary infection; presentation is typically with back pain; constitutional symptoms are not prominent in most cases.

Tuberculous meningitis—meningeal and leptomeningeal bacterial replication results in a robust inflammatory reaction that increases cerebrospinal fluid pressure and can cause cranial neuropathies. Common symptoms are headache, stiff neck, meningismus, and an altered mental status, including irritability, clouded thinking and malaise. The condition is not common, but usually fatal if untreated.

Miliary/disseminated tuberculosis—these describe widespread infection with absent or minimal host immune responses, usually arising as a result of primary infection, and seen more frequently in children and immunocompromised adults. Typical presentation is with fever and other constitutional symptoms over a period of several weeks.

Diagnosis

Tuberculin skin testing—intracutaneous injection of purified proteins of M. tuberculosis provokes a delayed hypersensitivity reaction which produces a zone of induration in those who are infected, but cannot distinguish disease from latent infection and may be falsely positive from BCG vaccination or nontuberculous mycobacterial infections.

Interferon-γ release-based assays—these detect *in vitro* responses to M. tuberculosis antigens. These appear to be more specific than tuberculin skin testing because false-positive reactions due to sensitization from BCG vaccination (see below) are less likely to occur. They may also be more sensitive, and are appealing because they do not require patients to return for reading of induration.

Detection of tubercle bacilli—microscopy staining of acid-fast bacilli in sputum or other tissue is the method most widely used to diagnose tuberculosis because it is inexpensive, rapid, and technologically undemanding. However, a relatively large number of bacilli are needed for a positive test, and up to 50% of patients with sputum cultures positive for M. tuberculosis have negative acid-fast smears. Culture of M. tuberculosis is the gold standard for confirming the diagnosis, but takes 10 to 40 days, depending on the method used. Nucleic acid amplification assays and other rapid diagnostic methods allow faster detection of both the presence of mycobacteria and assessment of drug resistance: these have promise in resource-limited settings, but further validation in endemic countries is needed.

Nucleic acid amplification—several new commercial assays that amplify M. tuberculosis DNA can result in rapid diagnosis of tuberculosis (<1 day). Some tests also can detect drug-resistance mutations, providing timely detection of multidrug-resistant (MDR) tuberculosis.

Particular issues—(1) Pulmonary tuberculosis—this can involve any portion of the lungs, hence radiographic findings are usually only suggestive, not diagnostic. (2) Pleural tuberculosis—diagnosis can be inferred from pulmonary findings when pulmonary parenchymal involvement is manifest, otherwise analysis of pleural fluid is essential. (3) Lymphatic tuberculosis—swelling of involved nodes accompanied by a positive tuberculin skin test and typical biopsy findings are strongly suggestive of tuberculosis and warrant presumptive therapy. (4) Tuberculous meningitis—diagnosis requires a high degree of suspicion; presumptive therapy is frequently necessary.

Treatment

Drug-susceptible tuberculosis—combination therapy with isoniazid and rifampin (and other antituberculosis drugs in the first 8 weeks) is highly effective. Treatment is usually once daily but can be given as infrequently as twice per week, with two major interventions to improve adherence and prevent bad outcomes being directly observed therapy (DOT) and the use of fixed-dose combination tablets. Modern 'short course' combination chemotherapy is curative in 6 months, except for bone and central nervous system tuberculosis, which require 12 months. Second-line agents are reserved for treatment of drug resistant tuberculosis and are generally less potent, more toxic and less readily available.

Drug-resistant tuberculosis—this significant challenge arises both through infection with drug-resistant strains (primary drug resistance) and by selection for drug-resistant strains due to ineffective therapy (secondary drug resistance). Multidrug resistant (MDR) tuberculosis is defined as resistance to at least rifampicin and isoniazid. Extensively drug-resistant (XDR) disease, which has been reported in more than 70 countries, is defined as MDR plus resistance to fluoroquinolones and at least one injectable second-line agent (capreomycin, amikacin, or kanamycin). Patients with drug-resistant tuberculosis should be managed by a physician who is a tuberculosis expert because of the complexity of their regimens and their high risk of failure of death.

Prevention

Strategies to control tuberculosis include: (1) Identification and treatment of infectious tuberculosis cases, which rapidly eliminates infectiousness. (2) Treatment of latent tuberculosis infection—the use of preventive therapy in high-risk individuals known or strongly suspected to be latently infected with *M. tuberculosis* can benefit not only the individual patient who does not fall ill with tuberculosis, but also potential contacts of that patient, who might become secondarily infected were disease to develop. (3) Prevention of exposure to infectious particles in air, especially in hospitals and other institutions—infected patients must be identified and managed in respiratory isolation. (4) Vaccination—the attenuated live vaccine, BCG (bacille Calmette-Guérin), is widely administered throughout the world, but remains controversial. Proponents argue that it provides about 50% protection against active tuberculosis disease and also diminishes haematogenous dissemination of primary tuberculosis infection, thereby reducing the incidence of miliary tuberculosis and tuberculous meningitis in children.

Introduction

Tuberculosis is one of the most important diseases in the history of humanity, and remains an extraordinary burden on human health today. Archaeological evidence demonstrates that tuberculosis was present in antiquity, and large epidemics of the disease emerged in Europe in the Middle Ages. While contemporary physicians consider tuberculosis to be one of the classic infectious diseases, recognition of the clinical manifestations of the disease has evolved over the past two millennia. The Greek term *phthisis* was used by Hippocrates to describe the wasting disease later known as tuberculosis. While the Greeks recognized various clinical manifestations of tuberculosis, understanding of the connection between the forms was limited. In the Middle Ages, the study of anatomy and the correlation of pathological findings with clinical syndromes led to a better understanding of the disease. The term 'tuberculosis' was used first only in the early 19th century, derived from the tubercles characterized in the study of pathological features of the disease.

The impact of tuberculosis on the humans population cannot be overstated, as the disease has killed hundreds of millions of people over the centuries and has had economic and social effects perhaps unparalleled in the history of medicine. Between 1700 and 1950, tuberculosis was a great killer in the developed world, earning the sobriquet "the captain of the men of death" from John Bunyan, and "the White Plague" from René and Jean Dubos. The inspiration that artists have drawn from tuberculosis, portrayed in literature, opera, and art, testifies not only to the importance of the disease within their contemporary societies, but also to the extent to which tuberculosis affected artists themselves. The annals of art are filled with those who succumbed to tuberculosis including Keats, Chopin, the Bronte sisters, Stevenson, Poe, and many, many others.

The conquest of tuberculosis through the development of vaccines, drugs, and diagnostics was a principal goal of biomedical research in the 19th and 20th centuries. The first description of the tubercle bacillus as the cause of tuberculosis by Robert Koch in 1882 was a scientific landmark. The postulates established by Koch for determining the microbial aetiology of disease have continuing influence today, and molecular correlates of those derived by Koch

further strengthen the ingenuity of his thesis. Koch also developed the microscopic and culture methods for detecting tubercle bacilli, still widely used today. Calmette and Guérin developed an effective vaccine for tuberculosis in the early 20th century, but use of the vaccine was not broad enough to control the disease and it may no longer be effective (see below). The discovery of streptomycin by Schatz and Waksman in 1943 was a major triumph; both Koch and Waksman received the Nobel Prize for their work. The development of additional antimicrobial agents against tuberculosis in the 1950s, 1960s, and 1970s, and the evaluation of chemotherapy in elegant studies conducted by the British Medical Research Council, the United States Public Health Service, and the United States Veterans Administration led to a marked apathy about tuberculosis in the closing decades of the 20th century.

Despite the availability of curative chemotherapy for more than half a century, however, tuberculosis continues to infect more than one-third of the world's population, causing 8.8 million new cases and 1.1 million deaths in 2010, and continuing to cause an enormous amount of suffering and disability. In 1994, the World Health Assembly declared that tuberculosis was a global health crisis, and the situation has only grown more serious since then. Epidemics of HIV-related tuberculosis and multidrug-resistant disease have expanded in recent years, and global control of tuberculosis remains a formidable challenge.

The unique biological properties of the causative organism, *Mycobacterium tuberculosis* complex, allow for a long incubation period between the time of infection and the development of symptoms. Latent tuberculosis infection can persist for decades before causing disease, or can persist for the lifetime of an infected person without ever causing clinically evident illness. Because latent infection creates a large reservoir of carriers of the infection, disease elimination is difficult to envisage.

Aetiology

Tuberculosis is a granulomatous disease caused by organisms of the *M. tuberculosis* complex, including *M. tuberculosis*, *M. bovis*, and *M. africanum*, of which *M. tuberculosis* is the most important. *M. tuberculosis* and the other mycobacteria are small rod-shaped or curved bacilli in the order Actinomycetales, family Mycobacteriaceae, with a unique thick cell wall composed of glycolipids and lipids. The lipid-rich coat of the mycobacteria renders these organisms resistant to acid decolorization following carbol-fuchsin staining, hence the term 'acid-fast bacilli'. Classification of the mycobacteria was based for many years on the staining and growth properties described by Runyon, but this unwieldy system has been largely replaced with modern techniques that identify mycobacteria by specific DNA sequences and, to a lesser extent, biochemical assays. Mycobacteria are frequently considered according to the diseases they cause more than their behaviour in the laboratory: *M. tuberculosis* complex causes tuberculosis; *M. leprae* causes leprosy; and the nontuberculous mycobacteria, including rapid growers, are associated with a wide range of manifestations, particularly in immunocompromised hosts.

The organisms of the *M. tuberculosis* complex are remarkably slow growing, with a generation time between 20 and 24 h. The exceedingly slow intrinsic reproductive rate of *M. tuberculosis* contributes both to its behaviour as a pathogen and to difficulties in recovering the organism in cultures. Moreover, *M. tuberculosis* is able to persist in a latent form within cells and granulomas for many years, and can reactivate to cause disease decades after infection is acquired. Tubercle bacilli are not known to form spores, but both typical bacilli and nonstaining forms of the bacteria persist in cells and tissues, as evidenced by detection of DNA, years after infection is acquired, and retain the capacity to replicate and produce clinical illness. These unique biological characteristics make the tubercle bacillus exceedingly difficult to combat and control.

Epidemiology

Global incidence

Despite the widely held belief that tuberculosis was waning during the 1980s, global tuberculosis incidence has been steady or increasing for several decades. In Western Europe and North America, the incidence of tuberculosis peaked in the 1700s and 1800s, and then declined over a period of years before the development of chemotherapy. Improvements in hygiene and nutrition, along with reductions in household crowding, were credited with these trends. Following the introduction of curative treatment for tuberculosis in the era following the Second World War the incidence of disease fell even further, and tuberculosis deaths were greatly decreased. The success in controlling tuberculosis experienced in the western nations was not replicated in developing countries, and increasing epidemics of the disease have been occurring in these areas. In addition, progress in tuberculosis control in the western nations ironically led to neglect of public health programmes that were responsible for reductions in morbidity. As a consequence of inattention to control, the United States of America experienced a resurgence of tuberculosis between 1985 and 1992, with a 21% increase in the annual number of reported cases during that time. In the United Kingdom, tuberculosis incidence has levelled off in recent years, with an annual incidence of 11 cases per 100 000 people since 1991. Worldwide, tuberculosis continues to kill more than 1.5 million people per year, making it the second leading infectious cause of death after HIV infection. In fact, tuberculosis is a leading cause of death in AIDS, and HIV-related tuberculosis deaths are attributed to AIDS not tuberculosis. If these deaths were attributed to tuberculosis, then tuberculosis would remain the leading infectious cause of death worldwide.

The World Health Organization (WHO) estimates that 2 billion people, or one-third of the world's population, are infected with *M. tuberculosis*. From this seedbed of latent infection, 8.8 million new cases of active disease and 1.1 million deaths were attributed to tuberculosis in 2010. The global distribution of tuberculosis case rates is shown in Fig. 6.25.1. Disease due to *M. tuberculosis* is most common in developing nations, both in absolute numbers and incidence of new cases. Twenty-two countries account for 80% of all cases of tuberculosis; India and China are responsible for 40% of cases. In general, the highest incidence of disease is found in the countries of sub-Saharan Africa where HIV infection has contributed to extraordinary increases in case rates. The greatest number of cases arise in the populous nations of Asia, which have moderately high rates of disease per capita. The global incidence of tuberculosis is increasing slightly, though population growth is resulting in higher numbers of cases each year. Declines in incidence in the developed world have been offset by increasing rates in the HIV-ravaged countries of Africa and by escalating incidence in Eastern Europe in the aftermath of the collapse of communism and its public health infrastructure.

Effect of age

Tuberculosis typically affects young adults, with peak incidence in those aged 25 to 44 years. The dynamics of tuberculosis within a particular country or region, however, reflect both historical trends in tuberculosis transmission and current risk factors and practices of disease control. For example, in Western Europe tuberculosis is seen in two demographic groups: elderly native Europeans who were presumably infected many years ago and who experience reactivation of latent infections as they age or become immunocompromised, and younger immigrants from high-incidence countries in the developing world. Interestingly, increasing age is not a risk factor for developing active tuberculosis *per se*; among ageing populations infected with *M. tuberculosis* earlier in life, the risk of developing disease decreases over time. In the United States of America tuberculosis is seen in young adults who have immigrated from endemic areas and in those with HIV infection, whereas reactivation tuberculosis in older people is increasingly uncommon. In the developing world, tuberculosis most commonly occurs in young adults, with rapidly escalating rates in those with HIV infection. In all countries where tuberculosis is prevalent, young children who acquire tuberculosis from adults account for a small proportion of all cases. Interestingly, children between the ages of 5 and 15 years have extremely low rates of tuberculosis, even in areas with a high disease burden.

Infection and disease

The epidemiology of tuberculosis can be considered as a function of two distinct but related phenomena: the likelihood of becoming infected with *M. tuberculosis* and the probability of developing disease once infection has occurred. Risk factors for becoming infected relate to exposure to infectious cases. Throughout the world, living with someone who has infectious tuberculosis is the most important risk factor for acquiring infection. The longer the duration of undiagnosed tuberculosis, the greater the severity of disease, and the more intimate the contact, the greater the chance of becoming infected. Exposure to infectious cases in other environments, including health care facilities, prisons, and the workplace, is another important route of infection. In areas of the world where tuberculosis is relatively widespread, exposure in the community is commonplace and probably unavoidable. In low prevalence countries, community exposure is most likely to occur in distinct pockets of increased incidence, such as poorer areas of large cities or neighbourhoods with high HIV prevalence.

Effect of host immunity

After *M. tuberculosis* infection is acquired, the risk of developing disease is dependent on host immunity. As discussed below, several conditions have been identified that increase the risk of active disease in a person with latent tuberculosis infection, most notably HIV infection. Reactivation from latent tuberculosis infection is an important mechanism for the development of adult tuberculosis. However, studies using DNA fingerprinting techniques show that a significant proportion of tuberculosis cases thought to be due to reactivation are actually recently acquired due to reinfection or new infection, particularly in high HIV prevalence settings.

Effect of *M. tuberculosis* strain

Interestingly, strain differences in *M. tuberculosis* have not been associated with the risk of disease, although inoculum size is associated

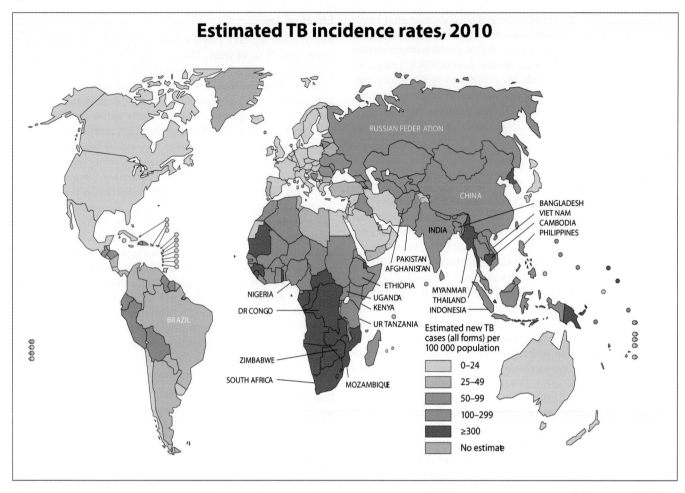

Estimated TB incidence rates, 2010

Estimated new TB cases (all forms) per 100 000 population

	0–24
	25–49
	50–99
	100–299
	≥300
	No estimate

The boundaries and names shown and the designations used on this map do not imply the expression of any opinion whatsoever on the part of the World Health Organization concerning the legal status of any country, territory, city or area or of its authorities, or concerning the delimitation of its frontiers or boundaries. Dotted lines on maps represent approximate border lines for which there may not yet be full agreement.

Source: *Global Tuberculosis Control 2011*. WHO, 2011.

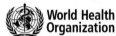

Fig. 6.25.1 WHO-estimated global tuberculosis incidence rates in 2010.

with probability of becoming ill. For example, household contacts of heavily sputum acid-fast bacilli smear-positive cases of tuberculosis who become infected have a higher incidence of active disease than contacts of acid-fast bacilli smear-negative cases who become infected. On the other hand, while there is some evidence that specific strains of *M. tuberculosis* may more successfully infect contacts than other strains, the risk of disease in those infected with these transmissible strains is not elevated. Genotyping of *M. tuberculosis* strains has demonstrated that a number of strains account for a large proportion of new tuberculosis cases in different geographic areas. On such strain is the W-Beijing strain which appears to have spread rapidly in regions with high tuberculosis incidence and has been associated with outbreaks of multidrug-resistant (MDR) organisms, extrapulmonary disease, and HIV infection.

Susceptibility

Tuberculosis is a disease traditionally associated with specific population groups, notably the poor, alcohol and drug abusers, and, more recently, those with HIV infection. The increased incidence of tuberculosis in impoverished populations is probably multifactorial, involving increased risk of infection (e.g. due to crowded living conditions and a higher background prevalence of disease in the community) and increased risk of developing disease after infection (e.g. due to malnutrition). Similar reasons may explain the higher rates of tuberculosis seen in cigarette smokers and alcohol and drug abusers, with suppression of host cellular immunity either directly or indirectly caused by substance abuse. The more recent association of tuberculosis and HIV infection is clearly related to development of cellular immunodeficiency in those with HIV, but in many settings those at highest risk for HIV infection are also more likely to be latently infected with *M. tuberculosis* than others. Genetic analysis of sibling pairs with tuberculosis using two-stage genome-wide linkage study identified potential susceptibility loci on chromosomes 15q and Xq.

Effect of the HIV epidemic

The impact of HIV infection on the epidemiology of tuberculosis is striking. As will be discussed below, HIV infection is the most potent known biological risk factor for tuberculosis. The relative risk of tuberculosis in an HIV-infected person is 200 to 1000 times greater than in someone without HIV infection. The risk of tuberculosis increases shortly after HIV seroconversion, doubling within the first year. As a result of the extraordinary risk conferred from HIV infection, the majority of tuberculosis patients in many sub-Saharan countries are HIV seropositive. The incidence of active tuberculosis in HIV-infected patients not receiving antiretroviral therapy (ART) in the United States of America, with latent tuberculosis infection defined by a positive tuberculin skin test, is about 10% per year. Even when ART is provided to individuals with HIV infection, the risk of tuberculosis remains substantially higher than in HIV-uninfected people from the same population. Of note, an annual incidence rate of about 10% is described in HIV-infected patients in South Africa regardless of tuberculin skin test status. In addition, HIV infection is the unifying theme in many nosocomial outbreaks of tuberculosis, as infection is spread among immuno-compromised patients receiving medical care at the same facility. It is increasingly apparent that control of tuberculosis will not be possible globally without control of HIV infection.

Effect of drug resistance

Another very important trend in tuberculosis epidemiology is the growing problem of drug-resistant tuberculosis. Drug-resistant tuberculosis is divided into two categories: primary resistance, which is the presence of drug resistance in someone who has never had treatment for tuberculosis, and secondary resistance, which is the presence of resistance in a patient who has previously been treated for tuberculosis. Primary resistance results from acquiring an infection that is already drug resistant, while secondary resistance is the result of inappropriate therapy that selects for resistant mutants of *M. tuberculosis*. A global survey of resistance performed by the WHO and the International Union Against Tuberculosis and Lung Disease found that the median prevalence of primary drug resistance was 10%, and the median prevalence of acquired resistance was 36%. Moreover, 'hot spots' of drug-resistant tuberculosis were identified on all continents. The most notable of these are in the former Soviet nations where MDR tuberculosis, defined as resistance to at least rifampicin and isoniazid, is identified in 10 to 20% of all cases. Multidrug-resistant tuberculosis treatment is exceedingly difficult, since the drugs used are less effective, more costly, and poorly tolerated due to drug-related side effects. Furthermore, failure to control the spread of drug-resistant tuberculosis has led to the outbreak of extensively drug-resistant (XDR) tuberculosis, which is defined as multidrug-resistant tuberculosis plus resistance to fluoroquinolones and at least one injectable second-line agent (capreomycin, amikacin, or kanamycin). Extensively drug-resistant tuberculosis been responsible for high rates of mortality in HIV-infected individuals in South Africa and is reported in more than 70 countries globally. Drug-resistant tuberculosis (MDR or XDR) will likely continue without effective implementation of directly observed therapy, short-course (DOTS) and development of more rapid diagnostic tests to detect drug resistance.

Pathogenesis

The development of active tuberculosis, like all infectious diseases, is a function of the quantity and virulence of the invading organism and the relative resistance or susceptibility of the host to the pathogen.

Indeed, one lineage of tuberculosis known as the W/Beijing family of strains is predominant in south-east Asia, but widely distributed in India and South Africa. W/Beijing strains of *M. tuberculosis* have been associated with outbreaks of drug-sensitive and drug-resistant tuberculosis and may be more virulent than other strains. Genetic host factors also play a key role in innate nonimmune resistance to *M. tuberculosis*. For example, the human gene *SLC11A1*, which has been mapped to chromosome 2q, may help determine susceptibility to tuberculosis, according to a study in Africa. But, like many infectious diseases, it is likely that resistance to tuberculosis is polygenic.

Transmission

Tubercle bacilli are transmitted between people by aerosols generated when an infectious person coughs or otherwise expels infectious pulmonary or laryngeal secretions into the air. *M. tuberculosis* bacilli excreted by this action are contained within droplet nuclei, extremely small particles (less than 1 μm) that remain airborne for long periods and are disseminated by diffusion and convection until they are deposited on surfaces, diluted, or inactivated by ultraviolet radiation. Individuals breathing air into which droplet nuclei have been excreted are at risk of acquiring tubercle bacilli by inhaling these nuclei and having them deposited in their alveoli, where a productive infection may occur. Transmission of tuberculous infection by other routes, such as inoculation in laboratories and aerosolization of bacilli from tissues in hospitals, has been documented, but these are an insignificant means of spread. *M. bovis* can be acquired from contaminated milk from tuberculous cows, but modern animal husbandry practices and the pasteurization of milk has substantially reduced this mode of infection throughout most of the world.

Natural history of tuberculosis in humans

People who are in contact with someone with infectious tuberculosis may acquire infection, as described above (see Fig. 6.25.2). Factors that affect the likelihood of infection being transmitted include the severity of the disease in the index case (e.g. extent of radiographic abnormalities, cavitation, frequency of cough), the duration and closeness of exposure, and environmental factors such as humidity, ventilation and ambient ultraviolet light. Several studies in diverse locations and circumstances have shown that approximately 20 to 30% of close contacts of an untreated tuberculosis patient become infected with *M. tuberculosis*, as demonstrated by the development of a reactive tuberculin skin test.

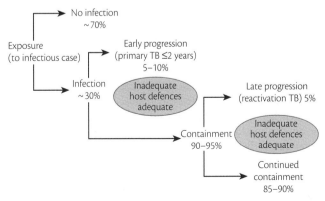

Fig. 6.25.2 Natural history of tuberculosis.

Immune response

Deposition of tubercle bacilli in the alveoli results in a series of protective responses by the cellular immune system that forestall the development of disease in the majority of infected people. Alveolar macrophages ingest tubercle bacilli, which then multiply intracellularly and eventually cause cell lysis with release of organisms. Killing of *M. tuberculosis* within macrophages is prevented by inhibition of phagolysosome formation by the tubercle bacilli through a process that is not understood. Additional alveolar macrophages engulf progeny bacilli, resulting in further intracellular growth and cell death. Over a period of weeks as tubercle bacilli proliferate within macrophages and are released, infection spreads to regional lymph nodes, elsewhere in the lungs, and systemically. Foci of tubercle bacilli can be established in multiple organs, including the lymph nodes, brain, kidneys, and bones. In most people, specific immunity is developed after several weeks and consists of activated T lymphocytes mediating a Th1 type response. Macrophages act as antigen-presenting cells, interacting with CD4 lymphocytes primed for *M. tuberculosis* antigens. Activated CD4 lymphocytes produce both IL-2, which promotes activation of additional T lymphocytes, and interferon-γ, which binds with receptors on macrophages and promotes intracellular killing of organisms. Tumour necrosis factor-α production is induced in macrophages, and this too promotes killing of intracellular bacilli. The specific role of CD8 cells in the control of tuberculosis has not been fully elaborated, although there is evidence that cytotoxic T lymphocytes may play a role in containing a tuberculous infection. In addition, CD8 lymphocytes also produce interferon-γ and participate in granuloma formation. Recent evidence also supports a role of innate immunity in combatting tuberculosis infection.

The classic immunological response to infection with tubercle bacilli is the walling off of viable bacilli in granulomas. Granulomas are collections of cells surrounding a focus of *M. tuberculosis*, usually within macrophages but sometimes extracellularly, that serve to contain the infection. Granulomas consist of macrophages, CD4 and CD8 lymphocytes, fibroblasts, giant cells, and epithelioid cells that produce an extracellular matrix of collagenous and fibrotic materials which are continually remodelled and can become calcified. A calcified granuloma at the initial site of infection in the lung is referred to as a Ghon complex, while the combination of a Ghon complex and a calcified regional lymph node is called Ranke's complex.

The development of the cellular immune response to *M. tuberculosis* is accompanied by the development of delayed-type hypersensitivity (DTH) to specific antigens from tubercle bacilli. While DTH is distinct from the cell-mediated immunity that provides protection from disease, this sensitivity to tubercle-derived proteins has proved enormously useful for diagnosing tuberculosis infection. The use of purified protein derivatives (PPD) of tuberculin is the basis for estimating the prevalence of latent tuberculosis infection in populations, is essential in studying the natural history of tuberculosis infection, and is frequently helpful in evaluating patients with suspected tuberculosis disease. The difference between DTH and immunity to tuberculosis is underscored by the observation that 80 to 90% of patients with active disease, and therefore clearly not immune, have positive tuberculin tests.

For the majority of people acquiring a new tuberculous infection, the development of cell-mediated immunity to the organism is protective and holds the bacilli in check, though viability is usually maintained. A small proportion of them will be unable to contain the infection and will progress to active tuberculosis disease, often referred to as primary tuberculosis. Factors associated with early progression of infection to disease include immunosuppression, particularly with HIV infection, a higher inoculum of organisms, malnutrition, and, perhaps, concomitant illness. While rates of active disease in young children who are contacts of cases are no higher than for older contacts, young children with primary tuberculosis do develop more severe forms of tuberculosis than adults, including disseminated disease and tuberculous meningitis.

Reactivation

Those who successfully contain the organism have a latent tuberculosis infection that may reactivate later in life. Based on studies of latent tuberculosis infection acquired in childhood or adolescence, the lifetime risk of reactivation of *M. tuberculosis* is about 10%. Table 6.25.1 lists conditions that are associated with an increased risk of reactivating latent tuberculosis infection. The most potent of these is HIV infection, which increases the rate of reactivation by as much as 1000-fold. Immunosuppression from malignancy, cytotoxic therapy, corticosteroids, and other agents that alter cellular immune responses also increase the likelihood that latent tuberculosis infection will reactivate. Other important factors that increase the risk of tuberculosis include diabetes and endstage renal disease, injection drug use (independent of HIV infection), low body weight, gastrointestinal surgery, and silicosis. Cigarette smoking is associated with increased tuberculosis incidence, as is alcohol abuse. Recently, the use of inhibitors of tumour necrosis factor-α for the treatment of rheumatoid arthritis or inflammatory bowel disease has been associated with increased risk

Table 6.25.1 Incidence of active tuberculosis in people with a positive tuberculin skin test, by selected risk factors

Risk factor	Number of tuberculosis cases/100 person-years
Recent tuberculosis infection:	
Infection <1 year past	2–8
Infection 1–7 years past	0.2
HIV infection	3.5–14
Injection drug use	
HIV seropositive	4–10
HIV seronegative	1
Silicosis	3–7
Radiographic findings consistent with prior tuberculosis	0.2–0.4
Weight deviation from standard:	
Underweight by ≥15%	0.26
Underweight by 10–14%	0.20
Underweight by 5–9%	0.22
Weight within 5% of standard	0.11
Overweight by ≥5%	0.07
Diabetes mellitus	0.3
Renal failure	0.4–0.9
None of the above factors	0.01–0.1

of tuberculosis. Rates of tuberculosis are usually higher in older people than in younger adults in developed countries, but this may represent a higher prevalence of latent infection in older cohorts, rather than immunological senescence.

Clinical features

Classification of tuberculosis infection and disease

Infection with *M. tuberculosis* can result in clinical manifestations ranging from asymptomatic carriage of latent bacilli to life-threatening pneumonia. Classification of the different stages of *M. tuberculosis* in humans by the American Thoracic Society (ATS) is shown in Table 6.25.2. This system is used more for public health purposes than for clinical management, but is useful because it reflects the natural history of *M. tuberculosis* and categorizes patients according to the type of evaluation and treatment they may need.

The ATS category 0 refers to someone without any tuberculosis exposure history and a negative tuberculin skin test (if performed). Category 1 includes those people exposed to an infectious case of tuberculosis but in whom no evidence of infection is found. This is a temporary category used during the evaluation of contacts of tuberculosis cases; repeat tuberculin testing several months after the exposure would result in these individuals being reclassified to another category. Category 2 is defined as latent tuberculosis infection without evidence of disease, and is based on a positive tuberculin skin test without clinical or radiographic signs of illness. Category 3 is confirmed active tuberculosis disease requiring treatment. As discussed below, this category is further divided according to site of disease and laboratory features, including results of acid-fast bacilli smears. Category 4 is defined as inactive tuberculosis. Patients in this category do not have active disease on the basis of clinical and laboratory evaluations, but are known to have previously had tuberculosis. This category includes those who have been treated and cured of active tuberculosis, as well as individuals who have spontaneously recovered from tuberculosis without treatment. Finally, category 5 refers to patients in whom tuberculosis is suspected, but who are still undergoing evaluation. Depending on the degree of suspicion of the diagnosis, such people might be started on presumptive therapy for tuberculosis pending the outcome of cultures and other laboratory assessments. Like category 1, this is a temporary category for patients in the middle of an evaluation, and all patients in this group are reclassified on the basis of diagnostic studies.

Table 6.25.2 American Thoracic Society classification system for tuberculosis

Classification	Description
TB0	No exposure, no infection
TB1	Exposed to tuberculosis, infection status unknown
TB2	Latent infection, no disease (positive PPD tuberculin test)
TB3	Active tuberculosis
TB4	Inactive tuberculosis, healed or adequately treated
TB5	Possible tuberculosis, status unknown ('rule out' tuberculosis)

PPD, purified protein derivative.

Clinical presentation of active tuberculosis

This is highly variable, depending on the site and extent of disease and the immune status of the host. Historically, active tuberculosis has been classified as 'primary' or 'post-primary' on the basis of both the presumed duration of infection and the clinical features of the disease. Recent studies using molecular epidemiological techniques, however, suggest that this classification may be unreliable. For example, the 'classic' presentation of reactivation tuberculosis has been seen in patients whose infection is clearly newly acquired, such as in nosocomial outbreaks where DNA fingerprinting confirms recent transmission. For practical purposes, tuberculosis is generally divided into pulmonary and extrapulmonary forms, with considerable clinical heterogeneity within these categories.

Pulmonary tuberculosis

Pulmonary tuberculosis is usually a subacute respiratory infection with prominent constitutional symptoms. The most frequent symptoms of pulmonary tuberculosis are cough, fever, night sweats, and malaise. Cough in pulmonary tuberculosis is initially nonproductive, but often progresses to sputum production and, in some instances, haemoptysis. The sputum is generally yellow in colour, and is neither malodorous nor thick. Haemoptysis may be seen in patients with untreated tuberculosis, but is also a feature of treated tuberculosis; damage from prior tuberculosis may result in bronchiectasis or residual cavities that can either become superinfected or erode into blood vessels or airways, producing haemoptysis. Extremely advanced tuberculosis may also present with bloody sputum. Rarely, the bleeding is massive leading to shock, asphyxia, and death.

Chest pain is not a prominent symptom in pulmonary tuberculosis, although musculoskeletal pain from coughing may be noted. In patients with tuberculous pleurisy, however, chest pain may be present, particularly on inspiration. Radicular pain across the chest may be associated with spinal tuberculosis. Dyspnoea alone may be a sign of extensive parenchymal destruction, large pleural effusions, endobronchial obstruction, or pneumothorax.

Patients with tuberculosis also experience loss of appetite and weight loss or cachexia, often out of proportion to their diminished intake of food. Elevations in tumour necrosis factor α are hypothesized to be the cause of cachexia in tuberculosis. Other symptoms with mild severity such as emotional liability, irritability, depression, and headache are frequent.

The duration of symptoms varies greatly, but most patients will report weeks to months of feeling ill before presentation. In surveys of populations with high rates of disease and poor access to medical care, a history of cough for more than 3 weeks was strongly associated with a diagnosis of active tuberculosis, but in HIV-infected patients any duration of cough predicts elevated risk for disease. Untreated tuberculosis is associated with high mortality, but many patients may have persistent symptoms for years. A study of untreated pulmonary tuberculosis in the pretherapy era found that after 5 years 50% of patients had died, 25% had spontaneously healed, and 25% were chronically ill with pulmonary disease. A subset of patients has rapidly progressive disease, the so-called 'galloping consumption' of old. Nowadays this is most often seen in patients with HIV infection or other forms of severe immunosuppression. These patients have an escalating course of severe pulmonary symptoms over a period of several weeks, often in the setting of disseminated disease. Failure promptly to diagnose and treat these patients results in death.

Physical findings in pulmonary tuberculosis are limited and not generally helpful in making a diagnosis. Fever is an irregular and unreliable feature, and while most patients complain of fevers before presentation, only one-half to three-quarters of patients with confirmed tuberculosis have a documented fever. Examination of the chest may reveal dullness to percussion and rales, although these findings are highly variable and nonspecific. Signs of consolidation are usually absent. The classic post-tussive rales described in the last century are not often present and are not specific to tuberculosis. Patients with disseminated tuberculosis may have lymphadenopathy, hepatomegaly, or evidence of central nervous system involvement, but these are not generally seen in typical pulmonary tuberculosis. Finger clubbing and cyanosis are findings associated with prolonged and advanced pulmonary disease. Thus, the diagnosis of tuberculosis almost always rests on the patient's history and epidemiological characteristics, in conjunction with laboratory studies described below. The most important step in making a timely diagnosis of tuberculosis is to think of it in the first place.

Radiological evaluations play a critical role in the diagnosis of pulmonary tuberculosis. Disease due to *M. tuberculosis* can involve any portion of the lungs, and radiographic findings are usually only suggestive, not diagnostic, of tuberculosis. The typical radiological manifestations of pulmonary tuberculosis are upper lobe infiltrates that may show cavitation. *M. tuberculosis* exhibits a unique predilection for the upper zones of the lungs for reasons that are not well understood. Latent infection characteristically reactivates in the apical segments of the upper lobes, or the superior segments of the lower lobes. The infiltrates are often fibronodular and irregular, and may be diffuse and associated with volume loss. Cavities, when present, are rarely symmetrical and do not usually have air–fluid levels, such as those seen in pyogenic lung abscesses. Several examples of the radiographic appearance of pulmonary tuberculosis are seen in Fig. 6.25.3.

The classic radiographic presentation described above is neither pathognomonic nor highly sensitive for pulmonary tuberculosis. Several other lung infections, notably the pulmonary mycoses, can present with similar findings. More importantly, one-third to one-half of patients with pulmonary tuberculosis lack the classic radiographic findings described. Lower lung zone infiltrates, mid-lung focal infiltrates, pulmonary nodules, and infiltrates with mediastinal or hilar adenopathy are also seen. HIV-infected tuberculosis patients, in particular, most often present with these 'atypical' findings, and up to 5% of them may have a normal chest radiograph in the setting of sputum cultures that yield *M. tuberculosis*. The lack of typical radiographic features should not, therefore, deter the clinician from considering the diagnosis in a patient with a clinical history compatible with and symptoms of tuberculosis.

CT is increasingly used to evaluate pulmonary disorders, including tuberculosis. While the classic findings described above do not usually require confirmation with a more sensitive test, CT scanning is sometimes used to evaluate radiographic findings that are not readily explained after an initial assessment. CT scans of the chest in patients with tuberculosis may reveal a greater extent of involvement than conventional radiographs, including multiple nodules, small cavities, and multilobar infiltrates. However, CT scanning can only suggest the possibility of tuberculosis in a patient

with other signs and symptoms consistent with the diagnosis, and further evaluation is still required.

The laboratory diagnosis of pulmonary tuberculosis relies on the microbiological evaluation of sputum or other respiratory tract specimens. A definitive diagnosis requires growth of *M. tuberculosis* from respiratory secretions, while a probable diagnosis can be based on typical clinical and radiographic findings with either acid-fast bacilli-positive sputum or other specimens, or typical histopathological findings on biopsy material. These latter approaches, however, have a variable lack of specificity depending on the prevalence of disease due to nontuberculosis mycobacteria in the population.

Throughout most of the world, sputum acid-fast staining is the sole test used to confirm the diagnosis of pulmonary tuberculosis. In the settings where it is utilized, the positive predictive value of the sputum acid-fast smear is very high, as the likelihood of nontuberculous mycobacterial disease is quite low. In industrialized countries, disease due to the nontuberculous mycobacteria is relatively more common and reliance on smears without cultures is potentially misleading. Despite the best efforts of clinicians, a confirmed diagnosis of tuberculosis cannot be established in some patients who have the disease, and a response to presumptive therapy forms the basis for establishing the diagnosis. Further details on the microbiological approach to diagnosis are provided below.

Extrapulmonary tuberculosis

In the United States of America extrapulmonary tuberculosis is defined as disease outside the lung parenchyma; in the United Kingdom it is defined as disease outside the lungs and pleura. This seemingly subtle distinction has considerable epidemiological impact, however, as pleural tuberculosis is the most common extrapulmonary site of disease in the United States of America.

During the initial seeding of infection with *M. tuberculosis*, described earlier, haematogenous dissemination of bacilli to several organs can occur. These localized infections, as in the lung, can progress into primary tuberculosis or become walled off in small granulomas where bacteria may remain dormant if they are not killed by cell-mediated immune responses. Extrapulmonary tuberculosis, therefore, can either be a presentation of primary or reactivation tuberculosis.

Extrapulmonary tuberculosis may be generalized or confined to a single organ. In otherwise immunocompetent adults, extrapulmonary tuberculosis is found in 15 to 20% of all tuberculosis cases. In young children and immunosuppressed adults, rates of extrapulmonary disease are substantially higher, appearing in more than one-half of HIV-related tuberculosis cases and one-quarter of tuberculosis cases under 15 years of age. Children less than 2 years old have high rates of miliary and meningeal disease.

The organs most frequently involved in extrapulmonary tuberculosis are listed in Table 6.25.3. To some extent the frequency with which specific organs are involved reflects the pathophysiology of the disease. Infection spreads from the lungs, the primary site of inoculation, by lymphatic and haematogenous routes. The tissues and organs most likely to be affected are the pleura, lymph nodes, kidneys and other genitourinary organs, bone, and central nervous system. Although infection is transiently spread in the blood, tuberculosis bacteraemia is unusual and is seen most often in patients with HIV infection and low CD4 lymphocyte counts.

The clinical presentation of extrapulmonary tuberculosis depends largely on the organ involved. Both pulmonary and extrapulmonary disease are found in up to 50% of patients with HIV-related

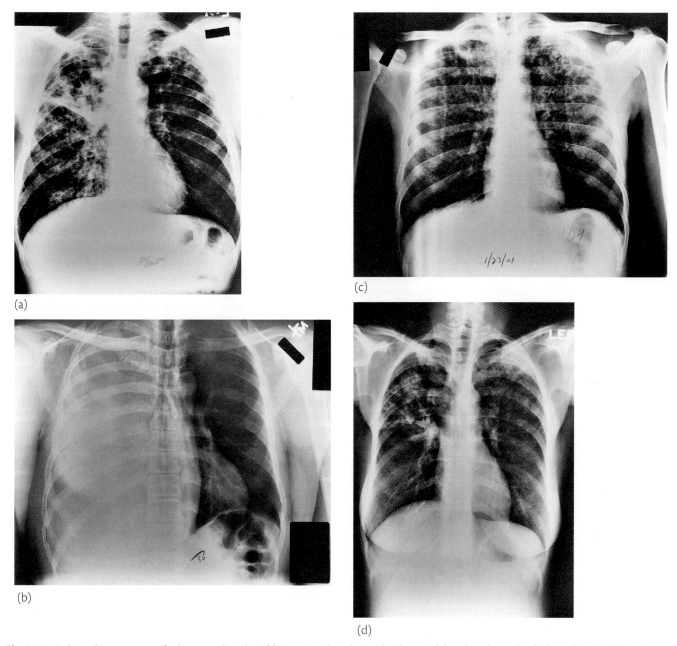

Fig. 6.25.3 Radiographic appearance of pulmonary tuberculosis. (a) Extensive tuberculosis with right upper lobe volume loss and multiple small cavities. This patient was the source of at least 14 secondary cases in contacts. (b) A 69-year-old man with right pleural tuberculosis. (c) Diffuse pulmonary nodules in an HIV-infected man with pulmonary tuberculosis. (d) Cavitary upper lobe disease in an HIV-infected woman.

Table 6.25.3 Common sites of extrapulmonary tuberculosis

Site	Percentage of extrapulmonary cases
Pleura	20–25
Lymphatics	20–40
Genitourinary	5–18
Bone/joint	10
Central nervous system	5–7
Abdominal	4
Disseminated	7–11

tuberculosis, so it is important to consider the possibility of extrapulmonary pathology when pulmonary tuberculosis is diagnosed in an HIV-infected patient (and vice versa). Pulmonary involvement is seen in up to one-quarter of patients with tuberculous meningitis and to lesser degrees with other sites of disease.

Pleural tuberculosis

This is the result of two distinct pathophysiological sequences, which present in strikingly different manners. Most pleural tuberculosis is associated with primary infection and is the result of seeding of the visceral pleura with relatively small numbers of tubercle bacilli via direct extension from adjacent lung tissue. A large proportion of patients with this form of tuberculous pleurisy will have obvious pulmonary disease, although findings may be subtle. The duration of symptoms is generally brief, e.g. several weeks, and patients complain of fever, chest pain, and nonproductive cough. Other constitutional and respiratory symptoms may be present. Unlike pneumococcal pneumonia, which presents abruptly, tuberculous pleurisy starts more insidiously.

The second form of pleural tuberculosis occurs when larger numbers of bacilli invade the pleural space and multiply, producing frank empyema. Tuberculous empyema is seen in older patients, almost all of whom have extensive pulmonary disease. Patients present with prolonged symptoms of cough, chest pain, fever, cachexia, and night sweats. Pneumothorax is a common complication of tuberculous empyema and may be associated with a more rapid disease course.

The radiographic picture in tuberculous pleurisy reflects the underlying pathophysiology of the disease. Patients with the primary type of pleurisy tend to have small unilateral effusions, and up to one-half have visible parenchymal lesions on plain radiographs. In patients with tuberculous empyema, the effusions are larger and more likely to be loculated, and adjacent pulmonary involvement is often evident.

The diagnosis of pleural tuberculosis can be approached along several lines. When pulmonary parenchymal involvement is manifest, sputum smears and cultures have a high yield, and the diagnosis of pleural disease can be inferred from the pulmonary findings. When pulmonary findings are minimal or the initial test results unrevealing, analysis of pleural fluid is essential. Acid-fast stains of pleural fluid are usually negative in patients with primary tuberculous pleurisy as the number of organisms in the pleural space is small. Repeated sampling will show organisms in less than one-half of cases. Similarly, culture results may be negative. The pleural fluid is usually serous and exudative, with a protein concentration that is more than 50% of the serum level, normal or low glucose, and a slightly acidic pH. The pleural fluid white blood cell count is usually in the range of 1000 to 10 000 per μL with a lymphocytic predominance. Lactate dehydrogenase levels are generally elevated, as are adenosine deaminase levels. All of these tests are nonspecific and cannot reliably distinguish tuberculosis pleurisy from other pleural diseases.

Pleural biopsy is frequently useful in establishing a diagnosis of tuberculous pleurisy. Percutaneous biopsy of the pleura reveals granulomatous inflammation in up to 80% of patients, and cultures obtained at the time of biopsy are positive in over one-half of patients. If a first attempt fails to provide a diagnosis, a second biopsy may be successful. More recently thoracoscopy has been utilized to improve the yield of biopsy by visualizing biopsy targets rather than blindly sampling with a percutaneous pleural needle.

Lymphatic tuberculosis

This can occur in any location, but classic scrofula involving the cervical or supraclavicular chains is the most common presentation. Mediastinal and hilar lymphatic tuberculosis is a feature both of primary and disseminated disease, but discovery of these lesions is usually incidental. The pathophysiology of lymphatic tuberculosis is thought to result from drainage of bacilli in the lungs into supraclavicular and posterior cervical lymph node chains. In contrast, lymphatic disease caused by nontuberculous mycobacteria usually involves anterior cervical, preauricular, or submandibular lymph nodes, suggesting acquisition through the oropharynx. In patients with HIV infection, multiple lymph node groups may be involved including axillary, inguinal, mesenteric, and retroperitoneal.

Symptoms in lymphatic tuberculosis are generally limited, unless the disease is disseminated. Painless swelling of a lymph node is the most common presentation. Constitutional symptoms are not prominent in most cases. Examination of the area may reveal several enlarged lymph nodes, as only about 20% of patients have disease of a solitary node.

The diagnosis of lymphatic tuberculosis usually depends on cultures from affected nodes. Biopsies may show granulomatous changes and acid-fast bacilli. Such findings are nonspecific, however, and cannot distinguish tuberculous from nontuberculosis lymphadenitis. As discussed elsewhere, the presence of a positive tuberculin skin test in the setting of typical biopsy findings is strongly suggestive of tuberculosis; in the setting of suspected lymphatic tuberculosis, these findings warrant presumptive therapy.

Genitourinary tuberculosis

This encompasses a broad array of clinical entities, ranging from disease of the kidneys to endometrial, prostatic, and epididymal disease. The most common of these is renal tuberculosis, which results from haematogenous seeding of the renal cortex during the primary infection. The pathogenesis of other genitourinary sites is either from downstream extension of renal infection over time or from haematogenous seeding at the time of the initial acquisition of *M. tuberculosis*.

Renal tuberculosis is probably underdiagnosed because it is frequently asymptomatic. Many cases of genitourinary tuberculosis are diagnosed as a result of routine urinalyses that detect sterile pyuria. The development of symptoms reflects a more advanced stage of disease, associated with considerable tissue destruction. When genitourinary tuberculosis is symptomatic, the most common symptoms are localized and include urinary symptoms and flank pain. In men, tuberculosis can cause prostatitis and epididymitis, both of which can present with pain resulting from swelling. In women, genital tract tuberculosis may be symptomatic when it involves the ovaries and Fallopian tubes; pelvic pain is also a feature of endometrial tuberculosis. Menstrual abnormalities and infertility may be the only signs of genital disease, however.

The diagnosis of genitourinary tuberculosis depends on the anatomical site of the disease. Renal tuberculosis, as noted, is suggested by sterile pyuria, and the diagnosis rests on isolation of organisms in the urine. Early morning urine samples are more likely to grow *M. tuberculosis* than spot samples obtained at other times. In patients with symptoms of upper urinary tract illness, radiological studies are often helpful. The kidneys may appear calcified on abdominal radiographs. Intravenous pyelography may show distorted or dilated calyces or renal pelvis, papillary necrosis, cavitation or abscesses of the renal parenchyma, or intrarenal or ureteral obstructions. Use of renal ultrasonography or CT scanning may be more sensitive for identifying the abnormalities of renal tuberculosis, but contrast radiography is the technique with which the greatest experience has accrued. When tuberculosis of the bladder is suspected, cystoscopy with biopsy may lead to the identification of granulomas before identification of organisms by culture. Diagnosis of prostatic, testicular, or epididymal tuberculosis is usually accomplished with cultures obtained by fine needle aspiration or transurethral resection of the prostate. Cervical and endometrial tuberculosis can be diagnosed by biopsy with culture.

Tuberculous meningitis (Oxford Textbook of Medicine 5e Chapter 24.11.1)

This is the most common central nervous system manifestation of tuberculosis. It is much more likely to occur in children under the age of 15 years and in HIV-infected patients than in immunocompetent adults. Although meningitis accounts for only a small fraction of all cases of tuberculosis, it is a devastating form of the disease that is uniformly fatal if left untreated.

The pathogenesis of meningeal tuberculosis varies with the age and immunological status of the patient. Reactivation of microscopic granulomas in the meninges was found by Rich to cause diffuse meningeal infection. These foci of infection are probably implanted at the time of primary bacillaemia. When these lesions rupture into the subarachnoid space they invoke an inflammatory response leading to tuberculous meningitis. Meningeal disease can also complicate miliary disease, especially in children. Likewise, adults can acquire meningeal disease during bacillaemia of miliary disease, but this is not the usual pathogenesis of meningeal infection. Rarely, invasion into the spinal canal from a paraspinous or vertebral focus can also be the source of central nervous system involvement.

The clinical features of tuberculous meningitis are the consequence of the pathophysiological process underlying the disease. Meningeal and leptomeningeal bacterial replication results in a robust inflammatory reaction, often localized to the base of the brain. The number of bacilli present is usually limited, and the severity of illness is a function of the host response. Meningeal inflammation causes increases in cerebrospinal fluid pressure and can also cause cranial neuropathies. Patients complain of headache, neck stiffness, meningism, and an altered mental status, including irritability, clouded thinking, and malaise; as the disease progresses, symptoms worsen considerably.

The clinical spectrum of tuberculous meningitis has historically been categorized in three stages, defined by the British Medical Research Council in 1948. Stage 1 consists of a prodrome lasting for 1 to 3 months. Nonspecific symptoms such as fever, malaise, and headache predominate. In this stage, patients are conscious and rational, but may have signs of meningism. Focal neurological signs are absent and there are no signs of hydrocephalus. In stage 2 disease, single cranial nerve abnormalities such as ptosis or facial paralysis appear, and paresis and focal seizures may occur. Kernig's and Brudzinski's signs have been noted as well as hyperactive deep tendon reflexes. Prominent signs include alterations in mentation, behavioural change, impaired cognitive ability, and increasing stupor. Headache and fever are also common features of this stage of disease.

In stage 3, patients are comatose (Glasgow coma scale 8 or below) or stuporous and often have multiple cranial nerve palsies and hemiplegia or paraplegia. By this stage, hydrocephalus is common and chronic inflammation in the enclosed space of the skull may result in significant intracranial hypertension. Seizures may be a prominent feature.

Fever, headache, altered level of consciousness, and meningism are present in the majority of patients in most large studies, although no one single sign or symptom has any reliable degree of sensitivity or specificity. Children can be especially difficult to diagnose as symptoms such as fever, vomiting, drowsiness, or irritability are commonly seen in many minor viral illnesses.

Transient tuberculous meningitis that presents as an aseptic meningitis and resolves without treatment has been described.

Benign presentations of meningeal tuberculosis are uncommon in clinical practice, and when the diagnosis is made, treatment is mandatory, even in the patient with seemingly trivial symptoms.

The diagnosis of tuberculous meningitis is often difficult and requires a high degree of suspicion. In the setting of disseminated disease, signs of tuberculosis in other organs, particularly the lungs, are often present. Between 25 and 50% of patients with meningitis in most series also have radiographic evidence of pulmonary tuberculosis, either active or healed. The critical features of tuberculous meningitis, however, are found in the cerebrospinal fluid. Patients with tuberculous meningitis usually have elevated cerebrospinal fluid pressure. An exudative fluid with a mononuclear cell pleocytosis is characteristic. Cerebrospinal fluid is usually clear and the protein is generally in the range of 100 to 500 mg/dl. Hypoglycorrhachia is typical, with cerebrospinal fluid glucose less than 50% of the serum value. The white blood cell count rarely exceeds 1000 per μL, and cell counts below 500 are typical. In early meningitis, the cells may be predominantly neutrophils, but mononuclear cells predominate in most instances. Acid-fast stains of concentrated cerebrospinal fluid are only positive in one-third or fewer of patients, and cultures are positive in only one-half, although repeated sampling increases the yield.

The disastrous consequences of failing to diagnose tuberculous meningitis, coupled with the low yield of cerebrospinal fluid acid-fast stains and cultures, has prompted the development of additional tests for establishing a diagnosis. Adenosine deaminase was initially reported to be exceptionally accurate for tuberculous meningitis. Subsequent experience, however, has found it to be insufficiently specific to distinguish tuberculosis from a variety of other acute and chronic meningitides. Several other tests based on identification of mycobacterial antigens or specific antibodies have been evaluated, but none has been found to be reliable. Nucleic acid amplification tests such as polymerase chain reaction (PCR) have great appeal, but the sensitivity and specificity of available assays are only moderately good. Thus, the diagnosis of tuberculous meningitis often rests on the astute judgment of a clinician with a high degree of suspicion based on epidemiological and clinical clues. Presumptive therapy is frequently necessary.

Central nervous system tuberculomas

These are an unusual manifestation and are seen in a small proportion of patients with tuberculous meningitis. Tuberculomas are the result of enlarging tubercles that extend into brain parenchyma rather than into the subarachnoid space. Patients with HIV infection appear to have an increased risk of central nervous system tuberculomas, but the disease is far less common than toxoplasmosis, even in areas where tuberculosis is highly prevalent. Central nervous system tuberculomas may appear with clinical features of meningitis or of intracranial mass lesions. In the absence of meningeal involvement, seizures or headaches may be the only symptoms. The diagnosis is suggested by brain imaging, with MRI scanning being more sensitive than CT scanning. Biopsy of the lesion is required for diagnosis, and material should be submitted for histopathological staining and culture.

Bone and joint tuberculosis

These may affect several areas, but vertebral tuberculosis (Pott's disease) is the most common form, accounting for almost one-half of cases. Haematogenous seeding of the anterior portion of vertebral bone during initial infection sets the stage for later development of Pott's disease. Infection grows initially within the anterior vertebral body, then may spread to the disc space and to paraspinous tissues. Destruction of the vertebral body causes wedging and eventual collapse. Patients usually complain of back pain, with constitutional symptoms less prominent. Neurological impairment is a late complication, but delays in diagnosis are common and many patients experience neurological sequelae. Imaging studies of the spine usually reveal anterior wedging, collapse of vertebrae, and paraspinous abscesses. The diagnosis is established with bone biopsy or curettage, or by culture of the drainage from a paraspinous abscess.

Miliary tuberculosis and disseminated tuberculosis

These are terms used interchangeably to describe widespread infection and the absence of minimal host immune responses. The term 'miliary tuberculosis' is derived from the classic radiographic appearance of haematogenous tuberculosis, in which tiny pulmonary infiltrates with the appearance of millet seeds are distributed throughout the lungs. Miliary tuberculosis is a more common consequence of primary tuberculosis infection than reactivation, and is seen more frequently in children and immunocompromised adults. Primary miliary tuberculosis presents with fever and other constitutional symptoms over a period of several weeks. Clinical evaluation may reveal lymphadenopathy or splenomegaly and choroidal tubercles on retinoscopy. Laboratory tests may show only anaemia. The chest radiograph is initially normal but later develops the typical miliary pattern. Involvement of multiple organ systems is the rule, usually liver, spleen, lymph nodes, central nervous system, and urinary tract. Patients with reactivation of latent infection who present with miliary disease may have a more fulminant course, although progression to severe disease without treatment is the rule in all patients. The diagnosis is made on tissue biopsy and culture, as sputum smears are usually negative, reflecting the small numbers of bacilli typically present in respiratory secretions.

Other forms of extrapulmonary tuberculosis are less common than those listed above, and the diagnosis is based on a combination of clinical suspicion and the results of biopsies and cultures. Abdominal, ocular, adrenal, and cutaneous tuberculosis are all rarely encountered in the modern era, even in immunocompromised patients.

Laboratory diagnosis

Evaluation of patients for *M. tuberculosis* infection or disease relies on both nonspecific and specific tests. Imaging studies, body fluid chemistries and cell counts, and histochemical staining, as described above, are useful and important tests for the diagnosis of tuberculosis. Specific studies for identifying mycobacterial infections include the tuberculin skin test, acid-fast microscopy, and mycobacterial culture.

Tuberculin skin testing

Tuberculin skin testing (TST) involves the intracutaneous injection of purified proteins of *M. tuberculosis* (purified protein derivative, or PPD tuberculin) that provokes a cell-mediated delayed-type hypersensitivity reaction which produces a zone of induration. Tuberculin originated with Robert Koch who prepared a tubercle sensitin that he thought would cure tuberculosis. Administration of

Koch's tuberculin, of course, did not cure the disease, and hypersensitivity reactions to the agent were sometimes severe or fatal, bringing Koch great discredit.

Fortunately, it was recognized that because tuberculin induced reactions in people who were infected with tuberculosis the substance might prove a better diagnostic test than treatment. Over a period of years refinements were made in the preparation of tuberculins, and in 1939 Seibert and Glenn produced the reference lot of tuberculin, called PPD-S, which has served as the international standard. Current tuberculin preparations are composed of a variety of small tuberculous proteins derived from culture filtrates and stabilized with a polysorbate detergent to prevent precipitation. The standard dose of tuberculin is 5 tuberculin units (TU) of PPD-S, equivalent to 0.1 mg tuberculin in a volume of 0.1 ml. Commercial and other tuberculin products are standardized against PPD-S to ensure bioequivalence.

Tuberculin testing is used to identify people with *M. tuberculosis* infection, and the test cannot distinguish those who have disease from those with latent infection. Injection of tuberculin into an infected individual invokes a delayed-type hypersensitivity response. Specific T lymphocytes sensitized to tuberculous antigens from prior *M. tuberculosis* infection cause a local reaction at the site of injection. Inflammation, vasodilation, and fibrin deposition at the site result in both erythema and induration of the skin. Induration is the key feature of a tuberculin response, and the result of tuberculin testing is categorized according to the amount of induration measured.

Tuberculin skin testing should be done by the Mantoux method, as this is the only technique that has been standardized and extensively validated. Using a tuberculin syringe and small gauge needle, 0.1 ml of PPD-S is injected intracutaneously in the volar surface of the forearm causing a small wheal. Injection into the subcutaneous space will result in uninterpretable results. Multipuncture devices should not be used. The amount of induration should be measured 2 to 5 days after the injection; measurements performed precisely 48 to 72 h later are not essential. The transverse diameter of induration should be measured in millimetres using a ruler. The edge of the induration can be seen and marked, or the margins can be detected using the ballpoint pen method, in which the pen is rolled over the skin with light pressure and its progress is stopped at the demarcation of the indurated area.

Criteria for the interpretation of tuberculin skin tests vary according to clinical and epidemiological circumstances. Cut-off points for positive tests developed by the ATS and the Centers for Disease Control and Prevention (CDC) are listed in Table 6.25.4. A cut-off point of 5 mm induration is used for individuals who are at high risk of tuberculosis infection, or at high risk of disease if infected. Such people include the close contacts of infectious patients and patients with radiographic abnormalities consistent with tuberculosis. The rationale for the 5-mm cut-off in these patients is that the prior probability of infection is high. A 5-mm cut-off is also used for HIV-infected patients and those immunocompromised by corticosteroids or other agents. Failure to diagnose tuberculosis infection in these people could be calamitous, so a lower threshold is used to maximize sensitivity. The use of control antigens such as candida or tetanus toxoid to aid the interpretation of tuberculin tests in HIV-infected patients has been shown to be of no value and is not recommended.

A cut-off point of 10 mm induration is used for people from populations with a high prevalence of tuberculosis or for individuals

Table 6.25.4 Criteria for tuberculin positivity, by risk group

Reaction ≥5 mm induration	Reaction ≥10 mm induration	Reaction ≥15 mm induration
HIV-positive persons	Recent immigrants (i.e. within the last 5 years) from high-prevalence countries or regions	Persons with no risk factors for tuberculosis
Recent contacts of infectious tuberculosis patients	Injection drug users	
Persons with fibrotic changes on chest radiograph consistent with prior tuberculosis	Residents and employees of the following high-risk congregate settings: Prisons and jails Nursing homes and other long-term facilities for older people Hospitals and other health care facilities Residential facilities for patients with AIDS Homeless shelters	
Patients with organ transplants and other immunosuppressed patients (receiving the equivalent of ≥15 mg/day prednisone for 1 month or more)	Persons with the following clinical conditions that place them at high risk: Silicosis Diabetes mellitus Chronic renal failure Some haematological disorders (e.g. leukaemias and lymphomas) Other specific malignancies (e.g. carcinoma of the head or neck and lung) Weight loss of ≥10% of ideal body weight Gastrectomy Jejunoileal bypass	
Others	Mycobacteriology laboratory personnel	
	Children <4 years of age or infants, children, and adolescents exposed to adults at high-risk	

with conditions that increase the risk of developing active disease if infected. This would include immigrants from endemic areas, residents of some inner cities, and health care workers, as well as patients with diabetes, renal disease, silicosis, and other medical conditions associated with an elevated risk of reactivation of latent tuberculosis. Finally, a cut off of 15 mm is used in people who have no risk factors for tuberculosis infection or disease. In most instances, these patients presumably would not be tested.

Tuberculin testing does have limitations in both sensitivity and specificity. The 5-TU dose of tuberculin used diagnostically is based on studies in the 1940s that showed that 99% of chronic tuberculosis patients responded to this dose, while fewer than 20% of those without disease and no history of tuberculosis exposure had a response. Subsequent research suggested that the lack of specificity of tuberculin testing may be the result of cross-reactions due to exposure to nontuberculous mycobacteria. For example, use of tuberculin derived from *M. avium intracellulare* (PPD-B) induces larger reactions than PPD-S in healthy people from areas where this organism is widespread in the environment. Another important cause of nonspecific reactions to tuberculin is vaccination with bacille Calmette-Guérin (BCG). While the reactogenicity of BCG vaccines differs according to the strain, immunization with BCG can produce falsely positive skin test results. Reactions induced by BCG tend to be smaller than true-positive reactions, and wane over a period of several years. Studies in populations with high rates of BCG coverage indicate that tuberculin testing can still be used to predict those who are most likely to be infected with *M. tuberculosis*, even though precision is reduced because of cross-reactions.

False-negative tuberculin tests result from both errors in applying and interpreting the test and from anergy. Errors in injection of tuberculin are common, and inter-reader variability in measuring results is high. Fortunately, if there is doubt about the interpretation of a skin test, multiple readers can measure the result over a period of days, or the test can be repeated and reinterpreted. Specific anergy to tuberculin is seen in several situations. Approximately 10 to 20% of patients with culture-confirmed pulmonary tuberculosis fail to respond to tuberculin as a result of anergy. These patients often will mount a response after their disease has been treated. HIV-infected patients have a high prevalence of anergy, both to tuberculin and other antigens. Only 10 to 40% of patients with low CD4 counts and confirmed tuberculosis respond to tuberculin. Transient anergy is associated with acute viral infections such as measles, live virus vaccinations, and other acute medical illnesses.

Alternative methods: interferon-γ production by sensitized T cells

Tuberculin skin testing is frustratingly crude and somewhat cumbersome, but despite its limitations has proved superior to numerous more 'modern' assays including antibody tests and other *in vitro* immunodiagnostics. Recently, however, the use of assays to detect interferon-γ production by sensitized T cells in response to challenge with specific antigens from the RD1 region of the *M. tuberculosis* genome has shown promise as an alternative to tuberculin testing. Two commercial interferon-γ release assays (IGRAs), one an enzyme-linked immunospot (T-SPOT-TB) and one an enzyme-linked immunosorbent assay (ELISA) (Quantiferon TB Gold-In Tube) are now approved in several countries for *in vitro* diagnosis of tuberculosis infection. These assays are more than 90% sensitive for active tuberculosis and more specific than tuberculin testing in BCG-vaccinated individuals, correlate better than tuberculin skin testing with exposure to a point source of infection, and may not be compromised by immunosuppression related to HIV infection. In some studies, these assays have greater sensitivity than tuberculin skin testing and almost always have better specificity. In evaluating individuals with latent tuberculosis infection, however, the lack of a gold standard of diagnosis makes comparisons difficult. However, emerging evidence suggests that interferon-γ release assays may be more accurate than tuberculin testing in predicting which people are at greatest risk of developing subsequent active tuberculosis disease. Thus, the assays have enormous potential and may contribute to improved detection of both active and latent tuberculosis infections.

Microscopic staining

Microscopic staining of acid-fast bacilli is the method most widely used to diagnose tuberculosis throughout the world. Acid-fast staining is inexpensive, rapid, and technologically undemanding, making it an attractive technique for identifying mycobacterial infections. The waxy glycolipid matrix of the mycobacterial cell wall is resistant to acid–alcohol decolorization after staining with carbol-fuchsin dyes, and red bacilli are visible after counterstaining. Both the Ziehl-Neelsen method (which requires heat fixation) and the Kinyoun method utilize methylene blue or malachite green counterstains, and have similar sensitivities for identifying acid-fast bacilli in clinical specimens.

The major limitation of acid-fast staining is that a relatively large number of bacilli must be present to be seen microscopically. Acid-fast smears are generally negative when there are fewer than 10 000 bacilli/ml of sputum, and many microscope fields need to be examined to identify bacilli even when there are 10 000 to 50 000 bacilli/ml. Thus, up to 50% of patients with sputum cultures positive for *M. tuberculosis* have negative acid-fast smears. In settings where the sputum smear is the only test done to confirm tuberculosis, a large number of smear-negative cases go undetected. This is a serious problem for patients without cavitary tuberculosis, who tend to have fewer bacilli in their sputum, including many HIV-infected tuberculosis patients in developing countries.

Improving the yield of sputum smears

Several techniques can be used to improve the yield of sputum smears. The most important method is enrichment of the specimen through concentration of the sputum. Centrifugation of sputum allows examination of the bacilli-rich pellet, which improves the sensitivity of smears substantially. Treatment of sputum with mucolytic agents is also helpful in identifying organisms by both smear and culture. Use of fluorochrome procedures to identify mycobacteria is more sensitive, but less specific, than acid-fast stains. Auramine O or auramine-rhodamine dyes are used on concentrated smears and examined under a fluorescence microscope. This technique allows much more rapid screening of slides than the traditional methods, but confirmation of positive results with Ziehl-Neelsen or Kinyoun staining is essential, as false-positive fluorochrome results are not uncommon. Fluorescence microscopy has been limited historically to well-equipped reference laboratories, but the introduction of light-emitting diode (LED)-based fluorescent microscopes has substantially lowered the cost of

this technology and increased its availability in resource-limited areas.

The proper collection of specimens is also important for optimizing the results of microscopy and culture. Early morning sputum specimens tend to have a higher yield than specimens collected at other times, and overnight sputum collections have provided even greater sensitivity. Morning gastric aspirates have a moderate yield for acid-fast bacilli in children, who generally have a difficult time producing sputum. Sputum induction with hypertonic saline is useful in evaluating patients with minimal or no sputum production, and the use of fibreoptic bronchoscopy is often advocated for patients with negative sputum smears. In several series, however, the yield of postbronchoscopy spontaneous sputum samples was higher than for the bronchoalveolar lavage fluid. While the goal of sputum collection is to collect a pure lower respiratory tract sample, specimens that appear to consist primarily of upper respiratory tract or oral secretions are often smear or culture positive in patients with pulmonary tuberculosis.

Examination of multiple specimens increases the sensitivity of sputum microscopy for acid-fast bacilli. The first smear identifies 70 to 80% of patients, the second another 10 to 15%, and the third another 5 to 10%. Review of additional specimens has little value.

In addition to the modest sensitivity of acid-fast staining, the specificity of this technique can also present problems. The morphological properties of the mycobacteria are sufficiently similar to make distinguishing *M. tuberculosis* from nontuberculous mycobacteria impossible on the basis of acid-fast smears. This is not a serious problem where tuberculosis is common and non-tuberculous mycobacterial infections are unusual. However, in many industrialized countries, disease due to the nontuberculous mycobacteria is relatively common, and distinguishing these types of infections has important therapeutic and public health implications. Thus, while sputum microscopy is useful because of its rapidity and low cost, it should be supplemented with culture or other more sensitive and specific tests whenever feasible.

Culture, nucleic acid amplification, and susceptibility testing

Culture of *M. tuberculosis*

This is the gold standard for confirming the diagnosis of tuberculosis. A variety of media are available that support the growth of mycobacteria, including egg-based and potato-based solid media and several broth-based media. The intrinsic growth rate of *M. tuberculosis* makes the recovery of the organism in culture a slow process. In traditional egg-based media such as Lowenstein–Jensen, growth of colonies of *M. tuberculosis* takes between 3 and 6 weeks, and 7H11 agar requires an average of 3 to 4 weeks to show colonies. Obviously, the slow pace of these traditional culture systems interferes with optimal patient management, and more rapid techniques are required.

Several faster (not rapid) systems for detection of mycobacteria in culture have been commercially developed. The Mycobacterial Growth Indicator Tube (MGIT) is a broth-based system that uses fluorescence detection to monitor growth. Both manual and automated systems are available. Once growth is detected, staining to identify acid-fast organisms and species identification need to be performed. The time to detection of mycobacteria using MGIT is considerably faster than conventional solid media, and the yield can be appreciably higher. Contamination of cultures with bacteria and fungi is common, and laboratory cross-contamination remains a concern. Nevertheless, the use of MGIT can increase case detection rates and speed the time to detection of tuberculosis.

Many clinical laboratories use more than one culture system for mycobacteria, both to increase the overall recovery rate and to provide quality control. In addition, if one culture becomes contaminated, alternative cultures can still be utilized.

Preparation of specimens for mycobacterial culture

This follows the same steps as outlined for acid-fast smears. In addition, specimens being submitted for culture also require decontamination to prevent overgrowth by more rapidly multiplying bacteria. Sodium hydroxide (NaOH) and N-acetyl-L-cysteine (NALC) are commonly used together for mucolysis and decontamination. By necessity, decontamination also inactivates >50% of mycobacteria in a specimen, thereby reducing the potential yield of the culture. Failure to decontaminate, however, leads to bacterial overgrowth and uninterpretable results. Lack of growth as a result of overdecontamination and bacterial overgrowth resulting from underdecontamination underscore the importance and utility of obtaining multiple specimens for culture, when possible. As with sputum smears, the yield of mycobacterial culture increases with evaluation of additional specimens.

Speciation

After mycobacterial growth has been identified, speciation of the organism is required. Conventional techniques for identification of mycobacterial species involve characterization of colony morphology, pigmentation, rate of growth, and biochemical tests. Niacin reduction, nitrate reduction, and lack of catalase activity at elevated temperatures are all characteristic of M. tuberculosis. Species identification using these methods is time consuming and tedious, and further delays the diagnosis of tuberculosis.

The use of nucleic acid probes has dramatically simplified speciation of mycobacteria in recent years. DNA probes that react with specific mycobacterial rRNA sequences to form DNA–RNA hybrids that can be readily detected by chemoluminescence are commercially available for M. tuberculosis, M. avium complex, M. kansasii, and M. gordonae. These probes can be performed within hours of detection of mycobacterial growth, and significantly accelerate the diagnosis of specific pathogens. The sensitivity of these probes is approximately 90 to 95%, depending on the species, with specificities approaching 100%. Cultures that fail to respond to any of the DNA–RNA probes are almost always due to another mycobacterial species, but final identification depends on the laborious biochemical techniques of old.

Nucleic acid amplification

The difficulties of identifying mycobacteria in patient specimens accentuate the need for rapid and sensitive diagnostic methods for tuberculosis. If any infection seems suited to diagnosis by nucleic acid amplification (NAA) assays, it would appear to be tuberculosis. Multiple studies of 'in-house' PCR assays for M. tuberculosis have shown modest sensitivity and specificity. PCR inhibitors in sputum have been a knotty problem in the molecular diagnosis of pulmonary tuberculosis, although sensitivity has been lower than culture in nonrespiratory specimens as well. Recently, several commercial NAA tests have been introduced or are nearing approval,

including assays based on reverse transcription (RT)-PCR, transcription-mediated amplification, ligase chain reaction, and strand displacement amplification. All of these techniques use specific M. tuberculosis DNA sequences (most use the M. tuberculosis transposon IS6110) as targets for NAA. The great advantage of these assays is that they can provide results within 1 day of the collection of specimens. Their disadvantage is that they are uniformly less sensitive than culture, particularly in sputum smear-negative patients. Early studies also suggested that specificity was excellent overall but was reduced in smear-positive samples; further refinements in these assays have resulted in improved sensitivity and specificity, but their diagnostic role in smear-negative sputum or extrapulmonary disease is limited by their moderate sensitivity. Furthermore, the cost of NAA tests may be too high for routine use in resource-limited settings where tuberculosis is endemic.

Recent advances in DNA amplification have made rapid detection of M. tuberculosis gene sequences more easily performed, marking a potentially revolutionary change in the diagnosis of tuberculosis. Line probe assays, using solid-phase PCR techniques to identify signature sequences from M. tuberculosis, can identify up to 99% of sputum smear-positive specimens and between 50 and 70% of smear-negative specimens. The turn-around-time for these assays is 4 to 8 h, and most results can be returned, in theory, within a few days, dramatically accelerating the diagnosis. In addition, as discussed below, line probe assays can also be used to detect resistance mutations associated with isoniazid, rifampicin, ethambutol, and a number of second-line antituberculosis drug resistance. Unfortunately, rapid genetic testing for pyrazinamide resistance, a key predictor of response to treatment of MDR and XDR tuberculosis, is not yet possible with these assays.

Another new addition to the diagnostic armamentarium is the GeneXpert MTB/RIF assay. This commercial kit uses molecular beacons to identify both M. tuberculosis gene sequences and specific mutations responsible for more than 95% of all rifampicin resistance. The test kit is contained in a small cartridge into which sputum is placed, and the entire process is automated within the cartridge and a tabletop machine, with results returned in 90 to 120 min. The sensitivity of the assay is greater than 98% for smear-positive sputum and 60 to 70% for smear-negative samples, with a sensitivity of over 95% for rifampicin resistance. The ability to provide a diagnosis of tuberculosis and determine rifampicin susceptibility within 2 h is of enormous importance, and this assay is now being rolled out through much of the world. Conventional drug-susceptibility testing is still required for patients found to have rifampicin resistance, but from a clinical perspective the diagnosis of rifampicin-resistant tuberculosis is tantamount to MDR tuberculosis in most settings, and treatment decisions may be based on the GeneXpert result.

Drug susceptibility testing

Susceptibility testing of M. tuberculosis isolates is essential for both clinical management and public health purposes. Susceptibility tests for the first-line antituberculosis drugs should be performed on at least one culture at the time of diagnosis for all patients. If the initial isolate is susceptible to the first-line agents and treatment proceeds without incident, additional susceptibility tests are not required. Susceptibility testing should be performed for patients who relapse with tuberculosis and for patients who are treatment failures after 3 to 4 months of therapy.

Susceptibility testing for *M. tuberculosis* uses standard concentrations of antituberculosis drugs to measure inhibition of bacterial growth in culture. Drugs tested routinely include isoniazid, rifampicin, pyrazinamide, ethambutol, and streptomycin. Testing of second-line antituberculosis drugs is only done when resistance to the first-line agents is documented or strongly suspected.

Conventional susceptibility testing is generally performed on subcultures of the primary isolate, though direct inoculation of sputum or other specimens can be performed in the case of a strongly positive acid-fast bacilli smear. The standard method for measuring susceptibility to antituberculosis drugs is the proportions method. The organism is grown on agar plates in the presence of known concentrations of specific drugs. Growth on the plates is then compared with growth on control plates. By convention, if the test plate shows a colony count that is >1% of the control value, the isolate is resistant. Laboratories will report the isolate as being susceptible or resistant to the concentration of the drug used in the assay.

Another method for susceptibility testing is to use the MGIT system, in which culture bottles contain antituberculosis drugs. Growth indices are compared to control cultures to determine susceptibility. The MGIT system provides results more quickly than the proportions method, is automated, but is more expensive. Recently, the microscopic examination of growth in wells that are filled with liquid culture medium (MODS) has been reported to enable detection within about 10 days and permit rapid assessment of drug resistance. This technique has some promise in resource-limited settings, but it is labour intensive and needs further validation in endemic countries.

As noted above, the use of molecular methods to determine tuberculosis drug susceptibility is a major advance. Specific mutations in *M. tuberculosis* have been identified which confer resistance to antituberculosis drugs. For example, mutations in a small region of the *rpo*B gene of *M. tuberculosis* are responsible for more than 90% of all rifampicin resistance. Sequencing of this portion of the genome using a variety of techniques has been shown to be feasible in research laboratories. Rapid identification of rifampicin resistance by molecular methods (line probe assay) would be of enormous clinical benefit, as almost all rifampicin-resistant *M. tuberculosis* isolates are also resistant to isoniazid and are, by definition, multidrug resistant. Thus early detection of resistance mutations would allow early initiation of appropriate treatment and infection control measures. A point of treatment nucleic acid amplification tests such as the GeneXpert MTB-RIF can detect at least rifampicin resistance. Among culture-positive patients, a single, Xpert MTB/RIF test done on spectrum directly had 98.2% and 72.5% sensitivity in smear-positive and negative tuberculosis respectively, and a 99.2% specificity in patients without tuberculosis. Molecular diagnosis of other types of resistance is more difficult, as the genetic basis of resistance to other drugs is either heterogeneous or not completely understood.

Treatment of active tuberculosis

The treatment of tuberculosis requires the use of a combination of antimycobacterial drugs active against the strain of *M. tuberculosis* causing the patient's disease. The use of multiple agents is necessitated by the emergence of drug resistance when single agents are used. Mutations that confer resistance to antimycobacterial drugs arise spontaneously in wild-type populations of *M. tuberculosis* in frequencies ranging from 1 in 10^5 to 1 in 10^8 bacilli. In the presence

of large numbers of organisms, such as are present during active pulmonary disease, a single agent will kill susceptible bacilli, but naturally drug-resistant mutants will survive and eventually emerge to cause drug-resistant disease. Since the mechanisms of resistance are genetically distinct and arise independently, multiple drug resistance within a single organism is exceedingly rare in nature. The use of two or more agents with different mechanisms of action assures that populations of drug-resistant bacilli are not selected for during therapy.

Antituberculosis drugs

These are divided into first-line and second-line agents. The first-line agents are widely available and used routinely in the treatment of tuberculosis, while the second-line agents are generally less potent, more toxic, and less readily available. Exceptions are the newer fluoroquinolones, such as moxifloxacin and levofloxacin, which appear to have good activity against *M. tuberculosis* in a mouse model. The ability of moxifloxacin to reduce the time to sputum conversion might shorten the duration of tuberculosis treatment, but this remains to be confirmed in ongoing clinical trials. Second-line drugs are reserved for the treatment of drug-resistant tuberculosis. Table 6.25.5 lists the first-line antituberculosis drugs, their activity in the treatment of tuberculosis, and common toxicities.

Regimens currently used for the treatment of tuberculosis have been developed on the basis of trials conducted by the United Kingdom Medical Research Council since the late1970s. By combining drugs that target both rapidly growing bacillary populations and slow-growing or semidormant organisms within cells, modern short-course chemotherapy can successfully cure drug-susceptible pulmonary tuberculosis in 6 months. The regimens recommended for treatment of drug-susceptible tuberculosis are shown in Table 6.25.6. Treatment of extrapulmonary tuberculosis is generally for the same duration as for pulmonary disease, with the exceptions of bone and joint and central nervous system tuberculosis, which are treated for 12 months.

The dynamics of mycobacterial growth are such that treatment need be administered only once daily, and can be given as infrequently as twice a week. The long generation time of *M. tuberculosis* and a post-antibiotic effect of antituberculosis drugs make more frequent drug dosing unnecessary. The dosages for drugs are listed

Table 6.25.5 Drugs for the treatment of tuberculosis

Agent	Activity	Toxicity
Isoniazid	Bactericidal	Liver, peripheral nerve, hypersensitivity
Rifampicin	Bactericidal and sterilizing	Liver, gastrointestinal, discoloration of body fluids, nausea, haematological
Rifapentine	Bactericidal and sterilizing	Liver, gastrointestinal, discoloration of body fluids, nausea, haematological
Pyrazinamide	Sterilizing	Liver, hyperuricaemia, gout, malaise, gastrointestinal
Ethambutol	Bacteriostatic (dose-dependent)	Liver, optic neuritis, skin
Streptomycin	Bactericidal	Ototoxicity, kidneys
Rifapentine	Bactericidal and steralizing	Liver, gastrointestinal, discoloration of body fluids, nausea, haematological

Table 6.25.6 Treatment regimens for tuberculosis in children and adults

	Frequency	Drugs
Option 1	Intensive phase, daily	Isoniazid, rifampicin, pyrazinamide, and ethambutol or streptomycin[b] for 8 weeks
	Continuation phase, daily or 2–3 times weekly[a]	Isoniazid and rifampicin for 16 weeks
	Continuation phase, once weekly	Isoniazid and rifapentine for 16 weeks
Option 2	Intensive phase, daily	Isoniazid, rifampicin, pyrazinamide, and ethambutol or streptomycin[b] for 2 weeks
	Intensive phase, twice weekly	Same drugs for 6 weeks[b]
	Continuation phase, twice weekly[a]	Isoniazid and rifampicin for 16 weeks
Option 3	Entire course of therapy, 3 times weekly[a]	Isoniazid, rifampicin, pyrazinamide, and ethambutol or streptomycin for 24 weeks

[a] Intermittent dosing should be directly observed. Patients with HIV infection should receive at least thrice-weekly dosing. Once weekly isoniazid/rifapentine is reserved for HIV-negative patients with negative sputum cultures at 2 months and without cavitation on chest radiograph.
[b] In areas where drug resistance is 4%, omit fourth drug.

in Table 6.25.7 according to the frequency with which they are administered.

Isoniazid remains a key component of treatment because of its high bactericidal activity. Rifampicin is essential for short-course therapy because it is active against all populations of bacilli, both within and outside of cells. Pyrazinamide is uniquely active during the first 2 months of therapy, but appears to have no activity thereafter. The addition of pyrazinamide to the treatment regimen allows the duration to be reduced from 9 to 6 months, however. Streptomycin has bactericidal activity against *M. tuberculosis*, and ethambutol has bacteriostatic activity at lower doses and bactericidal activity at high doses. These agents primarily are given to prevent the emergence of drug resistance, as they appear to add little activity to combination regimens against drug-susceptible tuberculosis.

Drug toxicities

Although antituberculosis therapy is remarkably well tolerated and almost always given on an ambulatory basis, important drug toxicities do exist. The most serious adverse drug reaction during tuberculosis treatment is liver toxicity, which may occur in up to 5 to 10% of treated patients. Isoniazid, rifampicin, and pyrazinamide are all associated with liver toxicity and use of these agents together increases the risk of a reaction. Isoniazid causes more hepatotoxicity than rifampicin or pyrazinamide, however, and is the agent most frequently implicated when reactions occur. Isoniazid can produce an idiosyncratic hepatocellular injury, manifested by elevated liver enzymes and clinical hepatitis. Elevation of transaminases does not always portend the development of hepatitis, but may serve as an important signal to anticipate clinical toxicity. The development of signs and symptoms of hepatitis, such as abdominal pain, nausea, vomiting, or jaundice, requires immediate discontinuation of isoniazid, as continuing treatment may result in death from hepatic failure. Risk factors for developing isoniazid hepatotoxicity include increasing age, chronic liver disease, alcohol abuse, daily dosing of isoniazid, and use of other hepatotoxic drugs, including rifampicin. In addition, individuals with a slow isoniazid acetylation genotype are significantly more likely to develop hepatotoxicity from the drug than intermediate or rapid acetylators. Isoniazid interferes with metabolism of pyridoxine (vitamin B_6) which can result in a sensory neuropathy. Coadministration of pyridoxine with isoniazid abrogates this effect without compromising the antimicrobial activity.

Rifampicin also causes hepatotoxicity, although the characteristic picture of liver disturbances due to rifampicin is cholestasis. However, the incidence of hepatotoxicity when rifampicin is given with isoniazid is substantially greater than when isoniazid is given alone. Rifampicin predictably causes a discoloration of body fluids, resulting in orange-tinted tears, sweat, and urine. Haematological toxicity from rifampicin includes thrombocytopenia and anaemia. Higher doses of rifampicin may produce a hypersensitivity reaction, with fever, rash, and joint swelling. It is for this reason that doses of rifampicin are not escalated during intermittent therapy, whereas the intermittent dosages of the other drugs are increased to deliver weekly doses that are equivalent to daily dosing.

Pyrazinamide is often associated with arthralgias, and may precipitate gout. Pyrazinamide inhibits renal tubular uric acid excretion, resulting in increased serum uric acid levels. Frank gouty arthritis is relatively uncommon with pyrazinamide use, and its frequency is reduced with intermittent dosing. Routine use of allopurinol to prevent gout is not recommended.

The major toxicity of ethambutol is optic neuritis, which is common at doses above 30 mg/kg daily and unusual at doses below 25 mg/kg daily. Patients receiving ethambutol should have baseline tests of visual acuity and colour discrimination, with monthly monitoring while on treatment. Ethambutol use is discouraged in children under 8 years old because of their inability reliably to

Table 6.25.7 Dosage recommendation for the initial treatment of tuberculosis in children and adults

Drugs	Daily dose		Twice-weekly dose		Thrice-weekly dose	
	Children	Adults	Children	Adults	Children	Adults
Isoniazid (mg/kg)	10–20 (max. 300 mg)	5 (max. 300 mg)	20–40 (max. 900 mg)	15 (max. 900 mg)	20–40 (max. 900 mg)	15 (max. 900 mg
Rifampicin (mg/kg)	10–20 (max. 600 mg)	10 (max. 600 mg)	10–20 (max. 600 mg)	10 (max. 600 mg)	10–20 (max. 600 mg)	10 (max. 600 mg)
Pyrazinamide (mg/kg)	15–30 (max. 2 g)	15–30 (max. 2 g)	50–70 (max. 4 g)	50–70 (max. 3.5 g)	50–60 (max. 3.5 g)	50–60 (max. 3.5 g)
Ethambutol (mg/kg)	15–25 (max. 1.5 g)	15–25 (max. 1.5 g)	50 (max. 4 g)	50 (max. 4 g)	25–30	25–30
Streptomycin (mg/kg)	20–40 (max. 1.0 g)	15 (max. 1.0 g)	25–30 (max. 1.5 g)	25–30 (max. 1.5 g)	25–?30 (max. 1.5 g)	25–30 (max. 1.5 g)

report visual disturbances. However, the incidence of optic neuritis with the doses of ethambutol typically used is so low that its use in young children is only relatively contraindicated.

Streptomycin was a staple of antituberculosis therapy for many years, but its use has been greatly curbed in recent years. Several studies have demonstrated that regimens containing isoniazid, rifampicin, and pyrazinamide are equally efficacious with or without streptomycin. Streptomycin is given by intramuscular injection, causing discomfort to patients and creating an infection risk for patients and health care workers. In addition, streptomycin can be ototoxic and nephrotoxic. Consequently, ethambutol has replaced streptomycin in many settings around the world.

Monitoring of therapy

Patients receiving therapy for tuberculosis require regular monitoring to assess adherence with therapy, clinical response, and adverse reactions. In the initial phase of therapy, monitoring by a nurse or other trained clinician at least weekly is recommended, and supervision of every dose of medication is suggested by the WHO and other authorities (see below). Patients should be observed for clinical responses, including defervescence, improvement in cough and appetite, and weight gain. Improvement in these symptoms and signs may take several weeks, but usually occurs within 3 weeks after starting treatment. Failure to improve suggests that the patient is not adhering to treatment, has drug-resistant tuberculosis, or has another illness in addition to or instead of tuberculosis.

Treatment response should also be documented with repeated sputum smears and cultures and a follow-up chest radiograph after 2 to 3 months (for pulmonary tuberculosis). All patients should have a repeat sputum smear and culture after 2 months of therapy; those who are smear or culture positive at 2 months should have another at 3 months. Failure to convert sputum smears and cultures to negative with 3 months of therapy is associated with a high risk of treatment failure; patients who are still smear or culture positive at 4 months of treatment are considered treatment failures and should be evaluated for drug-resistant disease. A culture at the end of therapy is recommended to document cure, while an end of therapy radiograph is not necessary.

Monitoring for drug toxicity is also required throughout therapy. At least monthly monitoring for symptoms and signs of liver toxicity is essential, and patients should be advised to stop therapy and seek care if evidence of hepatitis is noted. Routine liver enzyme monitoring is recommended primarily for patients with underlying liver disease or baseline abnormalities in liver enzymes. Patients with symptoms of hepatitis, of course, should have liver studies obtained. As noted above, monthly visual assessment is also recommended when ethambutol is given.

Adherence to therapy and directly observed therapy

Since the 1960s experts in tuberculosis have noted that the success of treatment depends largely on adherence to therapy. Poor adherence to therapy is responsible for treatment failures, early relapses, and the emergence of drug-resistant disease. Two major interventions to improve adherence and prevent poor outcomes are directly observed therapy (DOT) and the use of fixed-dose combination tablets. DOT was first promoted in the 1950s in India, and experience with DOT grew over the ensuing years. Intermittent dosing of tuberculosis therapy, along with the relatively short course of

treatment, make supervision of treatment feasible in many settings. Ecological and programmatic studies of DOT programmes have shown that the introduction of DOT improves cure rates for tuberculosis, reduces nonadherence, and reduces the emergence of drug-resistant disease. Two observational studies have shown better survival of HIV-infected tuberculosis patients who receive DOT.

On the other hand, two randomized trials of DOT in developing countries have not found improved treatment completion rates compared with self-administered treatment. These trials have been criticized for demonstrating only that DOT can be done badly, but the lack of randomized studies documenting that DOT *per se* leads to improved outcomes is of some concern. The data from observational studies are compelling, however, and DOT has been shown to be cost-effective in resource-limited settings and, therefore, is strongly encouraged by many experts and professional organizations.

The use of fixed-dose combination tablets is intended to reduce the risk of selecting for drug resistance, as opposed to improving adherence generally. By combining two, three, or four medications in the same tablet, depending on the regimen being used, the opportunity for patients to receive partial treatment that would select for drug resistance is avoided. The bioequivalence of fixed-dose combinations to individual medications has been established for some, but not all, of the combination products on the market.

The catastrophic state of global tuberculosis control led the WHO to develop the directly observed therapy, short-course (DOTS) strategy. This strategy is a series of policies related to national tuberculosis control practices. The five elements of the DOTS strategy are:

1 Governmental commitment to tuberculosis control

2 A reliable supply of tuberculosis drugs

3 Diagnosis of tuberculosis cases microscopically

4 A registration system for tracking the outcomes of treatment

5 Supervision (DOT) of at least the first 8 weeks of treatment

The DOTS strategy has been extremely successful in focusing attention on serious problems in tuberculosis treatment and control, and implementation of the programme in several countries has produced remarkable improvements in clinical outcomes for patients with tuberculosis. There is strong evidence that the use of the DOTS strategy results in lower rates of drug-resistant tuberculosis. Nonetheless, the WHO estimates that in 1999 only 21% of tuberculosis patients in the world were treated within a DOTS programme. Further expansion of the DOTS strategy and improvements in tuberculosis treatment programmes are clearly needed.

Treatment of multidrug-resistant tuberculosis

This is beyond the scope of this chapter. Patients with drug-resistant tuberculosis should be managed by a physician who is a tuberculosis expert. Effective treatment and cure of multidrug-resistant tuberculosis (MDR-TB) requires prolonged use (about 2 years) of a combination of drugs that include second-line drugs which are less effective than first-line agents, have a greater toxicity, or demonstrate both disadvantages. Supervised therapy is considered mandatory for patients with resistant tuberculosis. Physician mistakes remain one of the leading causes of the emergence of multidrug-resistant and extensively drug-resistant tuberculosis (XDR-TB), and the identification of a drug-resistant isolate of *M. tuberculosis* should result in immediate expert consultation. It is also clear that addressing drug-resistant tuberculosis cannot be accomplished without addressing the overall tuberculosis control effort.

Newer agents

Most of the agents that are currently used to treat tuberculosis have been in use for decades. In the past 5 years a number of novel agents have been developed and are being evaluated in clinical trials. Two fluoroquinolones, moxifloxacin and gatifloxacin, are currently being evaluated in a phase III trial of drug-sensitive pulmonary tuberculosis, to determine if duration of treatment can be shortened to 4 months. OPC-67683, a novel agent, is being evaluated in a randomized controlled trial of MDR tuberculosis. Bedaquiline (TMC207, a diarylquinoline), which inhibits mycobacterial ATP synthase is being evaluated in phase II clinical trials of drug-sensitive and MDR tuberculosis. PA824 (nitroimidazole) is also being evaluated in phase II trials. Other drugs in the drug development pipeline include the oxazolidinones (linezolid and, SQ109) and PNU-100480.

Treatment of tuberculosis in HIV-infected people

The United States (ATS/CDC/Infectious Disease Society of America) recommendations for the treatment of tuberculosis in HIV-infected adults are, with a few exceptions, the same as those for HIV-uninfected adults, i.e. standard 6-month rifampicin-based therapy. The continuation phase is extended from 6 to 9 months for any patient with cavitary tuberculosis and positive cultures at 2 months, regardless of the HIV status. The optional continuation phase regimen of isoniazid plus rifapentine once weekly is contraindicated in HIV-infected patients because of an unacceptably high rate of relapse, frequently with organisms that have acquired resistance to rifamycins. The development of acquired rifampicin resistance has also been noted among HIV-infected patients with advanced immune suppression treated with twice weekly rifampicin-based or rifabutin-based regimens. Consequently, patients with CD4 cell counts <100 cells/µl should receive daily or three-times weekly treatment. DOT and other adherence-promoting strategies are especially important for patients with HIV-related tuberculosis.

Recent randomized controlled trials have examined the question of optimal timing of antiteroviral therapy (ART) initiation in HIV-associated tuberculosis. A Cambodian trial (CAMELIA) showed that ART initiated within 2 weeks was beneficial in reducing mortality among all patients with tuberculosis with baseline CD4+ counts of 200 cells/mm3 or lower. Two other trials, one in South Africa (SAPIT) and one multinational (ACTG A5221) did not show a reduction in AIDS or death, apart from that among patients with baseline CD4+ counts less than 50 cells/mm3. Thus, earlier initiation of ART appears to be beneficial in patients with tuberculosis in whom immunosuppression is advanced. However, this benefit comes at the expense of an increase in the risks of immune reconstitution inflammatory syndrome (IRIS) and of adverse events that lead to the switching of ART drugs. In patients with higher CD4+ T-cell counts, the benefit of early initiation of ART is less clear, and it may be reasonable to defer initiation of ART until the continuation phase of tuberculosis treatment in order to simplify treatment and reduce the risk of complications. A fourth study conducted in HIV-infected patients with TB meningitis in Vietnam showed no mortality benefit with early initiation of ART but an increased frequency of adverse events.

Drug interactions

There are three possible complications that arise when tuberculosis treatment and antiretroviral drugs are coadministered: shared side effects and toxicity, drug interactions arising from the induction of metabolism (cytochrome P450 enzymes) and efflux pumps by rifampicin, and the immune reconstitution inflammatory syndrome. Rifamycins induce the activity of cytochrome P450 enzymes that are important in drug metabolism. Several key antiretroviral drug classes, protease inhibitors and non-nucleoside reverse transcriptase inhibitors, and integrase inhibitors, are substrates of cytochrome P450 enzymes. Protease inhibitors are also substrates of P-glycoprotein, which is also induced by rifamycins. The available rifamycins differ in potency as P450 enzyme inducers, with rifampicin and rifapentine being the most potent and rifabutin the least. Co-administration with rifampicin reduces the concentrations of non-nucleoside reverse transcriptase inhibitors and integrase inhibitors to a moderate extent, but dramatically reduces the concentrations of protease inhibitors. Rifabutin does not significantly affect the concentrations of ritonavir-boosted protease inhibitors and is recommended when protease inhibitors have to be used. However, the use of rifabutin in low resource settings is currently limited due to its very high cost and the widespread use of fixed-dose combination antituberculosis drugs that include rifampicin.

Immune reconstitution inflammatory syndrome

Between 8 and 45% of patients commencing ART while being treated for tuberculosis develop paradoxical deterioration of tuberculosis, the so-called IRIS. Paradoxical deterioration was well known in the pre-HIV era, but occurs much more frequently in HIV-infected patients starting ART. The pathogenesis of IRIS is not completely understood. The most common manifestations of tuberculosis-related IRIS are focal inflammatory exacerbations of tuberculosis (lymphadenitis, serositis, or abscesses, new infiltrates), 'unmasking' of tuberculosis or other subclinical diseases after ART initiation, etc. It typically occurs within 2 to 4 weeks after antiretroviral initiation. Risk factors associated with an increased risk of IRIS include shorter intervals between antituberculosis therapy and ART initiation, low baseline CD4 counts and high baseline viral load, and vigorous CD4/viral load response to antiretroviral therapy. However, new or worsening clinical features should be attributed to IRIS only after a thorough evaluation has excluded other possible causes, notably poor adherence to antituberculosis therapy, MDR tuberculosis, new opportunistic diseases, and systemic drug hypersensitivity reactions. The benefit of adjunctive corticosteroids in the management of patients with IRIS is suggested by results of at least one randomized controlled trial which showed that the use of 1.25 mg/kg prednisone for 2 weeks followed by 0.75 mg over 2 weeks in nonsevere IRIS was been associated with decreased hospitalization and morbidity.

Duration of therapy

Despite these complications, ART should not be withheld simply because the patient is being treated for tuberculosis. The optimal timing of initiation of ART in relation to initiation of antituberculosis treatment is unclear. Treatment for tuberculosis should always be initiated first, and it is prudent to wait at least until it is clear that the patient is improving and tolerating the antituberculosis therapy before beginning ART. While awaiting the results of ongoing controlled trials, a 2006 WHO expert opinion panel has suggested that the CD4 lymphocyte count should determine the initiation of ART, unless there is other serious HIV morbidity. These WHO guidelines state that patients with CD4 counts below 200 cells/µl should initiate ART after 2 to 8 weeks of antituberculosis therapy and those with CD4 counts 200 to 350 cells/µl after 8 weeks. Data from recent clinical trials support initiating ART for all patients with a CD4 count below 500 cells/µl within 2 months of starting tuberculosis therapy, as this reduces mortality by over 50%. Until there have been more controlled studies evaluating the optimal time for starting antiretroviral therapy in patients with HIV infection and tuberculosis, this decision should be individualized. Possible factors for consideration are a patient's initial response to treatment for tuberculosis, CD4 response to tuberculosis therapy, possible drug interactions, risk of IRIS, adherence, occurrence of side effects, and availability of ART. For patients who are already receiving an antiretroviral regimen when tuberculosis is detected, antiretroviral treatment should be continued during antituberculosis therapy.

Adjunctive steroid treatment

Corticosteroids are frequently advocated with tuberculosis treatment to reduce inflammation in tuberculosis, but evidence for this practice is often lacking, particularly in HIV infection. Mortality was reduced in a small trial of patients given prednisolone for tuberculous pericarditis. Also, dexamethasone reduced mortality in a large Vietnamese study of adults with tuberculous meningitis. The HIV-infected subgroup of the latter study appeared to gain a similar benefit, but this failed to achieve statistical significance. A Ugandan study of adjunctive prednisolone in HIV-infected patients with pleural tuberculosis found faster resolution with prednisolone, but no mortality benefit. Of great concern, however, was their finding of excess cases of Kaposi's sarcoma in the prednisolone arm. This sobering result is a reminder that the additive immunosuppressant effect of glucocorticoids can have severe consequences in HIV infection. Adjunctive glucocorticoids should only be used in HIV-infected patients when there is likely to be a mortality benefit, which may be the case for tuberculous meningitis and pericarditis, but there is still a need for definitive evidence from larger studies in both conditions.

Treatment of latent tuberculosis infection

Isoniazid chemoprophylaxis

Prevention of tuberculosis with isoniazid therapy was first documented in children in the mid-1950s. Subsequently, several controlled trials of isoniazid chemoprophylaxis were undertaken, and its efficacy firmly established. A meta-analysis of 11 placebo-controlled trials of isoniazid, involving more than 70 000 persons, found that treatment reduced tuberculosis incidence by 63%. Among patients who adhered to >80% of the isoniazid regimen, protection was 81%. These studies also showed that isoniazid chemoprophylaxis reduced tuberculosis deaths by 72%. The efficacy of isoniazid therapy to prevent tuberculosis in high-risk persons is incontrovertible.

Enthusiasm for isoniazid chemoprophylaxis was considerably dampened in the late 1960s and early 1970s when drug-related hepatotoxicity, including deaths, was observed. Several studies based on decision analysis or modelling suggested that the risks of chemoprophylaxis might outweigh the benefits, and use of preventive

therapy was curtailed or ignored in many settings. Because the risk of isoniazid-related hepatotoxicity increases with age, use of chemoprophylaxis in people older than 35 years was particularly discouraged.

Preventive therapy in high-risk individuals

The resurgence of tuberculosis in the developed world, particularly HIV-related tuberculosis, and the uncontrolled global epidemic have renewed interest in the use of preventive therapy in high-risk individuals known or strongly suspected to be latently infected with *M. tuberculosis*. The term 'treatment of latent tuberculosis infection' is now preferred, emphasizing that preventive treatment is really targeted at an established infection. The ATS and the CDC published guidelines in 2000 on screening for latent tuberculosis that stress the importance of targeting efforts on populations and patients who would benefit from treatment to prevent active disease. In the past, screening for tuberculosis infection has been unfocused and often directed at patients who, if found to be infected, would have little risk of progressing to active disease. The new guidelines propose that only people with a high risk of disease or high prior probability of latent tuberculosis be tested, and that treatment be offered to infected individuals regardless of age. Individuals who should be targeted for tuberculin testing are those listed in the first two columns of Table 6.25.4, i.e. those in whom a positive test is considered equal to or exceeding 5 or equal to or exceeding 10 mm induration. People without risk factors for tuberculosis (those in whom a positive test is equal to or exceeding 15 mm) should not be tested.

Treatment regimens for latent tuberculosis are listed in Table 6.25.8, along with the rating given to the regimen by the ATS and CDC. Isoniazid remains a favoured drug for tuberculosis preventive therapy because of its well-documented efficacy, low cost, and relatively low toxicity. The optimal duration of isoniazid therapy for latent tuberculosis has been the subject of extensive debate in recent years. The International Union Against Tuberculosis and Lung Disease conducted a landmark trial in Eastern Europe in the 1970s and 1980s that compared no treatment to 3, 6, or 12 months of isoniazid in adults with fibrotic changes on radiographs. The results showed that, compared to placebo, 12 months of isoniazid reduced the incidence of tuberculosis by 75%, compared to 66% for 6 months and 20% for 3 months. In addition, patients who completed the 12 months of therapy and were judged to be compliant experienced a 92% reduction in tuberculosis risk, compared to a 69% decrease for compliant patients completing a 6-month regimen.

Table 6.25.8 Treatment regimens for latent tuberculosis

Drug regimen	Duration (months)	Interval	Rating (HIV–)	Rating (HIV+)
Isoniazid	9	Daily	A II	A II
Isoniazid	9	Twice weekly	B II	B II
Isoniazid	6	Daily	B I	C I
Isoniazid	6	Twice weekly	B II	C II
Rifampicin	4	Daily	B II	B III
Rifapentine and isoniazid	3	Once weekly	A I	B I

A, strongly recommended; B, recommended; C, optional; I, randomized trials; II, data from other scientific studies; III, expert opinion.

An analysis by the Cochrane Collaborative found that 12 months of isoniazid was more effective than 6 months for prevention of tuberculosis. A recent analysis of varying durations of isoniazid therapy in Alaskan natives revealed that the effectiveness of isoniazid therapy was optimal after 9 months, and that further treatment conferred no additional benefit. Several studies of isoniazid in HIV-infected patients in Africa, however, have found that prolonged treatment for 3 or more years is more efficacious than shorter durations, presumably by preventing disease due to reinfection in these highly susceptible patients.

Several recent studies have demonstrated that shorter durations of preventive therapy using the combination of rifapentine and isoniazid given once a week under direct observation is an acceptable alternative to longer courses of isoniazid alone. A large study sponsored by the CDC's TB Trials Consortium found that the rifapentine/isoniazid 3-month regimen was not only non-inferior to isoniazid for 9 months in high-risk individuals, but almost reached superiority and was better tolerated, with significantly less hepatotoxicity. Another study in HIV-infected adults in South Africa found rifapentine/isoniazid to be of similar efficacy to isoniazid alone for 6 months.

Isoniazid hepatotoxicity

Although isoniazid is a well-tolerated drug, serious hepatotoxicity can occur in a small proportion of patients. Isoniazid may result in asymptomatic elevations in hepatic aminotransferase levels, but this does not always signal impending clinical toxicity. Hepatotoxicity is of concern when symptoms of hepatitis develop, including pain, nausea, vomiting, and jaundice. Continuing isoniazid in the presence of symptoms may lead to death from fulminant hepatic necrosis and liver failure, with a case fatality rate of 10 to 15%. Studies in the 1960s and 1970s found evidence of hepatotoxicity in 1 to 5% of recipients of isoniazid, with higher rates among older patients. More recent experience with isoniazid therapy that is closely monitored shows a risk of hepatotoxicity in the range of 0.1 to 0.3%. Thus, appropriate patient screening and follow-up makes the use of isoniazid for treating latent infection markedly safer.

Alternative regimens

In addition to the 3-month rifapentine/isoniazid treatment described above, other alternative regimens are sometimes used in selected situations. A 3-month regimen of rifampicin alone was found to reduce the incidence of tuberculosis by about 65% in men with silicosis, and was more effective than 6 months of isoniazid. The combination of rifampicin and isoniazid given for 3 to 4 months is widely used for treatment of latent tuberculosis in children and improves completion rates. This regimen has also been found to be equally effective as isoniazid in studies in adults.

The use of rifampicin does pose the risk of important drug interactions. For example, reduction in methadone concentrations caused by rifampicin can precipitate narcotic withdrawal. Moreover, rifampicin can lower levels of protease inhibitors and non-nucleoside reverse transcriptase inhibitors used to treat HIV infection. Substitution of rifabutin for rifampicin in patients receiving HIV drugs provides equally efficacious treatment of active tuberculosis and less effect on antiretroviral drugs. If multidrug-resistant tuberculosis is suspected, the recommended preventive therapy is pyrazinamide and ethambutol or pyrazinamide and a fluoroquinolone (e.g. moxifloxacin) for 6 to 12 months. Treatment for suspected exposure to multidrug-resistant tuberculosis should be routinely extended to 12 months in HIV-infected individuals.

Candidates for treatment of latent tuberculosis are listed in Table 6.25.4. Criteria for treatment include a positive tuberculin test according to the categories in Table 6.25.4, elevated risk for developing active tuberculosis if untreated, and exclusion of active tuberculosis by clinical evaluation and chest radiograph. In addition, HIV-infected and other severely immunocompromised persons who are contacts to an infectious tuberculosis patient should be treated for latent tuberculosis regardless of tuberculin skin test results.

Monitoring treatment

Patients receiving treatment for latent tuberculosis should be monitored for drug toxicity, as well as to promote adherence to therapy. As in treatment of active tuberculosis, patients receiving isoniazid should be warned about signs and symptoms of hepatotoxicity and advised to discontinue therapy and seek care if any of these occur. Patients with or at risk of chronic liver disease should have baseline liver enzymes obtained, with monthly monitoring if the results are abnormal. All patients should be clinically evaluated at least monthly to assess. Treatment using other preventive regimens (i.e. isoniazid) and treatment of patients with mild transaminase elevations (3 times upper limits of normal or less) can proceed with regular clinical and laboratory monitoring. Higher elevations of transaminases, or the development of symptoms or signs of hepatitis should be managed with discontinuation of therapy at least temporarily. Patients who complete therapy for latent tuberculosis do not need periodic monitoring for tuberculosis subsequently.

Prevention of tuberculosis

Strategies to control tuberculosis are aimed at the prevention of the spread of *M. tuberculosis* infection and the development of clinical tuberculosis. The principal approaches employed toward this end are:

- identification and treatment of infectious tuberculosis cases
- treatment of latent tuberculosis infection
- prevention of exposure to infectious particles in air, especially in hospitals and other institutions
- vaccination

Identification and treatment of infectious tuberculosis cases

Case identification and treatment reduces transmission by rendering patients with communicable tuberculosis noninfectious. Patients with pulmonary tuberculosis produce infectious aerosols that may transmit tubercle bacilli to contacts breathing the same air. When cases are identified and treated, infectiousness is rapidly eliminated. The duration of treatment required to prevent further transmission of infection is not known precisely, but experimental, clinical, and microbiological data suggest that the level of infectiousness is reduced enormously within several days of beginning effective treatment. The number of secondary infections generated by an infectious tuberculosis patient varies greatly depending on the duration of illness, the extent of pulmonary pathology, the amount of patient coughing, and the environment into which the patient expels infectious aerosols. Early diagnosis and treatment

446 CHAPTER 6 BACTERIA

reduces the number of secondary infections, while delays can result in ongoing transmission to large numbers of contacts. Failure to retain patients in treatment until they are cured also contributes to spread of infection.

Treatment of latent tuberculosis infection

This is discussed above. The benefit of treating latent infection is not only to the individual patient who does not fall ill with tuberculosis, but also accrues to the potential contacts of that patient, who might become secondarily infected were disease to develop. Targeting of high-risk groups for screening and treatment of latent tuberculosis thereby reduces tuberculosis incidence within communities. Groups that should be targeted for screening are listed in the first two columns of Table 6.25.4.

Prevention of exposure especially in hospitals and other institutions

Control of exposure to infectious aerosols can have a major impact on the spread of tuberculosis. In the late 1980s and early 1990s, transmission of tuberculosis, including multidrug-resistant tuberculosis, was widespread in hospitals, homeless shelters, and correctional facilities in New York City. More recently, the outbreak of extensively drug-resistant tuberculosis in the KwaZulu-Natal province of South Africa is a tragic reminder of the importance of infection control measures in institutions. The congregation of large numbers of highly susceptible people, especially HIV-infected persons, in closed environments with untreated tuberculosis patients has resulted in numerous microepidemics of both drug-susceptible and drug-resistant tuberculosis. Reversal of the resurgence of tuberculosis in New York at that time was attributable in large part to strengthening of infection control practices.

Identification and isolation of infected patients

Tuberculosis infection control involves prompt identification and isolation of patients with suspected tuberculosis. The decision to isolate a patient in a hospital setting is a function of epidemiological and clinical factors. Patients with known tuberculosis risk factors who present with symptoms and signs characteristic of pulmonary tuberculosis should be placed in respiratory isolation. Local epidemiological data should influence isolation practices. In settings where tuberculosis is prevalent, all HIV-infected patients with pneumonia may require isolation, whereas isolation can be more selective and based on individual patient features in low prevalence settings.

Respiratory isolation requires placement of the patient in a room with negative air pressure relative to adjoining areas, ventilation to the room should provide at least six complete air changes per hour, and air should not be recirculated without filtering or irradiation. Patients should be instructed to cover their coughs at all times, and should wear surgical face masks when outside the room to reduce aerosol generation. Anyone entering the patient's room should wear an appropriate face mask or respirator to prevent inhalation of droplet nuclei with tubercle bacilli. A considerable amount of debate has occurred in recent years in the United States of America regarding what constitutes appropriate protection for health care workers exposed to infectious tuberculosis. This debate is influenced as much by philosophy as by science, and will not be detailed here. Use of surgical masks for the protection against tuberculosis

is clearly inappropriate, even though these masks are useful when placed on patients to prevent creation of infectious aerosols. Tightly fitting face masks that filter out more than 99.7% of particles less than 0.5 μm in size (high-efficiency particle air (HEPA) filters) are effective. Other devices, including positive air pressure respirators (PAPRs), are also effective.

Use of ultraviolet germicidal irradiation can be useful for reducing the number of infectious particles in ambient air in settings where ventilation alone is not sufficient. Ultraviolet light must be concentrated in areas of rooms where exposure to people will not occur, such as upper air zones, in order to prevent skin and ocular toxicity. Areas where ultraviolet lights are often used include bronchoscopy suites, inside air circulation ducts, in emergency rooms, and in homeless shelters.

Criteria for discontinuation of respiratory isolation are listed in Box 6.25.1. Guidelines for taking patients out of isolation in the hospital are strict and are intended to protect other vulnerable patients and hospital staff from any exposure to the disease. Respiratory isolation is not usually required or practical in the home setting, and patients with infectious tuberculosis do not need to be hospitalized solely for respiratory isolation. It is assumed that contacts in the home environment will already have had significant exposure to tuberculosis by the time a diagnosis is made, and isolation of the patient affords no measurable benefit. Exceptions to this may include patients living in congregate living facilities or other special situations. The primary protective measures for contacts of cases are a clinical evaluation to identify and evaluate symptoms of tuberculosis and tuberculin skin testing with treatment of latent infection, if present. Instituting infection control measures is likely to be challenging in developing countries where the health care system is already overburdened and where facilities often lack negative pressure isolation rooms and air filtration systems. In such settings, work practice and administrative control measures have been emphasized and are considered to be more effective and less expensive. These measures consist of policies and procedures intended to promptly identify infectious tuberculosis cases so that additional precautions and health care steps can be taken.

BCG vaccination

Vaccination against tuberculosis with the bacille Calmette-Guérin (BCG) vaccine is widely administered throughout the world but is a practice mired in controversy. BCG is an attenuated live bacterial

---

Box 6.25.1 Criteria for discontinuing respiratory isolation for tuberculosis in hospital inpatients

- Alternative diagnosis established
- Infectious tuberculosis ruled out
- Tuberculosis diagnosed and:
  - Treatment given for at least 14 days *and*
  - Clinical response to therapy document, including improvement in fever and cough *and*
  - Acid-fast smears of sputum negative *or*
  - Patient discharged to home

vaccine developed in the early 20th century by Calmette and Guérin at the Institut Pasteur in Paris. After a series of uncontrolled and anecdotal assessments of the vaccine, a series of controlled trials of BCG was begun in the 1930s and continued through to the 1990s. The efficacy of BCG has varied greatly in these studies, ranging from more than 80% protection to complete lack of protection, with possibly increased risk in vaccine recipients. A meta-analysis of BCG trials performed in the early 1990s found that the weighted protective benefit of BCG was about 50% for both the prevention of active tuberculosis disease and death.

In addition to the protective efficacy observed in trials of BCG, there is evidence that BCG diminishes haematogenous dissemination of primary tuberculosis infection and thereby reduces the incidence of miliary tuberculosis and tuberculous meningitis in children. It is primarily for this reason that BCG is included in the Expanded Programme on Immunization of the WHO.

The current efficacy of BCG for preventing pulmonary tuberculosis is debated on the basis of several recent trials which have failed to show protection. Several hypotheses have been proposed for the variation in efficacy reported in various studies, including differences in susceptibility within populations, environmental exposure to mycobacteria which masks vaccine effect, and attenuation of vaccine immunogenicity. This last explanation is very compelling and fits well with clinical trial data. Unlike most vaccines, BCG is not standardized and there is no seedlot of vaccine from which new batches are derived. BCG is grown in several laboratories around the world and has not been re-passaged in animals since it was derived from cattle a century ago. Multiple commercial and noncommercial BCG products are in use presently, and comparative genomic analysis demonstrates considerable genetic heterogeneity in these strains, with many gene deletions and polymorphisms. One analysis of BCG trials found that protective efficacy was reduced in studies using multiply-passaged vaccine strains. The evidence supports the hypothesis that BCG has become further attenuated over time and no longer promotes immunity to *M. tuberculosis* infection and disease in adults. This position has not been universally accepted, however, and BCG remains one of the most widely administered vaccines in the world, largely for its perceived effects on paediatric tuberculosis.

Areas for further research

Effective global tuberculosis control will require a coordinated set of clinical and public health strategies that are based on a thorough understanding of the epidemiology, pathogenesis, and therapy of infection with *M. tuberculosis*. The WHO's DOTS strategy, which focuses on finding and effectively treating cases, has been augmented with additional strategies for intensified case-finding, use of preventive therapy, and infection control, particularly in countries with large HIV epidemics. Use of improved methods for the diagnosis and treatment of tuberculosis infection and disease, particularly drug-resistant tuberculosis, is urgently needed. Effective regimens for the treatment of MDR and extensively drug-resistant tuberculosis, with both existing and new agents, need to be developed. A better understanding of the pathogenesis of and natural immunity to tuberculosis may contribute to the development of a more effective vaccine. The sequencing of the genome of *M. tuberculosis* promises to open the door to a new generation of research

on tuberculosis and its control. Scientific progress alone, however, will be insufficient to combat tuberculosis worldwide. The willingness of societies and nations to pay for the deployment of the fruits of biomedical research, both past and future, to combat the disease where it is prevalent will be required for the conquest of tuberculosis.

Further reading

Abdool Karim SS, et al. (2011). Integration of antiretroviral therapy with tuberculosis treatment. *N Engl J Med*, **365**, 1492–501.

American Thoracic Society/Centers for Disease Control and Prevention/Infectious Disease Society of America. (2003). Treatment of Tuberculosis, 2003 ATS. CDC/IDSA Statement. *Am J Respir Crit Care Med*, **167**, 603–62.

Blanc FX, et al. (2011). Earlier versus later start of antiretroviral therapy in HIV-infected adults with tuberculosis. CAMELIA (ANRS 1295–CIPRA KH001) Study Team. *N Engl J Med*, **365**, 1471–81.

Boehme CC, et al. (2010). Rapid molecular detection of tuberculosis and rifampin resistant. *N Engl J Med*, **363**, 1005–15.

Davies PDO, Barnes P, Gordon SB (eds) (2008). *Clinical Tuberculosis*, 4th ed. Hodder Arnold.

Dooley KE, Chaisson RE (2009). Tuberculosis and diabetes mellitus: convergence of two epidemics. *Lancet Infect Dis*, **9**, 737–46.

Dorman SE, Chaisson RE (2007). From magic bullets back to the Magic Mountain: the rise of extensively drug-resistant tuberculosis. *Nat Med*, 13, 295–8.

Fox W, Ellard GA, Mitchison DA (1999). Studies on the treatment of tuberculosis undertaken by the British Medical Research Council tuberculosis units, 1946–1986, with relevant subsequent publications. *Int J Tuberc Lung Dis*, 3(10 Suppl 2), S231–79.

Gandhi NR, et al. (2006). Extensively drug-resistant tuberculosis as a cause of death in patients co-infected with tuberculosis and HIV in a rural area of South Africa. *Lancet*, **368**, 1575–80.

Havlir DV, et al.; AIDS Clinical Trials Group Study A5221 (2011). Timing of antiretroviral therapy for HIV-1 infection and tuberculosis. *N Engl J Med*, **365**, 1482–91.

Hopewell PC, et al. (2006). International standards for tuberculosis care. *Lancet Infect Dis*, **6**, 710–25.

Iseman MD (2000). *A Clinician's Guide to Tuberculosis*. Lippincott Williams & Wilkins, Philadelphia.

Lawn SD, Bekker L-G, Miller RF (2005). Immune reconstitution disease associated with mycobacterial infections in HIV infected individuals receiving antiretrovirals. *Lancet Infect Dis*, **5**, 361–73.

Maartens G, Wilkinson RJ (2007). Tuberculosis. *Lancet*, **370**, 2030–43.

Meintjes G, et al. (2010). Randomized placebo-controlled trial of prednisone for paradoxical tuberculosis-associated immune reconstitution inflammatory syndrome. *AIDS*, **24**, 2381–90.

Pai M, et al. (2009). Novel and improved technologies for tuberculosis diagnosis: progress and challenges. *Clin Chest Med*, **30**, 701–16, viii.

Rangaka M, et al. (2007). The effect of HIV-1 infection on T cell based and skin test detection of tuberculosis infection. *Am J Respir Crit Care Med*, **175**, 514–20.

Ryan F (1992). The Forgotten Plague: How the Battle Against Tuberculosis Was Won–And Lost. Little Brown, Boston.

Sterling TR, et al.; TB Trials Consortium PREVENT TB Study Team (2011). Three months of rifapentine and isoniazid for latent tuberculosis infection. *N Engl J Med*, **365**, 2155–66.

Török ME, et al. (2011). Timing of initiation of antiretroviral therapy in human immunodeficiency virus (HIV)-associated tuberculous meningitis. *Clin Infect Dis*, **52**, 1374–83.

World Health Organization (2007). *WHO Report 2007: Global tuberculosis control: surveillance, planning, financing.* Geneva, WHO/HTM/TB/2007.376

6.26 Disease caused by environmental mycobacteria

Jakko van Ingen

Essentials

Introduction—there are over 130 species of mycobacteria; species other than *M. tuberculosis* complex and *M. leprae* are collectively referred to as the nontuberculous or environmental mycobacteria (EM). Nontuberculous mycobacteria (NTM) are divided into two groups, the slow growers and the rapid growers. The most common organisms causing human disease are the slow-growing species *M. avium* complex and *M. kansasii* and, less commonly, *M. marinum*, *M. xenopi*, *M. simiae*, *M. malmoense*, and *M. ulcerans*. The rapid growers that are human pathogens are *M. abscessus*, *M. fortuitum*, and *M. chelonae*.

Ecology and epidemiology—NTM are ubiquitous in the environment and have been isolated from water, soil, domestic and wild animals, milk, and food products. Transmission to humans is though inhalation, ingestion, or traumatic inoculation. The prevalence of NTM infections is likely to have been underestimated, and appears to be increasing in developed countries.

Clinical features—four clinical syndromes have been described: (1) pulmonary disease; (2) lymphadenitis; (3) postinoculation mycobacteriosis; (4) disseminated disease. Cervical lymphadenitis is the most common presentation in children whereas chronic pulmonary disease is more frequent in adults.

Diagnosis—microscopic examination using acid fast stains and culture on appropriate media remain the cornerstone of diagnosis. The use of molecular techniques such as line probe assays, polymerase chain reaction restriction fragment length polymorphism (PCR-RFLP) analysis and 16S ribosomal DNA sequencing have enabled more accurate speciation of nontuberculous mycobacteria.

Treatment—this depends on the site and severity of the infection, the presence of predisposing conditions, and the species of mycobacterium. Therapy of disease due to slow growers is usually based on regimens containing a rifamycin, ethambutol, and either clarithromycin or azithromycin; that for rapid growers is largely empirical.

Introduction

Owing to the advent of molecular tools for identification, the genus *Mycobacterium* is now known to host over 130 species. The species other than the causative agents of tuberculosis and leprosy (Hansen's disease) are collectively referred to as nontuberculous mycobacteria or environmental mycobacteria (EM). The latter nomenclature reflects the habitats of these mycobacteria and the source of human infections. The EM are subdivided into slow and rapid growers, according to their rate of growth on subculture.

A small subset of the EM is capable of causing opportunistic infections in humans; most of these are slow growers. The bacteria of the *M. avium* complex (MAC, a complex that includes *M. avium*, *M. intracellulare*, and several rarely isolated species) are the most frequent causative agents of human infections, followed by *M. kansasii*, *M. ulcerans*, *M. marinum*, *M. malmoense*, *M. xenopi*, and *M. simiae*. Among the rapid growers, only the *M. abscessus* group, *M. chelonae*, and *M. fortuitum* are commonly associated with human infections. The relative frequency of disease caused by these species differs by geographical region. The principal pathogenic EM and the diseases associated with these species are listed in Table 6.26.1.

Ecology and epidemiology

The EM are particularly associated with soil and water. They have been isolated from various natural waters, varying from swamps to oceans, as well as from treated tap water. EM have also been isolated from domestic and wild animals, milk, and food products. Transmission to humans is by aerosol inhalation, ingestion, or traumatic inoculation. Skin test surveys have revealed that human infection is widespread and common, though overt disease is rare. Infection by EM may give rise to false-positive tuberculin skin test results and may affect the efficacy of BCG vaccination. This may explain, in part, the diversity of protection by BCG seen in various trials.

The incidence of overt disease likely results from an interplay between host susceptibility, virulence, and load of the various EM in the local environments and opportunities for infection.

Table 6.26.1 Principal pathogenic environmental mycobacteria and associated diseases

Species	Principal type of disease
Slow growers	
M. avium complex	Pulmonary disease, lymphadenitis, disseminated disease
M. kansasii	Pulmonary disease
M. xenopi	Pulmonary disease, spondylodiscitis in HIV-infected patients
M. malmoense	Pulmonary disease, lymphadenitis
M. szulgai	Pulmonary disease
M. simiae	Pulmonary disease
M. marinum	Cause of fish tank granuloma or swimming pool granuloma
M. ulcerans	Cause of Buruli ulcer disease
M. haemophilum	Lymphadenitis, skin disease in transplant recipients
M. terrae complex	Wound infections after soil contamination, tenosynovitis
M. gordonae	Common in the environment but rare cause of disease
Rapid growers	
M. abscessus	Pulmonary disease, disseminated skin disease
M. chelonae	Pulmonary disease, disseminated skin disease (both rare)
M. fortuitum	Pulmonary disease, postinoculation localized skin infections

Human transmission of overt disease is thought not to occur or to be highly exceptional.

The frequency of disease caused by different species of EM is unknown; this is because, unlike tuberculosis, reporting of cases is not mandatory. In the United States a nationwide survey of 32 000 mycobacterial isolates conducted in 1979 to 1980 indicated that 2/3 were EM. The estimated prevalence of disease caused by EM was 1.8 per 100 000 population in the 1980s. Clinical and laboratory studies from the United States, Canada, and Australia indicate that the burden of EM has been underestimated and is increasing in developed countries. This may be a result of increased clinical attention, improved laboratory techniques for detection, and a growing number of people at increased risk because of immunosuppressive drug use, chronic pulmonary diseases, and HIV infection.

Clinical features

The NTM cause four main types of disease: pulmonary, lymphadenitis, postinoculation, and disseminated.

Pulmonary disease

Chronic pulmonary disease

Chronic pulmonary infections are the most frequent disease manifestation of EM. Estimates of the incidence of pulmonary disease caused by EM differ from 1 per 100 000 population per year in Denmark to 4.3 per 100 000 population per year in Ontario, Canada. In many regions, the incidence of environmental mycobacterial disease in the middle-aged and elderly white population exceeds that of tuberculosis.

Two distinct disease entities exist; the cavitary disease type, radiologically similar to tuberculosis (see Fig. 6.26.1), affects patients with pre-existent pulmonary diseases, especially chronic obstructive pulmonary disease. As a result, it is more common among men and usually appears in their late 50s or 60s. The nodular-bronchiectatic disease type (Fig. 6.26.2) is a more subtle disease that mostly affects the lingula and middle lobe. This disease type is more common among female lifetime nonsmokers with no significant pulmonary history.

The symptoms of cough, malaise, weight loss, and reduced exercise tolerance develop over months or even years. Especially for the cavitary disease type, clinical distinction from tuberculosis is difficult, though its course is more prolonged. Diagnosis relies on isolation and accurate identification of the causative agents. Because these are environmental organisms, a single culture yielding EM is insufficient for diagnosis. Positive cultures from nonsterile samples such as those from the respiratory tract can result from accidental presence after environmental exposure or contamination during sample acquisition or handling. Hence, clinical and radiological as well as microbiological (i.e. multiple positive cultures yielding the same species) signs of infection must be obtained and other disease rigorously excluded to make a diagnosis of true environmental mycobacterial disease. Especially in the nodular-bronchiectatic disease type, bronchial washings and CT imaging are often required for diagnosis and follow-up.

Acute pulmonary disease

Environmental mycobacteria, especially MAC, can cause a hypersensitivity pneumonitis. Exposure is often from indoor spas, hence the name 'hot tub lung'. This acute or subacute disease results from either inflammation after antigen exposure, or true infection, or both. Dyspnoea, cough, and fever are the most common symptoms. Occasionally, hypoxemic respiratory failure may occur and require intervention. CT reveals diffuse infiltrates with prominent nodularity of all lung fields. The optimal treatment remains controversial and corticosteroids, antimycobacterial treatment, or both can be successful. Interrupting exposure to the mycobacteria is the most important intervention.

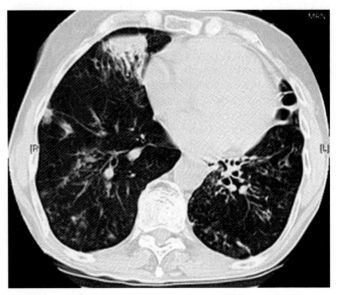

Fig. 6.26.1 Chest radiograph of a patient with right upper lobe cavitary *M. avium* disease

Fig. 6.26.2 CT image of nodular bronchiectatic *M. intracellulare* pulmonary disease.

Lymphadenitis

Lymphadenitis is the second most frequent environmental myco-bacterial disease. It predominantly, though not exclusively, affects immunocompetent children under the age of 8 years. Cervicofacial lymph nodes are most frequently affected, although infection of axillar and inguinal lymph nodes has been reported. Disease that involves the abdominal lymph nodes is observed in HIV-infected patients. In these patients, as well as in otherwise immunocompromised patients, lymphadenitis can be a sign of disseminated disease (see below).

Lymphadenitis is generally caused by slow-growing EM, mostly *M. avium* complex, *M. haemophilum*, *M. malmoense*, and *M. kansasii*. The different species seem to affect children of different ages, with *M. avium* affecting the youngest. The risk is reduced by neonatal BCG vaccination. Surgical treatment is curative and lymph node excision is preferred over incision and drainage, which may lead to sinus formation. A 3-month regimen of rifabutin and clarithromycin or a wait-and-see policy can be successful in selected cases.

Post-inoculation mycobacterioses

Postinoculation mycobacterioses affect the organs that have immediate interactions with the environment, i.e. the skin and the eyes. It remains unknown whether the mycobacteria are permanent members of the human skin microbiome. Skin disease caused by EM need not be a postinoculation disease; it may be a sign of disseminated disease (see below).

Localized skin infections

EM cause two named postinoculation skin diseases with characteristic clinical features: Buruli ulcer disease is a severe skin infection by *M. ulcerans*, presenting as nodular or, in later stages, ulcerative lesions and is endemic to parts of West Africa, Australia and Latin America, with minor pockets in East Asia. The source of *M. ulcerans* infection remains controversial, although water insects may be vectors. This disease is covered in Chapter 6.28. The swimming pool granuloma or fish tank granuloma is a localized nodular or pustular, sometimes ulcerative, skin lesion resulting from local infection of an existing skin abrasion by *M. marinum*. The infection is acquired during swimming or fish tank cleaning activities. There may be 'sporotrichoid' spread of lesions along the draining lymphatics. The disease can be self-limiting, but chemotherapy accelerates resolution. Local spread of the infection can occur and lead to tenosynovitis, osteomyelitis or even disseminated disease.

Most other cases of postinoculation environmental mycobacterioses are caused by rapid-growing *M. fortuitum* and *M. chelonae*. These include injection site abscesses and footbath-associated furunculosis. These diseases present as sporadic cases, though miniepidemics may be noted as a result of reusing of contaminated drug vials or needles or suboptimal hygiene measures in nail salons or other spas. Injection site abscesses may take months to develop and are either localized abscesses or multiple abscesses with spreading cellulitis. The latter occurs in patients who inject frequently, e.g. insulin-dependent diabetics. Surgical excision or drainage cures localized disease; 2 to 4 months of antibiotic treatment can be warranted for multiple or spreading lesions.

Tenosynovitis caused by EM is rare (Fig. 6.26.3); gardeners seem to be at increased risk and inoculation occurs in wounds from thorns or other plant material. Bacteria of the *M. terrae* -*M. nonchromogenicum* complex are the most frequent causative

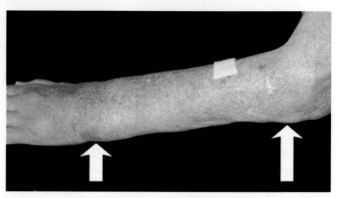

Fig. 6.26.3 Erythematous swelling in tenosynovitis caused by *M. malmoense*.

agents and related to wound contamination with soil. In rare cases, *M. kansasii*, *M. malmoense*, and rapid growers have been isolated.

Eye infections

Trauma to the cornea can lead to infection by rapid-growing *M. fortuitum* or *M. chelonae*. These localized infections respond well to topical treatment with combinations of macrolides, quinolones and aminoglycosides. Corneal grafting and systemic therapy may be warranted in severe cases.

Post-surgical infections

Accidental inoculation may occur during surgery with contaminated materials and can lead to severe infections. Osteomyelitis of the sternum and endocarditis with septicaemia has been reported after cardiac surgery. Again, causative agents are mainly rapid growers.

Disseminated disease

Prior to the HIV pandemic, disseminated infections by EM were rare and restricted to patients with congenital immune deficiencies. Disseminated disease caused by *M. avium* (or, less frequently, *M. genavense* or *M. simiae*) was an important and frequently lethal clinical entity during the early phase of the HIV pandemic, before the advent of highly active antiretroviral therapy (HAART). This was particularly true for countries with a low tuberculosis burden. Disseminated *M. avium* infection was far less frequent in HIV-infected patients in Africa. Dissemination of the causative mycobacteria was thought to start from the intestines, as many patients were known to harbour *M. avium* in their faeces before the onset of disseminated disease.

Since the introduction of HAART disseminated environmental mycobacterial disease has become infrequent in HIV-infected patients. At the same time, notification of this disease has not diminished, as more cases are now diagnosed in patients who are treated with immunosuppressive drugs, mostly after solid organ transplantation or in patients with haematological malignancies. In these 'new' patient categories, the dominant causative agents are *M. avium*, *M. genavense*, *M. haemophilum*, and *M. chelonae*. Disseminated disease presents with two distinct clinical syndromes. *M. avium* and the difficult to culture *M. genavense* cause a nonspecific disease with symptoms of fever, weight loss, night sweats, malaise, and anaemia (or, in *M. genavense* disease, pancytopenia); diarrhoea, abdominal lymph node enlargement and abdominal pain are frequent, especially in patients with HIV infection. The diagnosis is usually made by culture of bone marrow, liver or other biopsies, or by blood culture. *M. haemophilum* and the rapid growers cause a disseminated disease with subcutaneous abscesses, nodular lesions, or skin ulceration. This disease appears to be more common in patients with haematological malignancies. Their localization to the skin has been related to these species' preferences for lower temperatures. Diagnosis is usually made by culture and histological examination of biopsies of lesions, or blood cultures. Disease caused by *M. haemophilum* can be difficult to diagnose as the bacteria need an external iron source (e.g. blood, hence its name) for *in vitro* growth.

Diagnosis

Microscopic examination using acid fast stains and culture on appropriate media remain the cornerstone of diagnosis. Specimens may be stained with the Ziehl -Neelsen stain or one of its modifications, e.g. Kinyoun stain, and appear pink as a result of staining with carbol-fuschin. Microscopy is relatively insensitive as it requires at least 10 000 organisms per ml of sputum for smear positivity. The sensitivity of microscopy may be improved by use of a fluorochrome stain such as auramine-O or auramine-rhodamine and examination by fluorescence microscopy.

Mycobacterial culture is more sensitive but more time-consuming than microscopy as it requires specialized equipment and a containment level 3 facility. Non-sterile specimens such as sputum should be decontaminated before culture in order to eliminate more common bacteria or fungi that would overwhelm growth of mycobacteria. Sterile samples such as serous fluids, blood, or cerebrospinal fluid can be inoculated directly on to appropriate solid media (e.g. Middlebrook 7H11) or liquid media (e.g. BACTEC 12B broth or Mycobacteria growth indicator tube, MGIT).

Once cultures have grown speciation is performed by molecular tools such as line probe assays, polymerase chain reaction restriction fragment length polymorphism (PCR-RFLP) analysis, or 16S ribosomal DNA sequencing, which has enabled more accurate speciation of EM.

Susceptibility testing of EM is done in specialist reference laboratories.

Treatment

The choice of therapy depends on the causative agents and their *in vitro* susceptibility, the predisposing conditions and their prognosis, and the site of disease as well as its severity. In general, there is a lack of evidence for the efficacy of regimens as very few clinical trials have been performed.

For skin disease caused by *M. marinum*, drug susceptibility tests have a limited role as the disease usually responds to monotherapy with doxycycline, minocycline, or trimethoprim-sulfamethoxazole, or the combination of rifampicin and ethambutol. Multidrug therapy may be indicated in severe, spreading disease. Surgical excision, curettage, or drainage cures localized skin disease caused by rapid growers (see above) and surgical excision is the treatment of choice for lymphadenitis and even single nodular pulmonary lesions. For extrapulmonary disease by rapid growers where chemotherapy is needed, results of drug susceptibility tests should guide the selection of a regimen. A minimum of two active drugs is needed, based on the severity of disease and a treatment duration of 3 to 6 months may be indicated; timing of clinical improvement guides

Table 6.26.2 Recommended regimens for treatment of pulmonary infections caused by the more usually encountered slow-growing environmental mycobacteria in HIV-negative patients

Species	Regimen	Areas of uncertainty
M. avium complex	18–24 months of rifampicin, ethambutol and a macrolide *or* 24 months of rifampicin and ethambutol	Role of macrolides, role of aminoglycosides in severe disease
M. kansasii	9 months rifampicin and ethambutol	
M. xenopi	24 months rifampicin and ethambutol	Role of macrolides and quinolones
M. malmoense	24 months rifampicin and ethambutol	Role of macrolides and quinolones

the treatment duration. For extrapulmonary and disseminated disease caused by slow-growing species, mainly *M. avium*, treatment regimens should include a macrolide (clarithromycin, azithromycin), a rifamycin (rifampicin, rifabutin), and ethambutol.

Pulmonary disease by EM is difficult to treat; the long treatment duration and drug toxicities are a significant burden for patients. For disease caused by slow growers, mainly MAC, drug susceptibility results are only helpful for the macrolides. In case of macrolide susceptibility, most clinicians have adopted the use of macrolides, combined with rifampicin and ethambutol, despite limited evidence for additional efficacy of macrolides (Table 6.26.2). These regimens should be used for a total duration of 24 months or up to 1 year after culture conversion. The notable exception is *M. kansasii* for which short (9 month) regimens of rifampicin and ethambutol are highly effective. The role of quinolones in pulmonary disease by slow growers seems limited.

For pulmonary disease by rapid growers, mostly the *M. abscessus* group and *M. fortuitum*, drug susceptibility results guide the selection of drug regimens. For *M. abscessus* group infections, a macrolide combined with amikacin and cefoxitin, tigecycline or imipenem is often used. For *M. chelonae*, cefoxitin is inactive and tobramycin is more active than amikacin. Macrolides may not be effective against *M. fortuitum* owing to natural resistance and a multidrug regimen that combines a quinolone with doxycycline, trimethoprim-sulfamethoxazole, an aminoglycoside or imipenem can be used. Treatment duration in pulmonary disease by rapid growers is usually 4 to 6 months.

Cure rates of pulmonary disease by EM are limited, in the 50 to 70% range; *M. kansasii* disease has more favourable outcome. Adjunctive surgical resection of the affected areas of the lung improves outcomes in selected cases.

To achieve success in the treatment of environmental mycobacterial disease, optimal treatment of the underlying and predisposing conditions is vital.

Further reading

Griffith DE, *et al.* (2007). An official ATS/IDSA statement: diagnosis, treatment, and prevention of nontuberculous mycobacterial diseases. *Am J Respir Crit Care Med*, **175**, 367–416.

Falkinham JO III (2009). Surrounded by mycobacteria: nontuberculous mycobacteria in the human environment. *J Appl Microbiol*, **107**, 356–67.

Lindeboom JA, *et al.* (2007). Surgical excision versus antibiotic treatment for nontuberculous mycobacterial cervicofacial lymphadenitis in children: a multicenter, randomized, controlled trial. *Clin Infect Dis*, **44**, 1057–64.

Research Committee of the British Thoracic Society (2008). Clarithromycin vs ciprofloxacin as adjuncts to rifampicin and ethambutol in treating opportunist mycobacterial lung diseases and an assessment of *Mycobacterium vaccae* immunotherapy. *Thorax*, **63**, 627–34.

Subcommittee of the Joint Tuberculosis Committee of the British Thoracic Society (2000). Management of opportunist mycobacterial infections: Joint Tuberculosis Committee guidelines 1999. *Thorax*, **55**, 210–18.

van Ingen J, van Soolingen D (2011). Cervicofacial lymphadenitis caused by nontuberculous mycobacteria; host, environmental or bacterial factors? *Int J Pediatr Otorhinolaryngol*, **75**, 722–3.

Wolinsky E (1979). Nontuberculous mycobacteria and associated diseases. *Am Rev Respir Dis*, **119**, 107–59.

6.27 Leprosy (Hansen's disease)

Diana N.J. Lockwood

Essentials

Leprosy is a chronic granulomatous disease caused by *Mycobacterium leprae*, an acid-fast intracellular organism not yet cultivated *in vitro*. It is an important public health problem worldwide, with an estimated 4 million people disabled by the disease. Transmission of *M. leprae* is only partially understood, but untreated lepromatous patients discharge abundant organisms from their nasal mucosa into the environment.

Clinical features

These are determined by the degree of cell-mediated immunity towards *M. leprae*, with tuberculoid (paucibacillary) and lepromatous leprosy (multibacillary) being the two poles of a spectrum: (1) tuberculoid—well-expressed cell-mediated immunity effectively controls bacillary multiplication with the formation of organized epithelioid-cell granulomas; (2) lepromatous—there is cellular anergy towards *M. leprae* with abundant bacillary multiplication. Between these two poles is a continuum, varying from the patient with moderate cell-mediated immunity (borderline tuberculoid), through borderline, to the patient with little cellular response, borderline lepromatous.

Presenting symptoms—most commonly (1) anaesthesia—ranging from a small area of numbness on the skin due to involvement of a dermal nerve, to peripheral neuropathy with affected nerves tender and thickened; (2) skin lesions—most commonly macules or plaques; tuberculoid patients have few, hypopigmented lesions that are anaesthetic; lepromatous patients have numerous, sometimes confluent lesions.

Other manifestations—these include (1) type 1 (reversal reactions)—occur in borderline patients; characterized by acute neuritis and/or acutely inflamed skin lesions; often occur in the first 2 months after starting treatment; (2) type 2 (erythema nodosum leprosum reactions)—occur in up to 50% of patients with lepromatous leprosy; (3) neuritis—silent neuropathy is an important form of nerve damage, causing lifelong morbidity; (4) eye disease—blindness occurs in at least 2.5% of patients.

Diagnosis

This is made by recognition of typical skin lesions or thickened peripheral nerves, supported by the finding of acid-fast bacilli on slit skin smears that should be taken from at least four sites (earlobes, and edges of active lesions).

Treatment

There are six main principles of treatment: (1) stop the infection with chemotherapy—first-line antileprosy drugs are rifampicin, clofazimine, and dapsone, given in combination and duration as determined by whether disease is paucibacillary or multibacillary; these are highly effective in killing bacilli but may not halt nerve damage; (2) treat new nerve damage—a 6-month course of steroids should be given to those with nerve damage for less than 6 months; (3) treat reactions—steroids are likely to be required; (4) educate the patient about leprosy; (5) prevent disability; and (6) support the patient socially and psychologically—patients with leprosy the world over are frequently stigmatized; words such as 'leper' should be avoided; the disease can be referred to as 'Hansen's disease'.

Prevention

Vaccination with bacille Calmette–Guérin (BCG) can provide some protection against leprosy (20–80% in different trials).

Aetiology

Leprosy is caused by *Mycobacterium leprae*, an acid-fast intracellular organism not yet cultivated *in vitro*. It was first identified in the nodules of patients with lepromatous leprosy by Hansen in 1873. *M. leprae* preferentially parasitizes skin macrophages and peripheral nerve Schwann cells.

In vivo cultivation of *M. leprae*

M. leprae can be grown in the mouse footpad, but growth is slow, taking over 6 months to produce significant yields. The nine-banded armadillo is susceptible to *M. leprae* infection and develops lepromatous disease. The armadillo and mouse models of *M. leprae* infection have been useful for producing *M. leprae* for biological studies and studying drug sensitivity patterns, respectively.

Biological characteristics

M. leprae is a stable hardy organism that withstands drying for up to 5 months. It has a doubling time of 12 days (compared with 20 min for *Escherichia coli*). The optimum growth temperature is 27 to 30°C, consistent with the clinical observation of maximal *M. leprae* growth at cool superficial sites (skin, nasal mucosa, and peripheral nerves). *M. leprae* isolates from different parts of the world have similar biological characteristics. *M. leprae* possesses a complex cell wall comprising lipids and carbohydrates. It synthesizes a species-specific phenolic glycolipid and lipoarabinomannan.

Antibody and T-cell screening have identified numerous protein antigens and peptides that are important immune targets.

M. leprae genome

M. leprae has a 3.27-Mb genome that displays extreme reductive evolution. Less than one-half of the genome contains functional genes and many pseudogenes are present. One hundred and sixty-five genes are unique to M. leprae and functions can be attributed to 29 of them. These unique proteins are being identified and analysed to aid in development of new diagnostic tests. Comparison of biosynthetic pathways with Mycobacterium tuberculosis is giving new insights into M. leprae metabolism. For lipolysis M. leprae has only two genes (M. tuberculosis has 22); M. leprae has also lost many genes for carbon catabolism and many carbon sources (e.g. acetate and galactose) are unavailable to it. This gene loss leaves M. leprae unable to respond to different environments and under-lies the impossibility of growing the organism in vitro. Using comparative genomics and analysis of single nucleotide polymorphisms it has been shown that all extant cases of leprosy can be attributed to a single clone which then disseminated worldwide. Leprosy probably originated in India or eastern Africa and spread with successive human migrations.

Epidemiology

Leprosy continues to be an important public health problem worldwide. In 2010, 244 796 new cases were detected and registered. The highest numbers of cases were in India, Brazil, Indonesia, Bangladesh, and the Democratic Republic of Congo. India accounts for 64% of the global disease burden. From 1990, the World Health Organization (WHO) has led a leprosy elimination campaign and this defined elimination as less than 1 case per 10 000 population. Prevalence figures are highly influenced by operational activities such as reducing the length of treatment. The global focus is now on detecting new cases and providing sustainable care for leprosy patients. An estimated 4 million people are disabled by leprosy. Leprosy has not always been a tropical disease; it was widespread in medieval Europe and was endemic in Norway until the early 20th century. In North America, small foci of infection still exist in Texas and Louisiana. Nearly all new patients now seen in Europe and North America have acquired their infection abroad.

Risk factors

Leprosy is a chronic disease with a long incubation period. An average incubation time of 2 to 5 years has been calculated for tuberculoid cases and 8 to 12 years for lepromatous cases. American servicemen who developed leprosy after serving in the tropics presented up to 20 years after their presumed exposure. Most leprosy patients do not have known contact with a leprosy patient. Age, sex, and household contact are important determinants of leprosy risk; incidence reaches a peak at 10 to 14 years; the excess of male cases is attributed to women's reluctance to present to health workers with skin lesions. Poor nutritional status is cited as predisposing to leprosy but no good evidence substantiates this. Improved socioeconomic conditions, extended schooling, and good housing conditions reduce the risk of leprosy. Subclinical infection with M. leprae is probably common but the development of established disease is rare. Little work has been done on the early events in infection with M. leprae because there is no simple test that can establish whether an individual has encountered M. leprae and mounted a protective immune response.

HIV and leprosy

It was predicted that HIV infection would produce anergic, lepromatous leprosy, However HIV/leprosy coinfected patients have disease types across the leprosy spectrum with typical leprosy skin lesions and nerve involvement. Their skin lesions have typical leprosy histology with granuloma formation even in the presence of low circulating CD4 counts. Patients coinfected with HIV and leprosy are at higher risk of developing leprosy reactions and nerve damage. Leprosy may also present as an immune reconstitution syndrome (IRIS) in patients who have recently started on highly active antiretroviral therapy (HAART) and have rising CD4 counts and a falling viral load. These patients have borderline leprosy which is very immunologically active with inflamed skin lesions and reactions.

Transmission

The transmission of M. leprae is only partially understood. Untreated lepromatous patients discharge abundant organisms from their nasal mucosa into the environment. Studies in Indonesia and Ethiopia using polymerase chain reaction (PCR) primers to detect M. leprae DNA in nasal swabs have shown that up to 5% of the population in leprosy endemic areas carry M. leprae DNA in their noses. The organism is then inhaled, multiplies on the inferior turbinates, and has a brief bacteraemic phase before binding to and entering Schwann cells and macrophages. The combination of an environmentally well-adapted organism, high carriage rates, and a long incubation period means that, even with effective antibiotics, transmission will continue for a long time.

Pathogenesis

Leprosy is a bacterial infection in which the clinical features are determined by the host's immune response (Table 6.27.1).

Immune response to M. leprae and the leprosy spectrum

The Ridley–Jopling classification (Fig. 6.27.1) places patients on a spectrum of disease according to their clinical features, bacterial load, and histological and immunological responses. The two poles of the spectrum are tuberculoid (TT; paucibacillary) and lepromatous leprosy (LL; multibacillary). At the tuberculoid pole, well-expressed cell-mediated immunity effectively controls bacillary multiplication with the formation of organized epithelioid-cell granulomas; at the lepromatous pole there is cellular anergy towards M. leprae with abundant bacillary multiplication. Between these two poles is a continuum, varying from the patient with moderate cell-mediated immunity (borderline tuberculoid, BT) through borderline (BB) to the patient with little cellular response, borderline lepromatous (BL). The polar groups (TT, LL) are stable, but within the central groups (BT, BB, BL) the disease tends to downgrade to the lepromatous pole in the absence of treatment, and upgrading towards the tuberculoid pole may occur during or after treatment.

Both T cells and macrophages play important roles in the processing, recognition, and response to M. leprae antigens.

Table 6.27.1 Major clinical features of the disease spectrum in leprosy

Clinical features	Classification				
	Tuberculoid (TT)	Borderline tuberculoid (BT)	Borderline (BB)	Borderline lepromatous (BL)	Lepromatous (LL)
	Paucibacillary			Multibacillary	
Skin					
Infiltrated lesions	Defined plaques, healing centres	Irregular plaques with partially raised edges	Polymorphic, 'punched out centres'	Papules, nodules	Diffuse thickening
Macular lesions	Single, small	Several, any size, 'geographical'	Multiple, all sizes, bizarre	Innumerable, small	Innumerable, confluent
Nerve					
Peripheral nerve	Solitary enlarged nerves	Several nerves, asymmetrical	Many nerves, asymmetrical pattern	Late neural thickening, asymmetrical, anaesthesia and paresis	Slow symmetrical loss, glove and stocking anaesthesia
Microbiology					
Bacterial index	0–1	0–2	2–3	1–4	4–6
Histology					
Lymphocytes	+	++	±	++	±
Macrophages	–	–	±	–	–
Epithelioid cells	++	±	–	–	–
Antibody, anti-*M. leprae*	–/+	–/++	+	++	++

+, present, ++, present strongly, –, absent.

In tuberculoid leprosy, *in vitro* tests of T-cell function such as lymphocyte transformation tests show a strong response to *M. leprae* protein antigens with the production of Th1-type cytokines such as interferon-γ and interleukin 2 (IL-2). Skin tests with lepromin, a heat-killed *M. leprae* preparation, are strongly positive. Staining of skin biopsies from tuberculoid lesions with T-cell markers shows highly organized granulomas composed predominantly of CD4 cells and macrophages with a peripheral mantle of CD8 cells. This strong cell-mediated immune response clears bacilli but with concomitant local tissue destruction, especially in nerves.

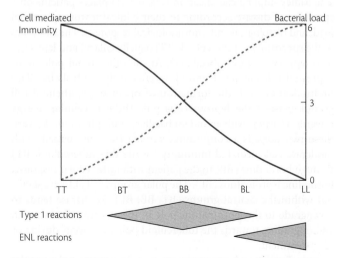

Fig. 6.27.1 Ridley–Jopling spectrum of bacterial load, cell-mediated immunity, and reactions.

Patients with lepromatous leprosy have no cell-mediated immunity to *M. leprae* with a failure of the T-cell and macrophage response. Tests for lepromin are negative. This anergy is specific for *M. leprae*. Patients with lepromatous disease respond to other mycobacteria such as *M. tuberculosis*, both *in vitro* and in skin tests. Identification of cell types in lepromatous granulomas shows a disorganized mixture of macrophages and T cells, mainly CD8 cells. The T-cell failure may be due to clonal anergy or active suppression. Defects in cytokine production have been demonstrated; intralesional injections of recombinant IL-2 reconstitute the local immune response with elimination of *M. leprae* from macrophages. There is low production of Th2-type cytokines. Macrophage defects described in lepromatous disease include defective antigen presentation and recognition, defective IL-1 production, a failure of macrophages to kill *M. leprae*, and a macrophage suppression of the T-cell response. Patients with lepromatous leprosy produce a range of autoantibodies that are both organ specific (against thyroid, nerve, testis, and gastric mucosa) and nonspecific, such as rheumatoid factors, anti-DNA, cryoglobulins, and cardiolipin.

Bacterial load

In lepromatous leprosy, bacilli spread haematogenously to cool superficial sites including eyes, upper respiratory mucosa, testes, small muscles, and bones of the hands, feet, and face as well as to peripheral nerves and skin. The heavy bacterial load causes structural damage at all these sites. In tuberculoid leprosy, bacilli are not readily found.

Nerve damage

Neural inflammation is pathognomonic of leprosy. Nerve damage occurs in small nerve fibres, both sensory and autonomic, in the skin and in peripheral nerve trunks. Nerve damage occurs before diagnosis, during treatment, and after treatment. In lepromatous infection, almost all the cutaneous nerves and peripheral nerve trunks are involved. Bacilli are found in Schwann, perineural, and endothelial cells. Extensive demyelination occurs and later wallerian degeneration. Despite large numbers of organisms in the nerve there is only a small inflammatory response, but ultimately the nerve becomes fibrotic and is hyalinized. At the tuberculoid end of the spectrum nerve damage is secondary to a granulomatous response to *M. leprae* antigens. Perineural inflammation and epithelioid granulomas destroy the Schwann cells and axons. In borderline leprosy the combination of *M. leprae* antigens and a cell-mediated immune response results in small granulomas abutting strands of normal-looking but heavily bacillated Schwann cells giving rise to the widespread nerve damage in borderline leprosy. The persistence of *M. leprae* antigens in Schwann cells means that immune-mediated nerve damage can occur after successful antibacterial treatment.

Leprosy reactions

Leprosy reactions are events superimposed on the Ridley–Jopling spectrum. Type 1 (reversal reactions) occur in borderline patients (BT, BB, BL) and are delayed hypersensitivity reactions caused by increased recognition of *M. leprae* antigens in skin and nerve sites. They are characterized by an increase in lymphocytes (CD4 and IL-2-producing cells) within lesions, severe oedema with disruption of the granuloma, and giant cell formation. There is local production of Th1-type cytokines such as interferon-γ and tumour necrosis factor-α.

Type 2 reactions, erythema nodosum leprosum (ENL), are partly due to immune complex deposition and occur in patients with borderline lepromatous and lepromatous leprosy who produce antibodies and have a large antigen load. There is vasculitis with lesional immunoglobulin deposition, complement activation, and polymorphs and circulating immune complexes. There is also enhanced T-cell activity with increased CD8 cells, increased circulating IL-2 receptors, and high levels of circulating tumour necrosis factor-α. After reaction, lepromatous patients revert to a state of immunological unresponsiveness.

Clinical features of leprosy

Patients commonly present with skin lesions, weakness or numbness due to a peripheral nerve lesion, or a burn or ulcer on an anaesthetic hand or foot. Borderline patients may present in reaction with nerve pain, sudden palsy, multiple new skin lesions, pain in the eye, or a systemic febrile illness. The cardinal signs are:

- typical skin lesions, anaesthetic at the tuberculoid end of the spectrum
- thickened peripheral nerves
- acid-fast bacilli on skin smears or biopsy

Early lesions

The commonest early lesion is an area of numbness on the skin or a visible skin lesion. The classic early skin lesion is indeterminate leprosy, which is commonly found on the face, extensor surface of the limbs, buttocks, or trunk. Indeterminate lesions consist of one or more slightly hypopigmented or erythematous macules, a few centimetres in diameter, with poorly defined margins. Hair growth and nerve function are unimpaired. A biopsy may show the perineurovascular infiltrate and only scanty acid-fast bacilli. The indeterminate phase may last for months or years before resolving or developing into one of the determinate types of leprosy.

Skin

The commonest skin lesions are macules or plaques; papules and nodules are more rare. Lesions may be found anywhere although rarely in the axillae, perineum, or hairy scalp. Skin lesions should be assessed for inflammation, colour, and sensation. Tuberculoid patients have few granulomatous hypopigmented lesions while lepromatous patients have numerous, sometimes confluent lesions. The few tuberculoid lesions are usually asymmetrical; more numerous lesions are likely to be distributed symmetrically.

Anaesthesia

Anaesthesia may occur in skin lesions when dermal nerves are involved or in the distribution of a large peripheral nerve. In skin lesions the small dermal sensory and autonomic nerve fibres supplying dermal and subcutaneous structures are damaged causing local sensory loss and loss of sweating within that area.

Peripheral neuropathy

Peripheral nerve trunks are vulnerable at sites where they are superficial or are in fibro-osseous tunnels. At these points a small increase in nerve diameter raises intraneural pressure causing neural compression and ischaemia. Damage to peripheral nerve trunks produces characteristic signs with dermatomal sensory loss and dysfunction of muscles supplied by that peripheral nerve. The predilection sites for peripheral nerve involvement are ulnar nerve (at the elbow) (Fig. 6.27.2), median nerve (at the wrist), radial nerve, radial cutaneous nerve (at the wrist), common peroneal nerve (at the knee), posterior tibial and sural nerves at the ankle, facial nerve as it crosses the zygomatic arch, and great auricular nerve in the posterior triangle of the neck (Fig. 6.27.3). All these

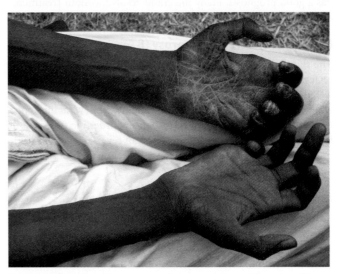

Fig. 6.27.2 The effects of ulnar and median nerve paralysis with wasting of the small muscles of the hand and evidence of neuropathic damage. (Copyright D A Warrell).

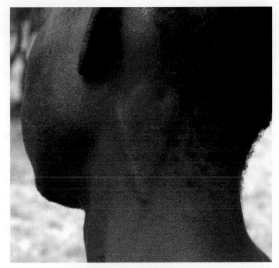

Fig. 6.27.3 Thickening of greater auricular nerve.
(Copyright D A Warrell.)

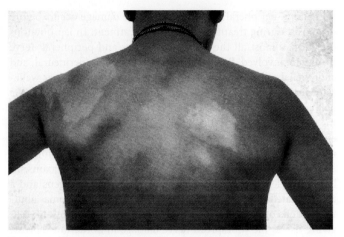

Fig. 6.27.4 BT leprosy. This Ethiopian woman was several hypopigmented patches. Testing for anaesthesia will confirm the diagnosis of BT leprosy.

nerves should be examined for enlargement and tenderness. Peripheral nerve function should be assessed by testing the motor function of the small muscles of the hands and feet using the Medical Research Council (MRC) grading scale. Sensory function is best assessed using graded nylon monofilaments (Semmes–Weinstein) as in diabetic screening. Patients should be asked about symptoms of neuropathy.

Tuberculoid leprosy (TT)

Infection is localized and asymmetrical. A typical tuberculoid skin lesion is a macule or plaque, single, erythematous, or purple, with raised and clear-cut edges sloping towards a flattened hypopigmented centre. The surface is anaesthetized, dry, and hairless. Sensory impairment may be difficult to demonstrate on the face where there are abundant nerve endings. If peripheral nerve trunk involvement is present, only one nerve trunk is enlarged. No *M. leprae* are found in skin smears. True tuberculoid leprosy has a good prognosis, many infections resolve without treatment, and peripheral nerve trunk damage is limited.

Borderline tuberculoid leprosy (BT)

The skin lesions are similar to tuberculoid leprosy and there may be few or many lesions (Figs. 6.27.4, 6.27.5). The margins are less well defined and there may be satellite lesions. Damage to peripheral nerves is widespread and severe, usually with several thickened nerve trunks. It is important to recognize borderline tuberculoid leprosy because these patients are at risk of reversal reactions leading to rapid deterioration in nerve function with consequent deformities.

Borderline leprosy (BB)

Borderline disease is the most unstable part of the spectrum and patients usually downgrade towards lepromatous leprosy if they are not treated or upgrade towards tuberculoid leprosy as part of a reversal reaction. There are numerous skin lesions which may be macules, papules, or plaques and they vary in size, shape, and distribution. The edges of the lesions may have streaming, irregular

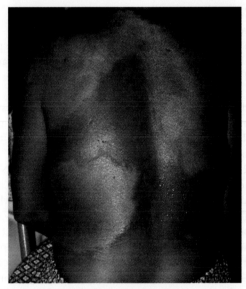

Fig. 6.27.5 Active tuberculoid lesions showing the sharp outer edge, thin raised erythematous dry rim, and the broad hypopigmented dry centre. The 'satellite' lesion at the lower outer edge indicates that this is borderline tuberculoid leprosy. Biopsies and smears should be taken from the raised active rim.
(Copyright D A Warrell.)

borders. Annular lesions with a broad irregular edge and a sharply defined punched-out centre are characteristic of borderline disease (Fig. 6.27.6). Nerve damage is variable.

Borderline lepromatous leprosy (BL)

This is characterized by widespread variable asymmetrical skin lesions. There may be erythematous or hyperpigmented papules, succulent nodules or plaques, and sensation in the lesions may be normal (Fig. 6.27.8). Peripheral nerve involvement is widespread. While patients with borderline lepromatous leprosy do not have the extreme consequences of bacillary multiplication that are seen in lepromatous disease, they may experience either or both reversal and ENL reactions.

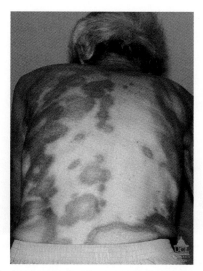

Fig. 6.27.6 Multiple, asymmetrical erythematous lesions. Sensation was intact inside the lesions.

Lepromatous leprosy (LL)

The patient with untreated polar lepromatous leprosy may be carrying 10^{11} leprosy bacilli. The onset of disease is frequently insidious, the earliest lesions being ill-defined, shiny, hypopigmented, or erythematous macules. Gradually the skin becomes infiltrated and thickened and nodules develop (Fig. 6.27.7); facial skin thickening causes the characteristic leonine facies (Fig. 6.27.9). Hair is lost, especially the lateral third of the eyebrows (madarosis). Dermal nerves are destroyed leading to a progressive glove and stocking anaesthesia. Position sense is preserved. Sweating is lost, which is uncomfortable in the tropics as compensatory sweating occurs in the remaining intact areas. Damage to peripheral nerves is symmetrical and occurs late in the disease. Infiltration of the corneal nerves causes anaesthesia of the cornea, which predisposes to injury, secondary infection, and blindness (Fig. 6.27.10).

Nasal symptoms can often be elicited early in the disease. Septal perforation may occur. There may be papules on the lips and nodules on the palate, uvula, tongue, and gums (Fig. 6.27.11). Bone involvement is common, with absorption of the terminal phalanges and pencilling of the heads and shafts of the metatarsals. Testicular atrophy results from diffuse infiltration compounded by acute orchitis that may occur during ENL reactions. The consequent loss of

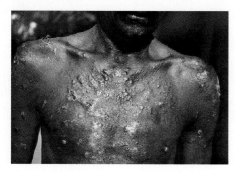

Fig. 6.27.7 Advanced nodular lepromatous leprosy. This Indian patient presented with ulcerating nodules all over his body.

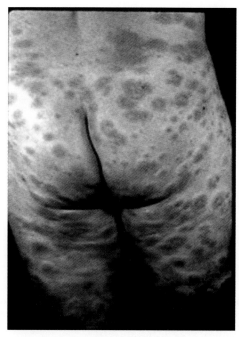

Fig. 6.27.8 BL leprosy with multiple erythematous lesions. No anaesthesia was present.

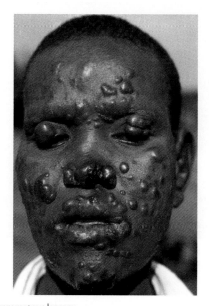

Fig. 6.27.9 Lepromatous leprosy.
(Copyright D A Warrell.)

testosterone leads to azoospermia and gynaecomastia (Fig. 6.27.12). The extremities become oedematous. The skin of the legs becomes ichthyotic and ulcerates easily.

Other forms of leprosy

There are several variant forms of leprosy. Pure neural leprosy occurs principally in India where it is the presenting form for 10% of patients. There is asymmetrical involvement of peripheral nerve trunks and no visible skin lesions. On nerve biopsy all types of leprosy have been found.

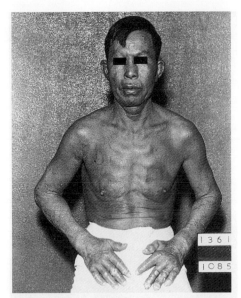

Fig. 6.27.10 Active, untreated lepromatous leprosy, showing generalized infiltration of the skin, swelling of fingers and lips, and thinning of eyebrows and eyelashes. The residual annular lesions visible in both pectoral regions indicate that this patient has 'downgraded' from borderline.

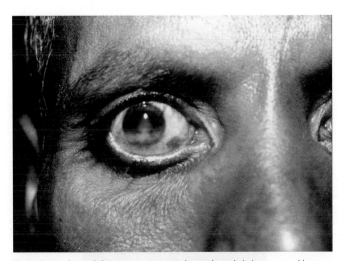

Fig. 6.27.11 Corneal damage to eye secondary to lagophthalmos caused by involvement of the zygomatic branch of the facial nerve.

Histoid lesions are distinctive nodules occurring in lepromatous patients who have relapsed due to dapsone resistance or noncompliance with chemotherapy.

Lucio's leprosy is a form of lepromatous leprosy found only in Latin Americans; it is characterized by a uniform diffuse shiny skin infiltration.

Eye disease in leprosy

Blindness due to leprosy, which occurs in at least 2.5% of patients, is a devastating complication for a patient with anaesthesia of the hands and feet. Eye damage results from both nerve damage and bacillary invasion. Lagophthalmos results from paresis of the orbicularis oculi due to involvement of the zygomatic and

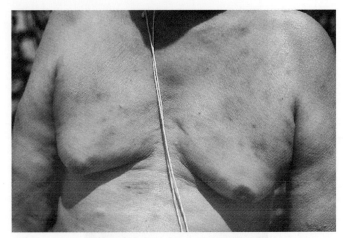

Fig. 6.27.12 Complications of lepromatous leprosy. Gynaecomastia is visible in this man, secondary to testicular involvement in lepromatous leprosy. Multiple nodules are present, many dark brown, due to clofazimine pigmentation. He also has new erythematous lesions of ENL.

temporal branches of the facial (VIIth) nerve. These superficial branches are frequently involved in borderline tuberculoid cases, particularly if there are facial skin lesions. In lepromatous disease, lagophthalmos occurs later and is usually bilateral. Damage to the ophthalmic branch of the trigeminal (Vth) nerve causes anaesthesia of the cornea and conjunctiva resulting in drying of the cornea and making the cornea susceptible to trauma and ulceration (Fig. 6.27.11). Lepromatous infiltration in corneal nerves produces punctate keratitis and corneal lepromas. Invasion of the iris and ciliary body makes them extremely susceptible to reactions.

Leprosy reactions

Type 1 (reversal reactions)

These are characterized by acute neuritis and/or acutely inflamed skin lesions. Nerves become tender with new loss of sensation or motor weakness. Existing skin lesions become erythematous or oedematous (Figs. 6.27.13 and 6.27.14); new lesions may appear (Fig. 6.27.15). Occasionally oedema of the hands, face, or feet is the

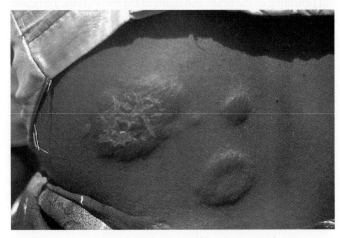

Fig. 6.27.13 Severe reversal (type 1) reaction. This Indian woman has erythematous, oedematous, and desquamating reactional lesions.

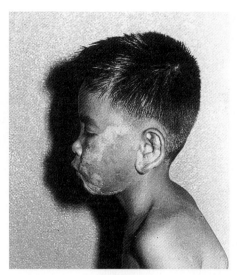

Fig. 6.27.14 Reversal-reaction plaque on the left cheek and ear. The edge of this borderline tuberculoid lesion has become very sharply defined, more raised, and erythematous, dry, and scaly. Treatment with corticosteroids is imperative as the patient is at grave risk of rapidly developing lagophthalmos due to associated involvement of branches of the facial nerve.

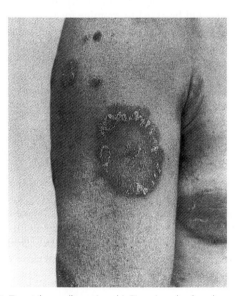

Fig. 6.27.15 Type 1 (reversal) reaction: this BL patient developed new, sharp-edged, well-defined, erythematous plaques with desquamating surfaces about 6 months after starting chemotherapy.

presenting symptom, but constitutional symptoms are unusual. Type 1 reactions occur in borderline patients; 35% of borderline lepromatous patients will experience a type 1 reaction. Patients often present with a skin lesion in reaction since a previously quiescent lesion has become active and visible. The peak time for reactions to develop is in the first 2 months after starting treatment and in the puerperium. Late reactions may occur years after finishing multidrug treatment. Some patient experience repeated reactions (Fig. 6.27.15).

Type 2 (ENL reactions)

These occur in lepromatous and borderline lepromatous patients. Up to 50% of lepromatous patients will experience ENL reactions and 5 to 10% of borderline lepromatous patients. Attacks are acute and may recur over several years. ENL manifests most commonly as painful red nodules on the face (Fig. 6.27.16) and extensor surfaces of limbs (Fig. 6.27.17). The lesions may be superficial or deep, with suppuration or brawny induration when chronic. Acute lesions crop and desquamate, fading over several days (Fig. 6.27.12). ENL is a systemic disorder producing fever and malaise and may be accompanied by uveitis, dactylitis (Fig. 6.27.18), arthritis, neuritis, lymphadenitis, and orchitis. ENL is often not recognized as a complication of leprosy outside endemic areas.

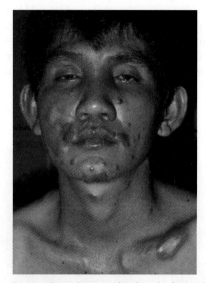

Fig. 6.27.16 Erythema nodosum leprosum (ENL) on the forehead of a patient with early lepromatous leprosy. The papules (and nodules) are firm and tender, with rather indefinite edges. In dark-skinned patients the ENL lesions are often easier to feel than to see, especially over the extensor surfaces of the arms and thighs.
(Copyright D A Warrell.)

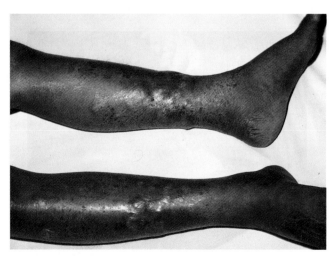

Fig. 6.27.17 Erythema nodosum leprosum (ENL) of the shins.
(Copyright D A Warrell.)

Neuritis

Silent neuropathy is an important form of nerve damage and presents as a functional neural deficit without a manifest acute or subacute neuritis (Figs. 6.27.2, 6.27.3, 6.27.19, and 6.27.20). An Indian study following a cohort of 2608 patients found that 75% of those developing deformity had no history of reactions. In Ethiopian and Bangladeshi cohort studies, silent neuritis accounted for most neuritis. This emphasizes the importance of regular nerve function testing so that new deficits can be detected.

Diagnosis

The diagnosis is made on the clinical findings of one or more of the cardinal signs of leprosy and supported by the finding of acid-fast bacilli on slit skin smears. The whole body should be inspected in a good light otherwise lesions may be missed, particularly on the buttocks. Skin lesions should be tested for anaesthesia to light touch, pin prick, and temperature. The peripheral nerves should be palpated systematically examining for thickening and tenderness

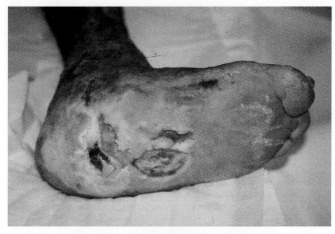

Fig. 6.27.20 This foot shows thick, dry cracked skin together with neuropathic damage in an anaesthetic foot. The toes are clawed, the foot arch has collapsed and there is evidence of a Charcot ankle joint.

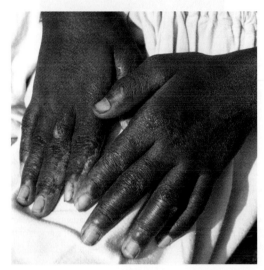

Fig. 6.27.18 Dactylitisas part of an ENL reaction. (Copyright D A Warrell.)

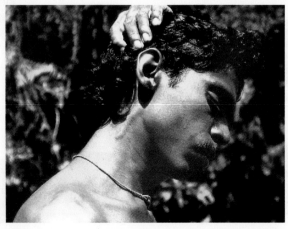

Fig. 6.27.19 Peripheral nerve thickening in leprosy. This young man had marked thickening of his great auricular nerve.

and peripheral nerve function should be assessed. Histological examination of a biopsy taken from the active edge of a lesion is helpful to support the diagnosis and confirm the classification. The pathologist should be asked to examine for neural inflammation which will differentiate leprosy from other granulomatous conditions. Serology is not usually helpful diagnostically because antibodies to the species-specific glycolipid PGL-1 are present in 90% of untreated lepromatous patients but only 40 to 50% of paucibacillary patients and 5 to 10% of healthy controls. Polymerase chain reaction for detecting *M. leprae* DNA has not proved sensitive or specific enough for routine diagnosis.

Outside leprosy endemic areas, doctors frequently fail to consider the diagnosis of leprosy. Of new patients seen from 1995 to 1999 at The Hospital for Tropical Diseases, London, diagnosis had been delayed in over 80% of cases. Patients had been misdiagnosed by dermatologists, neurologists, orthopaedic surgeons, and rheumatologists. A common problem was failure to consider leprosy as a cause of peripheral neuropathy in patients from leprosy endemic countries. These delays had serious consequences for patients; over one-half of them had nerve damage and disability.

Slit skin smears

The bacterial load is assessed by making a small incision through the epidermis, scraping dermal material, and smearing evenly onto a glass slide. At least four sites should be sampled (earlobes and edges of active lesions). The smears are then stained and acid-fast bacilli are counted. Scoring is done on a logarithmic scale per high-power field. A score of 1+ indicates 1 to 10 bacilli in 100 fields, 6+ over 1000 per field. Smears are useful for confirming the diagnosis and should be done annually to monitor response to treatment.

Differential diagnosis

Doctors should be aware of the normal range of skin colour and texture in their local population, and also of the common endemic skin diseases, such as onchocerciasis, that may coexist or mimic leprosy.

Skin

The variety of leprosy skin lesions means that a potentially wide range of skin conditions are in the differential diagnosis. At the tuberculoid end of the spectrum, anaesthesia differentiates leprosy from fungal infections, vitiligo, and eczema. At the lepromatous end the presence of acid-fast bacilli in smears differentiates leprosy nodules from onchocerciasis, Kaposi's sarcoma, and post-kala-azar dermal leishmaniasis (Fig. 6.27.21).

Nerves

Peripheral nerve thickening is rarely seen except in leprosy. Hereditary sensory motor neuropathy type III is associated with palpable peripheral nerve hypertrophy. Amyloidosis, which can also complicate leprosy, causes thickening of peripheral nerves. Charcot–Marie–Tooth disease is an inherited neuropathy that causes distal atrophy and weakness. The causes of other polyneuropathies such as HIV, diabetes, alcoholism, vasculitides, and heavy metal poisoning should all be considered where appropriate.

Treatment

There are six main principles of treatment:

1 Stop the infection with chemotherapy.

2 Treat new nerve damage.

3 Treat reactions.

4 Educate the patient about leprosy.

5 Prevent disability.

6 Support the patient socially and psychologically.

These objectives need the patient's cooperation and confidence and can be achieved through the leprosy outpatient clinic with appropriate support and patient education. On the first visit there should be a careful assessment of skin and mucosal involvement and accurate evaluation of nerve and eye function. Each patient should be classified using the Ridley–Jopling classification and assessed for evidence of a reaction of new nerve damage.

Chemotherapy

All patients with leprosy should be given an appropriate multidrug combination. The first-line antileprosy drugs are rifampicin, clofazimine, and dapsone. The drug combination and duration are determined by the classification of the patient. The WHO has recommended a simple classification for use in the field determined only by the number of skin lesions. Patients are classified as paucibacillary if they have up to five skin lesions and as multibacillary if they have six or more skin lesions. In the specialist clinic setting, where skin smears and skin biopsies can be combined with clinical data, patients can be classified into paucibacillary (skin smear-negative TT and BT) and multibacillary (skin smear-positive BT, all BB, BL, and LL). Table 6.27.2 gives the drug combinations, doses, and duration of treatment. Patients with multibacillary disease and an initial bacterial index greater than 4 will need longer treatment, and the duration should be guided by their clinical status and bacterial index.

Rifampicin is a potent bactericide for *M. leprae*. Four days after a single 600-mg dose, bacilli from a previously untreated patient with multibacillary disease were no longer viable in a mouse footpad test. It acts by inhibiting DNA-dependent RNA polymerase. Because *M. leprae* can develop resistance to rifampicin as a one-step process, this drug should always be given in combination with other antileprotics.

Dapsone (DDS, 4,4-diaminodiphenylsulphone) is weakly bactericidal. Oral absorption is good and it has a long half-life, averaging 28 h. It commonly causes mild haemolysis, but rarely anaemia. Glucose-6-phosphate dehydrogenase deficiency is seldom a problem. The 'DDS syndrome', which is occasionally seen in leprosy, begins 6 weeks after starting dapsone and manifests as exfoliative dermatitis associated with lymphadenopathy, hepatosplenomegaly, fever, and hepatitis.

Clofazimine is a red fat-soluble crystalline dye. The mechanism of its weakly bactericidal action against *M. leprae* remains unknown. The most troublesome side effect is skin discoloration, ranging from red to purple-black, the degree depending on the drug dose and extent of leprous infiltration (Fig. 6.27.22(a) and (b)). The pigmentation usually fades within 6 to 12 months of stopping clofazimine, although traces of discoloration may remain for up to 4 years. Urine, sputum, and sweat may become pink. Clofazimine also produces a characteristic ichthyosis on the shins and forearms.

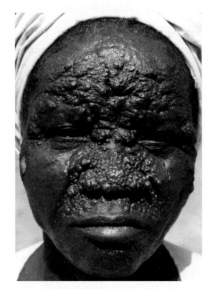

Fig. 6.27.21 African woman with facial epidermoid cysts superficially resembling lepromatous leprosy.
(Copyright D A Warrell.)

Table 6.27.2 WHO recommended multidrug therapy regimens

Type of leprosy[a]	Drug treatment		
	Monthly supervised	Daily self-administered	Duration of treatment
Paucibacillary	Rifampicin 600 mg	Dapsone 100 mg	6 months
Multibacillary	Rifampicin 600 mg	Clofazimine 50 mg	12 months
	Clofazimine 300 mg	Dapsone 100 mg	

[a] WHO classification for field use when slit skin smears are not available: paucibacillary—up to five skin lesions; multibacillary—more than six skin lesions.

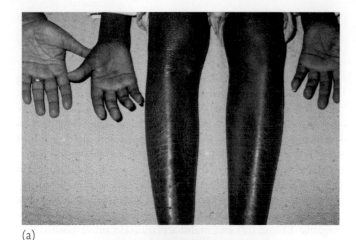

(a)

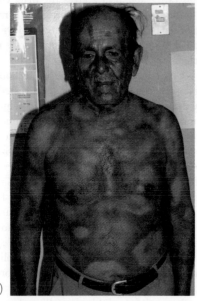

(b)

Fig. 6.27.22 Clofazamine pigmentation in Ethiopian (a) and Peruvian (b) patients.
(Copyright D A Warrell.)

Other drugs bactericidal for *M. leprae* include the fluoroquinolones pefloxacin and ofloxacin, minocycline, and clarithromycin. These agents are now established second-line drugs. Minocycline causes a black pigmentation of skin lesions and so may not be an appropriate substitute for clofazimine if pigmentation is to be avoided.

A single-dose triple-drug combination (rifampicin, ofloxacin, and minocycline) has been tested in India for patients with single skin lesions and improved 98% of patients. This regimen can also be used in patients who experience adverse effects of dapsone or clofazimine, even in patients with a high BI. Although the study had major flaws and single-dose treatment is less effective than the conventional 6-month treatment for paucibacillary leprosy, it is an operationally attractive field regimen or for use in patients with migrant lifestyles.

The principal outcome of treatment is improvement of skin lesions; nerve damage may also improve but to a lesser extent. At the end of a 6-month treatment of borderline disease there may

still be signs of inflammation, which should not be mistaken for active infection. Relapse is uncommon with a cumulative relapse rate of 1.07% for paucibacillary leprosy and 0.77% for multibacillary leprosy at 9 years after completion of multidrug therapy. *M. leprae* is such a slow-growing organism that relapse only occurs after many years. *M. leprae* isolates from relapsed patients who have received multidrug therapy are fully drug sensitive and patients can be retreated with the same regimen. The distinction between relapse and reaction may be difficult.

Since the introduction of multidrug therapy more than 16 million patients have been treated successfully. Clinical improvement has been rapid and toxicity rare. Monthly supervision of the rifampicin component has been crucial to success. Other benefits are reduced deformity rates and increased compliance in control schemes. Reactions may develop months or years after stopping chemotherapy, especially in patients with borderline lepromatous or lepromatous leprosy. It is therefore vital when discharging patients to warn them to return should new symptoms appear, especially in hands, feet, or eyes. Patients with reactions or physical or psychological complications will need long-term care.

Treatment of new nerve damage

Patients with nerve damage present for less than 6 months (assessed by patient history or testing) should receive a 6-month course of steroids starting at a dose of 40 mg prednisolone per day. A randomized controlled trial has shown that nerve damage present for more than 6 months is not improved by steroid treatment.

Management of reactions

Awareness of the early symptoms of reversal reactions by both patient and physician is important because, if left untreated, severe nerve damage may develop. The peak time for reversal reactions is in the first 2 months of treatment. Patients should be warned about reactions because the sudden appearance of reactional lesions after starting treatment is distressing and undermines confidence. The treatment of reactions is aimed at controlling acute inflammation, easing pain, reversing nerve and eye damage, and reassuring the patient. Multidrug therapy should be continued.

Type 1 (reversal) reactions

Simple anti-inflammatory drugs are rarely sufficient to control symptoms. If there is any evidence of neuritis (nerve tenderness, new anaesthesia, and/or motor loss), corticosteroid treatment should be started. Prednisolone should be given, starting at 40 to 60 mg/day, reducing to 40 mg after a few days, and then by 5 mg every 2 to 4 weeks. Patients with borderline tuberculoid leprosy in reaction commonly need 4 months of steroids while borderline lepromatous reactions may need 6 months or more.

Type 2 (ENL) reactions

This is a difficult condition to treat and frequently requires treatment with high-dose steroids (80 mg/day, tapered down rapidly) or thalidomide. Since ENL frequently recurs, steroid dependency can easily develop. Thalidomide (400 mg/day) is superior to steroids in controlling ENL and is the drug of choice for young men with severe ENL (Fig. 6.27.16). Women with severe ENL may benefit from thalidomide treatment. This is a difficult decision for the woman and her physician and needs careful discussion of the benefits and risks (phocomelia when thalidomide is taken in the first trimester). Women should use double contraception and report immediately if menstruation is delayed. Unfortunately, the problems with thalidomide mean that it is unavailable in several leprosy endemic countries despite its undoubted value. Clofazimine has a useful anti-inflammatory effect in ENL but takes 6 weeks to become effective and can be used at 300 mg/day for several months. Low-grade chronic erythema nodosum with iritis or neuritis will require long-term suppression, preferably with thalidomide or clofazimine. Acute iridocyclitis is treated with 1% hydrocortisone eye drops given 4 hourly and 1% atropine drops twice daily.

Neuritis

Silent neuritis should be treated similarly to reversal reactions with prednisolone at a dose of 40 mg/day which should be reduced slowly over a period of months.

Education of patients

Stigmatization due to leprosy occurs worldwide. Patients are frightened of social ostracization, physical rejection, and the development of deformities. It is often useful to ask them about their fears so that these can be addressed. They should be reassured that having started treatment they are not infectious to family or friends and can have a sex life. The importance of compliance with antibiotic therapy needs to be emphasized. The patient needs a careful explanation of the diagnosis, aetiology, and prognosis.

Prevention of disability

The morbidity and disability associated with leprosy is secondary to nerve damage. A major goal in prevention of disability is to create patient self-awareness so that damage is minimized. Monitoring sensation and muscle power in patient's hands, feet, and eyes should be part of the routine follow-up so that new nerve damage is detected early. The patient with an anaesthetized hand or foot needs to understand the importance of daily self-care, especially protection when doing potentially dangerous tasks and inspection for trauma. It is helpful to identify for each patient potentially dangerous situations, such as cooking, car repairs, or smoking. Soaking dry hands and feet followed by rubbing with oil keeps the skin moist and supple.

An anaesthetized foot needs the protection of an appropriate shoe. For anaesthesia alone, a well-fitting 'trainer' with firm soles and shock-absorbing inners will provide adequate protection. Once there is deformity, such as clawing, shoes must be made specially to ensure protection of pressure points and even weight distribution.

The patient should be taught to question the cause of an injury so that the risk can be avoided in the future. Plantar ulceration occurs secondary to increased pressure over bony prominences. Ulceration is treated by rest. Unlike ulcers in the feet of patients with diabetes or ischaemia, ulcers in leprosy heal if they are protected from weight-bearing. No weight-bearing is permitted until the ulcer has healed. Appropriate footwear should be provided to prevent recurrence.

Physiotherapy exercises should be taught to maximize function of weak muscles and prevent contracture. Contractures of hands and feet, foot drop, lagophthalmos, entropion, and ectropion are amenable to surgery.

Social, psychological, and economic rehabilitation

The social and cultural background of the patient determine the nature of many of the problems that may be encountered. The patient may have difficulty in coming to terms with leprosy. The community may reject the patient. Education, gainful employment, confidence from family, friends, and doctor, and plastic surgery to correct stigmatizing deformity all have a role to play.

Prognosis

The majority of patients, especially those who have no nerve damage at the time of diagnosis, do well on multidrug treatment with resolution of skin lesions. Left untreated, borderline patients will downgrade towards the lepromatous end of the spectrum and lepromatous patients will have the consequences of bacillary invasion. Borderline patients are at risk of developing type 1 reactions, which may result in devastating nerve damage. Treatment of the neuritis is currently unsatisfactory and patients with neuritis may develop permanent nerve damage despite corticosteroid treatment. It is not possible to predict which patients will develop reactions or nerve damage. Nerve damage and its complications may be severely disabling, especially when all four limbs and both eyes are affected.

Leprosy in women

Women with leprosy are in double jeopardy; not only may they develop postpartum nerve damage but also they are at particular risk of social ostracization with rejection by spouses and family.

Pregnancy and leprosy

There is little good evidence that pregnancy causes new disease or relapse. However, there is a clear temporal association between parturition and the development of type 1 reactions and neuritis when cell-mediated immunity returns to prepregnancy levels. In an Ethiopian study, 42% of pregnancies in borderline lepromatous patients were complicated by a type 1 reaction in the postpartum period. In the same cohort, patients with lepromatous leprosy experienced ENL reactions throughout pregnancy and lactation. ENL in pregnancy is associated with early loss of nerve function compared with nonpregnant individuals. Pregnant and newly delivered women should have regular neurological examination and steroid treatment instituted for neuritis. Rifampicin, dapsone, and clofazimine are safe during pregnancy. Clofazimine crosses the placenta and babies may be born with mild clofazimine pigmentation. Reactions can be managed with the steroid regimens given above but with a more rapid reduction in dose. Women should be warned before becoming pregnant of the risk that their condition may deteriorate after delivery. Ideally pregnancies should be planned when leprosy is well controlled.

Prevention and control

Leprosy control is now becoming more integrated into general services. Different models of providing leprosy control are used depending on the local facilities. In some endemic countries largely vertical programmes are being retained; in others such as Brazil leprosy services are provided within dermatological services. Effective treatment is not merely restricted to chemotherapy but also involves good case management with effective monitoring and supervision and prevention of disabilities. Treating patients with leprosy is a long-term enterprise involving patients, their families, and health workers.

Vaccines against leprosy

The substantial cross-reactivity between bacille Calmette–Guérin (BCG) and *M. leprae* has been exploited in attempts to develop a vaccine against leprosy. Trials of BCG as a vaccine against leprosy in Uganda, New Guinea, Burma, and South India showed it to confer statistically significant but variable protection, ranging from 80% in Uganda to 20% in Burma and this protective effect has been confirmed in a meta-analysis. A case-control study in Venezuela showed BCG vaccination to give 56% protection to the household contacts of patients with leprosy. Combining BCG and killed *M. leprae* has been tried, but in both a large population-based trial in Malawi and an immunoprophylactic trial in Venezuela there was no advantage for BCG plus *M. leprae* over BCG alone.

Areas of uncertainty and controversy

The optimum duration of treatment is a controversial area. The duration of treatment for multibacillary (MB) patients was reduced from 24 months to 12 months without good evidence. However, this occurred after the definition of MB patients was broadened and in India up to 60% of MB patients are smear-negative borderline tuberculoid patients. The concern regards patients with a high initial bacterial load. Data from India show that patients with a high initial bacterial load (bacterial index >4) treated with 2 years of rifampicin, clofazimine, and dapsone had a relapse rate of 8/100 person years, whereas patients treated to smear negativity had a relapse rate of 2/100 person years. The dilemma is that since skin smears are abandoned in many programmes those patients in need of longer treatment courses cannot be identified. A new treatment, uniform multidrug treatment (U-MDT), in which all leprosy patients are given 6-months of rifampicin, dapsone, and clofazimine are taking place. The problem is that this regimen adds in clofazimine for many patients who do not need it and will probably be inadequate for the small number of lepromatous leprosy patients with high bacterial loads who also maintain the infection in the community. These arguments illustrate the difficulty in providing sound evidence for policy decisions when a decade-long wait to establish relapse rates is needed.

Areas where further research is needed

The epidemiology of leprosy still poses unanswered questions. Why are 64% of all patients with leprosy in India? Is this due to living conditions, genetic susceptibility, or particular environmental conditions in India?

Early detection of cases is vital at both an individual and a population level. It is now recognized that substantial nerve damage occurs before diagnosis. A test for early infection might help detect individual cases before nerve damage is established and before the spread of infection. Leprosy-specific peptides for skin tests have been generated and are being evaluated.

The medical management of reactions and nerve damage is currently limited to steroids. These are not effective for about 30% of patients. Trials to determine the effectiveness of established and out-of-patent immunosuppressants such as azathioprine and ciclosporin are taking place.

The WHO started the 1990s with the bold slogan of 'Eliminating leprosy as a public health problem by 2000'. This initiative galvanized leprosy control programmes worldwide, but the unique biology of *M. leprae* and its interaction with the human host rendered this target unattainable. However, there is a strong perception that leprosy has been eliminated and this has hindered research and planning. The WHO policy for 2011–2015 focuses on sustaining leprosy work. Leprosy is a bacterial disease with challenging immunological complications and will be a global and individual problem for many decades. It is unlikely to be eradicated until there is considerable improvement in general health, wealth, living conditions, and education.

Further reading

Britton WJ, Lockwood DN (2004). Leprosy. *Lancet*, **363**, 1209–19.

Lockwood DNJ, Lambert S (2010). HIV and leprosy? Where are we at? *Lepr Rev*, **81**, 167–75.

Monot M, *et al.* (2005). On the origin of leprosy. *Science*, **308**, 1040–2.

Rodrigues L, Lockwood DNJ (2011). Leprosy now: epidemiology, progress, challenges, and research gaps. *Lancet Infect Dis*, **11**, 464–70.

Setia MS, *et al.* (2006). The role of BCG in prevention of leprosy: a meta-analysis. *Lancet Infect Dis*, **6**, 162–70.

Scollard DM (2008). The biology of nerve injury in leprosy. *Lepr Rev*, **79**, 242–53.

Ustianowski AP, *et al.* (2006). Interactions between HIV infection and leprosy: a paradox. *Lancet Infect Dis*, **6**, 350–60.

Van Brakel WH, *et al.* (2005). The INFIR Cohort Study: assessment of sensory and motor neuropathy in leprosy at baseline. *Lepr Rev*, **76**, 277–95.

World Health Organization (2006). *Global strategy for further reducing the leprosy burden and sustaining leprosy control activities 2006–2010*. World Health Organization, Geneva.

6.28 Buruli ulcer: *Mycobacterium ulcerans* infection

Wayne M. Meyers and Françoise Portaels

Essentials

Buruli ulcer is caused by *Mycobacterium ulcerans*, which secretes a cytotoxic and immunosuppressive toxin, mycolactone. The disease is characterized by necrosis of skin, subcutaneous tissue, and bone, and is re-emerging as a potentially disabling and stigmatizing affliction of inhabitants of tropical wetlands. Major foci are in West and Central Africa, but there are minor endemic foci in Australia, Mexico, South America, and South-East Asia. It is not contagious: environmental sources include water, vegetation, and insects, with humans probably becoming infected by traumatic introduction of the bacillus into the skin from the overlying *M. ulcerans*-contaminated surface in most instances. Clinical presentation may be as a cutaneous nodule, undermined ulcer, plaque or widely disseminated oedematous lesion. Clinical diagnosis is often accurate, but smears for acid fast bacilli, culture, polymerase chain reaction (PCR) assays, are confirmatory. Treatment was formerly by wide surgical excision and skin grafting, but antibiotics (rifampicin with streptomycin) have now been found effective; the best treatment approach remains to be clarified.

Introduction

Buruli ulcer is an indolent necrotizing infection of the skin, subcutaneous tissue, and bone caused by *Mycobacterium ulcerans*. In 1962 Clancey and Dodge described many patients from Buruli County, Uganda, with cutaneous ulcers reminiscent of those Cook described in 1897 from the same area, and named the disease Buruli ulcer. Since the World Health Organization (WHO) Buruli ulcer initiative there has been increased attention to efforts for the treatment and control of Buruli ulcer.

Aetiology

MacCallum and colleagues first isolated the causative agent in 1948 from patients in Australia. *M. ulcerans*, a slow-growing acid-fast bacillus (AFB), grows optimally at 32°C and elaborates mycolactone, a cytotoxic and immunosuppressive polyketide assembled by plasmid-encoded synthases of the aetiological agent. This toxin is the primary virulence factor of *M. ulcerans*. Data from 16S rRNA sequences define four major groups of *M. ulcerans*: African, American, Asian, and Australian strains. Phenolic mycosides of *M. ulcerans* and *Mycobacterium marinum* are identical and the 16S rRNA genes differ only slightly. Portaels *et al.* were the first to culture *M. ulcerans* from the environment, in 2008.

Epidemiology and transmission

Buruli ulcer is the third most common human mycobacterial infection worldwide, after tuberculosis (Chapter 6.25) and leprosy (Chapter 6.27). It occurs in humid, rural tropical or subtropical regions, and all endemic foci of Buruli ulcer are near rural freshwater wetlands, especially ponds and swamps. Major endemic areas are Benin, Cameroon, Democratic Republic of Congo, Gabon, Ghana, Ivory Coast, and adjacent countries. There are minor foci in southeast and northern Asia. Cases have also been reported in Mexico, South America, Papua New Guinea, and Australia (where it is known as Bairnsdale ulcer).

Documented environmental sources of *M. ulcerans* include irrigation systems, waterbugs dwelling in aquatic plant roots in swamps, and mosquitoes. In Australia, koalas, possums, potoroos, some domestic animals (cats, dogs, horses) and imported alpaca acquire the infection naturally.

The mode of transmission is not fully understood, although disease is known to be linked to contaminated water. Outbreaks of disease often follow environmental changes that promote flooding or alter water courses, such as deforestation or construction of dams and irrigation systems. Increased farming activities near wetlands and

global climatic changes may contribute to the rapid re-emergence of Buruli ulcer. In West Africa the peak age of onset is 5 to 15 years, although the disease can affect any age group. In Australia the median age at presentation is 55 to 65 years.

Transmission is probably via skin trauma, although insects may play a role. The trauma may be slight (e.g. hypodermic injection) or severe (land mine wound or snake bite). Biting insects (e.g. waterbugs) may serve as vectors. In Australia, risk for Buruli ulcer in humans is associated with the frequency of detection of *M. ulcerans* in mosquitoes, suggesting a possible role in transmission. Aerosols arising from ponds and swamp surfaces may disseminate *M. ulcerans*. Person-to-person transmission is rare.

Pathogenesis

Predisposing host factors are poorly understood. Putatively, severity and course of infection are related to pathogen virulence, mode of infection, inoculum size, host genetic factors, and immunological response of the host. A T-helper 1 cell (Th1) response tends to localize and heal infections while a T-helper 2 cells (Th2) type promotes dissemination. Once introduced, the small amount of mycolactone produced by inoculated *M. ulcerans* causes tissue necrosis and apoptosis, suppressing local immune responses and ensuring survival of the bacillus in necrotic tissue. Mycolactone targets subcutaneous fat cells, permitting necrosis to spread just superficial to fascial planes. *M. ulcerans* may invade lymphatic and blood vessels, causing metastatic spread of the mycobacterium.

Clinical features

Except for those with massive lesions, patients are usually surprisingly well without systemic symptoms or abnormal laboratory findings. Meyers and Portaels have published a schema for the natural history and inter-relationships of the forms of Buruli ulcer disease without specific therapy. Buruli ulcer may be localized or disseminated.

Localized disease

Typically, the initial cutaneous lesion is a single, firm, painless, nontender, movable, subcutaneous nodule up to 3 cm in diameter. Limbs are preferred sites, often around joints. The natural history of the disease is markedly variable, but nodules usually ulcerate within 1 to 3 months of inoculation. A whitish necrotic slough develops in the ulcer base with induration and hyperpigmentation of surrounding skin. Ulcer borders are undermined, sometimes extending widely (major ulcerative disease) (Fig. 6.28.1). Some small (1–2 cm in diameter) ulcerated lesions with shallow undermining self-heal (minor ulcerative disease). Without treatment, major ulcerative lesions tend to become inactive, after months or years, and heal by scarring. Scars are depressed and stellate, often causing disfiguring and crippling cicatricial contractures.

Disseminated disease

Disseminated disease may develop from nodules, arise from localized major ulcerative lesions, or disseminate directly and rapidly from the inoculation site, causing indurated plaques covering even an entire limb or vast areas of the trunk. Without treatment, such lesions will eventually slough, leaving a large ulcer with continuing

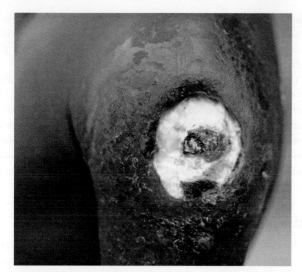

Fig. 6.28.1 Pristine Buruli ulcer on the left deltoid area in a 12-year-old Congolese boy who had received a hypodermic injection at this site 3 months previously. Note central necrotic slough in the base of the ulcer and undermined edges.

extension of disease at the borders. Eyes, breasts, and genitalia may be damaged or destroyed.

While metastatic spread may arise from localized disease, patients with the highly bacilliferous disseminated disease are most prone to metastatic lesions. Spread may be to distant skin sites or bone, especially bones of the limbs. In Africa, *M. ulcerans* osteomyelitis develops in approximately 10% of patients and often leads to amputations or other disabilities.

Differential clinical diagnosis

Diagnosis of nodular disease is often perplexing. Differential diagnoses include bacterial, mycotic, and parasitic infections, inflammatory lesions, and tumours. Ulcers resembling Buruli ulcer include tropical phagedenic ulcer (malodorous and not undermined), venous stasis ulcer (not undermined), and venomous snake bite or spider bite (history is helpful).

Pathology

Optimal biopsy specimens contain the necrotic base of ulcers and undermined edge of lesions including subcutaneous tissue and fascia. Histopathological sections reveal a contiguous coagulation necrosis (noncaseating) of the deep dermis, panniculus, and fascia. Vasculitis and mineralization are common. Clumps of extracellular acid-fast bacilli are most plentiful in the base of the ulcer; however, intracellular *M. ulcerans* may be seen in inflammatory cells at the edge of necrotic foci. Necrosis extends well beyond the location of bacilli. Local and regional lymph nodes are often invaded and sometimes necrotic. In bone, the marrow is necrotic and contains acid-fast bacilli, and trabeculae are eroded. These features are distinct from those of osteomyelitis of all other known aetiologies. Development of delayed-type hypersensitivity granulomas heralds healing by fibrosis.

Laboratory diagnosis

Fine needle aspirates are often employed for laboratory studies. Smears stained by the Ziehl-Neelsen method from the ulcer base

frequently reveal acid-fast bacilli in clumps. *M. ulcerans* is a slow-growing organism that can be cultured *in vitro* at 29 to 33°C. Polymerase chain reaction provides specific identification of *M. ulcerans*. Histopathological changes are characteristic.

Treatment

The former recommended treatment for most patients was wide surgical excision followed by skin grafting. Heating the lesion at 40°C was a useful adjunct. Today, antimicrobial therapy (rifampicin 10 mg/kg by mouth plus streptomycin 15 mg/kg by intramuscular injection) without surgery is recommended and heals most nodular and minor ulcerative disease, and some advanced lesions. An all-oral regimen of rifampicin plus clarithromycin is under study and seems effective. Physiotherapy is essential to prevent contracture deformities.

Prevention and control

Bacille Calmette–Guérin (BCG) vaccination provides short-lived protection. Practical control measures for inhabitants of endemic areas are usually ineffectual; however, use of a protected water supply is important. Tourists should avoid wetlands in endemic countries.

Socioeconomic impact

Patients are often stigmatized by disability or cosmetic damage, and may require welfare services for life (services are often locally limited or unavailable). They also require protracted hospital stays, taxing overburdened services.

Further reading

Alffenaar JW, *et al.* (2010). Pharmacokinetics of rifampin and clarithromycin in patients treated for *Mycobacterium ulcerans* infection. *Antimicrob Agents Chemother*, **54**, 3878–83. [Early results of an all-oral antibiotic therapeutic trial-using rifampin plus clarithromycin.]

Converse PJ, *et al.* (2011). Treating Mycobacterium ulcerans disease (Buruli ulcer): from surgery to antibiotics, is the pill mightier than the knife? *Future Microbiol*, **6**, 1185–98. [Review of status of antibiotic therapy, including experimental observations.]

Kiszewski AE, *et al.* (2006). The local immune response in ulcerative lesions of Buruli disease. *Clin Exp Immunol*, **143**, 445–51. [Delineates host response at tissue level.]

Lavender CJ, *et al.* (2011). Risk of Buruli ulcer and detection of Mycobacterium ulcerans in mosquitoes in southeastern Australia. *PLoS Negl Trop Dis*, **5**, e1305. [Detailed study of numbers of incident patients and numbers of *M. ulcerans*-positive mosquitoes.]

Meyers WM (1995). Mycobacterial infections of the skin. In: Doerr W, Seifert G (eds) *Tropical pathology*, pp. 291–377. Springer, Berlin. [Extensive coverage of the clinical and pathological features of Buruli ulcer.]

Meyers WM, *et al.* (2011). *Mycobacterium ulcerans* infection (Buruli ulcer). In: Guerrant RL, Walker DH, Weller PF (eds) *Tropical infectious diseases*, 3rd edition, pp. 248–52. Elsevier Saunders, Edinburgh. [Extensive update on *M. ulcerans* infection including epidemiology, pathogenesis and treatment.]

Portaels F, *et al.* (2008). First cultivation and characterization of *Mycobacterium ulcerans* from the environment. *PLoS Negl Trop Dis*, **2**, e178. [Cultivation and characterization of aetiological agent, in detail.]

Nienhuis WA, *et al.* (2010). Antimicrobial treatment for early, limited *Mycobacterium ulcerans* infection: a randomised controlled trial.

Lancet, **375**(9715), 664–72. {Results of large antibiotic therapy in West Africa.}

Schunk M, *et al.* (2009). Outcome of patients with Buruli ulcer after surgical treatment with or without antimycobacterial treatment in Ghana. *Am J Trop Med Hyg*, **81**, 75–81. [Evaluation of surgical and antibiotic therapy.]

Silva M, *et al.* (2009). Pathogenetic mechanisms of the intracellular parasite *Mycobacterium ulcerans* leading to Buruli ulcer. *Lancet Infect Dis*, **9**, 699–710. [Comprehensive review of pathogenesis.]

Walsh DS, *et al.* (2009). Buruli ulcer (*Mycobacterium ulcerans* infection): a re-emerging disease. *Clin Microbiol Newsletter*, **31**, 119-28. [Updated comprehensive review.]

6.29 Actinomycoses

K.P. Schaal

Essentials

Human actinomycoses are always synergistic polymicrobial infections in which fermentative actinomycetes—predominantly *Actinomyces israelii*, *A. gerencseriae*, or *Propionibacterium propionicum*—are the principal pathogens, usually needing the assistance of so-called concomitant microbes to produce disease. Nearly all of the members of the mixed actinomycotic microflora belong to the indigenous microbial community of human mucous membranes, hence actinomycoses present as sporadic endogenous infections which are not transmissible.

Clinical features—the initial actinomycotic lesion usually develops in tissue adjacent to a mucous membrane as a subacute to chronic process that is granulomatous as well as suppurative, typically giving rise to multiple abscesses and draining sinus tracts that are preferentially located in the cervicofacial region, thorax or abdomen. These characteristically progress slowly, penetrate tissues without regard to natural organ borders, and spread haematogenously, with symptoms remitting and exacerbating with and without antimicrobial treatment.

Diagnosis—this can be difficult as clinical symptoms, radiographic, or histopathological signs, and the results of serological tests may all be misleading. The finding of so-called sulphur granules is pathognomonic: these are macroscopically visible, yellowish or reddish to brownish particles that exhibit a cauliflower-like appearance under the microscope at low magnifications, and which may be found as free structures in pus or embedded in affected tissue. Reliable diagnosis chiefly rests on bacteriological culture.

Treatment and prognosis—antibacterial drugs used for treatment should be active against both the causative actinomycetes and all concomitant bacteria. For cervicofacial actinomycoses, the rare cutaneous processes, and most thoracic forms of the disease, this requirement is best fulfilled by amoxicillin plus clavulanic acid in medium to high doses: abdominal cases and the presence of unusually resistant concomitant bacteria may require the addition of further antimicrobials (e.g. an aminoglycoside plus either metronidazole or clindamycin). The prognosis of cervicofacial and cutaneous actinomycoses is good provided that treatment is adequate; thoracic and abdominal forms are more serious, with grave prognosis without proper treatment.

Definition

Actinomycoses are sporadically occurring endogenous polymicrobial inflammatory processes in which fermentative (facultatively anaerobic or capnophilic) actinomycetes of the genera *Actinomyces* and *Propionibacterium*, but rarely also *Bifidobacterium*, may act as the principal pathogens. Clinically, the subacute to chronic, granulomatous as well as suppurative disease tends to progress slowly and usually gives rise to multiple abscesses and draining sinus tracts. Because the term 'actinomycosis' denotes a polyaetiological inflammatory syndrome rather than a condition attributable to a single actinomycete species, it should only be used in the plural.

Aetiology of human actinomycoses

Actinomyces israelii and *A. gerencseriae* are by far the most frequent and most characteristic pathogens aetiologically involved in the human form of the disease. *A. gerencseriae* emerged from the former sero- and biovariety 2 of *A. israelii* in 1990. A third species of filamentous fermentative Gram-positive bacteria, *Propionibacterium propionicum* (formerly *Actinomyces propionicus*, *Arachnia propionica*), is a much less common cause of actinomycotic infections (Table 6.29.1).

Table 6.29.1 Fermentative actinomycetes isolated from human cervicofacial actinomycotic lesions at the Hygiene Institute of the University of Cologne and the Institute for Medical Microbiology and Immunology of the University of Bonn, Germany, between 1985 and 1999

Species identified	Number	Percentage of cases
One species per specimen:		
A. israelii	421	55.3
A. gerencseriae	111	14.6
A. naeslundii/A. oris/A johnsonii	122	16.0
A. odontolyticus	19	2.5
A. meyeri	5	0.7
A. georgiae	1	0.1
A. neuii subsp. neuii	1	0.1
P. propionicum	7	0.9
Bifidobacterium dentium	3	0.4
Corynebacterium matruchotii	12	1.6
Rothia dentocariosa	5	0.7
Not identified to species level	54	7.1
Two species per specimen:		
A. israelii + A. naeslundii/A. oris/A johnsonii	11	0.8
A. israelii + A. meyeri	2	0.1
A. israelii + A. odontolyticus	1	0.1
A. israelii + P. propionicum	2	0.1
P. propionicum + A. naeslundii/A. oris/A johnsonii	2	0.1
P. propionicum + A. neuii	1	0.1
Total number of isolates	761	100.0

Modified from Pulverer G, Schütt-Gerowitt H, Schaal KP (2003). Human cervicofacial actinomycoses: microbiological data of 1997 cases. *Clin Infect Dis*, **37**, 490–7.

Several other fermentative actinomycetes have occasionally been isolated from actinomycosis-like lesions (Table 6.29.1). In a given case, however, it is often difficult to decide whether these organisms are primary pathogens or merely contaminants, especially when the specimen has had contact with mucosal secretions or when two different actinomycete species have been isolated from the same specimen (Table 6.29.1). Nevertheless, *A. naeslundii, A. odontolyticus, A. viscosus, A. meyeri,* and *Bifidobacterium dentium* (formerly *Actinomyces eriksonii*) have all been reported to be capable of producing human infections clinically identical to those caused by *A. israelii, A. gerencseriae,* or *P. propionicum,* while *A. bovis,* the classic agent of bovine actinomycosis, has never been recovered with certainty from human infective processes (Table 6.29.1). Fermentative actinomycetes previously termed *A. naeslundii* and *A. viscosus* underwent considerable taxonomic and nomenclatural changes recently (Henssge *et al.,* 2009). According to these changes, organisms now named *A. viscosus* only occur in animals, particularly in hamsters. Human isolates of the former species *A. naeslundii* and *A. viscosus* have been assigned to *A. naeslundii* sensu stricto and the new species *A. oris* and *A. johnsonii,* but it is difficult to discriminate between these three species by routinely used diagnostic procedures.

Pathogenesis and pathology

Most of the fermentative actinomycetes pathogenic to humans are found regularly and abundantly in the mouths of healthy adults. However, these microbes occur only sporadically or in low numbers in the digestive, respiratory, and genital tracts, as well as in the mouths of babies before teething and of adults without any natural teeth or tooth implants. Therefore, these actinomycetes may be considered facultatively pathogenic commensals of the human mucous membranes, which, apart from the very rare actinomycotic wound infections following human bite or fist fight traumata, produce disease exclusively as endogenous pathogens.

For active invasion of the tissue, the classic pathogenic fermentative actinomycetes apparently require a negative redox potential, which may result either from insufficient blood supply (caused by circulatory or vascular diseases, crush injuries, or foreign bodies) or from the reducing and necrotizing capacity of other microbes in the lesion. Defective functions of the immune system do not specifically predispose to actinomycotic infections.

Synergistic polymicrobial infection

True actinomycoses are essentially always synergistic mixed infections, in which the actinomycetes act as the specific component, the so-called guiding organisms that decide on the characteristic course and the late symptoms of the disease. The so-called concomitant microbes (Table 6.29.2), which may vary considerably in composition (about 100 aerobic and anaerobic species) and number (up to 10 per case) of species from case to case, are often responsible for the clinical picture at the beginning of the infection and for certain complications; they are also part of the resident or transient surface microflora of the mucous membranes of humans.

Particularly pronounced synergistic interactions appear to exist between pathogenic fermentative actinomycetes, especially *Actinomyces israelii* and *A. gerencseriae,* and *Actinobacillus actinomycetemcomitans,* which has recently been reclassified as *Aggregatibacter actinomycetemcomitans.* The latter organism, the species designation of which refers to its characteristic association

Table 6.29.2 Concomitant actinomycotic flora isolated from cervicofacial actinomycotic lesions at the Hygiene- Institute of the University of Cologne and the Institute for Medical Microbiology and Immunology of the University of Bonn, Germany, between 1972 and 1999

Species/group identified	Number	Percentage of cases
Aerobically growing organisms		
Coagulase-negative staphylococci	781	39.1
Staphylococcus aureus	99	5.0
α-Haemolytic streptococci	206	10.3
β-Haemolytic streptococci	85	4.3
Other aerobically growing bacteria	104	5.2
Candida spp.	22	1.1
No aerobic growth	943	47.2
Anaerobes and capnophils		
Aggregatibacter (Actinobacillus) actinomycetemcomitans	283	14.2
'Microaerophilic' and anaerobic streptococci	992	49.7
Bacteroides ureolyticus/Campylobacter gracilis/Capnocytophaga spp./*Eikenella corrodens*	370	18.5
Black-pigmented *Bacteroidaceae*	501	25.1
Other *Bacteroides* spp. and *Prevotella* spp.	419	21.0
Fusobacterium spp.	753	37.7
Leptotrichia buccalis	160	8.0
Propionibacterium spp.[a]	549	27.5
Other anaerobic bacteria	72	3.6
Total number of cases examined	1997	100.0

[a] Other than *P. propionicum.*
Modified from Pulverer G, Schütt-Gerowitt H, Schaal KP (2003). Human cervicofacial actinomycoses: microbiological data of 1997 cases. *Clin Infect Dis,* **37**, 490–7.

with actinomycetes (Latin *actinomycetem comitans* = accompanying an actinomycete), may even sustain the inflammatory process under similar clinical symptoms after chemotherapeutic elimination of the causative actinomycete.

Histopathology

Initially an inflammatory granulation tissue develops, which usually breaks down to form either an acute abscess or chronic multiple abscesses with proliferation of connective tissue. The pathognomonic sulphur granules are formed primarily in the infected tissue, but may also appear as free structures in abscess content or sinus discharge. They are then of the highest diagnostic importance.

Sulphur granules, which were originally designated *Drusen* in Harz's first description of *Actinomyces bovis* in 1877, are macroscopically visible (up to 1 mm in diameter) yellowish or reddish to brownish particles that exhibit a cauliflower-like appearance under the microscope at low magnifications. They consist of a conglomerate of filamentous actinomycete microcolonies formed *in vivo* and surrounded by tissue reaction material, especially polymorphonuclear granulocytes (Fig. 6.29.1). At high magnification, a Gram-stained smear of the completely crushed granule reveals the presence of clusters of Gram-positive interwoven branching filaments with radially arranged peripheral hyphae and of a variety

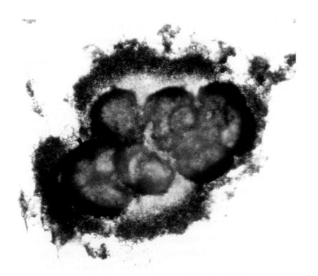

Fig. 6.29.1 Actinomycotic sulphur granule. Particle embedded in 1% methylene blue solution, after gently pressing on the coverslip (original diameter 0.8 mm). Note the spherical segment-like structures which represent actinomycete colonies formed *in vivo* and which are coloured brown because the blue dye has been reduced to its leuco base in the anaerobic centre of the particle. The blue-coloured structures surrounding the colonies are polymorphonuclear granulocytes. Magnification × 60.

of other Gram-positive and Gram-negative rods and cocci, which represent the concomitant flora (Fig. 6.29.2). A club-shaped layer of hyaline material may be seen on the tips of peripheral filaments, which can aid in the differentiation of actinomycotic sulphur granules from macroscopically similar particles of various other microbial and nonmicrobial origins.

Clinical manifestations

The primary actinomycotic lesion usually develops in tissue adjacent to a mucous membrane at sites such as the cervicofacial, thoracic, and abdominal areas. The infection tends to progress slowly and to penetrate without regard to natural organ borders, or to spread haematogenously even to distant sites. Remission and

exacerbation of symptoms with and without antimicrobial treatment is characteristic. As in other endogenous microbial diseases, the incubation period of actinomycoses is not defined.

Cervicofacial actinomycoses

In the vast majority of cases, actinomycotic lesions primarily involve the face or neck. Conditions predisposing to these cervicofacial infections include tooth extractions, fractures of the jaw, periodontal abscesses, foreign bodies penetrating the mucosal barrier (bone splinters, fish bones, awns of cereals), or suppurating tonsillar crypts.

Initially, the cervicofacial actinomycoses present either as an acute, usually odontogenic, abscess or cellulitis of the floor of the mouth, or as a slowly developing chronic hard painless reddish or livid swelling. Small acute actinomycotic abscesses may heal after surgical drainage alone. More often, however, the acute initial stage is followed by a subacute to chronic course if no specific antimicrobial treatment is given, thereby imitating the primarily chronic form, which is characterized by regression and cicatrization of central suppurative foci while the infection progresses peripherally producing hard painless livid infiltrations. These may lead to multiple new areas of liquefaction, fistulae (Fig. 6.29.3), which often discharge pus containing sulphur granules, and multilocular cavities with poor healing and a tendency to recur after temporary regressions of the inflammatory symptoms.

With inappropriate or no treatment, cervicofacial actinomycoses extend slowly, even across organ borders, and may become life-threatening by invasion of the cranial cavity, the mediastinum, or the bloodstream. In contrast, the so-called (peri)apical actinomycosis which is clinically indistinguishable from common apical periodontitis and which has been accused of being responsible for lack of healing after endodontic treatment or tooth implant surgery, essentially always remains localized, responds to usual periodontitis treatment and represents no serious threat to the patient's health or life. This condition should, therefore, not be termed 'actinomycosis', but possibly 'actinomycete periodontitis'.

Thoracic actinomycoses

Thoracic manifestations, which are much less common than the cervicofacial form (Table 6.29.3), usually develop after aspiration

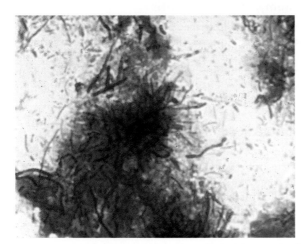

Fig. 6.29.2 Gram-stained smear prepared from a crushed sulphur granule. The causative actinomycetes appear as Gram-positive irregularly curved branching filaments which are partially arranged in nest-like structures. In addition, various other bacteria, in particular Gram-negative rods and Gram-positive cocci, can be seen representing the concomitant flora. Magnification ×1200.

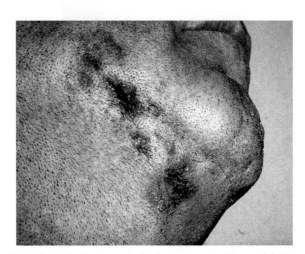

Fig. 6.29.3 Primarily chronic cervicofacial actinomycosis with several draining sinus tracts in a 42-year-old man.

or inhalation of material from the mouth (dental plaque or calculus, tonsillar crypt contents) or a foreign body that contains or is contaminated with the causative agents. Occasionally, this form of disease may result from extension of an actinomycotic process of the neck, from an abdominal infection perforating the diaphragm, or from a distant focus by haematogenous spread.

Primary pulmonary actinomycoses present as bronchopneumonic infiltrations that may imitate tuberculosis or bronchial carcinoma radiographically, appearing as single dense or multiple spotted shadows in which cavitations may develop (Fig. 6.29.4). If not diagnosed and treated properly, pulmonary infections may extend through to the pleural cavity producing empyema, to the pericardium, or to the chest wall; they may even appear as a paravertebral (psoas) abscess tracking down to the groin. Detailed aetiology, pathogenesis, and clinical relevance of a condition termed 'endobronchial actinomycosis' remain to be definitely clarified.

Abdominal actinomycoses

Actinomycoses of the abdomen and pelvis are rare (Table 6.29.3). They originate either from acute perforating gastrointestinal diseases (appendicitis, diverticulitis, various ulcerative diseases), from surgical or accidental trauma including injuries caused by ingested bone splinters or fish bones, or from inflammations of the female internal genital organs.

Women who wear intrauterine contraceptive devices (IUCD) or vaginal pessaries for long periods often show a characteristic colonization of the cervical canal and the uterine cavity, but particularly of the thread of the IUCD, by various fermentative actinomycetes and other anaerobes resembling the synergistic actinomycotic flora. However, this colonization only rarely results in an invasive actinomycotic process.

Most abdominal actinomycoses present as slowly growing tumours, which, in the absence of sinus tracts discharging pus with sulphur granules, are difficult to differentiate from malignant neoplasms such as colonic, rectal, ovarian, or cervical carcinomas. By direct extension, any abdominal tissue or organ may be involved including muscle, liver, spleen, kidney, fallopian tubes, ovaries, testes, bladder, or rectum. Haematogenous liver abscesses have been seen, especially associated with genital actinomycoses.

Actinomycotic infections of the central nervous system

Actinomycoses of the brain and the spinal cord are very rare. They may arise from direct extension of cervicofacial infections. Haematogenous spread is also possible, particularly from primary lesions in the lungs or abdomen. The spinal canal may be directly involved from these sites. Brain abscess is much more common than meningitis.

Actinomycoses of the bone

In contrast to bovine actinomycosis which usually affects the skeleton, bone involvement in humans is very rare. It usually develops by direct extension from soft tissue infection resulting in a periostitis with new bone formation visible by radiography. If the bone itself is invaded, localized areas of bone destruction surrounded by increased bone density usually develop. Mandible, ribs, and spine are most frequently involved.

Actinomycotic endocarditis

Endocarditis due to fermentative actinomycetes has occasionally been described. However, detailed bacteriological information on this condition is not yet available so that it remains to be seen whether it may rightly be termed actinomycosis or has merely to be considered an aetiological variant of the common form of endocarditis caused by indigenous oral microbes.

Cutaneous actinomycoses

Actinomycotic lesions of the skin are extremely rare. Usually, they originate from wounds that were contaminated with saliva or dental plaque following human bites or fist fights, but they may also result from haematogenous spread. Symptoms are similar to those of cervicofacial actinomycoses.

Diagnosis

Clinical symptoms are often misleading, especially in the early stages of the disease, histopathological appearances are unreliable, and diagnosis chiefly rests on bacteriological methods.

Table 6.29.3 Localization of human actinomycotic infections

Body site involved	Number	Percentage of cases
Cervicofacial area	3197	97.9
Thoracic organs	41	1.3
Abdominal organs including small pelvis	20	0.6
Extremities	4	0.1
Central nervous system	4	0.1
Total number of cases	3266	100.0

Modified from Schaal KP, Pulverer G (1984). Epidemiologic, etiologic, diagnostic, and therapeutic aspects of endogenous actinomycete infections. In: Ortiz-Ortiz L, Bojalil LF, Yakoleff V (eds) *Biological, biochemical, and biomedical aspects of actinomycetes*, pp. 13–32. Academic Press, Orlando.

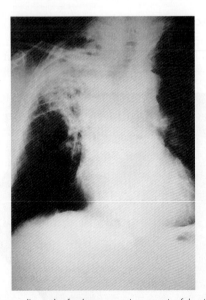

Fig. 6.29.4 Chest radiograph of pulmonary actinomycosis of the right upper lobe in a 62-year-old man. Initially, the disease was mistaken for bronchial carcinoma. It was diagnosed only after a huge subcutaneous abscess had developed covering the whole right shoulder blade.

Radiography

In cervicofacial cases, radiography is useful only for detecting bone involvement. A pulmonary infiltrate associated with a proliferative lesion or destruction of ribs is highly suggestive of either actinomycosis or a tumour. Radiography may also help to locate the abdominal processes and to identify the involvement of organs such as liver, kidney, urinary bladder, or ureter. In general, however, radiographic changes are not diagnostic.

Laboratory diagnosis

Clinical chemistry and haematology

Small localized actinomycotic lesions are not usually associated with abnormalities. In advanced cases, however, especially those in the thoracic or the abdominal area, a raised erythrocyte sedimentation rate and pronounced leucocytosis may be seen. When the central nervous system is involved, a polymorphonuclear or mononuclear pleocytosis is commonly found. The protein content of the cerebrospinal fluid is frequently elevated and the sugar content moderately depressed.

Bacteriology

Pus specimens containing sulphur granules and occasionally looking like semolina should prompt the clinician to ask and the bacteriologist to look specifically for actinomycetes using suitable cultural techniques and other methods.

Pus, sinus discharge, bronchial secretions, granulation tissue, or biopsy materials are suitable specimens. Precautions must be taken to prevent contamination of the specimen by the indigenous mucosal flora. In cases of cervicofacial actinomycoses, pus should therefore be obtained only by transcutaneous puncture of the abscesses or by transcutaneous needle biopsy after thorough skin disinfection. When abscesses have already been incised, a sufficient amount of pus should be collected instead of using only a swab. Because sputum always contains oral actinomycetes, bronchial secretions should be obtained by transtracheal aspiration, or material should be collected by transthoracic percutaneous needle biopsy. Percutaneous puncture of suspected abscesses, possibly under radiological control, is often the only way of obtaining suitable specimens for diagnosing abdominal actinomycoses.

The transport of specimens to the bacteriological laboratory should be as fast as possible, preferably by messenger. Alternatively, a reducing transport medium such as one of the modifications of Stuart's medium should be used. The specimen should arrive in the laboratory within 24 h, although it has occasionally proved possible to isolate actinomycetes from samples that took 7 days or more to get to the diagnostic laboratory by post.

A quick and comparatively reliable tentative diagnosis is possible microscopically when sulphur granules are present (Fig. 6.29.1). The demonstration of concomitant bacteria in Gram-stained smears prepared from crushed granule material (Fig. 6.29.2) allows the differentiation of actinomycotic granules from similar particles produced by *Nocardia* spp., *Actinomadura* spp., or *Streptomyces* spp.

Use of transparent culture media and careful microscopic examination of the cultures, preferably on Fortner plates, after at least 2, 7, and 14 days of incubation enables a specialized laboratory to detect possible actinomycete colonies and to subculture them for identification. Isolation and definite identification to the species level may require a further 1 to 2 weeks. Techniques such as the application of gene probes or the polymerase chain reaction (PCR) for detecting and identifying fermentative actinomycetes directly in clinical samples are not yet widely used; however, sequencing of the 16S rRNA gene often helps to identify actinomycete cultures to species level although this technique is intrinsically a phylogenetic and taxonomic rather than a diagnostic tool.

Serological diagnosis

None of the routine serological methods has yet provided satisfactory results because sensitivity and specificity have been found to be too low.

Treatment

As the aetiology of human actinomycoses is always polymicrobial, the antibacterial drugs used for treatment should in principle cover both the causative actinomycetes and all of the concomitant bacteria. This usually requires the administration of drug combinations in which aminopenicillins currently represent the therapeutic basis because they are slightly more active against the pathogenic actinomycetes than is penicillin G and because they are able to inhibit *Aggregatibacter (Actinobacillus) actinomycetemcomitans* which is usually resistant to narrow-spectrum penicillins. However, the presence of concomitant β-lactamase producers such as *Bacteroides fragilis*, *B. thetaiotaomicron*, or *Staphylococcus aureus* (β-lactamase producing) may impair the therapeutic efficacy of aminopenicillins and that of many other β-lactams so that the combination with a β-lactamase inhibitor is advisable or even necessary.

For cervicofacial actinomycoses, amoxicillin plus clavulanic acid has proved to be the treatment of choice. Three doses of 2.0 g amoxicillin plus 0.2 g clavulanic acid every day for 1 week and three doses of 1.1 g of the combination for an additional 7 days usually result in complete cure. Thoracic actinomycoses mostly respond to the same regimen. However, it is advisable to maintain doses of 2.2 g 3 times a day for 2 weeks, and to continue treatment for 3 to 4 weeks. Advanced pulmonary cases may require the addition of 2 g ampicillin three times a day in order to increase the tissue concentration of aminopenicillin and, depending on the composition of the concomitant flora, the use of an antimicrobial specifically active against resistant *Enterobacteriaceae*; the application of drugs such as metronidazole or clindamycin against strict anaerobes is only necessary as an adjunct to the aminopenicillins in chronic cases with reduced blood supply.

Since in abdominal actinomycoses *Enterobacteriaceae* and β-lactamase producing *Bacteroides* spp. are usually present and the correct diagnosis is mostly established late, suitable antimicrobial combinations for these cases are amoxicillin plus clavulanic acid plus metronidazole plus tobramycin (gentamicin) or ampicillin plus clindamycin plus an aminoglycoside. Imipenem might also be a good choice, but this drug has not yet been widely used for treating actinomycotic infections.

Neither clindamycin nor metronidazole should be used alone. Clindamycin is almost completely ineffective against *Aggregatibacter (Actinobacillus) actinomycetemcomitans* and metronidazole shows no activity at all against pathogenic actinomycetes. The use of further combinations, including additional aminoglycosides, cephalosporins, or β-lactamase-stable penicillins, may be necessary depending on the presence of unusual aerobic organisms. In patients allergic to penicillins, tetracyclines or possibly cephalosporins may be tried instead of aminopenicillins. Incision of abscesses and drainage of pus may still be necessary as an adjunct to the antimicrobial chemotherapy and may help to accelerate recovery and to decrease the risk of relapses.

Prognosis

The prognosis of cervicofacial and cutaneous actinomycotic infections is good provided that the diagnosis is established early and antimicrobial treatment is adequate. However, thoracic, abdominal, and systemic manifestations remain serious conditions that require all possible diagnostic and therapeutic efforts. Without proper treatment, the prognosis is grave.

Epidemiology

Actinomycoses are not transmissible and cannot be brought under control by vaccination or by measures that prevent spread. Sporadically, they occur worldwide. In Germany, the incidence of the disease was estimated to range from 1 in 40 000 (acute and chronic cases together) to 1 in 80 000 (chronic cases alone) per year, but appears to be decreasing in recent years.

Men are affected 2 to 4 times more frequently by cervicofacial actinomycoses than are women. However, the male to female ratio appears to vary with age. Although actinomycoses may be found in patients of any age, men are predominantly affected between their 20th and 50th years and women in the second to fourth decade of their lives. Before puberty and in old age, actinomycoses occur sporadically in patients of both sexes without the pronounced predisposition of men.

Other diseases caused by fermentative actinomycetes

Fermentative actinomycetes play some part in dental caries and periodontal disease, but are clearly not the most important microbes contributing to these important health problems. Lacrimal canaliculitis with and without conjunctivitis is commonly caused by fermentative actinomycetes, in particular *P. propionicum*, but less frequently also by *Actinomyces israelii*, *A. gerencseriae*, *A. naeslundii*, *A. oris*, or *A. odontolyticus*. The concomitant flora, when present, is usually less complex than that of typical actinomycoses. Removal of the lacrimal concretions that are usually present and local application of antimicrobials always result in prompt cure.

Trueperella pyogenes (formerly *Arcanobacterium*, *Actinomyces*, or *Corynebacterium pyogenes*, respectively) and *Arcanobacterium haemolyticum* (formerly *Corynebacterium haemolyticum*) cause acute pharyngitis, urethritis, cutaneous or subcutaneous suppurations, or bacteraemia. The recently described species *A. graevenitzii*, *A. europaeus*, *A. radingae*, *A. turicensis*, *A. funkei*, *A. cardiffensis*, *A. hongkongensis*, *A. oricola*, *A. urogenitalis*, *A. dentalis*, *A. massiliensis*, *A. timonensis*, and *A. hominis*, as well as *Trueperella* (*Arcanobacterium Actinomyces*) *bernardiae*, *Actinobaculum schaalii*, and *Varibaculum cambriense* have been isolated from various clinical sources including abscesses and blood cultures, and may also be associated with mixed bacterial flora. *A. neuii* subsp. *neuii* and *A. neuii* subsp. *anitratus* are most frequently involved aetiologically in abscesses and infected atheromas, but may also cause infections of skin structures, endophthalmitis, and bacteraemias including

endocarditis. *A. turicensis* and possibly *A. urogenitalis* seem to be particularly common in genital infections, while *A. radingae* was found only in patients with skin-related pathologies and *A. nasicola* was isolated from pus from the nasal antrum. *A. europaeus*, *A. turicensis*, and *A. urogenitalis* as well as *Actinobaculum schaalii*, *A. urinale*, and *A. massiliense* were detected in predominantly elderly patients with urinary tract or bloodstream infections, and *A. radicidentis* was isolated from infected root canals of teeth.

Further reading

Hall V (2011). Genus V. *Varibaculum* Hall, Collins, Lawson, Hutson, Falsen, Inganäs and Duerden 2003, 644[VP]. In: Whitman WB, *et al.* (eds) *Bergey's manual of systematic bacteriology*, 2nd ed., vol. 5: *Actinobacteria*, pp. 139–40. Springer-Verlag, Dordrecht.

Henssge U, *et al.* (2009). Emended description of Actinomyces naeslundii and description of Actinomyces oris sp. nov. and Actinomyces johnsonii sp. nov., previously identified as Actinomyces naeslundii genospecies 1, 2 and WVA 963. *Int J Syst Evol Microbiol*, **59**, 509–16.

Lawson PA (2011). Genus II. *Actinobaculum* Lawson, Falsen, Åkervall, Vandamme and Collins 1997, 902[VP]. In: Whitman WB, *et al.* (eds) *Bergey's Manual of systematic bacteriology*, 2nd ed., vol. 5: *Actinobacteria*, pp. 109–14. Springer-Verlag, Dordrecht.

McNeil MM, Schaal KP (1998). Actinomycoses. In: Yu VL, Merigan TC Jr, Barriere SL (eds) *Antimicrobial therapy and vaccines*, pp. 14–22. Williams and Wilkins, Baltimore.

Pulverer G, Schütt-Gerowitt H, Schaal KP (2003). Human cervicofacial actinomycoses: microbiological data of 1997 cases. *Clin Infect Dis*, **37**, 490–7.

Schaal KP (1986). Genus *Arachnia* Pine and Georg 1969, 269. In: Sneath PHA, *et al.* (eds) *Bergey's manual of systematic bacteriology*, vol. 2, pp. 1332–42. Williams and Wilkins, Baltimore.

Schaal KP (1986). Genus *Actinomyces* Harz 1877, 133. In: Sneath PHA, *et al.* (eds) *Bergey's manual of systematic bacteriology*, vol. 2, pp. 1383–418. Williams and Wilkins, Baltimore.

Schaal KP, Lee HJ (1992). Actinomycete infections in humans: a review. *Gene*, **115**, 201–11.

Schaal KP, Pulverer G (1984). Epidemiologic, etiologic, diagnostic, and therapeutic aspects of endogenous actinomycete infections. In: Ortiz-Ortiz L, Bojalil LF, Yakoleff V (eds) *Biological, biochemical, and biomedical aspects of actinomycetes*, pp. 13–32. Academic Press, Orlando.

Schaal KP, Yassin AF (2011). Family I. *Actinomycetaceae* Buchanan 1918, 403, emend. Stackebrandt, Rainey and Ward-Rainey 1997, 484. In: Whitman WB, *et al.* (eds) *Bergey's manual of systematic bacteriology*, 2nd ed., vol. 5: *Actinobacteria*, pp. 36–42. Springer-Verlag, Dordrecht.

Schaal KP, Yassin AF (2011). Genus I. *Actinomyces* Harz 1877, 133[AL], emend. Georg, Pine and Gerencser 1969, 292[VP]. In: Whitman WB, *et al.* (eds) *Bergey's manual of systematicn bacteriology*, 2nd ed., vol. 5: *Actinobacteria*, pp. 42–109. Springer-Verlag, Dordrecht.

Schaal KP, Yassin AF, Stackebrandt E (2006). The family Actinomycetaceae: the genera *Actinomyces*, *Actinobaculum*, *Arcanobacterium*, *Varibaculum*, and *Mobiluncus*. In: Balows A, *et al.* (eds) *The prokaryotes. A handbook on the biology of bacteria: ecophysiology, isolation, identification, applications*, 2nd edition, vol. 1, pp. 850–905. Springer, Berlin.

von Graevenitz A (2011). *Actinomyces neuii*: review of an unusual infectious agent. *Infection*, **39**, 97–100.

Yassin AF, Schaal KP (2011). Genus III. *Arcanobacterium* Collins, Jones and Schofield 1983, 438[VP]. In: Whitman WB, *et al.* (eds) *Bergey's manual of systematic bacteriology*, 2nd ed., vol. 5: *Actinobacteria*, pp. 114–26. Springer-Verlag, Dordrecht.

Yassin AF, *et al.* (2011). Comparative chemotaxonomic and phylogenetic studies on the genus *Arcanobacterium* Collins *et al.* 1982, emend. Lehnen *et al.* 2006: proposal for *Trueperella* gen. nov. and emended description of the genus *Arcanobacterium*. *Int J Syst Evol Microbiol*, **61**, 1265–74.

6.30 Nocardiosis

Roderick J. Hay

Essentials

Nocardia species—*Nocardia asteroides*, *N. brasiliensis*, and *N. otidiscaviarum*—are Gram-positive, filamentous, partially acid-fast bacteria. They are occasionally detectable in environmental sources such as soil, but they rarely cause infections in humans, although they can give rise to a variety of different diseases. In healthy individuals, most commonly in the tropics, they can present with cutaneous abscesses or subcutaneous infections (actinomycetoma) in which the organisms are present as clusters of filaments or grains. In immunocompromised patients they cause a disseminated or localized deep infection, with particular sites affected being the lungs or brain. Diagnosis of nocardial infection depends on culture, although histopathology is very useful in nocardial actinomycetomas. Antibiotic treatment is typically with a sulphonamide (often as co-trimoxazole for lung infections), but combinations of drugs are usually given because the responsiveness of *Nocardia* species is very variable.

Introduction

Nocardiosis (nocardiasis) is the infection caused by *Nocardia* species, at least 33 of which cause disease in humans. *N. asteroides*, formerly considered the most common species associated with human disease, has been redefined as *N. asteroides* complex which includes *N. asteroides* sensu stricto, *N. farcinica*, *N. nova*, and *N. transvalensis* complex. Of these, *N. farcinica* appears to be more virulent than the others as it is more likely to present with disseminated disease and is more resistant to antimicrobials. Molecular studies indicate that *N. brasiliensis*, *N.otitidiscavarium*, and *N. transvalensis* exhibit diverse characteristics and it is anticipated that new species will continue to emerge.

Nocardiosis most commonly affects the lungs (39% of cases) but may be systemic (≥2 sites involved, 32%), involve the central nervous system (9%); cutaneous (8%), or occur at a single extrapulomonary site (e.g. eyes, bone; 12%).

The nocardia are Gram-positive filamentous branching bacteria that ramify in infected tissues. They can also break up into bacillary forms and, in some conditions, aggregate into grains typical of mycetomas. These organisms are aerobic and partially acid fast. They grow readily on ordinary laboratory media.

Pathogenesis

Nocardia spp. are found in soil, particularly where there is decaying vegetation and in aquatic environments. They can also be isolated from the air and, in most cases, systemic infection is by the airborne route; rarely nocardiosis can be acquired after inoculation into the skin. The characteristic histopathological response to infection is the production of polymorphonuclear leucocyte abscesses without extensive fibrosis. Caseation and palisading granulomas are not generally seen. Dissemination to other organs such as brain and skin can occur. By contrast, in primary cutaneous infections the lesion is usually localized to an abscess containing filaments at the site of inoculation and is accompanied by local lymphadenopathy. Mycetoma grain formation may occur in some of these infections that follow inoculation. It is not known why, in some patients, transcutaneous infection with nocardia results in the development of a mycetoma whereas in others a subcutaneous abscess containing filaments is formed. The formation of mycetomas appears to be more common with *N. brasiliensis* infections.

Epidemiology

In the early 1970s the incidence of nocardiosis was estimated to be 500 to 1000 cases per year; this is likely to be an underestimate as nocardiosis is not a notifiable disease. The current incidence is likely to be much higher as the number of immunocompromised individuals at risk for nocardiosis (e.g. transplant recipients) increases. Otherwise healthy patients may be infected by nocardia, although the frequency of subclinical exposure and sensitization in normal populations is unknown. However, the majority of patients with systemic nocardiosis are immunocompromised, most commonly with a condition that affects the expression of T-lymphocyte-mediated immune responses. Underlying conditions include:

- malignancies, including cancer and lymphoma
- HIV infection and other immunodeficiency states such as chronic granulomatous disease
- solid organ transplantation
- other conditions that require high doses of corticosteroids, such as collagen vascular disease and rheumatoid arthritis
- pre-existing pulmonary disease; alveolar proteinosis, in particular, seems to predispose to nocardiosis
- tumour necrosis factor α inhibitors

Inhalation of the organism is thought to be the most common route of infection and is supported by evidence that the majority of infections involve the lung. Other modes of entry include ingestion of contaminated food, direct inoculation into the skin (causing cutaneous disease), and nosocomial transmission (e.g. a report of a cluster of postoperative sternal wound infection caused by *N. farcinica*). The usual site of primary infection is the lung and the disease may remain restricted to this site. It may also be disseminated to other organs, particularly to the brain and skin. Nocardiosis can occur at any age, although it is rare, particularly in childhood.

Clinical features

Primary cutaneous nocardiosis

This is an uncommon infection that appears to follow traumatic inoculation of organisms into a superficial abrasion. The usual primary lesion is a small nodule, ulcer, or abscess at the site of inoculation. There may be a small chain of secondary nodules (as in sporotrichosis, Chapter 7.1) along the course of a lymphatic and local lymphadenopathy is common (Fig. 6.30.1). Some such cases resolve spontaneously. This form of disease is usually caused by *N. asteroides*.

Nocardia mycetoma

This is discussed in Chapter 7.1; *N. brasiliensis* is the usual cause.

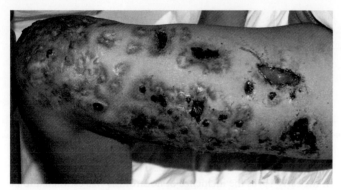

Fig. 6.30.1 Extensive chronic nocardiosis at site of injury in a 27-year-old Peruvian man, Instituto de Medicina Tropical 'Alexander von Humboldt', Universidad Peruana Cayetano Heredia, Lima, Peru.
(Copyright D A Warrell.)

Pulmonary nocardiosis

Pulmonary infection is seen in about 75% of cases of systemic nocardiosis, even where there are disseminated lesions elsewhere. Symptoms of pulmonary nocardiosis are variable with cough, fever, and leucocytosis. In otherwise healthy individuals the changes and signs may be very similar to pulmonary tuberculosis, whereas in the immunocompromised patient the lesions present as rapidly developing, single or multiple lung lesions. In HIV-infected patients with symptoms are often minimal, even in the presence of extensive disease. These changes are reflected by the course of the disease. In some patients progression is rapid, in others it is chronic.

Chest radiographs may show segmental or lobar infiltrates, cavitation, nodules, or diffuse miliary infiltrates; endobronchial infection has been recorded. Calcification is not common. The infection may spread locally to involve adjacent structures such as the pleural space and diaphragm or may spread to other sites. Very occasionally, *Nocardia* spp. can be isolated from sputum of otherwise healthy patients. Whether this reflects the process of asymptomatic sensitization is not known. Most cases of pulmonary nocardiosis are caused by *N. asteroides*.

Disseminated nocardiosis

Haematogenous spread is seen in the immunocompromised patient and may occur without evidence of pulmonary infection. The most common site for dissemination is the brain where it presents with localized abscesses without meningeal involvement. The signs are those due to an intracerebral space-occupying lesion. Spread to other sites is less common, although dissemination to skin, liver, kidneys, and bone may occur.

The acute disseminated forms and those with involvement of the central nervous system have the worst prognosis. Continued therapy with corticosteroids also appears to have bad prognostic significance. Infection in HIV-infected patients may not be recognized before death. Rapid diagnosis is therefore a key to successful management. By contrast, pulmonary infection in otherwise healthy patients is usually a chronic process and has to be distinguished from tuberculosis.

Laboratory diagnosis

The infection is often recognized initially by direct microscopy of pus, bronchial washings, or tissue. In Gram's stains the organisms

can be shown as fine branching filaments, although distinction from other bacteria may be difficult if short rod-like forms predominate. A modified acid-fast stain using weak acid can be used to demonstrate filaments.

Nocardia spp. grow on ordinary media but require prolonged incubation as colonies may take 5 to 21 days to appear. The laboratory should be informed if nocardiosis is suspected as cultures will need prolonged incubation. Growth may be enhanced by the use of selective media such as buffered charcoal yeast extract (BCYE) and Thayer–Martin medium. Nocardia have variable colonial morphology varying from chalky white to yellow, orange, or brown colonies.

Speciation of nocardia using conventional phenotypic methods is difficult and time-consuming. Polymerase chain reaction (PCR) for identification of nocardia species is more rapid and accurate the phenotypic tests but is not available in routine diagnostic laboratories.

Antimicrobial susceptibility testing should be performed for all clinically significant isolates. The optimal method is the broth microdilution method, but minimum inhibitory concentrations may be difficult to interpret.

Histopathological examination is useful in some cases. Filaments stain with modified acid-fast stains using an aqueous solution of a weak acid for decolorization, but can also be highlighted with the methenamine–silver stain (Grocott's modification). The branching nature of the organism is best appreciated in histopathological material. Other pathogens such as *Pneumocystis* spp. may also be present in histopathological material.

Serological tests (usually counter-immunoelectrophoresis or enzyme immunoassay) can be obtained in reference centres and are generally used to monitor the progress of therapy rather than establish the diagnosis.

Therapy

The mainstays of therapy are sulphonamides such as sulfadiazine and sulfafurazole, given in doses of 4 to 6 g daily. Co-trimoxazole is also effective, particularly in pulmonary forms, although the ratio of the trimethoprim to sulphonamide components is not ideal for intracerebral infections. In many cases, drainage of abscesses may hasten recovery. Non-*asteroides* species of nocardia often do not respond as well to sulphonamides. Much of the recommended drug therapy is derived from the personal experiences of a few cases. It is, for instance, the general practice to use two antibiotics.

Other drugs that have been used include amikacin, ampicillin, linezolid, and minocycline, although testing is necessary before using these. Experience of other drugs is similarly limited. For instance, ciprofloxacin, cefotaxime, and imipenem are all active *in vitro* but clinical experience with them is limited to a few cases.

Clustering of cases may occur occasionally, suggesting exposure to a common source of infection. In two such episodes there had been extensive construction work in the vicinity of the hospital involved. At present, no methods of prevention are known, although the existence of more than two cases in a single or adjacent wards should alert clinicians to the possibility of environmentally acquired infection.

Further reading

Boiron P, *et al.* (1992). Review of nocardial infections in France, 1987–1990. *Eur J Clin Microbiol Infect Dis*, **11**, 709–14.

Brown-Elliott BA, *et al.* (2006). Clinical and laboratory features of the *Nocardia* spp. based on current molecular taxonomy. *Clin Microbiol Rev*, **19**, 259–82.

Filice GA (2005). Nocardiosis in persons with human immunodeficiency virus infection, transplant recipients, and large, geographically defined populations. *J Lab Clin Med*, **145**, 156–62.

Georghiou PR, Blacklock ZM (1992). Infection with *Nocardia* species in Queensland. A review of 102 clinical isolates. *Med J Aust*, **156**, 692–7.

Hay RJ (1983). Nocardial infections of the skin. *J Hyg (Lond)*, **91**, 385–91.

Houang ET, *et al.* (1980). *Nocardia asteroides* infection: a transmissible disease. *J Hosp Infect*, **1**, 31–6.

Kilincer C, *et al.* (2006). Nocardial brain abscess: review of clinical management. *J Clin Neurosci*, **13**, 481–5.

Sakai C, Takagi T, Satoh Y (1999). *Nocardia asteroides* pneumonia, subcutaneous abscess and meningitis in a patient with advanced malignant lymphoma: successful treatment based on *in vitro* antimicrobial susceptibility. *Intern Med*, **38**, 683–6.

6.31 **Rat-bite fevers**

David A. Warrell

Essentials

Rat-bite fever is usually attributable to *Streptobacillus moniliformis* in the Americas, Europe, and Australia; in Asia, *Spirillum minus* is the commoner cause. Both bacteria are commensals of rodents and their predators. Haverhill fever follows ingestion of *S. moniliformis* in rat-contaminated milk or water. After an incubation period less than 1 week, *S. moniliformis* causes sudden high fever, rigors, myalgia, petechial rash, and migratory reactive or septic polyarthritis with synovial effusions. Complications include fulminant septicaemia, endocarditis, pneumonia, and metastatic abscesses. *S. minus* infection (sodoku) has a longer incubation period with similarly high fever but concomitant exacerbation of the bite wound, local lymphadenopathy, papular rash, and arthralgia without effusions. In both diseases, fever subsides after a few days but may relapse repeatedly over months. Untreated mortality is about 10% for *S. moniliformis* and 2 to 10% for *S. minus*. *S. moniliformis* can be cultured (with some difficulty) and the diagnosis confirmed by polymerase chain reaction (PCR) methods and serology. *S. minus* cannot be confirmed by culture or serology but can be demonstrated microscopically in the bite wound and other tissues or by isolation in animals. Penicillin is the treatment of choice for both infections. Prevention is by controlling peridomestic rats, avoiding bites by pet or laboratory rodents and pasteurising milk (Haverhill fever).

Introduction

Feral rodent populations are increasing worldwide and rat bites occur in impoverished infested rural and urban dwellings. Under these conditions, young children are often bitten while asleep and patients with diabetic or leprous neuropathy are particularly vulnerable. However, increasing numbers of rodents are now kept as pets and as laboratory animals, explaining why bites are becoming more common among pet owners and pet shop and laboratory workers. There are said to be at least 20000 rat bites in the United States of America each year. Wild rats harbour a variety of other zoonotic pathogens including cryptosporidium, pasteurella, yersinia, listeria, coxiella, salmonella, leptospira, toxoplasma, and hantaviruses.

Streptobacillus moniliformis infection (streptobacillary rat-bite fever and Haverhill fever)

Aetiology

Streptobacillus moniliformis is part of the normal pharyngeal flora of 50 to 100% of wild and 10 to 100% of laboratory rats. It can be recovered from their nasopharynx, middle ear, saliva, and urine. In rodents it can cause septicaemia, pneumonia, conjunctivitis, polyarthritis, and abortion. It has been isolated from rats, mice, guinea pigs, gerbils, squirrels, and animals that feed on rodents such as cats, dogs, pigs, ferrets, and weasels. *S. moniliformis* infection is reported in monkeys, koalas, and turkeys.

S. moniliformis is named after the necklace-like filaments and chains with yeast-like swellings seen in mature cultures on solid media. It is a nonmotile pleomorphic filamentous Gram-negative rod, 1 to 5 μm long. Although it can be grown in ordinary blood culture media, it is ultrafastidious, microaerophilic, and slow-growing making it difficult to isolate. However, it thrives on trypticase soy agar enriched with 20% horse or rabbit blood, serum, or ascitic fluid under 8% carbon dioxide. In liquid media, 'puff ball' colonies appear in 2 to 7 days. In concentrations as low as 0.0125%, sodium polyanethol sulphonate (liquoid), a laboratory anticoagulant added to most commercial aerobic media, inhibits the growth of *S. moniliformis*. On agar, 'fried-egg' colonies appearing after 5 days culture signify L-phase variants that lack a cell wall and are therefore resistant to penicillin.

Epidemiology

S. moniliformis infection occurs worldwide causing rat-bite fever and Haverhill fever.

Streptobacillary rat-bite fever

As a cause of rat-bite fever, *S. moniliformis* is apparently much commoner than *Spirillum minus* in the Americas, Europe, and Australia. Despite its name, there is no history of a bite in 30% of cases. Bites or scratches by rodents or their predators, contact with mucous membranes (e.g. when pet owners kiss or share food with their rodents), or other contact with these mammals whether living or dead may result in infection. In some countries, 10% of those bitten by wild rats are infected. Formerly, most people with rat bites were children of poor families living in urban areas. A bite might not be suspected because it was inflicted while they were asleep. In the United States of America, 55% of those infected are children younger than 12 years old. Increasing numbers of people with rat-bite fever are pet owners and pet shop and laboratory staff. Human-to-human transmission has not been reported.

Haverhill fever

Named after a town in Massachusetts where there was an outbreak involving 86 cases in 1926, Haverhill fever follows ingestion of raw milk, food, or water contaminated by rats. An outbreak in a boarding school in England in 1983 affected 304 people, 43% of the school's population, and was attributed to contamination of the water supply by rats.

Clinical features

Streptobacillary rat-bite fever

If transmission is by bite, the wound usually heals quickly with only trivial local inflammation or pustule formation.

The systemic illness starts suddenly after an incubation period that is usually less than 7 days, is often as short as 1 to 3 days, but is sometimes as long as 7 weeks. There is high fever with rigors, vomiting, severe headache, sore throat, myalgia, and muscle tenderness lasting 3 to 5 days. About 75% of patients develop a rash 1 to 8 days later. Discrete erythematous macules or papules, 1 to 4 mm in diameter, appear symmetrically on the lateral and extensor surfaces and over the joints. They are often most marked on the hands and feet (palms and soles) with associated petechiae, but may also occur on the face. Papules, vesicles, haemorrhagic vesicles, and pustules with scabs may develop. There is desquamation in about 20% of cases. Early in the illness, approximately one-half the patients develop an asymmetrical migratory subacute or chronic polyarthralgia or arthritis which is thought to be reactive (autoimmune). It usually involves the knees, ankles, elbows, shoulders, and hips and is often associated with sterile effusions. Far less commonly, a distinct streptobacillary septic (suppurative) arthritis affects single or multiple distal joints, most often the knee but also the fingers. Severe joint pain and tenderness may be the dominant symptom in patients with rat-bite fever. Diarrhoea and loss of weight are described in young children. Fever and other symptoms subside in a few days in treated cases, but fever may persist for 1 to 2 weeks, relapsing repeatedly over several months, and arthritis may persist for many months in those who are untreated. Severe infections can lead to bronchitis, pneumonia, pleural effusions, metastatic abscess formation (including cerebral abscess), endocarditis, myocarditis, pericarditis with effusion, subacute glomerulonephritis, interstitial nephritis, splenitis or splenic abscess, amnionitis, meningitis, hepatitis, systemic vasculitis, polyarteritis nodosa, and renal and multiorgan failure. Infective endocarditis, usually with underlying rheumatic or other valve disease, has been described.

Haverhill fever

Haverhill fever (erythema arthriticum epidemicum) follows a similar clinical course after the patient has drunk unpasteurized milk or contaminated water. Vomiting, stomatitis, and upper respiratory tract symptoms such as sore throat are said to be more prominent than in rat-bite fever.

Differential diagnosis

Unlike *Spirillum minus* infection (sodoku, see below), the other cause of rat-bite fever, the incubation period is usually short, the bite wound heals permanently with little local lymphadenopathy, the rash is morbilliform or petechial, and arthritis is common. Depending on the geographical area, *S. moniliformis* infection must be distinguished from other acute fevers associated with rodent bites and contact, including lymphocytic choriomeningitis and other arenaviruses, hantaviruses, leptospirosis, melioidosis, tularaemia, plague, murine typhus, trench fever, and *Pasteurella multocida*.

The polyarthritis may be confused with acute rheumatic fever, rheumatoid arthritis, systemic lupus erythematosus, or Still's disease. The acute febrile illness and exanthem may suggest other bacterial septicaemias such as meningococcaemia, rickettsial infections, and even secondary syphilis and in children, Kawasaki disease.

Fever after ingestion of raw milk should raise the possibility of brucellosis.

Diagnosis

The diagnosis can be confirmed by culture of bite wounds, blood, synovial and pericardial fluid, skin blister fluid, or pus from abscesses, but the organism is ultrafastidious and slow-growing (see above). In patients with infective endocarditis the differential diagnosis of these slow-growing microaerophilic organism includes *Haemophilus aphrophilus*, *Cardiobacterium hominis*, *Actinomyces actinomycetemcomitans*, and *Eikenella corrodens*. A high or rising titre of agglutinins, complement-fixing or fluorescent antibodies, may be detected between 2 and 3 weeks. Polymerase chain reaction based on 16S rRNA gene sequences, discriminated by BfaI restriction enzyme treatment, is promising. Patients sometimes show a moderate peripheral leucocytosis. The pleomorphic filamentous bacteria may be stained in peripheral blood leucocytes or tissue samples using Gram's, Wright's, or silver stains. In cases of streptobacillary septic arthritis, the synovial fluid contains many leucocytes (neutrophils around $50\,000 \times 10^9$/litre) and bacteria may be visible. False-positive serological tests for syphilis (Venereal Disease Research Laboratory (VDRL) test) are found in 15 to 25% of cases.

Treatment

S. moniliformis is sensitive to penicillin and can be treated with benzyl penicillin 1.2 million units/day for 5 to 7 days followed by oral penicillin or ampicillin 500 mg four times a day for 7 days if there is improvement. Procaine benzylpenicillin (adult dose 600 mg or 600 000 units) by intramuscular injection every 12 h for 7 to 14 days and penicillin V 2 g/day by mouth are also effective. Penicillin-resistant L-variants are susceptible to streptomycin (7.5 mg/kg intramuscularly twice daily), tetracycline (500 mg orally four times a day), and probably erythromycin. For patients hypersensitive to penicillin, erythromycin, chloramphenicol, tetracycline, or cephalosporins can be used. Erythromycin was used successfully in the boarding-school outbreak of Haverhill fever in England in 1983.

Patients with endocarditis should be treated with intravenous benzylpenicillin, 4.8 to 14.4 g (8–24 000 000 units) each day for between 4 and 6 weeks, or 4.8 000 000 units of procaine benzylpenicillin daily by intramuscular injection for 4 weeks if the cultured organism has a sensitivity of 0.1 µg/ml. The addition of streptomycin improves bactericidal activity and eliminates L-forms.

Affected joints may require aspiration or even surgical debridement.

Prognosis

The untreated case fatality was reported to be 10 to 13%. However, the overall mortality in patients with endocarditis, many of whom were untreated or treated late, exceeded 50%. Fulminant and rapidly fatal cases have been reported in immunocompetent children and adults. In survivors, residual arthralgia persisting for as long as 10 years has been described.

Spirillum minus infection (sodoku, sokosha)

Aetiology

The cause of sodoku, *Spirillum minus*, is a relatively thick tightly coiled Gram-negative rod or spirillum (not a spirochaete), between 2.5 and 5.0 μm long, with 2 to 6 (commonly 3) spirals, resembling campylobacters. It darts about under the power of its terminal flagella. Continuous culture on artificial media has not been achieved, but the organism can be demonstrated by inoculating material from the bite wound, regional lymph nodes, or blood intraperitoneally into mice or guinea pigs. Organisms usually appear in the rodent's blood within 5 to 15 days of inoculation. *Spirillum minus* may be found in the blood of up to 25% of apparently healthy rodents and in the eye discharge and mouths of rats with interstitial keratitis and conjunctivitis. In the 1930s, 'sodoku inoculata' (the blood of infected guinea pigs) was used to treat neurosyphilis.

Epidemiology

Sodoku is found worldwide but is particularly common in Japan. In Asia it is commoner than *S. moniliformis* as a cause of rat-bite fever. Infection results from bites, scratches, or mere contact with rodents or their predators including dogs, cats, and pigs.

Clinical features

The initial bite wound usually heals without signs of local inflammation. After an incubation period of 1 to 36 days, but usually 14 to 18 days, there is sudden fever which, in untreated cases, reaches its height in 3 days and resolves by crisis after a further 3 days. At the start of the illness the healed bite wound becomes inflamed, swollen, and indurated; it may break down to become a necrotic or suppurating ulcer. Regional lymph nodes are usually enlarged and tender. Other acute symptoms include rigors, myalgia, and prostration. A rash develops in approximately one-half of patients. It often spreads from the site of the bite and consists of angry purplish or reddish-brown indurated papules, plaques, or macules with urticarial lesions. Arthralgia may be severe but there are no joint effusions. Severe manifestations including meningitis, cerebral abscess, encephalitis, endocarditis, myocarditis, myocardial abscess, pleural effusion, chorioamnionitis, subcutaneous abscesses, and involvement of liver, kidney, and other organs are seen in about 10% of patients. Relapses of fever, rash, and other symptoms lasting 3 to 6 days may occur between remissions of between a week and 2 months and occasionally up to a year in untreated patients.

Differential diagnosis

Sodoku must be distinguishable from streptobacillary rat-bite fever (see above). Its tendency to relapse may suggest relapsing fever (*Borrelia* spp.) or trench fever (*Bartonella quintana*).

Diagnosis

The diagnosis can be confirmed by examining aspirates from the bite wound, lymph nodes, exanthem, or blood (thick and thin films) using dark-field microscopy or Wright's or Giemsa's stains. The organism can be detected in the blood, peritoneal fluid, or heart muscle of inoculated rodents but cannot be cultured on artificial media. No specific serological tests are available. False-positive serological tests for syphilis are found in 50 to 60% of cases, and reactions with Proteus OXK are also common.

Treatment

Penicillin is the drug of choice. For adults, procaine benzylpenicillin 600 mg (600 000 units) should be given every 12 h for 7 to 14 days. Penicillin V, 2 g/day by mouth, is also said to be effective. A Jarisch–Herxheimer reaction may complicate penicillin treatment.

Prognosis

Untreated case fatality is about 2 to 10%.

Prevention of rat-bite fevers

These infections can be prevented by controlling wild peridomestic rodents and by encouraging laboratory and pet shop workers to wear protective gloves and to handle rodents carefully, to avoid hand-to-mouth or hand-to-eye contact, to wash their hands, and to clean all rodent bite wounds. The efficacy of postexposure prophylaxis with antibiotics is unproven. Young children should be supervised when they handle pet rodents to avoid bites, kissing, sharing food, and hand-to-mouth or hand-to-eye contact. An enzyme-linked immunosorbent assay (ELISA) has been developed for surveillance of rodent colonies for *S. moniliformis*. Haverhill fever is prevented by avoiding the consumption of raw milk, by monitoring water supplies (especially those not derived from the mains), and by controlling rat populations.

Further reading

Dendle C, Woolley IJ, Korman TM (2006). Rat-bite fever septic arthritis: illustrative case and literature review. *Eur J Clin Microbiol Infect Dis*, **25**, 791–7.

Elliott SP (2007). Rat bite fever and *Streptobacillus moniliformis*. *Clin Microbiol Rev*, **20**, 13–22.

Gaastra W, Boot R, Ho HT, Lipman LJ (2009). Rat bite fever. *Vet Microbiol*, **133**, 211–28.

Kimura M, Tanikawa T, Suzuki M *et al.* (2008). Detection of Streptobacillus spp. in feral rats by specific polymerase chain reaction. *Microbiol Immunol*, **52**, 9–15.

McEvoy MB, Noah ND, Pilsworth R (1987). Outbreak of fever caused by *Streptobacillus moniliformis*. *Lancet*, **ii**, 1361–3.

Raffin BJ, Freemark M (1979). Streptobacillary rat bite fever: a pediatric problem. *Pediatrics*, **64**, 214–17.

Roughgarden JW (1965). Antimicrobial therapy of rat bite fever. A review. *Arch Intern Med*, **116**, 39–54.

Rupp ME (1992). *Streptobacillus moniliformis* endocarditis: case report and review. *Clin Infect Dis*, **14**, 769–72.

6.32 Lyme borreliosis

Gary P. Wormser, John Nowakowski, and Robert B. Nadelman

Essentials

Lyme borreliosis is a zoonotic bacterial infection caused by *Borrelia burgdorferi* sensu lato, a spirochaetal agent transmitted by certain species of *Ixodes* ticks. Small rodents and birds serve as reservoirs. It is the most common vector-borne infection in the United States of America and an important infection in many countries throughout the temperate regions of Europe and northern Asia, where a wider variety of borrelia species account for differences in clinical manifestations in Eurasia compared with the United States.

Clinical features—the commonest and earliest clinical manifestation is erythema migrans, a distinctive cutaneous lesion that occurs at the site of deposition of the spirochaete by the vector tick, beginning 7 to 14 days later as a red macule or papule, with the rash then expanding over days to weeks, with or without central clearing. This may be associated with 'viral' symptoms, fever and regional lymphadenopathy. Later manifestations include (1) carditis—usually manifested by fluctuating degrees of atrioventricular block; (2) neurological involvement—including cranial neuropathy (typically cranial nerve VII palsy), radiculopathy, and meningitis; (3) arthritis—typically migratory monoarthritis or asymmetric oligoarthritis; (4) acrodermatitis chronica atrophicans—a swollen, bluish-red appearing skin lesion in which the involved skin ultimately atrophies.

Diagnosis—the diagnosis of erythema migrans is purely clinical in geographical areas endemic for Lyme borreliosis: serological testing is not recommended because it is insufficiently sensitive on acute phase serum samples. In patients with suspected later clinical manifestations, serological testing is essential because clinical findings alone lack sufficient specificity. Polymerase chain reaction (PCR) testing of joint fluid and/or cerebrospinal fluid may be helpful in some cases.

Treatment—most people treated for Lyme borreliosis respond well to a 2-week course of antibiotic therapy (preferred oral regimen usually amoxicillin, doxycycline, or cefuroxime). Symptomatic treatment is recommended for patients who have or develop subjective complaints of unclear aetiology despite successful resolution of the objective manifestation of Lyme borreliosis following antibiotic therapy, since randomized double-blind placebo-controlled trials have shown that additional antibiotic treatment is not helpful.

Prevention—measures include avoiding exposure to ticks by limiting outdoor activities in tick-infested locations, using tick repellents, tucking in clothing to decrease exposed skin surfaces, and frequent inspection of the skin for early detection and removal of ticks.

Introduction

Lyme borreliosis (also called Lyme disease) is named after Lyme, Connecticut, United States of America. It is caused by the spirochaete *Borrelia burgdorferi* sensu lato which is transmitted to humans by the usually asymptomatic bite of certain ticks of the genus *Ixodes* (Fig. 6.32.1). *Borrelia burgdorferi* sensu stricto (hereafter referred to as *B. burgdorferi*) causes the disease in North America, while in Europe, several species of *Borrelia* in addition to *B. burgdorferi* cause this infection, including *B. garinii* which is probably the most common cause of classic Lyme neuroborreliosis (Bannwarth's syndrome) and *B. afzelii* the most common cause of acrodermatitis chronica atrophicans, a late cutaneous complication. The entire chromosome and associated plasmids of multiple different strains of *B. burgdorferi* have been completely sequenced.

Representative strains of other pathogenic species, such as *B. afzelii* and *B. garinii*, have also been sequenced.

Epidemiology

In North America, more than 25 000 new cases of Lyme borreliosis are reported each year, making it the most common vector-borne disease. It occurs in north-eastern, mid-Atlantic, north-central, and far western regions of the United States of America and in limited foci in Canada (mainly in eastern Ontario). Elsewhere, it occurs in much of the temperate regions of Europe and northern Asia. Ticks acquire this borrelial infection in a complex tick–vertebrate transmission cycle. The white-footed mouse is the most important reservoir for *B. burgdorferi* in North America. White-tailed deer, an important host for adult *Ixodes* ticks, are not a competent reservoir for Lyme borreliae. In Europe a wide variety of small rodents and birds serve as reservoirs. Migrating birds may play a role in the spread of *B. burgdorferi* to new geographical locations.

Lyme borreliosis occurs slightly more frequently in males than in females. There is a bimodal age distribution with the highest rates in children between 5 and 9 years old and in adults 55 to 59 years old.

Clinical manifestations

The somewhat different manifestations of Lyme borreliosis in Eurasia compared with North America (Table 6.32.1) may be explained by the wider variety of borrelia species causing infection in Eurasia. Clinical features are similar in adults and children.

Erythema migrans

Erythema migrans (EM) (Figs. 6.32.2, 6.32.3), the clinical hallmark of Lyme borreliosis, is recognized in approximately 90% of patients with objective clinical manifestations of *B. burgdorferi* infection. Typically, EM begins as a red macule or papule at the site of a tick bite that occurred 7 to 14 days earlier. The rash expands over days to weeks. Central clearing may or may not be present. Secondary cutaneous lesions may develop because of haematogenous spread of spirochaetes to other cutaneous sites. EM must be distinguished from local tick bite reactions, tinea, insect and spider bites, bacterial cellulitis, and plant dermatitis. Lesions eventually resolve spontaneously but may recur if antimicrobial therapy is not given.

Systemic symptoms, such as fatigue, myalgia, arthralgia, headache, fever and/or chills, and stiff neck, are less common in patients with EM caused by *B. afzelii* compared to either *B. burgdorferi* or *B. garinii*. Prominent respiratory and/or gastrointestinal symptoms are so infrequent that their presence should suggest an alternative diagnosis or coinfection with another tick-borne pathogen. Aside from the EM skin lesion itself, the most common objective physical findings are regional lymphadenopathy and fever. Occasional cases of a viral-like illness without EM have been attributed to Lyme borreliosis.

Carditis

Typically, cardiac disease develops within weeks to months after infection, sometimes together with EM. It is usually manifested by fluctuating degrees of atrioventricular block that may cause the patient to complain of dizziness, palpitations, dyspnoea, chest pain, or syncope. Myocarditis may be present but pericarditis with effusion is rarely observed, and endocarditis is absent. The incidence of

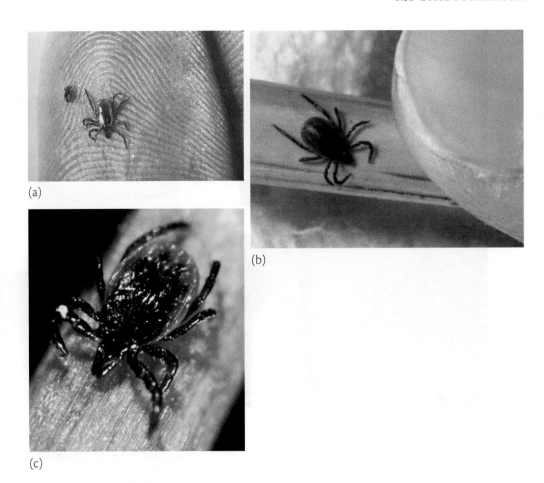

Fig. 6.32.1 (a) Adult female (right) and nymphal (left) *Ixodes scapularis* ticks. (b,c) Nymph of *Ixodes ricinus*, the vector tick in Europe.

Table 6.32.1 Lyme borreliosis in North America compared to Eurasia

	North American Lyme borreliosis	Eurasian Lyme borreliosis
Vector	*Ixodes(dammini) scapularis* or *Ixodes pacificus*	*Ixodes ricinus* or *Ixodes persulcatus*
Aetiological agent	*B. burgdorferi* sensu stricto	*B. burgdorferi* sensu stricto, *B. afzelii*, *B. garinii*, *B. spielmanii*
Clinical features	Erythema migrans is the most common manifestation.	Erythema migrans is the most common manifestation
	Systemic symptoms frequently present in patients with erythema migrans (up to 80%) Other skin manifestations such as borrelial lymphocytoma and acrodermatitis chronica atrophicans are much less common than in Europe	Systemic symptoms infrequently present in patients with erythema migrans (<35%) Other skin manifestations such as borrelial lymphocytoma and acrodermatitis chronica atrophicans are much more common than in North America
	Cranial nerve palsy (usually 7th) with or without meningitis is the most common neurological manifestation	Painful meningoradiculoneuritis with or without cranial palsy is the most common neurological manifestation

cardiac manifestations (as measured by ECG confirmed heart block) has been observed to be low in both the United States of America (<1%) and Europe (<4%).

Neurological disease

The incidence of neurological Lyme disease in Europe may be higher than in the United States of America. One explanation may be the greater neurotropism of *B. garinii* (a genospecies which has not been isolated in North America). The principal early neurological manifestations are cranial neuropathy (typically peripheral seventh nerve palsy which can be bilateral), radiculopathy, and meningitis, which may occur alone or together. EM may be present concomitantly. Late neurological manifestations are uncommon and include peripheral neuropathy, encephalopathy, and encephalomyelitis.

Antibiotics appear to hasten the resolution of meningitis but most studies are uncontrolled. The rate of resolution of motor dysfunction, which is fully reversible in the vast majority of cases, is not enhanced by antimicrobial therapy. Symptoms of encephalopathy and peripheral neuropathy improve or do not progress after treatment with antibiotics.

Rheumatological disease

Lyme arthritis occurs in both North America and Europe. In a study of 55 untreated patients with EM diagnosed in the United States of America between 1977 and 1979 and followed for a mean duration of 6 years, objective arthritis developed in more than one-half, occurring within 1 year for 90%. The majority of these patients developed intermittent attacks of migratory monoarthritis or

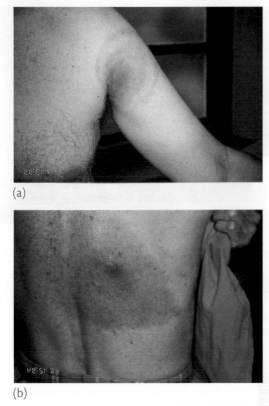

(a)

(b)

Fig. 6.32.2 (a) Erythema migrans rashes from patients who were culture positive for borrelia. (a) rash with typical central appearance; (b) rash with more homogeneous apparance.

asymmetric oligoarthritis, lasting a mean of 3 months per episode (range 3 days to 11.5 months). The knee was affected at some point in almost all patients, but other large and (less often) small joints could be affected. Temporomandibular joint involvement occurred in 11 (39%) of 28 patients with arthritis in one series. Although large effusions may occur, joint pain and erythema are often minimal. Baker's cysts may develop. Typically, synovial fluid analysis reveals a modestly elevated white cell count (median 24 250 white cells/mm^3 in one study) with a polymorphonuclear predominance and a normal glucose level. Synovitis lasting 1 year or more may ensue for a minority of United States patients, sometimes associated with joint destruction. Although *B. burgdorferi* DNA can be detected by polymerase chain reaction (PCR) in the synovial fluid of up to 85% of untreated patients with Lyme arthritis, *B. burgdorferi* has rarely been successfully cultured from joint fluid.

Acrodermatitis chronica atrophicans (ACA)

This cutaneous manifestation of late Lyme disease develops insidiously on a distal extremity, mainly in elderly women. It is a swollen bluish-red appearing skin lesion in which the involved skin ultimately atrophies. One-third of patients have an associated (usually sensory) polyneuropathy. *B. burgdorferi* has been recovered from a skin biopsy specimen of an ACA lesion of more than 10 years duration. Since the usual causative agent *B. afzelii* does not occur in the United States of America, ACA is essentially a European disease.

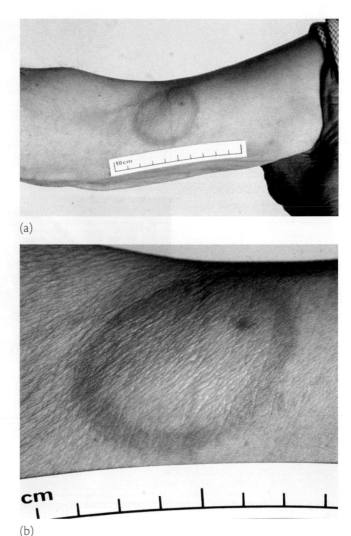

(a)

(b)

Fig. 6.32.3 English patient with typical erythema migrans. (Copyright D A Warrell.)

Miscellaneous clinical manifestations

Borrelia lymphocytoma, principally caused by *B. afzelii* and *B. garinii*, is a tumour-like nodule which typically appears on the pinna of the earlobe or on the nipple or areola of the breast. Lesions will eventually resolve spontaneously but disappear within a few weeks after antibiotic therapy. This lesion is extremely rare in North America.

Direct involvement of the eye (e.g. uveitis, keratitis, vitritis, optic neuritis) has been attributed to *B. burgdorferi* infection. However, since ophthalmological disorders have almost never been associated with the isolation of *B. burgdorferi* in culture, the actual pathogenesis in these cases is uncertain. Conjunctivitis, originally described in 11% of patients with EM, was rare (<5%) in recent studies of culture-positive patients and may be unrelated to borrelia infection.

Case reports have suggested that adverse outcomes may be associated with pregnancies complicated by maternal Lyme borreliosis. However, prospective and epidemiological studies suggest that the risk of transplacental transmission of *B. burgdorferi* is probably minimal when appropriate antibiotics (Tables 6.32.2, 6.32.3) are given to pregnant women with Lyme borreliosis. There are no published data to support a congenital Lyme borreliosis syndrome.

Table 6.32.2 Recommended antimicrobial regimens for treatment of patients with Lyme borreliosis

Drug	Dosage for adults	Dosage for children
Preferred oral regimens		
Amoxicillin	500 mg three times daily[a]	50 mg/kg per day in three divided doses (maximum 500 mg per dose)[a]
Doxycycline	100 mg twice daily[b]	<8 years: not recommended
		≥8 years: 4 mg/kg per day in two divided doses (maximum 100 mg/dose)
Cefuroxime axetil	500 mg twice daily	30 mg/kg per day in two divided doses (maximum 500 mg per dose)
Alternative oral regimens		
The following dosing regimens are specifically for patients with erythema migrans or borrelial lymphocytoma:		
Selected macrolides[c]	Azithromycin 500 mg orally daily for 7–10 days, clarithromycin 500 mg orally twice daily for 14–21 days (if not pregnant), or erythromycin 500 mg orally four times per day for 14–21 days	Azithromycin 10 mg/kg daily (maximum of 500 mg per day), clarithromycin 7.5 mg/kg twice daily (maximum of 500 mg per dose), or erythromycin 12.5 mg/kg four times daily (maximum of 500 mg per dose)
Preferred parenteral regimen		
Ceftriaxone	2 g intravenously once daily	50–75 mg/kg intravenously once daily (maximum 2 g)
Alternative parenteral regimens		
Cefotaxime	2 g intravenously every 8 h[d]	150–200 mg/kg per day intravenously in 3 or 4 divided doses (maximum 6 g per day)[d]
Penicillin G	3–4 million units intravenously every 4 h[d]	200 000–400 000 units/kg per day divided into six doses given every 4 h[d] (not to exceed 18–24 million units/day)

[a] Although higher dosage given twice daily might be equally as effective, in view of the absence of data on efficacy, twice daily administration is not recommended.

[b] Tetracyclines are relatively contraindicated in pregnant or lactating women and in children less than 8 years of age.

[c] Due to their lower efficacy, macrolides are reserved for patients who are unable to take or who are intolerant of tetracyclines, penicillins, and cephalosporins. Patients treated with macrolides should be closely followed to ensure resolution of the clinical manifestations.

[d] Dosage should be reduced for patients with impaired renal function.

(Modified from Wormser GP, *et al.* (2006). The clinical assessment, treatment, and prevention of Lyme disease, human granulocytic anaplasmosis and babesiosis. Clinical practices guidelines by the Infectious Diseases Society of America. *Clin Infect Dis*, **43**, 1089–134).

Laboratory diagnosis

Where Lyme borreliosis is endemic, the diagnosis of EM is purely clinical. Laboratory testing is neither necessary nor recommended.

In patients with suspected extracutaneous Lyme borreliosis, serological testing is essential to support the diagnosis. Culture of *B. burgdorferi* has been a highly insensitive diagnostic technique for this group of patients, presumably because of inaccessibility of tissues containing the microorganism. PCR testing of joint fluid and sometimes of cerebrospinal fluid may aid in diagnosis, provided appropriate care is taken in performing the assay accurately.

A two-step approach to serological diagnosis is used in both the United States of America and Europe to increase the accuracy of a positive test. A positive or equivocal first-step test (usually an enzyme-linked immunosorbent assay (ELISA) or an indirect immunofluorescence assay (IFA)) is followed on the same serum sample by a second-stage test (immunoblot). Two-step testing, however, is not indicated for those with little or no clinical evidence of Lyme borreliosis because of a low positive predictive value. Since IgM and IgG antibodies to *B. burgdorferi* may persist in serum for years after clinical recovery, serology has no role in measuring response to treatment.

Patients with extracutaneous Lyme borreliosis almost always have diagnostic serum antibodies at time of presentation. In some patients with early neuroborreliosis, however, antibodies to Lyme borrelia may be present in cerebrospinal fluid before they are detected in serum.

Coinfection

Ixodes scapularis ticks (Fig. 6.32.1a) are the vectors for several other infections that may be transmitted separately or simultaneously with *B. burgdorferi*, such as *Babesia microti* and the rickettsial agent *Anaplasma phagocytophilum* that causes human granulocytic anaplasmosis (HGA, formerly known as human granulocytic ehrlichiosis (HGE)). In Europe, species of *Babesia* and *Anaplasma* are present in *Ixodes ricinus* ticks (Fig. 6.32.1b,c), which are also vectors of the flavivirus causing tick-borne encephalitis. Coinfection may alter the clinical presentation and response to treatment of Lyme borreliosis.

Reinfections

Reinfection with Lyme borrelia can often be recognized clinically by the development of a repeat episode of EM occurring at a different skin site during the months when the vector tick is plentiful in the environment. The clinical manifestations of reinfection in Lyme borreliosis patients who have EM are indistinguishable from initial infection.

Treatment

Although most manifestations of Lyme borreliosis resolve spontaneously, antibiotics may speed the resolution of some and will almost certainly prevent the progression of disease. An approach to treatment is summarized in Tables 6.32.2 and 6.32.3. Presently available

Table 6.32.3 Recommended therapy for patients with Lyme borreliosis[a]

Indication	Treatment	Duration (days)	Range (days)
Tick bite in the USA	Doxycycline 200 mg (4 mg/kg in children ≥8 years of age) *and/or* observation	Single dose[b]	
Erythema migrans	Oral regimen[c,d]	14	10–21[e]
Early neurological disease			
Meningitis or radiculopathy	Parenteral regimen[c,f]	14	10–28
Cranial nerve palsy[g]	Oral regimen[c]	14	14–21
Cardiac disease	Oral regimen[c,h] or	14	14–21
	Parenteral regimen[c,h]	14	14–21
Borrelial lymphocytoma	Oral regimen[c,d]	14	14–21
Late disease			
Arthritis without neurological disease	Oral regimen[c]	28	28
Recurrent arthritis after oral regimen	Oral regimen[c,i]	28	28
	Parenteral regimen[c,i]	14	14–28
Antibiotic-refractory arthritis[j]	Symptomatic therapy[k]		
Central or peripheral nervous system disease	Parenteral regimen[c]	14	14–28
Acrodermatitis chronica atrophicans	Oral regimen[c]	21	14–28
Post-Lyme disease syndrome	Consider and evaluate other potential causes of symptoms, if none found then symptomatic therapy		

[a] Regardless of the clinical manifestation of Lyme disease, complete response to treatment may be delayed beyond the treatment duration. Relapse may occur with any of these regimens; patients with objective signs of relapse may need a second course of treatment.

[b] A single dose of doxycycline may be offered to adult patients and to children ≥8 years of age in the United States of America only when all of the following circumstances exist: (a) the attached tick can be reliably identified as an adult or nymphal *I. scapularis* tick that is estimated to have been attached for ≥36 h based on the degree of engorgement of the tick with blood or on certainty about the time of exposure to the tick; (b) prophylaxis can be started within 72 h of the time that the tick was removed; (c) ecological information indicates that the local rate of infection of these ticks with *B. burgdorferi* is ≥20%; and (d) doxycycline is not contraindicated. For patients who do not fulfil these criteria, observation is recommended.

[c] See Table 6.32.2.

[d] For adult patients intolerant of amoxicillin, doxycycline, and cefuroxime axetil, a macrolide may be given (Table 6.32.2). Patients treated with macrolides should be closely followed to ensure resolution of the clinical manifestations.

[e] If doxycycline is used, 10 days of therapy is effective; the efficacy of 10-day regimens with the other first-line agents is unknown.

[f] Data from European studies of neuroborreliosis indicate that oral doxycycline and parenteral antibiotic therapy are equally effective in Lyme meningitis. Similar studies have not been conducted in the United States of America. For nonpregnant adult patients intolerant of β-lactam agents, the recommended dosage of doxycycline, 200–400 mg/day orally (or intravenously if unable to take oral medications) in two divided doses, may be adequate. For children ≥8 years of age the recommended dosage of doxycycline for this indication is 4–8 mg/kg per day in two divided doses (maximum daily dosage of 200–400 mg).

[g] Most patients may be treated successfully with an oral regimen. Parenteral antibiotic therapy is recommended for patients with both clinical and laboratory evidence of coexistent meningitis. Systematic studies of oral antibiotic therapy in patients with cranial nerve palsy have only evaluated doxycycline. Other oral agents such as amoxicillin or cefuroxime axetil may be effective in patients who should not receive or cannot tolerate doxycycline, but clinical trials with these antibiotics are lacking. Most of the experience in the use of oral antibiotic therapy is for patients with seventh cranial nerve palsy. Whether oral therapy would be as effective for patients with other cranial neuropathies is unknown. The decision between oral and parenteral antimicrobial therapy for patients with other cranial neuropathies should be individualized.

[h] A parenteral antibiotic regimen is recommended at the start of therapy for patients who have been hospitalized for cardiac monitoring; an oral regimen may be substituted to complete a course of therapy or to treat ambulatory patients. A temporary pacemaker may be required for patients with advanced heart block.

[i] A second course of oral antibiotic therapy is preferred for the patient whose arthritis has substantively improved but has not yet completely resolved. Consideration of retreatment of such patients is often postponed for several months because of the anticipated slow resolution of inflammation after antibiotic treatment. During this interval use of nonsteroidal anti-inflammatory agents (NSAIDs) may be beneficial. Parenteral antibiotic therapy is reserved for those patients whose arthritis failed to improve at all or worsened.

[j] Antibiotic-refractory Lyme arthritis is operationally defined as persistent synovitis for at least 2 months after completion of a 1-month course of intravenous ceftriaxone (or at least 1 month after completion of two 4-week courses of an oral antibiotic regimen for patients unable to tolerate cephalosporins); in addition, PCR on synovial fluid (and synovial tissue if available) is negative for *B. burgdorferi* nucleic acids.

[k] Symptomatic therapy might consist of NSAIDs, intra-articular injections of corticosteroids, or other medications. If persistent synovitis is associated with significant pain or if it limits function, arthroscopic synovectomy should be considered.

Modified from Wormser GP, *et al.* (2006). The clinical assessment, treatment, and prevention of Lyme disease, human granulocytic anaplasmosis and babesiosis. Clinical practices guidelines by the Infectious Diseases Society of America. *Clin Infect Dis*, **43**, 1089–134.

fluoroquinolones, sulphonamides, first-generation cephalosporins, rifampicin, and aminoglycosides have no appreciable activity against *B. burgdorferi* and should not be used. There is no evidence to support combination antimicrobial therapy, prolonged (more than 1 month) or repeated courses of antibiotics, and 'pulse' or intermittent antibiotic therapy. Within 24 h after initiation of antibiotics, approximately 15% of patients with EM may develop transient intensification of signs (e.g. rash and fever) and symptoms

(e.g. arthralgias) consistent with a Jarisch–Herxheimer reaction. Treatment is symptomatic.

Most people treated for Lyme borreliosis have an excellent prognosis. Although a minority of patients treated for EM in recent series continue to have a variety of mild nonspecific complaints following antibiotic therapy, the development of objective extracutaneous disease after treatment is extremely rare. When such complaints are disabling and last for 6 months or more they have been referred to as post-Lyme disease syndrome (PLDS). Randomized double-blind placebo-controlled antibiotic treatment trials of patients with PLDS have failed to show evidence that the benefit of additional antibiotic therapy outweighs the complications of such treatment. Symptomatic therapy is recommended.

Patients with carditis and neurological disease tend to do well, but may sometimes have residual deficits (e.g. mild seventh nerve palsy) after treatment. In patients with arthritis, clinical recovery occurs typically with oral antibiotic therapy (often in conjunction with a nonsteroidal anti-inflammatory medication (NSAID)). Occasionally patients with Lyme arthritis with subtle signs of neuroborreliosis who are treated with oral antibiotics will develop overt late neuroborreliosis and require parenteral therapy. A small number of American patients with Lyme arthritis continue to have synovial inflammation for months or even several years after the apparent eradication of *B. burgdorferi* from the joint following antibiotic therapy (based on negative PCR testing). Such patients have improved after synovectomy. An immunological mechanism rather than active infection appears to be responsible for the continued inflammatory response in these patients.

In North America predominantly, but also in Europe, several patients with a variety of symptoms of uncertain aetiology, including pain and fatigue syndromes, have been labelled as having 'chronic Lyme disease', irrespective of tick exposure in an endemic area for Lyme borreliosis or credible clinical or laboratory evidence of infection due to Lyme borrelia. There is no scientific evidence that such patients have active infection due to borreliae.

Prevention

Preventive measures include avoiding exposure by limiting outdoor activities in tick-infested locations, using tick repellents, tucking in clothing to decrease exposed skin surfaces, and frequent skin inspections for early detection and removal of ticks. Use of acaricides on property and construction of deer fences have also been proposed.

Antibiotic prophylaxis with single-dose doxycycline given after recognized *I. scapularis* tick bites has been shown to be 87% effective in reducing further the low (less than 5%) risk of acquiring Lyme borreliosis after tick bites in the United States of America. Vaccination with a single recombinant outer surface protein A (OspA) preparation has been found to be safe and effective for preventing Lyme borreliosis in the United States of America, but this vaccine is no longer available. Canine vaccines for prevention of Lyme borreliosis, however, are widely used in North America.

Further reading

Aguero-Rosenfeld M, *et al.* (2005). Diagnosis of Lyme borreliosis. *Clin Microbiol Rev*, **18**, 484–509.

British Infection Association (2011). The epidemiology, prevention, investigation and treatment of Lyme borreliosis in United Kingdom patients: a position statement by the British Infection Association. *J Infect*, **62**, 329–38.

Cerar D, *et al.* (2010). Subjective symptoms after treatment of early Lyme disease. *Am J Med*, **123**, 79–86.

Eikeland R, *et al.* (2011). European neuroborreliosis: quality of life 30 months after treatment. *Acta Neurol Scand*, **124**, 349–54.

Feder HM Jr, *et al.* (2007). A critical appraisal of 'chronic Lyme disease'. *N Engl J Med*, **357**, 1422–30.

Halperin JJ, *et al.* (2007). Practice parameter: treatment of nervous system Lyme disease (an evidence-based review). Report of the Quality Standards Subcommittee of the American Academy of Neurology. *Neurology*, **69**, 91–102.

Klempner MS, *et al.* (2001). Two controlled trials of antibiotic treatment in patients with persistent symptoms and a history of Lyme disease. *N Engl J Med*, **345**, 85–92.

Mygland A, *et al.* (2010). EFNS guidelines on the diagnosis and management of European Lyme neuroborreliosis. *Eur J Neurol*, **17**, 8–16, e1–4.

Stanek G, *et al.* (2011). Lyme borreliosis: clinical case definitions for diagnosis and management in Europe. *Clin Microbiol Infect*, **17**, 69–79.

Wormser GP, *et al.* (2006). The clinical assessment, treatment, and prevention of Lyme disease, human granulocytic anaplasmosis, and babesiosis: clinical practice guidelines by the Infectious Diseases Society of America. *Clin Infect Dis*, **43**, 1089–134.

6.33 Relapsing fevers

David A. Warrell

Essentials

Louse-borne relapsing fever (LBRF) and tick-borne relapsing fevers (TBRF) are characterized by repeated episodes of high fever separated by afebrile period. They are caused by borrelia spirochaetes distinct from those responsible for Lyme borrelioses. Untreated patients may suffer as many as five (LBRF) or ten (TBRF) febrile relapses of decreasing severity.

Humans are the sole reservoir of epidemic LBRF caused by *Borrelia recurrentis* and transmitted by body lice (*Pediculus humanus corporis*). Endemic TBRFs are caused by at least 15 different borrelia species and have their own particular species of soft *Ornithodoros* tick vectors which also act as reservoirs. Transmission transplacentally, or by needlestick, blood transfusion, or laboratory accident is also possible.

LBRF is a classic historical epidemic disease of war, famine, and refugees, now largely confined to mountainous areas of the Horn of Africa and possibly Peru but still retaining its pandemic potential. TBRF is of increasing endemicity in sub-Sahelian West Africa and is common in Rwanda and Tanzania. It occurs sporadically in parts of North America, Europe, the Middle East, and central Asia.

The most distinctive feature of these infections, the relapse phenomenon, is explained by antigenic variation of borrelial outer-membrane lipoprotein (vmp). Starting 2–18 days after infection, there is acute fever, chills, headache, pain, and prostration. Petechial rash (thrombocytopenia), bleeding, jaundice, hepatosplenomegaly and liver dysfunction are common. In some forms of TBRF, there are neurological manifestations; lymphocytic meningitis, VII and other cranial nerve lesions, myelitis, radiculitis, etc.; and uveitis during relapses.

Dangerous complications are hyperpyrexia, shock, myocarditis causing acute pulmonary oedema, acute respiratory distress syndrome (ARDS), cerebral or massive external bleeding, ruptured spleen, hepatic failure, Jarisch–Herxheimer reactions (JHR), and typhoid or other complicating bacterial infections. Pregnant women are at high risk of aborting and perinatal mortality is high.

Diagnosis by microscopy of blood films is more difficult in TBRF than LBRF. Serology and polymerase chain reaction (PCR) are used increasingly. The most important differential diagnosis in residents and travellers from tropical endemic areas is falciparum malaria.

Untreated mortality, exceeding 40% in some epidemics, can be reduced to less than 5% by treatment with antibiotics such as penicillin, tetracycline, erythromycin, and chloramphenicol, but elimination of spirochaetaemia is often accompanied by a potentially fatal JHR.

Prevention of LBRF is by eliminating lousiness by sterilizing clothing, using insecticides, and improving hygiene. Improved house construction, control of peridomestic rodents, use of residual insecticides, protection of sleepers with impregnated bed nets, and a post-exposure course of doxycyline can reduce the risk of TBRF.

Historical background

A disease characterized by repeated episodes of several days of high fever separated by afebrile periods of about a week was first described by Rutty in Dublin in 1770, but Craigie in Edinburgh coined the name 'relapsing fever' and distinguished it from typhus in 1843. Obermeier discovered the cause, *Borrelia recurrentis* (Fig. 6.33.1), in 1867, and transmission by human body lice was proved by Mackie in 1907. The cause of African tick fever was discovered by Ross and Milne in 1904 and, independently, by Dutton and Todd in 1905. Some believe that Dutton died of *B. duttonii* infection (Fig. 6.33.2).

Aetiology

The bacteria that cause relapsing fevers are large, loosely coiled, motile spirochaetes (genus *Borrelia*, family Spirochaetaceae), 8 to 20 μm long and 0.2 to 0.6 μm thick, with between 3 and 15 coils and, in some strains, 15 to 30 axial filaments or flagella. They divide by transverse binary fission. Borrelia can be cultured on chick chorioallantoic membrane and maintained in rodents and ticks. *In vitro* culture of borrelia species, including *B. recurrentis*, *B. duttonii*, and *B. crocidurae*, is now possible using Barbour–Stoenner–Kelly medium. Rapidly increasing amounts of genomic data are available.

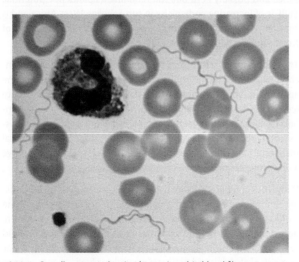

Fig. 6.33.1 *Borrelia recurrentis* spirochaetes in a thin blood film. (Copyright D A Warrell.)

Sequencing of flagellin and rrs genes suggests that there are three phylogenetic clusters of borrelia: (1) Lyme borreliae (*B. burgdorferi* sensu stricto, *B. garinii*, and *B. afzelii*, Chapter 6.32), (2) New World tick-borne relapsing fever borreliae (*B. parkeri*, *B. turicatae*, *B. hermsii*, etc.), and (3) Old World tick-borne relapsing fever and louse-borne relapsing fever borreliae (*B. crocidurae*, *B. duttonii*, *B. hispanica*, *B. recurrentis*, etc.). Molecular phylogenetic studies have shown close identity of *B. recurrentis* and *B. duttonii* suggesting only clonal difference and that *B. recurrentis* adapted rapidly to louse-transmission with genome reduction.

Epidemiology

Louse-borne (epidemic) relapsing fever (LBRF)

The vector of *B. recurrentis* is the human body louse *Pediculus humanus corporis* and, to a lesser extent, the head louse *P. humanus capitis*. Body lice, unlike head lice, retreat from the skin after feeding and hide and lay their eggs in clothing seams. More than 20 000 lice have been recovered from the clothes of one person. Lice are obligate blood-sucking human ectoparasites that ingest borreliae while feeding. Under conditions of crowding and poor hygiene they can move from person to person. When the host's body surface temperature deviates far from 37° C as a result of fever, climatic exposure, or death, or when infested clothing is discarded, the louse is forced to find a new host who can then be infected. Transmission of *B. recurrentis* is by scratching, which crushes lice so that their coelomic fluid is inoculated through broken skin or intact mucous membranes such as the conjunctiva, or inoculates infected louse faeces. Transplacental infection explains congenital infection. Blood transfusion, needlestick injuries, and contamination of broken skin by a patient's blood can also result in infection. Unlike ticks, lice cannot infect their progeny and are therefore not reservoirs and, since there is no known animal reservoir, the infection must persist in humans between epidemics in mild or asymptomatic forms.

Wars, famines, and other disasters that generate large numbers of refugees and prisoners favour the spread of lice and epidemic louse-borne infections such as relapsing fever and typhus. The yellow plague in Europe in AD 550, which halved the world's population, and the famine fevers of the 17th and 18th centuries in Ireland and elsewhere were probably LBRF. In the 20th century, a pandemic raged in North Africa, the Middle East, and Africa from 1903 to 1936, causing an estimated 50 million cases with 10% mortality. A second epidemic in 1943–6 created 10 million cases. An endemic focus persists in the Horn of Africa. Poor people with louse-infested clothes crowd together for shelter. In the Ethiopian highlands there are annual epidemics of thousands of cases coinciding with the small (*belg*) and big (*kiremt*) rains, but in the south the disease was perennial before its recent decline. Outbreaks have also occurred in Somalia and southern Sudan. In Ancash in the Peruvian Andes at altitudes above 3800 m, a cluster of 60 clinical cases was reported in 1983; 36 of the patients had *B. recurrentis* in their blood films. Serological evidence of *B. recurrentis* infection has been found in homeless people in Marseille.

Tick-borne (endemic) relapsing fever (TBRF)

In different parts of the world, particular species of borreliae and soft ticks (genus *Ornithodoros*, family Argasidae) are ecologically intimate, forming Borrelia–tick complexes (Table 6.33.1). At least 15 borrelia species are known to cause human TBRF. Ornithodoros

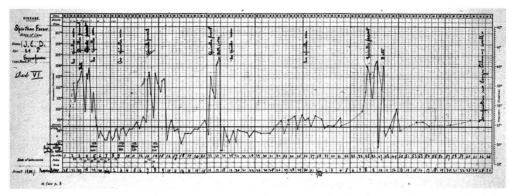

Fig. 6.33.2 Temperature chart of J. Everett Dutton who, with J L Todd, discovered the transmission of TBRF in the Congo. Dutton contracted TBRF at the beginning of November 1904. He had relapses of fever and spirochaetaemia on 7 and 16 December 1904 and 8 January 1905. His death on 27 February 1905 has been attributed by some, but not by Todd, to relapsing fever.
(From Dutton JE, Todd JL (1905). The nature of human tick-fever in the eastern part of the Congo Free State with notes on the distribution and bionomics of the tick. *Liverpool School of Tropical Medicine Memoir XVII.*)

tick vectors occur in dry savannah areas and scrub, caves, piles of timber and dead trees, or in holes in walls, roof spaces, and beneath the floors of log cabins, anywhere inhabited by small rodents. Unlike LBRF, TBRFs are zoonoses with the possible exception of *B. duttonii* infection that was thought to be transmitted only between humans. However, in central Tanzania, *B. duttonii* may infect domestic chickens and pigs. Vertebrate reservoir species include rodents (rats, mice, gerbils, squirrels, and chipmunks), insectivores, lagomorphs, bats, small carnivores, dogs, and birds. Ticks attack at night, remaining attached for less than 30 min before retreating back to their hiding places. Spirochaetes ingested while the tick sucks blood from an infected animal or human invade the tick's salivary and coxal glands and genital apparatus. Infection is transmitted to a new host either by a bite, introducing infected saliva, or by contaminating mucosal membranes with infected coxal fluid. Borreliae are not excreted in tick faeces. Ticks remain infected for life, even after being starved of blood for as long as 7 years. Spirochaetes can be transmitted venereally from male to female ticks and by females (but perhaps not those of the *O. moubata* complex) transovarially to their progeny. Some borreliae may be transmitted by hard ticks (Ixodidae), such as *B. lonestari* by *Amblyomma americanum* (United States) and *B. miyamotoi* by *Ixodes* spp. (Japan). TBRF, like LBRF, may be transmitted by blood transfusion, needlestick injuries, laboratory accidents, and transplacentally.

TBRF is endemic in most temperate and tropical countries except the Arctic, Antarctic, Australasian, and Pacific regions. In Europe, TBRF is caused by *B. hispanica*, especially in Spain, Portugal, and Greece, while *B. crocidurae* and at least three other *Borrelia* spp. are present in Turkey and other adjacent territories. In the West African savannah region, *B. crocidurae* is the most prevalent bacterial infection creating a medical problem second only to malaria. Its prevalence is 1% among children in western Senegal and it is increasing and spreading during the persisting drought (1970–2009). It is a common infection in Rwanda where, in one health centre alone, 1650 proven cases are treated each year (6% of all patients). In parts of East Africa, especially in Tanzania, *B. duttonii* is an important cause of abortion, perinatal mortality, and childhood infection. In Israel, the incidence of *B. persica* infection among military personnel is 6.4/100 000 per year. In North America, isolated sporadic outbreaks of *B. hermsii*, *B. turicatae*, and *B. parkeri* infection occur in mountainous areas of British Columbia, Arizona (especially along the north rim of the Grand Canyon), California (south of Lake Tahoe), Colorado, Montana, New Mexico, and Washington (Browne Mountain). Since the mid-1980s, 280 cases of TBRF have been identified in the United States of America. In Western countries, TBRF is occasionally diagnosed in returned travellers.

Table 6.33.1 Borrelia–tick complexes causing TBRFs

Borrelia spp.	*Ornithodoros* spp.	Geographical distribution
New World TBRF borreliae		
B. hermsii	O. hermsii	Canada, central and western USA, Mexico
B. turicatae	O. turicata	South-western USA, Mexico
B. parkeri	O. parkeri	Western USA, Baja California
B. mazzotti	O. talaje	Mexico, Central America
B. venezuelensis	O. (venezuelensis) rudis	Central America, Colombia, Venezuela, Argentina, Bolivia, Paraguay
Old World TBRF borreliae		
B. duttonii	O. moubata	Sub-Saharan Africa, Madagascar
B. crocidurae	O. (erraticus) sonrai	North, West, and East Africa, Middle East
B. graingeri	O. graingeri	East Africa
B. sp. nov.	O. porcinus	East Africa
B. tillae	O. zumpti	South Africa
B. persica	O. tholozani	Middle East, central Asia from Uzbekistan to western China
B. hispanica	O. erraticus	Iberian peninsula, Greece, Cyprus, North Africa
B. sp. nov.	O. erraticus	Southern Spain
B. latyschevii	O. tartakowskyi	Eastern Europe, Iran, Iraq, Afghanistan, central Asia
B. caucasica	O. (verrucosus) asperus	Eastern Europe, Iraq

Immunopathology and the relapse phenomenon

Symptomatic attacks of relapsing fever are terminated when specific bactericidal IgM antibodies generated by the B1b cell subset lyse spirochaetes in the blood, independently of complement and T cells. However, some spirochaetes persist between the relapses, extracellularly in various organs including spleen, liver, kidneys, eye, and especially in the brain and cerebrospinal fluid. Relapse of spirochaetaemia and symptoms is explained by antigenic variation, which has been investigated in the greatest detail in *B. hermsii*. Silent gene sequences from an archive stored in extra chromosomal plasmids are transposed to one end of an expression linear plasmid where their recombination leads to synthesis of a new variable major outer membrane lipoprotein (vmp). This new coat allows the borreliae to escape from the host's humoral immune response until antibodies are generated against the new serotypic vmp antigen; this explains the relapse phenomenon and the successive appearance of borreliae expressing different vmps during the course of an untreated infection. Borreliae also possess defences against the host's innate immunity. *B. hermsii* surface protein BhCRASP-1 binds factor H (FH), an inhibitor of the alternative pathway of complement activation, so protecting the pathogen against opsonophagocytosis by inhibiting C3b binding. Plasminogen is also bound and activated to plasmin by BhCRASP-1, stimulating fibrinolysis that frees spirochaetes to spread in the blood stream. Another protective mechanism is rosetting of erythrocytes around spirochaetes. This shields them, by masking or steric hindrance, from host antibody and may cause microcirculatory obstruction that is damaging to the host and reminiscent of cerebral malaria. Antigenic variation may also generate isogenic serotypes with properties that promote the spirochaete's survival in vector and reservoir species, e.g. invasiveness for vertebrates' cerebral vascular endothelium. These same vmps are the principal tumour necrosis factor-α (TNFα)-inducing factors in LBRF.

Pathophysiology

Physiological disturbances during the spontaneous crisis and the Jarisch–Herxheimer reaction (JHR) induced by antimicrobial treatment in LBRF are typical of an endotoxin reaction. Outer membrane vmps of *B. recurrentis* stimulate monocytes to produce TNFα through NF-κB. In patients treated with antibiotics, symptoms of the severe JHR are associated with a transient marked elevation in plasma concentrations of TNFα, interleukin (IL)-6, IL-8, and IL-1β (Fig. 6.33.3). The stimulus for cytokine release is the phagocytosis of spirochaetes made susceptible by the action of penicillin. Benzylpenicillin attaches to penicillin-binding protein I in *B. hermsii* spirochaetes. Large surface blebs are produced and the damaged spirochaetes are phagocytosed rapidly by neutrophils in the blood and by the spleen. Complement may enhance phagocytosis of spirochaetes, especially in the nonimmune host, but the complement system is not essential for elimination of spirochaetes whether or not specific immunoglobulins are present. *In vitro*, surface contact with spirochaetes induces mononuclear leucocytes to produce inflammatory cytokines and thromboplastin, which could be responsible for the fever and disseminated intravascular coagulation in LBRF. Kinins may be released during the JHR of syphilis and LBRF. The marked peripheral leucopenia that develops

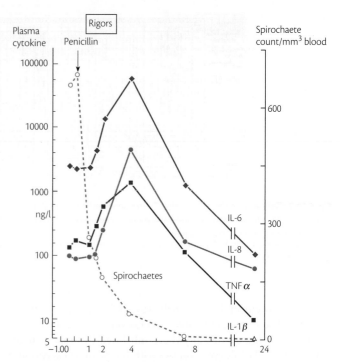

Fig. 6.33.3 Typical JRH in a patient with LBRF treated with intravenous penicillin. Following penicillin, the number of spirochaetes (dashed line referring to right hand axis) fell abruptly and circulating levels of TNFα, IL-6, IL-8, and IL-1β started to rise after about 1 h, peaking at 4 h. As cytokine levels were increasing, this patient experienced sustained rigors which subsided before peak levels were achieved.

during the reaction reflects sequestration, perhaps in the pulmonary blood vessels, rather than leucocyte destruction. Spirochaetes may be found in those organs that bear the brunt of the infection such as liver, spleen (Fig. 6.33.4), myocardium (Fig. 6.33.5), and brain (Fig. 6.33.6), but it is unclear how their pathological effects are produced. The petechial rash results from thrombocytopenia not vasculitis. The cardiorespiratory and metabolic disturbances in relapsing fever are principally the result of persistent high fever, accentuated by the JHR or spontaneous crisis.

Pathology

The vast majority of spirochaetes are confined to the lumen of blood vessels, but tangled masses are also found in the characteristic splenic miliary abscesses (Fig. 6.33.4) and infarcts as well as within the central nervous system adjacent to haemorrhages. Some strains of TBRF borreliae can invade the central nervous system, aqueous humour, and other tissues. In LBRF, a perivascular histiocytic interstitial myocarditis, found in the majority of cases, may be responsible for conduction defects, arrhythmias, and myocardial failure resulting in sudden death (Fig. 6.33.5). Splenic rupture with massive haemorrhage, cerebral haemorrhage (Fig. 6.33.6), and hepatic failure are other causes of death. The liver shows hepatitis with patchy midzonal haemorrhages and necrosis. There is meningitis and perisplenitis. Most serosal cavities and surfaces of viscera are studded with petechial haemorrhages (Figs. 6.33.5, 6.33.6) and there may be massive pulmonary haemorrhage (Fig. 6.33.7). Thrombi are occasionally found occluding small vessels, but the peripheral gangrene sometimes found in patients recovering from louse-borne typhus (Chapter 6.39, Fig. 6.39.7c) is not seen.

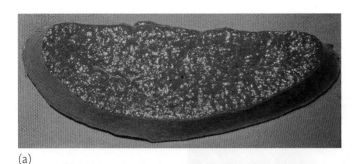

(a)

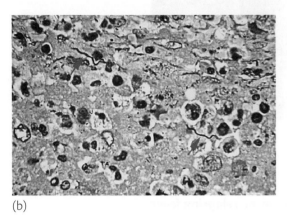

(b)

Fig. 6.33.4 Spleen in LBRF: (a) Section of spleen at autopsy; (b) Warthin Starry stain showing *Borrelia recurrentis* (arrows).
(a, copyright D A Warrell; b, courtesy of Dr Ken Fleming.)

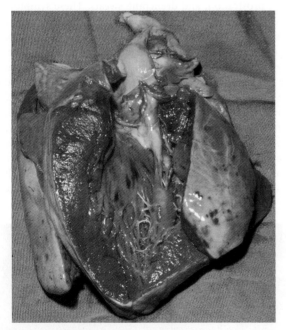

Fig. 6.33.5 Epicardial and endocardial haemorrhages.
(Copyright D A Warrell.)

Clinical features

Louse-borne relapsing fever

Adults

Prisoners and poor, malnourished street-dwellers are most likely to become infected, especially young men. After an incubation period of 4 to 18 (average 7) days, the illness starts suddenly with

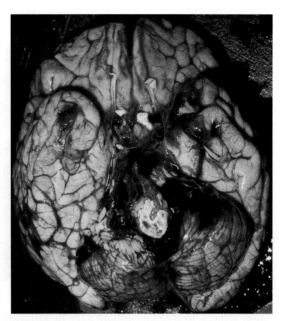

Fig. 6.33.6 Cerebral haemorrhage.
(Copyright D A Warrell.)

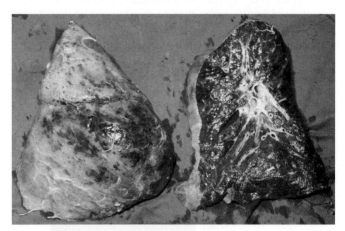

Fig. 6.33.7 Pulmonary haemorrhage.
(Copyright D A Warrell.)

rigors and a fever that mounts to nearly 40°C in a few days. Early symptoms are headache, dizziness, nightmares, generalized aches and pains (especially affecting the lower back, knees, and elbows), anorexia, nausea, vomiting, and diarrhoea. Later there is upper abdominal pain, cough, and epistaxis. Patients are usually prostrated (Fig. 6.33.8) and most are confused. Hepatic tenderness is the commonest sign (about 60%). The liver is palpably enlarged in approximately 50% of patients. Splenic tenderness and enlargement are slightly less common. Jaundice has been reported in 10 to 80% of patients. A petechial or ecchymotic rash is seen in 10 to 60% of patients (Figs. 6.33.9, 6.33.10); the lesions occur particularly on the trunk. Other sites of spontaneous bleeding include the conjunctivae (Fig. 6.33.11), nose in 25% (Fig. 6.33.9), and less commonly the lungs (Fig. 6.33.7), gastrointestinal tract, and retina. Many patients have tender muscles. Meningism occurs in about 40% of patients; other neurological features include cranial nerve lesions, monoplegias, flaccid paraplegia, and focal convulsions

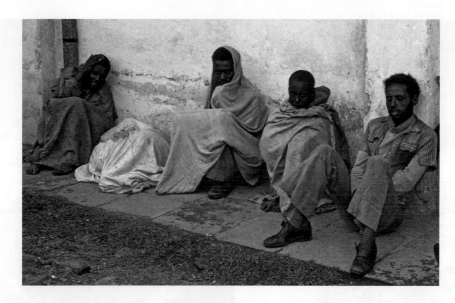

Fig. 6.33.8 Patients presenting with relapsing fever at a clinic in Addis Ababa. Most are febrile, confused, and prostrated.
(Copyright D A Warrell.)

attributable, perhaps, to cerebral haemorrhages. In untreated people, the first attack of fever resolves by crisis in 4 to 10 (average 5) days, followed by an afebrile remission of 5 to 9 days, and then a series of up to five relapses of diminishing severity, occasionally complicated by epistaxis. Petechial rashes are absent during relapses.

Pregnant women are especially susceptible to severe disease and abortions are frequent.

Children

In children older than 5 years, clinical features resemble those in adults but are generally less severe and the case fatality is lower. Fever, chills, headache, abdominal pain and tenderness, vomiting, cough, musculoskeletal pains, tachycardia, and petechial rash are common. In younger children, hepatosplenomegaly, cough, and

signs of consolidation may be more common. Reported case fatalities in children range from 1.9 to 5.5%.

Tick-borne relapsing fever

Adults

After an incubation period of 2 to 18 days, the illness starts with sudden fever, chills, headache, muscle and joint pains, extreme fatigue, prostration, and drenching sweats. These symptoms are similar to those in LBRF but the initial fever usually lasts about 3 days only to recur about 7 to 15 days later. Epistaxis, abdominal pain, diarrhoea, cough, and erythematous or petechial rashes may follow. Jaundice is less common than in LBRF. Several cases of acute respiratory distress syndrome (ARDS) have been described in the United States of America. Neurological disturbances are more common than in LBRF, varying in incidence with the borrelia species involved, from less than 5% in patients with *B. hispanica* and *B. persica* infections to as high as 40% in patients with *B. duttonii*. However, one careful study in northern Tanzania found no focal neurological abnormalities in patients with *B. duttonii* TBRF. The neurological features that have been described are reminiscent of

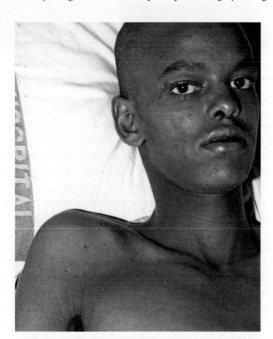

Fig. 6.33.9 Ethiopian patient with LBRF showing petechiae on the shoulder and epistaxis.
(Copyright D A Warrell.)

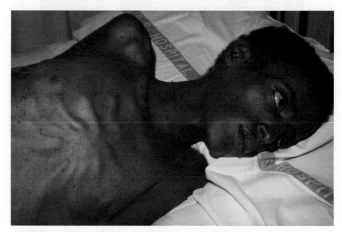

Fig. 6.33.10 Ethiopian patient with severe LBRF complicated by typhoid, showing jaundice, petechial haemorrhages, and emaciation.
(Copyright D A Warrell.)

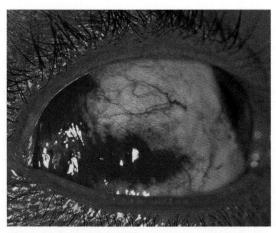

Fig. 6.33.11 Subconjunctival haemorrhage in a patient with LBRF. (Copyright D A Warrell.)

Lyme neuroborreliosis and include paraesthesias, visual symptoms, lymphocytic meningitis, cranial nerve palsies (especially VII), encephalitis, myelitis, sciatica, and radiculitis. Untreated patients may have up to 13 relapses (Fig. 6.33.2), becoming sequentially less severe. Ocular complications usually occur during the third and fourth relapses. They include conjunctival injection, eye pain, photophobia, eyelid oedema, keratitis, various degrees of anterior and posterior uveitis, optic neuritis, and blindness.

Spirochaetaemia is higher in pregnant than in nonpregnant women and abortion and perinatal mortality are common. In Tabora, Tanzania, parturition was precipitated in 58% of infected pregnant women. Perinatal mortality was 436/1000 births, its risk related to low birthweight and gestational age, and total fetal wastage was 475/1000.

Children

In endemic areas of *B. duttonii* TBRF in East Africa, most cases are in children, many of them under 5 years old, and pregnant women, implying that older nonpregnant people may acquire some immunity. Fever, splenomegaly, convulsions sometimes recurrent, meningism, petechiae, and jaundice are described. Neonates with congenital infection have fever, inability to suck, jaundice, and features of septicaemia. Reported case fatalities in children less than 1 year old are 2.3 to 73%, compared to 1.6 to 19% in older children.

Severe disease

Severe manifestations include hyperpyrexia, myocarditis with acute pulmonary oedema, ARDS, hepatic failure, ruptured spleen, and haemostatic failure attributable to thrombocytopenia, liver damage, and disseminated intravascular coagulation leading to cerebral, massive gastrointestinal, pulmonary, or peripartum haemorrhage. Dysentery, salmonellosis, typhoid, typhus, tuberculosis, bacterial pneumonia, and malaria are infections that can complicate relapsing fever, increasing the risk of death.

The spontaneous crisis and Jarisch–Herxheimer reaction

Whether or not treatment is given, attacks of relapsing fever usually end dramatically. On about the fifth day of the untreated illness, or about 1 to 2 h after antibiotic treatment, the patient becomes restless and apprehensive and suddenly begins to have distressingly intense rigors that last between 10 and 30 min. The ensuing phenomena have features of a classic endotoxin reaction. During the initial chill phase, temperature, respiratory and pulse rates, and blood pressure rise sharply. Delirium, gastrointestinal symptoms, cough, and limb pains are associated. Some patients die of hyperpyrexia at the peak of fever. The flush phase, which lasts many hours, is characterized by profuse sweating, a fall in blood pressure, and a slow decline in temperature. Deaths during this phase follow intractable hypotension, sudden postural hypotension prompted by the patient's standing up, or the development of acute pulmonary oedema attributable to myocarditis. The incidence of JHRs is highest in adults with LBRF treated with intravenous tetracycline (approaching 100% in some studies). It is lower when low-dose or slow-release penicillin is used and in children. JHR is less commonly observed in TBRF but can be severe and even fatal.

The classic JHR is in secondary syphilis in which the spirochaetes are in the tissues and the reaction is less frequent, more insidious, and much less severe than in relapsing fevers. Milder reactions have been described in Lyme disease and leptospirosis (treated with penicillin), sodoku (treated with arsenicals), *Brucella melitensis* (treated with tetracycline), and even in typhoid and meningococcal infections.

Laboratory findings

Spirochaete densities may exceed 500 000/mm³ of blood. There is a moderate normochromic anaemia and a neutrophil leucocytosis with marked leucopenia during the spontaneous crisis and JHR. Thrombocytopenia is usual and there is a mild coagulopathy with evidence of increased fibrinolysis. Biochemical evidence of hepatocellular damage (raised levels of aminotransferases, alkaline phosphatase, direct and total bilirubin, low albumin) and mild renal impairment are common. The cerebrospinal fluid shows a lymphocyte or neutrophil pleocytosis without visible spirochaetes.

There is ECG evidence of myocarditis including prolongation of the QTc interval, T-wave abnormalities, and ST-segment depression with transient acute right heart strain after the JHR. Chest radiographs may show pulmonary oedema or pneumonic consolidation.

Diagnosis

Thick and thin blood films should be taken while patients are febrile. Spirochaetes are demonstrated by Giemsa's, Wright's, Field's, or Diff-Quick staining (Fig. 6.33.1), dark-field examination, or a quantitative buffy coat technique (acridine orange). The sensitivity of thick films is 20 times greater than thin films. Misidentification of *Plasmodium vivax* microgametes as spirochaetes has led to the diagnosis of 'pseudoborreliosis'. In TBRF, spirochaetes may be difficult or impossible to find even at the height of a relapse and, increasingly, PCR and serology are being used. Lyme disease borreliae may produce cross-reacting antibodies due to expression of conserved antigenic epitopes, but an ELISA using the glycerophosphodiester phosphodiesterase (GlpQ) gene product can distinguish relapsing fevers from Lyme disease. In LBRF, the higher and more persistent spirochaetaemia is more easily detected. Borreliae can be isolated in mice and cultured *in vitro*.

The serum of patients with relapsing fever may give positive reactions with proteus OXK, OX19, and OX2 and false-positive serological responses for syphilis in 5 to 10% of cases.

Differential diagnosis

In a febrile patient with jaundice, petechial rash, bleeding, hepatosplenomegaly, thrombocytopenia, coagulopathy, and elevated serum aminotransferases, the most frequent and urgent differential diagnosis is falciparum malaria. Yellow fever and other viral haemorrhagic fevers such as Rift Valley Fever in the Horn of Africa, viral hepatitis, rickettsial infections (especially louse-borne typhus which shares LBRF's epidemiological predispositions), and leptospirosis may also cause confusion. Trench fever (*Bartonella quintana*) transmitted by lice, and sodoku (*Spirillum minus*) following a rat bite can also cause episodic recurrent fever. Although the diagnosis of relapsing fever can often be confirmed quickly by examining a blood smear, the possibility of complicating bacterial infection, particularly typhoid, or coinfection with malaria should never be forgotten.

Prognosis

During major LBRF epidemics, overall case fatalities of 40% or higher have been reported, but in treated cases they are less than 5%. TBRF is less dangerous and deaths during relapses are most unusual but have been reported. In both LBRF and TBRF, pregnant women and infants are at greatest risk of dying.

Treatment

Antibiotics

LBRF

LBRF is readily cured without relapses by a single oral dose of 500 mg tetracycline or 500 mg erythromycin stearate. However, since few patients with severe LBRF are able to swallow tablets without vomiting them up, a more reliable treatment is a single intravenous dose of 250 mg tetracycline hydrochloride or, for pregnant women and children, a single intravenous dose of 300 mg erythromycin lactobionate (children 10 mg/kg body weight). In mixed epidemics of LBRF and louse-borne typhus, a single oral dose of 100 mg doxycycline proved effective.

Benzylpenicillin (300 000 units), procaine penicillin with benzylpenicillin (600 000 units), and procaine penicillin with aluminium monostearate (600 000 units), all by intramuscular injection, are often effective but may fail to prevent relapses. Long-acting preparations clear spirochaetaemia slowly and the JHR is protracted. Some experienced clinicians prefer to use a low initial dose of penicillin (adult dose, 100 000–400 000 units by intramuscular injection) in severe cases and pregnant women because they believe that the incidence and severity of the JHRs will be less.

Chloramphenicol is effective in a single dose of 500 mg by mouth or intravenous injection in adults.

A recent meta-analysis of trials of chemotherapy of LBRF concluded that no clear superiority of any drug had been confirmed and that azithromycin should be tried in future.

TBRF

Although TBRF is usually milder than LBRF, it is more difficult to treat because spirochaetes persist in tissues, such as the central nervous system and eye, and produce relapses. Oral tetracycline, 500 mg every 6 h for 10 days is, however, effective. Oral erythromycin can be given to pregnant women (500 mg every 6 h for 10 days) and children (125–250 mg every 6 h for 10 days). In patients unable to swallow tablets, treatment can be initiated with 250 mg intravenous tetracycline hydrochloride or with 300 mg erythromycin lactobionate.

Chloramphenicol is effective in a dose of 500 mg every 6 h for 10 days in adults, and 250 mg every 6 h for 10 days in older children.

JHR

Antimicrobials have reduced the mortality of relapsing fevers from 30 to 70% to less than 5%. However, drugs such as tetracycline, which rapidly eliminate spirochaetes from the blood and prevent relapses, usually induce a severe JHR that may occasionally prove fatal. Clearly, in a disease with such a high natural mortality, treatment cannot be withheld, especially as severe spontaneous crises, which may also prove fatal, occur in a large proportion of LBRF cases after the fifth day of fever. There is no evidence, however, that the shorter and more intense reaction following tetracycline is more dangerous than the more prolonged but apparently milder reaction following slow-release penicillin. Neither hydrocortisone in doses up to 20 mg/kg nor paracetamol prevent the JHR but they reduce peak temperatures, hastens the fall in temperature, and lessens the fall in blood pressure during the flush phase. Pretreatment with oral prednisolone can prevent the JHR of early syphilis, but in LBRF neither an oral dose of 3 mg/kg prednisolone given 18 h beforehand nor an infusion of 3.75 mg/kg betamethasone prevented the reaction to tetracycline treatment. However, meptazinol, an opioid antagonist/agonist, diminishes the reaction when given in a dose of 100 mg by intravenous injection. The discovery of an explosive release of TNFα, IL-6, and IL-8 just before the start of the JHR prompted the testing of a polyclonal ovine Fab anti-TNFα antibody. When infused for 30 min before treatment with intramuscular penicillin, this antibody suppressed the JHR.

Supportive treatment

Patients must be nursed in bed for at least 24 h after treatment to prevent postural hypotensive collapse and the precipitation of fatal cardiac arrhythmias. Hyperpyrexia should be prevented with antipyretics, vigorous fanning, and tepid sponging. Although patients with acute LBRF have an expanded plasma volume, most are dehydrated and relatively hypovolaemic. Adults may need 4 litres or more of isotonic saline intravenously during the first 24 h. Infusion should be controlled by monitoring jugular venous or central venous pressures. Acute myocardial failure may develop, particularly during the flush phase of the JHR or spontaneous crisis. This is signalled by a rise in central venous pressure above 15 cmH$_2$O; 1 mg digoxin given intravenously over 5 to 10 min has proved effective in this emergency. Because of the intense vasodilatation, diuretics may accentuate the circulatory failure by causing relative hypovolaemia. Oxygen should be given during the reaction, particularly in severe cases. Vitamin K should be given to all patients with prolonged prothrombin times. Heparin is not effective in controlling coagulopathy and should not be used. Complicating infections (typhoid, salmonellosis, bacillary dysentery, tuberculosis, typhus, malaria) must be treated appropriately.

Prevention and control

No vaccines are available.

LBRF: delousing

Infested clothing should be deloused using heat (>60°C), chlorine bleach, or insecticide (10% dichlorodiphenyltrichloroethane (DDT), 1% malathion, 2% temephos, 1% propoxur, or 0.5% permethrin), and patients should be bathed with soap and 1% Lysol (cresol). Lice are abundant in hair, which should be washed or shaved off. Breaking transmission from lice to the susceptible population is essential for the control of an epidemic.

TBRF: tick control

Tick infestation of dwellings can be reduced by improved house construction (e.g. rodent-proofing of cabins on the North Rim of the Grand Canyon), control of peridomestic rodent hosts, and use of residual insecticides (pyrethroids, benzene hexachloride, λ-cyhalothrin, malathion, or DDT). Travellers should avoid sleeping in places where ticks and rodents are abundant, such as poorly maintained log cabins, should apply repellents to their skin (diethyl toluamide (DEET)), and should sleep under insecticide-impregnated bed nets. Postexposure prophylaxis with doxycycline (200mg followed by 100mg on the next 4 days) proved effective against *B persica* in Israel.

Further reading

Balicer RD *et al.* (2010). Post exposure prophylaxis of tick-borne relapsing fever. *Eur J Clin Microbiol Infect Dis*, [Epub ahead of print] PMID: 20012878.

Barbour AG, Hayes SF (1986). Biology of *Borrelia* species. *Microbiol Rev*, **50**, 381–400.

Brouqui P, Stein A, Dupont HT (2005). Ectoparasitism and vector-borne diseases in 930 homeless people from Marseilles. *Medicine (Baltimore)*, **84**, 61–8.

Bryceson ADM, *et al.* (1970). Louse-borne relapsing fever. A clinical and laboratory study of 62 cases in Ethiopia and a reconsideration of the literature. *QJM*, **39**, 129–70.

Burman N, Shamaei-Tousi A, Bergström S (1998). The spirochete *Borrelia crocidurae* causes erythrocyte rosetting during relapsing fever. *Infect Immun*, **66**, 815–9.

Cadavid D, Barbour AG (1998). Neuroborreliosis during relapsing fever: review of the clinical manifestations, pathology, and treatment of infections in humans and experimental animals. *Clin Infect Dis*, **26**, 151–64.

Fekade D, *et al.* (1996). Prevention of Jarisch-Herxheimer reactions by treatment with antibodies against tumor necrosis factor alpha. *N Engl J Med*, **335**, 311–5.

Felsenfeld O (1971). *Borrelia: strains, vectors, human and animal borreliosis*. Green, St Louis.

Guerrier G, Doherty T. (2011) Comparison of antibiotic regimens for treating louse-borne relapsing fever: a meta-analysis. *Trans R Soc Trop Med Hyg*, **105**, 483–90.

Hasin T, *et al.* (2006). Postexposure treatment with doxycycline for the prevention of tick-borne relapsing fever. *N Engl J Med*, **355**, 148–55.

Jongen VH, *et al.* (1997). Tick-borne relapsing fever and pregnancy outcome in rural Tanzania. *Acta Obstet Gynecol Scand*, **76**, 834–8.

LaRocca TJ, Benach JL (2008). The important and diverse roles of antibodies in the host response to borrelia infections. *Curr Top Microbiol Immunol*, **319**, 63–103.

Larsson C, *et al.* (2009). Current issues in relapsing fever. *Curr Opin Infect Dis*, **22**, 443–9.

Lescot M, *et al.* (2008). The genome of *Borrelia recurrentis*, the agent of deadly louse-borne relapsing fever, is a degraded subset of tick-borne *Borrelia duttonii*. *PLoS Genet*, **4**, e1000185.

Mayegga E, *et al.* (2005). Absence of focal neurological involvement in tick-borne relapsing fever in northern Tanzania. *Eur J Neurol*, **12**, 449–52.

McCall PJ, *et al.* (2007). Does tick-borne relapsing fever have an animal reservoir in East Africa? *Vector Borne Zoonotic Dis*, **7**, 659–66.

Negussie Y, *et al.* (1992). Detection of plasma tumor necrosis factor, interleukins 6, and 8 during the Jarisch-Herxheimer Reaction of relapsing fever. *J Exp Med*, **175**, 1207–12.

Parry EH, *et al.* (1970). Some effects of louse-borne relapsing fever on the function of the heart. *Am J Med*, **49**, 472–9.

Perine PL, Teklu B (1983). Antibiotic treatment of louse-borne relapsing fever in Ethiopia: a report of 377 cases. *Am J Trop Med Hyg*, **32**, 1096–100.

Rebaudet S, Parola P (2006). Epidemiology of relapsing fever borreliosis in Europe. *FEMS Immunol Med Microbiol*, **48**, 11–5.

Seboxa T, Rahlenbeck SI (1995). Treatment of louse-borne relapsing fever with low dose penicillin or tetracycline: a clinical trial. *Scand J Infect Dis*, **27**, 29–31.

Vial L, *et al.* (2006). Incidence of tick-borne relapsing fever in West Africa: longitudinal study. *Lancet*, **368**, 37–43.

Vidal V, *et al.* (1998). Variable major lipoprotein is a principal TNF-inducing factor of louse-borne relapsing fever. *Nat Med*, **4**, 1416–20.

Vuyyuru R, *et al.* (2011). Characteristics of *Borrelia hermsii* infection in human hematopoietic stem cell-engrafted mice mirror those of human relapsing fever. *Proc Natl Acad Sci U S A*, **108**, 20707–12.

Warrell DA, *et al.* (1970). Cardiorespiratory disturbances associated with infective fever in man: studies of Ethiopian louse-borne relapsing fever. *Clin Sci*, **39**, 123–45.

Warrell DA, *et al.* (1971). Physiologic changes during the Jarisch–Herxheimer reaction in early syphilis. A comparison with louse-borne relapsing fever. *Am J Med*, **51**, 176–85.

Warrell DA, *et al.* (1983). Pathophysiology and immunology of the Jarisch–Herxheimer-like reaction in louse-borne relapsing fever: comparison of tetracycline and slow-release penicillin. *J Infect Dis*, **147**, 898–909.

6.34 Leptospirosis

George Watt

Essentials

Leptospirosis is a worldwide zoonosis of greatest importance in the tropics that is caused by spirochaetes of the 16 species of the genus *Leptospira*. Rodents are the most important reservoir, with transmission of infection usually occurring through contact with contaminated water or moist soil. Organisms enter the human body through abrasions of the skin or through mucosal surfaces.

Clinical features—subclinical infection is common, but symptomatic disease typically begins with abrupt onset of intense headache, fever, chills, and myalgia. Conjunctival suffusion is a helpful diagnostic clue. Most patients recover within a week, but some then relapse, commonly with meningitis. Less than 10% of symptomatic infections result in severe, icteric illness (Weil's disease) that is characterized by jaundice, renal dysfunction, haemorrhagic manifestations, and high mortality. Leptospirosis-associated severe pulmonary haemorrhage syndrome, which can occur either with or without jaundice and renal failure, has a case fatality rate of about 50%.

Diagnosis—most cases go undiagnosed because serological confirmation is rarely available where most disease transmission occurs. The gold standard microscopic agglutination test is impracticable, and commercially available rapid serodiagnostic kits have unacceptably low sensitivities and lack specificity in regions of high endemic transmission.

Treatment and prognosis—aside from supportive care, antibiotics should be given to all patients with leptospirosis, regardless of age, the stage of their disease, or fear of a possible Jarisch–Herxheimer reaction. High-dose intravenous penicillin is the treatment of choice for adults and children with severe, late disease: doxycycline, ceftriaxone, cefotaxime, and azithromycin are effective in mild disease. Ensuring adequate renal perfusion prevents renal failure in most oliguric patients. Failure to make the diagnosis of leptospirosis is particularly unfortunate: severely ill patients with leptospirosis often recover completely with prompt treatment, but they may die if therapy is delayed or not given.

Introduction

Leptospirosis is a worldwide zoonosis of the greatest public health importance in the tropics. Infection may be asymptomatic, but 5 to 15% of cases are severe or fatal. Most cases go undiagnosed because symptoms and signs are often nonspecific and serological confirmation is rarely available where most disease transmission occurs. Failure to diagnose leptospirosis is particularly unfortunate as severely ill patients often recover completely with prompt treatment, but if therapy is delayed or not given death or renal failure are likely to ensue.

Aetiology

The organism responsible is a tightly coiled spirochaete with an axial filament and hooked ends, 0.1 to 0.2 µm wide, and 5 to 20 µm long. Leptospires are aerobic and travel with a corkscrew-like motion. Unstained organisms can be seen only by dark-field or phase-contrast microscopy. Silver staining is the method of choice for demonstrating leptospires in tissue specimens. Previously, the genus *Leptospira* contained two species, *Leptospira interrogans*, which was pathogenic, and *L. biflexa*, which was saprophytic. Stable antigenic differences allowed subclassification into serotypes, referred to in the literature as serovars (serovarieties). Antigens common to several serovars permitted arrangement into broader serogroups. More than 250 serovars belonging to 24 serogroups were identified for *L. interrogans*. Leptospirosis taxonomy is evolving, however, and the genus *Leptospira* has now been reclassified, based on DNA relatedness, into 16 species including at least 7 pathogenic species: *L. interrogans*, *L. borgpetersenii*, *L. inadai*, *L. noguchii*, *L. santarosai*, *L. weilii*, and *L. kirschneri*. The sequencing of the genome of *L. interrogans* was recently completed, and this advance should facilitate future advances in diagnosis and vaccine development, and provide insights into pathogenesis.

Epidemiology

Measuring incidence by active surveillance confirms that leptospirosis is a surprisingly common disease. Antibody positivity rates of 37% have been recorded in rural Belize and 23% in Vietnam. More than 2527 human cases and 13 deaths were reported for the first 9 months of 1999 by the Ministry of Public Health in Thailand. There was a sustained outbreak between 1998 and 2003. Multilocus sequence typing linked this outbreak to the emergence of a single dominant clone of *L. interrogans* serovar Autumnalis. Bandicoot rats (*Bandicota indica* and *B. savilei*) served as the reservoir. Human leptospirosis is an important disease in China, south-east Asia, India, Africa, and South and Central America. It is also of significance in eastern and southern Europe, Australia, and New Zealand. In the United States of America, the disease is primarily of veterinary importance, with only 50 to 150 human cases reported annually.

Leptospires nest in the renal tubules of mammalian hosts and are shed in the urine. They can survive for several months in the environment under moist conditions, particularly in the presence of warmth (above 22°C) and a neutral pH (pH 6.2 to 8.0). These conditions occur all year round in the tropics but only during the summer and autumn months in temperate climates. Roughly 160 animal species harbour organisms, but rodents are the most important reservoir. Carrier rates of over 50% have been measured in Norway rats, which shed massive numbers of organisms for life without showing clinical illness. Some serovars appear to be preferentially adapted to select mammalian hosts. For example, *L. interrogans* serovar Icterohaemorrhagiae is primarily associated with the Norway rat, *L. interrogans* serovar Canicola with dogs, and *L. interrogans* serovar Pomona with swine and cattle. However, a particular host species may serve as a reservoir for one or more serovars and a particular serovar may be hosted by many different animal species. A large epizootic occurred in Sri Lanka. In 2008, there were 7406 suspected cases (35.7 per 100 000 population) and 204 deaths; in 2009, 4980 cases and 145 deaths; and in 2010, 4553 cases and 121 deaths. Pyrogenes was the serovar in 80% of cases in Sri Lanka. The highest reported incidence was in the Seychelles, 43.2 per 100 000 population.

The transmission of infection from animals to humans usually occurs through contact with contaminated water or moist soil. Organisms enter humans through abrasions of the skin or through the mucosal surface of the eye, mouth, nasopharynx, or oesophagus. Crowded Asian or Latin American cities that are flood-prone and have large rat populations provide ideal conditions for disease transmission. Escalating migration of the rural poor to urban slums is likely to further exacerbate the risks of leptospirosis transmission. An outbreak in Nicaragua in 1995 and an urban epidemic in Salvador, Brazil in 1999 were associated with particularly heavy rains and flooding. Intense exposure to leptospires has been documented in rice, sugar cane, and rubber plantation workers. Less frequently, leptospirosis is acquired by direct contact with the blood, urine, or tissues of infected animals. Epidemiological patterns in the United States of America and the United Kingdom have changed. Recreational exposure to fresh water (canoeing, sailing, water skiing) and animal contact at home have replaced occupational exposure as the chief source of disease. During the 10-day Eco-Challenge-Sabah 2000 multisport endurance race, 26% of 304 athletes caught leptospirosis.

Pathology and pathogenesis

Leptospires are disseminated by the blood and may be recovered from all organs within 48 h of entering the host. Leptospiraemia lasts from 4 to 7 days and ends when agglutinating antibodies appear. Leptospires can persist for months in the kidneys and ocular tissue. Much of the pathogenesis of leptospirosis remains unexplained. There are only minor histopathological changes in the kidneys and livers of patients with marked functional impairment of these organs. Patients who survive severe leptospirosis have complete recovery of hepatic and renal function, which is consistent with the lack of structural damage to these organs.

Severely ill patients typically have marked leucocytosis but no leucocytic infiltrates in organs, a pattern produced by some toxins. Fatally infected animals and some human patients exhibit changes similar to those produced by the endotoxaemia of Gram-negative bacteraemia. An endotoxin-like substance is present in the cell wall of leptospires but lacks the ketodeoxyoctanoate of a true endotoxin.

Kidney

Renal failure is the most common cause of death in leptospirosis. Leptospires are frequently found in human renal tissue, but their role in mediating kidney damage is unknown. Interstitial nephritis is found primarily in individuals who have survived until inflammation has had an opportunity to develop, but is frequently absent in patients with fulminant disease.

Impaired renal perfusion constitutes the fundamental nephropathic change. Oliguria is rapidly reversed by administration of intravenous fluid in many patients, suggesting that volume depletion is frequent. Hypovolaemia is multifactorial and insensible water loss, diarrhoea, vomiting, reduced fluid intake, and haemorrhage can all contribute. A defect in the kidney's ability to concentrate urine increases fluid loss while renal potassium wasting can lead to hypokalaemia. This unique nonoliguric hypokalaemic renal insufficiency is characterized by impaired proximal sodium reabsorption, increased distal sodium delivery, and potassium wasting. Renal magnesium wasting has been demonstrated more recently but its clinical significance is not known. Widespread endothelial injury causes fluid to move from the intravascular to the extracellular space in some patients. Hypotension of cardiac origin is rare.

Liver

The pathogenesis of jaundice is unexplained; neither haemolytic anaemia nor hepatocellular necrosis are prominent features of leptospirosis. The most severe hepatic pathological changes are seen when organisms are difficult to demonstrate in tissue, suggesting subcellular toxic or metabolic insults.

Striated muscle

Myalgia is typical of early infection, and is presumably due to invasion of skeletal muscle by leptospires. Muscle biopsies in patients with early illness demonstrate vacuolation of the myofibrillar cytoplasm, loss of cellular detail, and fragmentation. Leptospiral antigen can be demonstrated by immunofluorescence within muscle tissue. Muscle pain resolves as antibody appears and organisms are cleared from the blood. Pathological changes are usually absent in muscle tissue from patients who have died, and myalgia is generally waning at the time of death.

Lungs

Localized or confluent haemorrhagic pneumonitis is the usual pulmonary finding, with petechial and ecchymotic haemorrhages noted throughout the lungs, pleura, and tracheobronchial tree. Early life-threatening pulmonary haemorrhage has long been reported from Asia, and is now being increasingly recognized in Latin America. Necropsy findings include massive intra-alveolar haemorrhage with or without diffuse alveolar damage. Leptospires can be demonstrated in lung tissue, but few intact organisms are seen at autopsy suggesting a possible immune-mediated process. Indeed, leptospirosis pulmonary haemmorrhage syndrome was recently shown to be associated with linear deposition of immunoglobulin and complement on the alveolar surface.

Haemorrhage

A progressive severe haemorrhagic diathesis is a prominent feature of experimental leptospirosis. In humans, bleeding is generally restricted to the skin or mucosal surfaces, although occasionally massive gastrointestinal or pulmonary haemorrhage occurs. Coagulopathy and/or thrombocytopenia are common in leptospirosis but do not adequately explain bleeding. By exclusion, capillary damage is the postulated mechanism, and toxins have been suggested as the mediators of endothelial injury.

Meningitis

Organisms easily enter the cerebrospinal fluid during leptospiraemia, and this is thought to explain the high incidence of meningitis. However, signs of meningeal irritation are not due to the invasion of the meninges by leptospires, a process that elicits little reaction. Organisms are frequently isolated from cerebrospinal fluid that is otherwise normal and from individuals without clinically detectable involvement of the nervous system. Symptoms of meningitis coincide with the development of antibody and disappearance of leptospires from the blood and cerebrospinal fluid, suggesting an immunological mechanism. Pathological changes are minimal or absent, and the prognosis is excellent.

Heart

Focal haemorrhagic myocarditis has been reported, but hypovolaemia, electrolyte imbalance, and uraemia are more frequent causes of cardiac dysfunction. Minor electrocardiographic changes such as first-degree heart block are common and reversible, but serious dysrhythmias also occur.

Eye

The aqueous humour provides a protective environment for leptospires, which readily enter the anterior chamber of the eye during the leptospiraemic phase of the disease. There they can remain viable for months, despite the development of serum antibodies. Uveitis is common. Inflammation of the anterior uveal tract begins weeks or even months after the onset of disease and has been attributed to the persistence of organisms in the anterior chamber.

Clinical manifestations

Subclinical infection is common and less than 10% of symptomatic infections result in severe icteric illness. Even relatively virulent serovars such as *L. interrogans* serovar Icterohaemorrhagiae lead more often to anicteric than to icteric disease. Old terms such as pea-picker's disease, swineherd's disease, and canicola fever, which linked specific serotypes with distinct disease manifestations, are misleading and should be abandoned. The median incubation period is 10 days, with a range of 2 to 26 days. The duration of the incubation period has no prognostic significance. Once symptoms develop (see Table 6.34.1), they are said to follow a biphasic course. After an initial febrile illness, there is defervescence of fever and symptomatic improvement, followed by a second period of disease. However, a clear demarcation between the first and second stages is atypical of icteric leptospirosis and in mild cases the distinction can be unclear, or the second stage may never occur. The diagnostic usefulness of a history of a biphasic illness has been overemphasized. HIV coinfection does not seem to affect the clinical presentation of leptospirosis in the few coinfected patients described thus far.

Anicteric leptospirosis

Symptoms and signs
Typically, the disease begins with the abrupt onset of intense headache, fever, chills, and myalgia. Fever often exceeds 40°C (103°F) and is preceded by rigors. Muscle pain can be excruciating and occurs most commonly in the thighs, calves, lumbosacral region, and abdomen. Abdominal wall pain accompanied by palpation tenderness can mimic an acute surgical abdomen. Nausea, vomiting, diarrhoea, and sore throat are other frequent symptoms. Cough and chest pain figure prominently in reports of patients from Korea and China.

Table 6.34.1 The most common clinical manifestations of 208 leptospirosis patients in Puerto Rico

Symptoms (% of cases)	Anicteric (106 cases)	Icteric (102 cases)
Fever	100	99
Myalgia	97	97
Headache	82	95
Chills	84	90
Sore throat	72	87
Nausea	71	81
Vomiting	65	75
Eye pain	54	38
Diarrhoea	23	30
Decreased urine	20	30
Cough	15	32
Haemoptysis	5	14
Signs (% of cases)		
Conjunctival injection	100	98
Muscle tenderness	70	79
Hepatomegaly	60	60
Pulmonary findings	11	36
Lymphadenopathy	35	12
Petechiae and ecchymoses	4	29

(Adapted from Diaz-Rivera RS et al. (1963). Zoonosis Research 2, 159.)

Conjunctival suffusion is a helpful diagnostic clue which usually appears 2 or 3 days after the onset of fever and involves the bulbar conjunctiva. Pus and serous secretions are absent, and there is no matting of the eyelashes and eyelids. Mild suffusion can easily be overlooked. Less common and less distinctive signs include pharyngeal injection, splenomegaly, hepatomegaly, lymphadenopathy, and skin lesions.

Within a week most patients become asymptomatic. After several days of apparent recovery, the illness resumes in some individuals. Manifestations of the second stage are milder and more variable than those of the initial illness and usually last 2 to 4 days. Leptospires disappear from the blood, cerebrospinal fluid, and tissues but appear in the urine. Serum antibody titres rise, hence the term 'immune' phase. Meningitis is the hallmark of this stage of leptospirosis. Pleocytosis of the cerebrospinal fluid can be demonstrated in 80 to 90% of all patients during the second week of illness, although only about 50% will have clinical signs and symptoms of meningitis. Meningeal signs can last several weeks but usually resolve within a day or two. Uveitis is a late manifestation of leptospirosis, generally seen 4 to 8 months after the illness has begun. The anterior uveal tract is most frequently affected, and pain, photophobia, and blurring of vision are the usual symptoms.

Laboratory findings
The white blood cell count varies but neutrophilia is usually found. Urinalysis may show proteinuria, pyuria, and microscopic haematuria. Enzyme markers of skeletal muscle damage, such as creatinine kinase and aldolase, are elevated in the sera of 50% of patients during the first week of illness. Chest radiographs from patients with pulmonary manifestations show a variety of abnormalities, but none is pathognomonic of leptospirosis. The most common finding is small patchy snowflake-like lesions in the periphery of the lung fields.

Icteric leptospirosis (Weil's disease)

Symptoms and signs
This dramatic and life-threatening illness is characterized by jaundice, renal dysfunction, haemorrhagic manifestations, and a high mortality rate. Although jaundice is the hallmark of severe leptospirosis, fatalities do not occur because of liver failure. The degree of jaundice has no prognostic significance, but its presence or absence does; virtually all leptospirosis renal deaths occur in icteric patients. Icterus first appears between the fifth and ninth days of illness, reaches maximum intensity 4 or 5 days later, and continues for an average of 1 month. Hepatomegaly is found in the majority of patients and hepatic percussion tenderness is a reliable clinical marker of continuing disease activity. There is no residual liver dysfunction in survivors of Weil's disease, consistent with the absence of structural damage seen on pathological examination of this organ.

Bleeding is occasionally seen in anicteric cases but is most prevalent in severe disease. Purpura, petechiae, epistaxis, bleeding of the gums, and minor haemoptysis are the most common haemorrhagic manifestations, but deaths occur from subarachnoid haemorrhage and exsanguination from gastrointestinal bleeding. Conjunctival haemorrhage is an extremely useful diagnostic finding and, when combined with scleral icterus and conjunctival suffusion, produces eye findings strongly suggestive of leptospirosis (Fig. 6.34.1). The frequency with which severe pulmonary haemorrhage

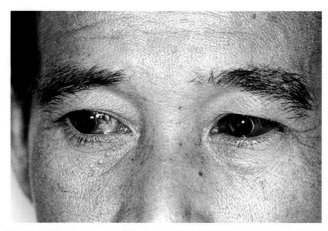

Fig. 6.34.1 Jaundice, haemorrhage, and conjunctival suffusion in acute leptospirosis.

complicates leptospirosis is variable, but is a cardinal feature of some outbreaks.

Life-threatening renal failure is a complication of icteric disease, although all forms of leptospirosis may be associated with mild kidney dysfunction. Oliguria or anuria usually develop during the second week of illness, but may appear earlier. Complete anuria is a grave prognostic sign, often seen in patients who present late in the course of illness with frank uraemia and irreversible disease. Because renal failure develops very quickly in leptospirosis, symptoms and signs of uraemia are frequently encountered. Anorexia, vomiting, drowsiness, disorientation, and confusion are seen early and progress rapidly to convulsions, stupor, and coma in severe cases. Disturbances of consciousness in a patient with severe leptospirosis are usually due to uraemic encephalopathy, whereas in anicteric patients aseptic encephalitis is the usual cause. Renal function eventually returns to normal in survivors of Weil's disease, although detectable abnormalities may persist for several months.

Leptospirosis-associated severe pulmonary haemorrhage syndrome (SPHS) is now recognized as a widespread public health problem with a case fatality rate of about 50% (Fig. 6.34.2).

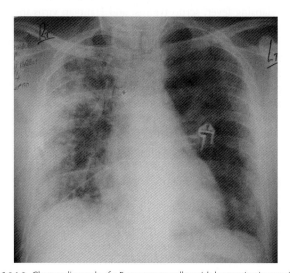

Fig. 6.34.2 Chest radiograph of a European traveller with leptospirosis-associated severe pulmonary haemorrhage syndrome acquired in Sabah (Malaysia). (Copyright D A Warrell.)

This lethal complication of leptospirosis can occur either with or without jaundice and renal failure. Haemoptysis is the cardinal sign, but may not be apparent until patients are intubated. Real-time polymerase chain reaction has shown that the apparent critical threshold for severe outcomes such as SPHS and death is a leptospiraemia of 10 000 or more bacteria/ml of blood.

Laboratory findings

Hyperbilirubinaemia results from increases in both conjugated (direct) and unconjugated (indirect) bilirubin, but elevations of the direct fraction predominate. Prolongations of the prothrombin time occur commonly but are easily corrected by the administration of vitamin K; modest elevations of serum alkaline phosphatase are typical. There is mild hepatocellular necrosis; greater than fivefold increases of transaminase (aminotransferase) levels are exceptional.

Jaundiced patients usually have a leucocytosis in the range of 15 to 30×10^9/litre, and neutrophilia is constant. Anaemia is common and multifactorial; blood loss and azotaemia contribute frequently, and intravascular haemolysis less often. Mild thrombocytopenia often occurs, but decreases in platelet count sufficient to be associated with bleeding are exceptional. The specific gravity of the urine is high. Hypokalaemia and hypomagnesaemia due to renal potassium and magnesium wasting can occur.

Diagnosis

Late disease can often be recognized by its typical clinical manifestations, but the presentation of early leptospirosis is usually nonspecific and is therefore difficult to identify clinically. Leptospirosis has long been acknowledged to be a frequent cause of undifferentiated febrile illness in developing countries. Coinfection with diseases such as malaria and scrub typhus have been reported and add to the diagnostic confusion of tropical fevers.

The laboratory diagnosis of leptospirosis remains problematic. Polymerase chain reaction (PCR) and culture are recommended during the first week of illness. The sensitivity of PCR is higher than culture but lower than standard microscopic agglutination test (MAT). The microscopic agglutination test is considered the serodiagnostic method of choice for leptospirosis, but its complexity limits its use to reference laboratories. Dilutions of patient sera are applied to a panel of live pathogenic leptospires. The results are viewed under dark-field microscopy and expressed as the percentage of organisms cleared from the field by agglutination. Inadequate quality controls of the live reference strain panels required can lead to frequent false-negative results. A new generation of commercially available rapid serodiagnostic kits that rely on whole leptospira antigen preparations have been developed. Unfortunately these assays seem to have unacceptably low sensitivities during acute-phase illness and persistent antibody produces low specificity in regions of high endemic transmission. The need for practical and affordable diagnostic kits to be available in areas where leptospirosis is common cannot be overemphasized. Polymerase chain reaction and urine antigen detection are research tools which would be of the greatest potential diagnostic value in patients who present early, before antibodies have reached detectable levels.

Isolation of leptospires from blood or cerebrospinal fluid is possible during the first 10 days of clinical illness, but specialized media are necessary. Serially diluted urine provides the highest yield. Unfortunately, culture results are only known 4 to 6 weeks later, too late to benefit hospitalized severely ill patients.

Treatment

The approach to the patient with possible leptospirosis is summarized in Fig. 6.34.3. Placebo-controlled double-blind trials have proved that doxycycline benefits patients with early mild leptospirosis, and that intravenous penicillin helps adults with severe late disease. The outcome of severe paediatric leptospirosis is also improved by penicillin therapy. Antibiotics should therefore be given to all patients with leptospirosis, regardless of age or when in their disease course they are seen. Doxycycline is given at doses of 100 mg orally twice a day for 1 week. Patients who are vomiting or are seriously ill require parenteral therapy. Intravenous penicillin G is administered as 1.5 million units every 6 h for 1 week. Recent trials from Thailand indicate that treatment with ceftriaxone, cefotaxime, and doxycycline had equivalent efficacy to penicillin in patients with mild to moderately severe disease. However, it is not known whether these antibiotics are as effective as high-dose penicillin for treatment of the most severely ill individuals. Doxycycline and azithromycin had comparable efficacy as presumptive treatment of mildly ill patients found later to have leptospirosis, scrub typhus, or duel infections.

There is controversy regarding the occurrence of a Jarisch–Herxheimer reaction in leptospirosis. If present, it is much less prominent in leptospirosis than in other spirochaetal illnesses. The important practical consideration is that antibiotics should not be withheld because of the fear of a possible Jarisch–Herxheimer reaction.

The management of pulmonary haemorrhage often requires prompt intubation and mechanical ventilation. Patients with SPHS have physiological and pathological evidence of acute respiratory distress syndrome, so ventilation using low tidal volumes and high postexpiratory end-pressures should be provided. Respiratory support to maintain adequate tissue oxygenation is essential because in nonfatal cases complete recovery of pulmonary function can be achieved. Ensuring adequate renal perfusion prevents renal failure in the vast majority of oliguric individuals. Continuous haemofiltration has been shown to be more effective than peritoneal dialysis in treating infection-associated hypercatabolic renal failure. Peritoneal dialysis, however, may be the only option in resource-limited settings. Whichever method of dialysis is chosen, however, it must be started promptly as delays increase mortality.

Prevention

Doxycycline, 200 mg taken once a week, prevents infection by *L. interrogans*. Widespread use of doxycycline prophylaxis is not indicated, but it can benefit those who are at high risk for a short time, such as military personnel and certain agricultural workers.

Infection by leptospires confers only serovar-specific immunity; second attacks due to different serovars can occur. The efficacy and safety of human leptospiral vaccines have yet to be conclusively demonstrated. Prevention of leptospirosis in the tropics is particularly difficult. The large animal reservoir of infection is impossible to eliminate, the occurrence of numerous serovars limits the usefulness of serovar-specific vaccine, and the wearing of protective clothing (e.g. rubber boots in rice fields) is both prohibitively expensive and impractical. Providing proper sanitation in urban slum communities would be the most effective control measure in this setting.

Prognosis

It is imperative to bring affordable tests to areas where leptospirosis is common because treatment (or lack of it) has a substantial impact on outcome. Atypical or mild cases are often confused with other entities such as aseptic meningitis, influenza, appendicitis, and gastroenteritis. Viral hepatitis is a common misdiagnosis in patients with Weil's disease. Leucocytosis, elevated serum bilirubin levels without marked transaminase elevations, and renal dysfunction are typical of leptospirosis but unusual in hepatitis. Malaria, typhoid fever, relapsing fever, scrub typhus, and Hantaan virus infection (haemorrhagic fever with renal syndrome) are important differential diagnoses in the tropics. Leptospirosis with prominent haemorrhagic manifestations is commonly misdiagnosed as dengue fever.

Case fatality rates are over 50% in SPHS and over 10% in Weil's disease. In addition to prompt diagnosis, efficient triage of high-risk patients is critical for the intensive monitoring and therapy required to manage complications. Acute renal failure and especially oliguria is a bad prognostic factor, as are respiratory insufficiency, hypotension, arrhythmias, and altered mental status.

Further reading

Abdulkader RCRM, *et al.* (1996). Peculiar electrolytic and hormonal abnormalities in acute renal failure due to leptospirosis. *Am J Trop Med Hyg*, **54**, 1–6.

Bharti AR, *et al.* (2003). Leptospirosis: a zoonotic disease of global importance. *Lancet Infect Dis*, **3**, 757–71.

Boonsilp S, *et al.* (2011). Molecular detection and speciation of pathogenic *Leptospira* spp. in blood from patients with culture-negative leptospirosis. *BMC Infect Dis*, **11**, 338.

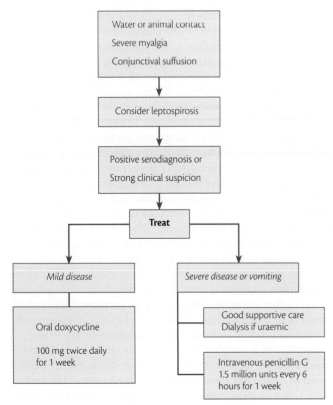

Fig. 6.34.3 Management of a febrile patient with possible leptospirosis.

Ko AI, *et al.* (1999). Urban epidemic of severe leptospirosis in Brazil. *Lancet*, **354**, 820–5.

Marchiori E, *et al.* (2011). Clinical and imaging manifestations of hemorrhagic pulmonary leptospirosis: a state-of-the-art review. *Lung*, **189**, 1–9.

McBride AJA, *et al.* (2005). Leptospirosis. *Curr Opin Infect Dis*, **18**, 376–86.

Nicodemo AC, *et al.* (1997). Lung lesions in human leptospirosis: microscopic, immunohistochemical, and ultrastructural features related to thrombocytopenia. *Am J Trop Med Hyg*, **56**, 181–7.

Sonthayanon P, *et al.* (2011). Accuracy of loop-mediated isothermal amplification for diagnosis of human leptospirosis in Thailand. *Am J Trop Med Hyg*, **84**, 614–20.

Thaipadungpanit J, *et al.* (2011). Diagnostic accuracy of real-time PCR assays targeting 16S rRNA and lipL32 genes for human leptospirosis in Thailand: a case-control study. *PLoS ONE*, **6**, e16236.

Thaipadungpanit J, *et al.* (2007). A dominant clone of *Leptospira interrogans* associated with an outbreak of human leptospirosis in Thailand. *PLoS Negl Trop Dis*, **1**, 1–6.

Watt G, *et al.* (1988). Placebo controlled trial of intravenous penicillin for severe and late leptospirosis. *Lancet*, **1**, 433–5.

Zaki SR, Shieh WJ, the Epidemic Working Group (1996). Leptospirosis associated with outbreak of acute febrile illness and pulmonary haemorrhage, Nicaragua. *Lancet*, **347**, 535–6.

6.35 Nonvenereal endemic treponematoses: yaws, endemic syphilis (bejel), and pinta

David A. Warrell

Essentials

The endemic treponematoses are chronic, granulomatous diseases caused by morphologically and serologically identical spirochaetes of the genus *Treponema*. They are spread by intimate but non-sexual contact and sometimes by fomites, mainly among children. *Treponema pallidum* subsp. *pertenue* causing yaws (framboesia), *T. pallidum* subsp. *endemicum* causing endemic syphilis (bejel) and *T. carateum* causing pinta (carate) are distinguishable from *T. pallidum* subsp. *pallidum*, causing venereal syphilis, by their epidemiology and pathological effects and genomic structure (e.g. the *arp* gene).

Despite the successful WHO/UNICEF mass penicillin treatment campaign (1952–64), there has been a resurgence of yaws, mainly in West Africa. Children living in rural areas in warm, humid climates in tropical countries are most affected by yaws. About 10% of untreated cases develop late, disfiguring, or crippling lesions of skin, bone, and cartilage.

Endemic syphilis occurs in arid areas of the Sahel and Arabian peninsula. It presents with buccal mucocutaneous lesions from contaminated cups. Late systemic effects are much less common than in venereal syphilis. Pinta persists in small foci in southern Mexico and South America, causing hypo- or hyper-pigmented skin lesions. Single-dose benzathine penicillin is effective treatment.

Prevention is by improving hygiene and eliminating the reservoir of infection by mass treatment.

Introduction

Syphilis (Chapter 6.36) and the nonvenereal treponematoses are distinguishable by their epidemiological characteristics and the pattern of infection produced in humans and experimentally infected laboratory animals (Table 6.35.1). Yaws is caused by *Treponema pallidum* subsp. *pertenue*, a spirochaete that is morphologically identical to *T. pallidum* subsp. *pallidum* (the cause of venereal syphilis), *T. pallidum* subsp. *endemicum* (the cause of nonvenereal syphilis or bejel), and *T. carateum* (the cause of pinta). None is cultivable *in vitro*. They share common antigens so that infection by one species produces varying degrees of cross-immunity to the others. They are serologically indistinguishable. Pathogenic treponemes can be differentiated by polymerase chain reaction using acidic repeat protein (*arp*) gene sequences. The genomes of eight treponemes have been compared. Restriction target site analysis revealed a high genome structure similarity of all strains.

Most of the genetic differences between *T. p. pallidum* and *T. p. pertenue* strains were accumulated in six genomic regions and are likely to contribute to the marked differences in pathogenicity between these strains. These regions of sequence divergence might be used for the molecular detection and discrimination of syphilis and yaws strains. The treponemes of yaws, syphilis, and pinta are fragile and readily killed by exposure to atmospheric oxygen, drying, mild detergents, or antiseptics. They cannot penetrate intact skin, but gain entry to the body through small abrasions and lacerations. They prefer cooler temperatures, below 37°C, which may explain their predilection for the skin and bones of the extremities. All cause chronic granulomatous diseases that exhibit primary, secondary, and tertiary (late) stages separated by quiescent or latent periods. Most of their pathological effects are immune-mediated, the peak of the immune response preceding healing. Some spirochaetes survive in tissues and can cause exacerbations as immunity declines.

Yaws

Epidemiology

Yaws is a chronic infection by *T. pallidum* subsp. *pertenue* of skin, bone, and cartilage and periodically the organism spreads systemically. It is nonvenereal and noncongenital and is predominantly a disease of children. Seventy-five per cent of those acutely infected are below the age of 15 years and the peak incidence is between the ages of 6 and 10 years. In endemic areas more than 80% of the population are infected. The organism is transmitted by direct contact of broken skin with an infectious lesion or by fingers or bites contaminated with lesion exudate or rarely indirectly through fomites. Spread is promoted by crowded, unhygienic conditions. In humid, warm environments the early lesion tends to proliferate and teems with spirochaetes, thus increasing the infectious reservoir, whereas

Acknowledgement: The author gratefully acknowledges inclusion of material from previous editions by his late friend and colleague Dr Peter L Perine.

Table 6.35.1 Major features of the treponematoses

Feature	Venereal syphilis	Yaws	Endemic syphilis	Pinta
Organism	*T. pallidum* subsp. *pallidum*	*T. pallidum* subsp. *pertenue*	*T. pallidum* subsp. *endemicum*	*T. carateum*
Age of infection (years)	20–40	5–15	2–10	10–30
Incubation period	10–90 days	14–28 days	?	2–6 months
Occurrence	Worldwide	Africa, South America, Oceania, Asia	Africa, Middle East	Central and South America
Climate	All	Warm, humid	Dry, arid	Warm, rural
Direct transmission:				
Venereal	Common	No	Rare	No
Nonvenereal	Rare	Common	Rare	Common
Congenital	Yes	No	?	No
Indirect transmission:				
Contaminated utensils	Rare	Rare	Common	No
Insects	No	Rare	No	?
Reservoir of infection	Adults	Infectious and latent cases; ?nonhuman primates	Infectious and latent cases	
Ratio infectious:latent cases	1:3	1:3–5	1:2	?
Late complications:				
Skin	+	+	+	+
Bone, cartilage	+	+	+	No
Neurological	+	No	?	No
Cardiovascular	+	No	?	No

in dry, arid climates or seasons the reverse is true. Yaws is rarely fatal but frequently disfiguring and debilitating.

During the 1952–64 World Health Organization UNICEF campaign, an estimated 152 million people were examined and 46.1 million clinical cases, latent infections, and contacts were treated with penicillin in 46 countries, reducing the global prevalence by 95% from 50 to 2.5 million cases and greatly diminishing the yaws reservoir in West and Central Africa, Central and South America, and Oceania. This campaign initiated development of primary health care in many countries. Unfortunately, since the late 1970s there has been a resurgence, initially after control was delegated to national authorities. Seven West African countries started new mass treatment campaigns in the 1980s, but by 1995 the estimated global prevalence of infectious cases was 460 000, with 400 000 of them being in West Africa. Yaws was eliminated in India by 2004, but it persists in rural populations in West Africa (e.g. 26 000 new cases in Ghana in 2005), Ethiopia, South-East Asia (5000 new cases in Indonesia, East Timor), Papua New Guinea (18 000 new cases), Solomon Islands, Vanuatu, and Ecuador. The current worldwide prevalence of infectious cases of yaws may be *c.*500 000. Some African countries such as Nigeria, previously rendered yaws-free by mass treatment campaigns, have experienced a sharp rise in the incidence of venereal syphilis, perhaps reflecting the decline of herd immunity to yaws. Yaws is also prevalent in some gorilla populations.

Pathogenesis

The lesions of yaws and the other treponematoses are due largely to the host's immune response to the treponeme. None of these treponemes carries or produces toxic substances. They have the ability to invade living cells without causing apparent injury. Cell destruction and tissue damage are probably due to the action of immune cells that injure normal tissue in the process of killing treponemes.

Host immunity reaches its highest level after several months of infection, just before disseminated lesions heal and latency begins. Thereafter the host is immune to reinfection and is not contagious, but since not all treponemes are killed, infectious lesions may reappear as immunity wanes over time. Most patients with yaws experience two or three infectious relapses during the first 5 years of infection.

Clinical features

Primary yaws

After an incubation period of 3 to 5 weeks, the initial lesion in yaws usually appears on the extremities. Characteristically, the primary lesion is a single painless papule that appears at the site of infection and enlarges to form a raspberry-like (framboesia) vegetative lesion called a papilloma. This is round to oval, elevated, and not indurated, ranging in size from 1 to 3 cm in diameter (Fig. 6.35.1).

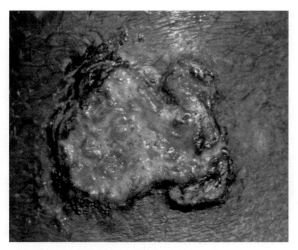

Fig. 6.35.1 Primary yaws lesion with ulceration and satellites.
(Courtesy of Dr B Hudson, Sydney, Australia.)

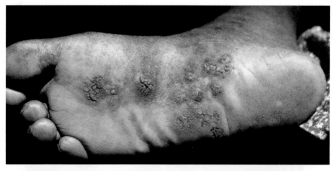

Fig. 6.35.3 Plantar papillomas with hyperkeratotic, macular, early plantar yaws ('crab yaws'). These lesions are painful.
(Courtesy of Dr B Hudson, Sydney, Australia.)

The surface teems with spirochaetes and is often covered by a thin yellow crust that is easily removed. It may ulcerate as it enlarges and becomes secondarily infected with other microorganisms. Lymph nodes draining the initial lesion may enlarge and become tender, but systemic symptoms are rare.

Secondary yaws

Secondary or disseminated ulceropapillomatous or maculopapular lesions appear after 2 to 6 months, often without any intervening latent period, on the skin of moist areas such as the axillae, joint flexures, genitalia, and the gluteal cleft (Fig. 6.35.2a,b). They also occur on the soles and palms and, because they are tender, may interfere with gait and use of the hands. Papillomas in different stages of development persist for 6 to 8 months and heal without scars unless they become secondarily infected. Despite the size and number of lesions, children with generalized papillomas experience little discomfort or other constitutional symptoms.

When the climate is arid, yaws lesions are commonly slightly raised scaly pigmented macules measuring between 1 and 4 cm in diameter. They have the same distribution as papillomas and may appear together with lesions of different morphology in the same patient (maculopapular yaws).

The periosteum and bones of the extremities are frequently inflamed during early yaws causing swelling, night pain, and tenderness. There is dactylitis of the proximal phalanges (Fig. 6.35.4). Painful osteoperiostitis of the legs, affecting mainly the tibias and fibulas, is especially common (Fig. 6.35.5). Hypertrophic osteitis of the maxilla, either side of the bridge of the nose, can cause grotesque swellings ('goundo'). Scaly tender hyperkeratotic lesions of the palms and soles also occur and may be incapacitating. Hyperkeratotic and bone lesions are not contagious, and macular lesions are only minimally so.

One or more relapses of secondary-type lesions usually occur during the first 5 years of infection, each separated by a period of latency. The lesions of late yaws occur thereafter in about 10% of untreated cases.

Late yaws

The lesions are not infectious because they contain few treponemes. Cutaneous plaques produce atrophic scars. Subcutaneous granulomatous nodules erode skin and produce deep ulcers that destroy underlying tissue and cause disfigurement. Hyperkeratotic palmar and plantar yaws (Fig. 6.35.3) are incapacitating and often prevent the use of the hands or the ability to walk normally. The weight is placed on the sides of the feet, which produces a gait much like that of a crab ('crab yaws').

The granulomas of late yaws have a histological appearance that is similar to the gummas of syphilis. These proliferative lesions may involve the palate and destroy the soft tissues of the nose, causing

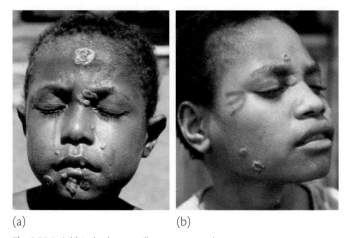

(a)   (b)

Fig. 6.35.2 (a,b) Early ulceropapillomatous secondary yaws.
(Courtesy of Dr B Hudson, Sydney, Australia.)

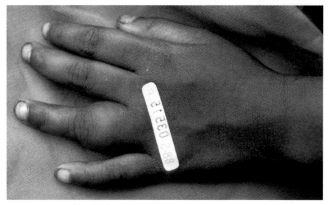

Fig. 6.35.4 Dactylitis.
(Courtesy of Dr B Hudson, Sydney, Australia.)

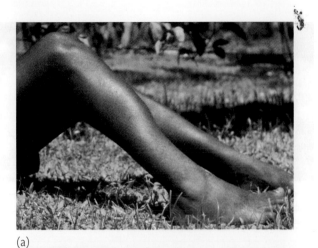

(a)

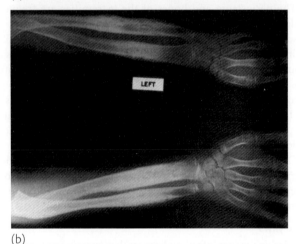

(b)

Fig. 6.35.5 (a,b) Osteoperiostitis.
(Courtesy of Dr B Hudson, Sydney, Australia.)

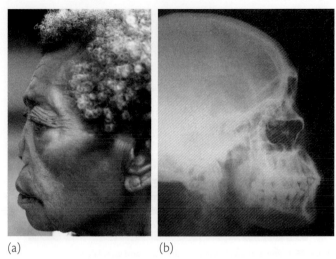

(a)   (b)

Fig. 6.35.6 (a,b) Gangosa (rhinopharyngitis mutilans) of endemic syphilis and yaws.
(Courtesy of Dr B Hudson, Sydney, Australia.)

a terrible disfiguration called gangosa (Fig. 6.35.6a,b). Gummatous periostitis of the skull, fingers, and long bones is erosive and often retards or stops growth. Active periostitis is occasionally found in young and middle-aged adults who had yaws in childhood. Burnt out osteitis leads to a characteristic deformity 'sabre tibia'.

Endemic syphilis

T. pallidum subsp. *endemicum* is transmitted by nonvenereal contact among children. In contrast to yaws, transmission by contaminated drinking vessels may be more common than by direct contact with infectious lesions. The disease tends to be familial, with spread of infection from children to adults rather than to the community in general. The lesions are virtually indistinguishable from early yaws, and the two diseases may occur at different times in the same population but not in the same person. Venereal syphilis can be acquired by children through social contact with adults who have venereal syphilis, and then be spread by nonvenereal person-to-person contact if levels of sanitation and personal hygiene are low.

Several variants of endemic syphilis are recognized by their geographical distribution: bejel of the eastern Mediterranean, North Africa, and Niger; and njovera or dichuchwa of Africa. Bejel is the only type of endemic syphilis still prevalent. It is found in seminomadic people such as the Tuareg, living in the Sahelian nations of Mauritania, Mali, Niger, Burkina Faso, and Senegal where dramatic increases in the number of cases of endemic syphilis have been reported. In Naimey (Niger), seroprevalence was 12% among children under 5 years of age. The disease is also prevalent among the nomadic tribes of the Arabian peninsula, where late complications such as osteoperiostitis predominate.

Clinical features

The initial lesions of endemic syphilis usually appear at the mucocutaneous borders of the mouth or on the oral mucous membranes (mucous patches) as the result of transmission by contaminated drinking vessels. Late ulceronodules and osteoperiostitis are seen in late endemic syphilis, but cardiovascular and neurological complications are extremely rare.

Pinta (carate)

T. carateum resides only in the skin. This peculiar tissue tropism is unexplained. It is probably an inherent property of the treponeme, acting in contact with climatic factors. Pinta is confined to remote parts of Central and South America, principally in the semiarid region of the Tepalcatepec Basin of southern Mexico and focal areas of Colombia, Peru, Ecuador, and Venezuela. Pinta is probably transmitted by direct skin or mucous membrane contact, by insect bites, and perhaps by tribal rituals resulting in skin scratches.

Clinical features

After an incubation period of 15 to 30 days, the primary lesions, single or few in number, are seen on the dorsal surfaces of the limbs, face, chest, or gluteal area, usually of children or young adults (Fig. 6.35.7). The lesion is an itchy erythematous papule or depigmented macule that enlarges slowly over a period of several weeks or months to form an erythematous plaque, sometimes with regional lymphadenopathy but without systemic symptoms. Satellite papules form at its edge and undergo a similar type of evolution. The plaques coalesce to form violaceous pigmented plaques that, in several years, slowly depigment from lighter shades of blue to white, leaving symmetrical atrophic depigmented scars.

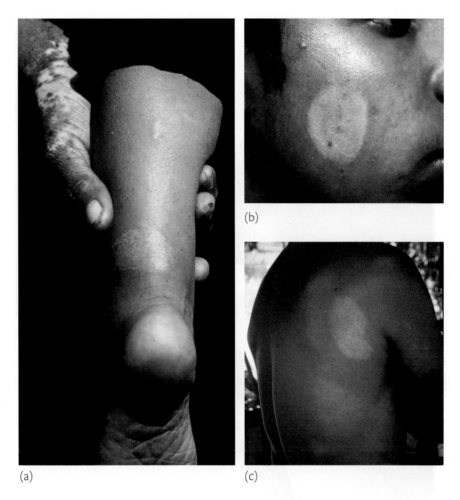

Fig. 6.35.7 (a–c) Early lesions of pinta in Yaruro people of north-western Venezuela.
(Courtesy of Prof. Rolando Hernández Pérez, Hospital Universitario 'Dr. Luis Razetti' Barinas, Universidad de los Andes, Venezuela.)

(a)   (b)   (c)

Rapid dissemination of lesions may occur months or up to about 4 years after the primary lesions, frequently affecting scalp, nails, and mucous membranes (Fig. 6.35.8). Depigmented, pigmented, and erythematous-desquamative lesions may occur simultaneously in the same patient. Late lesions are symmetrical, depigmented, atrophic, or hyperkeratotic.

Diagnosis

The diagnosis of yaws and other endemic treponematoses is made by a combination of clinical assessment, of positive dark-ground examination of early lesions and exudates which are usually teeming with treponemes, and of reactive serological tests for syphilis.

Early yaws, endemic syphilis, and pinta are not difficult to diagnose in endemic areas where the disease is familiar. The most difficult diagnostic problem arises when someone who had yaws as a child emigrates to an area of the world where the disease never existed. Such a person usually has reactive serological tests for syphilis and may have a few atrophic scars suggestive of earlier infection. What are the chances that this patient has or has had venereal syphilis? Should they be treated for latent yaws or syphilis? The patient's social and medical history should be carefully reviewed. Clinical findings suggestive of old yaws (scars, inactive tibial periostitis), and the absence of signs of congenital and venereal syphilis support the diagnosis of inactive or treated yaws.

If the patient has a reagin titre (Venereal Disease Research Laboratory (VDRL), rapid plasma reagin (RPR)) of less than 1:8 dilutions, they probably do not have active latent yaws or syphilis. If they received at least one therapeutic dose of long-acting penicillin in their native country during a yaws campaign, they require no further treatment. On the other hand, if the patient is a contact of a case of infectious venereal syphilis, they should be treated as being potentially infected with syphilis because *T. pallidum* subsp. *pallidum* occasionally superinfects people who had yaws as children. If treatment is given, the patient should receive a certificate stating the drug and dosage used and the results of their serological tests to prevent unnecessary future treatment.

Differential diagnosis

Ulceronodular skin lesions of yaws and endemic syphilis resemble tropical ulcers. Yaws lesions are not as painful, necrotic, or deep as tropical ulcers, which are usually singular and restricted to the lower one-third of the leg. Plantar warts are frequently confused with plantar papillomas of yaws, and both conditions may occur in the same patient. Pinta must be differentiated from other hypopigmented and hyperpigmented skin lesions including vitiligo, indeterminate leprosy, pityriasis alba, and psoriasis.

Treatment

Penicillin aluminium monostearate has been used for mass treatment in past campaigns, but benzathine penicillin is currently recommended because it is longer acting and more readily available.

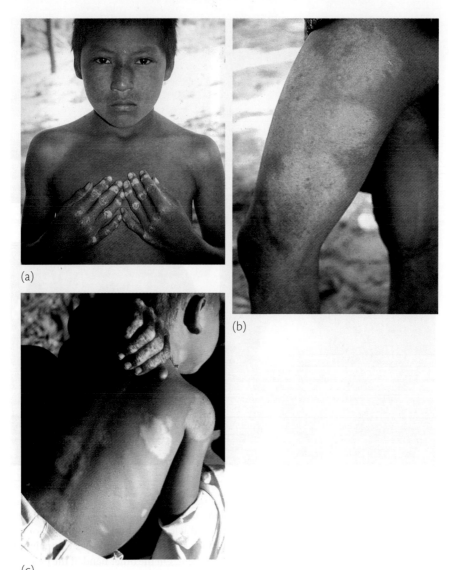

(a)

(b)

(c)

Fig. 6.35.8 (a–c) Disseminated lesions of pinta in Yaruro people of north-western Venezuela. (Courtesy of Prof. Rolando Hernández Pérez, Hospital Universitario 'Dr. Luis Razetti' Barinas, Universidad de los Andes, Venezuela.)

However, a single dose of oral azithromycin recently proved non-inferior to benzathine penicillin for treating yaws and may be preferred in future. People who have active infections or who are noninfectious should be given 1.2 mega units of benzathine penicillin in a single intramuscular injection; children under 10 years of age receive 0.6 mega units. Patients allergic to penicillin may be given tetracycline or erythromycin, 500 mg by mouth four times daily for 2 weeks; children under 10 years of age should be given erythromycin in dosages adjusted for their age. Treatment failures have been reported in Papua New Guinea.

Prevention and control

Transmission is reduced as personal hygiene among children improves. Prevention of yaws and other endemic treponematoses in a community requires elimination of the reservoir of infection, often by treating the entire population with penicillin. This has succeeded in some countries, notably recently with yaws in India.

Further reading

Antal GM, Lukehart SA, Meheus AZ (2002). The endemic treponematoses. *Microbes Infect*, **4**, 83–94.

Engelkens HJ, Vuzevski VD, Stolz E (1999). Non-venereal treponematoses in tropical countries. *Clin Dermatol*, **17**, 105–6, 143–52.

Farnsworth N, Rosen T (2006). Endemic treponematosis: review and update. *Clin Dermatol*, **24**, 181–90.

Hackett CJ, Loewenthal LJA (1960). *Differential diagnosis of yaws*. World Health Organization, Geneva.

Harper KN, *et al.* (2008). On the origin of the treponematoses: a phylogenetic approach. *PLoS Negl Trop Dis*, **2**, e148.

Harper KN, *et al.* (2008). The sequence of the acidic repeat protein (arp) gene differentiates venereal from nonvenereal *Treponema pallidum* subspecies, and the gene has evolved under strong positive selection in the subspecies that causes syphilis. *FEMS Immunol Med Microbiol*, **53**, 322–32.

Mitjà O, *et al.* (2012). New Treatment Schemes for Yaws: The Path Toward Eradication. *Clin Infect Dis*. [Epub ahead of print].

Padilha Gonçalves A, Basset A, Maleville J (1992). Tropical treponematoses. In: Canizares O, Harman RRM (eds) *Clinical tropical dermatology*, 2nd edition, pp. 129–50. Blackwell, Boston.

Perine PL, *et al.* (1984). *Handbook of endemic treponematoses: yaws, endemic syphilis and pinta*. World Health Organization, Geneva.

Smajs D, Norris SJ, Weinstock GM (2012). Genetic diversity in *Treponema pallidum*: Implications for pathogenesis, evolution and molecular diagnostics of syphilis and yaws. *Infect Genet Evol*, **12**, 191–202.

Walker SL, Hay RJ (2000). Yaws: a review of the last 50 years. *Int J Dermatol*, **39**, 258–60.

6.36 Syphilis

Basil Donovan and Linda Dayan

Essentials

Syphilis results from infection with the spirochaete *Treponema pallidum* subsp. *pallidum*, for which humans are the only known natural host. In adults it is transmitted primarily by sexual contact. The organism gains entry into the body through small breaks in the skin or the intact mucosal surfaces of the genitals, mouth, or anus, and is able to invade and survive in a wide variety of tissues.

Since the availability of penicillin, syphilis has become primarily (>90%) a disease of less affluent countries or of minority subpopulations in more affluent countries with poor access to health care. It is also a disease of people with rapid rates of partner change, e.g. men who have sex with men (MSM) and commercial sex workers.

Clinical features

Syphilis can manifest in three stages: (1) primary syphilis, which occurs within a few weeks to months after infection; (2) secondary syphilis, which presents after a few months up to a year; and (3) tertiary syphilis, which presents years to decades after primary infection. These stages can overlap, and they are frequently asymptomatic.

Primary syphilis—this appears 9 to 90 days after the organism gains entry via direct inoculation through the thin skin or mucosa of the anogenital tract or mouth during sexual exposure. The resulting lesion is typically a painless ulcer or 'chancre', sometimes indurated, that appears at the site of inoculation and is associated with regional lymphadenopathy, chancres can be multiple and atypical.

Secondary syphilis—occurs 3 to 6 weeks after the appearance of the chancre, with manifestations including fever, malaise, mucocutaneous lesions (rash, condyloma lata, mucous patches), generalized lymphadenopathy, and (uncommonly) visceral disease. Invasion of the central nervous system is common, but usually asymptomatic.

Latent syphilis—the lesions of both primary and secondary syphilis may wax and wane, but they eventually resolve; there are no signs or symptoms of active syphilis, but serological tests are positive for *T. pallidum*.

Tertiary syphilis—affects around one-third of infected people following a variable period of latent infection, with manifestations including (1) neurosyphilis—can present as (a) aseptic meningitis, with variable features, e.g. focal neurological deficits, cranial nerve palsies, hydrocephalus or psychiatric symptoms; (b) meningovascular disease, with endarteritis leading to cerebral infarction; (c) general paresis, involving changes in the parenchyma of the central nervous system that lead to the gradual onset of cognitive impairment, depression, and personality changes, later progressing to dementia, delirium, seizures, and delusions; (d) tabes dorsalis, with initial symptoms and signs including lightening pains and parasthesias, visceral crises, abnormal deep tendon reflexes, incontinence, ataxia with a wide-based gait, and pupillary abnormalities. (2) Gummatous syphilis—destructive granulomatous lesions most commonly present on skin, mucosal surfaces or in bone. (3) Cardiovascular syphilis—most commonly asymptomatic aortitis, aortic incompetence, aortic aneurysm, and coronary ostial stenosis.

Congenital syphilis—most pregnant women with early syphilis will transmit the condition to the fetus via the placenta, with congenital syphilis often resulting in fetal loss, stillbirth, or neonatal or childhood disease.

Diagnosis and treatment

Diagnosis—the transient nature of the lesions and the spirochetaemia limit the role of direct detection of *T. pallidum*, hence diagnosis usually relies on serology, with tests being (1) nonspecific (or nontreponemal or reagin)—e.g. rapid plasma reagin (RPR) and Venereal Disease Research Laboratory (VDRL) tests; detect phospholipid cardiolipin as an antigen; generally sensitive in early infection but tend to decline over the next several years without treatment; able to quantify disease activity and hence used for follow-up after treatment. (2) specific (or treponemal)—e.g. *T. pallidum* haemagglutination assay (TPHA); use *T. pallidum* as the antigen; may become positive shortly before the nonspecific tests; typically remain reactive for life after successful treatment and therefore have no role in assessing stage of infection, cure, or reinfection.

Treatment—parenteral penicillin G remains the preferred treatment for syphilis, with doxycycline providing an oral alternative. Successful treatment of early disease relies on demonstrating a fourfold decrease in reagin (RPR or VDRL) titres over the next 6 to 12 months. Sexual contacts of early syphilis should be treated presumptively, regardless of their test results, if the contact was within 90 days, usually with a single dose of benzathine penicillin G.

Prevention

The chance of acquiring syphilis following one act of intercourse with an infected person is 1 to 2%, which should be reduced by the use of condoms. Early treatment of disease decreases the duration of infectivity and thereby minimizes transmission to others, hence those at high risk of syphilis should be encouraged to undergo regular syphilis screening (as well as testing for HIV and other sexually transmissible infections).

Prevention of congenital infection and serious outcomes such as stillbirth and neonatal death rely on routine antenatal screening early in the pregnancy, with prompt treatment of infected mothers. Women in high-incidence settings should be rescreened later in pregnancy.

Introduction and historical perspective

In the 1490s, an epidemic of a new and virulent sexually transmissible disease appeared in Europe following the return of Christopher Columbus and his fleet from the Americas. This led many to believe that syphilis originated in the New World. There is now molecular phylogenetic evidence for this 'Columbian hypothesis'. Syphilis spread rapidly through Europe where it was known by a variety of names including *morbus gallicus* (the French disease), *lues venereum* (venereal disease), and the great pox.

The alternative theory proposes that syphilis was simply another variant of a preexisting treponemal infection that had adapted to sexual and congenital transmission and produced greater morbidity (the Unitarian hypothesis). A variety of yaws-like diseases that predominantly affected children were present in Europe and Africa at the time, and a few persisted in Europe into the 20th century.

Syphilus (the original spelling) was an afflicted shepherd in a poem by Girolamo Fracastoro published in 1530. The original text described the symptoms of syphilis, hypothesized about its origins, and mentioned the use of early remedies such as guaiacum, a compound derived from a Central American tree, and mercury.

Following an experiment by John Hunter in 1767 it was thought that gonorrhoea and syphilis were different manifestations of the same disease until Philippe Ricord, in 1838, clarified the differences between the two infections. Soon after, the three stages of syphilis were categorized and congenital and neurological syphilis were described.

Because of the toxicity and dubious benefit of the treatments available at the time, a prospective cohort study into the natural history of syphilis was conducted in Oslo between 1890 and 1920. This study followed 1978 initially symptomatic patients and demonstrated that approximately one-third developed late complications. Many of these complications proved fatal.

Rapid advances in knowledge occurred around the beginning of the 20th century. In 1905, Schaudinn and Hoffman demonstrated spirochaetes in secondary syphilitic lesions. One year later, Von Wasserman devised the first serological test for syphilis. In 1910, Paul Erlich announced results for his compound 606 (salvarsan), a form of arsenic that showed activity against syphilis.

The discovery of penicillin by Fleming, its development for therapeutic use by Florey and Chain, and the first clinical trial in 1943 by Mahoney revolutionized the treatment of syphilis. During the immediate post-war period the use of penicillin eclipsed other forms of therapy and by the mid-1950s the incidence of syphilis had fallen markedly throughout the industrialized world.

Aetiology, genetics, pathogenesis, and pathology

Treponema pallidum subsp. *pallidum*, a spiral-shaped bacterium, is a member of the order Spirochaetales and the cause of adult acquired and congenital syphilis. Humans are the only known natural host for all *T. pallidum* subspecies, although an unclassified and morphologically indistinguishable simian pathogen, the Fribourg–Blanc treponeme, was isolated from a baboon in Guinea in 1962. The inability to culture *T. pallidum in vitro* has retarded study of its biology.

T. pallidum subsp. *pallidum* is closely related to other pathogenic treponemes that cause nonvenereal disease: *T. pallidum* subsp. *carateum* (pinta), *T. pallidum* subsp. *pertenue* (yaws), and *T. pallidum* subsp. *endemicum* (endemic syphilis or bejel) (see Chapter 6.35). Subspecies *pertenue* and *endemicum* and the Fribourg–Blanc treponeme have recently been demonstrated to be genetically distinct from subspecies *pallidum*, consistent with the lack of cross-immunity. The spirochaete is 6 to 20 μm long and only 0.10 to 0.18 μm thick, making it invisible to ordinary light microscopy. Using dark-field microscopy, *T. pallidum* has 6 to 20 characteristic tightly wound spirals and it moves with corkscrew motility or by bending in the middle and popping back into place with a spring. Other nonpathogenic treponemes tend to have fewer coils or a jerkier motion. Commensal species of treponema (*T. denticola* and *T. oralis*) can mimic *T. pallidum*, limiting the usefulness of dark-field microscopy of oral and anal lesions.

The *T. pallidum* DNA genome was first published in 1998. It is small, with a single circular chromosome of 1 138 006 base pairs containing 1041 predicted protein coding sequences, consistent with its limited metabolic capabilities. The organism obtains most of its essential nutrients from the host environment, making it an obligate parasite. *In vivo*, *T. pallidum* has been grown in rabbits and reproduces itself slowly, doubling every 30 to 33 h. *T. pallidum* is able to survive better with low levels of oxygen (3–5%) and is sensitive to heat.

T. pallidum is able rapidly to invade and survive in a wide variety of tissues after gaining entry into the body through small breaks in the skin or the intact mucosal surfaces of the genitals, mouth, or anus. The organism has a reputation as a 'stealth' pathogen because its paucity of surface proteins and lipopolysaccharides helps it to evade the host immune response. *T. pallidum* induces humoral, cell-mediated, and local innate responses that appear to confer immunity to exogenous infection in the chronically infected person (chancre immunity). However, patients treated for early syphilis can become rapidly reinfected.

From the site of inoculation, *T. pallidum* replicates locally and spreads to regional lymph nodes, then into the blood stream from where it can traverse junctions between vascular endothelial cells. Lymphocyte, (CD4+) macrophage, and plasma cell infiltrates accompanied by vasculopathic changes, endarteritis and periarteritis, underlie the histology of syphilitic lesions of all stages. Silver staining of tissues may demonstrate the presence of spirochaetes, usually in the dermal–epidermal junction.

In secondary syphilis, treponemes are found in many sites including visceral organs, the central nervous system, and the skin. *T. pallidum* can remain clinically dormant in the aortic wall, producing an endarteritis in the vasa vasorum and varying degrees of thickening, scarring, and destruction of the arterial wall. This process results in the development of arterial plaques and calcification of the vessels found in cardiovascular syphilis.

In meningitis, perivascular infiltration of lymphocytes and plasma cells causes the meninges to become inflamed. In meningovascular syphilis, thickening of the intima, fibrous changes in the adventitia, and vascular narrowing cause changes in brain blood vessels with resultant infarction and cranial nerve palsies.

The gummas of late syphilis are chronic granulomatous lesions consistent with a hypersensitivity response with few treponemes present. Histologically, central necrosis, peripheral lymphocytosis, perivasculitis, and obliterating endarteritis are seen.

Epidemiology

Since the availability of penicillin, syphilis has become primarily (>90%) a disease of less affluent countries or of minority subpopulations in more affluent countries with poor access to health care. It is also a disease of populations with rapid rates of partner change such as men who have sex with men (MSM) and commercial sex workers.

The World Health Organization estimated that in 1999 syphilis continued to infect about 12 million new people a year globally. The greatest number of new infections, 5.8 million, is found in South-East and East Asia. Sub-Saharan Africa accounted for 3.4 million new cases and Latin America and the Caribbean 1.26 million. In Africa, between 4 and 17% of women are seropositive for syphilis in antenatal clinics, and many are coinfected with HIV. About a million pregnancies a year are seriously complicated or aborted by syphilis.

The incidence of syphilis in China has risen following the political and social changes that occurred in the last part of the 20th century. In the former Soviet Union, the incidence of syphilis among the young sexually active population rose rapidly after 1991 with the degradation of the public health system.

Since the beginning of the 21st century, syphilis rates in the United Kingdom, Europe, Asia, North America, Australia, and other developed countries have risen in MSM, especially in those who are HIV positive. Serosorting, the phenomenon of homosexual men of similar HIV status seeking each other for unsafe sex, has been a factor. Oral sex, considered to be relatively safe in terms of transmission of HIV infection, readily transmits syphilis.

Prevention

Syphilis in adults is transmitted primarily by sexual contact. The chance of acquiring the infection is estimated to be between 1 and 2% following one act of intercourse with an infected person. Syphilis is found in up to 60% of sexual partners.

As *T. pallidum* is present in mucosal or cutaneous lesions, infected adults are more likely to transmit the disease during primary or secondary stages. The use of condoms to prevent syphilis has not been evaluated in controlled trials. Intuitively, condoms should have some effect in reducing transmission, but they do not provide 100% protection as they do not cover all areas of anogenital skin during intercourse. Condoms should also be used for oral sex.

The early recognition and treatment of syphilis decreases the duration of infectivity thereby minimizing transmission to others. As symptoms are not always present, those who are at higher risk of syphilis such as MSM and commercial sex workers are encouraged to undergo regular syphilis screening, as well as testing for HIV and other sexually transmissible infections. In order to attract those most at risk of syphilis, health services need to be accessible and culturally appropriate, confidential, and provide free or affordable diagnosis and treatment. Presumptive treatment of sexual partners and early recognition and treatment of those who may be core transmitters in a sexual network is essential in any syphilis control programme.

Some authorities now use the internet to encourage MSM to have regular syphilis tests. The internet can also help these men to inform their sexual partners in a nonthreatening and confidential way.

Syphilis can be transmitted via donated blood or organs, although this is rare. Thus serological screening of donors is routine in most settings.

Mother-to-child transmission of syphilis usually occurs *in utero*. Prevention of congenital infection and serious outcomes such as stillbirth and neonatal death rely on screening and treating for syphilis in the mother early in the pregnancy. In high-incidence populations, rescreening around week 28 to 32 of the pregnancy and again at delivery is also recommended. With timely treatment of the mother, congenital syphilis is almost entirely preventable. Provision of comprehensive antenatal health care with affordable testing for syphilis should form part of a comprehensive syphilis control programme. Community education should encourage women to attend for health care early in pregnancy when treatment can be given with best effect. In high-prevalence areas, if a mother first presents at term, routine treatment of the neonate with a single dose of benzathine penicillin 50 000 units/kg is sometimes recommended if the mother has not been tested or adequate maternal treatment cannot be confirmed.

Clinical features

Clinical staging of syphilis is important to guide the process of contact tracing or partner notification. Primary, secondary, and early latent syphilis are collectively called 'infectious syphilis'. Late latent and tertiary syphilis are generally regarded as no longer infectious for sexual partners. However, pregnant women may pose an occasional risk to their offspring. Treatment for later stages of syphilis is typically longer than for early syphilis.

Primary syphilis

The chancre, or ulcer of primary syphilis, develops at the site of inoculation within 9 to 90 days (median 3 weeks) of infection, initially as a red macule that soon becomes papular before it ulcerates. The typical ulcer is painless, has fluid or grey slough in its centre, and a well-defined rolled edge. Mature ulcers may have a palpable indurated plaque deep to the lesion. However, chancres can occasionally be painful or multiple, and clinically indistinguishable from other causes of genital ulcers (Fig. 6.36.1). Mixed aetiologies are always possible (Fig. 6.36.2).

Common sites for chancres in men include the distal penis, while in women the posterior fourchette, labia, and vulva are the most commonly diagnosed sites (Fig. 6.36.3a). The anus, mouth, and lips are all possible sites for chancres, as well as other extragenital sites.

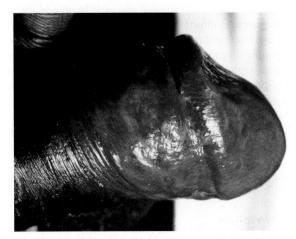

Fig. 6.36.1 Multiple painful chronic chancres in a man with HIV infection. (Courtesy of Dr David Bradford.)

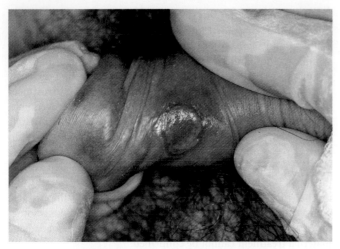

Fig. 6.36.2 Chancre against a background of primary genital herpes.

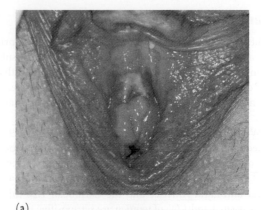

(a)

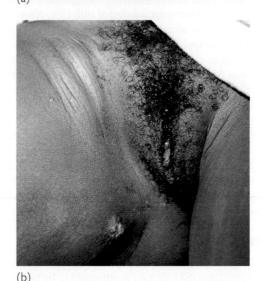

(b)

Fig. 6.36.3 (a) A periurethral chancre in a woman who presented with a painless lump. (b) Chancre on thigh and inguinal lymphadenopathy of primary syphilis.
((b) Copyright D A Warrell.)

If a chancre is small or hidden in the anal canal, vagina, cervix, or mouth, it usually passes unnoticed (Fig. 6.36.4). Most patients subsequently diagnosed with secondary syphilis do not recall the lesions of primary syphilis.

Painless and typically rubbery, small lymph nodes are often felt in the affected region within a week of the development of the chancre (Fig. 6.36.3b). The chancre usually heals spontaneously in 3 to 6 weeks, but it may occasionally recur ('chancre redux').

Secondary syphilis

This disseminated stage of the infection typically occurs between 3 and 6 weeks following the appearance of the chancre, and the two stages may overlap. However, up to 60% of patients do not recall any signs or symptoms of secondary syphilis at all.

The symptoms and signs of secondary syphilis are often described as protean, as listed in Table 6.36.1. Without treatment they resolve spontaneously only to reappear, usually in a milder form, in almost one-quarter (24%) of patients in the following 12 to 24 months (Fig. 6.36.5).

Latent syphilis

Latent syphilis is present when there are no signs or symptoms of active syphilis but serological tests are positive for *T. pallidum*. Latent syphilis is arbitrarily divided into early latent syphilis, when the asymptomatic infection has been present for less than 1 or 2 years, and late latent syphilis after this time. In practice, asymptomatic people diagnosed through screening are often deemed to have latent syphilis of unknown duration. As a precaution, such patients are treated with the longer courses of antibiotics that are used for late infections.

Before the antibiotic era, approximately two-thirds of adults remained in the latent phase throughout their lifetime and showed no signs of tertiary syphilis. These days many common antibiotics have some activity against *T. pallidum*, so it is likely that antibiotics used for other conditions are also altering the natural history of, if not accidentally curing, latent syphilis.

Tertiary syphilis

Tertiary syphilis occurred in 15 to 40% of those who remain untreated in the Oslo study, with some modest differences between

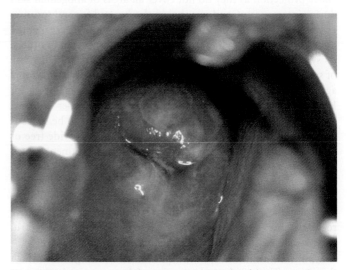

Fig. 6.36.4 An asymptomatic chancre on the anterior lip of the cervix in the same woman as Fig. 6.36.3a.

Table 6.36.1 Clinical manifestations of secondary syphilis

	Features	Frequency
Rash	Erythematous or coppery colour Nonpruritic or mildly pruritic Macular or maculopapular (50%) progressing to papular, papulosquamous, psoriasiform, annular (dark-skinned people), pustular, or follicular Usually symmetrical, round to oval lesions, 5 to 20 mm across (Fig. 6.36.5a,b) Trunk, palms, soles, and body flexures are most commonly involved Occasionally papules around the forehead hairline ('corona veneris')	Over 70%
Condyloma lata	Pale elevated moist plaques in warmer flexural areas such as perineum, perianal area, groin, axilla, perioral area, and nasolabial folds (Fig. 6.36.5c) Appear later than rash	15–50%
Mucous patches	Superficial erosions, papules, or plaques of mucosa of the oropharynx or anogenital area Involvement of the pharynx may result in hoarseness or sore throat	4–17%
Constitutional	Low-grade fever, malaise, headache, myalgias, arthralgias, anorexia, and nausea Occasionally severe	Common, but variable
Lymphadenopathy	Generalized, nontender, and characteristically rubbery and discrete (Fig. 6.36.3b)	Over 60%
Hepatitis	Mildly elevated transaminases Usually not clinically important	Up to 10%
Ocular	Iritis or uveitis	Occasional
Alopecia	Follicular disease can lead to patchy 'moth-eaten' alopecia of the scalp or, rarely, loss of the outer part of the eyebrows or beard	Occasional
Central nervous system	Asymptomatic neuroinvasion occurs in up to 25% Symptomatic meningitis or meningovascular disease may be more common in HIV infection Ocular and auditory cranial nerves most commonly involved	Up to 2%
Kidney	Asymptomatic proteinuria Nephritic syndrome Rapidly progressive glomerulonephritis	Rare
Heart	Myocarditis Ventricular arrhythmia	Rare
Parotitis		Rare
Gastritis	Gastritis and stomach ulcers resulting in nausea and abdominal pain	Rare
Periostitis, arthritis, or bursitis	Localized	Rare
Malignant syphilis ('lues maligna')	Rapidly progressive variant with marked constitutional symptoms and disfiguring crusted necrotic ulcers Possibly more common with HIV infection and in alcoholics	Rare

the sexes (Table 6.36.2). In part as a result of the wide availability of antibiotics used for other purposes, gummatous and cardiovascular syphilis are now relatively rare compared to neurosyphilis; most oral antibiotics are unlikely to achieve cidal levels in the central nervous system.

Neurosyphilis

The diagnosis of neurosyphilis frequently raises clinical dilemmas because of the nonspecific nature of its clinical presentations and the absence of definitive tests. Neurosyphilis may manifest as aseptic (basilar pattern) meningitis or meningovascular disease as early as the secondary stage or up to several years after infection. As well as the usual symptoms of meningitis, syphilitic meningitis may also present with focal neurological deficits such as hemiparesis, aphasia, seizures, or psychiatric symptoms. Cranial nerve palsies

accompany syphilitic meningitis in about 40% and hydrocephalus in 35% of patients.

Meningovascular syphilis stems from endarteritis leading to infarction, most commonly 5 to 12 years after infection. While any artery may be affected, the middle cerebral is the most frequently involved. Gradual onset and less extensive damage results from smaller arteries being involved than is usual in thrombotic stroke. Psychological changes can mimic the early stages of parenchymal disease (see below).

Confusing the diagnosis, up to 25% of individuals with early syphilis may have *T. pallidum* in the cerebrospinal fluid demonstrated by rabbit inoculation or polymerase chain reaction (PCR). This largely asymptomatic phenomenon is known as neuroinvasion and it is believed that most, but not all, will spontaneously clear *T. pallidum* from the cerebrospinal fluid. Studies in the

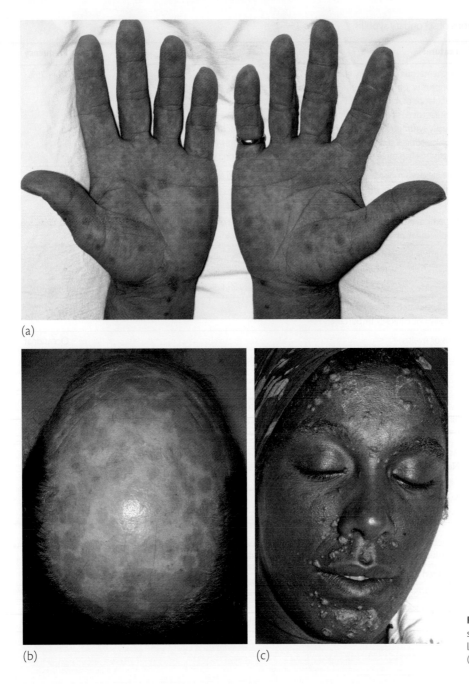

(a)

(b)   (c)

Fig. 6.36.5 (a,b) Rash of secondary syphilis on palms and scalp. (c) Papular lesions of secondary syphilis. (Copyright D A Warrell.)

preantibiotic era demonstrated that the degree of cerebrospinal fluid abnormalities (white cell count, raised protein, and reactive CSF-Venereal Disease Research Laboratory (VDRL) test) in asymptomatic neurosyphilis predicted later progression to symptomatic neurosyphilis.

Rarely, after 20 to 25 years, syphilitic meningitis or meningovascular disease can involve the spinal cord resulting in (often asymmetric) paresis, incontinence, hyper-reflexia, extensor plantar reflexes, and loss of position and vibration sense.

General paresis involves changes in the central nervous system parenchyma, characterized by fibrosis and atrophy, and occurs much later, approximately 15 to 25 years after the initial infection. Parenchymatous central nervous system lesions can present with usually gradual onset cognitive impairment, depression, and personality changes, later progressing to dementia, delirium, seizures, and delusions. Neurological signs can include irregular, often large, pupils that become unresponsive to light and accommodation (Argyll Robertson pupils), dysarthria, facial or hand tremor, loss of facial expression, hypotonia, and hyper-reflexia or loss of reflexes.

Table 6.36.2 Frequency of late complications of syphilis from the Oslo study in the preantibiotic era

Form of tertiary syphilis	Men (%)	Women (%)
Benign late (gummatous) syphilis	14.4	16.7
Cardiovascular syphilis	13.6	7.6
Neurosyphilis	9.4	5.0

Tabes dorsalis involves parenchymatous changes in the dorsal root tracts and posterior columns of the spinal cord 15 to 35 years after primary infection. Initial symptoms and signs may include lightening pains and paraesthesias, visceral crises, abnormal deep tendon reflexes, incontinence, ataxia with a wide-based gait, and papillary abnormalities. Rarely, gummas may involve the cerebrum or the spinal cord.

Gummatous (late benign) syphilis

Gummas are destructive granulomatous lesions that most commonly present on skin (70%), on mucosal surfaces (10%), or in bone (10%). They can occur a few years or decades after primary infection. On the skin gummas start as painless nodules that progressively necrose, leaving punched-out ulcers. The face, legs (Fig. 6.36.6), buttocks, trunk, and scalp are common sites. Gummatous involvement of the oropharynx can lead to perforations and severe scarring of the palate, pharynx, or nasal septum. Tongue involvement can lead to glossitis, swelling, and leucoplakia. Fractures can occur with gummas of bone.

Other organs occasionally affected include the liver, central nervous system, eyes, stomach, lungs, and testes.

Cardiovascular syphilis

Now rare, cardiovascular syphilis develops decades after primary infection. The most common forms are asymptomatic aortitis, aortic incompetence, (usually proximal) aortic aneurysm, and coronary ostial stenosis.

Congenital syphilis

Mother-to-child transmission occurs via the placenta at any stage of gestation. Because the transmission is haematogenous there is no primary lesion (chancre) and it is a disseminated infection from the outset. If the mother has early syphilis, transmission is almost certain; infectivity progressively declines to below 10% in late latent infection.

Fetal wastage from syphilis may manifest as first or second trimester abortion or still birth with a large pale fibrosed placenta or a macerated fetus. Of the infected babies that survive, only 30% have specific symptoms in the neonatal period, though almost all will exhibit symptoms by 3 months. Many of the early (at birth

or in the first 2 years) lesions resemble secondary syphilis in the adult (Fig. 6.36.7). Failure to thrive in the first few months may be the first sign. Affected infants tend to be small or premature, irritable, snuffly, and cry feebly. The skin is often dry and wrinkled. Generalized rubbery lymphadenopathy is common, often accompanied by hepatosplenomegaly and haematological abnormalities. Early deaths may be due to diffuse pulmonary infiltration.

Painful osteochondritis or epiphysitis of the long bones, and sometimes periostitis, can occur in the first 6 months with characteristic radiological appearances.

Late (after 2 years, but rarely beyond 30 years) congenital syphilis is analogous to tertiary syphilis in adults. However, gummatous disease may be more common while cardiovascular disease is rare compared to adult syphilis. Interstitial keratitis is the most common form of late congenital syphilis. From the fifth year of life onward, the child may develop bilateral eye pain and photophobia, and scleral vascularization. Gumma may lead to perforation of the palate. Periostitis may lead to deformity of the tibia (sabre tibia), the skull (Parrot's nodes), the scaphoid, and the clavicle.

The stigmata of congenital syphilis are permanent deformities or scars left by early or late disease. Sometimes stigmata may help to explain unexpected positive serological tests in adults, as the patient may be unaware of their prior infection. The bony deformities tend to persist, while *T. pallidum* can also invade tooth buds affecting the permanent teeth (Hutchinson's teeth) but not the milk teeth. The molars may be deformed with dwarfed cusps, while the incisors may be small, peg-shaped, and notched at the tip. Previous interstitial keratitis may be demonstrable for life on slit-lamp examination.

Differential diagnosis

Syphilis is often described as the great imitator due to the vast number of illnesses that it mimics. Screening for syphilis was once considered routine for medical and psychiatric hospital admissions. A high index of suspicion is required for the diagnosis.

Primary syphilis

Chancres can resemble anogenital ulcers from any cause, and more than one condition may be present (Fig. 6.36.2). Other causes of genital ulcers include herpes simplex virus infections, chancroid, lymphogranuloma venereum, and donovanosis. An anal chancre

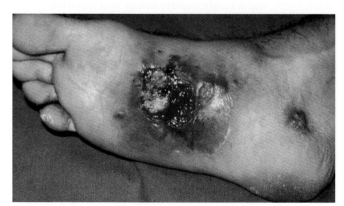

Fig. 6.36.6 Ulcerating nodular lesions of gummatous syphilis in a man with HIV infection. Initially thought to be Kaposi's sarcoma, the diagnosis was made by biopsy.
(Courtesy of Professor David Cooper.)

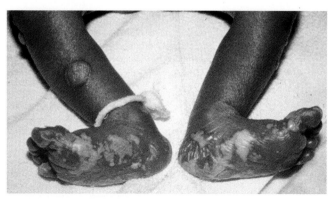

Fig. 6.36.7 Bullous syphilis lesions in a neonate.

can be painful and clinical indistinguishable from an ordinary anal fissure. Liberal use of the laboratory to exclude other causes of ulcers is essential. Alternatively, in resource-poor environments that have to rely on syndromic management of genital ulcers, antibiotic combinations need to cover all the common causes of genital ulcers in that region.

Secondary syphilis

The rash of secondary syphilis may resemble a drug eruption, pityriasis rosea, tinea versicolour, seborrhoeic dermatitis, erythema multiforme, scabies, lichen planus, psoriasis, fungal infections, and leprosy. Other infections causing generalized rashes include primary HIV infection, measles, rubella, and meningococcemia. Condyloma lata may be confused with genital warts. Syphilitic alopecia may resemble alopecia areata or fungal scalp infections.

Generalized lymphadenopathy, sore throat, and fever are also seen in infectious mononucleosis, rubella, toxoplasmosis, lymphoma, acute hepatitis, and, most importantly, primary HIV infection. Symptoms of meningitis may also be present in HIV infection, bacterial meningitis, enterovirus infections, and primary herpes simplex virus infection.

Latent syphilis

Childhood treponemal infections such as yaws and pinta, as well as prior congenital syphilis, may be serologically indistinguishable from adult-acquired syphilis and the specific tests are likely to remain positive for life. People from endemic treponemal areas or who may be at risk of congenital infection with positive syphilis serology should be examined for stigmata of these conditions. False-positive nonspecific tests (VDRL and rapid plasma reagin (RPR)) occur in 1 to 2% of the population (see 'Nonspecific serological tests'). Confirmation with a specific treponemal test is essential for asymptomatic people.

Neurosyphilis

Symptoms and signs of meningovascular syphilis are similar to those in other causes of stroke or cerebrovascular accidents due to haemorrhagic or thrombotic mechanisms. Gummas in the brain can be mistaken for tumours and abscesses, particularly in HIV infection. General paresis should be considered in the differential diagnosis of dementia, psychosis, seizures, delirium, and personality changes.

Gummatous syphilis

Other granulomatous diseases such as sarcoidosis, tuberculosis, and neoplastic lesions can be confused with gummatous syphilis.

Cardiovascular syphilis

Signs and symptoms of cardiovascular syphilis are similar to those of atherosclerotic disease and aortic aneurysms are more commonly due to hypertension. Other causes of aortic regurgitation without stenosis include Marfan's syndrome and infective endocarditis.

Clinical investigation

Direct detection of the organism

As with all bacterial infections, ideally *T. pallidum* should be directly detected (Table 6.36.3) because a serological response may take days to weeks to evolve. However, the transient nature of the lesions and the spirochaetaemia limit the role of direct detection, leading to reliance on serology or, in resource-poor environments, syndromic management. The role of PCR testing of the CSF has yet to be determined because asymptomatic and transient neuroinvasion by *T. pallidum* correlates poorly with standard criteria for diagnosing neurosyphilis.

Table 6.36.3 Methods of direct detection of *T. pallidum*

Method	Brief description	Role
Animal inoculation	Fresh (or flash-frozen to less than −78°C) lesion material or cerebrospinal fluid is usually inoculated by intratesticular or intradermal means into rabbits. The animals are then monitored for the development of skin lesions, orchitis, or serological response	The most sensitive test (approaching 100%), but only used as a gold standard to evaluate other tests in the research setting
Dark-field microscopy	Fresh serous fluid with motile organisms is collected by gentle pressure on the lesions and pressed under a coverslip. An on-site microscope with a reflecting dark-field condenser and a skilled microscopist are required. Diagnostic criteria include morphology and motion of the organisms	Only appropriate for specialist services. Not for oral or anal lesions. Patient must attend service in person. Immediate result
DFA test	Specimen collected as for dark-field microscopy, air dried on a glass slide, and stained with labelled anti-*T. pallidum* globulins immediately before fluorescence microscopy	Specimen does not need to be fresh, so can be transported to laboratory. High sensitivity (>90%) if the specimen is well collected. Suitable for oral lesions
DFAT test	DFA test adapted to histology specimens, usually transported in 10% buffered formalin	Skin, brain, placenta, umbilical cord, or gastrointestinal biopsy specimens can be tested
PCR test	Suspected chancres or lightly abraded lesion swabs in PCR transport medium. Possibly cerebrospinal fluid and placental blood	Very sensitive for moist primary and secondary lesions, but only available in referral laboratories

DFA, direct fluorescent antibody; DFAT, direct fluorescent antibody tissue; PCR, polymerase chain reaction.

Serology

Broadly there are two types of serological tests for syphilis, nonspecific (or nontreponemal or reagin) tests and specific (or treponemal) tests. Although less sensitive for some stages of syphilis as well as being less specific, nonspecific tests require less expertise, are cheaper, and are more indicative of active infection so they are often favoured for screening. Specific tests usually remain positive after treatment, limiting their role in screening in high-prevalence populations (Fig. 6.36.8). However, specific tests have an important place in screening in low-prevalence populations and in confirming nonspecific tests.

Nonspecific serological tests

The RPR and VDRL tests are flocculation tests targeting the phospholipid cardiolipin as an antigen. They are relatively sensitive in early infection (77 to 88% for primary syphilis and 100% for secondary syphilis) but tend to decline over the next several years without treatment (Fig. 6.36.8). Nonspecific tests are used for follow-up after treatment because they are readily able to quantify disease activity, nonspecific tests are used for follow-up after treatment. In general, a fourfold change in titre is taken as evidence of cure, relapse, or reinfection. Broadly equivalent, RPR tests can be read macroscopically while VDRL tests require a microscope. The toluidine red unheated serum test (TRUST) is a variant of the RPR test. The VDRL test is the only syphilis test recommended for CSF evaluation.

Such antilipoidal antibodies may be produced by other forms of acute or chronic tissue damage, so confirmation with a specific test is needed if there is no other sign of syphilis. Acute false-positive results are associated with acute infections such as hepatitis, herpes virus infections, measles, and malaria, as well as immunizations and pregnancy. Chronic (exceeding 6 months) false-positive reactions are associated with connective tissue disorders, immunoglobulin abnormalities, drug injecting, ageing, malaria, and malignancy.

Specific serological tests

These tests use *T. pallidum* as the antigen and may become positive shortly before the nonspecific tests. The specific tests typically (more than 85%) remain reactive for life after successful treatment and they do not provide meaningful quantitative results, so they

have no role in assessing stage of infection, 'cure', or reinfection. They are technically more difficult and expensive than nonspecific tests, so they may not be available for confirmation in resource-poor environments. Examples of specific tests include the *T. pallidum* haemagglutination assay (TPHA), the *T. pallidum* particle agglutination assay (TPPA), and the microhaemagglutination assay for antibodies to *T. pallidum* (MHA-TP). The fluorescent treponemal antibody absorption (FTA-ABS) test is often used as a confirmatory test and may be the first serological test to become positive in primary syphilis, so it may be added to the nonspecific test to investigate a genital ulcer.

Newer multiantigen enzyme immunoassays (EIAs) for IgG antibodies against *T. pallidum* are becoming increasingly common in high-volume laboratories because they are more objective and can be automated. The EIAs appear to have comparable sensitivity (70–90% for primary and 100% for secondary syphilis) and specificity to the other specific tests. There is considerable overlap in the causes of false-positive specific and nonspecific tests.

As IgM antibodies are large and considered unable to cross the placenta, FTA-ABS and EIA versions of the IgM test have been used on neonates to assess possible congenital infection. The use of IgM tests is not established, and a negative IgM test does not exclude congenital syphilis.

Available only in reference laboratories, western blot can detect IgG or IgM antibodies and appears to be at least as sensitive as other specific tests for syphilis. The IgM western blot looks promising as an aid to diagnosing congenital syphilis with a specificity over 90% and a sensitivity over 83%.

Criteria for diagnosis

Primary syphilis

The direct detection of *T. pallidum* (Table 6.36.3) from an ulcer confirms a diagnosis of primary syphilis. Alternatively, a clinically suspicious ulcer and any positive serological test are accepted as a confirmed diagnosis, although more than one serological test is normally ordered if resources permit. If initially seronegative, patients with suspicious ulcers should have repeat serology in 2 to 4 weeks.

Secondary syphilis

Treponemes may be demonstrated in moist mucocutaneous lesions of secondary syphilis, although suggestive symptoms or signs (Table 6.36.1) plus a positive RPR test are sufficient for the diagnosis. The nonspecific tests are normally reactive at high titres.

Latent syphilis

The diagnosis of latent syphilis requires two positive serological tests, at least one of them a specific test. Recent symptoms suggestive of primary or secondary (Table 6.36.1) syphilis, or a history of a negative test in the last 1 or 2 years, indicates early latent syphilis. The sexual risk history should be consistent with this clinical staging. Generally, nonspecific reactive test titres are higher in early latent than in late latent infection. In many cases a diagnosis of late latent syphilis or latent syphilis of unknown duration is a diagnosis of last resort after risk and symptom history, clinical examination, and serological picture are judged together. Past childhood treponemal infection can remain a possibility.

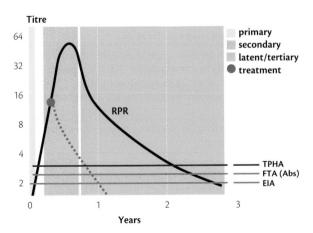

Fig. 6.36.8 Serological response to syphilis and its treatment.

Neurosyphilis

Neurosyphilis is defined as a reactive CSF-VDRL or a CSF mononuclear pleocytosis of more than 5 cells/μl, or both. While a reactive CSF-VDRL is very specific it has limited sensitivity (up to 70%) in detecting neurosyphilis. CSF protein concentration may be elevated. Because HIV can cause a CSF pleocytosis anyway, against a background of HIV infection a cut-off of >20 cells/μl has sometimes been used for a neurosyphilis diagnosis. A bloody tap may confound the diagnosis, while symptoms or signs of neurosyphilis add confidence to the diagnosis. CT or MRI of the brain or spinal cord may demonstrate lesions compatible with tertiary syphilis.

Gummatous syphilis

Gumma can be diagnosed clinically (Fig. 6.36.6) with reactive serology but, as clinical experience is limited, histological confirmation is usual.

Cardiovascular syphilis

Aortic valve disease or proximal aortic aneurysm with reactive syphilis serology strongly suggest cardiovascular syphilis. However, aneurysm and calcification of the aortic wall are found in other conditions such as hypertension. Coronary angiography demonstrates ostial stenosis.

Congenital syphilis

The diagnosis of congenital syphilis is often problematic, and many neonates are treated before it can be confirmed because of the high risk of serious disease. Direct detection of *T. pallidum* from the placenta or nasal discharge or skin lesions of a newborn infant is definitive but rarely achievable. Usually the diagnosis relies on clinical signs (if present) and serology. Positive serological tests in the neonate may reflect passive antibody transfer from the mother, but

a positive nonspecific test is useful if present in higher titres than the mother. An alternative approach to the management of a normal-looking baby of an infected mother is to perform serial quantitative nonspecific serology and treat if the titre rises. More experience is needed with PCR and western blot IgM antibody testing.

As clinically indicated, long-bone and chest radiology, lumbar puncture, cranial ultrasonography, and ophthalmic examination may contribute to the diagnosis where available.

Treatment

Choice of antibiotics

Parenteral penicillin G is the original and remains the preferred treatment for syphilis globally. In most parts of the world this takes the form of long-acting benzathine penicillin G injections, although some prefer daily injections with procaine penicillin, sometimes boosted with probenecid, because treponemicidal CSF levels may be achieved (Table 6.36.4). However, daily injections raise adherence and resource issues. No penicillin regime has demonstrated superiority in controlled trials.

Injectable ceftriaxone has been used with short-term success although the exact dose, frequency, and length of course are uncertain. Oral doxycycline provides an alternative for those with an allergy to penicillin, when there is no access to clean needles, or when the patient is averse to injections. Neither of these agents has been well studied.

Macrolides such as erythromycin and azithromycin have also been used, but the rapid emergence of high-level resistance on four continents, attributable to a single mutation in the *T. pallidum* genome makes this group of antibiotics inappropriate in most settings.

Some physicians may use oral corticosteroids to reduce the adverse effects of the Jarisch–Herxheimer reaction (see below)

Table 6.36.4 Treatment of syphilis

Form of syphilis	US Centers for Disease Control and Prevention (CDC)	Notable variations
Adult, early	Benzathine penicillin G 2.4 million units (equivalent to 1.8 g) intramuscularly in one dose	UK guidelines offer as an alternative: procaine penicillin G 750 mg intramuscularly once a day for 10 days; or if patient averse to injections, amoxicillin 500 mg plus probenecid 500 mg orally four times a day for 14 days; or if allergic to penicillin, doxycycline 100 mg orally twice a day for 14 days
Adult, late; excluding neurosyphilis	Benzathine penicillin G 2.4 million units intramuscularly weekly for three doses	UK alternative: procaine penicillin 750 mg intramuscularly once a day for 17 days; or if patient averse to injections, amoxicillin 2 g plus probenecid 500 mg orally four times a day for 28 days; or if allergic to penicillin, doxycycline 200 mg orally twice a day for 28 days
Neurosyphilis	Aqueous crystalline penicillin G 18–24 million units intravenously per day (as 3–4 million units every 4 h or as a continuous infusion) for 10–14 days	UK alternative: procaine penicillin 2 g intramuscularly once a day plus probenecid 500 mg orally four times a day for 17 days; or if patient averse to injections, amoxicillin 2 g plus probenecid 500 mg orally four times a day for 28 days; or if penicillin allergic, doxycycline 200 mg orally twice a day for 28 days
Syphilis in a pregnant woman	As per stage of adult syphilis	Desensitize if allergic to penicillin (see CDC guidelines); doxycycline is contraindicated in pregnancy
Congenital and childhood syphilis	Aqueous crystalline penicillin G 100 000–150 000 units/kg intravenously in divided doses for 10 days	UK and CDC alternative if active disease: procaine penicillin 50 000 units/kg intramuscularly once a day for 10 days; older children with primary or secondary syphilis, benzathine penicillin G 50 000 units/kg (up to 2.4 million units) in one dose; three doses if late infection or unknown duration of infection; child-protection assessment is essential

CDC, Centers for Disease Control and Prevention (United States of America).

in neurological and cardiovascular syphilis although there is no systematic evidence to support this practice.

Contacts

Sexual contacts of early syphilis should be treated presumptively regardless of their test results if the contact was within 90 days, usually with a single dose of benzathine penicillin G. Contacts beyond 90 days can be treated according to the clinical picture and serology results unless follow-up is uncertain.

Follow-up

The goals of treatment are to cure symptoms and signs of infection if present, to render the patient noninfectious, and to prevent late complications occurring or progressing. In primary or secondary syphilis, lesions and constitutional symptoms should be well on the way to resolving within days. However, some symptoms of early neurosyphilis may persist for several months. Antibiotic therapy halts further damage in cardiovascular, neurological, and gummatous syphilis but is usually unable to repair tissue damage that has already occurred.

Follow-up serology can be performed at 3, 6, and 12 months from treatment. Defining successful treatment of early syphilis relies on demonstrating a fourfold decrease in reagin (RPR or VDRL) titres over the next 6 to 12 months. If there is ongoing risk, reinfection may be impossible to separate from relapse; both are defined as a fourfold rise in reagin titres on at least two occasions. In late infections, where reagin titres are typically low, no drop in titre may be demonstrable. Frequently, a persistently low or nonreactive reagin test, an absence of current symptoms, and a history of adequate treatment have to be accepted as a cure.

Regular reagin testing is recommended for those at ongoing risk of reinfection.

Jarisch–Herxheimer reaction

The Jarisch–Herxheimer reaction may occur in up to 50% of those with primary syphilis and more than 70% of patients with secondary syphilis, but it is uncommon in late syphilis. This transient influenza-like reaction occurs between 4 and 24 h (median 8 h) after the first dose of antibiotics and lasts for several hours with malaise, low-grade fever, flushing, and tachycardia. Early and late lesions may transiently flare, secondary rashes may appear for the first time (and be mistaken for penicillin allergy), and cranial nerve and cardiovascular symptoms may worsen. In rare cases, premature labour and fetal distress have been induced. The reaction may result from the release of endotoxin-like substances from killed *T. pallidum*. Patients should be warned in advance and advised to stay home for the first night with paracetamol at hand.

Prognosis

Since the advent of penicillin the late complications of tertiary syphilis are relatively rare and adult mortality is almost never seen. However, in resource-poor environments or where antenatal screening is not routine, fetal wastage and serious congenital disease remain common.

With treatment all mucocutaneous syphilis lesions rapidly resolve, sometimes leaving an atrophic scar. Deformities of bones and teeth generally persist for life. The symptoms of early neurosyphilis usually resolve although this may take several months. The symptoms

and signs of late neurosyphilis generally persist but they should not progress. Follow-up CSF examination should document a declining pleocytosis (if present initially) by 6 months, although the CSF-VDRL may take longer to normalize.

Areas of controversy

The role of lumbar puncture

Lumbar puncture is indicated if neurological or ophthalmic symptoms or signs are present. The role of lumbar puncture in the diagnosis, treatment, and follow-up of other patients with syphilis has been debated. Resource and patient consent issues may be difficult. Many experts believe that if using a treatment regimen that is likely to enter the CSF such as daily procaine penicillin, then a lumbar puncture before treatment does not alter management of the case and can be omitted. Lumbar puncture can then be limited to cases where investigation might alter management, such as in cases of differential diagnosis. The United Kingdom guidelines recommend lumbar puncture when using a nonpenicillin regimen in people with HIV infection because of concerns about possible higher rates of neurosyphilis.

HIV infection

HIV and syphilis are both transmitted sexually so it is not surprising that both infections often coexist. Additionally, syphilis lesions can facilitate both the transmission and acquisition of HIV infection. Early syphilis can lead to a moderate decline in peripheral CD4 cell counts and an elevation of plasma HIV-1 viral load in HIV-infected people; both phenomena resolve with syphilis treatment.

No unique clinical syphilis syndromes have been reported in people with concurrent HIV infection. Limited, largely anecdotal, evidence suggests some more aggressive clinical manifestations of syphilis in HIV infection, but this is the exception rather than the rule. Early neurosyphilis may be more common but the diagnosis is compounded by the HIV infection itself causing neurological symptoms and CSF abnormalities. Higher CSF lymphocyte counts (20 rather than the usual 5 cells/μl) have been used to diagnose neurosyphilis because HIV commonly causes a CSF pleocytosis without syphilis. Higher serum RPR titres ($\geq$1:32) and a lower peripheral CD4 cell count (<350 cells/μl) have been shown to be predictive of neurosyphilis, making these tests relative indications for lumbar puncture particularly if both are present. Some have argued for routine lumbar puncture for HIV-infected people with syphilis, while others, noting that neurosyphilis remains uncommon even in this group, advocate limiting lumbar puncture to people with neurological or ocular symptoms, treatment failure, or late latent syphilis.

Despite some early reports of HIV-coinfected patients with negative serological tests in early syphilis, larger studies have failed to show any significant difference and standard syphilis testing procedures are recommended in HIV infection.

In general, authorities such as the United States Centers for Disease Control and Prevention recommend routine treatment with benzathine penicillin G (Table 6.36.4) in HIV infection.

A higher rate of serological treatment failure (defined as a fourfold decrease in RPR titre at 6–12 months) has been documented in HIV infection (*c.*20%) compared to HIV-uninfected people (5%). However, the clinical significance of this finding is unknown.

Likely developments in the near future

Nucleic acid amplification (NAA) tests such as PCR will aid the aetiological diagnosis of genital ulcers if they can be made widely available in multiplex form, i.e. testing for all serious causes of genital ulcers in a single test. PCR testing may also improve the diagnosis of congenital syphilis.

At a more mundane level, improving the availability of low-skill temperature-stable rapid syphilis tests that do not require refrigeration or even electricity could achieve a great deal in resource-poor environments where syphilis is most common. Early experience with immunochromatographic test strips coated with *T. pallidum* antigens that give results in 8 to 20 minutes have been encouraging.

The sequencing of the genome may eventually enable the development of a vaccine, but funding for syphilis research would need to be dramatically increased.

Further reading

British Association for Sexual Health and HIV (2008). *UK national guidelines on the management of syphilis.* www.bashh.org/guidelines

Cates W Jr, Rothenberg RB, Blount JH (1996). Syphilis control: the historical context and epidemiological basis for interrupting sexual transmission of *Treponema pallidum*. *Sex Transm Dis*, **23**, 68–75. [Review of the rationale of syphilis control programmes.]

Centers for Disease Control and Prevention (2010). Sexually transmitted diseases treatment guidelines 2010. *MMWR Recomm Rep*, **59** (RR-12), 26–39.

Centurion-Lara A, *et al.* (2006). Molecular differentiation of *Treponema pallidum* subspecies. *J Clin Microbiol*, **44**, 3377–80. [Evidence of genetic differences between subspecies of *T. pallidum*.]

Chakraborty R, Luck S (2007). Managing congenital syphilis again? The more things change…. *Curr Opin Infect Dis*, **20**, 247–52. [Up-to-date review of the epidemiology and clinical management.]

Chow EPF, *et al.* (2011). HIV and syphilis co-infection increasing among men who have sex with men in China: a systematic review and meta-analysis. *PLoS ONE*, **6**, e22768. [Reviews the emergence of both epidemics in this key population.]

Clark EG, Danbolt N (1964). The Oslo study of the natural course of untreated syphilis: an epidemiologic investigation based on a re-study of the Boeck-Bruusgaard material. *Med Clin North Am*, **48**, 613–23. [An analysis of the first natural history study.]

Drummond F, *et al.* (2010). The intersection between HIV and syphilis in men who have sex with men: some fresh perspectives. *HIV Therapy*, **4**, 661–73. [Reviews recent management debates and highlights potential control strategies.]

Gray RT, *et al.* (2010). Frequent testing of highly sexually active gay men is required to control syphilis. *Sex Transm Dis*, **37**, 298–305. [Models a novel approach to syphilis control.]

Fraser CM, *et al.* (1998). The genome sequence of *Treponema pallidum*, the syphilis spirochete. *Science*, **281**, 375–88. [First publication of the genome.]

Harper KN, *et al.* (2008). On the origin of the treponematoses: a phylogenetic approach. *PLoS Negl Trop Dis*, **2**, e148.

Hart G (1986). Syphilis tests in diagnostic and therapeutic decision making. *Ann Intern Med*, **104**, 368–76. [Reviews the use and limitations of syphilis tests.]

Holmes KK (2006). Azithromycin versus penicillin for early syphilis. *N Engl J Med*, **354**, 205. [Discusses trial data and implications of macrolide resistance by *T. pallidum*.]

Larsen SA, Steiner BM, Rudolf AH (1995). Laboratory diagnosis and interpretation of tests for syphilis. *Clin Microbiol Rev*, **8**, 1–21. [Comprehensive review.]

Lin CC, *et al.* (2006). China's syphilis epidemic: a systematic review of seroprevalence studies. *Sex Transm Dis*, **33**, 726–36. [Summarizes 174 studies that track the re-emergence of syphilis in China.]

Marra CM (2004). Neurosyphilis. *Curr Neurol Neurosci Rep*, **4**, 435–40. [An authoritative review of recent developments in diagnosis and management.]

Parkes R, *et al.* (2004). Review of current evidence and comparison of guidelines for effective syphilis treatment in Europe. *Int J STD AIDS*, **15**, 73–88.

Peeling RW, Ye H (2004). Diagnostic tools for preventing and managing maternal and congenital syphilis: an overview. *Bull World Health Organ*, **82**, 439–46.

Salazar JC, Hazlett KRO, Radolf JD (2002). The immune response to infection with *Treponema pallidum*, the stealth pathogen. *Microbes Infect*, **4**, 1133–40. [Review of recent developments in the pathophysiology and immunology of syphilis.]

Walker GJA (2001). Antibiotics for syphilis diagnosed during pregnancy. *Cochrane Database Syst Rev*, **3**, CD001143.

World Health Organization (2007). *The global elimination of congenital syphilis: rationale and strategy for action.* WHO, Geneva. [Highlights that congenital infection is the major cause of mortality and morbidity of syphilis.]

Zetola NM, Klausner JD (2007). Syphilis and HIV: an update. *Clin Infect Dis*, **44**, 1222–8. [A clinically-focused review.]

6.37 Listeriosis

H. Hof

Essentials

Listeriosis is caused by the Gram-positive bacillus *Listeria monocytogenes*, whose natural habitat is the soil. Consumption of soft cheeses, other dairy products, meat products, seafood, and vegetables is the principal route of infection. Patients at particular risk include those who are immunocompromised, very young, or very old. Pregnant women are also at risk, although they develop only mild disease, but the bacteria can be transmitted to the child either *in utero* or during birth, causing serious systemic disease.

Clinical features and diagnosis—the disease varies from a mild, influenza-like illness to fatal septicaemia and meningoencephalitis. Purulent, localized infections of any organ are sometimes seen. Diagnosis is confirmed by culture from blood, cerebrospinal fluid, or organ biopsies using enrichment and selective media. Immunoassays and nucleic acid amplification techniques are used in specialized laboratories; serology is nonspecific and not helpful.

Treatment, prognosis, and prevention—aside from supportive care, the usual treatment of choice is high-dose intravenous ampicillin combined with an aminoglycoside, which must be administered for at least 2 weeks. The prognosis is poor, with mortality of up to 30%. Prevention depends upon those that are vulnerable avoiding high-risk foods. There is no vaccine.

Introduction

Exposure of humans to *Listeria monocytogenes* is quite frequent, but infections are rare. Only a small proportion of exposed individuals are likely to become ill but for them, despite precise diagnosis and adequate therapy, the prognosis remains poor.

Historical perspective

In the 1920s, *L. monocytogenes* was shown to be capable of inducing systemic infections in experimental animals. About 40 years later, it became obvious that epidemics might occur in humans but it took a further 30 years before listeriosis was shown to be a foodborne disease in most instances. Today, listeria is an exciting research tool for studying the biology of intracellular microorganisms that trigger a cell-mediated immune response.

Aetiology, genetics, pathogenesis, and pathology

Among the various listeria species, *L. monocytogenes* is the major pathogen for humans (as well as for animals). *L. monocytogenes* has specific requirements for invading and surviving and replicating in host cells. Surface proteins such as internalins are critical for the adhesion to specific receptors on host cells. A pathogenicity island on the chromosome encoding for haemolysin (listeriolysin), phospholipases, and an actin polymerizing protein is crucial for intracellular survival, traffic in the cytoplasm, and cell-to-cell spread. By this means, listeria can cross anatomical barriers such as the intestinal mucosa, the blood–brain barrier, and the placenta. Humoral defence mechanisms are largely ineffective in coping with these bacteria. Rather, a cell-mediated immune response is required to overcome a listeria infection. Eventually, granulomas develop in infected organs, indicating a vigorous immune response. During the acute stage, when a massive multiplication of bacteria takes place intracellularly as well as extracellularly, a purulent inflammatory reaction is seen at the site of infection.

Epidemiology

Listeria species are widespread in nature and their natural habitat is the soil; they have been isolated from dust, food products, animal feed, water, sewage, and numerous animals. Infections of humans are mainly due to only a few special clones. Various food items of both plant and animal origin, contaminated either during growth or during processing, can give rise to an infection. Consumption of soft cheeses such as Brie, Camembert, and blue-vein types, other dairy products, meat products (e.g. sausages and delicatessen meat), seafood, and vegetables is the principal route of infection. However, tomatoes, apples, and carrots are practically free of listeria. The ability of listeria to multiply at temperatures from 0 to 40°C is of particular concern if infected foods are stored in the refrigerator and consumed without further cooking.

A study of foodborne illness in the United States of America between 2000 and 2008 estimated an annual incidence of 1600 cases of listeriosis, with a 16% mortality. In 2009 the estimated incidence of laboratory-confirmed listeriosis was 0.34 per 100 000 population. An increase in listeriosis has also been reported in several European countries, and decreased salt concentrations in prepared foods have been proposed as a possible cause. Transmission from infected animals to humans is unusual, but occupational infections in veterinary surgeons or farm workers are reported. Human-to-human transmission occurs only during pregnancy, when the bacteria colonizing the mother infect the fetus *in utero* or the neonate in the birth canal. In most cases disease occurs sporadically, but small epidemics are occasionally observed due to commercially distributed, highly contaminated food items. Predisposing conditions include glucocorticoid therapy, haematological or solid organ tumours, organ transplantation (especially renal), HIV infection, diabetes mellitus, endstage renal disease, chronic liver disease, collagen vascular diseases, and iron overload. Hospital-acquired listeriosis has been reported and has been associated with consumption of contaminated food. Nosocomial transmission between neonates has been associated with poor hand hygiene, close contact between infected patients and their mothers, skin care products, and instruments such as rectal thermometers or stethoscopes.

Prevention

A vaccine against *L. monocytogenes* has not yet been developed. Most infections are food-borne; food items are contaminated either intrinsically or during storage in the refrigerator. Foods such as salads should be avoided by people at special risk, and they should also not eat some preprepared food items unless they are thoroughly reheated to piping hot temperatures. Food items that commonly carry listeria, such as salads and mushrooms, should be kept separately in the refrigerator from those likely to be free of these bacteria, such as cold meats and other ready-to-eat food, otherwise there will be cross-contamination.

Improvement in the microbiological safety of food production processes and the continued education of the public will further reduce the risk of infection.

Inactivation of *L. monocytogenes* by radiation is readily achieved without changing the appearance or taste of foods. A combination of ultrasound treatment and rinsing of food stuff with 2% organic acids for 5 min is also able to reduce the contamination with these pathogens.

Clinical features

Listeriosis is generally an opportunistic infection of elderly people, with men more frequently affected than women. Furthermore immunocompromised patients such as those with haematological or solid organ tumours, organ transplant recipients, patients with severe underlying illness such as diabetes mellitus, endstage renal disease, liver cirrhosis, or iron overload, and pregnant women and newborn babies are at increased risk. Occasionally people without these risk factors can be infected, too. In a few cases, a mild gastroenteritis precedes the systemic infection. The clinical presentation varies from a mild influenza-like illness to fatal septicaemia and meningoencephalitis. Purulent localized infections of any organ occasionally occur.

Recognized syndromes include maternofetal and neonatal listeriosis, septicaemia, meningoencephalitis, cerebritis, gastroenteritis, and localized infections. Outbreaks of gastroenteritis with fever, diarrhoea, nausea, vomiting, and arthromyalgia have been described in immunocompetent adults who have ingested contaminated food. The diagnosis is usually missed because diarrhoeal stools are not cultured selectively for listeria.

Septicaemia occurs mainly in adult patients with malignancies, in transplant recipients, and in immunosuppressed and elderly people. Most present with fever, hypotension, and shock. Many patients also develop meningitis. Meningitis may start abruptly but, in adults, can also develop insidiously, with progressive neurological signs especially meningism. Fever may not be marked, particularly in elderly or immunosuppressed people. A purulent reaction is seen in the cerebrospinal fluid with most of the Gram-positive bacteria lying extracellularly.

Cerebritis in combination with meningitis or separately is increasingly recognized, particularly in immunosuppressed patient. Headache, fever, and varying degrees of paralysis and cerebral disorders such as dizziness or loss of consciousness may be observed. Rhombencephalitis begins with a headache, fever, nausea, and vomiting followed after several days with asymmetrical progressive cranial nerve palsies and decreased consciousness. Infection of the cerebellum may be followed by ataxia and problems of coordination. MRI or CT may show areas of uptake without ring enhancement. Sometimes a brain abscess is diagnosed. In such cases the cerebrospinal fluid may show few, if any, inflammatory cells, and protein and sugar concentrations are normal. Intracerebral foci may be sealed off, so that bacteria or even bacterial DNA are not detected in cerebrospinal fluid or blood, leading to a missed diagnosis.

Localized infections are rare, occurring mainly in immunosuppressed people. They include soft-tissue abscesses, osteomyelitis, septic arthritis, cholecystitis, peritonitis, endocarditis, endophthalmitis, and pneumonia. They usually result from seeding during an initial bacteraemic phase, but focal skin and eye infection can also result from direct occupational exposure.

In maternofetal listeriosis, the mother may develop fever, headache, myalgia, and low back pain due to the bacteraemic phase of the disease. Transplacental infection causes placentitis, amnionitis, and, depending on the time until delivery, spontaneous septic abortion or premature labour with delivery of a severely infected baby.

Neonatal listeriosis of early onset results from intrauterine infection and has a high mortality. The amniotic fluid is greenish and the baby septic and jaundiced, with signs of purulent conjunctivitis, bronchopneumonia, meningitis, and/or encephalitis. Granulomas affect many organs, hence the term 'granulomatosis infantisepticum'. Late-onset disease, developing several days to weeks after birth in a baby who was initially healthy, presents with meningitis. The infection may have been acquired from the mother's genital tract or through cross-infection as a nosocomial infection.

Differential diagnosis

Since various organs may be affected, listeriosis may mimic several quite different local or systemic infectious diseases. The septic manifestations are nonspecific, and particularly in immuno-compromised patients and elderly people one should think of listeriosis. Listeria meningitis develops insidiously in most instances, in contrast to other bacterial disorders. In particular, listeria encephalitis is difficult to recognize initially because it can resemble, for instance, a cerebrovascular accident. This infection should be considered in any patient with an acute brain stem or cerebellar disorder associated with fever, particularly if there are no risk factors for cerebrovascular disease.

Bacteraemia as well as meningitis are accompanied by fever and eventually shock. Encephalitis, which may develop slowly, can be confused in elderly people with cerebrovascular disease or even with brain metastases.

Criteria for diagnosis

Listeria are nonsporing, facultatively anaerobic, Gram-positive rods. Enrichment and selective methods are now well established for the isolation of these nonfastidious bacteria from the environment, food, or human specimen. Blood, cerebrospinal fluid, meconium, amniotic fluid, placental tissue, lochia, and swabs from purulent discharge from various organs can yield the pathogens. Gram-positive rods may be seen in a stained smear. Sometimes they are very short and thus can be mistaken for streptococci. A predominance of monocytes among the inflammatory cells, which might lead to early suspicion of listeria, is not regularly seen. Differentiation of the various species is generally possible by means of commercially available biochemical tests. Several typing methods are used to trace food sources, distinguish relapses from reinfections, and investigate outbreaks. Serovars 1/2a, 1/2b, and 4b are the most prominent among human isolates.

L. monocytogenes is the major pathogen, although occasional human infections with *L. ivanovii* and *L. seeligeri* have been reported. *L. welshimeri*, *L. innocua*, and *L. grayi* are not known to cause disease. The crucial difference is that pathogenic isolates display various virulence factors not present in nonpathogenic ones. In various isolates of *L. monocytogenes*, these properties can be differentially expressed, so that the pathogenicity will vary from strain to strain.

Immunoassays and nucleic acid amplification techniques have also been used in specialized laboratories to detect the bacteria. However, serology is nonspecific and does not aid diagnosis.

Treatment

Practically all strains of *L. monocytogenes* are susceptible to a large range of common antibiotics including ampicillin, gentamicin (which acts synergistically with ampicillin), co-trimoxazole, erythromycin, tetracycline, chloramphenicol, vancomycin, and rifampicin. On the other hand, *L. monocytogenes* is inherently resistant *in vitro* to the cephalosporins and fosfomycin. It is also resistant to nalidixic acid but susceptible to the newer quinolones such as moxifloxacin. It should be borne in mind, however, that many of the bacteria reside intracellularly where they are protected from some of the active antimicrobial agents.

There are no controlled trials of antibiotic treatment for listeriosis. According to clinical experience, high-dose intravenous ampicillin (i.e. 4×2–3 g/day) in combination with gentamicin (360 mg, or in a dose adjusted with the help of serum concentration measurements, once daily in a 60-min infusion) remains the treatment of choice for adults. This combination should be given for 2 weeks at least (it has been questioned, however, whether aminoglycosides really improves the clinical outcome). If necessary, ampicillin alone can be continued for another week or even longer, e.g. in case of endocarditis, until clinical resolution. For children, a daily dose of 200 to 300 mg/kg ampicillin, perhaps combined with 3 to 5 mg/kg gentamicin, is recommended. Gentamicin is best avoided in pregnancy, when ampicillin may be used alone, or erythromycin (2 g/day intravenously for 2–3 weeks) if the patient is allergic to penicillin. Recently, it has been questioned whether the combination is better than ampicillin alone. Intravenous co-trimoxazole (daily dose 20 mg/kg trimethoprim + 100 mg/kg sulfamethoxazole in four divided doses) is the best second-line treatment for meningoencephalitis. This drug can also be considered for oral sequence therapy after an intravenous ampicillin regimen. Since rifampicin is able to attack intracellular bacteria, a combination with this drug (600 mg intravenously daily for 14 days for adults but not for pregnant women or neonates) is theoretically helpful for cure.

It is very important to be aware that treatment with cephalosporins is likely to fail. Since acute pyogenic meningitis is usually treated initially with ceftriaxone or cefotaxime until the pathogen is known, ampicillin should also be given with this initial treatment whenever listeriosis is a clinical possibility, unless a Gram-stained cerebrospinal fluid sample shows good evidence of another bacterial cause. Carbapenems, such as meropenem and imipenem, have excellent *in vitro* activity against *Listeria* spp. Although they have not been approved for the treatment of listeriosis, meropenem is approved for the treatment of bacterial meningitis and has been successfully used to treat listeriosis.

Linezolid is also active against listeria, but clinical experience is limited to case reports.

Prognosis

Despite antibiotic therapy, the mortality of systemic listeriosis remains high at up to 30%. Since listeriosis occurs primarily in immunocompromised patients who lack normal defence mechanisms, relapses may occur if the antibiotic regimen is too short, allowing intracellular bacteria to survive. Such endogenous relapses are not attributable to resistant bacteria and so the same regimen can be applied for a second round. Sequelae may be serious.

Food industry

Today, the Hazard Analysis and Critical Control Points (HACCP) management system is now standard in the food industry in Western countries. Once it becomes clear that a working plant is permanently colonized with pathogenic listeria, laborious and expensive intervention and management procedures are necessary. When listeria are detected during screening of food items, the production company must withdraw the affected batches from the market.

Areas of uncertainty or controversy

So far, the infective dose required for induction of overt disease has not been defined. It may depend on cofactors such as concomitant enteric pathogens and in particular on the immune status of the host. Since so many foodstuffs are contaminated, it is practically impossible to guarantee in everyday life that all dishes are free from listeria. Some authorities therefore tolerate certain numbers of bacteria. However, zero tolerance is appropriate for food prepared for babies or sick people. An exact definition of the incubation period is not yet possible. After ingestion of a high inoculum, symptoms appear within a few hours, but it is likely that in some cases days may elapse before invasion occurs.

Likely developments in the near future

At least two different genetic lineages of *L. monocytogenes* isolates have been described in food items or in listeriosis cases. It is a matter of discussion whether this distinction might allow the health risk of contaminated food items to be evaluated.

Although the therapeutic value of moxifloxacin has not yet been assessed in human listeriosis, it can be deduced from cell culture experiments as well as from animal experiments that this quinolone, which is highly active *in vitro*, is able to penetrate into host cells and effectively kill intracellular *L. monocytogenes*, so that rapid cure may be achieved.

Further reading

Gellin BG, Broome CV (1989). Listeriosis. *JAMA*, **261**, 1313–18.

Hamon M, Bierne H, Cossart P (2006). *Listeria monocytogenes*: a multifaceted model. *Nat Rev Microbiol*, **4**, 423–34.

Hof H, Nichterlein T, Kretschmar M (1997). Management of listeriosis. *Clin Microbiol Rev*, **10**, 345–57.

Hof H, Lampidis R (2001). Retrospective evidence for nosocomial Listeria infection. *J Hosp Infect*, **48**, 321–2.

Lamont RF, et al. (2011). Listeriosis in human pregnancy: a systematic review. *J Perinat Med*, **39**, 227–36.

Liu D (2006). Identification, subtyping and virulence determination of *Listeria monocytogenes*, an important foodborne pathogen. *J Med Microbiol*, **55**, 645–59.

Mitjà O, et al. (2009). Predictors of mortality and impact of aminoglycosides on outcome in listeriosis in a retrospective cohort study. *J Antimicrob Chemother*, **64**, 416–23.

Nudelman Y, Tunkel AR (2009). Bacterial menigitis: epidemiology, pathogenesis and management update. *Drugs*, **69**, 2577–96.

Schlech WF (2000). Foodborne listeriosis. *Clin Infect Dis*, **31**, 770–5.

6.38 Legionellosis and legionnaires' disease

J.T. Macfarlane and T.C. Boswell

Essentials

Legionellaceae are Gram-negative bacilli, of which *Legionella pneumophila* is the principal cause of human infections. Their natural habitats are freshwater streams, lakes, thermal springs, moist soil and mud, but the principal source for large outbreaks of legionellosis is cooling systems used for air conditioning and other cooling equipment, with infection transmitted by contaminated water aerosols. Middle-aged men, smokers, regular alcohol drinkers, and those with comorbidity are most at risk.

Clinical features and diagnosis—(1) Legionnaires' disease (pneumonia)—typically presents with high fever, shivers, headache, and muscle pains; respiratory symptoms are sometimes minimal; confusion and diarrhoea may dominate the clinical picture. (2) 'Pontiac fever'—an acute nonpneumonic form that presents as a self-limiting, influenza-like illness. Detection of urinary antigen has become the mainstay for diagnosis.

Treatment, prognosis and prevention—aside from supportive care, the first choice antibiotics are macrolides (e.g. erythromycin, clarithromycin) and/or fluoroquinolones (especially levofloxacin). Case fatality is 5 to 15% in previously well adults, but much higher in those who are immunocompromised or develop respiratory failure. Prevention is by the correct design, maintenance, and monitoring of water systems. Notification of a case allows a public health investigation into the likely source and the detection, prompt treatment, and/or prevention of additional cases.

Introduction and historical perspective

In 1976, an outbreak of pneumonia affected 221 and killed 34 members of the American Legion who had attended a convention in a Philadelphia hotel. A newly identified organism, *Legionella pneumophila*, was discovered and named after the outbreak. Since then many different species of the family Legionellaceae have been discovered. Clinical illness is referred to as legionellosis, and there are two principal syndromes: legionnaires' disease (pneumonia) and Pontiac fever (a self-limiting influenza-like illness).

Aetiology and pathology

The organism

The Legionellaceae are aerobic nonsporing Gram-negative bacilli whose cell walls contain distinctive branched-chain fatty acids and lipo-oligosaccharide (LOS). They do not grow on routine media; specialized media such as buffered charcoal yeast extract (BCYE) are required for growth.

Of the 50 formally recognized *Legionella* species, *L. pneumophila* is the principal cause of human infections. Of the 70 or more serogroups (SG) of *L. pneumophila*, serogroups 1, 4, and 6 are the ones most frequently isolated in human infection. There are 17 species other than *L. pneumophila* that have been implicated in human infections; these include *L. micdadei*, *L. bozemanii*, *L. dumoffi*, and *L. longbeachae*.

Pathology

Legionellae are intracellular pathogens that are found within protozoa in the environment and in alveolar macrophages in humans. Following inhalation of contaminated aerosol droplets, legionellae reach the alveoli where they are internalized in macrophage endosomes. They block the development of the endosome into a phagolysosome, preventing the normal cellular bacterial killing mechanism through the action of an important virulence factor, the macrophage infectivity potentiator (mip) protein.

The lungs are the principal organ affected and show a severe inflammatory response. The alveoli and terminal bronchioles are distended by fibrin-rich debris, mononuclear inflammatory cells, and neutrophils. Organisms can be demonstrated within alveolar spaces by silver or immunofluorescence stains. In survivors, alveolar and interstitial fibrosis can result.

Epidemiology

The natural worldwide habitats of legionellae are freshwater streams, lakes, thermal springs, moist soil, and mud, where they are found in small numbers. They usually live and multiply within amoebae and other protozoa where they are protected from adverse condition and can survive and disseminate widely.

By contrast, in artificially constructed water systems, legionellae can multiply to extremely high numbers, encouraged by favourable temperatures (20–45°C) and water stagnation. As legionellae are associated with amoebae within the biofilm, complete eradication is difficult once systems are colonized.

The principal source for large outbreaks of legionellosis is wet (or evaporative) cooling systems (cooling towers) used for air conditioning and other cooling equipment. Cooling towers are commonly seen on the outside walls or roofs of buildings such as hotels, office blocks, hospitals, and factories. If poorly maintained, they can become heavily contaminated with legionellae leading to the emission of an infectious aerosol of legionella-containing droplets. Such aerosols can drift 500 m or more, depending on the position of the cooling tower and the climatic conditions.

Within buildings, legionellae commonly multiply in cold-water storage tanks, hot-water calorifiers, and in the hot and cold water distribution pipework, particularly if long and complicated runs of pipework lead to a loss of temperature control, or water stagnation ('dead-legs'). Contaminated aerosols are most commonly disseminated by showers, but other well-recognized sources include:

♦ whirlpool spas and other warm-water baths

♦ decorative fountains

♦ respiratory therapy equipment rinsed or topped up with contaminated tap water

♦ automatic car washes

♦ potting compost (for *L. longbeachae* SG1 in Australia).

In temperate countries, legionellosis is seasonal with most cases occurring in the summer and autumn. The same number are related to travel (either within the same country or more commonly abroad) as are acquired locally. A history of recent travel can be an important pointer to legionella infection. Locally acquired legionellosis is increasingly recognized as being domestically acquired.

Legionnaires' disease accounts for 2 to 9% of cases of community-acquired pneumonia. An increase in incidence of legionnaires' disease has been noted in the United States of America and the United Kingdom; this may be related to improvement diagnosis and reporting, but environmental influences such as increased rainfall and flooding have also been suggested.

Hospital-acquired legionellosis is uncommon, but occurs when hospital water supplies are contaminated with the organisms. Nosocomial infection may involve less pathogenic legionella strains affecting a highly susceptible or immunosuppressed patient population in small clusters.

Prevention

Several primary preventive measures can be taken to minimize the risks of acquiring legionellosis from water systems. Cooling towers must be registered with local authorities and regularly maintained, using biocide treatment to inhibit legionella growth; sampling for the presence of legionellae within the recirculating water must be carried out regularly. Hot and cold water systems must be adequately designed and maintained to minimize legionella growth, either through temperature control or use of chemicals, ozonation, or point-of-use filtration. In health care facilities, a balance needs to be struck between adequate water temperature at outlets and risks of scalding. Outlets that are not in regular use should be regularly flushed through to avoid water stagnation.

Although legionellosis is not a formally notifiable disease, even single cases should be reported to public health authorities for investigation of possible environmental sources. Continuing surveillance of legionellosis is important at local, national, and international levels. By collating data, coordinated European surveillance systems have been able to pinpoint outbreaks of legionnaires' disease associated with a particular holiday resort or hotel.

Clinical features

Legionella pneumonia

Legionella infection tends to lead to moderate or severe illness usually requiring hospital admission within 5 to 7 days. It causes 2 to 9% of cases of community-acquired pneumonia admitted to hospital (but with wide geographical and seasonal variation) and is the second commonest community-acquired pneumonia requiring intensive care.

The incubation period is usually 2 to 10 days. Men are 2 to 3 times more frequently affected than women. Infection in children and elderly people is unusual and the highest incidence is in 40- to 70-year-old people, with a mean age of 53 years. People particularly at risk include cigarette smokers, alcoholics, diabetics, and those with chronic illness or who are receiving corticosteroids or immunosuppressive therapy.

Clinical features

Typically, the illness starts fairly abruptly and progresses quickly with high fever, shivers, bad headache, and muscle pains. Respiratory symptoms such as cough and breathlessness can sometimes be minimal, with confusion and diarrhoea dominating the clinical picture, masking the true diagnosis of pneumonia. The patient commonly looks ill, with a high fever over 39°C, signs of pneumonia, and confusion (in one-half of patients).

Differential diagnosis

Table 6.38.1 compares features of *Legionella* pneumonia with other types of community-acquired pneumonia. No unique pattern allows the early clinical differentiation of *Legionella* infection from other, more common, causes of pneumonia. Important clues include epidemiological pointers (e.g. recent foreign travel or a local epidemic), high fever, confusion, multisystem involvement, absence of a predominant bacterial pathogen on sputum examination, and lack of response to β-lactam antibiotics.

Clinical investigation

The total white cell count is usually only moderately raised (to 15×10^9/litre), often with a lymphopenia. Hyponatraemia, hypoalbuminaemia, and abnormal liver function tests are detected in more than one-half of the cases (Table 6.38.1). Other nonspecific features may include raised blood urea and muscle enzymes, very high C-reactive protein, hypoxaemia, haematuria, and proteinuria. Gram's staining of sputum typically shows few pus cells and no predominant pathogen. Initial blood and sputum cultures are negative.

Radiographic features

Radiographic shadowing is usually homogeneous. Characteristically, radiographic deterioration occurs within the same or opposite lung (Fig. 6.38.1). Radiographic improvement is particularly slow. Only two-thirds of radiographs clear within 3 months and some take more than 6 months.

Prognosis and complications

A wide variety of complications have been reported, the most important being acute respiratory failure requiring assisted ventilation which occurs in up to 20% of patients. In addition to confusion, various neurological complications have been reported, leading to the suggestion of a neurotoxin. Acute but usually reversible renal failure may be seen in severe disease. Clinical recovery appears to be very slow in some patients, particularly of symptoms such as tiredness, weakness, breathlessness, memory and concentration impairment, and psychological sequelae. This can have medicolegal implications in those infected through negligent exposure to poorly maintained water systems.

Pontiac fever

This is the acute nonpneumonic form of *Legionella* infection that presents as an influenza-like illness. The attack rate is extremely high, with an incubation period of usually 36 to 48 h. Investigations and chest radiograph are normal, and the illness improves spontaneously, usually within 5 days.

Laboratory diagnosis

A variety of laboratory methods can be used to diagnose *Legionella* infection. In order of usefulness, they are:

1 Antigen detection:
  a Urinary antigen detection
  b Direct immunofluorescence
2 Culture
3 Serology
4 Molecular methods (e.g. polymerase chain reaction (PCR))

Urine is a readily available clinical sample. Diagnosis by urinary antigen detection has now become the mainstay of diagnosis in many centres, usually becoming positive at an early stage of infection and remaining positive for several weeks. Several well-validated commercial enzyme immunoassays and an immunochromatography test are available with excellent specificity and good sensitivity. Immunochromatography can give results in as little as 15 min. It is recommended that legionella urine antigen tests are performed for all patients with severe community-onset pneumonia. Their principal drawback is that only *L. pneumophila* SG1 infection is detected. This is an important limitation, particularly in immunocompromised patients in whom every effort should be made to obtain a positive culture. A negative urine antigen test does not exclude *Legionella* infection and the test should be repeated as clinically indicated.

Direct immunofluorescence with a monoclonal antibody specific for *L. pneumophila* can be used to detect bacteria in suitable respiratory specimens. This technique can provide a diagnosis early in the course of the infection, but is relatively time consuming and relies on the availability of a good respiratory tract sample (e.g. bronchoalveolar lavage (BAL) fluid).

Legionellae can be cultured from suitable respiratory samples (e.g. sputum, endotracheal aspirates, and BAL fluid) using appropriately enriched and permissive agar such as BCYE, supplemented with polymixin, anisomycin, vancomycin, and dyes. The presence of dyes makes identification of different species easier. Culture is diagnostic of infection, as colonization without infection has not been demonstrated, but it is time consuming, expensive, slow (culture can take up to 10 days), and relatively insensitive (especially once legionella active antibiotic therapy has been started). Culture does allow detection of species and serogroups other than *L. pneumophila* SG1, and comparison with isolates from suspected environmental sources. Such speciation and typing, using well-validated methods such as a DNA sequence-based typing scheme, is normally done in reference laboratories.

Table 6.38.1 Comparative clinical, laboratory, and radiological features of patients with community-acquired legionella, pneumococcal, staphylococcal, and mycoplasma pneumonia. Values are percentages unless otherwise stated

Feature	Pathogen			
	Legionella	Pneumococcal	Staphylococcal	Mycoplasma
Number of patients with data available	79	83	61	62
Patient				
Mean age (years)	53	52	47	34
Men	63	71	57	53
Comorbid disease	35	59	49	19
Symptoms				
Duration of symptoms before hospital referral (days)	7	5	14	13
Urinary tract infection symptoms	14	21	41	40
Productive cough	41	69	86	73
Pleural pain	36	72	56	38
Haemoptysis	14	16	37	3
Headache	27	56	31	26
Confusion	35	17	22	2
Rigors	14	62	7	40
Signs				
Altered mental state	43	25	22	2
Fever >39°C	72	25	43	15
Laboratory				
White cell count >15×10^9/litre	14	60	?	13
Serum sodium <130/dl	55	23	21	5
Blood urea >7 mmol/litre	60	55	52	16
Abnormal liver function tests	59	34	55	16
Radiographic features				
Number of patients with data available	49	91	26	46
Homogeneous consolidation	82	74	60	50
Multilobe involvement	39	39	59	52
Pleural fluid	24	34	32	20
Cavitation	2	4	26	0
Deterioration and spread of shadowing after admission	65	32	64	25

Data adapted from various references including: Macfarlane JT, *et al.* (1984). Comparative radiographic features of community acquired legionnaires' disease, pneumococcal pneumonia, mycoplasma pneumonia, and psittacosis. *Thorax*, **39**, 28–33; Woodhead MA, Macfarlane JT (1987). Comparative clinical and laboratory features of legionella with pneumococcal and mycoplasma pneumonias. *Br J Dis Chest*, **81**, 133–9; Macfarlane JT, Rose D (1996). Radiographic features of staphylococcal pneumonia in adults and children. *Thorax*, **51**, 539–40; Woodhead MA, Macfarlane JT (1987). Adult community acquired staphylococcal pneumonia in the antibiotic era: a review of 61 cases. *QJM*, **245**, 783–90.

In the past, serology (i.e. the detection of an antibody response to *Legionella*) was the mainstay of diagnosis, and this is still of value. Properly evaluated serological assays (especially those with sufficient specificity) are based on detecting antibodies to *L. pneumophila* SG1. Antibody responses can be delayed or absent in some patients, but about 40% of patients admitted to hospital will have raised antibodies on admission. A confirmed serological diagnosis involves demonstrating a fourfold or greater rise in antibody titre to 1:128 or more in suitably timed paired sera. A single high titre is suggestive but not confirmatory of infection. False-positive results can occur in some patients with recent campylobacter infection. In these cases, serology should be repeated in the presence of a campylobacter blocking fluid. Furthermore, single elevated antibody titres of 1:256 or more have been detected in 1 to 16% of healthy adults.

The detection of species and subtype-specific *Legionella* DNA in clinical samples by PCR is available in reference laboratories and offers good sensitivity. However, the lack of commercially available assays limits widespread diagnostic value.

Treatment

There are no randomized controlled trials of antibiotic therapy for legionellosis and evaluation of agents has been based on relatively

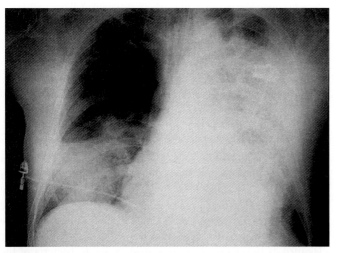

Fig. 6.38.1 Chest radiograph of a 58-year-old man who returned from a Mediterranean hotel holiday with legionella pneumonia. There is extensive, bilateral, homogeneous consolidation. He required assisted ventilation for worsening respiratory failure.

small case studies as well as *in vitro* and animal experiments. Macrolides (erythromycin and more recently clarithromycin) have for many years been regarded as the antibiotics of first choice, mainly based on clinical experience and retrospective analysis of outcome data. One of the key factors is the ability of an antibiotic to reach therapeutic concentrations within alveolar macrophages where the legionella bacteria multiplies. There have been increasing reports of the successful use of fluoroquinolone antibiotics, notably levofloxacin, and even some suggestion that, when combined with early diagnosis using urine antigen detection, they can reduce mortality and morbidity compared to traditional macrolide therapy. Fluoroquinolones demonstrate excellent bioavailability, bactericidal activity against legionellae, and very good intracellular penetration.

For nonsevere community-acquired legionella infection, our practice is to use an oral fluoroquinolone, with a macrolide as an alternative.

For the management of severe or life-threatening legionella pneumonia, we consider the use of a combination of antibiotics including a fluoroquinolone and a macrolide, especially during the crucial first few days, with rifampicin as an alternative if one of these agents cannot be used. Clinicians should be alert to the potential small risk of prolongation of the QT interval on the ECG with the recommended combination, particularly in the presence of other proarrhythmic risk factors. Parenteral rifampicin has a risk of hyperbilirubinaemia, which usually resolves on stopping the drug. There are also reports that the azalide antibiotic azithromycin and tetracyclines (e.g. doxycycline) may be useful.

Prognosis

The patient's previous health and appropriate early therapy are the two most important factors determining outcome. Mortality in previously fit patients is 5 to 15%. It is lower when early diagnosis by urine antigen detection allows prompt treatment. The mortality is approximately 30% in those requiring assisted ventilation, but in immunosuppressed individuals it can approach 75%.

Areas of uncertainty

Three main areas of uncertainty are the pathophysiology of multisystem involvement, (particularly of neuropsychological symptoms), optimal antibiotic management, and the long-term prognosis.

Likely future developments

Advances in bedside urine antigen testing create the possibility of early diagnosis and properly controlled trials of antibiotic therapy, together with controlled follow-up studies to assess long-term sequelae. Near-source rapid testing of water may enhance surveillance of water systems and outbreak investigations, especially if there is progress in detecting species other than *L. pneumophila* SG1.

Further reading

Blazquez Garrido RM, Parra FJE *et al.* (2005). Antimicrobial chemotherapy for legionnaires' disease: Levofloxacin versus Macrolides. *Clinical Infectious Diseases*, **40**, 800–6.

British Thoracic Society (2009). Guidelines for the management of community acquired pneumonia in adults: update 2009. *Thorax*, **64** Suppl III, iii1–55.

Cunha BA (1998). Clinical features of legionnaires' disease. *Semin Respir Infect*, **13**, 116–27.

Den Boer JW, Nijhof J, Friesema I (2006). Risk factors for sporadic community acquired legionnaires' disease. A 3-year national case-controlled study. *Public Health*, **120**, 566–71.

Greenberg D, *et al.* (2006). Problem pathogens: paediatric legionellosis—implications for improved diagnosis. *Lancet Infect Dis*, **6**, 529–35.

Health and Safety Commission (2000). Legionnaires' disease: the control of legionella bacteria in water systems. Approved code of practice and guidance L8. HSE Books, Sudbury, UK.

Lee JV, Joseph C (2002). Guidelines for investigating single cases of legionnaires' disease. *Commun Dis Public Health*, **5**, 157–62.

Lettinga KD, *et al.* (2002). Legionnaires' disease at a Dutch flower show: prognostic factors and impact of therapy. *Emerg Infect Dis*, **8**, 1448–54.

Macfarlane JT, *et al.* (1984). Comparative radiographic features of community acquired legionnaires' disease, pneumococcal pneumonia, mycoplasma pneumonia, and psittacosis. *Thorax*, **39**, 28–33.

Owens RC, Nolin TD (2006). Antimicrobial associated QT interval prolongation: points of interest. *Clin Infect Dis*, **43**, 1603–11.

Pedro-Botet L, Yu VL (2006). Legionella: macrolides or quinolones. *Clin Microbiol Infect*, **12** Suppl 3, 25–30.

Woodhead MA, Macfarlane JT (1985). The protean manifestations of legionnaires' disease. *J R Coll Physicians Lond*, **19**, 224–30.

Woodhead MA, Macfarlane JT (1987). Comparative clinical and laboratory features of legionella with pneumococcal and mycoplasma pneumonias. *Br J Dis Chest*, **81**, 133–9.

6.39 Rickettsioses

Philippe Parola and Didier Raoult

Essentials

Rickettsioses are zoonoses caused by obligate Gram-negative intracellular bacteria of the order Rickettsiales, comprising (1) rickettsioses due to bacteria of the genus *Rickettsia*, including spotted fever groups and typhus groups (Rickettsiaceae), (2) ehrlichioses and anaplasmoses due to bacteria of the Anaplasmataceae, and (3) scrub typhus due to *Orientia tsutsugamushi* (see Chapter 6.40).

Epidemiology, clinical features, and prognosis of particular rickettsioses

Tick-borne spotted fever group—20 species or subspecies of spotted fever group rickettsiae can infect humans following transmission from their natural vertebrate hosts by ixodid (hard) ticks, with many species having particular geographical restriction. Presentation is typically with fever, headache, muscle pain, rash, local lymphadenopathy, and—for some diseases—a typical inoculation eschar (the 'tache noire') at the tick bite site. These signs vary depending on the rickettsia involved and may allow distinction between different rickettsioses occurring at the same location. Diseases range in severity from mild to severe.

Murine (endemic) typhus—caused by *Rickettsia typhi*, whose natural host is rodents, between whom it is spread by the rat flea. Human infection usually results from contamination of disrupted skin or inhalation of flea faeces containing the organism. Disease is generally mild and self-limiting with non-specific features: less than 15% of cases present with the 'classic' triad of fever, headache, and rash.

Epidemic typhus—caused by *R. prowazekii*, for whom humans are the major (if not only) host, and transmitted by body lice, hence the disease is a particular problem during times of war, conflict, famine, and natural catastrophes. The most recent outbreak, the largest since the Second World War, occurred during the civil war in Burundi in the 1990s. Following a nonspecific prodrome, presentation is with fever, headache, myalgia and a wide range of other symptoms. Most patients develop a macular, maculopapular, or petechial rash. Mortality ranges from 4% (recent series) to 60% (without antibiotics).

Other rickettsioses—include (1) flea-borne spotted fever—cat flea typhus; (2) rickettsialpox—transmitted from mice by house mouse mites.

Diagnosis and treatment of rickettsioses

Diagnosis is by direct evidence of infection by culture or polymerase chain reaction (PCR), or by serological testing. Aside from supportive care, doxycycline remains the drug of choice for immediate empirical treatment of all rickettsioses on clinical suspicion, with many of these infections having high mortality if untreated.

Human ehrlichioses and anaplasmosis

These diseases are tick-borne zoonoses, whose causative agents are maintained through enzootic cycles between ticks and animals. Three species cause human diseases: (1) *Ehrlichia chaffeensis*—causes human monocytic ehrlichiosis; (2) *Anaplasma phagocytophilum*—causes human anaplasmosis; and (3) *E. ewingii*—causes granulocytic ehrlichiosis. These all present as undifferentiated seasonal febrile illnesses, ranging in severity from mild to severe, with multisystem organ failure. Diagnosis is by direct evidence of infection by culture or PCR, or (most commonly) by serological testing. Doxycycline is the antibiotic of choice.

Prevention

Prevention of rickettsioses in general is by (1) avoiding arthropod bites—by applying topical *N,N*-diethyl-*m*-toluamide (DEET) repellent to exposed skin, and treatment of clothing with permethrin; and (2) those staying in infested areas checking their bodies routinely for the presence of arthropods, and promptly removing ticks. In addition, (3) epidemic typhus—louse eradication is the most important preventive measure. No vaccines are available.

Introduction

Rickettsioses are zoonoses caused by obligate intracellular bacteria of the order Rickettsiales. These short Gram-negative rods retain basic fuchsin when stained by Gimenez's method. Their taxonomy has been radically reorganized in recent years. *Coxiella burnetii*, the cause of Q fever (Chapter 6.41), has been removed from the Rickettsiales. Currently, three groups of diseases are commonly classified as rickettsioses: (1) rickettsioses due to bacteria of the genus *Rickettsia*, including the spotted fever group (SFG) and the typhus group (Rickettsiaceae), (2) ehrlichioses and anaplasmoses due to bacteria of the Anaplasmataceae, and (3) scrub typhus due to *Orientia tsutsugamushi* (Chapter 6.40). Rickettsioses, ehrlichioses, and anaplasmoses are zoonoses associated with arthropods, including ticks, fleas, and mites, which have been implicated as their vectors, reservoirs, or amplifiers.

Rickettsioses (human infections attributable to *Rickettsia* spp.)

Bacteriology

Rickettsiae are 0.3 to 0.5 by 0.8 to 2.0 μm in size. Their cytoplasm contains ribosomes and strands of DNA, limited by a typical Gram-negative trilamellar structure consisting of a bilayer inner membrane, a peptidoglycan layer, and a bilayer outer membrane. Within host cells they are surrounded by an electron-lucent slime layer. The two main groups are the SFG and the typhus group. SFG rickettsiae are mainly associated with ticks, but also with fleas (*Rickettsia felis*) and mites (*R. akari*). Their optimal growth temperature is 32°C, their G+C content is 32 to 33, and they can polymerize actin and thus move into the nuclei of host cells causing spotted fevers in humans. Typhus group rickettsiae are associated with human body lice (*R. prowazekii*) or fleas (*R. typhi*), have an optimal growth temperature of 35°C and a G+C content of 29. They do not enter host cell nuclei but are confined to host cell cytoplasm, causing typhus in humans. Rickettsiae are rapidly inactivated at 56°C. They grow in eukaryotic cells where they live freely and divide by binary fission in the cytoplasm. They must be grown in tissue culture (L929 or Vero cells) or in yolk sacs of developing chicken embryos. Growth in cell monolayers is shown by plaque formation, representing disruption of massively infected cells. SFG rickettsiae form plaques of 2 to 3 mm diameter after 5 to 8 days, whereas typhus group rickettsiae form plaques 1 mm in diameter after 8 to 10 days. The major rickettsial antigens are lipopolysaccharides, lipoproteins, outer membrane proteins of the surface cell antigen (SCA) family, and heat shock proteins. Other antigens include a 17-kDa lipoprotein, and autotransporter family SCA proteins include the 120-kDa S-layer protein (OmpB or Sca5), OmpA (SGF only), and Sca4. Fourteen genes that may encode SCA proteins have been identified in sequenced rickettsial genomes, of which *sca1* is present in all species.

Taxonomy and genomics

Traditional bacteriological identification methods cannot be applied to rickettsiae because they are strictly intracellular. Immunofluorescence serotyping was used but has now been replaced by molecular methods. Genetic guidelines have been proposed for classifying rickettsial isolates at genus, group, and species levels using the sequences of five rickettsial genes, including 16S rRNA (*rrs*), *gltA*, *ompA*, *ompB*. This was validated using 20 uncontested *Rickettsia* spp. identified by serotyping with mouse antisera. Rules have also been proposed for creation of subspecies of rickettsiae that are genetically homogeneous but have distinct genotypic, serotypic, epidemiological, and clinical characteristics. The naming of rickettsiae detected or isolated from patients or arthropods in recent years has also been clarified. Variable intergenic spacers have been identified as the most suitable sequences for genotyping rickettsial strains. In 2001, the first genome of a tick-transmitted rickettsia (*R. conorii* strain Seven) was fully sequenced, revealing several characteristics that are unique among bacterial genomes, including long, irregularly distributed, palindromic repeat fragments. Comparison of their genomes suggests that *R. prowazekii* is a subset of *R. conorii*. The genomes of *R. felis*, *R. typhi*, and *R. bellii* have also been sequenced. These genomic data may provide insights into the mechanism of rickettsial pathogenicity and new tools for diagnostic, phylogenetic, and taxonomic studies.

Pathophysiology

When transmitted to a susceptible human host, pathogenic tick-borne SFG rickettsiae localize and multiply in endothelial cells of small to medium-sized blood vessels, causing a vasculitis which is responsible for the clinical and laboratory abnormalities that occur in tick-borne rickettsioses. Molecular characteristics and expression of particular rickettsial gene products probably contribute to differences in pathogenicity among species of SFG rickettsiae. Expression of OmpA allows adhesion to and entry into host endothelial cells. OmpB and new adhesins also contribute to adherence and invasion. After phagocytosis and internalization, the phagocytic vacuole is rapidly lysed and rickettsiae escape phagocytic digestion to multiply freely in the host's cytoplasm and nucleus (SFG species). Rickettsiae can move between cells by actin mobilization. A gene encoding a phospholipase D may be a key virulence factor. RickA, an *R. conorii* surface protein, activates the Arp2/3 complex *in vitro*, which is essential for actin polymerization.

Tick-borne SFG rickettsioses

Epidemiology

Ixodid (hard) ticks were first implicated as vectors of SFG rickettsioses in 1906, when the Rocky Mountain wood tick (*Dermacentor andersoni*) was shown to transmit *R. rickettsii*, the agent of Rocky Mountain spotted fever in the United States of America. In the 1930s, the role of the brown dog tick (*Rhipicephalus sanguineus*) in transmitting *R. conorii*, the causative agent of Mediterranean spotted fever, was described. However, between 1984 and 2008 at least 13 additional rickettsial species or subspecies causing tick-borne rickettsioses around the world were identified. Nine of these agents were initially isolated from ticks, often years or decades before a definitive association with human disease was established. Keys to the epidemiology of tick-borne diseases are the ecological characteristics of their tick vectors. For example, *Rhipicephalus sanguineus*, which is the vector of *R. conorii*, lives with dogs and has a low affinity for

people. However, the human affinity of *Rh. sanguineus* is increased in warmer temperatures. Cases of Mediterranean spotted fever are sporadic and occur mostly in urban endemic areas. In contrast, *Amblyomma hebraeum*, the vector of *R. africae* in southern Africa, actively attack animals and people that enter their biotopes. Numerous ticks can attack several hosts simultaneously, which explains why African tick-bite fever often occurs in groups of people entering the bush together.

However, the life cycles of most tick-borne rickettsiae are poorly understood. In their natural vertebrate hosts, infection may result in a rickettsaemia that allows noninfected ticks to become infected and for the natural cycle to be perpetuated. Ticks may also acquire rickettsiae through transovarial passage. Because ixodid ticks feed only once at each life stage, the rickettsiae acquired can only be transmitted to another host when the tick has moulted to its next developmental stage (trans-stadial passage) and takes its next blood meal. When rickettsiae are efficiently transmitted both trans-stadially and transovarially, the tick serves as a reservoir and the distribution of the rickettsiosis and its tick host will be identical. This has been demonstrated for only for some tick-borne rickettsiae. However, transmission of *R. rickettsii* by *Dermacentor andersoni* diminishes the ticks' survival and reproductive capacity of their filial progenies. *R. rickettsii* has been shown to be lethal for the majority of experimentally and transovarially infected *Dermacentor andersoni*. Similarly deleterious effects have been reported in *Rhipicephalus sanguineus* group ticks experimentally infected by *R. conorii conorii*. This has been suggested as a potential reason to explain a low prevalence of *Rh. sanguineus* infected with *R. conorii* in nature (usually <1%). However, naturally infected colonies of ticks have been maintained in laboratory conditions over several generations. External factors such as temperature may have an essential role in the survival of *Rh. sanguineus* naturally infected with *R.conorii* compared with uninfected, in liaison with the long-recognized phenomenon known as reactivation – that is, the change in temperature and physiology of the tick host induces the rickettsia to emerge from dormancy and attain infectivity with bad effects on ticks.

Agents and diseases throughout the world

Since 2005, three more SFG rickettsiae, first identified in ticks, have been found to be pathogenic for humans: 'Candidatus *Rickettsia raoultii*', 'Candidatus *Rickettsia kellyi*', and 'Candidatus *Rickettsia monacensis*'. A total of 20 species or subspecies of SFG rickettsiae have now been found to infect humans (Table 6.39.1). Geographical distributions are shown in Figs. 6.39.1 to 6.39.4. There are more rickettsiae 'of unknown pathogenicity' or 'suspected to be pathogens' to be identified as emerging pathogens in the near future.

Clinical features

Symptoms of tick-borne SFG rickettsioses begin 4 to 10 days after the bite and typically include fever, headache, muscle pain, rash, local lymphadenopathy, and, for some diseases, a typical inoculation eschar (the 'tache noire') at the site of the tick bite (Fig. 6.39.5). These signs vary depending on the rickettsia involved and may allow distinction between different rickettsioses occurring at the same location (Table 6.39.1). For example, there is no eschar in Rocky Mountain spotted fever, whereas they do occur in *R. parkeri* infections which have recently emerged in the United States of America. African tick-bite fever is characterized by the occurrence

Table 6.39.1 Characteristics of tick-borne rickettsiae identified in human infections by 2008

Rickettsia spp.	Recognized or potential tick vector(s)	First identification in ticks	Disease (first clinical description)	First microbiological documentation of human cases	Selected clinical and epidemiological characteristics
Confirmed pathogens					
Rickettsia rickettsii	*Dermacentor andersoni* *Dermacentor variabilis* *Rhipicephalus sanguineus* *Amblyomma cajennense* *Amblyomma aureolatum*	1906	Rocky Mountain spotted fever (1899)	1906[a]	Has the reputation of being the most severe tick-borne spotted fever rickettsiosis. However, case fatality has decreased dramatically in recent years in the USA, but fatal cases are still reported in South America. Peak occurrence during spring and summer. Eschars rarely reported. Broadly distributed in the western hemisphere and associated with several species of tick vectors
Rickettsia conorii conorii	*Rhipicephalus sanguineus*	1932	Mediterranean spotted fever (1910)	1932[a]	Disease occurs in urban (66%) and rural (33%) settings. Rash occurs in 97% of cases. Cases generally sporadic. Single eschar. Case fatality ratio approximately 2.5%
Rickettsia conorii israelensis	*Rhipicephalus sanguineus*	1974	Israeli spotted fever (1940)	1971[a]	Compared to Mediterranean spotted fever, eschars are rare (7%). Mild to severe illness
Rickettsia sibirica sibirica	*Dermacentor nuttalli* *Dermacentor marginatus* *Dermacentor silvarum* *Haemaphysalis concinna*	Unknown	Siberian tick typhus (1934)	1946[a]	Disease occurs in predominantly rural settings. Cases occur during spring and summer. Increasing reports of cases. Cases generally associated with rash (100%), eschar (77%), and lymphadenopathy
	Dermacentor sinicus	1974	North Asian tick typhus (1977)	1984[a]	
Rickettsia australis	*Ixodes holocyclus* *Ixodes tasmani*	1974	Queensland tick typhus (1946)	1946[a]	Disease occurs in predominantly rural settings. Cases occur from June to November. Vesicular rash (100%), eschar (65%), and lymphadenopathy (71%). Two fatal cases have been described
Rickettsia japonica	*Ixodes ovatus* *Dermacentor taiwanensis* *Haemaphysalis longicornis* *Haemaphysalis flava*	1996	Oriental or Japanese spotted fever (1984)	1985[a]	Disease occurs in predominantly rural settings. Agricultural activities, bamboo cutting. April to October. Eschar (91%) and rash (100%). May be severe. One fatal case reported
Rickettsia conorii caspia	*Rhipicephalus sanguineus* *Rhipicephalus pumilio*	1992	Astrakhan fever (1970s)	1991[a]	Disease occurs in predominantly rural settings. Associated with eschar (23%), maculopapular rash (94%), and conjunctivitis (34%)
Rickettsia africae	*Amblyomma hebraeum* *Amblyomma variegatum*	1990	African tick-bite fever (1934)	1992[1]	Disease occurs in predominantly rural settings and is associated with international travellers returning from safari, hunting, camping, or adventure races. Outbreaks and clustered cases common (74%). Symptoms include fever (88%), eschars (95%) which are often multiple (54%), maculopapular (49%) or vesicular (50%) rash, and lymphadenopathy (43%). No fatal cases reported
Rickettsia honei	*Aponomma hydrosauri* *Amblyomma cajennense* *Ixodes granulatus*	1993	Flinders island spotted fever (1991)	1992[a]	Disease occurs in predominantly rural settings. Peak in December and January. Symptoms include rash (85%), eschar (25%), and lymphadenopathy (55%)
Rickettsia sibirica mongolitimonae	*Hyalomma asiaticum* *Hyalomma truncatum*	1991	Lymphangitis associated rickettsiosis (1996)	1996[a]	Few cases described in southern France between March and July and in South Africa. Symptoms include eschar (75%), rash (63%), and lymphangitis (25%)
Rickettsia slovaca	*Dermacentor marginatus* *Dermacentor reticulatus*	1968	Tick-borne lymphadenopathy (1997) Dermacentor-borne necrosis and lymphadenopathy (1997)	1997[b] 2003[a]	Fever and rash rare. Typical eschar on the scalp with cervical lymphadenopathy. Illness mild

(Continued)

Table 6.39.1 (*Cont'd*) Characteristics of tick-borne rickettsiae identified in human infections by 2008

Rickettsia spp.	Recognized or potential tick vector(s)	First identification in ticks	Disease (first clinical description)	First microbiological documentation of human cases	Selected clinical and epidemiological characteristics
Rickettsia heilongjiangensis	*Dermacentor silvarum*	1982	Far Eastern spotted fever (1992)	1992, 1996[a]	Rash, eschar, and lymphadenopathy. No fatal cases reported
Rickettsia aeschlimannii	*Hyalomma marginatum marginatum* *Hyalomma marginatum rufipes* *Rhipicephalus appendiculatus*	1997	Unnamed (2002)	2002[b,c]	Few cases described in patients from Morocco and South Africa. Symptoms include eschar and maculopapular rash
Rickettsia parkeri	*Amblyomma maculatum* *Amblyomma americanum* *Amblyomma triste*	1939	Unnamed (2004)	2004[a]	One case reported in a patient in the USA. Symptoms include fever, multiple eschars, and rash
Rickettsia massiliae	*Rhipicephalus sanguineus* *Rhipicephalus turanicus* *Rhipicephalus muhsamae* *Rhipicephalus lunulatus* *Rhipicephalus sulcatus*	1992	Unnamed (2005)	2005[a]	The strain was obtained from the blood of a patient from Sicily in 1985, stored, and definitively identified in 2005. A second case has been reported in 2008 in a patient with fever, a chorioretinitis and rash in southern France.
'Candidatus Rickettsia marmionii'	*Haemaphysalis novaeguineae* *Ixodes holocyclus*	2003–2005	Australian spotted fever (2005)	2003–2005[a]	Between February and June. Six confirmed cases including one with eschar and two with a maculopapular rash
'Candidatus Rickettsia kellyi'	Unknown	Not done	Unnamed (2006)	2006[a,c]	A single case in a 1-year-old boy with fever and maculopapular rash
'Candidatus Rickettsia raoultii'	*Dermacentor reticulatus* *Dermacentor silvarum* *Dermacentor marginatus* *Rhipicephalus pumilio*	1999	Unnamed (2006)	2006[b]	Tick-borne lymphadenopathy including eschar on the scalp with cervical lymphadenopathy
'Candidatus Rickettsia monacensis'	*Ixodes ricinus*	1998	Unnamed (2006)	2006[a,c]	Two cases in tick-bitten patients from Spain with fever and a maculopapular rash
Rickettsia conorii indica	*Rhipicephalus sanguineus*	1950	Indian tick typhus	2001[b]	Compared to Mediterranean spotted fever, rash usually purpuric. Eschar rarely found. Mild to severe
Potential pathogens					
Rickettsia bellii	Various ixodid and argasid tick species	1966	–	–	None. Suspicions based on its pathogenicity on several animal species
Rickettsia canadensis	*Haemaphysalis leporispalustris*	1967	–	–	Possible Rocky Mountain spotted fever-like disease described in California and Texas. Suspected cause of acute cerebral vasculitis in Ohio
'Candidatus Rickettsia amblyommii'	*Amblyomma americanum* *Amblyomma cajennense* *Amblyomma coelebs*	1974	Unnamed (1993)	1993[c]	Possible cause of mild spotted fever rickettsiosis in the USA. Rickettsia also recently identified in Brazilian ticks
'Candiudatus Rickettsia texiana'	*Amblyomma americanum*	1943	Bullis fever (1942)	1943[d]	Possible agent of an epidemic which occurred among army personnel at Camp Bullis, Texas during 1942 and 1943. Maybe a strain of 'Candidatus *Rickettsia amblyommii*'
Rickettsia helvetica	*Ixodes ricinus* *Ixodes ovatus* *Ixodes persulcatus* *Ixodes monospinus*	1979	Unnamed (1999)	1999[b]	Although implicated in perimyocarditis and sarcoidosis, the validity of these associations has been debated or not accepted by rickettsiologists. Few cases documented by serology only in France and in Thailand. Rash and eschar seem to occur rarely

[a] Documentation by culture.
[b] Documentation by molecular tools.
[c] Documentation by serology.
[d] Documentation by animal or human inoculation.

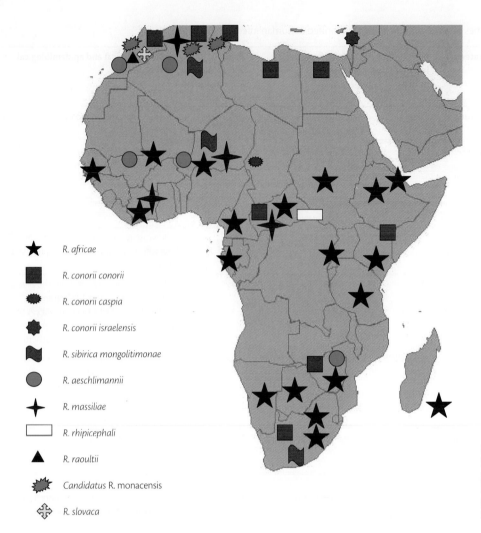

R. africae

R. conorii conorii

R. conorii caspia

R. conorii israelensis

R. sibirica mongolitimonae

R. aeschlimannii

R. massiliae

R. rhipicephali

R. raoultii

Candidatus R. monacensis

R. slovaca

Fig. 6.39.1 Tick borne rickettsiae in Africa. Coloured symbols indicate pathogenic rickettsiae. White symbols indicate rickettsiae of possible pathogenicity and rickettsiae of unknown pathogenicity.

of multiple inoculation eschars in groups of cases, explained by simultaneous mass attacks by infected amblyomma ticks at a particular geographical location. European Dermacentor ticks that bite humans are most active during early spring, autumn, and occasionally winter and are well known to bite on the scalp. Since *R. slovaca* is transmitted by Dermacentor ticks, the inoculation eschar of *R. slovaca* infection is characteristically located on the scalp during these seasons (Fig. 6.39.6).

SFG rickettsioses range in severity from mild to severe and fatal disease. An untreated case fatality exceeding 50% makes Rocky Mountain spotted fever the most dangerous SFG rickettsiosis. The case fatality of Mediterranean spotted fever is usually estimated at around 2.5% in diagnosed cases, but no severe complications or deaths have been reported with African tick-bite fever although the symptoms can be distressing.

Common nonspecific laboratory abnormalities in rickettsioses include mild leucopenia, anaemia, and thrombocytopenia. Hyponatraemia, hypoalbuminaemia, and hepatic and renal abnormalities may also occur. Several specific methods are available to confirm the diagnosis of tick-borne SFG rickettsioses and for other rickettsial diseases. Case definitions and diagnostic scores have been established for African tick-bite fever due to *R. africae* (Box 6.39.1) and Mediterranean spotted fever due to *R. conorii* (Table 6.39.2).

Flea-borne spotted fever

Flea-borne spotted fever (also called cat flea typhus) is an emerging rickettsiosis due to *R. felis*. It was probably first detected in cat fleas (*Ctenocephalides felis*) in 1918 and rediscovered in 1990. *R. felis* was initially characterized by molecular biology techniques and named the ELB agent for the EL Laboratory (Soquel, California, United States of America). In 1994, ELB agent DNA fragments were detected in blood samples from a Texan patient that had been kept since 1991. In 1994 and 1995, isolation of the ELB agent was reported and the name *R. felis* was proposed, but it was not cultivated definitively at low temperature and fully characterized until 2001 in Marseille, France. More evidence of the pathogenicity of *R. felis* was provided in 2000 in Mexico by three patients whose fever, exanthema, headache, and central nervous system involvement was attributed to *R. felis* infection using specific polymerase chain reaction (PCR) of blood and skin and seroconversion to rickettsial antigens. Two French patients with clinical rickettsial disease and 2 of 16 Brazilian patients with febrile rash showed high antibody titres to ELB agent and specific sequences of ELB agent were identified in the serum of one Brazilian patient. In 2002, two cases of typical spotted fever were reported in a married couple in Germany. Clinical features included fever, marked fatigue, headache, generalized maculopapular rash, and a single black

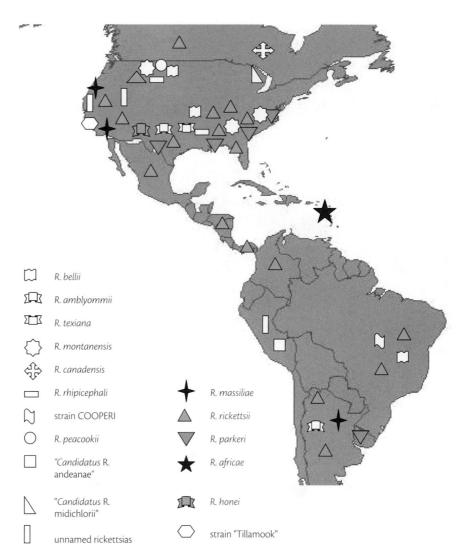

Fig. 6.39.2 Tick-borne rickettsiae in the Americas. Coloured symbols indicate pathogenic rickettsiae. White symbols indicate rickettsiae of possible pathogenicity and rickettsiae of unknown pathogenicity.

R. bellii	
R. amblyommii	
R. texiana	
R. montanensis	
R. canadensis	
R. rhipicephali	
strain COOPERI	
R. peacookii	
"*Candidatus* R. andeanae"	
"*Candidatus* R. midichlorii"	
unnamed rickettsias	

R. massiliae	
R. rickettsii	
R. parkeri	
R. africae	
R. honei	
strain "Tillamook"	

crusted cutaneous lesion surrounded by a livid halo on the thigh and abdomen associated with painful local lymphadenopathy. Serological techniques distinguished *R. felis* infection from several other rickettsiae in one of the patients. *R. felis* infection has been diagnosed serologically in Asia, Tunisia, and the Canary Islands. Rash and/or eschar were reported in most of the documented cases, making it difficult to distinguish from tick-borne spotted fevers.

R. felis is probably cosmopolitan. It has been found in New Mexico, Brazil, Uruguay, Algeria, Ethiopia, Thailand, Indonesia, Europe, New Zealand, and elsewhere in various species of fleas including *C. felis*, *C. canis*, *Pulex irritans*, *Archeopsylla erinacei*, and *Anomiopsyllus nudata*. Transovarial transmission of *R. felis* has been reported, suggesting that fleas could act as reservoirs of the rickettsiae but the role of mammals, including rodents, hedgehogs, cats, and dogs, in its life cycle and circulation remains unclear.

Rickettsialpox

Epidemiology
Rickettsialpox is a cosmopolitan mite-borne spotted fever rickettsiosis caused by *R. akari*. Originally described in New York in 1946, it is still reported mainly in the United States of America. It

was studied in the Ukraine in the early 1950s, but few cases have been confirmed in Europe. Serological surveys and occasional case reports identified low *R. akari* antibody titres in a few people in Albania, France, Germany, and Italy, but there have been no confirmed cases. *R. akari* was isolated from the blood of a patient from Zadar, Croatia, in 1991. Recently, rickettsialpox emerged in Turkey. However, the disease is probably ubiquitous but underdiagnosed, particularly in the tropics.

R. akari is associated with house mouse mites (*Liponyssoides sanguineus*), haematophagous arthropods that maintain *R. akari* in house mice (*Mus musculus*) and may transmit the disease when they bite people exposed by contact with house mice. This mite has been harvested from various other rodents in the United States of America, Eurasia, Africa, and Korea.

Clinical features
The first identified case in New York was an 11-year-old boy who presented with a high fever, a papulovesicular lesion on his back, and axillary lymphadenopathy and, over the next few days, developed a diffuse rash, a temperature of 40.5°C, and remained ill for about 1 week despite penicillin therapy. He made a complete recovery.

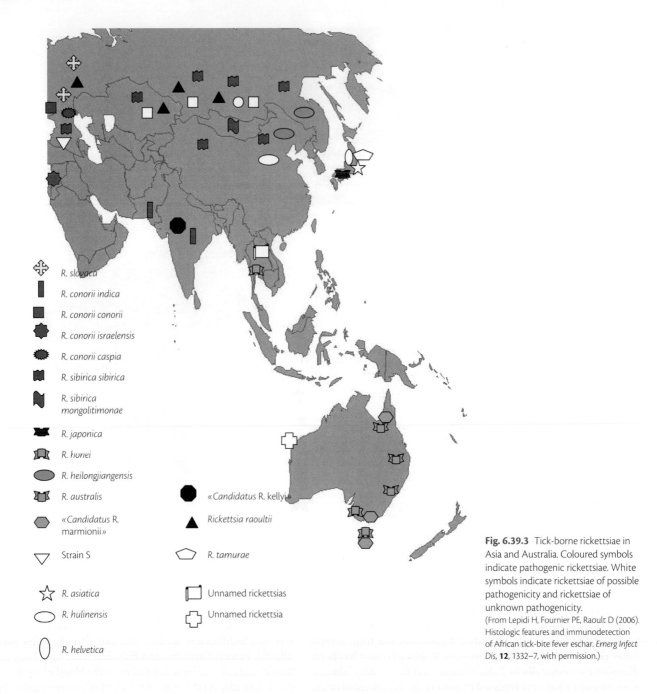

R. slovaca

R. conorii indica

R. conorii conorii

R. conorii israelensis

R. conorii caspia

R. sibirica sibirica

R. sibirica mongolitimonae

R. japonica

R. honei

R. heilongjiangensis

R. australis

«Candidatus R. marmionii»

Strain S

R. asiatica

R. hulinensis

R. helvetica

«Candidatus R. kellyi»

Rickettsia raoultii

R. tamurae

Unnamed rickettsias

Unnamed rickettsia

Fig. 6.39.3 Tick-borne rickettsiae in Asia and Australia. Coloured symbols indicate pathogenic rickettsiae. White symbols indicate rickettsiae of possible pathogenicity and rickettsiae of unknown pathogenicity.
(From Lepidi H, Fournier PE, Raoult D (2006). Histologic features and immunodetection of African tick-bite fever eschar. *Emerg Infect Dis*, **12**, 1332–7, with permission.)

During the next few months more than 100 more cases were recognized and the causative agent, named *R. akari* from the Greek word for mite, was described.

Rickettsialpox is often described as being like chickenpox because the rash is often vesicular. In 83 to 100% of cases, a primary eschar appears at the site of a mite bite, followed by fever, headache, and development of the papulovesicular rash. The eschar usually starts as a painless vesicle, often described by patients as a pimple, boil, or insect bite. Eventually, the vesicle ruptures and a dark brown or black crust develops over the lesion, forming the characteristic eschar. The exanthem consists of 2- to 10-mm-diameter discrete erythematous maculopapules distributed over the extremities, abdomen, back, chest, and face, but only rarely on palms and soles. After 2 to 3 days some lesions become indurated and develop a small vesicle containing cloudy fluid at their apices, described by the first investigators

as 'a window framed in the top of the papule'. Seventeen to 26% of patients have vesicular lesions on their buccal mucous membrane. Two to 7 days after the appearance of the primary lesion there is sudden fever, sweating, lassitude, myalgias, and headache which persist for 7 to 10 days in the absence of antibiotic treatment. Although it is generally described as being relatively benign and self-limiting, neurological symptoms such as photophobia, vertigo, pain on movement of the eyes, and nuchal rigidity may be severe enough to warrant lumbar puncture. *R. akari* has been isolated from eschar biopsy specimens from New York City patients with rickettsialpox.

Murine typhus

Epidemiology

Murine or endemic typhus was probably first reported by Bravo in Mexico in 1570, making it one of the oldest recognized

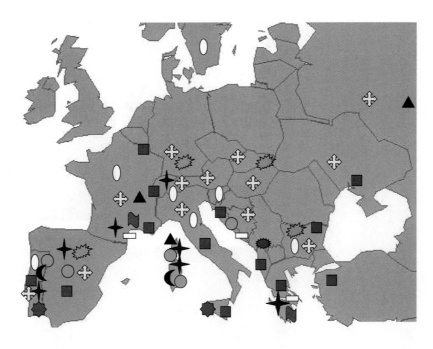

■	R. conorii conorii	☾	«Candidatus R. barbariae»
✴	R. conorii israelensis	✦	R. massiliae
✸	R. conorii caspia	✺	«Candidatus R. monacencis»
⬣	R. sibirica mongolitimonae	▲	R. raoultii
●	R. aeschlimannii	▭	R. rhipicephali
✛	R. slovaca	◯	R. helvetica

Fig. 6.39.4 Tick-borne rickettsiae in Europe. Coloured symbols indicate pathogenic rickettsiae. White symbols indicate rickettsiae of possible pathogenicity and rickettsiae of unknown pathogenicity.

arthropod-borne zoonoses. The first case was described clinically in grain silo workers in Australia and the disease distinguished from epidemic typhus in the 1920s. The causative organism was named *R. mooseri* and thereafter *R. typhi*. Its main vector is the rat flea (*Xenopsylla cheopis*) while rodents, mainly *Rattus norvegicus* and *Rattus rattus*, are its reservoirs. Other fleas or arthropods may also transmit *R. typhi*, including cat fleas (*C. felis*), mouse fleas (*L. segnis*), lice, mites, and ticks, and other rodents and wild and domestic mammals may be hosts. The classic cycle of infection is flea-borne between rats. *R. typhi* is only rarely transmitted transovarially in fleas. Rats are not fatally infected and rickettsaemia persists from day 7 to day 12 after inoculation. Fleas are infected for life, but their lifespan is not shortened. Rickettsiae are excreted in their faeces, where they remain viable for several years. Most people are thought to become infected when flea faeces containing *R. typhi* contaminate disrupted skin or are inhaled into the respiratory tract. Rarely, infections may result from flea bites.

Murine typhus is distributed worldwide but is often unrecognized especially in tropical countries. Cases are regularly documented in the United States of America, Mexico, and Europe, and it recently re-emerged in Japan. Ideas of prevalence are based principally on serosurveys and on cases in travellers from China, Indonesia, India, Morocco, Canary Islands, Africa, Malaysia, Thailand, and Vietnam. Serosurveys suggest that the disease is more prevalent in coastal areas of tropical countries, where rats are particularly common. It has been reported from Tunisia, Brazil (where it may be most prevalent in the south-east), and on the Thailand–Burma border.

Clinical features

Murine typhus is a mild disease with nonspecific features. The incubation period is 7 to 14 days. Fewer than 15% of cases present with the 'classic' triad of fever, headache, and rash. Later, fever and headache are more common than the rash, which is present in fewer than 50% of patients and is often transient or difficult to observe. Among 83 patients in Crete, 49 (59%) presented with rash and 17 additional patients (20%) developed rash subsequently. Fever (100%), headache (88%), and chills (87%) were also common. Nausea, abdominal pain, diarrhoea, jaundice, cough, confusion, and seizures have been reported and can lead to misdiagnosis. Fewer than 50% of patients report exposure to fleas or rats. In untreated

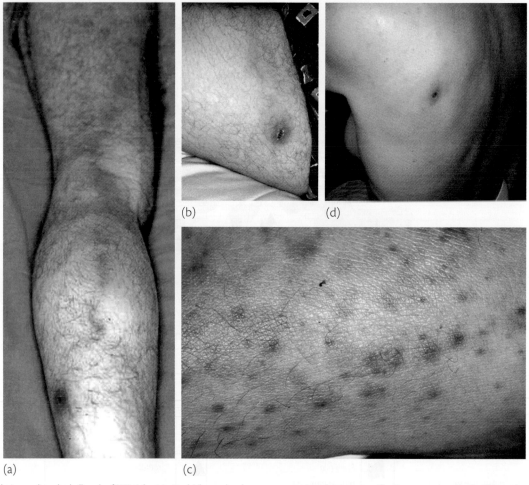

(a)   (b)   (d)   (c)

Fig. 6.39.5 Inoculation eschar, the hallmark of SFG rickettsiosis which may be absent or uncommon in some specific diseases, such as Rocky Mountain spotted fever, or associated with a lymphangitis, as in the case of *R. sibirica mongolitimonae* (a) and *R. africae* infection (b), or a rash, as in *R. africae* (c) and *R. heilongjiangensis* infection (d). (a, from Fournier PE, *et al.* (2000). *Rickettsia* mongolotimonae: a rare pathogen in France. *Emerg Infect Dis*, **6**, 290–2, with permission; b, copyright D A Warrell; c, copyright Dr Ed Dunbar, Manchester; d, from Mediannikov O, *et al.* (2004). Acute tick-borne rickettsiosis, caused by *Rickettsia heilongjiangensis* variant in the Russian Far East. *Emerg Infect Dis*, **10**, 810–17, with permission.)

patients, symptoms last for 7 to 14 days, after which there is usually a rapid return to health.

Epidemic typhus

Epidemiology

Epidemic typhus is caused by *R. prowazekii*, a typhus-group rickettsia. It is suspected to have been responsible for the 'Great Plague' of Athens in the 5th century BC. In 1909, Charles Nicolle discovered the role of lice in the transmission of typhus and later performed the first successful cultures in animals. He was rewarded with a Nobel Prize.

The vectors of epidemic typhus, body lice (*Pediculus humanus humanus* or *P. humanus corporis*), are a problem particularly during times of war, conflict, famine, and natural catastrophes. They live in clothes and thrive in cold weather when clothes may be washed infrequently and general hygiene declines. After the Second World War, foci persisted in the cooler mountainous countries in Africa

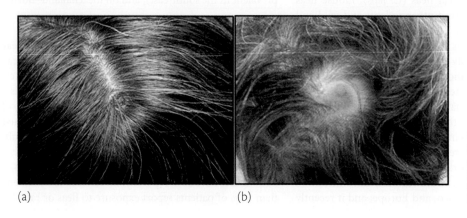

(a)   (b)

Fig. 6.39.6 Patients with *R. slovaca* infection. Inoculation lesion on the scalp (a), residual alopecia (b). (From Gouriet F, Rolain JM, Raoult D (2006). *Rickettsia slovaca* infection, France. *Emerg Infect Dis*, **12**, 521–3, with permission.)

Box 6.39.1 Diagnostic score for African tick-bite fever (ATBF)

A patient is considered as having ATBF when they meet the criteria A, B, or C:

A Direct evidence of *R. africae* infection by culture and/or PCR

Or

B Clinical and epidemiological features highly suggestive of ATBF such as multiple inoculation eschars and/or regional lymphadenitis and/or a vesicular rash and/or similar symptoms among other members of the same group of travellers coming back from an endemic area (sub-Saharan Africa or French West Indies)

and

Positive serology against SFG rickettsiae

Or

C Clinical and epidemiological features consistent with an SFG rickettsiosis such as fever and/or any cutaneous rash and/or a single inoculation eschar after travel to sub-Saharan Africa or French West Indies

and

Serology specific for a recent R. africae infection (seroconversion or presence of IgM >1:32), with antibodies to R. africae greater than those to *R. conorii* by at least two dilutions, and/or a western blot or cross-adsorption showing antibodies specific for *R. africae*.

Table 6.39.2 Diagnostic score for Mediterranean spotted fever due to *Rickettsia conorii*

Criteria	Score[a]
Epidemiological criteria	
Stay in endemic area	2
Occurrence in May–October	2
Contact (certain or possible) with dog ticks	2
Clinical criteria	
Fever more than 39°C	5
Eschar	5
Maculopapular or purpuric rash	5
Two of these criteria	3
All three criteria	5
Unspecific laboratory findings	
Platelets less than 150 × 10⁹/litre	1
AST or ALT more than 50 UI/litre	1
Bacteriological criteria	
Blood culture positive for *R. conorii*	25
Detection of *R. conorii* in a skin biopsy	25
Serological criteria	
Single serum and IgG more than 1:128	5
Single serum and IgG more than 1:128 and IgM more than 1:64	10
Fourfold increase in two sera obtained within a 2-week interval	20

ALT, alanine transferase; AST, aspartate transferase.
[a] The diagnosis is made when the score is 25 or more.

but epidemic typhus was considered a disease of the past. However, in recent years, intermittent outbreaks have occurred in Africa (Ethiopia, Nigeria, Burundi), Mexico, Central America, South America, eastern Europe, Afghanistan, northern India, and China. The most recent outbreak, the largest since the Second World War, occurred during the civil war in Burundi in the 1990s.

R. prowazekii is transmitted to people when infected louse feeding sites are contaminate by their faeces, or when the conjunctivae and other mucous membranes are exposed to crushed bodies or faeces of infected lice. Transmission may also result from the inhalation of infected faeces, which is thought to be the main route of infection in health workers attending patients. People who survive epidemic typhus remain infected with *R. prowazekii* for life; when stressed, they may experience a recrudescence (Brill–Zinsser disease), and may be the source of a new epidemic if they become infested with body lice. Humans were long considered the sole reservoir of *R. prowazekii* but its discovery in flying squirrels and their ectoparasites in North America indicate an alternative reservoir. Sylvatic (flying squirrel) typhus has not yet been associated with human fatalities, but North American flying squirrel strains of *R. prowazekii* appear similar to those isolated from patients during louse-borne outbreaks. A non-human typhus reservoir has also been reported in Ethiopia, where 10 isolates of *R. prowazekii* were obtained from hyalomma ticks recovered from livestock. The association of typhus-group rickettsiae with ticks has also been suggested.

Clinical features

After an incubation period of 10 to 14 days, patients develop malaise and vague symptoms before the sudden development of fever (all cases), headache (all cases), and myalgia (70–100%). In Burundi, a crouching attitude was observed, attributable to myalgia. Other common features are nausea or vomiting, coughing, and abnormalities of central nervous system function ranging from confusion to stupor and coma. Diarrhoea, pulmonary involvement, myocarditis, splenomegaly, and conjunctivitis may also occur. Most patients develop a macular, maculopapular, or petechial rash that classically begins on the trunk and spreads to the limbs (Fig. 6.39.7a,b). It is difficult to detect in pigmented skins. Gangrene of the distal extremities may occur in severe cases as mentioned in Thucydides' description of the Great Plague of Athens (Fig. 6.39.7c).

Case fatality ranges between 4% in the antibiotic era up to 60% before antibiotics were available. Brill–Zinsser disease can appear many years after the acute disease. It is less severe and the rash is less frequent.

Investigation and specific diagnosis

Serology

Serological tests are the most frequently used and widely available methods for diagnosis. The Weil–Felix test, the oldest test, is based on the detection of antibodies to various proteus antigens that cross-react with rickettsiae. Although it lacks specificity and sensitivity, it continues to be used in many developing countries. It has also provided the first diagnostic step towards recognition of emerging pathogens in countries with higher levels of technical development, as in the case of *R. japonica* in Japan. However, immunofluorescence assay (IFA) is currently considered the reference method. Acute-phase and convalescent-phase serum specimens must be collected, several weeks apart. One limitation of

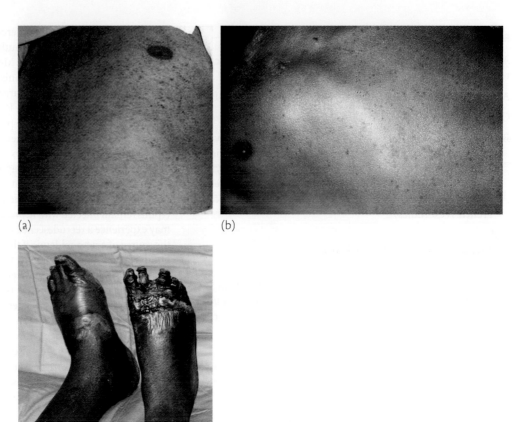

Fig. 6.39.7 (a) Rash in a patient with epidemic typhus due to *R. prowazekii* imported from Algeria to France. (b) Rash of epidemic typhus in an Ethiopian patient. (c) Peripheral gangrene in an Ethiopian patient with epidemic typhus.

(a, from Niang M, Brouqui P, Raoult D (1999). Epidemic typhus imported from Algeria. *Emerg Infect Dis*, **5**, 716–18, with permission; b, courtesy of the late Dr P L Perine; c, copyright D A Warrell.)

serology is cross-reactivity between antigens of pathogens within the same genus, and other genera. Most commercially available IFAs offer a very limited selection of antigens (e.g. *R. rickettsii* in the United States of America and *R. conorii*, *R. rickettsii*, and *R. typhi* in France). It is important to remind clinicians that IFA may be adequate to diagnose the class of infection (e.g. SFG rickettsiosis), but it is unlikely to provide a specific aetiological agent unless more sophisticated assays are performed. Serology should be considered an initial, but not the sole, method for recognizing and diagnosing 'emerging rickettsioses', particularly if no rickettsiae have been isolated or detected previously in that area. In the Unité des Rickettsies, Marseille, when cross-reactions are noted between several rickettsial antigens, a rickettsia is considered to be causal when titres of IgG or IgM antibody against this antigen are at least two serial dilutions higher than those against other rickettsial antigens. When differences in titres between several antigens are lower than two dilutions, western blot assays and, if necessary, cross-absorption studies are used.

Culture

Rickettsial isolation in culture is the definitive diagnostic method, but can be performed only in P3 facilities that can maintain living host cells or cell cultures. The centrifugation shell-vial technique using HEL fibroblasts has proved effective. Rickettsiae can be isolated from buffy coat preparations of heparinized or ethylenediaminetetraacetic acid (EDTA)-anticoagulated whole blood, skin biopsies, and from arthropods.

Histochemical and immunohistochemical procedures

Rickettsiae can been detected in tissue specimens by various histochemical methods, including Giemsa or Gimenez staining. Immunohistochemical methods are superior for SFG rickettsiae in formalin-fixed paraffin-embedded skin biopsies, particularly eschars (Fig. 6.39.8). Most available assays are SFG specific but not species specific.

Molecular tools

PCR and sequencing methods are sensitive and rapid tools for detecting and identifying rickettsiae in blood and skin biopsies. Primers amplifying sequences of several genes have been used. Arthropods are used as epidemiological tools to detect the presence of a pathogen in a specific geographical area. Nested PCR has been reported, but it must be remembered that standard nested PCR assays are highly susceptible to contamination and false-positive results. A PCR assay has been described that has increased sensitivity. This 'suicide PCR' is a nested PCR using single-use primers targeting a completely novel gene and so avoiding 'vertical' contamination by amplicons from previous assays, a limitation of the extensive use of PCR. The absence of a positive control does not impair the interpretation of positive results, which are validated by appropriate negative controls. All positive PCR products are sequenced to identify the causative agent. This technique has been successful with EDTA-blood, serum, lymph node specimens, and skin biopsies. Real-time quantitative PCR assays have been developed, as in the case of epidemic typhus. This could aid surveillance in public

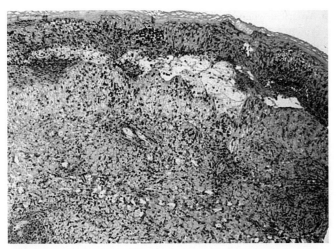

Fig. 6.39.8 Inoculation eschar from a patient with African tick-bite fever showing numerous dermal inflammatory infiltrates mainly composed of polymorphonuclear leucocytes. Immunoperoxidase staining with an anti-CD15 antibody; original magnification ×100.
(From Lepidi H, Fournier PE, Raoult D (2006). Histologic features and immunodetection of African tick-bite fever eschar. *Emerg Infect Dis*, **12**, 1332–7, with permission.)

health programmes, especially for countries where human cases are underdiagnosed.

Treatment and prognosis

Early empirical antibiotic is the rule for any suspected rickettsiosis, before confirmation of the diagnosis.

SFG rickettsioses

Doxycycline (200 mg/day) is the treatment of choice for all SFG rickettsioses, including Rocky Mountain spotted fever in young children. Duration of antibiotic therapy for SFG rickettsioses is governed more by clinical response than a statutory number of days. However, for most of these infections, therapy should continue for at least 3 days after the patient's fever has subsided. A single dose of 200 mg doxycycline has proved adequate for Mediterranean spotted fever, but patients with severe SFG rickettsioses should be given doxycycline intravenously for up to 24 hours after they become afebrile. Josamycin has also been used to treat some patients with SFG rickettsioses, including pregnant women with Mediterranean spotted fever. Newer macrolides such as azithromycin and clarithromycin are promising agents, particularly in children with Mediterranean spotted fever. Chloramphenicol is an alternative, but its use is limited by perceived side effects and it should be considered as empirical treatment of severe cases only if it is the only available drug, as in developing countries. Some fluoroquinolones may be effective against SFG rickettsiae. Many classes of broad-spectrum antibiotics including penicillins, cephalosporins, and aminoglycosides are ineffective against rickettsial diseases.

Murine typhus

Doxycycline is the drug of choice for nonpregnant adults and children. The optimal duration of therapy has not been assessed in clinical studies but 7 to 15 days, or for at least 48 h after the patient has become afebrile, has been recommended. A single dose of 200 mg doxycycline also proved adequate. Response to doxycycline is rapid with defervescence in 2 to 3 days. Chloramphenicol is an alternative, with the reservations discussed above, but relapses have

been reported. Fluoroquinolones proved effective *in vitro* against *R. typhi*, but the few clinical studies produced contradictory results. Other antibiotics effective against *R. typhi in vitro*, including rifampicin, thiamphenicol, macrolides, erythromycin, clarithromycin, josamycin, and telithromycin, have no clinical application, and amoxicillin, gentamicin, and trimethoprim/sulphamethoxazole are ineffective.

Epidemic typhus

Tetracycline and chloramphenicol are effective. Chloramphenicol is still widely used as empirical treatment of fever in tropical developing countries since its broad spectrum includes other serious infections such as meningococcaemia and typhoid fevers that can initially mimic epidemic typhus. Most patients improve markedly within 48 hours of starting treatment with either of these antibiotics. However, many physicians prefer to use tetracycline for all typhus diseases, as it is cheaper and safer. A single dose of 200 mg doxycycline, the reference treatment, is extremely efficient. Few or no relapses are observed with this treatment, which should be prescribed for any suspected case, including children, as no risk of tooth staining has been demonstrated with this regimen. Ciprofloxacin should be avoided.

Human ehrlichioses and anaplasmosis

These diseases are caused by bacteria of the family Anaplasmataceae, long thought to be of purely veterinary importance. Three species are now implicated in human diseases, *Ehrlichia chaffeensis* causing human monocytic ehrlichiosis, *Anaplasma phagocytophilum* causing human anaplasmosis, and *E. ewingii* causing granulocytic ehrlichiosis. These diseases are tick-borne zoonoses whose causative agents are maintained through enzootic cycles between ticks and animals.

Bacteriology, taxonomy, and genomics

The family Anaplasmataceae consists of intracellular alphaproteobacteria including human and mammal pathogens, whose host cells are of bone marrow or haematopoietic origin including erythrocytes, monocytes or macrophages, neutrophils, and platelets. Members of this family share a high degree of nucleotide sequence similarity in several chromosomal genes, such as *rrs*, *groESL operon*, *gltA*, *RpoB*, and *Ank*. The organisms grow within cytoplasmic vacuoles containing one to many individual organisms which resemble mulberries when observed by light microscopy, and have been called 'morulae' (Fig. 6.39.9). *Anaplasma marginale*, a cattle pathogen, was the first discovered, by Theiler in 1910. Since then, others have been described in animals and humans. In 2001, improvements in molecular phylogenetic methods modified the taxonomy of the Anaplasmataceae, based on comparison of sequences obtained from *rrs* (16s rRNA encoding gene) and the *groESL* operon. This contains a spacer region between *groES* and the *groEL* heat shock protein genes and is thought to be more informative phylogenetically than the coding regions. Four clades and four genera have been identified including *Anaplasma*, *Ehrlichia*, *Neorickettsia*, and *Wolbachia*, and some taxa, such as *Cowdria ruminantium* (now called *Ehrlichia ruminantium*) the cause of heart water in cattle, have been reclassified (Fig. 6.39.9). Analyses of other gene sequences and the complete genome sequencing of several species of the family (*A. phagocytophilum*, *E. chaffeensis*, *E. ruminantium*, *N. sennetsu*, and *W. pipientis*) have confirmed the

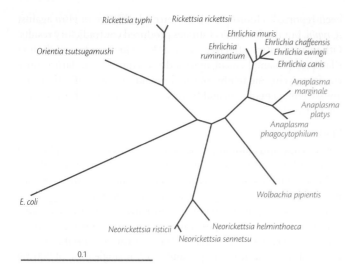

Fig. 6.39.9 Current phylogeny and taxonomic classification of genera in the family Anaplasmataceae. The distance bar represents substitutions per 1000 bp. *E. coli*, *Escherichia coli*.
(From Dumler JS, *et al.* (2005). Human granulocytic anaplasmosis and *Anaplasma phagocytophilum*. *Emerg Infect Dis*, **1**, 1828–34, with permission.)

new organization of the family Anaplasmataceae. Ehrlichia and anaplasma display a unique large expansion of immunodominant outer membrane proteins, facilitating antigenic variation. Unlike Rickettsiaceae, pathogenic Anaplasmataceae are capable of making all major vitamins, cofactors, and nucleotides, which could be beneficial to the invertebrate vector or the vertebrate host. Ehrlichia and anaplasma lack genes for biosynthesis of the lipopolysaccharide and peptidoglycan activating host leucocytes.

Human monocytic ehrlichiosis

Epidemiology
The first human case of monocytic ehrlichiosis (HME) was identified in 1986, when intracytoplasmic inclusions were seen in monocytes in the peripheral blood smear of a severely ill man bitten by ticks in Arkansas, United States of America. This case was first assumed to be due to *E. canis*, the agent of monocytic canine ehrlichiosis, but *E. chaffeensis* was later isolated.

E. chaffeensis is maintained in nature as a complex zoonosis, involving many vertebrate reservoirs for the bacterium and blood-meal sources for the tick vectors. The Lone Star tick (*Amblyomma americanum*) is its primary vector. All stages of this tick bite people. It is distributed in south, central, south-eastern, and mid-Atlantic areas of the United States of America, in meadows, woodlands, and hardwood forests. Primary hosts include many wild and domestic mammals, although deer are considered to be the definitive host. *E. chaffeensis* has been detected by PCR in other American ticks, but their role as vectors has not been demonstrated. There is no evidence of transovarial transmission, so ticks are not considered to be reservoirs. So far, the white-tailed deer (*Odocoileus virginianus*) is the sole recognized efficient reservoir of *E. chaffeensis* but domestic dogs (with mild to inapparent disease), red foxes, and domestic goats are potential reservoirs.

Between 1986 and 1997, more than 700 presumptive cases were reported to the Centers for Disease Control (CDC), and between 1999 and 2004, more than 1300 cases. Most cases of HME occur in the south, central, and south-eastern regions of the United States

of America, where *Amblyomma americanum* reaches its highest prevalence. HME is a seasonal disease whose incidence correlates with the activity of both nymphs and adult ticks. Most cases occur from May to July. Incidence based on active surveillance is 10 times higher than the highest rates reported using passive surveillance. HME seems to be prevalent in Brazil and has been reported from other parts of the world including Latin America, Europe, Africa, and Asia. These diagnoses were based on serological studies, so infection by closely related organism cannot be completely ruled out. Gene fragments closely related to those of *E. chaffeensis* have been detected by PCR in ticks and rodents trapped in continental Asia but, so far, the disease has been clearly identified only in the United States of America.

Clinical diagnosis
Tick bite or tick exposure is reported in 70 to 90% of patients with HME. It is more common in males and can affect individuals of all ages, including children and elderly people. The incubation period is 1 to 2 weeks (median 9 days). It presents as an undifferentiated febrile illness ranging in severity from a mild disease to multisystem organ failure. Apart from immunosuppression due to AIDS or other conditions, the most important risk factor for severe disease is age. The risk of life-threatening complications or death is higher in patients aged 60 years or more, but many severe or fatal cases have been described in apparently healthy children and young adults. More than one-half of patients have to be hospitalized and case fatality is estimated to be 3%.

Clinical features include fever (98%), headache (77%), myalgias (65%), vomiting (36%), rash (35%), cough (25%), and neurological findings with impaired consciousness (20%). The petechial, macular, maculopapular, or diffusely erythematous rash involves trunk, extremities, and, less commonly, the face. Malaise (30–80%), lymphadenopathy, gastrointestinal symptoms, pharyngitis, and, less frequently, conjunctivitis, dysuria, and peripheral oedema may also occur. Leucopenia, thrombocytopenia, and elevated hepatic transaminase levels are the most common laboratory findings. Asymptomatic infection may also occur and, since *Amblyomma americanum* is the vector of other tick-borne agents, coinfection is possible.

E. ewingii granulocytic ehrlichiosis
E. ewingii has been known since 1992 as the agent of canine granulocytic ehrlichiosis, first described in a dog in Arkansas in 1971. The disease was described subsequently in several other states in the south-eastern and south-central United States of America, where the recognized vector is the Lone Star tick, *Amblyomma americanum*. Dogs infected with *E. ewingii* showed fever, lameness, and/or neutrophilic polyarthritis, and/or unexplained ataxia, paresis, or other neurological abnormalities. Laboratory findings include thrombocytopenia, and may include reactive lymphocytes. White-tailed and South Carolina deer have also been shown to be infected with *E. ewingii*. Human infections with *E. ewingii* were first reported in 1999, when blood samples collected from 413 patients with possible ehrlichiosis in Missouri between 1994 to 1998 were analysed retrospectively. Molecular tools revealed that four tick-exposed patients were shown to be infected with *E. ewingii* and morulae were seen in neutrophils from two others. Clinical signs included fever, headache, and thrombocytopenia, with or without leucopenia. Three of them had underlying diseases and were receiving immunosuppressive therapy. More recently, four male

HIV-infected patients from Oklahoma and Tennessee were found to be infected using the same methods. Three were receiving highly active antiretroviral therapy (HAART) and their median CD4+ cell count was 176/µl. Symptoms included fever, malaise and myalgia, headache, and nausea and vomiting. They had leucopenia, thrombocytopenia, anaemia, elevated transaminases, and hyponatraemia. They all survived. It is not clear whether *E. ewingii* can cause disease in immunocompetent people.

Human granulocytic anaplasmosis

Epidemiology

Human granulocytic anaplasmosis was first identified in 1990 in a patient in Wisconsin, United States of America, who died with a severe febrile illness 2 weeks after a tick bite. Clusters of small bacteria, assumed to be phagocytosed Gram-positive cocci, were seen inside neutrophils in the peripheral blood, but a careful review suggested the possibility of human ehrlichiosis. Over the ensuing 2 years, 13 cases with similar intraneutrophilic inclusions were identified in the same region of north-western Wisconsin and eastern Minnesota. In 1994, through application of broad-range molecular amplification and DNA sequencing, the causative agent was recognized as distinct from *E. chaffeensis*. First known as the 'HGE agent', the organism was found to be closely related to *E. equi* and *E. phagocytophila* (pathogens of horses and ruminants, respectively). However, phylogenic studies suggested that they were a single species, *Anaplasma phagocytophilum*. The disease was renamed human granulocytic anaplasmosis (HGA).

HGA is increasingly recognized as an important and frequent cause of fever after tick bite in the upper Midwest, New England, parts of the mid-Atlantic states, and northern California. A total of 2963 cases of HGA have been recorded in the United States of America since 1994, and 700 cases in 2005 alone. Since 1997, the agent and disease have been recognized in Europe, where more than 60 cases have been documented. Seroepidemiological studies confirm that human *A. phagocytophilum* infection is highly prevalent in both the United States of America and in Europe.

Ixodes ticks are the recognized vectors. *A. phagocytophilum* is maintained in a transmission cycle with *Ixodes persulcatus* complex ticks, including *I. scapularis* in the eastern United States of America, *I. pacificus* in the western United States of America, and *I. ricinus* in Europe. A role for *I. persulcatus* in eastern Europe and Asia is also suggested. Tick infection is established after an infectious blood meal. The bacterium is transmitted in ticks trans-stadially but not transovarially, and so ticks are not reservoirs. The major mammalian reservoir for *A. phagocytophilum* in the eastern United States of America is the white-footed mouse *Peromyscus leucopus*, and other small mammals and white-tailed deer *Odocoileus virginianus* can also be infected. Other reservoirs may include ruminants and other mammals. In Europe, horses, cattle, sheep, goats, dog, cats, and small mammals, particularly rodents, may be reservoirs.

Clinical diagnosis

HGA presents most commonly as an undifferentiated febrile illness occurring in spring or summer. Most patients have a moderately severe febrile illness with headache, myalgia, and malaise. A review of clinical date from 10 studies across North America and Europe includes up to 685 patients (Table 6.39.3). The most frequent

Table 6.39.3 Meta-analysis of clinical manifestations and laboratory abnormalities in patients with human granulocytic anaplasmosis

Characteristics	All			North America		Europe	
	Median (%)[a]	Mean (%)	Number[b]	Mean (%)	Number	Mean (%)	Number
Symptom or sign							
Fever	100	92	480	92	448	98	66
Myalgia	74	77	514	79	448	65	66
Headache	89	75	378	73	289	89	66
Malaise	93	94	90	96	271	47	15
Nausea	44	38	256	36	207	47	49
Vomiting	20	26	90	34	41	19	49
Diarrhoea	13	16	90	22	41	10	49
Cough	13	19	260	22	207	10	49
Arthralgias	58	46	497	47	448	37	49
Rash	3	6	685	6	289	4	53
Stiff neck	11	18	22	22	18	0	4
Confusion	9	17	211	17	207	0	4
Laboratory abnormality							
Leucopenia	38	49	329	50	282	47	47
Thrombocytopenia	71	71	329	72	282	64	47
Elevated serum AST or ALT	74	71	170	79	123	51	47
Elevated serum creatinine	15	43	72	49	59	0	13

ALT, alanine aminotransferase; AST, aspartate aminotransferase.
[a] Median percentage of patients with feature among all reports.
[b] Number of patients with data available for meta-analysis.
Reprinted from Dumler JS, *et al.* (2005). Human granulocytic anaplasmosis and *Anaplasma phagocytophilum*. Emerg Infect Dis, **1**, 1828–34.

symptoms are malaise (94%), fever (92%), myalgia (77%), and headache (75%). A minority of patients have arthralgia, gastrointestinal symptoms (nausea, vomiting, diarrhoea), respiratory symptoms (cough, pulmonary infiltrates, acute respiratory distress syndrome (ARDS)), and liver or central nervous system disturbances. Rash was observed in 6%, but no specific rash has been described in HGA. A few patients were coinfected with other ixodes-borne agents such as Lyme borreliosis (Chapter 6.32) and babesiosis (Chapter 8.3) in Europe and the United States of America. Frequent laboratory abnormalities identified in up to 329 patients included thrombocytopenia (71%), leucopenia (49%), anaemia (37%), and elevated hepatic transaminase levels (71%). The case fatality of HGA is estimated as 0.5%.

Diagnosis

Laboratory confirmation of human ehrlichioses and anaplasmosis is based on several tests that are not yet widely available for routine use. Indirect immunofluorescence serology is the most widely available. However, limitations include delay in seroconversion and possible false-positive detection due to cross-reacting bacteria. Laboratory criteria for the diagnosis of both diseases have been defined by the Council of State and Territorial Epidemiologists (www.cste.org). They include a fourfold or greater change in antibody titre to *E. chaffeensis* or *A. phagocytophilum* antigen by IFA in paired serum samples, or a positive PCR assay and confirmation of *E. chaffeensis* or *A. phagocytophilum* DNA, or identification of morulae in leucocytes and a positive IFA titre, or immunostaining *E. chaffeensis* or *A. phagocytophilum* antigen in a biopsy or autopsy sample, or culture of *E. chaffeensis* or *A. phagocytophilum* from a clinical specimen (Fig. 6.39.10). Case definitions for HGA have also been proposed by the Study Group for *Coxiella*, *Anaplasma*, *Rickettsia*, and *Bartonella* of the European Society of Clinical Microbiology and Infectious Diseases, whose definition is more restrictive than that of the CDC in requiring sequence determination for confirmation of PCR amplicons (Box 6.39.2).

Treatment

Tetracyclines are the reference drugs in treating human ehrlichioses and anaplasmosis but optimal duration of doxycycline treatment has yet to be determined. It is recommended that the treatment be continued for 7 to 10 days, or for at least 3 to 5 days after defervescence. Most patients become afebrile within 1 to 3 days following treatment. *E. chaffeensis* is susceptible *in vitro* to rifampicin (without *in vivo* evidence) but resistant to aminoglycosides, macrolides and ketolides, co-trimoxazole, penicillin, cephalosporin, chloramphenicol, and quinolones. *In vitro* resistance of *E. chaffeensis* to fluoroquinolone was strongly correlated with the presence of a specific amino acid variation in part of the protein sequence of the A subunit of *GyrA*. When antibiotic susceptibilities of eight strains of *A. phagocytophilum* collected in various geographical areas of the United States of America were tested *in vitro*, doxycycline and rifampicin proved the most active. Levofloxacin was also active.

Prevention

Currently, no vaccines are available, including the epidemic typhus vaccine developed in the past. Prevention is based first on avoiding

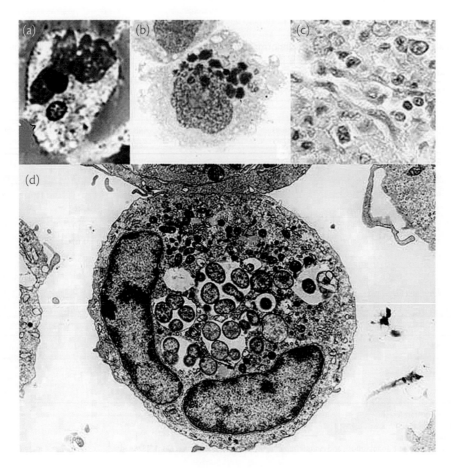

Fig. 6.39.10 *Anaplasma phagocytophilum* (a) in human peripheral blood band neutrophil (Wright's stain, original magnification ×1000), (b) in THP-1 myelomonocytic cell culture (LeukoStat stain, original magnification ×400),
(c) in neutrophils infiltrating human spleen (immunohistochemistry with haematoxylin counterstain, original magnification ×100), and
(d) ultrastructure by transmission electron microscopy in HL-60 cell culture (original magnification ×21 960).
(Courtesy of V Popov. From Dumler JS, *et al.* (2005). Human granulocytic anaplasmosis and *Anaplasma phagocytophilum. Emerg Infect Dis*, **1**, 1828–34, with permission.)

Box 6.39.2 Human granulocytic anaplasmosis (HGA) case definitions

Confirmed HGA

◆ Febrile illness with a history of a tick bite or tick exposure

and

◆ Demonstration of *A. phagocytophilum* infection by seroconversion or fourfold or more change in antibody titre (IFA)

or

◆ Positive PCR result (with subsequent sequencing of the amplicons demonstrating anaplasma-specific DNA in blood for European criteria)

or

◆ Isolation of *A. phagocytophilum* in blood culture

Probable HGA

◆ Febrile illness with a history of a tick bite or tick exposure

and

◆ Presence of stable titre of *A. phagocytophilum* antibodies in acute and convalescent sera if titre is more than 4 times above the cut-off value (IFA)

or

◆ Positive PCR result without sequencing confirmation

or

◆ Presence of intracytoplasmic morulae in a blood smear

(Bakken JS, Dumler JS (2006). Clinical diagnosis and treatment of human granulocytotropic anaplasmosis. *Ann N Y Acad Sci*, **1078**, 236–47; Brouqui P, *et al.* (2004). Guidelines for the diagnosis of tick-borne bacterial diseases in Europe. *Clin Microbiol Infect*, **10**, 1108–32)

---

arthropod bites. The best method for avoiding tick, flea, and chigger bites is topical *N,N*-diethyl-*m*-toluamide (DEET) repellent applied to exposed skin, and treatment of clothing (including army uniforms) with permethrin, which kills arthropods on contact. Those staying in infested area should routinely check their bodies for the presence of arthropods. Prompt tick removal using blunt rounded forceps is essential for the prevention of tick-borne illnesses. In the case of epidemic typhus, louse eradication (e.g. in refugee camps) is the most important preventive measure and is essential in the control of outbreaks. Since body lice live only in clothing, the simplest method of delousing is to remove and then destroy or wash and boil all clothing. Dusting of all clothing with insecticides kills body lice and reduces the risk of reinfestation. Weekly doxycycline, 200 mg, prevents scrub typhus, but the efficacy against rickettsial infections of doxycycline (100 mg daily), used for malaria chemoprophylaxis, is untested.

Likely future developments

Although they are among the oldest known vector-borne diseases, many new rickettsioses have emerged in recent years. What are the factors influencing their emergence and recognition? The role of the primary physician, including careful history taking and physical and laboratory examinations, has been emphasized, as it was essential for the description of some emerging SFG rickettsioses such as Flinders Island spotted fever, Japanese spotted fever, and Astrakhan fever. Molecular techniques have facilitated epidemiological studies of emerging human rickettsioses all over the world and, with the help of improved culture systems, have incriminated new species as causes of human diseases. People are undertaking more outdoor activities and tourism is developing in rural and remote areas, resulting in increased contact with arthropods and arthropod-borne rickettsial pathogens.

Changes in the host–vector ecology have influenced the emergence of HME, including increasing population densities and geographical distribution of *Amblyomma americanum*, increases in vertebrate host populations (wild turkeys, white-tailed deer) for this tick, the increases in reservoir host population for *E. chaffeensis* (e.g. white-tailed deer), increased human contact with natural foci of infection through recreational and occupational activities, the increased frequency or severity of disease in ageing or immunocompromised people, the increasing proportion of people older than 60 years of age, and immunocompromised people in the population in regions of enzootic infection, as well as available diagnostic procedures and improved surveillance and reporting. HME may occur outside the United States of America and numerous rickettsia, ehrlichia, or anaplasma species have been identified in arthropods, particularly ticks, throughout the world, although their pathogenicity for people has yet to be demonstrated. More studies throughout the world may lead to the description of emerging rickettsioses in the future.

Further reading

Bakken JS, Dumler JS (2006). Clinical diagnosis and treatment of human granulocytotropic anaplasmosis. *Ann N Y Acad Sci*, **1078**, 236–47.

Balraj P, *et al.* (2008). RickA expression is not sufficient to promote actin-based motility of *Rickettsia raoultii*. *PLoS ONE*, **3**, e2582.

Bechah Y, *et al.* (2008). Epidemic typhus. *Lancet Infect Dis*, **8**, 417–26.

Brouqui P, *et al.* (2004). Guidelines for the diagnosis of tick-borne bacterial diseases in Europe. *Clin Microbiol Infect*, **10**, 1108–32.

Chapman AS, *et al.* (2006). Rocky Mountain spotted fever in the United States, 1997–2002. *Vector Borne Zoonotic Dis*, **6**, 170–8.

Civen R, Ngo V (2008). Murine typhus: an unrecognized suburban vector-borne disease. *Clin Infect Dis*, **46**, 913–18.

Dantas-Torres F (2007). Rocky Mountain spotted fever. *Lancet Infect Dis*, **7**, 724–32.

Dumler JS, *et al.* (2005). Human granulocytic anaplasmosis and *Anaplasma phagocytophilum*. *Emerg Infect Dis*, **1**, 1828–34.

Dumler JS, *et al.* (2007). Ehrlichioses in humans: epidemiology, clinical presentation, diagnosis, and treatment. *Clin Infect Dis*, **45** Suppl 1, S45–51.

Dumler JS, *et al.* (2007). Human granulocytic anaplasmosis and macrophage activation. *Clin Infect Dis*, **45**, 199–204.

Fournier PE, Raoult D (2004). Suicide PCR on skin biopsy specimens for diagnosis of rickettsioses. *J Clin Microbiol*, **42**, 3428–34.

La Scola B Raoult D (1997). Laboratory diagnosis of rickettsioses: current approaches to diagnosis of old and new rickettsial diseases. *J Clin Microbiol*, **35**, 2715–27.

Lepidi H, Fournier PE, Raoult D (2006). Histologic features and immunodetection of African tick-bite fever eschar. *Emerg Infect Dis*, **12**, 1332–7.

Mouffok N, Parola P, Lepidi H, Raoult D (2009). Mediterranean spotted fever in Algeria–new trends. *Int J Infect Dis*, **13**, 227–35.

Paddock CD, *et al.* (2004). *Rickettsia parkeri*: a newly recognized cause of spotted fever rickettsiosis in the United States. *Clin Infect Dis*, **38**, 805–11.

Paddock CD, *et al.* (2006). Isolation of *Rickettsia akari* from eschars of patients with rickettsialpox. *Am J Trop Med Hyg*, **75**, 732–8.

Parola P, Raoult D (2001). Ticks and tickborne bacterial diseases in humans: an emerging infectious threat. *Clin Infect Dis*, **32**, 897–928. Erratum: *Clin Inf Dis*, **33**, 749.

Parola P, Paddock C, Raoult D (2005). Tick-borne rickettsioses around the world: emerging diseases challenging old concepts. *Clin Microbiol Rev*, **18**, 719–56.

Parola P, Rovery C, Rolain JM, Brouqui P, Davoust B, Raoult D (2009). *Rickettsia slovaca* and *R. raoultii* in tick-borne rickettsioses. *Emerg Infect Dis*, **15**, 1105–8.

Parola P, Socolovschi C, Jeanjean L, Bitam I, Fournier PE, Sotto A, Labauge P, Raoult D (2008). Warmer weather linked to tick attack and emergence of severe rickettsioses. *PLoS Negl Trop Dis*, **2**, e338.

Parola P, Socolovschi C, Raoult D (2009). Deciphering the relationships between *Rickettsia conorii conorii* and *Rhipicephalus sanguineus* in the ecology and epidemiology of Mediterranean spotted fever. *Ann N Y Acad Sci*, **1166**, 49–54.

Parola P, Labruna MB, Raoult D (2009). Tick-Borne Rickettsioses in America: Unanswered Questions and Emerging Diseases. *Curr Infect Dis Rep*, **11**, 40–50.

Pérez-Osorio CE, *et al.* (2008). *Rickettsia felis* as emergent global threat for humans. *Emerg Infect Dis*, **14**, 1019–23.

Raoult D, Parola P (2007). *Rickettsial diseases*. Informa Healthcare, New York.

Raoult D, Roux V (1999). The body louse as a vector of reemerging human diseases. *Clin Infect Dis*, **29**, 888–911.

Raoult D, Woodward T, Dumler JS (2004). The history of epidemic typhus. *Infect Dis Clin North Am*, **18**, 127–40.

Raoult D, *et al.* (1998). Outbreak of epidemic typhus associated with trench fever in Burundi. *Lancet*, **352**, 353–8.

Rikihisa Y (2006). New findings on members of the family Anaplasmataceae of veterinary importance. *Ann N Y Acad Sci*, **1078**, 438–45.

Roux V, Raoult D (1999). Body lice as tools for diagnosis and surveillance of reemerging diseases. *J Clin Microbiol*, **37**, 596–9.

Silveira I, *et al.* (2007). *Rickettsia parkeri* in Brazil. *Emerg Infect Dis*, **13**, 1111–13.

Vestris G, *et al.* (2003). Seven years' experience of isolation of *Rickettsia* spp. from clinical specimens using the shell-vial cell culture assay. *Ann NY Acad Sci*, **990**, 371–4.

Weissmann G (2005). Rats, lice, and Zinsser. *Emerg Infect Dis*, **11**, 492–6.

6.40 Scrub typhus

George Watt

Essentials

Scrub typhus (tsutsugamushi fever) is a zoonosis of rural Asia and the western Pacific islands that is caused by the obligate Gram-negative intracellular bacterium *Orientia* (formerly Rickettsia) *tsutsugamushi*, which is transmitted (typically from rats) to humans by the bite of a larval leptotrombidium mite (chigger). More than a billion people are at risk and more than a million cases are transmitted annually, making it the commonest rickettsial disease.

Clinical features—an eschar and regional lymphadenopathy often develop at the site of the chigger bite, and may by followed by a

systemic illness ranging in severity from inapparent to fatal. Many cases go undiagnosed, particularly those in which an eschar cannot be found. Diagnosis may be made serologically, but laboratory confirmation of infection is rarely available in rural areas where the disease is most frequently encountered. Aside from supportive care, treatment is with tetracycline, doxycycline, or chloramphenicol. Before antibiotics, mortality rates up to 35% were reported, but were generally much lower. Chemoprophylaxis with doxycycline can prevent infection. There is no vaccine.

Aetiology and epidemiology

Orientia tsutsugamushi differs in its cell wall structure and genetic makeup from rickettsiae, which it resembles under light microscopy. It is an obligate intracellular Gram-negative bacterium (Fig. 6.40.1). Infection with one of the multiple serotypes of *O. tsutsugamushi* confers transient cross-immunity to another. Scrub typhus is a zoonosis. Larval mites (of the *Leptotrombidium deliense* group) usually feed on small rodents, particularly wild rats of the subgenus *Rattus* (Fig. 6.40.2). Humans become infected when they accidentally encroach on a zone where there are infected mites (Fig. 6.40.3). These zones are often made up of secondary or 'scrub' growth, hence the term 'scrub typhus'. Infected chiggers are generally found in only very circumscribed foci within these zones. Large numbers of cases can occur when humans enter these so-called 'mite islands'. However, mite habitats as diverse as seashores and semideserts have been described. Many scrub typhus patients in south-east Asia are rice farmers. Disease transmission occurs when infected mites burrow into the skin, take a meal of tissue fluid, and inoculate the infectious organisms. Human-to-human transmission of scrub typhus via contaminated blood has never been documented. The endemic area forms a triangle of more than 5 million square miles bounded by northern Japan and south-eastern Siberia to the north, Queensland, Australia, to the south, and Pakistan to the west (Fig. 6.40.4). Increasing numbers of cases are being identified in India where, in the last few years, there

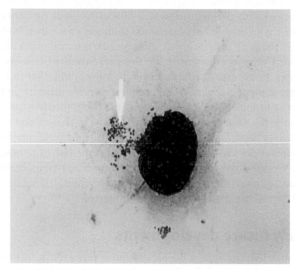

Fig. 6.40.1 Perinuclear clusters of Giemsa-stained *O. tsutsugamushi*.
(Courtesy of Dr Kriangrai Lerdthusnee, Department of Entomology, AFRIMS, Bangkok.)

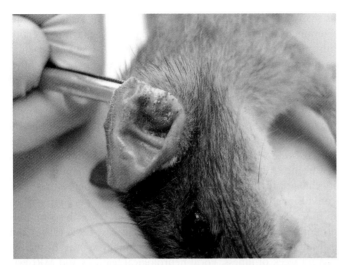

Fig. 6.40.2 Numerous reddish coloured chiggers attached to the earlobe of a wild rodent (*Rattus rattus*).
(Courtesy of Dr Kriangrai Lerdthusnee, Department of Entomology, AFRIMS, Bangkok.)

have been outbreaks with fatalities in Himachal Pradesh, Tamil Nadu, Meghalaya, Puducherry, Manipur, Nagaland, and Kerala. In one study from Vellore in Tamil Nadu, 47.5% of patients hospitalized for acute undifferentiated febrile illness were found to be suffering from scrub typhus. Disease transmission occurs in rural and suburban areas as well as in villages, but inhabitants of city centres are not at risk. In Thailand, *O. tsutsugamushi* Karp strain predominates with lower proportions of Gilliam and a single report of TA716.

Pathology and pathogenesis

Much remains unknown about the pathogenesis of scrub typhus, partly because most descriptions of severe cases pre-date advances made in immunohistology since the 1950s. Marked geographical variations in severity of the illness occur but determinants of severity are poorly characterized. Strains which differ in virulence, partial immunity, and regional differences in general health could affect disease presentation, but coinfection with the HIV-1 virus does not. Scrub typhus appears to be a vasculitis, but clinical and pathological findings do not correlate closely. The host cell of *O. tsutsugamushi* in humans has not been defined with certainty. The endothelial cell has been proposed because of findings in experimental animals and by analogy with other rickettsial diseases. However, in human liver infected with scrub typhus examined by electron microscopy, organisms predominate in Kupffer cells and hepatocytes rather than within endothelial cells. *O. tsutsugamushi* is present in peripheral white blood cells of patients with scrub typhus and is found within a variety of cell types. The HIV-1 viral load falls markedly in some AIDS patients who acquire acute *O. tsutsugamushi* infection, and sera from HIV-seronegative patients with scrub typhus inhibit HIV replication *in vitro*.

Clinical features

The painless chigger bite can occur on any part of the body, but is often in difficult to see in locations such as under the axilla or in the genital area. An eschar (Figs. 6.40.5, 6.40.6) forms at the bite site in about one-half of primary infections, but in a minority of secondary infections. The eschar begins as a small painless papule which develops during the 6- to 18-day (median 10 days) incubation period. It enlarges, undergoes central necrosis, and acquires a blackened scab to form a lesion resembling a cigarette burn. Regional lymph nodes are enlarged and tender. The eschar is usually well developed by the time fever appears and is often healing by the time the patient presents to hospital.

Fever, headache, myalgia, and nonspecific malaise are common symptoms. Hearing loss concurrent with fever is reported by

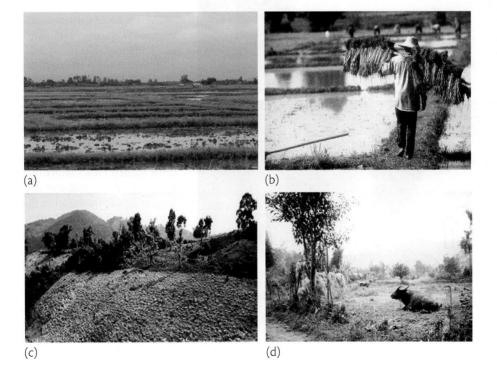

Fig. 6.40.3 Scrub typhus habitats.
(a) Transmission occurs in active rice fields. (b) Farmers intrude on the chigger–rodent cycle taking place on walkways between flooded fields. (c, d). Typical 'scrub' or secondary vegetation in Thailand.
(a, courtesy of Dr Kriangkrai Lerdthusnee, Department of Entomology, AFRIMS, Bangkok.)

(a)

(b)

(c)

(d)

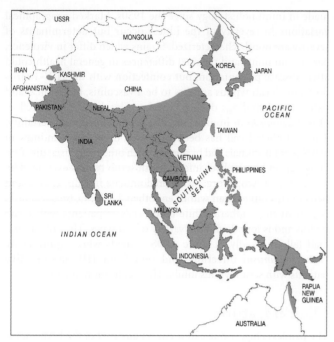

Fig. 6.40.4 Geographical distribution of scrub typhus.

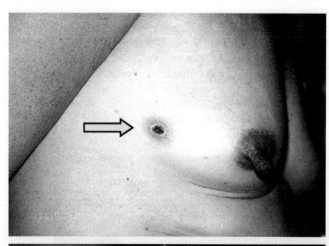

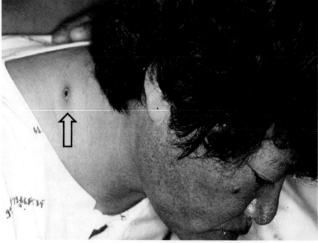

Fig. 6.40.5 Two typical eschars (blue arrows).

as many as one-third of patients and is a useful diagnostic clue. Conjunctival suffusion (Fig. 6.40.7) and generalized lymphadenopathy are common and helpful physical signs. A transient macular rash may appear at the end of the first week of illness but is often difficult to see (Fig. 6.40.8). The rash first appears on the trunk and becomes maculopapular as it spreads peripherally. Cough sometimes accompanied by bilateral reticular infiltrates on the chest radiograph is one of the commonest presentations of *O. tsutsugamushi* infection. In severe cases, tachypnoea progresses to dyspnoea, the patient becomes cyanotic, and full-blown acute respiratory distress syndrome (ARDS) may ensue. Apathy, confusion, and personality changes are not uncommon and only rarely progress to stupor, convulsions, and coma. Meningoencephalitis has been described in India, Taiwan, Korea, Japan, and Thailand. It was the commonest complication among children in north-east India (30%) and Taiwan (20%). Neurological symptoms usually appear during the second week of illness. Focal neurological features and MRI evidence of focal brain and spinal cord grey and white matter lesions have been observed. There may be a moderate mononuclear cell pleocytosis with mildly elevated protein and normal or slightly reduced glucose concentration. Meningoencephalitis was discovered at autopsy in almost all fatal cases including soldiers in the Second World War. Histopathological findings include diffuse or focal mononuclear cellular infiltration of the leptomeninges, typhus nodules (clusters of microglial cells), and cerebral haemorrhage. Abnormalities resolve completely in nonfatal cases.

Diagnosis

The eschar is the single most useful diagnostic clue and is pathognomonic when seen by a physician experienced in diagnosis of scrub typhus. Even typical eschars can be overlooked or misdiagnosed, however, and atypical presentations are common. Eschars in the genital area often lose their crust and can be confused with the ulcers of chancroid, syphilis, or lymphogranuloma venereum.

There is no constellation of laboratory test results which strongly suggests *O. tsutsugamushi* infection. Slight increases in the number of circulating white blood cells are common. Atypical lymphocytes and moderately elevated serum transaminase levels are not uncommon. Laboratory findings are chiefly useful to rule out other infections. A low white cell count and thrombocytopenia with a haemorrhagic rash suggest infection with dengue virus rather than *O. tsutsugamushi*. Haemorrhagic manifestations are more common in haemorrhagic fever with renal syndrome (HFRS) than in scrub typhus, and lumbar back pain, flank tenderness, and occult blood in urine suggest HFRS rather than *O. tsutsugamushi* infection. Raised serum creatinine and serum bilirubin levels with marked myalgia suggest leptospirosis rather than scrub typhus. Enteric fever rarely causes generalized lymphadenopathy or conjunctival suffusion.

Some occupations place individuals at increased risk of contracting not only *O. tsutsugamushi* infection but also other infections. For example, in Thailand most cases of scrub typhus and leptospirosis occur in rice farmers. Dual infections with scrub typhus and leptospirosis are not uncommon.

The Weil–Felix test using the proteus OXK antigen is a commercially available serodiagnostic test which has been used for many years, but is insensitive. The indirect immunofluorescent assay and the immunoperoxidase test are the confirmatory tests

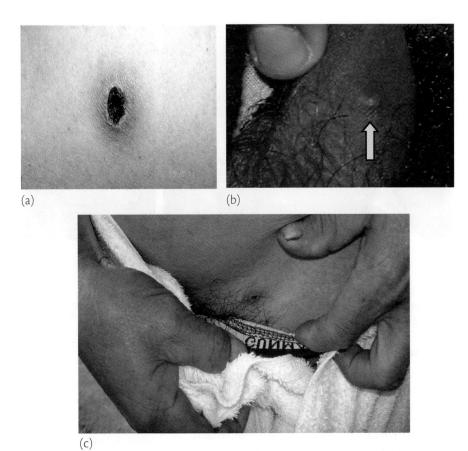

Fig. 6.40.6 Typical eschars (a) may be missed because they are located in difficult to examine areas (c). Eschars may be atypical and lose their crust in moist locales such as the scrotum (b). (b,c, courtesy of Dr Kriangkrai Lerdthusnee, Department of Entomology, AFRIMS, Bangkok.)

(a)   (b)   (c)

of choice but their complexity limits their use to a small number of reference centres. A rapid immunochromatographic test (ICT) showed high sensitivity and specificity in detection of *O. tsutsugamushi* IgM but for detection of total antibodies its specificity was much lower. Polymerase chain reaction (PCR) amplification of the *O. tsutsugamushi* 16S rRNA gene showed a diagnostic sensitivity and specificity of 44.8% and 99.7%, respectively, compared with IFA. Loop-mediated isothermal PCR assay (LAMP) targeting the

groEL gene, encoding the 60 kDa heat shock protein of *Orientia tsutsugamushi,* is a promising point of care method for diagnosing acute scrub typhus infection.

Treatment

Prompt antibiotic therapy shortens the course of the disease, lowers the risk of ARDS, and reduces mortality. Treatment must often be presumptive, but the benefits of avoiding severe scrub typhus by early antibiotic administration generally far outweigh the risks of a 1-week course of tetracycline, which is the treatment of choice. Either oral tetracycline 500 mg four times daily, or oral doxycycline 100 mg twice daily for 7 days is recommended. Oral chloramphenicol 500 mg four times a day is a cheaper alternative still widely used in endemic areas. Treatment for less than a week is initially curative, but may be followed by relapse. Parenteral doxycycline should be administered to patients who cannot swallow tablets or who are severely ill. In patients with meningoencephalitis, therapeutic levels of doxycycline may not be achieved when this drug is given orally or by nasogastric tube, especially if antacids are added. Parenteral chloramphenicol (50–75 mg/kg per day) is an alternative if parenteral tetracycline is unavailable.

Scrub typhus cases from northern Thailand which respond poorly to conventional therapy have been described, but neither the mechanism of resistance nor its geographical distribution have been defined. Scrub typhus has serious adverse effects on pregnancy but conventional therapy with tetracyclines or chloramphenicol for pregnant women and children poses problems.

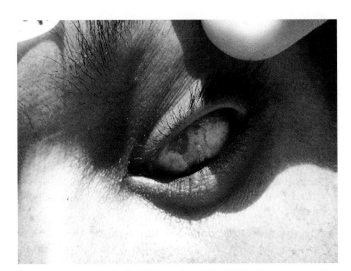

Fig. 6.40.7 Conjunctival suffusion in scrub typhus.

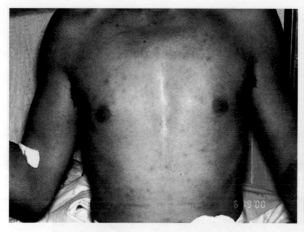
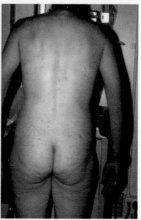

Fig. 6.40.8 The subtle rash of scrub typhus predominates on the trunk.

Both drug-sensitive and drug-resistant scrub typhus cases have been cured by azithromycin and this antibiotic appears to be the treatment of choice during pregnancy and early childhood.

Prevention and control

Weekly doses of 200 mg doxycycline can prevent *O. tsutsugamushi* infection. Chemoprophylaxis should be considered for nonimmune people sent to an enzootic area to perform work that places them at high risk of acquiring scrub typhus. Soldiers and road construction crews are typical examples, but chemoprophylaxis should also be considered in high-risk travellers such as trekkers. Contact with chiggers can be reduced by applying repellent to the tops of boots, socks, and on the lower trousers and by not sitting or lying directly on the ground. There is no vaccine for scrub typhus.

Prognosis

Scrub typhus was a dreaded disease in the preantibiotic era when case fatality rates reached as high as 50%. Prompt antibiotic therapy generally prevents death, but up to 15% of patients still die in northern Thailand. Deaths are attributed to a variety of factors including late presentation, delayed diagnosis, and drug resistance.

Further reading

Blacksell SD, *et al.* (2010). Accuracy of AccessBio immunoglobulin M and total antibody rapid immunochromatographic assays for the diagnosis of acute scrub typhus infection. *Clin Vaccine Immunol*, **17**, 263–6.

Dass R, *et al.* (2011). Characteristics of pediatric scrub typhus during an outbreak in the North Eastern region of India: peculiarities in clinical presentation, laboratory findings and complications. *Indian J Pediatr*, **78**, 1365–70.

Jeong YJ, *et al.* (2007). Scrub typhus: clinical, pathologic, and imaging findings. *Radiographics*, **27**, 161–72.

Kantipong P, *et al.* (1996). HIV infection does not influence the clinical severity of scrub typhus. *Clin Infect Dis*, **23**, 1168.

Kim DM, *et al.* (2011). Scrub typhus meningoencephalitis occurring during doxycycline therapy for *Orientia tsutsugamushi*. *Diagn Microbiol Infect Dis*, **69**, 271–4.

Olson JG, *et al.* (1980). Prevention of scrub typhus. Prophylactic administration of doxycycline in a randomized double blind trial. *Am J Trop Med Hyg*, **29**, 989.

Paris DH, *et al.* (2011). Diagnostic accuracy of a loop-mediated isothermal PCR assay for detection of *Orientia tsutsugamushi* during acute scrub typhus infection. *PLoS Negl Trop Dis*, **5**, e1307.

Silpapojakul K, *et al.* (1991). Rickettsial meningitis and encephalitis. *Arch Intern Med*, **151**, 1753–7.

Sonthayanon P, *et al.* (2006). Rapid diagnosis of scrub typhus in rural Thailand using polymerase chain reaction. *Am J Trop Med Hyg*, **75**, 1099–102.

Watt G, *et al.* (1996). Scrub typhus infections poorly responsive to antibiotics in northern Thailand. *Lancet*, **348**, 86–9.

Watt G, *et al.* (2003). HIV-1 suppression during acute scrub typhus infection. *Lancet*, **356**, 475–9.

Yum KS, *et al.* (2011). Scrub typhus meningo-encephalitis with focal neurologic signs and associated brain MRI abnormal findings: literature review. *Clin Neurol Neurosurg*, **113**, 250–3.

6.41 *Coxiella burnetii* infections (Q fever)

T.J. Marrie

Essentials

Q fever is a zoonosis caused by *Coxiella burnetii*, an intracellular Gram-negative spore-forming bacterium, the common animal reservoirs of which are cattle, sheep, and goats, although in a large outbreak in the Netherlands it appears that rats, *Rattus norvegicus* and *R. rattus*, may have played a role in the spread of the condition. *C. burnetii* is trophic for the endometrium and mammary glands of female animals, and during pregnancy the organism reaches very high concentrations in the placenta such that at the time of parturition organisms are aerosolized and contamination of the environment occurs. Inhalation of even one microorganism can result in infection.

Clinical features—there are two main forms of the disease: (1) acute—can present as inapparent infection, self-limited febrile illness, pneumonia, and hepatitis, or less commonly with a variety of organ-specific manifestations such as encephalitis, pericarditis, and pancreatitis; Q fever in pregnancy may be associated with unfavorable outcomes but recent data indicate the rate of unfavorable outcomes may be considerably less than previously thought. (2) Chronic—most often 'culture-negative' endocarditis or infection of aortic aneurysms, but occasionally osteomyelitis.

Diagnosis, treatment, and prevention—diagnosis is confirmed by serological testing: in acute disease antibodies to phase II antigen are higher than those to phase I, whereas the reverse is true in chronic disease. Acute Q fever is treated with doxycyline or a quinolone; chronic disease with long-term doxycycline and hydroxychloroquine; and Q fever in pregnancy with co-trimoxazole for the duration of the pregnancy and—for those with a chronic Q fever serological profile—1 year of doxycycline and hydroxyochloroquine after delivery. Vaccination should be offered to those whose occupation places them at high risk for *C. burnetii* infection.

History

In August 1935, Dr Edward Holbrook Derrick, Director of the Laboratory of Microbiology and Pathology of the Queensland Health Department in Brisbane, Australia, was asked to investigate an outbreak of undiagnosed febrile illness among workers at the Cannon Hill abattoir. Derrick realized that he was dealing with a type of fever that had not been previously described—he named it Q (for query) fever. Two years later, Sir Frank Macfarlane Burnet in Australia and Herald Rea Cox in the United States of America isolated the microorganism responsible for Q fever.

Coxiella burnetii

This microorganism, the sole species of its genus, has a Gram-negative cell wall and measures $0.3 \times 0.7\,\mu m$ (Fig. 6.41.1). It is an obligate phagolysosomal parasite of eukaryotes that sporulates, stains well with Gimenez's stain, and multiplies by transverse binary fission. *C. burnetii* undergoes phase variation akin to the smooth to rough transition in some enteric Gram-negative bacilli. In nature and laboratory animals it exists in the phase I state. Repeated passage of phase I virulent organisms in embryonated chicken eggs leads to the conversion from phase I virulent to phase II avirulent forms. Antibodies to phase I antigens predominate in chronic Q fever, while phase II antibodies are higher than phase I antibodies in acute Q fever. The genome of *C. burnetii* strain Nine Mile Phase I has 1 995 275 base pairs. There are many genes with potential roles in adhesion, invasion, intracellular trafficking, host-cell modulation, and detoxification. *C. burnetii* can now be grown in a cell-free medium, an advance that should lead to further insight into this complex microorganism.

Immune control of *C. burnetii* is T-cell dependent and it does not eliminate *C. burnetii* from infected humans. In 80 to 90% of bone marrow aspirates from those who have recovered from Q fever, polymerase chain reaction (PCR) assays for *C. burnetii* DNA are positive. The use of microarrays allows insight into the complexity of the host microorganism interaction in illnesses such as Q fever. In one such experiment 335 genes in the *C. burnetii*-infected human monocytic leukaemia cell line THP-1 were up- or down-regulated at least twofold.

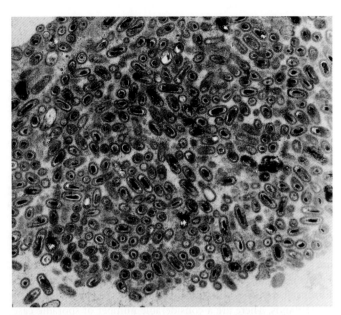

Fig. 6.41.1 Transmission electron micrograph showing *C. burnetii* cells within a macrophage in the heart valve of a patient with Q fever endocarditis. The dark material in the centre of each cell is condensed DNA. Magnification ×15 000.

C. burnetii has survived for 586 days in tick faeces at room temperature, 160 days or more in water, 30 to 40 days in dried cheese made from contaminated milk, and up to 150 days in soil.

Epidemiology

Q fever is a zoonosis. There is an extensive wildlife and arthropod (mainly ticks) reservoir of *C. burnetii*. Domestic animals are infected through inhaling contaminated aerosols or by ingesting infected material. These animals rarely become ill, but abortion and stillbirths may occur. *C. burnetii* localizes in the uterus and mammary glands of infected animals. During pregnancy there is reactivation of *C. burnetii* and it multiplies in the placenta, reaching 10^9 infective doses per gram of tissue. The organisms are shed into the environment at the time of parturition. Humans becomes infected after inhaling organisms aerosolized at the time of parturition, or later when organisms in dust are stirred up on a windy day. Infections have occurred up to 18 km downwind from a source. Infected cattle, sheep, goats, and cats are the animals primarily responsible for transmitting *C. burnetii* to humans. There have been several outbreaks of Q fever in hospitals and research institutes due to the transportation of infected sheep to research laboratories. Some studies have suggested that ingestion of contaminated milk is a risk factor for the acquisition of Q fever; volunteers seroconverted but did not become ill after ingesting contaminated milk.

Percutaneous infection, such as when an infected tick is crushed between the fingers, may occur but is rare. Transmission via a contaminated blood transfusion has rarely occurred. Vertical transmission from mother to child has been infrequently reported. A 1988 review documents 23 cases of Q fever in pregnant women. The authors found that Q fever was present in 1 in 540 pregnancies in an area of endemic Q fever in southern France. Person-to-person transmission has been documented on a few occasions.

To date, 45 countries on five continents have reported cases of Q fever. Q fever is estimated to cost $A1 million in Australia each year and results in the loss of more than 1700 weeks of work.

There are several studies where young age seems to be protective of infection with *C. burnetii*. In a large outbreak of Q fever in Switzerland, symptomatic infection was 5 times more likely to occur in those over 15 years of age compared with those younger than 15. In many outbreaks of Q fever, men were affected more commonly than women. It had been assumed that this was due to the fact that certain occupations in which men predominate were more likely to be associated with Q fever. However, in France, despite similar exposures, the male to female ratio is 2.45 to 1. The explanation for this gender difference is that female sex hormones are protective against Q fever infection.

Currently Q fever is common in several European countries with ongoing outbreaks in Germany and the Netherlands. There are a considerable number of sporadic cases of Q fever in England, France, and Spain. Currently Q fever is common in several European countries with ongoing outbreaks in Germany and the Netherlands. There are a considerable number of sporadic cases of Q fever in England, France, and Spain. The outbreak in the Netherlands is the largest to date, with over 4000 cases from 2007 to 2010, and many lessons can be learned from it. In 2007 a total of 168 individual human Q fever cases were notified, occurring after visits to dairy farms with abortion problems. The outbreak was concentrated around a single village, where a case-control study found that contact with manure, hay, and straw were risk factors. Moreover, people living in the eastern part of the village close to ruminant farms, one of which was a dairy goat farm with a recent history of abortion problems, were at higher risk than people living in other parts of the village. In 2008, 1000 human cases were notified, with average age 51 years (range 7–87 years), and 21% were hospitalized. In April 2009 a further sharp increase in human cases was observed, resulting in the total number of 2355. For patients reported in 2008 from whom clinical details were available, 545 were diagnosed with pneumonia, 33 with hepatitis, and 115 with other febrile illness. The gender ratio was 1 female to 1.7 males. In general, 59% of the notified human cases in 2009 lived within a 5-km zone around the notified dairy goat, dairy sheep farm, while 12% of the Dutch population lived within such as zones. Genotyping of *C. burnetii* isolates found that one unique genotype predominated in dairy goat herds and one sheep herd, and this genotype was similar to the human isolates.

Clinical features

Humans are the only species known consistently to develop illness following infection with *C. burnetii*. There is an incubation period of about 2 weeks (range 2–29 days) following inhalation of *C. burnetii*. A dose–response effect has been demonstrated experimentally and clinically. *C. burnetii* is one of the most infectious agents known; a single microorganism is able to initiate infection in humans. The resulting illness can be divided into acute and chronic varieties.

Acute Q fever

Self-limiting febrile illness

The most common manifestation of acute Q fever is a self-limiting febrile illness that is dismissed as a 'cold'. Serosurveys reveal that in most endemic areas 5 to 10% of the population have antibodies to *C. burnetii* but never remember the illness that resulted in seroconversion.

Q fever pneumonia

This is the most commonly recognized manifestation of Q fever. There is often a seasonal distribution, most of the cases occurring between February and May (consistent with the birthing season in the small ruminant reservoirs). The onset is nonspecific with fever, fatigue, and headache. The headache may be very severe, occasionally so severe that it prompts a lumbar puncture. A dry cough of mild to moderate intensity is present in 24 to 90% of patients. About one-third of patients have pleuritic chest pain. Nausea, vomiting, and diarrhoea occur in 10 to 30% of patients. Most cases of *C. burnetii* pneumonia are mild; however, about 10% are severe enough to require admission to hospital and, rarely, assisted ventilation is necessary. Death is rare in Q fever pneumonia and is usually due to comorbid illness. The white blood cell count is usually normal, but is elevated in one-third of patients. Liver enzyme levels may be mildly elevated at 2 to 3 times normal. Alkaline phosphatase is raised in up to 70% of patients and 28% are hyponatraemic. Reactive thrombocytosis is surprisingly common and microscopic haematuria is a common finding.

The chest radiographic manifestations of Q fever pneumonia are usually indistinguishable from those of other bacterial pneumonias (Fig. 6.41.2); however, rounded opacities are suggestive of this infection (Fig. 6.41.3). Some investigators have reported delayed clearing of the pneumonia; however, in our experience resolution is usually complete within 3 weeks.

Hepatitis

The liver is probably involved in all patients with acute Q fever. There are three clinical pictures:

- Pyrexia of unknown origin with mild to moderate elevation of liver function tests.

- A hepatitis-like picture: liver biopsy shows distinctive doughnut granulomas consisting of a granuloma with a central lipid vacuole and fibrin deposits. Prolonged fever unresponsive to antibiotics is common in these patients.

- 'Incidental hepatitis'.

Q fever in pregnancy

Acute Q fever occasionally complicates pregnancy. In 23 published cases 35% had premature birth, and 43% ended in abortion or neonatal death. In a serosurvey of 4588 pregnant women in Halifax, Nova Scotia, Canada, women seropositive for *C. burnetii* were 3 times more likely to have a current or previous neonatal death. Data from a large outbreak of Q fever in the Netherlands indicate that unfavorable outcomes due to Q fever during pregnancy are much lower than cited above from case reports.

Neurological manifestations

Encephalitis, encephalomyelitis, toxic confusional states, optic neuritis, and demyelinating polyradiculoneuritis are uncommon manifestations of Q fever.

Rare manifestations

These include myocarditis, pericarditis including constrictive pericarditis, bone marrow necrosis, rhabdomyolysis, glomerulonephritis, lymphadenopathy, pancreatitis, splenic rupture, acalculous cholecystitis, mesenteric panniculitis, erythema nodosum, epididymitis, orchitis, priapism, and erythema annulare centrifugum. Chronic fatigue may be a sequel of Q fever in some patients.

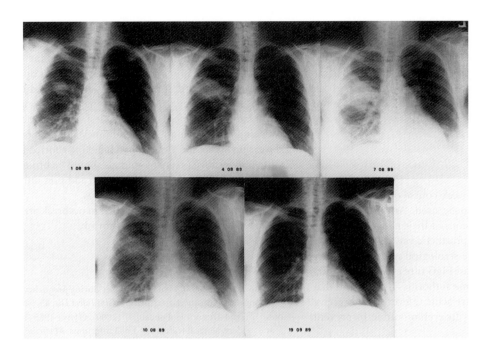

Fig. 6.41.2 Serial chest radiographs of a 35-year-old patient with Q fever pneumonia. The first radiograph (1 August 1989) shows a round opacity in the right upper lobe, which increases in size over the next 6 days. The pneumonia has completely cleared by 19 September 1989.

Chronic Q fever

The usual manifestation of chronic Q fever is that of culture-negative endocarditis. Some 70% of these patients have fever and nearly all have abnormal native or prosthetic heart valves. Hepatomegaly and or splenomegaly occur in about one-half of these patients and one-third have finger clubbing. A purpuric rash due to immune complex-induced leucocytoclastic vasculitis and arterial embolism occurs in about 20% of patients. Hyperglobulinaemia (up to 60 g/litre) is common and is a useful clue to chronic Q fever in a patient with the clinical picture of culture-negative endocarditis.

Other manifestations of chronic Q fever include osteomyelitis, infection of aortic aneurysm, and infection of vascular prosthetic grafts.

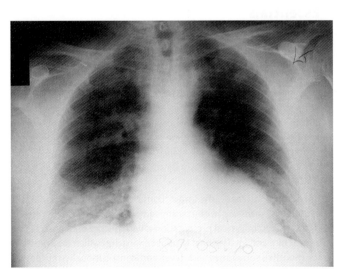

Fig. 6.41.3 Portable anteroposterior chest radiograph of a 72-year-old man with Q fever pneumonia. This radiographic picture is indistinguishable from pneumonia due to any other microbial agent.

The strains of *C. burnetii* that cause chronic Q fever do not differ from those that cause acute Q fever. Peripheral blood lymphocytes from patients with Q fever endocarditis are unresponsive to *C. burnetii* antigens *in vitro*, while responding normally to other antigens.

Diagnosis

A strong clinical suspicion based on the epidemiology and clinical features as outlined above is the cornerstone of the diagnosis of Q fever. This suspicion is confirmed by determining a fourfold or greater increase in antibody titre between acute and 2- to 3-week convalescent serum samples. A variety of serological tests are available including complement fixation, microimmunofluorescence, and enzyme immunoassay. The immunofluorescence antibody test is the best test. In acute Q fever the antibody titre to phase II antigen is higher than that to phase I antigen, while the reverse occurs in chronic Q fever. In chronic Q fever, antibody phase I titres are extremely high, in the order of 1:8192 and higher. In acute Q fever, antibody titres to phase I antigen are rarely in excess of 1:512 (usually 1:8 to 1:32), while peak antibody titres to phase II antigen are between 1:1024 and 1:2048. The microorganism can be isolated in embryonated eggs or in tissue culture; however, a biosafety level 3 laboratory is required. The PCR can be used to amplify *C. burnetii* DNA from tissues or other biological specimens.

Good laboratory practice, with known positive and negative controls is extremely important in the diagnosis of Q fever. Three different laboratories (in France, the United Kingdom, and Australia) tested the same serum samples using an IFA test. However, the antigen used in the test differed in each laboratory—Nine Mile strain in France; Nine Mile strain clone 4 as phase II antigen and Henzerling strain as phase 1 antigen in Australia; patient Lane strain ST 12 group for phase 1 and II antigens in the United Kingdom. Concordance was only 35%. The Australian and United Kingdom results had the greatest concordance and French and United Kingdom results the lowest. Serological testing revealed no chronic serological profiles when tested in either France or Australia but 10 when tested in the United Kingdom. Serological results from a patient with treated Q fever endocarditis suggested treated (France), chronic (United Kingdom), and borderline chronic (Australia) infection. How the antigens were prepared can also make a difference in the test results, and this paper does not indicate whether the strains were grown in tissue culture or egg yolk sac.

Treatment

Acute Q fever is treated with a 2-week course of tetracycline or doxycycline. Quinolones can also be used. Any patients who develop acute Q fever and have lesions of their native valves (e.g. congenital bicuspid aortic valve), prosthetic valves, or prosthetic intravascular material should have serological monitoring every 4 months for 2 years, and if the phase I IgG titre exceeds 1:800 further investigation is warranted. Some authorities recommend that patients with valvulopathy who have acute Q fever should receive 12 months of doxycycline and hydroxychloroquine to prevent chronic Q fever.

The duration of treatment for chronic Q fever is determined by monitoring the serum antibody titres to *C. burnetii*, although some authorities recommend lifelong therapy for chronic Q fever. In general, antibiotics can be discontinued when the IgA antibody titre to phase I antigen is less than 1:200. The treatment of choice for chronic Q fever is doxycycline 100 mg twice daily and hydroxychloroquine 200 mg three times daily to maintain a plasma level of between 0.8 and 1.2 µg/ml. This regimen is given for 18 months. Photosensitivity is a potential adverse reaction and patients should be warned to take preventive measures. In addition, an ophthalmologist must examine the optic fundus every 6 months for chloroquine accumulation. We have used rifampicin 300 mg twice a day and ciprofloxacin 750 mg twice a day to treat patients with chronic Q fever. Rifampicin and doxycycline or tetracycline and trimethoprim/sulfamethoxazole have also been used to treat chronic Q fever. Antibody titres should be measured every 6 months for the first 2 years. A progressive decline in antibody titre reflects the successful treatment of chronic fever. Cardiac valve replacement may be necessary as part of the management of chronic Q fever.

Many patients with granulomatous hepatitis due to Q fever have a prolonged febrile illness that does not respond to antibiotics. For these individuals treatment with prednisone 0.5 mg/kg has resulted in defervescence within 2 to 15 days. Once defervescence has occurred the dose of steroids is tapered over the next month.

Q fever occurring during pregnancy should be treated with co-trimoxazole for the duration of the pregnancy. In one retrospective study this approach reduced obstetrical complications from 81 to 44%. There were no intrauterine fetal deaths in the co-trimoxazole-treated group. Those with a chronic Q fever serological profile should be treated with doxycycline and hydroxychloroquine for 1 year following delivery.

Prevention

A formalin-inactivated *C. burnetii* whole-cell vaccine is protective against infection and has a low rate of side effects; 1% of vaccinees developed an abscess at the inoculation site and another 1% had a lump at this site 2 months after vaccination. The vaccine should be offered to those whose occupation places them at high risk for *C. burnetii* infection.

Good animal husbandry practices are important in preventing widespread contamination of the environment by *C. burnetii*. Prevention of zoonotic spread is best accomplished by isolating aborting animals for up to 14 days, raising feeding troughs to prevent contamination of feed by excreta, destroying aborted materials by burning and burying fetal membranes and stillborn animals, and wearing masks and gloves when handling aborted materials.

Only seronegative pregnant animals should be brought into the facilities where research is to be done. In addition only seronegative animals should be used in petting zoos.

Blood donation should be suspended in outbreak areas for up to 4 weeks following cessation of the outbreak.

Further reading

Carcopino X, *et al.* (2007). Managing Q fever during pregnancy: the benefits of long-term cotrimoxazole therapy. *Clin Infect Dis*, **45**, 548–55.

Raoult D, Tissot-Dupont H, Foucault C (2000). Q fever 1985–1998: clinical and epidemiological features of 1,383 infections. *Medicine (Baltimore)*, **79**, 110–23.

Raoult D, *et al.* (1999). Treatment of Q fever endocarditis: comparison of 2 regimens containing doxycycline and ofloxacin or hydroxychloroquine. *Arch Intern Med*, **159**, 167–73.

Roest HIJ, *et al.* (2011). The Q fever epidemic in the Netherlands: history, onset, response and reflection. *Epidemiol Infect*, **139**, 1–12.

6.42 Bartonellas excluding *B. bacilliformis*

Emmanouil Angelakis, Didier Raoult, and Jean-Marc Rolain

Essentials

Bartonella species are Gram-negative bacilli or coccobacilli belonging to the α2 subgroup of Proteobacteria that are closely related to the genera *Brucella* and *Agrobacterium*. Each persists in particular mammalian hosts, with transmission to humans primarily mediated by haematophagous arthropods. A remarkable feature of the genus *Bartonella* is the ability of a single species to cause either acute or chronic infection with either vascular, proliferative, or suppurative features, the pathological response to infection varying substantially with the host's immunocompetence.

Clinical features

Cat-scratch disease—the most common *Bartonella* zoonosis, caused by *B. henselae*, with transmission usually occurring directly by a cat scratch. Typical presentation is with history of a cat scratch and/or bite and locoregional lymphadenopathy (which may persist for months), sometimes with fever and constitutional symptoms. A few cases present with severe systemic symptoms indicating

disseminated infection. Encephalopathy and neuroretinitis are uncommon manifestations.

Trench fever—caused by *B. quintana*; transmitted by the body louse; typically presents as an acute febrile illness often accompanied by severe headache and pain in the long bones of the legs.

Bacillary angiomatosis—caused by *B. henselae* or *B. quintana*, particularly in immunocompromised patients (mainly those with HIV infection); presents with the gradual appearance of numerous brown to violaceous or colourless vascular tumours of the skin and subcutaneous tissues.

Bacillary peliosis—reported in immunosuppressed patients infected with *B. henselae*; causes vascular proliferation in solid internal organs with reticuloendothelial elements, particularly the liver (peliosis hepatis).

Bacteraemia and endocarditis—'culture-negative' and usually caused by *B. quintana* or *B. henselae*; patients with abnormal heart valves and those with chronic alcohol abuse are at particular risk.

Diagnosis, treatment, and prevention

Diagnosis—this is difficult because of the fastidious nature of bartonella and the nonspecific clinical manifestations; diagnostic techniques include culture from blood and other tissues, detection of organisms in lymph nodes by immunofluorescence, PCR amplification of bartonella genes, and serology.

Treatment—bartonella is susceptible to many antibiotics when grown in the laboratory, but this correlates poorly with *in vivo* efficacy. General recommendations are as follows: (1) cat-scratch disease—symptomatic treatment only, with azithromycin in severe or complicated cases; (2) trench fever—combination of doxycycline with gentamicin; (3) bacillary angiomatosis or peliosis—erythromycin; (4) endocarditis—gentamicin with ceftriaxone with or without doxycycline.

Prevention—*B. quintana* infections can be prevented by delousing, changing, or washing clothes. Immunocompromised patients should avoid contact with cats and cat fleas.

Historical perspective

Until 1990 the genus *Bartonella* contained only two species, *B. bacilliformis*, the cause of Carrión's disease (Chapter 6.43), and *B. quintana*, the cause of trench fever. In 1993, following the proposal of Brenner *et al.* based on comparison of 16S rDNA gene sequences, *Rochalimaea* spp. have been reclassified within the family Bartonellaceae and the genus *Bartonella*. In 1995, Birtles and colleagues proposed the unification of the genus *Grahamella* within the genus *Bartonella*. Numerous other *Bartonella* species have been described in humans and several other species. Human infections due to *Bartonella* species include old and newly described human infections. *Bartonella quintana* infection of humans was first described during the First World War as being responsible for trench fever, which caused more than 1 million deaths. Cat-scratch disease (CSD) was initially described in 1931 in France by Debré *et al.* but the aetiological agent (*B. henselae*) was first identified in 1992 and its role in bacillary angiomatosis was demonstrated using molecular methods.

Aetiology, genetics, pathogenesis, and pathology

The bacteria of the genus *Bartonella* are short, pleomorphic, fastidious aerobes that are oxidase and catalase negative. They are closely related phylogenetically to the genera *Brucella*, *Agrobacterium*, and *Rhizobium*. The 1.6-Mb genome of *B. quintana* was found to be a derivate of the 1.9-Mb genome of *B. henselae*. Prophages and horizontally acquired genomic islands have been identified in *B. henselae*, but are absent from *B. quintana*. It has been recently demonstrated that type IV secretion system located on plasmid in bartonella may act as a powerful system to transfer genes laterally between bacteria living in a sympatric lifestyle in amoeba. Because no distinguishing phenotypic characteristics have been described for bartonella species, their identification and phylogenetic classification have been based mainly on genetic studies. Many DNA regions and encoding gene sequences have been used, including the 16S rDNA gene, 16S–23S rRNA intergenic spacer region (ITS), citrate synthase gene (*gltA*), heat shock protein gene (*groEL*), genes encoding the PAP31 and 35-kDa proteins, and cell division protein gene (*ftsZ*). A phylogenetic neighbour-joining tree resulting from comparison of sequences of the concatenated genes of bartonella species is shown in Fig. 6.42.1. According to La Scola *et al.*, a new *Bartonella* isolate can be considered a new species if a 327-bp *gltA* fragment shares less than 96% sequence similarity with the existing species and if an 825-bp *rpoB* fragment shares less than 94% sequence similarity with the validated species. Bartonella are considered intracellular bacteria that target endothelial or red blood cells, resulting in a long-lasting intraerythrocytic bacteraemia and angiogenesis. The intraerythrocytic localization of bartonella has been demonstrated in several hosts (Table 6.42.1). Although intraerythrocytic infection by bartonella is host-specific, these pathogens can cause localized tissue manifestations in both reservoir and incidentally infected host(s). Bartonella species have the ability to colonize vascular tissues, which is considered to be a crucial step in the establishment of vasoproliferative lesions by *B. henselae* and *B. quintana* (bacillary angiomatosis and bacillary peliosis).

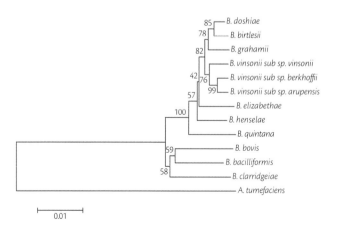

Fig. 6.42.1 Neighbour-joining tree based on the combined RNase P RNA, 16S and 23S rRNA sequence alignment.

Table 6.42.1 Species of *Bartonella* reported to date: epidemiological and clinical data

Bartonella spp.	Reservoir host	Vector detection in arthropods	Disease in humans	First cultivation	Detection in erythrocytes
B. bacilliformis	Human	Sand fly (*Lutzomyia* spp.)	CSD, END	1919	+
B. talpae	Mole	Unknown	Unknown	1911	
B. peromysci	Unknown	Unknown	Unknown	1942	
B. vinsonii subsp. *vinsonii*	Rodents	Unknown	Unknown	1946	
B. quintana	Human, cats	Human body lice and fleas	TF, BA, BAC, END	1961	+
B. henselae	Cats, rats, dogs	Fleas (*Ctenocephalides felis*)	CSD, BA, BAC, LMF, END, PH, RET	1990	+
B. elizabethae	Rodents, dogs	Fleas	END (1 case)	1993	
B. grahamii	Voles, rodents	Fleas?	RET (1 case)	1995	
B. taylorii	Rats	Fleas?	Unknown	1995	
B. doshiae	Voles	Fleas?	Unknown	1995	
B. clarridgeiae	Cats, dogs	*Ctenocephalides felis*	Unknown	1995	+
B. vinsonii subsp. *berkhoffii*	Dogs, coyotes, grey foxes	Fleas and ticks	END	1995	
B. vinsonii subsp. *arupensis*	Rodents, cattle	Deer ticks	BAC (1 case)	1999	
B. tribocorum	Rats	Unknown	Unknown	1998	
B. koehlerae	Cats	Fleas	END (1 case)	1999	+
B. alsatica	Rabbit	Fleas or ticks	END (2 cases) LMF (1 case)	1999	
B. bovis (*weissii*)	Cows, cats	Unknown	Unknown	1999	
B. washoensis	Rodents, dogs	Unknown	MYOC (1 case)	2000	
B. birtlesii	Rats	Unknown	Unknown	2000	
B. schoenbuchensis	Wild roe deer	Unknown	Unknown	2001	
B. capreoli	Wild roe deer	Unknown	Unknown	2002	
B. chomelii	Cows	Unknown	Unknown	2004	
B. rattimassiliensis	Rats	Unknown	Unknown	2004	
B. phoceensis	Rats	Unknown	Unknown	2004	

BA, bacillary angiomatosis; BAC, bacteraemia; CSD, cat-scratch disease; END, endocarditis; LMF, lymphadenopathy; MYOC, myocarditis; PH: peliosis hepatis; RET, retinitis; TF, trench fever.

Epidemiology

The most common *Bartonella* infection worldwide is CSD, caused by *B. henselae*. Human cases have been reported from several continents, including North America, Europe, and Australia, and from most countries where investigators looked for that infection. These bacteria are the most common bartonellas detected in cats worldwide and are highly prevalent. Transmission from cat to human mainly occurs directly by a cat scratch and possibly by a cat bite or possibly by cat flea or tick bite. Flea faeces may be the only infected material that can be inoculated by a cat scratch. Other *Bartonella* species have been detected in cat fleas (*B. clarridgeiae*, *B. koehlerae*, and *B. quintana*), and in rabbit fleas (*B. alsatica*).

B. quintana infections are transmitted by the body louse *Pediculus humanus*. Outbreaks of trench fever are linked mainly with poor socioeconomic conditions and wars, which predispose to body louse infestation. *B. quintana* infections decreased after the First World War and re-emerged during the Second World War. There have been sporadic outbreaks in Europe and the United States of America in poor people and alcoholics. *B. quintana* has been recently detected in head louse nits of a homeless man.

The epidemiology of the other *Bartonella* species is not well understood. They can cause asymptomatic bacteraemia in reservoir hosts: *B. henselae* and *B. clarridgeiae* in cats, *B. bovis* in cattle, *B. alsatica* in rabbits, and *B. tribocorum* in rats (Fig. 6.42.2).

Clinical features

A remarkable feature of bartonella is the ability of a single species to cause either acute or chronic infection with either vascular proliferative or suppurative features. The pathological response to infection with bartonella varies substantially with the host's immune status. There have been few clinical studies employing a standard case definition, culture confirmation, and rigidly defined

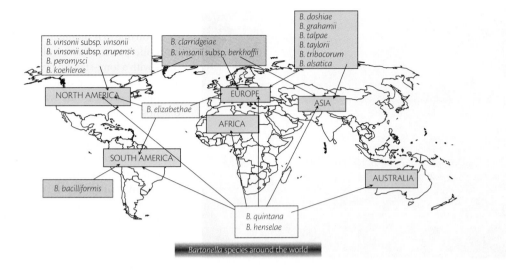

Fig. 6.42.2 *Bartonella* species isolated around the world.

disease outcomes in patients with similar immunocompetence. Therapeutic recommendations are often based on a few subjects.

Trench fever

Trench fever is also known as quintan fever, Wolhynia fever (because the disease was first observed by German medical officers on the East German front in Wolhynia), and 5-day fever (because of its tendency to relapse on the fifth day). After the bite of the body louse the incubation period ranges from 15 to 25 days, but in volunteers inoculated with a large volume of crushed infected lice it was less than 9 days. The illness varies from asymptomatic to severe. The classic clinical presentation among troops was an acute febrile illness, often accompanied by severe headache and pain in the long bones of the legs. The interval between attacks of pyrexia ranges from 4 to 8 days, but is usually 5 days. Trench fever often results in prolonged disability, but no fatalities have been recorded. The first 4 to 6 weeks of the illness are the most severe and, in a few cases, chronic fever, anaemia, loss of weight, and neuropsychiatric symptoms develop.

Cat-scratch disease (CSD)

CSD is a common infection. Cats are the main reservoir of *B. henselae*, and the bacterium may be transmitted between cats by the cat flea *Ctenocephalides felis*. Depending on the clinical manifestations, CSD has been characterized in two forms: classic typical clinical CSD with lymphadenopathy and a history of a cat scratch and/or bite, and atypical CSD. Classic CSD usually occurs in children and young adults but may also affect elderly people. Most patients with typical CSD remain afebrile. The main clinical manifestations in an immunocompetent host appear approximately 2 weeks after inoculation, although *B. henselae* DNA can be isolated from the peripheral blood of patients as long as 4 months after infection. One-third of the patients present with a history of fever lasting from 0 to 70 days (mean 14.8 days) with a maximum temperature between 37.9 and 42.0° C. The localization of lymphadenopathy is mainly axillary, cervical, or submaxillary, i.e. the lymph nodes that usually drain the area where the cat scratch occurs (Fig. 6.42.3). Lymphadenopathy may sometimes last for months, and in a few cases can be prolonged for as long as 12 to 24 months. General symptoms including malaise, headache, convulsion, sore throat, otalgia, vomiting, diarrhoea, anorexia, and tiredness can persist for

a long time. *B. henselae* has been identified in skin biopsy specimens of patients with CSD at the primary site of inoculation.

Atypical CSD occurs in a minority of cases, most of whom have severe systemic symptoms indicating disseminated infection. Patients with atypical CSD have prolonged fever (>2 weeks), myalgia, arthralgia/arthropathy, malaise, fatigue, weight loss, splenomegaly, and Parinaud's oculoglandular syndrome (POGS). POGS appears to be the most common ocular complication of CSD, affecting approximately 5% of symptomatic patients. Organisms from an infected cat are inoculated indirectly into the eye rather than by direct contact through a scratch.

Encephalopathy and neuroretinitis

These are less common manifestations of CSD. Two-thirds of patients with neuroretinitis have evidence of past infection by *B. henselae*. Other bartonellas causing retinitis include *B. quintana*, *B. grahamii*, *B. clarridgeiae*, and *B. elizabethae*. Retinitis is typically stellar. The onset of neurological complications varies from a few days to 2 months after the onset of lymphadenopathy and tends to occur more often in older school-age children. Features include headache, malaise, lethargy lasting for one to several weeks, impaired consciousness, acute hemiplegia, optic disc oedema and

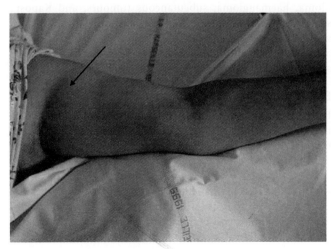

Fig. 6.42.3 Axillary lymphadenitis (CSD).

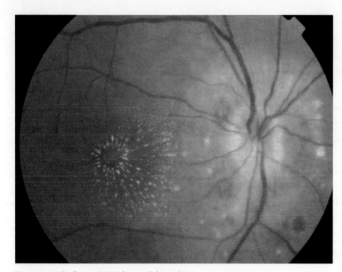

Fig. 6.42.4 Stellar retinitis due to *B. henselae*.
(Courtesy of Dr M J Dolan.)

macular star formation, loss of vision with central scotoma, and glaucoma (Fig. 6.42.4).

Bacillary angiomatosis

Bacillary angiomatosis, also called epithelioid angiomatosis, is a vascular proliferative disease most often involving the skin that occurs particularly in immunocompromised patients, mainly those infected with HIV. Without appropriate therapy, infection spreads systemically, can involve virtually any organ, and may be fatal. Rarely, it can also affect immunocompetent patients. Both *B. henselae* and *B. quintana* are considered aetiological agents. In the case of *B. quintana* there are associated subcutaneous and lytic bone lesions, and *B. henselae* is associated with peliosis hepatis. Bacillary angiomatosis is manifested by the gradual appearance of numerous brown to violaceous or colourless vascular tumours of the skin and subcutaneous tissues, numbering a few to several hundred and varying in size from a few millimetres to several centimetres. Three morphologically distinct cutaneous lesions have been described: (1) pyogenic granuloma-like lesions, the most common type; (2) subcutaneous nodules; and (3) hyperpigmented indurated plaques. The clinical differential diagnosis includes pyogenic granuloma, haemangioma, subcutaneous tumours, and Kaposi's sarcoma. The skin lesions are very similar to those reported for verruga peruana, the chronic form of Carrión's disease. Bacillary angiomatosis lesions can also involve the bone marrow, liver, spleen, or lymph nodes.

Bacillary peliosis

Bacillary peliosis is a condition affecting solid internal organs with reticuloendothelial elements, especially the liver in which bacillary peliosis causes vascular proliferation of sinusoidal hepatic capillaries resulting in blood-filled spaces (peliosis hepatis), but also the spleen, abdominal lymph nodes, and bone marrow. The disease was first described in patients with tuberculosis and advanced cancers and was associated with the use of anabolic steroids. It has also been reported in organ transplant recipients and HIV-infected patients with *B. henselae*.

Bacteraemia and endocarditis

Infection due to *B. quintana* should be suspected in indigent, chronic alcoholic patients with culture-negative endocarditis, especially those with a long-standing valve lesion. *B. quintana* bacteraemia has also been reported in other patients with endocarditis. Evidence of bartonella endocarditis was found in 0.5 to 12% of all patients diagnosed with endocarditis tested at reference centres in different countries in the old world, decreasing from north to south. Among cases of bartonella endocarditis in Europe, 75% were associated with *B. quintana* and 25% with *B. henselae*. In North Africa most cases were caused by *B. quintana*, which is also responsible for asymptomatic, prolonged, and intermittent bacteraemia in homeless people in cities both in Europe and in the United States of America.

Endocarditis due to *B. henselae* should be suspected in patients with previous valvulopathy and culture-negative endocarditis, especially those who have contacts with cats.

Endocarditis and/or bacteraemia caused by other bartonella species. are unusual but *B. elizabethae*, *B. vinsonii* subsp. *berkhoffii*, *B. vinsonii* subsp. *vinsonii*, *B. koehlerae*, and *B. alsatica* have been isolated from heart valves of patients with culture-negative endocarditis. One case of myocarditis has been attributed to *B. washoensis*.

Prolonged fever

Prolonged fever (>15 days) may occur in patients with atypical CSD.

Diagnosis

Diagnosis is difficult because of the fastidious nature of bartonella and the nonspecific clinical manifestations. Diagnostic techniques include culture and detection of organisms in lymph nodes by immunofluorescence, molecular techniques including polymerase chain reaction (PCR), and serology. Table 6.42.2 presents the most common clinical features caused by bartonella and the best techniques for their identification, and Fig. 6.42.5 presents the current diagnostic strategy.

Specimen collection

Various specimens, especially serum, blood, biopsy specimens, and arthropods, are useful. They should be sampled as soon as possible after the onset of disease. For serological diagnosis, serum samples should be collected early and during convalescence 1 to 3 weeks later. Serum samples can be stored easily at −20°C or below for long periods without degradation of antibodies. Blood should be sampled before antimicrobial therapy either in citrate-containing vials for culture or in ethylenediaminetetraacetic acid (EDTA) for PCR techniques. EDTA should be avoided for culture since it leads to detachment of cell monolayers. Biopsies of lymph nodes, cardiac valves, vascular aneurysms, or grafts should be taken in two parts, one in absolute alcohol for histopathology and immunodetection and another frozen and stored at −70°C in a sterile vial for culture and PCR analysis. These methods can be also used to detect bartonella in various arthropods including ticks, lice, and fleas (xenodiagnosis). The arthropod should be disinfected with iodinated alcohol and then crushed in medium before being inoculated into a shell vial for culture or processing using molecular methods. Arthropods can be easily stored dry in a box and sent by mail to a reference centre for analysis.

Table 6.42.2 Clinical manifestations and diagnostic methods for bartonella infections

Disease in humans	Commonly isolated	Rarely isolated	Specimen	Methods
Cat-scratch disease	B. henselae	B. quintana, B. clarridgeiae	Lymph nodes	PCR, serology
Endocarditis	B. henselae, B. quintana	B. elizabethae, B. koehlerae, B. vinsonii subsp. berkhoffii, B. alsatica	Blood, serum, valves	PCR, serology
Retinitis	B. henselae	B. grahamii	Serum, aqueous humour	PCR, serology
Bacillary angiomatosis	B. henselae, B. quintana		Blood, serum, cutaneous biopsy	PCR
Bacteraemia	B. quintana	B. henselae, B. vinsonii subsp. arupensis	Blood, serum	PCR, serology
Peliosis hepatitis	B. henselae		Blood, serum, hepatic biopsy	PCR, serology
Osteomyelitis	B. henselae		Blood, serum, bone biopsy	PCR, serology
Trench fever	B. quintana		Blood, serum	PCR

PCR, polymerase chain reaction.

Direct diagnosis

Culture

The most widely used methods for isolation are direct plating into solid media, blood culture in broth, and co-cultivation in cell culture. Bartonella can be grown on blood agar at 37°C in a 5% CO_2 atmosphere, except for *B. bacilliformis* which should be grown at 30°C. Primary isolates are typically obtained after 12 to 14 days, although an incubation period of up to 45 days may be necessary (Fig. 6.42.6). Subculture in blood broth in shell vials is the most efficient culture method in patients with endocarditis. Specimens are placed on human embryonic lung cells in shell vials and incubated at 37°C in an atmosphere of 5% CO_2. Culture may be successful using blood samples, skin, lymph nodes, or other organ biopsy samples. Lysis centrifugation and freezing have been shown to enhance the recovery of bartonella from blood. However, despite improved culture methods, the results of blood cultures may be negative if the patient has recently received antibiotics or if the organism is fastidious or requires special culture techniques. Bartonella-Alphaproteobacteria growth medium (BAPGM), may provide an improved or alternative method to isolate these fastidious microorganisms from patient samples. It has been recently demonstrated that MALDI-TOF mass spectrometry was an accurate and reproducible tool for the rapid and inexpensive identification of bartonella species.

Immunodetection

Detection of bartonella using specific antibodies has been achieved in various situations. Demonstration of microorganisms in valve tissues by the Warthin–Starry stain (Fig. 6.42.7) is a classic criterion for the histological diagnosis of infective endocarditis. Direct immunological detection in lymph nodes has been reported in patients with CSD, for patients with peliosis hepatis, in red blood cells of bacteraemic homeless people, in cardiac valves, and in skin biopsies. Immunohistochemistry is a convenient tool for detecting *B. quintana* in tissues but specific antibodies are often not available.

Molecular biology

PCR is a convenient method for detecting bartonella either in fresh or in formalin-fixed and paraffin-embedded tissues. The current target genes used for the detection and identification of bartonella are the citrate synthase gene (*gltA*), the 16S RNA gene, the 16S–23S rRNA *ITS*, the 60-kDa heat-shock protein (*groEL*), and the *pap31* gene. Although these methods are highly specific, their sensitivity varies according to the type of samples. Thus the current strategy for the diagnosis of bartonella infections is to use two different target genes (e.g. *ITS* gene and *pap31*), and if the results are discordant to use a third gene (*groEL*). Samples should be considered positive only if at least two genes are positive and if sequences obtained give the same identification. Improvement of molecular methods may increase the sensitivity especially the use of real-time

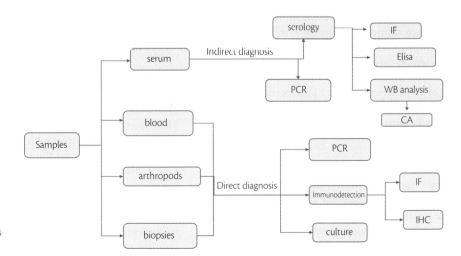

Fig. 6.42.5 Strategy for the diagnosis of *Bartonella* spp. infections.

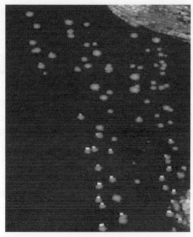

Fig. 6.42.6 Colony morphology of *B. henselae* on Columbia 5% sheep blood agar.

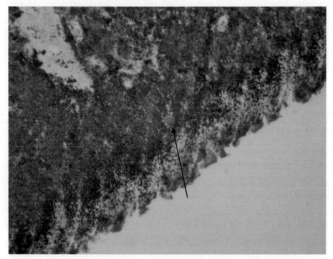

Fig. 6.42.7 Warthin–Starry staining of a cardiac valve of a patient with *B. quintana* endocarditis. Arrow shows the clumps of bacilli. Magnification ×400.

PCR with Taqman probes. Recently a new tool has been proposed for the diagnosis of bartonella endocarditis by real-time nested PCR assay performed on a LightCycler apparatus (LCN-PCR) using serum, which could shorten the delay in the diagnosis. For the typing and characterization of *B. henselae* isolates, multilocus sequence typing (MLST) is a relatively new typing method that groups bacteria based on comparison of nucleic acid sequences of 450 to 500 bp derived from the internal fragments of a number (typically seven) of housekeeping genes. More recently a molecular typing method based on the sequences of such noncoding zones rather than of housekeeping genes was developed and called multispacer typing (MST).

Indirect diagnosis

Serology is the only useful noninvasive method for the diagnosis of bartonella infections, especially for CSD, bacteraemia, and endocarditis. The sensitivity of serological tests varies between laboratories, from nearly 100% to less than 30% depending on the method used for preparation of antigens. Sources of antigens for serology can be either whole-cell lysates or outer membrane protein preparations and, more recently, recombinant proteins. The most widely used serological test for diagnosis is the indirect fluorescence assay (IFA) to detect antibodies against *B. henselae* whole cells. An IgG anti-*B. henselae* antibody titre of 1:64 or more is considered positive for infection when patients are tested at least 2 to 3 weeks after a suspected infection. Bartonella-associated endocarditis in humans and animals is usually associated with much higher IFA antibody titres (>1:800). False-negative results are due to either antigenic heterogeneity among *B. henselae* species or to other diseases such as mycobacterial infections, lymphoma, or Kaposi's sarcoma. Cross-reactions have been reported either with other bartonella species, or between bartonella species and *Coxiella burnetii* or chlamydia. Lepidi *et al.* have developed autoimmunohistochemistry, which is a peroxidase-based method with the patient's own serum as the source of antibodies directed against the aetiological microorganism, for the diagnosis of infective endocarditis. The rate of detection of bacteria by autoimmunohistochemistry was significantly higher than that by culture but was similar to that by PCR. The most sophisticated serological method, western blot analysis after cross-adsorption, has been shown to be a powerful tool for the identification of bartonella to species level in endocarditis (Fig. 6.42.8).

Treatment

In vitro susceptibility to antibiotics

This can be performed in either eukaryotic cells or axenic media. Bartonella species are susceptible to many antibiotics when they are grown axenically, including penicillin and cephalosporin compounds, aminoglycosides, chloramphenicol, tetracyclines, macrolide compounds, rifampicin, fluoroquinolones, and co-trimoxazole. However, these results correlate poorly with *in vivo* efficacy because antibiotics are not bactericidal, except for aminoglycosides. This has also been reported in cell-culture models for *B. henselae* in murine macrophage-like cells and for *B. quintana* in red blood cells. Recent *in vivo* data have demonstrated the benefit of a combination of doxycycline with gentamicin in the treatment of infections including endocarditis and bacteraemia in homeless peoples. Mutations in the 23S RNA gene and insertion of nine amino acids in the L4 ribosomal protein for *B. henselae* and *B. quintana*, respectively, can be selected *in vitro* by erythromycin. Mutations such as the A2059G transition have been detected directly in the lymph node of a patient with CSD, suggesting that natural erythromycin-resistant strains may infect humans.

In vivo in human patients

Trench fever

Most cases of trench fever were reported before the antibiotic era. However, successful treatment with tetracycline or chloramphenicol was reported during the Second World War. According to a recent placebo-controlled clinical trial, patients with chronic *B. quintana* bacteraemia should be treated with gentamicin (3 mg/kg intravenously once a day) for 14 days and with doxycycline (200 mg/day orally once a day) for 28 days. Patients with chronic bacteraemia should be carefully evaluated for endocarditis, which requires prolonged therapy under close monitoring. Those with

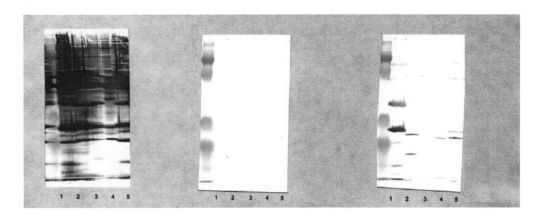

Fig. 6.42.8 Western blot of a patient with *B. quintana* endocarditis before (a) and after cross-adsorption with *B. quintana* (b) or *B. henselae* (c). Line 1: *B. quintana*; line 2: *B. henselae*; line 3: *B. elizabethae*; line 4: *B. vinsonii* subsp. *berkhoffii*; line 5: *B. alsatica*.

renal insufficiency or obesity need a twice-daily dosing schedule to avoid gentamicin nephrotoxicity.

CSD

CSD typically does not respond to antibiotic therapy. Management consists of analgesics for pain, follow-up, and drainage when necessary. Recent data re-emphasize that patients who do not improve clinically benefit from excision of affected lymph nodes and search for coexistent diseases such as tuberculosis and/or lymphoma. The only double-blind placebo-controlled study for the treatment of CSD with azithromycin in immunocompetent patients showed only a faster reduction of their lymph node volume as compared to placebo. Thus, the current recommendation for the treatment in mild to moderately ill immunocompetent patients with CSD is no antibiotic treatment. Treatment with azithromycin could help patients with bulky lymphadenopathy or those with complicated CSD with retinitis and central nervous system disease.

Endocarditis

Effective antibiotic therapy for suspected bartonella endocarditis should include an aminoglycoside (gentamicin) for at least 14 days together with ceftriaxone with or without doxycycline for 6 weeks to achieve a bactericidal effect. Valve replacement is necessary in the majority of patients because of extensive damage.

Bacillary angiomatosis and peliosis hepatis

Erythromycin is the first choice for bacillary angiomatosis and peliosis hepatis. Treatment should continue for at least 3 months for bacillary angiomatosis and 4 months for peliosis hepatis. Longer treatment should be given in HIV-infected and immunocompromised patients. An *in vitro* model of *B. quintana* cultured in endothelial cells has shown that erythromycin acts mainly antiangiogenically rather than as an antibiotic, explaining the often dramatic response to this antibiotic in bacillary angiomatosis. Bacillary peliosis hepatis responds more slowly than cutaneous bacillary angiomatosis, but hepatic lesions usually are improved after several months of treatment. Relapses of peliosis hepatis and bacillary angiomatosis lesions in bone and skin have been reported frequently, mostly in severely immunocompromised HIV-infected patients. Finally, patients who have relapses after the recommended treatment should receive secondary prophylactic antibiotic treatment with erythromycin or doxycycline as long as they are immunocompromised.

Prevention

B. quintana infections can be prevented by delousing, changing, or washing clothes. To avoid *B. henselae*, immunocompromised patients should avoid contact with cats and cat fleas. Only seronegative cats should be kept by immunocompromised people, but is better to avoid them altogether or to eradicate cat fleas.

Conclusions

Bacteria of the genus *Bartonella* are responsible for emerging and re-emerging infections worldwide and can present in many different ways, from benign and self-limited infections to severe and life-threatening diseases. Consequently, diagnosis and treatment of these infections should be adapted to each clinical situation, to the species involved, and to whether the disease is an acute or a chronic form.

Further reading

Alsmark CM, *et al.* (2004). The louse-borne human pathogen *Bartonella quintana* is a genomic derivative of the zoonotic agent *Bartonella henselae*. *Proc Natl Acad Sci U S A*, **101**, 9716–21.

Angelakis E, *et al.* (2010). *Bartonella henselae* in skin biopsy specimens of patients with cat-scratch disease. *Emerg Infect Dis*, **16**, 1963 6.

Birtles RJ, *et al.* (1995). Proposals to unify the genera *Grahamella* and *Bartonella*, with descriptions of *Bartonella talpae* comb. nov., *Bartonella peromysci* comb. nov., and three new species, *Bartonella grahamii* sp. nov., *Bartonella taylorii* sp. nov., and *Bartonella doshiae* sp. nov. *Int J Syst Bact*, **45**, 1–8.

Biswas S, Raoult D, Rolain JM (2006). Molecular characterization of resistance to macrolides in *Bartonella henselae*. *Antimicrob Agents Chemother*, **50**, 3192–3.

Breitschwerdt B, Kordick D (2000). *Bartonella* infection in animals: carriership, reservoir potential, pathogenicity and zoonotic potential for human infection. *Clin Microbiol Rev*, **13**, 428–38.

Brenner DJ, *et al.* (1993). Proposals to unify the genera *Bartonella* and *Rochalimaea*, with descriptions of *Bartonella quintana* comb. nov., *Bartonella vinsonii* comb. nov., *Bartonella henselae* comb. nov., and *Bartonella elizabethae* comb. nov., and to remove the family *Bartonellaceae* from the order *Rickettsiales*. *Int J Syst Bact*, **43**, 777–86.

Dehio C (2001). *Bartonella* interactions with endothelial cells and erythrocytes. *Trends Microbiol*, **9**, 279–85.

Foucault C, Brouqui P, Raoult D (2006). *Bartonella quintana* characteristics and clinical management. *Emerg Infect Dis*, **12**, 217–23.

Fournier PE *et al.* (2009). Rapid and cost-effective identification of *Bartonella* species using mass spectrometry. *J Med Microbiol*, **58**, 1154–9.

Greub G, Raoult D (2002). *Bartonella*: new explanations for old diseases. *J Med Microbiol*, **51**, 915–23.

Houpikian P, Raoult D (2001). 16S/23S rRNA intergenic spacer regions for phylogenetic analysis, identification, and subtyping of *Bartonella* species. *J Clin Microbiol*, **39**, 2768–78.

Houpikian P, Raoult D (2003). Western immunoblotting for *Bartonella* endocarditis. *Clin Diagn Lab Immunol*, **10**, 95–102.

Kernif T, *et al.* (2010). Molecular detection of *Bartonella alsatica* in rabbit fleas, France. *Emerg Infect Dis*, **16**, 2013–14.

La Scola B, Raoult D (1999). Culture of *Bartonella quintana* and *Bartonella henselae* from human samples: a 5-year experience (1993 to 1998). *J Clin Microbiol*, **37**, 1899–905.

La Scola B, *et al.* (2003). Gene-sequence-based criteria for species definition in bacteriology: the *Bartonella* paradigm. *Trends Microbiol*, **11**, 318–21.

Lepidi H, Fournier PE, Raoult D (2000). Quantitative analysis of valvular lesions during *Bartonella* endocarditis. *Am J Clin Pathol*, **114**, 880–9.

Lepidi H, *et al.* (2006). Autoimmunohistochemistry: a new method for the histologic diagnosis of infective endocarditis. *J Infect Dis*, **193**, 1711–17.

Maurin M, Raoult D (1996). *Bartonella (Rochalimaea) quintana* infections. *Clin Microbiol Rev*, **9**, 273–92.

Maurin M, Rolain JM, Raoult D (2002). Comparison of in-house and commercial slides for detection of immunoglobulins G and M by immunofluorescence against *Bartonella henselae* and *Bartonella quintana*. *Clin Diag Lab Immunol*, **9**, 1004–9.

Meghari S, *et al.* (2006). Anti-angiogenic effect of erythromycin in *Bartonella quintana*: *in vitro* model of infection. *J Infect Dis*, **193**, 380–6.

Musso D, Drancourt M, Raoult D (1995). Lack of bactericidal effect of antibiotics except aminoglycosides on *Bartonella (Rochalimaea) henselae*. *J Antimicrob Chemother*, **36**, 101–8.

Pitulle C, *et al.* (2002). Investigation of the phylogenetic relationships within the genus *Bartonella* based on comparative sequence analysis of the *rnpB* gene, 16S rDNA and 23S rDNA. *Int J Syst Evol Microbiol*, **52**, 2075–80.

Raoult D, *et al.* (2003). Outcome and treatment of *Bartonella* endocarditis. *Arch Intern Med*, **163**, 226–30.

Rolain JM, *et al.* (2001). Immunofluorescent detection of intraerythrocytic *Bartonella henselae* in naturally infected cats. *J Clin Microbiol*, **39**, 2978–88.

Rolain JM, *et al.* (2002). *Bartonella quintana* in human erythrocytes. *Lancet*, **360**, 226–8.

Rolain JM, *et al.* (2003). Molecular detection of *Bartonella quintana*, *B. koehlerae*, *B. henselae*, *B. clarridgeiae*, *Rickettsia felis* and *Wolbachia pipientis* in cat fleas, France. *Emerg Infect Dis*, **9**, 338–42.

Rolain JM, *et al.* (2004). Recommendations for treatment of human infections caused by *Bartonella* species. *Antimicrob Agents Chemother*, **48**, 1921–33.

Rolain JM, *et al.* (2006). Lymph node biopsy specimens and diagnosis of cat-scratch disease. *Emerg Infect Dis*, **12**, 1338–44.

Saisongkorh W, *et al.* (2010). Evidence of transfer by conjugation of type IV secretion system genes between Bartonella species and Rhizobium radiobacter in amoeba. *PLOS One*, **5**, e12666.

Sanguinetti-Morelli D, *et al.* (2011). Seasonality of cat-scratch disease, France, 1999-2009. *Emerg Infect Dis*, **17**, 705–7.

Zeaiter Z, *et al.* (2002). Phylogenetic classification of *Bartonella* species by comparing groEL sequences. *Int J Syst Evol Microbiol*, **52**, 165–71.

6.43 *Bartonella bacilliformis* infection

A. Llanos-Cuentas and C. Maguiña-Vargas

Essentials

Bartonellosis (Carrión´s disease, verruga Peruana, Oroya fever, Guaitará fever) is caused by the Gram-negative bacillus *Bartonella bacilliformis*. It is endemic in the western Andes and inter-Andean valleys of Peru, and is still occasionally reported in Ecuador, with infection resulting from the bite of various female sandflies.

Clinical features, diagnosis, management, prognosis and prevention—infection of red blood cells manifests with nonspecific 'viral-type' symptoms and haemolytic anaemia in the acute stage of disease. Following an asymptomatic phase, the late 'eruptive' stage is characterized by dermal nodules ('verrugas') that frequently heal spontaneously. Secondary opportunistic infections are common. Diagnosis in areas where the disease occurs is usually by demonstration of bacteria in the blood film. Ciprofloxacin is the treatment of choice in most cases. Mortality is 1.1 to 2.4% in endemic areas and around 9% in patients admitted to hospital. There is no satisfactory prevention for people living in endemic areas; tourists can take the usual precautions against being bitten by insects.

Aetiological agent

Barton, a Peruvian physician, described the causative organism in 1905. *Bartonella bacilliformis* is a small motile aerobic Gram-negative bacillus that stains deep red or purple with Giemsa (Fig. 6.43.1). This facultative intracellular haemotropic bacterium varies in morphology and quantity during various stages of the disease. Although it is a pleomorphic organism, two essential types are distinguishable, bacilli or rod-shaped forms and coccoid forms. Rod-shaped forms predominate in the acute stage of the disease and coccoid in the convalescent stage. *B. bacilliformis* may infect red blood cells (Fig. 6.43.2), endothelial cells of capillaries, and sinusoidal lining cells. The organism is 2 to 3 µm long and 0.2 to 2.5 µm thick. In cultures, 1 to 10 flagella, 3 to 10 µm long, may originate from one end of the organism. Bartonella can be cultured in Columbia agar supplemented with 5% defibrinated human blood or other supplemented media containing rabbit serum and haemoglobin at 28°C under aerobic conditions for up to 6 weeks. Multilocus sequence typing (MLST) of Peruvian isolates of *B. bacilliformis* showed wide genetic diversity. While seven of the eight sequence types were closely related, one exhibited profound evolutionary divergence suggesting that it might represent a new *Bartonella* genospecies.

Epidemiology

Bartonellosis has occurred since pre-Columbian times, as proven by artistic representations in pre-Inca pottery and lesions in an ancient mummy. It is an endemic disease mainly in inter-Andean valleys in west, central, and east Andean areas of Peru (Fig. 6.43.3)

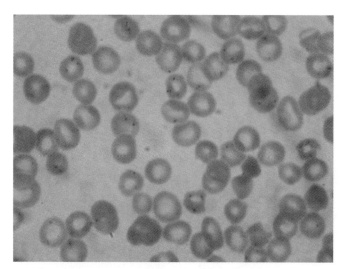

Fig. 6.43.1 *B. bacilliformis* in blood smear stained with Giemsa.

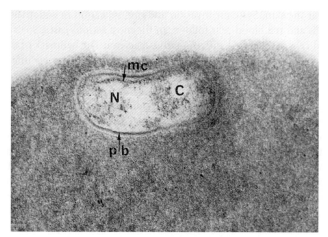

Fig. 6.43.2 *B. bacilliformis* in a red blood cell.

and increasingly in high jungle areas. This is an emergent disease, extensively distributed in Peru; 142 districts were affected in 2000 and 416 in 2006 (192% increase), and 18 of 24 departments of Peru have been involved (Fig. 6.43.4). Some cases have been reported during the last decade in Zumba (Chinchipe), Ecuador. The epidemiological pattern is endemic plus epidemic in the new areas. Transmission is usually in rural towns and around human dwellings. The disease occurs between 500 and 3200 m above sea level. Transmission varies throughout the year, being greatest towards the end of the rainy season (March to May). Interepidemic periods occur every 10 to 15 years. Incidence is greatly influenced by climatic, environmental, and ecological changes such as the El Niño phenomenon.

At present, 11 species and subspecies of the genus *Bartonella* have been associated with human infections but only three have epidemiological importance: *B. bacilliformis*, of which six antigenic variants have been described in Peru; *B. henselae*, the major cause of cat-scratch disease and peliosis (Chapter 6.42); and *B. quintana* (formerly *Rochalimaea*), the agent of trench fever (Chapter 6.42). Recently, a new bartonella named *B. rochalimae* has been described in tourists infected in Peru. Other bartonellas such as *B. vinsonii* subsp. *berkhoffii*, *B. vinsonii* subsp. *arupensis*, *B. elizabethae*, *B. koehlerae*, *B. alsatica*, *B. grahamii*, and *B. clarridgeiae* occasionally cause disease in humans. In immunocompromised people, especially those with the HIV/AIDS, *B. henselae* and *B. quintana* cause opportunistic infections, frequently manifested as cutaneous bacillary angiomatosis, resembling verruga peruana.

In endemic areas, 20.5% of those patients infected with *B. bacilliformis* remain asymptomatic, 31.5% develop the eruptive form (chronic phase) without evidence of an acute illness, and 37% develop the eruptive form preceded by some symptoms. Only 11% will develop the classic acute form; with a higher frequency in children. Outsiders generally develop acute severe forms of the disease (Oroya fever). Large epidemics have occurred when large groups of nonresidents have entered endemic areas. In 1870, an epidemic engulfed workers building the railroad from Lima to Oroya (Fig. 6.43.5); the estimated mortality was 7000.

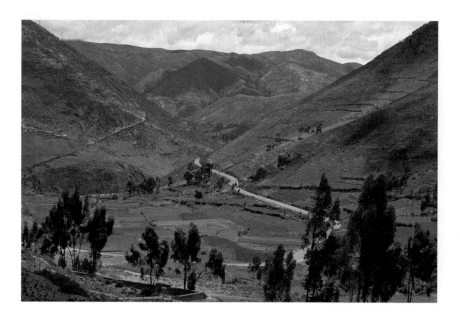

Fig. 6.43.3 Endemic area for bartonellosis; near Tarma, Peru. (Copyright D A Warrell.)

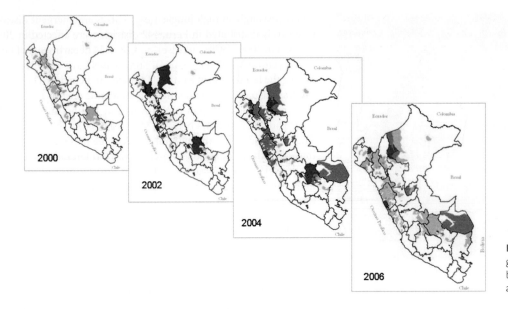

Fig. 6.43.4 Extension of the geographical distribution of bartonellosis in Peru between 2000 and 2006.

Infection results from the bite of females of several species of sandflies (*Lutzomyia*), especially *Lutzomyia verrucarum*. These vectors frequent human dwellings and, because they are active during twilight hours, humans are infected around sunrise and sunset. Although the reservoir is unknown, humans are regarded as being increasingly important. Asymptomatic *B. bacilliformis* infection has been demonstrated in endemic populations. However, since bartonellosis can be acquired in several Andean areas uninhabited by humans, other reservoirs for the disease may exist. Some domestic animals including horses, donkeys, mules, dogs, and cats are susceptible and develop lesions similar to verrugas. Bartonella-like isolates have been obtained from a mouse (*Phyllotis*, Cricetidae).

Pathogenesis

After inoculation of *B. bacilliformis* by sandfly bite, the bacteria multiply in endothelial cells of small vessels and phagocytic cells near the skin. Systemic invasion and multiplication in endothelial cells and red blood cells follows. In the most serious cases, 95% of red cells are infected with numerous bacteria. The hallmark of the disease is the severe haemolytic anaemia caused by massive infection of red blood cells and subsequent erythrophagocytosis. Several mechanisms contribute to anaemia: increased fragility, form and size alteration, and reduced half-life of infected and noninfected red cells. Some inhibition of haemoglobin synthesis, probably induced by toxic factors, has also been invoked, since red cell production increases dramatically with reduction of bacteraemia. Erythrophagocytosis contributes to lymphadenopathy and hepatosplenomegaly. 'Blockade' of the mononuclear phagocytic system and the presence of the circulating iron leads to superinfection, usually by enterobacteria, during the anaemia stage or early recovery from it. Transient depression of cellular immunity has been reported. During the anaemic phase, mild lymphopenia with a reduction of OKT4, a mild increase of OKT8, and decrease of the

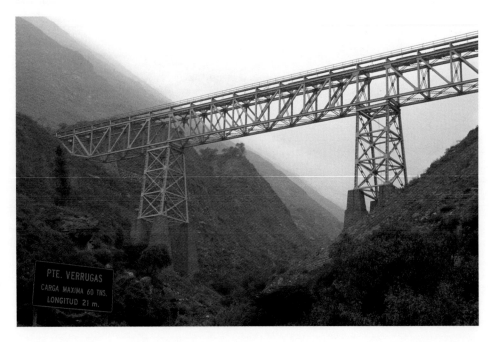

Fig. 6.43.5 Endemic area for bartonellosis; Rimac valley, Peru—Puente Verrugas. (Copyright D A Warrell.)

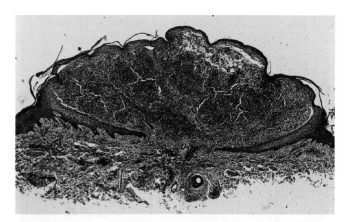

polyclonal stimulation of lymphocytes occurs. High levels of inter-leukin (IL)-10 were found in the acute phase. In Gram-negative sep-sis, an uncontrolled production of IL-10 may produce 'immunological paralysis' of antigen-presenting cells.

The eruptive form appears a few weeks to months after the acute illness has subsided, and in Peru is named 'verruga peruana' (Fig. 6.43.6a,b). The vascular skin lesions show endothelial pro-liferation and histiocytic hyperplasia (the cells contains degener-ate organisms; Fig. 6.43.7) and later show fibrosis and necrosis. Electron microscopy of verrucous tissue shows *B. bacilliformis* in the interstitial tissues, indicating that the presence of the bacteria is important for this unusual vascular response to occur. Verruga peruana results from persistent infection, an immune response that is probably insufficient, and a peculiar vascular reaction, which could be caused by an angiogenic bacterial factor.

Fig. 6.43.7 Verruga peruana: histology.

Clinical features

The disease has two stages, anaemic and eruptive, with an asymp-tomatic intermediate period. After an incubation period of around 60 days (range 10–210 days), nonspecific prodromal symptoms appear. The onset is usually gradual with malaise, mild chills, fever, and headache. Occasionally, high fever may develop rapidly or build up over a few days. It is accompanied by sweating and rigors. Common symptoms include weakness, aching of the head, back,

and extremities, prostration, and depression. The classical clinical picture is dominated by severe (haemolytic) anaemia and the patient rapidly become pale (Fig. 6.43.8), dyspnoeic, and jaundiced. There may be hepatosplenomegaly, generalized lymphadenopathy, tachycardia, myocarditis (Fig. 6.43.9), purpura, hepatitis, diarrhoea, pericardial effusion, exudates, anasarca, and retinal changes (Fig. 6.43.10); sometimes there is generalized oedema, drowsiness, and convulsions, and exceptionally meningoencephalomyelitis. The duration of this state is variable (generally 2–4 weeks). In pregnant women, the disease in this phase may cause abortion, fetal death, and transplacental transmission of the disease; maternal death is common. Fourteen per cent of the patients develop the classical symptoms (fever, anaemia, and frequently jaundice) and 86% develop fever alone.

In the intermediate period, patients are asymptomatic and recover from the anaemia through great bone marrow activity. This pre-eruptive period varies from weeks to months.

In the eruptive stage, many nodular lesions of varying size appear on the face, trunk, and limbs, over a period of a month or more and usually persist for 3 or 4 months. There is accompanying mild arthralgia, myalgia, and sometimes fever. The red or purplish skin lesions are papules a few millimetres across. Most often the eruption is miliary (miliary form) with many haemangioma-like lesions of the dermis (Fig. 6.43.6a,b). Nodular lesions (nodular

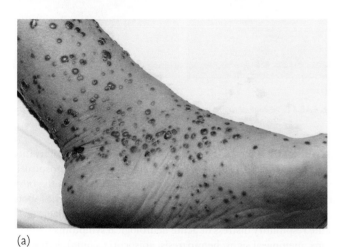

(a)

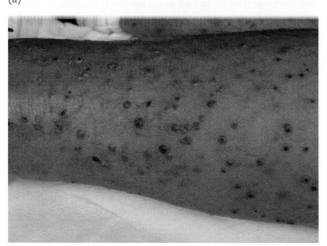

(b)

Fig. 6.43.6 Verruga peruana: miliary haemangioma-like lesions.

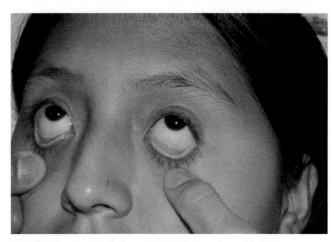

Fig. 6.43.8 Severe anaemia (haematocrit 9%) in a patient with acute bartonellosis.
(Copyright D A Warrell.)

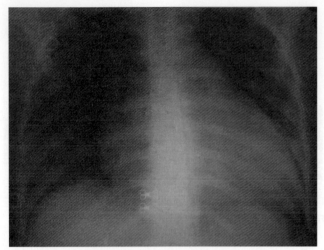

Fig. 6.43.9 Cardiomegaly due to myocarditis in a patient with acute bartonellosis.
(Copyright D A Warrell.)

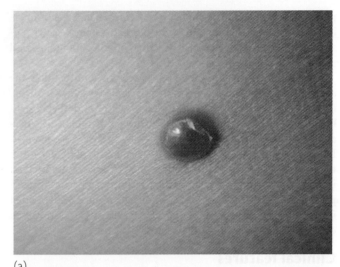

(a)

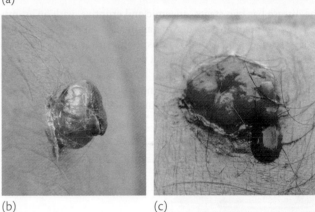

(b)   (c)

Fig. 6.43.11 Verruga peruana: nodular haemangiomatous lesions.

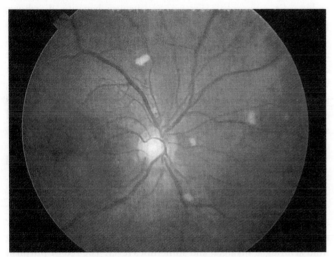

Fig. 6.43.10 Retinal changes.

form) are larger but fewer and more prominent on the extensor surfaces of arms and legs (Fig. 6.43.11a,b). They are painless and prone to bleeding (Fig. 6.43.11c), secondary infection, and ulceration. The appearance may resemble haemangioma, cutaneous bacillary angiomatosis, granuloma pyogenicum, Kaposi's sarcoma, fibrosarcoma, leprosy (histoid form), or yaws. Occasionally one to a few, large, deep-seated ulcerating lesions (mular form) may develop. These tend to appear near joints where they may be painful and limit motion. Apart from skin, the mucous membranes of the mouth, conjunctiva, and nose, serous cavities, and the gastrointestinal and genitourinary tracts may be involved. The eruptive phase frequently tends to heal spontaneously, although the course is often prolonged. A few patients develop a severe eruptive form, with dozens of bleeding and necrotic lesions which tend to become secondarily infected.

The severe acute form can develop infectious and/or noninfectious complications. The principal complication is superinfection leading to septicaemia, which occurs at different stages of the diseases but generally in the later part of the anaemic stage and during the intermediate stage. Formerly, salmonella, *Mycobacterium tuberculosis*,

and enterobacter were the most frequent pathogens. Reactivation of toxoplasmosis, histoplasmosis, pneumocystosis, leptospirosis, typhus fever, and staphylococcal infections are some of the other infections that are now frequent. A few patients develop the following syndromes: febrile haemorrhagic or ictero-haemorrhagic fever; acute respiratory distress or acute neurological symptoms (convulsions, meningeal signs, hemiparesis, anisocoria, coma). Refractory haemodynamic failure, severe respiratory distress, and renal failure are some of the noninfectious complications.

Diagnosis

Two elements must be considered: (1) travel or residence in an endemic area and (2) a compatible clinical picture with demonstration of the bacteria in the blood film (Fig. 6.43.1). Fluorescence antibody test, indirect haemagglutination, immunoblot (94% sensitive to chronic form and 70% sensitive to acute form), enzyme-linked immunosorbent assay (ELISA) and polymerase chain reaction (PCR) are new tests that are not generally available. PCR can detect *B. bacilliformis*-specific DNA from blood samples as well as skin biopsies. Antibodies are nonspecific due a cross-reaction with *B. henselae*, *B. quintana*, *Chlamydia psittaci*, and unknown antigens. The differential diagnosis in people living in endemic areas includes: leptospirosis, rickettsioses, toxoplasmosis, *P. vivax* malaria and louse-borne relapsing fever.

Laboratory features

Bartonella can be isolated from the blood during the anaemic stage and sometimes during the eruptive stage. The sensitivity of blood smear detection varies with the phase of the disease: 90% are positive during the acute phase, less than 10% in the verrucous phase, and less than 1% in asymptomatic people. The specificity varies from 75 to 98% and the positive predictive value is 71 to 94%. The enriched media may be positive in 4 to 28 days at 28°C. As fever develops, intraerythrocytic bacteria are visible in thick and thin films stained with Giemsa's, Wright's, or other Romanovsky stains. Organisms can also be seen and cultivated in verrucous skin lesions. The anaemia may be very severe (haematocrit <10%). It is haemolytic but Coombs' test negative. The blood picture is of a macrocytic and hypochromic anaemia with polychromasia, anisocytosis, and poikilocytosis. Reticulocytosis is marked (average 11%). The marrow is hyperactive and megaloblastic with erythrophagocytosis. The white cell count is not markedly elevated unless there is a secondary infection. Thrombocytopenia is quite common. After the crisis, the intracellular organisms become coccoid and later disappear, the white cell count rises, and there is lymphocytosis. Eosinophils, which are usually absent during the acute stage, reappear in the peripheral blood.

Prognosis

Deaths usually occur during the anaemic phase. In the preantibiotic era, case fatality varied between 20 and 95%. At present, it varies between 1.1 and 2.4% in endemic areas and around 9% in patients admitted to hospital. During outbreaks, especially when the disease is not promptly recognized and treated, the case fatality can reach around 88%. Alterations of consciousness (excitement, stupor, and coma) and progressive or focal neurological features, biochemical evidence of hepatic dysfunction (increased transaminases and alkaline phosphatase), pulmonary complications (noncardiogenic pulmonary oedema), severe neurological involvement, anasarca (severe hypoalbuminaemia), pregnancy, and not being indigenous are all associated with a higher mortality.

Treatment

Chloramphenicol, penicillin, erythromycin, co-trimoxazole, and ciprofloxacin are effective, usually eliminating the fever in around 48 h. Because of the common association with salmonellosis, ciprofloxacin is the treatment of choice in a dose of 500 mg orally twice a day for 14 days. The alternative is amoxicillin plus clavulanic acid 1 g orally twice a day for 14 days, which is the treatment of choice in pregnant women and children under 14 years of age. In severe acute disease, the drugs indicated are ceftriaxone 2 g intravenously daily plus ciprofloxacin 400 mg intravenously twice a day for 14 days. Supportive treatment includes transfusion of packed red cells and empirical dexamethasone if there is severe neurological involvement. Azithromycin 500 mg orally once a day for 7 days is the drug of choice for the verrucous form. The dose in children is 10 mg/kg daily orally for 7 days. The alternative is rifampicin (300 mg twice a day in adults or 10 mg/kg daily in children orally for 21–28 days).

Prevention

There is no satisfactory prevention for people who live in endemic areas. Sandflies can be eliminated temporarily by spraying inside and outside with dichlorodiphenyltrichloroethane (DDT) or pyrethroids, and this strategy is recommended during outbreaks. Spraying insecticides inside the house and mass use of long-lasting insecticide-impregnated bed nets are measures that reduce both incidence and secondary attack rate of the disease. Tourists can protect themselves with insect repellents, clothes impregnated with pyrethroids, and sleeping with nets impregnated with insecticides, or by avoiding sleeping in highly endemic areas.

Further reading

Birtles RJ, *et al.* (1999). Survey of *Bartonella* species infecting intradomicillary animals in the Huayllacallan valley, Ancash-Perú, a region endemic for human bartonellosis. *Am J Trop Med Hyg*, **60**, 799–805.

Chaloner GL, *et al.* (2011). Multi-locus sequence analysis reveals profound genetic diversity among isolates of the human pathogen *Bartonella bacilliformis*. *PLoS Negl Trop Dis*, **5**, e1248.

Chamberlin J, *et al.* (2002). Epidemiology of endemic *Bartonella bacilliformis*: A prospective cohort study in a Peruvian mountain valley community. *J Infect Dis* **186**, 983–90.

Maguiña C (1998). *Bartonellosis o Enfermedad de Carrión*. A.F.A. Editores Importadores S.A. Lima, Peru.

Maguiña C, Gotuzzo E (2000). Bartonellosis new and old. *Infect Dis Clin North Am*, **14**, 1–22.

Ministry of Health of Peru (2011) *Atención de la Bartonelosis o Enfermedad de Carrión en el Perú*. Norma técnica No. 048-MINSA/ DGSP-C .01.

Walker DH, Maguiña C, Minnick M (2006). Bartonellosis. In: Guerrant RL, Walker DH, Weller PF (eds) *Tropical infectious diseases: principles, pathogens and practice*, pp. 454–62. Elsevier, Churchill Livingstone, Philadelphia.

6.44 **Chlamydial infections**

David Taylor-Robinson and David Mabey

Essentials

Chlamydiae are pathogenic bacteria that probably evolved from host-independent, Gram-negative ancestors and are specialized for an intracellular existence. The chlamydial infectious elementary body binds to and enters the host cell by 'parasite-specified' endocytosis, with a new generation of elementary bodies being released 30 to 48 h later.

There are nine species of genus *Chlamydia* (which some would reclassify based on ribosomal sequence data into two genera, *Chlamydia* and *Chlamydophila*), of which *C. trachomatis* and *C. pneumoniae* are primarily human pathogens, and *C. psittaci*, *C. abortus*, and *C. felis* are species transmitted occasionally from animals.

Trachoma

Caused by *C. trachomatis* serovars A, B, Ba, and C. A disease of poor rural communities, mainly in Africa and Asia, where the reservoir of infection is the eye (and possibly nasopharynx) of children with active disease, with transmission from the eye of one individual to that of another via fingers, fomites, coughing and sneezing, and by eye-seeking flies.

Clinical features and diagnosis—the active (inflammatory) stage is a follicular conjunctivitis with characteristic subconjunctival follicles that are usually seen in children in endemic areas. Repeated infections lead to conjunctival scarring, with turned-in lashes rubbing against the cornea (trichiasis) and eventually causing severe damage (3.6% of global blindness, or 1.3 million cases). In endemic areas diagnosis is made on clinical grounds.

Treatment and prevention—inflammatory trachoma responds to either an appropriate course of 1% topical tetracycline ointment or a single oral dose of azithromycin. Community-based mass treatment is recommended when there is high prevalence of disease in children aged 1 to 9 years. Trichiasis requires surgical correction. A World Health Organization initiative to eliminate blinding trachoma by 2020 is based on the acronym 'SAFE': Surgery for trichiasis; Antibiotics for treatment; Face washing; Environmental improvement to reduce fly populations that transmit the organisms.

Genital tract infections

These are caused by *C. trachomatis* serovars D to K, which exist worldwide. In men they cause up to 50% of symptomatic nongonococcal urethritis and of acute epididymitis. In women they cause up to 50% of (mostly asymptomatic) urethritis and of (often asymptomatic) cervicitis; further spread leads to endometritis, salpingitis and (occasionally) perihepatitis, and infertility follows a single upper genital tract infection in about 10% of women. See the Oxford Textbook of Medicine 5e Chapter 8.5 for further discussion.

Other diseases caused by *C. trachomatis*

These include: (1) Adult paratrachoma and otitis media. (2) Reactive arthritis—at least one-third of sexually acquired reactive arthritis is initiated by genital *C. trachomatis* infection (see Oxford Textbook of Medicine 5e Chapter 19.8). (3) Neonatal infection—babies exposed to serovars D to K at birth often develop conjunctivitis, and some develop pneumonia. (4) Lymphogranuloma venereum—caused by *C. trachomatis* serovars L1, L2 or L3. Endemic in parts of Africa, Asia, South America, and the Caribbean; 2003 saw the start of an outbreak (serovar L2) across western Europe, the United Kingdom, North America, and Australia in homosexual men who were mainly HIV-positive. The clinical course comprises three stages: (a) primary—a small painless papule occurs at the site of inoculation; followed some weeks later by (b) secondary—inguinal and/or femoral lymphadenopathy with systemic features; anorectal involvement is usually seen in homosexual men; sometimes progressing to (c) tertiary—severe fibrosis, which is rarely seen because of earlier broad-spectrum antibiotic therapy. Diagnosis depends on serology or on identification of the organism in appropriate clinical samples. Treatment is usually with doxycycline or erythromycin.

Other chlamydiae

C. pneumoniae—transmitted directly from person to person by droplet spread and causes respiratory disease (pharyngitis, bronchitis, pneumonia), is a possible trigger for reactive arthritis and for some cases of juvenile chronic arthritis, and its DNA has been detected in atheromatous arteries, but without definite evidence that it contributes to heart disease. See the Oxford Textbook of Medicine 5e Chapter 18.4.2 for further discussion.

C. psittaci—transmitted from psittacine birds and causes psittacosis, which can range from a mild influenza-like illness to a fulminating toxic state with multiorgan involvement.

C. abortus—causes abortion in sheep and may do so in pregnant women exposed to infected animals during the lambing season.

Diagnosis and treatment

Diagnosis—depends on (1) culture—chlamydiae can be grown in cultured cells, but this is slow, labour intensive, and less sensitive than molecular methods; (2) antigen detection—enzyme immunoassays are easy to use, but insensitive; (3) nucleic acid detection—the 'gold standard' for routine diagnosis, screening, and for research into chronic or persistent disease; and—to a much lesser extent—(4) serology.

Treatment—chlamydiae are particularly sensitive to tetracyclines (e.g. doxycycline) and macrolides (e.g. erythromycin, and with azithromycin gaining popularity because it can be effective as a single dose: however, there is debate as to whether it is the most efficacious antibiotic).

Introduction

Trachoma is recognizable from historical in descriptions of blindness in ancient Chinese and Egyptian writings, but it was not until 1907 that L. Halberstaedter and S. von Prowazek first described intracytoplasmic inclusions in conjunctival scrapings from patients with trachoma and recognized the involvement of an infectious agent. In 1930, a chlamydial agent (*Chlamydia psittaci*) was first isolated from psittacosis; 27 years later the genomically and biologically different agent associated with trachoma, *C. trachomatis*, was isolated in fertile hens' eggs. The advent of the cell-culture technique paved the way for the isolation of *C. trachomatis* by this means in 1965 and, together with immunological developments, made it possible to explore the nature, range, prevalence, and pathogenesis of clinical conditions associated with chlamydial infection. The complete sequencing of the chlamydial genome in 1998 aided this progress.

Classification

Chlamydiae are ubiquitous pathogens infecting many species of mammals and birds. The family Chlamydiaceae, in the order Chlamydiales, was formerly classified as four species belonging to a single genus, *Chlamydia*. These species comprised *C. trachomatis* causing human ocular and genital infections; *C. pneumoniae* causing mainly human respiratory disease, but with some strains infecting horses and koalas; *C. psittaci* infecting birds and other animals, with occasional transmission to humans; and *C. pecorum*, the cause of pneumonia, polyarthritis, encephalomyelitis, and diarrhoea in cattle and sheep.

In the 21st century, a taxonomic reclassification was based on ribosomal sequence data, and the members of the family Chlamydiaceae were divided between two genera, *Chlamydia* and

Chlamydophila. This official taxonomy has not been fully implemented by researchers who favour a single genus *Chlamydia* now containing nine species: *C. trachomatis*, *C. pneumoniae*, *C. psittaci* (birds), *C. abortus* (sheep), *C. felis* (cats), *C. pecorum* (cattle), *C. suis* (pigs), *C. muridarum* (mice), and *C. caviae* (guinea pigs). The first two are primarily human pathogen; *C. psittaci*, *C. abortus*, and *C. felis* cause zoonotic infections which are transmitted occasionally to humans from infected animals. This classification is used here.

Growth cycle, serovars, and protein profile

Chlamydiae probably evolved from host-independent Gram-negative ancestors with peptidoglycan in their cell walls. They are bacteria specialized to exist intracellularly. The chlamydial envelope possesses bacteria-like inner and outer membranes. The infectious elementary body is electron dense, DNA rich, and approximately 300 nm in diameter. It binds to the host cell and enters by 'parasite-specified' endocytosis. Fusion of the chlamydia-containing endocytic vesicle with lysosomes is inhibited and the elementary body begins its unique developmental cycle within the eukaryotic cell. After about 10 h it differentiates into the larger (800–1000 nm) noninfectious, metabolically active, reticulate body. This divides by binary fission and by 20 h has begun to reorganize into a new generation of elementary bodies (Fig. 6.44.1). These reach maturity up to 30 h after entry into the cell and rapidly accumulate within the endocytic vacuole to be released from the cell between 30 and 48 h after the start of the cycle.

All species of *Chlamydia* contain a common heat-stable lipopolysaccharide antigen, which is exposed on the surface of the reticulate body but not on the elementary body. The major outer membrane protein (MOMP) is immunodominant in the elementary body and contains epitopes exhibiting genus, species, and serovar specificity. The serovar-specific epitope is the basis of the microimmunofluorescence (MIF) test by which *C. trachomatis* has been separated into 15 serovars: A, B, Ba, and C are responsible mainly for endemic trachoma; D to K for oculogenital infections; and L1, L2, and L3 for the genital disease lymphogranuloma venereum. Only one *C. pneumoniae* serovar has been identified, although minor geographical serovar variations have been described. *C. psittaci* is

loosely defined and likely to contain a wide variety of host-related serovars. Amino acid sequences of the MOMPs of all *C. trachomatis* serovars and epitope maps of different antigenic domains have been elucidated. The MOMP genes consist of five highly conserved regions punctuated by four short variable sequences. Serovar-specific epitopes have been demonstrated in variable sequence I and II, while species-specific epitopes have been found in variable sequence IV. It is also probable that these variable sequences influence chlamydial pathogenesis. *C. trachomatis*, *C. psittaci*, and *C. pneumoniae* species have been compared and although there is only 10% DNA homology between each of them, the MOMP genes show up to 65% amino acid homology, indicating a probable common ancestor. A common chlamydial 57-kDa protein has been described; its possible role in disease pathogenesis is considered below.

Immune response and pathogenesis

The immune response to chlamydial infections may be protective or damaging. Active trachoma is uncommon in adults in endemic areas, suggesting that protective immunity follows natural infection. Similarly, genital *C. trachomatis* infection is most prevalent in the youngest sexually active age groups, and the chlamydial isolation rate for men with nongonococcal urethritis is lower in those who have had previous episodes. The duration of ocular infection is shorter in adults than in children. Several trachoma vaccine trials in the 1960s used killed whole organism vaccines, which provided some degree of protection. Primates studies suggested that vaccination could provoke more severe disease on subsequent challenge, indicating immunopathological damage by *C. trachomatis*.

The lymphoid follicle is the hallmark of chlamydial infection and follicles contain typical germinal centres, consisting predominantly of B lymphocytes, with T cells, mostly CD8 cells, in the parafollicular region. The inflammatory infiltrate between follicles comprises plasma cells, dendritic cells, macrophages, and polymorphonuclear leucocytes, with T and B lymphocytes. Fibrosis is seen at a late stage, typically in trachoma and pelvic inflammatory disease. T lymphocytes are also present and outnumber B cells and macrophages. Biopsies from patients with cicatricial trachoma and persisting inflammatory changes show a predominance of CD4 cells, but those from patients in whom inflammation has subsided contain mainly CD8 cells.

A chlamydial heat-shock protein (hsp 60), homologous with the GroEL protein of *Escherichia coli*, elicits antibody responses which are associated with the damaging sequelae of *C. trachomatis* infections in both the eye and genital tract. *In vitro* studies show that interferon-γ interferes with the chlamydial development cycle, leading to persistent infection with continuing release of hsp 60. It is not known whether the immune response to hsp 60 is itself the cause of immunopathological damage, or merely a marker of more severe or prolonged infection.

Studies in trachoma-endemic communities suggest that T-helper 1 type cell-mediated responses are important in the clearance of ocular *C. trachomatis* infection. Gene expression at the site of infection, the conjunctival epithelium, is used to identify molecular pathways to fibrosis, in which matrix metalloproteinase 9 (MMP 9) appears be important. Case control studies have identified polymorphisms in several immune response genes (encoding TNFα, IFNγ, and IL-10) associated with the severe scarring of trachoma.

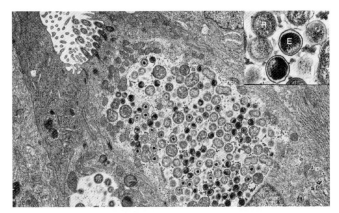

Fig. 6.44.1 Elementary bodies (E) and reticulate bodies (R) of *C. trachomatis*, forming an inclusion in an oviduct cell; shown by transmission electron microscopy.

Infectious chlamydial elementary bodies are actively taken up by epithelial cells, and develop inside an intracellular inclusion. Fusion of the chlamydial inclusion with lysosomes is inhibited while the organisms remain viable. An understanding of the pathogenesis of chlamydial infection has been enhanced by sequencing the complete genome of several *C. trachomatis* strains. The serovar D genome contains genes homologous with those coding for virulence factors in other bacteria, including a cytotoxin gene, and genes encoding a type III secretion pathway. A conserved chlamydial protease, proteasome-like activity factor (CPAF), is secreted into the host cell cytoplasm, where it interferes with the assembly and surface expression of HLA molecules and inhibits apoptosis. The serovar A genome has been found to be 99.6% identical to serovar D. The 'ocular' serovars (A, B, Ba, and C) differ from the 'genital' serovars (D–K) in lacking a functional tryptophan synthase gene, rendering them more sensitive to inhibition by interferon γ.

Trachoma

Trachoma is a chronic keratoconjunctivitis caused by the 'ocular' serovars A, B, Ba, and C of *C. trachomatis*. In the 19th century it was an important and common cause of blindness in Europe and North America, but it disappeared from more affluent parts of the world as living standards improved in the 20th century. In poor communities where hygiene standards are low, there is direct transfer of chlamydial organisms from eye to eye and trachoma is endemic. As standards of hygiene improve, this mode of transmission is no longer possible and trachoma tends to disappear. It is now a disease of poor rural communities, mainly in Africa and Asia, but it remains the leading infectious cause of blindness worldwide. A recent review by the World Health Organization (WHO) estimated that trachoma was responsible for 3.6% of global blindness, or 1.3 million cases.

Clinical features

The active (inflammatory) stage of trachoma is a follicular conjunctivitis, affecting chiefly the subtarsal conjunctiva, but follicles may be elsewhere on the conjunctiva and at the limbus. Such subconjunctival follicles are the characteristic sign of active disease (Fig. 6.44.2) and are usually seen in children in endemic areas. Limbal follicles resolve leaving characteristic shallow depressions known as Herbert's pits. New vessels (pannus) may be seen at this stage in the cornea (Fig. 6.44.3), usually at the superior margin, and punctate keratitis may also be a feature. Since symptoms are mild or absent, the disease may not be suspected unless the upper eyelid is everted. *C. trachomatis* can often be found in active cases, although

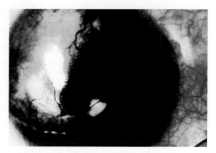

Fig. 6.44.3 Extensive neovascularization of the cornea (pannus) due to trachoma.

follicles can persist for some time after infection has been cleared. Intense inflammation is seen in the subtarsal conjunctiva in some cases (Fig. 6.44.4) in which the *C. trachomatis* organism loads are higher. The disease may progress over many years and, with repeated infection, result in conjunctival scarring (Fig. 6.44.5). As the scars contract, the lid margin turns inwards (entropion), and the lashes rub against the cornea, a condition known as trichiasis (Fig. 6.44.6). This damages the cornea, eventually rendering it opaque.

The WHO criteria for the clinical diagnosis of active trachoma, its potentially blinding sequelae, and for grading their severity is as follows:

1 Trachomatous inflammation, follicular (TF)—five or more follicles, each at least 0.5 mm in diameter, in the upper tarsal conjunctiva (Fig. 6.44.2)

2 Trachomatous inflammation, intense (TI)—pronounced inflammatory thickening of the tarsal conjunctiva that obscures more than one-half of the normal deep tarsal blood vessels (Fig. 6.44.4)

3 Trachomatous conjunctival scarring (TS)—easily visible scarring in the tarsal conjunctiva (Fig. 6.44.5)

4 Trachomatous trichiasis (TT)—at least one eyelash rubbing on the eyeball, or evidence of recent removal of inturned eyelashes (Fig. 6.44.6)

5 Corneal opacity (CO)—easily visible corneal opacity over the pupil, so dense that at least part of the pupil margin is blurred when viewed through the opacity

Epidemiology

Trachoma is a disease of poverty, which disappears as living standards improve. In the past, it has been endemic in urban communities such as in the East End of London, but it is now a disease of rural communities that lack access to water and sanitation, especially affecting marginalized groups. The reservoir of infection in

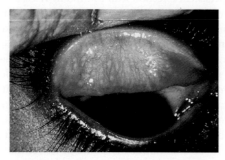

Fig. 6.44.2 Everted upper eyelid showing follicular trachoma (TF).

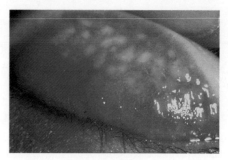

Fig. 6.44.4 Everted upper eyelid showing intense inflammatory trachoma (TI).

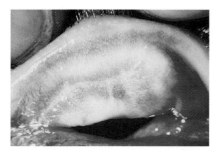

Fig. 6.44.5 Everted upper eyelid showing trachomatous scarring (TS).

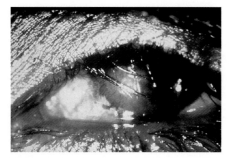

Fig. 6.44.6 Trachomatous trichiasis (TT).

endemic areas is the eye, and possibly the nasopharynx, of children with active disease. *C. trachomatis* may be transferred from the eye of one individual to that of another via fingers, fomites, coughing, and sneezing, and by eye-seeking flies. Active cases tend to cluster in households with prolonged intimate contact within the family. The higher prevalence of active disease and scarring in women than in men is probably due to their closer contact with children. Severe conjunctival scarring is associated with repeated exposure to reinfection.

Diagnosis

In trachoma-endemic areas, the diagnosis is made on clinical grounds, following the simplified WHO grading scheme (Figs. 6.44.2, 6.44.4–6.44.6). Trachomatous follicles (TF) may be confused with the giant papillae of vernal conjunctivitis, in which pannus may also be seen. Several viruses, notably adenoviruses, can cause a short lived follicular conjunctivitis. Intense cases of trachoma (TI), in which follicles may not be visible, should be distinguished from bacterial conjunctivitis. The diagnosis of trachomatous scarring (TS) is usually obvious, as few other conditions cause conjunctival scarring of the upper lid. Laboratory diagnosis of ocular *C. trachomatis* infection may help to direct treatment to communities with the greatest need, since clinical signs may persist for years after infection has been cleared. *C. trachomatis* may be found in about one-half of the cases of active inflammation (TF or TI), but in only a minority of those with scarring disease (TS). A portable dipstick test for chlamydial antigen detection has given promising results in trachoma endemic regions in Africa. Other diagnostic methods are discussed below.

Treatment

Inflammatory trachoma (TF and TI) responds to antimicrobial treatment (Table 6.44.1). The WHO recommends either 1% topical tetracycline ointment, to be applied to both eyes daily for 6 weeks, or a single oral dose of azithromycin (20 mg/kg, to a maximum

of 1 g). Community-based mass treatment is recommended when the prevalence of TF exceeds 10% in children aged 1 to 9 years. Reinfection is rapid if individual cases are treated separately. Trichiasis requires surgical correction. Several eyelid operations have been described, but few have been evaluated prospectively. Bilamellar tarsal rotation is probably the operation of choice.

Prevention

The WHO has launched a strategy for the global elimination of blinding trachoma by the year 2020, based on the acronym 'SAFE': Surgery for trichiasis, Antibiotics for the treatment of inflammatory disease and the elimination of the reservoir of infection, promotion of Face washing, and Environmental improvement to reduce fly populations. These procedures are likely to reduce the rate of transmission of ocular *C. trachomatis* infection and there is evidence that the prevalence of active trachoma has fallen in several countries in Africa and Asia in recent years.

Genital tract infections

Genital tract infections due to *C. trachomatis* serovars D to K (Table 6.44.2) occur worldwide. The highest prevalence is in women of 15 to 24 years of age and in men of 20 to 24 years of age. In developed countries, they are much more common than gonococcal infections. Their frequency imposes an enormous economic burden on health services. It is estimated that 2.8 million new cases of genital chlamydial infection occurred in the United States of America in the year 2000. In Sweden, widespread and effective diagnostic testing, coupled with aggressive contact tracing and treatment, reduced genital chlamydial infections in the decade from 1984, but subsequently there has been a slow increase. Screening programmes in some other developed countries, including the United Kingdom, have gradually been developed and implemented, but the reported chlamydial incidence has increased in most countries in Western Europe and North America since the mid 1990s. The extent to which this increase is due to more widespread testing using more sensitive assays is not clear.

Nongonococcal urethritis

The incubation period is 7 to 14 days compared to 2 to 5 days for gonococcal disease. *C. trachomatis* is detectable in the urethra of up to 50% of men with symptomatic nongonococcal urethritis and as many as 7% of those who are asymptomatic. It is also likely that chlamydiae are a cause of some cases of chronic (persistent/recurrent) nongonococcal urethritis. Treatment of gonococcal urethritis with an antibiotic ineffective against *C. trachomatis* may result in postgonococcal urethritis, which usually appears about 1 week after the treatment of gonococcal disease. *C. trachomatis* is responsible for a large proportion of such cases.

In women, chlamydial urethral infection may cause urethritis but, in contrast to men, infection and inflammation are almost always asymptomatic. The 'urethral syndrome' (dysuria and frequency with <10^5 organisms/ml urine) is rarely of chlamydial origin.

Prostatitis and epididymitis

There is no evidence that *C. trachomatis* causes acute symptomatic prostatitis. Transperineal biopsies from patients with chronic abacterial prostatitis show chronic inflammation, but chlamydiae have

Table 6.44.1 Recommended treatment schedules for chlamydial infections and associated diseases

Disease/infection	Antibiotic	Dose schedule[a]	Duration (days)
Trachoma	Topical tetracycline	1% ointment daily	42
	Azithromycin alone	20 mg/kg (up to 1 g)	Single dose
Adult inclusion conjunctivitis	Tetracycline HCl	500 mg 4 times daily	14
	Or doxycycline	100 mg twice daily	14
	Or erythromycin stearate	500 mg 4 times daily	14
	Or azithromycin	1 g	Single dose
NGU	Antibiotics and regimens as for treatment of adult inclusion conjunctivitis		7
Epididymo-orchitis	Ceftriaxone	250 mg	Single dose
	Then antibiotics as for NGU		10
Cervicitis/urethritis	Antibiotics and regimens as for NGU		7
Pelvic inflammatory disease (ambulatory patients)	Ceftriaxone	250 mg intramuscularly	
	Then doxycycline	100 mg twice daily	14
Pelvic inflammatory disease (patients admitted to hospital)	(a) Doxycycline	100 mg twice daily intravenously	≥4
	And cefoxitin	2 g three times daily intravenously	≥4
	Then doxycycline	100 mg twice daily	14
	And metronidazole	400 mg twice daily	14
	Or (b) clindamycin	600 mg 4 times daily intravenously	≥4
	And then Clindamycin	450 mg 4 times daily	10[b]
	And gentamicin	2 mg/kg intravenously	Single dose
	And then gentamicin	1.5 mg/kg 3 times daily	≥4
Neonatal infections	Erythromycin syrup	50 mg/kg daily in 4 divided doses	14
Lymphogranuloma venereum	Antibiotics and regimens as for NGU[c]		21
C. pneumoniae infections	Antibiotics and regimens as for NGU except doxycycline twice daily		7–21[d]
C. psittaci infections	Antibiotics and regimes as for NGU except doxycycline twice daily		≥14

NGU, nongonococcal urethritis
[a] All antibiotics orally unless otherwise indicated.
[b] Total duration of therapy 14 days.
[c] Azithromycin likely to be effective but multiple doses probably required.
[d] Relapse more often with short course.

not been detected by culture or direct immunofluorescence techniques, although polymerase chain reaction (PCR) tests are positive in about 10%. Such largely negative observations, and the failure to detect chlamydial antibody, suggest that *C. trachomatis* is not often implicated directly in the chronic disease. However, the predominance of CD8 cells in the tissues suggests that some cases of chronic disease might be of chlamydial origin.

C. trachomatis is responsible for up to 50% of cases of acute epididymitis or epididymo-orchitis occurring primarily in young men (≤35 years of age) in developed countries, and has been detected in at least one-third of epididymal aspirates. There is a strong correlation between IgM and IgG chlamydial antibodies, measured by MIF, and chlamydia-positive disease. In developing countries, although chlamydiae are important, *Neisseria gonorrhoeae* is the major cause of acute epididymitis. In patients older

than 35 years, epididymitis/epididymo-orchitis tends to be caused by urinary tract pathogens.

There is no good evidence that chlamydial epididymitis or chlamydial urethral infection leads to male infertility.

Bartholinitis, vaginitis, and cervicitis

C. trachomatis has been weakly associated with bartholinitis and should be considered in the absence of other known pathogens. Chlamydiae are often detected more frequently in women with bacterial vaginosis than in those without, but there is no evidence that they contribute to the disease. In prepubertal children, the vaginal epithelium is columnar and susceptible to chlamydial infection. In adults, the squamous epithelium of the vagina is not susceptible and the cervix is the primary target for *C. trachomatis*, where it is an established cause of mucopurulent/follicular cervicitis (Fig. 6.44.7)

Table 6.44.2 Assessment of the extent to which *C. trachomatis* is involved in various oculogenital and associated diseases

Disease	Evidence that C. trachomatis is a cause[a]	Proportion of disease due to C. trachomatis
In men		
Acute NGU	++++	Up to 50%
Postgonococcal urethritis	++++	Up to 90%
Persistent and recurrent NGU	++	?
Acute and chronic prostatitis	+	?
Acute epididymo-orchitis	++++	Up to 50%
Infertility	–	
In women		
Urethritis	+++	?
Bartholinitis	+	?
Vaginitis (prepuberty only)	+++	?
Bacterial vaginosis	–	
Cervicitis	++++	About 50%
Cervical dysplasia	+	
Endometritis	+++	?
Salpingitis	++++	? 40–60%
Periappendicitis	++	?
Perihepatitis	+++	?
Infertility	+++	≥10% due to chlamydial salpingitis
Ectopic pregnancy	+++	?
Early miscarriage	+	?
Abortion	–	
In men or women		
Conjunctivitis	++++	?
Otitis media	++	?
Arthritis (Reiter's syndrome)	+++	About 40%
Endocarditis	++	?
Pharyngitis	–	
Proctitis	+++	?
Lymphogranuloma venereum	++++	100% (by definition)
In infants		
Conjunctivitis	++++	Up to 50%
Pneumonia	++++	30%?
Chronic lung disease	++	?
Gastroenteritis	–	

NGU, nongonococcal urethritis.
[a]++++, overwhelming; +++, good; ++, moderate; +, weak; –, none.

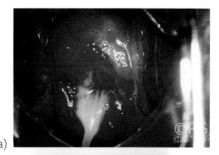

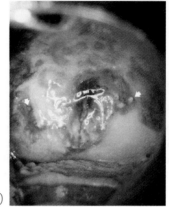

Fig. 6.44.7 (a) Mucopurulent cervicitis; (b) follicular cervicitis.

which is often asymptomatic. Women younger than 25 years, unmarried, using oral contraceptives, and who have signs of cervicitis are the most likely to have a chlamydial infection.

A significant association between cervical chlamydial infection and cervical squamous cell carcinoma, but not adenocarcinoma, has been established and it has been suggested that chlamydial infection may enhance the effect of oncogenic papillomaviruses.

Pelvic inflammatory disease

Canalicular spread of chlamydiae to the upper genital tract leads to endometritis, which is often plasma cell associated and sometimes intensely lymphoid. Further spread causes salpingitis (Fig. 6.44.8), seen in about 10% of women with cervical infection. Classic signs often ensue but inflammation may be subclinical. Spread to the peritoneum results in perihepatitis (the Fitz Hugh–Curtis syndrome) (Fig. 6.44.9), sometimes confused with acute cholecystitis in young women, in addition to periappendicitis and other abdominal symptoms. Surgical termination of pregnancy or insertion or removal of an intrauterine contraceptive device may predispose to dissemination of infection.

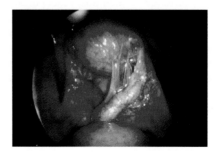

Fig. 6.44.8 Laparoscopic view of inflamed fallopian tube due to *C. trachomatis*. (Courtesy of P Greenhouse.)

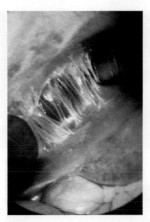

Fig. 6.44.9 Adhesions in perihepatitis (Fitz-Hugh–Curtis syndrome). (Courtesy of P Greenhouse.)

Chlamydial infection is the major cause of pelvic inflammatory disease in developed countries. Infertility may be the first indication of asymptomatic tubal disease. It occurs in about 10% of women following a single upper genital tract infection and in possibly one-half of those after two or three episodes. Infertility could result possibly from endometritis, and certainly from blocked or damaged tubes, or perhaps abnormalities of ovum transportation. Other consequences of salpingitis are chronic pelvic pain and ectopic pregnancy. The risk of ectopic pregnancy increases seven- to tenfold after chlamydial pelvic inflammatory disease.

There is conflicting evidence on the effect of *C. trachomatis* on pregnancy. Some studies have shown *C. trachomatis* infection to be associated with low birth weight and preterm delivery, but others have failed to confirm this. In general, *C. trachomatis* infection was diagnosed and treated at an earlier stage of gestation in those studies in which a correlation was found between infection and adverse birth outcome than in those in which this was not found.

Other diseases associated with *C. trachomatis*

Adult paratrachoma (inclusion conjunctivitis) and otitis media

Adult chlamydial ophthalmia is distinguished from trachoma by its causative *C. trachomatis* serovars D to K. It commonly results from the accidental transfer of infected genital discharge to the eye. In contrast to 'reactive' conjunctivitis seen in Reiter's syndrome (see below), chlamydiae can usually be detected in conjunctival specimens. It usually presents as a unilateral follicular conjunctivitis, acute or subacute in onset, with an incubation period of up to 21 days. The features are swollen lids, mucopurulent discharge, papillary hyperplasia, and, later, follicular hypertrophy and occasionally punctate keratitis. About one-third of patients have otitis media and complain of blocked ears and hearing loss. The disease is generally benign and self-limited. Pannus formation and corneal scarring are rare and not seen if systemic treatment is given. Patients and their sexual contacts should be investigated for genital chlamydial infection and managed appropriately.

Arthritis

Arthritis occurring with or soon after nongonococcal urethritis is termed 'sexually acquired reactive arthritis' (SARA). Conjunctivitis and

other features characteristic of Reiter's syndrome are seen in about one-third of patients. Evidence of chlamydial infection, by a specific serological response or by the presence of *C. trachomatis* elementary bodies or DNA and antigen in the joints, is found in at least one-third of patients. *C. trachomatis* has also been associated in the same way with 'seronegative' arthritis in women. Viable chlamydiae have not been detected in the joints of patients with SARA which is probably the result of immunopathology (see below). Despite this, early tetracycline therapy has been advocated by some investigators.

Immunocompromised patients

C. trachomatis has been isolated from the lower respiratory tract of a few immunocompromised adults with pneumonia, some after renal transplantation, but other pathogens are often also present. *C. pneumoniae* is not an especially important respiratory tract pathogen in AIDS patients. Genital *C. trachomatis* infection is likely to increase viral shedding from HIV-positive people, and enhance the susceptibility to HIV in the uninfected. Conversely, HIV infection increases the susceptibility of women to *C. trachomatis* genital infection. In contrast, hypogammaglobulinaemic patients do not appear to be especially prone to infection with any of the chlamydial species.

Neonatal infections

Although intrauterine chlamydial infection can occur, the major risk of infection to the infant is from passing through an infected cervix. The proportion of neonates exposed to infection depends, of course, on the prevalence of maternal cervical infection, which varies widely. Conjunctivitis appears in 20 to 50% of infants exposed to *C. trachomatis* (serovars D–K) infecting the cervix at birth. A mucopurulent discharge (Fig. 6.44.10) and occasionally pseudomembrane formation occur 1 to 3 weeks later. It usually resolves without visual impairment. Complications tend to be in untreated infants.

Approximately one-half of the infants who have conjunctivitis also develop pneumonia, although a history of recent conjunctivitis and bulging eardrums are found in only one-half of the infants. Chlamydial pneumonia usually begins between the 4th and 11th week of life, preceded by upper respiratory symptoms. There is tachypnoea, a prominent staccato cough, but no fever, and the illness is protracted. Radiographs show hyperinflation of the lungs with bilateral diffuse symmetrical interstitial infiltration and scattered areas of atelectasis. Finding serum IgM antibody to *C. trachomatis* in infants with pneumonia is pathognomonic. Children infected during infancy are more likely to develop obstructive lung

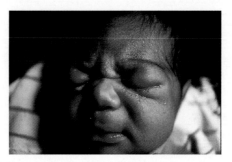

Fig. 6.44.10 Mucopurulent neonatal conjunctival discharge due to *C. trachomatis*.

disease and asthma than are those who have had pneumonia of other causes.

The vagina and rectum also may be colonized by *C. trachomatis* at birth, but this has not been associated with clinical disease. Rectal shedding might occur 2 to 3 months after birth, suggesting colonization of the gastrointestinal tract, but there is no evidence of infant chlamydial gastroenteritis.

Lymphogranuloma venereum

Lymphogranuloma venereum (LGV) is a systemic, sexually transmitted disease caused by serovars L1, L2, and L3 of *C. trachomatis*. These are more virulent in animal models than serovars A to K, and more invasive in humans. Serovars A to K are largely confined to mucosal columnar epithelial surfaces of the genital tract and eye, but the LGV serovars predominantly infect monocytes and macrophages, which pass through the epithelial surface to regional lymph nodes and may cause disseminated infection.

Clinical features

The clinical course of LGV can be divided into three stages. The primary stage at the site of inoculation, the secondary stage in the regional lymph nodes and/or the anorectum, and the tertiary stage of late sequelae affecting the genitalia and/or rectum.

After an incubation period of 3 to 30 days, the primary stage begins with a small, painless papule which may ulcerate. It occurs at the site of inoculation, usually the prepuce or glans in men; anorectal and rectosigmoid colon sites in homosexual men; or the vulva, vaginal wall, or occasionally the cervix in women. Extragenital primary lesions on fingers or tongue are rare. The primary lesion is self-healing and may pass unnoticed by the patient, especially if it is in the alimentary tract of homosexual men. Among patients with LGV presenting with buboes in Thailand, more than one-half had not been aware of an ulcer.

The secondary stage occurs some weeks after the primary lesion, which has usually healed. Chlamydiae are carried to regional or rectal lymph nodes. The inguinal form is more common in men than women, since the lymphatic drainage of the upper vagina and cervix is to the retroperitoneal rather than the inguinal lymph nodes. LGV proctitis occurs in those who practise receptive anal intercourse, probably due to direct inoculation.

The cardinal feature of the inguinal form of LGV is painful, usually unilateral, inguinal and/or femoral lymphadenopathy (bubo). Adenopathy above and below the inguinal ligament gives rise to the 'groove sign' in 10 to 20% of patients, once believed to be pathognomonic. Enlarged lymph nodes are usually firm and often accompanied by systemic signs of fever, chills, arthralgia, and headache. Biopsy reveals small discrete areas of necrosis surrounded by proliferating epithelioid and endothelial cells. These areas of necrosis may enlarge to form stellate abscesses, which may coalesce and break down to form discharging sinuses, although this phenomenon occurs in less than one-third of patients with inguinal disease. In women, signs include a hypertrophic suppurative cervicitis, backache, and adnexal tenderness. Anorectal involvement is seen predominantly in homosexual men. Clinical features include a purulent anal discharge, anorectal pain and bleeding due to an acute haemorrhagic proctitis or proctocolitis, and there may be pronounced systemic signs of fever, chills, and weight loss. Asymptomatic LGV is rare, according to a large study in the United Kingdom using molecular typing of chlamydial isolates. Early detection of LGV at a 'presymptomatic'

stage of disease might be found among people who are regularly screened for rectal *C. trachomatis*. Proctoscopy reveals a granular or ulcerative proctitis from which large numbers of polymorphonuclear leucocytes are seen in rectal smears. CT or MRI scans may show pronounced thickening of the rectal wall, with enlargement of iliac lymph nodes. Enlarged inguinal nodes may also be palpable.

Extragenital infection can cause lymphadenopathy outside the inguinal region. For example, cervical adenopathy due to LGV has been reported after oral sex, and laboratory workers who developed pneumonitis after accidental inhalation of LGV strains of *C. trachomatis* were found to have mediastinal and supraclavicular adenopathy. A follicular conjunctivitis has also been described following direct inoculation of the eye, which may be accompanied by preauricular lymphadenopathy. Other rare manifestations of the secondary stage include acute meningoencephalitis, synovitis, and cardiac involvement.

The tertiary stage appears after a latent period of several years, but all late complications are rare today because of the use of broad-spectrum antibiotics. Chronic untreated LGV leads to fibrosis, which may cause lymphatic obstruction and elephantiasis of the genitalia in either sex, or rectal strictures and fistulae. Rarely, it can give rise to the syndrome of esthiomene (Greek: 'eating away'), with widespread destruction of the external genitalia (Fig. 6.44.11).

Epidemiology

LGV is a rare disease in industrialized countries, but is endemic in parts of Africa, Asia, South America, and the Caribbean. The reported sex ratio is greater than 5:1 in favour of men, probably because of the easier recognition of disease. The epidemiology of infection is poorly defined because LGV is often indistinguishable clinically from chancroid and other causes of genital ulceration with bubo formation, and it has been difficult to obtain laboratory confirmation. LGV is an uncommon cause of genital ulceration in Africa. Ten per cent of patients with buboes presenting to a sexually transmitted disease clinic in Bangkok were found to have LGV, and an epidemic of LGV has been found among crack cocaine users

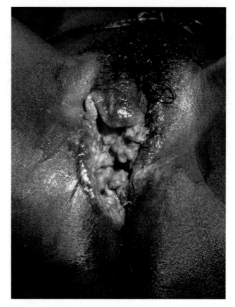

Fig. 6.44.11 Esthiomene: destruction of the female genitalia by lymphogranuloma venereum in a Nigerian patient.
(Copyright D A Warrell.)

in the Bahamas. In 2003, an outbreak of LGV proctitis due to the L2 serovar was reported among homosexual men in the Netherlands, and in the subsequent 3 years over 1000 cases were reported in homosexual men across Western Europe, the United Kingdom, North America, and Australia. The majority of affected men have been HIV positive.

Diagnosis

LGV may present as a genital ulcer or as inguinal lymphadenopathy (usually painful) without evidence of genital ulceration. The differential diagnosis of sexually acquired genital ulceration also includes chancroid, herpes, syphilis, and donovanosis (granuloma inguinale). Less common causes include trauma, nonvenereal infections such as cutaneous leishmaniasis or amoebiasis, and fixed drug eruption. The differential diagnosis of inguinal adenopathy includes chancroid, herpes, and syphilis, although there is usually a genital ulcer or at least a history of an ulcer in these conditions. Chronic sinus formation in the inguinal region may be due to tuberculosis of the lumbar spine, and bubonic plague should be considered in endemic areas where a patient with inguinal lymphadenopathy is acutely ill. LGV proctitis needs to be distinguished from inflammatory bowel disease due to ulcerative colitis or Crohn's disease, although clinical and histopathological features may be identical.

The laboratory diagnosis of LGV depends on serology or on identification of *C. trachomatis* in appropriate clinical samples. Because it is more invasive, LGV infection induces higher serum antibody titres than do uncomplicated genital infections with *C. trachomatis* serovars D to K. The MIF test can distinguish between infections with different chlamydial species. A MIF titre exceeding 1:128 strongly suggests LGV, particularly in a patient with typical signs and symptoms, although invasive genital infection with *C. trachomatis* serovars D to K, as in pelvic inflammatory disease, can also give rise to high antibody titres.

C. trachomatis can be identified in a smear of bubo material by direct fluorescence microscopy (Table 6.44.3) using commercially available conjugated monoclonal antibody, although bacterial contamination impedes detection. *C. trachomatis* can be isolated in cell culture from ulcer material, bubo aspirate, or endourethral or endocervical scrapings, but the success rate is poor. Commercially available nucleic acid amplification methods are much more sensitive and the diagnosis of LGV can be confirmed by amplification and restriction fragment length polymorphism (RFLP) typing or sequencing of the outer membrane protein 1 (*omp1*) gene.

Treatment

There has been no adequately powered study comparing antibiotic regimens for LGV. Recommended treatment for both bubonic and anogenital LGV is doxycycline 100 mg twice daily or erythromycin 500 mg four times daily for 21 days. Azithromycin has been used successfully in some cases, although a 1-g single oral dose is unlikely to be sufficient and the optimal regimen is unknown. Fever and bubo pain subside rapidly after antibiotic treatment is started, but buboes may take several weeks to resolve. Large collections of pus should be aspirated, using a lateral approach through normal skin. Rectovaginal fistulas, rectal strictures, and esthiomene require surgical correction with antibiotic cover.

C. pneumoniae infections

The prototype strains of *C. pneumoniae* were isolated in the 1960s from conjunctival samples collected from a child in Taiwan (strain TW-183) and another in Iran (strain IOL-207). In 1983, a third *C. pneumoniae* strain was isolated, this time from the throat of a patient with acute respiratory (AR) disease, i.e. pharyngitis (strain AR-39). This prompted the name TWAR (TW+AR) being coined for the isolates. The two original isolates (TW-183 and IOL-207) were serologically identical and distinct from *C. trachomatis* and *C. psittaci*. In 1989, *C. pneumoniae* was defined as the third species of the genus *Chlamydia*. Only one serovar of *C. pneumoniae* has been identified, although minor geographical serovar variations are described.

Table 6.44.3 Advantages and disadvantages of chlamydial detection procedures

Factor considered	Culture	Direct fluorescent antibody	Enzyme immunoassay[a]	Nucleic acid amplification
Speed/temperature for transport of specimen	Rapid or at low temperature	Unimportant if specimen fixed	Unimportant if specimen in buffer	Speed not crucial if at low temperature; may use fixed specimens
Storage requirements	4°C if overnight; liquid nitrogen if long term	4°C if short term; −20°C and fixed if long term	4°C if 3–5 days; freezing if longer	4°C if short term; −70°C if long term
Evaluation of adequacy of specimen	Not practical	Evaluate during test	Not practical	Determine whether DNA present
Special equipment or procedure	Centrifuge	Fluorescence microscope	ELISA reader	Thermocycling machine and electrophoresis equipment
Processing of specimen	Tedious	Simple	Relatively simple	Requires precautions against DNA contamination
Reading of test	Subjective and moderately tedious	Subjective and tedious	Objective and simple	Objective and simple
Duration of test	48–72 h	30 min	3 h	12–24 h
Sensitivity of test	<70%	70–100%	<50–70%	Up to 100%

ELISA, enzyme linked immunosorbent assay.
[a] Now rarely used.

Clinical features

Respiratory tract disease

After an incubation period of approximately 3 weeks, acute disease often begins with pharyngitis. More than 80% of patients with lower respiratory tract disease have a sore throat. A cough may develop later and fever is uncommon. Bronchitis sometimes appears and in young adults about 5% of primary sinusitis is associated with *C. pneumoniae*. Mild respiratory infections are probably frequent but pneumonia is most common. Radiographs usually reveal a unilateral pneumonia, but more severe infection causes bilateral signs. This is often difficult to distinguish clinically from *Mycoplasma pneumoniae* and other pneumonias. Up to one-fifth of exacerbations of chronic obstructive pulmonary disease (COPD) are associated with *C. pneumoniae* and it has been implicated in exacerbations of both adult and childhood asthma.

Arthritis

An exaggerated synovial lymphocyte response to *C. pneumoniae* has been found in some adults with reactive arthritis and *C. pneumoniae* DNA and high titres of specific antibody have been detected in synovial fluid from the joints of a few children with juvenile chronic arthritis, suggesting the possibility of a causal role.

Atherosclerosis

Finnish investigators in the 1980s observed an association between chronic coronary heart disease or acute myocardial infarction and antibody to *C. pneumoniae*. The idea of chronic infection was enhanced by the detection of chlamydiae or their DNA in at least 40% of atheromatous plaques in coronaries and other major arteries, but not normal tissue, of people as young as 15 years of age. Specific DNA was also found in peripheral blood mononuclear cells, suggesting that they transmit the organisms from the respiratory tract to the arterial wall. Euphoria about these findings has been dealt a blow by the results of three major antibiotic trials in the United States of America. Subjects who received long courses of azithromycin in two trials and gatifloxacin in the other, subsequently experienced untoward coronary events as often as those given a placebo. This outcome was not completely unexpected in patients with well-established, long-standing disease.

Other diseases

C. pneumoniae has been linked to Alzheimer's disease, stroke, and multiple sclerosis, as well as chronic secretory otitis media, cystic fibrosis, sarcoidosis, and primary biliary cirrhosis, but there is no evidence to suggest a causal association.

Epidemiology

C. pneumoniae genotypes have been detected in horses, koalas, bandicoots, amphibians, and reptiles but there is no evidence of transfer to humans. It is thought that human strains are transmitted directly from person to person. Serological evidence indicates that *C. pneumoniae* is widespread and endemic in many areas, although localized respiratory epidemics have been recorded in both military and civilian groups in Scandinavia, the United States of America, the United Kingdom, and elsewhere. *C. pneumoniae* probably causes many mild respiratory infections that were previously thought to be viral in origin and it is also likely that many infections labelled 'human psittacosis' or 'ornithosis' in the past were due to *C. pneumoniae*.

C. psittaci infections

The *C. psittaci* species forms a diverse group isolated from a variety of mammals, reptiles, and many avian species. There is a relatively low degree of homology between serovars exhibited in DNA–DNA hybridization analyses, with the possibility of further differentiation between organisms assigned to the species. The spectrum of animal diseases caused by *C. psittaci* and other chlamydiae includes conjunctivitis, pneumonia, enteritis, abortion, sterility, arthritis, and encephalitis, all of which result in economic loss. The organisms are occasionally transmitted to humans. Psittacosis is an avian and human infection by *C. psittaci* found in psittacine birds, and ornithosis is infection by strains from other birds. 'Psittacosis' is now often used indiscriminately when referring to infection from psittacine and nonpsittacine birds. It is a potential hazard to those who keep pet birds and those who work in poultry processing plants or in animal husbandry.

Clinical features

After an incubation period of 1 to 2 weeks, the presentation of psittacosis varies from a mild influenza-like illness to a fulminating toxic state with multiple organ involvement. The disease may begin insidiously over a few days, or start abruptly with high fever, rigors, and anorexia. A headache is common, a cough, often dry, occurs in over two-thirds of patients, and arthralgia and myalgia in over one-third of patients. Inspiratory crepitations are more usual than classic signs of consolidation. Chest radiographs show patchy shadowing, often in the lower lobes. Homogeneous lobar shadowing is less frequent, miliary and nodular patterns even less so, and significant pleural effusions are rare. Extrapulmonary complications, mostly rare, include endocarditis, myocarditis, pericarditis, a toxic confusional state, encephalitis, meningitis, tender hepatomegaly, splenomegaly, pancreatitis, haemolysis, and disseminated intravascular coagulation. Improved diagnostic tests should not allow *C. psittaci* infections to be confused with those caused by *C. pneumoniae*.

Other chlamydial infections

C. abortus is endemic among ruminants and colonizes the placenta, causing abortion in sheep and rarely in pregnant women. They are often farmers' wives exposed to sheep with enzootic abortion during the lambing season. *C. felis* is endemic among domestic cats worldwide causing feline keratoconjunctivitis, rhinitis, and pneumonitis, and it can be isolated from the genital tract of female cats. In humans it has caused follicular conjunctivitis similar to that caused by *C. trachomatis* serovars D to K.

Laboratory diagnosis of chlamydial infections

The laboratory identification of chlamydial infection depends on culture, antigen, or nucleic acid detection, and to a much lesser extent on serology. The advantages and disadvantages of the tests are summarized in Table 6.44.3. Certain swabs, e.g. those with cotton tips, are superior to others, and swabs provided in commercial enzyme immunoassay kits may be toxic if used for collecting specimens for culture. Examination of two or more consecutive swabs from patients improves the chlamydial detection rate, which may be achieved by pooling cervical and urethral specimens.

'First-catch' urine specimens are unsuitable for chlamydial culture, but the centrifuged deposits are unquestionably valuable samples from both men and women, if tested by molecular methods. This also applies to the use of meatal samples in men and of vulva/vaginal samples.

Culture and staining of chlamydiae

The growth of chlamydiae more than 40 years ago in cultured cells, rather than in embryonated eggs, revolutionized their detection and chlamydial research. *C. pneumoniae* is particularly difficult to isolate, but will grow in selected cell lines including Hep-2. The isolation *C. trachomatis* involves centrifugation of specimens onto cycloheximide-treated McCoy cell monolayers, followed by incubation and then staining with a fluorescent monoclonal antibody or with a vital dye, usually Giemsa's, to detect inclusions. One blind passage may increase sensitivity but cell-culture techniques are slow, labour intensive, and no more than 70% sensitive compared to molecular methods.

Staining of epithelial cells in ocular and genital smears with vital dyes to detect chlamydial inclusions is insensitive and often nonspecific. In contrast, detection of elementary bodies using species-specific fluorescent monoclonal antibodies is rapid, highly sensitive, and specific for *C. trachomatis* oculogenital infections, in the hands of skilled observers. This test is most suitable for dealing with a few specimens and for confirming positive results obtained with other tests.

Enzyme immunoassays and nucleic acid amplification techniques

Enzyme immunoassays that detect chlamydial antigens, usually the group lipopolysaccharide, are easy to use but insensitive. At least 30% of genital swab specimens and a larger proportion of urine samples from women contain less than 10 chlamydial organisms, so many chlamydia-positive patients have remained undiagnosed. Molecular methods have largely replaced these immunoassays.

The enormous amplification of specific nucleic acid sequences with the PCR assay, the strand displacement assay (SDA), and the transcription-mediated amplification (TMA) technique overcomes the lack of specificity and particularly the poor sensitivity of other tests. The first two assays detect the cryptic plasmid, present in multiple copies in each chlamydial elementary body. The TMA reaction is directed against rRNA, also present in multiple copies. These assays have replaced culture as the 'gold standard' and are now important in routine diagnosis, in maintaining effective screening programmes, and for research into chronic or persistent disease. A variant of *C. trachomatis* serovar E that had escaped detection by commonly used nucleic acid amplification systems was found in Sweden in 2006 and subsequently has been found widely throughout the country but scarcely outside. This underlines the importance of taking into account the structure and function of genomes when selecting appropriate target nucleic acid sequences for diagnostic tests.

A sensitive rapid 'point-of-care' dipstick test, mentioned previously in the section on trachoma, is not yet available commercially.

Serological tests

The traditional complement-fixation test (CFT) cannot distinguish between the chlamydial species. Most of the pertinent diagnostic information originates from the MIF test which measures class-specific antibodies (IgM, IgG, IgA, or secretory). A significant increase in IgM and/or IgG titre is so unusual that the test is of little value. The presence of *C. trachomatis* IgG and/or IgA antibody in tears correlates well with isolation from the conjunctiva in endemic trachoma and adult ocular paratrachoma. In genital infections, serum or local IgA-specific antibodies do not necessarily indicate a current cervical chlamydial infection. In pelvic inflammatory disease, especially in the Fitz-Hugh–Curtis syndrome, antibody titres tend to be higher than in uncomplicated cervical infections. A high IgG antibody titre (1:256 or greater), suggests causation in pelvic disease, but high titres do not always correlate with detection of chlamydiae and are associated more with chronic or recurrent disease. Specific *C. trachomatis* IgM antibody in babies with pneumonia is pathognomonic of chlamydia-induced disease.

In primary respiratory infections with *C. pneumoniae*, IgM antibody appears within a few weeks and IgG antibody by 2 months. In repeat infections, IgG but not IgM antibody develops more rapidly and to a greater titre. The interpretation of results on a single serum is confounded by cross-reacting antibodies to the other species. Finding *C. pneumoniae* antibody in a single serum sample is only an assurance of infection in children. It is unwise to use the CFT to diagnose LGV or psittacosis because of its lack of specificity.

Treatment of chlamydial infections

Chlamydiae are intracellular and hence insensitive to aminoglycosides and other antibiotics that do not penetrate cells efficiently. They are particularly sensitive to tetracyclines and macrolides, and also to a variety of other drugs. The rifamycins are probably more active than the tetracyclines *in vitro*, but there is evidence of chlamydial resistance to the rifamycins. These have only rarely been used to treat refractory chlamydial infections, and they are reserved for mycobacterial infections. Tetracycline resistance is not widespread enough to cause clinical problems but vigilance is needed to detect resistant strains, which would not be found by the new routine diagnostic procedures.

The macrolide erythromycin is often used particularly to treat chlamydial infections in infants, young children, and in pregnant and lactating women. A single dose of azithromycin is popular because it enhances compliance. The recent fluoroquinolones are among other active drugs but they are not used regularly.

Table 6.44.1 shows details of the doses and duration of antibiotic treatment. Systemic treatment is given as well as, or in preference to, topical treatment to eradicate nasopharyngeal carriage in trachoma and for neonatal chlamydial conjunctivitis, since topical treatment provides no additional benefit. Oral erythromycin should be used to treat conjunctivitis and to prevent the development of pneumonia.

Azithromycin in a single oral dose (20 mg/kg) is as effective as 6 weeks of topical tetracycline for active trachoma and it is the drug of choice. A single 1-g oral dose of azithromycin is recommended for nongonococcal urethritis, but there is debate about the extent of its effectiveness. Treatment is usually started before a microbiological diagnosis can be established in patients with complicated genital tract infections, including epididymo-orchitis and pelvic inflammatory disease, so additional broad-spectrum antibiotic cover may be needed. Adequate doses of antibiotics, strict compliance, and treatment of patients' partners are all essential to eradicate genital infections.

The treatment of *C. pneumoniae* and *C. psittaci* infections is the same as for *C. trachomatis*.

Further reading

Bauwens JE, *et al.* (2002). Epidemic lymphogranuloma venereum during epidemics of crack cocaine use and HIV infection in the Bahamas. *Sex Transm Dis*, **29**, 253–9.

Bavoil PM, Wyrick PB (eds) (2006). *Chlamydia: genomics and pathogenesis.* Horizon Bioscience, Norfolk, UK.

Brunham RC, Rey-Ladino J (2005). Immunology of chlamydia infection: implications for a *Chlamydia trachomatis* vaccine. *Nat Rev Immunol*, **5**, 149–61.

Carlson JH, *et al.* (2005). Comparative genomic analysis of *Chlamydia trachomatis* oculotropic and genitotropic strains. *Infect Immun*, **73**, 6407–18.

Chernesky MA (2002). *Chlamydia trachomatis* diagnostics. *Sex Transm Infect*, **78**, 232–4.

Grayston JT, *et al.* (1990). A new respiratory tract pathogen: *Chlamydia pneumoniae* strain TWAR. *J Infect Dis*, **161**, 618–25.

Herrmann B, *et al.* (2008). Emergence and spread of *Chlamydia trachomatis* variant, Sweden. *Emerg Infect Dis*, **14**, 1462–5.

Mabey D, Solomon A, Foster A (2003). Trachoma seminar. *Lancet*, **362**, 223–9.

Michel CEC, *et al.* (2006). A rapid point-of-care assay for targeting antibiotic treatment to eliminate trachoma. *Lancet*, **367**, 1585–90.

Rasmussen SJ (1998). Chlamydial immunology. *Curr Opin Infect Dis*, **11**, 37–41.

Resnikoff S, *et al.* (2004). Global data on visual impairment in the year 2002. *Bull World Health Organ*, **82**, 844–51.

Schachter J, *et al.* (2010). *Proceedings of 12th International Symposium on Human Chlamydial Infections.* International chlamydia symposim, San Francisco, California.

Solomon A, *et al.* (2004). Mass treatment with single-dose azithromycin for trachoma. *N Engl J Med*, **351**, 1962–71.

Stephens RS, *et al.* (1998). Genome sequence of an obligate intracellular pathogen of humans: *Chlamydia trachomatis. Science*, **282**, 754–9.

Taylor-Robinson D (1991). Genital chlamydial infections: clinical aspects, diagnosis, treatment and prevention. In: Harris JRW, Forster SM (eds) *Recent advances in sexually transmitted diseases and AIDS*, pp. 219–62. Churchill Livingstone, Edinburgh.

Taylor-Robinson D, Thomas BJ (1998). *Chlamydia pneumoniae* in arteries: the facts, their interpretation, and future studies. *J Clin Pathol*, **51**, 793–7.

Thylefors B, *et al.* (1987). A simple system for the assessment of trachoma and its complications. *Bull World Health Organ*, **65**, 477–83.

Van der Bij AK, *et al.* (2006). Diagnostic and clinical implications of anorectal lymphogranuloma venereum in men who have sex with men: a retrospective case-control study. *Clin Infect Dis*, **42**, 186–94.

Viravan C, *et al.* (1996). A prospective clinical and bacteriologic study of inguinal buboes in Thai men. *Clin Infect Dis*, **22**, 233–9.

Wang SP, *et al.* (1967). Trachoma vaccine studies in monkeys. *Am J Ophthalmol*, **63**, 1615–20.

6.45 **Mycoplasmas**

David Taylor-Robinson and Jørgen Skov Jensen

Essentials

Mycoplasmas are the smallest self-replicating prokaryotes. They are devoid of cell walls, with the plasticity of their outer membrane favouring pleomorphism, although some have a characteristic bottle-shaped appearance. Mycoplasmas recovered from humans belong to the genera *Mycoplasma* (14 species) and *Ureaplasma* (2 species). They are predominantly found in the respiratory and genital tracts, but sometimes invade the bloodstream and thus gain access to joints and other organs.

Respiratory infection

Clinical features—*Mycoplasma pneumoniae* is the most important mycoplasmal respiratory pathogen, with presentations ranging from inapparent infection and mild, afebrile, upper respiratory-tract disease to severe pneumonia. It is responsible for 15 to 20% of all pneumonias in the United States of America, and is particularly common in older children and younger adults. Extrapulmonary manifestations include Stevens–Johnson syndrome and haemolytic anaemia.

Diagnosis and treatment—diagnosis is made by culture (slow and of limited value in clinical diagnosis), molecular methods (rapid detection by PCR is routine in some settings) and/or serology. Aside from supportive care, treatment is usually with tetracyclines or erythromycin. There is no commercially available effective vaccine.

Genitourinary and related infections

Clinical features—(1) Men—*M. genitalium* causes nongonococcal urethritis (NGU) in men, and ureaplasmas may play a role in some cases. (2) Women—*M. genitalium* causes urethritis, cervicitis, endometritis, and possibly salpingitis; *M. hominis* and (to a lesser extent) ureaplasmas are associated with bacterial vaginosis; *M. hominis* may contribute to salpingitis. (3) Pregnancy—ureaplasma infection of amniotic fluid is associated with preterm labour; ureaplasmas may be involved in the chronic lung disease of very low birthweight babies.

Diagnosis and treatment—diagnosis of infection by ureaplasmas and *M. hominis* is usually by culture of swabs from the urethra or cervix/vagina; PCR is used to detect *M. genitalium*. Patients with NGU should receive an antibiotic with activity against *C. trachomatis*, ureaplasmas, and *M. genitalium*, e.g azithromycin, with moxifloxacin used if *M. genitalium* becomes resistant and chronic disease develops.

Rheumatological manifestations

(1) Chronic arthritides—*M. fermentans* has been detected in the joints of patients with, e.g. rheumatoid arthritis, but the significance of this is unknown. (2) Reiter's syndrome—sexually acquired reactive arthritis (SARA) is not uncommon after *M. genitalium*-positive NGU, but no causal link has been established. (3) Arthritis in patients with hypogammaglobulinaemia is often caused by mycoplasmas (particularly ureaplasmas).

Introduction

Mycoplasmas, the trivial name for members of the class Mollicutes, are the smallest (0.3 µm diameter) free-living microorganisms. They lack the rigid cell wall of other bacteria, making them resistant to penicillins and related antimicrobials. Instead, they have a pliable trilaminar unit membrane (Fig. 6.45.1) enclosing the cytoplasm, DNA, RNA, and other components necessary for propagation in cell-free media. The small size of the mycoplasma genome (as little as 580 kbp) restricts metabolic capabilities, making culture of some mycoplasmas difficult or impossible. Despite their general

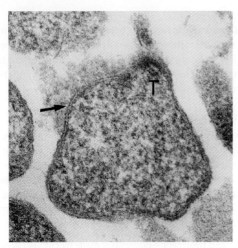

Fig. 6.45.1 Electron micrograph of *M. pulmonis* (murine origin), illustrating that the organism does not have a bacterial cell wall but has a trilaminar unit membrane (arrow); also note what appears to be a terminal structure (T). Magnification ×66 000.

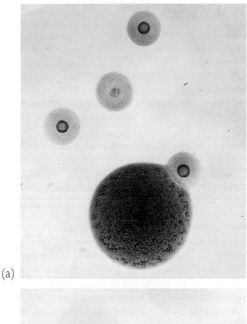

(a)

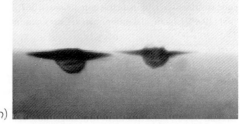

(b)

Fig. 6.45.2 (a) Fried-egg-like mycoplasma colonies (one ill-formed) and a larger bacterial colony. Transmission light microscopy, magnification ×43. (b) Section through mycoplasma colonies illustrating growth in the depth of the agar. Magnification ×78.

similarity, mycoplasmas are a heterogeneous group with differing host specificities, nutritional requirements, metabolic reactions, and DNA and antigenic composition. Mycoplasmas are divided into four orders: Mycoplasmatales, Entomoplasmatales comprising those from insects and plants, Acholeplasmatales, and the strictly anaerobic Anaeroplasmatales. The last two do not need sterol for growth. The mycoplasmas isolated commonly from humans belong to the family Mycoplasmataceae within the order Mycoplasmatales. This family includes the genus *Mycoplasma*, the organisms of which metabolize glucose or arginine or both, and the genus *Ureaplasma*, the organisms (ureaplasmas) of which uniquely hydrolyse urea. Ureaplasmas were originally termed T-strains or T-mycoplasmas because of the tiny (T) colonies (15–60 μm diameter) they form on agar medium, in contrast to the larger (≥90 μm diameter) characteristic fried-egg-like colonies produced by most other mycoplasmas (Fig. 6.45.2).

Historical perspective

The first mycoplasma to be recognized, *Mycoplasma mycoides* subsp. *mycoides*, was isolated in 1898 from cattle with pleuropneumonia. As other pathogenic and saprophytic isolates accumulated from veterinary and human sources, they became known as pleuropneumonia-like organisms (PPLO), a term later superseded by mycoplasmas. The first mycoplasma of human origin, *M. hominis*, was recovered from a Bartholin's gland abscess in 1937 and the first of undoubted pathogenicity, *M. pneumoniae*, from the respiratory tract in 1962. Ureaplasmas were first detected in the urethras of men with nongonococcal urethritis (NGU) in 1954 and *M. genitalium* was isolated from this site in 1981. The mycoplasma of human origin recognized most recently is *M. amphoriforme*, isolated in 1995. Over more than a century, numerous other mycoplasmas have been isolated from various animals and have been shown to be of economic importance because of the pneumonia, arthritis, keratoconjunctivitis, and mastitis they cause among livestock and poultry. This is apart from the plant diseases recognized as being due to mycoplasmas in recent years. In humans, as in other animal species, mycoplasmas cause respiratory and genital

tract diseases and escape from these sites to cause disease elsewhere, e.g. in joints.

Mycoplasmas are also notorious for contaminating cell cultures, particularly continuous cell lines. Various species of animal or human origin are responsible, e.g. porcine *M. hyorhinis* and human *M. orale* or *M. fermentans*. The contamination may affect almost any property under investigation in a totally unpredictable way and may lead to misinterpretation of any result based on studies in cultured cells.

Occurrence of mycoplasmas in humans

Fourteen species of mycoplasmas and two ureaplasmas have been isolated from humans, and constitute the normal flora or behave as pathogens (Tables 6.45.1, 6.45.2); in addition, several case reports have described infection with species of animal origin. Most of the human flora is found in the oropharynx. There is little information about the distribution or significance of *M. amphoriforme*, *M. penetrans*, *M. pirum*, and *M. spermatophilum*.

Respiratory infections

Relationship between mycoplasmas and respiratory disease

M. pneumoniae is the most important mycoplasma found in the respiratory tract (see below); most of the others behave as

Table 6.45.1 Biological features, occurrence, and disease association of mycoplasmas of human origin[a]

Mycoplasma	Metabolism of:	Haemadsorption	Frequency of detection in the:					Cause of disease
			Respiratory tract	Genitourinary tract	Rectum	Eye	Blood	
M. amphoriforme	Glucose	Yes	Rare[b]	–[c]	–[c]	–[c]	–[c]	?Yes
M. buccale	Arginine	No	Rare	–	–	–	–	No
M. faucium	Arginine	Yes[d]	Rare	–	–	–	–	No
M. fermentans	Glucose, arginine	No	Common	Rare	–	–	Rare	?Yes
M. genitalium	Glucose	Yes	Rare	Common	Rare	Rare	?	Yes
M. hominis	Arginine	No	Rare	Common	Common	Rare	Very rare	Yes
M. lipophilum	Arginine	No	Rare	–	–	–	–	No
M. orale	Arginine	Yes[d]	Common	–	–	–	–	No
M. penetrans	Glucose, arginine	Yes	–	Rare	Very rare	–	?	?
M. pirum	Glucose	?	?	–	Rare	?	Very rare	?
M. pneumoniae	Glucose	Yes	Rare[e]	Very rare	–	–	–	Yes
M. primatum	Arginine	No	–	Rare	–	–	–	No
M. salivarium	Arginine	No	Common	Rare	–	–	–	No[f]
M. spermatophilum	Arginine	No	–		?Rare	?	?	?
Ureaplasma parvum[g]	Urea	Serotype 3 only	Rare	Common	Common	Rare	Very rare	Yes
Ureaplasma urealyticum[g]	Urea	No	Rare	Common	Common	Rare	Very rare	Yes

[a] Occasional isolations of mycoplasma species of nonhuman origin not included.
[b] Except in immunocompromised patients.
[c] No reports of detection.
[d] With chick erythrocytes only.
[e] Except in disease outbreaks.
[f] Except in hypogammaglobulinaemia.
[g] Ureaplasmas have been divided into two species formerly described as biovars.

commensals (Table 6.45.1). *M. genitalium* was found originally in the male genitourinary tract but was isolated subsequently from a few respiratory specimens, which also contained *M. pneumoniae*. *M. genitalium* is not an important pathogen in the respiratory tract. *M. fermentans* has been detected in the throat more often since the use of polymerase chain reaction (PCR) (see below) and has been recovered from adults with an acute influenza-like illness, which sometimes deteriorates rapidly with development of a rare but often fatal respiratory distress syndrome. *M. hominis* is occasionally recovered from the respiratory tract. However, although it caused a mild pharyngitis in adult male volunteers inoculated orally, it is not known to do this naturally in children or adults. *M. amphoriforme* is a newly described species isolated from patients with chronic bronchitis, primarily those with B-cell deficiencies, and is phylogenetically related to pathogenic species such as *M. pneumoniae* and *M. genitalium*. The clinical importance of *M. amphoriforme* in the general population is unknown.

In the late 1930s, nonbacterial pneumonias or primary atypical pneumonia were distinguished from typical lobar pneumonia. Patients from whom the 'Eaton agent' had been isolated in embryonated eggs often developed cold agglutinins. This agent was presumed to be a virus until it was found to be sensitive to chlortetracycline and gold salts. Its mycoplasmal nature was established by cultivation on a cell-free agar medium. The agent, *M. pneumoniae*, was established as a respiratory pathogen by studies based on isolation, serology, volunteer inoculation, and vaccine protection.

Clinical features of *M. pneumoniae* disease

M. pneumoniae produces a range of effects from inapparent infection and mild afebrile upper respiratory tract disease to severe pneumonia. The most typical clinical syndrome is tracheobronchitis, often accompanied by upper respiratory tract manifestations such as acute pharyngitis. A clinical diagnosis of *M. pneumoniae* pneumonia is impossible as it shares features of other nonbacterial pneumonias. Malaise and headache often precede chest symptoms by 1 to 5 days, and pneumonia is seen radiographically before physical signs such as rales are detectable. Usually, only one of the lower lobes is involved and the radiograph shows patchy opacities. Pneumonia develops in about one-third of those infected and about 20% of patients have bilateral pneumonia. Pleurisy and pleural effusions are unusual. The course of the disease is variable but often protracted. Symptoms may persist for several weeks and may relapse. The organisms can persist in respiratory secretions despite antibiotic therapy, particularly in patients with hypogammaglobulinaemia where excretion may continue for months or years rather than weeks. Although a few very severe infections have been reported, usually in patients with immunodeficiency or sickle cell anaemia, death is rare. In children, illness may be prolonged with paroxysmal cough followed by vomiting, simulating whooping cough. *M. pneumoniae* has been implicated in bronchial asthma, but this is controversial (see below).

Table 6.45.2 Summary of the relationship between mycoplasmas and disease. Evidence for an association (A) between the indicated mycoplasma[a] and disease, and for the causation (C) of disease

	M. pneumoniae		M. fermentans		Ureaplasmas		M. hominis		M. genitalium	
	A	C	A	C	A	C	A	C	A	C
Upper respiratory tract disease	+++	+++	-		-		+++	-	-	
Bronchitis	+++	+++	-		-		-		-	
Pneumonia	++++	++++	++	+	-		-		-	
Asthma	++	+	NE		NA		-		-	
Extrapulmonary sequelae of M. pneumoniae infection (see text)	+++	+++	NA		NA		NA		NA	
Nongonococcal urethritis	NA		-		+++	+++	-		++++	++++
Chronic prostatitis	NA		NE		++	+	-		+	-
Epididymitis	NA		NE		++	++	-		++	++
Bartholinitis	NA		NE		-		+	-	NE	
Bacterial vaginosis	NA		NE		++	-	++++	+	-	
Cervicitis	NA		-		-		-		+++	+++
Pelvic inflammatory disease	NA		NE		+		+++	++	+++	+++
Infertility	NA		NE		++	-	-		++[b]	++
Urinary calculi	NA		-		++	+	-		NE	
Pyelonephritis	NA		NE		+	-	+++	++	NE	
Chorioamnionitis	NA		++	+	++	++	-		NE	
Preterm labour/birth	NA		NE		+++	++	++	++	+	+
Spontaneous abortion	NA		+	-	+++	+	++	+	+	-
Postabortal fever	NA		NE		++	+	++++	+++	NE	
Postpartum fever	NA		NE		++	+	++++	+++	NE	
Postpartum arthritis	NA		NE		-		+++	+++	NE	
Low birthweight	NA		NE		++	+	-		NE	
Neonatal chronic lung disease	NA		NE		+++	++	++	+	NE	
Rheumatoid arthritis	+	-	+++	-	++	-	-		+	-
Juvenile chronic arthritis	++	+	NE		-		-		NE	
Sexually acquired reactive arthritis/Reiter's disease	-		-		++	++	-		++	++
Arthritis in hypogammaglobulinaemia	++++	++++	NE		++++	++++	++++	+++	NE	
Wound infections	NA		NE		++	+	+++	+++	NE	
HIV infection	-		++	-	-		-		-	

NA, not appropriate to examine; NE, not examined; ++++, strong; +++, good; ++, moderate; +, weak; -, none.
[a] See text for M. amphoriforme and other mycoplasmas.
[b] Tubal factor infertility.

Extrapulmonary manifestations of *M. pneumoniae* infection

Disease caused by *M. pneumoniae* is usually limited to the respiratory tract, but various extrapulmonary conditions may occur during the course of the respiratory illness or subsequently (Table 6.45.3). Whether any are due to *M. genitalium* is uncertain. Haemolytic crisis is precipitated by cold agglutinins (anti-I antibodies). Mycoplasmas apparently alter the I antigen on erythrocytes sufficiently to stimulate an autoimmune response. A similar mechanism may be responsible for neurological and other complications. Invasion of the central nervous system cannot be discounted as *M. pneumoniae* has been isolated from cerebrospinal fluid.

Epidemiology of *M. pneumoniae* infections

Pathology is age dependent. About one-quarter of infections in children aged 5 to 15 years result in pneumonia, whereas only about 7% of infections in young adults do so. Pneumonia is less frequent thereafter, but is more severe the older the patient.

M. pneumoniae causes inapparent or mild upper respiratory tract symptoms more often than severe disease. It is responsible for a minority of all upper tract infections, usually attributable to viruses or streptococci. *M. pneumoniae* causes many lower respiratory tract infections, e.g. about 15 to 20% of all pneumonias in the United States of America. In populations such as military

Table 6.45.3 Extrapulmonary manifestations of *M. pneumoniae* infections

System	Manifestations	Estimated frequency
Cardiovascular	Myocarditis, pericarditis	<5%
Dermatological	Urticaria, erythema multiforme, Stevens–Johnson syndrome, other rashes	Some skin involvement in about 25%
Gastrointestinal	Anorexia, nausea, vomiting, and transient diarrhoea	15–45%
	Hepatitis	?
	Pancreatitis	?
Genitourinary	Acute glomerulonephritis	Insignificant
Haematological	Cold agglutinin production	About 50%
	Haemolytic anaemia	?
	Thrombocytopenia	?
	Intravascular coagulation	>50 reported cases
Musculoskeletal	Myalgia, arthralgia, arthritis	15–45%
Neurological	Meningitis, meningoencephalitis, ascending paralysis, transient myelitis, cranial nerve palsy, poliomyelitis-like illness	<5% in a few studies based on serology

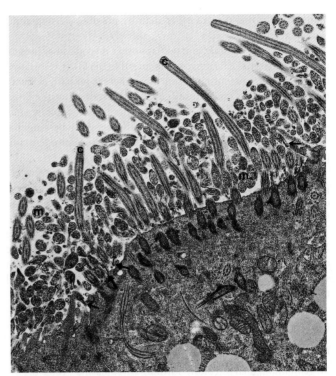

Fig. 6.45.3 Electron micrograph of ciliated epithelial cells in the tracheal mucosa of a hamster infected with *M. pneumoniae*. Note cilia (c) and individual organisms (m), some with specialized terminal structure oriented towards the membrane of the host cell (arrows). Magnification ×9880.

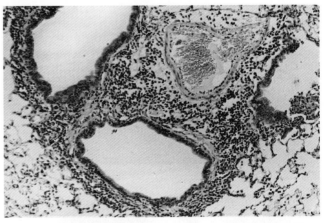

Fig. 6.45.4 Pneumonia 2 weeks after intranasal inoculation of a hamster with *M. pneumoniae*. Note peribronchiolar and perivascular infiltration of mononuclear cells, predominantly lymphocytes. Haematoxylin and eosin, magnification ×98.

recruits it has been responsible for up to 40% of acute pulmonary illness.

M. pneumoniae infections appear to occur globally. Infection is endemic in most areas and throughout the year, with a predilection for late summer and early autumn. Epidemic peaks have been observed about every 4 to 7 years. The incubation period ranges from 2 to 3 weeks. Spread from person to person occurs slowly, usually where there is continual or repeated close contact, as within a family.

Immunopathological factors in the development of *M. pneumoniae* pneumonia

The crucial step of adherence of *M. pneumoniae* organisms to respiratory mucosal epithelial cells, cytadsorption (Fig. 6.45.3), is mediated by P1 and other specialized adhesins on the mycoplasmal surface. This is often followed by cellular invasion. In animals, there is peribronchiolar and perivascular pulmonary infiltration mostly by T lymphocytes (Fig. 6.45.4). The pneumonia caused by *M. pneumoniae* is largely an immunopathological process since immunosuppression prevents pneumonia or diminishes its severity. A mycoplasmal polysaccharide–protein fraction is involved in the cell-mediated immune response, whereas the main antigenic determinant in complement fixation and other serological reactions is a glycolipid. After the initial lymphocyte response, polymorphonuclear leucocytes and macrophages appear in the bronchiolar exudate. The slow evolution of the primary disease contrasts with an accelerated and often more intense host response to reinfection. Children between 2 and 5 years old show serological evidence of infection at an early age. The pneumonia that occurs in older people is considered to be an immunological over-response to reinfection, with lung infiltration by previously sensitized lymphocytes.

Chronic respiratory disease

Animal mycoplasmas are frequently associated with chronic illnesses, and so the possible role of mycoplasmas has been considered in human chronic respiratory disease. *M. pneumoniae* often persists in the respiratory tract long after clinical recovery and occasionally the disease is protracted but there is no evidence that *M. pneumoniae* is a primary cause of chronic bronchitis, or that it maintains chronic disease other than by possibly causing some acute exacerbations.

M. salivarium, *M. orale*, and perhaps other mycoplasmas present in the oropharynx of healthy people spread to the lower respiratory tract of people with chronic bronchitis. There is no hard evidence that these mycoplasmas cause acute exacerbations, but they may perpetuate an episode. Specific antibody responses follow such exacerbations more frequently than at other times, suggesting that mycoplasmas multiply and contribute to the tissue damage that is primarily due to viruses and bacteria.

M. amphoriforme was recovered from the respiratory tract of patients with chronic bronchitis, most of whom were B-cell deficient. Recovery may depend on the eradication of this organism but its role in the general population is unknown.

The role of *M. pneumoniae* in asthma is controversial. Acute *M. pneumoniae* infection is associated with wheezing and the organism has been found, mainly by PCR, more frequently in subjects with asthma than in those without. However, no causal relationship has so far been established.

Genitourinary and related infections

Nongonococcal urethritis (NGU) and its complications

M. genitalium, a large-colony-forming mycoplasma (Table 6.45.1, Fig. 6.45.5a), is strongly associated with acute NGU (Table 6.45.4). It has been detected almost independently of *Chlamydia trachomatis* by PCR in about 25% of cases compared with significantly fewer

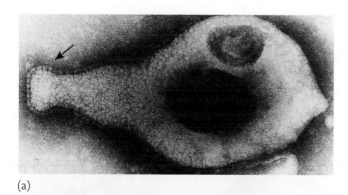

(a)

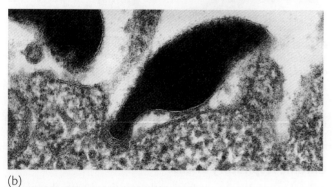

(b)

Fig. 6.45.5 (a) Electron micrograph of *M. genitalium*, negatively stained to show flask-shaped appearance and terminal specialized structure (arrow). Magnification ×90 000. (b) Electron micrograph of *M. genitalium* adhering to a Vero cell by the terminal structure. Magnification ×60 000.

(From Tully JG, *et al*. (1983) *Mycoplasma genitalium*, a new species from the human urogenital tract. *Int J Syst Bacteriol*, **33**, 387, with permission.)

(about 6%) healthy controls. It also causes urethritis experimentally in male chimpanzees and adheres to and enters epithelial cells (Fig. 6.45.5b). Intracellular *M. genitalium* may be partially protected from antimicrobials, particularly tetracyclines, resulting in persistent or recurrent nongonococcal urethritis. Most recently, *M. genitalium* has been associated with balanoposthitis in men with acute NGU.

Although *M. hominis* has been isolated from about 20% of patients with acute NGU, it has not been implicated as a cause.

The role of ureaplasmas in NGU has been contentious for many years. The results of most qualitative studies have failed to demonstrate a significant difference between the prevalence of ureaplasmas in men with or without acute NGU, but there are some quantitative data indicating higher titres of organisms in men with disease. There are two species of human ureaplasmas, *U. urealyticum* and *U. parvum*. PCR assays of clinical specimens tend to show a stronger association between *U. urealyticum* and NGU, but most studies did not consider clinical histories. Intraurethral inoculation of first-passage ureaplasma strains produced a mild urethritis and an antibody response in male chimpanzees. The disease responded to tetracycline therapy. Four investigators who inoculated themselves intraurethrally developed urethritis. In one study, two received cloned *U. urealyticum*, serotype 5, isolated from patients with acute NGU in whom no other potentially pathogenic microorganisms could be detected, although *M. genitalium* was not sought at that time. Both developed symptoms and signs of urethritis which responded to treatment with minocycline. Another volunteer experiment suggested that ureaplasmas may cause disease the first few times they gain access to the urethra but later insults result in colonization without disease, accounting perhaps for their frequent occurrence in the urethras of healthy men.

Some patients with hypogammaglobulinaemia develop a prolonged urethrocystitis with persistent ureaplasmal infection. Treatment is often complicated by antimicrobial resistance and a combination of different classes of antibiotics is recommended.

Epididymitis and chronic prostatitis

Ureaplasmas may be a rare cause of epididymitis since they have been recovered from the urethra and epididymal aspirate fluid of a patient with acute nonchlamydial, nongonococcal epididymitis, with a specific antibody response. *M. genitalium* has not been sought in aspirates, but it has been found in the urethra without other known pathogens (Table 6.45.4).

Information linking prostatic infection with acute ureaplasmal urethral infection is scanty, although ureaplasmas have been isolated more frequently and in greater numbers from patients with acute urethroprostatitis than from controls. Most of those with more than 10^3 organisms in expressed prostatic fluid responded to tetracycline therapy. In contrast, ureaplasmas have not been found, and *M. genitalium* only rarely found in prostatic biopsy specimens from patients with chronic abacterial prostatitis. *M. hominis* is not associated with prostatitis.

Pelvic inflammatory disease (Oxford Textbook of Medicine 5e Chapter 8.5)

Microorganisms in the vagina and lower cervix may ascend to and cause inflammation of the fallopian tubes and adjacent pelvic structures (Table 6.45.4). Large-colony-forming mycoplasmas,

Table 6.45.4 Association of *M. genitalium*, *M. hominis*, and ureaplasmas with human genitourinary, reproductive, and perinatal disease

Disease	Evidence suggesting a causal relationship of:			Comments on the relationship
	M. genitalium	*M. hominis*	Ureaplasmas	
Nongonococcal urethritis	Strong	None	Good	The proportion of nongonococcal urethritis caused by ureaplasmas is unknown
Chronic prostatitis	Weak	None	Weak	None of the microorganisms appears to be a cause
Epididymitis	Some (not published)	None	Some	Ureaplasmas involved in one case of acute disease
Urinary calculi	?	None	Weak	Experimentally, ureaplasmas cause bladder calculi in male rats but so far little evidence for a cause of natural human disease
Pyelonephritis	?	Some	None	*M. hominis* possibly causes some cases of acute pyelonephritis and exacerbations
Reiter's disease/sexually acquired reactive arthritis	Some	None	Some	*M. genitalium* detected in joint of one patient; ureaplasmas are related on the basis of lymphocytic response to specific antigen
Bartholinitis	?	Very weak	None	Doubtful whether *M. hominis* is involved
Bacterial vaginosis	None	Weak	None	*M. hominis* and to a lesser extent ureaplasmas are associated with bacterial vaginosis, but a causal relationship is unproved
Cervicitis	Good	None	None	*M. genitalium* is associated with nongonococcal, nonchlamydial cervicitis
Pelvic inflammatory disease	Good	Some	Weak	*M. genitalium* is associated serologically and has been detected in the upper genital tract of patients with endometritis and salpingitis; *M. hominis* probably causes a small proportion of cases, but very doubtful that ureaplasmas do
Postabortal fever	?	Good	Weak	*M. hominis*, and to a much lesser extent ureaplasmas, are responsible for some cases, but the proportion is unknown
Postpartum fever	?	Good	Weak	*M. hominis*, and to a much lesser extent ureaplasmas, are responsible for some cases, but the proportion is unknown
Infertility	Some	None	None	*M. genitalium* is associated serologically to tubal factor infertility; ureaplasmas are associated with reduced sperm motility, but a causal relationship is unproved
Preterm birth	Weak	Some	Some/good	*M. genitalium* associated in a few studies, but not in others. Considerable evidence for the involvement of ureaplasmas, less so for *M. hominis*; both possibly as part of bacterial vaginosis
Spontaneous abortion and stillbirth	?	Weak	Weak	Maternal and fetal infections are associated with spontaneous abortion, but a causal relationship is unproved
Chorioamnionitis	?	None	Some	An association exists with ureaplasmas, but a causal relationship is unproved
Low birth weight	?	None	Weak	An association exists with ureaplasmas in some studies, but a causal relationship is unproved
Neonatal meningitis	?	Some	Some	A rare event
Neonatal lung disease	?	Weak	Some	*M. hominis* has been involved in pneumonia soon after birth; ureaplasmas possibly involved in premature infants weighing less than 1000 g

predominantly *M. hominis*, have been isolated from inflamed fallopian tubes, tubo-ovarian abscesses, and pelvic abscesses or fluid. Laparoscopy samples yielded *M. hominis* from the tubes of about 10% of women with salpingitis but not from those of healthy women. This might occur with bacterial vaginosis since large numbers of the organisms are in the vagina (Oxford Textbook of Medicine 5e Chapter 8.4). Hysterosalpingography may also precipitate inflammation of the fallopian tubes in women who carry *M. hominis* in the lower genital tract. *M. hominis* antibody was found in approximately one-half of salpingitis patients, but in only

10% of healthy women. Antibody was found in one-half of the patients who had *M. hominis* present in the lower genital tract.

Although ureaplasmas have been isolated directly from the fallopian tubes of a very small proportion of patients with acute salpingitis, from pelvic fluid, and from a tubo-ovarian abscess, it seems that they are of little importance in acute pelvic inflammatory disease.

PCR testing has established that *M. genitalium* is involved in at least some cases of pelvic inflammatory disease. It is a cause of cervicitis and its presence in the cervix or upper genital tract is associated significantly with histological endometritis. It has rarely been detected in tubes but in one study of women with pelvic inflammatory disease, an antibody response was detected to *M. genitalium* but not to *M. hominis* or *C. trachomatis* in one-third of the patients. Other studies have not shown this association but *M. genitalium* has been related serologically to tubal factor infertility.

Fallopian-tube organ culture, in which the tissues are maintained in a condition similar to that *in vivo*, show that gonococci destroy the epithelium, *M. genitalium* causes some damage, *M. hominis* organisms multiply but only produce swelling of some cilia, and human ureaplasmas cause no damage. This differential effect may be a true reflection of the pathogenic potential of these microorganisms *in vivo* but, as the immune system is not operational, failure to demonstrate damage does not confirm avirulence. Inoculation of *M. hominis* or *M. genitalium* into primates caused a self-limiting acute salpingitis and parametritis with an antibody response, whereas ureaplasmas had no effect.

Effects of mycoplasmas on pregnancy

Preterm birth

The involvement of genital mycoplasmas is debated but ureaplasma infection of the amniotic fluid is associated with preterm labour. *M. hominis* probably plays a part through its involvement with bacterial vaginosis, a known cause of preterm labour. *M. hominis* and ureaplasmas are unlikely to cause low birthweight in otherwise normal full-term infants. The role of *M. genitalium* is controversial; it has been associated with preterm birth in some but not all studies.

Postabortal and postpartum fever

M. hominis has been isolated from the blood, with an antibody response, in up to 10% of women with fever after abortion but not from those without fever. However, a pure culture of *M. hominis* in blood is needed before it can be accepted as a cause of fever. The role of ureaplasmas is unclear. Patients with postabortal or postpartum fever of mycoplasmal origin usually recover without antibiotic treatment.

Neonatal infections

Whether transmitted *in utero* or during birth, ureaplasmas may be isolated from the throats and tracheal aspirates of some neonates. Ureaplasma-infected infants of very low birthweight (<1000 g) have died or have developed chronic lung disease twice as often as uninfected infants of similar birth weight or those of over 1000 g. However, the pathogenicity of ureaplasmas is uncertain since erythromycin treatment has failed to prevent disease in two trials. *M. hominis* has very rarely been implicated in pneumonia soon after birth but the other bacteria present could be responsible.

Mycoplasmal infection should be considered in cases of neonatal disease of the central nervous system in which the results of bacteriological staining and culture are negative. *M. hominis* or ureaplasmas have been found in the cerebrospinal fluid of neonates with meningitis or brain abscess.

Joint infections

Rheumatoid arthritis

Mycoplasmas cause several animal arthritides, and gold salts (used to treat rheumatoid arthritis) inactivate mycoplasmas. However, the search for mycoplasmal infection of joints was unfruitful until PCR testing showed *M. fermentans* and ureaplasma DNA in more than 20% of patients with rheumatoid arthritis and other chronic inflammatory disorders, in contrast to those with noninflammatory disorders. The significance of these findings is unknown.

M. pneumoniae and other mycoplasmal infections

In mycoplasmal arthritides of animals, organisms isolated from the joints are often found in the respiratory tract. Human *M. pneumoniae* respiratory infection is often accompanied by nonspecific arthralgia or myalgia (Table 6.45.3) during the acute phase, and occasionally it leads to migratory polyarthritis affecting middle-sized joints in adults. A fourfold or greater rise in the titre of antibody to *M. pneumoniae* has been seen occasionally in juvenile chronic arthritis, but an aetiological association has not been demonstrated.

M. hominis has been isolated from septic joints, usually hip, that have developed in mothers after childbirth. The arthritis responds to tetracycline therapy and the diagnosis should be considered in a postpartum arthritis which is unaffected by penicillin.

Reiter's disease

Arthritis may occur soon after or concomitant with NGU (sexually acquired reactive arthritis; SARA) or the arthritis may be associated with conjunctivitis and urethritis (Reiter's disease). *M. genitalium* causes uncomplicated NGU and ureaplasmas may do so to a lesser extent, but previous antimicrobial treatment usually prevents adequate investigation of patients with arthritis. *M. genitalium* has been detected in the synovial fluid of a patient with SARA and clinical experience has shown that SARA is not uncommon after *M. genitalium*-positive NGU, but no causal link has been established. The latter is also true in the case of some patients whose synovial lymphocytes have been shown to proliferate *in vitro* in response to ureaplasmal antigens.

Wound infections

M. hominis has rarely been linked to fever in patients with burns, trauma, or wound infections. It is most common in fever after surgery on the urogenital tract; ureaplasmas are also likely to be present, but neither these nor *M. hominis* will be found unless specifically sought. Kidney transplant patients occasionally develop mixed infections with ureaplasmas and *M. hominis*, which in severe cases may create fistulas.

A rare wound infection is 'seal finger' or 'blubber finger' which is well known in Arctic regions where the handling of sea mammals is part of daily living. A few days after a seal bite, oedema of the affected finger develops with swelling of the interphalangeal joint adjacent to the lesion. It is extremely painful, suppuration can occur, extensive surgery may be needed, and residual dysfunction is possible. The infection usually responds rapidly to tetracyclines but macrolides are inefficient. Rapidly growing mycoplasmas, some of which have not been speciated, can be recovered from the lesion.

Mycoplasmas in immunosuppressed patients

Arthritis in patients with hypogammaglobulinaemia

Arthritis of mycoplasmal aetiology (Fig. 6.45.6a,b) should be considered in patients with hypogammaglobulinaemia who develop an abacterial septic arthritis. *M. pneumoniae*, *M. hominis*, *M. salivarium*,

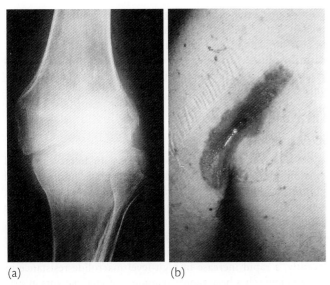

Fig. 6.45.6 (a) Damage to the knee joint of a hypogammaglobulinaemic patient caused by *U. urealyticum* infection. (b) Sinus connected with the shoulder joint of a patient with hypogammaglobulinaemia; ureaplasmas were isolated repeatedly from the sinus exudate.
(Courtesy of A D B Webster.)

and, in particular, ureaplasmas have been isolated from synovial fluids of at least two-fifths of these patients. Vigilance should be kept for infection by mycoplasmas of nonhuman origin. The arthritis usually responds to tetracyclines or other antimicrobials to which the organisms are sensitive. Intravenous and combination therapy should be considered to avoid antimicrobial resistance developing due to suboptimal drug concentrations at the infection site. Administration of specific antiserum against the mycoplasma in question may be helpful in a few patients when antimicrobial therapy fails.

Mycoplasmas in patients with HIV-infection

Although *M. fermentans* was distributed widely in tissues taken at autopsy from some patients with AIDS, no association has been found with the stage of the disease, CD4 count, plasma HIV-1 viral load, or rate of progression of the illness.

M. penetrans, which avidly invades eukaryotic cells, was isolated from urine sediments of a few HIV-1-positive men who have sex with men. While it is possible that *M. fermentans*, *M. penetrans*, or other mycoplasmas might proliferate in this immunodeficiency state, there is no convincing evidence that they are important for the development of AIDS.

Conditions of rare or equivocal mycoplasmal aetiology

Bacterial vaginosis (Oxford Textbook of Medicine 5e Chapter 8.4)

M. hominis organisms may well have a role in the pathogenesis of bacterial vaginosis in which they occur in very large numbers, but proof is impossible due to the variety of other bacteria present in profusion. Ureaplasmas are less likely to be pathogenic and *M. genitalium* does not seem to be involved at all.

Pyelonephritis

Over 30 years ago *M. hominis* was isolated, sometimes in pure culture, from the upper urinary tract of almost 10% of patients with acute pyelonephritis, occasionally accompanied by an antibody response, but not from patients with noninfectious urinary tract diseases. However, there has never been confirmation that *M. hominis* is responsible for a few cases of acute pyelonephritis or acute exacerbations of chronic pyelonephritis.

Urinary calculi

Animal model and human isolation studies have suggested that ureaplasmas, which have a urease, could be involved in the development of urinary calculi, but proof is lacking.

Other conditions

There is no confirmation that ureaplasmas are associated with male or female infertility, nor is there any credible evidence that mycoplasmas are related to fibromyalgia, chronic fatigue syndrome, or the Gulf War syndrome.

Laboratory diagnosis of mycoplasmal infections

M. pneumoniae infection

The diagnosis is made by culture, molecular methods, and/or serology. The complex culture media for *M. pneumoniae* isolation contain glucose, selective antibiotics, and a pH indicator (phenol red). The fluid medium, inoculated with sputum, throat washing, pharyngeal swab, or other specimen, is incubated at 37°C and a colour change (red to yellow) signals the fermentation of glucose (Table 6.45.1) with production of acid, due to multiplication of the organisms. This preliminary identification may be confirmed by subculturing to agar medium and demonstrating inhibition of colony development by specific antiserum (Fig. 6.45.7) or by immunofluorescence of colonies with an *M. pneumoniae*-specific antibody.

Culture may take as long as 5 weeks, and consequently it is of limited value in clinical diagnosis. Rapid detection of *M. pneumoniae* by PCR has become routine in some settings. Serological testing by complement fixation is still undertaken in some laboratories. Recent infection is indicated by a fourfold or greater rise in antibody

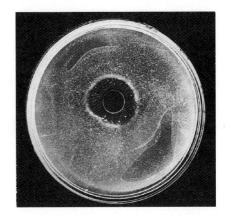

Fig. 6.45.7 Mycoplasma identification by agar growth inhibition. Colony development inhibited around a filter-paper disc impregnated with specific antiserum. Note also antibody–antigen precipitation at edge of inhibition zone.

titre with a peak at about 3 to 4 weeks after disease onset, but this occurs in only about 80% of cases. A high titre (1:128 or greater) in a single serum is suggestive but not proof of infection in the previous few weeks or months; a fourfold or greater fall in antibody titre, perhaps over 6 months, may be helpful, but may be difficult to relate to a particular prior illness. The complement-fixation test does not distinguish between *M. pneumoniae* and *M. genitalium*. A more accurate diagnosis is made using a specific IgM microimmunofluorescence test which confirms a current infection or one within the previous few weeks. IgM detection is much less reliable in reinfection, which is most often the case in adults. This also applies to commercially available enzyme immunoassays specific for IgM which are used more routinely. Cold agglutinins, detected by agglutination of O Rh-negative erythrocytes at 4°C, also correlate with specific IgM and are suggestive of a recent *M. pneumoniae* infection, but the test is rarely used as it is not specific.

Genitourinary and other infections

Swabs from the urethra or cervix/vagina provide a slightly more sensitive means of collecting specimens for mycoplasmal isolation than urine specimens. Ureaplasmas and *M. hominis* usually show evidence of growth in culture media within 1 to 5 days. Primary isolation of *M. genitalium* is difficult and may take 50 days or more, so that PCR is used to detect this mycoplasma. A PCR assay also identifies *M. fermentans* and *U. urealyticum*/*U. parvum*.

M. hominis cultured on agar medium produces colonies of c. 200 to 300 μm diameter, whereas ureaplasma colonies are tiny (15–60 μm) (Fig. 6.45.8a) but can be seen more easily on medium containing manganous sulphate (Fig. 6.45.8b). *M. hominis* may grow on ordinary blood agar where it produces nonhaemolytic pinpoint

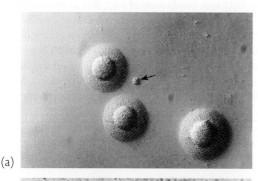

(a)

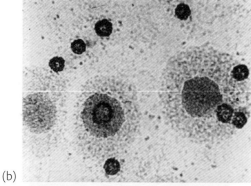

(b)

Fig. 6.45.8 (a) A ureaplasma colony (15 μm diameter) (arrow) adjacent to colonies of *M. hominis* (90 μm diameter) grown from urethral exudate. Oblique light, magnification ×68. (b) Dark ureaplasma colonies with colonies of *M. hominis* on agar containing manganous sulphate. Magnification ×136.

colonies after extended incubation. Ureaplasma colonies are too small to be detected on blood agar, but occasionally a scrape from the agar surface will yield ureaplasmas when inoculated into ureaplasma medium. In a few research laboratories only, serological tests have been used to detect antibodies to *M. hominis*, *M. genitalium*, and the ureaplasmas.

Treatment

M. pneumoniae infections

M. pneumoniae is sensitive to the bacteriostatic tetracyclines and erythromycin. The newer macrolides, such as clarithromycin and azithromycin, are very active *in vitro*, but their clinical effect is not documented extensively in randomized clinical trials. The newer quinolones, such as moxifloxacin, are also highly active *in vitro*. They should not be used as first-line therapy but, as they are bactericidal, they may have a role in immunosuppressed patients. Recently, a rapid increase in high-level macrolide resistance in *M. pneumoniae* has been reported among infected patients in Asia but there have been only sporadic cases in Europe.

The value of tetracyclines was shown first in a controlled trial in military recruits in the United States of America in whom demethylchlortetracycline significantly reduced the duration of fever, pulmonary infiltration, and other signs and symptoms. In civilian practice, antimicrobials may prove less effective, probably because disease is often well established before treatment begins. In addition, the intracellular location of organisms may hinder their elimination, particularly from immunodeficient patients. Nevertheless, treatment with an antimicrobial is worthwhile. Erythromycin rather than a tetracycline is often used for pregnant women and children, although with reluctance by some. The newer antibiotics should not be ignored. Successful treatment of disease with bacteriostatic drugs does not always correlate with eradication of intracellular organisms from the respiratory tract. Relapse may be avoided by giving antibiotics for at least 10 days. It is uncertain whether early treatment prevents complications but it should start as soon as possible, even if there is only clinical evidence and a suggestive single antibody titre.

Corticosteroids in conjunction with antimicrobials appear to have been helpful in patients with severe pneumonia and erythema multiforme.

Genitourinary and other infections

Antimicrobial susceptibility of the mycoplasma species found most commonly in the urogenital tract is presented in Table 6.45.5 as a combination of *in vitro* susceptibility data and clinical experience. Treatment must take into account the fact that several different microorganisms may be involved and that a precise microbiological diagnosis is not available. Patients with NGU should receive an antibiotic with activity against *C. trachomatis*, ureaplasmas, and *M. genitalium*. Azithromycin is being used increasingly for chlamydial infections and is also active against a wide range of mycoplasmas, including *M. genitalium* and, to a lesser extent, ureaplasmas. However, in settings where azithomycin 1 g single dose is used as the first-line therapy for NGU and cervicitis, development of high-level macrolide resistance may be common. Such development of resistance is less common where azithromycin is given as 500 mg day 1 followed by 250 mg o.d. days 2–5. This is a better option than using one of the tetracyclines since *M. genitalium* is less sensitive to

Table 6.45.5 Susceptibility of some genital mycoplasmas to various antibiotics. A combination of *in vitro* susceptibility data and clinical efficacy is given where such experience is available

Antibiotic	M. hominis	M. fermentans	U. urealyticum	M. genitalium
Tetracyclines				
Tetracycline	+	+	+	±
Doxycycline	++	++	++	±
Macrolides				
Erythromycin	−	±	+	+
Clarithromycin	−	±	++	++
Azithromycin	−	±	+	+++[a]
Lincosamides				
Clindamycin	+++	++	±	±
Quinolones				
Ciprofloxacin	+	++	+	+
Ofloxacin	+	++	+	+
Moxifloxacin	++	+++	++	+++

+++, extremely sensitive; ++, highly sensitive; +, moderately sensitive; ±, weakly sensitive; −, insensitive; [a], high-level macrolide resistance may be common in settings where azithomycin 1 g single dose is commonly used.

these antibiotics and 10% or more of ureaplasmas are resistant to tetracyclines. If resistance does occur, patients may require a quinolone with a good Gram-positive spectrum, such as moxifloxacin.

A broad-spectrum antibiotic should also be included in the treatment of pelvic inflammatory disease to cover *C. trachomatis*, *M. hominis*, and *M. genitalium*. Since 20% or more of *M. hominis* strains are resistant to tetracyclines, other antibiotics such as clindamycin or fluoroquinolones may be needed.

Prevention of infection

M. pneumoniae infection or disease may occur despite high titres of serum mycoplasmacidal antibody. The correlation between the presence of IgA in respiratory secretions and resistance to *M. pneumoniae* disease endorses the importance of local immune factors in resistance. IgA could prevent attachment of organisms to respiratory epithelial cells. Protective immunity also depends on the severity of infection. Thus, in one study, patients with nonpneumonic illness were susceptible to an epidemic occurring 5 years later, whereas those with *M. pneumoniae* pneumonia were protected until the following epidemic 10 years later.

No effective vaccine has been developed for human use. Vaccination against *M. pneumoniae* has been attempted. Formalin-inactivated vaccines prevented mycoplasmal pneumonia in only one- to two-thirds of subjects, perhaps because they failed to stimulate cell-mediated immunity and/or local antibody. Live attenuated vaccines, containing temperature-sensitive mutants of *M. pneumoniae*, have not been considered safe for general human use. Recombinant DNA vaccines involving P1 and other proteins, or a recombinant vaccine developed by cloning part of the *M. pneumoniae P1* gene into an adenovirus vector, may offer greater success in the future.

Further reading

Haggerty CL (2008). Evidence for a role of *Mycoplasma genitalium* in pelvic inflammatory disease. *Curr Opin Infect Dis*, **21**, 65–9.

Herrmann R, Ruppert T (2006). Proteome of *Mycoplasma pneumoniae*. *Methods Biochem Anal*, **49**, 39–56.

Jensen JS (2006). *Mycoplasma genitalium* infections. Diagnosis, clinical aspects, and pathogenesis. *Dan Med Bull*, **53**, 1–27.

Maniloff J (ed) (1992). Mycoplasmas. *Molecular biology and pathogenesis*. ASM Press, Washington, DC.

McGarrity GJ, Kotani H, Butler GH (1992). Mycoplasmas in tissue culture cells. In: Maniloff J (ed) *Mycoplasmas. Molecular biology and pathogenesis*, pp. 445–54. ASM Press, Washington, DC

Razin S, Tully JG (ed) (1996). *Molecular and diagnostic procedures in mycoplasmology*, vol. **1**. *Molecular characterization*. Academic Press, London.

Razin S, Yogev D, Naot Y (1998). Molecular biology and pathogenicity of mycoplasmas. *Microbiol Mol Biol Rev*, **62**, 1094–156.

Sutherland ER, Martin RJ (2007). Asthma and atypical bacterial infection. *Chest*, **132**, 1962–6.

Taylor-Robinson D (1996). Infection due to species of *Mycoplasma* and *Ureaplasma*: an update. *Clin Infect Dis*, **23**, 671–84.

Taylor-Robinson D (1996). Mycoplasmas and their role in human respiratory tract disease. In: Myint S, Taylor-Robinson D (eds) *Viral and other infections of the human respiratory tract*, pp. 319–39. Chapman & Hall, London.

Taylor-Robinson D (2007). The role of mycoplasmas in pregnancy outcome. *Best Pract Res Clin Obstet Gynaecol*, **21**, 425–38.

Taylor-Robinson D, Jensen JS (2011). *Mycoplasma genitalium*: from chrysalis to multicolored butterfly. *Clin Microbiol Rev*, **24**, 498–514.

Taylor-Robinson D, Keat A (2001). How can a causal role for small bacteria in chronic inflammatory arthritis be established or refuted? *Ann Rheum Dis*, **60**, 177–84.

Taylor-Robinson D, Gilroy CB, Jensen JS (2000). The biology of *Mycoplasma genitalium*. *Venereology*, **13**, 119–27.

Tully JG, Razin S (ed) (1996). *Molecular and diagnostic procedures in mycoplasmology*, vol. **2**. *Diagnostic procedures*. Academic Press, London.

Waites KB, Taylor-Robinson D (2011). *Mycoplasma* and *Ureaplasma*. In: Murray PR, *et al.* (eds) *Manual of clinical microbiology*, vol. 1, Chapter 59. ASM Press, Washington, DC.

6.46 A checklist of bacteria associated with infection in humans

J. Paul

Essentials

In addition to the relatively small number of well-known pathogenic bacteria that are able to infect otherwise healthy people, e.g. *Staphylococcus aureus*, *Mycobacterium tuberculosis*, and *Streptococcus pyogenes*, there is a steadily growing list of less well known organisms, many of which are able to cause disease only under special circumstances.

All bacteria associated with infections in humans are listed in the table that forms the bulk of this chapter, which has been designed to serve as a single port of call for clinicians who seek concise information on the less well known clinically significant bacteria. Every name in the table has been checked to see that it has 'standing in nomenclature': widely used names that do not have standing in nomenclature (at the time of writing) are included, but written in inverted commas (e.g. 'Spirillum minus'—one of the causes of rat bite fever). For an up-to-date check on nomenclature, the reader is referred to http://www.bacterio.cict.fr/. Reported antibiotic susceptibilities and treatments are listed as a rough guide only: for some organisms the only available published information consists of *in vitro* test results for small numbers of strains, or apparent clinical response to therapy for a single case. There is no substitute for the determination of the susceptibilities of organisms as they are cultured on a case-by-case basis in tandem with the monitoring of therapeutic response.

Geographical restriction and particular exposures—some pathogenic bacteria, e.g. *Burkholderia pseudomallei* (the cause of melioidosis), are associated with special geographical areas; others are associated with particular forms of exposure, e.g. some *Actinobacillus* species with animal bites, and *Rickettsia* species with tick bites.

Bacterial commensals and usually harmless environmental organisms as causes of disease—given the right kind of help, bacteria that live usually as harmless human commensals can cause disease, e.g. skin commensals such as *Staphylococcus epidermidis* can cause line sepsis and infect prosthetic devices; gut commensals such as *Bacteroides* species can grow in abscesses; and oral commensals such as *Streptococcus salivarius* can cause endocarditis. Immunosuppressed patients, ventilated patients, and patients undergoing continuous ambulatory peritoneal dialysis are vulnerable to infection by a wide range of otherwise harmless environmental organisms.

Improved understanding of disease processes and discovery of 'new' pathogens—a refined understanding of, e.g. periodontal disease, has resulted in the characterization of new organisms such as *Pseudoramibacter alactolyticus*, *Johnsonella ignava*, *Centipeda periodontii*, and *Capnocytophaga gingivalis*: some of these have subsequently been identified in systemic infections such as bacteraemia.

Impact of new laboratory techniques—these have revealed the presence of new species and new disease associations, e.g. *Tropheryma whipplei* was associated with Whipple's disease by molecular methods before the organism was cultured; molecular methods have detected oddities like *Bradyrhyzobium elkanii* in aortic aneurysm tissue, although its role as potential pathogen is doubtful.

Changes in nomenclature—amidst the discovery of new bacteria, taxonomic rearrangements and changes in nomenclature pile on additional layers of confusion for the clinician. For example, it has been recognized that organisms formerly known as *Burkholderia cepacia* are actually a complex of several genomospecies, which have been given individual names. It is also confusing when a well-known genus is split to reflect the recognition that its composite species are a number of groups that are only distantly related, e.g. many organisms that were once known as *Bacteroides* species. New organisms will continue to be described and name changes will continue to occur.

For an up-to-date check on nomenclature, the reader is referred to http://www.bacterio.cict.fr/.

Table 6.46.1 A checklist of bacteria associated with infection in humans

Nomenclature		Associated infections	Reported susceptibilities and treatments	Notes
Genus	**Species and subspecies**			
(synonyms, CDC alphanumeric groups)				
A				
Abiotrophia adiacens—see *Granulicatella adiacens*]				
Abiotrophia	*A. defectiva*	Endophthalmitis, brain abscess, osteomyelitis, peritonitis, endocarditis	Vancomycin, ceftriaxone (plus gentamicin or rifampicin)	Previously known as nutritionally deficient or variant streptococci
[*Abiotrophia elegans*—see *Granulicatella elegans*]				
[*Abiotrophia para-adiacens*'—see *Granulicatella* notes]				
Achromobacter (*Alcaligenes*)	*A. denitrificans* *A. insolitus* *A. piechaudii* *A. ruhlandii* *A. spanius* *A. xylosoxidans*	Septicaemia, CAPD peritonitis, pneumonia, ear infection, pulmonary infection in cystic fibrosis, keratitis, vascular line sepsis	Ureidopenicillins, ceftazidime, carbapenems	
[*Achromobacter* CDC group Vd and *Achromobacter* groups A, C, and D—see *Ochrobactrum*]				
[*Achromobacter* groups B and E—see *Pannonibacter*]				
Acidaminococcus	*A. fermentans*	Abscesses, postsurgical infections	Metronidazole	
Acidovorax (*Pseudomonas*)	*A. avenae* *A. delafeldii* *A. facilis* *A. temperans*	Wound infection, UTI, bacteraemia, meningitis, septic arthritis		
Acinetobacter	*A. baumannii* *A. calcoaceticus* *A. haemolyticus* *A. johnsonii* *A. junii* *A. lwoffi* *A. parvus* *A. radioresistens* *A. schindleri* *A. ursingii*	Septicaemia, UTI, wound infections, abscesses, endocarditis, meningitis, osteomyelitis	Aminoglycosides, ureidopenicillins, ceftazidime, carbapenems, tigecycline	May be multidrug-resistant. Nosocomial outbreaks reported. Infections associated with debilitated patients
Actinobacillus	*A. equuli* *A. lignieresii* *A. suis*	Wound infection, abscesses, endocarditis, meningitis	Ampicillin (plus gentamicin for endocarditis)	Associated with animal contact and bites
	A. hominis	Septicaemia, empyema	Amoxicillin–clavulanate	
	A. ureae (*Pasteurella ureae*)	Meningitis, pneumonia, endocarditis, hepatitis, peritonitis	Ampicillin (plus gentamicin for endocarditis), chloramphenicol	Respiratory tract commensal in humans

(Continued)

Table 6.46.1 (*Cont'd*) A checklist of bacteria associated with infection in humans

Nomenclature		Associated infections	Reported susceptibilities and treatments	Notes
Genus	**Species and subspecies**			
(synonyms, CDC alphanumeric groups)				
Actinobaculum	A. *massiliense* A. *schaalii* A. *urinale*	Pyelonephritis, UTI, septicaemia, superficial skin infection	Penicillin, cefuroxime, nitrofurantoin, tetracycline, clindamycin	
Actinomadura	A. *latina* A. *madurae* A. *pelletieri* A. *vinacea*	Actinomycetoma, Madura foot	Co-trimoxazole, dapsone	
Actinomyces	A. *cardiffensis* A. *dentalis* A. *europaeus* A. *funkei* A. *georgiae* A. *gerencseriae* A. *graevenitzii* A. *hongkongensis* A. *israelii* A. *meyeri* A. *naeslundii* A. *neuii neuii* A. *neuii anitratus* A. *odontolyticus* A. *oricola* A. *radicidentis* A. *radingae* A. *turicensis* A. *urogenitalis* A. *viscosus*	Actinomycosis	β-Lactams	
Advenella	A. *incenata*	Pulmonary infection, bacteraemia		
Aerococcus	A. *sanguinicola* A. *urinae* A. *urinaehominis* A. *viridans*	Endocarditis, UTI, wounds, meningitis, abscesses, CAPD peritonitis, lymphadenitis, spondodactylitis	Penicillin, vancomycin (plus gentamicin for endocarditis)	
Aeromonas	A. *allosaccharophila* A. *bestiarum*A. *Caviae* A. *enteropelogenes* A. *hydrophila* A. *jandaei* A. *media* A. *salmonicida* A. *schubertii* A. *trota* (A. *tructi*) A. *veronii*	Wound infection, abscesses, septicaemia, meningitis, leech-bite infection, alligator-bite infection, acute diarrhoea	Aminoglycosides, chloramphenicol, ceftazidime, co-trimoxazole	Infections associated with aquatic exposure. A. *veronii*includes biovars Veronii and Sobria. The taxonomic status of some species is unclear. The status of A. *allosaccharophila* is controversial. A. *trota* may be a synonym of A. *enteropelogenes*

		Infection	Treatment	Comments
Afipia	*A. felis*	Cat-scratch disease	Imipenem, aminoglycosides	Cat-scratch disease is associated also with *Bartonella* spp.
	A. broomeae	Bone marrow infection, septic arthritis	Imipenem, aminoglycosides	Role as pathogen uncertain
	A. clevelandensis	Bone infection	Imipenem, aminoglycosides	Role as pathogen uncertain
	A. birgiae	Pneumonia	Imipenem, aminoglycosides	Roles as pathogens uncertain
	A. massiliensis			
Aggregatibacter	*A. actinomycetemcomitans (Actinobacillus actinomycetemcomitans, Haemophilus actinomycetemcomitans)*	Periodontitis, endocarditis, abscesses, pericarditis, meningitis	Penicillin (plus gentamicin for endocarditis), ceftriaxone, coamoxiclav	Human oral commensal. Some strains reported to be penicillin-resistant
	A. aphrophilus (Haemophilus aphrophilus, H.paraphrophilus)	Sinusitis, otitis media, pneumonia, abscesses, endocarditis	Ceftriaxone, cefotaxime, chloramphenicol, ampicillin, aminoglycosides	
	A. segnis (Haemophilus segnis)			
Agrobacterium	*A. radiobacter (A. tumefaciens)*	Endocarditis, CAPD peritonitis, UTI, line sepsis	Co-trimoxazole, gentamicin, amikacin, piperacillin–tazobactam	The nomenclature of this taxon is unsettled. The names A. tumefaciens and A. radiobacter both have standing in nomenclature. Transfer of *Agrobacterium* to *Rhizobium* has been proposed
[*Alcaligenes denitrificans*—see *Achromobacter denitrificans*]				
Alcaligenes	*A. faecalis*	Pneumonia, otitis, UTI, osteomyelitis, bacteraemia	Amoxicillin–clavulanate, cephalosporins, fluoroquinolones	
	A. latus			
[*Alcaligenes xylosoxidans*—see *Achromobacter xylosoxidans xylosoxidans*]				
[*Alcaligenes piechaudii*—see *Achromobacter piechaudii*]				
[*Alcaligenes ruhlandii*—see *Achromobacter ruhlandii*]				
Alishewanella	*A. fetalis*	From fetal necropsy specimen		Clinical significance uncertain
Alistipes	*A. finegoldii (Bacteroides finegoldii)*	Appendicitis, peritonitis, abdominal abscess	Metronidazole, ertapenem	β-Lactamase producers. Abdominal infections, found in association with other anaerobes
	A. onderdonkii			
	A. putredinis (Bacteroides putredinis)			
	A. shahii			
Alloiococcus	*A. otitis (Alloiococcus otitis)*	Otitis media	Vancomycin	
[*Amycolata autotrophica*—see *Pseudonocardia cutotrophica*]				
Amycolatopsis	*A. orientalis (Nocardia orientalis)*			Role as pathogen uncertain
	A. palatopharyngis	Palatopharyngeal infection		Clinical significance poorly defined
Anaerobiospirillum	*A. succiniproducens*	Diarrhoea, bacteraemia	Cefuroxime, tetracycline, chloramphenicol	Infection may be related to exposure to cat or dog faeces
	A. thomasii			
Anaerococcus (Peptostreptococcus)	*A. hydrogenalis*	Mixed anaerobic infections, abscesses	β-Lactams, metronidazole	
	A. lactolyticus			
	A. octavius			
	A. prevotii			
	A. tetradius			
	A. vaginalis			
Anaeroglobus	*A. geminatus*	From postoperative collection		Role as pathogen uncertain
Anaerorhabdus (Bacteroides)	*A. furcosus*	Lung abscess, appendix and abdominal abscesses		

(Continued)

Table 6.46.1 (*Cont'd*) A checklist of bacteria associated with infection in humans

Nomenclature		Associated infections	Reported susceptibilities and treatments	Notes
Genus	Species and subspecies			
(synonyms, CDC alphanumeric groups)				
['Anguillina coli'—see Serpulina pilosicoli]				
Anaplasma	A. phagocytophilum	Anaplasmosis	Doxycycline	Previously known as human granulocytic ehrlichiosis
[Arachnia propionica—see Propionibacterium propionicus]				
Arcanobacterium	A. haemolyticum (Corynebacterium haemolyticum)	Tonsillitis, cellulitis, lymphadenopathy, brain abscess, septicaemia, osteomyelitis	Penicillin, erythromycin	
	A. bernardiae (Actinomyces bernardiae)	UTI, septicaemia, septic arthritis	β-Lactams	
	A. pyogenes (Actinomyces pyogenes)	Septic arthritis	β-Lactams	
Arcobacter (Campylobacter)	A. butzleri	Abdominal cramps, diarrhoea		Self-limiting
	A. cryaerophilus			
Arthrobacter	A. albus	UTI, bacteraemia, skin infection	Vancomycin, penicillins	Arthrobacter sp. has been implicated in Whipples syndrome, a disease usually associated with Tropheryma whipplei
	A. creatinolyticus			
	A. cumminsii			
	A. luteolus			
	A. oxydans			
	A. scleromae			
	A. woluwensis			
Atopobium	A. minutum (Lactobacillus minutus)	UTI, dental abscesses, pelvic abscesses, wound infection		Isolates from periodontal sites suggest possible role in periodontal disease
	A. parvulum (Streptococcus parvulus)			
	A. rimae (Lactobacillus rimae)			
	A. vaginae	Bacterial vaginosis		
[Aureobacterium—see Microbacterium]				
Azospirillum	A. brasilense (Roseomonas fauriae)	CAPD peritonitis, line sepsis	Imipenem, aminoglycosides, ceftriaxone, ciprofloxacin	
B				
Bacillus	B. anthracis	Anthrax	Penicillin, erythromycin	Ciprofloxacin for postexposure prophylaxis
[Bacillus brevis—see Brevibacillus agri]				
	B. circulans	Pneumonia, septicaemia, corneal infections, meningitis, food poisoning, eye infection, lung infection	Vancomycin, clindamycin, aminoglycosides, imipenem, penicillin	Other than the well-known B. anthracis and B. cereus, Bacillus spp. are rare causes of focal and systemic sepsis. Some isolates are resistant to vancomycin. Isolates may represent specimen or laboratory contamination. B. thuringiensis is a biological insecticide which has caused corneal infection
	B. coagulans			
	B. megaterium			
	B. mycoides			
	B. sphaericus			
	B. thuringiensis			
	B. cereus	Food poisoning, wound infection, cutaneous lesions, bacteraemia, endocarditis, eye infection	Clindamycin, vancomycin, gentamicin	Diarrhoea is self-limiting. B. cereus is resistant to β-lactams
	B. licheniformis			
	B. pumilus			
	B. subtilis			

Genus	Species	Infection	Treatment	Comments
Bacteroides	B. caccae B. capillosus B. coagulans B. eggerthii B. finegoldii B. fragilis B. massiliensis B. nordii B. ovatus B. pyogenes B. salyersae B. splanchnicus B. stercoris B. tectus B. thetaiotaomicron B. uniformis B. ureolyticus B. vulgatus	Abscesses, bacteraemia, bite infections, wound infections, chronic otitis media, pelvic inflammatory disease, neonatal sepsis	Ureidopenicillins, carbapenems, metronidazole	Resistance to metronidazole and β-lactams has been reported. Many species previously classified as Bacteroides have been transferred to other genera: see Alistipes, Anaerorhabdus, Campylobacter, Dialister Mitsuokella, Parabacteroides, Prevotella, Porphyromonas, and Tannerella
Balneatrix	B. alpica	Pneumonia, bacteraemia, meningitis	Ceftriaxone, ofloxacin, amoxicillin, netilmicin	Infection associated with exposure to hot spring water
Bartonella	B. bacilliformis	Oroya fever, verruga peruana	Chloramphenicol, streptomycin	
	B. elizabethae (Rochalimaea elizabethae)	Endocarditis	Gentamicin, imipenem, co-trimoxazole	
	B. clarridgeiae B. henselae (Rochalimaea henselae)	Cat-scratch disease, bacillary angiomatosis	Aminoglycosides, doxycycline	Cat-scratch disease is associated also with Afipia felis
	B. quintana (Rochalimaea quintana)	Trench fever, bacillary angiomatosis	**Aminoglycosides, doxycycline**	
	B. schoenbuchensis	Deer ked dermatitis		Evidence to associate this organism with deer ked dermatitis is circumstantial
	B. vinsonii arupensis	Bacteraemia	Ceftriaxone	Zoonosis from rodents
Bergeyella	B. zoohelcum (Weeksella zoohelcum)	Wound infection, septicaemia, meningitis	Cefotaxime, penicillins, ciprofloxacin, tetracycline	Associated with dog and cat bites
Bifidobacterium	B. adolescentis B. angulatum B. bifidum B. dentium B. longum (B. infantis) B. pseudocatenulatum	Bacteraemia, abscesses, peritonitis, otitis, paronychia	Clindamycin, penicillins, cefoxitin	Reported risk factors include surgery, malignancy, steroid therapy, intravenous drug use, and acupuncture. Some strains used as probiotics
[Bifidobacterium inopinatum—see Scardovia inopinata]				
Bilophila	B. wadsworthia	Appendicitis, abscesses, bacteraemia, biliary tract sepsis, mastoiditis	Metronidazole, amoxicillin/clavulanate, ureidopenicillins, cephalosporins	
Bordetella	B. bronchiseptica B. hinzii B. holmesii B. trematum	Respiratory tract infection Bacteraemia, otitis, wound infection	Tetracycline, fluoroquinolones	Zoonosis from dogs and other animals. B. hinzii is a pathogen of poultry

(Continued)

Table 6.46.1 (*Cont'd*) A checklist of bacteria associated with infection in humans

Nomenclature		Associated infections	Reported susceptibilities and treatments	Notes
Genus	**Species and subspecies**			
(synonyms, CDC alphanumeric groups)				
	B. parapertussis	Whooping cough, respiratory tract infection	Erythromycin	*B. parapertussis* causes less severe disease
	B. pertussis			
Borrelia	*B. afzelii*	Lyme disease	Amoxicillin, doxycycline, ceftriaxone	
	B. andersoni			
	B. bissettii			
	B. burgdorferi			
	B. garinii			
	B. japonica			
	B. lusitaniae			
	B. sinica			
	B. spielmanii			
	B. tanukii			
	B. turdi			
	B. valaisiana			
	B. caucasica	Relapsing fever	Tetracycline, erythromycin, chloramphenicol, penicillin	*B. recurrentis* is louse-borne; other agents are tick-borne
	B. crocidurae			
	B. duttonii			
	B. graingeri			
	B. hermsii			
	B. hispanica			
	B. latyschewii			
	B. mazzottii			
	B. parkeri			
	B. persica			
	B. recurrentis			
	B. turicatae			
	B. venezuelensis			
Bosea	*B. massiliensis*	Linked with ventilator-associated pneumonia	Doxycycline, telithromycin	Amoeba-resisting bacterium from hospital water supplies
Brachyspira	*B. aalborgi*	Intestinal spirochaetosis		Of uncertain significance
	B. pilosicoli (*Serpulina pilosicoli*, '*Anguillina coli*')			
Bradyrhizobium	*B. elkanii*	Detected in tissue from aortic aneurysm		Potential role as pathogen uncertain
[*Branhamella catarrhalis*—see *Moraxella catarrhalis*]				
Brevibacillus	*B. centrosporus*	Bacteraemia	Vancomycin	Previously confused with *B. laterosporus* and reported as such in clinical literature
	B. parabrevis	Bacteraemia, abscess	Vancomycin	
Brevibacterium	*B. casei*	Bacteraemia, endocarditis, meningitis, chest infection, pericarditis, vascular catheter sepsis	Glycopeptides	
	B. epidermidis			
	B. luteolum (*B. lutescens*)			
	B. mcbrellneri			
	B. otitidis			
	B. paucivorans			

Genus	Species	Disease	Treatment	Notes
Brevundimonas (Pseudomonas)	B. diminuta, B. vesicularis	Septicaemia, endocarditis	Cefazolin, ceftriaxone, piperacillin (plus gentamicin for endocarditis)	
Brucella	B. abortus, B. canis, B. melitensis, B. suis	Brucellosis	Doxycycline (plus streptomycin or rifampicin)	The four species names used for clinical purposes represent biovars of a single species, B. melitensis
Bulleidia	B. extructa	Necrotizing ulcerative periodontitis in HIV patients		
Burkholderia (Pseudomonas)	B. ambifaria, B. anthina, B. cenocepacia, B. cepacia (Pseudomonas cepacia), B. dolosa, B. multivorans, B. pyrrocinia, B. stabilis, B. vietnamiensis	Lung infection in cystic fibrosis, bacteraemia, endocarditis, septic arthritis, UTI	Ureidopenicillins, ceftazidime, aztreonam, carbapenems, fluoroquinolones, co-trimoxazole	B. cepacia sensu stricto and other taxa listed are genomospecies of the B. cepacia species complex (B. cepacia sensu lato). Hard to differentiate by routine methods. Differences in disease progression in cystic fibrosis may relate to different genomospecies
	B. gladioli (Pseudomonas glacioli)	Lung infection in cystic fibrosis	Ureidopenicillins, ceftazidime, aztreonam, carbapenems, fluoroquinolones, co-trimoxazole	
	B. fungorum	Septic arthritis, bacteraemia, meningitis	Amoxicillin, cefuroxime, ceftazidime, ciprofloxacin, meropenem, co-trimoxazole	
	B. mallei (Pseudomonas mallei)	Glanders	Sulfadiazine, co-amoxiclav, tetracycline, co-trimoxazole	
	B. pseudomallei (Pseudomonas pseudomallei)	Melioidosis	Ceftazidime, co-trimoxazole, chloramphenicol, imipenem	
Buttiauxella	B. agrestis, B. noackiae	Appendicitis, wound infection	Aminoglycosides, doxycycline	Cephalosporin resistance reported
Butyrivibrio	B. fibrisolvens	Endophthalmitis	Penicillin, chloramphenicol	From rumina of farm animals

C

[Calymmatobacterium granulomatis—see Klebsiella granulomatis]

[Campylobacter butzleri—see Arcobacter butzleri]

[Campylobacter cinaedi—see Helicobacter cinaedi]

[Campylobacter fennelliae—see Helicobacter fennelliae]

[Campylobacter pyloridis—see Helicobacter pylori]

Genus	Species	Disease	Treatment	Notes
Campylobacter	C. coli, C. jejuni jejuni, C. jejuni doylei, C. mucosalis	Gastroenteritis, bacteraemia	Erythromycin, fluoroquinolones	Infections are usually self-limiting

(Continued)

Table 6.46.1 (*Cont'd*) A checklist of bacteria associated with infection in humans

Nomenclature		Associated infections	Reported susceptibilities and treatments	Notes
Genus (synonyms, CDC alphanumeric groups)	**Species and subspecies**			
	C. concisus C. curvus (*Wolinella curva*) C. gracilis (*Bacteroides gracilis*) C. rectus (*Wolinella recta*) C. showae C. sputorum	Periodontitis, appendicitis, peritonitis, head and neck infections, abscesses	Ureidopenicillins, amoxicillin/clavulanate, carbapenems, fluoroquinolones, metronidazole	
	C. fetus fetus	Fever, diarrhoea, meningoencephalitis, endocarditis, abscesses	Erythromycin, ampicillin, chloramphenicol, gentamicin	
	C. fetus venerealis	Bacterial vaginosis		Role as human pathogen poorly defined. Reported from faeces of homosexual men
	C. hyointestinalis C. lari (*C. laridis*) C. upsalensis	Diarrhoea, bacteraemia, abscess	Erythromycin, ampicillin, gentamicin	Zoonoses from mammals and birds
Capnocytophaga	C. canimorsus (CDC DF-1) C. cynodegmi (CDC DF-2) C. gingivalis C. granulose C. haemolytica C. ochracea C. sputigena	Wound infection, septicaemia, abscesses, meningitis, endocarditis Periodontitis, septcaemia	Penicillin Penicillins, ciprofloxacin, tetracycline, chloramphenicol	From dog bites From oral flora. Infections associated with malignancy and neutropenia
Cardiobacterium	C. hominis C. valvarum	Endocarditis, meningitis	Penicillin (plus gentamicin for endocarditis)	
Catonella	C. morbi	Periodontitis, endodontic infection		Role as pathogen unclear
CDC EF-4		Bite infections	β-Lactams	
Cedecea	C. davisae C. lapagei C. neterii	Bacteraemia	Chloramphenicol, cefamandole, gentamicin	Two other species (sp. 3 and sp. 5) have been isolated from clinical specimens
Cellulomonas	C. denverensis C. hominis (CDC coryneform group A-3)	Bacteraemia, meningitis, pilonidal abscess, wound infection, homograft valve infection	Clarithromycin, clindamycin, imipenem, minocycline, rifampicin, vancomycin	
[Cellulomonas cellulans—see Cellulosomicrobium]				
[Cellulomonas turbata—see Oerskovia turbata]				
Cellulosimicrobium	C. cellulans (*Cellulomonas cellulans, Oerskovi xanthineolytica*) C. funkei	Meningitis, pyonephrosis, CAPD peritonitis, endophthalmitis	Vancomycin and gentamicin or rifampicin	
Centipeda	C. periodontii	Periodontitis		Role as pathogen unclear. Shown to inhibit lymphocytes

Chlamydia			
C. trachomatis	Trachoma, genital infection, neonatal infection, lymphogranuloma venereum	Erythromycin, tetracycline, azithromycin	Includes 18 serovars clustered into two biovars: trachoma and lymphogranuloma venereum
Chlamydophila			
C. abortus (*Chlamydia psittaci*)	Abortion		Associated with contact with infected ruminants
C. pneumoniae (*Chlamydia pneumoniae*)	Chest infection	Tetracycline	Infections in humans associated with biovars TWAR
C. psittaci (*Chlamydia psittaci*)	Psittacosis	Tetracycline	Zoonosis from birds
Chromobacterium			
C. violaceum	Septicaemia, osteomyelitis, abscesses, eye infection	Erythromycin, tetracycline, chloramphenicol, gentamicin	Associated with exposure to soil and water
Chryseobacterium (*Flavobacterium*)			
C. gleum	Bacteraemia, abdominal sepsis, vascular catheter sepsis	Piperacillin-tazobactam, minocycline, fluoroquinolones, rifampicin	Susceptibilities vary. Often multiresistant
C. indologenes			
[*Chryseobacterium meningosepticum*—see *Elizabethkingia meningoseptica*]			
[*Chryseomonas luteola*—see *Pseudomonas luteola*]			
Citrobacter			
C. amalonaticus	UTI, meningitis, bacteraemia, haemolytic–uraemic syndrome	Aminoglycosides, β-lactams	Variable susceptibility. May be multiresistant. Nosocomial outbreaks of infection reported. *Citrobacter spp. are part of the normal faecal flora*
C. braakii			
C. diversus			
C. farmeri			
C. freundii			
C. gilenii			
C. koseri			
C. murliniae			
C. rodentium			
C. sedlakii			
C. werkmanii			
C. youngae			
Clostridium			
C. argentinense	Wound infection, bacteraemia, abscesses	Penicillin, clindamycin, metronidazole	Many *Clostridium* spp. have been isolated form clinical specimens. For most, their clinical significance is poorly defined. *C. baratii* and *C. butyricum* are rare causes of botulism. *C. fallax, C. histolyticum, C. novyi, C. septicum,* and *C. sordelli* are gas-gangrene agents. Treatment of gas gangrene includes debridement and penicillin, clindamycin, or metronidazole
C. baratii			
C. beijerinckii			
C. bifermentans			
C. bolteae			
C. butyricum			
C. cadaveris			
C. carnis			
C. celatum			
C. clostridioforme			
C. cochlearium			
C. cocleatum			
C. fallax			
C. ghonii			
C. glycolicum			
C. haemolyticum			
C. histolyticum			
C. indolis			
C. innocuum			
C. irregulare			

(Continued)

Table 6.46.1 (*Cont'd*) A checklist of bacteria associated with infection in humans

Nomenclature		Associated infections	Reported susceptibilities and treatments	Notes
Genus	**Species and subspecies**			
(synonyms, CDC alphanumeric groups)				
	C. leptum			
	C. limosum			
	C. malenominatum			
	C. novyi			
	C. oroticum			
	C. paraputrificum			
	C. piliforme			
	C. putrefasciens			
	C. ramosum			
	C. sardiniense (C. absonum)			
	C. septicum			
	C. sordelli			
	C. sphenoides			
	C. sporogenes			
	C. subterminale			
	C. symbiosum			
	C. tertium			
	C. botulinum	Botulism		Antitoxin and respiratory support as treatment
	C. difficile	Diarrhoea, pseudomembranous colitis	**Metronidazole, vancomycin**	Infection associated with antibiotic exposure
	C. perfringens	Food poisoning, necrotizing enterocolitis, gas gangrene		Debridement and penicillin, clindamycin, or metronidazole for treatment of gas gangrene
	C. tetani	Tetanus	**Metronidazole, penicillin**	Antitoxin and supportive treatment
Collinsella	*C. aerofaciens*			From faecal flora. Clinical significance is undefined
[*Comamonas acidovorans*—see *Delftia acidovorans*]				
Comamonas (*Pseudomonas*)	*C. terrigena*	Bacteraemia, UTI, conjunctivitis, endocarditis, wound infection, abdominal abscess, peritonitis, meningitis	Ureidopenicillins, ceftazidime, ciprofloxacin, aminoglycosides, imipenem	Infections in neutropenic patients. Infections associated with animal bite and exposure to tropical fish
	C. testosteroni			
Corynebacterium	*C. accolens*	Septicaemia, peritonitis, UTI, eye infection, wound infection, endocarditis, osteomyelitis, septic arthritis, meningitis, abscesses	Glycopeptides, β-lactam, erythromycin, rifampicin	More than 40 *Corynebacterium* spp. have been isolated from clinical specimens. For many of them, clinical significance and empirical therapy are poorly defined. Many isolates are susceptible to β-lactams. Multiresistant, vancomycin-susceptible isolates of CDC coryneform group G-2, *C. jeikeium* and *C. urealyticum* have been reported. Nosocomial outbreaks have been reported. *Corynebacterium* spp. may be specimen or laboratory contaminants. CDC coryneform groups 1, E, F-1, and G-2 await designation of scientific names
	C. afermentans			
	C. amycolatum			
	C. appendicis			
	C. argentoratense			
	C. atypicum			
	C. aurimucosum (C. nigricans)			
	C. auris			
	C. bovis			
	C. confusum			
	C. coyleae			
	C. durum			
	C. falsenii			
	C. freneyi			

Organism	Infection	Treatment	Comments
C. glucuronolyticum			
C. imitans			
C. jeikeium			
C. kroppenstedtii			
C. kutscheri			
C. lipophilum			
C. macginleyi			
C. matruchotii			
C. mucifaciens			
C. pilosum			
C. propinquum			
C. renale			
C. resistens			
C. riegelii			
C. sanguinis			
C. singulare			
C. striatum			
C. sundsvallense			
C. thomssenii			
C. tuberculostearicum			
C. tuscaniense			
C. urealyticum			
C. xerosis			
C. diphtheriae	Diphtheria, cutaneous infection	Penicillin, erythromycin	Toxigenic infection requires treatment with antitoxin
C. minutissimum	Erythrasma, bacteraemia, endocarditis		Role as an agent of erythrasma is poorly defined
C. mycetoides	Tropical ulcer, septicaemia		
C. pseudodiphthericum	UTI, endocarditis, lymphadenopathy, necrotizing tracheitis	Penicillin	
C. pseudotuberculosis	Lymphadenitis, pulmonary infection	Penicillin, erythromycin	Associated with sheep contact. May require drainage or excision
C. ulcerans	Diphtheria-like disease, pharyngitis	Penicillin, erythromycin	Toxigenic infection requires treatment with antitoxin
C. vitaeruminis	Associated with aortic aneurysm		Role as pathogen uncertain
[Corynebacterium group A-3—see Cellulomonas]			
[Corynebacterium groups A-4 and A-5—see Microbacterium]			
[Corynebacterium group 2—see Arcanobacterium bernardice]			
Coxiella			
C. burnetii	Q fever	Tetracycline, ciprofloxacin, co-trimoxazole, rifampicin	
Cryptobacterium			
C. curtum	Periodontitis		

(Continued)

Table 6.46.1 (*Cont'd*) A checklist of bacteria associated with infection in humans

Nomenclature		Associated infections	Reported susceptibilities and treatments	Notes
Genus	**Species and subspecies**			
(synonyms, CDC alphanumeric groups)				
Cupriavidus (*Ralstonia*) (*Wautersia*)	C. gilardii, C. pauculus, C. respiraculi, C. taiwanensis	Meningitis, pulmonary infection in cystic fibrosis, line sepsis	Cephalosporins, imipenem, co-trimoxazole, quinolones, amikacin	
D				
Delftia	D. acidovorans (Comamonas acidovorans)	Bacteraemia, endocarditis	Ureidopenicillins, fluoroquinolones	
Dermabacter	D. hominis	Brain abscess, bacteraemia, wound infection	Cephalosporins, glycopeptides	
Dermacoccus	D. sp.	Associated with aortic aneurysm		Role as pathogen uncertain. Found on skin and mucous membranes
Dermatophilus	D. congolensis	Cutaneous infection	Penicillin	Zoonosis from cattle, sheep, goats, and horses
Desulfomicrobium	D. orale	Periodontitis		
Desulfomonas	D. piger (D. pigra)	Pilonidal cyst abscess, peritonitis		From faecal flora
Desulfovibrio	D. desulfuricans, D. vulgaris, 'D. fairfieldensis'	Bacteraemia, liver abscess. Cultured from urine of patient with UTI and meningoencephalitis	Penicillin, clindamycin	
Dialister	D. invisus, D. micraerophilus, D. pneumosintes, D. propionicifaciens	Periodontitis, endodontic infection, bacteraemia		
Dichelobacter	D. nodosus (Bacteroides nodosus)	Pilonidal cyst, rectal fistula, wound infection		Cause of ovine footrot. Isolates reported from humans may not be D. nodosus
Dietzia	D. maris	Prosthetic hip infection, bacteraemia	Vancomycin, teicoplanin, rifampicin, amoxicillin, gentamicin, clindamycin, co-trimoxazole	Papillomatosis has been associated with 'Dietzia strain X'
Dolosicoccus	D. paucivorans	Bacteraemia	Cephalosporins	
Dolosigranulum	D. pigrum	Spinal cord infection, eye infection		Significance as a pathogen poorly defined.
Dysgonomonas	D. capnocytophagoides (CDC group DF-3), D. gadei, D. mossii	Diarrhoea, bacteraemia, abscess	Tetracycline, clindamycin, imipenem	
E				
Edwardsiella	E. hoshinae, E. ictaluri, E. tarda	Wound infection, abscesses, gastroenteritis	β-Lactams, aminoglycosides, fluoroquinolones	Aquatic exposure, penetrating fish injury

Genus	Species	Infection	Treatment	Comments
Eggerthella	E. hongkongensis E. lenta (Eubacterium lentum) E. sinensis	Rectal abscess, bacteraemia	Penicillin, metronidazole	Variable susceptibility to cefotaxime
Ehrlichia	E. chaffeensis E. ewingii	Ehrlichiosis	Tetracycline, doxycycline	Antibodies to E. muris detected in healthy humans in Japan
[Ehrlichia sennetsu—see Neorickettsia sennetsu]				
Eikenella	E. corrodens	Septicaemia, endocarditis, abscesses, septic arthritis	Penicillin (plus gentamicin for endocarditis)	
Elizabethkingia	E. meningoseptica (Chryseobacterium meningosepticum, Flavobacterium meningosepticum)	Meningitis, bacteraemia, endocarditis, necrotizing fasciitis, pneumonia	Quinolones, co-trimoxazole, minocycline, rifampicin	Treatment with vancomycin is controversial
Empedobacter	E. brevis (Flavobacterium breve)	Endophthalmitis, bacteraemia, UTI	Broad-spectrum cephalosporins	Carbapenem-resistant
Enterobacter	E. aerogenes E. amnigenus E. asburiae E. cancerogenus E. cloacae E. gergoviae E. hormaechei E. kobei E. ludwigii E. sakazakii	Bacteraemia, respiratory tract infections, UTI	Carbapenems, fluoroquinolones, aminoglycosides, ureidopenicillins	May be multiresistant. Common cause of nosocomial infection
Enterococcus	E. avium E. casseliflavus (E. flavescens) E. cecorum E. dispar E. durans E. faecalis E. faecium E. gallinarum E. gilvus E. hirae E. malodoratus E. mundtii E. pallens E. pseudoavium E. raffinosus E. solitarius	Bacteraemia, abscesses, endocarditis, meningitis, UTI, peritonitis, osteomyelitis, wound infection	Penicillins, glycopeptides	May be resistant to penicillins and glycopeptides. Nosocomial outbreaks reported
Erwinia	E. persicinus	UTI	Cephalosporins, fluoroquinolones, aminoglycosides	The causative agent of necrosis of bean pods
Erysipelothrix	E. rhusiopathiae	Erysipeloid, septicaemia, endocarditis	Penicillin	Animal contact
[Escherichia adecarboxylata—see Leclercia adecarboxylata]				

(Continued)

Table 6.46.1 (*Cont'd*) A checklist of bacteria associated with infection in humans

Nomenclature		Associated infections	Reported susceptibilities and treatments	Notes
Genus	**Species and subspecies**			
	(synonyms, CDC alphanumeric groups)			
Escherichia	*E. albertii*	Diarrhoea		Previously known as *Hafnia alvei*-like strains
	E. coli	UTI, bacteraemia, wound infection, meningitis, enteric infection, haemolytic uraemic syndrome	β-Lactams, aminoglycosides, fluoroquinolones, co-trimoxazole	Susceptibilities variable
	E. fergusonii	Bacteraemia, wounds, UTI	Chloramphenicol, gentamicin	Ampicillin-resistant
	E. hermanii	Wounds	Chloramphenicol, cephalosporins, gentamicin	
	E. vulneris	Wounds	Ampicillin, cephalosporins, gentamicin	
Eubacterium	*E. brachy*	Wounds, abscesses, septicaemia, periodontitis	Penicillins, clindamycin, metronidazole	
	E. combesii			
	E. contortum			
	E. cylindroids			
	E. infirmum			
	E. limosum			
	E. minutum			
	E. moniliforme			
	E. multiforme			
	E. nitrogenes			
	E. nodatum			
	E. plautii			
	E. rectale			
	E. saburreum			
	E. saphenum			
	E. sulci			
	E. tenue			
	E. timidum			
	E. tortuosum			
	E. ventriosum			
	E. yurii yurii			
	E. yurii mararetiae			
	E. yurii schtitka			
Ewingella	*E. americana*	Septicaemia, wounds, UTI	Ureidopenicillins, aminoglycosides	
Exiguobacterium	*E. acetylicum*	Wound infection, bacteraemia		
	E. aurantiacum			
F				
Facklamia	*F. hominis*	UTI, bacteraemia, abscess		
	F. ignava			
	F. languida			
	F. sourekii			

Genus	Species	Infection	Treatment/Comment
Filifactor	*F. alocis*	Gingivitis, periodontitis	
	F. villosus		
Finegoldia	*F. magna (Peptostreptococcus) magnus*		
[*Flavimonas oryzihabitans*—see *Pseudomonas oryzihabitans*]			
Flavobacterium	*F. mizutaii (Sphingobacterium mizutae)*		
[*Flavobacterium gleum*—see *Chryseobacterium gleum*]			
[*Flavobacterium indologenes*—see *Chryseobacterium indologenes*]			
[*Flavobacterium meningosepticum*—see *Elizabethkingia meningoseptica*]			
'Flexispira'	*'F. rappini'*	Bacteraemia, diarrhoea	Not in approved lists of bacterial names. There is a growing consensus that 'Flexispira' actually represents several *Helicobacter* spp.
[*Fluoribacter bozemanae*—see *Legionella bozemanae*]			
[*Fluoribacter dumoffii*—see *Legionella dumoffii*]			
[*Fluoribacter gormanii*—see *Legionella gormanii*]			
Francisella	*F. philomiragia (Yersinia philomiragia)*	Septicaemia, invasive systemic infection	Fluoroquinolones, aminoglycosides, chloramphenicol, cefoxitin
	F. tularensis	Tularaemia	Streptomycin, tetracycline
Fusobacterium	*F. gonidiaformans*	Abscesses, bacteraemia, periodontitis, endocarditis, necrobacillosis	Metronidazole, penicillins, carbapenems, cephalosporins
	F. mortiferum		
	F. naviforme		
	F. necrogenes		
	F. necrophorum necrophorum		
	F. necrophorum fundiliforme		
	F. nucleatum nucleatum		
	F. nucleatum fusiforme		
	F. nucleatum polymorphum		
	F. nucleatum vincentii		
	F. periodonticum		
	F. russii		
	F. ulcerans		
	F. varium		

G

Genus	Species	Infection	Treatment/Comment
Gardnerella	*G. vaginalis*	Intrauterine and neonatal sepsis	β-Lactams, clindamycin. Associated with bacterial vaginosis

(Continued)

Table 6.46.1 (*Cont'd*) A checklist of bacteria associated with infection in humans

Nomenclature		Associated infections	Reported susceptibilities and treatments	Notes
Genus	**Species and subspecies**			
(synonyms, CDC alphanumeric groups)				
Gemella	*G. bergeri* *G. haemolysins* *G. morbillorum* (*Streptococcus morbillorum*) *G. sanguinis*	Bacteraemia, endocarditis	Penicillin or vancomycin (plus gentamicin for endocarditis)	
Globicatella	*G. sanguinis*	Bacteraemia, UTI, meningitis	Vancomycin	
Gordonia (*Gordona*) (*Rhodococcus*)	*G. aichensis* *G. araii* *G. bronchialis* *G. effuse* *G. otitidis* *G. polyisoprenivorans* *G. rubropertinctus* *G. sputi* *G. terrae*	Pulmonary infection, cholecystitis, breast abscess, sternal wound sepsis, brain abscess, bacteraemia, otitis	Co-trimoxazole, ceftriaxone, imipenem, fluoroquinolones	
Granulicatella	*G. adiacens* (*Abiotrophia adiacens*) *G. elegans* (*Abiotrophia elegans*)	Endocarditis, septic arthritis, endodontic infection	Penicillin or cefazolin or vancomycin plus gentamicin (plus rifampicin)	Previously known as nutritionally deficient or variant streptococci; the proposed name 'Abiotrophia para-adiacens' for strains allied to what is now known as *Granulicatella adiacens* does not have standing in nomenclature
Grimontia	*G. hollisae* (*Vibrio hollisae*)	Diarrhoea	β-Lactams, quinolones	Infection associated with ingestion of shellfish
H				
[*Haemophilus aphrophilus*—see *Aggregatibacter aphrophilus*]				
[*Haemophilus paraphrophilus*—see *Aggregatibacter aphrophilus*]				
[*Haemophilus segnis*—see *Aggregatibacter segnis*]				
Haemophilus	*H. aegyptius*	Brazilian purpuric fever	Ampicillin, cephalosporins, chloramphenicol	Treated by some authors as a biotype of *H. influenzae*
	H. aphrophilus *H. parainfluenzae* *H. pittmaniae*	Sinusitis, otitis media, pneumonia, abscesses, endocarditis	Cefotaxime, chloramphenicol, ampicillin, aminoglycosides	The genus *Aggregatibacter* has been proposed to accommodate *H. aphrophilus* (including *H. paraphrophilus* as a heterotypic synonym of *H. aphrophilus*), *H. segnis*, and *Actinobacillus actinomycetemcomitans*
	H. ducreyi	Chancroid	Macrolides, ceftriaxone, fluoroquinolones	
	H. influenzae	Bacteraemia, meningitis, epiglottitis	Cephalosporins, penicillins, fluoroquinolones	Many strains produce penicillinases
Hafnia	*H. alvei*	Bacteraemia		Doubtful enteropathogen. Susceptibility variable. Includes two genomospecies. '*Hafnia alvei*-like' strains from Bangladesh have been described as *Escherichia albertii*
Helcococcus	*H. kunzii* '*H. pyogenica*' *H. sueciensis*	Sebaceous cyst infection, breast abscess, wound infection	Penicillins, vancomycin	From skin flora. The name *H. pyogenica* does not have standing in nomenclature

Organism	Infection	Treatment	Comments
Helicobacter			
H. bilis (Flexispira rapini corrig. taxon 9)	Cholecystitis, bacteraemia		Zoonosis from rodents
H. canis	Gastroenteritis		Zoonosis from dogs
H. cinaedi (Campylobacter cinaedi)	Proctitis in homosexual men, septicaemia	Ampicillin, gentamicin	Zoonoses from hamsters
H. fennelliae (Campylobacter fennelliae)			
H. bizzozeronii	Gastritis		Zoonoses from domestic and farm animals.
H. felis			Some organisms known as 'Flexispira rapini' may belong to this group of Helicobacter spp.
H. salomonis			
'Candidatus H. bovis'			
'Candidatus H. heilmannii' ('Gastrospirillum hominis')			
'Candidatus H. suis'			
('H. heilmannii-like organisms')			
H. canadensis	Gastroenteritis		Zoonoses from birds (or possibly rodents)
H. pullorum			
H. pylori (Campylobacter pyloridis)	Gastritis	Omeprazole plus clarithromycin and metronidazole	Numerous similar treatment combinations have been recommended
'H. westmeadii'	Bacteraemia in AIDS		Name does not have standing in nomenclature
'H. winghamensis'	Gastroenteritis		Name does not have standing in nomenclature. Possibly a zoonosis from rodents
Herbaspirillum			
H. sp.	Associated with aortic aneurism		Detected by 16S gene analysis. Of doubtful clinical significance
Holdemania			
H. filiformis			From faecal flora. Clinical significance is unclear
I			
Ignatzschineria I. arvae	Bacteraemia	Penicillins, cephalosporins, quinolones	Associated with myiasis
Ignavigranum I. ruoffiae	Wound infection, ear abscess		Role as pathogen poorly defined
Inquilinus I. limosusI. sp.	Pulmonary infection in cystic fibrosis, endocarditis	Imipenem, quinolones, gentamicin	
J			
Janibacter J. melonis	Bacteraemia	Vancomycin, β-lactams, fluoroquinolones	An undescribed Janibacter sp. was isolated from a leukaemia patient
Johnsonella J. ignava	Periodontitis		
K			
Kerstersia K. gyiorum	Wound infection		
Kingella K. denitrificans, K. kingae, K. oralis, K. potus	Septic arthritis, endocarditis, bite infection	Penicillins (plus gentamicin for endocarditis)	
[Kingella indologenes—see Suttonella indologenes]			
Klebsiella K. granulomatis (Calymmatobacterium granulomatis)	Donovanosis	Tetracycline, co-trimoxazole	
[Klebsiella ornitholytica, K. planticola, K. terrigena—see Raoultella]			

(Continued)

Table 6.46.1 (*Cont'd*) A checklist of bacteria associated with infection in humans

Nomenclature		Associated infections	Reported susceptibilities and treatments	Notes
Genus	Species and subspecies			
(synonyms, CDC alphanumeric groups)				
Klebsiella	*K. oxytoca* *K.pneumoniae* ssp. *pneumoniae* *K. pneumoniae* ssp. *ozaenae* *K. varicola*	UTI, bacteraemia, wound infection, respiratory tract infection	β-Lactams, aminoglycosides, fluoroquinolones	Susceptibilities vary. Nosocomial outbreaks reported
	K. pneumoniae ssp. *rhinoscleromatis*	Rhinoscleroma	Ciprofloxacin, rifampicin, co-trimoxazole	
Kluyvera	*K. ascorbate* *K. cryocrescens* *K. georgiana* *K. intermedia* (*Enterobacter intermedius*)	Bacteraemia. UTI, mediastinitis, line sepsis	Aminoglycosides, ceftazidime, imipenem, ciprofloxacin	
Kocuria (*Micrococcus*)	*K. kristinae* *K. rosea* *K. varians*	Cholecystitis, line-related sepsis	Penicillin, clindamycin, vancomycin	
[*Koserella trabulsii*—see *Yokenella regensburgei*]				
Kurthia	'*K. bessonii*' *K. gibsonii* *K. zopfii*	Bacteraemia endocarditis	Penicillin	Not in approved lists of bacterial names Isolated from faeces of patients with diarrhoea
Kytococcus (*Micrococcus*)	*K. schroeteri* *K. sedentarius*	Endocarditis cerebral cyst infection	Imipenem, vancomycin, rifampicin	
L				
Lactobacillus	*L. acidophilus* *L. brevis* *L. casei* *L. catenaformis* *L. coleohominis* *L. crispatus* *L. fermentum* *L. gasseri* *L. iners* *L. jensenii* *L. leichmannii* *L. oris* *L. paracasei* *L. paraplantarum* *L. plantarum* *L. rhamnosus* *L. salivarius* *L. vaginalis*	Abscesses, bacteraemia, endometritis, endocarditis. lung infection, UTI	Cephalosporins, vancomycin, penicillins, aminoglycosides, clindamycin	Reported risk factors for infection include surgery, malignancy, diabetes, and immunodeficiency. May be vancomycin-resistant
Lactococcus (*Streptococcus*)	*L. garviae* *L. lactis*	Bacteraemia, endocarditis, UTI	Penicillin (plus gentamicin for endocarditis)	

Genus	Species	Infection	Treatment	Comments
Lautropia	*L. mirabilis*			Role as potential pathogen unclear. From oral flora of HIV patients and sputum of cystic fibrosis patient
Leclercia	*L. adecarboxylata* (*Escherichia adecarboxylata*)	Bacteraemia, wound infection		Variable susceptibility
Legionella	*L. anisa* *L. birminghamensis* *L. bozemanae* (*L. bozemanii*) *L. cincinnatiensis* *L. dumoffii* *L. feeleii* *L. gormanii* *L. hackeliae* *L. israelensis* *L. jordanis* *L. lansingensis* *L. longbeachae* *L. lytica* *L. maceachernii* *L. micdadei* *L. oakridgemsis* *L. pneumophila* *L. quinlivanii* *L. rubrilucens* *L. sainthelersi* *L. tucsonensis* *L. wadsworthia* *L. worsleiensis*	Legionnaires' disease, Pontiac fever	Macrolides, fluoroquinolones, rifampicin	Infections caused by species other than *L. pneumophila* and *L. micdadei* are seldom reported
Leifsonia	*L. aquatica* (*Corynebacterium aquaticum*)	UTI, endocarditis, meningitis, CAPD peritonitis	Ampicillin, chloramphenicol, gentamicin	Previously confused with *Aureobacterium* (which has been united with *Microbacterium*)
Leminorella	*L. grimontii* *L. richardii*	UTI, bacteraemia, surgical site infection, peritonitis	Imipenem, chloramphenicol, tetracycline, gentamicin	
Leptospira	*L. biflexa* *L. borgpetersenii* *L. broomii* *L. inadai* *L. interrogans* *L. kirschneri* *L. noguchii* *L. santarosai* *L. weilii*	Leptospirosis	Penicillin, tetracycline	*L. interrogans* is composed of severalnamed serogroups, including: australis, bataviae, canicola, copenhageni, cynopteri, hurstbridge, hardjo, grippotyphosa, icterohaemorrhagiae, panama, pomona, pyrogenes, sejroe, tarassovi

(Continued)

Table 6.46.1 (*Cont'd*) A checklist of bacteria associated with infection in humans

Nomenclature		Associated infections	Reported susceptibilities and treatments	Notes
Genus	**Species and subspecies**			
(synonyms, CDC alphanumeric groups)				
Leptotrichia	*L. buccalis* *L. goodfellowii* *L. shahii* *L. trevisanii*	Bacteraemia, endocarditis	β-Lactams, metronidazole	Associated with dental plaque and gingivitis. 'L. amnionii' from amniotic fluid does not have standing in nomenclature and may belong in the genus Sneathia
Leuconostoc	*L. citreum* *L. lactis* *L. mesenteroides* ssp. *cremoris* *L. mesenteroides* ssp. *dextranicum* *L. mesenteroides* ssp. *mesenteroide* *L. pseudomesenteroides*	Meningitis, bacteraemia, pulmonary infection	Penicillin and gentamicin or clindamycin	Vancomycin-resistant
Listeria	*L. ivanovii* *L. grayi* *L. monocytogenes* *L. seeligeri*	Septicaemia, meningitis, intrauterine infection, enteric infection	Ampicillin and gentamicin	
[*Listonella damsela*—see *Photobacterium damselae*]				
Luteococcus	*L. peritonei* *L. sanguinis*	Peritonitis, bacteraemia		
M				
Massilia	*M. timonae*	Bacteraemia, wound infection		
Megasphaera	*M. elsdenii* *M. micronuciformis*	Endocarditis, abscess	Metronidazole	
Mesorhizobium	*M. amorphae*	Pneumonia		
Methylobacterium	*M. extorquens* *M. mesophilicum* (*Pseudomonas mesophilica*)	Bacteraemia, CAPD peritonitis, UTI, septic arthritis	Ureidopenicillins, imipenem, am noglycosides, chloramphenicol, fluoroquinolones	Detected in aortic aneurysm
Microbacterium (*Aureobacterium*)	*M. arborescens* *M. imperiale* (CDC coryneform groups A-4 and A-5) *M. liquefaciens* (*Aureobacterium liquefaciens*) ('*Corynebacterium aquaticum*') *M. oxydans* *M. paraoxydans* *M. resistens* *M. trichothecenolyticum*	Endophthalmitis, UTI, endocarditis, soft tissue infection, hypersensitivity pneumonitis, meningitis, CAPD peritonitis, bacteraemia	Glycopeptides, β-lactams, chloramphenicol, gentamicin	*M. resistens* is vancomycin-resistant. *Microbacterium* isolates have been misidentified as '*Corynebacterium aquaticum*' a taxon now known as *Leifsonia aquatica*
Micrococcus	*M. luteus* *M. lytae*	Bacteraemia, endocarditis, septic arthritis	Vancomycin, penicillin, rifampicin	From skin flora. Common specimen contaminants

Genus	Species	Infection	Treatment	Comments
Mitsuokella	M. multacida (Bacteroides multiacidus)			Role as human pathogen poorly defined
Mobiluncus	M. curtisii curtisii M. curtisii holmesii M. mulieris	Endometritis, chorioamnionitis	Ampicillin, cephalosporins, clindamycin	Associated with bacterial vaginosis
Moellerella	M. wisconsensis	Diarrhoea		Of uncertain significance
Mogibacterium	M. diversum M. neglectum	Endodontic infection		
Moraxella	M. atlantae M. catarrhalis (Branhamella catarrhalis) M. lacunata M. nonliquefaciens M. osloensis	Conjunctivitis, wound infection, endocarditis, abscesses, osteomyelitis, respiratory infections, endocarditis, bacteraemia	Penicillin, cefuroxime	Penicillin resistance has been reported. Some authors retain Branhamella catarrhalis
[Moraxella phenylpyruvica—see Psychrobacter phenylpyruvicus]				
[Moraxella urethralis—see Oligella urethralis]				
Morganella	M. morganii morganii M. morganii sibonii	Bacteraemia, UTI, wound infection	β-Lactams, aminoglycosides	Susceptibilities vary
Moryella	M. indoligenes			
Mycobacterium	M. abscessus M. africanum M. alvei M. asiaticum M. arupense M. aubagnense M. aurum M. avium M. barrassiae M. boenickei M. bohemicum M. bolletii M. bovis M. branderi M. brisbanense M. brumae M. canariasense M. celatum M. chelonae M. chimaera M. chubuense M. colombiense M. conceptionense M. confluentis M. conspicuum M. cookii M. cosmeticum		Isoniazid, rifampicin, ethambutol, pyrazinamide, streptomycin, azithromycin, clarithromycin, ciprofloxacin, dapsone, clofazimine, imipenem, co-trimoxazole, amikacin	Many Mycobacterium spp. have been associated with infection. M. tuberculosis, M. africanum, and M. bovis are the agents of tuberculosis. M. scrofulaceum causes cervical adenitis. The agent of Buruli ulcer is M. ulcerans. M. marinum causes fish-tank granuloma. M. lepraecauses leprosy. M. malmoense, M. szulgai, M. shimoidei, M. kansasii, and M. xenopi cause pulmonary infection. M. intracellulareand M. avium cause systemic infection mainly in immunocompromised patients. The rapid growers, M. chelonae,M. abscessus, and M. fortuitum cause local postinoculation injury and systemic infection

(Continued)

Table 6.46.1 (*Cont'd*) A checklist of bacteria associated with infection in humans

Nomenclature		Associated infections	Reported susceptibilities and treatments	Notes
Genus	**Species and subspecies**			
(synonyms, CDC alphanumeric groups)				
	M. doricum			
	M. elephantis			
	M. flavescens			
	M. florentinum			
	M. fortuitum			
	M. gadium			
	M. gastri			
	M. genavense			
	M. goodii			
	M. gordonae			
	M. haemophilum			
	M. hassiacum			
	M. heckeshornense			
	M. heidelbergense			
	M. hodleri			
	M. holsaticum			
	M. houstonense			
	M. immunogenum			
	M. interjectum			
	M. intracellulare			
	'M. jacuzzii'			
	M. kansasii			
	M. kubicae			
	M. kumamotonense			
	M. lacus			
	M. lentiflavum			
	M. leprae			
	M. mageritense			
	M. malmoense			
	M. marinum			
	M. massiliense			
	M. microgenicum			
	M. microti			
	M. monacense			
	M. mucogenicum			
	M. neoaurum			
	M. nebraskense			
	M. neworleansense			
	M. nonchromogenicum			
	M. novocastrense			
	M. palustre			
	M. parascrofulaceum			
	M. parmense			
	M. peregrinum			
	M. phlei			
	M. phocaicum			
	M. porcinum			

Organism	Infection	Treatment	Comments
	M. saskatchewanense		
	M. scrofulaceum		
	M. seoulense		
	M. septicum		
	M. shimoidei		
	M. simiae		
	M. smegmatis		
	M. szulgai		
	M. terrae		
	M. thermoresistibile		
	M. triplex		
	M. triviale		
	M. tuberculosis		
	M. tusciae		
	M. ulcerans		
	M. vaccae		
	M. wolinskyi		
	M. xenopi		
Mycoplasma	*M. amphoriforme*	Respiratory infection, postpartum fever, pyelonephritis, pelvic inflammatory disease, myocarditis, pericarditis, meningitis	Tetracycline, macrolides, fluoroquinolones	May be resistant to macrolides. *M. pneumoniae* infection may be complicated by haemolytic anaemia, intravascular coagulation, Stevens–Johnson syndrome, or erythema multiforme
	M. buccale		
	M. faucium		
	M. fermentans		
	M. genitalium		
	M. hominis		
	M. lipophilum		
	M. orale		
	M. penetrans		
	M. pirum		
	M. pneumoniae		
	M. primatum		
	M. salivarium		
	M. spermatophilum		
	M. phocicerebrale (*M. phocacerebrale*)	Seal finger	Tetracycline	Other *Mycoplasma* spp. from seals are *M. phocae* and *M. phocirhinis*
Myroides (*Flavobacterium*)	*M. odoratimimus*	UTI, wound infection	Minocycline	May be multiresistant
	M. odoratus			
N				
Neisseria	*N. animaloris* (CDC group EF-4a)	Wound infections, abscesses, endocarditis, meningitis, bacteraemia	Amoxicillin	Zoonoses from animal bites
	N. canis			
	N. weaveri (CDC group M-5, '*Neisseria parelongata*')			
	N. zoodegmatis (CDC group EF-4b)			

(Continued)

Table 6.46.1 (*Cont'd*) A checklist of bacteria associated with infection in humans

Nomenclature		Associated infections	Reported susceptibilities and treatments	Notes
Genus	**Species and subspecies**			
(synonyms, CDC alphanumeric groups)				
	N. bacilliformis	Meningitis, bacteraemia, endocarditis, osteomyelitis	Penicillin, cephalosporins	Bacteraemia in AIDS reported for several species. Penicillin resistance rarely reported in commensal *Neisseria* spp. *N. subflava* includes bicvars flava, perflava, and subflava
	N. cinerea			
	N. elongata elongata			
	N. elongata glycolytica			
	N. elongata nitroreductens			
	N. flavescens			
	N. lactamica			
	N. mucosa			
	N. polysaccharea			
	N. sicca			
	N. subflava			
	N. gonorrhoeae	Gonorrhoea, septicaemia, ophthalmia neonatorum	Cephalosporins	Susceptibility varies geographically. The name '*Nesseria gonorrhoeae* ssp. *kochii*' was proposed for isolates from conjunctivitis cases in rural Egypt
	N. meningitidis	Septicaemia, meningitis, conjunctivitis, genital infection, epiglottitis	Penicillin, cefotaxime	Rifampicin, ciprofloxacin, or ceftriaxone to clear carriage
Neorickettsia	N. sennetsu (*Ehalichia sennetsu*)	Sennetsu fever	Doxycycline	Associated with eating raw fish in Asia
Nocardia	N abscessus	Nocardiosis (including bacteraemia, pulmonary and soft tissue infections)	Sulphonamides, co-trimoxazole, amikacin, imipenem	
	N. africana			
	N. anaemiae			
	N. aobensis			
	N. araoensis			
	N. arthritides			
	N. asiatica			
	N. asteroides			
	N. beijingensis			
	N. brasiliensis			
	N. brevicatena			
	N. carnea			
	N. concave			
	N. cyriacigeorgica			
	N. elegans			
	N. exalbida			
	N. farcinica			
	N. higoensis			
	N. inohanensis			
	N. kruczakiae			
	N. mexicana			
	N. niigatensis			
	N. ninae			
	N. nova			
	N. otitidiscaviarum			

Organism	Infection	Treatment	Comments
N. pauclvorans *N. pneumoniae* *N. pseudobrasiliensis* *N. puris* *N. sienata* *N. takedensis* *N. thailandensis* *N. testaceus* *N. transvalensis* *N. vermiculeta* *N. veterana* *N. yamanashiensis*			
Nocardiopsis *N. dassonvillei* *N. synnemataformans*	Mycetoma, cutaneous infection, pulmonary infection, conjunctivitis	Fluoroquinolones, piperacillin	
O			
Ochrobactrum (*Achromobacter* CDC group Vd; *Achromobacter* groups A, C, and D) *O. anthropi* *O. intermedium*	Bacteraemia, endophthalmitis, liver abscess	Imipenem, fluoroquinolones, aminoglycosides	Nosocomial infections in debilitated patients
Oerskovia *O. turbata* (*Cellulomonas turbata*)	Bacteraemia, endocarditis	Amikacin, co-trimoxazole, chloramphenicol	Vancomycin resistance reported
Oligella *O. ureolytica* (CDC IVe) *O. urethralis* (*Moraxella urethralis*)	UTI, septicaemia	Aminoglycosides, cephalosporins	Associated with urinary catheters
Olsenella *O. uli* (*Lactobacillus uli*)			
Orientia *O. tsutsugamushi* (*Rickettsia tsutsugamushi*)	Scrub typhus	Tetracycline, chloramphenicol	
P			
Paenibacillus *P. alvei* *P. macerans* *P. polymyxa* *P. popilliae*	Septicaemia, meningitis, pneumonia	Vancomycin	
Pannonibacter *P. phragmitetus* (*Achromobacter* groups B and E)			
Pantoea *P. agglomerans* (*Enterobacter agglomerans*) *P. ananatis* *P. dispersa*	Bacteraemia, endocarditis, wound infection, cellulitis, alligator-bite infection, endophthalmitis	Carbapenems, fluoroquinolones, ureidopenicillins, aminoglycosides	Susceptibilities vary. May be multiresistant
Parabacteroides *P. distasonis* *P. goldsteinii* (*Bacteroides goldsteinii*) *P. merdae*	Abscesses	Metronidazole	

(Continued)

Table 6.46.1 (Cont'd) A checklist of bacteria associated with infection in humans

Nomenclature		Associated infections	Reported susceptibilities and treatments	Notes
Genus	**Species and subspecies**			
(synonyms, CDC alphanumeric groups)				
Parachlamydia	P. acanthamoebae	Humidifier fever		
Paracoccus	P. yeei	Bacteraemia	Ampicillin, cephalosporins, ciprofloxacin	
Parvimonas	P. micra (Peptostreptococcus micros)			
Pasteurella	P. aerogenes P. bettyae P. canis P. dagmatis P. gallinarum P. haemolytica P. multocida multocida P. multocida gallicida P. multocida septica P. pneumotropica P. stomatis	Wound infection, septicaemia, abscesses, pneumonia, endocarditis, meningitis	Penicillin, tetracycline, ciprofloxacin	Pasteurella infections in humans relate to species usually associated with animals. There may be no history of an animal bite or contact
[Pasteurella ureae—see Actinobacillus ureae]				
Pediococcus	P. acidilactici P. damnosus P. dextrinicus P. parvulus P. pentosaceus	Bacteraemia, abscesses, pulmonary infection	Imipenem, gentamicin, chloramphenicol	Debilitated hospital patients. Resistant to vancomycin
Peptococcus	P. niger	Abdominal sepsis	Penicillin, clindamycin	
Peptoniphilus (Peptostreptococcus)	P. asaccharolyticus P harei P. indolyticus P. ivorii P. lacrimalis	Mixed anaerobic infections, abscesses	β-Lactams, metronidazole, chloramphenicol	
Peptostreptococcus	P. anaerobius P. stomatis 'P. trisimilis'	Mixed anaerobic infections, abscesses, endocarditis	β-Lactams, metronidazole, chloramphenicol	See also Peptoniphilus, Anaerococcus, Finegoldia
Photobacterium	P. damselae (Listonella damsela and Vibrio damsela)	Necrotizing wound infection, bacteraemia	Penicillins, tetracycline, chloramphenicol	Infection associated with penetrating fish injury. May require debridement
Photorhabdus (Xenorhabdus)	P. luminescens	Bacteraemia, wound infection	Cefoxitin, oxacillin, gentamicin	
Plesiomonas	P. shigelloides	Gastroenteritis, septicaemia, meningitis, endophthalmitis	Ciprofloxacin, trimethoprim, cephalosporins	Infections associated with contaminated food and water

Genus/species	Infection/disease	Treatment	Comments
Porphyromonas (Bacteroides)			
P. asaccharolytica	Mixed anaerobic infections at various sites, periodontitis, human and animal bites	Metronidazole, ureidopenicillins, amoxicillin/clavulanate, carbapenems, cephalosporins, chloramphenicol	Members of the oral flora of humans and animals
P. cangingivalis			
P. canoris			
P. cansulci			
P. catoniae			
P. circumdentaria			
P. crevioricanis			
P. endodontalis			
P. gingivalis			
P. gingivicanis			
P. levii			
P. macacae			
P. somerae			
P. uenonis			
Prevotella (Bacteroides)			
P. bergensis	Abscesses, bacteraemia, wound infection, bite infections, genital tract infections, periodontitis, endodontic infection	Metronidazole, amoxicillin/clavulanate, ureidopenicillins, carbapenems, cephalosporins, clindamycin, chloramphenicol	A genus that includes the well-known former *Bacteroides melaninogenicus* and allied species of anaerobes
P. bivia			
P. buccae			
P. buccalis			
P. corporis			
P. dentalis			
P. denticola			
P. disiens			
P. enoeca			
P. heparinolytica			
P. intermedia			
P. loeschii			
P. melaninogenica			
P. multiformis			
P. multisaccharivorax			
P. nigrescens			
P. oralis			
P. oris			
P. oulorum			
P. tannerae			
P. timonensis			
P. veroralis			
P. zoogleoformans			
Propionibacterium			
P. acnes	Abscesses, endocarditis, bacteraemia, septic arthritis, endophthalmitis	Glycopeptides, penicillin, macrolides	Associated with acne vulgaris
P. avidum			
P. granulosum			
P. propionicum (Arachnia propionicus)			
Propionimicrobium			
P. lymphophilum (Propionibacterium lymphophilum)	UTI		Isolated from lymph nodes in Hodgkin's disease
Proteus			
P. mirabilis	UTI, bacteraemia, wound infection, abscesses	β-Lactams, aminoglycosides, fluoroquinolones	Susceptibilities vary
P. penneri			
P. vulgaris			

(Continued)

Table 6.46.1 (*Cont'd*) A checklist of bacteria associated with infection in humans

Nomenclature		Associated infections	Reported susceptibilities and treatments	Notes
Genus	**Species and subspecies (synonyms, CDC alphanumeric groups)**			
Providencia	*P. alcalifaciens* *P. rettgeri* *P. rustigianii* *P. stuartii*	UTI, wound infection, bacteraemia	β-Lactams, aminoglycosides, fluoroquinolones	Susceptibilities vary. *P. alcalifaciens* has been associated with gastroenteritis
	[*Pseudomonas acidivorans*—see *Delftia acidivorans*]			
Pseudomonas	*P. aeruginosa* *P. alcaligenes* *P. chlororaphis* *P. fluorescens* *P. mendocina* *P. monteilii* *P. mosselii* *P. otitidis* *P. pertocinogena* *P. pseudalcaligenes* *P. putida* *P. stutzeri*	Bacteraemia, UTI, wound infection, abscesses, septic arthritis, conjunctivitis, endocarditis, meningitis, otitis	Ureidopenicillins, aminoglycosides, cefazidime, fluoroquinolones, carbapenems	Nosocomial infections associated with invasive devices in debilitated patients. Nosocomial outbreaks reported. May be multiresistant
	[*Pseudomonas cepacia*—see *Burkholderia cepacia*]			
	[*Pseudomonas diminuta*—see *Brevundimonas diminuta*]			
	[*Pseudomonas mallei*—see *Burkholderia mallei*]			
	[*Pseudomonas maltophilia*—see *Stenotrophomonas maltophilia*]			
	[*Pseudomonas mesophilica*—see *Methylobacterium mesophilicum*]			
	P. luteola (*Chryseomonas luteola*)	Bacteraemia, endocarditis, CAPD peritonitis	Ureidopenicillins, ceftazidime, ciprofloxacin, aminoglycosides	
	P. oryzihabitans (*Flavimonas oryzihabitans*)	Septicaemia, eye infection, CAPD peritonitis	Ampicillin, tetracycline, gentamicin, cefotaxime	
	[*Pseudomonas paucimobilis*—see *Sphingomonas paucimobilis*]			
	[*Pseudomonas pickettii*—see *Ralstonia pickettii*]			
	[*Pseudomonas pseudomallei*—see *Burkholderia pseudomallei*]			
	[*Pseudomonas putrefaciens*—see *Shewanella putrefaciens*]			
	[*Pseudomonas terrigena*—see *Comamonas terrigena*]			
	[*Pseudomonas testosteroni*—see *Comamonas testosteroni*]			
	[*Pseudomonas vesicularis*—see *Brevundimonas vesicularis*]			
Pseudonocardia	*P. autotrophica* (*Amycolata autotrophica*)			Role as pathogen uncertain
Pseudoramibacter	*P. alactolyticus*	Periodontal disease, wound infection, abscesses	Penicillin, clindamycin, chloramphenicol	

Organism	Infection	Treatment	Comment
Psychrobacter *P. immobilis* *P. phenylpyruvicus* (*Moraxella phenylpyruvica*)	Meningitis, bacteraemia, eye infection	Penicillins, aminoglycosides, chloramphenicol	Immunocompromised patients
R			
Rahnella *R. aquatilis*	UTI, septicaemia	Ciprofloxacin	
Ralstonia *R. insidiosa* *R. mannitolilytica* *R. pickettii* (*Pseudomonas pickettii*) *R. taiwanensis*	Meningitis, peritonitis, bacteraemia, UTI, pulmonary infection	Co-trimoxazole, imipenem, ceftazidime, quinolones	
Raoultella (*Klebsiella*) *R. ornithinolytica* *R. planticola* *R. terrigena*	Bacteraemia, UTI, surgical sepsis, pancreatitis	Cephalosporins, carbapenems, aztreonam, quinolones, aminoglycosides	β-Lactamase producers. Associated with histamine (scombrotoxin) fish poisoning
'Rasbo' *'R. bacterium'*	Pneumonia, pericarditis		Proposed name does not have standing in nomenclature
Rhodococcus *R. equi* (*Corynebacterium equi*)	Bacteraemia, osteomyelitis, lung abscesses	Vancomycin, erythromycin, aminoglycosides	In immunocompromised patients, including AIDS
Rickettsia *R. africae* *R. akari* *R. australis* *R. conorii* *R. felis* *R. honei* *R. japonica* *'R. mongolotimonae'* *R. prowazekii* *R. rickettsiae* *R. sibirica* *R. slovaca* *R. typhi*	Rickettsial spotted fever, tick typhus, tick-bite fever, rickettsialpox	Tetracycline	Transmitted by arthropods. Agents of Astrakhan fever, Israeli tick typhus, and Thai tick typhus await designation of scientific names. Other *Rickettsia* spp. are of uncertain clinical significance
Roseomonas *R. cervicalis* *R. gilardii* ssp. *gilardii* *R. gilardii* ssp. *rosea* *R. mucosa*	Bacteraemia, wound infection, peritonitis	Aminoglycosides, imipenem, ciprofloxacin, ticarcillin-clavulanate	
[*Roseomonas fauriae*—see *Azospirillum brasilense*]			
Rothia *R. dentocariosa* *R. mucilaginosa* (*Micrococcus mucilaginosus*) (*Stomatococcus mucilaginosus*)	Endocarditis, abscesses Endocarditis, meningitis, neutropenic sepsis, necrotizing fasciitis	Penicillin and gentamicin Glycopeptides, imipenem, rifampicin, ceftriaxone	

(*Continued*)

Table 6.46.1 (*Cont'd*) A checklist of bacteria associated with infection in humans

Nomenclature		Associated infections	Reported susceptibilities and treatments	Notes
Genus	**Species and subspecies**			
(synonyms, CDC alphanumeric groups)				
Ruminococcus	*R. flavefaciens* *R. hansenii* (*Streptococcus hansenii*) *R. luti* *R. productus* (*Peptostreptococcus productus*)	Abdominal sepsis, abscesses	Penicillins	
S				
Salmonella	*S. bongori* *S. choleraesuis* ssp. *arizonae* *S. choleraesuis* ssp. *choleraesuis* *S. choleraesuis* ssp. *diarizonae* *S. choleraesuis* ssp. *houtenae* *S. choleraesuis* ssp. *indica* *S. choleraesuis* ssp. *salamae* *S. enteritidis* *S. paratyphi* *S. subterranea* *S. typhi* *S. typhimurium* *S. enterica* ssp. *arizonae* *S. enterica* ssp. *diarizonae* *S. enterica* ssp. *enterica* *S. enterica* ssp. *houtenae* *S. enterica* ssp. *indica* *S. enterica* ssp. *salamae* *S. subterranea*	Gastroenteritis, enteric fever, osteomyelitis	β-Lactams, fluoroquinolones, chloramphenicol	Salmonella nomenclature is complicated by the existence of two sets of names, both of which have standing in nomenclature. Both sets of names are listed in the table. The first scheme listed is perhaps more helpful for clinicians because it treats the clinically important taxa *S. typhi* (the agent of typhoid fever), *S. paratyphi*, *S. enteritidis*, and *S. typhimurium* as species. In the alternative scheme, these taxa are treated as serovars of *S. enterica* ssp. *enterica* (e.g. *Salmonella enterica* ssp. *enterica* serovar Typhi) although as a form of shorthand the serovars can be written thus: *Salmonella* Typhi, *Salmonella* Paratyphi etc. As yet, *S. subterranea* has not been associated with infection. It should be noted that bacteriologists widely adhere to the practice of writing serotype names in the form of Linnaean binomials (e.g. '*S. virchow*') and that such names do not have standing in nomenclature
Scardovia	*S. inopinata* (*Bifidobacterium inopinatum*)	Dental caries		
Selenomonas	*S. artemidis* *S. dianae* *S. flueggei* *S. infelix* *S. noxia* *S. sputigena*	Bacteraemia, lung abscess	Clindamycin, chloramphenicol, metronidazole	Malignancy and alcohol abuse reported as risk factors for infection
[*Serpulina—see* Brachyspira]				
Serratia	*S. ficaria* *S. fonticola* *S. grimesii* *S. liquefaciens* *S. marcescens* *S. odorifera* *S. plymuthica* *S. proteamaculans* *S. quinivorans* *S. rubidaea*	Septicaemia, abscesses, burn infections, osteomyelitis	Imipenem, aminoglycosides, fluoroquinolones, ureidopenicillins, ceftazidime	Nosocomial outbreaks reported. May be multiresistant. At time of writing a proposal to use the name *S. rubidae* in place of *S. rubidaea* has not been validly published

Genus	Species	Infection	Antibiotics	Comments
Shewanella	S. algae; S. putrefaciens (Alteromonas putrefaciens) (Pseudomonas putrefaciens)	Abdominal sepsis, meningitis, bacteraemia	Ampicillin, cefotaxime, gentamicin, chloramphenicol	Debilitated patients
Shigella	S. boydii; S. dysenteriae; S. flexneri; S. sonnei	Enteric infection	Co-trimoxazole, fluoroquinolones	
Simkania	S. negevensis	Bronchiolitis, pneumonia		
Slackia	S. exigua (Eubacterium exiguum)	Periodontitis		
Sneathia	S. sanguinegens (Leptotrichia sanguinegens = L. microbii)			
Sphingobacterium (Flavobacterium)	S. multivorum; S. spiritivorum; S. thalpophilum	Bacteraemia, pulmonary infection	Co-trimoxazole, chloramphenicol, tetracycline, cephalosporins, quinolones	
[Sphingobacterium mizutae—see Flavobacterium mizutaii]				
Sphingomonas	S. parapaucimobilis; S. paucimobilis (Pseudomonas paucimobilis); S. sanguinis (S. sanguis); S. yanoikuyae	Septicaemia, UTI, wound infections, CAPD peritonitis	Ceftazidime, aminoglycosides	Nosocomial infections
Spirillum	'S. minus'	Rat-bite fever	Penicillin	Streptobacillus moniliformis is also a rat-bite fever agent. The name 'Spirillum minus' does not have standing in nomenclature
Staphylococcus	S. aureus; S. auricularis; S. capitis capitis; S. capitis ureolyticus; S. caprae; S. cohnii cohnii; S. cohnii urealyticus; S. delphini; S. epidermidis; S. equorum; S. gallinarum	Bacteraemia, wound infection, endocarditis, catheter-related sepsis, UTI, toxic shock syndrome, food poisoning, eye infection, osteomyelitis	Glycopeptides, β-lactams, aminoglycosides, tetracycline, macrolides, rifampicin, fluoroquinolones, daptomycin, linezolid, fusidic acid, mupirocin	Staphylococci are surface commensals of humans and animals. S. aureus is also a major pathogen, causing focal and systemic sepsis, toxic shock syndrome, and food poisoning. S. epidermidis infection is often associated with foreign bodies (e.g. catheters and implants).S. saprophyticus causes UTI. S. lugdunensis is a rare cause of endocarditis.S. intermedius, S. hyicus, and others are from animals. Susceptibilities are variable but glycopeptide resistance is as yet rare

(Continued)

Table 6.46.1 (*Cont'd*) A checklist of bacteria associated with infection in humans

Nomenclature		Associated infections	Reported susceptibilities and treatments	Notes
Genus	**Species and subspecies**			
(synonyms, CDC alphanumeric groups)				
	S. haemolyticus			
	S. hominis hominis			
	S. hominis novobiosepticus			
	S. hyicus			
	S. intermedius			
	S. lugdunensis			
	S. pasteuri			
	S. saccharolyticus			
	S. saprophyticus			
	S. schleiferi schleiferi			
	S. schleiferi coagulans			
	S. sciuri			
	S. simulans			
	S. vitulinus (S. pulvereri)			
	S. warneri			
	S. xylosus			
Stenotrophomonas	S. maltophilia (Pseudomonas maltophila) (Xanthomonas maltophila) (Stenotrophomonas africana)	Bacteraemia, meningitis, wound infection, UTI, pneumonia	Fluoroquinolones, chloramphenicol, co-trimoxazole	Resistance to aminoglycosides, penicillins, and carbapenems reported
[Stomatococcus mucilaginosus—see Rothia mucilaginosa]				
Streptobacillus	S. moniliformis	Rat-bite fever, Haverhill fever	Penicillin, erythromycin	'Spirillum minus' is also a causative agent of rat-bite fever
Streptococcus	S. acidominimus	Pneumonia, pericarditis, meningitis	β-Lactams	From cattle
	S. agalactiae	Pharyngitis, bacteraemia, pyogenic infection, necrotizing infection, septic arthritis, UTI, glomerulonephritis, meningitis	β-Lactams, macrolides	S. pyogenes (Lancefield group A), S. agalactiae (group B), and S. dysgalactiae equisimilis (groups C and G) are commensals and pathogens of humans. S. iniae is from fish. Others are from mammals
	S. canis			
	S. dysgalactiae dysgalactiae			
	S. dysgalactiae equisimilis			
	S. equi equi			
	S. equi zooepidemicus			
	S. iniae (S. shiloi)			
	S. porcinus			
	S. pseudoporcinus			
	S. pyogenes			
	S. urinalis			

Genus	Species	Infection	Treatment	Comments
	S. anginosus S. constellatus constellatus S. constellatus pharyngis S. intermedius	Abscesses, bacteraemia, endocarditis, pharyngitis	β-Lactams, macrolides	Often termed 'S. milleri' or microaerophilic streptococci. From human oral flora
	S. equinus (S. bovis) S. gallolyticus ssp. gallolyticus S. gallolyticus ssp. pasteurianus S. infantarius ssp. coli S. infantarius ssp. infantarius S. lutetiensis S. pasteurianus	Endocarditis, CAPD peritonitis	β-Lactams (plus gentamicin for endocarditis)	Intestinal streptococci from animals and humans. Some taxonomic problems relating to this group (the 'bovis' streptococci) await resolution
	S. criceti S. mutans S. ratti S. sobrinus	Dental caries, endocarditis	β-Lactams	From the tooth-surface flora of humans and mammals
	S. cristatus S. gordonii S. massiliensis S. mitis S. oralis S. parasanguinis S. salivarius S. sanguinis S. sinensis S. vestibularis	Bacteraemia, endocarditis, wound infection	β-Lactams, macrolides	Human oral streptococci including taxa sometimes known as the 'viridans streptococci'
	S. pneumoniae S. pseudopneumoniae	Pneumonia, bacteraemia, sinusitis, peritonitis, otitis, conjunctivitis	β-Lactams, macrolides, chloramphenicol	Penicillin resistance locally common
	S. suis	Meningitis	β-Lactams	Associated with pig contact
Streptomyces	S. albus S. anulatus 'S. paraguayensis' S. somaliensis	Actinomycetoma	Dapsone, co-trimoxazole	
	S. bikiniensis S. griseus	Bacteraemia, abscess, pericarditis, endocarditis	Vancomycin, tetracycline, penicillin	Treatment options poorly defined
Succinivibrio	S. dextrinosolvens	Bacteraemia, pneumonia	Penicillin	From faecal and gingival flora
Sutterella	S. wadsworthensis	Appendicitis, peritonitis, abscesses, osteomyelitis	Amoxicillin/clavulanate, ticarcillin/clavulanate, meropenem, ceftriaxone	One-third of isolates reported to be metronidazole resistant
Suttonella	S. indologenes (Kingella indologenes)	Endocarditis, eye infection	Penicillin (plus gentamicin for endocarditis)	
T				
Tannerella	T. forsythensis (T. forsythia, T. forsythus)	Endodontic infection		

[Tatlockiamaceachernii—see Legionella maceachernii]

(Continued)

Table 6.46.1 (Cont'd) A checklist of bacteria associated with infection in humans

Nomenclature		Associated infections	Reported susceptibilities and treatments	Notes
Genus	**Species and subspecies**			
(synonyms, CDC alphanumeric groups)				
[*Tatlockia micdadei*—see *Legionella micdadei*]				
Tatumella	*T. ptyseos*	Bacteraemia, UTI	Ampicillin, tetracycline, chloramphenicol, gentamicin	The significance of isolates from sputum is unclear
Tissierella	*T. praeacuta* (*Bacteroides praeacuta*) (*Clostridium hastiforme*)	Bacteraemia	Metronidazole	
Trabulsiella	*T. guamensis*	Diarrhoea	Co-trimoxazole, gentamicin, chloramphenicol	Role as possible pathogen uncertain
Treponema	*T. amylovorum* *T. denticola* *T. lecithinolyticum* *T. maltophilum* *T. medium* *T. parvum* *T. pectinovorum* *T. putidum* *T. scoliodontum* *T. socranskii* *T. vincentii*			Associated with periodontal disease. Role as potential pathogens unclear
	'*T. carateum*'	Pinta	Penicillin	Name does not have standing in nomenclature
	T. minutum '*T. phagedenis*' '*T. refringens*'			From genital flora. Considered nonpathogenic but have been isolated from genital lesions
	T. pallidum	Syphilis	Penicillin	
	'*T. pallidum endemicum*'			*T. pallidum endemicum*' is the agent of nonvenereal endemic syphilis
	T. pertenue ('*T. pallidum pertenue*')	Yaws	Penicillin	
Tropheryma	*T. whipplei* (*T. whippelii*)	Whipple's disease		Uncultured organism
Tsukamurella	*T. inchonensis* *T. paurometabola* *T. pulmonis* *T. strandjordii* (*T. strandjordae*) *T. tyrosinosolvens*	Septicaemia, cutaneous infections, lung infections	β-Lactam (plus aminoglycoside)	Line-associated infections in debilitated patients. *T. pulmonis* isolated from the sputum of a tuberculosis patient
Turicella	*T. otitidis*	Otitis, cervical abscess	Glycopeptides, β-lactams	
U				
Ureaplasma	*U. parvum* *U. urealyticum*	Urethritis	Tetracycline, erythromycin	

V

Vagococcus	*V. fluvialis*		Ampicillin, vancomycin cefotaxime	Possible role as pathogen poorly defined
Varibaculum	*V. cambriensis*	Abscesses		
Veillonella	*V. atypical* *V. dipsar* *V. montpellierensis* *V. parvula*	Abscesses, bacteraemia	Metronidazole	
Vibrio	*V. alginolyticus*	Wound infection, ear infection	Chloramphenicol, tetracycline	Infection associated with aquatic exposure
	V. cholerae	Cholera	Tetracycline	
	V. cincinnatiensis	Bacteraemia	Moxalactam, chloramphenicol, cephalosporins	Risk factors for infection not defined
[*Vibrio damsela*—see *Photobacterium damselae*]				
	V. fluvialis *V. furnissii* *V. metschnikovii* *V. mimicus* *V. parahaemolyticus*	Diarrhoea, septicaemia	Tetracycline, chloramphenicol	Infection associated with ingestion of contaminated water or shellfish
	V. harveyi (V. carchariae)	Wound infection	Cephalosporins, chloramphenicol, gentamicin	Infection associated with shark bite. May require debridement
[*Vibrio hollisae*—see *Grimontia hollisae*]				
	V. vulnificus	Wound infection, septicaemia, meningitis, endometritis	Tetracycline, penicillins, gentamicin, chloramphenicol	Risk factors include aquatic exposure and penetrating fish injury. May require debridement

W

Wautersiella	*W. falsenii*	Bacteraemia, wound infection		
Weeksella	*W. virosa*	Peritonitis	Imipenem, ampicillin	From vaginal flora
[*Weeksella zoohelcum*—see *Bergeyella zoohelcum*]				
Weissella	*W. confusa*	Endocarditis		
Williamsia	*W. muralis*	Pulmonary infection		
Wohlfahrtiimonas	*W. chitiniclastica*	Bacteraemia	Ceftriaxone	Associated with myiasis
Wolbachia	*W. sp.*	filariasis	doxycycline	Endosymbiont of filarial nematodes
[*Wolinella curva*—see *Campylobacter curvus*]				
[*Wolinella recta*—see *Campylobacter rectus*]				

X

Xanthomonas	*X. campestris*	Bacteraemia		
[*Xenorhabdus luminescens*—see *Photorhabdus luminescens*]				

(*Continued*)

Table 6.46.1 (*Cont'd*) A checklist of bacteria associated with infection in humans

Nomenclature		Associated infections	Reported susceptibilities and treatments	Notes
Genus	**Species and subspecies**			
(synonyms, CDC alphanumeric groups)				
Y				
Yersinia	*Y. aldovae* *Y. bercovieri* *Y. enterocolitica* *Y. frederiksenii* *Y. intermedia* *Y. kristensenii* *Y. mollaretii* *Y. pseudotuberculosis* *Y. rohdei*	Enterocolitis, soft tissue infections, mesenteric lymphadenitis	Tetracycline, chloramphenicol, aminoglycosides, fluoroquinolones, cephalosporins	Medical significance of many *Yersinia* spp. is unclear. Antibiotic treatment is not indicated for uncomplicated enteric infection
	Y. pestis	Plague	Streptomycin, tetracycline	
Yokenella	*Y. regensburgei* (*Koserella trabulsii*)	Bacteraemia, wound infection	Aminoglycosides, chloramphenicol	

CAPD, continual ambulatory peritoneal dialysis; sp. species; ssp. subspecies; UTI, urinary tract infection.

7

Fungi (mycoses)

Contents

7.1 Fungal infections

Roderick J. Hay

Essentials

The mycoses are disorders caused by fungi, which are saprophytic or parasitic organisms found in every continent and environment. Many are common commensals in nature, but others cause agricultural disease. The mycoses that are human infections include diseases ranging from those that are worldwide and common, such as dermatophytosis and candida infections, to those that are rare and often potentially life threatening, e.g. histoplasmosis. In humans, fungi usually adopt one of two morphologies: (1) the yeast form—where individual cells produce daughter cells by a process of budding and subsequently separate; or (2) the hyphal form—where cells do not separate but multiply to produce chains of cells joined end to end.

Diagnosis

Mycological diagnosis is often complex because many fungi are also commensals or transiently carried in humans, hence it is necessary to show both that the organisms are present and that they are causing disease, which is particularly difficult in the context of opportunistic fungal infection. The main laboratory diagnostic tests involve (1) visualization of fungi in tissue—by direct microscopy or histopathology; (2) culture—often using a glucose peptone agar (Sabouraud's agar); (3) detection of antibody, fungal antigens, or DNA—assimilation of genetic tests such as PCR-based methods into routine diagnosis has been slow, and they are offered by few laboratories.

Superficial infections

Superficial fungal infections may reach prevalence rates of 15 to 25% in some communities, with the common infections being dermatophytosis or ringworm, pityriasis versicolor, and superficial candidiasis.

Dermatophytoses—otherwise known as tinea infections—commonly affect the feet (tinea pedis), the body (tinea corporis), the scalp (tinea capitis) and the finger and toe nails (onychomycosis). They occur in all climates and usually present in primary care as scaly rashes. Diagnosis is made by direct microscopy of skin scales mounted in potassium hydroxide (20%) to demonstrate hyphae, and by culture.

Pityriasis versicolor—caused by a skin surface commensal, *Malassezia globosa*, and often triggered by sun exposure. Presentation is with hypo– or hyperpigmented scaling on the trunk. Laboratory diagnosis (if required) is by demonstration of the yeasts and hyphae in skin scales removed by scraping.

Superficial candidiasis—these infections affect the mouth, vagina, and body folds, often in the context of some form of predisposition, e.g. recent antibiotic therapy or, in the case or severe oral infection, immunosuppression including that associated with HIV/AIDS. Infections are diagnosed by microscopy and culture, the latter being particularly important where non-*albicans Candida* species may be involved.

Treatment—the main treatments for superficial mycoses are topical agents that include imidazole preparations (e.g. ketoconazole, clotrimazole), but for widespread infections or those involving hair or nails, oral imidazoles (e.g. itraconazole, fluconazole) or the allylamine, terbinafine, are employed.

Subcutaneous mycoses

Subcutaneous fungal infections, e.g. mycetoma (Madura foot), chromoblastomycosis and sporotrichosis, are not common and usually restricted to the tropics and subtropics. They may present in immigrants from tropical areas, sometimes years after the person has left the tropics, and hence cause diagnostic confusion. Diagnosis is by histological examination of affected tissues or culture. Treatment is often difficult, with only partial responses being achieved, but oral imidazole drugs or terbinafine are helpful in some cases.

Systemic mycoses

Systemic mycoses are deep and often disseminated infections that involve many different sites, including the blood and bone marrow. They may be caused by organisms which invade normal hosts (endemic mycoses) and those which only cause disease in compromised patients (opportunistic mycoses).

Endemic mycoses—these include histoplasmosis, coccidioidomycosis (see Chapter 7.3) and infections due to *Penicillium marneffei* (see Chapter 7.6), all of which may occur in healthy people, although many are also common complications of HIV/AIDS. Initial manifestations are as respiratory infections, but they can spread haematogenously to other sites, e.g. skin, liver, and brain. Diagnosis is made on culture or biopsy of affected areas.

Opportunistic mycoses—these occur in those who are immunocompromised, e.g. patients with neutropenia secondary to cancer. The routes of fungal entry into the body are very variable, e.g. skin, gastrointestinal tract, lung. Infections include systemic candidiasis, aspergillosis, and zygomycosis, but in severely compromised patients, e.g. those with profound neutropenia, many organisms not usually associated with human disease can cause invasive infections, e.g. *Fusarium* species. *Cryptococcus neoformans*, a yeast that can invade the lungs, often presents with meningitis or other signs of intracranial infection.

Prognosis and treatment—the endemic mycoses are often fatal if untreated, and even with treatment the mortality of opportunistic fungal infection can be high, e.g. over 40% for the severely neutropenic patient with aspergillosis. Aside from supportive care, oral or parenteral agents such as amphotericin B, fluconazole, itraconazole, voriconazole, posaconazole, and caspofungin are the treatments of choice, but detecting the organisms and successfully treating the infections remains a challenge.

Introduction

Fungi are saprophytic or parasitic organisms that are normally assigned to a distinct kingdom. As eukaryotes, they have the complex subcellular organization and highly organized genetic material seen in both animal and plant cells. The cell wall is a distinctive feature of fungi and has a complex cytoskeleton based on mannan, glucan, or chitin subunits. The arrangement and reproduction of individual cells is also characteristic. Most fungi form new cells terminally, which remain connected to form long, branching filaments or hyphae (the mould fungi). Some reproduce in a similar manner but each new cell separates from the parent by a process of budding (the yeast fungi). It is a feature of certain fungi to be yeast-like during one phase of their life history but hyphal at another, a phenomenon known as dimorphism. In culture, mould fungi usually form a cottony growth on laboratory media while yeasts normally have a smooth, shiny appearance.

Fungi adversely affect humans in a number of ways. They cause disease indirectly by spoilage and destruction of food crops, with subsequent malnutrition and starvation. Many of the common moulds produce and release spores, which may act as airborne allergens to produce asthma or hypersensitivity pneumonitis. Fungi elaborate complex metabolic by-products, some of which are useful to humans, such as the penicillins. However, others are toxic. Disease caused by the ingestion of fungal toxins includes both poisoning by eating certain mushrooms (mycetism) and damage caused by the ingestion of minute quantities of toxin (mycotoxicosis), e.g. in contaminated grain. The contribution of the latter mechanism to human disease remains largely unexplored, as does the question of whether inhalation of toxic fungal spores may cause pathology. Finally, fungi may invade human tissue. Medical mycology is largely concerned with this last group. Invasive fungal diseases are normally divided into three groups: the superficial, subcutaneous, and deep mycoses. In superficial infections, such as ringworm or thrush, fungi are confined to the skin and mucous membranes. Extension deeper than the surface epithelium is rare. Subcutaneous infections are usually tropical: the main site of involvement is within subcutaneous tissue, although secondary invasion of adjacent structures such as bone or skin may occur. In deep or systemic infections, deep organs such as the lung, spleen, or brain are invaded. This classification of mycoses is based on the main 'sphere of involvement' by the causal organisms, but there are exceptions. For instance, brain involvement has been recorded in patients with chromoblastomycosis, which is normally a subcutaneous infection.

The fungi causing systemic mycoses are often classified in two groups: the opportunists and the endemic pathogens. The former cause disease in overtly compromised individuals. These contrast with the true pathogens, which cause infection in all subjects inhaling airborne spores.

Superficial fungal infections

The main superficial mycoses are the dermatophyte infections, superficial candidiasis, and tinea versicolor (see Oxford Textbook of Medicine 5e Section 23). These are both common and widespread. Rare superficial infections include tinea nigra, and black or white piedra.

Dermatophyte infections (dermatophytoses)

Aetiology

The dermatophyte or ringworm infections are caused by a group of organisms capable of existing in keratinized tissue such as stratum corneum, nail, or hair. The mechanism of invasion is thought to be linked to production of extracellular enzymes; three distinct metalloproteinase genes are found in *Microsporum canis*.

Epidemiology

Some dermatophyte fungi have a worldwide distribution; others are more restricted. The most common and most widely distributed is *Trichophyton rubrum*, which causes different types of infection in different parts of the world. It is commonly associated with athlete's foot (tinea pedis) in temperate areas as well as tinea corporis or tinea cruris in the tropics. This distinction is not based solely on climatic factors, as immigrants from tropical countries, particularly eastern Asia, may still have tinea corporis caused by *T. rubrum* when living in northern Europe. Certain dermatophytes are limited to defined areas. For instance, tinea imbricata caused by *T. concentricum*, is found in hot, humid areas of the eastern Asia, Polynesia, and South America. Scalp ringworm tends to occur in well-defined endemic areas in Africa and elsewhere. In different regions, different species of dermatophytes may predominate. Thus, in North Africa, the most common cause of tinea capitis is *T. violaceum*; in southern parts of the continent, the major agents may be *Microsporum audouinii*, *M. ferrugineum*, and *T. soudanense*. Not all dermatophyte infections are endemic and dominant species may disappear to be replaced by others. *M. audouinii*, once endemic and common in the United Kingdom, is now infrequent but associated with infections in African Caribbean children. By contrast, *T tonsurans* is now established as a major cause of tinea capitis in urban areas in the United Kingdom, parts of Europe, and the United States of America. Dermatophytes may be passed from person to person (anthropophilic infections), from animal to person (zoophilic), or from soil to person (geophilic). Sources of zoophilic organisms in Europe include cats and dogs, cattle, hedgehogs, and small rodents. Rarer sources include horses, monkeys, and chickens. Lesions produced by zoophilic species may be highly inflammatory.

Factors governing the invasion of stratum corneum are largely unknown, but heat, humidity, and occlusion have all been implicated. Susceptibility to certain infection, such as tinea imbricata, may be genetically determined.

Clinical features

The clinical features of dermatophyte infections are best considered in relation to the site involved. Often the term tinea, followed by the Latin name of the appropriate part (such as *corporis*, meaning 'body') is used to describe the clinical site of infection.

Tinea pedis

Scaling or maceration between the toes, particularly in the fourth interspace, is the most common form of dermatophytosis seen in temperate countries. Itching is variable, but may be severe. Sometimes blisters may form both between the toes and on the soles of the feet. The causative organisms are commonly *T. rubrum* and *T. interdigitale*, the latter being responsible for the vesicular forms. Similar appearances can be caused by *Candida albicans* and in the bacterial infection, erythrasma. Gram-negative bacterial infection causes erosive interdigital disease associated with discomfort.

'Dry type' infections of the soles and palms

These are normally caused by *T. rubrum*. Palms (Fig. 7.1.1) or soles have a dry, scaly appearance, which in the soles may encroach on to the lateral or dorsal surfaces of the foot. The palmar involvement is often unilateral, an important diagnostic feature. Nail invasion is often seen (see below). Itching is not prominent, and infections are usually chronic.

Tinea cruris

Infections of the groin, most often caused by *T. rubrum* or *Epidermophyton floccosum*, are relatively common. They occur in

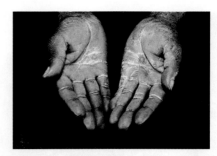

Fig. 7.1.1 Palmar scaling due to *Trichophyton rubrum*.

both tropical and temperate climates, although in the former the infection may spread to involve the whole waist area in both males and females. Tinea cruris in females is uncommon in Europe. An erythematous and scaly rash with a distinct margin extends from the groin to the upper thighs or scrotum. Itching may be severe. Coincident tinea pedis is common, and patients should be examined for this. The rash of crural erythrasma shows uniform scaling without a margin, whereas in candidiasis, satellite pustules occur distal to the rim.

Onychomycosis (caused by dermatophytes)

Invasion of the nail plate is most often seen with *T. rubrum* infections. The plate is invaded distally and becomes thickened and friable with terminal loss of the nail plate. Onycholysis may be seen. More rarely, and most often with *T. interdigitale*, the dorsal surface of the plate is invaded, causing superficial white onychomycosis.

Tinea corporis (body ringworm)

Dermatophyte or ringworm infection on the trunk or limbs may produce the characteristic annular plaque with a raised edge and central clearing (Fig. 7.1.2). Scaling and itching is variable. Lesions caused by zoophilic organisms may be highly inflammatory and in certain cases, particularly those caused by *T. verrucosum*, intense itching, oedema, and pustule formation (kerion) may develop. This reaction is seldom secondarily infected by bacteria but is a response to the fungus on hairy skin. Infections of the beard, tinea barbae, are often highly refractory to treatment. Facial dermatophyte infections may mimic a variety of nonfungal skin diseases, including acne, rosacea, and discoid lupus erythematosus. However, the underlying annular configuration can usually be distinguished. The term tinea incognito is used to describe such atypical lesions.

Tinea capitis (scalp ringworm)

In the United Kingdom as in the United States of America, the most common cause of scalp ringworm is *T. tonsurans*, an anthropophilic fungus which mainly occurs in inner cities, particularly in

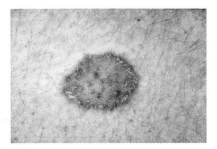

Fig. 7.1.2 Tinea corporis due to *Microsporum gypseum*.

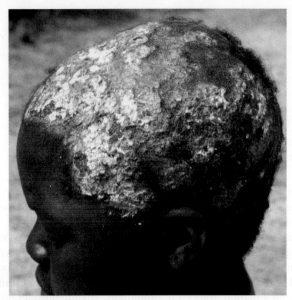

Fig. 7.1.3 Advanced favus of scalp in a Nigerian cattle herd caused by *Trichophyton schoenleinii*.
(Copyright D A Warrell.)

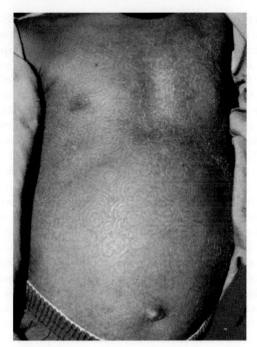

Fig. 7.1.4 Tinea imbricata, Papua New Guinea.
(Courtesy of Dr B Hudson, Sydney.)

black Caribbean or African children. This has now replaced *Microsporum canis*, originating from an infected cat or dog, although this dermatophyte is dominant elsewhere in the United Kingdom and Europe. Scalp ringworm is mainly a disease of childhood, but infections may occur in adult women. Spontaneous clearance at puberty is the rule. *M. canis* causes an 'ectothrix' infection where spores form on the outside of the hair shaft and the scalp hair breaks above the skin surface. Scaling, itching, and loss of hair occur. Other causes of ectothrix infection include *M. audouinii*, which is becoming more common in Europe, and is still seen in West Africa. This infection can be spread from child to child and causes serious social handicap. The infection may occur in epidemic form, particularly in schools. By contrast, infections with *M. canis* are acquired from a primary animal source rather than by spread from human lesions. In endothrix infections where sporulation is within the hair shaft, scaling is less pronounced and hairs break at scalp level (black dot ringworm). Examples include *T. tonsurans* and *T. violaceum*, the latter being most prevalent in the Middle East, parts of Africa, and India, although it also is being recognized with increasing frequency in Europe.

Favus, now most often seen in isolated foci in the tropics, is a particularly chronic form of ringworm caused by *T. schoenleinii* or *T. violaceum* where hair shafts become surrounded by a necrotic crust or scutulum (Fig. 7.1.3). Individual crusts coalesce to form a pale, unpleasant-smelling mat over parts of the scalp. Such infections may cause extensive and permanent hair loss.

Tinea imbricata (tokelau)

This infection is endemic in parts of eastern Asia, West Pacific, and Central and South America, and is caused by *T. concentricum*. In many cases the trunk is covered with scales laid down in concentric rings producing a ripple effect (Fig. 7.1.4). Alternatively, large, loose scales may form (hence the name; *imbricata* is the Latin word for 'tiled'). The infection is often chronic, and may constitute a serious social handicap. There is some evidence that susceptibility of this disease in Papua New Guinea may be inherited as an autosomal recessive trait.

Infection in HIV and immunocompromised patients

While dermatophyte infections are no more common in the immunocompromised patient, they may differ clinically. In patients with HIV infections there may be (1) more tinea facei, (2) more widespread and atypical skin lesions, and (3) a distinct pattern of nail infection characterized by white discoloration spreading rapidly through the nail plate from the proximal nail fold.

Laboratory diagnosis

The mainstays of diagnosis are direct microscopy of skin scales mounted in potassium hydroxide (20%) to demonstrate hyphae, and culture. Scalp hairs may also be examined in a similar way, and the site of arthrospore formation, inside or outside the shaft, determined. Fluorescent whitening agents (Calcofluor) or chlorazol black stain have been used to highlight fungi in scales. Further tests, such as the ability to penetrate hair, may be used to separate similar cultures. Identification of organisms is important, as it will indicate the source of infection in scalp ringworm, for example. When large numbers of children are involved, screening of scalp infections with a filtered ultraviolet lamp (Wood's light) is useful. Certain species, including *M. canis* and *M. audouinii*, cause infected hair to fluoresce with a vivid greenish light. Scalps can also be screened for infection by passing a sterile brush or scalp massager through the hair and plating this directly on to an agar plate.

Treatment

The treatment of dermatophyte infections depends to an extent on the nature and severity of infection. Topical therapy is reserved for circumscribed infections such as athlete's foot and tinea corporis, not involving hair or nail keratin. Scalp and nail infections, severe or widespread ringworm, and failures of topical therapy are usually treated orally with griseofulvin, itraconazole, or terbinafine.

Specific antifungal drugs in topical form are effective and well tolerated. The important compounds in this group are miconazole, clotrimazole, ketoconazole, and econazole, which are imidazole derivatives, undecenoic acid, and tolnaftate and the allylamine, terbinafine. Generally treatment is given for 7 to 30 days. They are all very similar in their clinical efficacy, but topical terbinafine is particularly rapid in foot infection (≤7 days). Adverse reactions are rare.

For oral therapy the main alternatives are terbinafine, itraconazole, or fluconazole. Terbinafine (250 mg/day) is rapidly effective in most forms of dermatophytosis that require oral therapy and also produces rapid responses in toe nail (12 weeks) and sole infections (2 to 4 weeks), without a high rate of relapse. Side effects include headache and nausea, but loss of taste may also occur. Itraconazole is somewhat similar in its profile, but is given intermittently (200 mg twice daily for 7 days). This course is given once for sole infections but repeated three times at monthly intervals for toe nail infections, as pulsed therapy. Side effects include nausea and abdominal discomfort. Fluconazole is also active and is given in a dose of 150 mg weekly; 300 mg may be necessary for toe nail infections. This side effect profile is similar to itraconazole. All three drugs are extremely rare causes of hepatic toxicity. Griseofulvin is still used for tinea capitis in a dose of 10 to 20 mg/kg daily. Treatment should be continued for at least 6 weeks in tinea capitis. Side effects are not common, but include headache, nausea, and urticaria. The drug can also precipitate acute intermittent porphyria and systemic lupus erythematosus in predisposed subjects.

Scytalidium infections

The organisms *Scytalidium dimidiatum* (*Hendersonula toruloidea*) and *S hyalinum*, can cause a superficial scaly condition that resembles the 'dry type' of dermatophyte infection on the palms or soles. Nail plate destruction may also occur, the lateral border of the nail being the initial site of invasion. The disease has been seen in Europe, almost invariably in immigrants from the tropics, particularly the Caribbean, West Africa, India, or Pakistan. Its prevalence in the tropics is unknown, although in some surveys it has been shown to be relatively common. In skin scrapings the tortuous hyphae may resemble those of a dermatophyte, but the organisms do not grow on media containing cycloheximide, which is often incorporated into agar for routine dermatophyte isolation.

Treatment is difficult, but some improvement may follow the use of keratolytic compounds such as salicylic acid. Nail infections do not respond to terbinafine, griseofulvin, or azoles.

Miscellaneous nail infections

Occasionally, fungi other than dermatophytes or *Scytalidium* species are isolated from dystrophic nails. These include *Scopulariopsis brevicaulis*, *Onychocola canadensis*, acremonium, and fusarium species, and certain types of aspergillus. These infections are usually seen in elderly or immunosuppressed individuals. It is often difficult, particularly with aspergillus species, to establish that the organism is playing a pathogenic role.

Pityriasis versicolor (tinea versicolor)
Aetiology
Pityriasis versicolor is a superficial infection caused by *Malassezia* species, usually *M. globosa*. Although most common in tropical countries, it has a worldwide distribution. Dermal penetration does not occur.

There are six species of malassezia that can be found on normal skin, the commonest of which are *M. sympodialis* and *M. globosa*. In pityriasis versicolor there is transformation of yeast cells to produce hyphae. It is likely that the state of host immunity plays some part in pathogenesis and depression; for instance, endogenous or exogenous corticosteroids potentiate the disease in some individuals. However, it is also commonly seen in normal individuals, and climatic factors or sun exposure are believed to trigger the infection in many cases. There is no effective animal model for studies of this disease.

Epidemiology
Pityriasis versicolor is very common in the tropics, where it may be widespread on the body. Its incidence in temperate climates has increased over the last 20 to 30 years. It is not more common in HIV-infected individuals.

Clinical features
The rash of pityriasis versicolor is asymptomatic or mildly pruritic. Its presents with scaling, confluent macules on the trunk, upper arms, or neck. These may be hypopigmented or hyperpigmented. In some people and in the tropics, other areas including face, forearms, and thighs may be involved.

The diagnosis is rarely confused with other complaints, although eczema or ringworm infections are sometimes considered. Patients are often anxious to exclude leprosy, but the two are unlikely to be mistaken. In vitiligo, depigmentation is complete and there is no scaling.

Laboratory diagnosis
The diagnosis is made by demonstration of the yeasts and hyphae of malassezia in skin scales removed by scraping. Culture is difficult and unnecessary.

Treatment
Topical ketoconazole, miconazole, clotrimazole, or econazole is effective. Oral itraconazole may be used in recalcitrant cases. Whatever the treatment, relapse is common.

Other malassezia-associated conditions
Malassezia yeasts have been implicated in the pathogenesis of a number of other skin diseases such as seborrhoeic dermatitis and a form of itchy folliculitis, malassezia folliculitis. The evidence connecting seborrhoeic dermatitis, one of the most common of skin diseases, and malassezia is largely concerned with the response of antifungal drugs and the observation that improvements in the rash mirror disappearance of organisms from the skin. Severity of the skin condition does not appear to reflect the numbers of yeasts on the skin surface.

Superficial candidiasis
Aetiology
Superficial candidiasis is a term used to describe a group of infections of skin or mucous membranes caused by species of the genus *Candida*. They range in severity from oral thrush to chronic mucocutaneous candidiasis, a chronic infection refractory to conventional antifungal treatment.

Candida albicans is the species most frequently involved. It is a saprophytic yeast often found as a commensal in the mouth

---

Box 7.1.1 Predisposing factors in superficial candidiasis

♦ Local epithelial defects, occlusion, constant immersion in water, e.g. damaged nail folds, beneath dentures

♦ Defects of immunity (primarily T cell or phagocytosis)
  • Primary immunological disease, e.g. chronic granulomatous disease
  • Immunodefects secondary to intercurrent illness, e.g. leukaemia
  • Immunodefects secondary to therapy, e.g. cytotoxic therapy in organ transplantation

♦ Drug therapy, e.g. antibiotics

♦ Carcinoma or leukaemia

♦ Endocrine disease
  • Diabetes mellitus
  • Hypothyroidism, hypoparathyroidism, hypoadrenalism (all in chronic mucocutaneous candidiasis)

♦ Physiological changes, e.g. infancy, pregnancy, old age

♦ Miscellaneous disorders, e.g.
  • Iron deficiency
  • Zinc deficiency
  • Malabsorption

---

and gastrointestinal tract, and is commonly present in the vagina. Several factors may influence the incidence of carriage. For instance, oral colonization is more common in hospital staff than in equivalent nonhospital employees. Vaginal carriage is more common in pregnancy. Other factors (Box 7.1.1) are known that predispose to conversion from a commensal to a parasitic role with the causation of disease—candidiasis. The list includes factors that influence host immunological response, such as carcinoma, AIDS, or cytotoxic therapy; those that disturb the population of other microorganisms, such as antibiotics; and those that affect the character of the epithelium, such as dentures.

Other species of *Candida* may also cause superficial infections, but are less common. They include *C. glabrata*, *C. dubliniensis*, and *C. parapsilosis*. There is evidence that the first two species are more common in oral infection in patients with HIV and *C. glabrata* in vaginal candidiasis.

Epidemiology
Superficial candida infections are seen in all countries.

Clinical features
There are a number of clinically distinct types of superficial infection caused by candida species, as follows.

Oral candidiasis (thrush)
Oral infection by candida is fairly common, particularly in infancy and old age, or in association with antibiotic or cytotoxic therapy, or in diseases where the neutrophil or T-lymphocyte responses may be impaired. In older people, the wearing of dentures is a predisposing factor. The lesions present with discomfort both in the mouth and at the corners of the lips. The mouth and buccal mucosa show patchy or confluent, white adherent plaques; less commonly the mucosa and tongue are sore and glazed—erythematous candidiasis. Angular cheilitis usually accompanies the oral lesions. In long-standing cases, the plaque may become hypertrophic, with oedema of the mucosal surfaces, or the mucosa may appear glazed and raw.

There is a significant correlation between leucoplakia and oral candidiasis, and it has been suggested that the infection may lead to epithelial dysplasia.

The diagnosis is made by the demonstration of yeasts and hyphae of candida in smears, and by culture.

Vaginal candidiasis (thrush)
See Oxford Textbook of Medicine 5e Chapter 8.4 for further detail.

Paronychia
Infection around the nail fold is seen in people whose occupations involve frequent wetting of the hands (such as cooks) or in those with eczema or psoriasis. The aetiology is complicated and there may be a mixture of bacterial infection and irritant or allergic contact dermatitis as well as candida infection. The condition presents with painful, red swelling of the nail fold. Pus may be discharged. Secondary invasion of the lateral border of the nail plate by candida may occur from this site.

Candida intertrigo
Infection of the moist folds of the skin in the groin or under the breasts causes itching and discomfort. The area becomes macerated and erythematous. Candida may contribute to this condition, but is certainly not the only factor. It may also superinfect the napkin area in infants. The presence of satellite pustules (see above) is a useful indicator of involvement by candida in the disease process.

Direct invasion of toe-web folds by candida closely resembles 'athlete's foot' caused by dermatophytes. A similar erosive infection may occur in the finger webs—interdigital candidiasis—and is seen most commonly in the tropics.

Chronic superficial candidiasis
Chronic candida infections of the mouth, vagina, and nail present problems in management. Chronic oral candidiasis, for instance, is associated with leucoplakia. Predisposing causes should be searched for. The most serious of this group of infections is chronic mucocutaneous candidiasis, a rare condition in which chronic skin, nail, and mucosal infection coexist (Fig. 7.1.5). A series of underlying genetic, endocrine (hypoparathyroidism, hypoadrenalism, or hypothyroidism), and immunological abnormalities has been found; in some cases it has been associated with mutations in an

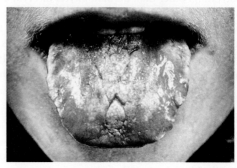

Fig. 7.1.5 Oral candidiasis in a patient with chronic mucocutaneous candidiasis.

autoimmune regulator gene (*AIRE*). Extensive human papillomavirus (wart) or dermatophyte infections may also be present in these patients, whose condition is normally diagnosed in childhood.

Oral candidiasis is one of the earliest signs of untreated AIDS, occurring in a high proportion of patients. The appearances are similar to those seen with other groups, although plaque formation may be very extensive. Oesophageal infection is common in this group.

Laboratory diagnosis

All these infections are diagnosed by microscopy and culture. When associated with the condition, candida cells are always evident on microscopy. Culture establishes the specific identity and is important particularly where species other than *Candida albicans* may be involved.

Treatment

Two groups of drugs are effective in superficial candidiasis. The polyenes such as nystatin and amphotericin B are topically active in many forms of candidiasis. They are often less effective in oral candidiasis in immunodeficient patients, including those with AIDS. Likewise, topical azole drugs such as miconazole and clotrimazole are usually effective in superficial candidiasis. For unresponsive cases, oral therapy with fluconazole and itraconazole may be necessary. Fluconazole resistance can occur and *C. glabrata* is seldom responsive to this drug.

For vaginal infections, topical creams or vaginal preparations should be used—many requiring only a single treatment. Single-dose oral fluconazole is an alternative. In recalcitrant cases it may be necessary to use longer courses of fluconazole or itraconazole.

Miscellaneous superficial mycoses

There are a number of relatively rare, superficial fungal infections such as tinea nigra, and black or white piedra. They never cause invasive disease, and are mainly confined to the tropics.

Tinea nigra

Tinea nigra is a superficial infection confined to the epidermis of the palms or soles, and more rarely elsewhere. The initial lesion is a dark macule without scaling, which resembles a brown stain on the skin and spreads slowly over the palmar or plantar surface. The disease is normally asymptomatic.

On scraping the skin, brown pigmented hyphae can be seen by direct microscopy, and the causative organism, *Phaeoanellomyces werneckii*, isolated. The lesions respond to Whitfield's ointment.

Black piedra

Black piedra is a disease of the tropics in which small, dark nodules form on hair shafts in the scalp or, less commonly, elsewhere. There are no symptoms. Each nodule consists of a dense mat of hyphae containing the sexual spores (ascospores) of the fungus.

The diagnosis is made by direct microscopy of infected hair, and the isolation of *Piedraia hortae*. Treatment using a 1% azole solution or amphotericin B lotion is usually effective.

White piedra

White piedra occurs in both temperate and tropical climates, and is rare. It produces pale nodules on the hair of the beard, groin, or scalp. The hair shaft may fracture. The nodule consists of hyphae, arthrospores (spores formed by fragmentation of hyphae), and blastospores (budding yeast cells). The organism *Trichosporon*

species can be readily cultured. The treatment is similar to that for black piedra.

Subcutaneous mycoses

Subcutaneous infections caused by fungi are rare, and are mainly seen in the tropics. The organisms gain entry via the skin; in mycetoma, organisms may be implanted subcutaneously via a thorn. The majority of the causative organisms in this group of infections can be isolated from vegetation or soil. Involvement of deep viscera is rare. Attempts to establish experimental infections that resemble the human diseases have been largely unsuccessful. A clearer understanding of the pathogenesis therefore awaits such a model system. These infections tend to be chronic, chemotherapy may be lengthy, and in the case of mycetoma, often unsuccessful.

Mycetoma (Madura foot)

Aetiology

Mycetoma is a chronic infection involving subcutaneous tissue, bone, and skin, in which colonies of infecting fungi or actinomycetes (grains) are found within a network of burrowing abscesses and sinuses (Fig. 7.1.6).

The more common organisms that cause mycetoma are listed in Box 7.1.2. The organisms are divided into two groups, the actinomycetomas and the eumycetomas, caused by actinomycetes and fungi, respectively. The size and colour of the grains (red, pale, or dark) are important clues to their identification. The organisms can be found in the natural environment such as soil, and some have even been identified in association with acacia thorns in an endemic area. The infection is initiated when an infected thorn is implanted in deep tissue. However, many years may elapse before the formation of a clinically apparent mycetoma.

Epidemiology

The disease is seen primarily in the tropics, although rare cases, apart from imported ones, may occur in temperate areas. Countries with the most reported cases include India, Mexico, Senegal, Sudan, and Venezuela. However, the disease is widely distributed in the tropics, particularly in Africa to the south and east of the Sahara Desert.

The pattern of prevalence of infections caused by certain organisms differs strikingly in different parts of the world. For instance, *Streptomyces somaliensis* is most common in the Sudan and Middle East, but *Madurella grisea* is mainly found in the New World. Altogether about 60% of reported infections are caused by

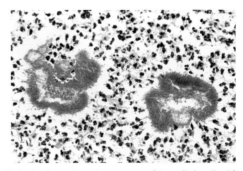

Fig. 7.1.6 Grains in abscess in actinomycetoma (*Nocardia brasilensis*) (haematoxylin and eosin stain).

Box 7.1.2   Causes of mycetoma

♦ Fungi, e.g.
  • *Madurella mycetomatis*
  • *Madurella grisea*
  • *Scedosporium apiospermum*
  • *Exophiala jeanselmei*
  • *Leptosphaeria senegalensis*
  • *Species of Acremonium, Aspergillus, Fusarium*
♦ Actinomycetes, e.g.
  • *Nocardia brasiliensis*
  • *Actinomadura madurae*
  • *Actinomadura pelletieri*
  • *Streptomyces somaliensis*

---

actinomycetes, of which *Nocardia brasiliensis* is the most common (Chapter 6.30).

Clinical features

Early mycetomas may present with a circumscribed area of hard painless subcutaneous swelling (Fig. 7.1.7). Later, sinus tracts open on to the skin surface and visible grains may be discharged, along with serosanguinous fluid (Fig. 7.1.8). Bone erosion and destruction, leading to deformity, may occur. However, severe pain is rarely a problem. Local lymph node invasion may occur, but more widespread involvement is very rare.

Feet and lower legs are the areas most commonly involved, but the arms, buttocks, chest, and head may all be sites of infection. Mycetoma caused by *N. brasiliensis* may occur in any site, but one favoured area is the chest wall.

The radiological features of mycetoma are cortical erosion, followed by the development of lytic deposits in bone. Periosteal proliferation and destruction, leading to deformity, may follow. MRI provides a clearer picture of bone involvement and may be positive earlier than radiography.

Laboratory diagnosis

The diagnosis is made by the demonstration and identification of grains obtained from the sinus openings by gentle pressure or curettage. If these measures are not successful, tissue should be obtained by deep surgical biopsy. Grains can be mounted in potassium hydroxide and examined microscopically. Those containing

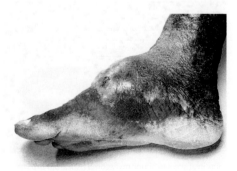

Fig. 7.1.7 A mycetoma caused by *Madurella grisea*.

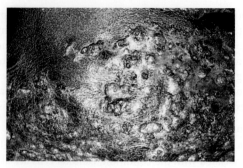

Fig. 7.1.8 *Nocardia brasiliensis* actinomycetoma draining sinus.

filaments 3 to 4 μm or more in diameter are caused by true fungi (eumycetomas), and those with filaments of less than 1 μm by actinomycetes (actinomycetomas). These features can usually be distinguished by direct microscopy.

The morphology of grains fixed, sectioned, and stained with haematoxylin and eosin is typical. Special stains are less helpful. Grains can be used for culture, although several attempts at isolation may have to be made. Serology (such as immunodiffusion) can also be helpful, although the tests are not widely available.

Treatment

Actinomycetomas may respond to sulphones such as dapsone (50-100 mg daily) or sulphonamides such as sulphadiazine. The treatment of choice for many is long-term co-trimoxazole (2-3 tablets twice daily) with an initial 2 to 3 months of streptomycin or rifampicin. Treatment may have to be continued for many months or years. Dapsone is an effective and cheaper alternative to co-trimoxazole. Extensive actinomycetomas may respond poorly and additional treatment with amikacin or fucidin may be necessary. The eumycetomas seldom respond to antifungal therapy. About 20% of *Madurella mycetomatis* infections respond to ketoconazole. In other infections griseofulvin, amphotericin B, voriconazole, ketoconazole, and itraconazole have rarely produced remission or cure. A trial of therapy may be attempted, where the patient can be monitored closely in outpatient departments. Otherwise, radical surgery or amputation is usually necessary. Small, local excisions are rarely successful.

Mycetoma is slowly progressive and increasingly disabling. However, wider dissemination is very rare, and therefore cases are seldom fatal, except where the skull is involved. However, the deformity caused by the disease may be severely disabling.

Chromoblastomycosis (chromomycosis)

Aetiology

Chromoblastomycosis, one of the intermediate subcutaneous mycoses, is a chronic granulomatous fungal infection characterized histologically by the presence of brown, spherical fungal cells known as sclerotic cells or fumagoid bodies. In most cases, the lesions are confined to the skin and subcutaneous tissues. In the past there has been great confusion over nomenclature of the aetiological agents of chromoblastomycosis. At present, five agents assigned to four genera are recognized as causing chromoblastomycosis – most are due to the first two. They are:

♦ *Fonsecaea pedrosoi*, which occurs in high-rainfall areas and is found worldwide

♦ *Cladophialophora carrionii*, the sole cause of chromoblastomycosis in arid areas

- *Phialophora verrucosa*, the first agent to be described
- *Fonsecaea compactum*, an uncommon cause and isolated only a few times
- *Rhinocladiella aquaspersa*, a rare cause.

Sporadic cases caused by other dematiaceous fungi such as *Cladosporium trichoides* and *Taeniolella boppii* have been reported from Uganda and Brazil.

Epidemiology

The principal endemic areas for chromoblastomycosis are tropical and subtropical countries including Central and South America, Costa Rica, Africa, Japan, Australia, Madagascar, and Indonesia. Curiously, sporadic cases have been reported from Finland and Russia.

Although soil itself does not seem to be a particularly good substrate, the various agents of chromoblastomycosis occur as saprobic fungi in the environment and have been isolated from soil, decaying vegetation and rotting wood. Strains of *F. pedrosoi* and *P. verrucosa* have been isolated from the atmosphere but proved less virulent than those isolated from human lesions or organic material.

Infection occurs as a result of trauma, however minor, the fungi gaining entrance through a cut, abrasion, or thorn prick. Farmers and labourers in agricultural areas are most likely to be exposed to contaminated material. Although lesions on exposed areas may be accounted for in this way, it was suggested by Wilson in 1958 that lesions on nonexposed areas may result from a previously unrecognized pulmonary focus. Bacquero later demonstrated the presence of *F. pedrosoi* in bronchial washings and subsequently proved their pathogenicity by inoculating those strains into normal skin of human volunteers and recovering the fungus from the ensuing skin lesions. Other methods of transmission have included metal particles from automobiles, and acupuncture. Person-to-person and animal-to-human transmission have not so far been reported. Chromoblastomycosis has rarely been reported in children, and it may be that factors other than trauma and exposure to contaminated material are necessary for its development.

Pathogenesis

Host resistance and virulence of the organism are the two main factors associated with the pathogenesis of this disease. Chromoblastomycosis occurs mainly in healthy individuals. However, it has been found in immunosuppressed patients. Although the mechanism of granuloma formation is not well understood, it appears that lipids extracted from these fungi and cell-wall constituents may be responsible for this reaction.

Clinical features

The initial lesion of chromoblastomycosis is a small papule at the site of trauma, which gradually enlarges (Fig. 7.1.9). Nodules and tumours develop, producing a malodorous discharge; eventually, over a period of years, a wide variety of morphological patterns may emerge including dry, hyperkeratotic plaques, verrucose lesions, and large, cauliflower-like masses (Fig. 7.1.10). Extensive cicatricial plaques, surrounded by peripherally spreading vegetative lesions, may also be present. Evolution is slow and lesions usually involve the lower limb. However, any part of the body may be involved and the sites may be multiple.

Dissemination occurs by (1) surface spread; (2) the lymphatics, the most common method; (iii) autoinoculation from scratching;

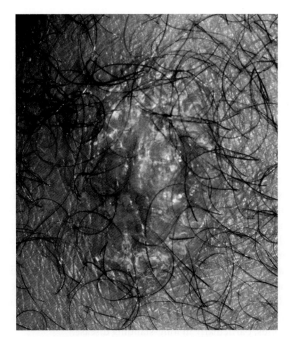

Fig. 7.1.9 Chromoblastomycosis. Early lesion in a Brazilian patient. (Copyright D A Warrell.)

and (iv) haematogenously, resulting in subcutaneous lesions at sites distant from the primary. Visceral metastases are known to occur and involvement of the central nervous system, respiratory system, larynx, and vocal folds has been recorded. Therapeutically, therefore, early diagnosis is important.

Complications of long-standing chromoblastomycosis include lymphoedema, flexion deformity of joints, and development of squamous carcinoma.

Diagnosis

Although the history and clinical presentation may suggest the diagnosis, the varied clinical presentation of chromoblastomycosis necessitates consideration of other granulomatous diseases such as sporotrichosis, cutaneous tuberculosis, Hansen's disease, blastomycosis, candidiasis, leishmaniasis, paracoccidioidomycosis,

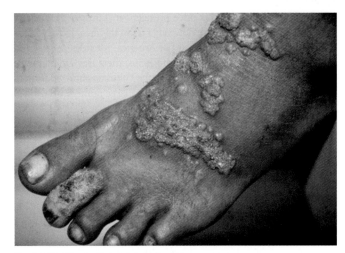

Fig. 7.1.10 Chromoblastomycosis: late lesion. (Courtesy of João LC Cardoso, São Paulo, Brazil.)

rhinosporidiosis, tertiary syphilis, squamous carcinoma, and even psoriasis, sarcoidosis, and discoid lupus erythematosus.

Therefore, to establish a definitive diagnosis, histological and mycological investigations are essential. Diagnosis is confirmed by the presence of the characteristic brown, sclerotic bodies in histological sections. From both epidemiological and therapeutic points of view, culture is necessary as *F. pedrosoi* is the most difficult of the causative fungi to eradicate whereas *C. carrionii* responds rapidly to treatment.

Treatment

Small, single, localized lesions are satisfactorily eradicated by cryo-surgery, but long-term follow-up is needed to assess accurately the success of this treatment. Thermotherapy has been found effective by some, again principally in the management of small, single, lesions, but here the possibility of a burn must be borne in mind. Rapid spread of the disease has been associated with inadequate surgery, curettage, and electrodesiccation.

Oral monotherapy has been unsuccessful in some cases and drug resistance remains a problem. However itraconazole and terbinafine have both been reported as effective agents. A combination of 5-flucytosine with either thiabendazole or itraconazole may also be efficacious, particularly in long-standing disease.

Whatever method of treatment is used, chromomycosis although clinically healed, should be followed-up for at least 2 years before its total eradication can be assumed.

Sporotrichosis

Aetiology

The most common clinical form of sporotrichosis is a subcutaneous infection, which may spread proximally from its initial site in a series of nodules along the course of a lymphatic (Fig. 7.1.11a, b). More rarely, systemic involvement is seen, e.g. in the lung (see 'Systemic mycoses', below).

The causative organism *Sporothrix schenckii* can be found in soil, in vegetation, or in association with plants or bark. People who develop the subcutaneous infection may have had contact with material that harbours the organism, such as moss or flowers (e.g. florists). It is assumed that the pathogen gains entry via an abrasion and in some endemic areas there is often a preceding history of a cat scratch or insect bite.

Epidemiology

Although sporotrichosis was once prevalent in Europe, particularly France, nonimported cases are now very rare in this area. However, the disease is seen in the United States of America, Mexico, Central and South America, and Africa. In the late 1930s, there was a remarkable epidemic of sporotrichosis in workers in the Witwatersrand gold mines (South Africa). The source of infection was a large number of wooden pit props contaminated with the organism. Other, smaller 'epidemics' have been described in certain groups, such as Mexican pottery workers packing ceramics in straw. Normally, however, cases are sporadic in incidence. There are also 'hyperendemic' areas where there is an unexpectedly high incidence of this infection, e.g. Rio de Janeiro State, Brazil.

Systemic sporotrichosis is much rarer, and cases have mainly been described from the United States.

Clinical features

There are two main clinical types of subcutaneous sporotrichosis.

The first, the fixed type, presents with a solitary cutaneous ulcer or nodule. In this form of the disease, infection does not spread

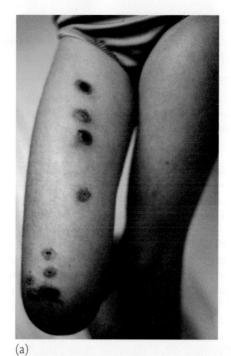

(a)

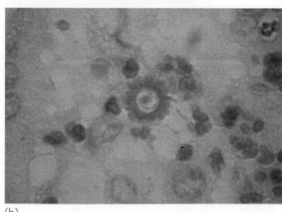

(b)

Fig. 7.1.11a (a) Sporotrichosis. (b) Histopathological appearances. (a, courtesy of João LC Cardoso, São Paulo, Brazil; b, copyright Professor R Hay.)

along lymphatics. It has been suggested that it is most common in children, and it has been described most frequently in Central and South America.

In the lymphangitic form, an initial nodule forms on a limb or extremity, such as a finger. This may break down and ulcerate. Subsequently, one or more secondary nodules develop along the draining lymphatic channel, which may ulcerate through the skin (Fig. 7.1.11a). Other variants include the psoriasiform or verrucous types or a superficial granuloma that resembles lupus vulgaris. These usually represent chronic infection.

Rarer forms include secondary spread via scratching, which may present with multiple widespread ulcers or multiple cutaneous lesions secondary to systemic disease. In HIV-positive individuals, widespread cutaneous lesions may develop.

Fixed-type sporotrichosis may resemble many other forms of cutaneous ulceration. However, in endemic areas a major source of confusion is cutaneous leishmaniasis. The lymphangitic variety may also resemble other infections, notably atypical mycobacterial infections, particularly fish-tank granuloma, or 'sporotrichoid' leishmaniasis.

Treatment

Some cases of sporotrichosis may heal spontaneously. However, treatment is usually advised to prevent scar formation. The cheapest treatment is potassium iodide, which is administered in a saturated aqueous solution. The starting dose is 0.5 to 1 ml, given three times daily, and this is increased drop by drop per dose to 3 to 6 ml, three times daily. The mixture is more palatable if given with milk. Treatment should be given for a month after clinical resolution. However, both itraconazole and terbinafine are also effective; minimal durations of treatment for these agents have not been defined.

Subcutaneous mucoromycosis due to basidiobolus

Subcutaneous mucoromycosis is an infection primarily seen in children in Africa or eastern Asia (Indonesia). It is characterized by the development of localized woody swellings on the limbs or trunk. The swelling is rarely inflammatory, but has a well-defined leading edge, and is hard. Progression is slow. The causative organism *Basidiobolus haptosporus* can be cultured or demonstrated histologically in biopsy material. Although resolution has been recorded without treatment, therapy is normally given. Potassium iodide solution is the treatment of choice, and is given in as high a dose as possible (see 'Sporotrichosis', above). Itraconazole may also be effective.

Subcutaneous mucoromycosis due to conidiobolus (conidiobolomycosis or rhinoentomophthoromycosis)

Conidiobolomycosis is a similar infection confined to subcutaneous tissue and presenting with painless swelling. The infection is mainly seen in West Africa, but a case has been seen in the Caribbean. There are important differences from the subcutaneous mucoromycosis caused by basidiobolus. The disease is most common in young adults, and is confined to facial tissues around the nose, the forehead, and the upper lip (Fig. 7.1.12). The initial site of infection is in the region of the inferior turbinate in the nose. The diagnosis is established by biopsy or culture. The causative organism is *Conidiobolus coronatus*. Treatment with itraconazole or ketoconazole is effective, but an alternative is high-dose potassium iodide. Relapse after treatment is common, and residual fibrosis may be severely disfiguring.

Lobo's disease (lobomycosis)

Lobo's disease is a subcutaneous infection. The organism, *Lacazia loboi* in tissue, appears to be a yeast. It has a tendency to form chains of four to six yeast cells with prominent nucleoli, joined by a narrow intercellular bridge. However, the organism has never been cultured from human cases and can only be identified by biopsy and histology. The disease is seen in countries of South America around and to the north of the Amazon basin, and cases are also seen in Central America. Apart from humans, the only other species affected are freshwater dolphins. Often, exposed sites (such as earlobes) are invaded and small nodules containing the organisms develop. These may resemble keloids (Fig. 7.1.13). More diffuse plaques may also be seen. Deep invasion has not been documented. The treatment is excision, and there is no effective chemotherapy, although there have been recent reports that posaconazole may be effective.

Systemic mycoses

The systemic or deep visceral mycoses include some of the rare and more serious fungal infections. There are two main types of infection in this group: (1) the endemic mycoses, caused by organisms that invade normal hosts, and (2) the opportunistic mycoses, which cause disease only in compromised patients. The fungi associated with these two types of infection differ in their innate levels of pathogenicity, but an element of opportunism, depending on host susceptibility, is usually recognizable in all cases of systemic mycoses.

The endemic pathogens cause infections such as histoplasmosis or coccidioidomycosis. These diseases have well-defined endemic zones and the majority of those exposed remain symptomless but usually develop positive skin tests. However, in certain patients, chronic local or disseminated disease may occur. In the systemic infections caused by opportunistic fungi, there is usually a serious underlying abnormality in the patient affecting T lymphocytes

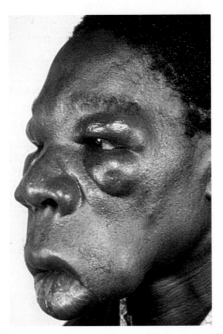

Fig. 7.1.12 Subcutaneous mucoromycosis (*Conidiobolus coronatus*). (Copyright Professor R Hay.)

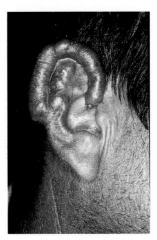

Fig. 7.1.13 Lobo's disease in a Brazilian man. (Copyright D A Warrell.)

(such as HIV) or neutrophils (such as cancer chemotherapy). Such infections are worldwide in occurrence: where tissue invasion occurs the mortality is high. Cryptococcosis, a systemic yeast infection, has features of both types of systemic disease and occurs in both normal and immunosuppressed subjects (Chapter 7.2).

The systemic endemic infections are histoplasmosis, coccidioidomycosis (Chapter 7.3), blastomycosis, paracoccidioidomycosis (Chapter 7.4), and infections due to *Penicillium marneffei* (Chapter 7.6). The significance of various laboratory tests in these infections is shown in Table 7.1.1.

Histoplasmosis (see Oxford Textbook of Medicine 5e Chapter 18.4.2)

There are two forms of histoplasmosis. In both types, the organism is present in tissue in its yeast phase. In small-form or classic histoplasmosis, the diameter of the yeast cells is between 3 and 4 µm. Infections are most common in the United States of America, but sporadic cases are reported widely from the New World, Africa, and eastern Asia. By contrast, large-form or African histoplasmosis is most common in Central Africa, south of the Sahara and north of the Zambezi river. Yeast forms in infected tissue are much larger, 10 to 15 µm in diameter. Both infections are clinically distinct (see below), but cultural isolates are indistinguishable.

Histoplasmosis (classic or small-form histoplasmosis)

Aetiology

Histoplasmosis is a systemic infection caused by *Histoplasma capsulatum*. The main route of infection is pulmonary. The majority of those exposed are sensitized without overt signs of infection, but

more rarely chronic pulmonary or disseminated forms of the disease are seen.

The organism, *H. capsulatum*, can be found in soil in endemic areas. Its growth is facilitated by the presence of bird excreta, e.g. in old chicken houses, bird roosts, and barns. In tropical and some temperate areas, bat guano plays a similar role. Exposure to a suitable source, such as a cave containing bats, is often recorded in acute epidemic histoplasmosis (see below). It is rarely identified in more slowly evolving cases.

The condition of the host is important in determining the clinical course and manifestations of histoplasmosis. Slowly evolving (chronic), disseminated disease may occur in normal individuals. However, infants, elderly people, or those with untreated AIDS appear to be more likely to develop the more rapidly progressive forms of disseminated infection.

Epidemiology

The major endemic area, as shown by skin testing, is in the central region of the United States around the Ohio and Mississippi valley basins. Prevalence is highest in the states of Tennessee, Kentucky, and Ohio. Up to 95% of those skin-tested in certain parts of these areas have positive delayed reactions to intradermal histoplasmin. Scattered cases of active disease, healed calcified foci in chest radiographs, and foci found at autopsy representing inactive histoplasmosis also provide evidence of spread within this area. However, the disease also occurs in other parts of the United States, Mexico, Central and South America, Africa, eastern Asia, and Australia. Outside the major endemic areas in the United States, human cases are less frequent, and much of the evidence of the endemicity comes from positive skin tests or the presence of the organism in

Table 7.1.1 Laboratory tests in systemic mycoses[a]

	Direct microscopy	Significance of positive cultures	Serology	Histopathology
Histoplasmosis				
Classic (small form)	Sometimes positive	Significant	ID, CIE, CFT Urine antigen detection	Yeasts (3–4 µm)
African histoplasmosis	Positive in pus (valuable)	Significant	ID, CFT	Yeasts (10–15 µm)
Coccidioidomycosis	Positive in pus, sputum, etc. (valuable)	Significant NB Handle with caution	ID, CFT, TP, CIE	Spherules (50–150 µm)
Blastomycosis	Positive in pus, sputum, etc. (valuable)	Significant	ID, CFT, CIE (unreliable)	Yeasts (4–10 µm) Broad-based buds
Paracoccidioidomycosis	Positive in pus, sputum etc. (valuable)	Significant	ID, CFT, TP Antigen detection	Yeasts (5–15 µm) Multiple buds
Cryptococcosis	Often positive in CSF (rare in urine, pus) NB Indian ink	Significant	Latex agglutination or ELISA for antigen (ID, CFT, WCA, IF)	Encapsulated yeasts (5–10 µm) Mucicarmine positive
Systemic candidiasis	Positive in oral smzears, sputum, etc. (interpret with caution)	Significance depends on site and presence of positive microscopy	ID, CFT, WCA, CIE Antigen detection	Yeasts (5–10 µm) and hyphae
Invasive aspergillosis	Rarely positive, depends on site	Positive sputum cultures not always significant	ID, CIE, rarely positive Antigen detection e.g. Pasteurex	Hyphae—dichotomous branching
Invasive mucoromycosis	Rarely positive	Depends on site	Rarely positive	Hyphae—broad and aseptate

CFT, complement fixation test; CIE, counterimmunoelectrophoresis; CSF, cerebrospinal fluid; ID, immunodiffusion; IF, immunofluorescence; RIA, radioimmunoassay; TP, tube precipitation; WCA, whole-cell agglutination.
[a] Molecular diagnostic techniques are increasingly used but are not standardized.

selected sites, such as caves. Although there has been considerable discussion on the nature of soil factors responsible for the growth of *H. capsulatum*, the conditions limiting its occurrence to certain areas are largely unknown.

Clinical features

The clinical forms of histoplasmosis can be placed in several groups:

- asymptomatic
- acute symptomatic pulmonary:
  - acute epidemic
  - acute reinfection
- chronic pulmonary
- disseminated (acute, subacute, and chronic)
- primary cutaneous (by inoculation)

Asymptomatic infection

Over 99% of patients becoming infected in endemic areas record no overt symptoms but develop a positive skin test. The incidence of positive skin tests declines in individuals above the age of 60 years.

Acute (symptomatic) pulmonary histoplasmosis

Acute epidemic histoplasmosis Groups of people exposed to a source of infection, e.g. during cave exploration, or those who may have inhaled a large infecting dose, often develop a symptomatic illness 12 to 21 days after exposure. The main features are pyrexia, cough, chest pain, and malaise. Flitting arthralgia and, less commonly, erythema nodosum or multiforme may occur. The radiological appearances may be much more severe than would be supposed from the symptoms, and enlargement of hilar lymph nodes and diffuse or patchy consolidation suggesting pneumonitis may occur (Fig. 7.1.14).

These patients develop precipitating or complement-fixing antibody, but this often follows the peak of illness. About 50% of

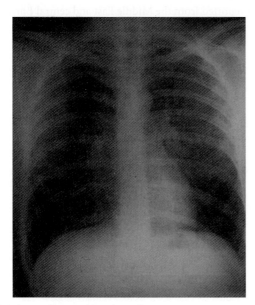

Fig. 7.1.14 Acute pulmonary histoplasmosis.
(Copyright Professor R Hay.)

those with symptoms do not develop positive antibody responses. Likewise, skin-test conversion is often too late to be of diagnostic value, and its use is normally contraindicated, as a single histoplasmin test may cause the development of false-positive serological results. Cultures are often negative. The symptoms and history of exposure to a suitable source, combined with a rising antibody titre, are often the best evidence of infection.

The majority of cases require no specific therapy apart from rest. Those with severe or prolonged symptoms or impaired gas exchange require intravenous amphotericin B or itraconazole. The lung lesions often heal to leave multiple scattered pulmonary calcifications.

Acute reinfection histoplasmosis Massive acute exposure to *H. capsulatum* in sensitized individuals is believed by some physicians to cause a less severe infection associated with bilateral pulmonary infiltrates. The incubation period is shorter than with acute epidemic histoplasmosis, namely 5 to 10 days.

Chronic pulmonary histoplasmosis

Chronic pulmonary disease caused by *H. capsulatum* is mainly seen in the United States. It is more common in men and smokers, and there is often underlying pulmonary disease such as emphysema. Early cases may present with pyrexia and cough, but malaise and weight loss occur later. Lesions may heal initially, but relapse is common, leading to established consolidation and cavitation. The most common radiological appearance of early lesions is of unilateral, wedge-shaped, segmental shadows in the apical zones. Subsequently, the disease may become bilateral, with fibrosis and cavitation. In some cases, extensive and progressive destruction of lung tissue may occur.

Culture and serology are both helpful methods of diagnosis in this form of histoplasmosis, but repeated attempts may be required before positive results are obtained.

In early cases, resolution may occur on rest alone. However, relapse occurs in at least 25% of cases, and these patients may require amphotericin B therapy or itraconazole. Although chemotherapy may virtually sterilize lesions, fibrosis persists and relapse may occur. Surgical excision or lobectomy is sometimes effective.

Solid lung tumours may persist after the primary infection. These may be single (coin lesions) or multiple, and have to be distinguished from carcinomas. The diagnosis is normally made at surgery, although the presence of calcification may give a clue to the nature of the lesion (histoplasmoma). The organisms can be demonstrated by histopathology, but they are seldom viable.

Disseminated histoplasmosis

There is considerable variation in the rate of progression of histoplasmosis that has spread beyond the initial focus in the lung. In rapid or acutely disseminated cases, widespread infiltration of reticuloendothelial cells of bone marrow, spleen, and liver may occur. Gastrointestinal lesions, endocarditis, and meningitis are less common, and meningitis is more usually associated with a slower course of disseminated disease. Infants, elderly people, or immunosuppressed patients are more susceptible to acute dissemination. The most prominent symptoms are fever and weight loss, with accompanying hepatosplenomegaly. Extensive purpura and bruising secondary to thrombocytopenia may occur. The blood picture may reflect marrow infiltration with organisms, leading to pancytopenia. Disseminated histoplasmosis is also seen in patients with AIDS. The clinical manifestations are not significantly different, although skin papules and ulcers have been reported in many (Fig. 7.1.15); isolation of histoplasma from blood has also been reported more frequently in these patients. Cultures, including sputum or bone marrow, should be taken. Serology is often positive, with high titres of complement-fixing antibodies occurring in some patients. However, new antigen detection systems in serum or urine provide a better means of confirming the diagnosis and monitoring treatment.

A much more slowly progressive form of disseminated histoplasmosis may present with fewer localized lesions, such as persistent oral ulcers, chronic laryngitis, or adrenal insufficiency. Granulomas, few of which contain organisms, can be found in the liver in some patients. Such cases may present up to 30 years after the patient has left an endemic area. Outside endemic areas this form is the most widely recognized presentation of histoplasmosis, occurring in Europeans, for instance, who have worked in Africa or eastern Asia.

The diagnosis of disseminated histoplasmosis is made on culture or biopsy of affected areas. Antibodies may only be positive in low titres and in all cases adrenal involvement should be looked for.

Treatment is required in all forms of disseminated histoplasmosis. Itraconazole is preferred by most physicians, although amphotericin B may be necessary in some patients. Posaconazole is an alternative. In patients with AIDS who are acutely ill, the disease is often controlled by a short (2-week) course of amphotericin B and thereafter patients receive continuous itraconazole indefinitely.

Primary cutaneous histoplasmosis

Primary infection sometimes follows accidental inoculation of viable organisms in a laboratory or autopsy room. This type of infection is normally associated with a chancre at the site of inoculation and regional lymphadenopathy. The condition is self-limiting.

African histoplasmosis

Overt pulmonary involvement is rare in this form of histoplasmosis, and the normal portal of entry of the pathogen is not known. The most common presenting features are skin lesions (papules, nodules, abscesses, or ulcers) (Fig. 7.1.16) or lytic bone deposits. Solitary or multiple foci may be present, and in the latter instances rapid progression and death may occur. In such cases, gastrointestinal and lung lesions may develop.

The diagnosis is normally made by culture, smear, or biopsy. The organism *H. capsulatum* var. *duboisii* is identical to that causing classic histoplasmosis in culture, but in lesions the yeast forms are considerably larger (10–15 µm).

Although local excision of skin nodules has been reported to be curative, treatment with itraconazole, ketoconazole, or amphotericin B is usual. Some patients will respond to co-trimoxazole. A skeletal scan should be made to detect occult foci of infection.

Blastomycosis (see also Oxford Textbook of Medicine 5e Section 23)

Blastomycosis (North American blastomycosis) caused by *Blastomyces dermatitidis* is a systemic fungal infection in which skin and lung involvement are common features.

The infective organism, *B. dermatitidis*, has only been isolated from the environment on rare occasions. Positive sites have included soil and rotten timbers. The organism infects humans and domestic animals, particularly dogs.

Epidemiology

Blastomycosis was originally thought to be confined to North America, where it occurs sporadically throughout the south and east-central area, and in areas of central Canada. 'Epidemics' of acute disease are rare, and where these occur a source of infection is rarely demonstrated. There is evidence that sources may include areas exposed to flooding.

More recently, cases have been found in Africa. Again, these are widely scattered from the north coast to the southern parts of the continent, and are rare in all areas. Patients with the disease have also been reported from the Middle East and central Europe.

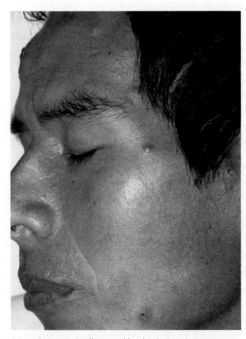

Fig. 7.1.15 Histoplasmosis. Molluscum-like skin lesions in an HIV-immunosuppressed Peruvian patient.
(Copyright D A Warrell.)

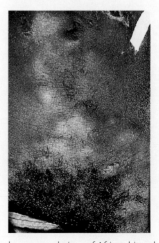

Fig. 7.1.16 Nodular subcutaneous lesions of African histoplasmosis in a Nigerian man.
(Copyright D A Warrell.)

Clinical features

The clinical forms of blastomycosis differ from histoplasmosis in a number of important aspects. The existence of an asymptomatic form has not been proved conclusively, because there is no reliable skin test. Acute infections or infections in groups are rare, and the features are often similar to histoplasmosis (acute pulmonary). However, specific serological tests may be negative in 30 to 50% of cases. The demonstration of the organisms in sputum and positive cultures are more reliable diagnostic criteria. Although some cases undoubtedly resolve without sequelae, some physicians advise chemotherapy, with a short course of amphotericin B in acute cases of blastomycosis.

Chronic pulmonary blastomycosis

Chronic consolidation or cavitation of the upper or mid zones occur with chronic pulmonary infections. Fever, malaise, and cough with sputum are seen. Weight loss may be prominent. Culture is again the most reliable method of diagnosis.

The mainstays of treatment are itraconazole or amphotericin B.

Disseminated blastomycosis

Although generalized infiltration in skin, lungs, and liver may occur over a short period, leading to rapid death, signs of chronic extrapulmonary dissemination are more usual.

The skin is an area that is frequently involved (chronic cutaneous blastomycosis). The face or forearms and hands are common sites for skin lesions. These are slow, spreading, verrucose plaques with central scarring. The initial lesion is often a dermal nodule. Many such cases have underlying pulmonary consolidation, or cavities. The diagnosis is established by biopsy and culture. Bone deposits in the form of lytic lesions, and involvement of the genitourinary tract, particularly the epididymis, are also seen in chronic disseminated blastomycosis. Unlike tuberculosis, the kidneys are often spared.

In slowly progressive forms of blastomycosis, itraconazole (200–400 mg daily) has proved to be very effective. Alternatively, amphotericin B can be given intravenously and is indicated where there is rapidly progressive disease.

Coccidioidomycosis

See Chapter 7.3.

Paracoccidioidomycosis

See Chapter 7.4.

Systemic sporotrichosis

In addition to causing cutaneous disease, *Sporothrix schenckii* may be responsible for a systemic mycosis. The infection is rare and has been mainly reported from the United States of America. Involvement may be confined to a single site such as a lung or a joint, or it may be multifocal. Cavitation in the lung associated with weight loss and pyrexia is probably the most common variety of systemic sporotrichosis. Unlike cutaneous forms of the disease, systemic sporotrichosis responds poorly to potassium iodide, and amphotericin B is the treatment of choice.

Rare systemic infections

These include pulmonary invasion by *Geotrichum candidum* (geotrichosis) and adiaspiromycosis, a respiratory infection caused by *Emmonsia crescens* or *E. parva*. Isolated examples of human disease caused by fungi are consistently reported and almost always occur in the immunosuppressed host. In these patients many fungi that are normally saprophytes in the environment may invade and cause disease.

Systemic mycoses caused by opportunistic fungi

The opportunistic mycoses are a worldwide problem, although fortunately rare in most countries. In recent years they have been recognized more frequently with the increase in transplantations of organs such as heart or bone marrow and in the more effective but immunocompromising regimes of cancer chemotherapy. Opportunistic invasion by organisms such as *Candida* or mucoromycetes (rhizopus, absidia) may also occur in cases of malnutrition. One of the recent trends in the management of the patient with neutropenia has been the emergence of new pathogens such as non-*albicans* species of *Candida* or other organisms such as fusarium, trichosporon, or scedosporium species.

The opportunists present particular problems in diagnosis and management. Because many of the organisms are normally saprophytic, it has to be positively established that they have assumed an invasive role. Mere isolation may not provide sufficient evidence and in some instances low titres of antibody may be present even in normal hosts. The significance of various laboratory tests in these infections is shown in Table 7.1.1. Treatment is also difficult and it is important in most cases to attempt to reverse the process that led to the establishment of the infection.

Systemic candidiasis

Aetiology

In addition to their role in superficial infections, *Candida* yeasts may also cause invasive systemic disease. The clinical forms described range from bloodstream isolation or candidaemia to disseminated invasive disease, sometimes with involvement of a single organ, site, or body cavity (deep focal candidiasis) as may occur in peritonitis or meningitis. Urinary tract infections may also be caused by candida species.

The factors underlying systemic candida infections are shown in Box 7.1.3. All these factors are important in disrupting the balance

---

Box 7.1.3 Predisposing factors in deep candida infections

- Local defects, foreign bodies, e.g. prosthetic heart valves, intravenous lines
- Defects of immunity (primarily T cell or phagocytosis), e.g. cytotoxic therapy or systemic lupus erythematosus
- Drug therapy, e.g. antibiotics
- Carcinoma or leukaemia
- Endocrine disease, e.g. diabetes mellitus in urinary tract candidiasis
- Physiological changes, e.g. infancy, old age, and pregnancy (urinary tract)
- Miscellaneous disorders, e.g.
  - Malnutrition
  - Surgery such as gastrointestinal resections
  - Drug addiction

by which candida is maintained as a saprophyte. Intravenous or central venous pressure lines may serve as a portal of entry or as a nidus for circulating yeasts in a candidaemia. Antibiotic therapy may upset the balance by inhibiting a potentially competitive bacterial flora.

Candida albicans is the most common species involved but other species may be isolated, particularly in cases of endocarditis, e.g. *C. parapsilosis*. *C. tropicalis* has been implicated in infections of patients with neutropenia. These non-*albicans Candida* species are now more frequent causes of systemic infection and are important to recognize as their antifungal susceptibility may differ from that of *C. albicans*. Portals of entry include the gastrointestinal tract (common), skin, and urinary tract (rare). However, superficial candidiasis or saprophytic colonization of mouth, skin, or airways may also occur in compromised patients and does not necessarily indicate systemic invasion.

Epidemiology

Systemic infections caused by *Candida* species are worldwide in distribution. However, they are particularly associated with a number of predisposing factors such as neutropenia, antibiotic usage, indwelling lines, and abdominal surgery.

Clinical features

Candidaemia

The isolation of candida in blood culture may be linked to any of the factors listed in Box 7.1.3. Common predisposing features are the presence of intravenous lines, previous surgery (mainly gastrointestinal), antibiotic therapy, hepatic failure, or neutropenia. Patients develop a swinging fever and feel generally unwell. Clinical shock may occur.

Some such cases resolve following removal of predisposing factors, particularly the intravenous lines. Generally, however, all such patients receive treatment and a careful investigation should be made to identify the presence of established invasive disease. Other sites should be searched for evidence of infection; e.g. urine by culture or the presence of white cells. Signs of muscle invasion (tenderness) or metastatic skin nodules should be excluded (Fig. 7.1.17). Other signs of invasion include the development of new cardiac murmurs or of soft, white, retinal plaques caused by candida. Persistently positive blood cultures or serum candida antigen levels or high antibody titres may also indicate possible deep invasion.

Disseminated candidiasis

Although multiorgan invasive candidiasis may follow candidaemia, at least 50% of disseminated infections develop in patients without initially positive blood cultures. The features of some forms of invasive candidiasis are listed above (under candidaemia). Although

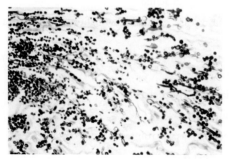

Fig. 7.1.17 Candidiasis disseminated to skin (methenamine silver, × 516).

candida may be isolated from the sputum in these patients, there is rarely objective evidence of lung invasion. Moreover, there is no radiological appearance that is diagnostic of pulmonary candidiasis and, indeed, chest radiographs may even appear normal. General localizing signs may be a late feature of disseminated candidiasis.

Laboratory diagnosis of disseminated candidiasis

The diagnosis may be made by culture or PCR, and repeated attempts to isolate should be made where cultures are initially negative. Numerous techniques have been used to detect antibody or antigen in disseminated candidiasis. However, in many patients, particularly those with neutropenia, it may not be possible to confirm the diagnosis using laboratory tests and treatment is often initiated on the basis of clinical suspicion (empirical therapy) as the risk of delaying antifungal therapy is great.

By themselves, positive cultures, particularly from sputum, or the presence of antibodies do not necessarily prove the existence of deep-seated candidiasis. A positive isolation may simply indicate the presence of colonization and normal individuals may have low titres of antibody to candida. If there is a readily accessible lesion from which to take a biopsy, such as a skin nodule or even a pulmonary infiltrate, this may provide the best evidence of invasion, although such procedures may carry their own risk (Fig. 7.1.16).

Treatment of disseminated candidiasis

Untreated disseminated candidiasis is normally progressive and fatal. The signs must be separated from, for instance, bacterial septicaemia, which may coexist with the candida infection.

The treatment of invasive candidiasis is intravenous amphotericin B or caspofungin or intravenous or oral fluconazole given until there is a clinical and mycological response. This may take between 2 and 20 weeks depending on the site of infection and the underlying state of the patient. Fluconazole is usually used in infections where the patient is not neutropenic. Lipid-associated forms of amphotericin B are also useful and carry a lower risk of renal impairment. An alternative approach is to add flucytosine in doses of 150 to 200 mg/kg body weight daily to amphotericin B in serious infections or where cure may be hampered by poor penetration of amphotericin B, such as in the eye. A biologic, Mycograb, which is an antibody against *Candida* heat shock protein 70 has been shown to improve treatment responses in candidaemia when used in combination with amphotericin B.

Deep focal candidiasis

Candida infections in the peritoneum or meninges most often follow direct implantation after dialysis or surgery. Alternatively, secondary invasion from the middle ear or a perforated bowel is also possible. The signs and symptoms are similar to bacterial meningitis or peritonitis but *Candida* is isolated. Sometimes these infections clear spontaneously, but normally treatment is instituted with fluconazole, which penetrates areas such as peritoneum, or amphotericin B.

Candida endocarditis

Invasion of heart valves, mainly the mitral or aortic valves, most commonly follows homograft replacement, but it may occur also in patients with neutropenia or drug addicts. The symptoms are similar to bacterial endocarditis. However, *Candida* vegetations may reach considerable size. Embolic phenomena may involve obstruction of large vessels including the femoral artery or large cerebral vessels. The detection of large vegetations using an echocardiography, particularly in cases with negative blood cultures, should raise the possibility of fungal endocarditis. Blood cultures are usually positive at some stage in the illness but repeated sampling may be necessary. High antibody titres are usually seen in such cases and serological tests are therefore of considerable value.

Untreated candida endocarditis is uniformly fatal. There is also a high mortality associated with cases in which early surgical intervention is precipitated by impending heart failure. Normally, treatment consists of amphotericin B given intravenously and, where possible, valve replacement. There is no evidence to suggest that the addition of flucytosine to the regimen increases the effectiveness of treatment. However, the relapse rate is high and combination therapy may therefore be a reasonable approach on theoretical grounds.

Urinary tract candidiasis

Candida species may be isolated from the urine, particularly in conditions associated with urinary stasis such as neurogenic bladder or where there is an indwelling catheter. Type 2 diabetes is another predisposing factor. There is no value in using the presence of pyuria or quantitative yeast-colony counts to assess the significance of infection. Treatment is normally given where there are symptoms such as dysuria or frequency or where there is a potential risk of invasion such as in immunosuppressed patients. Fluconazole is very useful in these patients as urinary levels are above inhibitory concentrations.

Aspergillosis (see also Chapter 2.4 and Oxford Textbook of Medicine 5e Section 18)

Aspergillosis is the name given to diseases associated with species of mould fungi of the genus *Aspergillus*. As such, it comprises a series of clinically distinct infections: aggressive pulmonary infections with angio-invasion and the potential for widespread systemic haematogenous spread (invasive pulmonary aspergillosis); slow but progressive paranasal sinus infection mainly seen in the tropics (paranasal aspergillus granulom); and colonization of a pre-existing space or cavity (aspergilloma) which may give rise to medical problems including severe haemorrhage. They are also associated with both superficial and subcutaneous fungal infections. *Aspergillus* species cause a number of different allergic disorders including asthma and allergic bronchopulmonary aspergillosis (Oxford Textbook of Medicine 5e Chapter 18.14.2). Box 7.1.4 indicates the range of diseases associated with aspergillus.

Aspergillus species are ubiquitous and have established themselves in every conceivable terrain and environment. As they propagate through the production of large number of airborne spores, exposure is difficult to avoid. Production of spores is also determined by local and environmental conditions. For example, construction or destruction of buildings and turnover of soil have been associated with focal outbreaks of infection in predisposed and immunosuppressed individuals. Susceptibility to aspergillus infections is dependent, to a large extent, on defective immunity or structural abnormalities, and therefore the major diseases caused by these organisms are usually seen in immunosuppressed individuals, including, in particular, neutropenic patients or people with anatomocal abnormalities such as lung cavities. The incidence of infection can reach high levels in certain populations such as patients following bone marrow transplantation (Chapter 2.4).

Aspergillus can produce a number of potent metabolic byproducts or myxotoxins, such as the aflatoxins produced by *A. flavus* which, if present in contaminated food, can induce liver necrosis.

Box 7.1.4 Diseases caused by aspergillus species

Superficial infections

♦ Onychomycosis
♦ Otitis externa
♦ Keratomycosis

Subcutaneous infections

♦ Mycetoma
♦ Systemic infections
♦ Localized invasive aspergillosis:
  · Aspergilloma, chronic aspergillosis of the paranasal sinuses, chronic pulmonary aspergillosis, paranasal aspergillus granuloma
♦ Invasive aspergillosis with potential for systemic spread:
  · Invasive (pulmonary) aspergillosis (common sites for dissemination are brain, liver, skin)
  · Aspergillus endocarditis

Allergic disease

♦ Asthma, allergic rhinitis,
♦ Extrinsic hypersensitivity pneumonitis (*A. clavatus*)
♦ Allergic bronchopulmonary aspergillosis
♦ Allergic aspergillus sinusitis

Toxicosis

♦ Mycotoxin-producing aspergilli, e.g. *A. flavus*—aflatoxins

---

The commonest human pathogen amongst the aspergillus species is *A. fumigatus*, followed by *A. flavus* which causes infections more commonly in warmer climates. *A. niger* causes aspergilloma rather than invasive disease but *A. nidulans* rarely causes mycetoma. *A. terreus* is sometimes found as a cause of onychomycosis. Hence aspergillus infections may present to a wide range of different specialities and, in the severely immunocompromised patient, dissemination of aspergillus through the blood stream may result in infection of almost any organ.

Cryptococcosis

See Chapter 7.2.

Invasive mucoromycosis (mucoromycosis, zygomycosis phycomycosis)

Aetiology

Invasive disease caused by mucor-like (mucoromycete) fungi is rare. In the compromised host it may lead to paranasal destruction, necrotic lung or skin lesions, and disseminated disease.

The causative organisms commonly belong to three genera: *Absidia*, *Rhizopus*, and *Rhizomucor*. More rarely other organisms such as *Cunninghamella* or *Saksenaea* have been implicated. Most of the agents are associated with decaying vegetable matter and are common airborne moulds. The route of infection is highly variable: they may invade via the lungs, paranasal sinuses, gastrointestinal tract, or damaged skin. The predisposing illness may in some way determine the site of clinical invasion. Underlying factors include diabetic ketoacidosis (rhinocerebral involvement), leukaemia and immunosuppressive therapy (lung and disseminated infection), malnutrition (gastrointestinal infection), and burns or wounds (cutaneous invasion). These patterns are not always strictly followed.

Epidemiology

Mucoromycosis is rare but has a worldwide distribution. Its invasive nature, particularly the tendency to involve blood vessels and its selection of compromised hosts, distinguishes this form of infection from subcutaneous mucoromycosis, which is also caused by mucoromycete species.

Clinical features

The most characteristic features of this type of infection are the extensive necrosis and infarction that may follow blood vessel invasion leading to thrombosis. A similar type of invasion may occur with invasive aspergillosis, but is usually less prominent. Invasive mucoromycosis follows a number of different patterns.

The infection may initially localize in one of several sites. The most common is in the paranasal sinuses and this is most often seen in diabetic patients with ketoacidosis. The patient presents with fever and unilateral facial pain. Subsequently, there may be facial swelling with nasal obstruction and proptosis. There may be invasion into the orbit leading to blindness, into the brain, and into the palate. Palatal ulceration should be searched for. Widespread dissemination with infarction of major organs or limbs may occur subsequently. A similar pattern of invasion of surgical wounds or burns may occur and has on occasions been associated with contamination of dressing packs. Infections are initially localized causing extensive necrosis around the original wound. Gastrointestinal invasion may be heralded by perforation of viscera, and diarrhoea or haemorrhage.

Alternatively, a patient may present with established pulmonary or widespread dissemination. Such patients are usually leukaemic or are severely immunosuppressed. Neutropenia is often seen.

Once infection has spread beyond the original site, mucoromycosis is almost invariably fatal with or without treatment.

Laboratory diagnosis

The diagnosis is suggested by the combination of infection and extensive infarction, particularly if it occurs in any of the sites mentioned. The organisms may be difficult to culture even from biopsy and histology is often the quickest way of establishing the diagnosis. Serology is frequently negative.

Treatment

Treatment should be initiated as soon as possible and extensive surgical debridement combined with intravenous amphotericin B in maximum daily dosage offers the best chance of success. Local instillations of amphotericin B may also be used where appropriate (such as nasal sinuses). Some physicians also recommend anticoagulation with heparin to forestall thrombosis. Despite therapy, the mortality remains high. Liposomal amphotericin B also has been used with some success is cases of mucoromycosis.

Rhinosporidiosis

Rhinosporidiosis is an infection found in India, Sri Lanka, parts of East Africa, and South America. It is characterized by polypoid growth from the nose or conjunctiva. The causative organism can be demonstrated in tissue and consists of aggregates of large sporangia containing spores in various phases of development. However, they have never been successfully cultured and they appear to be related genetically most closely to aquatic protista, members of the Mezomycetozoa and not fungi. The treatment is surgical excision.

Otomycosis and oculomycosis

External otitis is often multifactorial, but in some cases dense fungal colonization can contribute to the picture. In severe cases, the external ear may be plugged by a dense mat of mycelium. Aspergillus species are the most common organisms cultured, particularly *A. niger*, but candida, penicillium, and mucor may all contribute. Intensive ear toilet may eradicate the infection without recourse to antifungal agents.

Infections of the eye, particularly the cornea, caused by fungi (oculomycosis) are rare. They often follow penetrating injuries to the globe or contamination of lacerations. An opacity develops within the cornea with associated pain and chemosis. An exudate is usually present in the aqueous humour. Prompt treatment with intensive topical instillation of drugs containing an antifungal drug such as miconazole or econazole is necessary every 2 to 4 h. Perforation of the eye may occur in advanced cases.

Approaches to management of fungal infections

Antifungal agents can be considered in four main groups: the polyenes, azoles, morpholines, and allylamines, and an assortment of unrelated drugs with specific activity.

Polyenes

The polyene antifungals are macrolide substances derived originally from streptomycetes. They include amphotericin B, natamycin, and nystatin. More recent additions to this group are partricin and mepartricin. Amphotericin B is the only one widely used as a parenterally administered drug. Nystatin and natamycin are purely topical. Amphotericin B is metabolized in the liver with low penetration of body cavities, cerebrospinal fluid, and urine. The polyenes have broad activity against a wide range of fungi. The mode of action of the polyenes appears to involve inhibition of sterol synthesis in the fungal cell membrane.

The combination of an amphotericin B with a lipid, for instance a liposome, has been proposed as a means of reducing the nephrotoxicity of this drug. Three commercial lipid amphotericins are available: AmBisome (a true liposome), amphotericin B lipid complex—ABLC or Abelcet (a ribbon-like lipid binding amphotericin B), and amphotericin B colloidal dispersion (ABCD) (a dispersion of lipid discs).

Azoles

The imidazoles are synthetic antifungal agents. They include miconazole, clotrimazole, econazole, isoconazole, ketoconazole, tioconazole, and bifonazole. The triazole series contains two potent oral agents, fluconazole and itraconazole. Voriconazole and posaconazole are newer additions Most are used topically except for ketoconazole (oral), itraconazole (oral), voriconazole (oral and intravenous and posaconazole (intravenous). These are metabolized in the liver and, like amphotericin B, affect fungal cell-membrane synthesis and penetrate cerebrospinal fluid and urine in low concentrations. The imidazoles have a broad spectrum of activity against many fungi, particularly those causing superficial infectiond. Fluconazole is less active against moulds and there are instances of both primary (*Candida krusei*, *C. glabrata*) and secondary resistance to this compound. New triazoles, voriconazole and posaconazole, are now available; voriconazole is an effective treatment for invasive aspergillosis. The allylamines such as terbinafine are primarily active against superficial fungi, but *in vitro* appear to have fungicidal activity at low concentrations.

Other antifungals in this category include flucytosine, which is a synthetic pyrimidine analogue. Given either intravenously or orally it is mainly useful for chromomycosis and certain yeast infections. Drug resistance is a major problem with flucytosine, particularly with cryptococcus. The drug shows a number of modes of action including disruption of RNA transcription following uptake by the cell. Caspofungin an echinocandin, is an effective treatment for deep candida, including fluconazole-resistant, infections. Newer echinocandins are anidulafungin and micafungin. Griseofulvin is derived from a species of penicillium. It can be given orally and is only useful against dermatophytes. It is best absorbed when given with a meal and selectively accumulates in stratum corneum in concentrations approximately 10 times greater than serum levels. Griseofulvin acts by inhibiting intracellular microtubule formation.

Management of superficial infections

Specific details of therapy are included under the separate diseases. Benzoic acid compound (Whitfield's ointment), which contains 2% salicylic acid and 2% benzoic acid, acts as a keratolytic agent by causing exfoliation of the superficial layers of the stratum corneum. Other topical agents with only weak antifungal activity include gentian violet (candidiasis or dermatophytosis); Castellani's paint, which contains magenta and resorcinol (candidiasis or dermatophytosis); and brilliant green (dermatophytosis). Selenium sulphide (2%) remains a highly effective method of treating pityriasis versicolor by application once daily for 2 weeks.

The more specific antifungals such as the polyenes, amphotericin B, nystatin, and natamycin (candidiasis) or the imidazoles (candidiasis, dermatophytosis, and pityriasis versicolor) are highly effective and probably quicker than the keratolytics or dyes, although more expensive. Local irritancy can be a problem, particularly with Whitfield's ointment, which is usually given as a half-strength preparation. Allergic contact dermatitis is rare but has been recorded from some imidazoles (miconazole, clotrimazole, tioconazole) and tolnaftate. Topical terbinafine is highly active in tinea pedis with cures being effected with less than 1 week of therapy.

Terbinafine or itraconazole is more effective in many forms of dermatophytosis requiring oral therapy than griseofulvin. In onychomycosis they are preferred. Terbinafine has occasional side effects, mainly related to gastrointestinal intolerance, although it may also cause transient loss of taste. It is given in daily doses of 250 mg. Itraconazole is usually given in 'pulses', e.g. 200 mg twice daily for 1 week monthly. Itraconazole likewise can cause gastrointestinal discomfort and nausea. Both drugs rarely cause hepatic injury, with a frequency of less than 1 in 70 000 to 1 in 120 000. This is in contrast with ketoconazole, which also causes hepatitis but in around 1 in 8000 cases. Liver function tests should be monitored if ketoconazole is used extensively over any length

of time. In high doses, ketoconazole may block human androgen biosynthesis causing side effects such as gynaecomastia. Fluconazole is also effective in dermatophytosis and is given in weekly doses of 150 to 300 mg. Griseofulvin is still the principal treatment for tinea capitis (10 to 20 mg/kg per day).

In onychomycosis caused by dermatophytes both terbinafine and itraconazole lead to remission of toe-nail infections in only 3 months. Terbinafine is used on a daily basis, whereas itraconazole is given in a pulsed regimen, 200 mg twice daily for 1 week every month for 3 to 4 months. There is one study which shows better responses with terbinafine for toe-nail disease. Amorolfine, a morpholine drug, is used in the topical treatment of nail disease where there is less than complete involvement of the nails. It can be given together with other drugs, such as terbinafine.

Management of deep mycoses

Very few drugs are effective in systemic fungal infections, and those that are used should always be accompanied by supportive measures and, if possible, an attempt to eliminate any predisposing conditions. For instance, if their condition permits, patients who have developed a candidaemia while a central venous line is in place should be managed by removal of the line. However, fluconazole is also usually given as well. In the patient with neutropenia, a positive blood culture would be regarded as evidence of dissemination and antifungal therapy would be required.

Amphotericin B is given intravenously in a 5% dextrose infusion not containing additional drugs, if possible. A test dose of 1 to 5 mg is given over 2 h and this is followed by gradually increasing doses over the next 3 to 9 days to the normal maximum of 0.6 to 1.0 mg/kg body weight daily depending on the infection. In some cases this slow approach may help the patient to tolerate the drug better, or may define the dose at which side effects such as pyrexia start. In severely ill patients, half of the full dose may be given 4 h after a test dose of 5 mg, usually under hydrocortisone cover. The full dose is given 24 h later. Side effects include thrombophlebitis, nausea, hypotension, and pyrexia. Renal clearance may fall in the initial period but this usually returns to normal after a temporary halt in therapy. More permanent renal tubular damage may follow a total dose of 4 g or more. Amphotericin B does not penetrate urine, cerebrospinal fluid, or peritoneal fluid in significant concentrations. Local instillations (such as the peritoneum) can be used, but can be highly irritant. Amphotericin B is normally given until clinical or mycological cure is induced. This is often difficult to judge accurately and in many of the mycoses caused by the systemic pathogens a course of at least 2 g is often used on an empirical basis. In the opportunistic infections, lower total doses are probably effective and the length of treatment should depend on the clinician's judgement.

This approach is not necessary with the lipid-associated amphotericin B formulations, which can be given without the slow buildup. The initial dose is usually 1 mg/kg but standard daily doses of 3 mg/kg are common. Patients are less likely to develop renal impairment although it can occur. There have been a few clinical trials comparing these formulations with amphotericin B and these show equal efficacy with less toxicity; however, these formulations are expensive. The main lipid-associated formulations are given above.

The azole drugs are also used in systemic mycoses. Fluconazole is given in systemic candidiasis, urinary tract infections, and as a long-term suppressive, in addition to primary therapy, in cryptococcosis in patients with AIDS. Side effects are uncommon, although it can cause nausea and vomiting. Fluconazole can be given orally or intravenously. It penetrates urine in effective concentrations. Its daily dosage varies from 100 to 200 mg for oropharyngeal infections to 600 to 800 mg for disseminated candidiasis. It is highly active in candida infections. It can also be used in some endemic mycoses such as histoplasmosis. Resistance to fluconazole has mainly been recorded with oropharyngeal candidiasis, principally in HIV-positive patients, although it can occur with other candida infections; e.g. *C. krusei* and *C. glabrata* are often primarily resistant to this drug.

Itraconazole has been evaluated in a variety of systemic mycoses from aspergillosis to cryptococcosis. Its active range includes histoplasmosis, sporotrichosis, chromoblastomycosis, blastomycosis, coccidioidomycosis, and paracoccidioidomycosis. Itraconazole is used as an oral preparation, but an intravenous formulation is now available. Oral absorption is often defective in individuals with AIDS and patients after bone marrow transplantation and in these groups the mean daily dosage is doubled (200 mg). An itraconazole suspension is also available for treatment of oral infections.

Voriconazole is now the treatment of choice for aspergillosis and for some other systemic mycosis. Long-term administration may lead to photosensitivity and increased incidence of skin cancers. The indications for posaconazole include fluconazole unresponsive infections but it also appears be effective in some mould infections including some cases of fusarium infection.

Flucytosine (5-fluorocytosine) is an effective oral and intravenous antifungal agent that is primarily active against yeasts such as candida and cryptococcus. It enters urine, cerebrospinal fluid, and peritoneal fluid. Its excretion is reduced in renal failure and the daily dose should be reduced accordingly and blood levels monitored. The main disadvantage of flucytosine is the development of either primary or secondary drug resistance in a significant number of isolates, and when given in toxic doses it may cause bone marrow depression. The serum level should not be allowed to rise above 100 to 120 μg/ml.

Combination amphotericin B and flucytosine therapy may offer an alternative but effective method of treatment. Theoretically, as the drugs synergize, the dose of amphotericin B may be reduced. In cryptococcal meningitis, combination therapy using a dose of 0.3 to 0.6 mg/kg body weight of amphotericin B with the normal dose of flucytosine is more effective at sterilizing the cerebrospinal fluid and preventing relapse. In other forms of systemic infection such as candidiasis there is little evidence that it is more effective than amphotericin B alone, although this may be the case. Combinations of other drugs have not been critically evaluated *in vivo*.

Caspofungin is used in fluconazole-resistant deep candidiasis.

A new 'biological' antibody therapy (Mycograb) directed against a candida heat shock protein has recently been developed and shows considerable promise as adjunctive therapy for patients with systemic candidiasis.

Further reading

General

Dismukes WE, Pappas PG, Sobel J (2006). *Clinical mycology*. Oxford University Press, New York.

Merz W, Hay RJ (eds) (2005). *Mycology. Topley and Wilson's microbiology and microbial infections*, 10th edition, Vol. 4. Arnold, London.

Kibbler CC, MacKenzie DWR, Odds FC (1996). *Principles and practice of clinical mycology*. John Wiley & Sons, Chichester.

Midgley G, Clayton YM, Hay RJ (1997). *Diagnosis in colour. Medical mycology*. Mosby-Wolfe, London.

Dermatophytosis

Aly R (1994). Ecology and epidemiology of dermatophyte infections. *J Am Acad Dermatol*, **31**, S21–25.

Hay RJ (2005). Fungal infections. In: Bos JD (ed.) *Skin immune system (SIS)*, pp. 593–604. CRC Press, Boca Raton, FL.

Hay RJ, *et al*. (1996). Tinea capitis in south-east London—a new pattern of infection with public health implications. *Br J Dermatol*, **135**, 955–8.

Munoz-Perez MA, *et al*.(1998). Dermatological findings correlated with CD4 lymphocyte counts in a prospective 3 year study of 1161 patients with human immunodeficiency virus disease predominantly acquired through intravenous drug abuse. *Br J Dermatol*, **139**, 33–9.

Scytalidium

Hay RJ, Moore MK (1984). Clinical features of superficial fungal infections caused by *Hendersonula toruloidea* and *Scytalidium hyalinum*. *Br J Dermatol*, **110**, 677–83.

Malassezia

Ashbee, H.R (2006). Recent developments in the immunology and biology of *Malassezia* species. *FEMS Immunol Med Microbiol*, **47**, 14–23.

Candidiasis

Bodey GP (ed.) (1993). *Candidiasis. Pathogenesis, diagnosis and treatment*. Raven Press, New York.

Greenspan D, *et al*. (2000). Oral mucosal lesions and HIV viral load in the Womens Interagency HIV study (WIHS). *J Acquir Immune Defic Syndr*, **25**, 89–104.

Pappas PG, *et al*. (2009). Clinical practice guidelines for the management of candidiasis: 2009 update by the Infectious Diseases Society of America. *Clin Infect Dis*, **48**, 503–35.

Sobel JD (1992). Pathogenesis and treatment of recurrent vulvovaginal candidiasis. *Clin Infect Dis*, **14**, S148–153.

Mycetoma

Hay RJ (2005). Eumycetomas. In: Merz WG, Hay RJ (eds.) *Mycology. Topley and Wilson's Microbiology and Microbial Infections*, 10th edition, Vol. 5, pp. 385–95. Arnold, London.

Fahal AH (2004). Mycetoma: a thorn in the flesh. *Trans Roy Soc Trop Med Hyg*, **98**, 3–11.

Chromoblastomycosis

Banks IS, *et al*. (1985). Chromomycosis in Zaire. *Int J Dermatol*, **24**, 302–7.

Bayles MAH (1989). Chromomycosis. In: *Tropical fungal infections, Baillière's clinical tropical medicine and communicable diseases*, Vol. 4, pp. 45–70. Baillière Tindall, London.

Esterre P, *et al*. (1997). Natural history of chromo-blastomycosis in Madagascar and the Indian Ocean. *Bull Soc Pathol Exot*, **90**, 312–17.

Minotto R, *et al*. (2001). Chromoblastomycosis: a review of 100 cases in the state of Rio Grande do Sul, Brazil. *J Am Acad Dermatol*, **44**, 585–92.

Silva JP, *et al*. (1999). Chromoblastomycosis: a retrospective study of 325 cases on Amazonic Region (Brazil). *Mycopathologia*, **143**, 171–5.

Sporotrichosis

Carvalho MT, *et al*. (2002). Disseminated cutaneous sporotrichosis in a patient with AIDS: report of a case. *Rev Soc Bras Med Trop*, **35**, 655–9.

da Rosa AC, *et al*. (2005). Epidemiology of sporotrichosis: a study of 304 cases in Brazil. *J Am Acad Dermatol*, **52**, 451–9.

Kauffman CA (1999). Sporotrichosis. *Clin Infect Dis*, **29**, 231–236.

Systemic mycoses

de Pauw BE, Meunier F (1999). The challenge of invasive fungal infection. *Chemotherapy*, **45**, Suppl 1, 1–14.

Histoplasmosis

Ashford DA, *et al.* (1999). Outbreak of histoplasmosis among cavers attending the National Speleological Society Annual Convention, Texas, 1994. *Am J Trop Med Hyg*, **60**, 899–903.

Barton EN, *et al.* (1988). Cutaneous histoplasmosis in the acquired immunodeficiency syndrome: a report of three cases from Trinidad. *Trop Geogr Med*, **40**, 153–7.

Khalil MA, Hassan AW, Gugnani HC (1998). African histoplasmosis: report of four cases from north-eastern Nigeria. *Mycoses*, **41**, 293–5.

Wheat LJ, Kaufman CA (2003). Histoplasmosis. *Infect Dis Clin North Am*, **17**, 1–19.

Wheat J, *et al.* (2000). Practice guidelines for the management of patients with histoplasmosis. Infectious Diseases Society of America. *Clin Infect Dis*, **30**, 688–95.

Blastomycosis

Chapman SW, *et al.* (2000). Practice guidelines for the management of patients with blastomycosis. Infectious Diseases Society of America. *Clin Infect Dis*, **30**, 679–83.

Emerson PA, Higgins E, Branfoot A (1984). North American blastomycosis in Africans. *Br J Dis Chest*, **78**, 286–91.

Lemos LB, *et al.* (2000). Blastomycosis: organ involvement and etiologic diagnosis. A review of 123 patients from Mississippi. *Ann Diagn Pathol*, **4**, 391–406.

Opportunistic systemic mycoses

Magill SS, *et al.* (2006). The association between anatomic site of Candida colonization, invasive candidiasis, and mortality in critically ill surgical patients. *Diagn Microbiol Infect Dis*, **55**, 293–301.

De Pauw BE (2006). Increasing fungal infections in the intensive care unit. *Surg Infect*, **7** Suppl 2, S93–6.

Wingard JR (1999). Fungal infections after bone marrow transplant. *Biol Blood Marrow Transplant*, **5**, 55–68.

Aspergillosis

Marr KA (2008). Fungal infections in hematopoietic stem cell transplant recipients. *Med Mycol*, **46**, 293–302.

Pini G, *et al.* (2008). Invasive pulmonary aspergillosis in neutropenic patients and the influence of hospital renovation. *Mycoses*, **51**, 117–22.

Walsh TJ, *et al.* (2008). Treatment of aspergillosis: clinical practice guidelines of the Infectious Diseases Society of America. *Clin Infect Dis*, **46**, 327–60.

Mucoromycosis

Nenoff P, *et al.* (1998). Rhinocerebral zygomycosis following bone marrow transplantation in chronic myelogenous leukaemia. Report of a case and review of the literature. *Mycoses*, **41**, 365–72.

Rhinosporidiosis

Fredericks DN, *et al.* (2000). *Rhinosporidium seeberi*: a human pathogen from a novel group of aquatic protistan parasites. *Emerg Infect Dis*, **6**, 272–6.

Therapy

Bassetti M, *et al.* (2006). Candida infections in the intensive care unit: epidemiology, risk factors and therapeutic strategies. *Expert Rev Anti-Infect Ther*, **4**, 875–85.

Bennett JE (2006). Echinocandins for candidemia in adults without neutropenia. *N Engl J Med*, **355**, 1154–9.

Elweski B (ed.) (1996). *Cutaneous fungal infections*. Marcel Dekker, New York.

Gupta AK, *et al.* (2006). Onychomycosis therapies: strategies to improve efficacy. *Dermatol Clin*, **24**, 381–6.

Maertens J, *et al.* (2009). Antifungal prophylaxis in leukemia patients; 2009 update of the ECIL-1 and 2 guidelines. https://www.eortc.be/home/IDG/ECIL/ECIL3_Antifungal_prophylaxis_update_2009.pdf (accessed 7/11/2011).

Vanden Bossche H *et al.* (1998). Antifungal drug resistance in pathogenic fungi. *Med Mycol*, **36** Suppl 1, 119–28.

7.2 Cryptococcosis

William G. Powderly

Essentials

Cryptococcus neoformans, which is found worldwide as a soil organism and thought to be transmitted by inhalation, most often causes disease in patients with abnormal cell-mediated immunity, notably patients with HIV infection and solid-organ transplant recipients, but the infection also occurs rarely in apparently immunocompetent people in restricted geographical areas, especially involving *C. neoformans* var. *gattii*.

The most common presentation is with subacute meningoencephalitis, but other manifestations, e.g. isolated pulmonary disease, are well described. Diagnosis is by culture or serology. Untreated cryptococcal meningitis is fatal: aside from supportive care (including monitoring for raised intracranial pressure), the therapy of choice is an initial period (at least two weeks) of amphotericin B, followed by at least 3 months of fluconazole. Most immunocompromised patients subsequently require maintenance suppressive therapy, usually with fluconazole.

Aetiology and epidemiology

Infection with the fungus *Cryptococcus neoformans* occurs mainly in patients with impaired cell-mediated immunity. It is the most common systemic fungal infection in patients infected with HIV and is also seen as a complication of solid-organ transplantation, lymphoma, and corticosteroid therapy. *C. neoformans* is found worldwide as a soil organism; it is an encapsulated yeast measuring from 4 to 6 μm with a surrounding polysaccharide capsule ranging in size from 1 to over 30 μm. Two varieties exist, distinguishable by serology: *C. neoformans* var. *neoformans* (serotypes A and D) and *C. neoformans* var. *gattii* (serotypes B and C). Virtually all HIV-associated infection is caused by *C. neoformans* var. *neoformans*. About 5% of HIV-infected patients in the Western world develop disseminated cryptococcosis; the disease is more prevalent in sub-Saharan Africa and South-East Asia. *C. neoformans* var. *gattii* infection is more common in tropical and subtropical areas (Australia, New Guinea, and the Philippines) in apparently immunocompetent people. Recent outbreaks of *C. neoformans* var. *gattii* infection have occurred in the Pacific Northwest of North America. It has only rarely been reported in HIV-immunosuppressed patients.

The exact mechanism of infection is unknown. It is assumed that transmission occurs via inhalation of the organism leading to colonization of the airways and subsequent respiratory infection. Throughout the world, the excreta of birds such as pigeons are the richest environmental source of *C. neoformans* var. *neoformans*.

The ecological association of *C. neoformans* var. *gattii* is with river red and forest river gum trees (*Eucalyptus camaldulensis* and *E. tereticornis*) and with mammals such as koalas. It has been suggested that infective basidiospores are released at flowering.

In the case of *C. neoformans* var. *neoformans*, the absence of an intact cell-mediated response results in ineffective clearance with subsequent dissemination. The polysaccharide capsule, composed mainly of glucuronoxylomannan, is thought to be its primary virulence factor. It is not clear whether cryptococcal infection in immunocompromised patients represents acute primary infection or reactivation of previously dormant disease.

Clinical features

The most common presentation of cryptococcosis is a subacute meningitis or meningoencephalitis with fever, malaise, headache, and altered behaviour and level of consciousness. Symptoms are usually present for 2 to 4 weeks before diagnosis. Classic meningeal symptoms and signs (such as neck stiffness or photophobia) (Fig. 7.2.1) occur in only about a quarter to a third of patients. Papilloedema and cranial nerve palsies (especially VI and VII) are common (Fig. 7.2.2). Patients may present with encephalopathic symptoms such as lethargy, altered mentation, personality changes, and memory loss. Analysis of the cerebrospinal fluid usually shows a mildly elevated serum protein, normal or slightly low glucose, and a lymphocytic pleocytosis. India ink staining of the cerebrospinal fluid will usually reveal the yeast. Cryptococcal antigen is almost invariably detectable in the cerebrospinal fluid. The opening pressure in the cerebrospinal fluid is elevated in a majority of patients.

Infection with *C. neoformans* can involve sites other than the meninges. Isolated pulmonary disease has been well described and usually presents as a solitary nodule in the absence of other symptoms. Cryptococcal pneumonia also occurs. In immunocompromised patients, especially those with AIDS, subsequent dissemination is common but presentations such as cough or dyspnoea, and abnormal chest radiographs may be the initial finding. Many patients have positive blood cultures. Skin involvement

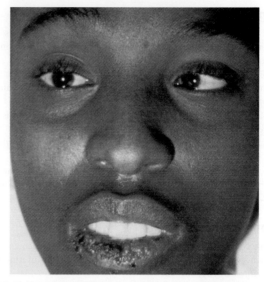

Fig. 7.2.2 Right cranial VI (abducens) nerve paralysis in an African HIV-seropositive patient with *Cryptococcus neoformans* var. *neoformans* meningitis. (Copyright D A Warrell.)

is common; several types of skin lesion have been described (Fig. 7.2.3) but the most common form is that resembling molluscum contagiosum. Osteolytic bone lesions and prostatic involvement have also been described.

In New Guinea, *C. neoformans* var. *gattii* is the commonest cause of chronic meningitis (Fig. 7.2.1). Immunocompetent people are affected. Compared to *C. neoformans* var. *neoformans* meningitis in AIDS patients, patients with *C. neoformans* var. *gattii* have more aggressive retinal involvement with papilloedema and haemorrhagic papillitis in more than a half of patients, leading to blindness in one-third of survivors.

Emergence of *Cryptococcus gattii* in British Columbia, Canada, and the Pacific Northwest

Cases of *Cryptococcus gattii*, were described on Vancouver Island, British Columbia, Canada, in 1999. The Pacific Northwest of North America (British Columbia in Canada, and Washington and Oregon in the United States) now has one of the highest incidences of this infection worldwide. Although not as clearly associated with classic immunosuppressed states such as HIV/AIDS or transplantation, infection with *C. gattii* in this region of the world is more likely to

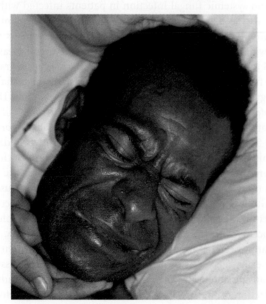

Fig. 7.2.1 Neck stiffness in a Papua New Guinean patient with *Cryptococcus neoformans* var. *gattii* meningitis. (Copyright D A Warrell.)

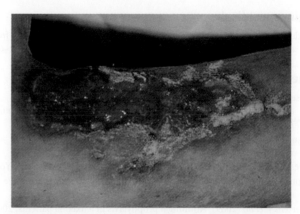

Fig. 7.2.3 Cryptococcal cutaneous ulcer. (Courtesy of Professor R Hay.)

occur in older patients with other comorbid conditions. Infection with *C. gattii* appears to cause cryptococcomas in the lung and brain (often large, multifocal lesions) more commonly than *C. neoformans*.

Diagnosis

The latex agglutination test for cryptococcal polysaccharide antigen in the serum is highly sensitive and specific in the diagnosis of infection with *C. neoformans* and a positive serum cryptococcal antigen titre of greater than 1:8 is presumptive evidence of cryptococcal infection. Such patients should be evaluated for possible meningeal involvement. Culture of *C. neoformans* from any site should also be regarded as significant and is an indication for further evaluation and initiation of therapy.

Treatment

Management of patients with cryptococcal infection depends on the extent of the disease and the immune status of the patient. The finding of a solitary pulmonary nodule in a normal host may not need treatment, provided patients have careful follow up. Fluconazole (200–400 mg/day) can be given for 3 to 6 months in most patients with localized pulmonary disease. Extrapulmonary disease is generally managed in the same way as meningitis. In patients who are not known to be immunosuppressed, a search for underlying problems should be initiated. An HIV antibody test should be performed, as cryptococcal meningitis may be the initial AIDS-defining event. Additionally, a CD4+ lymphocyte count should be considered, as cryptococcal infection has been described as one of the manifestations of so-called 'isolated CD4 T lymphocytopenia'.

Untreated, cryptococcal meningitis is fatal. In patients with AIDS, amphotericin B (0.7 mg/kg intravenously) given for 2 weeks followed by fluconazole (400 mg orally) for a further 8 weeks is associated with the best outcome to date in prospective trials, with a mortality of less than 10% and a mycological response of approximately 70%. This regimen is also reasonable for treatment of meningitis in other circumstances. Concomitant use of flucytosine (100 mg/kg per day in four divided doses) with amphotericin B may be considered. In patients with AIDS, it does not improve immediate outcome but may decrease the risk of relapse. In other hosts, more prolonged use (4–6 weeks) of amphotericin B and flucytosine may be curative but is also toxic. In this circumstance (e.g. solid-organ transplant patients requiring immunosuppressive therapy), lipid or liposomal formulations of amphotericin B may be less toxic options.

Clinical deterioration in patients with meningitis may be due to cerebral oedema, which may be diagnosed by a raised opening pressure of the cerebrospinal fluid. All patients with cryptococcal meningitis should have the opening pressure measured when a lumbar puncture is performed; if the opening pressure is high (>25 cmH$_2$O), pressure should be reduced by repeated lumbar punctures, a lumbar drain, or a shunt.

Cryptococcosis in the immunocompetent patient

Provided HIV infection and isolated CD4 lymphopenia have been excluded, immunocompetent patients with cryptococcal meningitis can be generally managed with a shorter (3–4 months) course of treatment. An approach similar to that recommended for immunosuppressed patients is still recommended; i.e. an initial (2–4 weeks) of amphotericin B-based induction therapy followed by 8 to 10 weeks of fluconazole.

Cryptococcal meningitis in AIDS requires lifelong suppressive therapy unless the immunosuppression is reversed with effective treatment of HIV infection. In that circumstance, treatment can be discontinued if the CD4+ lymphocyte count increases to over 200 cells/mm^3. In other immunocompromised patients, suppressive treatment for 6 to 12 months may be given. Effective antiretroviral therapy may also sufficiently improve the immune system such that there is an immunological response to the fungal infection. This may be associated with clinical deterioration and apparent relapse of symptoms; this immune reconstitution syndrome should not prompt change in antifungal therapy and patients should receive anti-inflammatory therapy, as needed. It has also been described in transplant patients whose immunosuppressive therapy is decreased during management of the cryptococcal infection.

All patients should receive antiretroviral therapy, although the timing of initiation of antiretroviral therapy in relation to treatment of cryptococcal meningitis remains unclear. A recent randomized trial examining the timing of antiretroviral therapy (ACTG 5164) showed that early initiation of antiretroviral therapy (within 2 weeks of diagnosis) was associated with a survival benefit (compared to later initiation). Cryptococcal infection was the second most common infection in that study. By contrast, a small study from Zimbabwe showed increased mortality in patients with cryptococcal meningitis who received early antiretroviral therapy.

Fluconazole, 200 mg daily, is the suppressive treatment of choice. Fluconazole, in dosages ranging from 400 mg weekly to 200 mg daily, and itraconazole, 100 mg twice daily, are very effective in preventing invasive cryptococcal infections, especially in HIV-positive patients with CD4 counts less than 50 to 100 cells/mm^3. However, because of the relative infrequency of invasive fungal infections, antifungal prophylaxis does not prolong life and is not routinely recommended where antiretroviral therapy is readily available.

Further reading

Bicanic T, Harrison TS (2005). Cryptococcal meningitis. *Br Med Bull*, **72**, 99–118.

Datta K, *et al.* (2009). Spread of Cryptococcus gattii into Pacific Northwest region of the United States. *Emerg Infect Dis*, **15**, 1185–91.

Ellis DH, Pfeiffer TJ (1990). Ecology, lifecycle, and infections propagule of *Cryptococcus neoformans*. *Lancet*, **36**, 923–5.

Graybill JR, *et al.* (2000). Diagnosis and management of increased intracranial pressure in patients with AIDS and cryptococcal meningitis. *Clin Infect Dis*, **30**, 47–54.

Makadzange AT, *et al.* (2010). Early versus delayed initiation of antiretroviral therapy for concurrent HIV infection and cryptococcal meningitis in sub-Saharan Africa. *Clin Infect Dis*, **50**, 1532–8.

Perfect JR, *et al.* (2010). Clinical Practice guidelines for the management of cryptococcal disease: 2009 update by the Infectious Diseases Society of America. *Clin Infect Dis*, **50**, 291–322.

Shelbourne S, *et al.* (2005). The role of immune reconstitution inflammatory syndrome in AIDS-related *Cryptococcus neoformans* disease in the era of highly active antiretroviral therapy. *Clin Infect Dis*, **40**, 1049–52.

Sorrel TC (2001). *Cryptococcus neoformans* variety *gattii*. *Med Mycol*, **39**, 155–68.

Speed B, Dunt D (1995). Clinical and host differences between infection of the two varieties of *Cryptococcus neoformans*. *Clin Infect Dis*, **21**, 28–34.

Zolopa AR, *et al.* (2009). Early antiretroviral therapy reduces AIDS progression/death in individuals with acute opportunistic infections: a multicenter randomized strategy trial. *PLoS One*, **4**, e5575.

7.3 Coccidioidomycosis

Gregory M. Anstead and John R. Graybill

Essentials

Coccidiodomycosis results from inhalation of arthroconidia of *Coccidioides* spp., which are soil fungi endemic to the south-western United States of America and parts of Latin America. Most infections are asymptomatic, but primary infection may resemble community-acquired pneumonia, sometimes with hypersensitivity manifestations such as erythema nodosum, erythema multiforme, and arthritis. Acute pulmonary infection usually resolves spontaneously, but—especially in immunocompromised patients, African Americans, and Filipinos—it may progress to persistent pulmonary disease or disseminate to skin, soft tissues, the osteoarticular system and the central nervous system. Diagnosis is by culture, histopathologic exam or serology. Fluconazole and itraconazole are usually the initial drugs of choice, with amphotericin B reserved for severe pulmonary and disseminated disease, and in pregnancy. In refractory cases, posaconazole and voriconazole are alternative antifungal agents.

Introduction

Coccidioidomycosis results from inhalation of arthroconidia of dimorphic fungi of the genus *Coccidioides*, of which the two species are *C. immitis* (Californian isolates) and *C. posadasii* (non-Californian isolates). Both species produce similar clinical effects. These soil fungi inhabit semiarid to arid areas in the south western United States of America and parts of Latin America. Hyperendemic areas include the San Joaquin Valley (California) and Pima, Pinal, and Maricopa counties in Arizona. There are approximately 150 000 infections per year in the United States of America, and about one-third of those infected become symptomatic.

Persons at risk

Residence in or travel to endemic areas is the key risk factor for acquiring coccidioidomycosis. Arizona accounts for about 60% of reported American cases. At increased risk of more serious disease are people of Filipino or African American descent, those with blood group B, those exposed to soil, and the immunocompromised (organ transplant recipients, HIV infection, cancer, and diabetes; pregnancy; recipients of tumour necrosis factor α antagonists). Outbreaks may follow dust storms, earthquakes, droughts, and activities causing soil disruption, such as archaeological digs. Recent data from Arizona have defined a primary exposure season with peaks in May and September, which correlates with seasonal rainfall.

Pathogenesis

Inhaled coccidioides arthroconidia are ingested by pulmonary macrophages and, over 3 days or more, convert to thick-walled round spherules containing hundreds of endospores. When spherules rupture, the endospores may disseminate to meninges, bones, skin, or other soft tissues. Resolution of coccidioidomycosis depends on intact cell-mediated immunity.

Diagnosis

This is based on clinical findings supported by microbiological, histopathological, and/or serological evidence. *Coccidioides* mycelia grow readily on many culture media. They are formed by barrel-shaped arthroconidia, with intercalated 'ghost' cells. The mycelia are extremely fragile, and the minimum infective dose approaches one arthroconidium, so these fungi must be handled with great caution by laboratory personnel. *Coccidioides* is considered a potential agent for bioterrorism, and there are strict rules for its handling in the United States. Histopathological findings may vary, from abscesses with many spherules, large endospores, and neutrophils (in uncontrolled disease) to well-formed granulomas with few organisms (in patients with competent cell-mediated immunity). These findings are readily seen with haematoxylin and eosin staining.

Serological methods are often used for the diagnosis of coccidioidomycosis. IgM antibodies, detected by the tube precipitin (TP) test or immunodiffusion TP, appear within the first few weeks of infection and clear within 1 or 2 months. IgG is detectable by complement fixation (CF) or immunodiffusion CF after several months and persists for years. Serum CF titres of 1:16 or higher suggest deterioration or dissemination. In coccidioidal meningitis, any positive titre confirms the diagnosis; the cerebrospinal fluid IgG titre is positive more than 75% of the time, whereas cerebrospinal fluid cultures are positive in less than 50% of patients.

More recently, enzyme-linked immunosorbent assay (ELISA) has been used for the detection of coccidioidal IgG and IgM antibodies. ELISA optical density correlates roughly with immunodiffusion CF titre. Negative ELISA results do not require confirmation by other tests. However, positive tests may not be entirely specific, and should be confirmed by immunodiffusion or complement fixation tests. A diagnostic test based on the detection of coccidioidal antigens in the serum and urine has been commercialized by Miravista Laboratories. However, problems with this test include low sensitivity and cross-reaction with histoplasma and blastomyces antigens.

Clinical presentation

Primary infection

About 60% of subjects are asymptomatic. Symptomatic primary infection presents from 1 to 3 weeks after exposure, with fever, cough, and pulmonary infiltrates, and may be accompanied by hypersensitivity manifestations, such as erythema nodosum, erythema multiforme, and arthritis. Eosinophilia or eosinophilic pleocytosis (in meningitis) may be present. Usually, however, the clinical syndrome of primary coccidioidal pneumonia is similar to other forms of community-acquired pneumonia (CAP), and this contributes to the difficulty of making a specific diagnosis. In high-incidence areas, such as Pima or Maricopa Counties in Arizona, coccidioides is the cause of up to 29% of CAP. It is now recommended that patients presenting with CAP in highly endemic areas should be tested for coccidioidomycosis. Although antifungal therapy is not required for the treatment of primary infection, it is now understood that primary coccidioidal pneumonia can be an infection with significant morbidity, resulting in prolonged respiratory symptoms and delays in return to normal activity levels. Treatment of primary disease should be undertaken with immunocompromised patients. Recent appreciation of the clinical significance of primary coccidioidomycosis makes up a substantial percentage of community acquired pneumonias in Arizona again raises the question whether fluconazole should be used more routinely for primary disease.

In addition to uneventful resolution, there are various outcomes of primary coccidioidomycosis, which include those given below.

Coccidioma formation

Pulmonary infiltrates may contract into an asymptomatic mass (coccidioma), which may persist for years. In an immunocompetent person, antifungal therapy is unnecessary.

Progressive/persistent pneumonia

Heavily exposed immunosuppressed patients may develop acute respiratory failure. Amphotericin B treatment is recommended. Pneumonia persists more than 2 months, with extensive infiltrates and, often, cavitation. Initial treatment with amphotericin B is recommended if the patient is severely ill. The Infectious Diseases Society of America guidelines suggest between 3 and 6 months for the duration of therapy, but we would favour treatment for more than 6 months after resolution of symptoms, and for more than a year with diffuse miliary disease. Conversion to an oral azole is appropriate when the patient is improving.

Chronic pulmonary coccidioidomycosis

This occurs in about 5% of patients with symptomatic primary coccidioidomycosis and may have a fluctuating course over years. Nodular lesions may cavitate, with surrounding infiltrates and fibrosis. Cavitary disease may be asymptomatic or be associated with rupture and pneumothorax, haemorrhage, or secondary infection. Cavities smaller than 2.5 cm in diameter tend to resolve, while cavities larger than 5 cm persist. Cavities may remain stable for years or become infected with *Aspergillus*, or fluctuate with intermittent infiltrates and fibrocavitary disease. Chronic pulmonary coccidioidomycosis can progressively destroy the lungs and requires medical therapy with either fluconazole or itraconazole. The appropriate duration of therapy is uncertain. If large asymptomatic cavities persist for several years, resection should be considered. Coccidioidal mycetoma may occur in pre-existing cavities and is treated by resection.

Disseminated coccidioidomycosis

Pleura and pericardium may be invaded during pulmonary coccidioidomycosis. Haematogenous dissemination occurs within a few months after infection and may involve skin, soft tissue, osteoarticular tissue, and meninges (Figs. 7.3.1–7.3.3). Papules, nodules,

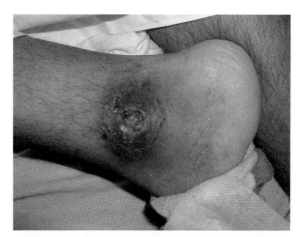

Fig. 7.3.2 Ulcerative ankle lesion with underlying osteomyelitis in a patient with coccidioidomycosis.

abscesses, verrucous plaques, or ulcers are seen. Medical therapy is often combined with surgical therapy to debulk lesions.

In chronic coccidioidomycosis, fluconazole at 400 or 800 mg/day or itraconazole at 200 mg twice daily are used but death may ensue despite intensive medical and surgical intervention.

Osteoarticular disease

Any bone or joint may be targeted, but those that are weight-bearing are more vulnerable (Fig. 7.3.4). Infection can destroy the vertebral body, with collapse and joint instability. Paraspinous abscesses should be drained and, if necessary, the joint(s) stabilized.

Central nervous system involvement

Coccidioidal meningitis may be accompanied by coccidioma, vasculitis, infarction, and hydrocephalus. Most clinicians initiate treatment of meningitis with high-dose fluconazole (800–2000 mg/day), which may be reduced as the patient improves. Lifelong treatment is necessary. Obstructive hydrocephalus requires ventriculoperitoneal shunting.

Selection of antifungal agents

Antifungal therapy of primary coccidioidomycosis remains controversial, with no randomized trials comparing different

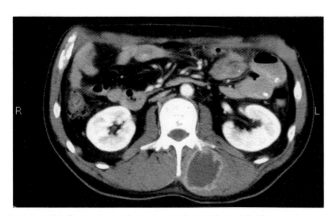

Fig. 7.3.1 CT of paraspinous abscess in a patient with coccidioidomycosis.

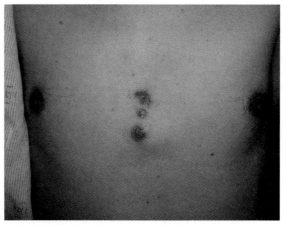

Fig. 7.3.3 Abscesses on the chest in a patient with coccidioidomycosis.

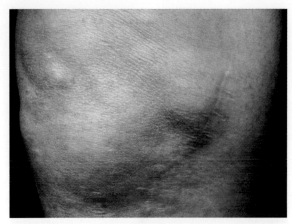

Fig. 7.3.4 Coccidioidal arthropathy.
(Copyright R. Hay.)

treatments. One observational study indicated that clinicians were more likely to treat patients with more severe disease or culture positivity. Disseminated disease developed in 10% of the treated patients, indicating that treatment of primary disease does not guarantee a benign future course. Azoles are preferred for treating most forms of coccidioidomycosis. Fluconazole and itraconazole appear similarly effective, but fluconazole is usually chosen because of fewer adverse reactions. For either drug, 400 mg/day is usually given for a year or more after clinical cure. In HIV-infected patients with nonmeningeal disease, antifungal therapy may be stopped if their fungal disease is quiescent and their CD4 count has increased above 250 cells/μL due to antiretroviral therapy. In meningitis, fluconazole has replaced intrathecal amphotericin B. Intrathecal amphotericin B is difficult to administer, and can cause arachnoiditis and vasculitis. A case-controlled study of coccidioidal meningitis comparing treatment with amphotericin B (primarily intrathecal) to fluconazole indicated that the neurologic complication rate (strokes, hydrocephalus, etc.) and the overall mortality (39 to 40%) were similar in both groups, with survivors commonly having persistent neurological deficits. Thus, fluconazole therapy for coccidioidal meningitis, although better tolerated and easier to administer, has not been associated with an improved prognosis.

Posaconazole has also been used for primary therapy in a series of 20 patients with chronic pulmonary or nonmeningeal disseminated disease. Of these 20 patients treated for up to 6 months, 17 had a satisfactory clinical response. Posaconazole is licensed in Europe for salvage therapy of coccidioidomycosis, based on limited clinical experience. Posaconazole may succeed in cases of disseminated nonmeningeal coccidioidomycosis in which other azoles and amphotericin B have failed. The dose is 200 mg four times daily, given orally with a high-fat containing meal. Voriconazole has been used successfully in cases of refractory coccidioidomycosis, including meningitis.

Amphotericin B should be used largely as salvage therapy and in pregnancy, since azoles are teratogenic. If amphotericin B is toxic or not successful, in the last two trimesters of pregnancy fluconazole may be used with less risk of teratogenicity. After therapy has been stopped, the patient should be observed for years as coccidioidomycosis has an unpleasant propensity to relapse. *In vitro* testing of antifungals in coccidioidomycosis typically shows susceptibility, and such testing is not helpful. The echinocandins have not been shown to be of value for the treatment of coccidioidomycosis.

Recently, antifungal prophylaxis has been recommended for transplant recipients living in highly endemic areas. Nevertheless, the mortality rate remains high (29%) for transplant recipients who develop coccidioidomycosis while receiving prophylaxis. Patients with a history of coccidioidomycosis may receive solid organ transplants when the disease is inactive and if they maintain lifelong azole therapy (e.g. fluconazole 400 mg/day). Antifungal prophylaxis for transplant recipients visiting the endemic zone is not recommended.

Further reading

Ampel NM (2010). New perspectives on coccidioidomycosis. *Proc Am Thorac Soc*, **7**, 181–5. [Review addressing the epidemiology of coccidioidomycosis and controversies regarding the diagnosis of coccidioidomycosis and the treatment of primary pulmonary infection.]

Crum NF, *et al.* (2004). Coccidioidomycosis: a descriptive survey of a reemerging disease. *Clinical characteristics and emerging controversies. Medicine* (Baltimore), **83**, 149–75. [Cohort study of the characteristics of 223 patients with coccidioidomycosis.]

Galgiani JN, *et al.* (2005). Coccidioidomycosis. *Clin Infect Dis*, **41**, 1217–23. [The 2005 guidelines of the Infectious Diseases Society of America for the treatment of coccidioidomycosis.]

Limper AH, *et al.* (2011). An official American Thoracic Society statement: treatment of fungal infections in adult pulmonary and critical care patients. *Am J Resp Crit Care Med*, **183**, 96–128. [Review of the diagnosis and treatment of invasive fungal infections, including coccidioidomycosis.]

Mathisen G, *et al.* (2010). Coccidioidal meningitis: clinical presentation and management in the fluconazole era. *Medicine* (Baltimore), **89**, 251–84. [Study comparing amphotericin B and fluconazole for the treatment of coccidioidal meningitis.]

7.4 **Paracoccidioidomycosis**

M.A. Shikanai-Yasuda

Essentials

Paracoccidioidomycosis is a systemic mycosis caused by the dimorphic fungus *Paracoccidioides brasiliensis*, which is found in soil and in a variety of animals, and transmitted to humans by inhalation. It is restricted geographically to Central and South America, where it is the commonest endemic chronic human mycosis, acquired in rural and periurban areas, equally distributed among prepubescent boys and girls, but more frequent in men than women (10:1).

Clinical features—manifestations range from an asymptomatic course to severe and potentially fatal disseminated disease. (1) Acute form (juvenile type)—1 to 20% of cases; presentation is with progressive lymphadenopathy; fever and weight loss are common; liver and spleen are usually moderately enlarged; other manifestations include mucocutaneous lesions and bone and small bowel involvement. (2) Chronic form—usually occurs in men aged 30 to 50 years who have worked in agricultural areas; frequently involves the lung, skin and mucous membranes (mainly pharynx, larynx, and trachea); may involve lymph nodes and adrenals, also (less frequently) intestine, spleen, bones, central nervous system (brain, cerebellum, meninges) and genitourinary system. Complications include microstomia, laryngeal/tracheal/bronchial stenosis, pulmonary emphysema/fibrosis, respiratory insufficiency and cor pulmonale.

Diagnosis and treatment—diagnosis is by (1) direct microscopy or culture from sputum, pus or other lesions; (2) histopathology—silver or periodic acid–Schiff staining reveals granulomas containing fungal cells with either proliferative and/or exudative reactions; or (3) serological testing. Treatment of mild cases is with sulfamethoxazole–trimethoprim or itraconazole; severe cases of acute or chronic disease require intravenous amphotericin B or other amphotericin formulations, followed by oral drugs. Long courses of treatment (6–36 months) are required until stabilization or disappearance of antibodies detected by immunodifusion or counterimmunoelectrophoresis tests.

Definition

Paracoccidioidomycosis is a systemic granulomatous disease caused by a dimorphic fungus, *Paracoccidioides brasiliensis*, that involves mainly the lungs, phagocytic mononuclear system, mucous membranes, skin, and adrenals.

History

The disease was first described in 1908 by Lutz, a Brazilian scientist. In 1912, Splendore classified the organism as a yeast of the genus *Zymonema* and, in 1928, Almeida and Lacaz suggested the name *Paracoccidioides*. In 1930, Almeida named the fungus *Paracoccidioides brasiliensis*. Formerly, the disease was known as South American blastomycosis or Lutz–Splendore–Almeida disease. In 1977, it was renamed paracoccidioidomycosis.

Epidemiology

Paracoccidioidomycosis is the most common endemic human mycosis in Latin America but is restricted geographically to Central and South America, ranging from Mexico to Argentina. The disease is prevalent in Brazil, Colombia, Venezuela, Argentina, Uruguay, Paraguay, Guatemala, Ecuador, Peru, and Mexico. Imported cases have been recorded in the United States of America, Europe, and Asia. Paracoccidioidomycosis is the eighth most important cause of mortality from chronic infectious diseases in Brazil, the highest among systemic mycoses.

Prevalence, inferred from the result of intradermal paracoccidioidin testing, ranges from 6 to 60.6% among rural and urban populations of endemic and nonendemic areas; lower rates were observed in the same region when a more specific antigen, 43 kDa glycoprotein, was employed in comparison with paracoccidioidin. The disease is equally distributed among prepubescent boys and girls but among adults the sex ratio of clinical cases is 10 or more men to each woman. This may be explained by the ability of oestrogens to inhibit the transformation of mycelium or conidia to yeast. The disease is most common among 20- to 50-year-old agricultural workers or those who have lived in rural endemic areas. Spouses of patients are rarely affected by the disease, which suggests that hormonal and genetic factors play a part in the distribution of this mycosis. Transmission from one person to another has not been shown.

Ecology

The geographical regions where paracoccidioidomycosis is most prevalent are humid with more acidic soils and a temperature range from 15 to 30°C. *P. brasiliensis* has been isolated from soil, animals such as armadillos and bats, dog food, penguin faeces, and the intestinal contents of bats. Efforts to maintain the fungus in bat intestines have been unsuccessful. The saprophytic habitat of *P. brasiliensis* has yet to be discovered.

Aetiology

Phylogenetic studies of eight regions in five nuclear loci of 65 *P. brasiliensis* isolates indicated initially that this fungus consisted of at least three distinct, previously unrecognized species: S1 (species 1 with 38 isolates from Brazil, Argentina, Paraguay, Peru, and Venezuela isolates), PS2 (phylogenetic species 2 with five Brazilian and one Venezuelan isolates), and PS3 (phylogenetic species 3 with 21 Colombian isolates). Additionally, other Brazilian isolate 'Pb01-like' species exhibit great sequence and morphological divergence from the S1/PS2/PS3 species clade and was named as *Paracoccidioides lutzii*.

Mycology

P. brasiliensis is a dimorphic fungus that can be cultivated either as a mould or a yeast. When cultured at 25°C, it appears after 15 to 30 days as white colonies. When Sabouraud's dextrose agar is used, the mycelium shows hyaline septate hyphae with branches.

P. brasiliensis grows as a yeast in human and animal tissues (Fig. 7.4.1) and in cultures maintained at 37°C. Colonies can be observed after 7 to 20 days. Under direct microscopy, yeast forms are seen as oval or spherical cells with doubly refractile walls; the cells vary in size from buds of 2 to 10 μm in diameter

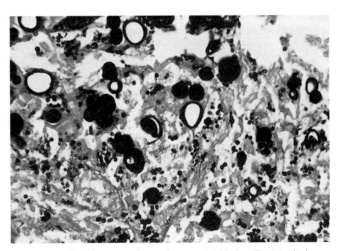

Fig. 7.4.1 Small and large yeast forms of *Paracoccidioides brasiliensis* in the lung of a transplant recipient (methenamine silver stain).
(Courtesy of C S Lacaz.)

to mature cells of 20 to 30 μm. Mother cells may produce 10 to 12 uniform or variably sized buds (Fig. 7.4.2), forming the characteristic 'pilot wheel' shape observed in biological samples or in infected tissues.

Conidia produced by mycelium represent the infectious form and are inhaled through the respiratory tract.

Analysis of 6022 assembled groups from mycelium and yeast phase expressed sequence tags of about 80% of the estimated genome of *P. brasiliensis*. The transcriptome analysis reported information about sequences related to the cell cycle, stress response, drug resistance, and signal transduction pathways of the pathogen.

Virulence

Virulence, defined as the ability to produce disseminated infection in experimental animals, varies between different fungal isolates but little is understood of the biochemical basis for these differences. The presence of higher levels of α-1,3-glucan in virulent strains of *P. brasiliensis* compared with avirulent strains was initially related to virulence, but no correlation has been shown between glucans and virulence in experimentally induced infections. Binding of laminin to yeast cells (possibly through binding to gp43) enhanced their pathogenicity in the hamster testicle model.

Pathogenesis

Experimental and clinicopathological observations indicate that the respiratory route is the main portal of entry and the lung is the primary site of infection.

The first fungus–host contact occurs through inhalation of airborne conidia. When mice are experimentally infected through the respiratory route, conidia have been observed in the alveoli soon after inoculation. Some 12 to 18 h after the exposure, yeast forms can be observed in the alveoli. There is an initial inflammatory response, which is mediated by polymorphonuclear cells, followed by granuloma formation.

The primary infective complex develops at the inoculation site and involves the surrounding lymphatic vessels and regional lymph nodes. The fungus spreads to other parts of the lung through peribronchial lymphatic vessels and drains into regional lymph nodes. Haematogenous dissemination to a variety of organs and tissues may occur at this time. The lesions usually undergo involution and

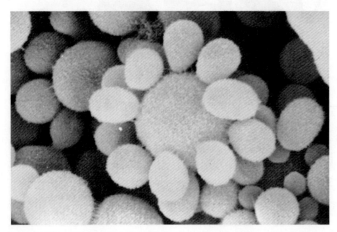

Fig. 7.4.2 Scanning electron micrograph of a multiple budding yeast cell of *Paracoccidioides brasiliensis*.
(Courtesy of C S Lacaz.)

the fungi remain dormant if the host's immune response can control their proliferation. A balanced host–fungus relationship is associated with the absence of symptoms, although, in some children or young adults, acute disease may arise, primarily affecting the phagocytic mononuclear system. In adult life, previously quiescent lesions may become reactivated, especially in the lungs, leading to the adult or chronic form of the disease.

Pathology

The characteristic lesion is a granuloma containing *P. brasiliensis* cells. The infected tissue may exhibit a predominantly proliferative, granulomatous inflammatory response and/or an exudative reaction, sometimes resulting in necrosis, with variable numbers of neutrophils and large numbers of extracellular yeast cells, leading to a chronic epithelioid granuloma.

Autopsy studies, mainly of adult patients, indicate that the organs most frequently involved are the lungs (42–96%), adrenals (44–80%), lymph nodes (28–72%), pharynx/larynx (18–60%), and skin/other mucosal surfaces (2.7–64%).

Host–fungal interaction

Nonspecific immune response

The influence of genetic factors on the individual susceptibility to this mycosis is suggested by the observation of higher rates of HLA phenotypes A9, B13, B40, and Cw3 among patients than in controls and higher rates of HLA DRB1*11 in patients with unifocal disease than with other forms of the. In isogenic mice, resistance to *P. brasiliensis* is controlled by a single autosomal gene.

The ability of circulating human neutrophils obtained by bronchoalveolar washing to digest the yeast forms of fungi was impaired in severe cases, while this defect was absent in uninfected family members of patients.

Specific immune response

Host–fungal interaction in infection and disease was analysed through *in vivo* intradermal tests for ubiquitous fungal antigens, *in vitro* lymphoblastic transformation tests, and intra- and extracellular cytokines secretion, chemokines and regulatory T cell activity after stimulation with mitogens or *P. brasiliensis* antigens (PbAg). Infected people (asymptomatic individuals without disease) showed a positive skin test to PbAg, absence of specific antibodies, a vigorous lymphoproliferative response to PbAg, and a typical T-helper (Th) type 1 pattern of cytokines (see Table 7.4.1). They had a higher expression of CD80 monocytes and lower expression of CD86 monocytes compared to patients with chronic or acute disease. Patients with acute disease showed impairment of proliferative response to PbAg and Th2 cytokine pattern. This pattern is associated with poor granuloma formation, spreading of the fungus and high levels of antibody production (immunoglobulins IgG 1, IgG 4, and IgE). Patients with chronic disease had intermediate profiles. The specific lymphoproliferative response was lower than in asymptomatic paracoccidioidomycosis-infected patients but higher than in patients with acute disease (see Table 7.4.1).

More recent research indicates that regulatory T cells exhibiting suppressive activity in patients' cells seem to play a role in controlling local and systemic immune response. In mice, treatment of dendritic cells with gp43 plus lipopolysaccharide was followed by increase of fungal colony forming units in the lungs in comparison with controls, suggesting that gp43 might reduce effectiveness

Table 7.4.1 Host–fungal interaction in paracoccidioidomycosis: cytokine secretion and *P. brasiliensis* antigenaemia/antigenuria in infection and disease

Groups	Cytokine secretion and antigenaemia/antigenuria	Intracellular cytokines
Infection[a]	IFγ, Ab undetectable	IFγ↑, TNFα↑, IL-2↑
Acute disease	IFγ↓, IL-4↑↑, IL-5↑↑, IL-10↑, Ab↑ (IgG 4), antigenaemia/antigenuria↑	IFγ↓, TNFα↓, IL-2↓
Chronic disease	IFγ↓, IL-4↑, IL-5↑, IL-10↑, Ab↑ (IgG 2)	IFγ↓, TNFα↓, IL-2↓
Immunosuppressed patients	? IFγ↓, IL-10↑, ? IL-4, ? IL-5↓, Ab increased or lower levels, antigenaemia/antigenuria ↑	?[b]

Ab, antibodies; IF, interferon; IL, interleukin; TNFα, tumour necrosis factor α; ↓, decrease; ↑, increase.

[a] Asymptomatic individuals sensitized by *P. brasiliensis* antigens without signs and symptoms.

[b] Decrease in lymphoproliferation in response to *P. brasiliensis* antigens: intracellular cytokines unknown.

of the immune response in the primary infection. In pulmonary murine paracoccidioidomycosis, a dual role of interleukin 4 (IL-4, a Th2 cytokine) was observed in IL-4-depleted mice depending on the host genetic pattern: isogenic resistant mice showed better control of the disease. Conversely, susceptible mice showed enhanced pulmonary infection, suggesting a role for IL-4 in the modulation of immune response, not only as Th2 cytokine.

Antibodies may enhance phagocytosis through opsonization of the fungus, but their role in resistance is not established. The importance of late hypersensitivity in protection has been observed recently in patients receiving cytotoxic therapy for associated neoplasms and in those with AIDS presenting severe disease.

Clinical features

The range is from an asymptomatic course to severe and potentially fatal disseminated disease. The incubation period is unknown except in a laboratory worker, who developed a skin lesion some days after an accidental inoculation. The disease has been reported in children 3 years of age or older who had lived for some years in the endemic area.

A proposed classification of clinical forms of paracoccidioidomycosis is shown in Box 7.4.1.

> **Box 7.4.1** Paracoccidioidomycosis: proposed classification of clinical forms
>
> ◆ Paracoccidioidomycosis infection
> ◆ Regressive (self-healing) paracoccidioidomycosis
> ◆ Paracoccidioidomycosis disease
> • Acute form (juvenile type)—moderate or severe
> • Chronic form (adult type)—mild, moderate, or severe
> ◆ Sequelae

Localization in a particular tissue or organ and the degree of severity of the disease according to established criteria make this classification easily and uniformly applicable. General and nutritional debility and organ dysfunction (lung, brain, adrenals, bone marrow) indicate the severity of the disease. In immunosuppressed patients, signs of chronic and acute disease are observed simultaneously, with dissemination of fungi through phagocytic mononuclear cells.

Acute form (juvenile type)

Children, adolescents, and young adults (under 30 years of age) are affected, men and women equally. Only 1 to 20% of patients fall into this group. There is progression for 2 or 3 months or longer, characterized by involvement of the phagocytic mononuclear system. Cervical, axillary, and inguinal nodes are the most commonly enlarged (Fig. 7.4.3). Nodes are initially hard but are sometimes fluctuant and drain pus rich in fungi. Less frequently, deep-seated lymph nodes may also be affected. When the hepatic perihilar lymph nodes are enlarged, they may produce symptoms of obstructive jaundice.

The liver and spleen are usually moderately enlarged. Bones (clavicle, scapulae, ribs, skull, long, and flat bones) and, rarely, the bone marrow may be involved. Radiographs show lytic lesions without periosteal reaction. Involvement of the small bowel may be asymptomatic or produce abdominal pain, diarrhoea, constipation, and even intestinal obstruction. Radiological studies of the digestive tract reveal intestinal tract involvement in about 50% of clinical cases. Fever and weight loss are common. Multiple mucocutaneous lesions are more frequent in some geographical areas (Fig. 7.4.4). High transient blood eosinophilia (up to 30 000/mm³) has sometimes been described.

Clinical lung involvement is rarely described in this form of paracoccidioidomycosis. In some case reports, either bronchopneumonia or primary complex-like disease have been observed.

Chronic form

This form of the disease usually occurs in 30- to 50-year-old men who have worked in agricultural areas. The male to female ratio varies from 10:1 to 25:1. The evolution is insidious and, in many cases, clinically mild.

The organ most frequently involved is the lung, followed by skin and mucous membranes, mainly pharynx, larynx, and trachea.

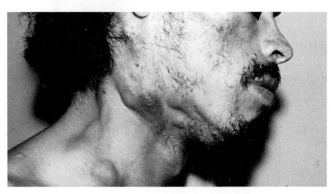

Fig. 7.4.3 Lymph node and skin involvement in a patient with the acute form of paracoccidioidomycosis.
(Courtesy of C S Lacaz.)

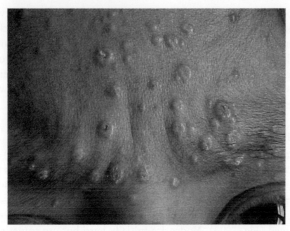

Fig. 7.4.4 Multiple molluscum-like lesions in a young Peruvian patient.
(Copyright Francisco Bravo, Lima.)

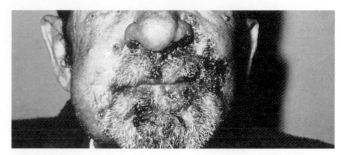

Fig. 7.4.6 Mucocutaneous lesions in a patient with chronic paracoccidioidomycosis.
(Courtesy of C S Lacaz.)

Lymph nodes and adrenals may be compromised. More than one organ or tissue is usually involved. Less frequently, intestine, spleen, bones, central nervous system (brain, cerebellum, meninges), eyes, genitourinary system, myocardium, pericardium, and arteries are involved.

The patients may be asymptomatic or complain of dyspnoea, cough, sometimes purulent sputum, and, rarely, haemoptysis. Fever is unusual. Physical examination is frequently normal or there may be scattered rales. In contrast, chest radiography commonly reveals bilateral, asymmetrical, reticulonodular infiltrates in the middle and lower parts of the lungs (Fig. 7.4.5). Apical cavities and pleural effusions are less frequently observed.

Cutaneous lesions include papules, pustules, ulcers, crusted ulcers, vegetations, tuberculoids, verrucoids, or acneiform lesions mainly on the face (Fig. 7.4.6) or limbs. Multiple, scattered lesions result from haematogenous dissemination (Fig. 7.4.7). Subcutaneous cold abscesses, more commonly associated with bone lesions, can occur.

Mucosal lesions are usually in the mouth and/or oropharynx, including the palate (Fig. 7.4.8), uvula, and tonsils, or in the respiratory tract, involving mainly the larynx (vocal cords, glottis, and epiglottis) and trachea. Pain is usually intense and may hamper mastication and swallowing. Hoarseness and dysphonia result from laryngeal lesions and may lead to obstruction of the upper respiratory tract. Examination shows ulcerative, verrucous, vegetant, and infiltrative 'moriform' stomatitis, resembling a raspberry, with papules, vesicles, and haemorrhagic spots. The last is characteristic of this mycosis and appears as shallow ulcers, with a granular surface showing multiple, fine, haemorrhagic points.

Few lymph nodes may be involved, in contrast to the acute form of the disease.

Uni- or bilateral lesions in the adrenal glands have been found in about half of patients coming to autopsy. Partial adrenal insufficiency has been documented in about 40% of the cases but only 7.4% were symptomatic.

Concomitant tuberculosis is observed in about 10 to 15% of cases of pulmonary paracoccidioidomycosis and has also been described

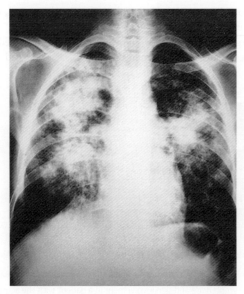

Fig. 7.4.5 Alveolar and interstitial infiltrates in both lungs in a patient with chronic paracoccidioidomycosis.
(Department of Infectious and Parasitic Diseases, School of Medicine, University of São Paulo.)

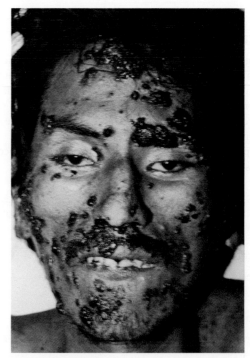

Fig. 7.4.7 Disseminated skin lesions.
(Courtesy of Universidad Peruviana Cayetano Heredia.)

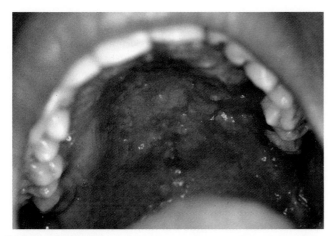

Fig. 7.4.8 Palatal lesion.
(Copyright D A Warrell.)

in cases of lymph node involvement by *P. brasiliensis*. Carcinomas may arise in pulmonary or mucosal mycotic lesions.

Sequelae

Nowadays, sequelae constitute one of the most important problems in the management of paracoccidioidomycosis. Although fungal multiplication can been controlled by chemotherapy, impairment of vital functions might prove fatal.

Acute form

Lesions in the small intestine and mesenteric lymph nodes may fibrose, causing lymphatic obstruction, intestinal malabsorption, or protein-losing enteropathy. A clinical picture of severe malnutrition and immunodeficiency has been reported (Fig. 7.4.9).

Chronic form

As the lesions usually tend to heal by fibrosis, sequelae such as microstomia and laryngeal, tracheal, or even bronchial stenosis may be observed. Corrective surgery is indicated.

Pulmonary emphysema, fibrosis, respiratory insufficiency, and, finally, cor pulmonale are frequent sequelae. Obstructive and restrictive patterns of ventilatory defect have been found in about 36 and

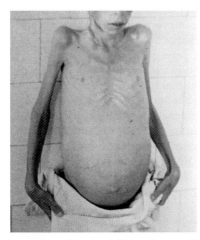

Fig. 7.4.9 Ascites, cachexia, and immunodeficiency due to malabsorption and protein-losing enteropathy as sequelae of acute paracoccidioidomycosis.
(Courtesy of M. Shiroma.)

16% of patients, respectively. As many as 30% of these patients may die as a result of respiratory or cardiorespiratory failure. Adrenal reserve is decreased in 15 to 50% of patients and there is central nervous system dysfunction in about 6 to 25% of patients.

Diagnosis

Microbiological identification

Isolated or budding (single or multiple) mother cells are observed under direct microscopy in sputum, pus from lymph nodes, and material from the skin or mucous membrane lesions.

Specimens are cultured at 37°C on blood, chocolate, or yeast extract agar. The colonies are produced after 7 days, usually in 10 to 20 days. Cultures can be maintained at 25°C on Sabouraud's dextrose agar, where the colonies may be noticed after 15 to 30 days.

Histopathology

Silver or periodic acid–Schiff staining is required to detect the fungus on sputum. Diagnostic features are the variable size (1–30 μm) of the yeast cells, and their multiple budding. Proliferative or exudative reactions, as described in the section on pathology, may be observed.

Immunological tests

Serological reactions

Immunodiffusion (Ouchterlony) and counterimmunoelectrophoresis are the best techniques initially. Sensitivities and specificities are as high as 95%. Cross reactions are mainly with other deep mycoses such as histoplasmosis, aspergillosis, cryptococcosis, and candidiasis.

Complement fixation and indirect immunofluorescence are less reliable tests for diagnosis but they can be employed in patients under treatment.

Recently, enzyme immunoassays employing PbAgs, including a 43 kDa glycoprotein, have shown high sensitivity and specificity. Antibody titres tend to decrease about 3 to 6 months after starting specific therapy and to disappear after 9 months to 5 years or more.

Antigenaemia and antigenuria have been considered useful indications in patients presenting low levels of antibodies in the sera, both for diagnosis and follow-up after treatment, particularly in an immunocompromised host. Circulating gp43 and gp70 antigens were detected in 100% of cerebrospinal fluid and almost all serum samples of patients with neuroparacoccidioidomycosis.

The correlation between immunological and histopathological findings and clinical forms is outlined in Table 7.4.1.

Treatment

Clinically active disease is treated for between 6 and 36 months until stabilization or disappearance of antibodies detected by immunodiffusion or counterimmunoelectrophoresis tests. In milder cases, co-trimoxazole (160 mg of trimethoprim and 800 mg of sulphamethoxazole) or imidazoles (itraconazole 100–400 mg/day) have been shown to be effective. In a randomized trial, sulphadiazine (150 mg/kg per day), itraconazole (50–100 mg/day), and ketoconazole (200–400 mg/day) were equally effective in patients with moderately severe disease. Voriconazole has been used in a randomized study in comparison with itraconazole with similar results and, since it achieves high levels in cerebrospinal fluid, it could be useful in neuroparacoccidioidomycosis.

Severe cases of acute or chronic disease should be treated with intravenous infusion of amphotericin B. The daily dose begins at 0.1 to 0.2 mg/kg, increasing up to 1.0 mg/kg. The total dose ranges from 1 to 3 g or more. Toxic reactions to amphotericin B include fever, chills, headache, anaemia, and nephrotoxicity characterized by tubular acidosis and potassium urinary excretion and resultant hypokalaemia and azotaemia. In most cases, these reactions can be controlled until the end of the course of therapy. Liposomal amphotericin has been used in severe cases of paracoccidioidomycosis, but a short period of treatment was followed by relapses.

Prognosis

Even though the disease is easily controlled in the majority of cases, the course of treatment is long and abandonment of treatment is the most important cause of therapeutic failure, e.g. in Brazil. Normalization of cellular specific responses, particularly of the skin test (paracoccidioidin) indicates a good prognosis.

Death may occur in severe acute or chronic cases and severe cases with sequelae.

Further reading

Borges-Walmsley MI, *et al.* (2002). The pathobiology of *Paracoccidioides brasiliensis*. *Trends Microbiol*, **10**, 80–7.

Calich VLG, *et al.* (1985). Susceptibility and resistance of inbred mice to *Paracoccidioides brasiliensis*. *Br J Exp Pathol*, **66**, 585–94.

Felipe MS, *et al.* (2005). Transcriptional profiles of the human pathogenic fungus *Paracoccidioides brasiliensis* in mycelium and yeast cells. *J. Biol Chem*, **280**, 24706–14.

Matute DR, *et al.* (2006). Cryptic speciation and recombination in the fungus *Paracoccidioides brasiliensis* as revealed by gene genealogies. *Mol Biol Evol*, **23**, 65–73.

Oliveira SJ, *et al.* (2002). Cytokines and lymphocyte proliferation in juvenile and adult forms of paracoccidioidomycosis: comparison with infected and non-infected controls. *Microbes Infect*, **4**, 139–44.

Shikanai-Yasuda MA (2005). Pharmacological management of paracoccidioidomycosis. *Expert Opin Pharmacother*, **6**, 385–97. [Critical revision on treatment.]

Teixeira MM, *et al.* (2009). Phylogenetic analysis reveals a high level of speciation in the Paracoccidioides genus. *Mol Phylogenet Evol*, **52**, 273–83.

7.5 *Pneumocystis jirovecii*

Robert F. Miller and Laurence Huang

Essentials

The ascomycete fungus *Pneumocystis jirovecii* (previously called *Pneumocystis carinii*) is the cause of pneumocystis pneumonia (PCP) in humans, which occurs largely among people with impaired CD4+ T-lymphocyte function or numbers, e.g those infected with HIV, or organ transplant recipients taking therapeutic immunosuppressive agents. The organism is restricted to humans, and disease is now thought to arise from *de novo* infection by inhalation from an exogenous source.

Clinical features and diagnosis—presentation of PCP is nonspecific, with progressive dyspnoea and nonproductive cough. Examination of the chest is typically normal, but fine bibasal end-inspiratory crackles may be heard. Diagnosis is usually by demonstration of organisms on microscopy (preferably with immunofluorescence staining) of induced sputum or bronchoalveolar lavage fluid.

Treatment and prognosis—aside from supportive care, first-line therapy of PCP is sulphamethoxazole–trimethoprim (co-trimoxazole, which has a high rate of treatment-limiting adverse drug reactions), with adjunctive corticosteroids indicated for those with severe disease. In patients whose disease is failing to respond, or those intolerant of co-trimoxazole, the main alternatives are intravenous pentamidine or clindamycin with primaquine. Among HIV-infected patients, recent data suggest that early initiation of antiretroviral therapy is beneficial.

Prevention—primary prophylaxis is recommended for (1) HIV-infected patients—when the CD4 count falls below 200 cells/µl or they have HIV-constitutional features or other AIDS-defining diagnoses; and (2) other at risk groups—e.g. some organ transplant recipients. Secondary prophylaxis is given after an episode of PCP. The first-choice prophylactic agent is co-trimoxazole; alternative options include nebulized pentamidine.

Introduction

What is *Pneumocystis jirovecii*?

Pneumocystis species are ascomycetous fungi which infect a wide variety of mammalian hosts asymptomatically but sometimes cause pneumonia, which is known as pneumocystis pneumonia (PCP). *Pneumocystis jirovecii* (previously called *Pneumocystis carinii*) is the cause of PCP in humans.

Who gets PCP?

Most patients have abnormalities of T-lymphocyte function or numbers but, rarely, PCP develops in patients with isolated B-cell defects and in people without evidence of immunosuppression. In non-HIV-infected people, glucocorticoid administration is an independent risk factor for development of PCP irrespective of the type or intensity of immunosuppression or the nature of the underlying disease process. In HIV-infected people, those at greatest risk of PCP have CD4+ T lymphocyte counts less than 200 cells/ µl. In the early years of the AIDS epidemic, PCP was the AIDS-defining diagnosis for almost two-thirds of patients. Since the introduction of highly active antiretroviral therapy (HAART), although there has been a marked decline in incidence of PCP, it remains the most common serious opportunistic infection in HIV-infected people in Europe, the United States of America, and Australasia. Patients living in countries without access to PCP prophylaxis or HAART remain at high risk of PCP.

Aetiology

Pneumocystis cannot be cultured *in vitro*. *Pneumocystis* organisms from different mammalian host species show antigenic, karyotypic, and genetic heterogeneity. Cross-infection between host species has not been successful, suggesting host specificity and that pneumocystis infection in humans is not a zoonosis. The demonstration of antibodies against pneumocystis in the majority of healthy children and adults has been regarded previously as supportive of the hypothesis that PCP arises in an immunocompromised individual by reactivation of a childhood-acquired latent infection. However, this hypothesis is challenged by the failure to demonstrate pneumocystis in bronchoscopic alveolar lavage (BAL) fluid or necropsy lung tissue of immune competent people and the observation that pneumocystis DNA is detectable only at low levels in less than 25% of HIV-infected people with low CD4+ T-lymphocyte counts presenting with respiratory episodes and with diagnoses other than PCP. Human pneumocystis infection is now thought to arise from *de novo* infection from an exogenous source. Finding different genotypes in each episode in patients with recurrent PCP supports the reinfection model.

Pathogenesis

After inhalation, the organism reaches the alveoli where the trophic form attaches to type 1 pneumocytes. In an immune competent person, the organism is eliminated; in the immunodeficient, PCP will develop.

The major surface glycoprotein of pneumocystis binds to macrophages and induces T-lymphocyte proliferation and increased secretion of L1 (L1CAM, CD171), L2 and tumour necrosis factor-α. Monocytes respond to major surface glycoproteins by releasing interleukin 8 and tumour necrosis factor α. Pneumocystis induces changes in the quantity and quality of pulmonary surfactant; total cholesterol, glycerol, and phospholipase A2 are increased while phospholipid is reduced.

Clinical presentation

Patients typically present with progressive exertional dyspnoea, a nonproductive cough, and fever of several days or weeks duration. They often report an inability to take in a deep breath that is not due to pleural pain. Purulent sputum, haemoptysis, and pleural pain are atypical for PCP and suggest a bacterial or mycobacterial pathogen. In HIV-infected patients, the presentation is usually more indolent than in patients immunosuppressed for other reasons. However, in a small proportion of HIV-infected patients, the disease course of PCP is fulminant with an interval of 7 days or less between onset of symptoms and progression to respiratory failure. Occasionally, PCP may present as pyrexia of undetermined origin.

Examination of the chest is usually normal; occasionally fine bibasal end-inspiratory crackles are heard. Signs of focal consolidation or pleural effusion suggest an alternative diagnosis.

Pathology

Within the lung, *Pneumocystis* infection is characterized by an eosinophilic, foamy intra-alveolar exudate, associated with a mild plasma-cell interstitial pneumonitis. Morphologically, two forms of pneumocystis may be identified: thick-walled cystic forms (6–7 μm diameter) that lie freely within the alveolar exudate are demonstrated by Grocott's methenamine silver, toluidine blue O, or cresyl violet stains (Fig. 7.5.1). The exudate consists largely of thin-walled, irregularly shaped, single-nucleated trophic forms (2–5 μm diameter) that are shown by Giemsa stain but lack

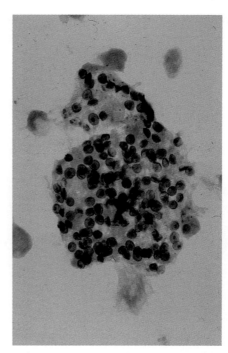

Fig. 7.5.1 Cysts of *Pneumocystis jirovecii* in lung tissue. The walls of the cysts are stained black (silver stain).

distinctive features. Rarely, interstitial fibrosis, diffuse alveolar damage, granulomatous inflammation, nodular and cavitary lesions, and pneumatocele formation may occur. Rarely, pneumocystis infection extends beyond the airspaces; extrapulmonary pneumocystosis involving liver, spleen, gut, or eye may occur and is strongly associated with use of nebulized pentamidine for prophylaxis.

Investigations

Chest radiograph

The chest radiograph may be normal in early or mild PCP. With more severe disease or later presentation, bilateral perihilar interstitial or reticular infiltrates are seen (Fig. 7.5.2). These may progress to diffuse bilateral alveolar (air space) consolidation that mimics pulmonary oedema. In the late stages, the lungs may be massively consolidated and almost airless. Radiographic deterioration from near normal at presentation to being markedly abnormal may occur over 48 h or less. Up to 20% of chest radiographs are atypical, showing intrapulmonary nodules, cavitary lesions, lobar consolidation, pneumatoceles (Fig. 7.5.3), or hilar/mediastinal lymphadenopathy. All of these typical and atypical radiographic appearances may also be seen in bacterial, mycobacterial, and fungal infections and in nonspecific pneumonitis and pulmonary Kaposi's sarcoma.

With treatment and clinical recovery, the chest radiograph in some individuals may remain abnormal for many months in the absence of symptoms. In others, postinfectious bronchiectasis or fibrosis occurs.

Arterial blood gases/oximetry

Less than 10% of patients with PCP have a normal partial pressure of oxygen (Pao_2) and a normal A–a gradient ($P(A–a)o_2$). These

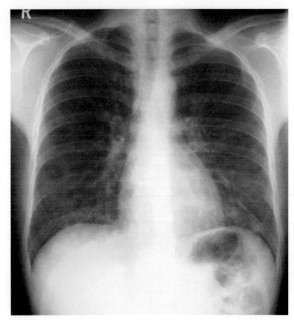

Fig. 7.5.2 Chest radiograph showing bilateral interstitial infiltrates typical of pneumocystis pneumonia.

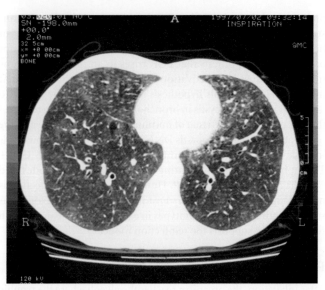

Fig. 7.5.4 CT of thorax showing diffuse bilateral 'ground-glass' shadowing typical of pneumocystis pneumonia.

measures are sensitive though not specific for PCP and may also occur in bacterial pneumonia, pulmonary Kaposi's sarcoma, and tuberculosis.

CT

High-resolution CT of the chest may be useful in the symptomatic patient with a normal or equivocal chest radiograph. Areas of 'ground-glass' shadowing indicate active pulmonary disease (Fig. 7.5.4). These appearances may be caused by other fungal infection and by cytomegalovirus as well as by PCP.

Induced sputum

Spontaneously expectorated sputum is inadequate for diagnosis of PCP. Sputum induction by inhalation of ultrasonically nebulized hypertonic (2–5 mol/litre) saline may provoke a suitable sample. Pneumocystis is usually found in clear saliva-like samples. Purulent samples suggest an alternative diagnosis. The sensitivity varies between 55 and 90% and a negative result for pneumocystis should prompt further diagnostic tests.

Bronchoscopy

Fibre-optic bronchoscopy with BAL has a sensitivity exceeding 90% for detection of pneumocystis. Immunofluorescence staining increases the diagnostic yield compared to conventional histochemical staining. Transbronchial biopsies add very little to the diagnostic yield and are associated with a relatively high complication rate (c.8%). As *Pneumocystis* persists in the lung for many days (and even weeks) after the start of antimicrobial therapy, bronchoscopy may be performed up to 1 week after commencing antimicrobial therapy without a reduction in diagnostic yield.

Molecular detection tests

Detection of pneumocystis-specific DNA by the polymerase chain reaction (PCR) on BAL fluid and induced sputum is superior to conventional histochemical methods but specificity is less than 100%. Detection of *Pneumocystis* DNA by PCR may also be achieved on oropharyngeal samples obtained by gargling with 10 ml normal saline. These molecular techniques are not widely available.

Empirical therapy

Many centres in the United Kingdom and North America seek to confirm a diagnosis in every suspected case of PCP. Others treat HIV-infected patients empirically when they present with features typical of PCP: symptoms and signs, chest radiographic abnormalities, and hypoxaemia. Bronchoscopy is reserved for those who fail to respond to empirical therapy by day 5 or who have atypical presentations. Both strategies are equally effective in clinical practice.

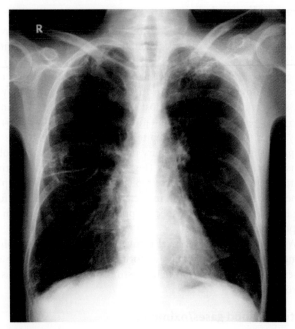

Fig. 7.5.3 Chest radiograph showing atypical appearances for pneumocystis pneumonia, including bilateral apical shadowing and a right mid-zone thin-walled pneumatocele.

Treatment

It is important to stratify PCP as mild (Pao_2 on air >11.0 kPa, Sao_2 >96%), moderate (Pao_2 8.0–11.0 kPa, Sao_2 91–96%), or severe (Pao_2 >8.0 kPa, Sao_2 >91%) as some drugs are unproven or ineffective in severe disease.

First-choice treatment is high-dose co-trimoxazole (sulphamethoxazole 100 mg/kg per day and trimethoprim 20 mg/kg per day, in two to four divided doses orally or intravenously). In HIV-infected patients with PCP, 21 days are recommended; in those with other causes of immunosuppression, from 14 to 21 days are frequently given. In mild disease, oral medication may be given throughout; in moderate or severe disease, intravenous therapy is usually given for the first 7 to 10 days, then orally.

Other treatment in patients with severe disease is clindamycin (450–600 mg three to four times daily orally or intravenously) with primaquine (15–30 mg once daily orally). Despite its toxicity, pentamidine (4 mg/kg per day intravenously) may be used if other treatments have failed. In patients with mild or moderate disease, alternatives to co-trimoxazole include clindamycin with primaquine (doses as above), dapsone (100 mg once daily orally) with trimethoprim (20 mg/kg per day orally), or atovaquone (750 mg twice daily orally). Nebulized pentamidine has no role in treatment of PCP; treatment response is delayed, early relapse is common, and extrapulmonary dissemination of pneumocystosis is not suppressed.

HIV-infected patients presenting with PCP pneumonia should receive antiretroviral therapy but face the risk of immune reconstitution inflammatory syndrome (IRIS). A recent randomized controlled trial of early versus late initiation of antiretroviral therapy in patients presenting with opportunistic infections other than tuberculosis has shown a mortality benefit with early initiation; 63% of patients included this trial had pneumocystis pneumonia.

Adjuvant steroids

HIV-infected patients with moderate or severe PCP and Pao_2 less than 9.3 kPa, on air, benefit from adjuvant corticosteroids, which reduce the need for mechanical ventilation and risk of death. Many non-HIV-infected patients with PCP are already receiving glucocorticoids as part of their regimen of immunosuppression and the benefits of dose increases have not clearly been demonstrated. Adjunctive glucocorticoid regimens include prednisolone (40 mg twice daily orally for 5 days, then 40 mg once daily on days 6 to 10, then 20 mg once daily on days 11 to 21) or methylprednisolone (intravenously at 75% of these doses). An alternative regimen is methylprednisolone (1 g intravenously for 3 days, then 0.5 g intravenously on days 4 and 5) followed by prednisolone (reducing from 80 mg once daily orally to zero over 16 days).

Adverse reactions

Adverse reactions to co-trimoxazole, which usually occur between days 6 and 14 of treatment, are more common in HIV-infected patients than in patients with other causes of immunosuppression. Anaemia and neutropenia (≤40% of patients), rash and fever (≤30% each), and biochemical hepatitis (≤15%) are the most frequent adverse reactions. Coadministration of folic or folinic acid does not attenuate haematological toxicity. Diarrhoea and rash (≤30% each) are the most frequent adverse reactions to clindamycin. Stool should be examined for *Clostridium difficile* in patients developing diarrhoea on clindamycin.

Glucose-6-phosphate dehydrogenase deficiency

Patients with glucose-6-phosphate dehydrogenase deficiency should not receive co-trimoxazole, dapsone, or primaquine.

Prophylaxis

HIV-infected patients are at increased risk of PCP as the CD4+ T lymphocyte count decreases. Primary prophylaxis (to prevent a first episode of pneumocystis pneumonia) is given when the CD4 count falls below 200 cells/μl or the CD4: to total lymphocyte ratio is less than 1:5 to patients with HIV-constitutional features (unexplained fever of 3 or more week's duration or oral candida irrespective of CD4 count), and to patients with other AIDS-defining diagnoses, for example Kaposi's sarcoma. Secondary prophylaxis is given after an episode of PCP.

The first-choice agent for primary and secondary prophylaxis is co-trimoxazole (960 mg daily: 800 mg sulphamethoxazole and 160 mg trimethoprim). A lower dose (i.e. 960 mg three times weekly or 480 mg daily) may be equally effective and have fewer side effects. Co-trimoxazole may also protect against bacterial infections and reactivation of cerebral toxoplasmosis. Alternative, less effective options include nebulized pentamidine (300 mg once monthly, or once per fortnight if the CD4 count is 50 μl or less), dapsone (100 mg daily) with pyrimethamine (25 mg once weekly (and folinic acid)), atovaquone (750 mg twice daily), and azithromycin (1.25 g once weekly).

Non-HIV-infected patients with high attack rates of PCP should receive prophylaxis (drug choice and doses as above). At-risk groups include those with acute lymphoblastic leukaemia, severe combined immunodeficiency syndrome, Hodgkin's lymphoma, rhabdomyosarcoma, primary and secondary central nervous system tumours, Wegener's granulomatosis, and organ transplantation including allogenic bone marrow, renal, heart, heart/lung, and liver.

Areas of uncertainty/future research

The mode of transmission of human pneumocystis infection is unclear but recent molecular data suggests that transmission from infected patients to susceptible immunocompromised individuals may occur and that patients with minor immune suppression, including those with moderate to severe chronic obstructive lung disease, and those receiving long-term corticosteroids (prednisolone 20 mg/day or more), irrespective of the cause of underlying immune suppression, may be colonized by pneumocystis, thus acting as a potential infectious reservoir. The drug target for sulphamethoxazole and dapsone is dihydropteroate synthase (DHPS). Mutations in the *DHPS* gene of pneumocystis occur more commonly in individuals who have prior exposure. There is conflicting evidence as to whether *DHPS* mutations are associated with poor outcome (failure to respond to co-trimoxazole or death) from PCP.

Further reading

Kaplan JE, *et al.* (2009). Guidelines for prevention and treatment of opportunistic infections in HIV-infected adults and adolescents: recommendations from CDC, the National Institutes of Health, and the HIV Medicine Association of the Infectious Diseases Society of America. *MMWR Recomm Rep*, **58** (RR-4), 1–207. [Evidence-based guidelines for use of prophylaxis against Pneumocystis jirovecii pneumonia.]

Morris A, *et al.* (2004). Current epidemiology of *Pneumocystis* pneumonia. *Emerg Infect Dis*, **10**, 1713–20. [A comprehensive review of the epidemiology of human pneumocystis infection.]

Redhead SA, *et al.* (2006). *Pneumocystis* and *Trypanosoma cruzi*: nomenclature and typifications. *J Eukaryot Microbiol*, **53**, 2–11. [A detailed account of the taxonomy of *Pneumocystis* and the reasons behind the re-naming of infection in humans as *Pneumocystis jirovecii*.]

Thomas CF, Limper AH (2004). *Pneumocystis* pneumonia. *N Engl J Med*, **350**, 2487–98. [A detailed summary of information about human pneumocystis infection.]

Walzer PD, Cushion MT (eds) (2004). *Pneumocystis carinii* pneumonia, 3rd edition. Marcel Dekker, New York. [The definite, fully comprehensive, text on the basic biology, clinical presentation and treatment of pneumocystis infection.]

Zolopa A, *et al.* (2009). Early antiretroviral therapy reduces AIDS progression/death in individuals with acute opportunistic infections: a multicenter randomized strategy trial. *PLoS One*, **4**, e5575.

7.6 *Penicillium marneffei* infection

Thira Sirisanthana

Essentials

Penicillium marneffei infection is very rare in the immunocompetent but one of the most common opportunistic infections in HIV-infected people in South-East Asia, north-eastern India, southern China, Hong Kong, and Taiwan. Presentation is usually with fever, chills, lymphadenopathy, hepatomegaly, and splenomegaly, with skin lesions—most commonly papules with central necrotic umbilication—in two-thirds of cases. Diagnosis is made by microscopy of bone marrow aspirate or biopsy specimens. Standard treatment, which is usually effective, is with amphotericin B followed by itraconazole.

Introduction

Penicillium marneffei was first isolated from Chinese bamboo rats *Rhizomys sinensis* in Vietnam in 1956. The fungus is endemic in South-East Asia, north-east India, south China, Hong Kong, and Taiwan. Less than 40 cases of infection with *P. marneffei* were reported before the HIV epidemic. Since then, the incidence of disseminated *P. marneffei* infection has increased markedly. This increase is mainly due to infection in patients immunocompromised by HIV. Most patients have been reported from Thailand, Hong Kong, and Taiwan. Cases have also been reported in HIV-infected individuals from the United States of America, Europe, Japan, and Australia following visits to the endemic region. *P. marneffei* infections have also been reported in HIV-negative immunosuppressed patients, e.g. solid organ and bone marrow transplant recipients.

Aetiology

P. marneffei is the only dimorphic fungus of the genus *Penicillium*. The fungus grows in a mycelial phase at 25°C on Sabouraud dextrose agar. Mould-to-yeast conversion is achieved by subculturing the fungus on to brain-heart-infusion agar and incubating at 37°C. Microscopic examination of the mycelial form shows typical structures of the genus *Penicillium*; examination of the yeast form reveals unicellular, pleomorphic, ellipsoidal-to-rectangular cells (*c.*2 μm × 6 μm in dimension) that divide by fission and not by budding.

Natural history

Many features of the natural reservoir, mode of transmission, and natural history of *P. marneffei* infection remain unknown. The fungus was isolated from several species of bamboo rats in the endemic area. Since the bamboo rats usually live near the forest and have limited contact with people, it is believed that both humans and bamboo rats are infected with *P. marneffei* from a common source, rather than patients' being infected by rats. By analogy with other endemic systemic mycosis, such as histoplasmosis, it is likely that *P. marneffei* conidia are inhaled from a contaminated reservoir in the environment and subsequently disseminate from the lungs if and when the host becomes immunosuppressed. The disease is significantly more likely to occur in the rainy season, suggesting that there may be an expansion of the environment reservoirs with favourable conditions for growth during these rainy months.

In endemic areas, it is likely that a certain proportion of the population is infected, but remains asymptomatic. Patients have been reported with long periods of asymptomatic infection before presentation with clinical *P. marneffei* infection. In other cases, the clinical manifestation of *P. marneffei* infection occurred within weeks of exposure to the fungus.

Clinical features

The majority of patients with *P. marneffei* infection have already been infected with HIV. Commonly, they present with symptoms and signs of infection of the reticuloendothelial system. These include fever, chills, lymphadenopathy, hepatomegaly, and splenomegaly. Cough, dyspnoea, and lung crepitations may be present. Other manifestations are secondary to dissemination of the fungus via the bloodstream. Cutaneous and subcutaneous lesions are observed in up to two-thirds of the patients. As in other systemic mycoses such as histoplasmosis or paracoccidioidomycosis, skin lesions resemble molluscum contagiosum (Fig. 7.6.1). They may break down and bleed (Fig. 7.6.2) while some larger lesions become indurated and appear infarcted. Mucosal and palatal lesions are also seen (Fig. 7.6.3). Arthritis and osteomyelitis are not uncommon. Cases with mesenteric lymphangitis, colitis, genital or oropharyngeal ulcer, retropharyngeal abscess, or pericarditis have been reported.

In HIV-infected patients, *P. marneffei* infection occurs late in the course of the disease. The patient's CD4+ cell count at presentation is typically 50 cells/μl or less. HIV-infected patients with *P. marneffei* infection have a more acute onset and higher fever. They are more likely to have fungaemia and their skin lesions are more numerous and tend to be papules with central necrotic umbilication. Non-HIV-infected patients are more likely to have one or several subcutaneous nodules, which may develop into abscesses and cause skin ulceration.

Biochemical and haematological laboratory findings are nonspecific and include elevation of liver enzymes, anaemia, and leukocytosis. The chest radiograph may show diffuse interstitial, localized alveolar

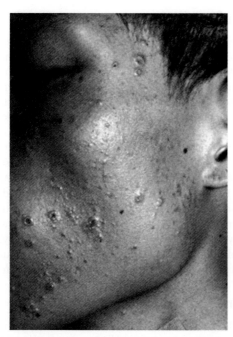

Fig. 7.6.1 *P. marneffei* in an HIV-infected Thai patient: typical molluscum-like lesions.
(Copyright G Watt, Bangkok, Thailand.)

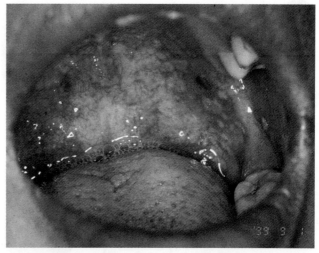

Fig. 7.6.3 *P. marneffei* palatal lesions.
(Copyright D Walsh.)

or diffuse alveolar infiltrates. Cases with chest radiographs showing cavitary lesions or lung masses have been reported (Fig. 7.6.4).

Diagnosis

Diagnosis depends on familiarity with the clinical syndrome and a high index of suspicion. Presumptive diagnosis can be made by

microscopic examination of Wright-stained samples of bone-marrow aspirate, touch smears of the skin-biopsy specimen, and/or the lymph-node biopsy specimen. Many intracellular and extracellular basophilic, spherical, oval, and elliptical yeast cells can be seen with this technique, some of which have clear central septation, a characteristic feature of *P. marneffei* (Fig. 7.6.5). The diagnosis is confirmed by histopathological sections and/or by culturing the fungus from the blood, skin biopsy specimens, bone marrow, or lymph nodes. Cases of *P. marneffei* infection can clinically resemble tuberculosis, histoplasmosis, and cryptococcosis. Tests to detect the antibody or antigen of *P. marneffei* as well as tests based on the polymerase chain reaction (PCR) have been developed. Clinical trials are needed to show their usefulness in the diagnosis of active *P. marneffei* infection and in predicting relapses. They may also be used to identify HIV-infected individuals, who are infected with *P. marneffei* but are still asymptomatic. These individuals may then benefit from pre-emptive treatment with an antifungal agent.

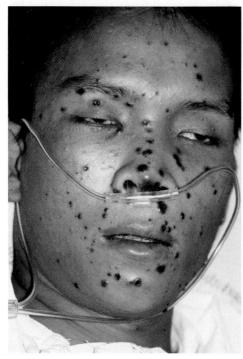

Fig. 7.6.2 Bleeding into *P. marneffei* skin lesions.
(Copyright D Walsh.)

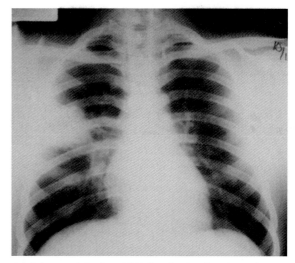

Fig. 7.6.4 Pulmonary lesion in an HIV-infected patient from Hong Kong.
(Copyright D A Warrell.)

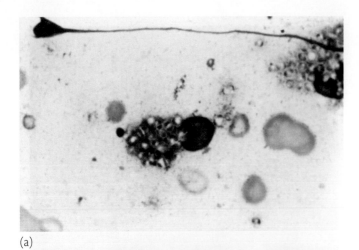

(a)

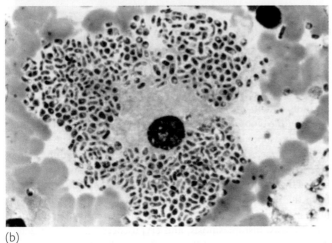

(b)

Fig. 7.6.5 Microscopic appearance of *P. marneffei* yeasts in (a) skin biopsy and (b) bone marrow biopsies, showing characteristic septation.
(Copyright Thira Sirisanthana.)

Treatment

P. marneffei infection is a potentially fatal disease. The mortality rate is high if the diagnosis has not been made promptly. The fungus is sensitive to ketoconazole, fluconazole, itraconazole, and amphotericin B. The recommended treatment is to give amphotericin B intravenously in the dose of 0.6 mg/kg per day for 2 weeks, followed by itraconazole 400 mg/day orally in two divided doses for the next 10 weeks. Patients with less severe symptoms may be treated with itraconazole in the same dosage for 12 weeks without the initial treatment with amphotericin B. The majority of patients respond well, with resolution of fever and other signs of infection within the first 2 weeks. After initial treatment, HIV-infected patients should be given 200 mg/day of itraconazole orally as secondary prophylaxis for life in countries where antiretroviral treatment is not available. In patients who are treated with highly active antiretroviral drugs, secondary prophylaxis with itraconazole can be stopped after their CD4$^+$ cell counts reach 100 cells/μl and remain at or above that level for at least 6 months.

Further reading

Chaiwarith R, *et al.* (2007). Discontinuation of secondary prophylaxis against penicilliosis marneffei in AIDS patients after HAART. *AIDS*, **21**, 365–7. [When can secondary prophylaxis be stopped?]

Deng Z, *et al.* (1988). Infection caused by *Penicillium marneffei* in China and Southeast Asia: review of eighteen published cases and report of four more Chinese cases. *RevInfect Dis*, **10**, 640–52. [Review of *P. marneffei* infection in patients not infected with the human immunodeficiency virus.]

Sirisanthana T, Supparatpinyo K (1998). Epidemiology and management of penicilliosis in human immunodeficiency virus-infected patients. *Int J InfectDis*, **3**, 48–53. [Review of the epidemiology and management of penicilliosis.]

Supparatpinyo K, *et al.* (1994). Disseminated *Penicillium marneffei* infection in Southeast Asia. *Lancet*, **344**, 110–13. [Report of the clinical findings in patients with disseminated *P. marneffei* infection.]

Supparatpinyo K, *et al.* (1998). A controlled trial of itraconazole to prevent relapse of *Penicillium marneffei* infection in patients infected with the human immunodeficiency virus. *N Engl J Med*, **339**, 1739–43. [Report on the means to prevent relapse of *P. marneffei* infection.]

8

<hr/>

Protozoa

Contents

<hr/>

8.1 Amoebic infections

Richard Knight

Essentials

Two very different groups of amoebic species infect humans.
(1) Obligate anaerobic gut parasites—including the major
pathogen *Entamoeba histolytica*, *Dientamoeba fragilis* (which
causes relatively mild colonic involvement with diarrhoea),
and eight non-pathogenic species including *Entamoeba
dispar*. (2) Aerobic free-living, water and soil amoebae—these can
become facultative tissue parasites in humans after cysts or trophozoites are inhaled, ingested, or enter damaged skin or mucosae.

Entamoeba histolytica *infection*

The term amoebiasis (when unqualified) generally refers to *E. histolytica* infection, which is common in Mexico, South America, Natal,
the west coast of Africa, and South-East Asia; nearly all amoebic disease seen in temperate countries is acquired elsewhere. Transmission
is by the faecal–oral route; following ingestion of infective cysts, a
population of trophozoites becomes established in the caecum and
proximal colon.

Clinical features—clinical features range from minimal changes in
bowel habit to severe dysentery. Onset is usually gradual or intermittent, with initially mild constitutional upset, colicky abdominal
pain, and foul-smelling stools that always contain visible or occult
blood. Less typical presentations of amoebic colitis include (1) fulminant; (2) amoebic colitis without dysentery; (3) amoeboma—
presenting as an abdominal mass, most frequently in the right iliac
fossa; (4) localized perforation and amoebic appendicitis; (5) rectal
bleeding. The most significant complication is hepatic amoebiasis.

Diagnosis, treatment, and prognosis—examination of dysenteric
stool, bowel-wall scrapings, liver abscess aspirate, or other samples
in temporary wet mounts is critical, with identification of live erythrocytophagous trophozoites confirming the diagnosis of invasive
amoebic disease. Other diagnostic methods include (1) demonstration of amoebal DNA in faeces/tissues by PCR; (2) serology—but

seropositivity does not distinguish current and past tissue invasion. Aside from supportive care, metronidazole for 5 days is usually the first-choice treatment, with the addition of diloxanide to eliminate infection from the bowel and so prevent recurrence of tissue invasion or transmission to others. Uncomplicated invasive intestinal disease (and uncomplicated hepatic amoebiasis) should have mortality less than 1%, but this may reach 40% for amoebic peritonitis with multiple gut perforation.

Hepatic amoebiasis—less than 50% of patients give any convincing history of dysentery and few have concurrent dysentery. Presentation is typically with fever, sweating, liver or diaphragmatic pain, weight loss, and tender hepatomegaly. Diagnosis is usually achieved by demonstration of a (most often solitary) liver abscess on ultrasonography or CT and positive serological testing, with a therapeutic amoebicide trial generally being preferable to diagnostic needling of the liver.

Prevention—simple hygienic measures and health education provide considerable protection: boiling water for 5 min kills cysts. Travellers to endemic areas may need a medical check on their return; but chemoprophylaxis is not appropriate.

Free-living amoebae

Three genera of free-living amoebae, *Naegleria*, *Acanthamoeba*, and *Balamuthia*, cause human disease. *Naegleria* causes a primary meningoencephalitis after bathing or diving in fresh water; Amphotericin B is an effective drug, but most cases are fatal, partly because of diagnostic delays. *Acanthamoeba* causes a painful keratitis, mainly in contact lens users, which usually responds to intensive local amoebicides, although corneal grafting may be needed; it also causes a highly fatal granulomatous encephalitis in immunocompromised patients. *Balamuthia* causes an granulomatous encephalitis similar to that of *Acanthamoeba* in both immunocompromised and immunocompetent individuals; primary skin or facial lesions are common.

Introduction

The amoebic species infecting humans belong to two very different groups. The obligate anaerobic gut parasites include the major pathogen *Entamoeba histolytica*, which ranks second to malaria as the most dangerous parasite in humans; *Dientamoeba fragilis*, a minor pathogen; and eight nonpathogenic species including the common and important *Entamoeba dispar*. The second group includes certain aerobic free-living, water and soil amoebae which produce cytopathic changes in cultured cell monolayers and cerebral invasion after intranasal inoculation into mice. They can become facultative tissue parasites in humans after cysts or trophozoites are inhaled, ingested, or enter damaged shin or mucosae.

All motile feeding amoebae are called 'trophozoites'; they move with pseudopodia and divide by binary fission. The hyaline external cytoplasm, the 'ectoplasm', is a contractile gel that surrounds the sol endoplasm containing numerous phagocytic and pinocytic vacuoles. Noninvasive trophozoites feed on bacteria. Most species can form environmentally resistant transmissive cysts by rounding up and secreting a chitinous cyst wall.

The definitive taxonomic separation of *E. dispar* as a nonpathogenic species separate from *E. histolytica* was made in 1993. This was based upon genomic and biochemical differences. This distinction is of fundamental importance because their cysts and noninvasive

trophozoites are morphologically indistinguishable, but they are now separated by specific antigen and PCR assays. All strains of *E. histolytica* are now regarded as pathogenic, whereas the commoner *E. dispar* is never pathogenic.

Entamoeba histolytica infection

Biology and pathogenicity

Following ingestion of infective cysts, a population of trophozoites becomes established in the caecum and proximal colon. Some degree of tissue invasion occurs in all subjects with at least low-titre seroconversion. Tissue invasion is frequently mild, self-limiting, and with minimal symptoms, but at the other end of the clinical spectrum it can lead to extensive destruction of the colonic mucosa. Parasite genotype may partly determine clinical outcome. Invasive trophozoites have a characteristic morphology; they may reach 30 to 40 μm in diameter and are very active with apparently purposeful, unidirectional movements during which they become considerably elongated. Their most important diagnostic characteristic is the presence of host erythrocytes within the endoplasm, which otherwise appears clear and contains no bacteria. Trophozoites containing red blood cells are described as erythrocytophagous. Progression through tissues is by active movement, facilitated by secreted collagenase; leucocytes are drawn chemotactically towards the amoebae but most are rapidly destroyed on contact.

The transmissive cystic form of the parasite is derived entirely from a commensal population within the colonic lumen. Live commensal amoebae measure from 10 to 20 μm in diameter, the endoplasm is granular and contains bacteria, and the pseudopodia are blunt and movement is sluggish. Intestinal hurry from any cause, including the use of laxatives, can lead to the appearance of commensal trophozoites in the faeces. Cysts are spherical and measure from 11 to 14 μm in diameter; when mature, they contain four nuclei, several chromatoid bodies that are ribosome aggregates, and a glycogen vacuole.

Host factors may increase susceptibility to overt disease. Steroid therapy given systemically or locally into the rectum carries great risk, as may cytotoxic therapy. Severe amoebic bowel disease is particularly common in late pregnancy and the puerperium. Before puberty, both sexes are equally susceptible to hepatic amoebiasis, but in adults this condition is much more common in males. Local disease can also favour tissue invasion; thus amoebic ulceration may be superimposed upon colonic and rectal cancers, or those of the uterine cervix. Colonic disease is favoured by concurrent *Trichuris* infection or intestinal schistosomiasis. Infection with HIV appears to have little effect on colonic disease but may facilitate liver involvement.

Epidemiology

The incidence of disease is particularly high in Mexico, South America, Natal (South Africa), the west coast of Africa, and South-East Asia. In most temperate countries, *E. histolytica* is now rare and nearly all amoebic disease seen in such countries will have been acquired elsewhere. Symptomless or convalescent carriers are the main source of infection; patients with dysentery normally pass only trophozoites in their stool and are therefore noninfectious. Cysts remain viable in the environment for up to 2 months. The infection is eventually self-limiting and rarely exceeds 4 years. Tissue invasion can occur at any time during an infection but is much more common during the first 4 months; the incubation period may be as short as 7 days. *E.histolytica*-associated diarrhoea can retard growth in preschool children.

The incidence of amoebiasis in a population is best estimated from seropositivity surveys. Surveys for cysts are of no value as their differentiation from *E. dispar* is impossible. All modes of faeco-oral transmission occur in amoebiasis. Of special importance are the food handler and contaminated vegetables; transmission by flies and drinking-water is less common. Drinking-water can be contaminated in the home or at surface-water sources. Direct spread can produce outbreaks; it occurs within institutions for children and people with learning difficulties and with contaminated colonic irrigation equipment. Household clustering is common; hand-fed infants are frequently infected from the fingers of their mother. Contamination of piped water supplies can lead to serious disease outbreaks, as happened in the Chicago hotels epidemic in 1933. Interruption of piped water supplies probably caused the recent outbreak in Georgia. *Entamoeba* infections are common among male homosexuals, but most are due to *E. dispar*; oro-anal contact is probably responsible. However, invasive amoebiasis in HIV-positive homosexual men is an emerging problem in east Asia.

Pathology

The basic lesion is cell lysis and tissue necrosis, which, by creating locally anoxic and acidic conditions, favours further penetration of the parasite; most amoebae are seen at the advancing edge of the lesion with little inflammatory cell response. In tissue sections, amoebae stain indistinctly with haematoxylin and eosin but appear bright red with periodic acid–Schiff stain; iron haematoxylin is necessary to show nuclear detail. Cysts of *E. histolytica* are never seen in tissue.

Amoebic lesions of the gut are most common in the rectosigmoid and caecum but can occur anywhere in the large bowel; involvement may be patchy or continuous. Less commonly, the appendix or terminal ileum are affected. The initial lesions are either small, discrete erosions of the mucosa or minute crypt lesions (Fig. 8.1.1). Unrestrained, the lesions extend through the mucosa, across the muscularis mucosa and into the submucosa, where they expand laterally to produce lesions that are typically flask shaped in cross-section (Fig. 8.1.2). Further lateral spread of the submucosal lesions leads to their coalescence and, later, to denudation of overlying mucosa. The bowel wall may become appreciably thickened. Blood vessels involved in the disease may thrombose, bleed into the gut lumen, or, in the case of portal-vein radicles,

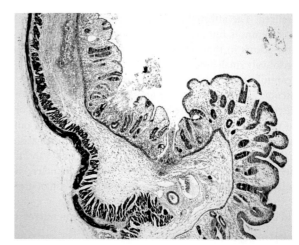

Fig. 8.1.2 Amoebic colitis. Superficial ulcer breaching the muscularis mucosae. (Copyright Viqar Zaman.)

enable dissemination of amoebae to the liver. In very severe lesions, and usually in association with toxic megacolon, there is an irreversible coagulative necrosis of the bowel wall.

Amoebomas are tumour-like lesions of the colonic wall measuring up to several centimetres in length; they are most common in the caecum and may be multiple. Histologically there is tissue oedema, with a mixed picture of healing and new areas of epithelial loss and tissue destruction; round-cell infiltration is patchy. Lesions may be annular and rarely an amoeboma initiates an intussusception; narrow, stricture-like amoebomas may occur in the anorectal region.

Amoebae reach the liver in the portal vein. Once initiated, the amoebic lesion extends progressively in all directions to produce the liver-cell necrosis and liquefaction that constitute an amoebic liver abscess. The lesions are well demarcated from surrounding liver tissue; untreated nearly all will eventually extend into adjacent structures. Secondary bacterial infection is rare and usually follows rupture or aspiration.

Clinical manifestations

Invasive intestinal amoebiasis

The clinical features show a wide spectrum from minimal changes in bowel habit to severe dysentery. Lesions may be limited to a small part of the large bowel or extend throughout its length. A relapsing course is common.

Amoebic colitis with dysentery

Dysentery, the passage of loose or diarrhoeal stools containing fresh blood, occurs when there is generalized colonic ulceration or when more localized lesions occur in the rectum or rectosigmoid. Onset may be gradual, intermittent, or, much less commonly, acute. Typically, constitutional upset is initially mild and the patient remains ambulant; mild or moderate abdominal pain is common, often colicky and maximal over affected parts of the gut. Tenesmus can occur but is rarely severe. Stools vary in consistency from semiformed to watery. They are foul smelling and always contain visible or occult blood; even when they are watery, faecal matter is nearly always present. Symptoms frequently wax and wane over a period of weeks or even months and such patients can become debilitated and wasted. In a few patients the disease runs a fulminating course. The most frequent physical sign is abdominal tenderness in one or both iliac fossae, but tenderness may be

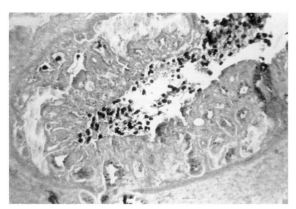

Fig. 8.1.1 Amoebic colitis. Crypt abscess. Periodic acid–Schiff stains amoebae red.
(Copyright Viqar Zaman.)

generalized. The affected gut may be palpably thickened. A low fever is common, but dehydration is uncommon. Abdominal distension occurs in the more severely ill patients, who sometimes pass relatively small amounts of stool.

A careful proctoscopy or sigmoidoscopy should be done. The endoscopic appearances may be nonspecific in early, acute, or very severe colitis; the findings are hyperaemia, contact bleeding, or confluent ulceration. In more chronic cases, the presence of normal-looking intervening mucosa is highly suggestive of amoebiasis. Early lesions are often elevated, with a pouting opening only 1 to 2 mm in diameter; later, ulcers may reach 1 cm or more in diameter, with an irregular outline and often a loosely adherent, yellowish or grey exudate. Mucosal scrapings or superficial biopsies taken at endoscopy should be examined immediately by wet-preparation microscopy.

Special forms of amoebic colitis

Fulminant colitis This may arise *de novo*, e.g. in pregnant women or during steroid therapy, or it may evolve during a dysenteric illness. Patients show progressive abdominal distension, vomiting, and watery diarrhoea. Bowel sounds are absent and there may be little or no abdominal tenderness, guarding, or rigidity. Plain radiographs may reveal free peritoneal gas, together with acute gaseous dilatation of the colon; affected segments of bowel may appear relatively narrow and show visible mucosal pathology. Barium enema and full sigmoidoscopy are contraindicated. Stools contain erythrocytophagous trophozoites.

Amoebic colitis without dysentery When ulceration is limited to the caecum or ascending colon, or when early, mild, or localized lesions occur elsewhere in the colon, there may be no dysenteric symptoms. Patients complain of change in bowel habit, blood-staining of the stool, flatulence, and colicky pain. Often the only physical sign is tenderness in the right iliac fossa or elsewhere along the course of the colon. Some patients eventually go into complete remission; others progress to a dysenteric illness.

The most important diagnostic measure is repeated stool examination for erythrocytophagous amoebae; the finding of cysts or commensal trophozoites is of little diagnostic value, especially in endemic areas. Sigmoidoscopy is often normal when the distal bowel is not involved but colonoscopy may reveal typical lesions.

Amoeboma This presents as an abdominal mass, most frequently in the right iliac fossa. The lesion may be painful, tender, and associated with fever. Bowel habit is altered and some patients have intermittent dysentery, especially if lesions are multiple or distal. Evidence of partial or intermittent bowel obstruction may be present, particularly when lesions are distal and annular.

Localized perforation and amoebic appendicitis Sudden perforation with peritonitis can occur from any deep amoebic ulcer; alternatively, leakage may lead to a pericolic abscess or retroperitoneal cellulitis. Amoebic appendicitis is an uncommon but important condition that occurs when amoebic lesions are confined to the appendix and caecum. The clinical presentation can resemble that of simple appendicitis, often with some clinical evidence of dysentery. If it is unrecognized at appendicectomy the outcome can be disastrous, with gut perforation; fresh smears should be made from the resected appendix and examined immediately.

Rectal bleeding Some patients with amoebiasis present with rectal bleeding, with or without tenesmus; this occurs particularly in children. Massive bleeding into the gut lumen can occur in any form of amoebic colitis but is rare.

Differential diagnosis

Amoebic colitis must be differentiated from other causes of infective colitis. High-volume diarrhoea, copious mucus, and severe tenesmus are all uncommon in amoebiasis. In temperate countries, nonspecific ulcerative colitis, *Clostridium difficile* colitis, and colorectal carcinoma create the greatest diagnostic problems. Parasitic conditions to be considered are intestinal schistosomiasis, heavy *Trichuris* infection, and balantidiasis. More chronic amoebic pathology may clinically resemble Crohn's disease, ileocaecal tuberculosis, diverticulitis, or anorectal lymphogranuloma venereum.

Hepatic amoebiasis

Less than half of all patients give any convincing history of dysentery and few have concurrent dysentery. In those with no dysenteric history, the interval between presumed infection and presentation may be as short as 3 weeks or as long as 15 years; for most, it is between 8 weeks and 1 year.

The dominant symptoms are fever and sweating, liver or diaphragmatic pain, and weight loss. Onset of constitutional symptoms is often insidious, but pain may begin abruptly. Most patients seek medical help between 1 and 4 weeks. Fever is typically remittent, with a prominent evening rise, brief rigors, and very profuse sweating. Liver pain may be poorly localized initially and later become pleuritic, referred to the right shoulder tip or localized to the abdominal wall. Within a few weeks, patients lose much weight and often become anaemic; a painful dry cough is common.

The most important clinical finding is liver enlargement (Fig. 8.1.3) with localized tenderness, which should be searched for in the right hypochondrium, the epigastrium, and along all the intercostal spaces overlying the liver. Liver pain, on compression or heavy digital percussion, is a less useful sign. Left-lobe lesions can present as an epigastric mass. Hepatomegaly may be difficult to detect by abdominal palpation when enlargement is mainly upwards, but bulging of the right chest wall may be noted, together with a raised upper level of liver dullness on percussion. Reduced breath sounds or crepitations may be heard at the right lung base.

Important radiological findings are a raised or locally upward-bulging right diaphragm (Fig. 8.1.4) with immobility on screening, areas of lung collapse or consolidation, and sometimes a pleural effusion. A neutrophil leukocytosis is almost invariable, the ESR is raised, and normochromic normocytic anaemia is common. Liver function tests are frequently completely normal or there may be a raised alkaline phosphatase; less commonly the serum transaminase or bilirubin is elevated. Liver scanning to demonstrate a filling defect is of great value; about 70% of lesions are solitary, but multiple lesions are common in children and those with concurrent dysentery. Ultrasonographic and CT scans are the most useful. Lesions appear round or oval and are usually between 4 and 10 cm in diameter at the time of presentation. On ultrasonography most are hypoechoic with well-defined walls without enhanced echoes. Even when concurrent dysentery is absent, the stools are frequently, but not always, positive for *E. histolytica*. Colonoscopy may reveal unsuspected lesions.

Complication

Most complications involve extension of hepatic lesions into adjacent structures: usually the right chest, the peritoneum, and the pericardium. Upward extension usually produces adhesions between the liver, the diaphragm, and the lung; in consequence, subphrenic rupture and amoebic empyema are rare, although a right serous pleural effusion is not uncommon. Untreated, the disease process

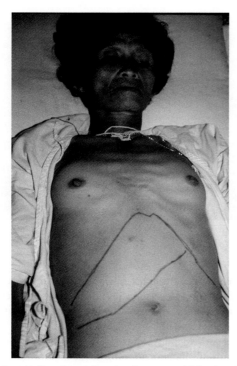

Fig. 8.1.3 Amoebic liver abscess. Hepatic enlargement with focal tenderness in a Thai woman.
(Courtesy of the late Professor Sornchai Looareesuwan.)

advances upwards through lung tissue leading to hepatobronchial fistula and expectoration of brownish, necrotic liver tissue, the so-called 'anchovy sauce' sputum. Rupture into the peritoneum can occur at any time; it is sometimes the mode of presentation of an amoebic liver abscess, the cause of peritonitis being discovered only at laparotomy. Amoebic pericarditis usually results from upward extension of a left-lobe liver lesion. Initially patients have retrosternal pain and a pericardial friction rub; later rupture or large serous effusion produces cardiac tamponade. The diagnosis is most difficult when an underlying liver abscess was not suspected.

Less commonly the lesion extends through the skin, producing a sinus and cutaneous lesion. The gut, stomach, vena cava, spleen, and kidney are occasionally involved by direct spread. Blood-borne spread to the lung produces a lesion resembling an isolated pyogenic lung abscess. Amoebic brain abscesses due to *E. histolytica* are rare; most are discovered postmortem (Fig. 8.1.5). Jaundice occurs when a large lesion compresses the common bile duct or when multiple lesions compress several intrahepatic bile ducts. Rupture into a major bile duct can cause haemobilia. Portal-vein compression occasionally produces portal hypertension and congestive splenomegaly.

Differential diagnosis
Amoebic serology and scanning have now greatly simplified diagnosis. However, a few patients, generally less than 5%, are initially seronegative; scanning patterns may be atypical before lesions have liquefied. Pyogenic abscess, especially when cryptogenic, may be clinically indistinguishable and this condition is quite common in some Asian countries. Other conditions to be distinguished are primary and secondary carcinoma of the liver, lesions of the right lung base and right pleura, subphrenic abscess, cholecystitis, septic cholangitis including that resulting from aberrant *Ascaris* worms, and liver hydatid cysts.

Needle aspiration of the liver (Fig. 8.1.6) may be necessary for diagnostic or therapeutic purposes (see below). Suspected pyogenic abscess is the main indication for the former; blood cultures should also be taken. Typically the aspirate in hepatic amoebiasis is pinkish-brown, odourless, and bacteriologically sterile (Fig. 8.1.7); a thinner, malodorous, or frothy aspirate suggests bacterial infection. A therapeutic amoebicide trial is generally preferable to diagnostic needling of the liver.

Cutaneous and genital amoebiasis
Skin ulceration due to *E. histolytica* produces deep, painful, and foul-smelling lesions that spread rapidly. Secondary bacterial infection is common and may mask the amoebic pathology. Lesions are most frequent in the perianal area, but also occur at colostomy stomas, laparotomy scars, and at the site of skin rupture by a hepatic lesion.

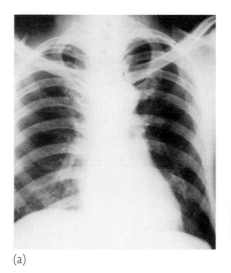

(a)

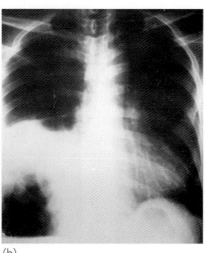

(b)

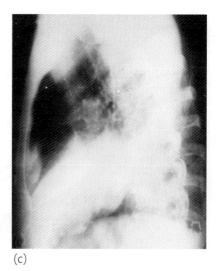

(c)

Fig. 8.1.4 Amoebic liver abscess. Radiographic changes showing (a) elevated right diaphragm; (b) enormous abscess in the right lobe of the liver outlined with air (fluid level) and contrast medium introduced during the aspiration of more than 1 litre of pus; and (c) same patient as (b), lateral view.
(Courtesy of the late Professor Sornchai Looareesuwan.)

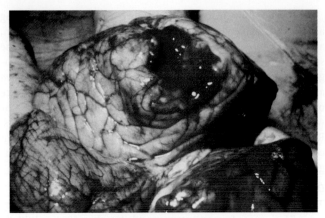

Fig. 8.1.5 Metastatic brain abscess in a patient with an amoebic liver abscess.
(Courtesy of the late Professor Sornchai Looareesuwan.)

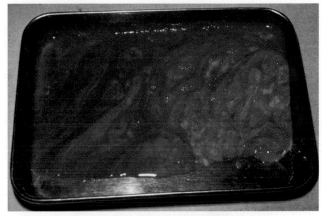

Fig. 8.1.7 'Anchovy sauce' pus drained from and amoebic liver abscess.
(Copyright Viqar Zaman.)

Female genital involvement results from faecal contamination, the extension of perianal lesions, or by the formation of internal fistulae from the gut, which can involve the bladder. Lesions of the vulva and uterine cervix may resemble carcinoma. Male genital lesions follow rectal coitus, the lesion beginning as a balanoposthitis and progressing rapidly.

Laboratory diagnosis

Microscopy and culture

The identification of live erythrocytophagous trophozoites in temporary wet mounts is of prime importance because it confirms the diagnosis of invasive amoebic disease. Amoebae should be sought in dysenteric bowel-wall scrapings, the last portion of aspirate from a liver abscess (Fig. 8.1.8), sputum, and tissue scrapings from skin lesions. In nondysenteric stools, flecks of pus, blood, or mucus should be looked for and examined. The amoebae remain active for about 30 min at room temperature. Other microscopical features of faeces in amoebic colitis are scanty or absent leucocytes, clumped or degenerating red cells, and, sometimes, Charcot–Leyden crystals. If wet preparations are not made or are negative, a portion of the specimen should be preserved in polyvinyl alcohol or sodium

acetate–acetic acid–formalin fixative for later smear preparation; alternatively, drying faecal smears should be fixed in Schaudinn's solution. In either case, fixed smears should be stained with Gomori trichrome or Heidenhain's iron haematoxylin.

Cysts and commensal trophozoites of *E. histolytica* found in wet faecal mounts are indistinguishable from those of *E. dispar*. The cysts of both species are four-nucleated and can be differentiated from the smaller *E. hartmanni* using an eyepiece micrometer. Direct mounts are made by emulsifying a small portion of stool in 1% eosin and in Lugol's iodine; however, the diagnostic sensitivity, per specimen, is only about 30%. Concentration methods for cysts such as formol-ether sedimentation give a 70% sensitivity per specimen. Cultivation of intestinal amoebae from faeces in Robinson's medium is relatively easy. Species identification requires immunofluorescent staining. Amoebae are often difficult to find microscopically in liver aspirates. Positive cultures from extraintestinal sites do confirm invasive *E. histolytica*.

DNA and immunological tests

Polymerase chain reaction (PCR) methods can now be used for both *E. histolytica* and *E. dispar* using either faecal or tissue material. *E. histolytica* antigen can be detected in faecal specimens, and assays for antigen in serum have also been used in extraintestinal disease. These new

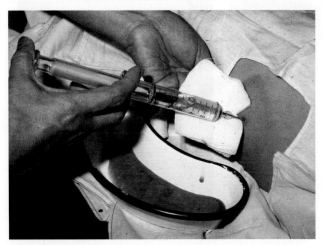

Fig. 8.1.6 Diagnostic/therapeutic aspiration of 'anchovy sauce' pus from a patient with amoebic liver abscess. Contrast medium is being injected after aspiration of the abscess.
(Copyright D A Warrell.)

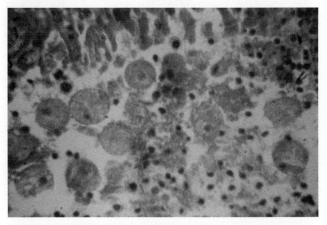

Fig. 8.1.8 Aspirate from amoebic liver abscess showing margin of hepatocytes and erythrocytophagous trophozoites of *E. histolytica*.
(Copyright Viqar Zaman.)

methodologies have excellent sensitivity and specificity. Where they are available, they greatly simplify diagnosis in both amoebic disease and in carriers. They are already revolutionizing our ideas on epidemiology. *E. histolytica* DNA can now be detected in the blood, urine, and saliva of patients with invasive disease using real-time PCR assay.

Many serodiagnostic methods have been applied to amoebiasis. The most detectable antibody is IgG, with some IgM in active disease. However, seropositivity does not distinguish current and past tissue invasion. The more sensitive methods are indirect haemagglutination, enzyme immunoassay, and indirect immunofluorescence. Latex agglutination and gel-diffusion precipitation are also used, the former being commercially available as a slide test, taking only minutes to perform. Using sensitive tests, over 95% of patients with liver abscess are seropositive, as are about 60% of those with invasive bowel disease; patients with amoeboma are nearly all seropositive. All patients with tissue invasion eventually become seropositive. Titres decline after therapy but may remain positive for 2 years or more with the most sensitive tests.

Patient management
Chemotherapy

Metronidazole for 5 days will be the first choice in most patients. The usual adult dose of metronidazole is 800 mg thrice daily for 5 or 8 days; the paediatric dose is 35 to 50 mg/kg in three divided doses. The alternative is tinidazole, which has the advantage of a single daily dose, 2 g in adults and 50 to 60 mg/kg in children. A 5- or even a 3-day course may be sufficient for tissue amoebae but rates of parasite elimination from the intestine are low. When nitroimidazoles are contraindicated, or not available, erythromycin is useful in nonsevere colitis.

The synthetic derivative dehydroemetine is a potent tissue amoebicide. It has less cumulative cardiotoxicity than the alkaloid emetine and is more rapidly excreted in the urine. Where appropriate nitroimidazoles are unavailable, as continues to be the case in many tropical contexts, this drug will continue to be life saving, especially when a parenteral drug is needed. A daily intramuscular dose of dehydroemetine of 1.25 mg/kg (maximum 90 mg) is given for 5 days.

Cutaneous and genital amoebiasis responds well to metronidazole, partly perhaps because the lesions often contain anaerobic bacteria. Amoebiasis at other sites is nearly always secondary to hepatic lesions and the chemotherapy will be the same. Metronidazole crosses the blood–brain barrier and should be used in the desperate situation of amoebic brain abscess due to *E. histolytica*.

All patients with *E. histolytica* infection treated with a tissue amoebicide should also be given diloxanide to eliminate infection from the bowel and so prevent recurrence of tissue invasion or transmission to others. The dosage of diloxanide for adults is 500 mg thrice daily for 10 days; the daily dose in children is 20 mg/kg daily in three divided doses. Alternatives to diloxanide when it is not available are paromomycin 30 mg/kg daily for 5 to 10 days or iodoquinol 650 mg thrice daily for 20 days, but iodoquinol may cause optic or peripheral neuropathy if the dose is exceeded. Early reinfection with *E. histolyica* after diloxanide is reported to be a problem among male homosexuals in Japan.

Convalescent carriers, and also infected family contacts, should always be treated. Persons entering temperate countries from the tropics or new residents from such countries should be screened if there is a significant risk of infection; those with *E. histolytica* faecal antigen, or who are seropositive and have four-nucleated *Entamoeba* cysts in their stools, should be treated. In these contexts diloxanide is the drug of choice. Metronidazole is less effective even using an

8-day course and side-effects are troublesome. Unfortunately cure rates with tinidazole are very low when followed up at 1 month.

Supportive and surgical management
Intestinal amoebiasis

Supportive management plays a major role in patients with complicated amoebic colitis, with emphasis on fluid and electrolyte replacement, gastric suction, and blood transfusion as necessary. Gut perforation complicating extensive colitis carries a very poor prognosis; management may have to be medical. Parenteral metronidazole is invaluable in these situations because of its activity against anaerobic bacteria in the peritoneum and blood stream. Gentamicin plus a cephalosporin will normally be given as well.

Amoebomas respond well to metronidazole; a slow response should arouse suspicion that the amoebic lesion is superimposed upon other pathology, particularly a carcinoma. Surgical management is important in several situations. Acute colonic perforation in the absence of diffuse colitis or ruptured amoebic appendicitis may be amenable to local repair. In the case of diffuse colitis, local repair, or end-to-end anastomosis, may not be possible because of the poor condition of the gut wall: temporary exteriorization with an ileostomy may be necessary. In fulminant colitis with multiple perforation the viability of the gut wall is uncertain and the only definitive option is total colectomy.

Hepatic amoebiasis

A favourable response to medical treatment alone can be expected in about 85% of patients. Liver abscesses may rupture before, during, or after oral chemotherapy; this requires parenteral metronidazole or dehydroemetine. Intra-abdominal rupture will always require laparotomy. Extension into the pleural or pericardial cavities necessitates drainage of these structures, together with aspiration of the liver lesion; pericardial drainage is most urgent when tamponade is present. Hepatopulmonary lesions generally require drainage of the liver lesion but medical treatment alone has been successful in some cases. Antibiotics will always be needed when the abscess ruptures into the peritoneum or lung.

The most common management problem is slow response to the amoebicide. Patients whose pain and fever do not subside by 72 h are at significantly greater risk of rupture or therapeutic failure, and aspiration is generally to be recommended. A likely explanation of poor initial response is a tense lesion that restricts drug entry. Regular ultrasonographic monitoring is of great value as it will indicate the risk of rupture and guide the aspiration procedure. No change in lesion size on ultrasound can be expected during the first 2 weeks, although its outline may become clearer. Percutaneous aspiration with a wide-bore needle will be possible in most patients; if unsuccessful or anatomically contraindicated, then surgical help should be sought. Catheter drainage is a possible alternative to repeated needle aspiration with very large abscesses. Resolution times for small or moderate lesions are unaffected by aspiration. All patients with hepatic amoebiasis should be give diloxanide to eliminate bowel infection.

Prognosis

Uncomplicated invasive intestinal disease and uncomplicated hepatic amoebiasis should normally have a mortality rate of less than 1%. In complicated disease, the mortality is much greater and may reach 40% for amoebic peritonitis with multiple gut perforation. Prognosis is usually better in centres where the disease is common and more likely to be recognized early. Late diagnosis increases the probability of complicated disease and mortality rises accordingly.

Unless parasitological cure is achieved and the gut completely freed of *E. histolytica*, clinical relapse is quite common, although probably limited by immunological responses. There is, so far, no evidence of naturally occurring strains of *E. histolytica* being resistant to normally used drugs. Hepatic scans show that nearly all liver abscesses completely disappear within 2 years; the median resolution time is 8 months. In secondarily infected lesions, bizarre hepatic calcification may be seen years afterwards. Healing of the bowel is remarkably rapid and complete; occasionally fibrous strictures persist after severe dysentery,

Prevention

Chlorination of water supplies does not destroy amoebic cysts, but adequate filtration will remove them. Regular stool screening of food handlers and domestic staff is of no value, but health education is important with encouragement to have a medical check if diarrhoea occurs.

Visitors to the tropics should not attempt chemoprophylaxis; in particular, long-term unsupervised use of hydroxyquinoline drugs must be strongly deprecated. Simple hygienic measures provide considerable protection. Boiling water for 5 min kills cysts. Routine examinations in temperate countries for returning visitors from the tropics or for new residents coming from such countries is of no value unless *E. histolytica* can be differentiated from *E. dispar*. Amoebic serology is particularly useful in those with gut symptoms or a history of dysentery.

Other parasitic gut amoebae including *Dientamoeba fragilis*

The nuclei of *Entamoeba* species have a fine ring of peripheral chromatin and a small central endosome. *E. gingivalis* has no cystic stage and lives in the mouth within gingival pockets and tonsillar crypts. It is spread by kissing or more indirect oral contact. Its possible role in periodontal disease was formerly dismissed but there is now renewed interest following recognition of its high prevalence in individual lesions in people with this condition; it may act as a bacterial vector within the lesions. It has been found on intrauterine devices that have been removed because of symptoms. Both in the uterus and in the mouth, this amoeba occurs in association with the bacterium *Actinomyces israelii*.

Five other *Entamoeba* species are nonpathogenic colonic commensals. *Entamoeba coli* has eight-nucleated cysts and is the commonest species in most surveys. *E. dispar* and *E. hartmanni* both have cysts with four nuclei; the former was previously known as 'nonpathogenic *E. histolytica*' and the latter as 'small race *E. histolytica*'. Size is the only simple diagnostic criterion for *E. hartmanni*; its cysts are less than 10 μm in diameter. The relative prevalence of *E. dispar* and *E. histolytica* varies greatly, but the former is usually much more common, especially where sanitation and water supplies are better. *E. chattoni* is primarily a pig and primate parasite; the cyst has one nucleus and an 'inclusion body'. Human infections are common in highland Papua New Guinea where humans and pigs may share a peridomestic environment; elsewhere it is rare. Lastly there is *E. moshkovskii*, which normally lives in soil and sewage; it infects and can be transmitted between humans. It was previously incorrectly referred to a low-temperature variant of *E. histolytica*.

Endolimax nana and *Iodamoeba bütchlii* both have nuclei with large endosomes and no visible peripheral chromatin. Cysts of the former are oval in shape with four nuclei; those of the latter are somewhat irregular in shape with a single nucleus and a large glycogen vacuole that stains prominently with iodine. Neither species is pathogenic.

Dientamoeba fragilis is overlooked in most parasitological laboratories and most reports are from developed countries. There is good evidence that it can cause colonic inflammation; however, this is not severe and there is no ulceration or systemic spread. It has no cystic stage and, unless this organism is specifically looked for, it will be missed. In fixed stained smears, about 60% of trophozoites have two nuclei; the endosome is large and lobulated and there is no peripheral chromatin. Infected patients may shed the parasite intermittently. Alternatively *D. fragilis* may be identified in faeces or cultures using immunofluorescence with specific antibody or of parasite DNA by PCR; some patients are seropositive. Transmission is direct but possibly within eggs of the threadworm *Enterobius*. It causes a relatively mild diarrhoeal illness that may persist for several weeks and sometimes there is a superficial eosinophilic colitis. Irritable bowel syndrome may be suspected. Protein-losing enteropathy is reported and blood eosinophilia is quite common. This infection is frequent in some institutional contexts. It is found within some resected appendices but a causal role is unlikely. Electron micrographs and genetic studies indicate that *D. fragilis* is a trichomonad rather than a true amoeba. The infection responds to metronidazole, but a single dose of ornidazole is also effective. Series of symptomatic patients who improve after treatment continue to be reported.

Free-living amoebae

A shared feature of these species is the very large central nuclear endosome, quite different from that of *E. histolytica*, from which differentiation may be necessary in tissue sections. Under dry conditions, trophozoites form resistant cysts that permit survival and also airborne dispersal; cysts can resist chlorination. Many species are thermophilic and they are one of the causes of 'humidifier fever', a form of extrinsic allergic alveolitis presenting with fever, cough, and dyspnoea. Some bacteria including *Legionella* and *Parachlamydia acanthamoebae* may live symbiotically within these amoebae persisting within the phagosome, being resistant to lysosomal enzymes. Surprisingly, *Legionella* can survive encystment: the amoebae provide a refuge for these bacteria when chlorination or other antibacterial measures are applied. Three genera of free-living amoebae cause human infections:

1 *Naegleria* is an amoeboflagellate with two trophozoite forms. The amoeba moves rapidly with a single pseudopodium, it can transform into a nonfeeding flagellate in hypotonic media, and these free-swimming forms facilitate dispersal. Cysts are thin walled and spherical.

2 *Acanthamoeba* has no flagellate form. The small pseudopodia are multiple, thin, and spike-like; they are called acanthopodia (Fig. 8.1.9). Cysts are thick walled, angulated, and buoyant (Fig. 8.1.10); their dispersal may be wind borne. Several species are pathogenic but morphological classification is unsatisfactory; rRNA sequences differentiate 15 genotypes. *Acanthamoeba* is sometimes isolated from throat or nasal swabs or from stool specimens.

3 *Balamuthia* is closely related to *Acanthamoeba* and not a leptomyxid amoeba; it shows little directional movement and has an irregular or branched shape. Cysts are thick walled and spherical. Human infections formerly attributed to *Hartmanella* are now all thought to be due to *Balamuthia mandrillaris*, a species described in 1993 from a mandrill baboon that died of

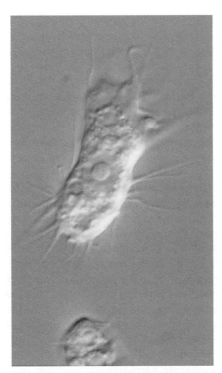

Fig. 8.1.9 *Acanthamoeba* trophozoite showing spike-like acanthopodia. (Courtesy of the late Professor Sornchai Looareesuwan.)

meningoencephalitis in San Diego zoo. *Balamuthia* can only be cultured on tissue culture monolayers. About 150 cases have been reported worldwide, but many are from Latin America.

Primary amoebic meningoencephalitis due to *Naegleria fowleri*

Epidemiology and pathology

Nearly all patients give a history of swimming or diving in warm fresh water or spa water between 2 and 14 days before the illness began. Common-source outbreaks occur during warm summer months in temperate countries. Amoebic trophozoites cross the cribriform plate from the nasal mucosa to the olfactory bulbs and subarachnoid space. At autopsy the brain shows cerebral softening and damage to the olfactory bulbs; cysts are never formed in the tissues. The first human case was reported in 1965, but retrospective analysis showed that there were 112 cases between 1937 and 2007 in the United States of America, with only one survivor. A recent report of

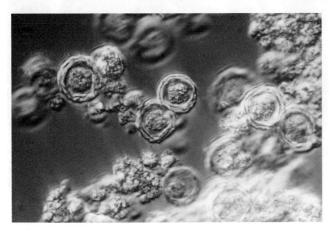

Fig. 8.1.10 *Acanthamoeba* cysts. (Copyright Viqar Zaman.)

13 patients seen in Karachi, Pakistan, over a 17-month period suggests that this should be regarded as an emerging infection. Some are undoubtedly missed clinically and are discovered at autopsy or in preserved pathological material. Specific antisera enable amoebae to be recognized by immunofluorescence staining.

Clinical features and diagnosis

Patients are immunocompetant; most are young adults and children. Initial nasal symptoms and headache are soon followed by fever, neck rigidity, coma, and, later, convulsions; most die within a few days. Cerebrospinal fluid is often turbid and bloodstained with high protein, low glucose and neutrophils. Amoebae must be urgently looked for in wet specimens using phase-contrast microscopy. Unless amoebae are seen, bacterial meningitis will be suspected; on Gram staining amoebae appear as indistinct smudges. Fixed preparations stained with iron haematoxylin will show full details of nuclear structure. Confirmation is by culture at 37°C using a bacterial lawn on non-nutrient agar. Amphotericin B can be an effective drug, it should be given by daily intravenous infusion, and intrathecally; other additional drugs that have been used are miconazole or fluconazole, and rifampicin; in mouse models, azithromycin is effective. So far, very few patients have survived but this may partly be due to diagnostic delays.

Amoebic keratitis due to *Acanthamoeba*

Most patients, but not all, are contact lens users, some are using disposable lenses. Among contact lens users, annual incidence rates of 1.49 and 0.33 per 10 000 are reported from Scotland and Hong Kong, respectively, but most figures are lower. Risk factors include poor hygiene when handling lenses and their cases, use of chlorine-based disinfectants, swimming or washing eyes while wearing lenses, handling lenses after gardening, and too prolonged use of plastic or unwashed lenses. The most appropriate disinfectants are chlorhexidine and hydrogen peroxide.

Corneal lesions are painful and present as indolent and progressive ulcers leading eventually to perforation. Recognition may be in the context of lesions unresponsive to antibiotics or corticosteroids. Differentiation must be made from commoner causes of microbial keratitis, including *Pseudomonas*, *Staphylococcus*, and herpes simplex. Inflammatory cells are mainly neutrophils. Infection may be by wind-borne cysts upon a damaged epithelium or from contact lenses. Solutions used to store or wash lenses can be contaminated by these amoebae, many of which are resistant to some antiseptics, especially as cysts. Amoebae are found in corneal scrapings or histologically in corneal tissue, but can be missed unless stained with iron haematoxylin or immunofluorescence. PCR methods are now available. Cysts may be seen in tissue. Cultures from fresh material, using a bacterial lawn on non-nutrient agar, should be at 30°C. The majority (90%) of cases are due to genotype T4.

Early aggressive topical treatment using a biguanide together with a diamidine is usually successful, however only the former is cysticidal. Alternatives are topical fluconazole plus miconazole with oral itraconazole. Initially, hourly application is needed, and courses may last a month. Additional topical neomycin or chloramphenicol may be necessary. Regular surgical debridement may be needed and sometimes corneal grafting. Corneal grafting may be needed.

Granulomatous amoebic encephalitis due to *Acanthamoeba* and *Balamuthia*

The main route of infection is the lower respiratory tract followed by haematogenous spread to the brain. Other routes of entry are the

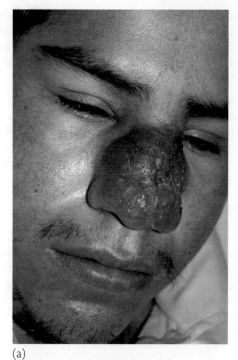

(a)

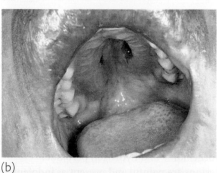

(b)

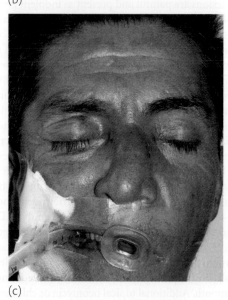

(c)

Fig. 8.1.11 *Balamuthia mandrillaris* infection. Cases at Instituto de Medicina Tropical 'Alexander von Humboldt' Universidad Peruana Cayetano Heredia, Lima, Peru: (a) cutaneous lesion in a 26-year-old man from Ica, (b) perforating lesion of palate in 16-year-old boy from Piura, and (c) encephalitis in a 57-year-old man from Piura showing the skin lesion that was the likely portal of entry. (Copyright D A Warrell.)

skin (Fig. 8.1.11a), the nasopharynx (Fig. 8.1.11b), the lungs and the stomach. Primary lesions have been described at all these sites. Soil contamination of skin and craniofacial wounds is an important risk factor.

Almost all patients infected by *Acanthamoeba* are immunocompromised; this is associated with malignancy, collagen disorder, alcoholism, diabetes mellitus, AIDS, and steroid or immunosuppressant therapy, including that used in transplant patients. Many patients with *B. mandrillaris* are also immunocompromised, but in Peru, most of the patients have no obvious cause for immunosuppression.

These infections are now important in transplantation medicine. *Acanthamoeba* encephalitis has been reported in immunosuppressed transplant recipients of liver or haematopoietic stem cells. Transplant donors can also be the source of infection, In 2009 two patients with *B. mandrillaris* were reported who received kidney graft from the same donor. In 2010 four patients received organs from a presumed stroke patient. Two recipients developed *B. mandrillaris* encephalitis and died but two others who received heart and kidney transplants remained asymptomatic; the donor had had a large chronic skin lesion on his back and this was the presumed source of the infections.

Pathologically lesions resemble chronic bacterial brain abscesses or localized subacute haemorrhagic necrosis; involvement of the meninges is common. Some patients present with headache and meningism, others with evidence of a focal brain lesion (Fig. 8.1.11c, Fig. 8.1.12).

Unless these amoebae are found in wet tissue preparations or cerebrospinal fluid, the diagnosis will be usually based on histology, often at autopsy. Cysts may be seen in tissue but trophozoites may be missed unless stained with iron haematoxylin or immunofluorescence using specific antisera. Cultural diagnosis at 37°C from fresh biopsies or cerebrospinal fluid is sometimes possible. PCR methods are becoming available.

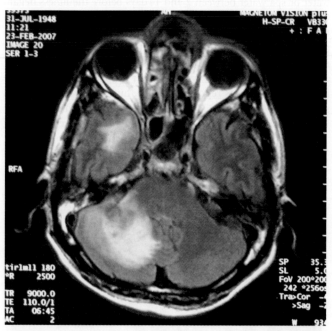

Fig. 8.1.12 *Balamuthia mandrillaris* infection. MRI scan in same patient as in Fig. 8.1.11c. (Copyright D A Warrell.)

Survival of patients with this condition is still only rarely reported; of about 150 patients with *B. manrillaris* reported worldwide by 2008 only 7 are known to have survived. Intracranial pressure can be relieved by mannitol and CSF drainage, and total excision of cerebral lesions is occasionally possible. Drug treatment with combinations of fluconazole with pentamidine, 5-fluorocytosine, sulphadiazine, and azithromycin may be successful. *Acanthamoeba* encephalitis has been successfully treated with cotrimoxazole plus rifampicin in a liver transplant recipient.

Further reading

Gut amoebae (*Entamoeba*)

Ali IKM, *et al.* (2007). Evidence for a link between parasite genotype and outcome with *Entamoeba histolytica*. *J Clin Microbiol*, **45**, 285–89.

Barwick RS, *et al.* (2002). Outbreak of amebiasis in Tbilisi, Republic of Georgia, 1998. *Am J Trop Med Hyg*, **67**, 623–31.

Calderaro A, *et al.* (2006). *Entamoeba histolytica* and *Entamoeba dispar*: comparison of two PCR assays for the diagnosis in a non-endemic setting. *Trans R Soc Trop Med Hyg*, **100**, 450–7.

Diamond LS, Clark CG (1993). A redescription of *Entamoeba histolytica* Schaudinn, 1903 (emended Walker 1911) separating it from *Entamoeba dispar* Brumpt, 1925. *J Eukaryot Microbiol*, **40**, 340–4.

Fotedar R, *et al.* (2007). Laboratory techniques for *Entamoeba* species. *Clin Microbiol Rev*, **20**, 511–32.

Haque R, *et al.* (2010). Diagnosis of ambic liver abscess and amebic colitis by detection of *Entamoeba histolytica* DNA in blood, urine, and saliva by a real-time PCR assay. *J Clin Microbiol*, **48**, 2798–801.

Mondal D, *et al.* (2006). *Entamoeba histolytica*-associated diarrheal illness is negatively associated with the growth of preschool children: evidence from a prospective study. *Trans R Soc Trop Med Hyg*, **100**, 1032–8.

Pritt BS, Clark CG (2008). Amebiasis. *Mayo Clin Proc*, **83**, 1154–60.

Ravdin JI, ed. (2000). *Amebiasis (tropical medicine: science and practice)*. Imperial College Press, London.

Singh O, *et al.* (2009). Comparative study of catheter drainage and needle aspiration in management of large liver abscess. *Ind J Gastroenterol*, **28**, 88–92.

Stanley SL Jr. (2003). Amoebiasis. *Lancet*, **361**, 1025–34.

Watanabe K, *et al.* (2011). Amebiasis in HIV-1 infected Japanese man: clinical features and response to therapy. *PLOS Neglect Trop Dis*, **5**, e1318.

Dientamoeba fragilis

Ginginkardesler KO, *et al.* (2008). A comparison of metronidazole and single dose ornidazole for the treatment of dientamoebiasis. *Clin Microbiol Infect*, **14**, 601–4.

Johnson EH, *et al.* (2004). Emerging from obscurity: biological, clinical, and diagnostic aspects of *Dientamoeba fragilis*. *Clin Microbiol Rev*, **17**, 553–70.

Stark D, *et al.* (2005). Detection of *Dientamoeba fragilis* in fresh stool specimens using PCR. *Int J Parasitol*, **35**, 57–62.

Stark D, *et al.* (2006). Dientamoebiasis: clinical importance and recent advances. *Trends Parasitol*, **22**, 92–6.

Stark D, *et al.* (2010). A review of the clinical presentation of dientamoebiasis. *Am J Trop Med Hyg*, **82**, 614–19.

Windsor JJ, Macfarlane L (2005). Irritable bowel syndrome: the need to exclude *Dientamoeba fragilis*. *Am J Trop Med Hyg*, **72**, 501–2.

Free-living amoebae

Bravo SG, Alvarez PJ, Gotuzzo E. (2011). *Balamuthia mandrillaris* infection of the skin and central nervous system: an emerging disease of concern to many specialities in medicine. *Curr Opin Infect Dis*, **24**, 112–17.

Carter R.F. (1972). Primary amoebic meningo-encephalitis. *Trans R Soc Trop Med Hyg*, **66**, 193–208.

Centres for Disease Control and Prevention (2008). Primary amoebic meningencephalitis—Arizona, Florida, and Texas, 2007. *MMWR Mort Mort Wkly Rep*, **57**, 573–7.

Centres for Disease Control and Prevention (2010). Notes from the field: transplant-transmitted Balamuthia mandrillaris—Arizona 2010. *MMWR Morb Mort Wkly Rep*, **59**, 1182.

Dart JKG, Saw VPJ, Kilvington, S (2009). *Acanthamoeba* keratitis: diagnosis and treatment update 2009. *Am J Ophthalmol*, **148**, 487–99.

Fung KT-T, *et al.* (2008). Cure of Acanthamoeba cerebral abscess in a liver transplant patient. *Liver Transplant*, **14**, 308–12.

Greub GD, Raoult D (2004). Microorganisms resistant to free-living amoebae. *Clin Microbiol Rev*, **17**, 413–33.

Heggie TW (2010). Swimming with death: *Naegleria fowleri* infections in recreational waters. *Travel Med Infect Dis*, **8**, 201–6.

Jung SRL, *et al.* (2004). *Balamuthia mandrillaris* meningoencephalitis in an immunocompetent patient: an unusual clinical course and a favorable outcome. *Arch Pathol Lab Med*, **128**, 466–8.

Khan NA. (2008). *Acanthamoeba* and the blood brain-barrier: the breakthrough. *J Med Microbiol*, **57**, 1051–57.

Khan NA, ed. (2009). *Acanthamoeba: biology and pathogenesis*. Caister Academic Press, Norwich, UK.

Martinez DY, *et al.* (2010). Successful treatment of Balamuthia mandrillaris amoebic infection with extensive neurological and cutaneous involvement. *Clin Infect Dis*, **51**, 7–11.[A summary of the management of all 7 known survivors of this condition is given.]

Matin A, *et al.* (2008). Increasing importance of *Balamuthia mandillaris*. *Clin Microbiol Rev*, **21**, 435–48

Mutoh T, *et al.* (2010). A retrospective study of nine cases of Acanthamoeba keratitis. *Clin Ophthalmol*, **4**, 1189–92.

Orozco L, *et al.* (2011). Neurosurgical intervention in the diagnosis and treatment of *Balamuthia mandrillaris*. *J Neurosurg*, **115**, 636–40.

Paltiel ME, *et al.* (2004). Disseminated cutaneous acanthamebiasis: a case report and review of the literature. *Cutis*, **73**, 241–8.

Shakoor S, *et al.* (2011). Primary amebic meningencephalitis caused by *Naegleria fowleri*, Karachi, Pakistan. *Emerg Infect Dis*, **17**, 258–61.

Visvesvara GS, Moura H, Schuster FL (2007). Pathogenic and opportunistic free-living amoebae: *Acanthamoeba* spp., *Balamuthia mandrillaris*, *Naegleria fowleri*, and *Sappinia diploidea*. *FEMS Imm Med Microbiol*, **50**, 1–26.

Visvesvara GS, Schuster FL, Martinez AJ. (1993). *Balamuthia mandrillaris*, N.G., N. Sp., *agent of amebic meningoencephalitis in humans and other animals*. *J Eukaryot Microbiol*, **40**, 504–14.

8.2 Malaria

David A. Warrell, Janet Hemingway, Kevin Marsh, Robert E. Sinden, Geoffrey A. Butcher, and Robert W. Snow

Essentials

In 2010, WHO estimated 216 million cases of malaria worldwide with 655,000 deaths, 26% fewer than in 2000. 91% of the deaths were in Africa and 86% in children aged less than 5 years. However, the Institute for Health Metrics and Evaluation estimated a global total of 1,238,000 malaria deaths in the same year. Malaria remains endemic in 106 countries. Nigeria, Democratic Republic of Congo, Burkina Faso, Mozambique, Ivory Coast, and Mali account for 60% of malaria deaths.

Acknowledgement: The authors and editors acknowledge the inclusion in this chapter of material contributed by Professor D J Bradley to the 4th edition of the *Oxford Textbook of Medicine*.

Human malaria parasites, mosquitoes, and transmission of malaria

Malaria parasites and their impact on the human genome—six species of *Plasmodium* commonly cause malaria in humans: *P. falciparum*, *P. vivax*, *P. ovale* (two species), *P. malariae* and *P. knowlesi*. The genome of *P. falciparum*, the most pathogenic species, has been completely sequenced. This parasite has exercised immense selection pressure on the human genome, as is evident from the global distribution of the many human genes that constrain malarial development, such as a point mutation in position 6 of the β-globin chain (sickle cell haemoglobin), and deletion of α-globin genes (α thalassaemia).

Biology of the parasite and mosquito vector—sporozoites are injected into humans during the female anopheles mosquito's blood meal. They invade hepatocytes. Hepatic schizogony releases merozoites into the blood stream where they invade red blood corpuscles (RBCs) and undergo further asexual multiplications before gametocytes form. If these are ingested by mosquitoes, male and female gametes fuse, resulting in ookinetes that penetrate the mosquito's midgut and develop into oocysts. Daughter sporozoites are released. They invade the mosquito's salivary glands, ready to infect a new human host. Persistent latent forms (hypnozoites) of *P. vivax* and *P. ovale* remain in the liver to give rise to later relapses of parasitaemia and symptoms. All the stages express distinct antigen, repertoires excite different immune responses, and are equipped survive in different microenvironmants.

Mosquito biology—species of the *Anopheles gambiae* complex, the most effective malaria vectors, prefer to feed on humans to whom they are attracted by smell: other species are less particular. They vary in their choice of breeding habitats. MacDonald's equation for vectorial capacity and the related basic reproduction number (R_0) allows prediction of the impact of vector control methods under different conditions. The genome sequence of *An. gambiae* is known. Important mosquito phenotypes that have a genetic basis include blood feeding preference, habitat choice, insecticide susceptibility, and vectorial capacity.

Other mechanisms of transmission—malaria can be transmitted by transfusion of blood products, marrow transplants, and contaminated needles.

Epidemiology

In 2007, 2.4 billion people were exposed to *P. falciparum* infection across 87 countries, and 3.18 billion people were exposed to *P. vivax* across 63 countries. Intensity of malarial transmission depends on the varying efficiencies of the local anopheline vectors and their frequency of contact with humans.

Malarial endemicity expresses the amount or intensity of transmission in an area or community. Epidemic malaria implies a periodic or sharp increase in the amount of malaria. Stable transmission implies persistently high prevalence, insensitive to aberrations in climate or local habitats as in holoendemic areas of Africa; unstable malaria is characterised by great variability in space and time, as in South-East Asia. Prevalence of infection in children aged 2 to 9 years is described as hypoendemic (<10%), mesoendemic (11–50%), hyperendemic (51–75%), or holoendemic (>75%).

The epidemiological background to clinical malaria—is changing due to population growth, environmental changes (often human-induced, whether local or global), changing resistance of parasites to drugs, the HIV epidemic and the consequences of attempts at malaria control. An estimated 550 million clinical attacks of *P. falciparum* occurred worldwide in 2002: 71% in Africa, 23% in the low-transmission but densely populated countries of South-East Asia, and 3% in the Western Pacific. In Africa in 2005, *P. falciparum* is estimated to have caused 1.1 million deaths directly, 71 000 to 190 000 infant deaths following placental infection *in utero*, and over 3000 newly acquired persistent epilepsies through brain insults among patients surviving an episode of cerebral malaria in childhood.

Innate resistance and immunity

More human genetic polymorphisms have been associated with innate protection from malaria than for any other infectious disease. Duffy blood group negative RBCs are resistant to *P. vivax* infection, explaining the prevalence of the DARC(Fy) −46C/C genotype especially in West Africa, but there may be an associated susceptibility to HIV-1 infection.

In most stably endemic areas, acquisition of immunity, although never complete, ensures that death due to malaria is rare after the age of 5 years and hardly ever occurs in normally immune competent adults. Immunity allows tolerance of levels of parasitisation that would cause illness in a naive individual by neutralizing parasite toxins or down-regulating the cytokine response to challenge. However, a key aspect of immunity to malaria is control of parasite growth by interfering with parasites' replication or accelerating their removal from the circulation. There is progressive acquisition of both 'strain'-specific and cross-protective responses to a range of potential malarial epitopes. Immunity is stage-specific but probably acts predominantly at the blood stages. Antibody-mediated protection against blood-stage parasites is demonstrated by the relative protection of children in endemic areas during their first few months of life by passively transferred maternal antibody and by experimental amelioration of acute malaria by immune gammaglobulin. Malnutrition increases the risk of severe falciparum malaria in children.

HIV–malaria interaction—in pregnant women, HIV and *P. falciparum* infections are mutually synergistic. Consequences of malaria, especially anaemia, are more severe in HIV-positive women. In areas of unstable malarial transmission, HIV-positive nonimmune adults are at increased risk of severe and fatal malaria. In malaria endemic areas, HIV-positive children are at increased risk of severe malaria.

Molecular pathology, organ pathology, and pathophysiology

Molecular pathology—intravascular, asexual forms are responsible for all the pathological effects of malaria in humans. Fever and inflammation are probably initiated by interaction between parasite products and pattern recognition receptors on host cells, leading to cytokine release by macrophages. The relative virulence of *P. falciparum* is attributed to cytoadherence and sequestration of parasitized RBCs to venular endothelium, especially in the lungs, brain, intestines and muscles, resulting in reduced perfusion and tissue damage. Local release of potentially toxic/pharmacologically active compounds such as reactive oxygen species or nitric oxide may also be involved.

Organ pathology—the brain may be oedematous, especially in African children. Small blood vessels are congested with tightly sequestered parasitized RBCs (PRBCs) containing pigmented mature trophozoites and schizonts, making the brain slate-grey in colour. The cerebrovascular endothelium shows pseudopodial projections, closely apposed to electron-dense, knob-like protruberances on the surface of PRBCs. Other changes include petechial haemorrhages in the white matter, ring haemorrhages and Dürck's granulomas. Among other organs and tissues, retina, bone marrow, lung, heart, liver, intestine, spleen, kidney, and placenta show variable evidence of PRBC sequestration and some other distinctive features.

Pathophysiology—anaemia results from destruction/phagocytosis of both normal red cells and PRBCs as well as from dyserythropoiesis; autoimmune haemolysis is rare. Thrombocytopenia is attributable to splenic sequestration, dysthrombopoiesis, and immune-mediated lysis. Cerebral malaria is associated with inappropriately low cerebral blood flow, increased cerebral anaerobic glycolysis and microcirculatory obstruction. In African children, plasma concentrations of TNF-α, IL-1α and other cytokines correlate with disease severity. Cytokines may be involved in hypoglycaemia, coagulopathy, dyserythropoiesis, and leucocytosis in falciparum malaria. Pulmonary oedema may result from fluid overload, but more often there is increased pulmonary capillary permeability associated with neutrophil sequestration in the pulmonary capillaries. In African children, a syndrome of respiratory distress is associated with metabolic acidosis and severe anaemia. Hypoglycaemia is caused by impaired gluconeogenesis, reduced hepatic glycogen or hyperinsulinaemia secondary to quinine/quinidine treatment. In malarial acute kidney injury, there is evidence of PRBC sequestration, and pigment (haemoglobin and myoglobin) toxicity may contribute.

Clinical features

Classic periodic febrile paroxysms with afebrile asymptomatic intervals are uncommon unless treatment is delayed.

Severe falciparum malaria—this is defined by (1) clinical features—prostration, impaired consciousness, respiratory distress/ acidotic breathing, multiple convulsions, circulatory collapse, pulmonary oedema (radiological), abnormal bleeding, jaundice, and haemoglobinuria; and (2) laboratory tests—severe anaemia, hypoglycaemia, acidosis, renal impairment, and hyperlactataemia, that are of proven prognostic significance.

Cerebral malaria is defined by impaired consciousness in patients with acute P. falciparum infection in whom other causes of coma, including hypoglycaemia and transient postictal coma, have been excluded. Convulsions, dysconjugate gaze, retinal changes, symmetrical upper motor neuron signs, and abnormal posturing are common. Neurological manifestations are different in adults and children. African children surviving cerebral malaria may suffer persistent neurological, cognitive, and learning defects.

So-called benign malarias, P. ovale, P. malariae, and particularly P. vivax, can cause even more severe feverish symptoms than falciparum malaria. Splenic rupture is more common with vivax malaria. P. knowlesi, one of the monkey malarias, has recently been recognized as an important and potentially fatal zoonosis in humans in several South-East Asian countries.

Malaria in pregnancy—malaria is an important cause of maternal anaemia and death, abortion, stillbirth, premature delivery, low birth weight, and neonatal death. RBCs infected with strains of P. falciparum expressing Var2CSA bind to chondroitin sulphate A expressed on the surface of the syncytiotrophoblast. Placental dysfunction, fever, and hypoglycaemia contribute to fetal distress.

Chronic immunological complications of malaria—these include quartan malarial nephrosis, tropical splenomegaly syndrome (hyperreactive malarial splenomegaly) and endemic Burkitt's lymphoma.

Diagnosis

Repeated thick and thin blood smears and rapid antigen detection over a period of 72 h are necessary to confirm or exclude the diagnosis of malaria. Differential diagnoses include other acute febrile illness: falciparum malaria has been misdiagnosed as influenza, viral hepatitis, epilepsy, viral encephalitis, or traveller's diarrhoea, sometimes with fatal consequences.

Laboratory investigation

In falciparum malaria, blood glucose must be checked frequently, especially in children, pregnant women, and severely ill patients, whether or not the patient is receiving quinine/quinidine treatment.

Treatment

The efficacy of antimalarial chemotherapy is threatened by emerging resistance of P. falciparum to available drugs. The World Health Organization (WHO) now advocates the combination of two or more different classes of antimalarial drugs with unrelated mechanisms of action to delay emergence of resistance.

P. vivax, P. ovale, P. malariae, P. knowlesi malarias—these are treated with chloroquine. Resistant P. vivax (New Guinea, Indonesia) is treated by increasing the dose of oral chloroquine.

Uncomplicated P. falciparum malaria in malarious areas—WHO recommends the replacement of monotherapy with the combination of an artemesinin with another drug (artemisinin-based combination therapy, ACT), even in Africa, although this is more expensive and resistance to artemisinins has recently emerged in Cambodia. ACTs include artemether-lumefantrine ("Riamet" or "Coartem"), artesunate-amodiaquine, dihydroartemisinin-piperaquine ("Eurartesim") and artesunate-sulphadoxine pyrimethamine. For presumed nonimmune travellers returning to nonendemic areas, artemether–lumefantrine, atovaquone–proguanil, or quinine with doxycycline or clindamycin (pregnant women and children) are recommended.

Severe falciparum, vivax, and knowlesi malaria—urgent appropriate, parenteral chemotherapy is necessary, initiated with a loading dose. Intravenous artesunate is the drug of choice. Intramuscular artemether, or quinine by intermittent or continuous intravenous infusion or intramuscular injection are less effective. Artemisinin by rectal suppository has proved effective. Resistance to artemisinins is emerging in Cambodia, Thailand, and Burma.

Supportive care—patients with severe malaria should be transferred to the highest possible level of care. Convulsions must be controlled; fluid, electrolyte, and acid–base homeostasis restored; and organ/ tissue failure treated (e.g. haemofiltration for acute renal failure). Harmful ancillary remedies of unproven value, such as corticosteroids and heparin, have no role in the treatment of cerebral malaria.

Prevention

Modern malaria control and prevention aims to limit human–vector contact by indoor residual spraying (IRS) and insecticide (pyrethroid) treated nets (ITNs). ITNs can reduce all-cause childhood mortality by 17%, averting 5.5 deaths for every 1000 African children protected, preventing over 50% of clinical cases, and reducing prevalence by 13%. Repellents such as diethyltoluamide (DEET) are used for personal protection. Vectors can also be controlled by environmental modification or manipulation, and human contact can be reduced by zooprophylaxis and by modifying human dwellings and behaviour.

Intermittent preventive treatment in pregnant women (IPTp) and infants (IPTi) with sulphadoxine–pyrimethamine—efficacy is likely to decrease because IPTp works less well in HIV-positive women and there is no proven safe alternative to sulphadoxine–pyrimethamine in areas where resistance to this combination is rapidly expanding.

Malarial vaccines—obstacles to developing a malaria vaccine are the multistage complexity of the parasite, polymorphism of potential immune targets, and the parasite's capacity for evolving evasive strategies, such as antigenic variation and diversity. However, candidate pre-erythrocytic, blood-stage, and transmission-blocking vaccines have been developed. A subunit vaccine (RTS,S) comprising a fusion protein combining part of the circumsporozoite protein of *P. falciparum* with HBsAg and a complex adjuvant (AS02) has achieved 53% protective efficacy against malaria disease.

Travellers—prevention of malaria in people from nonmalarious areas who are visiting endemic regions, including those visiting their friends and relatives (VFRs), has become more difficult because of resistance to antimalarial drugs. Travellers are advised to (1) be aware of the risk; (2) prevent exposure to anopheline mosquitoes; (3) take chemoprophylaxis where appropriate—malarone, mefloquine, or doxycycline is appropriate in areas of chloroquine-resistant falciparum malaria; (4) seek immediate medical advice in case of any feverish illness developing while abroad, or within 3 or more months of returning, and to mention malaria as a possibility—regardless of the precautions taken—to any doctor who sees them. Up-to-date advice is important, as the global distribution and intensity of malarial transmission is changing. Pregnant women are best advised to avoid malarious areas. Travellers spending time in the jungles of South-East Asia should be alert to the risk of contracting knowlesi malaria.

Introduction

Malaria is the most important human parasitic disease globally and has had large effects on the course of history and settlement in tropical regions. Following the discovery in the 19th century of both the causative protozoan parasite, *Plasmodium*, and its mosquito vector, the disease was brought under control in many countries through the application of antimalarial drugs, insecticides such as dichlorodiphenyltrichloroethane (DDT), and other environmental interventions including urbanization. In the United States of America, Europe, the Mediterranean region, the Middle East, most Caribbean islands, some South American countries, northern Australia, and most of China, elimination or a high degree of control was largely achieved. Even in Sri Lanka in the early 1960s, cases had fallen from 1.1 million annually to just 18, but failure to maintain surveillance and react to outbreaks resulted in a return to previous levels.

In recent years, malaria has been subject to increased control efforts, with varying degrees of success, but the disease was resurgent in the 1980s and 1990s. Malaria remains the dominant tropical vector-borne disease but, after decades of neglect, international interest in its control has recently revived. There is now a global effort to develop new methods to intervene against parasite dissemination, stimulated by the emergence of drug resistant parasites in South-East Asia and Africa, mosquitoes resistant to DDT and other insecticides, and by the recognition that malaria has a considerable economic impact: in Africa, total gross domestic product losses due to malaria amount to US$12 billion per year, and the global cost is US$18 billion. With over 500 million malaria cases annually and more than a million deaths in more than 100 countries, there remains a clear and urgent need for improved control and treatment.

Biology of the malaria parasite

Life cycle and parasite cell strategies

Six of the 147 known species of protozoan parasites genus *Plasmodium* that cause malaria (*mal aria*, Italian, literally 'bad air') commonly infect humans: *P. falciparum*, *P. vivax*, *P. ovale curtisi*, *P. ovale wallikeri*, *P. malariae*, and *P. knowlesi* (Fig. 8.2.1). The biological organization and life cycle of *P. falciparum*, the species most pathogenic to humans, are distinct from that of all but *P. reichenowi*. A new species (*P. gaboni*) was discovered recently in two chimpanzees in Gabon. It is close to *P. falciparum* and *P. reichenowi* and might infect humans.

Animal models

Notwithstanding their significance as sources of human infection, plasmodia infections of animals, adapted to laboratory species, have proved essential to progress in all aspects of malaria. In addition to well-known activities, such as drug development, experimental animals have contributed to our basic understanding of host–parasite interactions. The importance of antibody in acquired immunity, to give one example, was demonstrated in monkeys many years before the equivalent demonstration in humans. Despite the limitations—practical, legal, and ethical—animal experimentation continues in importance to the present day.

Genomic organization of *Plasmodium* and consequences for the human host

Plasmodium is diploid only until the first (meiotic) division of the genome following fusion of the male and female gametes and is haploid for the rest of its life cycle. The 23-Mb genome of *P. falciparum* has been completely sequenced: it contains from 5000 to 6000 genes distributed between 14 chromosomes ranging in size from about 1 Mb to 2.4 Mb. Considering its comparatively small number of genes, it is remarkable that it not only maintains a complex life cycle but survives in the face of the overwhelming number (20000–30000) of genes available to its human host. The parasite has exercised immense selection pressure on the human genome as is evident from the global distribution of the many human genes that constrain malarial development (Box 8.2.1).

Development in the mosquito

After the blood meal, ingested intraerythrocytic gametocytes (Fig. 8.2.2) in the midgut of the female mosquito are triggered to undergo gamete formation (exflagellation) by a drop in temperature of more than 5°C and the presence of raised concentration of mosquito-derived xanthurenic acid. The gametocytes escape out of the red blood cell (RBC) into the lumen of the midgut, where the female gamete can be fertilized within minutes by a microgamete released from microgametocytes (Fig. 8.2.2). Major zygote/ookinete surface proteins are detectable on the zygote surface within 1 h of fertilization, particularly P48/45, P230, P25, and P28, which are potential components of a transmission-blocking vaccine.

Within about 8 h of fertilization, the briefly diploid genome has undergone meiosis producing a single nucleus containing four haploid genomes. Over the ensuing 9 to 12 h, the zygote becomes a motile and invasive banana-shaped ookinete (Figs. 8.2.2 and 8.2.3). The extracellular gametes, zygotes, and ookinetes are exposed to

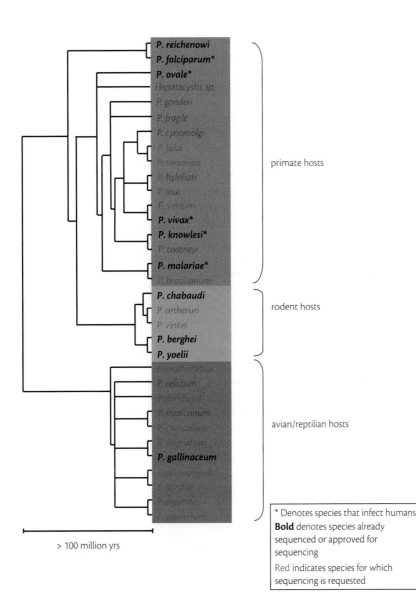

* Denotes species that infect humans
Bold denotes species already sequenced or approved for sequencing
Red indicates species for which sequencing is requested

Fig. 8.2.1 A cartoon of the evolutionary relationships of malarial parasites derived from analysis of multiple genomes. The branch lengths are not to scale and do not represent the evolutionary distance between species.
(D Neafsey and S Volkman, unpublished data.)

potentially lethal components in the blood meal, such as complement to which the parasite is initially resistant, antibodies, and mosquito proteases. Then, 24 to 36 h after the blood meal was ingested, the ookinete penetrates the chitinous peritrophic membrane, newly secreted by the mosquito to defend itself against parasitic invasion, and the plasma membrane of midgut epithelial cells. Unlike sporozoites and merozoites (Fig. 8.2.3), the ookinete lacks rhoptries and consequently does not form a parasitophorous vacuole (PV) when it invades the epithelial cells. On meeting the collagen-containing basal lamina on the outer wall of the midgut, the ookinete transforms into a vegetative replicating form, the oocyst, protected from the mosquito's immune system by a thick proteinaceous wall containing proteins P380 and circumsporozoite protein (CSP). Commonly, fewer than five of the thousands of gametocytes originally present in the blood meal form oocysts (Fig. 8.2.4).

Parasite movement
The motile ookinete, merozoite, and sporozoite are impelled by an unconventional actomyosin motor (Fig. 8.2.5).

Development of the oocyst into sporozoites
Depending partly on ambient temperature, the oocyst nucleus undergoes from 10 to 13 endomitotic divisions over a period of

10 to 25 days, until finally a single cytokinetic division results in the simultaneous production of between 2000 and 10 000 daughter sporozoites (Fig. 8.2.2). Mature sporozoites secrete a protease (ECP-1) to digest the proteinaceous oocyst wall to escape into the mosquito's haemocoelomic fluid. Only those capable of invading the salivary glands survive. They bind to salivary gland receptors via ligands such as CSP, TRAP, and MAEBL (apical membrane antigen/erythrocyte binding-like), penetrate the plasma membrane of the acinar cells, and come to lie in the salivary ducts. *P. falciparum* sporozoites can remain infectious in the glands for up to 55 days, many times longer than the natural lifetime of the infected mosquito, which delivers 10 to 100 sporozoites per bite.

Development of the exo-/pre-erythrocytic (liver) stages
CSP, the dominant surface protein on the sporozoite, is critical to this phase of the life cycle and has been the most popular vaccine candidate. Most of the sporozoites deposited in the dermis by the biting mosquito cross the capillary epithelium and are rapidly transported in the bloodstream to the liver, where they invade phagocytic Kupffer cells. A few sporozoites may enter the lymphatic system, where they may prime antigen-presenting cells in the lymph nodes. Kupffer cells tolerate microbes and their

Box 8.2.1 Some human genetic polymorphisms associated with resistance to malaria

- α –Thalassaemia
- β –Thalassaemia
- Haemoglobin S
- Haemoglobin E
- Haemoglobin F
- Haemoglobin C
- South-East Asian ovalocytosis
- Hereditary sphero-, ellipto-, pyropoikilo-cytoses[a]
- G6PD deficiency
- Pyruvate kinase deficiency
- Duffy blood group
- ABO blood groups
- S-s-U blood group
- Glycophorin B deficiency
- Complement receptor-1
- MHC class I
- MHC class II
- HLA Bw53
- HLA DRB1*1302
- TNF-α promoter
- IFN-γ receptor

G6PD, glucose-6-phosphate deydrogenase; IFN, interferon; MHC, major histocompatibility complex; TNF, tumour necrosis factor (see also http://www.malariagen.net).

[a] *In vitro* evidence only.

products (portal vein tolerance), but intracellular sporozoites also inhibit phagocytes' oxidative burst. CSP inhibits fusion of lysosomes with the parasite-containing vacuoles (PV). Sporozoites then escape from the Kupffer cells into the space of Disse and invade adjacent hepatocytes. CSP, secreted from the micronemes,

binds to heparin sulphate proteoglycans on the hepatocytes and, with TRAP and a perforin-like molecule, enables penetration of the hepatocyte membrane. The parasite may migrate through several hepatocytes, killing them in the process and inducing the production of hepatocyte growth factor that contributes to parasite nutrition. The sporozoites form PVs in hepatocytes where they differentiate into replicating exo-erythrocytic (EE) schizonts.

Parasites inhibit apoptosis, a host cell defence mechanism, so that hepatocyte mitochondria remain available for recruitment by the PV. Down-regulation of hepatocyte proteosomal activity reduces presentation of secreted parasite antigens to major histo-compatability complex molecules, compromising recognition of the infected hepatocyte by cytotoxic T cells. However, EE-stage parasites remain a prime target for potential vaccines. Within the infected hepatocyte, sporozoites undergo schizogony, each producing from 10 000 to 30 000 daughter cells (Table 8.2.1), or merozoites (Fig. 8.2.3). They are released in large cellular masses (merosomes) containing hepatocyte cytoplasm that are attacked by macrophages and neutrophils in the liver. However, individual merozoites escape into the circulation where they invade red blood cells (RBCs). Infection of the liver is without clinical consequences, possibly because only a small number of parasites complete development and little toxic waste is released. The cell cycles of *P. vivax* and *P. ovale* can become arrested with formation of quiescent hypnozoites that can persist in the hepatocyte for long periods, enabling these parasites to survive seasonal absences of mosquitoes. Reactivation of hypnozoites by unknown factors produces 'relapse' infection in the blood. Latencies and frequencies of hypnozoite relapses are very variable, suggesting that the

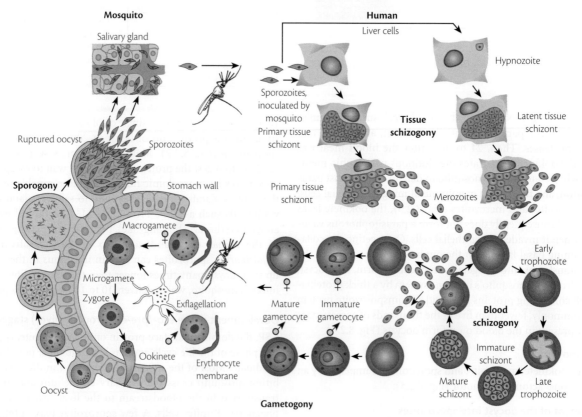

Fig. 8.2.2 Developmental cycle of *Plasmodium* species.
(Redrawn by permission of F. Hoffman-la- Roche Ltd, Basel, Switzerland.)

Fig. 8.2.3 Diagram of invasive stages, ookinete, sporozoite, and merozoite, illustrating their extensively conserved subcellular architecture.
(From Sinden RE (1978). Cell biology. In: Killick-Kendrick R, Peters W (eds) *Rodent malaria*, pp. 85–168. Academic Press, London.)
Ap, Apicoplast; AR, Apical ring; Co, collar; cr, crystalloid; IM, inner membrane vacuole; M, mitochondrion; MN, micronemes; Nu, nucleus; OM, plasmamembrane; P, pigment; PR, polar ring; R, ring; Rh, rhoptry.

strains responsible had their origins in both tropical and temperate zones (Table 8.2.1). Hypnozoites do not grow and are therefore susceptible only to 'causal prophylactic' drugs such as primaquine and atovaquone that target mitochondrial enzyme pathways responsible for essential energy metabolism. Relapse must not be confused with a recrudescence, which occurs as a result of the amplification of a chronic subpatent blood-stage infection of *P. falciparum* or *P. malariae*.

Development in the erythrocyte

The underlying mechanism of merozoite invasion of the RBC is highly conserved across *Plasmodium* species, whereas host cell recognition and binding is species limited. Different *Plasmodium* species invade RBCs of different ages. *P. vivax* invades reticulocytes

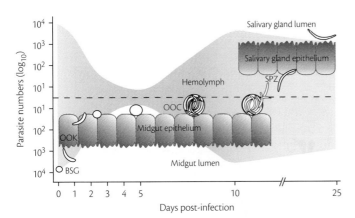

Fig. 8.2.4 Diagram illustrating the population bottleneck experienced by *Plasmodium* as it passes from the vertebrate host into the mosquito vector, with the nadir in number being experienced at the oocyst stage.
(Modified from Christophides GK (2005). Transgenic mosquitoes and malaria transmission. *Cell Microbiol*, **7**, 325–33.)

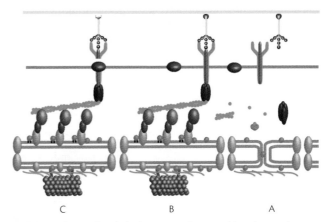

Fig. 8.2.5 Mechanism by which the actomyosin motor drives the parasite (ookinete, sporozoite, and merozoite) into host cells and through tissues.
(a) On binding the host receptor (yellow), the parasite ligand (green) recruits aldolase (red), which binds to fibrous actin (green spiral). (b) This short actin fibre is moved by myosin A (orange), anchored to the cytoskeleton through myosin A tail domain-interacting protein (purple) and glideosome-associated protein (grey), to the posterior of the cell. (c) At the posterior of the cell, rhomboid protease cleaves the ligand transmembrane domain liberating the parasite from the host cell ligand.

Table 8.2.1 Distinguishing characteristics of malaria parasites infecting humans

Parasite	P. falciparum	P. vivax	P. ovale curtisi and P. ovale wallikeri	P. malariae	P. knowlesi
Development of liver stages (days)	5–7	6–8	9	14–16	5.5
Merozoite number in exo-erythrocytic schizont	<30 000	<10 000	<15 000	<15 000	Unknown
Hypnozoite	No	Yes	Yes	No	No
Maximum period to first relapse	–	<3 yrs	<100 days	–	
Blood parasites detected by microscopy (days)	9–10	11–13	10–14	15–16	9–11[b]
Days/years to first symptoms[a]	12	15/< 1[a]	17/<4[a]	28	9–11[h]
RBC Cycle (hours)	48	48	49–50	72	24
Merozoite number in blood schizonts	16	16	8/16[c]	8–12	10
Distinguishing characteristics of species by microscopy[d]	Commonly rings only; Maurer's clefts; crescentic gametocytes,	Schuffner's dots, trophozoites irregular	Large nuclei; Schuffner's dots, trophozoites irregular	Band forms	Light stippling; sometimes band forms; resembles P. malariae
Maximum RBC infected (%)	>60	0.01	<0.3	<0.2	12
Oocyst development at 28°C (days)	9–10	8–10	12–14	14–16	8–10
Oocyst size (μm)	55	50	45	40	65

[a] Exceptional cases of P. vivax and P. ovale took nearly 1 year and 4 years, respectively.

[b] From Chin, et al. (1968). Experimental mosquito-transmission of Plasmodium knowlesi to man and monkey. Am J Trop Med Hyg, **17**, 355–8.

[c] Merozoite numbers in schizonts from relapses of P. ovale are increased.

[d] See Garnham PCC (1966). Malaria parasites and other haemosporidia. Blackwell, Oxford, and Coatney GR, et al. (1971). The primate malarias. US Department of Health, Education and Welfare, Bethesda, Maryland, USA.

Data from Garnham PCC (1966). Malaria parasites and other haemosporidia. Blackwell, Oxford; Coatney GR, et al. (1971). The primate malarias. US Department of Health, Education and Welfare, Bethesda, MD; and Bruce-Chwatt LJ (1985). Essential malariology, 2nd edition, Heinemann Medical, London.

and P. ovale also prefers younger RBCs; P. falciparum and P. malariae invade mature RBCs. Antibodies recognizing the various parasite ligands can inhibit merozoite invasion, thus offering potential targets for prophylactic vaccines. Invasion is a complex active process, taking less than a minute, that involves modification of both the merozoite surface and RBC membrane (Fig. 8.2.6). Following the discovery that most strains of P. vivax invade red cells carrying the Duffy blood group (Duffy antigen receptor for chemokines, DARC), two multi-

gene families of P. falciparum parasite proteins involved in invasion have been described. Erythrocyte binding proteins (EBPs; EBP-1 -181) with receptor ligands known as Duffy-binding-like domains interact with Glycophorins or Band 4.1 on the erythrocyte (Table 8.2.2). A second family homologous with the P. vivax reticulocyte binding Protein (PvRBP) known as (Pf RH15) may interact with sialic acid on some receptors, though as yet not all are known (Table 8.2.2) while evidence from southern Africa indicates that some strains

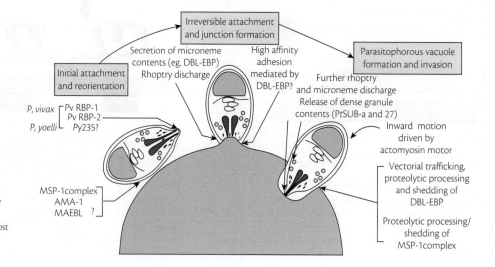

Fig. 8.2.6 Merozoite invasion of the red blood cell.
(From Chitnis CE, Blackman MJ. (2000). Host cell invasion by malaria parasites. *Trends Parasitol*, **16**, 411–16.)

of *P. vivax* may invade Duffy-negative erythrocytes. In a recent report, it is claimed that PfRH5 binds to a blood group antigen, basigin, and that this interaction is common to all parasite strains. If confirmed, this provides the opportunity for new therapies, especially in the arena of vaccine design.

Inside the RBC, a PV is created to contain the merozoite. After successful invasion of the RBC, proteins such as *P. falciparum* reticulocyte-like binding homologue proteins (PfRh) 1 to 4 are released into the PV (Table 8.2.2).

Following invasion, phagocytosis of RBC cytoplasm by the growing trophozoite occurs through a cytostome or micropore in the parasite's plasma membrane, forming intracytoplasmic digestive vacuoles into which digestive enzymes such as plasmepsins and dipeptide aminopeptidase are secreted. Digestion of RBC proteins yields toxic haem that is sequestered as haematin crystals in membrane-bound vesicles, to be discarded when schizonts divide into merozoites. The rapid growth of the asexual parasite within the RBC demands new permeability pathways in erythrocyte membranes to facilitate entry of essential nutrients and the egress of toxic metabolites, especially lactic acid. *P. falciparum* builds membranous transport structures in the RBC cytoplasm including Maurer's clefts, originally described in 1903, and the recently described tubulovesicular network. Parasite nutrient transporters

Table 8.2.2 Interactions of some of the major erythrocyte receptors and the merozoite proteins to which they bind

Parasite ligand	Location	Red blood cell receptor	Binding phenotype
P. falciparum			
PfMSP-1 [42]	MS	Band 3	–
PfMSP9	MS	Band 3	–
AMA-1	MN/MS		–
EBA-175	MN	Glyc A	NsTaCr
EBL-1	?MN	Glyc B	NsTrCs
EBA-140	MN	Glyc C	NsTsCr
EBA-181	MN	Band4.1	NsTrCs
PfRH-1	RH/MN	?	NsTrCr
PfRH-2	RH/MN	?	NrTrCs
PfRH-4	RH/MN	Comp.Rec.1	NrTsCs
PfRH-5	RH/MN	Basigin	NrTrCr
P. vivax			
PvDBP	–	Duffy antigen	–
PvRBP1	RH	?	
PvRBP2	RH	?	

AMA-1, apical membrane antigen 1; Comp.Rec.1, Complement receptor 1, DBP: Duffy binding protein (a group of proteins that includes the *P. vivax* Duffy-binding proteins); EBA, erythrocyte binding protein; Gylc., glycophorin; MN, micronemes; MS, merozoite surface; PfMSP, *P. falciparum* merozoite surface proteins (1$_{42}$ is 42k Da fragment) PvRBP, *P. vivax* reticulocyte binding proteins; RH, rhopteries. There is some evidence that in limited areas of East Africa *P. vivax* strains are not dependent on PvDBP.
Binding phenotype, based on enzyme treatment of red cells: N, neuraminidase; T, trypsin; C, chymotrypsin; r, resistant; s, sensitive
Source: based on Oh SS, Chishti AH (2005). Host receptors in malaria merozoite invasion. *Curr Top Microbiol Immunol*, **295**, 203–302; Guar D, Chitnis CE (2011). Molecular interactions and signalling mechanisms during erythrocyte invasion by malaria parasites. *Curr Opin Microbiol*, **14**, 422–8; Crosnier C, *et al.* (2011). Basigin is a receptor essential for erythrocyte invasion by *Plasmodium falciparum*. *Nature*, **480**(7378), 534–7.

in the infected RBC (iRBC) membrane are important targets for new antimalarial compounds. *P. falciparum* erythrocyte membrane protein 1 (PfEMP1) is the major parasite protein and is exposed on the RBC membrane as discrete warts (knobs). Energy metabolism of the asexual blood stages is critically dependent upon the mitochondrion. The recently discovered apicoplast is a vestigial chloroplast originating from red algae. It is responsible for pathways in lipid metabolism distinct from those of either vertebrates or mosquitoes and can, therefore, be targeted by drugs such as fosmidomycin, doxycycline, and clindamycin. These drugs are slow acting, taking two generations of parasite growth (96 h) before inhibition takes effect. Over the next 24 to 72 h, depending on the species, the parasite develops within the PV, eventually forming schizonts containing up to 30 merozoites (Table 8.2.1). Just before merozoite release, schizont volume increases and bursts the iRBC explosively. When blood-stage infections are synchronous, iRBC destruction, release of merozoites, and parasite toxic products into the bloodstream result in typical periodic patterns of fever in the human host.

Sexual development (gametocytes)

The asexual parasites themselves are a developmental dead end, but their expansive growth in the blood increases the potential for differentiation into the sexual forms that are responsible for continuing the life cycle by infecting female mosquitoes. Stress on the developing asexual forms, e.g. antimalarial drugs, immune pressure, and metabolic stress induced by the asexual population itself, stimulates gametocyte production. The progeny of each schizont are all asexual, all male, or all female. Males (microgametocytes) accumulate the proteins required for rapid DNA replication and flagellar motility during gametogenesis and then shut down protein synthesis with the loss of ribosomes and endoplasmic reticulum (ER). In contrast, the mature females (macrogametocytes) retain protein synthetic machinery (ER and Golgi), although shutting down active protein synthesis. Because mature gametocytes of both sexes have ceased protein synthesis, they are less susceptible than asexual parasites to many antimalarial compounds. However, they remain vulnerable to inhibitors of energy metabolism such as primaquine and artemisinin combination therapy. The sexual stages of most malarial parasites mature in the same time as the asexual parasites, but *P. falciparum* is atypical in requiring not 48 h but about 10 days to mature (Table 8.2.1). Like the asexual parasites, immature gametocytes of *P. falciparum* express PfEMP1, have knobs, and adhere to receptors. Normally, only mature gametocytes are released into the peripheral bloodstream, where they may persist for 22 days, with a population half-time of 2.2 to 7 days. Most gametocytes are not taken up by mosquitoes but are removed by the spleen, where they stimulate antibody responses to the 'stored' gametocyte proteins, some of which are subsequently expressed on the surface of the gametes (e.g. P230, P48/45) and are now considered possible targets for transmission-blocking vaccines.

Biology of the mosquito vector

The first indication that mosquitoes might be involved in human disease cycles was in 1876, when Patrick Manson found that culex mosquitoes transmitted filarial worms. Ross and Grassi's discoveries of malaria transmission by anopheles mosquitoes followed in the 1890s. The Dipteran order of insects, to which the more than 3500 species and subspecies of mosquitoes belong, has many blood-feeding members and contains the insects of greatest medical and veterinary importance. Mosquitoes have coevolved with their vertebrate hosts, extending their feeding range from reptiles to mammals. The adaptation of malaria parasites to their mosquito hosts probably occurred about 20 000 years ago. From the human perspective, the most devastating link is that between *P. falciparum* and the African mosquito *Anopheles gambiae*, which is estimated to have been in place for as little as 10 000 years.

Blood feeding and host preference

Unlike many haematophagous insects, it is only adult female mosquitoes that have piercing and sucking mouthparts, adapted for taking a blood meal from vertebrate hosts to nourish the development of a single egg batch. Of the three groups of mosquitoes—anophelines, culicines, and aedines—only about 50 anophelines are malaria vectors. Many mosquitoes are part of complexes of sibling species, distinguishable only by modern molecular methods. The *An. gambiae* and *An. funestus* groups contain the most important African malaria vectors. Within the *An. gambiae* complex, *An. gambiae sensu stricto*, the best of the human malaria vectors, prefers to feed on humans, while *An. quadriannulatus*, a nonvector, feeds on cattle and *An. arabiensis*, a secondary vector in many parts of Africa, preferentially feeds on cattle but will take a human blood meal. Olfaction plays a vital role in the host-seeking behaviour of mosquitoes. The segmented antennae and, to a lesser extent, the maxillary palps have numerous sensillae, mostly olfactory, which are responsible for detecting stimuli and eliciting specific behaviour patterns from the mosquito. Feeding selectivity is based on attraction by warmth, moisture, carbon dioxide, and constituents of sweat. Human odour contains 33 chemical signalling compounds, but at least 5 are repellent to mosquitoes.

Preferred habitat for breeding

Mosquitoes have exploited a wide range of aquatic breeding habitats. In Africa, *An. gambiae* breeds extensively in any small, open, clean water body, including standing water in cattle hoofprints, while *An. funestus* breeds in larger, open, clean water bodies such as small ponds. Female mosquitoes lay one to three batches of 30 to 200 eggs during their lifespan, allowing an explosive increase in mosquito numbers from a relatively small number of females once breeding conditions become favourable.

Vectorial capacity and transmissibility

Mosquitoes are most efficient as vectors when the interval between parasite ingestion and its transmission to the next human host (extrinsic incubation period) coincides with the periodicity of female mosquito blood feeds associated with egg production. Vectorial capacity is defined as the average number of potentially infective bites delivered by all the mosquitoes feeding on a single host within 1 day. The numbers of mosquitoes feeding depends on mosquito density in relation to host density and the probability that the mosquito feeds on a host in any 1 day. The feeding frequency on humans is related to the proportion of meals taken on humans compared to other potential hosts. These factors were incorporated into MacDonald's equation for vectorial capacity:

$$V = [ma] \times [p^n] \times [(a/-\log_e n(p))]$$

subsequently modified by Garrett-Jones in 1964 and 1974 to

$$V = [ma]^2 \, (p^n/-\log_e p)$$

where *m* is relative vector density (i.e. number of mosquitoes per human), *a* is human-biting frequency (i.e. number of human blood meals per vector per day), *ma* is the number of bites per person per night, *p* is the proportion of vectors surviving per day, and *n* is the latent period (days) of the parasite in the mosquito (extrinsic incubation period).

A measure of the proportion of mosquitoes taking a meal from an infected human that actually become infective is often added to this equation. This is a measure of the genetic and physiological competence of the mosquito. Small changes in the probability that the vector feeds on a host in 1 day (*a*), the duration of the extrinsic incubation period (*n*), and the probability that the mosquito will survive 1 day (*p*) produce large changes in vectorial capacity. This outcome led MacDonald to predict, as early as 1957, that adulticides would be more effective than larvicides in reducing malaria transmission rates, a lesson that has been relearned many times since by successive generations of entomologists. A related measure of the transmissibility or ability of an infectious agent to spread in a population is the basic reproduction number (R_0). R_0 is generally defined as the expected number of hosts who would be infected after one generation of the parasite by a single infectious person who had been introduced into an otherwise naive population. If R_0 is greater than 1, the number of people infected by the parasite increases; and if R_0 is less than 1, the number declines. The value of R_0 and the proportion of the mosquito population that is refractory to infection ultimately explain whether malaria will spread or be eliminated.

To monitor insect infection rates a number of different techniques can be deployed. The gold standard is the dissection and microscopical examination of blood-fed female mosquitoes (Fig. 8.2.7), but the polymerase chain reaction (PCR) is used increasingly. The recent discovery of a much higher level of human transmission of *P. knowlesi* in Borneo also shows how reliant techniques such as microscopy are on the ability of microscopists to differentiate between what they believe they should see and what they actually see. New molecular techniques that track specific single nucleotide polymorphism (SNP) patterns now make it practicable to follow the emergence and spread of a disease outbreak and should reduce the level of parasite misclassification in both humans and mosquitoes. However, the specificity and sensitivity of such tests needs careful analysis and is often poorly understood by field practitioners. Sensitivity is the probability that a test will correctly identify an infected host; specificity is the probability that a test will correctly identify organisms. PCR-based tests are available for the four human malaria parasites and *P. knowlesi*. A valid concern with this type of molecular method is that, although they detect the presence of pathogen nucleic acids with great sensitivity, they may not be well correlated with the presence or abundance

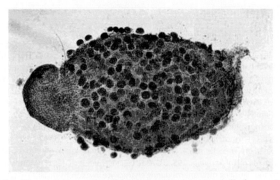

Fig. 8.2.7 Dissected *Plasmodium falciparum* oocysts on gut wall of mosquito. (Courtesy of WHO/MAP/TDR.)

of viable pathogens. This may be complicated by issues of vector competence, when the mosquito is infected with the parasite but is incapable of transmitting it.

Distribution and density of mosquito populations

Mapping mosquito populations is important for guiding epidemiological activities within a study area. Advances in remote sensing should improve this process. In Kenya, multitemporal meteorological satellites have been used to predict periods when malaria transmission is likely to increase, based on correlations between advanced high-resolution satellite-derived indices of vegetation biomass and mosquito abundance. Use of such remote sensor data will allow studies of large, remote geographical areas to which access is difficult. Logistical growth models have been used to estimate the mosquito population carrying capacity of a given environment. Within this model, the extent to which mosquito births and deaths are conditioned by density is referred to as density dependence. However, the role of density dependence in natural populations is controversial. Other factors, such as predation, interspecies competition, and disease, may intervene to regulate population size long before it reaches its carrying capacity. Density-independent factors that influence population growth include environmental conditions such as food availability, adverse weather, extremes of temperature and relative humidity, and insecticide treatment programmes aimed at changing the age structure/size of mosquito populations. However, some insecticide-based interventions act only at a personal level, failing to reduce insect populations sufficiently to produce a herd or population protection effect on humans.

Mosquito genetics and insecticide resistance

The genome sequence of *An. gambiae* was published in 2002. Important mosquito phenotypes that have a genetic basis include blood feeding preference, habitat choice, insecticide susceptibility, and vectorial capacity. Blood feeding involves expression of salivary gland proteins that promote vasodilatation, inhibit platelet aggregation, and prevent blood coagulation in the host. Vector competence is a complex trait involving ingestion, replication, and transmission of plasmodium. The absence of any one of several structural or biochemical properties of the female mosquito could render her incapable of supporting successful completion of the parasite's life cycle. An important advance towards genetic characterization of mosquito refractoriness to parasite invasion in *An. gambiae* was the construction of a microsatellite map for quantitative trait loci. Insecticide resistance is genetically inherited. DNA-based systems are now available for identifying species, determining whether they are infected, identifying the source of their blood meal, and finding the most common insecticide resistance mechanisms. Microarray technology has speeded up the process of identification of metabolic genes that are over- or underexpressed in resistant insects. Different target site resistances can be detected by simple PCR, e.g. a simple SNP-based PCR assay can be deployed to detect the *kdr*-type pyrethroid resistance mechanism, which results from a single nucleotide change in the sodium channel of the insect's nervous system and results in phenotypic resistance to DDT and to all pyrethroids in homozygotes. Heterozygous insects are phenotypically susceptible to all the insecticides. The resistance can be selected by exposure to either DDT or pyrethroids. Retrospective analysis of specimens in laboratory or museum collections demonstrated that the *kdr* mutation was first selected in the 1940s to 1960s by the use of DDT in West and East Africa but remained completely undetected. In West Africa, resistance spread dramatically and was heavily reselected by the introduction of the pyrethroids in the late 1970s. Today, *kdr* in *An. gambiae* in West Africa has been selected almost to completion. It has managed to move between the sibling species of the *An. gambiae* complex and is still spreading. In one longitudinal study in Senegal, the Leu1014Phe *kdr* resistance mutation in *Anopheles gambiae* mosquitoes increased from 8% in 2007 to 48% in 2010 (p = 0.0009). In East Africa, resistance had been confined to small areas of Kenya but *An arabiensis* populations of southwestern Ethiopia now show a high frequency of the West African kdr mutation. In southern Africa, despite the extensive use of DDT in indoor residual spraying programmes over many years, there is no evidence of *kdr*-type resistance in either *An. gambiae* or *An. funestus*.

There has been spectacular progress in producing transgenic mosquitoes in recent years. At least five mosquito species (*An. gambiae*, *An. stephensi*, *An. albimanus*, *Aedes aegypti*, and *Culex quinquefasciatus*) can be transformed using at least four transposable elements (Fig. 8.2.8). Effector genes can abolish the mosquito's vectorial ability. Introduction of such mosquito strains might reduce malaria transmission by replacing wild-type mosquitoes.

Mosquito immunity to malaria

For many years, it was assumed that the insects did not possess an immune system. However, mosquitoes express several elements of vertebrate-specific immune responses. The ookinetes penetrating the mosquito midgut epithelial cells induce some *Anopheles* species to produce nitric oxide synthetase; defensin, a Gram-negative bacterial binding protein; and a thioester-containing protein TEP-1, and to initiate several other enzymatic pathways that may ultimately lead to parasite death. As a result, only a small percentage of mature ookinetes manage to reach the basal lamina to form oocysts, which are themselves vulnerable to melanization and destruction.

Epidemiology

Spatial limits of malaria

The probable maximum preintervention distribution of malaria (*c.*1900) is shown in Fig. 8.2.9, reaching latitudinal extremes of 64° north and 32° south. Human efforts to control malaria have

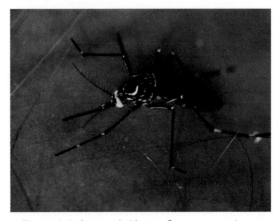

Fig. 8.2.8 Transgenic *Aedes aegypti* with green fluorescent protein expressed in the eyes.

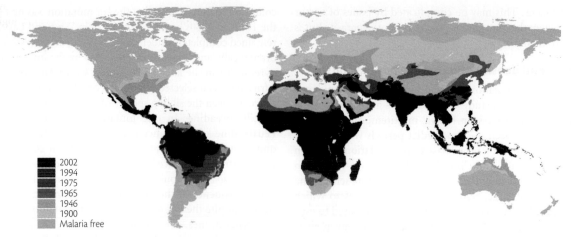

Fig. 8.2.9 Global distribution of malaria from pre-intervention to the present (c.1900–2002).
Hay SI, et al. (2004). The global distribution and population at risk of malaria: past, present and future. *Lancet Infectious Diseases*, **4**, 327–336.

restricted its distribution dramatically during the 20th century as shown by the reported limits in 1946, 1965, 1975, 1992, 1994, and 2002. These distribution maps were compiled largely from country reports and expert opinion arising from the network of regional offices of the World Health Organization (WHO). Although they are imperfect representations of the distribution of global malaria infection risk in space and time, they do highlight the progress of malaria control in the 20th century. Between 1900 and 2002, the combined effects of development and control have halved the area of human malaria risk from 53 to 27% of the Earth's land surface. The number of countries and territories with populations of over 100 000 inhabitants exposed to some level of malaria risk fell from 140 to 106 during this time. However, population growth has increased the total number of people exposed to malaria risk from approximately 1 billion in 1900 to approximately 3 billion in 2002.

Renewed interest in global malaria control has been associated with a renaissance in mapping malaria risks. The Malaria Atlas Project has synthesized all available medical intelligence on areas of the world reportedly free from malaria risk and adjusted these limits to other factors that would not support transmission of either *P. falciparum* or *P. vivax*, including human settlement patterns, climate, and altitude. It has been estimated that in 2007 2.4 billion people were exposed to some risk of infection with *P. falciparum* across 87 countries (Fig. 8.2.10). The true biological and medical extent of *P. vivax* is harder to map and estimate; adaptations of work published in 2006 suggest that 3.18 billion people may be exposed to *P. vivax* in 2007 across 63 countries. No efforts have yet been made to map the distributions of the other two human malarias, *P. malariae* and *P. ovale*. *P. malariae* is widespread and often overlooked and *P. ovale* largely replaces *P. vivax* in West Africa, where the population is resistant.

The variation in intensity of malaria transmission worldwide

Mosquito-related factors

Only mosquitoes that become infected and then survive for longer than the duration of the extrinsic cycle of the parasite (say 10 days) can pass on the infection. As mosquitoes of a given species have a relatively constant probability of dying during a day, regardless of

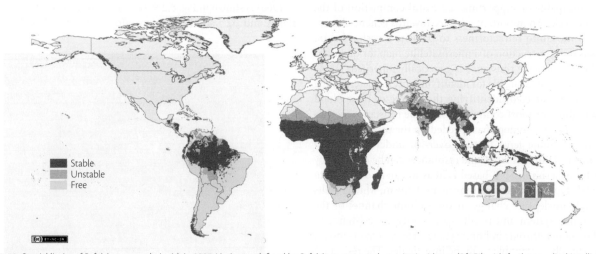

Fig. 8.2.10 Spatial limits of *P. falciparum* malaria risk in 2007. Limits are defined by *P. falciparum* annual parasite incidence (*Pf*API) with further medical intelligence, temperature, and aridity masks. Areas were defined as stable (dark red areas, where *Pf*API ≥0.01% per year), unstable (medium grey areas, where *Pf*API <0.01% per year), or no risk (light grey, where *Pf*API = 0).
(From Guerra CA, et al. (2008). The limits and intensity of *Plasmodium falciparum* transmission: Implications for malaria control and elimination worldwide. *PLoS Med*, **5**, e38.)

their age, the longevity may be described by the probability of surviving through 1 day. It varies greatly between mosquito species and environments. Rainfall, temperature, ecology, human settlement patterns, and prevalence of effective control measures largely govern the abundance of malaria mosquito vectors and the development of the parasite in their salivary glands. The behavioural characteristics of mosquitoes make some of them more efficient vectors of malaria than others. The ability of An. gambiae to breed opportunistically in small collections of water in rural areas, feed and rest indoors, take frequent blood meals, and live for a relatively long period makes it the world's most efficient malaria vector. However, urban areas provide environments that are less suited to the breeding of An. gambiae and so malaria transmission in the rapidly expanding conurbations of Africa is very low. In Africa, An. arabiensis is better adapted to semiarid areas but is a less efficient vector than An. gambiae, accounting for the lower transmission of P. falciparum observed at the fringes of the Sahara, southern Africa, and the Horn of Africa. In South Asia, An. culicifacies may feed only every third day. As few as 10% of its meals may be from people, resulting in a human-biting habit that is 15-fold lower than An. gambiae. The diversity of vectors is driven by habitat preferences and adapted behaviours ('bionomics'), e.g. An. sundaicus, An. maculatus, An. balabacensis, and An. subpictus occupy specific geographical niches in Java (Indonesia). Their varying efficiencies as vectors of malaria account for most of the diversity of malaria in that archipelago.

Transmission and malarial endemicity

Within the geographical ranges of dominant vector species, there are huge variations in the likelihood that a mosquito is infected with malaria and the frequency with which they feed on humans. Across the central belt of tropical Africa, individuals may be challenged from less than once to over 1500 times each year. In other parts of the world, where malaria vectors are less efficient than in Africa, an individual might expect to be infected from once a year to every 10 years. Exceptions are found in New Guinea, several states in India, and smaller foci at forest fringes of Thailand, Vietnam, Cambodia, and Burma (Myanmar).

The frequency of contact between humans and malaria-infected vectors is a fundamental epidemiological concept that drives the health impact of malaria and the choice of control strategies. The frequency of malaria parasite encounters experienced by communities (transmission) is expressed using a variety of epidemiological terms and measured using field studies of contact and infection in mosquitoes and humans. The term 'endemicity' is a general expression of the amount or intensity of malaria transmission in an area or community. 'Epidemic malaria' indicates a periodic or sharp increase in the amount of malaria in a given indigenous community. Precise information about the degree of endemicity must be based on quantitative and statistical concepts. Malaria transmission is also classified as stable or unstable. 'Stable' implies equilibrium; the prevalence of infection is persistently high and endemicity is relatively insensitive to aberrations in climate or local habitats. Under stable endemic conditions, variation in transmission is minimal over many years although seasonal fluctuations still do occur and transmission can continue even with very few vectors. Conversely, 'unstable' malaria is characterized by great variability in space and time.

R_0 is often the benchmark epidemiological measure of malaria transmission but it is rarely measured empirically in the field.

Two related measures, more commonly used, are derived from sampling mosquitoes or young children. The entomological inoculation rate (EIR) measures the average number of infected bites that an individual might experience from local vectors in a unit of time (often expressed per year) and measured by catching mosquitoes inside and outside people's houses and dissection of mosquito salivary glands to see if they are infected. The parasite rate (PR) represents the proportion of individuals (usually children aged 2–9 years) who have evidence of infection in their peripheral blood when sampled during a cross sectional study in the community. It is not strictly a rate but a proportional ratio of infected persons. The PR has been widely used to classify P. falciparum endemicity since the 1950s. Four commonly used terms indicate the prevalence of infection in children aged between 2 and 9 years: hypoendemic (< 10%); mesoendemic (11–50%); hyperendemic (51–75%); and holoendemic (>75%, when measured in infants but routinely measured in children aged 2–9 years). Most measures of malaria transmission are related, often nonlinearly. Classical epidemiological models of malaria transmission, based largely on infection and vectors, are gradually accommodating new concepts related to pathogenesis, virulence, disease outcomes, and heterogeneity of susceptibility and transmission. These new suites of mathematical models should provide a more elaborate framework for understanding the diversity of malaria as a public health problem and how best to tailor control methods to meet specific short and long-term transmission-dependent needs.

The changing epidemiology of malaria
Population growth and environmental change

In most parts of the world, the epidemiological background to clinical malaria is likely to change due to population growth, environmental changes (often the result of human activity, whether local or global), changing resistance of parasites to drugs, and the consequences of attempts at malaria control. Predicting the resources needed to meet international malaria control objectives in the near future must take account of increasing populations at risk of malaria and the changing pattern and intensity of land use. The rate of population growth is significantly higher in urban than rural areas; sometime before 2025, most Africans will live in cities. Urban growth will reduce malaria risk. The pressure on agricultural land as populations grow can lead to deforestation, while increases in irrigation and dams together with poor land management can lead to desertification. In Africa, deforestation rates in the 1990s exceeded those in South America and are projected to increase with the growing capacity of humans to exploit forest habitat. The impact of deforestation on malaria transmission depends on which vector is dominant locally. In Africa, deforestation could create a habitat favouring An. gambiae, a more efficient malaria vector than the forest mosquito An. moucheti. Deforestation is also benefiting An. darlingi, the most efficient malaria vector in the Americas, but in South-East Asia deforestation may reduce malaria transmission by An. dirus. In Africa, most of the 525 large and 45594 small dams have been built since 1950. Their number will increase in the near future and may aggravate malaria transmission, e.g. the restoration of An. funestus to the Sahel, after a prolonged period of drought and desertification, has been attributed to irrigation.

Population movements

Human migration has been associated with malaria epidemics when population pressure in hilly areas drives the inhabitants down into malarious regions, when congregation of workers at new sites mixes infected with susceptible people, or when malnourished refugees, with impaired resistance to infection, camp where public health measures have collapsed. Regional conflicts result in large-scale population movements to avoid the ravages of war. During the mid-1990s, the exodus of nonimmune refugees from the nonmalarious highlands of Burundi to endemic areas of Tanzania resulted in an epidemic of severe malaria.

HIV epidemic

In sub-Saharan Africa, an HIV epidemic has been superimposed on an established malaria pandemic. Considering the wide geographical overlap and concurrent high prevalence of both infections, even a modest interaction could have substantial public health implications. HIV-infected adults in malaria-endemic areas and HIV patients of all ages in areas of unstable malaria transmission are at increased risk of malaria infection and death. In endemic areas, the case fatality of malaria is also higher in HIV-infected children. The impact of HIV on malaria depends on the level of malarial endemicity and, hence, the age patterns of clinical malaria and on the geographical distributions of HIV. Populations in southern Africa and urban areas of Africa are most vulnerable to this interaction.

The public health burden of malaria

Direct and indirect consequences of infection

The relationship between *P. falciparum* infection and disease outcome is complex. People born into areas of stable *P. falciparum* transmission frequently have periods when they are being infected with the parasite and periods when they remain uninfected. Most will, at some stage in their lives, develop a clinical response to infection, usually an attack of fever. This may resolve without any medical intervention, progress to severe disease with natural resolution,

resolve through medical intervention, or end fatally. In areas where transmission is stable, less than 0.05% of infections prove fatal. This low case fatality is largely a result of combinations of innate genetic protection and acquired clinical immunity. There are, however, indirect consequences of malaria infection that are less effectively controlled by immunity. Chronic subclinical infections, e.g. due to incomplete parasite elimination with failing drugs, may lead to anaemia or other forms of malnutrition that independently increase susceptibility to severe effects of future infections. Subclinical infections may increase the severity of other infectious diseases. Asymptomatic infection of the placenta of a pregnant woman may significantly reduce the weight and hence the chances of survival of her newborn child. Patients who survive severe disease may be left with debilitating sequelae, such as spasticity or epilepsy, or more subtle consequences including behavioural disturbances or cognitive impairment. The combined direct, indirect, and consequential impacts of *P. falciparum* on health are summarized in Fig. 8.2.11.

Epidemiological patterns of stable and unstable malaria

The epidemiological features of human malaria differ markedly even between endemic areas. At one extreme, as in holoendemic areas of tropical Africa, everyone is infected shortly after birth, parasitaemia is almost universal throughout childhood, and the brunt of mortality falls in early childhood; epidemics do not occur except at high altitude or during aberrant rainfall in semiarid areas.

Children living in the *An. gambiae* belt of tropical Africa will usually have their first malaria infection during their first 3 months of life when they still have maternal antibodies. The disease is very mild, consisting of just one or two peaks of fever that usually resolve without treatment. When they are between 4 and 6 months old, when maternal antibodies have waned, each new infection leads to more severe febrile illnesses. The repeated infection–fever cycle progressively increases the loss of RBCs to the parasite plus a suppressed ability to replace them. Combined with other severe

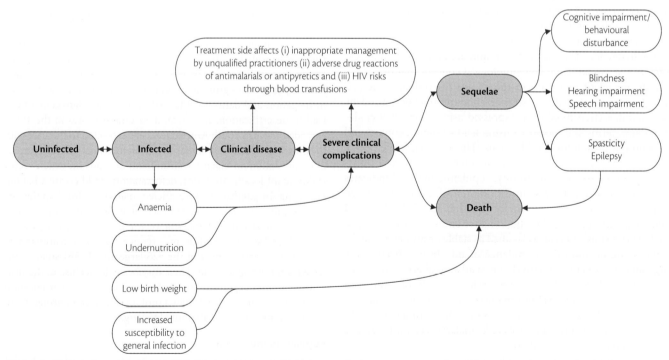

Fig. 8.2.11 Direct, indirect, and consequential clinical consequences of *P. falciparum* infection.
(Redrawn from Snow RW, Gilles HM (2002). The epidemiology of malaria. In: Warrell DA, Gilles HM (eds) Bruce-Chwatt's essential malariology, 4th edition, pp. 85–106. Arnold, London.)

pathological consequences such as metabolic acidosis and coma, approximately 1% of all children living in these areas will die before their third birthday. The survivors will continue to have frequent attacks of fever until about the onset of puberty. Many will experience between 20 and 50 malaria attacks before reaching their fifth birthday. Thereafter, the frequency of attacks of fever and the intensity parasitaemia slowly wanes until levelling out sometime in early adolescence.

From that point forward, people have an almost constant low parasitaemia despite an almost complete absence of symptoms. In adults, episodes of fever due to malaria occur only once in 2 to 10 years, and last only a few hours even without treatment. The one exception to this rule is malaria in pregnant women, especially those pregnant for the first time.

Malaria in pregnancy

It is estimated that, each year, over 30 million women become pregnant in malarious areas of Africa. In mesoholoendemic areas, pregnant women experience relatively little malaria-specific morbidity but have an increased risk of infection and higher density parasitaemia leading to anaemia and placental sequestration of parasites. Maternal anaemia is an important contributor to maternal mortality and it is estimated that 9% of the excess risk is directly attributed to *P. falciparum* infection. Prematurity and low birth weight (<2500 g) associated with maternal malaria have been reported indirectly to contribute to 3 to 8% of infant mortality. Interactions between malaria and HIV are particularly important among pregnant women who, when coinfected, have an increased risk of clinical attacks of malaria, anaemia and giving birth to a low birth weight baby. It is estimated that 500 000 women will develop clinical malaria in Africa as a result of their HIV infection. It remains uncertain whether malaria during pregnancy increases the vertical transmission of HIV.

Areas of unstable malaria

At the other end of the spectrum, as in parts of South-East Asia, where malaria is unstable or hypoendemic disease affects all ages, the risk of clinical illness is almost directly proportional to the risk of infection, and the risks of acquiring the parasite and developing a clinical event are time and space dependent throughout heterogeneous foci. Despite differences in the age patterns of disease with differing levels of endemicity, there is a much lower overall incidence of clinical disease and death in communities located in areas of low transmission intensity (hypomesoendemic) than in those experiencing moderate-to-high transmission (hyperholoendemic). However, during epidemics, disease burdens in lower transmission areas can be devastating, disrupting livelihoods. Overall, as the annual risk of new infections increases from zero, through to low-to-moderate risks of new infections (say one or two new infections per year), the rates of disease increase proportionately and probably linearly. As transmission intensity increases through hyper- to holoendemic conditions, the relationship between the annual risk of infection and the rates of disease is less clear, probably nonlinear and may reach a plateau after about 10 new infections per year. To understand the clinical spectrum of malaria seen in patients from a given locality, it is essential to understand the local epidemiology.

Global malarial morbidity and mortality

Although it is convenient to classify entire regions of the world by levels of endemicity, the low intensity transmission characteristics of most areas of South-East Asia resemble large swathes of Africa. Similarly, there are areas of South-East Asia that might be regarded as typical of the central *An. gambiae* belt of Africa. Precise estimates of the numbers of clinical cases and deaths due to malaria are notoriously poor in all malaria endemic countries. National data on malarial illness and death are characterized by gaps and inaccuracies due to under-reporting and misdiagnosis. Deaths usually occur outside the formal health sector and many clinical events are self medicated.

Given the weaknesses in international malaria disease reporting, estimations have been made of the public health burden using modified historical and climate-driven maps of malaria transmission, projected population human settlement counts, and endemicity-specific epidemiological survey data of clinical attacks and deaths due to *P. falciparum*. These approaches suggest that there were approximately 550 million clinical attacks of *P. falciparum* worldwide in 2002, distributed by WHO regions as follows: 71% in the Africa region, 23% in the low-transmission but densely populated countries of South-East Asia, 3% in the western Pacific, 0.7% in the Americas; 2.3% in the eastern Mediterranean (including Somalia and Sudan), and 0.1% in the European region. Less is known about global *P. falciparum* mortality and still less about the neglected disease burdens posed by *P. vivax*, despite its wider distribution. In Africa, application of similar epidemiological disease burden models to assess the wider public health consequences of *P. falciparum* (Fig. 8.2.11) suggested that in 2005 *P. falciparum* caused 1.1 million deaths directly, between 71 000 and 190 000 infant deaths following placental infection *in utero*, and over 3000 newly acquired persistent epilepsies through brain insults among patients surviving an episode of cerebral malaria in childhood.

Estimates of annual mortality of malaria in India have been particularly confusing, varying from 2000 (Government of India) to 16 000 (WHO) or 125 000 to 277 000 (as assessed by 'verbal autopsy').

Susceptibility to infection and innate resistance

In endemic areas, malaria is thought to account for around one-quarter of all childhood deaths so that this infection has been a major selective force in human evolution. More human genetic polymorphisms have been associated with innate protection from malaria than with any other infectious disease (Table 8.2.1). The best known is sickle cell haemoglobin, due to a point mutation in position 6 of the β-globin chain. Here, the mutant-gene frequency is stabilized because the enhanced survival of AS heterozygotes is counterbalanced by the lethal consequences of homozygosity (SS). The protection afforded to AS heterozygotes seems to act predominately on the development of clinical disease. Although infection rates are similar for AA and AS genotypes, the AS genotype is almost completely protected against life-threatening *P. falciparum* malaria. α-Thalassaemia, resulting from deletion of α-globin genes, is less strongly protective against *P. falciparum* malaria but, as most forms are virtually asymptomatic, very high gene frequencies have developed in some parts of the world such as Oceania. However, in Africa, where the selective pressure is greatest, the gene frequency is less (typically *c*.40%). This may be explained by the fact that when sickle cell trait and α-thalassaemia coexist, far from acting synergistically, they cancel out each other's protection, a striking example of negative epistasis.

Many other genetic variants affecting the RBC have been associated with protection from malaria, including other variants of the β-globin gene (HbC and HbE), polymorphisms of the RBC enzymes glucose-6-phosphate dehydrogenase (G6PD) and pyruvate kinase, and variants of structural proteins (erythrocyte band 3), which cause South-East Asian ovalocytosis.

The Duffy (blood group) antigen receptor for chemokines (DARCFy), expressed on the surface of RBCs, is also a receptor for penetration of RBCs by merozoites of *P. vivax*. The extreme rarity of the DARC +46C/C genotype is responsible for the striking resistance to this parasite of people of West African origin. However, these same receptors influence plasma levels of HIV-1 suppressive and proinflammatory chemokines such as CCL5/RANTES and are the site of HIV-1 attachment to RBCs, affecting by HIV adsorption the transinfection of target cells. In African Americans, possession of the prevalent DARC −46C/C genotype was found to be associated with a 40% increase in the risk of acquiring HIV-1. If extrapolated to all Africans, approximately 11% of the HIV-1 burden in Africa may be linked to this genotype.

Many potentially protective polymorphisms affecting other key aspects of malaria–human interaction have now been identified. These include polymorphisms affecting endothelial receptors, cytokines, and other key molecules of the immune system. Any listing of putative protective polymorphisms, such as Table 8.2.1, is bound to become quickly out of date. There is now an international coordinated effort to apply whole genome scanning approaches to identify key polymorphisms conferring protection against malaria. Regularly updated information can be found at http://www.malariagen.net.

Acquired resistance

Different aspects of the acquisition of immunity in endemic populations are illustrated in Fig. 8.2.12. Such immunity is often described as being slow to acquire and incomplete. From the figure, it can be seen that the prevalence of asymptomatic infection remains high for many years and even in adulthood a substantial proportion of people are infected at a single time point. It is unlikely that anyone ever achieves sterilizing immunity. However, the most important aspects of immunity, the ability to avoid severe disease and death, develop much faster. In most stably endemic areas, death due to malaria is rare after the age of 5 and hardly ever occurs in normally immunocompetent adults.

A characteristic of immunity to malaria is the early acquisition of the ability to tolerate levels of parasitization that would cause illness in a naive individual. This presumably involves either, or both, a immune response to neutralize parasite toxins or a down-regulation of the host's normal cytokine response to challenge. However, it is important to recognize that such 'antitoxic' responses cannot of themselves be the mainstay of protection against serious morbidity, for if the parasite population continued to expand, the host's RBC population would soon be overwhelmed leading to severe anaemia. Thus, even at an early stage, the key aspect of immunity to malaria is an acquired ability to control parasite growth, either by interfering with the replication of parasite or by accelerating the removal from the circulation.

Emphasis is often given to the strain-specific nature of malarial immunity, with the idea that immunity depends on having to acquire a repertoire of responses to different 'strains' of the parasite. However, because the parasite population is constantly

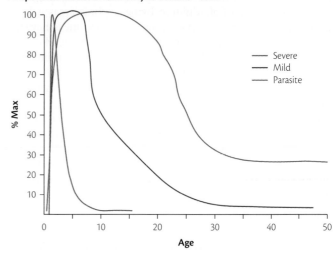

Population indices of immunity to malaria – Kilifi

— Severe
— Mild
— Parasite

Fig. 8.2.12 Acquisition of immunity to malaria with age. The figure shows the period prevalence of three markers of immunity to malaria: the susceptibility to severe (life threatening) malaria, susceptibility to mild febrile episodes due to malaria, and the susceptibility to asymptomatic parasitization. Data are taken from an endemic population in Kilifi District on the coast of Kenya and normalized to a percentage of the maximum achieved in the population.

outbreeding, it is more accurate to think of polymorphism in key molecular targets of protective immune responses rather than of fixed 'strains'. For some of these polymorphic targets, i.e. parasite-derived molecules expressed on the outside of the infected RBC membrane, children do build up a repertoire of responses. New infections tend to be those that the individual has not yet seen. However, there is also considerable evidence that some protective responses are cross-protective from an early stage. It is likely that the development of immunity involves the progressive acquisition of both strain-specific and cross-protective responses to a range of potential targets.

Potentially, effective immune responses could act at any point in the parasite's life cycle (Fig. 8.2.2). Immunity is largely stage specific, i.e. immunity induced by the sporozoite stage that can prevent infection probably has little effect on the blood stages. Similarly the targets and mechanisms responsible for immunity to gametocytes (which prevent transmission) are separate from those responsible for immune response to pre-erythrocytic and erythrocytic stages. Experimental infection of humans and animals with attenuated sporozoites leads under some circumstances to complete immunity to infection (see 'Malarial vaccines', below). However, there is little evidence that such responses play a major role in naturally acquired immunity to malaria and, in fact, adults in endemic areas become infected at similar rates to children (albeit without progressing to clinical illness).

Naturally acquired immunity to malaria probably acts predominantly at the blood stages of the parasite's cycle. Here, the parasite is present briefly as a free merozoite before spending most of its time apparently hidden inside the host RBC. Effective responses are likely to depend either on antibody-mediated mechanisms or on indirect cellular effects involving the release of a range of mediators. The potential importance of antibody mediated responses to blood-stage parasites was demonstrated in classical studies in which gammaglobulin from immune adults was shown to markedly ameliorate attacks of malaria in children.

Similarly, the relative protection of children in the first few months of life in endemic area is thought to be due in part to passively transferred maternal antibody. A number of potentially key targets for protective immune responses have been identified. These tend to be either molecules involved in the invasion of RBCs by merozoites or parasite-induced molecules inserted on the surface of the infected RBC during the second half of its blood stage. Most of these antigens show considerable antigenic polymorphism and those growing up in endemic areas develop a wide range of antibodies to many antigenic types. Increasingly it appears that protection from clinical malaria may stem from multiple mechanisms and that the breadth and quality of the immune response to a number of antigens may be more important than responses to any single antigen. Humans also make immune responses to several gametocyte specific antigens. However, although experimental approaches to interrupting transmission in animal models hold promise for transmission blocking vaccines, the evidence that such responses play an important role in nature is controversial.

Immunity is diminished after long periods of absence from endemic areas and in pregnancy. Previously immune pregnant women are at risk of parasitization of the placenta, resulting in spill-over peripheral parasitaemia, increasing anaemia, and impairment of placental function leading to low birth weight babies. This results not from a breakdown in previously established immunity but from the specific appearance of a new site for sequestration of parasites. Parasitized RBCs (PRBCs) recovered from the placenta express a specific subset of PfEMP1 molecules that bind to chondroitin sulphate A (CSA) on the syncytiotrophoblast, leading to the accumulation of sometimes massive numbers of metabolically active parasites. The PfEMP1 molecules responsible for this adhesion are rarely encountered in infections outside pregnancy and so women enter their first pregnancy without specific antibodies. These are acquired during the course of the first and subsequent pregnancies so that effects of placental parasitization and its consequences decrease progressively with ensuing pregnancies.

Malaria and HIV immunosuppression

HIV infection modifies the response to malaria under a number of situations. In pregnant women, the two conditions seem to be mutually synergistic with the prevalence and consequences (particularly anaemia) being more severe in HIV-positive women. In nonimmune adults in areas of unstable transmission, HIV positivity is associated with an increased risk of clinical malaria and with increased risk of death in those who develop it. Recently it has become clear that HIV positivity in children in endemic areas is strongly associated with increased risk of being admitted to hospital with severe malaria.

Malaria and complicating bacterial infections

Immunosuppression and vulnerability to bacterial infections in children with severe P. falciparum malaria was predicted by B M Greenwood in 1971, based on studies of murine *P. berghei* infection. Subsequently, an association between *P. falciparum* malaria and nontyphoid salmonella was discovered in children in The Gambia and with Gram-negative rod septicaemias in adults in Thailand. A series of cross-sectional and longitudinal case–control studies in Kilfi, Kenya have demonstrated convincingly that the protective effect of HbAS against invasive bacterial disease is mediated by the known protection of HbAS against malaria, and that, therefore, malaria is a cause of invasive bacterial disease. As a result,

interventions to control malaria will have the important additional benefit by reducing the burden of invasive bacterial disease, a major cause of childhood illness and death in sub-Saharan Africa. In the case of invasive nontyphoid salmonella (NTS) infection, the commonest cause of bacteraemia in many parts of sub-Saharan Africa and a frequent and often fatal complication of *Plasmodium falciparum* infection, a possible mechanism by which tolerance to malaria impairs resistance to NTS has been suggested. Induction of haem oxygenase-1 (HO-1) mediates tolerance to the cytotoxic effects of haem during malarial haemolysis but might impair resistance to NTS by limiting production of bactericidal reactive oxygen species. In mice infected with *Salmonella typhimurium*, phenylhydrazine-induced haemolysis, haemin administration or coinfection with a nonlethal strain of *P. yoelii* caused acute, fatal hyperbacteraemia. However, this could be prevented by inhibiting HO-1 with tin protoporphyrin, allowing oxidative burst activity of granulocytes and macrophages, the normal mechanism of protection against invasive salmonella disease.

Malaria and malnutrition

For many years the relationship between malnutrition and malaria was contentious, with claims that it was associated with protection from severe disease. Although there may be situations where very severe nutritional deficiencies may be associated with reduced risk, in general malnutrition is an important risk factor for severe malaria in children in endemic areas.

Molecular pathology

All the pathology associated with malaria infection is attributable to asexual parasite multiplication in the bloodstream. The consequences to the host of the intraerythrocytic multiplication of parasites range from a variety of severe, but not life-threatening, symptoms common to all the species that infect humans, to the potentially lethal complications particularly associated with acute *P. falciparum* infection.

The characteristic symptom of malaria is fever and this is probably initiated by a combination of stimuli involving parasite products interacting with pattern recognition receptors, such as Toll-like receptors, and cell surface receptors, such as CD36, on host cells. Parasite products involved include variant parasite molecules expressed on the surface of PRBCs, such as PfEMP1, glycosylphosphatidylinositol anchors which are found on many plasmodium membrane proteins, and haemozoin. These interactions lead to the stimulation of both pro- and anti-inflammatory cytokine cascades, the balance of which may determine the relative outcome in terms of antiparasite effect and host pathology. At one end of the spectrum lies a relatively mild, self-limiting illness; at the other is an attack of severe disease that shares many of the pathological features of sepsis, in which overvigorous or disordered immune responses play a key role. Thus, while tumour necrosis factor (TNF) is protective against the parasite, many studies show an association between severe disease and exaggerated proinflammatory cytokine responses, including TNF, interleukin (IL) IL-1β, IL-6, IL-10, and interferon-γ as well as the macrophage inflammatory protein chemokines MIP1α and MIP1β.

Infection with all species of malaria induces fever, but the acute illness with *P. malariae* or *P. ovale* species is relatively self-limiting. Although *P. vivax* is traditionally considered a relatively benign parasite, the acute illness can be quite severe and it is increasingly realized that deaths due to *P. vivax* infection do occur. However, it is *P. falciparum* that is responsible for the majority of severe disease and death. The principal life-threatening complications of *P. falciparum* in African children are cerebral malaria and severe anaemia often associated with metabolic acidosis and respiratory distress. The clinical picture in nonimmune adults is more complex and can include single or multiple organ failure. A key difference in the biology of *P. falciparum* believed to play a central role in its enhanced virulence is its propensity to undergo sequestration (Figs. 8.2.13–8.2.15). Only the younger developmental stages of the parasite circulate, as the more mature forms adhere to specific receptors on venular endothelium. Parasite sequestration occurs in many capillary beds and is often particularly intense in the lungs, brain, intestines, and muscles. The resultant reduction in, or obstruction of, local blood flow probably results in reduced perfusion and tissue damage. However it seems likely that this is just one part of a complex set of responses set in train by the interaction of sequestered cells and endothelial cells and the cells of the immune system leading to local release of a number of potentially toxic or pharmacologically active compounds (such as reactive oxygen species or nitric oxide).

Several endothelial receptors for infected RBC cytoadherence have been identified, including CD36 (formerly platelet glycoprotein IV), thrombospondin, ICAM-1, VCAM-1, and E-selectin. No clear correlation has yet emerged between the ability of parasites to bind to individual receptors and disease pattern (other than in the case of pregnancy-associated malaria), though there is suggestive evidence that severe disease in children maybe associated with the ability of parasites to utilize multiple receptors. Some parasite isolates show two other adhesive properties: the rosetting of uninfected erythrocytes around RBCs containing mature developmental forms of the parasite (Fig. 8.2.16) and autoagglutination of infected erythrocytes in the absence of immune serum. Both phenomena have been linked to severe malaria and it is presumed that the multicellular aggregates, if they occur *in vivo*, may exacerbate vascular obstruction caused by sequestration.

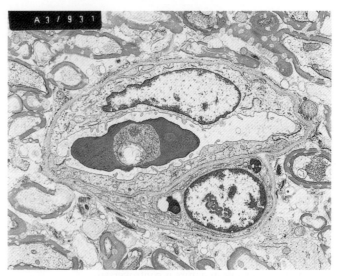

Fig. 8.2.14 Human cerebral malaria. Electron micrograph showing endothelial cell microvilli making contact with a parasitized erythrocyte.
(Copyright Dr N Francis.)

On the parasite side of the equation, PfEMP1 plays a key role in cytoadherent interactions, with binding to different receptors localized to different domains of the molecule. The case of pregnancy-associated malaria offers one example where a specific set of PfEMP1 molecules with the ability to bind to a specific receptor (chondroitin sulphate) forms the basis of organ specific biology and pathology. It remains to be seen whether similar subsets of PfEMP1 molecules will be identified associated with other clinical syndromes.

Severe anaemia is a common part of the picture of severe malaria, especially in young children. Although destruction of parasitized RBCs *per se*, especially in a heavy infection, may lead to a significant fall in haemoglobin, it has long been recognized that this cannot account for the often profound degree of anaemia. Two additional processes seem to be important: the sensitization of RBCs with immune complexes and activated components of the complement system leading to immune mediated removal of non-infected cells and a degree of dyserythropoiesis.

Although an episode of *P. falciparum* malaria is potentially life threatening, in endemic areas the large majority of clinical episodes resolve (albeit after an unpleasant illness) without producing severe disease and death. Clearly behavioural factors such as treatment-seeking behaviour are important, but it also seems likely that the

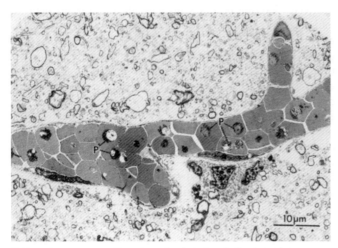

Fig. 8.2.13 Brain section of a patient who died of cerebral malaria. The image shows a blood vessel packed with red blood corpuscles, the majority of which were identified as being infected by the presence of parasites (P) or, at a higher magnification, the presence of knobs.
(Courtesy of Professor D Ferguson.)

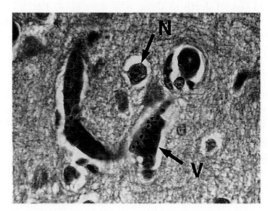

Fig. 8.2.15 Section of frontal cortex from a Vietnamese patient who died of cerebral malaria, showing sequestration of parasitized red blood corpuscles in blood vessels. N, neuron; V, vessel.
(Courtesy of Dr Gareth Turner, Oxford.)

wide range of outcomes represent a balance between host and parasite specific factors. In the end, it may be that severe disease represents the unfortunate coincidence of the wrong host with the wrong parasite.

Organ pathology

Brain

Probably only falciparum malaria causes cerebral pathology although *P. vivax*-infected RBCs may also be sequestered. At autopsy, the brain may be oedematous, especially in African children, but there is rarely any evidence of cerebral, cerebellar, or medullary herniation. Small blood vessels, including those of the leptomeninges, are congested with PRBCs. Many of the parasites are schizonts and mature trophozoites containing malaria pigment (Figs. 8.2.13 and 8.2.14), giving the surface of the brain a characteristic leaden or plum-coloured appearance. Its cut surface is slate grey. In larger vessels, PRBCs form a layer along the endothelium ('margination'). Up to 70% of RBCs in the cerebral vessels are parasitized and are more tightly packed than in other organs. The cerebrovascular endothelium shows pseudopodial projections, closely apposed to electron-dense, knob-like protruberances on the surface of PRBCs (Fig. 8.2.14). Numerous petechial haemorrhages are seen in the white matter, the result of bleeding from end arterioles, proximal to occlusive plugs of PRBCs, and fibrin. Ring haemorrhages are centred on small subcortical vessels. They may organize, attracting small collections of microglial cells around an area of demyelination without inflammatory cells (Dürck's granulomas).

Retina

Retinal whitening is associated with swelling of neurons secondary to local hypoxia and haemorrhages are caused by blockage of small retinal vessels with PRBCs and microthrombi.

Bone marrow

In the acute phase of falciparum malaria, there is iron sequestration, erythrophagocytosis, dyserythropoiesis, and cytoadherence with plugging of sinusoids. Maturation defects are present in the

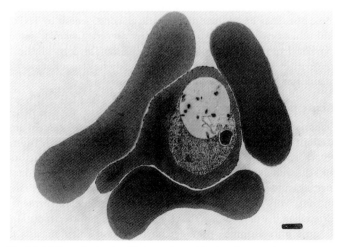

Fig. 8.2.16 Rosetting *in vitro*. The central parasitized erythrocyte shows many electron-dense protruberances (knobs) beneath its membrane (bar = 1 μm). (Copyright Professor D Ferguson.)

marrow for at least 3 weeks after clearance of parasitaemia. Increased numbers of large, abnormal-looking megakaryocytes have been found in the marrow and the circulating platelets may also be enlarged, suggesting dysthrombopoiesis. Malarial pigment and parasites may be found in monocytes and phagocytes in the marrow, even when they are not detectable in peripheral blood.

Liver

The liver is most severely affected in *P. falciparum* malaria. It becomes enlarged and oedematous and is coloured brown, grey, or even black from deposition of malaria pigment. Hepatic sinusoids are dilated, containing hypertrophied Kupffer cells and PRBCs obstructing the circulation. Parasitized and uninfected RBCs are phagocytosed by Kupffer cells, endothelial cells, and sinusoidal macrophages. The small areas of centrilobular necrosis present in severe cases may be attributable to shock or disseminated intravascular coagulation. Hepatocytes appear only mildly abnormal but are depleted of glycogen in some hypoglycaemic patients. Lymphocytic infiltration of portal tracts has been described in some cases of tropical splenomegaly syndrome, a chronic immunological complication of malaria.

Gastrointestinal tract

Cytoadherent, sequestered, PRBCs may be found in the small and large bowel, especially in capillaries of the lamina propria and larger submucosal vessels. The bowel may appear congested, with mucosal ulceration and haemorrhage.

Kidney

Renal failure, with or without 'blackwater fever', is a common and serious complication of severe falciparum malaria in some populations. It is usually associated with acute tubular injury rather than glomerulonephritis. Glomerular lesions consist of mild accumulations of monocytes within glomerular capillaries (acute transient glomerulonephritis) without immune complex deposition. There is PRBC sequestration in glomerular and tubulointerstitial vessels, with fibrin thrombi and pigment-laden macrophages. Tubular pigment casts are prominent in cases of blackwater fever and severe rhabdomyolysis.

Levels of parasite sequestration in the kidney are usually relatively low. They correlates with premortem renal failure, and are significantly higher in malaria-associated renal failure than in fatal cases without renal failure. In quartan malarial nephrosis, a chronic immunological complication of malaria, a distinctive chronic glomerulonephritis develops.

Lung

At autopsy, the lungs are found to be oedematous in almost every case. Pulmonary capillaries and venules are packed with PRBCs and inflammatory cells: neutrophils, plasma cells, and pigment-laden macrophages. The capillary lumen is narrowed by oedema of vascular endothelium and there is interstitial oedema and hyaline-membrane formation. Secondary bronchopneumonia is commonly found.

Spleen

The spleen is enlarged, engorged, and coloured dark red or grayish black. The red and white pulp is congested and hyperplastic, and the splenic cords and sinuses are filled with phagocytic cells containing pigment, PRBCs, and noninfected RBCs. Macrophages may extract the parasites from PRBCs, a process known as 'pitting'. Tropical splenomegaly syndrome is a chronic immunological complication of malaria (see below).

Heart

Myocardial capillaries are congested with pigment-laden macrophages, lymphocytes, plasma cells, and PRBCs but these are not tightly packed or cytoadherent. Subendocardial and epicardial petechial haemorrhages are unusual and there is no myocarditis.

Placenta

Sinusoids are packed with PRBCs and pigment-laden macrophages, giving the placenta a black or slate-grey hue. Necrosis of the syncytiotrophoblast, fibrinoid necrosis, loss of villi, proliferation of cytotrophoblastic cells, and thickening of the trophoblastic membrane may explain impaired fetal nutrition. Although transmission of infection across an intact placenta is considered uncommon, PRBCs are sometimes visible in fetal–placental vessels.

Pathophysiology

Anaemia and thrombocytopenia

Malarial anaemia results from destruction/phagocytosis of PRBCs and dyserythropoiesis. Hyperferritinaemia, an acute-phase reaction, explains the initial iron sequestration and hypoferraemia. Immune-mediated haemolysis occurs in some populations. Erythrocyte survival is reduced even after the disappearance of parasitaemia and there is increased splenic clearance of non-parasitized RBCs and PRBCs. Evidence of Coombs' test-positive haemolysis was found in the Gambia. Intravascular haemolysis occurs in patients whose erythrocytes are congenitally deficient in enzymes such as G6PD in response to oxidant drugs such as primaquine. In classic blackwater fever, G6PD levels are, by definition, normal and the mechanism of haemolysis is unknown. Quinine-mediated haemolysis is suspected but has never been satisfactorily demonstrated. Thrombocytopenia is attributable to splenic sequestration, dysthrombopoiesis, and immune-mediated lysis.

Cerebral malaria

In Thai adults with cerebral malaria, global cerebral blood flow was inappropriately low and there was evidence of cerebral anaerobic glycolysis with increased lactate concentrations in the cerebrospinal fluid. Recently, in Bangladeshi patients with severe malaria, orthogonal polarization spectral imaging was used directly to observe the rectal mucosa, as a surrogate for the cerebral microcirculation. Microcirculatory obstruction (proportion of vessels involved and the degree of obstruction) correlated with disease severity and decreased on clinical recovery. Vessels with little or no blood flow were often seen adjacent to vessels with hyperdynamic blood flow.

In African children with cerebral malaria, plasma concentrations of TNFα, IL-1α, and other cytokines correlate closely with disease severity, as judged by parasitaemia, hypoglycaemia, case fatality, and the incidence of neurological sequelae. Cytokines may have other effects on cerebral function, perhaps by releasing nitric oxide, which interferes with neurotransmission, or by leading to the generation of free oxygen radicals. Cytokines may also cause fever, hypoglycaemia, coagulopathy, dyserythropoiesis, and leucocytosis in falciparum malaria.

In South-East Asian adults, the opening pressure of cerebrospinal fluid at lumbar puncture was usually normal. Cerebral oedema was demonstrable by CT during life in only a small minority, usually as an agonal phenomenon. In these patients, there was little evidence of increased blood–cerebrospinal fluid barrier permeability or that brain swelling was responsible for coma. However, in African children with cerebral malaria, intracranial pressure, as reflected by cerebrospinal fluid opening pressure at lumbar puncture, is usually elevated and the majority have swollen brains. In fatal cases, the brain shows evidence of increased vascular permeability. Ischaemic damage, resulting from a critical reduction in cerebral perfusion pressure, hypoglycaemia, and status epilepticus, probably contributes to brain damage in these children.

Pulmonary oedema

This may be provoked by fluid overload, in which case, central venous and pulmonary artery wedge pressures will be elevated. More commonly, the clinical picture is of acute respiratory distress syndrome (ARDS), with normal or low hydrostatic pressures in the pulmonary vascular bed. In these cases, the mechanism is likely to be increased pulmonary capillary permeability resulting from leucocyte products and cytokines, consistent with the histological appearances of neutrophil sequestration in the pulmonary capillaries, increased permeability, and hyaline membrane formation.

Hypoglycaemia and other metabolic disturbances

Cinchona alkaloids (quinine or quinidine) are potent stimulators of insulin secretion by the pancreatic β-cells, causing hyperinsulinaemia. The resulting reduction in hepatic gluconeogenesis and increased peripheral glucose uptake by tissues causes hypoglycaemia. In malaria, glucose consumption is increased by fever, infection, anaerobic glycolysis, and the metabolic demands of the malaria parasites. Glycogen reserves may be depleted, especially in children and pregnant women, as a result of fasting and 'accelerated starvation'. In African children with severe malaria, adult patients with severe disease, and pregnant women, hypoglycaemia develops spontaneously (without treatment with cinchona alkaloids) and is associated with appropriately low plasma insulin concentrations. Plasma lactate and alanine concentrations are elevated and ketone bodies are moderately increased. Counter-regulatory hormone levels are usually very high. The mechanism of hypoglycaemia in these cases may be inhibition of hepatic gluconeogenesis by TNFα and other cytokines. In African children, severe anaemia, tissue hypoxia, hypoperfusion, and increased anaerobic glycolysis by host and parasites contribute to profound metabolic (lactic) acidosis, manifesting clinically as respiratory distress.

Acute renal failure

Oliguria and renal dysfunction reversible by fluid replacement are attributable to hypovolaemia resulting from dehydration. Hyperparasitaemia, jaundice, and haemoglobinuria are risk factors for acute tubular necrosis. Renal cortical perfusion is reduced during the acute stage of the disease but renal cortical necrosis is rare and survivors rarely show evidence of chronic renal impairment. Cytoadherence of PRBCs in the renal microvasculature, deposition of fibrin microthrombi, prolonged hypotension ('algid malaria'), haemoglobinuria in 'blackwater fever' and myoglobinuria may contribute to acute renal failure. Quartan malarial nephrosis is a chronic immunological complication of malaria (see below).

Hyponatraemia

In patients with relatively normal plasma osmolalities, hyponatraemia has been attributed to the inappropriate secretion of ADH triggered by fever or reduced effective plasma volume. However, in Thai patients, ADH levels were appropriate to their gross hypovolaemia. This has been confirmed in Bangladeshi patients. In those who are salt depleted and dehydrated, mild hyponatraemia is often attributable to intravenous therapy with 5% dextrose.

Hypovolaemia and 'shock' ('algid malaria')

Hypotension may be explained by hypovolaemia (dehydration and, rarely, haemorrhagic shock following splenic rupture or gastrointestinal haemorrhage) but is most often associated with a secondary Gram-negative bacteraemia. The source may be an intravenous cannula, urethral catheter, aspiration pneumonia, or invasion of the bloodstream by an enteric pathogen such as salmonella. Transient immunosuppression, impaired macrophage function, or 'blockade' of the reticuloendothelial system may increase the susceptibility of patients to severe secondary bacterial infections.

Clinical features in adults and children

Malaria is typically an acute febrile illness that, if incompletely treated, tends to recrudesce or relapse over periods of months or even years. The classic periodic febrile paroxysms—occurring every 24 h (quotidian), 36 h (subtertian), 48 to 50 h (tertian), or 72 h (quartan) with afebrile asymptomatic intervals—are rarely observed unless treatment is delayed. Severity depends on the species and strain and, hence, on the geographical origin of the infecting parasite, on the age, genetic constitution, state of immunity, general health, and nutritional state of the patients, and on the speed and appropriateness of antimalarial treatment.

Falciparum malaria ('malignant' tertian or subtertian malaria)

The 'prepatent period', the shortest interval between an infecting mosquito bite and detectable parasitaemia, is usually 9 or 10 days but may be as short as 5 days (Table 8.2.1). The incubation period, the interval between infection and the first symptom, usually ranges from 7 to 14 days (mean 12 days) but may be prolonged by immunity, chemoprophylaxis, or partial chemotherapy. In Europe and North America, 98% of patients with imported falciparum malaria present within 3 months of arriving back from the malarious area. A few present up to 1 year later, but none after 4 years.

Several days of prodromal symptoms such as malaise, headache, myalgia, anorexia, and mild fever are interrupted by the first paroxysm. Suddenly the patient feels inexplicably cold (in a hot climate) and apprehensive. Mild shivering quickly turns into violent shaking with teeth chattering. There is intense peripheral vasoconstriction and gooseflesh. Some patients vomit. The rapid increase in core temperature may trigger febrile convulsions in young children. The rigor lasts up to 1 h and is followed by a hot flush with throbbing headache, palpitations, tachypnoea, prostration, postural syncope, and further vomiting while the temperature reaches its peak. Finally, a drenching sweat breaks out and the fever defervesces over the next few hours. The exhausted patient sleeps. The whole paroxysm is over in 8 to 12 h, after which the patient may feel remarkably well. These symptoms are typical of a classical 'endotoxin reaction' produced by infection with Gram-negative bacteria or the release of TNFα and other cytokines by other agents. Classic tertian or subtertian periodicity is rarely seen with falciparum malaria. A high irregularly spiking, continuous, or remittent fever or daily (quotidian) paroxysm is more usual. Other common symptoms are headache, backache, myalgias, dizziness, postural hypotension, nausea, dry cough, abdominal discomfort, diarrhoea, and vomiting. Nonimmune patients with falciparum malaria are usually severely unwell. Commonly, there is anaemia and mild jaundice, with moderate tender enlargement of the spleen and liver. Useful negative findings are the lack of lymphadenopathy, rash (apart from herpes simplex 'cold sores'), and focal signs.

Severe falciparum malaria

WHO (2000) has defined severe disease by the clinical and laboratory features shown in Box 8.2.2.

Cerebral malaria

The global average case fatality of falciparum malaria is about 1%, or 1 to 3 million deaths per year. Cerebral malaria is an important severe manifestation of *P. falciparum* infection, accounting for a large proportion of adult deaths. Patients who have been feverish and ill for a few days may have a generalized convulsion from which they do not recover consciousness, or their level of consciousness may decline gradually over several hours. High fever alone can impair cerebral function causing drowsiness, delirium, obtundation, confusion, irritability, psychosis, and, in children, febrile convulsions. The term 'cerebral malaria', implying

---

Box 8.2.2 Features of severe falciparum malaria

Clinical manifestations

- Prostration
- Impaired consciousness
- Respiratory distress (acidotic breathing)
- Multiple convulsions
- Circulatory collapse
- Pulmonary oedema (radiological)
- Abnormal bleeding
- Jaundice
- Haemoglobinuria

Laboratory tests

- Severe anaemia (haemoglobin <5 g/dl or haematocrit <15%)
- Hypoglycaemia (blood glucose <2.2 mmol/litre or 40 mg/dl)
- Acidosis (plasma bicarbonate <15 mmol/litre, or base excess more than −10, or arterial pH <7.35)
- Renal impairment (urine output <12 ml/kg/h, or plasma creatinine above age-related normal range; persisting after rehydration)
- Hyperlactataemia (plasma lactate >5 mmol/litre)

encephalopathy specifically related to *P. falciparum* infection, should be restricted to patients: (1) who are unrousable and comatose, showing no appropriate verbal response and no purposive motor response to noxious stimuli (Glasgow Coma Scale ≤9/14); (2) who have evidence of acute *P. falciparum* infection; and (3) in whom other encephalopathies, including hypoglycaemia and transient postictal coma, have been excluded. Mild meningism may be elicited but neck rigidity and photophobia are rare. Retinal abnormalities (Fig. 8.2.17) are best seen with the pupils dilated with 0.5 to 1% tropicamide and 2.5% phenylephrine. Haemorrhages like Roth spots, papilloedema, or exudates are present in about 15% of South-East Asian adults with cerebral malaria. In African children with cerebral malaria, retinal changes include macular and peripheral retinal whitening, vessel changes (orange vessels, tramlining, capillary whitening), retinal haemorrhages, papilloedema, and cotton wool spots. Of these changes, the whitening and vessel changes are specific ('malarial retinopathy') and are associated with a case fatality of about 18%, compared with 44% in children with papilloedema and 7% in those with normal fundi.

In adult patients, pupillary, corneal, oculocephalic, and oculovestibular reflexes are normal. Dysconjugate gaze is common. Muscle tone and tendon reflexes are usually increased and there is ankle clonus. Plantar responses are extensor and abdominal reflexes are absent. In African children, brainstem reflexes may be abnormal and there may be neurological evidence of severe intracranial hypertension with rostrocaudal progression suggesting cerebral, cerebellar, and medullary herniation. Hypotonia is more common than in adults. Patients of all ages may show abnormal flexor or extensor posturing (decerebrate or decorticate rigidity), associated with sustained upward deviation of the eyes, pouting, and grunting respiration (Fig. 8.2.18). Hypoglycaemia must be excluded. Most children with cerebral malaria and about half the adult patients experience generalized convulsions. In children, seizures may be covert and difficult to detect. Twitching of the facial muscles or the corner of the mouth, deviation of gaze with nystagmus, irregularities of breathing, and stereotyped posturing of one arm may provide the only clue (Fig. 8.2.19). Fewer than 5% of adult survivors have persisting neurological sequelae: these include cranial nerve lesions, extrapyramidal tremor, and transient paranoid psychosis. However, more than 10% of African children who survive an attack of cerebral malaria have sequelae such as hemiplegia, cortical blindness, epilepsy, ataxia, or cognitive and learning disabilities.

Other severe manifestations and complications

Anaemia (see above) is an inevitable consequence of all but the mildest infections. It is most common and severe in pregnant women, children (Fig. 8.2.20), and in patients with high parasitaemia, schizontaemia, secondary bacterial infections, and renal failure. Spontaneous bleeding from the gums (Fig. 8.2.21) and gastrointestinal tract is seen in fewer than 5% of adult patients with severe malaria and is rare in children. Jaundice (Fig. 8.2.22) is common in adults but rare in children. Biochemical evidence of severe hepatic dysfunction is most unusual and hepatic failure suggests concomitant viral hepatitis or another diagnosis.

Hypoglycaemia is an important complication. Quinine or quinidine treatment can cause hypoglycaemia in pregnant women with severe or uncomplicated falciparum malaria and in any patient with severe disease. This develops a few hours to 6 days after starting this

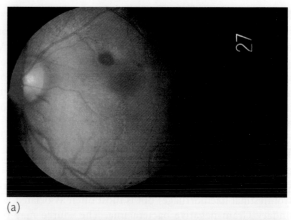

(a)

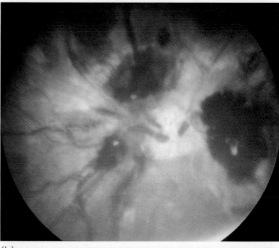

(b)

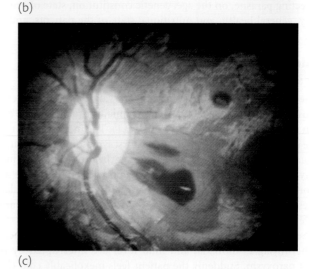

(c)

Fig. 8.2.17 Retinal abnormalities. (a) Retinal haemorrhages close to the macula in a Thai patient with cerebral malaria; (b), (c) multiple large haemorrhages and areas of retinal whitening in Kenyan children with cerebral malaria. (a, copyright D A Warrell; b, c courtesy K Marsh).

treatment, even after the parasitaemia has cleared. However, even in the absence of quinine or quinidine treatment, pregnant women and children with falciparum malaria and patients with hyperparasitaemia or complicating bacteraemia may become hypoglycaemic early in their illness. Clinical features of hypoglycaemia include

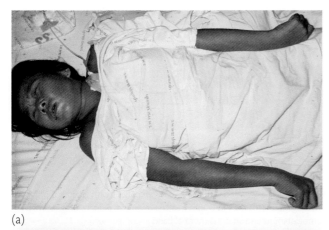

(a)

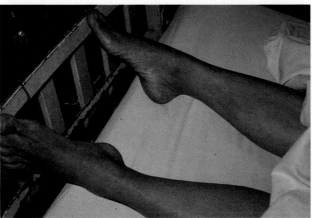

(b)

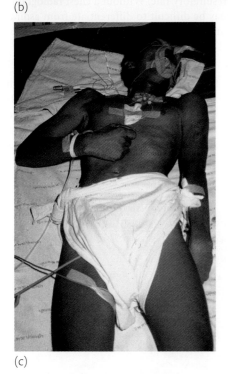

(c)

Fig. 8.2.18 (a, b) Extensor posturing (decerebrate rigidity) in a Thai woman with cerebral malaria and profound hypoglycaemia; and (c) extensor posturing (decorticate rigidity) in a Thai man with cerebral malaria. (Copyright D A Warrell.)

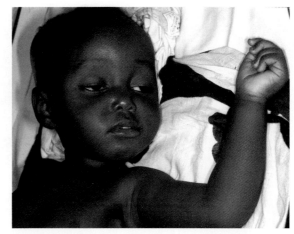

Fig. 8.2.19 Covert seizure in a child with cerebral malaria. Note deviation of eyes to the left, retraction of the corner of the mouth, and posturing of the left arm. (Copyright D A Warrell.)

anxiety, tachycardia, breathlessness, feeling cold, confusion, sweating, light-headedness, restlessness, fetal bradycardia or other signs of fetal distress, coma, convulsions, and extensor posturing. All may be misinterpreted as manifestations of malaria *per se*.

Hypotension and shock ('algid malaria') is a consequence of pulmonary oedema, metabolic acidosis, gastrointestinal haemorrhage, and complicating Gram-negative bacteraemias. Mild supine hypotension with postural drop in blood pressure is caused by vasodilatation and relative hypovolaemia. Cardiac arrhythmias are rare but may be precipitated by too rapid intravenous infusion or excessive doses of chloroquine, quinine, or quinidine. Patients with coronary insufficiency may develop angina during febrile crises of malaria.

Renal dysfunction, indicated by oliguria and increased blood urea and serum creatinine concentrations, occurs in about one-third of adults with severe malaria but is uncommon in children. Most patients respond to cautious rehydration, but 10% develop renal failure requiring dialysis.

In patients whose RBCs are congenitally deficient in G6PD or other enzymes, intravascular haemolysis and haemoglobinuria (Fig. 8.2.23) may be precipitated by oxidant antimalarial drugs such as primaquine and tafenoquine, whether or not they have malaria. Classic blackwater fever is the association of haemoglobinuria from massive intravascular haemolysis, not explicable by G6PD deficiency,

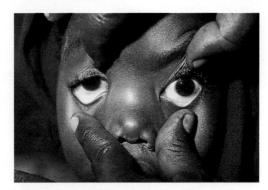

Fig. 8.2.20 Profound anaemia (haemoglobin 1.2 g/dl) in a Kenyan child with *P. falciparum* parasitaemia. (Copyright D A Warrell.)

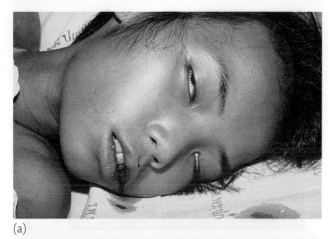

(a)

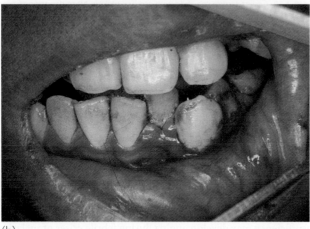

(b)

Fig. 8.2.21 Cerebral malaria. (a), (b) Spontaneous systemic bleeding from a gingival sulci in a Thai patient with disseminated intravascular coagulation. (Copyright D A Warrell.)

with severe manifestations of falciparum malaria, such as renal failure, hypotension, and coma, in a nonimmune patient.

Metabolic acidosis is seen in association with hyperparasitaemia, hypoglycaemia, and renal failure. It is usually lactic acidosis.

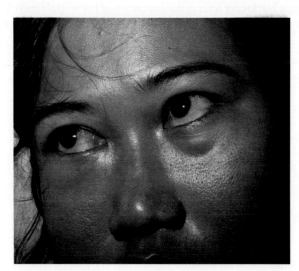

Fig. 8.2.22 Jaundice in a Thai woman with severe malaria. (Copyright D A Warrell.)

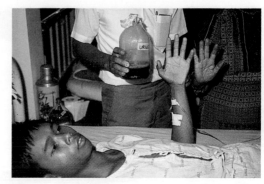

Fig. 8.2.23 Intravascular haemolysis in a Karen patient with glucose-6-phosphate dehydrogenase deficiency in whom treatment with an oxidant drug resulted in haemoglobinuria and anaemia (normal hand in comparison). (Copyright D A Warrell.)

In African children, respiratory distress with deep (Kussmaul) breathing (Fig. 8.2.24), associated with severe anaemia and metabolic acidosis, is a syndrome that carries an even higher case fatality than cerebral malaria.

Pulmonary oedema (Fig. 8.2.25) is the terminal event in many adults dying of falciparum malaria. It may be precipitated by fluid overload late in the clinical course but pulmonary oedema can also develop in patients with severe disease in normal fluid balance, in which case jugular venous, central venous, or pulmonary artery wedge pressures are normal, as in ARDS. In pregnant women, pulmonary oedema may evolve suddenly after delivery. The earliest sign is an increase in respiratory rate. Without a chest radiograph, pulmonary oedema may be difficult to differentiate from aspiration pneumonia, a common complication in comatose patients, or metabolic acidosis.

Cerebellar dysfunction

A rare presentation of falciparum malaria is cerebellar ataxia with unimpaired consciousness. Similar signs may be seen in patients recovering from cerebral malaria. In Sri Lanka, a syndrome of delayed cerebellar ataxia has been described 3 to 4 weeks after an attack of fever attributed to falciparum malaria. Complete recovery is the rule.

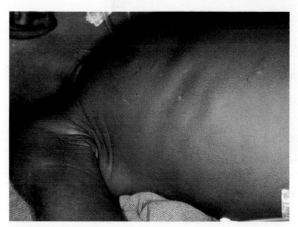

Fig. 8.2.24 Respiratory distress with acidotic 'Kussmaul' breathing in a child with severe malaria. (Copyright D A Warrell.)

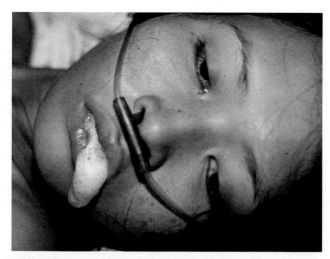

Fig. 8.2.25 Pulmonary oedema in a Thai woman developing soon after delivering a stillborn baby.
(Courtesy of the late Professor Sornchai Looareesuwan.)

Malarial psychosis

The term 'malarial psychosis' has been uncritically applied, often without proven aetiology. Acute psychiatric symptoms in patients with malaria may be attributable to their drug treatment, including antimalarial drugs such as chloroquine, mefloquine, and the obsolete mepacrine, and to exacerbation of pre-existing functional psychoses. However, in some patients, organic mental disturbances associated with malaria infection have been the presenting feature or, more often, have developed during convalescence after attacks of otherwise uncomplicated malaria or cerebral malaria. Depression, paranoia, delusions, and personality changes associated with malaria are classified as brief reactive psychoses. These symptoms rarely last for more than a few days.

Vivax, ovale, and malariae malarias

The prepatent and incubation periods are given in Table 8.2.1. Some strains of *P. vivax*, especially those from temperate regions (*P. v. hibernans* from Russia, *P. v. multinucleatum* from China) may have very long incubation periods (250–637 days). Only about one-third of imported cases of vivax malaria present within a month of returning from the malarious area; between 5 and 10% will present more than 1 year later.

The inappropriately termed 'benign' malarias cause paroxysmal, feverish symptoms even more hectic and distressing than those of falciparum malaria. Prodromal symptoms may be more severe with *P. malariae* infection. The characteristic tertian interval between fever spikes in *P. vivax* and *P. ovale* infections and the quartan pattern in *P. malariae* infections is established after several days of irregular fever if treatment is delayed. Vivax and ovale malarias have a persistent hepatic cycle, which may give rise to relapses every 2 or 3 months for 5 to 8 years in untreated cases. *P. malariae* does not relapse but a persisting, undetectable parasitaemia may cause recrudescences for more than 50 years.

Vivax malaria

People of West African origin are inherently resistant to *P. vivax* infection. Although symptoms may be severe and temporarily incapacitating, especially in nonimmunes, the acute mortality of vivax malaria is very low. During the 1967–9 Sri Lankan epidemic of predominantly vivax malaria, there were more than 500 000 cases with a case fatality of only 0.1%. Acutely, vivax malaria can cause anaemia, thrombocytopenia, and mild jaundice with tender hepatosplenomegaly. Rarely, the anaemia may be severe enough to be life threatening in debilitated patients and it may contribute to chronic malaise, wasting, malnutrition, and underperformance. Splenic rupture, which carries a mortality of 80%, may be more common with vivax than falciparum malaria. It results from acute, rapid enlargement of the spleen, with or without trauma. Chronically enlarged spleens are less vulnerable. Splenic rupture presents with abdominal pain and guarding, signs of haemorrhagic shock, fever, and a rapidly falling haematocrit. These features may be misattributed to malaria itself. In pregnancy, vivax malaria contributes to maternal anaemia and reduced birth weight.

Severe vivax malaria

Plasmodium vivax generally produces a relatively benign, nonfatal disease but in areas such as Rajasthan in India, Papua Indonesia, Papua New Guinea. and Brazil, cerebral malaria, pulmonary oedema, acute kidney injury, and fatalities have been described. Cerebral vivax malaria has also been reported with *P. v. multinucleatum* infection in China. Acute noncardiogenic pulmonary oedema is an increasingly recognized complication of vivax malaria in nonimmune people. Clearly, the pathogenicity and clinical consequences of vivax malaria deserve re-evaluation.

Ovale and malariae malarias

Acute symptoms may be as severe as those of vivax infection, but anaemia is less severe and the risk of splenic rupture is lower although splenomegaly may be particularly gross in areas where *P. malariae* is prevalent. *P. ovale* causes negligible mortality, but *P. malariae* causes chronic morbidity and mortality from nephrotic syndrome and tropical splenomegaly syndrome. The same strictures apply to cerebral *malariae* malaria as to cerebral vivax malaria, especially as *P. malariae* coexists with *P. falciparum* throughout most of its range. Recently it was confirmed that *P. ovale* parasites worldwide belong to two genetic haplotypes: classic and variant. Application of molecular techniques has also led to the discovery of these species in many regions not previously known to have *P. ovale*, particularly many Asian countries. The dimorphic forms have been named *P. ovale curtisi* (classic type) and *P. ovale wallikeri* (variant type). Infection by the latter is associated with higher parasite densities. It is not known whether these two species result from a monkey–hominid switch or whether they have different exclusive mosquito vectors. Because of misdiagnosis, the frequency and severity of infections by the *P. ovale* species may have been massively underestimated.

Monkey malarias

Knowlesi malaria

Recently, *P. knowlesi* infection in humans has been recognized as an important zoonosis in several South-East Asian countries. It is probably not new but has been overlooked. It is transmitted among long-tailed macaques *Macaca fascicularis* and related cercopithecine monkeys by jungle mosquitoes of the *An. leucosphyrus* group (notably *An. latens*) and causes fatal malaria in rhesus monkeys *M. mulatta*. *P. knowlesi* was first identified as an important cause of human malaria in Kapit Division, Sarawak (Malaysia), in 2000–2, where 120 (58%) of malaria cases were found to be infected. It had been confused microscopically with *P. malariae* because early trophozoites may appear as band forms, although these are not always seen (Fig. 8.2.26). Using *P. knowlesi*-specific PCR primers, about 30% of human cases of malaria in Sarawak, together with cases in Sabah, Palawan (Philippines), Pahang (peninsular Malaysia), Thailand, Burma, and Singapore, have been identified. Increasing human encroachment into the jungle habitat in South-East Asia and possibly an adaptive switch in pathogenicity suggest that *P. knowlesi* infection may become more important. It is currently regarded as a zoonosis because human-to-human transmission has not yet been demonstrated.

Clinical features

There are daily spikes of fever (quotidian periodicity). Four fatal cases in Sarawak had fever and chills, abdominal pain and other gastrointestinal and pulmonary symptoms, jaundice, hypotension, acute renal failure, and hyperparasitaemia (764 720 parasites/µl in one case). In Malaysian Borneo, about 10% of patients develop potentially fatal complications and the case fatality is 1.8%.

Other monkey malarias

Human erythrocytes can be infected with at least five other species of simian plasmodia. There have been rare cases of natural infections or accidental laboratory infections by *P. brasilianum*, *P. cynomolgi*, *P. inui*, *P. schwetzi*, and *P. simium*. Severe feverish and systemic symptoms have been described, but no cerebral or other severe complications. No patient has died. Parasitaemia may remain undetectable for 2 to 6 days after the start of symptoms. Periodicity is tertian in *P. simium* and *P. cynomolgi* infections. Infectivity and virulence may be enhanced by repeated passage in humans.

Malaria in pregnancy and the puerperium

Malaria is an important cause of maternal anaemia and death, abortion, stillbirth, premature delivery, low birth weight, neonatal death, and congenital malaria in areas of unstable malaria transmission where women of reproductive age have little acquired immunity. In nonimmune women, hyperpyrexia, hypoglycaemia, anaemia, cerebral malaria, and pulmonary oedema are more common in pregnancy. During the great epidemic of falciparum malaria in Sri Lanka in 1934–5, case fatality among pregnant women was 13%, twice that in nonpregnant women. In Thailand, where malaria was at one time the leading cause of maternal mortality, cerebral malaria in late pregnancy had a case fatality of 50%. In some parts of Africa, one-quarter to one-half of all placentas are parasitized. The incidence is highest in primiparae. Changes in humoral and cell mediated immunity in pregnancy do not explain this vulnerability. It is clear that the placenta is a privileged site for parasite multiplication. RBCs infected with strains (genotypes) of *P. falciparum* expressing Var2CSA, a member of the PfEMP1 family, bind to chondroitin sulphate A, a receptor expressed on the surface of the syncytiotrophoblast. Other host receptors, such as hyaluronic acid and the neonatal Fc receptor, may also support placental binding. This may explain sequestration in the placenta. Placental dysfunction, fever, and hypoglycaemia contribute to fetal distress, which is common when malaria strikes in the last trimester of pregnancy. Painless uterine contractions are often detectable by monitoring. They may subside as the patient is cooled.

Special risks to the mother of malaria during pregnancy

Severe anaemia, exacerbated by malaria, is an important complication of pregnancy in many tropical countries that may persist into the puerperium and beyond. Especially in communities where chronic hookworm anaemia is prevalent, high-output anaemic cardiac failure may develop in late pregnancy.

Asymptomatic hypoglycaemia may occur in pregnant women with malaria, without provocation by cinchona alkaloids, and pregnant women with severe uncomplicated malaria are particularly vulnerable to quinine-induced hypoglycaemia. There is an increased risk of pulmonary oedema, precipitated by fluid overload and the sudden increase in peripheral resistance and autotransfusion of hyperparasitaemic blood from the placenta that occurs just after delivery (Fig. 8.2.25).

Interaction between malaria and HIV in pregnancy

In HIV-infected pregnant women, the beneficial effects of parity on severity of malaria are attenuated and peripheral and placental parasitaemia and risk of having an episode of malaria and anaemia during pregnancy are increased. Malaria–HIV coinfection is associated with an increased risk of low birth weight, preterm birth, intrauterine growth retardation, and postnatal infant mortality. Malaria transiently increases peripheral blood and placental HIV viral load but whether this affects the risk of vertical transmission of HIV infection or accelerates HIV disease progression is unknown.

Prevention

Whenever possible, pregnant women should avoid living in and, especially, sleeping in malarious areas. Otherwise, they should sleep under insecticide-treated bed nets, should be monitored for infection in an antenatal clinic and should receive intermittent preventive treatment with sulphadoxine–pyrimethamine or antimalarial prophylaxis extending into the early puerperium.

Congenital and neonatal malaria

Congenital or vertically transmitted malaria is diagnosed by detecting parasitaemia in the neonate within 7 days of birth, or later if there is no possibility of postpartum mosquito-borne infection. Save for a few discordant reports, most evidence from malarious parts of the world indicates that congenital malaria is rarely symptomatic, despite the high prevalence of placental infection. This confirms the adequacy of protection provided by IgG from the immune mother, which crosses the placenta, by active immunization from exposure to soluble malarial antigens *in utero* and by the high proportion of fetal haemoglobin in the neonate, which retards parasite development. Congenital malaria is, however, much more common in infants born to nonimmune mothers. Its incidence increases during malaria epidemics and it can cause stillbirth or perinatal death. All four species can produce congenital infection, but, because of its very long persistence, *P. malariae* causes a disproportionate number of cases in nonendemic countries. Fetal plasma quinine and chloroquine concentrations are about one-third of the simultaneous maternal levels. Thus, antimalarial concentrations adequate to cure the mother may be subtherapeutic in the fetus. Quinine and chloroquine are excreted in breast milk, but the suckling neonate would receive only a few milligrams per day. Maternal hypoglycaemia, a common complication of malaria, or its treatment with quinine may produce marked fetal bradycardia and other signs of fetal distress.

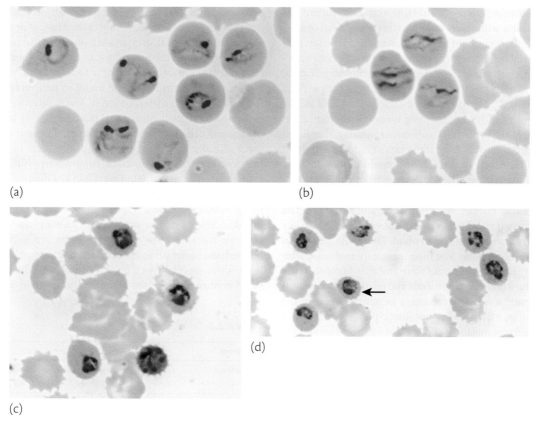

Fig. 8.2.26 *P. knowlesi* from human patient on Geimsa-stained blood films. Showing (a) rings and early trophozoites, (b) band forms resembling *P. malariae* (these are not always seen), (c) trophozoites and early schizonts, and (d) trophozoites, early schizonts, and possible gametocyte (arrow). (Copyright Professor J Cox-Singh.)

Differential diagnosis

Clinical features of congenital malaria are nonspecific: irritability, feeding problems, hepatosplenomegaly, anaemia, and jaundice. Unless parasites are found in a smear from a heel prick or cord blood, the patient may be misdiagnosed as having rhesus incompatibility or another congenital infection such as cytomegalovirus, herpes simplex, rubella, toxoplasmosis, or syphilis.

Transfusion malaria, 'needlestick', and nosocomial malaria

Malaria can be transmitted in blood from apparently healthy donors. Exceptionally, donors may remain infective for up to 5 years with *P. falciparum* and *P. vivax*, 7 years with *P. ovale*, and 46 years with *P. malariae*. Because the infecting parasites are erythrocytic forms (not sporozoites), no exoerythrocytic (hepatic) cycle will be established and so vivax and ovale malarias will not relapse. Theoretically, parasitaemia might be detectable immediately and, hence, the incubation period should be shorter than with mosquito-transmitted malaria. However, the incubation period tends to be longer because of the time needed to build up parasitaemias sufficient to cause symptoms. Mean incubation periods are 12 days (range 7–29 days) for *P. falciparum*, 12 days (range 8–30 days) for *P. vivax*, and 35 days (range 6–106 days) for *P. malariae*. Whole blood, packed cells (blood products), leucocyte or platelet concentrates, fresh plasma, marrow transplants, and haemodialysis have been responsible for transfusion malaria. As patients requiring transfusion are likely to be debilitated and

may be immunosuppressed, and there may be a long delay before making the diagnosis because malaria is not suspected, unusually high parasitaemias may develop with *P. falciparum* and *P. malariae*, but with *P. ovale* and *P. vivax* infections, the parasitaemia is usually limited to 2% because only reticulocytes are invaded. Severe manifestations are common and mortality may be high, e.g. 8 out of 11 infections in a group of heroin addicts and even acute *P. malariae* infections may prove fatal.

Nosocomial malaria has resulted from contamination of saline used for flushing intravenous catheters, contrast medium, and intravenous drugs. Malaria has complicated parenteral drug abuse.

Prevention

Outside the malaria endemic area, donors who have been in the tropics during the previous 5 years should be screened for malarial antibodies (indirect fluorescent antibody). In the endemic area, recipients of blood transfusions can be given antimalarial prophylaxis, or at least they should be watched carefully for evidence of infection. Addition of antimalarial drugs to stored blood is not justified.

Diagnosis

Since malaria can present with a wide range of symptoms and signs, none of them diagnostic, it must be excluded by repeated thick and thin blood smears and rapid antigen detection in any patient with acute fever who has history of possible exposure. Until malaria is confirmed or an alternative diagnosis emerges, at least three smears should be taken over a period of 72 h. However, if the patient has symptoms compatible with severe malaria, a therapeutic trial of antimalarial chemotherapy must not be delayed. Antimalarial drugs may make microscopical diagnosis more difficult and so chemoprophylaxis should be stopped while the patient is under investigation for malaria. A history of travel to malarious areas during the previous year must be obtained. Malaria cannot be excluded just because the patient took prophylactic drugs, for none is completely protective. Short airport stopovers, even on the runway, or working in or living near an international airport, may allow exposure to an imported infected mosquito. Small outbreaks of autochthonous malaria (transmission of malaria imported into areas from which malaria has been eliminated but where competent vector mosquitoes exists) have been reported in Europe, North America, and elsewhere. The possibility of transmission by blood transfusion, 'needlestick', or nosocomial infection should be kept in mind. Those who grew up in an endemic area will probably lose their immunity to disease after living for a few years in a temperate zone and they become newly vulnerable on return home to visit friends and relations, especially in rural areas. In malaria endemic regions, a large proportion of the immune population may have asymptomatic parasitaemia and it cannot be assumed that malaria is the cause of a patient's symptoms even if parasitaemia is detected. In malarious countries, the diagnosis of malaria may be missed in the heat of an epidemic of some other infection such as meningitis, pneumonia, or cholera.

Differential diagnosis (Table 8.2.3)

Malaria must be included in the differential diagnosis of any acute febrile illness unless it can be excluded by: (1) impossibility of exposure, (2) repeated negative blood smears, and (3) a therapeutic trial of antimalarial chemotherapy. In Europe and North America, imported malaria has been misdiagnosed as influenza, viral hepatitis, viral haemorrhagic fever, epilepsy, viral encephalitis, or travellers' diarrhoea, sometimes with fatal consequences. Cerebral malaria must be distinguished from other infective meningoencephalitides. Examination of the cerebrospinal fluid will identify most of these infective causes (Oxford Textbook of Medicine 5e Chapters 24.11.1 and 24.11.2). Abdominal reflexes are absent in cerebral malaria but are brisk in patients with psychotic stupor and hysteria. Overdose of antimalarial drugs (chloroquine and quinine) has been confused with cerebral malaria. Intravenous drug abusers are at risk from both severe malaria and drug overdose. Alcoholism may be confused with cerebral malaria, whether the patient presents inebriated, with delirium tremens, or with Wernicke–Korsakoff syndrome.

Suspicion of viral haemorrhagic fever may lead to patients with imported fevers being isolated in a high-containment unit where basic investigations, such as examination of a blood smear, may be delayed for fear of infection. Jaundice is a common feature of yellow fever but unusual in other viral haemorrhagic fevers.

Malaria in pregnancy may be confused with viral hepatitis, acute fatty liver with liver failure or eclampsia, and in the puerperium with puerperal sepsis or psychosis.

Laboratory diagnosis

Microscopy

Parasites may be found in blood smears (Fig. 8.2.27) taken by venepuncture, finger-pulp or earlobe stabs, and from the umbilical cord and impression smears of the placenta. In fatal cases, cerebral malaria can be confirmed rapidly as the cause of death by making a smear from cerebral grey matter obtained by needle necropsy through the superior orbital fissure, the foramen magnum, the ethmoid sinus via the nose, or a fontanelle in young children. Sometimes no parasites can be found in peripheral blood smears from patients with malaria, even in severe infections. This may be explained by partial antimalarial treatment or by sequestration of parasitized cells in deep vascular beds. In these cases, parasites or malarial pigment may be found in a bone marrow aspirate. Pigment may be seen in circulating neutrophils. A number of Romanowski stains, including Field's, Giemsa, Wright's, and Leishman's, are suitable for malaria diagnosis. The rapid Field's technique, which can yield a result in minutes, and Giemsa are recommended. Smears may be unsatisfactory for any one of a number of reasons: the slides are not clean; stains are unfiltered, old, or infected; the buffer pH is incorrect (it should be pH 7.0–7.4); drying is too slow, especially in a humid climate (producing heavily crenated erythrocytes); or the blood has been stored in anticoagulant

Table 8.2.3 Differential diagnosis of malaria

Symptom	Diagnosis
Acute fever	Heat stroke, hyperpyrexia of other causes, other infections, other causes of fever
Fever and impaired consciousness (cerebral malaria)	Viral, bacterial, fungal, protozoal (e.g. African trypanosomiasis, amoebic) or helminthic meningoencephalitis, cerebral abscess. Head injury, cerebrovascular accident, intoxications (e.g. insecticides), poisonings (e.g. antimalarial drugs), metabolic (diabetes, hypoglycaemia, uraemia, hepatic failure, hyponatraemia). Septicaemias, cerebral typhoid
Fever and convulsions	Encephalitides, metabolic encephalopathies, hyperpyrexia, cerebrovascular accidents, epilepsy, drug and alcohol intoxications, poisoning, eclampsia, febrile convulsions, and Reye's syndrome (children)
Fever and haemostatic disturbances	Septicaemias (e.g. meningococcaemia), viral haemorrhagic fever, rickettsial infection, relapsing fevers, leptospirosis
Fever and jaundice	Viral hepatitis, yellow fever, leptospirosis, relapsing fevers, septicaemias, haemolysis, biliary obstruction, hepatic necrosis (drugs, poisons)
Fever with gastrointestinal symptoms	Travellers' diarrhoea, dysentery, enteric fever, other bacterial infections, inflammatory bowel disease
Fever with haemoglobinuria ('blackwater fever')	Drug-induced haemolysis (e.g. oxidant antimalarials in glucose 6-phosphate-dehydrogenase-deficient patient), favism, transfusion reaction, dark urine of other causes (e.g. myoglobinuria, urobilinogen, porphobilinogen)
Fever with acute renal failure	Septicaemias, yellow fever, leptospirosis, drug intoxications, poisonings, prolonged hypotension
Fever with shock ('algid malaria')	Septicaemic shock, haemorrhagic shock (e.g. massive gastrointestinal bleed, ruptured spleen), perforated bowel, dehydration, hypovolaemia, myocarditis

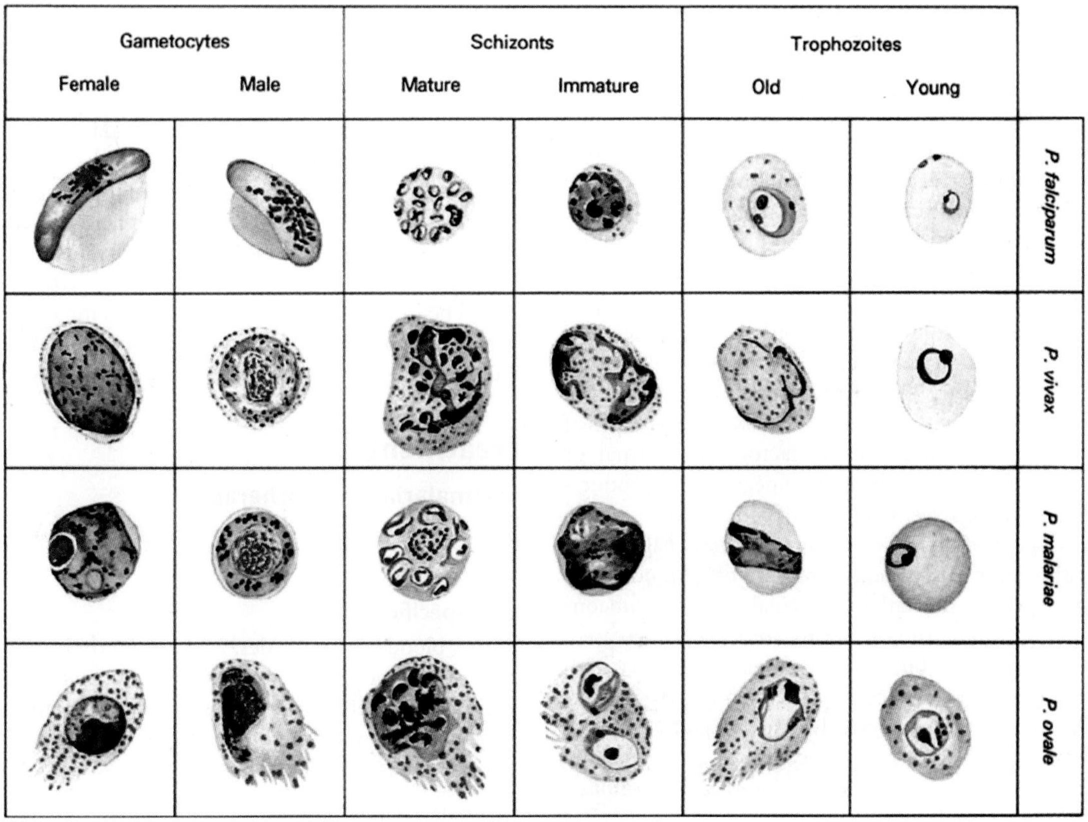

Fig. 8.2.27 Malaria parasites developing in red blood cells.
(Courtesy of the Wellcome Trust.)

causing lysis of parasitized erythrocytes. It is difficult to make a good smear if the patient is very anaemic. Common artefacts resembling malaria parasites are superimposed platelets, particles of stain and other debris, and pits in the slide. Other erythrocyte infections such as bartonellosis and babesiosis may be misdiagnosed as malaria. Parasites should be counted in relation to the total white cell count (on thick films when the parasitaemia is relatively low) or erythrocytes (on thin films). An experienced microscopist can detect as few as 5 parasites/μl (parasites in 0.0001% of circulation RBCs) in a thick film and 200/μl (0.004% parasitaemia) in a thin film.

Fluorescent microscopy

The quantitative buffy coat method involves spinning blood in special capillary tubes in which parasite DNA is stained with acridine orange and a small float presses the PRBCs against the wall of the tube where they can be viewed by ultraviolet microscopy. In expert hands, the sensitivity of this method can be as good as with conventional microscopy of thick blood films but species diagnosis is difficult and the method is much more expensive.

Rapid malarial antigen detection

Malaria dipstick antigen-capture assays employ monoclonal antibodies to detect *P. falciparum* histidine-rich protein 2 (PfHRP-2) or parasite-specific lactate dehydrogenase or aldolase from the glycolytic pathway found in all species. They are a convenient addition or alternative to microscopy as they are quick (taking about 20 min), sensitive (detecting >100 parasites/μl or 0.002%

parasitaemia), and species specific. However, false positivity has been a problem and only the parasite-specific lactate dehydrogenase tests detect *P. ovale* and *P. malariae*. The NOW malaria test (Inverness Medical) is available in the United Kingdom. Currently, Paracheck Pf (Orchid Biomedical Systems, Goa, India) and SD Bioline malaria antigen test (Standard Diagnostics, South Korea) are not available in the United Kingdom but are recommended. ParaSight F (Becton-Dickinson), ICT Malaria Pf (ICT Diagnostics), and OptiMAL (Flow Laboratories) are also available.

Other methods

Enzyme- and radioimmunoassays, DNA probes (using chemiluminescence for detection), and PCR now approach the sensitivity of classical microscopy. They take much longer (up to 72 h), are much more expensive, and are unlikely to replace microscopy for routine diagnosis. However, some of these newer methods could be automated for screening blood donors or for use in epidemiological surveys. PCR can distinguish parasite strains.

Serological techniques

Malarial antibodies can be detected by immunofluorescence, enzyme immunoassay, or haemagglutination, for epidemiological surveys, for screening potential blood donors, and occasionally for providing evidence of recent infection in nonimmune individuals. These tests are not useful in making an acute diagnosis of malaria. In future, detection of protective antibodies will be important in assessing the response to malaria vaccines.

Other clinical laboratory investigations

Anaemia is usual, with evidence of haemolysis. Serum haptoglobins may be undetectable. The direct antiglobulin (Coombs') test is usually negative. Neutrophil leucocytosis is common in severe infections whether or not there is a complicating bacterial infection, but the white cell count can also be normal or low. The presence of visible malarial pigment in more than 5% of circulating neutrophils is associated with a bad prognosis. Thrombocytopenia is common in patients with *P. falciparum*, *P. vivax*, and *P. knowlesi* infections; it does not correlate with severity. In the *P. knowlesi*-endemic area, low platelet counts are strongly suggestive of *P. knowlesi* infections when blood film is positive with *P. malariae*-like parasites. Prothrombin and partial thromboplastin times are prolonged in up to one-fifth of patients with cerebral malaria. Concentrations of plasma fibrinogen and other clotting factors are normal or increased, and serum levels of fibrin(ogen) degradation products are normal in most cases. Fewer than 10% of patients with cerebral malaria have evidence of disseminated intravascular coagulation. However, antithrombin III concentrations are often moderately reduced and have prognostic significance. Total and direct (unconjugated) plasma bilirubin concentrations are usually increased, consistent with haemolysis, but in some patients with very high total bilirubin concentrations there is a predominance of conjugated bilirubin, indicating hepatocyte dysfunction. Some patients have cholestasis. Serum albumin concentrations are usually reduced, often grossly. Serum aminotransferases, 5′-nucleotidase, and, especially, lactic dehydrogenase are moderately elevated, but not nearly as much as in viral hepatitis. Hyponatraemia is the most common electrolyte disturbance. There may be mild hypocalcaemia (after correction for hypoalbuminaemia) and hypophosphataemia, especially after patients have been given blood or a glucose infusion. Biochemical evidence of generalized rhabdomyolysis (elevated serum creatine kinase concentration, myoglobinaemia, and myoglobinuria) is sometimes found. In about one-third of patients with cerebral malaria, the blood urea concentration is increased above 80 mg/dl (13 mmol/litre) and serum creatinine above 2 mg/dl (176 μmol/litre). Lactic acidosis is common in severely ill patients, especially those with hypoglycaemia and renal failure. It may be suspected if there is a wide 'anion gap', i.e. $[Na^+] - [Cl^-] + [HCO_3^-]$ is greater than 12 meq/litre.

Blood glucose must be checked frequently, especially in children, pregnant women, and severely ill patients, even if the patient is not receiving quinine treatment and is fully conscious. A bedside dipstick method, with or without photometric quantification, is rapid and convenient. Microscopy and culture of cerebrospinal fluid is important in patients with cerebral malaria to exclude other treatable encephalopathies. In cerebral malaria the cerebrospinal fluid may contain up to 15 lymphocytes/μl and an increased protein concentration. Pleocytosis of up to 80 cells/μl, mainly leucocytes, may be found in patients who have had repeated generalized convulsions. The cerebrospinal fluid glucose level will be low in hypoglycaemic patients and this result may be the first hint of hypoglycaemia. In view of the finding of cerebral compression and high opening pressures in many African children with cerebral malaria, some paediatricians prefer to delay lumbar puncture, while covering the possibility of bacterial meningoencephalitis with empirical antimicrobial treatment. Blood cultures should be performed in patients with a high white cell count, shock, persistent fever, or an obvious focus of secondary bacterial infection. Gram-negative rod bacteria (*Escherichia coli*, *Pseudomonas aeruginosa*, etc.) have been cultured from the blood of adult patients with 'algid' malaria and in African children an association was found between malaria and nontyphoid salmonella septicaemia.

Urine should be examined by microscope and dipsticks. Common abnormalities are proteinuria, microscopic haematuria, haemoglobinuria, and RBC casts. The urine is literally black in patients with severe intravascular haemolysis. Urine specific gravity should be measured: the optical method is most convenient when urine output is small. Monitoring plasma concentrations of antimalarial drugs such as quinine is rarely possible but can be useful.

Treatment

Antimalarial chemotherapy

Classes of drugs that have antimalarial activity are shown in Box 8.2.3.

Stage specificity

Among blood schizonticides, artemisinin derivatives can prevent the development of rings or trophozoites, but quinine and mefloquine cannot stop development before the stage of mature trophozoites and pyrimethamine–sulphadoxine combinations do not prevent the development of schizonts.

Antimalarial drugs
Arylaminoalcohols

The antimalarial properties of cinchona alkaloids were discovered in Peru around 1600 but their mode of action remains unknown. Quinine became the first-line treatment of severe falciparum malaria after the emergence of chloroquine resistance but is now being replaced by artemisinin derivatives. Intravenous injection of

---

Box 8.2.3 Classes of antimalarial drugs

- Arylaminoalcohols—quinoline methanols (quinine and quinidine extracted from the bark of the cinchona tree), mefloquine, and lumefantrine
- 4-Aminoquinolines—chloroquine and amodiaquine
- Bisquinolines—piperaquine
- Folate-synthesis inhibitors—type 1 antifolate drugs that compete for dihydropteroate synthase (sulphones and sulphonamides); type 2 antifolate drugs that inhibit malarial dihydrofolate reductase (the biguanides proguanil and chlorproguanil and the diaminopyrimidine pyrimethamine)
- 8-Aminoquinolines—primaquine and tafenoquine (Etaquine, WR-238605, or SB-252263)
- Antibiotics—tetracycline, doxycycline, clindamycin, azithromycin, and fluoroquinolones
- Peroxides (sesquiterpene lactones)—artemisinin (*qinghaosu*) derivatives and semisynthetic analogues (artemether, arteether, artesunate, and artelinic acid)
- Naphthoquinones—atovaquone

quinine is dangerous as high plasma concentrations may result during the distribution phase, causing fatal hypotension or arrhythmias. However, quinine can be given safely if it is diluted and infused intravenously over 2 to 4 h, or, if intravenous infusion is not possible and parenteral treatment is needed, it may be given by intramuscular injection divided between the anterolateral parts of both thighs. For intramuscular injection, the stock solution of quinine dihydrochloride (300 mg/ml) should be diluted to 60 mg/ml. It is well absorbed from this site. Historically, intramuscular quinine carried the risk of tetanus but it is safe provided that strict sterile precautions are observed. Because most deaths from severe falciparum malaria occur within the first 96 h of starting treatment, it is important to achieve parasiticidal plasma concentrations of quinine as quickly as possible. This can be accomplished safely with an initial loading dose of twice the maintenance dose (Table 8.2.4). The initial dose of quinine should not be reduced in patients who are severely ill with renal or hepatic impairment, but in these cases the maintenance dose should be reduced to between 3 and 5 mg/kg if parenteral treatment is required for longer than 48 h.

Minimum inhibitory concentrations of quinine for *P. falciparum* in South-East Asia and other areas of the tropics have increased. Longer courses of quinine and combination with pyrimethamine–sulphonamide combinations, tetracycline, or clindamycin have been required for cure. Quinine need not be withheld or stopped in patients who are pregnant. In therapeutic doses, it does not stimulate uterine contraction or cause fetal distress. Hypoglycaemia is the most important complication of quinine treatment. Plasma quinine concentrations above 5 mg/litre cause 'cinchonism': transient high-tone deafness, giddiness, tinnitus, nausea, vomiting, tremors, blurred vision, and malaise. Rarely, quinine may give rise to haemolysis, thrombocytopenia, disseminated intravascular coagulation, hypersensitivity reactions, vasculitis, and granulomatous hepatitis. Self-poisoning with quinine causes blindness, deafness, and central nervous depression. These features are rarely seen in patients being treated for malaria, even though their plasma quinine concentrations may exceed 20 mg/litre. This may be explained by the increased binding of quinine to α_1-acid glycoprotein (orosomucoid) and to other acute-phase reactive serum proteins associated with acute infection.

Quinidine, the dextrorotatory stereoisomer of quinine, is more effective against resistant strains of *P. falciparum* but is more cardiotoxic than quinine. Because it was widely stocked for treating cardiac arrhythmias, quinidine gluconate injection was once more generally available than parenteral quinine. The Centers for Disease Control in the United States of America formerly supplied it for the parenteral treatment of malaria, but it has now been replaced by artesunate.

Table 8.2.4 Antimalarial chemotherapy in adults or children with uncomplicated malaria who can swallow tablets

Option and age of patient	Chloroquine-resistant *P. falciparum* or where the origin of the infection is unknown	Chloroquine-sensitive *P. falciparum* or *P. vivax*, *P. ovale*, *P. malariae*, or monkey malarias
1	**Artemether with lumefantrine**	**Chloroquine**[a]
Adult	4 tablets (each containing 20 mg artemether and 120 mg lumefantrine)	600 mg base on the 1st and 2nd days; 300 mg on the 3rd day
	Twice daily for 3 days	
Child	<15 kg body weight, 1 tablet	*c.* 10 mg base/kg on the 1st and 2nd days; 5 mg base/kg on the 3rd day
	15<25 kg, 2 tablets	
	25<35 kg, 3 tablets	
	All twice daily for 3 days	
		For radical cure of *P. vivax*/*P. ovale* (except pregnant and lactating women or G6PD-deficient patients), add:
2	**Proguanil with atovaquone**	**Primaquine**
Adult	4 tablets (each containing 100 mg proguanil and 250 mg atovaquone)	15 mg base/day on days 4–17; or 45 mg/week for 8 weeks[b]
	Once daily for 3 days	
Child	11–20 kg, one tablet	0.25 mg/kg per day on days 4–17; or 0.75 mg/kg per week for 8 weeks[b]
	21–30 kg, 2 tablets	
	31–40 kg, 3 tablets	
	All once daily for 3 days	
3	**Quinine**	
Adult	600 mg salt, 3 times daily for 7 days[c]	
Child	Approx. 10 mg salt/kg, 3 times daily for 7 days[c]	

[a] For chloroquine-resistant *P. vivax*, repeat the course.

[b] For Chesson-type strains (South-East Asia, western Pacific), use double the dose or double the duration up to a total dose of 6 mg base/kg in daily doses of 15–22.5 mg for adults.

[c] In areas where 7 days of quinine is not curative (e.g. Thailand), add tetracycline 250 mg four times each day or doxycycline 100 mg daily for 7 days, except for children under 8 years and pregnant women, or add clindamycin 5 mg/kg three times daily for 7 days.

Mefloquine is a synthetic drug, effective against some *P. falciparum* strains resistant to chloroquine, pyrimethamine–sulphonamide combinations, and quinine. It cannot be given parenterally, but is well absorbed when given by mouth, reaching peak plasma concentrations in 6 to 24 h, with an elimination half-time of 14 to 28 days. The drug can be given as a single dose but, to reduce the risk of vomiting and other gastrointestinal side effects, the dose is best divided into two halves given 6 to 8 h apart. Gastrointestinal symptoms occur in 10 to 15% of patients but are usually mild. Less frequent side effects include nightmares and sleeping disturbances, dizziness, ataxia, sinus bradycardia, sinus arrhythmia, postural hypotension, and an 'acute brain syndrome' consisting of fatigue, asthenia, seizures, and psychosis. These unpleasant symptoms, whose incidence has probably been exaggerated, have made the drug unpopular. Those taking β-blockers or with a past history of epilepsy or psychiatric disease should avoid the drug. Unfortunately, *in vitro* resistance to mefloquine and treatment failures have now been reported in South-East Asia, Africa, and South America. One large observational study in Thailand suggested an increased risk of stillbirth associated with mefloquine but this was not found in Malawi. Mefloquine treatment should be avoided in pregnant women, especially during the first trimester, and pregnancy should be avoided within 3 months of stopping mefloquine.

Lumefantrine (benflumetol) is an arylaminoalcohol that, despite its structural similarity to halofantrine (now withdrawn), is not cardiotoxic. It is combined with artemether as a co-artemether (see below).

4-Aminoquinolines

Chloroquine, a synthetic antimalarial, is concentrated in the parasite's lysosomes where haemoglobin is digested, and may act by inhibiting the haempolymerase that converts toxic haemin into insoluble haemozoin (malarial pigment). Alternatively, the drug may interfere with parasite feeding by disrupting its food vacuole. From the original foci in Thailand and Colombia, chloroquine-resistant *P. falciparum* has spread to most parts of the tropics. The observation that chloroquine resistance could be reversed *in vitro* by high concentrations of calcium channel blockers, which in other situations could reverse the multidrug resistance (mdr) phenotype acquired by tumour cells, focused attention on a malarial homologue of the human *MDR* gene. Genes involved in the development of resistance include *P. falciparum* chloroquine resistance transporter on chromosome 7 and loci on chromosome 5, which harbours the *MDR* gene homologue *PfMDR1*, and chromosome 11. Despite the widespread resistance of *P. falciparum* to this drug and the recent emergence of chloroquine-resistant *P. vivax* in New Guinea and adjacent areas of Indonesia, chloroquine remains the most widely used antimalarial drug worldwide. It is the treatment of choice for *P. vivax*, *P. ovale*, *P. malariae*, and *P. knowlesi* infections and for uncomplicated falciparum malaria acquired in the few areas where the parasite remains sensitive to this drug (Central America northwest of the Panama Canal, Hispaniola (Haiti and the Dominican Republic, and parts of the Middle East). Elsewhere, the emergence of chloroquine resistance has had a devastating effect on malarial morbidity and mortality. In Senegal, mortality from malaria in children under 5 years old increased up to 11-fold between 1984 and 1995. Absorption of chloroquine after intramuscular or subcutaneous injection is very rapid. Unless small doses are given frequently, this can produce dangerously high plasma concentrations, probably accounting for the deaths of some children soon after they had received intramuscular injections of chloroquine. Therapeutic blood concentrations persist for 6 to 10 days after a single dose. Plasma concentrations above about 250 ng/ml cause dizziness, headache, diplopia, disturbed visual accommodation, dysphagia, nausea, and malaise. Chloroquine, even in small doses, may cause pruritus in dark-skinned races. It may exacerbate epilepsy and photosensitive psoriasis. Cumulative, irreversible retinal toxicity from chloroquine has been reported after lifetime prophylactic doses of 50 to 100 g base (i.e. after 3–6 years of taking 300 mg of base per week), although this is most unusual. Chloroquine overdose is described in Oxford Textbook of Medicine 5e Chapter 9.1. Chloroquine is safe during pregnancy and lactation.

Amodiaquine, although structurally similar to chloroquine, retains activity against chloroquine-resistant strains of *P. falciparum* in some geographical areas. Unlike chloroquine, it is metabolized to a toxic quinoneimine capable of causing toxic hepatitis and potentially lethal agranulocytosis (which occurred in up to 1 in 2000 people taking amodiaquine prophylactically). Amodiaquine is still used, but, because of its risks and the limited therapeutic advantage over chloroquine, its use for prophylaxis and repeated treatment is now discouraged by WHO.

Bisquinolines

Piperaquine was used extensively as prophylaxis and treatment in China and Indochina from the 1960s until emergence of piperaquine-resistant strains of *P. falciparum* during the 1980s. More recently, it has been combined with artemisinins, as an artemisinin-based combination therapy (ACT) as: dihydroartemisinin (DHA), trimethoprim, piperaquine phosphate, and primaquine phosphate (China-Vietnam (CV), CV4 and CV8); DHA, trimethoprim, and piperaquine phosphate (Artecom), and DHA and piperaquine phosphate only (Artekin, Duo-Cotecxin), which have proved effective and safe in mainland South-East Asia. Piperaquine is highly lipid soluble with a large volume of distribution at steady state/bioavailability, long elimination half-life, and a clearance that is markedly higher in children than in adults. Its tolerability, efficacy, pharmacokinetic profile, and low cost make it suitable as a constituent of ACT.

Folate-synthesis inhibitors

Pyrimethamine–sulphonamide combinations The mode of action of the antifolate drugs is well understood. Pyrimethamine 75 mg and sulphadoxine 1500 mg (Fansidar), once valuable in the treatment of chloroquine-resistant falciparum infections worldwide, is no longer marketed in the United Kingdom, but it and other pyrimethamine combinations such as with dapsone (Maloprim) and with sulphalene (Metakelfin) are still used elsewhere. Unfortunately, resistance to these synergistic combinations has spread to most malarious continents, resulting from mutations at residues 108, 51, 59, 16, and 164 of the parasite's dihydrofolate reductase gene. Pyrimethamine is a folate inhibitor that may cause folic acid deficiency in pregnant women and others unless folinic acid supplements are given. The sulphonamide components of these combinations may cause systemic vasculitis (Stevens–Johnson syndrome), or toxic epidermal necrolysis. Fansidar caused fatal reactions in 1 in 18 000 to 26 000 prophylactic courses. Aplastic anaemia and agranulocytosis can also occur. Both pyrimethamine and sulphonamide cross the placenta and are excreted in milk. In the fetus and neonate, sulphonamides can displace bilirubin from plasma protein-binding sites, thus causing kernicterus. For these reasons, pyrimethamine–sulphonamide combinations are not recommended for treatment during pregnancy or lactation unless no alternative drug is available, and should never be used for prophylaxis.

Chlorproguanil–dapsone This combination was developed as an alternative to pyrimethamine–sulphonamide combinations to replace chloroquine for the treatment of uncomplicated falciparum malaria in Africa. It proved more effective than pyrimethamine–sulphonamide combinations in treating parasites with *DHFR* mutations at bases 108, 51, and 59, but should probably be further combined with an artemisinin to extend its useful therapeutic life.

8-Aminoquinolines
Primaquine is the only readily available drug effective against hepatic hypnozoites of *P. vivax* and *P. ovale*. It is essential for the radical cure of these infections. Primaquine is gametocytocidal for all species of malaria. Mass treatment of patients with *P. falciparum* infection could eliminate the sexual cycle in mosquitoes by sterilizing gametocytes. Its elimination half-time is 7 h. Primaquine causes haemolysis in patients with congenital deficiencies of erythrocyte enzymes, notably G6PD, but severe intravascular haemolysis is unusual except in areas such as the Mediterranean (e.g. Sardinia) and Sri Lanka. Primaquine can cross the placenta and cause severe haemolysis in a G6PD-deficient fetus, most commonly a boy, and is also excreted in breast milk. It should therefore not be used during pregnancy or lactation in areas where G6PD deficiency is prevalent. Like sulphonamides and sulphones (i.e. dapsone), primaquine can produce severe haemolysis and methaemoglobinaemia in patients with congenital deficiency of NADH methaemoglobin reductase. Those affected quickly develop dusky cyanosis, noticed first in the nail beds. In patients with G6PD deficiency, weekly dosage with 45 mg of primaquine is better tolerated than the usual daily dose of 15 mg. In the Solomon Islands, Indonesia, Thailand, and Papua New Guinea, a total dose of 6.0 mg/kg (twice the usual dose) or even more may be needed to eliminate the primaquine-resistant Chesson-type strain of *P. vivax*. This is usually given as 15 mg base/day for 28 days.

Tafenoquine is a newer 8-aminoquinoline; it has a longer half-life (2 weeks) than primaquine and is over 10 times more active as a hypnozoiticide. It is also a potent schizonticide.

Peroxides (sesquiterpene lactones)
Artemisinins Artemisinin or *qinghaosu* (pronounced 'ching-how-soo') from the Chinese medicinal herb *Artemisia annua* (sweet wormwood), family Compositae, has been used to treat fevers in China for more than 1000 years. It is a sesquiterpene lactone, with an endoperoxide (trioxane) active group that was isolated in China in 1971–2. Iron within the parasite probably catalyses the cleavage of the endoperoxide bridge leading to the generation of free radicals, which then form covalent bonds with parasite proteins (alkylation). Artemisinins destroy the blood stages of *P. falciparum* from trophozoite to schizont, including those of multiresistant strains. They clear parasitaemia more rapidly than other antimalarial drug.

Artemisinin resistance Resistance of *P. falciparum* to artemisinins has been documented at Thailand's borders with Cambodia (2008) and Burma (2012). This was a discovery of enormous significance for the present campaign to improve antimalarial therapy worldwide and to eradicate rather than just eliminate malaria. Elimination of all the *P. falciparum* parasites from that area according to WHO's new Global Plan for Artemisinin Resistance Containment will succeed only if emerging resistance is not already more widespread. A possible consequence of reduced artemisinin sensitivity is also exposing the artemisinin-based combination treatment (ACT) partner drug to development of resistance. An effective partner drug will conceal for a while the emergence of reduced artemisinin responsiveness. Delayed parasite clearance may also affect recrudescence, gametocyte-carriage rates and mosquito infectivity. Artemisinin resistance seems to affect ring-stage parasites more than trophozoite and schizont stages. Molecular mechanisms of resistance are so far unknown but are a subject of intense research interest.

Artesunate Dihydroartemisinin (DHA) is the active metabolite, which has a short half-life. In severe falciparum malaria, intravenous artesunate is the treatment of choice but this drug can also be given by intramuscular injection. Multicentre trials enrolling 1461 patients in South-East Asia demonstrated a case fatality of 15% in patients treated with intravenous artemether, compared to 22% in those treated with intravenous quinine, a reduction in mortality of 34.7% in the artesunate-treated group. Studies of 5425 African children showed a relative reduction in case fatality of 22.5% (95% CI 8.1–36.9%, p = 0.0022)

Systematic review of 11 randomized controlled trials comparing intramuscular artemether with parenteral quinine showed lower mortality with artemether, but this was not significant in an analysis of adequately blinded trials. Within these, in an individual patient data analysis of 1919 adults and children, the odds ratio for deaths in artemether recipients was 0.8. In the prospectively defined subgroup analysis of adults with multisystem failure, there was a significant difference in mortality in favour of artemether but intramuscular artemether is erratically absorbed in patients with severe malaria especially those with shock. Artemotil (arteether) is similar to artemether but has been far less used.

Artemisinin suppositories Rectal artesunate proved superior to intravenous/intramuscular quinine in reducing parasite densities 12 and 24 h after administration. Suppository formulations of artemisinin should prove particularly valuable in treating children at peripheral levels of the health service where access to medical care and to intravenous therapy are negligible. In a large placebo controlled trial in Bangladesh, Ghana, and Tanzania, prereferral rectal artesunate significantly reduced death or permanent disability in children who arrived in clinic between 6 and 15 h later. Subsequently, various aspects of this trial have been criticized but its message is a very important one for much of the malaria endemic region.

Artemether with lumefantrine combination (co-artemether) and other ACTs are effective for the oral treatment of multiresistant falciparum malaria.

The severe neurotoxicity reported in animals given large doses of artemisinins has not been detected in any of the tens of thousands of human patients treated with these compounds. Artemisinins have proved safe in the second and third trimesters of pregnancy but there are insufficient data to support their use in the first trimester.

Hydroxynaphthoquinones
Naphthoquinones, such as atovaquone, act on the electron-transport chain in malarial mitochondria through their structural

similarity to coenzyme Q. Atovaquone is marketed in combination with proguanil for the treatment and prevention of multiresistant *P. falciparum*. It inhibits the parasite's mitochondrial respiration by binding to the cytochrome *bc* complex. The drug is poorly and variably absorbed, but bioavailability is greatly enhanced by a fatty meal. Its elimination half-life is between 50 and 70 h.

Antibiotics

All antimalarial antibiotics inhibit ribosomal protein synthesis and probably act on the parasite's mitochondria. Tetracycline, clindamycin, azithromycin, quinolones, and sulphonamides such as co-trimoxazole have some antimalarial activity. They kill parasites too slowly to be used alone but are useful in combination for the treatment of uncomplicated *P. falciparum* malaria.

Treatment of falciparum malaria

Despite discovery of the rapidly effective, easily used, and safe artemisinin derivatives, treatment of falciparum malaria remains challenging in many parts of the world. The use of antimalarial drugs is poorly controlled, there are supply problems resulting from expense, inadequate distribution and erratic and incomplete dosing. Fake antimalarial drugs are penetrating increasingly into the markets in Africa and Asia. A worrying recent development has been the documentation of reduced *in vivo* susceptibility to artemisinins with delayed parasite clearance in Pailin, western Cambodia, and possibly in adjacent countries.

Combination antimalarial treatment

The combination of two or more different classes of antimalarial drugs with unrelated mechanisms of action to delay emergence of resistance was proposed by Wallace Peters in the early 1970s but was not effectively implemented because of the difficulty of identifying drugs that were still active against multidrug resistant *P. falciparum* and whose elimination half-times were similar. To counter the threat of resistance of *P. falciparum* to monotherapies, and to improve treatment outcome, combinations of antimalarials are now recommended by WHO (2006) for the treatment of falciparum malaria.

Artemisinin-based combination therapy (ACT)

The rapid clearance of parasitaemia and resolution of symptoms by artemisinin derivatives provides strong theoretical support for their use in combination with drugs such as mefloquine, amodiaquine, or pyrimethamine–sulphonamide. A meta-analysis of 11 randomized controlled trials confirmed that, in patients with uncomplicated malaria, addition of 3 days of artesunate to these drugs significantly reduced treatment failure, recrudescence, and gametocyte carriage. This lead to WHO's 2006 recommendation to replace monotherapy with ACT. This has proved effective, except in South-East Asia (Cambodia and possibly in Thailand and Burma), where resistance to artemisinins has recently been reported.

Treatment of uncomplicated P. falciparum malaria (Table 8.2.4)

For treating adults, infants, and children in malarious areas, WHO (2006) recommends ACTs even in Africa, where the deployment of artemisinins cannot yet be justified by published evidence. The drug combined with artesunate depends on the resistance of local strains of *P. falciparum*. In South-East Asia, lumefantrine or mefloquine might be added. In Africa, lumefantrine, amodiaquine, or sulphadoxine–pyrimethamine might be added. For presumed nonimmune travellers returning to nonendemic areas, WHO recommends artemether–lumefantrine, atovaquone–proguanil, or

quinine + doxycycline or clindamycin. Doxycycline should not be given to pregnant women or children under 8 years old.

Patients with uncomplicated malaria can usually be given antimalarial drugs by mouth. However, feverish patients may vomit the tablets. The risk of vomiting can be reduced if the patient lies down quietly for a while after taking an antipyretic such as paracetamol. Otherwise, the initial dose of antimalarial drug may have to be given by injection or suppository.

Treatment of severe falciparum malaria (Table 8.2.5)

Urgent parenteral chemotherapy, initiated with a loading dose, is the priority as there is a highly significant relationship between delay in chemotherapy and mortality. Severely ill or deteriorating patients who have been exposed to malaria should be given a therapeutic trial even if the initial smears are negative. Dosage should be calculated according to the patient's body weight and drugs should be administered parenterally both to patients with severe falciparum malaria and to those who are vomiting and unable to retain swallowed tablets. The treatment of choice is artesunate given by intravenous bolus injection. It can also be given by intramuscular injection. Artemether by intramuscular injection or quinine by intermittent or continuous intravenous infusion or intramuscular injection is less effective. If patients with severe malaria cannot swallow and retain tablets and antimalarial treatment by intramuscular/intravenous injection/infusion is likely to be delayed for several hours, insertion of a single artesunate suppository substantially reduces the risk of death or permanent disability.

Therapeutic response and vital signs must be monitored clinically (temperature, pulse, blood pressure) and by examination of blood films. Patients should be switched to oral treatment as soon as they are able to swallow and retain tablets. They must be watched carefully for signs of drug toxicity. In the case of quinine, the most common adverse effect is hypoglycaemia. Therefore, the blood sugar should be checked frequently.

General management

Patients with severe malaria should be transferred to the highest level of care available, preferably a high dependency area or intensive care unit. They must be nursed in bed because of their postural hypotension and because of the risk of splenic rupture were they to fall. Body temperatures above 38.5°C are associated with febrile convulsions, especially in children, and between 39.5 and 42°C with coma and permanent neurological sequelae. In pregnant women, hyperpyrexia contributes to fetal distress. Therefore, temperature should be controlled by fanning, tepid sponging, a cooling blanket, or antipyretic drugs, such as paracetamol (15 mg/kg in tablets by mouth, or powder washed down a nasogastric tube, or as suppositories) and ibuprofen (tablets or parenteral).

Cerebral malaria

Convulsions, vomiting, and aspiration pneumonia are common, so patients should be nursed in the lateral position with a rigid oral airway or endotracheal tube in place. They should be turned at least once every 2 h to avoid bedsores. Vital signs, Glasgow Coma Score, and convulsions should be recorded. Convulsions can be controlled with diazepam given by slow intravenous injection (adults 10 mg, children 0.15 mg/kg) or intrarectally (0.5–1.0 mg/kg), or with midazolam given initially by intravenous injection of small doses every 2 min and then, when the seizure is controlled, by continuous intravenous infusion diluted in 5% dextrose or normal saline (dosage is adjusted for age and response, in the range of 30 to

Table 8.2.5 Antimalarial chemotherapy in adults or children with severe malaria who cannot swallow tablets

Chloroquine-resistant P. falciparum or the origin of the infection is unknown	Chloroquine-sensitive P. falciparum or P. vivax, P. ovale, P. malariae, or monkey malarias
1. Artesunate[a]	**1. Chloroquine**[b]
2.4 mg/kg (loading dose) IV on the first day, followed by 1.2 mg/kg daily for a minimum of 3 days until the patient can take oral therapy or another effective antimalarial	25 mg base/kg diluted in isotonic fluid by continuous IV infusion over 30 h (or 5 mg base/kg over 6 h every 6 h)
OR	OR
2. Artemether	**2. Quinine (see left-hand column below)**
3.2 mg/kg (loading dose) IM on the first day, followed by 1.6 mg/kg daily for a minimum of 3 days until the patient can take oral treatment or another effective antimalarial. In children, the use of a 1 ml tuberculin syringe is advisable since the injection volumes will be small	
OR	
3. Quinine	
Adults: 20 mg salt/kg (loading dose)[c] diluted in 10 ml/kg isotonic fluid by IV infusion over 4 h, followed 8 h after the start of the loading dose with 10 mg salt/kg over 4 h, every 8 h until patients can	
Children: 20 mg salt/kg (loading dose)[c] diluted in 10 ml/kg isotonic fluid by IV infusion over 2 h, followed 12 h after the start of the loading dose with 10 mg salt/kg over 2 h, every 12 h until patients can swallow[d]	
The 7-day course should be completed with quinine tablets, approximately 10 mg salt/kg (maximum 600 mg) every 8–12 h[e]	
OR	
4. Quinine (in intensive care unit)	
7 mg salt/kg (loading dose)[c] IV by infusion pump over 30 min, followed immediately with 10 mg salt/kg (maintenance dose) diluted in 10 ml/kg isotonic fluid by IV infusion over 4 h, repeated every 8 h until patient can swallow, etc.[d,e]	
OR	
5. Quinidine (in intensive care unit)	
15 mg base/kg (loading dose)[c] IV by infusion over 4 h, followed 8 h after the start of the loading dose with 7.5 mg base/kg over 4 h every 8 h, until the patient can swallow,[d] then quinine tablets to complete 7 days of treatment[e]	
If it is not possible to give drugs by intravenous infusion	
1 Artesunate	**1. Chloroquine**[b]
Same dosage as for IV above given IM	Total dose 25 mg base/kg given as either:
	IM or SC 2.5 mg base/kg, every 4 h
OR	IM or SC 3.5 mg base/kg, every 6 h
2 Artemether	
As above	
OR	OR
3. Quinine	**2. Quinine**
20 mg salt/kg diluted to 60–100 mg/ml (loading dose)[c] IM into anterolateral thigh (half given into each leg), followed by 10 mg salt/kg, every 8 h until patient can swallow etc.[d,e]	IM (see above left-hand column)
If it is not possible to give drugs by injection (IM/IV) or infusion	
1. Suppositories	**1. Chloroquine**
Artemisinin[f]	
40 mg/kg loading dose as suppositories intrarectally, followed by 20 mg/kg at 4, 24, 48, and 72 h followed by an oral antimalarial drug[g]	10 mg base/kg of body weight as tablets/syrup by mouth or nasogastric tube, then refer the patient to a higher level of healthcare for parenteral treatment
	OR
	Continue 5 mg base/kg 5, 24, and 48 h later[g]

Table 8.2.5 *(Cont'd)* Antimalarial chemotherapy in adults or children with severe malaria who cannot swallow tablets

Artesunate[f]	
One 200 mg suppository intrarectally at 0, 4, 8, 12, 24, 36, 48, and 60 h followed by an oral antimalarial drug[h]	
OR	OR
2. Tablets of artemisinin (artesunate, artemether, artemether with lumefantrine), quinine, mefloquine, or other appropriate antimalarials[g] Given by mouth or crushed and given via naso-gastric tube	**2. Suppositories of artemisinin or artesunate, oral quinine, mefloquine, or sulphadoxine/pyrimethamine (see left-hand column)**[g]

IM, intramuscular; IV, intravenous; SC, subcutaneous.

[a] Artesunic acid 60 mg is dissolved in 0.6 ml of 5% sodium bicarbonate diluted to 3–5 ml with 5% (w/v) dextrose and given immediately by intravenous ('push') bolus injection.

[b] Parenteral chloroquine should be used with great caution in young children.

[c] Loading dose must not be used if the patient has received quinine, quinidine, or halofantrine within preceding 24 h.

[d] In patients requiring more than 48 h of parenteral therapy, reduce the dose to 5.7 mg salt/kg every 8 h or 3.75 mg quinidine base/kg every 8 h.

[e] In areas where 7 days of quinine is not curative (e.g. Thailand), add tetracycline 250 mg four times each day or doxycycline 100 mg daily for 7 days except for children under 8 years and pregnant women, or add clindamycin 5 mg/kg three times daily for 7 days.

[f] Artemisinin and artesunate suppositories are registered for use in a few countries. If suppository formulations are not available, tablets of artemisinins should be given orally if possible, or crushed and given by nasogastric tube.

[g] Transfer the patient to hospital as soon as possible after initiating chemotherapy.

[h] In Vietnam, 4 mg/kg of artesunate in suppository form (China) intrarectally as a loading dose, followed by 2 mg/kg at 4, 12, 48, and 72 h followed by an oral antimalarial drug, proved as effective as artemisinin suppositories.

300 μg/kg per h). Prophylactic use of phenobarbital was associated with increased case fatality in a placebo-controlled study in African children and is not recommended. Stomach contents should be aspirated through a nasogastric tube to reduce the risk of aspiration pneumonia. Elective endotracheal intubation is indicated if coma deepens and the airway is jeopardized. Deepening coma with signs of cerebral herniation is an indication for CT or MRI, or a trial of treatment to lower intracranial pressure, such as an intravenous infusion of mannitol (1.0–1.5 g/kg of a 10–20% solution over 30 min) or mechanical hyperventilation to reduce the arterial P_{CO_2} to below 4.0 kPa (30 mmHg).

A number of potentially harmful ancillary remedies of unproven value have been recommended for the treatment of cerebral malaria. Two double-blind trials of dexamethasone (2 mg/kg and 11 mg/kg intravenously over 48 h) in adults and children in Thailand and Indonesia showed no reduction in mortality but prolongation of coma and an increased incidence of infection and gastrointestinal bleeding. Low-molecular-weight dextrans, osmotic agents, heparin, adrenaline (epinephrine), ciclosporin A, prostacyclin, pentoxifylline, malarial hyperimmune globulin, anti-TNFα monoclonal antibodies, desferrioxamine, dichloroacetate, and N-acetyl cysteine have proved ineffective in the treatment of cerebral and other forms of severe malaria. Some of these interventions were associated with serious side effects. There is some evidence that levamisole inhibits sequestration of PRBCs in patients with falciparum malaria and clinical trials are planned.

Anaemia
Indications for transfusion include a low (<20% or rapidly falling) haematocrit, severe bleeding, or predicted blood loss (e.g. imminent parturition or surgery), hyperparasitaemia, and failure to respond to conservative treatment with oxygen and plasma expanders. When the screening of transfused blood is inadequate and infections such as HIV, HTLV-1, and hepatitis viruses are prevalent in the community, the criteria for blood transfusion must be even more stringent. Exchange transfusion is a safe way of correcting the anaemia without precipitating pulmonary oedema in those who are fluid overloaded or chronically and severely anaemic. The volume of transfused blood must be recorded on the fluid balance chart. Transfusion must be cautious, with frequent observations of the jugular or central venous pressure and auscultation for pulmonary crepitations. Survival of compatible donor RBCs is greatly reduced during the acute and convalescent phases of falciparum malaria.

Disturbances of fluid and electrolyte balance
Fluid and electrolyte requirements must be assessed individually in patients with malaria. Circulatory overload with intravenous fluids or blood transfusion may precipitate fatal pulmonary oedema, but untreated hypovolaemia may lead to fatal shock, lactic acidosis, and renal failure. Hypovolaemia may result from salt and water depletion through fever, diarrhoea, vomiting, insensible losses, and poor intake. The state of hydration is assessed clinically from the skin turgor, peripheral circulation, postural change in blood pressure, peripheral venous filling, and jugular or central venous pressure. The history of recent urine output and measurement of urine volume and specific gravity may be useful. In tropical climates, adult patients with severe falciparum malaria may require 1 to 3 litres of intravenous fluid during the first 24 h of hospital admission. Fluid replacement should be controlled by observations of jugular, central venous, or pulmonary artery wedge pressures. Hyponatraemia (plasma sodium concentration 120–130 mmol/litre) usually requires no treatment, but these patients should be cautiously rehydrated with isotonic saline if they are clinically dehydrated, have low central venous pressures, a high urinary specific gravity, and a low urine sodium concentration (<25 mmol/litre).

Renal failure
Patients with falling urine output and elevated blood urea nitrogen and serum creatinine concentrations can be treated conservatively at first, but established acute renal failure must be treated with haemofiltration or dialysis. Hypovolaemia is corrected by the cautious infusion of isotonic saline until the central venous pressure is in the range +5 to +15 cmH₂O. If urine output remains low after rehydration, increasing doses of slowly infused intravenous furosemide up to a total dose of 1 g and finally an intravenous infusion of dopamine (2.5–5 μg/kg per min) can be tried. If these measures fail to achieve a sustained increase in urine output, strict fluid balance should be enforced with particular emphasis on fluid restriction. Indications for haemoperfusion/dialysis include a rapid increase in

serum creatinine level, hyperkalaemia, fluid overload, metabolic acidosis, and clinical manifestations of uraemia (diarrhoea and vomiting, encephalopathy, gastrointestinal bleeding, and pericarditis). Haemofiltration is the most effective technique in malaria but haemodialysis or peritoneal dialysis is also effective. The initial doses of antimalarial drug should not be reduced in patients with renal failure but, after 48 h of parenteral treatment, the maintenance dose should be reduced by one-third or one-half.

Metabolic acidosis

Lactic acidosis is an important life-threatening complication, especially in anaemic children. It should be treated by improving perfusion and oxygenation by blood transfusion and correcting hypovolaemia, clearing the airway, increasing the inspired oxygen concentration, and by treating septicaemia, a frequently associated complication.

Pulmonary oedema

This must be prevented by propping the patient up at an angle of 45° and controlling fluid intake so that the jugular or central venous pressure is kept below +5 cmH$_2$O. Those who develop pulmonary oedema should be propped upright and given oxygen to breathe. In a well-equipped intensive care unit, the judicious use of vasodilator drugs can be controlled by monitoring haemodynamic variables, fluid overload can be corrected by haemoperfusion, and oxygenation can be improved by mechanical ventilation with positive end-expiratory pressure.

Hypotension and 'shock' ('algid malaria')

This should be treated as for bacteraemic shock. The circulatory problems should be corrected with blood transfusion (e.g. in anaemic children with respiratory distress and acidosis), plasma expanders, dopamine, and broad-spectrum antimicrobial treatment (such as gentamicin with ceftazidime or cefuroxime plus metronidazole) should be started immediately, bearing in mind that likely routes of infection include the urinary tract, lungs, and the gut. Other causes of shock in patients with malaria include dehydration, blood loss (i.e. following splenic rupture), and pulmonary oedema.

Hypoglycaemia

This may be asymptomatic, especially in pregnancy, and its clinical manifestations may be confused with those of malaria. Blood sugar must be checked every few hours, especially in patients being treated with cinchona alkaloids. Hypoglycaemia may arise despite continuous intravenous infusions of 5 or even 10% dextrose. A therapeutic trial of dextrose (1 ml/kg by intravenous bolus injection) should be given if hypoglycaemia is proved or suspected. This should be followed by a continuous infusion of 10% dextrose. Glucose may be given by nasogastric tube to unconscious patients or by peritoneal dialysis in those undergoing this treatment for renal failure. Among agents that block insulin release, diazoxide was ineffective, but octreotide, a synthetic somatostatin analogue, proved effective in some severe cases of quinine-induced hypoglycaemia.

Hyperparasitaemia and exchange blood transfusion

In nonimmune patients, case fatality exceeds 50% with parasitaemias above 500 000/µl. In Western countries, exchange blood transfusion, haemopheresis (and even plasmapheresis) have been used in presumed nonimmune patients with 'hyperparasitaemia' variously defined as parasitaemias exceeding 5 to 10%. Apart from reducing parasitaemia, these procedures might remove harmful metabolites, toxins, cytokines, and other mediators and restore normal RBC mass, platelets, clotting factors, and albumin. Potential dangers are electrolyte disturbances (e.g. hypocalcaemia), cardiovascular complications including ARDS, and infection from the blood or through infection of intravascular lines. Among more than 100 patients reported, some improved clinically soon after the procedure and most survived. However, there was reporting bias and a meta-analysis discovered no advantage. The efficacy of exchange transfusion is never likely to be put to the test of a randomized controlled trial. Artemisinins clear parasitaemia so rapidly that additional reduction of parasite load by exchange transfusion may not be important.

Splenic rupture

Acute abdominal pain and tenderness with left shoulder-tip pain and haemodynamic deterioration in patients with vivax and falciparum malaria suggests splenic rupture, especially if there is a history of recent abdominal trauma. Free blood in the peritoneal cavity and a torn splenic capsule can be detected by ultrasound or CT examination and confirmed by needle aspiration of the peritoneal cavity, laparoscopy, or laparotomy. Conservative management with blood transfusion and close observation in an intensive care unit is sometimes successful but access to surgical help is essential in case of sudden deterioration.

Disseminated intravascular coagulation

Patients with evidence of a coagulopathy should be given vitamin K (adult dose 10 mg by slow intravenous injection). Prothrombin complex concentrates, cryoprecipitates, platelet transfusions, and fresh-frozen plasma should be considered. Anticoagulants such as heparin and dalteparin are absolutely contraindicated.

Management of pregnant and lactating women with malaria

Chemotherapy

Unjustified fears of abortifacient and fetus-damaging effects of antimalarial drugs have led to the delay or even withdrawal of treatment, but experience since the 19th century has confirmed the safety of quinine in pregnancy. Chloroquine, proguanil, pyrimethamine, and sulphadoxine–pyrimethamine are also considered safe in the first trimester of pregnancy. Inadvertent exposure to other antimalarials in pregnancy is not an indication for termination of the pregnancy. Concerns about mefloquine in pregnancy have not been confirmed but doxycycline and other tetracyclines should be avoided during pregnancy and breastfeeding. Artemisinin derivatives have proved safe in the second and third trimesters of pregnancy, but there are insufficient safety data about their use in the first trimester.

For pregnant women with uncomplicated falciparum malaria, WHO (2006) recommends quinine ± clindamycin in the first trimester and ACTs in the second and third trimesters with artesunate + clindamycin or quinine + clindamycin as alternatives.

For severe falciparum malaria, WHO (2006) recommends artesunate and artemether above quinine in the second and third trimesters of pregnancy because they do not cause recurrent hypoglycaemia. However, blood glucose must be checked at least once a day in pregnant women with malaria, whether or not they are receiving quinine. In the first trimester, the risk of hypoglycaemia associated with quinine is lower, and uncertainties over the safety of the artemisinin derivatives are greater.

In lactating women, only tetracyclines, dapsone-containing antimalarials and possibly primaquine are contraindicated.

Ancillary treatments

Maternal fever should be reduced as soon as possible. Induction of labour, caesarean section, or accelerating the second stage of labour with forceps or vacuum extractor should be considered in patients with severe falciparum malaria. Fluid balance is particularly critical in these patients. If possible, the central venous pressure should be monitored. Exchange transfusion of 1000 to 1500 ml of blood in late pregnancy proved an effective way of managing severe anaemia with high-output cardiac failure in Nigeria. Circulating volume could be reduced and the risk of postpartum pulmonary oedema lessened by replacing exfused blood with a smaller volume of packed cells.

Prevention of malaria during pregnancy

As malaria during pregnancy can result in severe consequences for both the mother and child, therapeutic courses of antimalarials are effective as an intermittent preventive treatment and can be considered (see 'Control and prevention', below).

Treatment of *P. vivax*, *P. ovale*, *P. malariae*, and *P. knowlesi* malarias (Tables 8.2.4 and 8.2.5)

Chloroquine is the treatment of choice for vivax, ovale, malariae, knowlesi, and uncomplicated falciparum malarias in the few geographical areas where this drug can still achieve a satisfactory clinical response. Severe infections will require parenteral treatment (Table 8.2.5). Chloroquine-resistant *P. vivax* (New Guinea, Indonesia) is treated by increasing the dose of oral chloroquine. The usual 3-day course of chloroquine is well tolerated. In patients with vivax or ovale malarias, this should be followed by radical cure with primaquine to destroy hepatic hypnozoites, but caution is needed if there is a risk of a congenital enzyme deficiency (see '8-Aminoquinolines', above), especially in pregnant or lactating women.

Prognosis

Case fatality of acute vivax, ovale, and malariae malarias is negligible except in the circumstances mentioned above. In knowlesi malaria, case fatality appears to be about 2%. Strictly defined cerebral malaria has a mortality of about 10 or 15% when medical facilities are good and may be less than 5% in Western intensive care units. Antecedent factors that predispose to severe falciparum malaria include the lack of acquired immunity or lapsed immunity, splenectomy, pregnancy, and immunosuppression (e.g. HIV infection). There is a strong correlation between the density of parasitaemia and disease severity. Severe falciparum malaria is defined by clinical criteria such as impaired consciousness, renal failure, hypoglycaemia, haemoglobinuria, metabolic acidosis, and pulmonary oedema. The case fatality of pregnant women with cerebral malaria, especially primiparae in the third trimester, is several times greater than in nonpregnant patients. The following laboratory findings carry a poor prognosis: peripheral schizontaemia, malarial pigment in more than 5% of circulating neutrophils, high cerebrospinal fluid lactate or low glucose, low plasma antithrombin III, serum creatinine exceeding 265 μmol/litre or a blood urea nitrogen of more than 21.4 mmol/litre, haematocrit less than 20%, blood glucose less than 2.2 mmol/litre, and elevated serum enzyme concentrations (e.g. aspartate and alanine aminotransferases, lactate dehydrogenase).

Chronic immunological complications of malaria

Quartan malarial nephrosis

In parts of East and West Africa, South America, India, South-East Asia, and Papua New Guinea, epidemiological evidence links *P. malariae* infection to immune-complex glomerulonephritis that leads to nephrotic syndrome. Few of those exposed to repeated *P. malariae* infections develop nephrosis, suggesting that additional factors are involved. Histological changes, which are not entirely specific, are progressive focal and segmental glomerulosclerosis with fibrillary splitting or flaking of the capillary basement membrane, producing characteristic lacunae. Electron microscopy reveals electron-dense deposits beneath the endothelium. Immunofluorescence confirms glomerular deposits of immunoglobulins, C3, and *P. malariae* antigen in about 25% of cases. More than half the patients present by the age of 15 years with typical features of nephrotic syndrome. *P. malariae* is frequently found in blood smears and *P. malariae* antigen in renal biopsies in children but not in adults. The renal lesions may be perpetuated by autoimmune mechanisms. The pattern of immunofluorescent staining has some prognostic significance. Few patients respond to corticosteroids, but some are helped by azathioprine and cyclophosphamide, especially those whose renal biopsies show the coarse or mixed patterns of immunofluorescence. Antimalarial treatment is not effective. This condition could be prevented by antimalarial prophylaxis and has disappeared in countries such as Guyana following malaria eradication.

Tropical splenomegaly syndrome (hyperreactive malarial splenomegaly)

Transient splenomegaly is a feature of acute attacks of malaria in nonimmune or partially immune patients, while progressive splenomegaly is seen in children resident in malarious areas while they acquire immunity. However, a separate entity has been described in Africa (especially Nigeria, Uganda, and Zambia), the Indian subcontinent (Bengal, Sri Lanka), South-East Asia (Vietnam, Thailand, and Indonesia), South America (Amazon region), Papua New Guinea, and the Middle East (Aden). Defining features are: (1) residence in a malarious area, (2) chronic splenomegaly, (3) persistently elevated serum IgM and malarial antibody levels, (4) hepatic sinusoidal lymphocytosis, and (5) a clinical and immunological response to antimalarial prophylaxis. This condition is thought to result from an aberrant immunological response to repeated infection by any of the species of malaria parasite. Though requiring exposure to malaria and responding to antimalarial therapy, there is no association with the actual level of malarial endemicity. However, major differences in incidence in different ethnic groups suggest genetic predisposition.

Immunopathology

The essential feature is the dysregulation of IgM production leading to the formation of macromolecular aggregates of IgM (cryoglobulins), the clearance of which leads to progressive splenomegaly and hepatomegaly. This may stem in part from the production of lymphocytotoxic antibodies specific for suppressor T lymphocytes, which normally control B cell production of IgM. In African patients, there is often an increase in circulating B lymphocytes. Distinction from chronic lymphatic leukaemia may be difficult.

In Ghana, clonal rearrangements of the JH region of the immunoglobulin gene were found in patients with tropical splenomegaly who failed to respond to proguanil chemoprophylaxis, suggesting that the syndrome may evolve into a malignant lymphoproliferative disorder. Some of these patients had features of splenic lymphoma with villous (hairy) lymphocytes.

Clinical features

In malaria endemic areas, patients with tropical splenomegaly syndrome are distinguishable by their progressive splenic enlargement persisting beyond childhood. The spleen may be enormous, filling the left iliac fossa, extending across the midline and anteriorly, and producing a visible mass with an obvious notch. The liver is usually enlarged, especially the left lobe. The massive splenomegaly causes a vague dragging sensation and occasional episodes of severe pain with peritonism, suggesting perisplenitis or infarction. Anaemia may become severe enough to cause the features of high-output cardiac failure. Acute haemolytic episodes are described. These patients are vulnerable to infections, especially of the skin and respiratory system, and most deaths are attributable to overwhelming infection.

Laboratory findings

Severe chronic anaemia is the result of destruction and pooling in the spleen and dilution in an increased plasma volume. Thrombocytopenia may also be caused by splenic sequestration; it rarely causes bleeding. There is neutropenia and, in African patients, peripheral lymphocytosis and lymphocytic infiltration of the bone marrow. Serum IgM is greatly elevated (>2 standard deviations above the population mean, and often very much higher).

The essential histopathological feature is lymphocytosis of the hepatic sinusoids with Kupffer-cell hyperplasia. In some cases, round-cell infiltration of the portal tracts is associated with fibrosis, leading to portal hypertension. In the spleen there is dilatation of the sinusoids, hyperplasia of the phagocytic cells with erythrophagocytosis, and infiltration with lymphocytes and plasma cells. In patients with splenic lymphoma and villous lymphocytes, more than 30% of circulating lymphocytes are villous. These cells can be distinguished from hairy-cell leukaemia by their lack of CD25, CD11c, and tartrate-resistant acid phosphatase markers.

Differential diagnosis

Tropical splenomegaly syndrome must be distinguished from other causes of chronic, painless, massive splenomegaly, including leukaemias, lymphomas, myelofibrosis, thalassaemias, haemoglobinopathies, visceral leishmaniasis (by examination of bone marrow or splenic aspirates), and schistosomiasis (by liver biopsy, rectal snip, and stool examination). Lymphomas (especially chronic lymphatic leukaemia and follicular lymphoma) and even leukaemias may develop in patients with tropical splenomegaly syndrome. Nontropical idiopathic splenomegaly (normal serum IgM) and Felty's syndrome produce a similar histological picture in the liver. Many cases of splenomegaly in the tropics remain undiagnosed.

Treatment

Prolonged antimalarial chemoprophylaxis is the most important element of treatment. The majority of patients improve within 12 months of chemotherapy. The choice of drug will depend on the local sensitivity of whichever species or group of species of malaria parasite are thought to be responsible for this syndrome. The short- and long-term dangers of splenectomy rule out this procedure in the rural tropics. Folic acid may be needed. Diagnosis of patients with splenic lymphoma with villous lymphocytes (Ghana) is important as, in this condition, the risks of splenectomy are outweighed by the benefits.

Endemic Burkitt's lymphoma (Chapter 5.3)

Endemic Burkitt's lymphoma, a tumour of the jaw, abdomen, and other areas that spreads to the bone marrow or meninges, is the most common type of childhood malignant disease in many parts of East and West Africa and Papua New Guinea. It has also been reported from Brazil, Malaysia, and the Middle East. Burkitt noticed that its distribution (by altitude, temperature, and rainfall) and even its seasonal incidence followed that of falciparum malaria. Outside malaria endemic areas, Burkitt's lymphoma occurs sporadically. There is a suggestion that the B-cell line in cases in whites comes from lymphoid tissue, whereas in cases in Africans it comes from the bone marrow. Epstein–Barr virus (EBV) produces a lifelong infection of B lymphocytes. Normally this is controlled by specific, HLA-restricted, cytotoxic T cells, which recognize a virus-induced, lymphocyte-detected membrane antigen on B cells. Immunosuppression, as in recipients of renal allografts, allows uncontrolled proliferation of the EBV-infected B-cell line, which may give rise to one of the three chromosomal translocations [t(8;14), t(2;8), t(8;22)] that activate the c-myc oncogene on chromosome 8 responsible for malignant transformation. Acute P. falciparum infection leads to a reduction in the numbers of suppressor T (CD8) lymphocytes allowing proliferation and increased immunoglobulin secretion by EBV-infected B cells. In highly malaria endemic areas of Kenya, well children aged between 5 and 9 years (the age of maximum incidence of the tumour) have reduced EBV-specific interferon-γ responses. These tumours may grow so rapidly that massive local tissue destruction results in urate nephropathy and acute renal failure. Cyclophosphamide, vincristine, methotrexate, and prednisolone are used in chemotherapy, producing remissions in 80 to 90% of patients and a long-term survival of 20 to 70%. Breakdown of large tumours during the first week of chemotherapy may be so dramatic that the acute tumour lysis syndrome may be precipitated. This consists of metabolic acidosis, hyperuricaemia, hyperphosphaturia, hyperphosphataemia, hyperproteinaemia, and hyperkalaemia, which may result in fatal cardiac arrhythmia and acute uric-acid nephropathy with renal failure.

Control and prevention

General principles of control

The intensity of malaria parasite transmission is spatially heterogeneous. This has important implications for overall risks of disease and the age patterns of disease, disability, and death. Endemicity is a measure of the intensity of malaria transmission in a human population and determines the average age of first exposure, the rate of development of immunity, and, thus, the expected clinical spectrum of disease. It follows that interventions should be tailored to these basic epidemiological foundations, e.g. intermittent preventive treatment in infants (IPTi) is likely to have little impact on the incidence of clinical malaria and anaemia in areas of exceptionally low transmission. Optimizing the introduction of diagnostics to rationalize the use of new, expensive therapies will require better tools to target where this is cost-efficient and where presumptive treatment remains appropriate. Deciding the strategy and optimal mixture of interventions depends on an understanding of the epidemiological patterns in a given area: one size will not fit all.

Across the central belt of sub-Saharan Africa, interventions that minimize loss of life must be directed to young children and their mothers. In addition, careful thought must be given to measures that have a profound impact on the burden of malaria, particularly in the few areas where people might receive one new infection every night and immunity is acquired very early in life. Perhaps reducing human–vector contact might compromise the natural immunity prevalent in the community. In communities infrequently exposed to malaria, a focus on case management alone is a dangerous strategy where the lack of immunity means that each infectious bite carries a far greater risk of severe disease and death compared to many areas of Africa. Preventing the infectious bite carries little risk of compromising immunity and delivers benefit to all in the community.

The cornerstones of contemporary malaria control, case management, indoor residual house spraying (IRS), and insecticide (pyrethroid) treated nets (ITNs) will remain effective only as long as the drugs and pesticides remain effective. Case management is undermined by the evolution of parasite resistance to antimalarial drugs. IRS and ITNs lose their effectiveness as the vectors evolve behavioural or physiological resistance. How we use new chemical agents to minimize resistance is key but there is always a risk that, as resistance develops (or donors lose interest), malaria control will fail and populations that have lost their functional immunity will be more vulnerable to malaria.

Contemporary malaria control has a fundamentally different mission from the Global Malaria Eradication Campaign (1955–69) that was coordinated by WHO. That campaign did not eradicate malaria everywhere, as planned, but did reduce malaria morbidity and mortality and the global extent of the disease. The focus of eradication was on the use of indoor residual spraying with DDT (dichlorodiphenyltrichloroethane) accompanied by effective case detection and management with effective drugs. In some places, malaria remains absent today. In other places, elimination was only a remote possibility because the starting basic reproductive number of infection was so high. After 1974, when resistance began to emerge to widely used insecticides and drugs, the international political and financial commitment to global control waned. In areas where malaria persisted, populations had reduced functional immunity as malaria transmission increased, so malaria morbidity and mortality rebounded. Resistance of *P. falciparum* to most antimalarial drugs had reached epidemic proportions in South-East Asia. In Africa, mortality from malaria in children doubled from the 1980s through to the mid-1990s coincidentally with the rapid expansion of *P. falciparum* resistant to chloroquine and sulphadoxine–pyrimethamine.

Against a rising malaria disease burden, new global programmes such as WHO's Roll Back Malaria (RBM) initiative have emerged and aspire to reduce malaria morbidity and mortality by 75% by 2015. Because of malaria's intrinsic links to development and poverty, malaria also forms part of the United Nations Millennium Development Goal that aims to halt and then reverse the rising incidence of malaria by 2015.

A number of strategies can be combined to reduce the burden of malaria effectively. Most are regarded as cost-effective solutions in resource-poor counties and affordable within the constraints of international financial support. The interventions can be grouped into those that limit human–vector contact (including indoor residual house spraying and insecticide-treated nets), those that aim to reduce vector abundance by targeting breeding sites or adult vector populations and those that target the parasite (including intermittent presumptive treatment and prompt case management).

Limiting human–vector contact

So far, two methods for large-scale operational vector control—indoor residual spraying and long-lasting insecticide-containing nets (LLINs)—have proved capable of reducing malaria transmission. Both are adulticide measures, targeted at reducing the number of adult infective female mosquitoes. Unfortunately, uptake and acceptance of both interventions is poor among local populations in malaria endemic regions, although the situation may be improving. Perversely, coils, aerosols, and insecticide-impregnated mats sold through the private sector have greater acceptance rates, but have little or no demonstrable affect on disease transmission.

Insecticide-treated nets (ITNs)

The use of bed nets impregnated with pyrethroids such as permethrin, cyhalothrin, or deltamethrin gives substantial protection against malaria in endemic areas. In some areas, insecticide-treated door and window curtains are used instead of bed nets. The current combined evidence indicates that ITNs can reduce all-cause childhood mortality by 17%, averting 5.5 deaths for every 1000 African children protected. Over 50% of clinical attacks can be prevented through the wide-scale use of ITNs and infection prevalence can be reduced by 13% in areas of stable endemic transmission. The effect is due to a combination of reduced access of mosquitoes to people because of the net, a repellent and lethal effect of the insecticide on the mosquitoes trying to bite, and, sometimes, an effect on local mosquito densities so that even those outside the nets may get some protection. Thus, health impacts are maximized when large sectors of a community are using ITNs, thereby providing a 'public good' by reducing local transmission. Nets are obviously most effective when mosquito biting is concentrated late at night and indoors.

ITNs appear to be one of the most promising means of control while the development of an operational vaccine is awaited. Although initial coverage in many malaria endemic countries was poor, it has increased in recent years through free distribution linked to mass vaccine campaigns or availability of heavily subsidized nets at clinics. This is crucial for reaching vulnerable and impoverished rural populations. Retreatment of nets has proved difficult to maintain in many parts of Africa. However, the recent launch of two registered brands of permanently treated nets aims to circumvent this problem. LLINs retain 50% of their original anopheline knockdown efficacy after 2 years and cost approximately US$4.80 each in 2005. Currently only one class of insecticides, pyrethroids, are recommended by the WHO Pesticide Evaluation Scheme (WHOPES) for use on nets because of their rapid action, low mammalian toxicity relative to their insect toxicity, and lack of odour. The efficacy of pyrethroids on LLINs is, however, threatened by the rapid increases in pyrethroid resistance among mosquito vectors in many parts of the world. In any insecticide-based vector control activity, insecticide resistance should be monitored at least annually as resistance is dynamic and can evolve rapidly.

Repellents

Repellents are used for personal protection. Compounds such as diethyltoluamide (DEET) applied directly to the skin or to clothes can reduce the amount of mosquito–human biting contact for several hours after they are applied. However, their main use is against day-biting mosquitoes such as *Aedes aegypti* rather than malaria vectors. Some insecticides, such as DDT, have strong repellent properties.

Indoor residual house spraying (IRS)

During the global eradication era, IRS was instrumental in breaking malaria transmission in many parts of the world including Sri Lanka and South America. DDT at $2\,g/m^2$ will remain toxic to endophilic anophelines for 6 months or more on nonabsorbent wall materials, with cyhalothrin or deltamethrin at a much lower dosage giving up to 4-month protection, while organophosphorus insecticides such as malathion, propoxur, and fenitrothion at the same dosage last about 3 months. This approach relies on killing the mosquito after it has fed and is thus a more community-focused intervention than ITN, requiring coverage of all houses and shelters. It requires a strong national organization to manage the routine spraying of houses and the compliance of householders to allow spray teams access and to remove their possessions from the house before spraying. There are few community-wide randomized controlled trials of IRS across Africa upon which to base an informed choice about the likely benefits of this approach in reducing morbidity and mortality. Most studies have been undertaken in areas of low transmission, with results similar to those with ITN. It is accepted, however, that interruption of transmission is harder to achieve under conditions of intense perennial transmission. In remote rural areas, the logistics of IRS are more difficult, but community cooperation has been achieved and mean parasitaemia was reduced by 80% in one remote area of Mozambique.

Reducing vector abundance

Mosquitoes are highly selective in their choice of larval habitat. The World Health Organization defines environmental management as the implementation of activities related to the modification or manipulation of environmental factors to minimize vector propagation in order to reduce human-vector interaction. Three accepted strategies are as follows:

- Environmental modification—making sites unsuitable for vector breeding by draining, changing the rate of water flow, and adding or removing shade, cutting emergent vegetation, and altering the margins of bodies of water. Near the sea, salinity changes may be relevant. For small reservoirs and irrigation canals, cyclical changes in water level by means of a large siphon may control larvae by alternately stranding and flushing. Intermittent drying out of irrigation channels may also be of value

- Environmental manipulation—filling holes, e.g. with polystyrene beads or soil, or using the Bti toxin derived from the bacteria *Bacillus thuringiensis*

- Reducing human contact—using infective vectors by zooprophylaxis, modifying of human habitations, or purposely changing human behaviour

The basic epidemiology of local mosquito populations must be understood before control programmes are initiated. Mosquitoes cannot be eradicated because of the cost, ecological impact, or logistics and so the target threshold for the vector population is set at or below acceptable levels of potential disease transmission. Where habitats cannot be drained or rendered structurally unsuitable for mosquito breeding, chemical larvicides may be used. Historically, diesel oil, at 40 litre/ha of water surface with or without the addition of insecticides, prevented the larvae breathing when it was applied to the water surface with a spreading agent. Paris Green (1 kg/ha), temephos granules (2–20 kg/ha), or less than one-tenth of the amount of pyriproxyfen are effective and safer.

Intermittent preventive treatment

As an intermittent preventive treatment in pregnancy (IPTp), it was shown during the late 1990s that a therapeutic course of sulphadoxine–pyrimethamine given on two or three occasions during the second and third trimesters of pregnancy was effective in preventing infection of the placenta, reducing the incidence of anaemia in pregnant mothers, and increasing the birth weights of newborn children. This strategy continues to be implemented in many African countries but it is likely to become decreasingly effective because IPTp works less well in HIV-positive women and there is no proven safe alternative to sulphadoxine–pyrimethamine for IPTp in areas where resistance to this combination is rapidly expanding. DHA–mefloquine, DHA–piperaquine, and mefloquine–azithromycin combinations have been proposed as potential replacements subject to successful trials.

The concept of IPT has recently been extended to target infants (IPTi) by providing therapeutic courses of antimalarials at the same time as vaccination. Studies in Africa have shown that sulphadoxine–pyrimethamine or amodiaquine reduces the incidence of malaria and severe anaemia during the first year of life by 50 to 67%. The combined effects of IPTi and ITNs are currently being investigated.

Access to effective medicines

Even though preventive strategies may halve the incidence of clinical malaria, effective and prompt case management remains a fundamental adjunct to control, particularly among African children who experience at least 20 clinical attacks during their first 5 years of life. Cheap drugs such as chloroquine and sulphadoxine–pyrimethamine was the basis of malaria management in Africa and, during the early 1990s, resistance to both drugs increased rapidly and malaria mortality rose to levels similar to those witnessed in the colonial era despite a general decline in childhood deaths not attributable to malaria. Possible replacements for failing drugs are existing drugs combined with artemisinin derivatives. ACTs have the additional public health benefit of reducing transmission, like wide-scale use of ITNs. Introduction of combination mefloquine–artesunate therapy among refugees on the Thai–Burmese border was associated with an 18.5-fold reduction in gametocyte carriage rates, halving frequency of *P. falciparum* transmission in the area.

Control strategies based on case management depend on prompt treatment of appropriate patients with effective medicines. Since clinical criteria for diagnosing malaria have low specificity, parasitological diagnosis remains the gold standard. However, in many remote rural communities diagnostic facilities are inadequate and WHO's Integrated Management of Childhood Illnesses (IMCI) recommends that all children living in malaria endemic areas (where >5% of fevers are due to malaria) should be given presumptive antimalarial treatment if they are febrile. The logic is that misdiagnosis, even in a small proportion of febrile children with malaria, can be serious because of the rapidity of progression to severe disease. Recommendations for older children and adults in malaria endemic areas are more ambiguous, posing a problem at a time when new, more expensive drugs are being deployed and malaria continues to be a diagnosis of convenience or a diagnosis by default, leading to massive overdiagnosis and overtreatment of malaria in these age groups.

Access to medicines remains poor in many malarious countries. In Kenya, less than 5% of children received an antimalarial within 24 h of the onset of symptoms. Increasing accessibility to new ACTs for the most vulnerable groups, largely African children, will require innovative methods of delivery. Operational approaches to improve access to effective medicines include training mothers or community-resource persons to administer medicines in the home, better training of shopkeepers to deliver advice when selling over-the-counter antimalarials, and improving community awareness of the need to get children to clinic early.

The aim of wide-scale use of ACT in Africa by 2015 is confronted by several problems. First, new ACT drugs cost 10 times as much as current failing drugs, putting them beyond the essential drugs budgets of most poor countries. International funding has been assembled through the Global Fund to Fight AIDS, Tuberculosis and Malaria but this will be effective only if there are guarantees of long-term sustainable financing. Secondly, the agricultural sector must produce sufficient *Artemisia annua*, the source of artemisinins. In the longer term, synthetic artemisinin compounds might eventually alleviate the dependence on natural products.

Malarial vaccines

Difficulties facing vaccine development

Vaccines offer one of the most effective public health tools for controlling infectious diseases. The obstacles to developing a malaria vaccine are formidable: the malaria parasite is complex and multi-staged, with a large genome (25–30 Mb with 5000–6000 genes). Many of the potential immune targets are polymorphic and the parasite has a large capacity for evolving evasive strategies. Most effort has gone into developing subunit vaccines based usually on single antigens thought to be critical in the parasite's biology. There are now a large number of potential vaccine candidates and one of the barriers to moving from concept to vaccine is the lack of appropriate animal models or *in vitro* correlates of immunity against which to select candidates for field trials. In the case of pre-erythrocytic vaccines, the development of centres for experimental immunization and challenge has offered a way of identifying effective candidates and it is likely that this approach will be extended to blood-stage vaccines.

Pre-erythrocytic vaccines

The aim of a pre-erythrocytic vaccine is either to block the establishment of an infection by preventing sporozoites from invading hepatocytes or to target the intrahepatic parasite to prevent progression to a blood-stage infection. Such infection-blocking immunity can be established in murine and human malaria by the repeated injection of irradiated sporozoites. Although establishing an important proof of principle, the apparent impracticality of using live attenuated sporozoites led to a focus on achieving the same effect using subunit vaccines. This led to the cloning in the 1980s of the first malaria gene, for the circumsporozoite protein, a major component of the coat of the sporozoite. This provided the basis for the development of a subunit vaccine, RTS,S, a fusion protein combining part of the circumsporozoite protein of *P. falciparum* with HBsAg with a complex adjuvant (AS02). RTS,S has consistently provided 30 to 40% protection against sporozoite

challenges in nonimmune volunteers. Recent trials in infants and young children in Kenya and Tanzania showed a protective efficacy of 53% against malaria disease and large-scale phase III trials in infants across Africa are underway. Interim results were published in 2011of this candidate malaria vaccine RTS,S/AS01. By the 14th month after the first dose, the vaccine efficacy was 50.4% against malaria attacks and 45.1% against severe malaria (34.8% for the whole targeted population during an average follow-up of 11 months). This announcement was criticized by some as premature and did not encourage the early deployment of this vaccine. The demonstration of efficacy (albeit not complete) of a subunit vaccine (RTS, S) based on one part of a single molecule from such a complex parasite has been important in giving confidence to the idea of developing antimalarial vaccines. Many investigators feel that given the complexity of the parasite and the high degree of antigenic polymorphism, the eventual ideal vaccine will involve combinations of antigens, probably from both pre-erythrocytic and erythrocytic stages. An extension of the same idea has recently seen a return of interest in the possibility of whole parasite vaccines. Remarkably, it has been shown that many of the apparent logistic objections to the production of attenuated sporozoite vaccines can in fact be overcome. However, needle inoculation in the skin of a purified irradiated *P. falciparum* sporozoites in 80 volunteers proved poorly immunogenic. Animal studies demonstrated that intravenous immunization was critical for inducing a high frequency of sporozoite-specific CD8(+), IFN-γ-producing T cells in livers of nonhuman primates and mice and conferring protection to mice.

Blood-stage vaccines

The aims of blood-stage vaccines are to limit parasite replication and prevent clinical disease. A number of candidate vaccines based on key molecules on the merozoite surface or released from the merozoite at the time of RBC invasion (e.g. MSP1, MSP2, MSP3, AMA1) are at various stages of development and several candidate vaccines are in early field trials. Particular problems likely to be faced involve the high degree of antigenic polymorphism shown by most of the candidate vaccine molecules. Antigenic variation of proteins on the surface of schizont-infected red cells has stood in the way of developing vaccines based on the obvious target for protective immune responses, the parasite-derived antigens expressed on the infected RBC surface. However, a recent report that the interaction between an erythrocyte membrane protein, basigin, a receptor for a merozoite protein (PfRH5) is essential for all strains tested gives new encouragement to the development of a blood-stage antimerozoite vaccine. In the particular case of pregnancy-related malaria, the RBC expressed parasite molecules are of much more limited diversity and efforts are under way to develop a vaccine based on this subset of PfEMP1 antigens. These efforts have not yet reached the stage of human trials.

Transmission-blocking vaccines (TBVs)

TBVs aim to prevent the transmission of malaria by blocking the parasite's development in the mosquito by inducing antibodies targeting either antigens present on the sexual stages of the parasites or mosquito antigens that are required for the successful development of the parasite in the midgut of its vector. Candidate vaccines have been shown to induce antibodies that completely block transmission of *P. falciparum* and *P. vivax*.

The malaria vaccine field is rapidly changing and updated information on the range of candidate vaccines can be obtained at http://www.malariavaccine.org and http://www.who.int/immunization.

Prevention of malaria in travellers

Advice to travellers

The prevention of malaria in travellers, particularly those usually resident in nonmalarious areas but visiting endemic regions, including those visiting their friends and relatives ('VFR's), has become more difficult because of resistance to antimalarial drugs. As a result, prevention can never be complete. Travellers must be advised to: (1) be aware of the risk; (2) reduce exposure to being bitten by anopheline mosquitoes; (3) take chemoprophylaxis where appropriate; and (4) seek immediate medical advice in the event of any fever or influenza-like illness developing while in the area, or within 3 months or more of leaving it, and to mention malaria as a possibility regardless of the precautions taken.

Preventive advice is subject to uncertainty because unequivocal data on efficacy are often unavailable, published studies are conflicting, the distribution of resistance to many prophylactics is changing and not well mapped, and experts disagree on the balance between the risk of malaria and the risk of side effects. Travellers may obtain conflicting opinions from different sources, jeopardizing their adherence to any one regimen. The WHO list of malarious areas, updated annually, and other publications are inevitably directed towards prophylaxis for areas of greatest transmission. Advice from someone who knows the country and the traveller's itinerary is more specific and therefore more reliable.

No prophylactic regimen will give total protection, but many will reduce substantially the risk of malaria. Strict adherence, even to a suboptimal prophylactic regimen, is more important than vacillation in search of the ideal.

Diagnosis of imported malaria is a medical emergency as, exceptionally, falciparum malaria can be fatal within 24 h of the first symptom and the disease is often misdiagnosed (see Table 8.2.3). Several fatal cases are reported in the United Kingdom and the United States of America each year. Expert diagnosis and appropriate drugs may not be readily available. Useful guidelines are published by Centres for Disease Control in the United States of America and the Health Protection Agency and National Travel Health Network and Centre in the United Kingdom.

When falciparum malaria is diagnosed in a traveller, the rest of their tour group should be screened as a matter of urgency, as they can be presumed to have shared the same exposure risk.

Prevention of mosquito bites

Bed nets without tears or other holes through which mosquitoes might enter, impregnated with a pyrethroid insecticide such as permethrin, deltamethrin, or cyhalothrin, should be used and properly tucked in. These also afford protection against other arthropod vectors, ectoparasites and even night-biting kraits (snakes). A well-screened bedroom and other accommodation, combined with use of a knock-down insecticide after the doors have been closed before dusk, gives substantial protection. Clothes (long sleeves and trousers) that deter mosquito bites, repellent sprays and soaps (containing DEET or permethrin), and avoiding exposure to bites in the evenings will also help.

Chemoprophylaxis

Choice and dosage of chemoprophylaxis

Detailed maps of the distribution of malaria in different countries and the recommended chemoprophylaxis for each area are listed in 'Further reading'. Where there is a substantial risk of chloroquine-resistant falciparum malaria, atovaquone–proguanil, mefloquine, or doxycycline are appropriate (Box 8.2.4). Of these, mefloquine

and atovaquone–proguanil are licensed for children and doxycycline should not be given to children under 8 years old (British National Formulary: 12 years) (Table 8.2.6). Pregnant women are best advised to avoid malarious areas. Apart from proguanil–chloroquine, no drug has been proved safe for prophylaxis during pregnancy but, if exposure is unavoidable in a high-risk area, mefloquine is recommended.

Atovaquone–proguanil

This combination has two great advantages: adverse effects are less frequent and less serious than for mefloquine and doxycycline; and it is a causal prophylactic, attacking pre-erythrocytic stages of malarial parasites. Consequently, it need be continued for only 7 days after leaving the malarious area, improving the chance of adherence. However, resistance is emerging and atovaquone–proguanil is expensive. The cost for short visits is similar to that of mefloquine or doxycycline but the differential cost rises greatly for longer visits.

Mefloquine

Mefloquine has a long half-life and on a weekly dosage schedule the blood level rises to a plateau from about 7 weeks. Most of its side effects, the main problem with its use, are associated with the initial three doses. The drug should therefore be started 2.5 weeks before departure to a malarious area, to allow a switch to an alternative if side effects prove troublesome. It can be used safely for at least 2 or 3 years. The most serious early side effects of mefloquine are neuropsychiatric: anxiety, depression, delusions, fits, and psychotic attacks. Their incidence is disputed. Airline passenger surveys have shown a frequency of 1:10 000, but experienced doctors in the United Kingdom assert a much higher frequency.

Box 8.2.4 Recommended malaria prophylaxis (adult dose) in addition to general measures specified in text

- Where chloroquine-resistant *P. falciparum* is absent:
  - Chloroquine 300 mg base weekly (best for short-term visitors)
  - Proguanil 200 mg daily (best for long-term residents)
- Where chloroquine-resistant *P. falciparum* is not widespread and is predominantly of low degree:
  - Chloroquine 300 mg base weekly plus proguanil 200 mg daily
- Where highly chloroquine-resistant *P. falciparum* occurs:[a]

  (1) Atovaquone–proguanil 1 tablet daily

  or

  (2) Mefloquine 250 mg weekly

  or

  (3) Doxycycline 100 mg daily

  or

  (4) [Chloroquine 300 mg base weekly plus proguanil 200 mg daily]

[a]Regimens (1), (2), and (3) are more effective in some areas of South-East Asia, Africa, and South America, but there is a low but significant risk of severe side effects with (2) and (3). Regimen (4) will give only limited protection but is the least likely of the four regimens to cause toxic side effects and is preferred for pregnant women and, at reduced dosage, for young children (Table 8.2.6).

Table 8.2.6 Doses of prophylactic antimalarial drugs for children

Age	Weight (kg)	Drug and tablet size		
		Chloroquine (150 mg) weekly with proguanil (100 mg) daily	Mefloquine 250 mg	Doxycycline 100 mg
Fraction of tablet				
Term to 12 weeks	<6.0	1/4	NR	NR
3–11 months	6.0–9.9	1/2	1/4	NR
1–3 years 11 months	10.0–15.9	3/4	1/4	NR
4–7 years 11 months	16–24.9	1	1/2	NR
8–12 years	25–44.9	1 1/2	3/4	NR
>12 years	>44.9	2	1	1

NR, not recommended.

For children aged under 2 years in areas of chloroquine resistance, the appropriate medication is chloroquine plus proguanil. Chloroquine is available as a syrup but the proguanil has to be powdered on to jam or food. Measures against mosquito bites are specially important.

It is not recommended for those in the first trimester of pregnancy or at risk of pregnancy during the 3 months after the end of chemoprophylaxis. In later pregnancy, the uncertain risk of stillbirth rate must be balanced against the considerable risks of malaria. Mefloquine is contraindicated in people with a history of epilepsy or psychiatric disease. Mefloquine resistance is reported from Africa, South-East Asia, and the Amazon region.

Doxycycline

Doxycycline proved to give good protection against drug-resistant falciparum malaria in trials in Oceania and it is being increasingly used, especially for those who cannot or are unwilling to take mefloquine. It should not be used in children or pregnant women. The main side effects are photosensitization, which occurs in up to 3% of users, a tendency to precipitate vaginal thrush in women (preventable with a one-dose therapy for candidal infections), and the rare risk of *Clostridium difficile* diarrhoea. However, doxycycline may reduce the risk of travellers' diarrhoea. 'Heartburn' and gastrointestinal discomfort from doxycycline itself is not uncommon. The drug is taken daily with food, taking care not to miss any days and avoiding lying down too soon after taking it to avert a real risk of acute pain from ulceration of the lower oesophagus. To get accustomed to taking daily medication, it should be taken a few days before departure.

Chloroquine and/or proguanil

In malarious areas where chloroquine-resistant *P. falciparum* is rare or absent, mainly in western Asia, North Africa, and Central America, chloroquine 300 mg (base), two tablets taken once a week, gives good protection. Since it suppresses only the blood forms, it will not prevent relapses of *P. vivax* or *P. ovale*. Continuous chloroquine prophylaxis is limited to 6 years because of a low risk of irreversible retinopathy. Beyond this, proguanil may be substituted. Proguanil 200 mg daily will act as a true causal prophylactic but is poorly protective against *P. vivax*. The extremely low incidence of adverse effects from proguanil makes it acceptable to long-term residents in endemic areas.

Where the prevalence and degree of chloroquine resistance is low, in parts of India and the rest of South Asia, the combination of chloroquine and proguanil (Table 8.2.7) remains effective and has the advantage of low toxicity and safety in pregnant women and in young children. However, it no longer provides adequate protection in sub-Saharan Africa, parts of India, South-East Asia, or the Amazon region.

Continuation after leaving the malarious area

All antimalarial agents except atovaquone–proguanil must be continued for 4 weeks after leaving the malarious area so that merozoites are killed when they emerge late from the liver into the blood stream.

Chemoprophylaxis in people with epilepsy

Proguanil, atovaquone–proguanil, and doxycycline do not increase the risk of fits in people with epilepsy.

Rejected chemoprophylactic drugs

The following drugs are unsuitable for chemoprophylaxis: amodiaquine because of the high risk of agranulocytosis; Fansidar (25 mg pyrimethamine and 100 mg sulphadoxine per tablet) because of the frequency of severe skin reactions; pyrimethamine on its own because it is ineffective in most malarial areas; and halofantrine because of its cardiotoxicity.

Geographical risk of malaria

The risk of malaria is much higher in sub-Saharan Africa than elsewhere. Prophylaxis must be taken except where the altitude is too great for transmission to occur or in the nonendemic southern parts of the continent (Fig. 8.2.10). In Asia, the risk is usually much lower. Visitors to the air-conditioned hotels of the larger cities of South-East Asia do not need prophylaxis but elsewhere in Asia there may be urban malaria. Mefloquine does not protect adequately against malaria in South-East Asia; travellers to areas of higher transmission will need regimens (1) or (3) in Box 8.2.4. Those living for long periods in such areas may prefer to adopt vigilance and the early treatment of fevers, but awareness of the risk is essential. Freedom from malaria in Asia by travellers does not mean that they will escape infection in Africa!

Travellers in remote areas away from prompt medical assistance should carry a therapeutic dose of atovaquone–proguanil, mefloquine, or lumefantrine-artemether in case they develop an acute fever.

Acknowledgements

Thanks to Dr Janet Cox of St George's University of London for information about *P. knowlesi* infection.

Further reading

General

Russell PF (1955). *Man's mastery of malaria*. Oxford University Press, London.

Warrell DA, Gilles HM (eds) (2002). *Essential malariology*, 4th edition. Arnold, London.

Wernsdorfer WH, McGregor IA (1988). *Malaria. Principles and practice of malariology*. Churchill Livingstone, Edinburgh.

World Health Organization (2011). *World malaria report 2010*. http://www.who.int/malaria/world_malaria_report_2010/en/index.html

Parasite biology

Coatney GR, *et al.* (1971). *The primate malarias*. US Department of Health, Education and Welfare, Bethesda, MD.

Collins WE, Jeffrey GM (2005). *Plasmodium ovale*: parasite and disease. *Clin Microbiol Rev*, **18**, 570–81.

Collins WE, Jeffrey GM (2007). *Plasmodium malariae*: parasite and disease. *Clin Microbiol Rev*, **20**, 579–92.

Crosnier C, *et al.* (2011). Basigin is a receptor essential for erythrocyte invasion by *Plasmodium falciparum*. *Nature*, **480**(7378), 534–7.

Garnham PCC (1966). *Malaria parasites and other haemosporidia*. Blackwell, Oxford.

Gaur D, *et al.* (2004). Parasite ligand-host receptor interactions during invasion of erythrocytes by *Plasmodium* merozoites. *Int J Parasitol*, **34**, 1413–29.

Kats LM, *et al.* (2008). Protein trafficking to apical organelles of malaria parasites—building an invasion machine. *Traffic*, **9**, 176–86.

Kwiatkowski D (2006). Host genetic factors in resistance and susceptibility to malaria. *Parassitologia*, **48**, 450–67.

Loscertales MP, *et al.* (2007). ABO blood group phenotypes and *Plasmodium falciparum* malaria: unlocking a pivotal mechanism. *Adv Parasitol*, **65**, 1–50.

Oh SS, Chishti AH (2005). Host receptors in malaria merozoite invasion. *Curr Top Microbiol Immunol*, **295**, 203–32.

Ollomo B, *et al.* (2009). A new malaria agent in African hominids. *PLoS Pathog*, **5**, e1000446.

Prugnolle F, Durand P, Neel C, *et al.* (2010). African great apes are natural hosts of multiple related malaria species, including *Plasmodium falciparum*. *Proc Natl Acad Sci USA*, **107**, 1458–63.

Sinden RE (1978). Cell biology. In: Killick-Kendrick R, Peters W (eds) *Rodent malaria*, pp. 85–168. Academic Press, London.

Sutherland CJ, *et al.* (2010). Two nonrecombining sympatric forms of the human malaria parasite Plasmodium ovale occur globally. *J Infect Dis*, **201**, 1544–50.

Mosquito biology

Fine PEM (1981). Epidemiological principles of vector mediated transmission. In: McKelvey JJ, *et al.* (eds) Vectors of disease agents, pp. 77–91. Praeger Scientific, New York.

Hemingway J, *et al.* (2006). The Innovative Vector Control Consortium: improved control of mosquito borne diseases. *Trends Parasitol*, **22**, 308–12.

James AA, *et al.* (1999). Controlling malaria transmission with genetically engineered *Plasmodium* resistant mosquitoes: Milestones in a model system. *Parasitologia*, **41**, 461–71.

Mongin E, *et al.* (2004). The *Anopheles gambiae* genome: an update. *Trends Parasitol*, **20**, 49–52.

Trape JF, *et al.* (2011). Malaria morbidity and pyrethroid resistance after the introduction of insecticide-treated bednets and artemisinin-based combination therapies: a longitudinal study. *Lancet Infect Dis*, **11**, 925–32.

Epidemiology and control

Chandramohan D, Jaffar S, Greenwood BM (2002). Use of clinical algorithms for diagnosing malaria. *Trop Med Int Health*, **7**, 45–52.

Guerra CA, *et al.* (2008). The limits and intensity of *Plasmodium falciparum* transmission: Implications for malaria control and elimination worldwide. *PLoS Med*, **5**, e38.

Guyatt HL, Snow RW (2004). The impact of malaria in pregnancy on low-birth weight in sub-Saharan Africa. *Clin Microbiol Rev*, **17**, 760–9.

Hay SI, *et al.* (2004). The global distribution and population at risk of malaria: past, present and future. *Lancet Infectious Diseases*, **4**, 327–336.

Hay SI, *et al.* (2005). Urbanization, malaria transmission and disease burden in Africa. *Nat Rev Microbiol*, **3**, 81–90.

Hay SI, *et al.* (2009). A world malaria map: Plasmodium falciparum endemicity in 2007. *PLoS Medicine*, **6**, e1000048

Lengeler C (2005). Insecticide treated bednets and curtains for preventing malaria. *Cochrane Database Syst Rev*, CD000363.

MacDonald, G (1957). *The epidemiology and control of malaria*. Oxford University Press, London.

Murray CJ, *et al.* (2012). Global malaria mortality between 1980 and 2010: a systematic analysis. *Lancet*, **379**, 413–31.

Snow RW, *et al.* (2005). The global distribution of clinical episodes of *Plasmodium* falciparum malaria. *Nature*, **434**, 214–17.

Snow RW, Omumbo JA (2006). Malaria. In: Jamison DT, *et al.* (eds) *Disease and mortality in sub-Saharan Africa*, 2nd edition, pp. 195–214. World Bank, Washington, DC.

Snow RW, *et al.* (2012). The changing limits and incidence of malaria in Africa: 1939–2009. *Advances in Parasitology*, **78**, 169–262.

Clinical features, immunology, pathology, diagnosis, treatment, and prevention in travellers

Anstey NM, *et al.* (2009). The pathophysiology of vivax malaria. *Trends in Parasitology*, **25**, 20–27.

Artemether-Quinine Meta-analysis Study Group (2001). A meta-analysis using individual patient data of trials comparing artemether with quinine in the treatment of severe falciparum malaria. *Trans R Soc Trop Med Hyg*, **95**, 637–50.

Beare NA, *et al.* (2006). Malarial retinopathy: a newly established diagnostic sign in severe malaria. *Am J Trop Med Hyg*, **75**, 790–7.

Cunnington AJ, *et al.* (2011). Malaria impairs resistance to Salmonella through heme- and heme oxygenase-dependent dysfunctional granulocyte mobilization. *Nat Med*, **18**, 120–7.

Daneshvar C, *et al.* (2009). Clinical and laboratory features of human *Plasmodium knowlesi* infection. *Clin Infect Dis*, **49**, 852–60.

Dondorp A, *et al.* (2005). Artesunate versus quinine for treatment of severe falciparum malaria: a randomised trial. *Lancet*, **366**, 717–25.

Dondorp AM, *et al.* (2008). Direct in vivo assessment of microcirculatory dysfunction in severe falciparum malaria. *J Infect Dis*, **197**, 79–84.

Ekland EH, Fidock DA (2007). Advances in understanding the genetic basis of antimalarial drug resistance. *Curr Opin Microbiol*, **10**, 363–70.

Gomez MF, *et al.* (2009). Pre-referral rectal artesunate to prevent death and disability in sever malaria: a placebo-controlled trial. *Lancet*, **373**, 557–66.

Hanson J, *et al.* (2009). Hyponatremia in severe malaria: evidence for an appropriate anti-diuretic hormone response to hypovolemia. *Am J Trop Med Hyg*, **80**, 141–5.

He W, *et al.* (2008). Duffy antigen receptor for chemokines mediates trans-infection of HIV-1 from red blood cells to target cells and affects HIV-AIDS susceptibility. *Cell Host Microbe*, **17**, 52–62.

Kochar DK, *et al.* (2005). Plasmodium vivax malaria. *Emerg Infect Dis*, **11**, 132–4.

Lalloo DG, *et al.* (2007). UK malaria treatment guidelines. *J Infect*, **54**, 111–21.

MacPherson GG, *et al.* (1985). Human cerebral malaria: a quantitative ultrastructural analysis of parasitized erythrocyte sequestration. *Am J Pathol*, **119**, 385–401.

Marsh K, *et al.* (1995). Indicators of life-threatening malaria in African children: clinical spectrum and simplified prognostic criteria. *N Engl J Med*, **332**, 1399–404.

Moody A (2002). Rapid diagnostic tests for malaria parasites. *Clin Microbiol Rev*, **15**, 66–78.

Noedl H, *et al.* (2009). Evidence of artemisinin-resistant malaria in western Cambodia. *N Engl J Med*, **359**, 2619–20.

Phyo AP, *et al.* (2012). Emergence of artemisinin-resistant malaria on the western border of Thailand: a longitudinal study. *Lancet*, **379**, 1960–6.

Scott JA, *et al.* (2011). Relation between falciparum malaria and bacteraemia in Kenyan children: a population-based, case-control study and a longitudinal study. *Lancet*, **378**, 1316–23.

Turner GDH, *et al.* (1994). An immunohistochemical study of the pathology of fatal malaria. *Am J Pathol*, **145**, 1057–69.

Vallely A, *et al.* (2007). Intermittent preventive treatment for malaria in pregnancy in Africa: what's new, what's needed? *Malar J*, **6**, 16.

Warrell DA, *et al* (1982). Dexamethasone proves deleterious in cerebral malaria. A double-blind trial in 100 comatose patients. *N Engl J Med*, **306**, 313–19.

World Health Organization (2000). Severe falciparum malaria. *Trans R Soc Trop Med Hyg*, **94** (Suppl. 1), S1–90.

Internet resources

Centers for Disease Control and Prevention. *Malaria.* http://www.cdc.gov/malaria/index.htm

Chiodini P, *et al.* (2007). *Guidelines for malaria prevention in travellers from the United Kingdom 2007.* Health Protection Agency, London. http://www.hpa.org.uk/webw/HPAweb&HPAwebStandard/HPAweb_C/1203496943315?p=1153846674367

Lalloo DG, *et al.* (2007). UK malaria treatment guidelines. *J Infect*, **54**, 111–21. http://www.hpa.org.uk/web/HPAwebFile/HPAweb_C/1194947343507.

Malaria Atlas Project. http://www.map.ox.ac.uk

Malaria Vaccine Initiative. *Accelerating malaria vaccine development.* http://www.malariavaccine.org

MalariaGen. *Genomic epidemiology network.* http://www.malariagen.net

National Travel Health Network and Centre. *Protecting the health of British travellers.* http://www.nathnac.org/

RDT info. *Commercially available rapid tests for malaria.* http://www.rapid-diagnostics.org/rti-malaria-com.htm

VectorBase. *An NIAID bioinformatics resource center for invertebrate vectors of human pathogens.* http://www.vectorbase.org/index.php

World Health Organization (2006). *Guidelines for the treatment of malaria.* http://www.who.int/malaria/docs/TreatmentGuidelines2006.pdf

World Health Organization (2008). *International travel and health.* http://www.who.int/ith/chapters/en/index.html

World Health Organization. *Immunization, vaccines and biologicals.* Available from: http://www.who.int/immunization

8.3 Babesiosis

Philippe Brasseur

Essentials

Babesia are intraerythrocytic, tick-transmitted, protozoan parasites that infect a broad range of wild and domesticated mammals including cattle, horses, dogs, and rodents. Human babesial infection is uncommon, caused by *B. microti* in North America and *B. divergens* in Europe, with most infections occurring in asplenic people. Presentation is typically with nonspecific 'viral-type' symptoms. Haemolytic anaemia is a characteristic feature and can be severe, particularly with *B. divergens*. Diagnosis is by discovering babesia organisms in Giemsa-stained blood smears, or detection of its DNA in blood by PCR. Aside from supportive care, treatment is usually with combinations of clindamycin, quinine, atovaquone and azithromycin. Mortality ranges from 5 to 40%. Prevention is by use of repellents, removing ticks from the skin, and avoidance of exposure in asplenic and immunocompromised individuals: there is no vaccine.

Epidemiology

Although several species of babesia may infect humans, two species, *Babesia microti* and *B. divergens*, are responsible for most cases of human babesiosis. In the United States of America, thousands of cases of *B. microti* infections have been reported since 1988, mostly from the north-east coast including Nantucket, Martha's Vineyard, and Block Island. *B. microti* is transmitted by *Ixodes scapularis* (previously *I. dammini*) and its reservoir host is the common white-footed mouse *Peromyscus leucopus*. *B. duncani*,

a new species has been identified in 9 patients in Washington State. *B. equi* cases have been identified in California and a single fatal case of *B. divergens* infection in Missouri. The zoonotic *Borrelia burgdorferi*, causing Lyme disease, is also transmitted by *I. scapularis* and coinfections are documented. The risk of both babesiosis and Lyme disease is highest in June when nymphal *I. scapularis* are most abundant. More than 20 cases of transfusion-transmitted babesiosis have been reported in the United States of America. A number of cases have been reported of infection exported to other countries in visitors from the United States.

Since the first description of human babesiosis in Europe in 1957, more than 40 cases have been reported. Most of them were due to *B. divergens*, a common cattle pathogen transmitted by *I. ricinus*. France, the United Kingdom, and Ireland account for more than 50% of the cases reported in Europe. Farmers, foresters, campers, and hikers are affected, usually between May and October, the season of activity of *I. ricinus*. Most infections (83%) occur in asplenic people. No transfusion-transmitted case has been reported in Europe, but the risk exists, since *B. divergens* may survive in packed red blood cells for several weeks at 4°C. *B. venatorum*, closely related to but distinct from *B. odocoilei* that infects white-tail deer in United States of America has been isolated in 3 asplenic patients in Italy, Austria and Germany.

Pathogenesis

Ticks infected with babesia inoculate parasites while feeding on a vertebrate. Babesia enter red blood cells directly and multiply by budding to form two or four parasites, rarely more, in 8 to 10h. They are released and invade other erythrocytes. The spleen plays a major role in resistance to babesial infections, especially in the case of *B. divergens* babesiosis.

Clinical features

B. microti infection

In humans, *B. microti* babesiosis is characterized by gradually developing malaise, anorexia, and fatigue with subsequent development of fever, sweats, and generalized myalgia, starting from 1 to 4 weeks after a tick bite; 95% of those infected have intact spleens. Headache, shaking chills, nausea, depression, and hyperaesthesia are less frequent. Mild hepatomegaly and splenomegaly may be detected and spontaneous splenic rupture may occur. A mild to severe haemolytic anaemia sometimes complicated by acute kidney injury, thrombocytopenia and normal white blood cell count are generally present. Lactate dehydrogenase, liver enzymes, and unconjugated bilirubin levels may be increased. Parasites are found in peripheral blood of 1 to 20% of patients with intact spleens, but in up to 80% of those who are asplenic. The illness is usually more severe in asplenic and older patients. Complications are more likely in the immunocompromised. Acute illness lasts from 1 to 4 weeks, but weakness and malaise often persist for several months. A low, asymptomatic parasitaemia may persist for several weeks after recovery. Case fatality is about 5%.

B. divergens infection

In Europe, *B. divergens* infections are usually more severe than those caused by *B. microti*, with a case fatality up to 42%. After an incubation period of 1 to 3 weeks, there is sudden severe intravascular haemolysis resulting in haemoglobinuria, severe anaemia, and jaundice, associated with nonperiodic high fever (40–41°C), hypotension, shaking chills, intense sweats, headache, myalgia, lumbar pain, vomiting, and diarrhoea. Peripheral blood *B. divergens* parasitaemia varies from 5 to 80%. Patients rapidly develop renal failure, which may be associated with pulmonary oedema, coma, and death.

Diagnosis

Babesiosis should be suspected in any patient from any area who presents with fever and a history of tick bite. Initially, *Plasmodium falciparum* malaria may be suspected, but lack of recent travel in malaria-endemic areas or recent blood transfusion and lack of a spleen should lead to suspicion of babesiosis. Diagnosis is based on discovering babesia in Giemsa-stained blood smears (Fig. 8.3.1). Babesia can be distinguished from plasmodia by the absence of gametocytes and pigment in erythrocytes.

B. microti is characterized by multiple basket-shaped parasites. In some cases, parasitaemia is sparse and detection of antibodies, using an indirect fluorescent antibody assay, may be useful for diagnosis. Antibody titres rise during the first weeks and fall after 5 months, but correlation between antibody titre and severity of the disease is poor. A real-time polymerase chain reaction (RT-PCR) assay targeting the 18S rRNA gene of *B. microti* has been developed.

B. divergens is characterized in Giemsa-stained blood smears by double piriform intraerythrocytic parasites or tetrads, but annular, punctiform, and filamentous forms may also be encountered. Serology cannot be used for a rapid diagnosis of *B. divergens* infection. Amplification of babesial DNA by polymerase chain reaction, using species-specific primers may establish the diagnosis of both *B. microti* and *B. divergens* within 24 h. These assays are more sensitive than, but equally specific as, smear detection. Clearance of DNA seems to be related to disappearance of parasites.

Treatment and prevention

Chloroquine, sulphadiazine, co-trimoxazole, pentamidine, or diminazene aceturate appear ineffective in completely eliminating babesia parasites. For *B. microti* infection, the standard treatment is a combination of atovaquone (750 mg every 12 h) and azithromycin (500–1000 mg orally on day 1, and 250–1000 mg therafter) for 7 days. Alternatively, a combination of clindamycin (600 mg intravenously or orally) with quinine (650 mg orally) every 6 to 8 h for at least 7 days in adults; treatment for children is atovaquone (20 mg/kg every 12 h, maximum 750 mg/dose) and azithromycin (10 mg/kg per day on day 1 and 5 mg/kg per day thereafter) or alternatively a combination of clindamycin (7–10 mg/kg) and quinine (8 mg/kg) every 6 to 8 h for at least 7 days. For immunocompromised patients, a treatment for 6 weeks and 2 additional weeks after blood parasite clearance is recommended. For patients with high parasitaemias (≥ 10%), haemolysis, or renal failure or those that are immunocompromised, these therapies might not be sufficient and exchange transfusion should be considered.

In Europe, babesiosis should be treated as a medical emergency. Immediate chemotherapy with either a combination of clindamycine and quinine or clindamycin alone reduces parasitaemia and prevents extensive haemolysis and renal failure. Exchange transfusion should be used in fulminating *B. divergens* cases. Imidocarb dipropionate, which has been used for treatment of cattle babesiosis, has been successfully used in two patients in Ireland, although this drug is not approved for human treatment.

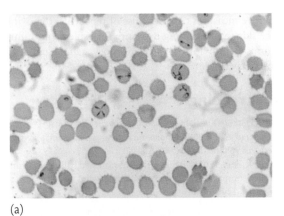

(a)

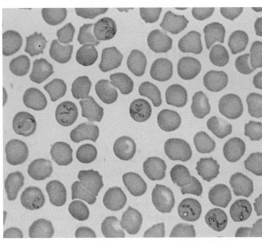

(b)

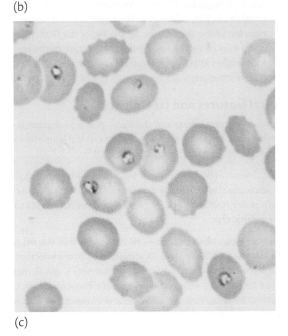

(c)

Fig. 8.3.1 (a) *Babesia divergens* infection in a 29-year-old Frenchman infected in Normandy. He had been splenectomized 4 months previously for idiopathic thrombocytopenia . Parasitaemia reached 30%. He was successfully treated with exchange transfusion, clindamycin, and quinine. (b) *Babesia microti* in a male patient, Missouri, United States of America (×100). (c) *Babesia microti* in a 72-year-old female patient, Massachusetts, United States of America (×150). (a, copyright P Brasseur; b, c, courtesy of Centers for Disease Control, Atlanta, GA.)

Preventive measures consist of use of repellents, removing ticks from the skin, and avoiding exposure for asplenic and immuno-compromised individuals. To date, no vaccine against human babesiosis is available.

Further reading

Homer MJ, et al (2000). Babesiosis. *Clin Microbiol Rev*, **13**, 451–69.

Vannier E, Krause PJ (2009). Update on babesiosis. *Interdiscip Perspect Infect Dis*; **984568**. Epub 2009 Aug 27.

Wudhikarn K, et al. (2011). Transfusion-transmitted babesiosis in an immunocompromised patient: a case report and review. *Am J Med*, **124**, 800–5.

8.4 Toxoplasmosis

Oliver Liesenfeld and Eskild Petersen

Essentials

Toxoplasma gondii is a protozoan parasite with worldwide distribution that infects up to one-third of the world's population. Human infection is acquired through ingestion in water or food of oocysts shed by cats, or by ingestion of bradyzoites released from cysts contained in uncooked or undercooked meat (e.g. sheep, swine, cattle). Following invasion in the intestine, tachyzoites rapidly disseminate throughout the host. Immune mechanisms mediate the formation of cysts, primarily in the brain, eye, and skeletal and heart muscles, where they persist for the life of the host. Presence of infection may be established by direct detection of the parasite in clinical samples (often by polymerase chain reaction, PCR) or by serological techniques.

Clinical features and treatment

Immunocompetent adults and children—primary infection is usu-ally subclinical, but some patients develop cervical lymphadenopa-thy; specific treatment is not usually required.

Ocular disease—choroidoretinitis; treatment with pyrimethamine and sulphadiazine is usually recommended if there are severe inflammatory responses and/or proximity of retinal lesions to the fovea or optic disk.

Immunocompromised patients—the central nervous system is the most commonly affected site. Reactivation of latent infection can cause life-threatening encephalitis. Empirical anti-*T. gondii* therapy is given to patients with single or multiple ring-enhancing brain lesions on imaging, positive serology, and advanced immunodefi-ciency, most commonly with the combination of pyrimethamine/sulphadiazine and folinic acid.

Congenital toxoplasmosis—infection acquired in early pregnancy may cause severe damage to the fetus or intrauterine death; infec-tion in the second and third trimesters goes unnoticed in the newborn in most cases, but signs of disease, e.g. chorioretinitis, may occur later in life. Suspected or established maternal infec-tion acquired during pregnancy must be confirmed by prenatal

diagnosis of fetal infection using PCR on amniotic fluid: if this is posi-tive it is highly probable that the fetus is infected and pyrimethamine/sulphadiazine and folinic acid should be given and continued throughout the pregnancy.

Prevention

Prevention of infection by avoiding ingestion is the strategy of choice in seronegative people. Pyrimethamine sulphadiatine can be used for primary and secondary prophylaxis of seropositive immunocompromised patients or seronegative recipients of organ transplants from seropositive donors. Spiramycin can be used for secondary prevention of transmission from the acutely infected mother to her fetus.

Historical perspective

The first human case ascribed to infection with *Toxoplasma gondii* was a child with hydrocephalus reported by Janku in 1923. Sabin reported the first case of encephalitis due to *T. gondii* in 1941. Lymphadenopathy was recognized as a key symptom by Siim and Gard and Magnusson (1951). Encephalitis due to *T. gondii* in immunocompromised patients was first reported from patients with Hodgkin's disease during immunosuppressive treatment in 1967.

Aetiology, genetics, pathogenesis, and pathology

Aetiology

T. gondii is an obligate intracellular protozoan of the phylum Apicomplexa, subclass Coccidiasina. The parasite exists in three basic forms of medical importance: the oocyst ($10 \times 12\,\mu m$ in size), which is the product of the parasite's sexual cycle in the intestine of all members of the cat family; the tachyzoite (2–$4\,\mu m$ wide and 4–$8\,\mu m$ long), which is the asexual invasive form; and the cyst, which contains hundreds or thousands of bradyzoites in tissues (Fig. 8.4.1). Tissue cysts (the latent stage) remain viable through-out life of the host.

Ingestion of *T. gondii* cysts or oocysts (the natural route of infec-tion) results in cyst (or oocyst) rupture and release of bradyzoites (or sporozoites) into the intestinal lumen, followed by rapid entry into intestinal cells and multiplication as tachyzoites. Tachyzoites are spread by disruption of infected cells, invasion of neighbouring cells, and via the bloodstream. In intermediate hosts and extrain-testinal tissues of the cat, cysts containing bradyzoites are formed and persist lifelong. Immunodeficiency may result in reactivation of latent infection and severe disease, whereas reinfection does not appear to cause clinically apparent disease. A single case of symp-tomatic infection with an exotic strain despite previous infection with a type II strain has been published.

T. gondii consists of three clonal lineages designated types I, II, III, and archetypes, which differ in virulence and geographical distribution. Archtypes not belonging to type I, II or III, are more common in Brazil compared to Europe and the United States of America, and clinical toxoplasmosis is more severe in Brazil compared to Europe (Gilbert *et al.* 2008). The recent description of strain-specific pep-tides has allowed typing of strains using serum. The generation of

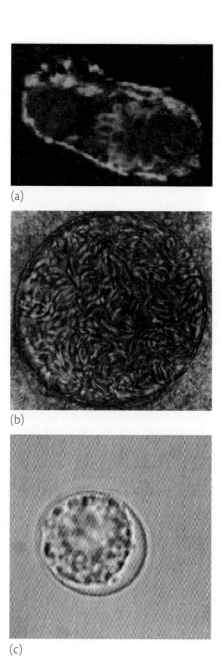

(a)

(b)

(c)

Fig. 8.4.1 *Toxoplasma gondii*: (a) Rosette-forming tachyzoites inside a macrophage, (b) bradyzoites inside a tissue cyst, and (c) oocyst in cat faeces.

specific gene-deficient strains of *T. gondii* and the sequencing of the *Toxoplasma* genome (http://toxodb.org) will provide further insight into parasite virulence factors and specific host immune responses.

Pathogenesis

The inoculum size and virulence of the organism and the genetic background and immunological status of the individual appear to influence the course of the infection in humans. Following active invasion, *T. gondii* induces the formation of a parasitophorous vacuole containing secreted parasite proteins but excluding host proteins that would normally promote phagosome maturation, thereby preventing lysosome fusion. The molecular characterization and function of a number of proteins from organelles

including rhoptries, micronemes, and dense granules have been reported. These molecules and the immunodominant tachyzoite surface antigen SAG1 are among the most promising vaccine candidates. Following intracellular replication and host cell disruption, parasites are disseminated via the blood stream and infect multiple organs including the central nervous system, eye, skeletal and heart muscle, and placenta. The developing immune response causes the formation of cysts in the central nervous system and skeletal muscle during the first week of infection. These persist lifelong. In immunocompromised hosts, cysts may disrupt and cause recrudescence of the infection, which then presents as life-threatening toxoplasmic encephalitis. Infection with *T. gondii* results in a strong and persistent Th1 response characterized by the production of interleukin 12 (IL-12), interferon-γ, and tumour necrosis factor α (TNF-α). Strain-specific differences in the modulation of host-cell transcription are mediated by a protein kinase, ROP16, released from rhoptries and injected into the host, resulting in the activation of signalling pathways and IL-12 production. The combined action of these cytokines and specific antibodies protects the host against rapid replication of tachyzoites and subsequent pathological changes. Dendritic cells and their capacity to produce IL-12 were identified as the main activators of Th1 immune reactions. Granulocytes may also contribute to the early production of IL-12. The activated macrophage inhibits or kills intracellular *T. gondii*, which counteract these actions by down-regulating surface molecules and interfering with apoptosis pathways in antigen-presenting cells, suggesting a role for these cells as 'Trojan horses' in early stages of infection. Sensitized CD4+ and CD8+ T lymphocytes are cytotoxic for *T. gondii*-infected cells. Both proinflammatory (e.g. interferon-γ and TNF-α) and down-regulatory cytokines (e.g. IL-10 and transforming growth factor β) are involved in balancing this response. Within 2 weeks after infection, IgG, IgM, IgA, and IgE antibodies against multiple *T. gondii* proteins can be detected. Reinfection may occur but does not appear to result in disease or in congenital transmission of the parasite. The production of IgA antibodies on mucosal surfaces appears to protect the host against reinfection.

Pathology

Histopathological changes in toxoplasma lymphadenitis in immunocompetent people are frequently distinctive and often diagnostic. They consist of reactive follicular hyperplasia, irregular clusters of epithelioid histiocytes encroaching on and blurring the margins of the germinal centres, and focal distension of sinuses with monocytic cells. Eye infection in immunocompetent patients produces acute choroidoretinitis characterized by severe inflammation and necrosis. The pathogenesis of recurrent choroidoretinitis is controversial. Rupture of cysts may release viable organisms that induce necrosis and inflammation; alternatively, choroidoretinitis may result from a hypersensitivity reaction of unknown cause. Damage to the central nervous system by *T. gondii*, toxoplasmic encephalitis (TE) is characterized by multiple foci of enlarging necrosis and microglia nodules. In infants, periaqueductal and periventricular vasculitis and necrosis are distinctive of congenital toxoplasmosis. The necrotic areas may calcify and lead to radiographic findings suggestive but not pathognomonic of toxoplasmosis. Hydrocephalus may result from obstruction of the aqueduct of Sylvius or foramen of Monro. Tachyzoites and cysts are seen in and adjacent to necrotic foci. The presence of multiple brain abscesses

is the most characteristic feature of TE in severely immunodeficient patients and is especially characteristic of AIDS. At autopsy in
AIDS patients with TE, there is almost universal involvement of
the cerebral hemispheres and a remarkable predilection for the
basal ganglia. In cases of congenital toxoplasmosis, necrosis of the
brain is most intense in the cortex and basal ganglia.

Epidemiology

Infection with *T. gondii* in humans is naturally acquired through
ingestion of cysts or oocysts. Humans can be infected by ingestion
of undercooked or raw meat (e.g. sheep, swine, cattle) containing
tissue cysts, or of water or food containing oocysts excreted in the
faeces of infected cats. The differences in seroprevalence of *T. gondii* depend on eating habits and customs that support the ingestion
of cysts as the major source of infection. Epidemics of toxoplasmosis in humans and sheep attributed to exposure to infected cats
indicate the importance of oocyst excretion by cats. Several outbreaks of toxoplasmosis through contamination of drinking water
by oocysts have been reported. This is a major route of transmission under poor socioeconomic conditions, where untreated surface water is drunk. Transmission of *T. gondii* in organs transplanted
from seropositive donors to seronegative recipients remains an
important cause of infection in immunocompromised patients.
T. gondii may also be transmitted by blood or leucocytes from
immunocompetent or immunocompromised donors.

In congenital transmission, the parasite gains access to the fetal
circulation by infection of the placenta following maternal parasitaemia. The reported birth prevalence of congenital toxoplasmosis
ranges from 1 to 10 per 10 000 live births in Europe and North
America. The frequency of congenital transmission depends on
the time during gestation when the mother acquired her infection
(Fig. 8.4.2). Maternal infection acquired weeks or a few months
before gestation poses very little or no risk to the fetus. Infection
acquired around the time of conception and within the first
2 weeks of gestation in most cases does not result in transmission,
whereas rates of transmission are above 60% in the last trimester.
There is an inverse relationship between frequency of transmission
and severity of disease. Infection in the first and second trimester, although less frequent than infection in the third trimester,
results in severe congenital toxoplasmosis more often (Fig. 8.4.3).
In contrast, maternal infection during the third trimester, although
more frequent than infection in the first or second trimester, usually results in subclinical infection of the newborn. It is important
to be aware that the overall frequency of subclinical infection in
newborns with congenital toxoplasmosis is as high as 85%. The
vast majority of these neonatal infections are initially unnoticed,
of which a fraction of later develop choroidoretinitis. Treatment
of the mother during pregnancy aims to reduce the frequency
and severity of fetal infection. However, the efficacy of such treatment is debatable (see below). Treatment aimed at preventing
mother-to-child transmission should be given within 3 weeks of
infection. In practice, this is very difficult because most infections
are asymptomatic.

Seroprevalence increases with age. It does not vary significantly
between sexes and tends to be less in cold, hot, and arid areas and
at high altitudes. Incidence of infection varies with the population
group and geographical location. In El Salvador and France, seropositivity is as high as 40% to 50% by the fourth decade of life,
compared with an overall seroprevalence of 15% in the United
States of America. In various countries, seroprevalence of *T. gondii*
has decreased by approximately one-third over the past decades.

Prevention

Since the infection is naturally acquired through ingestion of
undercooked cyst-containing meat or food contaminated with
oocysts, infection is preventable in almost all cases. Primary prophylaxis (prevention of infection) by avoiding ingestion is the strategy of choice in seronegative people, whereas in seropositive
immunocompromised patients (e.g. people with AIDS) or seronegative recipients of organ transplants (e.g. heart, bone marrow)

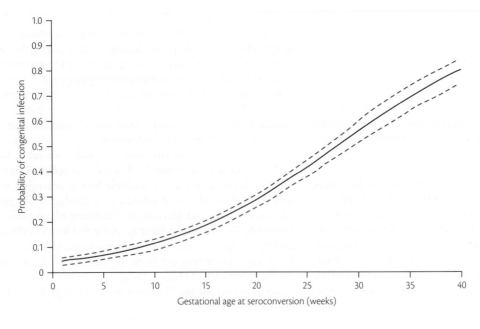

Fig. 8.4.2 Risk of mother-to-child
transmission of *T. gondii* by gestational
age at maternal seroconversion.
(From Thiebaut R, *et al.* (2007). Effectiveness
of prenatal treatment for congenital
toxoplasmosis: a meta-analysis of individual
patients' data. *Lancet,* **369**, 115–22, with
permission.)

(a) Risk of intracranial lesions (n-473)

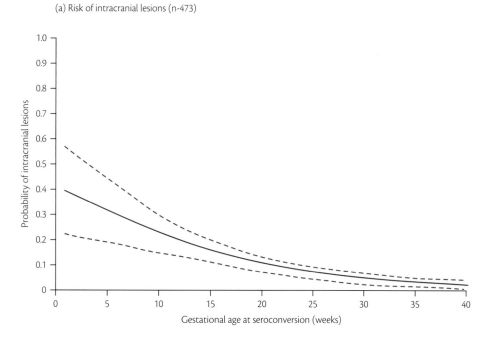

(b) Risk of eye lesions (n-526)

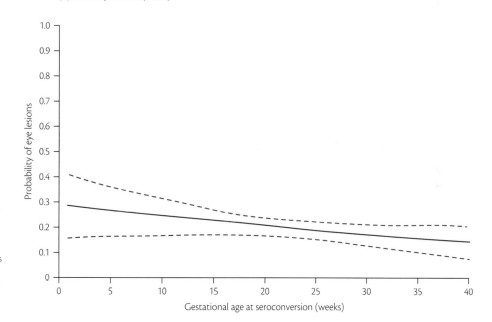

Fig. 8.4.3 Risk of intracranial and eye lesions in children infected with *T. gondii* by gestational age at maternal seroconversion.
(From Thiebaut R, *et al.* (2007). Effectiveness of prenatal treatment for congenital toxoplasmosis: a meta-analysis of individual patients' data. *Lancet*, **369**, 115–22, with permission.)

from seropositive donors, primary prophylaxis using pyrimethamine sulphadiatine has proved effective. Secondary prevention is employed to prevent transmission from the acutely infected mother to her fetus using spiramycin in immunocompromised patients following treatment of reactivated toxoplasmosis (maintenance therapy) using pyrimethamine/sulphadiazine. Systematic serological screening of all pregnant women is performed only in some countries. Uncertainty about the incidence of congenital infection, problems with the sensitivity and specificity of serological tests especially in the first trimester, and doubts of the benefit of treating newborns with asymptomatic congenital toxoplasmosis has hampered attempts to implement screening programmes in several countries. Neonatal screening programmes have allowed the identification of as many as 80% of infected newborns.

Clinical features

Infection with *T. gondii* may be subclinical or it may cause clinical signs and symptoms that vary according to the immune status of the patient and their clinical situation ('toxoplasmosis'). Four clinical situations can be distinguished: the immunocompetent patient, patients with ocular disease, the immunocompromised patient, and the patient with congenital toxoplasmosis.

Immunocompetent adults and children

Primary *T. gondii* infection in children and adults is generally asymptomatic. In approximately 10% of the patients, it causes a self-limited and nonspecific illness that very seldom requires treatment. The most frequently observed clinical manifestation is isolated cervical or occipital lymphadenopathy. Lymph nodes are not tender, do not suppurate, are usually discrete, and stay enlarged for less than 4 to 6 weeks. Very infrequently, chronic lymphadenitis, myocarditis, polymyositis, pneumonitis, hepatitis, or encephalitis can occur in otherwise healthy individuals. Acute toxoplasma infection during pregnancy is asymptomatic in the vast majority of women.

Ocular toxoplasmosis

Toxoplasma choroidoretinitis can be observed in congenital or postnatally acquired disease where it results from acute infection or reactivation. Choroidoretinitis may present in infancy or early childhood or reactivate later. It is uncommon after the age of 40. Bilateral disease, old retinal scars, and involvement of the macula are hallmarks of retinal disease in these cases. In contrast, in patients who present with toxoplasma choroidoretinitis in acute toxoplasmosis typically only one eye is involved, the macula is spared, and there is no old scarring.

AIDS and non-AIDS immunocompromised patients

In contrast to the relatively favourable course of toxoplasmosis in most immunocompetent people, it is life threatening in the immunosuppressed. Toxoplasmosis almost always occurs as a result of reactivation of chronic infection. It occurs when a heart, kidney, or liver from a seropositive donor is transplanted into a seronegative recipient. The central nervous system is the most common affected site. TE may present subacutely, gradually evolving over weeks, or as an acute confusional state with or without focal neurological deficits, evolving over days. Clinical features include changes in level of consciousness, seizures, focal motor deficits, cranial nerve disturbances, sensory abnormalities, cerebellar signs, movement disorders, bacterial abscess, and neuropsychiatric disturbances. The differential diagnosis of TE lesions includes central nervous system lymphoma, progressive multifocal leukoencephalopathy, and infection with cytomegalovirus, *Cryptococcus neoformans*, aspergillus, and *Mycobacterium tuberculosis*. In immunocompromised patients, toxoplasmosis can also present as choroidoretinitis, pneumonitis, or multiorgan disease, presenting with acute respiratory failure and haemodynamic abnormalities resembling septic shock.

Congenital toxoplasmosis

Prenatal ultrasound examination often fails to detect a fetus with congenital toxoplasmosis. Abnormalities include intracranial calcification, ventricular dilatation, hepatic enlargement, ascites, and increased placental thickness. Approximately 85% of newborns with congenital infection appear normal at birth. Psychomotor retardation and intellectual disability develop only in those children who showed overt features of brain damage at birth. However, if untreated, congenital toxoplasmosis may result later in loss of vision, children born with symptoms of congenital infection may or later develop psychomotor retardation, intellectual disability, and hearing loss. Fetal and neonatal disease is more severe the earlier in gestation the acute infection was acquired. The classic triad of chorioretinitis, hydrocephalus, and cerebral calcification is rather rare. None of the signs described in newborns with congenital disease are pathognomonic for toxoplasmosis and may be mimicked by other congenital infection such as cytomegalovirus, herpes simplex virus, rubella, and syphilis. Early maternal infection may result in death of the fetus *in utero* and spontaneous abortion.

Clinical investigation and criteria for diagnosis

Infection in the immunocompetent host

Immunocompetent adults and children with toxoplasma lymphadenitis are usually not treated unless symptoms are severe or persistent. Characteristic histological criteria and a panel of serological tests (IgG, IgM, IgG avidity index) consistent with recently acquired infection establish the diagnosis of toxoplasma lymphadenitis in older children and adults. If required, treatment is usually administered for 2 to 4 weeks, followed by reassessment of the patient's condition. The combination of pyrimethamine, sulphadiazine, and folinic acid for 4 to 6 weeks is the most common drug combination used (Table 8.4.1).

Management of maternal and fetal infection

The IgG and IgM antibody status of a pregnant woman should be obtained before or early in pregnancy. The absence of high-avidity IgG antibodies before or early in pregnancy allows identification of those women at risk of acquiring the infection. The presence of IgG and IgM antibodies indicates recent infection in approximately 40% of patients. The presence of high avidity antibodies essentially rules out an infection acquired in the previous 3 or 4 months, whereas low avidity antibodies can persist for more than 3 months after infection. Detection of IgG and IgM antibodies establishes that the patient has been infected, whereas seronegative women should be provided with necessary information to prevent primary infection (see above). Absence of IgM antibodies during the first two trimesters virtually rules out recently acquired infection unless the sera were obtained too early for the IgM antibody response to be detectable or too late after IgM antibodies had become nondetectable. The definitive diagnosis of acute toxoplasma infection or toxoplasmosis requires demonstration of a rise in titres in serial specimens (either conversion from a negative to a positive titre or a significant rise from a low to a higher titre). Treatment of women with acute acquired infection using spiramycin was thought to reduce the incidence and severity of fetal infection by approximately 60%, but a recent meta-analysis of data from children diagnosed by prenatal screening showed an effect only on intracranial lesions and not on choroidoretinitis at birth. Therapy should be started as soon as possible after diagnosis of recently acquired maternal infection (Table 8.4.1). Since maternal infection does not necessarily result in fetal infection, suspected or established maternal infection acquired during pregnancy (based on ultrasonography or serology) must be confirmed by prenatal diagnosis of fetal infection using polymerase chain reaction (PCR) on amniotic fluid. PCR has an overall reported sensitivity of between 64 and 98.8%. When the PCR is positive or it is highly probable that the fetus is infected, pyrimethamine/sulphadiazine is given in combination with folinic acid after gestational week 12 and continued throughout the pregnancy. Spiramicin is used before gestational week 20. If the initial ultrasound reveals no abnormalities, it should be repeated at least monthly until term. Hydrocephalus is an indication for therapeutic abortion. Since fetal infection is undetected in 85% of newborns, serology is commonly performed for neonatal diagnosis. The presence of IgG antibodies in the neonate's serum may reflect maternal and/or its own antibodies. Testing for IgM and IgA antibodies will identify up to 75% of infected newborns. Maternally transferred IgG antibodies usually decline and

Table 8.4.1 Suggested regimens for the treatment of infection with *T. gondii*

	Therapy/drug	Dosage	Duration
Acute acquired infection	Symptomatic[a]		
Acute toxoplasmosis in pregnant women[b]	Spiramycin	3 g once a day in three divided doses without food	Until term[c] or until fetal infection is documented
Documented fetal infection (after 12 weeks of gestation)[d]	Pyrimethamine	Loading dose: 100 mg once a day in two divided doses for 2 days, then 50 mg once a day	Until term
	plus		
	Sulphadiazine	Loading dose 75 mg/kg once a day in two divided doses (max. 4 g once a day) for 2 days, then 100 mg/kg once a day in two divided doses (max. 4 g once a day)	Until term
	plus		
	Leucovorin (folinic acid)	5–20 mg once a day	During and for 1 week after pyrimethamine therapy
Congenital Toxoplasma infection in the infant[e]	Pyrimethamine	Loading dose 2 mg/kg once a day for 2 days, then 1 mg/kg once a day for 2–6 months, then this dose every Monday, Wednesday, Friday	1 year
	plus		
	Sulphadiazine	100 mg/kg once a day in two divided doses	1 year
	plus		
	Leucovorin	10 mg three times weekly	During and for 1 week after pyrimethamine therapy
	Corticosteroids (prednisone)[f]	1 mg/kg once a day in two divided doses	Until resolution of signs and symptoms
Choroidoretinitis in adults	Pyrimethamine	Loading dose 200 mg once a day, then 50–75 mg once a day	Usually 1–2 weeks after resolution of symptoms
	plus		
	Sulphadizine	Oral, 1–1.5 g once a day	Usually 1–2 weeks after resolution of symptoms
	plus		
	Leucovorin	5–20 mg three times weekly	During and for 1 week after pyrimethamine therapy
	Corticosteroids[f]	1 mg/kg once a day in two divided doses	Until resolution of signs and symptoms
Acute/primary therapy of toxoplasmic encephalitis in AIDS-patients	Standard regimens:		
	Pyrimethamine	Oral, 200 mg loading dose, then 50–75 mg once a day	At least 4–6 weeks after resolution of signs and symptoms
	Leucovorin	Oral, IV, or IM, 10–20 mg once a day (up to 50 mg once a day)	During and for 1 week after pyrimethamine therapy
	plus		
	Sulphadiazine	Oral, 1–1.5 g four times daily	[g]
	or		
	Clindamycin	Oral or IV, 600 mg four times daily (up to IV 1200 mg four times daily)	[g]
	Possible alternative regimens:		
	(1) Co-trimoxazole	Oral or IV, 3–5 mg (trimethoprim component)/kg four times daily	[g]
	(2) Pyrimethamine plus leucovorin	As in standard regimens	[g]
	plus one of the following:		

Table 8.4.1 *(Cont'd)* Suggested regimens for the treatment of infection with *T. gondii*

Therapy/drug	Dosage	Duration
Atovaquone	Oral, 750 mg four times daily	g
Clarithromycin	Oral, 1 g two times daily	g
Azithromycin	Oral, 1200–1500 mg once a day	g
Dapsone	Oral, 100 mg once a day	g

IM, intramuscular; IV, intravenous; q6h, every 6 h; q12h, every 12 h.

[a] Acute acquired infection in immunocompetent patients does not require specific treatment unless there are severe or persistent symptoms or evidence of damage to vital organs. If such signs or symptoms occur, treatment with pyrimethamine/sulphadiazine, and leucovorin should be initiated (for dosages, see 'Toxoplasmic choroidoretinitis in adults').

[b] Practices vary widely between centres.

[c] German and Austrian guidelines recommend to use spiramycin prophylaxis until 17 weeks of pregnancy followed by a 4-week course of pyrimethamine plus sulphadiazine plus leucovorin.

[d] Practices vary widely between centres (pyrimethamine plus sulphadoxine is used in some centres, monthly alternating cycles of pyrimethamine plus sulphadiazine and spiramycin).

[e] Practices vary widely between centres (monthly alternating cycles of pyrimethamine plus sulphadiazine and spiramycin).

[f] When cerebrospinal protein is more than 1 g/dl and when active choroidoretinitis threatens vision.

[g] Duration of treatment as for pyrimethamine in patient with TE.

disappear within 6 to 12 months. Immunoblots can in most but not all cases distinguish maternal and fetal *T. gondii* specific IgG and IgM antibodies. Treatment of the fetus is followed by treatment of the symptomatic newborn throughout the first year of life, but the benefit of treating asymptomatic newborns with congenital toxoplasmosis after birth is debatable (Table 8.4.1).

Choroidoretinitis

The decision to treat active toxoplasma choroidoretinitis should be based on examination by an experienced ophthalmologist. Low titres of IgG antibody are usual in patients with active choroidoretinitis due to reactivation of congenital *T. gondii* infection. IgM antibodies are usually not detected. Patients with retinochoroiditis due to postnatally acquired disease usually have serological tests results consistent with an infection acquired in the recent past. PCR performed on aqueous humour has shown sensitivities of up to 55% that increased to 85% when used in combination with serological tests. Most ophthalmologists recommend treatment if there are severe inflammatory responses and/or proximity of retinal lesions to the fovea or optic disk (Table 8.4.1). The combination of pyrimethamine and sulphadiazine is the most commonly used regimen. Prednisolone is added if the lesion threatens the macula. The incidence of recurrent toxoplasma retinochoroiditis has been significantly reduced by using long-term intermittent co-trimoxazole.

Infection in the immunocompromised host

In immunocompromised patients with suspected reactivation, PCR rather than serological methods are strongly recommended. Pre-emptive antiparasitic therapy should be considered in all symptomatic seropositive immunosuppressed patients suspected to have toxoplasmosis. If the clinical features suggest central nervous system and/or spinal cord involvement, CT or MRI is mandatory. In most studies PCR performed on cerebrospinal fluid showed sensitivities between 60 and 75% while PCR on blood samples did not achieve sensitivities greater than 30% in most studies. Empirical anti-*T. gondii* therapy is accepted practice for patients with multiple ring-enhancing brain lesions (usually established by MRI), positive IgG antibody titres against *T. gondii*, and advanced immunodeficiency. Clinical and radiological response to specific anti-*T. gondii* therapy supports the diagnosis of central nervous system toxoplasmosis. The most commonly used and successful regimen

continues to be the combination of pyrimethamine/sulphadiazine and folinic acid (Table 8.4.1). Clindamycin can be used instead of sulphadiazine in patients intolerant of sulphonamides. Duration of treatment is recommended for 4 to 6 weeks after resolution of all signs and symptoms (often for several months or longer). After treatment of the acute phase (primary or induction treatment) in immunosuppressed patients, maintenance treatment (secondary prophylaxis) should be instituted using the same regimen as for the acute phase but at half the dose. In patients with AIDS, secondary prophylaxis is usually discontinued when the patient's CD4 count has returned to above 200 cells/mm^3 and HIV PCR peripheral blood viral load has been reasonably controlled for at least 6 months.

Areas of uncertainty and future developments

◆ Epidemiology:
  · Sources of infection, relative importance, e.g. water, meat, cats

◆ Pathogenesis/pathology:
  · Susceptibility of the host to infection, e.g. HLA types
  · Strain differences and clinical presentation
  · Virulence factors

◆ Diagnosis:
  · Improved avidity testing using recombinant antigens
  · Increased sensitivity of PCR on amniotic fluid

◆ Treatment/prophylaxis:
  · Clinical treatment trials in different clinical situations, e.g. eye disease and congenital toxoplasmosis using new drugs, e.g. atovaquone

◆ Prevention strategies/screening:
  · Co-trimoxazole for prevention of multiple episodes of recurrent episodes of chorioretinitis
  · Atovaquone for prophylaxis of toxoplasmic encephalitis
  · Prophylaxis and treatment in bone marrow transplant recipients

- Effectiveness of prevention strategies in pregnancy
- Cost-effectiveness of routine screening programmes
- Vaccination: proteins, DNA, adjuvants, and mucosal strategies

Further reading

Cook AJ, *et al.* (2000). Sources of toxoplasma infection in pregnant women: European multicentre case–control study. European Research Network on Congenital Toxoplasmosis. *BMJ*, **321**, 142–47.

Elbez-Rubinstein A, *et al.* (2009). Congenital toxoplasmosis and reinfection during pregnancy: case report, strain characterization, experimental model of reinfection, and review. *J Infect Dis*, **199**, 280–5.

Gilbert RE, *et al.* (2008). The European Multicentre Study on Congenital Toxoplasmosis (EMSCOT). Ocular Sequelae of Congenital Toxoplasmosis in Brazil Compared with Europe. *PLoS Negl Trop Di*, **2**, e277.

Gras L, *et al.* (2005). Association between prenatal treatment and clinical manifestations of congenital toxoplasmosis in infancy: a cohort study in 13 European centres. *Acta Paediatr*, **94**, 1721–31.

Holland GN (2003). Ocular toxoplasmosis: a global reassessment. Part I: epidemiology and course of disease. *Am J Ophthalmol*, **136**, 973–88.

Holland GN (2004). Ocular toxoplasmosis: a global reassessment. Part II: disease manifestations and management. *Am J Ophthalmol*, **137**, 1–17.

Luft BJ, *et al.* (1984). Toxoplasmic encephalitis in patients with acquired immune deficiency syndrome. *JAMA*, **252**, 913–17.

McLeod R, *et al.* (2006). Outcome of treatment for congenital toxoplasmosis, 1981–2004: the National Collaborative Chicago-Based, Congenital Toxoplasmosis Study. *Clin Infect Dis*, **42**, 1383–94.

Montoya JG, Liesenfeld O (2004). Toxoplasmosis. *Lancet*, **363**, 1965–76.

Remington JS, Thulliez P, Montoya JG (2004). Recent developments for diagnosis of toxoplasmosis. *J Clin Microbiol*, **42**, 941–5.

Saeij JP, *et al.* (2006). Polymorphic secreted kinases are key virulence factors in toxoplasmosis. *Science*, **314**, 1780–3.

Schmidt DR, *et al.* (2006). Treatment of infants with congenital toxoplasmosis: tolerability and plasma concentrations of sulfadiazine and pyrimethamine. *Eur J Pediatr*, **165**, 19–25.

SYROCOT (2007). Effectiveness of prenatal treatment for congenital toxoplasmosis: a meta-analysis of individual patients' data. *Lancet*, **369**, 115–22.

Thalib L, *et al.* (2005). Prediction of congenital toxoplasmosis by polymerase chain reaction analysis of amniotic fluid. *BJOG*, **112**, 567–74.

Thiebaut R, *et al.* (2007). Effectiveness of prenatal treatment for congenital toxoplasmosis: a meta-analysis of individual patients' data. *Lancet*, **369**, 115–22.

8.5 *Cryptosporidium* and cryptosporidiosis

S.M. Cacciò

Essentials

Cryptosporidia are small coccidian parasites that infect the mucosal epithelia of a variety of vertebrate hosts, including humans, affecting the health, survival, and economic development of millions of people and animals worldwide. Human infection is mainly caused by two species: (1) *Cryptosporidium parvum*—also prevalent in young livestock; can be transmitted from animals to humans (zoonotic transmission, particularly important in children), from person to person ('urban' cycle, due to faecal–oral spread), through contamination of public drinking-water supplies (which can produce massive outbreaks) or food (prepared by a sick food handler), and nosocomially. (2) *C. hominis*—essentially a human parasite; may produce large waterborne outbreaks.

Clinical features—infection involves either children or adults, but is a major cause of diarrhoea in children under 5 years old in both developed and developing countries. Patients may be asymptomatic or experience acute or chronic diarrhoea, depending on their age and immune status. (1) immunocompetent humans—infection usually results in acute self-limiting diarrhoea; (2) patients immunocompromised by drugs or AIDS, and those with concurrent infections such as measles or chickenpox—clinical symptoms are more severe and persistent and may become chronic, leading to electrolyte imbalance, wasting and even death. Since 2004, *Cryptosporidium* has been included in the WHO 'Neglected Diseases Initiative', in recognition of the importance of this infection in developing countries.

Diagnosis and treatment—diagnosis is usually made by detection of oocysts in stool, often by use of direct fluorescent-antibody tests. Detection of soluble cryptosporidium antigens in faecal samples by enzyme-linked immunosorbent assay (ELISA) is useful for the screening of large numbers of specimens. Molecular methods allow reliable identification of species and genotypes, and are therefore of paramount importance for environmental or epidemiological research purposes. Patients who are immunocompetent are usually managed symptomatically: there is no very effective anticryptosporidial treatment, but those with persistent disease can be given nitazoxanide. Management of patients who are immunocompromised is difficult: aside from supportive care, highly active antiretroviral therapy (HAART) is effective, both by immune reconstitution (in patients with HIV/AIDS) and by direct inhibition of parasite proteases.

Prevention—primary control is by limiting the opportunity for faecal–oral transmission, both direct and indirect, with maintenance of drinking-water quality and general hygiene (especially in hospitals, wards, etc.) essential for the prevention of the infection. Secondary control, when water supplies are contaminated, can be achieved by boiling water or filtering it (using an appropriate device) before drinking.

Acknowledgement: The author and editors acknowledge the inclusion of material from the chapter by Dr D P Casemore in the 4th edition of this textbook. Plates for this chapter were kindly provided from photographs by A. Curry and D.P. Casemore.

Introduction

The cryptosporidia are obligate intracellular parasites of many species from all vertebrate classes. In humans, infection is caused mainly by two species, *Cryptosporidium parvum*, which is also prevalent in young livestock and can be transmitted zoonotically, and *C. hominis*, which is essentially a human parasite. First described in laboratory mice by Tyzzer in 1912, cryptosporidium was recognized as a cause of human infection in 1976. In the 1980s it emerged worldwide as a common cause of severe or life-threatening infection in severely immunocompromised patients, especially those with AIDS, and of acute, self-limiting gastroenteritis in otherwise healthy subjects, especially children.

Biology

Cryptosporidium species have been traditionally considered as members of the coccidia (phylum Apicomplexa), but recent investigations have revealed a closer phylogenetic affinity with the Gregarinae, which are parasites of invertebrates. The oocyst, containing four sporozoites, is an environmentally robust transmissible stage and is fully sporulated and infective upon excretion with the host faeces. Cryptosporidia are monoxenous, i.e. they complete their lifecycle in a single host (Fig. 8.5.1). *C. parvum* is not tissue specific but shows a predilection for the lower ileum during the primary stages of infection.

Following ingestion of oocysts, the motile sporozoites are released, through a suture in the oocyst wall, in the lumen of the small bowel. They quickly attach superficially to cells, rounding up to form fixed trophozoites (meronts). The initial site of infection is the brush border of enterocytes in the small bowel, but the parasite is able to infect other epithelial and parenchymal cells. The complex life cycle includes both asexual and sexual stages of replication (Figs. 8.5.1 and 8.5.2). The endogenous (tissue) stages develop within a parasitophorous vacuole, the outer layer of which is derived from the host cell's outer membranes, in a unique intracellular but extracytoplasmic location.

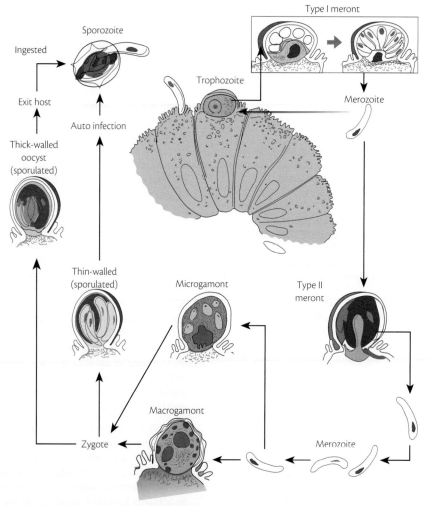

Fig. 8.5.1 Diagrammatic representation of the lifecycle of *C. parvum*. Following ingestion of oocysts, the motile sporozoites are released, attach to cells, and develop into fixed trophozoites (uninucleate meronts) in an intracellular but extracytoplasmic location. These undergo schizogony (asexual multiple budding), the first-stage meronts producing 8 merozoites, some of which recycle to form further type I meronts. Type II meronts produce 4 merozoites, which form gamonts (sexual stages) that mature as either macrogametes or as microgamonts containing 16 motile microgametes. Most of the zygotes formed after fertilization develop into thick-walled, environmentally resistant, transmissible oocysts, which then sporulate, usually by the time they are excreted. Some have only a thin unit membrane, which ruptures to release the sporozoites *in situ* to produce an autoinfective cycle.
(Adapted from a drawing by Kip Carter, University of Georgia, and shown by courtesy of W I Current and CRC Press, Inc., Boca Raton, FL.)

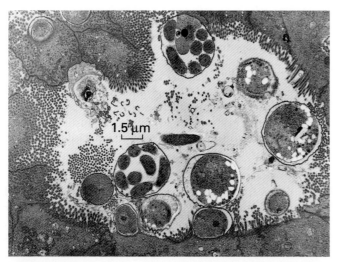

Fig. 8.5.2 Electron micrograph of a transverse section of small bowel of a mouse infected with *C. parvum*. The section shows numerous developmental stages: uninucleate meronts (trophozoites); type I meronts (schizonts) containing merozoites in which may be seen the darker granules of the apical complex organelles; the degenerate remains of a schizont and a free-swimming merozoite within the lumen; and macrogamonts showing dark wall-forming granules and electron-lucent amylopectin (polysaccharide) food-storage granules. The parasitophorous vacuole can be clearly seen surrounding the parasite stages. Some of the intracellular stages appear to be free within the lumen because of the plane of sectioning.

Molecular biology

The sequences of the genome of both *C. parvum* and *C. hominis* have been described and have revealed many peculiar characteristics. The genomes are very compact, about 10 Mb organized in six chromosomes, and are essentially composed of genes. Unusual biochemical pathways and genes have been described and these may serve as novel targets for drug development.

Protocols based on nucleic acid amplification of specific genes are available to differentiate cryptosporidium species and genotypes in both clinical and environmental samples.

Epidemiology

C. parvum occurs worldwide and is common in humans and in young livestock animals, especially lambs and calves, and has been reported in goats, horses, pigs, and farmed deer as well as in mammalian wildlife. Prevalence in humans varies both geographically and temporally. Because of the diversity of host species that can infect humans, the epidemiology of the infection is complex and involves both direct and indirect routes of transmission from animals to man (zoonotic transmission) and from person to person (urban cycle). A recent study has demonstrated that respiratory involvement commonly occurs in HIV-seronegative children with intestinal cryptosporidiosis and cough, suggesting the potential for respiratory transmission of the infection.

Zoonotic transmission

Transmission from livestock is common, particularly in children, including those from urban homes and schools visiting educational farms and rural activity centres. Companion animals have long been considered potential sources for human cryptosporidiosis.

However, they appear to be most commonly infected with host-specific nonzoonotic cryptosporidium species; they are therefore not considered important reservoirs of infection. Cryptosporidiosis is rarely seen in adults in rural areas, presumably as a result of frequent exposure and the development of immunity.

Human-to-human transmission

Cases of human-to-human transmission have been reported between family members, sexual partners, children in daycare centres, and hospital patients and staff. Outbreaks in daycare centres have been reported in the United Kingdom and the United States of America, mainly as a result of direct (person-to-person) faecal–oral transmission, although the infection may be introduced in the first instance through zoonotic contact. Affected adults may acquire infection from young children in the home or occupationally. Infection may be transmitted sexually where this involves faecal exposure. Cryptosporidium is a cause of traveller's diarrhoea, although apparently not as frequently as giardia.

Waterborne transmission

In the United Kingdom, the United States of America, and elsewhere, there have been numerous well-documented outbreaks resulting from contamination of public drinking-water supplies. Outbreaks, which can be massive, have been associated with *C. hominis*, which indicates contamination of the supply by human sewage, or with *C. parvum*, which suggests an animal source of contamination. Isolates from endemic (sporadic) cases, some of which will be waterborne, fall into both categories. Oocysts have been demonstrated widely in both raw and treated water and legislation has been introduced in the United Kingdom and the United States of America in an attempt to limit the latter.

Cryptosporidium is also one of the most commonly recognized causes of recreational waterborne disease. Most outbreaks are the result of faecal accident or cross-connection in swimming pools. Faecal contamination coupled with oocyst resistance to chlorine, low infectious dose, and high bather densities facilitate transmission. The potential for intentional contamination of water supplies has led to inclusion of cryptosporidium as a Category B priority pathogen for biodefence.

Foodborne transmission

Cryptosporidiosis has been attributed to ingestion of contaminated apple juice, chicken salad, milk, and food items prepared by sick food handlers. Food-borne transmission is probably underestimated, because the long incubation period (3–7 days or more) makes the relationship between cryptosporidiosis and a possibly contaminated food item difficult to establish. Methods for the detection of oocysts in fruits and vegetables have been developed and validated.

Nosocomial transmission

Transmission has been reported between health care staff and patients and between patients, particularly the immunocompromised. Large numbers of oocysts may be present in patients' stools and in vomit; transmission via fomites occurs, although this route is limited by the susceptibility of oocysts to desiccation. Poor hand-washing practice has been identified as an important factor. In an outbreak with high mortality in a ward of immunocompromised patients in Denmark, transmission was probably by patients' hands via a ward ice-making machine.

Demography

Age and sex distribution

In the United Kingdom, approximately two-thirds of cryptosporidium-positive samples are from children between 1 and 10 years of age, with a secondary peak in adults under 45 years; the infection is uncommon in infants less than 1 year old and in older people. Distribution appears to be the same in both sexes. A relative increase in adult cases is often seen in waterborne outbreaks. In developing countries, infection is common in infants less than 1 year old and asymptomatic infection is common in older subjects.

Temporal distribution

In the United Kingdom, a marked bimodal seasonal pattern of disease has been described: one peak during spring and the second during late summer/early autumn. The spring peak, which coincides generally with lambing and calving, is almost exclusively due to *C. parvum*, while both *C. parvum* and *C. hominis* occur in the late summer/early autumn peak. In the United States of America, the peak onset of cryptosporidiosis occurs annually from early summer to early autumn and, as it coincides with the summer recreational water season, it might reflect the increased use of communal swimming venues, particularly by susceptible hosts like young children.

Frequency of occurrence

Laboratory rates of detection in immunocompetent subjects average about 2% in developed countries (range <1–5%) and about 8% in developing countries (range 2–30%), and cryptosporidium is about fourth in the list of pathogens detected in stools submitted to the laboratory. In the United Kingdom, from about 5000 to 6000 confirmed cases are reported annually; it is generally somewhat less frequent than giardiasis. Among young children in the United Kingdom, cryptosporidiosis is more common than salmonellosis and detection rates may exceed 20% during peak periods.

Cryptosporidiosis is one of the most common causes of diarrhoea in patients with AIDS and in some studies prevalence has exceeded 50%. The infection rate in patients with AIDS in the United Kingdom has been falling in recent years, which has been attributed to infection control advice and the use of multiple antiretroviral therapy. Infection rates are not generally increased for most other immunocompromised groups.

Clinical aspects

Pathology

Histopathology

There is mucosal involvement of the small bowel, other parts of the gastrointestinal tract, and sometimes beyond. Moderate to severe abnormalities of villous architecture occur, with stunting and fusion of villi and lengthening of crypts. There may be evidence of mild inflammation, with some cellular infiltration into the lamina propria.

The endogenous stages of the parasite in the luminal surface are generally inconspicuous and appear as small (2–8 μm) bodies, apparently superficially attached to the brush border, unevenly distributed over the apical cells, and within the crypts of the villi (Figs. 8.5.1 and 8.5.2). Peaking and apoptosis of infected cells have been reported. There is usually little intracellular change at the ultrastructural level beyond the attachment zone of the parasite. Rectal biopsy may reveal mild nonspecific proctitis. Extensive and chronic involvement of the bile duct and gallbladder is seen in some patients with AIDS.

Immunological response

T cells play a crucial role in the elimination of cryptosporidial infections. In humans, T-cell immunosuppression caused by other infection or chemotherapy increases susceptibility to infection. Moreover, severe cryptosporidiosis has been reported in individuals with mutations affecting the costimulatory CD40 or CD40L required for T-cell activation. In particular, CD4+ T cells are necessary to control infection and achieve sterile immunity in adults, whereas the role of CD8+ T cells is not fully established. In agreement with these findings, low levels of CD4+ T cells counts (<100 cells/mm3) indicates a poor prognosis if infection occurs. The most important cytokine in resistance to cryptosporidum is interferon-γ and the principal source are CD4+ T cells. Therefore, it appears that a Th1 immune response is involved in the clearance of the infection. IL12, produced by dendritic cells and macrophages upon exposure to antigens, plays an important role in the activation of interferon-γ production by T cells. During infection, antigen-specific antibodies can be detected in serum, including IgG, IgA, and IgM. If the infection is brought under control, the IgM titre declines very soon, whereas IgG may persist for several months. Experimental studies in the murine model and data from studies involving AIDS patients have shown that, although antibodies may contribute to the protective immune response against cryptosporidia, they are not normally essential for establishing host resistance.

Possible pathogenic mechanisms

The watery diarrhoea is characteristic of noninflammatory infection of the small bowel, especially that associated with toxin-producing organisms and enteric viruses. Several mechanisms have been suggested to explain the symptoms: reduction in absorptive capacity, particularly for water and electrolytes; increase in secretory capacity from crypt hypertrophy; osmotic effects from loss of brush-border enzymes (e.g. disaccharidases) resulting in malabsorption of sugars, increased osmolality of chyme, and subsequent microbial fermentation of sugars in the colon (which may account for the characteristic offensive smell); and toxic activity.

Clinical presentation in otherwise healthy (immunocompetent) people

Cryptosporidiosis in the immunocompetent person is a self-limiting, acute gastroenteritis with a variety of presenting symptoms. In cases where the time of exposure has been known, the incubation period was about 5 to 7 days (range probably 2–14 days; wider limits have been suggested but are unlikely). There may be a prodrome of 1 day to a few days, with malaise, abdominal pain, nausea, and loss of appetite. Gastrointestinal symptoms start suddenly, the stools being described as watery, greenish with mucus in some cases, without blood or pus, and very offensive. Patients may open their bowels more than 20 times a day but more usually 3 to 6 times. Other symptoms include colicky, abdominal pain, especially after meals, anorexia, nausea, and vomiting, abdominal distension, and marked weight loss. Influenza-like systemic effects, including malaise, headache, myalgias, and fever, commonly occur. Gastrointestinal symptoms usually last about 7 to 14 days, but weakness, lethargy, mild abdominal pain, and intermittent loose bowels sometimes persist for up to a further month.

There is no evidence of transplacental transmission but infection during late pregnancy may cause metabolic disturbances in the mother, leading to the infant's failure to thrive. Failure to thrive has also been observed in older infants and children and may be associated with persistent infection and enteropathy, especially in developing countries.

Reported sequelae include pancreatitis (associated with severe abdominal pain), toxic megacolon, and reactive arthritis. In immunocompetent patients, deaths are rarely attributable to cryptosporidiosis.

Recent studied in the United Kingdom have further demonstrated that the impact of cryptosporidiosis on public health extends beyond that of acute diarrhoeal illness. Notably, an increased risk of nonintestinal sequelae (joint pain, eye pains, recurrent headache, and fatigue) is associated with infection with *C. hominis* but not with *C. parvum*.

Clinical presentation in immunocompromised patients

Susceptibility to cryptosporidiosis and the severity of the disease is increased in patients who are immunocompromised as a result of AIDS, hypo- or agammaglobulinaemia, severe combined immunodeficiency, leukaemia, malignant disease, and bullous pemphigoid. Disease susceptibility and severity are also increased during immunosuppressive treatment with cyclophosphamide and corticosteroids, as in patients undergoing bone marrow transplantation, and in children immunosuppressed by measles and chickenpox, especially where there is associated malnutrition. Infection in patients with leukaemia may be unusually severe and has sometimes proved fatal, particularly when associated with aplastic crisis, and may then require modification of chemotherapy to control the infection.

Symptoms of cryptosporidiosis are generally similar to those in immunocompromised patients but often develop insidiously. In those with late-stage AIDS with very low CD4 cell counts or in some other profound deficiency states, diarrhoea may be frequent, profuse, and watery, like cholera. Patients may open their bowels frequently, passing up to 20 litres of infected fluid stool per day; persistent nausea and vomiting is usually associated with severe diarrhoea and suggests a poor prognosis. Associated symptoms include colicky, abdominal pain often associated with meals, severe weight loss, weakness, malaise, anorexia, and low-grade fever. Cryptosporidial infection in immunocompromised patients may involve the pharynx, oesophagus, stomach, duodenum, jejunum, ileum, appendix, colon, rectum, gallbladder, bile duct, pancreatic duct, and the bronchial tree. Cryptosporidial cholecystitis (presenting with severe right upper quadrant abdominal pain), sclerosing cholangitis, pancreatitis, hepatitis, and respiratory-tract symptoms may occur, with or without diarrhoea. The clinical picture may include other features of HIV infection and there is often coinfection with other pathogens such as cytomegalovirus, *Pneumocystis jiroveci*, and *Toxoplasma gondii*.

Patients with less severe impairment of immunity may experience resolution or a more chronic course, with less profuse diarrhoea, sometimes with remission and then recurrence, possibly associated with biliary tract involvement. Except in those patients whose immune suppression can be relieved by stopping immunosuppressant drugs, or, in the case of HIV, intensifying antiretroviral therapy, severe symptoms may persist until the patient dies. This is either as a result of dehydration, acid–base or electrolyte disturbances, and cachexia, from some other opportunistic infection or malignant disease, or a combination of these.

Laboratory investigations

In early acute cases the stools are usually watery, greenish with mucus in some cases, without blood or pus. Peripheral leucocytosis and eosinophilia are found rarely. Serum electrolyte abnormalities will develop in patients who become severely dehydrated. In immunocompromised patients with cryptosporidial cholecystitis, serum alkaline phosphatase and γ-glutamyl transpeptidase levels are raised, while aminotransferase and bilirubin levels may remain normal.

In patients with AIDS, commonly associated infections are with cytomegalovirus and *Isospora belli*. Mixed infection with *Campylobacter*, *Giardia*, and *Cyclospora* species may be found in immunocompetent patients.

In the bowel mucosa, there is histological evidence of enterocyte damage, villous blunting, and inflammatory-cell infiltration of the lamina propria; cell peaking and apoptosis have been reported. Histopathological appearances of the affected biliary tract resembles primary sclerosing cholangitis. Radiographic abnormalities include dilatation of the small bowel, mucosal thickening, prominent mucosal folds, and abnormal motility and, in the biliary system, dilated distal biliary ducts, stenosis with an irregular lumen, and other changes reminiscent of primary sclerosing cholangitis.

Differential diagnosis

The absence of blood, pus, cells, or Charcot–Leyden crystals may distinguish cryptosporidiosis from some acute bacterial diarrhoeas and that associated with amoebiasis and isosporiasis. In immunocompetent patients, the symptoms of cryptosporidiosis resemble those of giardiasis or cyclosporiasis. Intense abdominal pain and cramps are generally more common in cryptosporidiosis, but bloating and weakness less common. In immunocompromised patients, especially in those with AIDS, isosporiasis is clinically indistinguishable, but can be diagnosed by finding the organisms in the stool, where Charcot–Leyden crystals may also be found. This infection responds to treatment with co-trimoxazole, as does cyclosporiasis.

Treatment of cryptosporidiosis

Several groups may benefit from an effective treatment, particularly patients with HIV/AIDS, transplant recipients, patients undergoing cancer chemotherapy, and those with severe malnutrition. However, existing therapeutics for other apicomplexan diseases are largely ineffective against cryptosporidium infection, probably because of the unique intracellular, extracytoplasmic location of cryptosporidians and limited understanding of the host -parasite interaction. Hundreds of drugs have been tested in the laboratory, but results have suggested that only paromomycin, azithromycin, spiramycin, and albendazole are partially effective. The failure to develop effective therapy for cryptosporidiosis is also related to the limited attempts undertaken by health agencies and the private sector, mostly because of a perceived limited market for such drugs in developed countries. Recent developments, which include the sequencing of the genomes of *C. parvum* and *C. hominis*, have led to the identification of new molecular targets for drug development. The availability of a substantial number of chemical libraries for drug discovery should also facilitate screening for effective drugs.

Today, the therapy of choice is nitazoxanide (2-acetyloloxy-*N*-(5-nitro-2-thiazolyl, NTZ) benzamide), a synthetic agent that has a demonstrated activity against a broad range of parasites as well as some bacteria. *In vitro* studies showed inhibition of growth at concentrations of less than 10 µg/ml, and studies in adults have shown that single doses of up to 4 g are well tolerated without important adverse effects. NTZ has been approved for the treatment of cryptosporidiosis in the United States and South America. The efficacy of NTZ in children and in immunocompromised patients has not been fully investigated.

Immunocompromised patients with persistent severe diarrhoea, malabsorption, and other complications may require prolonged palliative treatment. They should avoid excess milk, as lactose intolerance may develop. Parenteral feeding and fluid, electrolyte, and nutrient replacement may be needed. Antiperistaltic agents such as loperamide, diphenoxylate, or opiates may increase abdominal pain and bloating. Antiemetics may be needed for symptomatic relief. Temporary relief of biliary obstruction has been achieved by endoscopic papillotomy and of cholecystitis by cholecystectomy. Diarrhoea and vomiting may, however, prove intractable.

Highly active antiretroviral therapy (HAART) is the treatment of choice for cryptosporidiosis in immunocompromised patients, and can be used not only prophylactically but also as a treatment and

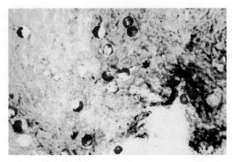

Fig. 8.5.4 Modified Ziehl-Neelsen-stained faecal smear showing oocysts of *C. parvum* examined with × 100 oil-immersion objective lens. The uniformity of size (4.5–5 µm) but variability of staining of oocysts can be seen.

secondary prophylaxis for established infections. HAART therapy is effective against cryptosporidiosis and acts both by immune reconstitution and direct inhibition of parasite proteases.

Laboratory detection and diagnosis

The characteristic endogenous stages (Figs. 8.5.1 and 8.5.2) may be found in histological sections, using light and electron microscopy, but diagnosis is usually by detection of oocysts in stools. Oocysts have also been found in vomit and sputum in some cases, especially those associated with AIDS. The oocysts of *C. parvum* are spherical or slightly ovoid, about 4 to 6 µm, and appear refractile in wet faecal preparations with a highly refractile inner body, the cytoplasmic residuum; the four sporozoites within may be distinguished with difficulty using special optical systems (Figs. 8.5.3–12).

Several conventional stains have been adapted for diagnostic purposes, such as the modified Ziehl–Neelsen method and phenol–auramine fluorescent stain.

Direct fluorescent-antibody tests, which detect intact organisms through the use of monoclonal antibodies that label the oocyst wall, are widely used due to their excellent sensitivity and specificity. Detection of cryptosporidium soluble antigens in faecal samples by an enzyme-linked immunosorbent assay (ELISA) is very easy to perform and particularly useful for the screening

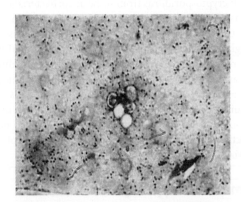

Fig. 8.5.3 Modified Giemsa-stained faecal smear showing oocysts of *C. parvum*, examined with × 100 oil-immersion objective lens. The uniformity of size (4.5–5 µm) but variability of staining of oocysts can be seen. The eosinophilic nuclei and basophilic bodies of the sporozoites can be clearly seen within the oocysts that have taken up the stain.

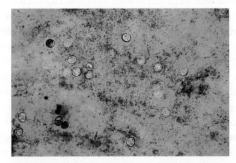

Fig. 8.5.5 Modified Ziehl-Neelsen-stained faecal smear showing oocysts of *C. parvum*. The uniformity of size (4.5–5 µm) is apparent but the oocysts in this preparation show a definite increase in refractility and marked failure to take up the stain (identity confirmed by immunofluorescence and electron microscopy).

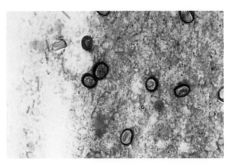

Fig. 8.5.6 Modified Ziehl-Neelsen-stained faecal smear showing oocyst-like bodies (mushroom spores) examined with × 100 oil-immersion objective lens (from specimen submitted to Reference Unit for identification).

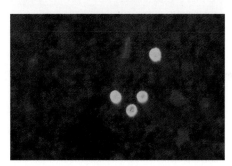

Fig. 8.5.8 Phenol-auramine/carbol fuchsin-stained faecal smear showing oocysts of *C. parvum*, examined with × 720 dry objective lens (screening magnification) on a fluorescence microscope.

of large numbers of specimens, albeit its specificity is limited by cross-reactions with other antigens of parasitic and nonparasitic origin that can generate false positives. None of the above-mentioned methods can differentiate cryptosporidium species and genotypes. Therefore, molecular methods, including conventional and real-time PCR, are increasingly used for environmental or epidemiological research purposes. The high specificity and sensitivity of PCR-based methods and the possibility of detecting multiple gastrointestinal pathogens in a single reaction, suggest that these methods may find application in routine diagnostics in the close future.

Standardization of approach to screening and of reporting is essential for epidemiological purposes. Ideally, all stool samples from cases of diarrhoea should be screened; restriction, where unavoidable, should be based on age group (see demography) and not on factors such as stool consistency. Concentration of stool specimens is not usually required for diagnosis in acute cases.

Fungal spores, yeasts, cysts of *Balantidium*, sporocysts of *Isospora*, and oocysts of *Cyclospora* may readily be mistaken for cryptosporidial oocysts.

Infectivity, resistance, and control

Infectivity

In studies using monkeys and lambs, the infective dose for *C. parvum* was fewer than 10 oocysts. In human volunteer studies in the United States of America, the minimum infective dose for *C. parvum* and *C. hominis* appeared to be similar (ID_{50} was 132 and 83, respectively). In contrast to *C. parvum*, however, *C. hominis* elicited a serum IgG response in most infected persons. A recent study has demonstrated the infectivity of *Cryptosporidium meleagridis* in healthy adult volunteers.

Resistance and disinfection

Oocysts can survive for several months in a cool, moist environment but are highly susceptible to desiccation, prolonged freezing, and moderate heat (pasteurization temperatures). They are remarkably resistant to most disinfectants and antiseptics, including chlorine at concentrations far greater than those used in water treatment and even to glutaraldehyde under normal use conditions. Some disinfectants may be more effective if used at elevated temperature (37°C or higher). Oocysts are sensitive to 10 volume (3%) hydrogen peroxide, to appropriate levels of ozone, and to medium or high-pressure ultraviolet.

In hospitals, adequate disinfection of faecal contamination or of endoscopes is difficult. If such instruments have been used for patients with cryptosporidiosis, prolonged immersion in

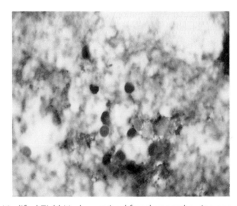

Fig. 8.5.7 Modified Ziehl-Neelsen-stained faecal smear showing oocyst-like bodies (mould spores) examined with × 100 oil-immersion objective lens. The spores are uniform in size but a little smaller (4.0 μm) than oocysts of *C. parvum*. They are generally more uniform in their acid-fast staining (identity confirmed by mycological culture and electron microscopy).

Fig. 8.5.9 Phenol-auramine/carbol fuchsin-stained faecal smear showing oocysts of *C. parvum*, examined with × 100 oil-immersion objective lens on a fluorescence microscope.

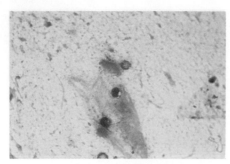

Fig. 8.5.10 Fluorescent dye-tagged monoclonal antibody-stained faecal smear showing oocysts of *C. parvum*, examined with × 50 oil-immersion objective lens (screening magnification) on a fluorescence microscope. The suture or associated surface cleft or fold, through which the sporozoites are released, can be seen

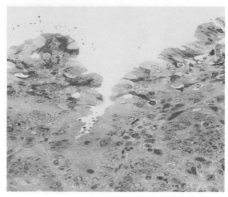

Fig. 8.5.12 Toluidine blue-stained semithin section of human rectal biopsy tissue of an AIDS patient with cryptosporidiosis. The apparent pseudo-external location of the parasite can be seen, the true location being intracellular but extracytoplasmic.

glutaraldehyde at a temperature higher than 37°C, or in hydrogen peroxide, after careful cleaning, may be required to ensure safety.

Control of transmission

Primary control is by limiting the opportunity for faecal–oral transmission, both direct and indirect. Symptom-free subjects not in contact with immunocompromised patients can normally be permitted to work if their hygiene is scrupulous. Spread via fomites is possible but this route is limited by the susceptibility of oocysts to desiccation. Patients with AIDS are more susceptible to infection with uncommon species or genotypes and advice may be needed to limit exposure.

Contamination of water supplies is inevitable, even in developed countries, and may be the source of some sporadic cases as well as outbreaks. When a public advisory notice is issued to boil water, raising the water just to boiling point is sufficient. In general, bottled water and water from point-of-use filters are unlikely to contain parasites but may carry an increased bacterial load, the health significance of which is uncertain for the immunocompromised. Patients with AIDS and others who are profoundly compromised should be advised never to drink water that has not been boiled or filtered through a suitable device. Users of filters should remember that these devices may concentrate potential pathogens and care is needed in replacing and disposing of filter elements.

Hospitals involved in the care of profoundly immunocompromised patients should be particularly vigilant in the management of patients with cryptosporidiosis. Long-term arrangements should be made for the provision of safe water for the immunocompromised to avoid difficulties when a notice to boil water is issued.

Further reading

Cacciò SM, Pozio E (2006). Advances in the epidemiology, diagnosis and treatment of cryptosporidiosis. *Expert Rev Anti Infect Ther*, **4**, 429–43.

Casemore DP (1991). ACP Broadsheet 128. Laboratory methods for diagnosing cryptosporidiosis. *J Clin Pathol*, **44**, 445–51.

Collinet-Adler S, Ward HD (2010). Cryptosporidiosis: environmental, therapeutic, and preventive challenges. *Eur J Clin Microbiol Infect Dis*, **29**, 927–35.

Hunter PR, Nichols G (2002). Epidemiology and clinical features of *Cryptosporidium* infection in immunocompromised patients. *Clin Microbiol Rev*, **15**, 145–54.

Meinhardt PL, Casemore DP, Miller KB (1996). Epidemiologic aspects of human cryptosporidiosis and the role of waterborne transmission. *Epidemiol Rev*, **18**, 118–36.

Xiao, L (2010). Molecular epidemiology of cryptosporidiosis: an update. *Exp Parasitol*, **24**, 80–9.

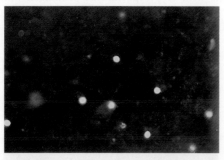

Fig. 8.5.11 Modified Ziehl-Neelsen-stained sputum smear from an AIDS patient with respiratory involvement (examined with × 100 oil-immersion objective lens). The *C. parvum* bodies present may include endogenous (tissue) stages attached to exfoliated cells. For this reason, oocyst wall-specific indirect immunofluorescence may show a poor reaction. There may also be less uniformity of size and differences in the staining appearance of the internal structures.

8.6 *Cyclospora* and cyclosporiasis

R. Lainson

Essentials

Most species of *Cyclospora* (Protozoa: Apicomplexa: Eimeriidae) are parasites of various reptiles and mammals. *C. cayetanensis*, which probably infects only humans, is transmitted by way of resistant oocysts voided in the faeces and contaminating food or water. Distribution is worldwide, particularly in regions with a low level of hygiene. Clinical presentation is with explosive outbreaks of acute diarrhoea, with this infection now regarded as an important causative agent of traveller's diarrhoea. Diagnosis is dependent on detection of oocysts in faeces by direct examination or in stained faecal smears. Aside from supportive care, treatment with trimethoprim–sulfamethoxazole has proved effective in eliminating the parasite in immunocompetent patients, but relapses are common in those with AIDS. Prevention is by ensuring good general hygiene, and in areas of high endemicity water should be boiled before drinking or use in preparation of fruits/vegetables that are to be eaten raw.

Introduction

Species of the coccidian genus *Cyclospora* (Protozoa: Apicomplexa: Eimeriidae) have been recorded in invertebrates (millipedes), reptiles (principally snakes), insectivores (moles), rodents, and primates (monkeys and humans).

Endogenous development of most species is within the epithelial cells of the small intestine, culminating in the production of oocysts, which are voided in the faeces and serve as the means of transmission.

Small, bisporocystic coccidial oocysts detected in the faeces of patients with diarrhoea in Papua New Guinea almost certainly represented the first discovery of cyclospora in humans in 1979, but due to difficulties in determining the number of sporozoites in each sporocyst, the parasite was not identified to generic level. What were clearly unsporulated oocysts of the same parasite, seen by other authors in patients with diarrhoea, were for many years referred to as 'cryptosporidium-like oocysts', 'cyanobacterium-like bodies' (bodies resembling blue-green algae), or even 'fungal spores', and it was not until 1992 that the exact nature of the cysts was established and the parasite named as *Cyclospora cayetanensis*.

Life cycle

Cyclospora species have been most extensively studied in nonhuman hosts, in which stages of development are typically intracytoplasmic in the epithelial cells of the small intestine. An exception is *C. talpae* of the mole *Talpa europaea*, which develops within the nucleus of the epithelial cells of the bile ducts and cells of the capillary sinusoids in the liver.

Asexual reproduction (merogony) (Fig. 8.6.1a) is followed by the production of female gametocytes (macrogamonts) (Figs. 8.6.1b–f) and male gametocytes (microgamonts) that produce a large number of flagellated gametes (Figs. 8.6.1g–j). Following fertilization of the female parasites, the zygotes develop a resistant membrane (Fig. 8.6.1k). The resulting oocysts are voided, unsporulated, in the host's faeces. The extracellular stages are illustrated in Figs. 8.6.2.

During periods varying from a few days to 1 or 2 weeks, depending on the species of *Cyclospora* and the temperature of the contaminated environment, the zygote within the oocyst (Fig. 8.6.3a) undergoes division to produce two sporoblasts (Fig. 8.6.3b), each of which develops a resistant membrane, the sporocyst (Fig. 8.6.3c). Division of each sporoblast then gives rise to two elongate sporozoites, leaving a conspicuous residual body (Figs. 8.6.2b and 8.6.3c). The sporozoites are the stages that infect further animals of the same species when oocysts are ingested with contaminated food or water.

Epidemiology

Failure to experimentally infect a variety of animals or to detect *C. cayetanensis* in those living in or near houses with human infection has led to the conclusion that humans are the specific host of this coccidian and the sole source of its oocysts.

The parasite is globally distributed, although risk of infection is greatest in developing countries with low standards of hygiene where prevalence rates up to 40% (Peru) have been reported. It is particularly prevalent in Central America and southern Asia. Serious outbreaks of acute diarrhoea have been reported, however, among guests at social events in the United States of America and Canada, with the source of infection traced to imported raspberries from Guatemala. Another outbreak, in Germany, occurred among a group of 34 people who had eaten a salad of imported lettuce spiced with fresh leafy herbs. In other countries, oocysts of *C. cayetanensis* have been detected on green leafy vegetables, in sewage, and even in tap water. Transmission is most common when humans are exposed to cyclospora oocysts in faecally contaminated environmental water, food, or soil. Airborne and zoonotic transmission is suspected but not confirmed.

Clinical features

An acute, watery, and nonbloody diarrhoea is variously accompanied by abdominal pain, steatorrhoea, headache, fever, nausea, and general malaise. The diarrhoea may be persistent and last for several weeks. Asymptomatic infections are known to occur, notably in the indigenous population of developing countries.

Diagnosis

Diagnosis is dependent on the demonstration of oocysts of *C. cayetanensis* in the faeces by direct microscopic examination. Flotation methods, using saturated sugar or aqueous zinc sulphate solutions, are useful in concentrating the oocysts, which measure from 8.0 to 10.0 μm in diameter (average 8.6 μm).

The living oocysts are autofluorescent using ultraviolet illumination, which is useful for rapid diagnosis. In addition,

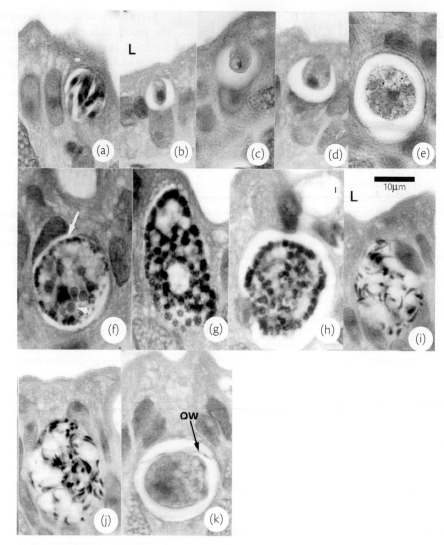

Fig. 8.6.1 Intracellular development in epithelial cells of the ileum (haematoxylin and eosin stained sections) in a typical life cycle of a *Cyclospora* species:(a) segmented meronts; (b–e) developing macrogamonts; (f) mature macrogamont with small wall-forming bodies (arrow) and large wall-forming bodies (arrowhead); (g, h) developing microgamonts; (i, j) mature microgamonts shedding microgametes; (k) intracellular zygote, with developing oocyst wall (OW). (From Lainson R (2004). The genus *Cyclospora* (Apicomplexa: Eimeriidae), with a description of *Cyclospora schneideri* n.sp. in the snake *Anilius scytale scytale* (Aniliidae) from Amazonian Brazil—a review. *Mem Inst Oswaldo Cruz*, **100**, 103–110, with permission).

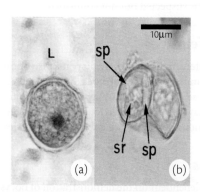

Fig. 8.6.2 Extracellular stages in a typical life cycle of a *Cyclospora*: (a) unsporulated oocyst in the intestinal lumen; (b) sporulated and ruptured oocyst in faeces. L, lumen; Sp, sporozoite; Sr, sporocystic residuum. Bar, 10 μm (all figures). (From Lainson R (2004). The genus *Cyclospora* (Apicomplexa: Eimeriidae), with a description of *Cyclospora schneideri* n.sp. in the snake *Anilius scytale scytale* (Aniliidae) from Amazonian Brazil—a review. *Mem Inst Oswaldo Cruz*, **100**, 103–110, with permission).

most diagnostic laboratories use a variety of staining methods to colour the oocysts in faecal smears fixed in 10% formalin: notably, modified Ziehl–Neelsen acid-fast staining, and safranin stain. These do not reveal details of the oocyst contents (Fig. 8.6.4), but their size and spherical shape readily distinguishes them from other coccidian oocysts or sporocysts that may be stained by the same methods. The polymerase chain reaction with primers specific for *C. cayetanensis* also affords a highly sensitive, but more costly, diagnostic technique.

There are four other intestinal coccidia that infect humans and may produce similar symptoms, but they are morphologically readily differentiated from *C. cayetanensis* when viewed unstained (Fig. 8.6.5). The oocysts of cryptosporidium, also an important cause of acute diarrhoea, are spherical but are only from 4.5 to 5.0 μm in diameter (half the size of *C. cayetanensis* oocysts) and they contain four naked sporozoites. *Isospora belli* oocysts are elongated, measure from 25 to 33 μm in length and from 12 to 16 μm in width, and have two sporocysts, each of which contains four sporozoites. Humans are the definite host of two species of *Sarcocystis*,

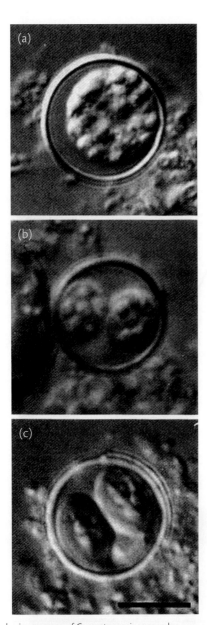

Fig. 8.6.3 Developing oocysts of *C. cayetanensis* as seen by Nomarski interference-contrast microscopy: (a) unsporulated oocyst; (b) formation of the two sporoblasts; (c) formation of the two sporocysts. Bar, 5 μm.
(From Ortega YR, Gilman RH, Sterling CR (1994). A new coccidian parasite (Apicomplexa: Eimeriidae) from humans. *J Parasitol*, **80**, 625–9, with permission).

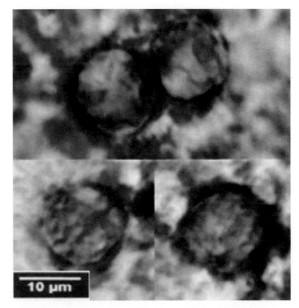

Fig. 8.6.4 Safranin-stained oocysts of *C. cayetanensis*. Bar, 10 μm.
(From Eberhard ML, Pieniazak NJ, Arrowood MJ (1997). Laboratory diagnosis of *Cyclospora* infections. *Arch Pathol Lab Med*, **121**, 792–7, with permission.)

the noncystic *Dientamoeba fragilis*, all of which commonly cause abdominal pain and diarrhoea.

Pathology

Histology of jejunal biopsies from patients with cyclosporiasis has shown blunting and widening of infected villi and an intense lymphocytic infiltration in the lamina propria and overlying epithelium (Fig. 8.6.6). There is a diffuse oedema, together with reactive hyperaemia and vascular dilation that is accompanied by congestion of the villous capillaries.

Treatment

Co-trimoxazole (960 mg two times daily for 1 week) has proved effective in eliminating the parasite in immunocompetent patients and has been shown successfully to control relapses in those with AIDS by the administration of 960 mg three times a week, indefinitely. Ciprofloxacin (500 mg two times daily for 1 week) is recommended for patients who react badly to sulphonamides.

Prevention

As with all other organisms dependent on faecal–oral transmission, simple precautions will help prevent infection with *C. cayetanensis*. Water should be boiled before drinking or when used to wash fruits (although these are best peeled) or green leafy vegetables that are to be eaten raw. These measures are not only important in the endemic areas of developing countries, but need to be taken when consuming fruit or vegetables that are imported from such regions, as seen with the serious outbreaks of cyclosporiasis in the United States of America due to unwashed raspberries imported from Guatemala.

S. hominis and *S. suihominis*: unlike *C. cayetanensis*, their oocysts undergo endogenous sporulation and contain two sporocysts, each containing four sporozoites. The oocysts are very fragile and usually rupture, so that only free sporocysts may be found in the faeces. These are easily differentiated from *C. cayetanensis* oocysts by their larger size (average 16 μm × 10.5 μm) and ellipsoidal shape.

A well-trained microscopist will have no difficulty in distinguishing other protozoa of the human intestine. Among these are the cystic stages of *Entamoeba histolytica* and *Giardia lamblia* and

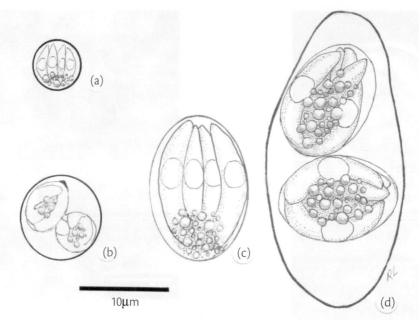

Fig. 8.6.5 Faecal stages of the five intestinal coccidia that infect humans: (a) oocyst of *Cryptosporidium parvum*, (b) oocyst of *Cyclospora cayetanensis*, (c) sporocyst of *Sarcocystis hominis* or *S. suihominis* (the two are morphologically indistinguishable), and (d) oocyst of *Isospora belli*. Bar, 10 μm.

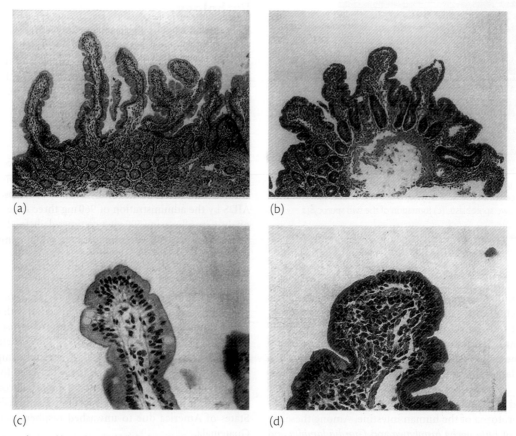

Fig. 8.6.6 Comparison of normal human jejunal villi (a,c) and villi infected with *C. cayetanensis* (b,d): low-power appearance (a,b) and high-power appearance (c,d). Note the blunting and widening of the villi, with inflammatory lymphocytic infiltrate in the lamina propria and infiltration of overlying epithelium.
(From Ortega YR, *et al.* (1997). Pathologic and clinical findings in patients with cyclosporiasis and a description of intracellular parasite life-cycle stages. *J Infect Dis*, **176**, 1584–9, with permission.)

Further reading

Ashford RW (1979). Occurrence of an undescribed coccidian in man in Papua New Guinea. *Ann Trop Med Parasitol*, **73**, 497–500.

Chacín-Bonilla L (2010). Epidemiology of Cyclospora cayetanensis: a review focusing in endemic areas. *Acta Trop*, **115**, 181–93.

Eberhard ML, Pieniazak NJ, Arrowood MJ (1997). Laboratory diagnosis of *Cyclospora* infections. *Arch Pathol Lab Med*, **121**, 792–7.

Lainson R (2005). The genus *Cyclospora* (Apicomplexa: Eimeriidae), with a description of *Cyclospora schneideri* n.sp. in the snake *Anilius scytale* scytale (Aniliidae) from Amazonian Brazil—a review. *Mem Inst Oswaldo Cruz*, **100**, 103–110.

McDonald V, Kelly MP (2005). Intestinal coccidia: cryptosporidiosis, isosporiasis, cyclosporiasis. In: Cox FEG, *et al.* (eds) *Topley & Wilson's Microbiology & Microbial Infections: Parasitology*, 10th edition, pp. 399–421. Hodder Arnold ASM Press, London.

Ortega YR, Sanchez R (2010). Update on Cyclospora cayetanensis, a food-borne and waterborne parasite. *Clin Microbiol Rev*, **23**, 218–34.

Ortega YR, *et al.* (1992). *Cyclospora cayetanensis*: a new protozoan pathogen of humans. Abstract 289 in Proceedings of the 41st Annual Meeting of the American Society of Tropical Medicine and Hygiene. *Am J Trop Med Hyg*, (Suppl), p. 210.

Ortega YR, Gilman RH, Sterling CR (1994). A new coccidian parasite (Apicomplexa: Eimeriidae) from humans. *J Parasitol*, **80**, 625–9.

Ortega YR, *et al.* (1997). Pathologic and clinical findings in patients with cyclosporiasis and a description of intracellular parasite life-cycle stages. *J Infect Dis*, **176**, 1584–9.

8.7 Sarcocystosis (sarcosporidiosis)

John E. Cooper

Essentials

Sarcocystosis is characterized by the invasion of muscles and sometimes other tissues by protozoa of the genus *Sarcocystis*, of which *S. hominis* (intermediate host domestic cattle) and *S. suihominis* (domestic pig) are the most significant to humans, to whom they are transmitted by ingestion of uncooked beef or pork. Humans serve as either intermediate or final host: (1) intermediate host—presence of cysts in muscle is usually asymptomatic, but may cause myositis or myopathy; detected on clinical examination or muscle biopsy; (2) final host—may be asymptomatic or cause fever and gastrointestinal upset; oocysts or sporocysts can be detected in faeces. There is no specific treatment. Prevention is by not eating uncooked meat from any animal.

Acknowledgement: I am most grateful to Dr Sarah Cooper for reading and commenting on an early draft of the text.

Introduction

Although often described as uncommon in humans, Sarcocystosis appears to be widespread but undetected. It has been reported from most continents but the exact distribution of the different species remains uncertain, largely on account of the absence of definitive clinical signs in many cases. In 2011, 9 travellers who had stayed on Tioman island (east coast of west Malaysia) presented in Germany 4 to 41 days later with fever, pruritus, myalgia, fatigue, nausea, and headache. Laboratory abnormalities included eosinophilia (15 to 20%) and mildly elevated serum creatine kinase concentrations. Muscle biopsies demonstrated sarcocystis-like bradyzoites. The epizootiology of this possible outbreak has not yet been discovered (GeoSentinel). Over the past decade, veterinary studies, especially serological surveys, have indicated that *Sarcocystis* species are present in a wide range of domesticated and wild mammals and other animals, often at a high prevalence (Fig. 8.7.1). Snakes and their rodent prey are definitive and intermediate hosts for many species of *Sarcocystis*; there is evidence of coevolution of the parasites with their vertebrate hosts. Equine protozoal myeloencephalitis, a disease of domestic horses due to *S. neurona*, has prompted a considerable body of research on *Sarcocystis* in recent years because of its great economic importance.

Sarcocystosis presents both actual and perceived public health problems. Some species, such as *S. hominis* and *S. suihominis*, can

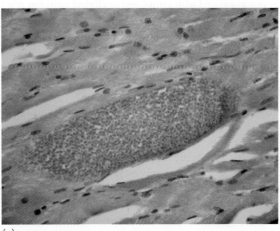

(a)

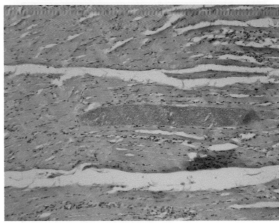

(b)

Fig. 8.7.1 *Sarcocystis* in skeletal muscle of a little penguin *Eudyptula minor* (haematoxylin and eosin).
(Courtesy of Dr Richard Norman.)

be transferred from animals to humans but others, while often causing alarm among those who encounter them, do not appear to be transmissible. For example, *S. rileyi*, which commonly affects ducks and geese in North America, presents with readily visible cream-coloured cysts generally running in parallel lines in the muscles of affected birds. This condition, often termed 'rice breast disease', is familiar to hunters and to those who skin waterfowl before they are cooked. Many affected carcasses are discarded, but meat containing the cysts presents no known hazard to people who eat it.

However, the role of host resistance in sarcocystosis has not been fully investigated and it is possible that immunosuppression may render humans susceptible to species of *Sarcocystis* that are primarily parasites of wild birds, reptiles, or mammals.

Clinical features

Humans as the final host

Depending on the species of parasite and the previous health of the host, infection in humans who have ingested meat containing cysts of *Sarcocystis* can have effects that range from gastrointestinal disorders and pyrexia to an asymptomatic state.

Humans as the intermediate host

The presence of cysts in human skeletal, visceral, or cardiac muscle is usually not associated with symptoms or clinical signs but it is likely that large numbers may, as in animals, cause myositis or myopathy, especially if calcification occurs, sometimes with vasculitis.

Diagnosis

Humans as the final host

Oocysts or sporocysts can be detected in faeces in smears (especially using Heine's method), in wet saline preparations, or, better, using a sodium chloride or sucrose flotation method (Fig. 8.7.2). The oocysts/sporocysts are usually readily recognized by an experienced parasitologist but can easily escape the attention of those who are less familiar with the organism. *Sarcocystis* must be distinguished from other sporozoal organisms that are either being produced in the intestine or are in transit in the lumen following ingestion.

Humans as the intermediate host

Occasionally, tissue cysts are detected during routine clinical examination, especially if calcification has occurred. They may also be seen in muscle biopsies, either as an incidental finding or because samples have been taken specifically for diagnostic purposes. Calcified cysts found in biopsies or located at autopsy have a gritty texture when cut.

Sarcocystosis of muscle (Figs. 8.7.1 and 8.7.3) must be differentiated from toxoplasmosis, in which tissue cysts can also be found. The morphology of the two protozoa differs. In particular, cysts of *Sarcocystis* have a distinct wall, which is thick and striated in some species, and do not stain with periodic acid–Schiff stain, which usually gives *Toxoplasma* cysts a magenta colour.

Treatment

There is no specific therapy for sarcocystosis in humans or animals, although albendazole has been reported to ameleriorate symptoms in a human patient with skeletal cysts and ponazuril has been shown to prevent infection of the central nervous system of mice experimentally given sporocysts of *S. neurona*. When humans are the final host, symptomatic and supportive treatment is indicated.

Prevention

Sarcocystosis can be prevented by not eating uncooked meat from any animal. Vaccines, at present experimental, have been shown to produce cellular immunity to certain *Sarcocystis* species in horses.

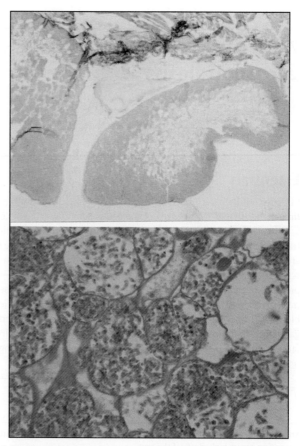

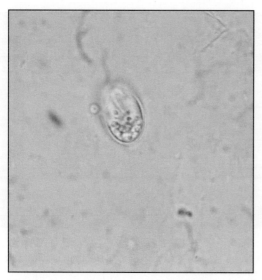

Fig. 8.7.2 Sporocyst containing sporozoites in faeces of a fox *Vulpes vulpes*. There are two within the oocyst when freshly passed but single sporocysts are often seen. (Courtesy of Dr John McGarry.)

Fig. 8.7.3 Cysts of bovine origin, containing crescent-shaped bradyzoites that are infective in the definitive host. (Courtesy of Dr John McGarry.)

Further reading

Arness MK, et al. (1999). An outbreak of acute eosinophilic myositis attributed to human Sarcocystis parasitism. Am J Trop Med Hyg, **61**, 548–53.

Bunyaratvej S, Bunyawongwiroj P, Nitiyanant P (1982). Human intestinal sarcosporidiosis: report of six cases. Am J Trop Med Hyg, **31**, 36–41.

Dangoudoubiyam S, Oliveira JB, Víquez C, et al. (2011). Detection of antibodies against Sarcocystis neurona, Neospora spp and Toxoplasma gondii in horses from Costa Rica. Journal of Parasitology, **97**(3), 522–4.

Fayer R (2004). Sarcocystis spp. in human infections. Clin Microbiol Rev, **17**, 894–902.

Houk AE, Goodwin DG, Zajac AM, et al. (2010). Prevalence of antibodies to Trypanosoma cruzi, Toxoplasma gondii, Encephalitozoon cuniculi, Sarcocystis neurona, Besnoitia darlingi, and Neospora caninum in North American opossums, Didelphis virginiana, from Southern Louisiana. J. Parasitol, **96**(6), 1119–22.

Marsh AE, et al. (2004). Evaluation of immune responses in horses immunized using a killed Sarcocystis neurona vaccine. Vet Ther, **5**, 34–42.

Mehrotra R, et al. (1996). Diagnosis of human Sarcocystis infection from biopsies of the skeletal muscle. Pathology, **28**, 281–2.

Olias P, Gruber AD, Kohls A, et al. (2010). Sarcocystis species lethal for domestic pigeons. Emerg Infect Dis., **16**(3), 497–9.

Slapeta JR, et al. (2003). Evolutionary relationships among cyst-forming coccidia Sarcocystis spp. (Alveolata: Apicomplexa: Coccidea) in endemic African tree vipers and perspective for evolution of heteroxenous life cycle. Mol Phylogenet Evol, **27**, 464–75.

Tian M, Chen Y, Wu L, Rosenthal BM, et al. (2011). Phylogenetic analysis of Sarcocystis nesbitti (Coccidia: Sarcocystidae) suggests a snake as its probable definitive host. Available online 28 July 2011. Journal of Veterinary Parasitology (doi:10.1016/j.vetpar.2011.07).

Velásquez JN, et al. (2008). Systemic sarcocystosis in a patient with acquired immune deficiency syndrome. Hum Pathol, **39**, 1263–7.

Wong KT, Pathmanathan R (1992). High prevalence of human skeletal muscle sarcocystosis in south-east Asia. Trans R Soc Trop Med Hyg, **86**, 631–2.

Wünschmann A, Rejmanek D, Conrad PA, et al. (2010). Natural fatal Sarcocystis falcatula infections in free-ranging eagles in North America. Journal of Veterinary Diagnostic Investigation, **22**(2), 282–9.

Zaman V, Colley FC (1975). Light and electron microscopic observations of the life cycle of Sarcocystis orientalis sp. n. in the rat (Rattus norvegicus) and the Malaysian reticulated python (Python reticulatus). Z Parasitenkd, **47**, 169–85.

8.8 Giardiasis, balantidiasis, isosporiasis, and microsporidiosis

Martin F. Heyworth

Essentials

Giardiasis

Infection with Giardia intestinalis, a flagellate protozoan that colonizes the lumen of the small intestine, is acquired by ingesting environmentally resistant cysts of the parasite, typically in water or food. Strains of the parasite that can potentially infect humans are harboured by various mammals, including domestic dogs and cattle.

Clinical features—manifestations include watery diarrhoea, abdominal discomfort and distension, weight loss, and malabsorption, with the infection typically being persistent and severe in individuals with genetic impairment of antibody production. G. intestinalis infection can lead to impairment of growth, and possibly of intellectual development, in children.

Diagnosis and treatment—diagnosis is by faecal examination for evidence of G. intestinalis infection, including (1) parasite antigen—by enzyme-linked immunosorbent assay (ELISA); (2) cysts—by microscopy (a historic approach that lacks sensitivity); or (3) parasite DNA—by polymerase chain reaction (PCR) amplification. Aside from supportive care, treatment is with metronidazole (although the parasite is becoming increasingly resistant), tinidazole and nitazoxanide.

Prevention—cysts of G. intestinalis in water can be killed by boiling or removed by filtration.

Balantidiasis

Balantidium coli is a ciliate protozoan that invades the colonic mucosa. Infection—which may or may not be acquired from pigs or other animals—may be asymptomatic or cause diarrhoea that can be watery or contain blood and mucus. Perforation of the colon can occur, leading to peritonitis, and the parasite can also spread to the liver and lungs. Diagnosis is by recognition of the parasite on microscopic examination of diarrhoeal stools, colonic mucus, or rectal biopsies. Aside from supportive care, treatment with metronidazole or tetracycline has reportedly eradicated infection in some instances. Prevention is by filtration or boiling of drinking-water, hand washing before handling food, and careful cleaning and cooking of food.

Isosporiasis

Cystoisospora belli is a coccidian protozoan that colonizes epithelial cells of the small intestine. Infection is presumed to occur by ingestion of parasite oocysts in water or food, but vehicles for transmission to humans are unknown, although the organism has been found on cockroaches. Clinical features include watery diarrhoea, dehydration, fever, and weight loss, with isosporiasis being an opportunistic infection associated with HIV infection. Diagnosis is by microscopic examination of faecal specimens for oocysts of C. belli, which show blue autofluorescence under ultraviolet light. Aside from supportive care, trimethoprim–sulphamethoxazole is partially effective.

Microsporidiosis

Microsporidia are minute intracellular parasites, now regarded as fungi which infect various animals and birds. About a dozen species can cause human infection (some only rarely). In at least some cases, microsporidiosis appears to be acquired by ingestion of spores of the causative organism(s) in water.

Clinical manifestations are most frequently reported in HIV-infected patients, and include diarrhoea ascribed to colonization of the small intestinal mucosa by Enterocytozoon bieneusi or Encephalitozoon intestinalis. Other manifestations of microsporidial infection include acalculous cholecystitis, sinusitis, cough/dyspnoea, urethritis, and keratitis.

Diagnosis, treatment, and prevention—intestinal microsporidiosis is diagnosed by microscopic examination of faecal specimens (after appropriate staining) for microsporidian spores, or by detection of microsporidian DNA in faecal specimens. Aside from supportive care, albendazole is an effective drug for treating Encephalitozoon infections, although Ent. bieneusi does not respond. In HIV-infected patients, remission of Ent. bieneusi infection can be achieved by antiretroviral drug treatment that reduces the HIV load. Prevention can be achieved by killing spores in water by boiling or exposure to ultraviolet light.

Introduction

The organisms that cause the diseases covered in this chapter are not closely related to each other. Of these infections, the first three are caused by protozoa: giardiasis by a flagellate, balantidiasis by a ciliate, and isosporiasis by a coccidian. The term 'microsporidiosis' encompasses a group of infections caused by approximately a dozen species of minute parasites (microsporidia) that are now classified as fungi.

Transmission of the organisms covered in this chapter mainly occurs by drinking or eating water or food containing environmentally resistant life-cycle stages of the parasites. Two of the diseases, isosporiasis and, particularly, microsporidiosis, have become more widely recognized since the start of the HIV/AIDS pandemic in the early 1980s and are included among the opportunistic infections seen in patients with AIDS. The four diseases occur worldwide; although most published reports of balantidiasis and isosporiasis are from tropical countries, these two diseases also occur in nontropical locations.

Historical perspective

Before the 1990s, literature on human giardiasis emphasized a relationship between drinking unfiltered water in wilderness areas and acquiring this infection, as well as occurrence of giardia species in beavers and muskrats. Although it is possible that faeces from these animals were sources of *G. intestinalis* cysts that could infect human subjects, it is also possible that cysts of human origin could have infected the amphibious mammals. The range of hosts for organisms morphologically classifiable as *G. intestinalis* is wide (birds and various terrestrial and marine mammals). *G. intestinalis* organisms have been divided into eight assemblages (designated A–H), on the basis of their DNA sequences. Assemblages A and B cause human infection; the other assemblages infect nonhuman hosts. Besides human subjects, hosts for assemblages A and B include domestic pets (dogs and cats) and livestock (cattle, sheep, and pigs). Proving that an assemblage A or B organism from a nonhuman host can cause human infection is difficult; although giardiasis is classified as a zoonosis, evidence of animal-to-human (and vice versa) transmission is largely circumstantial. In this chapter, the terms 'assemblage' and 'genotype', as applied to *G. intestinalis*, are used interchangeably.

Historically, balantidiasis and isosporiasis were recognized sufficiently rarely that they were the subjects of anecdotal case reports. This apparent rarity made it difficult to perform clinical trials to identify drugs useful for treating these diseases. In the 1980s, however, such a trial established the utility of co-trimoxazole in treating isosporiasis.

Before the HIV/AIDS pandemic, most of the literature on microsporidian infections dealt with such infections in nonhuman hosts (e.g. silk moths, honeybees, fish, and rabbits). The burgeoning literature on human microsporidiosis in HIV-infected individuals was complemented by increased awareness of microsporidia that typically infect immunocompetent people, notably organisms that cause keratitis.

Because they lack mitochondria and some other features of 'higher' eukaryotic (nucleated) cells, giardia and microsporidia were formerly considered to be primitive. Following the discovery in these organisms of gene sequences homologous with mitochondrial DNA and of organelles (mitosomes) that appear to be derived from mitochondria, the organisms are now regarded as highly specialized rather than primitive. The apparently primitive features are almost certainly adaptations to the parasitic lifestyle, reflecting the colonization of an anaerobic niche (vertebrate intestinal lumen) by giardia species and of host intracellular environments by microsporidia.

Giardiasis

Aetiology, pathogenesis, and pathology

G. intestinalis (synonyms *G. lamblia* and *G. duodenalis*) colonizes the lumen of the small intestine. The parasite's life cycle comprises two stages: motile trophozoites (Fig. 8.8.1) and thick-walled ellipsoidal cysts that are excreted in the faeces. *G. intestinalis* trophozoites are dorsoventrally flattened organisms with eight flagella, two nuclei, and a ventral adhesive disc that enables them to become attached to the luminal surface of intestinal epithelial cells. Trophozoites absorb nutrients in the small intestinal lumen and multiply in this environment. New hosts become infected by ingesting *G. intestinalis* cysts; exposure of cysts to gastric acid leads to emergence of trophozoites from the cysts. Trophozoites encyst in the intestinal lumen and the resulting cysts are excreted from the host. The environmentally resistant cyst wall consists of protein and a polymer of *N*-acetylgalactosamine.

The mechanisms responsible for diarrhoea and malabsorption in giardiasis are partially understood. Shortening of microvilli on the luminal surface of intestinal epithelial cells has been observed in small intestinal biopsies from patients with giardiasis. Reduced activity of intestinal disaccharidases has been reported in giardia-infected human subjects and rodents. This functional enzyme deficiency might lead to osmotic diarrhoea (via the presence of undigested disaccharides in the intestinal lumen).

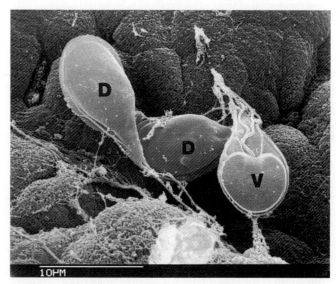

Fig. 8.8.1 Scanning electron micrograph of three *Giardia intestinalis* trophozoites on a jejunal biopsy specimen from a patient with giardiasis.
The dorsal surfaces of two trophozoites are visible (D), and the ventral adhesive disc of the other trophozoite is shown (V).
(Courtesy of Dr Robert L. Owen; modified from Carlson JR, Heyworth MF, Owen RL (1984). Giardiasis: Immunology, diagnosis and treatment. *Survey of Digestive Diseases*, **2**, 210–23, with permission.)

Study of immunity against giardia species has been more feasible in rodents than in human subjects. In mice, clearance of giardia infection appears to be dependent on CD4+ (helper) T lymphocytes and to follow the generation of an intestinal IgA response against the parasite. Genetically altered knock-out mice that are unable to produce intestinal IgA have an impaired ability to clear giardia infection. In human volunteers who were deliberately infected with *G. intestinalis*, an intestinal IgA response to the parasite occurred. IgA directed against trophozoites binds to these organisms and may, conceivably, inhibit their attachment to the intestinal epithelium, such that they are susceptible to peristaltic expulsion from the host. Giardia infection in mice and in human subjects leads to intestinal hypermotility, which may promote clearance of the parasite.

Epidemiology

G. intestinalis infection is acquired by drinking water that contains cysts. Other modes of spread include faecal–oral transmission of cysts, as in day-care centres for small children, and foodborne transmission of cysts. Waterborne giardiasis occurs as a result of drinking unfiltered, unboiled water from streams and lakes containing *G. intestinalis* cysts. Swimming in (and inadvertently drinking) water in lakes and rivers containing the cysts is also a risk factor for giardiasis. Outbreaks of this infection have resulted from the unintended presence of *G. intestinalis* cysts in public drinking water supplies and in swimming pools. Giardiasis is one of several parasitic and bacterial diseases that are potentially or actually transmitted by eating raw vegetables grown on fields irrigated or contaminated with untreated human sewage or animal manure. Aquatic molluscs, such as mussels grown commercially in estuarine water, concentrate particulate materials (including giardia cysts) from water by filter feeding, thus posing a potential infection hazard to human subjects who eat the molluscs raw.

From the 1990s onwards, there have been numerous comparisons of genome sequences of *G. intestinalis* isolated from human and nonhuman hosts. Close similarity between DNA sequences of *G. intestinalis* from different host species suggests, rather than proves, interspecies transmissibility of the parasite.

Genotyping of *G. intestinalis* organisms has revealed genetic similarity between giardia isolates from people and from dogs occupying the same households in India, a finding that suggests transmission of *G. intestinalis* between dogs and people. Approximately 10% of giardia isolates from cattle belong to genotypes that can potentially cause human infection. Flies that feed on garbage and sewage are able to carry giardia cysts on their exoskeletons and in their alimentary tracts and may therefore contaminate human food with viable cysts.

Immunodeficiency predisposes to the occurrence of severe and persistent giardiasis. Human immunodeficiency states that are associated with giardiasis include conditions that impair host antibody responses, notably 'common variable' hypogammaglobulinaemia and X-linked immunoglobulin deficiency. Impairment of intestinal IgA production is a feature of these particular immunodeficiency diseases and may explain how they predispose to chronic giardiasis (via impaired production of antitrophozoite IgA).

Prevention

G. intestinalis cysts can be removed from water by filtration, for example using membrane filters with a pore diameter of less than 5 μm. Cysts in water are killed by boiling. Exposure of water to ultraviolet light can inactivate giardia cysts and other organisms in the water. Water intended for human consumption can be screened for *G. intestinalis* cysts by exposure to magnetic beads coated with an antibody directed against cyst antigens (to capture cysts from suspension) followed by immunofluorescence microscopy using a fluorescent antibody to detect any cysts, or polymerase chain reaction (PCR) testing to detect *G. intestinalis* DNA. Viable and dead cysts retrieved from water can be distinguished by staining with fluorescent dyes that selectively stain living or dead cysts, respectively.

If domestic pets and farm animals are sources of human giardiasis (a likely, though not rigorously proven, scenario), avoidance of unhygienic interactions with these animals would help to avoid interspecies transmission of *G. intestinalis*.

Clinical features

Giardia infection can be asymptomatic (as shown by cyst excretion in the absence of symptoms) and also causes various clinical problems. These include abdominal discomfort, tenderness, and distension, a sensation of fullness, nausea, anorexia, and watery diarrhoea. Other clinical features include heartburn, flatulence, steatorrhoea, and weight loss. In immunologically normal persons, untreated giardiasis typically lasts for several weeks, with symptoms that fluctuate in severity. Clinical sequelae that have occasionally been reported include megaloblastic anaemia resulting from impaired absorption of vitamin B_{12} or folic acid, and postgiardiasis irritable bowel syndrome. *G. intestinalis* infection can lead to growth impairment, and possibly impaired cognitive development, in children. This aspect of giardiasis has been described particularly in resource-limited tropical environments.

Laboratory diagnosis

The traditional approach to diagnosing giardiasis (faecal light microscopy to detect *G. intestinalis* cysts) is subjective and insensitive. Sensitivity can be increased by using immunofluorescence microscopy, although this is (also) a labour-intensive and subjective approach. ELISA for faecal *G. intestinalis* antigen(s) is an objective method that is more sensitive than traditional light microscopic examination for cysts. Though currently more a research tool than a reality in clinical diagnostic laboratories, it is likely that PCR testing to diagnose giardiasis (by detection of *G. intestinalis* DNA) will be routinely available within a few years. A PCR diagnostic platform that simultaneously detects DNA of several human parasites (including *G. intestinalis*) in faecal material has been described.

Treatment

Table 8.8.1 summarizes various drug regimens for treating giardiasis. Metronidazole resistance of *G. intestinalis* is increasingly recognized and has prompted a continuing search for alternative therapeutic agents. In recent years, nitazoxanide has been introduced for treating giardiasis.

Methods to develop new drugs for treating giardiasis include (1) modifying the structure of a historically effective drug, such as metronidazole, by attaching 'novel' side chains to the nucleus of the drug molecule, and testing the resulting compounds for antitrophozoite activity; (2) designing inhibitor molecules for enzymes (and processes) that are features of giardia species, though not of human cells, e.g. arginine deiminase (and cyst formation);

Table 8.8.1 Various drug regimens for treating giardiasis

Drug	Dose	Treatment duration
Metronidazole	250 mg, three times daily (adult)	5 days
	15 mg/kg body wt per day, in 3 doses (paediatric)	5 days
Albendazole	400 mg daily	5 days
Tinidazole	2 g (adult)	Single dose
	50 mg/kg (paediatric)	Single dose (2 g maximum)
Ornidazole	2 g (adult)	Single dose
Furazolidone	100 mg, four times daily (adult)	7–10 days
	6 mg/kg per day, in 4 doses (paediatric)	7–10 days
Quinacrine	100 mg, three times daily	5 days
Nitazoxanide	500 mg, twice daily (adult)	3 days
	100 mg, twice daily (age 1–3 years)	3 days
	200 mg, twice daily (age 4–11 years)	3 days

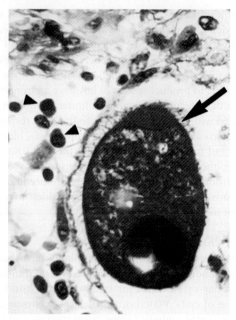

Fig. 8.8.2 Light micrograph of *Balantidium coli* trophozoite (arrow) in colonic tissue (×705). Cilia are visible on the surface of the organism. Arrowheads indicate tissue plasma cells.
(Modified from Neafie RC (1976). Balantidiasis. In: Binford CH, Connor DH (eds) *Pathology of tropical and extraordinary diseases*, vol. 1, pp. 325–7. Armed Forces Institute of Pathology, Washington DC, with permission.)

(3) empirical testing of other drugs and/or plant products for antitrophozoite activity. Efficient testing of such activity involves high-throughput automated in vitro systems, such as multiwell microtitre plates containing cultured trophozoites, and screening for the ability of candidate drugs to kill these organisms. Clinical trials of drugs that show promise during in vitro testing may then be warranted, in human subjects with giardiasis. Polyphenols extracted from various berries (including strawberries, blackberries, and cloudberries) are toxic to *G. intestinalis* trophozoites when incubated with the organisms at concentrations of the polyphenols that would be achievable by oral administration to human subjects. 'Probiotic' bacteria of the genus *Lactobacillus* reduce the intensity and/or duration of giardia infection in mice and in gerbils.

Balantidiasis

Aetiology, pathogenesis, and pathology

Balantidium coli, the cause of balantidiasis, is the largest protozoan parasite of man. *B. coli* has a two-stage life cycle comprising motile trophozoites that invade the colonic mucosa (Fig. 8.8.2) and non-motile cysts. Spread of the infection to new hosts occurs by ingestion of the parasite. *B. coli* trophozoites invade and cause ulceration of the colonic mucosa. The mechanisms responsible for tissue invasion by these organisms are not known.

Epidemiology

There is circumstantial evidence that humans can acquire *B. coli* infection from animals. This infection has been described in pigs and in many species of nonhuman primates. A high prevalence of the infection has been seen in human communities that live in close proximity to *B. coli*-infected pigs (e.g. in New Guinea). Consequently, there has been speculation that pigs are a reservoir for spread of *B. coli* to humans. Balantidiasis has also occurred in human subjects who had no known contact with pigs or other animals. Clusters of cases of balantidiasis have been seen in long-stay psychiatric hospitals. In India, *B. coli* cysts have been found in

water available for either drinking or use in cooking, and cysts of the organism have been found on cockroaches in Nigeria.

Clinical features

Human subjects with *B. coli* infection can be asymptomatic or can develop diarrhoea with stools that are either watery or that consist of blood and mucus. In severe *B. coli* infection, patients can develop colonic perforation, peritonitis, gangrene of the appendix (resulting from the presence of *B. coli* in the appendiceal wall), and spread of the parasite to the liver or lungs. Balantidiasis is a rare cause of liver abscess and of pulmonary haemorrhage. As is evident from the clinical features outlined above, balantidiasis may be clinically indistinguishable from amoebiasis, bacillary dysentery, ulcerative colitis, and Crohn's disease, and can be fatal. *B. coli* infection in the lungs has been described in occasional patients with concurrent malignant disease (including chronic lymphocytic leukaemia).

Laboratory diagnosis

Balantidiasis can be diagnosed by microscopic examination of diarrhoeal stools or colonic mucus obtained at sigmoidoscopy. Examination may show motile trophozoites or, less frequently, cysts of *B. coli*. Histological examination of rectal biopsies may reveal *B. coli* trophozoites. Pulmonary balantidiasis can be diagnosed by bronchoalveolar lavage and finding the parasite in the lavage fluid.

Prevention and treatment

Prevention of balantidiasis involves avoidance of *B. coli* cyst ingestion, via filtration or boiling of drinking-water, hand washing before handling food, and careful cleaning and cooking of food.

Patients with balantidiasis have been treated empirically with various antimicrobial drugs. There is, however, little interpretable information about the effectiveness of such treatment, although eradication of *B. coli* has been reported in some individuals treated with metronidazole or tetracycline. Surgical intervention may be necessary in patients with liver abscess or clinical evidence of appendicitis or colonic perforation.

Isosporiasis

Aetiology, pathogenesis, and pathology

The organism that causes isosporiasis was formerly known as *Isospora belli*. Organisms formerly included in the genus *Isospora* that are parasitic to mammals have now been assigned to the genus *Cystoisospora* (the generic name *Isospora* has been retained for avian parasites). *Cystoisospora belli* is a parasite of the human small intestine. There is limited evidence that *C. belli* infects nonhuman hosts: oocysts of *C. belli* have been isolated from dog faeces in India and the parasite has been transmitted experimentally to gibbons.

C. belli oocysts are ellipsoidal structures that are excreted in the faeces of infected individuals (Fig. 8.8.3). Studies of cystoisospora species that parasitize nonhuman hosts indicate that infection occurs via ingestion of oocysts and that sporozoites (which emerge from oocysts) penetrate epithelial cells of the small intestine. Subsequent development of cystoisospora species comprises: (1) an asexual pathway, with production of merozoites, which can infect additional epithelial cells; and (2) a sexual pathway, in which fusion of gametes produces oocysts that are excreted from the host.

Mechanisms responsible for the watery diarrhoea that occurs in isosporiasis are unknown. Presumably, the parasitization of epithelial cells in the small intestine contributes to the diarrhoea.

Epidemiology

C. belli infection has been documented in immunosuppressed and, rarely, in immunocompetent individuals. Among 397 HIV-infected patients in Venezuela, 56 (14%) were found to have *C. belli* infection (as judged by the presence of oocysts in faecal specimens). Of these 56 patients with *C. belli* infection, 98% had diarrhoea. Vehicles for transmission of *C. belli* oocysts to human subjects have not been identified, but presumably include water and food. Oocysts of this parasite are among the human pathogens found on

cockroaches in Nigeria. *C. belli* infection appears to be an occasional cause of travellers' diarrhoea.

Clinical features

In patients infected with HIV, *C. belli* infection is associated with chronic watery diarrhoea, abdominal cramps, nausea, fever, and weight loss. Severe dehydration can result from diarrhoea attributable to *C. belli* infection in HIV-infected patients. In immunocompetent individuals, symptoms ascribed to isosporiasis are similar to those that occur in AIDS-associated *C. belli* infection. Isosporiasis has been described in a few patients with haematological malignancy (including Hodgkin's disease, non-Hodgkin's lymphoma, and adult T-cell leukaemia), in whom immunosuppression was presumably a risk factor for *C. belli* infection.

Rarely, extraintestinal *C. belli* infection has been described in patients with AIDS; in the relevant patients, tissues parasitized by *C. belli* have included gallbladder epithelium, liver, spleen, and mesenteric lymph nodes.

Laboratory diagnosis

Isosporiasis can be diagnosed by microscopic examination of faecal specimens for *C. belli* oocysts. Although these structures are relatively large (*c.*20 to 30 μm in length), they are translucent and may be difficult to see in unstained samples. Their visibility is increased by incubation with carbol fuchsin, which stains oocyst internal structures red, or by incubation with lactophenol cotton blue. An alternative approach is to examine faecal smears under ultraviolet light; with this type of illumination, *C. belli* oocysts show blue autofluorescence.

Treatment and prognosis

The efficacy of oral co-trimoxazole in treating *C. belli*-induced diarrhoea was demonstrated in a study of patients with AIDS and isosporiasis in Haiti. Recognition of adverse drug reactions to co-trimoxazole, and less than 100% efficacy of this drug combination in treating isosporiasis, have prompted alternative therapeutic approaches. Diclazuril, albendazole–ornidazole, and pyrimethamine–sulphadiazine are three such alternatives that have shown anecdotal promise in treating isosporiasis associated with HIV infection.

In immunocompetent patients without HIV infection, isosporiasis can persist for weeks or months if untreated. The overall prognosis in patients with isosporiasis and HIV infection is determined by the HIV infection.

Microsporidiosis

Aetiology, pathogenesis, and pathology

Microsporidia are obligate intracellular parasites, whose lifecycle comprises an extracellular stage (spore) and stages that occur in host cells. Spores (Fig. 8.8.4) are shed into the environment by infected hosts and infect other members of the host species. The spores induce infection by high velocity extrusion of a hollow tube that penetrates a host cell and forms a channel for delivering sporoplasm (spore contents) into this cell. Replication of the parasite and subsequent production of spores occur in host cells. Some species of microsporidia invade and survive in macrophages and can become anatomically disseminated within the host in these mobile

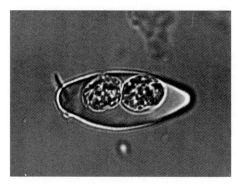

Fig. 8.8.3 Light micrograph of a *Cystoisospora belli* oocyst (×2500).
(Courtesy of Dr William L. Current. From Garcia LS (2001). *Diagnostic medical parasitology*, 4th edition. ASM Press, Washington DC, with permission.)

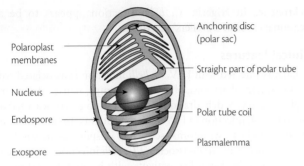

Fig. 8.8.4 Diagram of a microsporidian spore, showing internal structure. (Courtesy of Professor Elizabeth U. Canning. Modified from Canning EU, Hollister WS (1992). Human infections with microsporidia. *Rev Med Microbiol*, **3**, 35–42, with permission.)

cells. Microsporidia have a small genome (e.g. 2.9×10^6 bp in the case of *Enceph. cuniculi*).

In HIV-infected patients, diarrhoea is the clinical feature that has been most frequently associated with microsporidiosis. In particular, this symptom has been historically ascribed to infection with *Ent. bieneusi* and with *Enceph. intestinalis*. The diarrhoea reported in these microsporidian infections possibly results from the presence of microsporidia in the small intestinal mucosa. As discussed below, however, a causal role has not been unambiguously established for intestinal microsporidiosis in diarrhoea that is associated with HIV infection. Microsporidian parasitization of the intestinal mucosa can be seen on microscopic examination of biopsy specimens (Fig. 8.8.5).

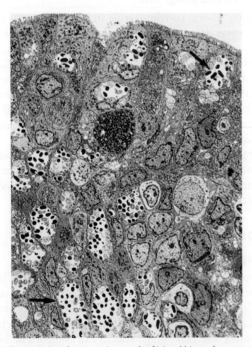

Fig. 8.8.5 Transmission electron micrograph of jejunal biopsy from a patient with AIDS and *Encephalitozoon intestinalis* infection. The microvillus border (epithelial surface) is at the top of the photograph. Epithelial cells and lamina propria leukocytes are heavily infected with *Enceph. intestinalis* (arrows). (Courtesy of the Electron Microscopy and Histopathology Unit, London School of Hygiene and Tropical Medicine. From Croft SL, Williams J, McGowan I (1997). Intestinal microsporidiosis. *Semin Gastrointest Dis* **8**, 45–55, with permission.)

Microsporidia that infect human subjects are listed in Table 8.8.2. Authenticated human infections with microsporidia other than *Ent. bieneusi*, *Enceph. intestinalis*, *Enceph. hellem*, and *Vittaforma corneae* are rare and some of the microsporidian species have been found in one or two patients only. 'Microsporidium' is a nontaxonomic genus created for microsporidia of unclear identity.

In mice at least, interferon-γ contributes to protective immunity against *Enceph. intestinalis* and *Enceph. cuniculi* infections.

Epidemiology

Most of the documented clinical experience with microsporidiosis has occurred in patients with HIV infection. Microsporidian infections have been described in immunosuppressed recipients of solid organ or bone marrow transplants.

Although intestinal microsporidiosis has been frequently documented in HIV-infected patients (e.g. by examination of intestinal biopsy specimens and by finding microsporidian spores in faecal material), such documentation does not prove that microsporidia cause HIV-related diarrhoea. In 31 HIV-infected patients with duodenal *Ent. bieneusi* infection, 18 had diarrhoea and 13 did not. Work in the Czech Republic has shown that intestinal

Table 8.8.2 Species of microsporidia that infect humans

Species	Reported sites of infection
Enterocytozoon bieneusi	Small intestinal epithelium, gallbladder epithelium, rarely in respiratory tract and maxillary sinus
Encephalitozoon (formerly *Septata*) *intestinalis*	Intestinal epithelium, gallbladder epithelium, paranasal sinuses, respiratory tract, liver, kidney, pituitary, conjunctiva. Colonizes macrophages
Encephalitozoon hellem	Corneal epithelium, respiratory tract, kidney, paranasal sinuses
Encephalitozoon cuniculi	Kidney, urinary bladder, duodenal mucosa, conjunctiva, respiratory tract, adrenal glands, brain, heart, spleen, lymph nodes, cerebrospinal fluid
Vittaforma corneae (formerly *Nosema corneum*)	Corneal stroma, urinary tract
Trachipleistophora hominis	Skeletal muscle, conjunctiva, corneal stroma, nasopharynx (washings)
Trachipleistophora anthropophthera	Brain, kidney, heart, pancreas, thyroid, parathyroid glands, liver, spleen, lymph nodes, bone marrow, cornea
Pleistophora ronneafiei	Skeletal muscle
Anncaliia algerae[a]	Skeletal muscle, skin, corneal stroma
Anncaliia vesicularum[a]	Skeletal muscle
Anncaliia connori[a]	Generalized
Tubulinosema sp.	Skeletal muscle
Nosema ocularum	Corneal stroma
'*Microsporidium ceylonensis*'	Corneal stroma
'*Microsporidium africanum*'	Corneal stroma

[a] Organisms in the genus *Anncaliia* were formerly designated by the generic names *Brachiola* and *Nosema*.

infection with *Ent. bieneusi* and *Encephalitozoon* species is common in HIV-negative, asymptomatic individuals. An outbreak of food-borne *Ent. bieneusi* infection (characterized by abdominal pain, nausea, and diarrhoea) occurred in Sweden in 2009.

Experimental work with animals suggests that human infection with some species of microsporidia occurs via ingestion of spores. Environmental sources of microsporidian spores that can infect human subjects include water and, possibly, nonhuman hosts. Spores of *Enceph. intestinalis* have been detected in river water in Spain and DNA of this species has been found in drinking-water in Guatemala by PCR testing. Risk factors for *Ent. bieneusi* infection, in a population of HIV-infected patients surveyed in France, included swimming in a pool in the 12 months before the survey. In rural Mexican households, faecal excretion of *Encephalitozoon* spores was associated with the use of unboiled water for drinking and for preparing food. Heavy parasitization of respiratory tract epithelial cells with *Enceph. hellem*, in at least one HIV-infected patient examined at autopsy, raises the possibility that some microsporidian infections can be acquired by inhaling spores.

Some species of microsporidia listed in Table 8.8.2 are known to infect nonhuman hosts: for example, DNA of three microsporidian species (*Ent. bieneusi*, *Enceph. intestinalis*, and *Enceph. hellem*) has been identified in faecal specimens from urban pigeons in Spain. Spores of *Enceph. intestinalis* have been identified in faecal specimens from nonhuman mammals (dogs, pigs, goats, cows, and donkeys). *Ent. bieneusi* can infect dogs, cats, pigs, goats, and cows. House mice in central Europe have been found to be infected with *Ent. bieneusi*, *Enceph. hellem*, and *Enceph. cuniculi*. At least two species of human pathogenic microsporidia, *Anncaliia algerae* and *Trachipleistophora hominis*, can infect mosquitoes, although it is not known whether mosquitoes can transmit these microsporidia to human subjects.

There has been speculation that microsporidiosis in immuno-deficient subjects might sometimes reflect (re)activation of micro-sporidian infection acquired before the onset of immunodeficiency, and meanwhile latent.

Prevention

Water can be screened for microsporidian spores by immunocapture of spores on magnetic beads coated with antispore antibody, followed by PCR to detect microsporidian DNA. Microsporidian spores in water can be killed by boiling or by exposure of water to ultraviolet light.

A gene chip method has been developed for detecting and discriminating between DNA of *Ent. bieneusi* and of all three *Encephalitozoon* species simultaneously. This method is potentially applicable to environmental screening of drinking-water samples and to diagnostic testing of clinical material, such as human faecal specimens, to look for evidence of microsporidian infection in a patient.

Given uncertainty about the clinical significance of intestinal microsporidian infections, it is doubtful whether efforts to remove microsporidian spores from drinking-water would be justified.

Clinical features

Clinical features of microsporidian infections reflect the anatomical site colonized by the microsporidia (Table 8.8.2). Besides watery diarrhoea, weight loss and fat malabsorption have been reported in HIV-infected patients with intestinal microsporidiosis. As noted above, however, the clinical significance of microsporidian infection of the intestine is uncertain. Microsporidian infection of the gallbladder has been described in occasional HIV-infected patients who had acalculous cholecystitis, who were treated by cholecystectomy. Symptoms of sinusitis, cough, and dyspnoea have been reported in patients with microsporidian infection of the paranasal sinuses and respiratory tract. Symptomatic urethritis has been ascribed to microsporidian infection in occasional HIV-infected patients. Pulmonary *Ent. bieneusi* infection, though rarely reported, has occurred in patients with HIV infection.

Microsporidian infection of the conjunctiva and corneal epithelium causes symptoms of keratoconjunctivitis (foreign body sensation in the eye, ocular discomfort and redness, photophobia, blurred vision, and sometimes reduced visual acuity). Microsporidian infections of the corneal stroma lead to reduced visual acuity, with or without corneal ulceration. Microsporidian keratitis, in individuals without HIV infection, has been recognized increasingly in Asia. Exposure to mud after recent rainfall appears to be a risk factor for this microsporidian eye infection. In India, *Vittaforma corneae* DNA has been demonstrated (by PCR testing) in corneal scrapings from patients with keratitis. In the present chapter, the terms 'keratitis' and 'keratoconjunctivitis' are used interchangeably. Clinical features in patients with actual or presumed cerebral microsporidiosis have included headache, cognitive impairment, nausea, vomiting, and epileptic seizures. Symptoms of myositis (muscle pain, tenderness, weakness, and wasting) have been described in patients with microsporidian infection of skeletal muscles.

Laboratory diagnosis

Intestinal infection with *Ent. bieneusi* or *Enceph. intestinalis* can be diagnosed by finding microsporidian spores in faecal samples, for example by microscopic examination after exposure to various stains. The spores (which are ovoid) can be detected by microscopy after incubation with crystal violet plus iodine and chromotrope 2R (leading to violet staining of the spores), with optical brighteners such as Uvitex 2B and Calcofluor White M2R (which bind to chitin in the spores, resulting in fluorescence), or with fluorescent antibodies directed against the spores. Spores of *Ent. bieneusi* are smaller ($c.1.5\,\mu m \times 0.9\,\mu m$) than those of *Enceph. intestinalis* ($c.2.5\,\mu m \times 1.5\,\mu m$).

Detection of microsporidian DNA in clinical specimens is a more sensitive *ex vivo* method than microscopy for diagnosing microsporidiosis.

Approaches to diagnosis of microsporidian keratitis include examining conjunctival/corneal scrapings or biopsies for spores and (noninvasively) *in vivo* examination of the cornea with a scanning confocal microscope to look for spore-filled epithelial cells.

Treatment and prognosis

Encephalitozoon infections can be treated with albendazole. In a small controlled trial, HIV-infected patients with *Enceph. intestinalis* infection were treated with albendazole (400 mg orally twice daily) or with placebo. Albendazole treatment led to clearance of gastrointestinal *Enceph. intestinalis* infection in this study. Uncontrolled trials and anecdotal case reports describe partial or complete resolution of symptoms (diarrhoea, sinusitis, and keratoconjunctivitis) in patients with *Enceph. intestinalis*, *Enceph. hellem*, or *Enceph. cuniculi* infection following albendazole treatment. Pregnancy is a contraindication to albendazole treatment. Albendazole is not an effective treatment for *Ent. bieneusi* infection.

In HIV-infected patients with *Ent. bieneusi* infection, remission of this microsporidian infection can be achieved by treatment of the HIV disease with combined antiretroviral therapy (cART). This treatment involves simultaneous administration of several drugs directed against HIV, including HIV protease inhibitors, and leads to restoration of immune competence, as evidenced by a raised CD4+ (helper/inducer) T-cell count and reduced HIV load. When effective in HIV-positive *Ent. bieneusi*-infected patients, cART leads to reduction of HIV load, elevation of the circulating CD4+ T-lymphocyte count, clearance of *Ent. bieneusi* infection, and cessation of diarrhoea. Fumagillin is active against *Ent. bieneusi* and *Encephalitozoon* species, although its clinical attractiveness for systemic administration is limited by toxicity to human subjects (manifested by thrombocytopenia and neutropenia).

Introduction of cART has influenced the natural history of HIV infection in those parts of the world where cART is available. The prevalence of AIDS-related microsporidiosis (e.g. intestinal infection with *Ent. bieneusi* and *Enceph. intestinalis*) has fallen since the introduction of cART has 'converted' HIV infection into a chronic condition in some countries. Maintenance of a relatively high CD4+ (helper/inducer) T-cell count (as a result of cART) protects against HIV-related microsporidiosis.

Successful treatment of microsporidial keratitis with fumagillin, or voriconazole, eye drops has been reported.

HIV-negative patients with microsporidian infection of the corneal stroma have been treated by corneal transplantation, with results that have ranged from failure (opacification of the transplant) to apparent success, as judged by transparency of the graft 6 months after transplantation.

Individual patients infected with *Trachipleistophora hominis* or *Anncaliia vesicularum* reportedly showed some clinical improvement after treatment with albendazole–sulphadiazine–pyrimethamine, or albendazole–itraconazole, respectively.

In HIV-infected patients with microsporidiosis, the overall prognosis is determined by the HIV infection.

Likely future developments

It is likely that the mechanisms by which anti-giardia antibodies protect against *G. intestinalis* infection will be understood during the next 10 years. Such understanding would include the molecular characterization of giardia target antigens that are recognized by protective antibody. Further clarification of the importance of domestic pets and agricultural livestock as sources for human giardiasis and microsporidiosis is likely by genotyping of morphologically identical parasites from human and nonhuman hosts. Selective survival and geographical spread of metronidazole-resistant *G. intestinalis* strains are predictable challenges to the effective treatment of giardiasis.

Further reading

Anonymous (2010). Drugs for parasitic infections. *Treatment Guidelines from The Medical Letter*, Vol. **8**(Suppl). [Survey of treatment options for parasitic diseases, including the infections discussed in this chapter.]

Didier ES, *et al.* (2005). Therapeutic strategies for human microsporidia infections. *Expert Rev Anti Infect Ther*, **3**, 419–34. [Review of drug treatment of microsporidiosis.]

Didier ES, Weiss LM (2011). Microsporidiosis: not just in AIDS patients. *Curr Opin Infect Dis*, **24**, 490–5. [Concise review of human microsporidiosis.]

Eckmann L (2003). Mucosal defences against *Giardia*. *Parasite Immunol*, **25**, 259–70. [Review of *Giardia* infections, with emphasis on host protective mechanisms against *Giardia* organisms.]

Feng Y, Xiao L (2011). Zoonotic potential and molecular epidemiology of *Giardia* species and giardiasis. *Clin Microbiol Rev*, **24**, 110–40. [Comprehensive review of genomic aspects and host range of giardia species.]

Field AS (2002). Light microscopic and electron microscopic diagnosis of gastrointestinal opportunistic infections in HIV-positive patients. *Pathology*, **34**, 21–35. [Review that includes photomicrographs of *Cystoisospora* (*Isospora*) *belli* and of microsporidia in human intestinal mucosa.]

House SA, *et al.* (2011). *Giardia* flagellar motility is not directly required to maintain attachment to surfaces. *PLOS Pathog*, **7**, e1002167. [Study of wild-type and genetically modified giardia trophozoites, to define mechanism of trophozoite attachment to surfaces. Online article includes links to video clips showing trophozoite movement and attachment *in vitro*.]

Lindsay DS, Dubey JP, Blagburn BL (1997). Biology of *Isospora* spp. from humans, nonhuman primates, and domestic animals. *Clin Microbial Rev*, **10**, 19–34. [Review of *Cystoisospora* (*Isospora*) species, including the human parasite *Cystoisospora* (*Isospora*) *belli*.]

Schuster FL, Ramirez-Avila L (2008). Current world status of Balantidium coli. *Clin Microbiol Rev*, **21**, 626–38. [Review of microbiological and clinical aspects of *Balantidium coli* infections.]

Sharma S, *et al.* (2011). Microsporidial keratitis: need for increased awareness. *Surv Ophthalmol*, **56**, 1–22. [Review of ocular microsporidiosis.]

Tejman-Yarden N, Eckmann L (2011). New approaches to the treatment of giardiasis. *Curr Opin Infect Dis*, **24**, 451–6. [Discussion of methods to develop new drugs for treating giardiasis.]

8.9 *Blastocystis hominis* infection

Richard Knight

Essentials

Blastocystis hominis is an anaerobic unicellular noninvasive colonic parasite of animals and humans. It is transmitted faeco-orally, with human infection associated with travel, institutions, animal handlers and immunodeficiency. Case reports strongly suggest that it causes a self-limited diarrhoeal illness. Diagnosis is by microscopic examination of faecal smears or concentrates. A trial of treatment with metronidazole is justified in patients who are immunocompromised, also when symptoms are prolonged.

Aetiology and biology of the parasite

Molecular and ribosomal RNA studies now indicate that *Blastocystis hominis* is a stramenopile (a synonym for kingdom Chromista). *Blastocysti* has no flagella, unlike other stramenopiles, which slime nets, water moulds, and brown algae. The form commonly described in faeces and also in cultures is spherical, from 4 to 15 μm in diameter, with one prominent central vacuole surrounded by peripheral cytoplasm (Fig. 8.9.1) that electron microscopy shows to contain a nucleus, a Golgi complex, and mitochondrion-like organelles (Fig. 8.9.2). It grows readily in cultures with mixed bacteria but axenic cultures can also be established; division is by binary fission. Transmission is by small, resistant, faecal cysts, from 3 to 8 μm in diameter. The basic life cycle alternates between the univacuolar and cystic stages. However electron microscopy of faeces and cultures may also show multivacuolar, granular, and amoeboid forms of uncertain significance. Bizarre environmentally induced forms with huge vacuoles may develop in cultures (Fig. 8.9.3). The common 'univacuolar' form was named *Blastocystis* by Brumpt in 1912 as a yeast, although it was first described by Alexieff in 1911 as a protozoan cyst.

Epidemiology

Prevalence may exceed 35% in some human populations associated with high faeco-oral transmission. This infection is associated with travel, institutions, animal handlers, and immunodeficiency. *Blastocystis* is genetically diverse and occurs in a wide range of domesticated and wild animals including invertebrates. Currently only one species, *B. hominis*, is recognized, but at least nine subtypes (genotypes) infect humans; important zoonotic sources are pigs, cattle, nonhuman primates, and birds, including chickens and ducks. Human-to-human transmission usually involves subtype 3. The resistant cysts can occur in both sewage influents and effluents.

Diagnosis

B. hominis is usually recognized as univacuolar forms in direct wet faecal smears or formol ether concentrates. Wet mounts can be stained with iodine, giving a brownish central body, or with toluidine blue. The organism is often numerous in symptomatic subjects. Permanent mounts stain well with trichrome. *Blastocystis* can

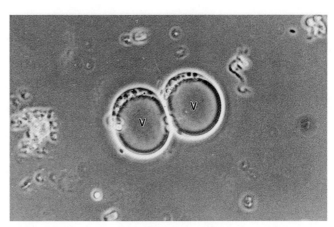

Fig. 8.9.1 *B. hominis* from culture showing binary fission; the cytoplasm is at the periphery. v, vacuole. Phase contrast, ×400.

resemble amoebic cysts but lack their characteristic nuclei. In fixed smears stained specifically for *Cryptosporidium*, there is no oocyst wall. Special techniques are used to concentrate and identify cysts in environmental samples. Inflammatory cells in faecal exudates or inflammation seen at endoscopy should promote search for an additional invasive pathogen.

Clinical features and treatment

A noninvasive diarrhoeal illness lasting from 3 to 10 days is attributed to this organism, sometimes symptoms continue for weeks or months. Associated features are abdominal bloating, flatulence, and anorexia. Symptoms are more prolonged in immunocompromised subjects. There is no definite association with irritable bowel syndrome or urticaria. Illnesses are self-limiting in most persons but infection and symptoms can usually be eliminated with metronidazole or tinidazole; the organism is also sensitive to cotrimoxazole, furazolidine, and hydroxyquinoline.

Blastocystis has been reported once in a liver abscess aspirate but the patient was later shown to have amoebiasis. Another patient with faecal blastocystis and rectocolitis responded rapidly to metronidazole but it appears that amoebiasis was not properly excluded.

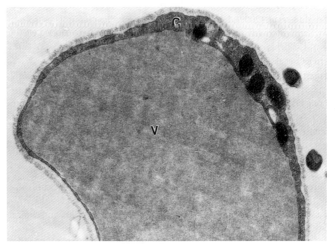

Fig. 8.9.2 *B. hominis*. Electron micrograph showing the peripheral cytoplasm (c) and the central vacuole (v); the inclusions in the cytoplasm are mitochondria. ×5000.

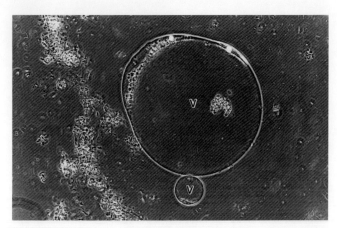

Fig. 8.9.3 *B. hominis* from culture showing the great variation in size. v, vacuole. Dark field, ×400.

Evidence for pathogenicity

Definite histopathology in humans is still lacking, although serum antibody has been reported in symptomatic subjects. A good laboratory animal model remains elusive; mice are not normal hosts for this parasite and pathology is not reported in any of its normal hosts. A convincing *in vitro* cytopathic model awaits discovery although cultured colonic epithelial cells release cytokines in the presence of blastocystis. Cysteine proteinase has been postulated as a virulence factor.

The genetic heterogeneity of blastocystis isolates correlates weakly with host species. In a recent human study, genotype determined by PCR, correlated with symptoms. Clinical response to metronidazole is hardly compelling evidence for pathogenicity since concurrent infection with other enteropathogens is common and this drug has a wide spectrum of activity including an effect upon small bowel bacterial overgrowth. More well-documented outbreaks and cytopathic evidence are needed.

Further reading

Chen Te-Li, *et al.* (2003). Clinical characteristics and endoscopic findings associated with *Blastocystis hominis* in healthy adults. *Am J Trop Med Hyg*, **69**, 213–16.

Eroglu F, *et al.* (2009). Identification of *Blastocystis hominis* isolates from asymptomatic and symptomatic patients by PCR. *Parasitol Res*, **105**, 1589–92.

Hu KC, et al. (2008). Amoebic liver abscess or is it? *Gut*, **57**, 627.

Janarthanan S, *et al.* (2011). An unusual case of invasive *Blastocystis hominis*. *Endoscopy*, **43**, E185–6.

Long HY, *et al.* (2006). *Blastocystis hominis* modulates immune responses and cytokine release in colonic epithelial cells. *Parasitol Res*, **87**, 1029–30.

Stensvold CR, *et al.* (2009). Pursuing the clinical significance of *Blastocystis*-diagnostic limitations. *Trends Parasitol*, **25**, 23–9.

Suresh K, Smith HV (2004). Comparison of methods for detecting *Blastocystis hominis*. *Eur J Clin Microbiol Infect Dis*, **23**, 509–11.

Suresh K, Smith HV, Tan TC (2005). Viable *Blastocystis* cysts in Scottish and Malaysian sewage samples. *Appl Environ Microbiol*, **71**, 5619–20.

Tan KSW (2008). New insights on classification, identification, and clinical relevance of *Blastocystis* spp. *Clin Microbiol Rev*, **21**, 639–65.

8.10 Human African trypanosomiasis

August Stich

Essentials

Human African trypanosomiasis (HAT, sleeping sickness) is caused by two subspecies of the protozoan parasite *Trypanosoma brucei*: *T. b. rhodesiense* is prevalent in East Africa among many wild and domestic mammals; *T. b. gambiense* causes an anthroponosis in Central and West Africa. The disease is restricted to tropical Africa where it is transmitted by the bite of infected tsetse flies (*Glossina* spp.).

Although well under control in the mid 20th century, HAT has returned to Africa in epidemic proportions since the 1980s, causing a severe public health problem in countries such as the Democratic Republic of Congo, Angola, Sudan, and Uganda. A joint effort by national, international, and nongovernmental organizations, as well as the pharmaceutical industry, is required to reverse this trend.

Clinical features

HAT progresses through distinct clinical stages that invariably lead to death if left untreated. Progress is fast in rhodesiense HAT, often resembling the clinical picture of malaria or septicaemia, and slow—sometimes lasting years—in gambiense HAT.

(1) Trypanosomal chancre—a papule at the site of the bite, surrounded by an intense local erythematous/oedematous reaction and with regional lymphadenopathy, healing without treatment after 2 to 4 weeks.

(2) Haemolymphatic stage (HAT stage 1)—manifests with fever, chills, rigors, headache and joint pains; hepatosplenomegaly and generalized lymphadenopathy are common

(3) Meningoencephalitic stage (HAT stage 2)—insidious onset of headache, sometimes with change in behaviour and personality; convulsions are common; sleep pattern becomes fragmented, eventually leading to somnolence and coma, with inability to drink and eat leading to dehydration and wasting.

Outside Africa, HAT is a rare diagnosis as an imported infection in travellers, but has to be considered in any patient with fever, chronic lymphadenopathy, or neurological changes returning from HAT endemic areas.

Diagnosis, staging, and treatment

Diagnosis—this is established by the detection of trypanosomes (usually by direct microscopy) in chancre aspirate, blood, lymph, or cerebrospinal fluid. Serology is useful for rapid screening under field conditions, but does not necessarily imply overt disease.

Staging—this is crucial for correct management: the cerebrospinal fluid must be examined in every patient found positive for trypanosomes in blood or lymph aspirate.

Treatment—HAT is curable, but many factors make this difficult: the disease is found in remote places, diagnosis is difficult, treatment is costly and complicated, and many drugs are not easily available. Aside from supportive care, specific treatment depends on the trypanosome subspecies and the stage of the disease, including (1) stage 1—pentamidine, and suramin; (2) stage 2—melarsoprol, eflornithine, and nifurtimox. There are no generally accepted recommendations on drug combinations, but—especially in late stages—treatment is difficult and dangerous to the patient; all of the drugs used are toxic and have many side effects, some potentially lethal.

Prevention

Control can be achieved by a combination of mass screening programmes, treatment of patients, and vector control, which together can lead to a complete break of the transmission cycle. There is no vaccine.

Introduction

Sleeping sickness or human African trypanosomiasis (HAT) is caused by subspecies of the protozoan haemoflagellate *Trypanosoma brucei* transmitted to humans and animals by tsetse flies (*Glossina* spp.). The distribution of the vector restricts sleeping sickness to the African continent between 14° north and 29° south (Fig. 8.10.1). Human disease occurs in two clinically and epidemiologically distinct forms, gambiense or West African and rhodesiense or East African sleeping sickness (Table 8.10.1). A third subspecies of the parasite, *T. b. brucei*, causes disease in cattle but is nonpathogenic in humans. In Uganda, the only country where all three forms occur, gambiense and rhodesiense sleeping sickness are currently about to overlap.

The first case reports of the disease go back to the 14th century. In the past, its impact on health in Africa has been enormous. Many areas were long rendered uninhabitable for people and livestock. During the early decades of the 20th century, millions may have died in Central Africa around Lake Victoria and in the Congo basin (Fig. 8.10.2). The success of control programmes in the 1960s

Table 8.10.1 The principal features of West and East African sleeping sickness

Disease	West African sleeping sickness	East African sleeping sickness
Parasite	*Trypanosoma brucei gambiense*	*Trypanosoma brucei rhodesiense*
Vector	Transmitted by riverine tsetse flies (*Palpalis* group)	Transmitted by savannah tsetse flies (*Morsitans* group)
Clinical course	Insidious onset, slow progression, death in stage II after many months or years	Acute onset, chancre frequent, rapid course, death frequently in stage I (cardiac failure)
Diagnosis	Parasitaemia scanty, Winterbottom's sign, serology	Parasitaemia usually higher and easily detectable, serological tests unreliable
Treatment	See Table 8.10.3	
Epidemiology	Tendency for endemicity, humans as main reservoir with evidence for several other mammal species, severe public health problem in many West and Central African countries	Wild (antelopes e.g. bushbuck) and occasionally domestic animals as reservoir and source of case clusters and epidemic outbreaks

promised the disappearance of sleeping sickness as a public health problem. However, recent epidemics in the Democratic Republic of Congo, northern Angola, southern Sudan, the Central African Republic, Uganda, and other countries have confirmed a major resurgence of HAT. According to estimates by the World Health Organization (WHO) at the turn of the millennium, the achievements in sleeping sickness control during colonial times had been nearly completely reversed. However, recent successes of control programmes run by national institutions and various nongovernmental organizations could again reduce its prevalence and transmission in many accessible areas of central Africa.

Today, about 60 million people in 36 African countries are exposed to the potential risk of HAT. In some 300 currently existing active foci, up to 100 000 people are still believed to be infected, almost all with *T. b. gambiense*. If left untreated, they are doomed. For tourists and expatriates, sleeping sickness has always been a rare disease, although several clusters of cases have been reported

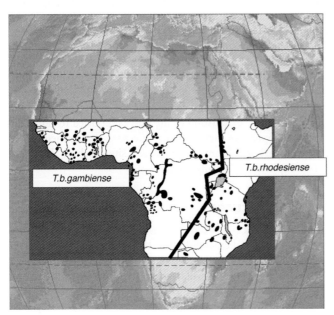

Fig. 8.10.1 The geographical distribution of human African trypanosomiasis.

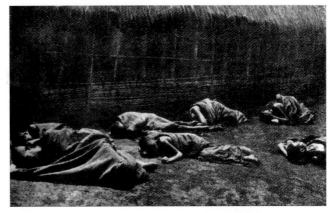

Fig. 8.10.2 Sleeping sickness patients on an island in Lake Victoria; historical photograph taken during Robert Koch's research expedition to East Africa.

in tourists to Tanzania, Zambia, and Malawi. The role of trypanosomes recently diagnosed in patients in some areas of the Indian subcontinent caused by *T. evansi* is currently under investigation.

Aetiology

In 1895, Sir David Bruce (1855–1931) suggested an association between trypanosomes and 'cattle fly fever', a major problem for livestock in southern Africa. In 1902, Robert M Forde and Everett Dutton from the Liverpool School of Tropical Medicine identified trypanosomes in the blood of a patient during a research expedition in the Gambia (see Fig. 8.10.6b), and in 1903, Aldo Castellani isolated trypanosomes from the cerebrospinal fluid. In the same year, tsetse flies were identified as the vector.

Trypanosoma brucei (phylum Sacromastigophora, order Kinetoplastida) is an extracellular protozoal parasite. Like leishmania, it possesses a centrally placed nucleus and a kinetoplast, a distinct organelle containing extranuclear DNA. The kinetoplast is the insertion site of an undulating membrane, which extends over nearly the whole cell length and ends as a free flagellum.

The three subspecies of *T. brucei* are indistinguishable morphologically. However, they differ considerably in their interaction with their mammalian host and the epidemiological pattern of the diseases they cause. Formerly, *T. b. gambiense* and *T. b. rhodesiense* isolates were characterized either by isoenzyme analysis or by animal inoculation. The advent of molecular techniques created expectations of more reliable tools for their differentiation. However, genomic characterization has revealed several more subdivisions than the three that were expected. Whereas West African isolates proved relatively homogeneous, East African isolates from humans and animals did not simply conform to what is still called *T. b. rhodesiense* and *T. b. brucei* but showed a complex relationship with evidence of sexual genetic exchange in the vector. Further molecular research may lead to a comprehensive phylogenetic tree and a deeper insight into trypanosomal evolution and biology.

Transmission

Although congenital, blood-borne, and mechanical transmission have been reported and may play an occasional role, the main mode of transmission is through the bite of infected tsetse flies (*Glossina* spp., order Diptera; Fig. 8.10.3). These are biologically unique insects, which occur only in Africa, with 31 distinct species and subspecies of which less than half are potential vectors of HAT. Their distinctive behaviour, ecology, and chosen habitat explain many epidemiological features of sleeping sickness. Tsetse flies can live for many months in the wild, are viviparous, and give birth to only about eight larvae per lifetime. Both sexes feed on blood.

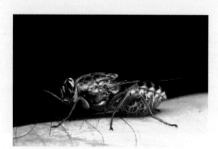

Fig. 8.10.3 Adult tsetse fly *Glossina morsitans.*

They are fastidious in requiring warm temperatures, shade, and humidity for resting and larviposition and so their distribution is highly localized. Recently, the mapping and monitoring of possible HAT transmission foci has become possible with the use of satellite imaging techniques.

During the blood meal on an infected mammalian host, the tsetse fly takes up trypanosomes ('short-stumpy form') into its mid-gut, where they develop into procyclic forms and multiply. After about 2 weeks, they migrate to the salivary glands as epimastigotes where they finally develop into infective metacyclic forms. At the next blood meal, they are injected into a new vertebrate host where they appear as 'long-slender' trypomastigotes and multiply by binary fission. In contrast to leishmania and *T. cruzi*, *T. brucei* is an exclusively extracellular parasite.

Molecular and immunological aspects

The cyclic changes of the trypanosome into different developmental stages are accompanied by variations in morphology, metabolism, and antigenicity. Several unique metabolic pathways have been described in trypanosomes, distinct from their host and thus qualifying as potential drug targets.

The bloodstream forms of *T. brucei* are covered with a dense coat of identical glycoproteins with up to about 500 amino acids per molecule. Being highly immunogenic, they stimulate the production of specific antibodies, mainly of the IgM subclass. Once the surface glycoproteins have been recognized by host antibodies, the parasite will be attacked and destroyed through complement activation and cytokine release, giving rise to local and systemic inflammatory reactions.

However, about 2% of *T. brucei* in each new generation change the expression of their specific surface glycoprotein. The 'coat' will then be different in the new clone (thus called variant surface glycoprotein, VSG). This phenotypic switch is done mainly by programmed DNA rearrangements, moving a transcriptionally silent VSG gene into an active, telomerically located expression site. Each *T. brucei* parasite already has the information for hundreds of different VSG genes, and within a whole trypanosome population, the potential repertoire for such different VSG copies seems to be virtually infinite.

Every new VSG copy is antigenically different, thus stimulating the production of a new IgM population. This antigenic variation is the major immune evasion strategy of the parasite, enabling the trypanosome to persist in its vertebrate host. It also reduces parasite load and prolongs the infection. But the inevitable outcome is immune exhaustion of the host (supported by additional immunosuppressive metabolites of the parasites), penetration of trypanosomes into immune-privileged sites such as the central nervous system, and finally death.

Clinical features

Sleeping sickness is a dreadful disease, causing great suffering to patients, their families, and the affected community. The infection often has an insidious onset, but *T. brucei*, whether the East or West African subspecies, will invariably kill unless treated in time. The natural course of HAT can be divided into different and distinct stages. Their recognition and differentiation is important for the clinical management of the patient.

Trypanosomal chancre

Tsetse bites can be quite painful, usually leaving a small and self-healing mark. In the case of a trypanosomal infection, the local reaction can be quite pronounced and longer lasting. A small raised papule will develop after about 5 days. It increases rapidly in size, surrounded by an intense erythematous tissue reaction (Fig. 8.10.4) with local oedema and regional lymphadenopathy. Although some chancres have a very angry appearance, they are not usually very painful unless they become ulcerated and superinfected. They heal without treatment after 2 to 4 weeks, leaving a permanent, hyperpigmented spot.

Trypanosomal chancres occur in about half the cases of *T. b. rhodesiense*. In *T. b. gambiense*, they are much less common and often go undetected in endemic populations.

Haemolymphatic stage (HAT stage I)

After local multiplication at the site of inoculation, the trypanosomes invade the haemolymphatic system, where they can be detected after 7 to 10 days. There they are exposed to vigorous host defence mechanisms, which they evade by antigenic variation. This continuous battle between antigenic switches and humoral defence results in a fluctuating parasitaemia with parasites frequently becoming undetectable, especially in gambiense HAT. The cyclic release of cytokines during periods of increased cell lysis results in intermittent, nonspecific symptoms: fever, chills, rigors, headache, and joint pains. These can easily be misdiagnosed as malaria, viral infection, typhoid fever, or many other conditions. Hepatosplenomegaly and generalized lymphadenopathy are common, indicating activation and hyperplasia of the reticuloendothelial system.

A reliable sign, particularly in *T. b. gambiense* infection, is the enlargement of lymph nodes in the posterior triangle of the neck (Winterbottom's sign). Other typical signs are a fugitive patchy or circinate rash, a myxoedematous infiltration of connective tissue ('puffy face syndrome'), and an inconspicuous periostitis of the tibia with delayed hyperaesthesia (Kérandel's sign).

In *T. b. rhodesiense* infection, this haemolymphatic stage is very pronounced with severe symptoms, often resembling falciparum malaria or septicaemia. Frequently, patients die within the first weeks after the onset of symptoms, mostly through cardiac involvement (myocarditis). In the early stage of *T. b. gambiense* infection, symptoms are usually infrequent and mild. Febrile episodes become less severe as the disease progresses.

Meningoencephalitic stage (HAT stage II)

Within weeks in *T. b. rhodesiense* and months in *T. b. gambiense* infection, cerebral involvement will invariably follow; trypanosomes cross the blood–brain barrier.

The onset of stage II is insidious. The exact time of central nervous system involvement cannot be determined clinically. Histologically, perivascular infiltration of inflammatory cells ('cuffing') and glial proliferation can be detected, resembling cerebral endarteriitis. As the disease progresses, patients complain of increasing headache, and their families may detect a marked change in behaviour and personality. Neurological symptoms, which follow gradually, can be focal or generalized, depending on the site of cellular damage in the central nervous system. Convulsions are common, usually indicating a poor prognosis. Periods of confusion and agitation slowly evolve towards a stage of distinct perplexity when patients lose interest in their surroundings and their own situation. Inflammatory reactions in the hypothalamic structures lead to a dysfunction in circadian rhythms and sleep regulatory systems. Sleep pattern become fragmented and finally result in a somnolent and comatose state. Progressive wasting and dehydration follows the inability to eat and drink.

In children, HAT progresses even more rapidly towards this meningoencephalitic stage. Parents often notice insomnia and behavioural changes long before the diagnosis is established.

There is no unique clinical sign of late HAT, opening up a wide range of possible neurological and psychiatric differential diagnoses. However, the appearance of the patient with apathy, the typical expressionless face, and swollen lymph nodes at the posterior triangle of the neck, is very suggestive for HAT in endemic areas (Fig. 8.10.5).

Clinical features of stage II patients with *T. b. rhodesiense* infections were compared in two locations in East Africa. Nonspecific signs of infection were more common in Uganda, whereas classic neurological manifestations dominated the clinical picture in Tanzania. Coinfections with malaria and HIV

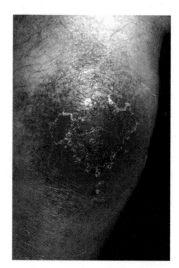

Fig. 8.10.4 Trypanosomal chancre on the calf of a missionary returning from the Congo.

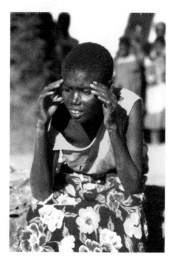

Fig. 8.10.5 Patient with late-stage trypanosomiasis.

influenced neither clinical presentation nor response to treatment in Tanzania.

Diagnosis

HAT can never be diagnosed with certainty purely on clinical grounds alone. Definitive diagnosis requires the detection of the parasite in chancre aspirate, blood, lymph, or cerebrospinal fluid using various parasitological techniques.

Lymph node aspirate

Lymph node aspiration is widely used, especially for the diagnosis of gambiense HAT. Fluid of enlarged lymph nodes, preferably of the posterior triangle of the neck (Winterbottom's sign), is aspirated and examined immediately at ×400 magnification without additional staining. Mobile trypanosomes can be detected for a few minutes between the numerous lymphocytes.

Wet preparation, thin, and thick blood film

During all stages of the disease, trypanosomes may appear in the blood where they can be detected in unstained wet or in stained preparations. The yield of detection is highest in the thick blood

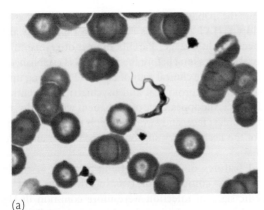

(a)

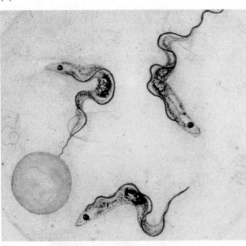

(b)

Fig. 8.10.6 (a) Trypanosomes in thin human blood film (Giemsa stain, ×1000). (b) Everett Dutton's painting of trypanosomes.

film, a technique widely used for the diagnosis of blood parasites such as plasmodium or microfilaria. Giemsa or Field staining techniques are appropriate (Fig. 8.10.6).

Especially in gambiense HAT, parasitaemia is usually low and fluctuating, often even undetectable. Repeated examinations on successive days are sometimes necessary until trypanosomes can be documented.

Concentration methods

To increase the sensitivity of blood examinations, various concentration assays have been developed. Trypanosomes tend to accumulate in the buffy coat layer after centrifugation of a blood sample. The best results have been obtained with the mini anion exchange column technique (mAECT), where trypanosomes are concentrated after passage through a cellulose column, the quantitative buffy coat (QBC) method, which was originally developed for the diagnosis of malaria, or the capillary tube centrifugation (CTC) method, which is widely used in the field.

Nucleic amplification techniques

Several specific primers have been described to detect trypanosomal DNA using the polymerase chain reaction (PCR). They had been successfully applied to samples from blood, lymph, and cerebrospinal fluid, mostly in research laboratory conditions. Although some of these techniques are able to detect fewer than 10 trypanosomes per probe, in the real situation of clinical diagnosis PCR assays are inferior to conventional parasitological techniques.

Serological assays

Serology is a useful tool to detect antibodies against trypanosomiasis. Various test methods have been described, some of them are now commercially available. They are mainly based on the enzymelinked immunosorbent assay (ELISA) technique or immunofluorescence, but provide reliable results only in gambiense HAT.

For rapid screening under field conditions, the card agglutination test for trypanosomiasis (CATT) is an excellent tool in areas of *T. b. gambiense* infestation. It is easy to perform and delivers results within 5 min. A visible agglutination in the CATT suggests the existence of antibodies, but does not necessarily imply overt disease. Still, any positive serological result requires parasitological confirmation.

Nonspecific laboratory findings

Anaemia and thrombocytopenia are caused by systemic effects of cytokine release, especially of tumour necrosis factor α (TNFα). Hypergammaglobinaemia can reach extreme levels as a result of polyclonal activation of plasma cells. IgM levels detected in HAT are among the highest observed in any infectious disease.

Diagnosis of stage II

Stage determination is crucial for the correct management of a patient. This cannot be done on clinical grounds alone. Cerebrospinal fluid must therefore be examined in every patient found positive for trypanosomes in blood or lymph aspirate. A lumbar puncture should also be performed in all patients in whom HAT is suspected clinically even if peripheral examinations had proved negative. A minimum of 5 ml of cerebrospinal fluid is required to examine for:

- Leucocytes—cerebral involvement in HAT stage II is accompanied by pleocytosis, mostly lymphocytes, in the cerebrospinal fluid. By convention a number of five cells or more per mm³ cerebrospinal fluid defines central nervous system involvement even if the patient does not (yet) have neurological symptoms. Pathognomonic for HAT is the appearance of activated plasma cells with eosinophilic inclusions in the cerebrospinal fluid, the morular cells of Mott (Fig. 8.10.7).

- Trypanosomes—the chances of detecting trypanosomes in the cerebrospinal fluid increase with the level of pleocytosis and the technique used. The highest yield is obtained by cerebrospinal fluid double centrifugation and rapid microscopy at the bedside.

- Protein—in patients with HAT, a level of 37 mg of protein per 100 ml cerebrospinal fluid (dye-binding protein assay) or more is highly suggestive of the advanced stage. Stage II HAT is characterized by an autochthonous production of IgM antibodies in the cerebrospinal fluid, which can be selectively detected if suitable laboratory facilities exist (e.g. latex IgM test).

Treatment

General considerations

HAT is curable, especially if the diagnosis is made at an early stage of the disease. In the stark reality of the African situation, however, there are many major obstacles to successful patient management:

- Sleeping sickness is a disease of rural, remote places. The active foci of sleeping sickness are usually in faraway and insecure places, which are difficult to reach. Many treatment centres work under emergency conditions with extremely restricted resources. Numerous affected patients, without proper access to health care, are left unattended.

- The diagnosis is difficult. Initial diagnosis and exact staging of trypanosomiasis requires sophisticated methods that are often dangerous to the patient and justified only in the hands of experienced personnel. Repetitive training programmes, constant supervision, and continuous quality control are necessary but in reality rarely available.

- The treatment of trypanosomiasis is extremely costly, although the drugs themselves are now covered by a donation programme. Invariably, demand exceeds the locally available resources. External funding and sustainable donor commitments for rural Africa are generally decreasing.

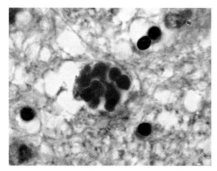

Fig. 8.10.7 Morular cell of Mott in a histological brain section of a stage II HAT patient (haematoxylin and eosin stain, ×1000).

- The treatment is complicated. Treatment of HAT is dangerous, prolonged, and usually requires hospitalization. Most patients with late-stage trypanosomiasis are severely ill and malnourished. Adverse drug reactions during treatment are difficult to assess because of concomitant pathologies. Their management requires considerable medical skill and good nursing care. Hospitals in rural Africa are often inadequately equipped and staffed to accomplish good patient care.

- Many drugs are not easily available. Many trypanosomicidal agents are on the verge of disappearance, despite increasing demand. The range of drugs is diminishing, and hardly any new treatments are in sight. This is especially worrying in view of the reported spread of drug resistance.

- HAT treatment is not standardized. Trypanosomiasis treatment regimens vary considerably between countries and treatment centres. Results from different centres are comparable to only a very limited extent. Few properly conducted and sufficiently powered clinical trials are available to evaluate duration, dosage, and possible combinations of drugs. Sufficient infrastructure for carrying out clinical research exists in only a handful of places.

The price for cure of HAT is high: dangerous drugs with limited availability and prolonged treatment schedules administered in many places by poorly trained personnel in rudimentary medical facilities. Little progress has been achieved in the last 30 years.

Stage I drugs

The treatment of HAT depends on the trypanosome subspecies and the stage of the disease (Table 8.10.2).

Pentamidine

Since its introduction in 1937, pentamidine has become the drug of choice for gambiense HAT stage I, achieving cure rates as high as 98%. However, there are frequent failures in rhodesiense HAT. Lower rates of cellular pentamidine uptake in *T. b. rhodesiense* may explain these differences. Some cures of stage II infections have also been reported, but cerebrospinal fluid drug levels are usually not sufficiently high to guarantee a reliable trypanosomicidal effect in the central nervous system.

Pentamidine is usually given by deep intramuscular injection, often to outpatients. If hospital care and reasonable monitoring conditions are available, an intravenous infusion, given in normal saline over 2 h, might be used instead. The main advantage of pentamidine over other drugs is the short treatment course and ease of administration. Adverse effects are related to the route

Table 8.10.2 The choice of drugs in the treatment of sleeping sickness

		Gambiense sleeping sickness		Rhodesiense sleeping sickness
HAT	1st line	Pentamidine	1st line	Suramin
Stage I	2nd line	Eflornithine	2nd line	Melarsoprol
HAT	1st line	Eflornithine (+ nifurtimox?)	1st line	Melarsoprol
Stage II	2nd line	Melarsoprol	2nd line	Melarsoprol + nifurtimox

of administration or its dose and are usually reversible (Table 8.10.3).

Pentamidine is also used as second-line therapy for visceral leishmaniasis and especially in the prophylaxis and treatment of opportunistic *Pneumocystis jiroveci* pneumonia in AIDS. Since the start of the HIV pandemic, the cost of pentamidine has been increased more than tenfold by producers, making it unaffordable by health institutions in low-income countries. After an intervention by WHO, a limited amount of pentamidine is now made available for use in HAT as part of a donation programme.

Suramin

In the early 20th century, the development of suramin, resulting from German research on the trypanosomicidal activity of various dyes ('Bayer 205'), was a major breakthrough in the field of tropical medicine. For the first time, African trypanosomiasis, at least in its early stages, became treatable without causing major harm.

Even today, suramin is still used to treat stage I HAT, especially rhodesiense. Like pentamidine, it does not reach therapeutic levels in cerebrospinal fluid. Suramin is injected intravenously after dilution in distilled water.

Adverse effects depend on nutritional status, concomitant illnesses (especially onchocerciasis), and the patient's clinical condition. Although life-threatening reactions have been described, serious adverse effects are rare (Table 8.10.3).

Stage II drugs

Melarsoprol

Until the systematic introduction of the arsenical compound melarsoprol in 1949, late stage trypanosomiasis was virtually untreatable. Since then, it has remained the most widely used stage II antitrypanosomal drug both for gambiense and rhodesiense infections. It has saved many lives, but has a high rate of dangerous

Table 8.10.3 Dosage and principal adverse reactions of antitrypanosomal agents

Drug	Dosage regimen	Adverse drug reactions
Pentamidine	4mg/kg body weight intramuscular daily or on alternate days for 7 to 10 injections (3 dose regimen currently under investigation)	Hypotensive reaction with tachycardia, dizziness, even collapse and shock, especially after intravenous administration, close monitoring of pulse rate and blood pressure after injection is mandatory
		Inflammatory reactions at the site of injection (sterile abscesses, necrosis)
		Renal, hepatic, and pancreatic dysfunction
		Neurotoxicity: peripheral polyneuropathy
		Bone marrow depression
Suramin	Day 1: Test dose of 4–5 mg/kg body weight	Pyrexia (very common)
	Day 3, 10, 17, 24, and 31: 20 mg/kg body weight, maximum	Early hypersensitivity reactions such as nausea, circulatory collapse, urticaria
	Dose per injection 1 g	Late hypersensitivity reactions: skin reactions (exfoliative dermatitis), haemolytic anaemia
		Renal impairment: albuminuria, cylinduria, haematuria (high renal tissue concentrations); regular urine checks during treatment are mandatory
		Neurotoxicity: peripheral neuropathy
		Bone marrow toxicity: agranulocytosis, thrombocytopenia
Melarsoprol	New regimen:	Treatment-induced encephalopathy
	Day 1–10: 2.2 mg/kg body weight	Pyrexia
		Neurotoxicity: peripheral motor or sensory polyneuropathy
		Dermatological reactions: pruritus, urticaria, exfoliative dermatitis,
		Cardiotoxicity
		Renal and hepatic dysfunction
Eflornithine	Most commonly used dosage regimen:	Gastrointestinal symptoms such as nausea, vomiting and diarrhoea
	100 mg/kg body weight at 6-hourly intervals for 14 days	Bone marrow toxicity: anaemia, leucopenia, thrombocytopenia
		Alopecia, usually towards the end of the treatment cycle
		Neurological symptoms such as convulsions
Nifurtimox	5mg/kg body weight 3 times daily for 30 days	Abdominal discomfort such as nausea, pains, and vomiting in half of the treated patients, often leading to a disruption of the treatment course
		Neurological complications: convulsions,
		Impairment of cerebellar function, polyneuropathy
		Skin reactions

adverse effects. Increasing frequency of relapses and resistance has been reported in some parts of Congo, Angola, Sudan, and Uganda.

Melarsoprol clears trypanosomes rapidly from the blood, lymph, and cerebrospinal fluid. Its toxicity usually restricts its use to late-stage disease. It is given by slow intravenous injection; extravascular leakage must be avoided.

A new, simpler regimen is based on recently acquired knowledge of the drug's pharmacokinetics (Table 8.10.3). The most important adverse effect is an acute encephalopathy, provoked around day 5 to 8 of the treatment course in 5 to 14% of all patients. There are severe headache, convulsions, rapid neurological deterioration, or deepening of coma. Characteristically, the comatose patient's eyes remain open. Most probably, this is an immune-mediated reaction precipitated by release of parasite antigens in the first days of treatment. The overall case fatality under treatment ranges between 2 and 12%, depending on the stage of disease and the quality of medical and nursing care. Simultaneous administration of glucocorticosteroids (prednisolone 1 mg/kg body weight; maximum 40 mg daily) reduces mortality, especially in cases with high cerebrospinal fluid pleocytosis. However, in areas where tuberculosis, amoebiasis, and strongyloidiasis are highly prevalent, corticosteroids have dangers of their own.

Eflornithine (DFMO)

Initially developed as antitumour agent, eflornithine (α-difluoromethylornithine) was introduced in 1980 as an antitrypanosomal drug, in the hope that it might replace melarsoprol for treatment of stage II trypanosomiasis. However, exorbitant costs and limited availability have restricted its use mostly to melarsoprol-refractory cases of gambiense sleeping sickness. *T. b. rhodesiense* is much less sensitive, because of a much higher turnover rate of the target enzyme ornithine decarboxylase, and therefore cannot be treated with eflornithine.

The drug can be taken orally, but intravenous administration is preferred as it achieves a much higher bioavailability and success rate. Eflornithine should be administered slowly over a period of at least 30 min. Continuous 24-h administration is preferable if facilities allow.

The range of adverse reactions to eflornithine is wide, as with other cytotoxic drugs in cancer treatment. Their occurrence and intensity increase with the duration of treatment and the severity of the patient's general condition (Table 8.10.3).

In the late 1990s no pharmaceutical company produced eflornithine for use against HAT, despite pressure by WHO. The discovery of its therapeutic effect in cosmetic creams against facial hair helped to restimulate production and thus had a beneficial 'spin-off' effect for HAT. In 2001 agreements were signed between WHO and two major drug companies which led to a 'public–private partnership' (PPP) and helped to assure a sufficient supply of eflornithine and other drugs essential for the treatment of HAT. In 2006, the agreement was prolonged until 2011.

Nifurtimox

Ten years after its introduction for the treatment of American trypanosomiasis in 1967, nifurtimox was found to be effective in the treatment of gambiense sleeping sickness. It has a place as second-line treatment in melarsoprol-refractory cases or in combination chemotherapies.

Nifurtimox is given orally and generally not well tolerated, but adverse effects are usually not severe. They are dose-related and rapidly reversible after discontinuation of the drug (Table 8.10.3).

Combination treatments in HAT

Melarsoprol, eflornithine, and nifurtimox interfere with trypanothione synthesis and activity at different stages. There is also experimental evidence that combinations of suramin and stage II drugs might be beneficial. Therefore, by reducing the overall dosage of each individual component, drug combinations have the potential to reduce the frequency of serious side effects and the development of resistance, which are such common problems in the treatment of sleeping sickness.

Recent prospective clinical trials have shown a beneficial effect of nifurtimox eflornithine combination therapy (NECT). This has the potential to develop into the preferred first-line treatment of stage II gambiense HAT in the future.

Individual protection

Tsetse flies have a very patchy distribution. Infested strips of land are often well known to the local population and should be avoided as far as possible. HAT among tourists and occasional visitors to endemic areas is a rare event. Pentamidine or suramin chemoprophylaxis is historical, and can no longer be recommended. Long-sleeved, brightly coloured clothing and insecticide repellents are the best defence against attacking tsetse flies.

Prevention and control

In the past, tremendous efforts were undertaken to control the threat posed by sleeping sickness to human lives and economic development in rural Africa. Control programmes are based on the five complementary pillars given in Box 8.10.1.

The most important strategy is active case finding. This requires mobile teams, which regularly visit villages in endemic areas. Mostly based on the results of CATT screening, patients, preferably in the early stage of the disease, are identified and treated. Gradually, the parasite reservoir is depleted. As glossina is a relatively incompetent vector, with infectivity rates usually below 0.1% and susceptible to control measures such as insecticide application, trapping, or even the release of sterile males, the combination of various approaches can lead to a complete break of the transmission cycle. In the past this was achieved in many places. However, the resurgence of sleeping sickness in areas ridden by war and civil unrest during the last decades of the 20th century, in combination with the decreasing availability of drugs on the international market and the general loss of interest in health issues of the developing world, gives rise to the fear that HAT will always be a problem in many rural parts of Africa (Fig. 8.10.8).

Trypanosomiasis in the 21st century

There is hardly any other tropical disease that demonstrates more clearly the dichotomy characterizing our modern age. On one side,

---

Box 8.10.1 Control of human African trypanosomiasis

- Diagnosis and treatment of patients
- Active case finding
- Vector control
- Implementation and continuation of a surveillance system
- Training, health education, and community participation

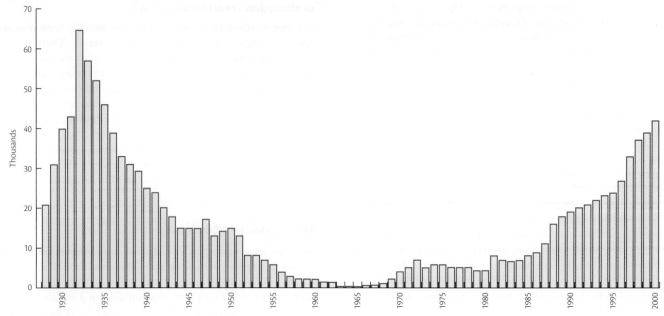

Fig. 8.10.8 Number of annually reported cases of human African trypanosomiasis.
(source: *WHO Report on Global Surveillance and Epidemic-prone Infectious Diseases*); according to WHO, the actual patient numbers are about 10-fold higher.

trypanosomes are kept in culture and studied extensively in numerous research laboratories. Their genome is sequenced, and many molecular, biochemical, and immunological phenomena have been discovered as a result of basic science research.

General interest in this disease is usually restricted only to its research aspects, however. Diagnostic and especially therapeutic tools are increasingly unavailable, because the tens of thousands of infected people in Africa are not commercially viable consumers. The prospects for the fight against trypanosomiasis look grim, although some recent successes have been accomplished usually through the work of committed nongovernmental organizations (e.g. in Sudan and Angola). Global concern about the crisis of human trypanosomiasis in Africa is a question of scientific ethics and international solidarity.

Further reading

Brun R, *et al.* (2009). Human African trypanosomiasis. *Lancet*, **375**, 148–59.

Burri C (2010). Chemotherapy against human African trypanosomiasis: is there a road to success? *Parasitology*, **137**, 1987–94.

Dumas M, Bouteille B, Buguet A (eds) (1999). *Progress in human African trypanosomiasis, sleeping sickness*. Springer-Verlag, Paris.

Jannin J, Cattand P (2004). Treatment and control of human African trypanosomiasis. *Curr Opin Infect Dis*, **17**, 565–70.

Kuepfer I, *et al.* (2011). Clinical presentation of T. b. rhodesiense sleeping sickness in second stage patients from Tanzania and Uganda. *PLoS Negl Trop Dis*, **5**, e968.

Maudlin I (2006). African trypanosomiasis. *Ann Trop Med Parasitol*, **100**, 679–701.

Pepin J, *et al.* (1989). Trial of prednisolone for prevention of melarsoprol-induced encephalopathy in gambiense sleeping sickness. *Lancet*, **i**, 1246–50.

Priotto G, *et al.* (2009). Nifurtimox-eflornithine combination therapy for second-stage African *Trypanosoma brucei gambiense* trypanosomiasis: a multicentre, randomised, phase III, non-inferiority trial. *Lancet*, **374**, 56–64.

Stich A, Barrett MP, Krishna S (2003). Waking up to sleeping sickness. *Trends Parasitol*, **19**, 195–7.

World Health Organization (1998). *Control and surveillance of African trypanosomiasis*. WHO Technical Report Series 881. WHO, Geneva.

8.11 **Chagas disease**

M.A. Miles

A poeira de Curvelo não az mal para ninguém não

Do pulmão lá ninguém morre

O que mata é o coração

The dust of Curvelo does not harm anybody

No one dies there of lung disease

What kills is the heart

(From the poem *O galo cantou na serra* by Luiz Claudio and Guimarães Rosa)

Essentials

Trypanosoma cruzi, the protozoan parasite which causes Chagas disease, is a zoonosis with many mammal host and vector species. It is transmitted to humans by contamination of mucous membranes or abraded skin with infected faeces of bloodsucking triatomine bugs, also by blood transfusion, organ transplantation, transplacentally, and orally by food contaminated with infective forms. It multiplies intracellularly (pseudocysts) as amastigotes in mammalian cells, particularly heart and smooth muscle, from which flagellated trypomastigotes emerge to reinvade cells or circulate in blood. Around 10 million people are infected in Latin America; imported cases and congenital cases may occur elsewhere.

Clinical features

There are classically three phases. (1) Acute—may be asymptomatic, or with manifestations including fever, myalgia, headache, vomiting, diarrhoea, anorexia, facial or generalized oedema, rash, generalized lymphadenopathy, and hepatosplenomegaly; there may be a lesion at the portal of entry; fatal in less than 10%. (2) Meningoencephalitic—rare in adults, excepting those who are immunocompromised (most typically with HIV/AIDS); also seen in congenital cases. (3) Chronic—occurs in up to 30% of those recovering from the acute phase; most often with cardiac involvement (typically cardiomyopathy leading to congestive cardiac failure, with risk of arrhythmia and ECG abnormalities due to focal inflammatory lesions of the conducting system), also megaoesophagus and megacolon. Infection is opportunistic, relapsing in the immunocompromised.

Diagnosis

(1) Acute phase—parasitaemia is scanty, but circulating trypomastigotes may be detectable in the acute phase by microscopy of blood, enhanced by concentration methods. (2) Chronic phase—multiple blood cultures or feeding and subsequent dissection of laboratory-reared triatomines (xenodiagnosis) may reveal infection. (3) Serological testing—can demonstrate evidence of infection, but needs to be standardized with reference sera and by external quality control.

Treatment

(1) Acute phase—proven cases should be treated promptly with nifurtimox or benznidazole, but there is no guarantee that a full course of treatment will eliminate the infection. (2) Chronic phase—the value of drug treatment for adults is still debated; supportive care may include the following (a) for heart disease—conventional drug treatment for cardiac failure and arrhythmias; cardiac pacemaker; (b) for megaoesophagus—dilatation; segmentary removal of stomach muscle; replacement of the distal oesophagus; (c) megacolon—resection and anastomosis with the rectal stump.

Prevention

Proven methods of controlling domestic triatomine bugs include insecticide spraying (with pyrethroids), health education, community support, and house improvement. Serological surveillance of children detects residual endemic foci or congenital transmission and is vital for monitoring the success of control programmes. The Southern Cone programme against *Triatoma infestans* is considered a model for international cooperation in disease control. There is no vaccine.

Introduction and aetiology

In 1907, in the space of a few months, the Brazilian scientist Carlos Chagas discovered the disease that bears his name and described the entire lifecycle of the causative organism. Chagas first found the protozoan agent *Trypanosoma cruzi* in the gut of the large blood-sucking insect vector, the triatomine bug (order Hemiptera, family Reduviidae, subfamily Triatominae) (Fig. 8.11.1). Later he returned to bug-infested houses and detected *T. cruzi* in the blood of sick children.

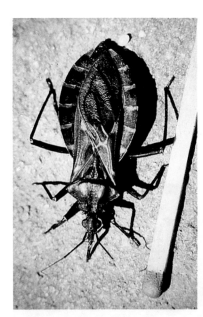

Fig. 8.11.1 Adult female triatomine bug (*Panstrongylus megistus*), with a single egg shown adjacent to the tip of the abdomen.
(Courtesy of Dr T V Barrett.)

T. cruzi is a kinetoplastid protozoan. In addition to the nucleus, it has a second, microscopically visible DNA-containing organelle, the kinetoplast. The main lifecycle stages (trypomastigote, amastigote, epimastigote) are distinguished by the position of the kinetoplast relative to the nucleus and by the presence or absence of a free flagellum.

Vector-borne transmission of *T. cruzi* is by contamination of the mammal host with infected faeces of triatomine bugs, not by their bite. During or shortly after feeding, bugs release blackish liquid faeces and urine on to the skin of the host. Infective forms (metacyclic trypomastigotes) penetrate mucous membranes or abraded skin. Inside the mammal, *T. cruzi* is primarily an intracellular parasite. Trypomastigotes enter nonphagocytic or phagocytic cells, in which they transform to ovoid or round aflagellate amastigotes that multiply inside the cell by binary fission to produce a pseudocyst (Fig. 8.11.2). After 5 days or more, the pseudocyst ruptures to release numerous new trypomastigotes, which reinvade cells or circulate in the blood. Multiplication may occur at the site of infection, but pseudocysts subsequently predominate in muscle, especially heart and smooth muscle. In the blood, trypomastigotes are small, often C-shaped, with a large terminal kinetoplast (Fig. 8.11.3). In fulminating or experimental infections, slender highly motile trypomastigotes may also sometimes be seen. Trypomastigotes do not multiply in the blood. Triatomine bugs become infected by taking a blood meal from an infected mammal; birds and reptiles are not susceptible to infection. Infection in the bug is confined to the alimentary tract, where *T. cruzi* multiplies by binary fission as epimastigotes (kinetoplast adjacent to the nucleus). Metacyclic trypomastigotes are produced in the hindgut and rectum of the bug. All stages of the *T. cruzi* lifecycle can be cultured *in vitro*. *T. cruzi* can also be transmitted by blood transfusion and organ transplantation, across the placenta, via breast milk (rarely), and orally through food contaminated by triatomine faeces and the raw meat of infected mammals. Sexual transmission has not been documented.

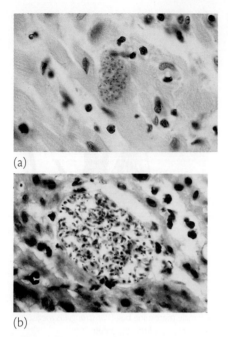

(a)

(b)

Fig. 8.11.2 Pseudocyst of *Trypanosoma cruzi*. Pseudocyst in (a) heart muscle and (b) umbilical cord, from a congenital case of Chagas disease. (a, courtesy of J E Williams; b, courtesy of Dr Hipolito de Almeida.)

Epidemiology

T. cruzi is confined to the Americas, although closely related organisms of the same subgenus (*Schizotrypanum*) are cosmopolitan in bats. The vast majority of the 140 triatomine bug species are also restricted to the Americas. Their natural habitats are the refuges of mammals, birds, and reptiles, in trees, in burrows, and among rocks. All mammals are thought to be susceptible to *T. cruzi*, which has been reported from at least 150 mammal species. The opossum (*Didelphis* spp.) is the most common sylvatic host. A few triatomine species thrive as domestic colonies. More than 10 000 bugs have been found in a single house. Before the recent Southern Cone initiative to control *Triatoma infestans*, the species was widespread in rural housing of the Southern Cone countries of South America (Argentina, Bolivia, Brazil, Chile, Paraguay, Uruguay, and southern Peru). *Rhodnius prolixus* is the common vector in northern South America and also occurs in Central America, with *Triatoma dimidiata* as secondary vector in the same regions. *Panstrongylus*

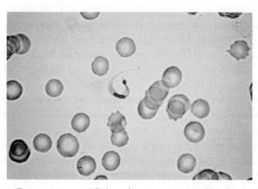

Fig. 8.11.3 *Trypanosoma cruzi* C-shaped trypomastigote in blood. Note the large posterior kinetoplast.

megistus (Fig. 8.11.1) infests central and eastern Brazil, and *Triatoma brasiliensis* north-eastern Brazil. Animals that share human dwellings, such as guinea pigs (cuy), dogs, cats, rats, and mice are domestic reservoirs of *T. cruzi* infection. Chickens, although not susceptible to *T. cruzi*, encourage bug infestation and can sustain large colonies.

Serological surveys suggest that about 10 million people may now be infected with *T. cruzi* in South and Central America, a figure which is reduced from up to 20 million around four decades ago. In some communities, seropositivity rates may still exceed 50%. As expected from the precarious contaminative route of transmission, prevalence rises with age. Based on prevalence, before recent control initiatives, it was estimated that up to 300 000 new infections might occur in Latin America each year; this is now reduced to around 60 000/year. Only approximately 1000 cases are known from the Amazon basin, about half of these due to oral transmission by drinking fruit juices (e.g. from berries of açaí or bacaba palms or cane sugar garapa) in which infected bugs have been accidentally ground up. Oral outbreaks may also occur elsewhere: one among schoolchildren in Caracas, Venezuela, due to guava juice, involved 103 cases. There are relatively few Amazonian cases because the local forest vectors do not colonize houses. For the same reason, autochthonous infection is very rare in the United States of America. but a recent report emphasized its endemicity in Texas with an autochthonous canine cycle, abundant vectors (*Triatoma* species) in many counties, and established domestic and peridomestic cycles providing competent reservoirs throughout the state. It has been suggested that Chagas disease should be made reportable in Texas, as it is in Arizona and Massachusetts. In south Texas, blood donor screening should be mandatory, and the serological profiles of human and canine populations should be established.

Not surprisingly, sporadic *T. cruzi* infections may be found among migrants from Latin America to the United States of America and elsewhere. This gives rise to occasional cases of transmission by blood or organ donors and to rare congenital cases. Fear of blood transfusion transmission suggests a need to screen some blood donors outside traditional endemic areas. In 2007, the World Health Organization (WHO) launched a 'Global Network for Chagas Elimination' to raise global awareness and coordinate prevention of transmission.

Initial acute infections are frequently asymptomatic or overlooked. It is thought that less than 10% of acute infections in children are fatal. Morbidity due to Chagas disease arises primarily from the chronic infection. Once acquired, infection is usually carried for life. Around 30% of those infected will subsequently display ECG abnormalities and chagasic cardiomyopathy, and a proportion of those have associated megaoesophagus or megacolon.

There are marked regional differences in the epidemiology of Chagas disease. Megasyndromes are common in central and eastern Brazil but seldom described in northern South America and Central America. Research in molecular genetics has shown that *T. cruzi* is not a Single entity, but a species with at least six genetic lineages. Until Recently these were divided into TCI and TCIIa–e, but they have now, more logically, been re-designated as six distinct groups TCI, TCII, TCIII, TCIV, TCV, and TCVI, with differences between ecologies, hosts, vectors, geographical, and disease distributions. The common opossum Didelphis is the most ubiquitous host of TCI, whereas TCIII is associated with the armadillo

Dasypus. North of the Amazon the principal agent of Chagas disease is TCI, which causes severe and fatal cardiomyopathy. In contrast, in the Southern Cone countries, where megaoesophagus and megacolon are common, Chagas disease is predominantly caused by TCII, TCV, and TCVI. It has been proved that *T. cruzi* has an extant capacity for genetic exchange, and TCV and TCVI are natural TCII /TCIII hybrids, which are particularly prevalent in humans in Paraguay, Chile, Bolivia, and adjacent regions.

Pathogenesis and pathology

At the portal of entry, local multiplication of *T. cruzi* may lead to unilateral conjunctivitis or to a skin lesion (Fig. 8.11.4). Unruptured pseudocysts in muscle apparently generate no inflammatory response. Pseudocyst rupture is followed by infiltration of lymphocytes, monocytes, and/or polymorphonuclear cells. Antigens released from pseudocysts may spread and be adsorbed on to adjacent uninfected cells. Such uninfected cells may be attacked by the immune response of the host and be destroyed. In this way, expanded focal lesions may be produced. Postmortem histology of human hearts and experimental studies in dogs has demonstrated a clear association between ECG abnormalities and focal lesions in the conducting system of the heart. Much damage may occur in the acute phase of infection, particularly if pseudocysts are numerous. Postmortem histology has demonstrated that neuron loss is a feature of chagasic cardiopathy and of megasyndromes that is exacerbated by further disease or age-related loss. Thus, a threshold may be reached, often many years after the acute infection, at which organ function is perturbed. Further ECG abnormalities, aperistalsis, and organ enlargement may ensue. This 'neurogenic' pathogenesis has been linked to sudden death.

It is proposed that pathological exposure of normal host-sequestered antigens, or sharing of antigens between *T. cruzi* and its host, may precipitate autoimmune pathogenesis. Some chronic chagasic cardiomyopathy is said to display a renewed intense inflammatory response and a progressive diffuse myocarditis, and a slow decline in cardiac function.

The contribution of the lifelong infection to the pathogenesis of chronic Chagas disease is somewhat controversial, although published studies suggest that elimination of residual infection may improve long-term prognosis. After the initial acute phase, trypomastigotes are detectable in the blood only by sensitive indirect methods. Similarly, pseudocysts in the tissues are infrequent, but are detectable immunologically and by amplification of *T. cruzi* DNA.

T. cruzi infection is controlled primarily by a cell-mediated immune response, especially the Th1 arm of the immune response. Patients immunocompromised by AIDS have impaired Th1 responses. Thus HIV-positive patients chronically infected with *T. cruzi* may suffer reactivated acute Chagas disease, with microscopically patent parasitaemia and poor prognosis.

At the level of gross pathology, substantial megacardia may be seen. Thinning of the myocardium may be present, with focal aneurysms visible upon transillumination, especially at the apex of the left ventricle (Fig. 8.11.5) and thrombus in the right atrial appendage (Fig. 8.11.6). Apical aneurysm is considered to be a pathognomonic sign of chronic chagasic cardiomyopathy. Megaoesophagus (Fig. 8.11.7) and megacolon (Fig. 8.11.8) may show enormous dilatation and thinning of the wall. Chagasic megaoesophagus is more frequent than chagasic megacolon, but both may occur in the same patient and are often accompanied by chagasic heart disease. Chagasic megaoesophagus may be a prelude to carcinoma. Occasionally megasyndromes may arise in infants, following congenital infection.

Clinical features

Classically, there are three clinical phases of Chagas disease. In the acute phase, symptoms include fever, myalgia, headache, hepatosplenomegaly, generalized lymphadenopathy, facial or generalized oedema, rash, vomiting, diarrhoea, and anorexia. If *T. cruzi* has been inoculated through the conjunctiva, Romaña's sign may be present: unilateral conjunctivitis, chemosis, and periophthalmic oedema (Fig. 8.11.4). If the portal of entry is the skin, an indurated oedematous cutaneous lesion (chagoma) may be seen. Regional

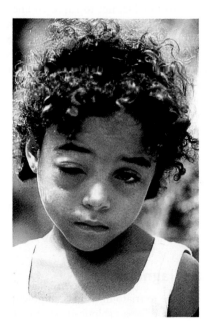

Fig. 8.11.4 Romaña's sign in acute Chagas disease.

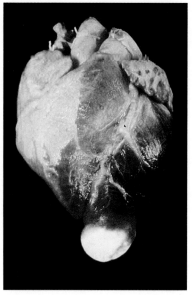

Fig. 8.11.5 Apical aneurysm of the left ventricle in chronic Chagas disease.
(Courtesy of Dr J S de Oliveira.)

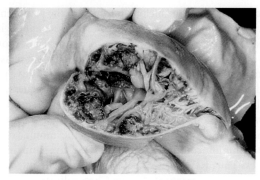

Fig. 8.11.6 Mural thrombus filling the right atrial appendage.
(Copyright D A Warrell.)

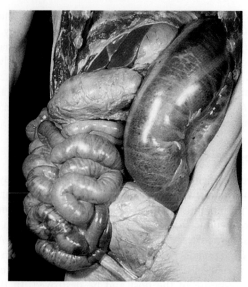

Fig. 8.11.8 Megacolon postmortem in chronic Chagas disease.
(Courtesy of Dr J. S. de Oliveira.)

lymphadenopathy may be present. Multiple chagomas may occasionally occur in acute-phase infections in infants. ECG abnormalities may include sinus tachycardia, increased PR interval, T-wave changes, and low QRS voltage. The incubation period may be as short as 2 weeks or as long as several months if infection is due to transfusion of contaminated blood. General lymphadenopathy and splenomegaly are frequent in blood transfusion-acquired infections.

Congenital acute infection may cause fever, oedema, metastatic chagomas, neurological signs such as convulsions, tremors, and weak reflexes, and apnoea. Hepatosplenomegaly is frequent. The ECG is usually normal but low-voltage complexes, reduced T-wave height, and longer atrioventricular (AV) conduction time may be present.

Meningoencephalitis is rare in adults, more frequent in infants, and common in immunocompromised patients. It carries a poor prognosis.

The clinical picture of AIDS-associated chagasic meningoencephalitis may be similar to toxoplasmosis. Haemorrhagic necrotic encephalitis is described in the nests of trypanosomes in microglia. Congenital infection may resemble toxoplasmosis, cytomegalovirus infection, or syphilis, with an increased likelihood of abortion and premature birth. Congenital infection is well known in Bolivia but less frequently reported from Venezuela and Brazil.

Symptomatic or asymptomatic acute infection may be followed by a symptom-free indeterminate phase of unpredictable length, which may be life long.

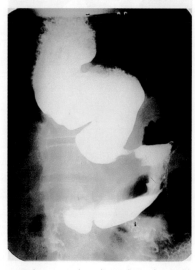

Fig. 8.11.7 Megaoesophagus seen by radiography in chronic Chagas disease.
(Courtesy of Dr J S de Oliveira.)

Chronic-phase symptoms may emerge in up to 30% of patients recovering from the acute phase. Cardiac symptoms include arrhythmias, palpitations, chest pain, oedema, dizziness, syncope, and dyspnoea. The cardiac enlargement may be massive with chronic congestive cardiac failure, apical aneurysm (Fig. 8.11.5), and thrombus in the right atrial appendage (Fig. 8.11.6). The cardiac conducting system is involved, especially the sinus node, bundle of His and AV node, in which there is mononuclear and mast-cell infiltration, inflammation, and fibrosis. Characteristic ECG abnormalities are right bundle branch block (RBBB) and left anterior hemiblock (LAH). AV conduction abnormalities, including AV block, may be present. Arrhythmias may include sinus bradycardia, sinoatrial block, ventricular tachycardia, primary T-wave changes, and abnormal Q-waves. The severity of heart disease is graded by the degree of disturbance. Sudden death is attributable, not to ruptured aneurysm, but to arrhythmias often precipitated by exercise (e.g. on the football field). Radiography may reveal megacardia (Fig. 8.11.9). Signs of oesophageal involvement include loss of peristalsis, regurgitation, and dysphagia (Fig. 8.11.7). Parotid enlargement may be associated.

In megacolon, there may be failure of defaecation, constipation, and faecaloma (Fig. 8.11.8). Progressive dilatation of either organ can be graded clinically according to severity and may be detectable by radiography. Megaduodenum and megaureter are also described. The lymph nodes between the pulmonary trunk and the aorta are frequently enlarged.

The differential diagnosis includes other types of heart disease and causes of ECG abnormalities. RBBB and LAH are indicative, but a history of exposure to *T. cruzi* infection and laboratory diagnostic evidence must be considered (see below).

Laboratory diagnosis

A history of exposure to triatomine bugs, to potentially contaminated transfused blood, or a prolonged stay in endemic regions must be considered.

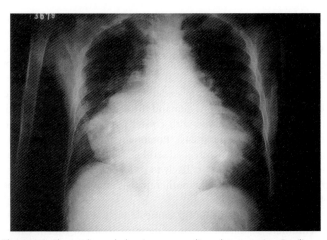

Fig. 8.11.9 Chest radiograph showing gross cardiac enlargement in a Brazilian woman with chronic Chagas disease.
(Copyright D A Warrell.)

Motile trypomastigotes might be seen in unstained, wet blood preparations examined by microscopy (Fig. 8.11.3). Nevertheless, parasitaemia is often scanty or undetectable by this method. The sensitivity of parasitological diagnosis may be enhanced by microscopy of samples prepared with concentration methods, such as the centrifugation pellet from separated serum (Strout's method), the haematocrit buffy coat layer, Giemsa-stained thick films, or the centrifugation sediment after lysis of red blood cells with 0.87% ammonium chloride. All these tests may be negative if parasitaemia is low. Potentially infected blood must be handled with care, especially during haematocrit centrifugation, as a single trypomastigote can cause infection. Multiple blood cultures may also be performed, with a sensitive blood agar-based medium and physiological saline overlay. Even more sensitive than blood culture is xenodiagnosis, in which hungry fourth or fifth instar bugs from a clean triatomine colony, raised from bug eggs and fed only on birds, are allowed to feed on the patient. Bugs are applied in a plastic pot contained discretely in a black bag, which is tied beneath the patient's forearm. The bugs are dissected 20 to 25 days later. The hindgut and rectum are drawn out into a drop of sterile physiological saline, mixed with a blunt instrument (microspatula), and observed microscopically for motile epimastigotes and trypomastigotes. Dissection should be performed behind a small, Perspex safety screen or in a microbiological safety cabinet. *R. prolixus* is the most avid feeder for xenodiagnosis but may cause delayed hypersensitivity reactions in sensitized patients. Anaphylaxis is rare but two cases are known. The local vector should be used as the susceptibility of triatomine species varies with the strain of *T. cruzi*.

After the acute-phase infection, all the above methods of parasitological diagnosis will fail except xenodiagnosis and, possibly, multiple blood cultures. Up to 50% of patients in chronic phase may yield a positive xenodiagnosis, providing at least 10 triatomine bugs are used. Although polymerase chain reaction amplification of *T. cruzi* DNA is sensitive and specific, it is not yet available as a routine diagnostic test. Serum antibody is produced within a few days of *T. cruzi* infection and persists for life in untreated patients. There is an early IgM response, but it is not sustained at the high levels seen in African trypanosomiasis. Persistent IgG may be detected by the enzyme-linked immunosorbent assay, the indirect fluorescent-antibody test, or the indirect haemag-glutination test. Complement fixation, developed in 1913, is effective but now seldom used. Crossreactions may occur with visceral and mucocutaneous leishmaniasis, with treponematoses, and possibly with other hyperimmune responses or autoimmune diseases. Recombinant antigens have been used to improve species specificity and some are commercially available; rapid tests have also been introduced. The majority of diagnostic kits are prepared from *T. cruzi* II preparations but are presumed to be equally applicable to other lineages. Serological assays must be standardized with negative and positive control sera and by reference to experienced external reference centres to check reproducibility. Quality of commercial tests should not be presumed without reference to authoritative comparative studies. Transplacentally acquired IgG may persist for up to 9 months in infants born of seropositive mothers. However, IgM-specific seropositivity in such infants is an indicator of congenital infection. Note that IgM may decline rapidly in filter paper blood spots if they are used as the source of serum. Serology may be performed post mortem using pericardial fluid.

Treatment

Proven acute cases must be treated promptly in an effort to minimize tissue damage and neuron loss. The synthetic oral nitrofuran, nifurtimox was the first successful drug for the treatment of Chagas disease. Bayer has recently safeguarded supply by restarting production in El Salvador. Nifurtimox is given in three divided daily doses at 8 to 10 mg/kg for 90 days, up to double doses for infected children. Adverse effects, which may lead to interruption of treatment, can include anorexia, loss of weight, psychological disturbances, excitability, nausea, and vomiting. Benznidazole is an oral nitroimidazole. The adult dosage is 5 to 7 mg/kg in two divided doses for 60 days; for children, 10 mg/kg also in two divided doses for 60 days. Adverse effects may also demand interruption of treatment. These include rashes, fever, nausea, peripheral polyneuritis, leukopenia, and, rarely, agranulocytosis. Double or even higher doses have been used for immunocompromised patients, especially if meningoencephalitis is present. There is no guarantee that a full course of treatment will eliminate the infection. Although the value of drug treatment for chronic infections is still debated, it is favoured for children under 12 years or by some for those under 15 years, because children tolerate treatment better than adults. Favourable access to these drugs may be obtained via WHO.

Chemotherapy is an important part of supportive treatment. It has been argued that the chronic phase should treated more aggressively to eliminate T. cruzi and so prevent new inflammatory foci and the extension of tissue lesions, to prevent cardiomyopathy and megaorgans and reduce cardiac block and arrhythmia. Not only children and recently infected cases but all cases of the indeterminate chronic form of Chagas disease including chronic Chagas cardiomyopathy grade II of the New York Heart Association classification should be treated unless this is contraindicated by concomitant diseases or pregnancy. A suggested regimen is repeated 30 consecutive day treatments for 6 to 12 months with intervals of 30 to 60 days using combinations of drugs with different mechanisms of action, such as benznidazole + nifurtimox, benznidazole or nifurtimox + allopurinol, or triazole antifungal agents such as posaconazole, inhibition of sterol synthesis. Results of the Benznidazole Evaluation for Interrupting Trypanosomiasis trial (BENEFIT; ClinicalTrials.gov number, NCT00123916) are awaited.

In acute-phase heart failure, sodium intake is restricted and diuretics and digitalis may be indicated. Meningoencephalitis may require anticonvulsants, sedatives, and intravenous mannitol. Heart failure due to Chagas disease may require vasodilatation (angiotensin-converting enzyme inhibitors) and maintenance of normal serum potassium levels; digitalis is a last resort because it may aggravate arrhythmias. A pacemaker may be fitted to improve bradycardia not responding to atropine, or for atrial fibrillation with a slow ventricular response that is not responsive to vagolytic drugs, or for complete AV block. Amiodarone has been suggested as the most useful drug to treat arrhythmias but it may still be aggravating. For ventricular extrasystoles lidocaine, mexiletine, propafenone, flecainide, and β-adrenoreceptor antagonists may be effective. Lidocaine may be used intravenously in emergencies. It is essential to consult detailed WHO expert reports and physicians with substantial experience in the management of chagasic heart disease.

Surgery is a vital part of case management for Chagas disease. Resection of ventricular aneurysms has been suggested. Specialized surgery has been developed in Brazil for the treatment of megaoesophagus and megacolon. Early megaoesophagus may respond to balloon dilatation. The Heller–Vasconcelos operation, in which a portion of muscle at the junction of the oesophagus and stomach is removed, may alleviate megaoesophagus. Severe megaoesophagus requires replacement of the distal oesophagus, e.g. with a portion of jejunum. The modified Duhamel–Haddad operation has been considered the most successful surgery for correction of a megacolon: after resection, the colon is lowered through the retrorectal stump as a perineal colostomy. Subsequent suturing, under peridural anaesthesia, gives a wide junction between the colon and the rectal stump.

Prognosis, even in treated patients who show serological reversion, is unpredictable as the sequelae of damage due to the acute phase of Chagas disease cannot be foreseen.

Prevention and control

There is no vaccine against Chagas disease and no immunotherapy.

With the aim of activating a Th1 immune profile with stimulation of CD8+ T cells, several experimental vaccines, including recombinant proteins, DNA and viral vectors, and heterologous prime-boost combinations have been developed and proved immunogenic and protective in mice. However, there have been no clinical trials.

Chagas disease flourishes where there is poverty and poor housing conditions. There are proven methods of controlling domestic triatomine bugs. These depend on insecticide spraying, health education, community support, and house improvement. Synthetic pyrethroids are the insecticides of choice and several commercial sources are available. Vector control programmes consist of preparatory, attack, and vigilance phases. In the preparatory phase, the distribution of all dwellings must be mapped, the presence of infested houses assessed, and the attack and vigilance phases costed and planned. The attack phase involves spraying all houses and peridomestic buildings, irrespective of whether bugs have been found. During the vigilance phase, the community plays an essential role in reporting residual bug infestations, which elicit a rapid respraying response for the affected sites. Serology is vital for monitoring the success of control programmes. Children born after control programmes begin should be serologically negative beyond 9 months of age (to exclude transplacental transfer of IgG) except for infrequent cases of congenital transmission.

Blood donors in or from endemic areas should be screened serologically. If conditions demand the use of seropositive blood, it can be decontaminated with crystal violet (250 mg/litre) and storage at 4°C for at least 24 h. Potentially infected organ donors or recipients should be screened serologically. Seropositive immunosuppressed recipients are likely to suffer reactivated acute-phase infection. Prophylactic chemotherapy with benznidazole may be effective.

The Southern Cone programme launched a massive effort to eliminate T. infestans from Argentina, Bolivia, Brazil, Chile, Paraguay, Uruguay, and southern Peru. Domestic infestation in Brazil has been reduced by 85%. Uruguay and Chile are essentially free of vector-borne and blood-transfusion transmission. Substantial progress has also been made in the other participating countries. Similar international collaborations have been initiated in Central America and the Andean Pact countries. Reinvasion of sylvatic bugs into domestic habitats may complicate vector control in some regions. One example is T. brasiliensis in north-eastern Brazil, which reinvades houses from adjacent rock piles. A second example is R. prolixus, which, in some regions of Venezuela and Colombia, has the capacity to reinvade houses from adjacent infested palm trees, as demonstrated by comparative population genetics. A surveillance programme and rapid responses to new domestic triatomine populations has been planned to protect the Amazon against domiciliation of vectors.

Unanswered questions and future research

T. cruzi is of immense research interest. It is not entirely clear how the organism evades the host immune response. Furthermore, the pathogenesis of Chagas disease is not fully understood. Molecular methods have radically changed our understanding of the epidemiology of T. cruzi infection. Molecular features unique to trypanosomatids (trypanosomes and leishmanias) make T. cruzi an attractive model for molecular biologists. Further research is required to produce a nontoxic, low-cost oral drug, which would eliminate the reservoir of infection in humans, and to clarify further the population genetics and epidemiological significance of diverse strains. The origins and evolution of the organism and its vectors are also of considerable academic interest.

Trypanosoma rangeli

The second human trypanosomiasis in the New World is due to T. rangeli infection. T. rangeli is also transmitted by triatomine bugs, in particular the genus Rhodnius. In Rhodnius species, however, T. rangeli traverses the wall of the alimentary tract, infects the haemocoel, and reaches the salivary glands, in which the metacyclic infective trypomastigotes are produced. T. rangeli is thus transmitted by the bite of the triatomine bug and not by contamination with bug faeces. Although enzootic T. rangeli infection is widespread in Latin America, transmission to humans is virtually confined to areas in which R. prolixus is the domestic vector of T. cruzi. Coinfections of T. cruzi and T. rangeli may occur. The organism

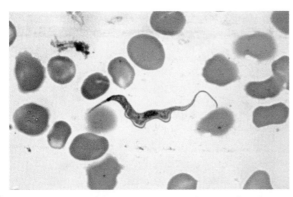

Fig. 8.11.10 *Trypanosoma rangeli* in a blood smear from an infected mouse. (Courtesy of J Williams.)

appears to be nonpathogenic in humans. *T. rangeli* can be pathogenic to *Rhodnius* species The importance of *T. rangeli* lies in the fact that it may confuse xenodiagnosis to detect *T. cruzi*. With care and experience, *T. rangeli* can be distinguished from *T. cruzi* either by its long slender epimastigotes (up to 80 μm in length) and its smaller kinetoplast or by its presence in the haemolymph or salivary glands of some xenodiagnosis bugs. The lifecycle in the mammalian host is uncertain, but *T. rangeli* is thought to divide in the peripheral blood. Trypomastigotes are rarely seen in human blood: they are much larger than *T. cruzi*, with a small subterminal kinetoplast (Fig. 8.11.10). Antibodies to *T. cruzi* certainly crossreact strongly with *T. rangeli*. Based on experimental work in mice, *T. rangeli* infections are thought to induce very low crossreactive antibody titres to *T. cruzi*. As with *T. cruzi*, there is subspecies genetic heterogeneity, with at least two and up to four distinct *T. rangeli* lineages, thought to be linked to two species groups within the triatomine genus *Rhodnius*.

Further reading

Bern C (2011). Antitrypanosomal therapy for chronic Chagas' disease. *N Engl J Med*, **364**, 2527–34.

Bethony JM, et al. (2011). Vaccines to combat the neglected tropical diseases. *Immunol Rev*, **239**, 237–70.

Castro JA, de Mecca M M, Bartel LC (2006). Toxic side effects of drugs used to treat Chagas disease (American trypanosomiasis). *Hum Exp Toxicol*, **25**, 471–9. [The potential side effects of treatment.]

Coura JR, Borges-Pereira J. (2011). Chronic phase of Chagas disease: why should it be treated? A comprehensive review. *Mem Inst Oswaldo Cruz*, **106**, 641–5.

Gaunt MW, et al. (2003). Mechanism of genetic exchange in American trypanosomes. *Nature*, **421**, 936–39. [The first experimental proof that *T. cruzi* has an extant capacity for genetic exchange.]

Maudlin I, Holmes P, Miles MA (eds) (2004). *The Trypanosomiases*. CABI Publishing, Wallingford, UK. [A detailed review of diverse aspects of both the South American and the African trypanosomiases.]

Miles MA (2004). The discovery of Chagas disease: progress and prejudice. *Infect Dis Clin North Am*, **18**, 247–60. [An account of historical and political aspects of the unusual discovery of Chagas disease.]

Miles MA, Feliciangeli MD, Arias AR (2003). American trypanosomiasis (Chagas disease) and the role of molecular epidemiology in guiding control strategies. *Br Med J*, **326**, 1444–8. [A synthesis of the application of molecular epidemiology to elucidate transmission of *T. cruzi* and guide interventions.]

Raia AA (1983). *Manifestações digestivas da moléstia de Chagas*. Sarvier, São Paulo, Brazil. [For the surgeon, fascinating accounts of the

development of lifesaving procedures, especially correction of megaoesophagus and megacolon (in Portuguese).]

Quijano-Hernandez I, Dumonteil E. (2011). Advances and challenges towards a vaccine against Chagas disease. *Hum Vaccin*, **7**, 1184–91.

Riera C, *et al.* (2006). Congenital transmission of *Trypanosoma cruzi* in Europe (Spain): a case report. *Am J Trop Med Hyg*, **75**, 1078–81. [A case history of congenital transmission in Europe.]

Sarkar S, *et al.* (2010). Chagas disease risk in Texas. *PLoS Negl Trop Dis*, **4**, pii: e836.

Schmuniz GA (2007). Epidemiology of Chagas disease in non endemic countries: the role of international migration. *Mem Inst Oswaldo Cruz*, **30** (Suppl. 1), 75–85. [Forewarning on the occurrence of Chagas disease outside traditional endemic regions.]

World Health Organization (2002). *Control of Chagas disease*, Technical Report Series 905. WHO, Geneva. [Not strictly on control, but one of the best clinical reviews of Chagas disease in the English language.]

Miles MA, *et al.* (2009). The molecular epidemiology and phylogeography of Trypanosoma cruzi and parallel research on Leishmania: looking back and to the future. *Parasitology*, **136**, 1509–28.

8.12 **Leishmaniasis**

A.D.M. Bryceson and Diana N.J. Lockwood

Essentials

Leishmaniasis is caused by parasites of the genus *Leishmania*, which are transmitted to humans from human or animal reservoirs by the bites of phlebotomine sandflies. In places the disease is common and important, with perhaps 500 000 cases of visceral leishmaniasis and 1.5–2 million cases of cutaneous leishmaniasis worldwide each year. As an imported disease, cutaneous leishmaniasis is common in travellers, military personnel, and immigrants coming from endemic areas, while the diagnosis of the less common visceral leishmaniasis is frequently overlooked.

Cutaneous leishmaniasis

Clinical features—at the site of the infected sandfly bite, an erythematous nodule typically develops into a sore which fails to heal spontaneously in (1) diffuse cutaneous leishmaniasis; (2) leishmaniasis recidivans; and (3) American mucosal leishmaniasis (espundia)—a condition in which mucosal lesions develop in 4 to 40% of patients with untreated cutaneous ulcers due to *L. brasiliensis*; the nose is most commonly involved, and eventually the whole nose and mouth may be destroyed.

Diagnosis and treatment—diagnosis is by demonstration of leishmania organisms in tissue smears or biopsy material by microscopy, culture, or polymerase chain reaction (PCR). Many leishmanial sores can be left to heal naturally, but treatment is indicated for those that are severe, or failing to heal spontaneously, or due to particular species (e.g. *L. brasiliensis*). Treatment may be (1) local—e.g. surgery/curettage; infiltration with a pentavalent antimonial; or (2) systemic—most cutaneous species of leishmania are sensitive to pentavalent antimonials.

Visceral leishmaniasis

Zoonotic disease is common around the Mediterranean littoral, across the Middle East and central Asia, in northern and eastern China, and in South and Central America. Anthroponotic disease causes large outbreaks in North Eastern India and the Sudan.

Clinical features—most infections are subclinical, but clinical presentation is with gradual onset of fever, discomfort from an enlarged spleen, abdominal swelling, weight loss, cough, or diarrhoea. The illness may be associated with HIV infection.

Diagnosis and treatment—diagnosis is by isolation of leishmania from spleen, bone marrow, liver, lymph node, or buffy coat. Serology is useful for diagnosis, and may replace direct demonstration of parasites in remote areas. The best treatment is intravenous liposomal amphotericin B, but (much cheaper) pentavalent antimonials are most often used in countries where visceral leishmaniasis is endemic.

Prevention

Prevention is by controlling reservoir hosts and sandfly vectors, or by avoiding bites by vectors. There is no vaccine.

Introduction

Leishmaniasis is caused by parasites of the genus *Leishmania*, which are transmitted by sandflies of the genus *Phlebotomus* in the Old World and *Lutzomyia* in the New World. The infection may be anthroponotic or zoonotic, having respectively human or animal reservoirs. In humans, the disease is usually either cutaneous or visceral. The most important variant is mucosal leishmaniasis of South and Central America. In places the disease is common and important, but there are few accurate statistics. The World Health Organization (WHO) estimates 500 000 cases of visceral leishmaniasis and 1.5 to 2 million cases of cutaneous leishmaniasis occur annually, with 200 million people at risk of each disease, but these figures may underestimate the problem. As an imported disease, cutaneous leishmaniasis is common in travellers, military personnel, and immigrants coming from endemic areas, while the diagnosis of the less common visceral leishmaniasis is frequently overlooked.

Aetiological agent and lifecycle

In its vertebrate host, the oval amastigote form of the parasite (2–3 μm in diameter) is found in cells of the reticuloendothelial system (Fig. 8.12.1). In the sandfly or in culture medium, it is in the elongated, motile, promastigote form with an anterior flagellum.

The most important species of *Leishmania* that cause disease in humans and their own reservoir hosts are shown in Table 8.12.1. Isoenzyme patterns and DNA hybridization are used to distinguish species.

Sandflies require a precise microclimate that is provided in certain places in each endemic focus at particular seasons of the year. Transmission is often seasonal. Amastigotes are ingested from blood or tissues of the mammalian host by the female fly and transform into promastigotes in the gut, rendering the fly infective after about 10 days.

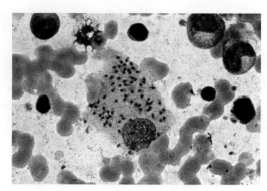

Fig. 8.12.1 Amastigotes of *L. donovani* in a reticuloendothelial cell. From the splenic aspirate of a child with visceral leishmaniasis in Kenya. (Copyright A D M Bryceson.)

Cutaneous leishmaniasis

Epidemiology

The vectors of *Leishmania major* live in rodent burrows. Visiting hunters, travellers, soldiers, and tourists, and dwellers at oases or in new settlements, are affected. The disease may be sporadic or epidemic, as recently among Afghan refugees in camps in Pakistan. The vectors of *L. tropica* live in crevices in buildings and walls. The disease may be endemic or epidemic. The vector of *L. aethiopica* bites people sleeping in their huts. The disease is endemic and most people are affected by early adulthood. *L. infantum* causes simple, self-healing skin lesions in some parts of southern Europe and North Africa. *L. donovani* causes post-kala-azar dermal leishmaniasis (PKDL) in India.

In the New World, transmission is usually in the forest. *L. brasiliensis*, the major cause of American cutaneous and mucosal leishmaniasis, is the most widely distributed of the New World species. Its vectors are highly anthropophilic and human infection is common. Periurban and urban foci of infection are increasing. Malnutrition is a risk factors for mucosal leishmaniasis. Infection with *L. peruviana* occurs in high Andean valleys, where it may be locally common.

Pathogenesis and pathology

Leishmania, when inoculated by the sandfly, invade and multiply in macrophages in the skin. The parasitized macrophage granuloma is infiltrated by lymphocytes and plasma cells. Piecemeal or focal necrosis destroys parasitized cells. The overlying epidermis shows hyperkeratosis and ulcerates. In chronic lesions, epithelioid cells and Langhans giant cells produce a picture similar to that of noncaseous tuberculosis. Rarely, the cellular immune response is suppressed and histology shows heavily parasitized macrophages with little or no lymphocytic infiltrate, characteristic of diffuse cutaneous leishmaniasis.

L. aethiopica, *L. mexicana*, and *L. brasiliensis* may invade cartilage. Cartilaginous lesions are extremely chronic. *L. brasiliensis*, and occasionally *L. panamensis* or *L. guyanensis*, may metastasize through the bloodstream to sites deep in the mucosa of the upper respiratory tract, where they may lie dormant. After months or years a lesion develops, characterized by necrosis, vasculitis, and tissue destruction.

Immunity to a given species of leishmania is usually lifelong. Second infections occur occasionally, especially in older people or immunosuppressed.

Table 8.12.1 Epidemiology of leishmaniasis

Organism	Geographical location	Reservoir	Main vectors
Old World			
L. donovani	North-east India, Bangladesh, Nepal	Humans	*Phlebotomus argentipes*
L. infantum	Mediterranean basin, Sudan, West Africa, Middle East, China, central Asia	Dogs, foxes, jackals	*P. perniciosus, P. perfiliewi, P. chinensis,* etc.
L. donovani (Africa)	Sudan, Kenya, Horn of Africa	Humans	*P. orientalis, P. martini*
L. major	Semideserts in North Africa and Middle East, north India, Pakistan, central Asia	Gerbils (especially *Rhombomys, Meriones*)	*P. papatasi*
L. major	Sub-Saharan savannah, Sudan	Rodents (especially *Arvicanthis, Tatera*)	*P. duboscqi*
L. tropica	Towns in Middle East, Mediterranean basin, central Asia	Humans, ?dogs	*P. sergenti*
L. aethiopica	Highlands of Kenya, Ethiopia, Uganda	Hyraxes (*Procavia, Heterohyrax*)	*P. longipes, P. pedifer*
New World			
L. chagasi (=*L. infantum*)	Most of Central and South America, especially Brazil	Dogs, foxes, opossums (*Didelphis*)	*Lutzomyia longipalpis, Lu. evansi*
L. mexicana	Central and northern South America	Forest rodents (especially *Ototylomys*)	*Lu. olmeca*
L. amazonensis	Tropical forests of South America	Forest rodents (especially *Proechimys, Oryzomys*)	*Lu. flaviscutellata*
L. brasiliensis	Tropical forests and cultivated land throughout South and Central America	Rodents, opossums, dogs, and equines	*Lu. wellcomei, Lu. whitmani,* etc.
L. guyanensis	Northern South America	Sloths (*Choleopus*), arboreal anteaters (*Tamandua*)	*Lu. umbratilis*
L. panamensis	Central America, Ecuador, Colombia	Sloths (*Choleopus*)	*Lu. trapidoi,* etc.
L. peruviana	West Andes of Peru	Dogs, rodents, opossums	*Lu. verrucarum, Lu. peruensis*

Clinical features

After an incubation period of a few days to several months, an erythematous nodule develops at the site of the infected sandfly bite. A golden crust forms (Fig. 8.12.2). The sore reaches its final size, usually 1 to 5 cm in diameter, over weeks or months. The crust may fall away, leaving an ulcer with a raised edge (Fig. 8.12.3). Satellite

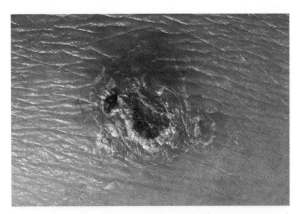

Fig. 8.12.2 Nodular lesion of cutaneous leishmaniasis. Showing crusting and small satellite papules, typical of early lesions of all species, in this case *L. brasiliensis*. (Copyright A D M Bryceson.)

papules are common. After months or years, the lesion starts to heal leaving a depressed, mottled scar. Any secondary bacterial infection is superficial and unimportant. The lesion is not normally painful, but may disfigure or disable if scarring is severe or over a joint. Draining lymphatic vessels may be thickened or nodular.

There are many variations on this classical pattern. Sores due to *L. major* form and heal rapidly (mean 3–5 months) and may be inflamed and exudative: the so-called wet or rural sore. Sores due to *L. tropica* tend to be less inflamed and to heal more slowly (mean 10–14 months): the so-called dry or urban sore (Fig. 8.12.4). Lesions due to *L. infantum* have an incubation period of many months and may persist over several years. In *L. aethiopica* infections, lesions are usually central on the face. Satellite papules accumulate to produce a slowly growing, shiny tumour or plaque that may not crust or ulcerate, taking between 2 and 5 years to heal (Fig. 8.12.5); mucocutaneous leishmaniasis may develop, producing swelling of the lips and expansion and elongation of the nose. Leishmanial lymphangitis may accompany sores of any species but

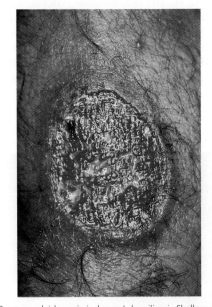

Fig. 8.12.3 Cutaneous leishmaniasis due to *L. brasiliensis*. Shallow ulcer with raised edge. (Copyright A D M Bryceson.)

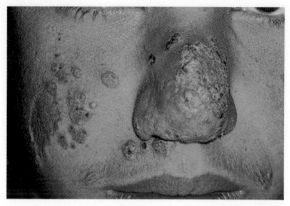

Fig. 8.12.4 Cutaneous leishmaniasis due to *L. tropica* in a young man in Kabul. Crusty nodular lesions are spreading on the face. There is a typical depressed scar of a previous lesion on the right cheek.
(Copyright Dr Mark Bailey.)

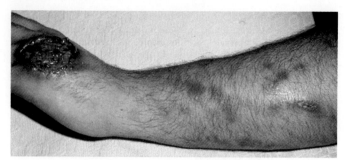

Fig. 8.12.6 Leishmanial lymphangitis in a man with cutaneous leishmaniasis from Belize. On occasion, hard thickened lymphatics may accompany an insignificant cutaneous lesion.
(Copyright A D M Bryceson.)

is commoner in the New World than the Old World (Fig. 8.12.6). On occasion, hard thickened lymphatics may accompany an insignificant cutaneous lesion.

L. brasiliensis often causes deep, spreading ulcers, which heal over 6 to 24 months. Up to 15% of patients will relapse after spontaneous or therapeutic cure. *L. mexicana* lesions are commonly on the limbs or side of the face and heal in 6 to 8 months. Sores on the pinna of the ear may invade the cartilage, persist for many years, and destroy the pinna.

Three forms of cutaneous leishmaniasis do not heal spontaneously: diffuse cutaneous leishmaniasis, leishmaniasis recidivans, and American mucosal leishmaniasis.

Diffuse cutaneous leishmaniasis

This occurs with *L. aethiopica* and *L. amazonensis* infections but is rare. The primary nodule spreads locally without ulceration and secondary blood-borne lesions appear at other sites in the skin, affecting especially the face and the cooler extensor surfaces of the limbs (Fig. 8.12.7). The eye, mucosae, viscera, and peripheral nerves are spared, which differentiates it clinically from lepromatous leprosy. The infection proceeds gradually over many years.

Leishmaniasis recidivans (lupoid leishmaniasis)

This is a rare complication of *L. tropica* infection. The initial sore heals, but papules recrudesce in the edge of the scar and the lesion spreads slowly over many years (Fig. 8.12.8).

American mucosal leishmaniasis (espundia)

Depending on the geographical location, between 4 and 40% of patients with untreated cutaneous ulcers due to *L. brasiliensis* develop mucosal lesions, half of them within 2 years of the appearance of the original lesion and 90% within 10 years. About one in six patients gives no history of a previous skin lesion. In most cases the nasal mucosa is affected, and in one-third another site is also involved: in order of frequency, the pharynx, palate, larynx, or upper lip. The initial lesion is a nodule and the initial symptom is of nasal obstruction. It commonly presents as protuberant new growth of the nose or lips (Figs. 8.12.9 and 8.12.10), or cicatrization, which causes an elongated 'tapir' nose. Mucosal leishmaniasis is slowly destructive, the septum perforates, and eventually the whole nose and mouth may be destroyed. Death may result from secondary sepsis, starvation, or laryngeal obstruction. Mucosal leishmaniasis is occasionally seen in travellers returning from South America.

Mucosal lesions are occasionally seen with Old World species, usually in the mouth or larynx, and tend to be associated with old age, corticosteroid medication, or other forms of mild immunosuppression (Fig. 8.12.11).

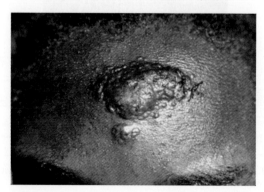

Fig. 8.12.5 Spreading nodular lesion typical of *L. aethiopica*, Kenya.

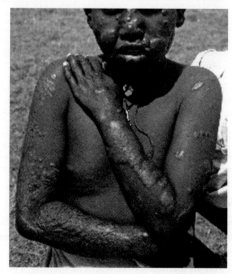

Fig. 8.12.7 Diffuse cutaneous leishmaniasis caused by *L. aethiopica*, Ethiopia.

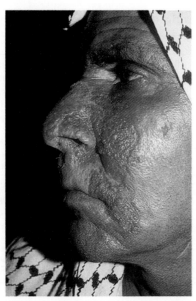

Fig. 8.12.8 Lupoid or recidivans leishmaniasis in a citizen of Baghdad. (Courtesy of Dr Ahmed.)

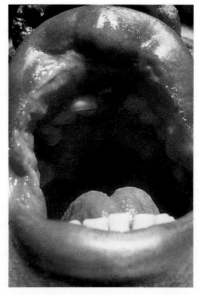

Fig. 8.12.10 Infiltration of lip and palate due to mucosal leishmaniasis in Peru.

Laboratory findings

Parasitological diagnosis

Normally, leishmania organisms may be isolated from 80% of sores during the first half of their natural course. The nodular part of the lesion is grasped firmly between the finger and thumb until it blanches. An incision a few millimetres long is made into the dermis with the point of a scalpel, which is used to scrape dermal tissue and juice. Material obtained may be used to inoculate special diphasic culture medium and to prepare smears for staining with Giemsa, Wright's, or Leishman's stains (Fig. 8.12.1). Biopsy material may be used to make impression smears, for culture and for histology for differential diagnosis. Polymerase chain reaction (PCR) using kinetoplast DNA primers is nearly 99% sensitive and 93% specific. Diagnosis of mucosal leishmaniasis requires a deep punch biopsy specimen. Species diagnosis by PCR is desirable for American parasites to assess the risk of mucosal leishmaniasis.

Immunological diagnosis

The leishmanin test is occasionally useful in differential diagnosis. It is an intradermal test of delayed hypersensitivity that indicates previous exposure to leishmanial parasites. It becomes positive in over 90% of cases of self-healing forms of cutaneous leishmaniasis and mucosal leishmaniasis. Evaluation of a positive test must take into account naturally acquired positivity in the population at risk. Serology is unhelpful.

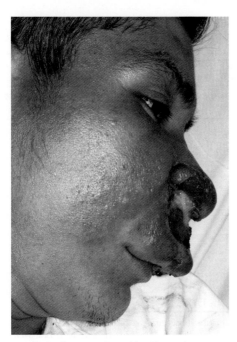

Fig. 8.12.9 Espundia. Swollen upper lip and 'tapir' nose due to mucosal leishmaniasis, at Instituto de Medicina Tropical 'Alexander von Humboldt' Universidad Peruana Cayetano Heredia, Lima, Peru. (Copyright D A Warrell.)

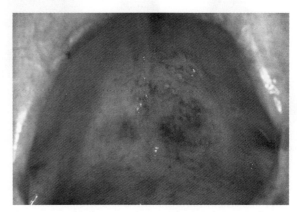

Fig. 8.12.11 Mucosal leishmaniasis due to *L. infantum*. Showing erythematous infiltration of the hard palate in an elderly British expatriate living in southern Spain and taking steroids for asthma. (Copyright A D M Bryceson.)

Treatment

Old World sores, or those due to *L. mexicana*, *L. amazonensis*, and *L. peruviana* that are not troublesome, may be left to heal naturally. But those that are disfiguring, potentially disabling, inconvenient, or around the ankle where they heal slowly, should be treated either locally or systemically. Systemic treatment is required when there is risk that the sore may be due to *L. brasiliensis*, *L. panamensis*, or *L. guyanensis*, when the sore is too large or badly sited for local treatment, when there is lymphatic spread, and for mucosal leishmaniasis, diffuse cutaneous leishmaniasis, and recidivans leishmaniasis.

Local treatment

Surgery, curettage, CO_2 laser, cryotherapy, and thermotherapy are effective methods of removing small sores. Infiltration into the lesion with a pentavalent antimonial, weekly for 2 or 3 weeks or longer, may be successful. The technique needs practice and the infiltration is transiently painful (Fig. 8.12.12). An ointment containing 12% paromomycin and 15% methylbenzethonium chloride cures 70% lesions due to *L. major* in 20 days and may be suitable for lesions caused by other species, except *L. brasiliensis*, but is not always well tolerated.

Systemic treatment

All cutaneous species of leishmania are sensitive to pentavalent antimonials in conventional dosage except *L. aethiopica*, where paromomycin may be used. Pentamidine is effective but seldom warranted because of toxicity. Ketoconazole or fluconazole may be useful for *L. major* and *L. mexicana* infections. Miltefosine is effective for *L. major*, *L. mexicana*, *L. guyanensis*, and *L. panamensis* infections. Patients with diffuse cutaneous leishmaniasis should be treated with two drugs for at least 2 months longer than it takes to clear parasites from the skin, and relapses should be treated again promptly. Relapsed cases of mucosal leishmaniasis have usually become unresponsive to antimonials and should be treated with amphotericin B deoxycholate for at least 4 to 6 weeks or liposomal amphotericin B for 3 weeks. See Tables 8.12.2 and 8.12.3 for dosage regimens. In addition, they may require antibiotics for secondary sepsis, attention to nutrition, and, later, plastic surgery.

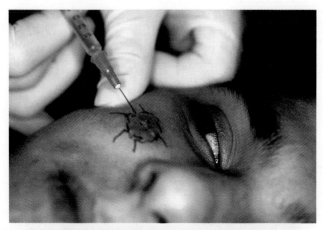

Fig. 8.12.12 Infiltrating a lesion of cutaneous leishmaniasis with sodium stibogluconate. The edge of the lesion is demarcated using a ballpoint pen and infiltrated radially from several points on its perimeter using an intradermal syringe and needle.
(Copyright A D M Bryceson.)

Table 8.12.2 Dosage regimens for the treatment of leishmaniasis

Drug	Dose
Sodium stibogluconate or meglumine antimoniate	By body surface area, so that: 10–20 mg Sb/kg body weight is given once daily for 21 days (visceral or cutaneous disease) or 28 days (visceral or mucosal disease)—PKDL may need treatment for 2–4 months. See Table 8.12.3 for dosage. By body weight: 20 mg/kg per dose as above, but less well tolerated by adults
Amphotericin B desoxycholate	1 mg/kg body weight on alternate days for 2 weeks (visceral disease) or 4–6 weeks (mucosal disease)
Liposomal amphotericin B	Ampoules of 50 mg, 3–5 mg/kg body weight per daily dose over a period of 3–6 days, to a total of 21 mg/kg. In India a total dose of 15 mg/kg is sufficient. A single dose of 10 mg/kg has a comparable cure rate. A 20-day regimen of 2.5 mg/kg cures PKDL in Sudan
Miltefosine	Adult dose 100–150 mg daily for 28 days; paediatric dose 2.5 mg/kg body weight daily for 28 days
Paromomycin	15 mg/kg body weight daily for 21 days
Ketoconazole	60 mg (11 mg base)/day (adult) for 4–6 weeks
Coadministered combinations	Two of the three drugs liposomal amphotericin B, miltefosine, and paromomycin, given in the doses above for 7–10 days

See text for choice of drug regimen.

Visceral leishmaniasis

Epidemiology

Visceral leishmaniasis is found in four main zoogeographical zones: the Ganges Brahmaputra plains, the Mediterranean basin extending into West and Central Asia, Sudan and East Africa, and Brazil (see Table 8.12.1).

Table 8.12.3 Simplified dosage regimens for pentavalent antimonials

Nearest weight of patient (kg)	Calculated dose (mg Sb)	Recommended dose in ml (mg Sb)	
		Sodium stibogluconate[a]	Meglumine antimoniate[b]
90	1088	11.0 (1100)	13.0 (1105)
80	1006	10.0 (1000)	12.0 (1220)
70	925	9.5 (950)	11.0 (935)
60	832	8.5 (850)	10.0 (850)
50	737	7.5 (750)	9.0 (765)
40	635	6.5 (650)	7.5 (637)
30	524	5.0 (500)	6.0 (510)
20	400	4.0 (400)	5.0 (425)
10	252	2.5 (250)	3.0 (255)
5	159	2.0 (200)	2.5 (212)

Calculations are based on body surface area according to the formula: body surface area in $m^2 = 0.13/kg^2$, whereby a 20 kg child receives 20 mg Sb/kg at 542 mg Sb/m^2.
[a] Sodium stibogluconate solution containing 100 mg Sb/ml.
[b] Meglumine antimoniate solution containing 85 mg Sb/ml.
(Adapted from Anabwani GM, Bryceson AD (1982). Visceral leishmaniasis in Kenyan children. *Indian Pediatr*, **19**, 819–22.)

Around the Mediterranean littoral, across the Middle East and central Asia, and in northern and eastern China, zoonotic visceral leishmaniasis is endemic in many places, where as many as 50% of domestic and stray dogs may be infected. Children under 5 years of age are especially affected. It is the second most common infectious cause of fever of unknown origin in children in the Balkan countries. HIV infection is a risk factor for adults. In other places, the disease is sporadic. Nonimmune adults such as tourists, hunters, and soldiers are susceptible.

The Ganges and Brahamputra river valleys of India and Bangladesh are the home of epidemic anthroponotic visceral leishmaniasis, or kala-azar, which returns approximately every 15 to 20 years. The majority of cases are in young people under 15 years of age and are found in clusters. The annual incidence is about 250 per 100 000. About 50% of household contacts of cases in Bihar India are seropositive, one in four of whom will develop disease. Malnutrition predisposes to clinical disease. In the interepidemic period, the parasite survives in patients with post-kala-azar dermal leishmaniasis.

Visceral leishmaniasis is endemic in parts of Sudan, where it may be both anthroponotic and zoonotic, and in adjacent parts of Ethiopia and Kenya. Older children and teenagers are most commonly affected. Sporadic cases also occur in nomads and visitors. In Sudan, an epidemic that began in the south in the late 1980s and caused over 100 000 deaths between 1984 and 1994 is still raging. It has been especially severe among refugees from the civil war. In remote areas, half the cases do not reach a medical facility and 90% of deaths go unreported.

In South America, the disease is most common in north-eastern Brazil, where older children are affected. Previously a rural disease, it is becoming increasingly important in towns.

Visceral leishmaniasis may appear unexpectedly in immunosuppressed patients, e.g. after renal transplantation, with haematological malignancies, while receiving immunosuppressive drugs, and in pregnant women. In endemic areas, it is an opportunistic infection in patients with HIV infection.

Visceral leishmaniasis may be transmitted by blood transfusion from subclinical cases; parasites were cultured from 2 to 4% of donor blood samples in endemic areas of France and Spain.

Pathogenesis and pathology

For every case of classical visceral leishmaniasis, there are about 30 subclinical infections that cause leishmanin positivity and lifelong immunity to the infecting species. Established visceral infections are characterized by the failure of specific cell-mediated immunity. The leishmanin test is negative. The parasite multiplies freely in macrophages in the spleen, bone marrow, lymphoid tissues, jejunal submucosa, and Kupffer cells of the liver. Histology shows a variable degree of granuloma formation and interstitial inflammation in the liver that may lead to fibrosis. In the spleen especially, there is massive reticuloendothelial hyperplasia and infiltration with plasma cells. Small splenic infarcts may develop.

Antibodies, polyclonal IgG, and immune complexes circulate at high concentration but rarely cause complications. About half of the patients have mild malabsorption but seldom diarrhoea. When present, jaundice usually has another cause such as viral hepatitis. Spontaneous bleeding is unusual and is associated with hypoprothrombinaemia. Visceral leishmaniasis is characterized by anaemia, leukopenia, thrombocytopenia, and hypoalbuminaemia. The anaemia results mainly from shortened red-cell survival with destruction of cells in the spleen, together with splenic pooling and sequestration (hypersplenism). In young children, profound anaemia may develop rapidly as a result of severe haemolysis. Death is usually due to secondary infection.

Clinical features

The male/female ratio is between 3:1 and 4:1. The incubation period is usually 2 to 8 months. In endemic areas, the onset is usually ill defined. The patient develops fever, discomfort from an enlarged spleen, abdominal swelling, weight loss, cough, or diarrhoea. Classically, the fever spikes twice daily, usually without rigors, but daily, irregular, or undulant fevers are common. During an epidemic or in visitors to an epidemic area, symptoms may start abruptly with high fever and rapid progression of illness with toxaemia, weakness, dyspnoea, and acute anaemia.

Physical examination of early cases may show only symptomless splenomegaly. Patients with advanced disease are wasted, with hair changes and pedal oedema typical of hypoalbuminaemia. Hyperpigmentation is characteristic of visceral leishmaniasis in India (kala-azar means 'black disease'). The spleen is huge, smooth, and nontender unless there has been a recent infarct. The liver is moderately enlarged in one-third of cases. In African patients, a generalized lymphadenopathy is common.

Over months or years the patient becomes emaciated, with a distended abdomen (Fig. 8.12.13). Intercurrent infections are common, especially pneumococcal otitis media, pneumonia, septicaemia, tuberculosis, measles, dysentery, other locally important infections, and rarely, cancrum oris. Untreated, between 80 and 90% of patients die.

Post-kala-azar dermal leishmaniasis (PKDL)

About up to 10% of Indian patients and up to 50% of Sudanese and East African patients develop a rash on the face, extensor surfaces of the arms and legs, and trunk after recovery from visceral leishmaniasis. In India, the rash begins after an interval of 1 or 2 years and progresses over many years: pale macules become erythematous plaques, papules, or nodules resembling lepromatous leprosy, and almost the entire body surface may be involved, including buccal and genital mucosa, and conjunctiva (Fig. 8.12.14). In Kenya, the rash usually appears while the patient is still recovering, as discrete nodules, which show a granulomatous histology with scanty parasites. It heals spontaneously within 6 months (Fig. 8.12.15). Sudanese patients show a mixture of these two forms. PKDL is rarely seen after *L. infantum* infections.

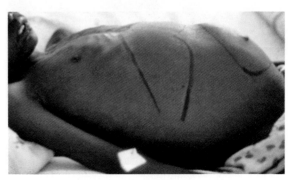

Fig. 8.12.13 Visceral leishmaniasis in a Kenyan child. Note the wasting, massive enlargement of liver and spleen, and increased pigmentation.

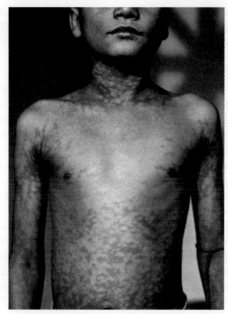

Fig. 8.12.14 Post-kala-azar dermal leishmaniasis in an Indian child. Showing the typical hypopigmented macular rash. Note also the nodules on the lower lip.

Visceral leishmaniasis and HIV infection

Visceral leishmaniasis may be associated with HIV infection, especially in southern Europe, where it is commonest among intravenous drug users. It may be due to reactivation of latent infection with leishmania or to a recent infection. In Spain, over 50% of adults with visceral leishmaniasis are HIV positive, and it is estimated that 9% of HIV-infected people will acquire visceral leishmaniasis. In northern India, during 2004/05, about 6% of all cases were coinfected with HIV. The presentation may not be typical and there may be unusual skin lesions. Antiretroviral treatment has greatly reduced the clinical impact of coinfection, but in some patients leishmaniasis now presents as an immune reconstitution inflammatory syndrome. Often the parasite is found by chance, e.g. in a rectal or skin biopsy taken for other purposes, or in bronchoscopic lavage. The bone marrow is teeming with parasites but two-thirds of cases have no detectable antileishmanial antibodies. In 90% of cases, the CD4 count is less than 0.2×10^6/litre. Response

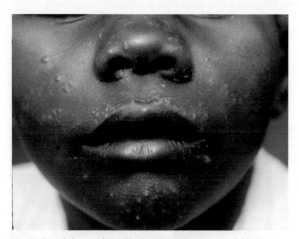

Fig. 8.12.15 Post-kala-azar dermal leishmaniasis in a Kenyan child. Showing the typical collection of small discrete nodules on the face.
(Copyright A D M Bryceson.)

to treatment is poor and relapse usual (see 'Treatment' below). HIV coinfected people are infective to sandflies and may also transmit parasites by sharing needles.

Laboratory diagnosis

Parasitological diagnosis

Leishmania organisms may be isolated from reticuloendothelial tissue. Yields are of the order of: spleen, over 95% cases; bone marrow or liver, 85%; lymph node in Sudan, 65%; and buffy coat, 70%. Bone marrow aspiration is most commonly used, but splenic aspiration is simple, painless, and safe if the prothrombin time is normal and the platelet count above 40×10^9/litre. Occasionally, the diagnosis is made accidentally on biopsy of bone marrow, liver, lymph node, or bowel mucosa. PCR for leishmanial DNA in bone marrow is even more sensitive. PCR for leishmanial DNA in blood is useful for follow up HIV co-infected patients.

Serological diagnosis

Except in HIV coinfections, antibodies are present in high titre, useful for diagnosis, and may replace parasite diagnosis in the remote areas. Indirect immunofluorescence is the gold standard but, for fieldwork, it has been replaced by enzyme-linked immunosorbent assay, direct agglutination, and the rK39 antigen dipstick. All give comparable results with sensitivities of about 90% and specificities above 95% (positive predictive value c.99% and negative predictive value c.70%). The leishmanin skin test is negative.

Other findings

There is normochromic, normocytic anaemia without reticulocytosis, and neutropenia, eosinopenia, and thrombocytopenia. Serum albumin is low (c.20 g/litre) and globulin high (c.70 g/litre), IgG and IgM being approximately thrice and twice the normal population values. Hepatic enzymes and prothrombin and partial thromboplastin times are usually normal.

Treatment

Chemotherapy

Liposomal amphotericin B by intravenous infusion is the best drug for visceral leishmaniasis in adults and children. It is concentrated and retained in reticuloendothelial cells and is not toxic. Over 99% patients respond promptly, but HIV-coinfected patients relapse. The drug is also effective against PKDL in India and Sudan and it is the drug of choice in pregnancy. The drug is becoming affordable in endemic countries where WHO has recently negotiated a 90% reduction in price. Otherwise, a pentavalent antimonial remains the drug of choice in most situations, except in Bihar, India. See Tables 8.12.2 and 8.12.3 for dosage regimens.

Conventional amphotericin B deoxycholate is cheaper than liposomal amphotericin B and just as effective, though more toxic, and is useful for patients unresponsive to antimonials.

Sodium stibogluconate containing 100 mg Sb/ml and meglumine antimoniate containing 85 mg Sb/ml are of equal efficacy and toxicity. The drug is administered by intramuscular injection, which may be painful, or by intravenous injection through a fine-gauge needle, slowly or by infusion in 50 to 100 ml of 5% dextrose over 20 min to reduce the risk of venous thrombosis. Treatment is given daily for 28 days. Usually the drug is well tolerated but towards the end of treatment there may be malaise, anorexia, nausea, vomiting, and muscle pains. Should toxic effects develop, rest for 1 day and reduce each dose by 2 mg Sb/kg. Hepatic and pancreatic enzyme levels may rise and haemoglobin levels fall, but they return to normal when treatment is stopped. The electrocardiogram develops unimportant T-wave changes. At higher doses, the corrected QT interval may be prolonged, heralding the development of a serious arrhythmia. Cure rates exceed 95% except in Bihar, north of the river Ganges where primary antimony resistance is spreading and up to 60% patients do not respond to antimonials.

The aminoglycoside antibiotic paromomycin, or aminosidine, is equally effective and well tolerated, but cure rates vary between countries and endemic foci. It is given by intramuscular injection or intravenous infusion over 90 min. Renal function and hearing should be monitored. Paromomycin is not readily available outside countries with control programmes.

The sole oral drug, miltefosine, cures from 90 to 94% of HIV-negative adults and children with visceral leishmaniasis in Sudan and India, even in areas of parasite resistance to antimonials.

Trials in Bihar have shown that 7 to 10-day courses of combined treatment with any two of liposomal amphotericin B, paromomycin, and miltefosine are highly effective.

Patients who are immunosuppressed as a result of HIV coinfection or immunosuppressive drugs respond slowly, require longer treatment, and are more liable to relapse than immunocompetent patients. Ideally, treatment of such patients should be monitored by splenic aspirate counts of parasites and continued for 2 or 3 weeks beyond parasitological cure. Antimonials cause adverse effects in two-thirds of HIV coinfected patients and may precipitate clinical pancreatitis. Liposomal amphotericin B and paromomycin are effective and well tolerated. Relapse may be prevented by secondary prophylaxis with pentamidine given every 2 weeks. Highly active retroviral therapy (HAART) reduces the number of relapses and delays their onset.

PKDL may be treated in India with miltefosine for 12 weeks or amphotericin B deoxycholate for 3 to 4 months; and in Sudan and East Africa with pentavalent antimonials for 30 to 60 days or liposomal amphotericin B for 20 days.

Supportive treatment

Intercurrent infection must be sought and treated and nutritional deficiencies corrected. Blood transfusion is rarely needed.

Response to treatment

Fever, splenic size, haemoglobin, serum albumin, and body weight are useful monitors of progress. Proof of parasitological cure is not usually necessary. Reassessment at 6 weeks and 6 months will detect over 90% of relapses. Serology is unhelpful in monitoring progress. Relapse rates should be under 4%. Relapsed patients are slower to respond and run a 40% chance of further relapses and of becoming unresponsive to antimony.

Economic impact

Visceral leishmaniasis is a major economic burden on affected families. The direct costs of an episode of visceral leishmaniasis in rural India or Bangladesh, where the drug is, in principle, provided free, are equivalent to the household's annual income.

Prevention and control of cutaneous and visceral leishmaniasis

Prevention is a matter of controlling reservoir hosts and sandfly vectors or of avoiding bites by vectors. Successful control requires an accurate knowledge of transmission in each ecological focus.

In the Old World, urban cutaneous leishmaniasis is controlled by case-finding and treatment, better housing, and domestic spraying with residual insecticides, while rural leishmaniasis is controlled in the Middle East and North Africa by poisoning or destruction of gerbil colonies. Mediterranean and urban visceral leishmaniasis in South America may be controlled by the destruction or treatment of dogs, but dogs are infectious to flies before they become symptomatic and screening of dogs is problematic. Dog collars impregnated with permethrin reduce the numbers of flies that become infected. In India, mass campaigns to spray houses and cattle sheds are needed in addition to case-finding and treatment. In the interepidemic period, cases of PKDL should be sought and treated. Currently no nation has an effective control programme in place.

In endemic populations, infection may be prevented during the season of transmission by the use of insect repellent creams and of fine mesh bed nets, top sheets or chadors (women's outer garments or cloaks) impregnated with permethrin during the hours of biting, usually around dusk and dawn. In endemic foci, a higher level of education in households is associated with lower rates of disease. Vaccines have proved disappointing.

Further reading

Blum J, et al. (2004). Treatment of cutaneous leishmaniasis among travellers. *J Antimicrob Chemother*, **53**, 158–66.

Cruz I, et al. (2006). *Leishmania*/HIV co-infections in the second decade. *Indian J Med Res*, **123**, 357–88.

den Boer M, Davidson RN (2006). Treatment options for visceral leishmaniasis. *Expert Rev Anti Infect Ther*, **4**, 187–97.

Desjeux P (2001). The increase in risk factors for leishmaniasis worldwide. *Trans R Soc Trop Med Hyg*, **95**, 239–43.

Lockwood DNJ, Sundar S (2006). Serological tests for visceral leishmaniasis. *Br Med J*, **333**, 711–12.

Murray HW, et al. (2005). Advances in leishmaniasis. *Lancet*, **366**, 1561–77.

Sundar S, et al. (2011). Comparison of short-course multidrug treatment with standard therapy for visceral leishmaniasis in India: an open-label, non-inferiority, randomised controlled trial. *Lancet*, **377**, 477–86.

Weisser M, et al. (2007). Visceral leishmaniasis: a threat to immunocompromised patients in non-endemic areas? *Clin Microbiol Infect*, **8**, 751–3.

WHO (2010). *Control of the leishmaniases: report of a meeting of the WHO Expert Committee on the Control of Leishmaniases, Geneva, 22–26 March 2010*. WHO technical report series; no. 949. World Health Organization, Geneva.

Websites

Centres for Disease Control. http://www.cdc.gov/parasites/leishmaniasis/index.html

World Health Organization. *Leishmaniasis*. http://www.who.int/leishmaniasis/en/ [Both have good summaries on leishmaniasis and links to new research findings.]

8.13 Trichomoniasis

Sharon Hillier

Essentials

Trichomonas vaginalis is a sexually transmitted protozoan pathogen that may cause more than one-half of all curable sexually transmitted genital infections worldwide. Women with trichomoniasis are often asymptomatic, but they may develop vaginal malodour, discharge, erythema, or itching, and their male or female sexual partners may also be infected, although urethritis in men is less likely to cause symptoms. Women with trichomoniasis have an increased risk of HIV acquisition, HIV shedding, pelvic inflammatory disease, and preterm birth. For diagnosis, rapid antigen detection, culture, and polymerase chain reaction (PCR) methods have advantages over conventional microscopy, but are more expensive. Oral metronidazole is usually an effective treatment, with both sexual partners needing to be treated to prevent reinfection.

Introduction

Trichomoniasis is an infection of the human urogenital tract caused by the protozoan *Trichomonas vaginalis*. There are about 170 million new cases each year, making it the world's commonest nonviral sexually transmitted infection and, according to the World Health Organization (WHO), it accounts for more than one-half of all curable sexually transmitted infections worldwide. Pregnant women who have trichomoniasis are at increased risk of preterm delivery as well as HIV acquisition and shedding.

Historical perspective

T. vaginalis was first described in 1836. In the preantibiotic era, it was considered a frequent unwanted outcome of sexual activity associated with symptoms but with few adverse health outcomes. With diagnosis and treatment, this infection has become less prevalent in wealthier countries but has remained highly prevalent in the developing world.

Aetiology, genetics, pathogenesis, and pathology

Although there are more than 100 species of this protozoan, only *T. vaginalis* parasitizes the human genital tract. *In vitro*, *T. vaginalis* has a well-defined, contact-mediated, cytotoxic effect, but its relationship to pathogenesis *in vivo* is unknown. It activates complement and attracts neutrophils, which may kill the parasite

Acknowledgement: The editors acknowledge the inclusion of material from Dr J P Ackers' chapter in the previous edition of the *Oxford Textbook of Medicine*.

but, in large numbers, may also contribute to the pathology. The organism produces several proteolytic enzymes which degrade genital tract mucins. Several potential *T. vaginalis* adhesions have been identified but, apart from its surface lipophosphoglycan, there is little evidence supporting a role in adhesion. Availability of the *T. vaginalis* genome sequence has allowed wider search for surface, soluble, and secreted proteins involved in host–parasite interactions. In women, *T. vaginalis* may be found in the vagina and the exterior cervix in over 95% of infections, but is recovered from the endocervix in 13%. The urethra and Skene's glands are also commonly infected. In men, the urethra is the most common site of infection but the organism has also been recovered from epididymal aspirates. Dissemination beyond the lower urogenital tract is extremely rare even in severely immunocompromised patients.

Trichomoniasis in women was previously regarded as unpleasant but harmless; however, epidemiological studies have now linked it with a modest increase in the risk of heterosexual HIV transmission, and with complications in pregnancy.

Epidemiology

Understanding the epidemiology of trichomoniasis has been limited by the variability in the sensitivity and accuracy of diagnostic methods used. Although it is often difficult to isolate the organism from male contacts of infected women, epidemiological evidence suggests that *T. vaginalis* is transmitted almost exclusively by sexual intercourse, both during heterosexual intercourse and in sexual activity between female sexual partners. Although the organism can survive for many hours at room temperature if kept damp, there is only limited evidence that this pathogen is transmitted among household members in the absence of sexual exposure. A very small proportion of female babies of infected mothers will become infected during birth, but this infection is transient and trichomoniasis discovered in a child should immediately raise the suspicion of sexual abuse.

Very few studies have been made of genuinely unselected populations; the majority have examined either pregnant women or those attending sexually transmitted disease clinics. Usually cases in women are observed 5 or 10 times more than those in men. *T. vaginalis* has been reported in 18 to 24% of women attending sexual health clinics in the United States of America and in 3 to 34% of women in four African cities. The epidemiology of this pathogen is less well understood among men, but has been reported in 3 to 20% of men attending sexually transmitted disease clinics. Factors associated with trichomoniasis include coinfection with other sexually transmitted pathogens, past infection with *Trichomonas*, being unmarried, having more than one sexual partner, and not using condoms.

In several developed countries, there has been a steady decline in the incidence of trichomoniasis in the past few decades, but this has not occurred in less-developed countries nor in deprived inner-city areas in industrialized nations. Human trichomoniasis is becoming a disease of the underprivileged.

Prevention

Because up to one-half of infected individuals are asymptomatic, the only way to reduce the population prevalence of this pathogen is through screening of individuals and providing treatment to individuals and their sexual partners. Several studies have documented improved cure rates in women whose male partners received treatment. Persons who report use of male or female condoms have a reduced incident of recurrent trichomoniasis. There is no effective vaccine against *T. vaginalis*.

Clinical features

In women, *T. vaginalis* can infect the vagina, urethra, and the Bartholin's and Skene's glands. From 10 to 50% of cases are asymptomatic but acute inflammatory diseases may occur, with copious and malodorous vaginal discharge, vulvovaginal soreness and irritation, dysuria, and dyspareunia. Trichomoniasis is significantly associated with purulent yellow vaginal discharge, vulvar itching, and colpitis macularis (strawberry cervix) detectable by colposcopy, with vulval and vaginal erythema. Vaginal pH is usually elevated and concomitant bacterial vaginosis is common. The discharge fluctuates with time and, if untreated, may disappear spontaneously or persist for months or even years.

Most men with trichomoniasis are asymptomatic, but the parasite is responsible for a small but increasing proportion of cases of nongonococcal urethritis.

Differential diagnosis

In women, vaginal discharge syndromes including bacterial vaginosis, yeast vulvovaginitis, and trichomoniasis should be considered (see Oxford Textbook of Medicine 5e Chapter 8.4). Women who present with vaginal discharge, vulvar itching, and/or vaginal malodour may have no infection, or could have any combination of these common vaginal infections. In men, other causes of urethritis should be ruled out.

Criteria for diagnosis

An accurate diagnosis cannot be made based upon signs or symptoms elicited during the clinical evaluation.

Trichomoniasis in women

The most commonly used method for diagnosis is identification of the pathogen in vaginal (not endocervical) secretions examined under the microscope at ×400 magnification. In clinical specimens or culture, *T. vaginalis* is a motile and round or oval flagellate, 10 to 13 μm long and 8 to 10 μm wide. Fixed and stained, it is about 25% smaller (Fig. 8.13.1). Diagnostic features include the jerky motility, undulating membrane, and microtubular rod (axostyle), which runs through the body and projects as a thin spine from the posterior end. In contact with vaginal epithelial cells *in vitro*, the organism becomes extremely flattened and adherent. The life cycle is simple; no resistant cysts are formed and there are no intermediate or reservoir hosts. Two other trichomonads, *T. tenax* and *Pentatrichomonas hominis*, are uncommon and probably harmless human parasites of the mouth and large bowel, respectively. All three species are site specific. Urogenital trichomoniasis is not due to contamination from other sites.

Microscopy is inexpensive and can be used as a bedside diagnostic test, allowing immediate treatment of infected people. However, its sensitivity is only 65 to 80% and it requires a microscope. Broth culture methods for detection of *T. vaginalis* have the advantage of

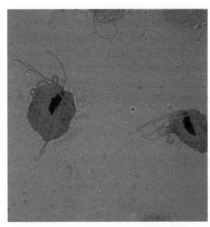

Fig. 8.13.1 Trichomonads in vaginal secretions (Giemsa stain). (Copyright J P Ackers.)

greater sensitivity, but require up to 5 days' incubation. Diamond's TYM and the very convenient if rather expensive InPouch system are among the best. Rapid antigen tests can be performed within the clinic in a few minutes. Their sensitivity and specificity are equivalent to those of culture, with the advantage of providing results during the clinic visit. The polymerase chain reaction (PCR) has the highest sensitivity and specificity for diagnosis of *T. vaginalis* but is expensive and requires specialized equipment, limiting its implementation. Specimens for PCR can be obtained less invasively with self-administered tampons.

Trichomoniasis in men

For diagnosis of urethritis due to trichomonas in men, culture or PCR is essential as the sensitivity of microscopy with urethral swab or scrapings, centrifuged urine sediment, or prostatic fluid is only 10 to 20%.

Treatment

The first, and the so-far only effective, drugs are 5-nitroimidazoles. A single 2 g dose of oral metronidazole is most widely used. The alternative is 250 mg three times a day for 7 days. Recurrence occurs in 8 to 20% of women in the first month after therapy. About half the occurrences are attributed to reinfection by the same or a new sexual partner. Women who experience treatment failure are more likely to have isolates of *T. vaginalis* that show reduced susceptibility to metronidazole *in vitro*. Single-dose metronidazole may not be adequate to treat these patients. Sexual partners must also be treated. Only the 7-day regimen has been extensively evaluated in men, in whom it appears as effective as in women. In pregnant women, single-dose metronidazole treatment probably achieves parasitological cure but one trial suggested increased risk of preterm and low-birthweight deliveries.

Prognosis

In most women who receive appropriate treatment, symptoms will resolve but they are at increased risk of becoming infected with *Trichomonas* in the future. Men may spontaneously clear their infections, but unless both sexual partners are treated, reinfection is common.

Areas of uncertainty or controversy

Trichomonisis has been linked with preterm birth, pelvic inflammatory disease (Oxford Textbook of Medicine 5e Chapter 8.5), and an increased risk of HIV. However, metronidazole treatment has failed to reduce the risk of preterm delivery or acquisition of HIV. No study has yet documented that accurate diagnosis and treatment of trichomoniasis provides a long-term health benefit for men and women.

Likely developments in the near future

Broader implementation of specific and sensitive screening tests and prospective studies of treatment should reveal whether routine screening and treatment of T. vaginalis reduces morbidity.

Further reading

Gülmezoglu AM, Azhar M. (2011). Interventions for trichomoniasis in pregnancy. *Cochrane Database Syst Rev*, **5**, CD000220.

Hobbs MM, et al. (2008). *Trichomonas vaginalis and trichomoniasis.* In: Holmes KK, et al. (eds) *Sexually transmitted diseases*, 6th edition, pp. 773–93. McGraw-Hill, New York.

Honigberg BM (ed) (1989). *Trichomonads parasitic in humans.* Springer-Verlag, New York.

Huppert JS, et al. (2007). Rapid antigen testing compares favorably with transcriptase-mediated amplification assay for the detection of *Trichomonas vaginalis* in young women. *Clin Infect Dis*, **45**, 194–8.

Johnston VJ, Mabey DC (2008). Global epidemiology and control of *Trichomonas vaginalis. Curr Opin Infect Dis*, **21**, 56–64.

Kissinger P, et al. (2008). Early repeated infections with *Trichomonas vaginalis* among HIV-positive and HIV-negative women. *Clin Infect Dis*, **46**, 994–9.

Klebanoff M, et al. (2001). Failure of metronidazole to prevent preterm delivery among pregnant women with asymptomatic Trichomonas vaginalis infection. *New Engl J Med*, **345**, 487–93.

Krieger JN (1995). Trichomoniasis in men: old issues and new data. *Sex Transm Dis*, **22**, 83–96.

Petrin D et al. (1998). Clinical and microbiological aspects of *Trichomonas vaginalis. Clin Microbiol Rev*, **11**, 300–17.

Ryan CM, et al. (2011). *Trichomonas vaginalis*: current understanding of host-parasite interactions. *Essays Biochem*, **51**, 161–75.

Van der Pol B, et al. (2008). *Trichomonas vaginalis* infection and human immunodeficiency virus acquisition in African women. *J Infect Dis*, **197**, 548–54.

Nematodes (roundworms)

Contents

9.1 Cutaneous filariasis

Gilbert Burnham

Essentials

Filarial infections are transmitted by simulium flies, some of which bite humans almost exclusively, whereas others are to varying degrees zoophilic. They are found worldwide in humans and animals, the filariae which cause cutaneous infections being *Onchocerca volvulus*, *Loa loa*, and the mansonellas.

Onchocerciasis

Onchocerciasis (river blindness), caused by *O. volvulus*, infects perhaps 20 million people, mostly in Africa.

Clinical features—larvae introduced into the body when the vector takes a blood meal develop into male or female adult worms within palpable nodules, commonly located over bony prominences. Other important manifestations are: (1) Eye damage—microfilariae enter the cornea from the skin and conjunctiva; manifestations include sclerosing keratitis, iridocyclitis and (sometimes) choroidoretinal lesions; without treatment permanent visual impairment or blindness are common. (2) Skin disease—ranging from itching with a localized maculopapular rash, to intensely itching with a chronic generalised papular rash or lichenified hyperkeratotic lesions.

Diagnosis, treatment, and prevention—diagnosis is usually made by finding microfilariae in skin snips. Treatment is with ivermectin, often given as a single annual dose, which has dramatically reduced the eye and skin lesions that ravaged many communities in Africa and Latin America. Methods of prevention include adding insecticides to rivers to interrupt simulium breeding and mass distribution of ivermectin.

Loa loa

This filaria, for which humans are the only host, is transmitted by the chrysops fly in West and Central Africa. Clinical manifestations include transient localized inflammatory oedema (Calabar swellings), the appearance of a migrating worm under the skin or (most dramatically) crossing the eye, and (rarely) meningoencephalitis. Diagnosis is based on typical clinical findings, or traditionally by finding microfilariae in a daytime blood sample. Treatment is usually with diethylcarbamazine, although both ivermectin and albendazole are effective. All treatments risk serious adverse reactions in the heavily affected. The best prevention is avoiding chrysops fly bites.

Mansonellas

This group of filarial infections is transmitted by culicoides midges and is common to many countries, but of negligible clinical importance under most circumstances. Only *Mansonella streptocerca* produces clear-cut manifestations, most typically chronic papular skin lesions. Diagnosis is by finding characteristic microfilariae in the blood or skin. People who are asymptomatic do not require treatment, but *M. streptocerca* responds well to ivermectin.

Onchocerciasis

Onchocerciasis, or river blindness, occurs in 34 countries in Africa, Latin America, and the Arabian Peninsula (Fig. 9.1.1). Perhaps 18 million people are infected and 125 million at risk of infection. The vast majority of these are in Africa. In 1995 it was estimated that infection with *Onchocerca volvulus* had caused blindness in 270 000 people, and left another 500 000 with severe visual impair-

ment. Mass treatment with ivermectin has now greatly lessened the ocular burden of infection. Besides eye changes, onchocerciasis has chronic systemic effects, causing extensive and disfiguring skin changes, musculoskeletal complaints, weight loss, changes to the immune system, and perhaps also epilepsy and growth arrest. Skin lesions are the most common manifestation of onchocerciasis. Changes include acute and chronic itchy papular disease, and intensely pruritic lichenification. Lesions may be localized or widespread. In the later stages severe degenerative skin disease develops, with a loss of elastic tissue, and extensive pigmentary changes.

The disease, endemic to some of the world's poorest areas, has a great impact on the economic and social fabric of communities. A complex human–parasite tolerance allows people who host millions of parasites to continue daily existence. Mass treatment with ivermectin has controlled the public health consequences of this disease in many heavily infected areas.

Epidemiology

The microfilariae of *O. volvulus* were first observed by O'Neill in Ghana in 1875 in an intensely pruritic chronic skin condition called 'craw-craw'. Leuckart described the adult worm 20 years later, and in 1923 Blacklock in Sierra Leone showed the blackfly *Simulium damnosum* to be the vector. Hissette in the Congo and Robles in Guatemala linked blindness with onchocerciasis. Long before, Ghanaians along the Red Volta river had associated the biting flies with skin lesions and blindness.

The Onchocerciasis Control Programme controlled vector breeding in West Africa's Volta basin between 1974 and 2002, and is thought to have prevented 600 000 cases of blindness. Today, the largest numbers of infected people live in Nigeria, Cameroon, Chad, Ethiopia, Uganda, Angola, and the Democratic Republic of the Congo. In the Americas, onchocerciasis was most common in the highland areas of Guatemala, but also present in Mexico, Venezuela, Colombia, Brazil, and Ecuador. Within foci, the disease may be distributed unevenly. An aggressive and efficient mass treatment of foci in these countries should eliminate onchocerciasis from the Americas by 2013.

In Africa, blindness was traditionally noted to be more common in savannah and woodland than rainforest areas, but people in forest areas had more depigmented skin disease. Different strains or forms of the parasite were shown to be present in savannah and woodland areas, particularly in West Africa. Environmental changes and migrations have now lessened these distinctions. Onchocercal skin disease reduces marital prospects (and dowry size), disrupts social relationships, and decreases the productivity of agricultural workers.

Parasitology

The larvae of *O. volvulus* enter the human during a blood meal taken by an infected female simulium fly. Within 1 to 3 months, larvae develop into male or female adult worms within palpable nodules commonly located over the bony prominences of the thorax, pelvic girdle, or knees (Fig. 9.1.2). Nodules may also be found on the head, particularly among children. These average 3 cm in diameter and are easily palpable, but some are deep, particularly around the pelvis.

A female worm may release 1300 to 1900 microfilariae per day for 9 to 11 years. From the nodules, these microfilariae find their way mainly to the skin and eyes. In the skin they are found

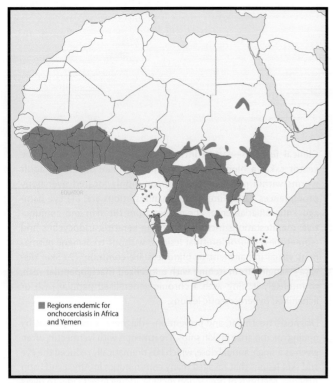

(a)

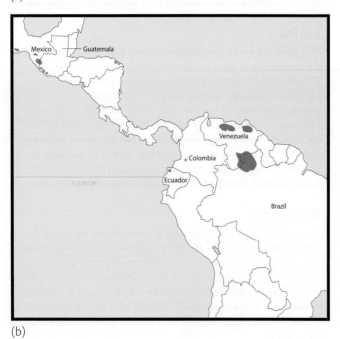

(b)

Fig. 9.1.1 Distribution of onchocerciasis in Africa and the Middle East (a), and Latin America (b).

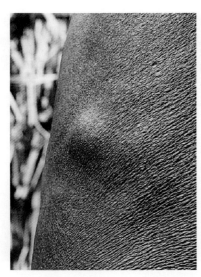

Fig. 9.1.2 A 3-cm subcutaneous nodule.

predominantly in the subepidermal lymphatics. In the eye, most microfilariae are in the anterior chamber, but are also found in the retina and optic nerve. When an infected human is bitten, anticoagulants from the simulium fly create a pool of blood from which blood and microfilariae are ingested. Within the fly, those microfilariae that survive moult twice over the following 6 to 12 days to become infective larvae.

Microfilariae are about 250 to 300 μm in length and may live for up to 2 years. They move easily through the skin and connective tissue, ordinarily remaining within lymphatic vessels and provoking little reaction while alive. They have been seen in blood, urine, cerebrospinal fluid, and internal organs. Millions of microfilariae may be present in a heavily infected person. Although live microfilariae are tolerated by their human hosts, dead and dying microfilariae may evoke intense inflammatory reactions, which are responsible for the eye and skin damage.

Important *Simulium* spp. are complexes made up of sibling species, identifiable through the banding patterns of their larval chromosomes. In Africa, the main vectors are members of the *S. damnosum* complex or *sensu lato* (*s.l.*), which can fly long distances. The vectors in areas of Uganda, Tanzania, Ethiopia, and the Congo are members of the *S. neavei* complex. In the Americas, complexes of *S. ochraceum*, *S. metallicum*, and *S. exiguum* are the principal vectors; these cover shorter distances. Some simulium flies will bite humans almost exclusively, whereas other species are to varying degrees zoophilic.

Simulium develop in water courses varying in size from broad rivers to small streams, depending on the individual sibling species. Rapidly flowing water provides the oxygenation needed for the development of the immature stages. Most larvae and pupae develop on rocks or vegetation just below the water surface, but those of *S. neavei* develop on amphibious *Potamonautes* crabs. During this development period the larvae are susceptible to insecticides. These breeding patterns have made the larviciding of water sources an effective control approach. Unique relationships have developed between the simulium fly and local parasites, so that flies from one geographical area do not efficiently transmit parasites from other areas. Simulium flies of the Americas are in

general less efficient at transmission than those of Africa, particularly those in savannah regions.

Clinical features

The manifestations of onchocerciasis are almost entirely caused by localized host inflammatory responses to dead or dying microfilariae. In a heavily infected person, 100 000 or more microfilariae die every day. The predominant immune response in onchocerciasis is antibody mediated, but with an important cellular component. Inflammatory responses may vary considerably between groups of people, depending on the length of exposure to antigens and the down-regulating activities of the host's immune system.

Eosinophils play an important role in the inflammatory response. Cellular proteins derived from eosinophils are deposited in connective tissues throughout the dermis, and bind to elastic fibres causing their destruction and, thereby, skin damage (see 'Skin disease' below).

An important discovery was that filarial parasites host endosymbiotic wolbachia bacteria. The inflammatory response to onchocerciasis seems largely attributable to the wolbachia rather than to the parasite itself. When the parasites were depleted of their wolbachia by doxycycline they did not induce corneal lesions. Further studies showed that inflammatory changes in the cornea in response to wolbachia were dependent on the expression of myeloid differentiation factor 88. Doxycycline may prove an alternative treatment for onchocerciasis in certain circumstances.

Exposure of the fetus to antigens associated with the parasite *in utero* and through breast milk may induce immune tolerance in residents of endemic areas. This could explain the difference in the disease patterns seen in people from nonendemic areas who become infected.

Among those coinfected with HIV there is a lessened reactivity to *O. volvulus* antigens, but no difference in adverse reactions following ivermectin treatment.

Eye damage

The risk of visual impairment increases as the prevalence and intensity of infection rises in a community. Microfilariae enter the cornea from the skin and conjunctiva. Punctate keratitis develops around dead microfilariae, and clears when inflammation settles. In those exposed to years of heavy infection, sclerosing keratitis and iridocyclitis are likely to develop, causing permanent visual impairment or blindness.

The first sign of sclerosing keratitis (Fig. 9.1.3a) is haziness at the medial and lateral margins of the cornea. This is followed by the migration of pigment onto the cornea, accompanied by a progressive ingrowth of vessels. Gradually the cornea becomes opacified. The central and superior areas are the last involved. Although eye lesions can be found wherever onchocerciasis occurs, blindness is most common in the West African savannah. Before control efforts began in Burkina Faso, 46% of men and 35% of women would eventually become blind.

Posterior segment lesions, which can coexist with anterior eye lesions, may be caused by inflammation around microfilariae entering the retina along the posterior ciliary vessels (Fig. 9.1.3b). Chorioretinal lesions are commonly seen at the outer side of the macula, or encircling the optic disc. Posterior segment changes are an important cause of loss of vision in Liberia. Optic atrophy

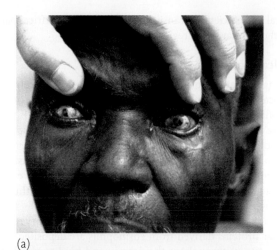

(a)

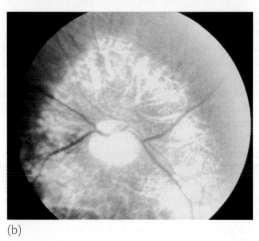

(b)

Fig. 9.1.3 (a) Bilateral sclerosing keratitis in a man blinded by onchocerciasis in Nigeria and (b) onchocerciasis producing a Hissette–Ridley fundus and optic atrophy in a person with central keyhole vision remaining.
(a, courtesy of Professor A D M Bryceson; b, courtesy of the Royal Tropical Institute, Amsterdam.)

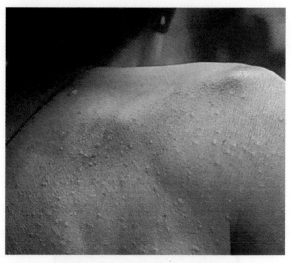

Fig. 9.1.4 Maculopapular rash.
Courtesy of Mauricio Sauerbrey.

Light-skinned expatriates infected while visiting an endemic area may present 1 year or more later with intensely itchy and red macular or maculopapular lesions. These may be confined to one area of the body or be more generalized, and may be associated with fever, muscle and joint pain, and sometimes oedema. Rash may sometimes persist for several months following ivermectin treatment.

In endemic areas, degenerative skin changes may develop in some people with long-standing infection. Elastic fibres are destroyed, leaving the skin thinned with a wrinkled cigarette-paper appearance. The atrophied skin begins to sag, the most extreme state being 'hanging groin' with its apron-like skin folds (Fig. 9.1.7). Depigmentation of the pretibial areas, or 'leopard skin', is a characteristic finding in older people living in endemic areas (Fig. 9.1.8).

has been reported in 1 to 4% of people with onchocerciasis in Cameroon, and 6 to 9% in northern Nigeria. Loss of peripheral vision is well recognized in onchocerciasis.

Skin disease

Of all the consequences of onchocerciasis, skin lesions are the most pervasive. Surveys of seven endemic sites in five African countries found that between 40 and 50% of adults had troublesome itching, which was so intense in some cases that the victims slept on their elbows and knees to minimize the symptoms.

In its mildest form, onchocerciasis presents as itching with a localized maculopapular rash (Fig. 9.1.4). These reactive lesions and itching may be evanescent, clearing completely without treatment in a few months. In other instances, the papular lesions may become chronic, generalized, and accompanied by severe itching (Fig. 9.1.5). Oedema and excoriations can be associated, and lesions may heal with hyperpigmentation. Particularly distressing are lichenified hyperkeratotic lesions, which may be widespread and intensely itchy (Fig. 9.1.6). A localized form of chronic papular dermatitis, often confined to one extremity, is known as 'sowda', Arabic for dark. In this condition, first described from Yemen, there is an exceptionally strong IgG antibody response.

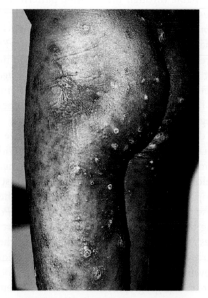

Fig. 9.1.5 Excoriated papular lesions of onchocerciasis with hyperpigmentation.

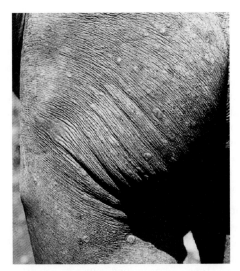

Fig. 9.1.6 Lichenified skin lesions with atrophy.

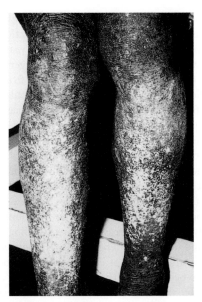

Fig. 9.1.8 Depigmented 'leopard skin'.

Other conditions associated with onchocerciasis

Both men and women with onchocerciasis weigh less than uninfected people and report more musculoskeletal pains. Evidence, first from Uganda and more recently from other African countries, has suggested a possible association between epilepsy and onchocerciasis. There is also evidence for an association between increasing microfilarial load and excess mortality.

A peculiar pattern of growth arrest beginning around the age of 6 to 10 years was reported from a Ugandan onchocerciasis focus near Jinja in 1951. This Nakalanga syndrome now seems to have disappeared from the area following the elimination of onchocerciasis, but has been noted in western Uganda, and may be present in Burundi. A condition of children in South Sudan, known as 'nodding disease', occurs in areas of onchocerciasis endemicity, though its pathogenesis is unknown. 'Nodding disease' has also affected small areas of Uganda and Tanzania. Clinical features include head nodding, mental retardation, stunted growth, blindness, body stiffness, endless running nose and saliva, and faecal and

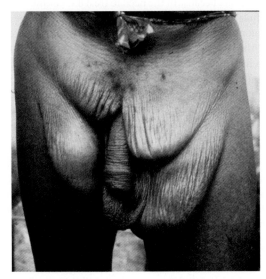

Fig. 9.1.7 'Hanging groins'.
(Courtesy of the late Dr B O L Duke.)

urinary incontinence. Onchocerciasis and neurocysticercosisare unlikely to be the cause and attention is turning to possible toxic contamination of food.

Diagnosis

Finding microfilariae in skin snips has been the time-honoured method of diagnosis. Microfilariae lie close to the surface, and are most plentiful in the iliac crest area, except in Latin America, where they are more common in the shoulder and scapular areas. Using either a scalpel blade or a sclerocorneal punch, four to six snips (about 5 mg each) are taken under sterile conditions and immersed in normal saline. Microfilariae swimming free of the skin fragments can be counted easily with a dissecting microscope within 24 h. The examination of excised onchocercal nodules shows sections of adult worms. Enzyme immunoassay and polymerase chain reaction (PCR) diagnostic methods have a high degree of sensitivity and specificity. Eosinophilia is common in onchocerciasis.

The Mazzotti test, in which people with onchocerciasis react with itching and a skin rash to 50 mg of oral diethylcarbamazine, is seldom needed for diagnosis, and can be dangerous in heavy infections.

For community assessment, the prevalence of nodules in 30 to 50 men over the age of 20 years, multiplied by 1.5, gives the approximate community prevalence of onchocerciasis. Where the prevalence of nodules is more than 40% the risk of blinding disease is high.

Treatment

The introduction of ivermectin for onchocerciasis in 1987 was one of the milestones of tropical disease treatment. The symptoms of onchocerciasis can be effectively controlled by the treatment of individuals attending clinics, or through the mass treatment of endemic communities.

Ivermectin is derived from *Streptomyces avermitilis*. A single dose of 150–200 µg/kg clears microfilariae from the skin for several months. Annual treatment controls microfilarial counts, and prevents the progression of clinical findings, although in some locations it is given twice yearly, with the intention of interrupting transmission. Treatment can be repeated if itching returns before the next dose is due. In the absence of reinfection, individual treatment should probably be continued for 10 years or more, or until microfilariae are no longer detectable. In Nigeria, after 8 years of treatment, gross visual impairment decreased from 16% to 1%, nodule prevalence fell from 59% to 18%, and papular skin dermatitis reduced from 15% to 2%. Treatment in pregnancy and under the age of 5 years is not recommended, although there has been no clear evidence of harm (increased risk of malformations or abortions) where treatment has been given inadvertently.

Limiting the numbers of microfilariae through annual ivermectin treatment improves early and advanced anterior segment eye lesions, halts the development of optic nerve disease, and improves severe onchocercal skin lesions. Adverse reactions to ivermectin commonly consist of increased itching, swelling of the face or extremities, and headache and body pains. Hypotension has been reported rarely after treatment in heavily infected people. Bullae have been seen occasionally. The most pronounced adverse reactions occur after the first ivermectin treatment, decreasing after subsequent treatment cycles. Ivermectin has no adverse effects in uninfected people. Although ivermectin temporarily reduces the release of microfilariae by adult worms, it does not destroy the adults. Those coinfected with *Loa loa*, are at risk of developing potentially fatal central nervous system events after treatment with ivermectin. Although most severe reactions occur with *L. loa* counts more than 30 000 microfilariae/ml, caution should be observed when treating anyone with counts greater than 8000 microfilariae/ml. It has been suggested that treatment with ivermectin in coinfected people be preceded by a 3-week course of albendazole to bring the *L. loa* count to less than 8000 microfilariae/ml.

Ivermectin appears to have several separate actions against the parasite. In microfilariae it acts primarily on parasite neurotransmitters, producing paralysis. This action appears to be mediated by the potentiation or direct opening of glutamate-gated chloride channels. The prolonged disappearance of microfilariae after a single treatment is the result of the drug's effect on embryogenesis in the adult female worm. There is also a poorly understood direct effect on the adult worm, which may be greatest against male worms. Treatment with ivermectin does not prevent the development of new infections by additional larvae introduced by bites of infected flies.

Resistance to ivermectin has been reported where veterinary parasites have been exposed to high and prolonged selection pressures. In 2007, in an area in Ghana under treatment for many years where many treatments had been given, the ivermectin effect of reducing embryogenesis was noted to have lessened, although ivermectin still retained its microfilaricidal effects. Further study found that people in this area of Ghana had received irregular treatment, with low coverage levels achieved. This has not been seen elsewhere, and may reflect irregular treatment patterns among some persons in these Ghana foci. As ivermectin is the only agent currently available for the control of onchocerciasis, the development of widespread parasite resistance would be of very serious consequence.

Prevention and control

Methods have included insecticides added to rivers to interrupt simulium breeding, mass distribution of ivermectin, and nodulectomy in an attempt to prevent blindness.

Vector control

Killing simulium larvae by adding the insecticide dichlorodiphenyltrichloroethane (DDT) to rivers eliminated onchocerciasis in Kenya and the Mabari forest of Uganda. In 1974, the Onchocerciasis Control Programme was formed to control simulium by larviciding rivers in the Volta basin of West Africa using ecologically suitable compounds. This highly successful vector control programme, later supplemented with ivermectin distribution, has now permitted tens of millions of people to live free of disease. Mass distribution of ivermectin is now the principal method for onchocerciasis control, although vector control may still be appropriate in a few locations, especially where transmission is with *S. naevi*.

Ivermectin mass distribution

After the effectiveness of ivermectin had been shown, its manufacturer Merck & Co. established the Mectizan Donation Program to provide the drug free 'for as long as necessary to as many as necessary'. Between 1988 and 2011, 900 million ivermectin treatments had been approved for endemic countries by the Mectizan Donation Program which oversees drug approvals.

The goal of a control programme in Latin America has been the elimination of disease through twice yearly treatment. This has effectively interrupted transmission in 7 of 13 foci with as few as 11 six-monthly treatments. It is anticipated that by 2012 transmission of onchocerciasis will be interrupted and treatment may be stopped, though with post-treatment surveillance in place. In Africa follow-up of three foci in Mali and Senegal where treatment was stopped after 15 to 17 years have shown that only a few cases of onchocerciasis remain, and that any black fly transmission is below the level necessary to sustain disease in the community. This has raised interest in elimination of onchocerciasis in Africa, previously thought not to be possible. Based on data from the Americas, twice or even four times yearly ivermectin treatment could greatly shorten the time needed to reach a point where transmission of onchocerciasis cannot be sustained in a community. Other models are not quite as optimistic. Treatment programs in Africa have focused on meso- and hyperendemic areas of disease, originally with a goal of reducing blindness. Elimination programmes would have to greatly expand treatment to include very large areas where onchocerciasis is hypoendemic. Because of the need to treat 85% or more of the eligible population for 15 to 20 years, initial efforts would be to focus on 'shrinking the map', with wide-scale elimination a more distant goal for Africa. However, the use of community-based distributors in Africa has proved a highly efficient and cost-effective approach which could take treatment to many new areas with treatment for other conditions included as well. The areas of Angola and northern Democratic Republic of Congo, which are heavily coinfected with *Loa loa*, present a great challenge to mass treatment.

Nodulectomy

A third form of onchocerciasis control has been the nodulectomy programmes of Mexico and Guatemala. For many years, health workers have moved from village to village removing nodules, especially around the head. The evidence for this preventing blindness is not strong.

Eliminating infections

Although ivermectin brings great relief to the individual, and has a clear impact on the disease in mass distribution programmes for affected populations, it does not kill adult worms. While symptoms and risks are controlled through annual treatment, the disease itself is not eliminated, and the potential for the development of drug resistance remains. A number of macrofilaricidal drugs capable of eliminating the disease through the killing of adult worms have been tested, but none has so far proved suitable for either individual or mass treatment. However, the search continues. It is the availability of a safe, inexpensive macrofilaricidal drug that is most likely to make the elimination of onchocerciasis possible.

Loiasis

Loa loa is a filaria transmitted by *Chrysops* spp. flies in West and Central Africa. The adult worm migrates beneath the skin, and sometimes across the eye, moving at about 1 cm per minute. Periodically, the infection causes sudden but transient localized inflammatory oedema known as Calabar swellings.

Parasitology

The larvae of *L. loa* burrow into human skin during feeding of the chrysops or mangrove fly (*C. silacea* or *C. dimidiata*). In humans, the parasites mature and live in the fascial layers. After 1 year or more, microfilariae are produced. Microfilariae are most heavily present in the blood in the daytime, between 10.00 and 15.00, when the chrysops fly bites. Once taken up by the fly, microfilariae go through developmental stages in the fly's thoracic muscles. After 10 days the fly is able to infect a human, and can do so for another 5 days.

Epidemiology

Infection is most common around the Gulf of Guinea, particularly in Nigeria and Cameroon, but extends through Central Africa into Chad, Sudan, and Uganda, and south to the Congo and Angola (Fig. 9.1.9). Humans are the only host, although a similar parasite is found in monkeys in the same areas. The fly lives in the rainforest canopy, and descends to bite humans, attracted perhaps by movement. Transmission may be most intense during the rainy season, when flies are breeding on the muddy banks of forest streams.

Clinical features

The first clinical symptoms of loiasis may appear as soon as 5 months after infection, or as late as 13 years. Calabar swellings appear suddenly, most commonly on the forearms or wrists, and sometimes following heavy exercise or exposure to heat. These oedematous lesions are red and itchy, and may be associated with fever and irritability, but are generally nontender.

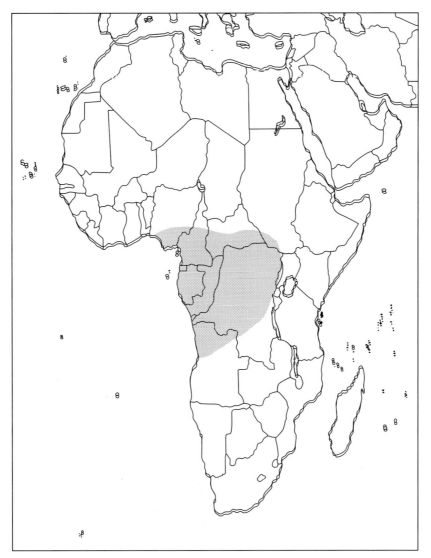

Fig. 9.1.9 Map of the approximate distribution of *Loa loa*.

After several days the affected part returns to normal. However, recurrence is common at irregular intervals. Swellings are not confined to the arms, but may be present in the face, breasts or legs. Calabar swellings are a hypersensitivity reaction to worm antigens, which may be released in the process of migration or perhaps during the maturation of the worm. A high proportion of eosinophils are seen in peripheral blood smears, often exceeding 70%.

A second common feature is the appearance of a migrating worm (Fig. 9.1.10). This may be under the skin in any location, but is most dramatic when it crosses the eye ('eye worm'; Fig. 9.1.11). Other than local irritation of the conjunctiva while the worm is passing, and the obvious concern of the host, there are no serious consequences. The time of passage may last from 30 min to more than 1 day.

Rare but potentially serious consequences of *L. loa* are meningoencephalitis, renal disease, and endomyocardial fibrosis. Arthralgias have also been noted. The meningoencephalitis may occur spontaneously, although usually after treatment with diethylcarbamazine or ivermectin. Fatalities have been reported following treatment. The renal and endocardial complications of loiasis may have an immune origin.

Laboratory diagnosis

Diagnosis has traditionally been by the finding of microfilariae in a daytime blood sample, or by a history or typical clinical findings. The use of more sensitive PCR methods has shown that many, even perhaps most, of those infected do not have microfilariae in their peripheral blood.

Treatment

The standard treatment has been diethylcarbamazine, which kills microfilariae and many adult worms. The treatment is commonly given in doses of 5 mg/kg divided into 3 daily doses for 21 days. Fever, arthralgia, and itching can occur during treatment. Ivermectin at 200 μg/kg dramatically decreases the number of microfilariae and some of the loiasis symptoms, but has little macrofilaricidal effect. Two courses of treatment may be required. As with diethylcarbamazine, there is a risk of potentially fatal meningoencephalitis in those with high microfilarial counts. It is prudent not to treat those with concomitant onchocerciasis until *L. loa* counts have been reduced below 8000 microfilariae/ml with albendazole. Treatment with smaller doses of ivermectin does not offer any advantages.

Since many people with loiasis also have onchocerciasis, careful monitoring for severe eye and skin inflammation is important when giving diethylcarbamazine. A single treatment is unlikely to eradicate all adult worms, and in endemic areas reinfection is probable. Blood films for microfilariae or PCR tests should be followed to indicate the need for retreatment. Ivermectin is very active against microfilariae, but like diethylcarbamazine, poses the risk of a serious meningoencephalitis. As *L. loa* does not harbour wolbachia, treatment with doxycycline is ineffective.

Prevention

The best prevention is avoiding chrysops fly bites. Having window screens on dwellings, wearing clothing to protect the legs and forearms, and avoiding areas where biting is frequent can reduce the risk. Chemoprophylaxis with diethylcarbamazine has been suggested, using either 5 mg/kg on three consecutive days in a month, or a weekly dose of 300 mg while living in an area of transmission.

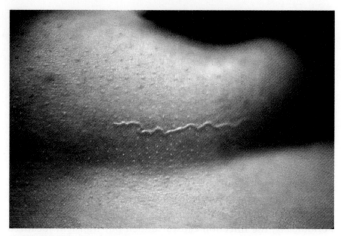

Fig. 9.1.10 Migrating *Loa loa*.

Mansonellosis

Mansonella spp. are a group of filarial species common to many countries, but are of negligible clinical importance under most circumstances. Infection is transmitted by *Culicoides* spp. midges.

Epidemiology

Mansonella (formerly *Dipetalonema*) *perstans* is found in much of tropical Africa, as well as Trinidad and several parts of South America. The adult worms live free in the abdominal cavity, and microfilariae are found in the blood and skin. *Mansonella ozzardi* is found in the West Indies and Central and South America. In addition to culicoides, simulium flies have been reported to transmit *M. ozzardi* in the Amazon basin. *Mansonella streptocerca* is a common infection in West and Central Africa, extending into western Uganda. Both microfilariae and adult worms are found in the skin, but without the nodules seen in onchocerciasis. Unless *M. streptocerca* microfilariae are differentiated parasitologically from those of *O. volvulus*, inappropriate mass onchocerciasis treatment programmes could be implemented.

Clinical manifestations

Of the mansonellas, only *M. streptocerca* produces clear-cut symptoms, although even these can be confused with those of *O. volvulus*, which may be a coinfection. Chronic papular lesions are commonly present, often associated with postinflammatory hyperpigmentation. Lichenification may occur less commonly. Hypopigmentation has been noted in areas of skin overlying the

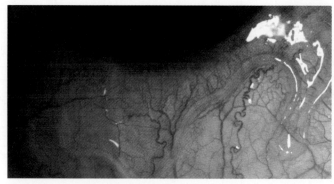

Fig. 9.1.11 *Loa loa* crossing the bulbar conjunctiva.

location of adult worms in the skin. In general, these findings are not easily distinguishable from those of onchocerciasis. Eosinophilia is common.

M. perstans has been reported to produce Calabar-like swellings, pruritus, fever, and headache. *M. ozzardi* infections are generally asymptomatic, although fever, arthralgia, headache, and itching have been associated with infection in the Amazon area.

Diagnosis

Diagnosis is by finding characteristic microfilariae in the blood or skin. The tails of the microfilariae have a distinctive walking-stick shape, and contain four prominent nuclei, distinguishing them from microfilariae of *O. volvulus*. A PCR assay as been described for *M. streptocerca*, and both quantitative buffy coat fluorescent staining and enzyme immunoassay methods for *M. perstans*. Eosinophilia is a characteristic finding.

Treatment

In asymptomatic people no treatment is required. *M. streptocerca* responds well to ivermectin, producing prolonged suppression of circulating microfilariae. Mild reactions similar to those in onchocerciasis may be seen. The treatment of *M. perstans* with doxycycline is effective, consistent with the effect of drug on wolbachia. A combination of both diethylcarbamazine and mebendazole is highly effective against *M. perstans*, while ivermectin has little effect.

Further reading

Boussinesq M (2006). Loiasis. *Ann Trop Med Parasitol*, **100**, 715–31.
Bregani ER, *et al.* (2006). Comparison of different anthelminthic drug regimens against *Mansonella perstans* filariasis. *Trans R Soc Trop Med Hyg*, **100**, 458–63.
Brieger WR, *et al.* (1998). The effects of ivermectin on onchocercal skin disease and severe itching: results of a multicentre trial. *Trop Med Int Health*, **3**, 951–61.
Chan CC, *et al.* (1989). Immunopathology of ocular onchocerciasis. I. Inflammatory cells infiltrating the anterior segment. *Clin Exp Immunol*, **77**, 367–73.
Cooper PJ, *et al.* (1999). Eosinophil sequestration and activation are associated with the onset and severity of systemic adverse reactions following the treatment of onchocerciasis with ivermectin. *J Infect Dis*, **179**, 738–42.
Cupp EW, *et al.* (2011). Importance of ivermectin to human onchocerciasis: past, present, and future. *Res Rep Trop Med*, **2**, 81–92.
Cupp EW, *et al.* (2011). Elimination of human onchocerciasis: History of progress and current feasibility using invermectin (Mectizan®) monotherapy. *Acta Trop*, **120S**, S100–S108.
Diawara L, *et al.* (2009). Feasibility of onchocerciasis elimination with ivermectin treatment in endemic foci in Africa: First evidence from studies in Mali and Senegal. *PLOS Negl Trop Dis*, **3**, e497.
Emukah EC, *et al.* (2004). A longitudinal study of impact of repeated mass ivermectin treatment on clinical manifestations of onchocerciasis in Imo State, Nigeria. *Am J Trop Med Hygiene*, **70**, 556–61.
Fischer P, *et al.* (1997). Occurrence and diagnosis of *Mansonella streptocerca* in Uganda. *Acta Trop*, **63**, 43–55.
Garcia A, *et al.* (1995). Longitudinal survey of *Loa loa* filariasis in southern Cameroon. *Am J Trop Med Hyg*, **52**, 370–5.
Gillette-Ferguson I, *et al.* (2006). *Wolbachia*- and *Onchocerca volvulus*-induced keratitis (river blindness) is dependent on myeloid differentiation factor 88. *Infect Immun*, **74**, 2442–5.
Kaiser C, *et al.* (1996). The prevalence of epilepsy follows the distribution of onchocerciasis in a west Ugandan focus. *Bull World Health Organ*, **74**, 361–7.
Little MP, *et al.* (2004). Association between microfilarial load and excess mortality in onchocerciasis: an epidemiological study. *Lancet*, **363**, 1514–21.
Mackenzie CD, *et al.* (2012). Elimination of onchocerciasis from Africa: possible? *Trends Parasitol*, **28**, 16–22.
Mectizan and onchocerciasis: a decade of accomplishment (1998). *Ann Trop Med Parasitol*, **92** Suppl 1, S1–174.
Murdoch ME, *et al.* (2002). Onchocerciasis: the clinical and epidemiological burden of skin disease in Africa. *Ann Trop Med Parasitol*, **96**, 283–96.
Osei-Atweneboana MY, *et al.* (2007). Prevalence and intensity of *Onchocerca volvulus* infection and efficacy of ivermectin in endemic communities in Ghana: a two-phase epidemiology study. *Lancet*, **369**, 2021–9.
Ottesen EA (1995). Immune responsiveness and the pathogenesis of human onchocerciasis. *J Infect Dis*, **171**, 659–71.

9.2 Lymphatic filariasis

Richard Knight and D.H. Molyneux

Essentials

Wuchereria bancrofti, *Brugia malayi*, and *B. timori* are mosquito-borne nematode parasites that are important causes of morbidity, disability, and social stigma in tropical and subtropical countries. Bancroftian filariasis due to *W. bancrofti*, which has no animal reservoir, accounts for 90% of human infections worldwide.

Clinical features

Acute lymphatic filariasis—(1) lymphadenitis and lymphangitis—most common in the inguinal and femoral nodes; (2) acute genital—usually tender fusiform or cylindrical swelling of the spermatic cord; (3) abscess and fever—affected nodes may break down to produce an open ulcer.

Chronic lymphatic filariasis—(1) lymphoedema and elephantiasis—initially transient pitting oedema occurs during acute inflammatory episodes in proximal nodes; eventually brawny, nonpitting oedema becomes permanent; (2) chronic genital—most commonly hydrocele; (3) chronic lymphadenitis and lymphangitis; (4) chyluria and lymphuria; (5) nonlymphatic pathology—including tropical pulmonary eosinophilia, filarial arthritis, and filarial glomerulonephritis.

Diagnosis and treatment

Diagnosis—microfilariae are typically found in Giemsa-stained blood films, the sample is best taken at night (22.00–02.00), except in Oceania and parts of South-East Asia. Microfilariae are also sometimes found in aspirates from lymph varix, hydrocele, lymphocele of the cord, or in urine. A rapid antigen detection test allows the mapping of prevalence and assessment of the impact of mass drug distribution.

Treatment—diethylcarbamazine, which may provoke both local and systemic reactions, or doxycycline are needed in some situations, including infected visitors, people leaving infected areas, and those with tropical pulmonary eosinophilia or other clinical features where elimination of adult worms is a priority. Concurrent bacterial infection requires prompt treatment with antibiotics, and supportive bandaging can reduce chronic oedema.

Prevention

The Global Programme for the Elimination of Lymphatic Filariasis involves annual rounds of drug administration to all eligible persons to interrupt transmission, by reducing the numbers of circulating microfilariae, together with (in appropriate circumstances) vector control.

Introduction

Wuchereria bancrofti, *Brugia malayi*, and *B. timori* are mosquito-borne nematode parasites. They are important causes of morbidity, disability and social stigma in tropical and subtropical countries (Fig. 9.2.1). The total population at risk is estimated to be 1.307 billion in some 72 countries where these infections are endemic. Bancroftian filariasis due to *W. bancrofti* infects 120 million people of whom about 40 million have clinical disease and some 80 million have hidden lymphatic damage; it was introduced into the Americas from Africa by the Atlantic slave trade. The two *Brugia* species infect about 13 million people in South and South-East Asia. *B. timori* has a localized distribution in Timor Leste and Indonesia.

Aetiology: the biology of the parasite

The adult worms live in the larger lymphatic vessels and lymph nodes; many live as 'worm nests' within dilated lymphatics of the limbs and male genitals. The worms are smooth, creamy-white, and threadlike; females measure 8 to 10 cm in length and males 4 cm. Their lifespan is estimated to be 4 to 6 years, but may be longer—a critical issue for planning, implementation, and duration of elimination programmes. Mated females produce numerous microfilariae throughout their life; these actively motile embryonic worms are sheathed by the remnants of the egg shell. They are 180 to 290 μm in length and 7 to 10 μm in diameter, with diagnostic species morphologies in stained blood films.

Microfilariae migrate via the lymphatic system to the blood, where they have an estimated lifespan of up to 12 months. Their numbers in the peripheral blood vary during the day and night, a phenomenon known as periodicity, and when not circulating they are sequestered in lung and reticuloendothelial capillaries. Maximum counts in the blood coincide with the biting cycle of the vector. The species and strain of parasite determine the periodicity. Most common is the nocturnally periodic form, with maximum microfilarial counts found between 22.00 and 02.00, and virtual absence during the day. Alternatively, microfilariae may be present throughout the 24-h cycle, with prominent peaks during the day or the night; referred to as diurnal or nocturnal subperiodicity, respectively.

After ingestion by the mosquito, microfilariae penetrate the midgut and migrate to the thoracic muscles, where they mature over 9 to 15 days to infective third-stage larvae. These then migrate to the head of the mosquito and escape through the arthrodial membranes around the proboscis during a blood meal. Larval worms enter the puncture wound made by the vector, enter the peripheral lymphatic system, and most eventually reach the lymph vessels of the proximal limb and male genitalia. Sexual maturity and the appearance of microfilariae in the blood usually take 8 to 18 months, but sometimes only 3 months.

Both adult worms and microfilariae harbour *Wolbachia* bacterial endosymbionts that are essential for the reproduction and survival of the parasite.

Epidemiology and transmission

In endemic areas microfilaria prevalence rates increase steadily from early childhood and often reach a maximum in early adult life, when a

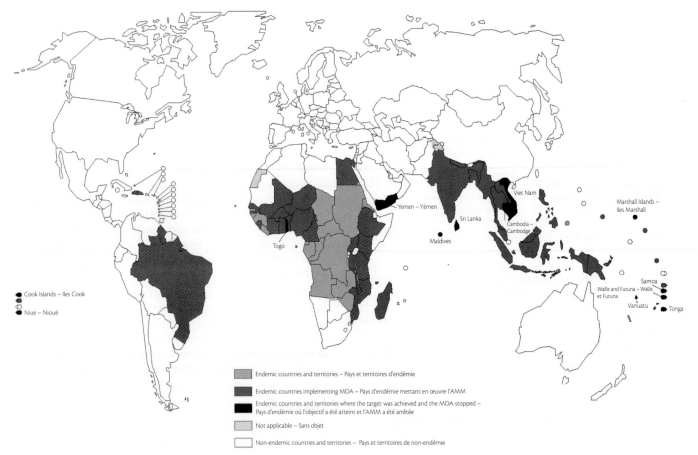

Fig. 9.2.1 Lymphatic filariasis endemic countries and territories by mass drug administration (MDA), 2010.
(Reproduced with kind permission of the World Health Organization.)

prevalence of 10 to 30% is not unusual in highly endemic areas. However, a recent meta-analysis suggests that prevalence, in the absence of a decline in transmission, may often continue to rise with age. Prevalence in males is generally higher, perhaps as a result of greater vector exposure. The cord blood of some infants shows microfilariae. Recent studies using an immunochromatographic card test (ICT) to detect adult worm antigen showed that in a population of Haitian children prevalence reached 25% by the age of 4 years. The ICT test is used to map the distribution of *Wuchereria bancrofti* and gives a prevalence of approximately double that detected by night blood films. Detailed mapping, using districts, assists in defining programme implementation units for the purposes of planning mass drug distribution.

W. bancrofti has no animal reservoir. *Brugia malayi*, however, is a zoonosis in some areas of its distribution (southern Thailand, Indonesia, and Malaysia), with a reservoir in cats and leaf monkeys, although their importance in maintaining the cycle in humans is not known; elsewhere it is an anthroponosis with only a human source of infection.

Mosquito vectors and geographical distribution

W. bancrofti infection

Culex spp. transmission

This vector, mainly *C. quinquefasciatus*, breeds mostly in organically polluted water, usually in urban and suburban areas, but also villages where there are suitable latrine and cesspit habitats. *Culex* is the most widely distributed vector and is increasing with urbanization; it occurs in India, Sri Lanka, Central and South America, some Caribbean islands, urban and coastal villages in East Africa and Egypt, and formerly in parts of China, where transmission has been eliminated. *Culex* bites at night; the microfilariae are nocturnally periodic. *Culex* is the most efficient vector and can maintain transmission at low microfilarial densities, making control difficult.

Anopheles spp. transmission

The same species of *Anopheles*, notably *An. gambiae* sensu lato and *An. funestus*, commonly transmit both filariasis and malaria in East and West Africa. In Papua New Guinea and Vanuatu the vectors are *Anopheles* of the *punctulatus* complex. *Anopheles* bites at night, mainly on the legs; microfilariae are nocturnally periodic.

Aedes spp. transmission

This is limited to southern Oceania, especially Fiji, Samoa, Tonga, the Cook Islands, and New Caledonia; but also patchily in Thailand, the Philippines, Vietnam, and the Nicobar islands. *Aedes* feeds throughout the 24-h cycle, but predominantly with a daytime biting peak, and bites all over the body; the microfilariae are diurnally subperiodic.

Ochlerotatus spp. transmission

This genus of mosquito transmits subperiodic and aperiodic strains of *W. bancrofti* in Asian forest habitats and in the Philippines, Samoa, and New Caledonia. Until recently this genus was classified in the genus *Aedes*.

B. malayi infection

Zoonotic *Mansonia* spp. transmission in swamp forests

This occurs in Malaysia, Indonesia, and southern Thailand. *Mansonia* bites mainly by night, but also during the day, usually on the legs below the knee; the microfilariae are nocturnally subperiodic.

Transmission in agricultural areas

In parts of Malaysia, Buru in Indonesia, and southern Thailand a mixed anthroponosis and zoonosis occurs in transitional zones, with monkeys and cats as reservoirs, and both *anopheles* and *mansonia* as vectors. Microfilariae have periodicities intermediate between nocturnally periodic and nocturnally subperiodic.

In India (mainly Kerala), Malaysia, Sulawesi, southern Thailand, and Vietnam infection involves humans only, with *anopheles* as the main vector and *mansonia* as an accessory vector; the microfilariae are nocturnally periodic.

B. timori infection

This is confined to Timor Leste and islands in the Lesser Sundas group in eastern Indonesia. *Anopheles barbirostris* is the vector, and the microfilariae are nocturnally periodic.

Pathogenesis

Local immunological reactions to worm antigens provoke acute and subacute responses, with dilatation of lymphatics and infiltration of tissues with eosinophils and monocytes. The antigens derive from the moulting fluids of developing worms, excretory products, microfilariae trapped within the lymphatic system, and also dying worms, including those killed by chemotherapy. *Wolbachia* lipoproteins from living and dying worms also provoke inflammation; thus, living worms can create lymph vessel dilatation and stasis. Several immunological mechanisms and cytokines are involved including vascular endothelial growth factors. Living worms also induce suppressive immunomodulatory responses that facilitate worm survival so that subjects with high blood microfilaraemias may have no evident clinical disease.

Dead and disintegrating worms become surrounded by granulation tissue with giant cells and epithelioid cells. Stasis and blockage of lymph vessels leads to distal dilatation, with varicosities and valve incompetence. Worms also cause local noninflammatory lymph vessel dilatation. Prolonged or recurrent lymph stasis leads to the accumulation of protein-rich interstitial tissue fluid, fibroblast proliferation, dilated dermal lymphatics, and epithelial acanthosis and hyperkeratosis.

Determinants of pathology include the duration of exposure, intensity of transmission, anatomical sites of infective mosquito bites, human genetic factors, and the species and strain of parasite. Prenatal exposure to filarial antigen is of great importance and induces immunological tolerance. Residents in high-transmission areas often show patent microfilaraemia, but little immunopathology. However, in some adults a later decline in microfilarial prevalence parallels increased host immunological reactivity and pathology. New residents and visitors show marked local reactivity to worms, and often no blood microfilariae; the latter situation was well documented among American troops in the Pacific in the Second World War, and French troops in former Indochina.

Clinical manifestations

Acute lymphatic filariasis

In endemic areas acute episodes are recurrent from the age of 10 years, and most frequent 4 to 8 months after the peak of seasonal transmission.

Episodes last several days or weeks; fever and malaise are common, but blood eosinophilia is not marked. Persons leaving endemic areas cease to have acute episodes after 1 year, although they may experience recurrent pain in previously affected tissues, especially after unusual exercise.

Filarial lymphadenitis and lymphangitis

Tender lymphadenopathy is most common in the inguinal and femoral nodes, but axillary and epitrochlear nodes are also affected. Tender retrograde lymphangitis typically spreads peripherally below the node.

Acute genital filariasis

This is uncommon in boys before puberty, but common thereafter. The typical lesion is funiculitis, with a tender fusiform or cylindrical swelling of the spermatic cord; epididymitis and orchitis are less common.

Filarial abscess and filarial fever

Affected nodes in the groin or elsewhere may break down producing an open ulcer that heals slowly leaving characteristic scars. Pelvic and retroperitoneal lymphadenitis can produce a febrile illness that is difficult to diagnose.

Chronic lymphatic filariasis

Lymphoedema and elephantiasis

Initially, transient pitting oedema occurs during acute inflammatory episodes in proximal nodes. Bacterial infection, often caused by *Streptococcus pyogenes*, is common in those with compromised lymphatics, especially when the skin is fissured, breached in an interdigital cleft, or when there is minor injury, an ulcer, or insect bite; this presents as cellulitis and ascending lymphangitis. Later, oedema persists between episodes, becoming distally nonpitting. Eventually, brawny nonpitting oedema becomes permanent (Fig. 9.2.2). In patients with leg involvement, epidermal thickening, papillomatosis, and fissuring are common (Fig. 9.2.3).

Chronic genital filariasis

Hydrocele (Fig. 9.2.4) is the most common lesion, and prevalence rates may reach 30% in men over 35 years in highly endemic areas; many patients give a history of preceding episodes of funiculitis or epididymitis. Hydrocele fluid is usually a transudate, but lymph or blood may be present. The tunica vaginalis is often thickened. Nodular lesions of the spermatic cord and epididymis are common, and the testis itself may become enlarged and indurated. Lymphoceles occur on the cord. Dilated dermal lymphatics in the scrotal wall associated with atrophic epidermis produce lymph scrotum, the skin having a velvety appearance. Rupture of these lymphatics leads to weeping skin lesions and often secondary infection, occasionally complicated by Fournier's gangrene caused by anaerobic bacterial sepsis.

Lymphoedema of the scrotum is a late sequel; often the testes are unaffected, and penile lesions are rare. Vulval lymphoedema is underrecognized; it is associated with dilated retroperitoneal lymphatics, and must be distinguished from lymphogranuloma venereum.

Chronic lymphadenitis and lymphangitis

Recurrent episodes of acute inflammation lead to persisting and sometimes massive lymph node enlargement. Thickened lymphatic cords may be palpable connecting the axillary and epitrochlear, or the femoral and popliteal nodes. Varicose lymph vessels may be visible in these areas. Lymph varices are fluctuant sacs of lymphatic tissue derived usually from the capsule of a node, hence the alternative term lymphadenocele. They partially empty when the part is

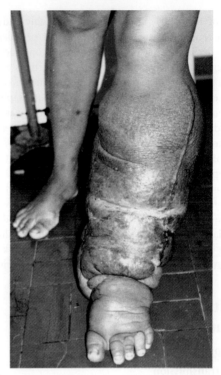

Fig. 9.2.2 Chronic elephantiasis in a man in Belém, northern Brazil. Note the scars of unsuccessful surgery.
(Copyright Pedro Pardal.)

raised, and aspiration reveals lymph or occasionally chyle. They occur in the medial thigh, groin, axilla, and sometimes even the neck.

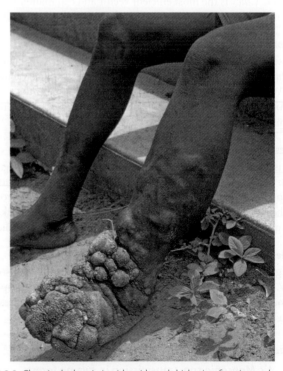

Fig. 9.2.3 Chronic elephantiasis with epidermal thickening, fissuring, and papillomatosis in a man in north-east Nigeria.
(Copyright D A Warrell.)

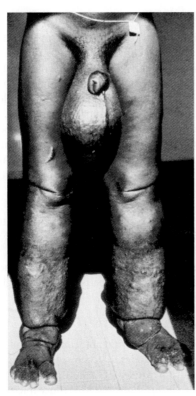

Fig. 9.2.4 Gross hydrocele in a patient with chronic filariasis.
(Courtesy of the late P E C Manson-Bahr.)

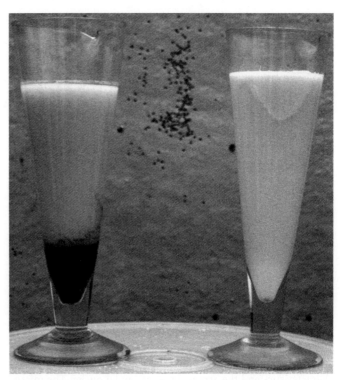

Fig. 9.2.5 Chyluria and haematuria in a patient with chronic filariasis.
(Courtesy of the late P E C Manson-Bahr.)

Chyluria and lymphuria

Dilated pelvic and retroperitoneal lymphatics may rupture into the urinary tract in the renal pelvis, ureter, or bladder. When there is lymph stasis above the cisterna chyli then small-bowel chyle may reflux into the urine postprandially. Chyluria is often intermittent and blood stained (Fig. 9.2.5). Continued loss of protein and lipids in the urine may lead to weight loss and cachexia. Chyluria may eventually be self-limiting.

Nonlymphatic pathology

Tropical pulmonary eosinophilia

This presents as a subacute or chronic illness with cough, wheezing, and reticular or miliary pulmonary shadowing. Microfilariae are absent from the blood, but eosinophilia is marked, and titres of filarial antibody are very high. Some patients have features of lymphadenopathic or genital filariasis, but many do not. Loss of lung function is restrictive. The response to antifilarial treatment is good, but untreated the condition can lead to pulmonary fibrosis and pulmonary hypertension. The syndrome is the result of a heightened immunological response to dead microfilariae, which may be found in biopsies of lung and other tissue surrounded by eosinophilic microabscesses. It occurs in most endemic areas, but is rare in Africa. It is more common in men, and rare in children, and many patients are not long-term residents.

Filarial arthritis

Joint involvement is subacute, and often recurrent with effusion; it usually affects the knee.

Filarial glomerulonephritis

This results from filarial and streptococcal immune-complex deposition on the glomerular basement membrane, but there is also tubular damage. Clinical findings include proteinuria and haematuria, which usually respond to chemotherapy. The incidence of clinically significant disease and its prognosis are uncertain.

Diagnosis

Clinical

Many patients will have several clinical features that, together with a history of preceding acute episodes, will be strongly suggestive diagnostically—manifestations such as varicose lymphatics, lymphadenocele, retrograde lymphangitis, and lymph scrotum are highly specific to filariasis. Genital lesions are rare in *Brugia* infections, which usually present with lymphoedema below the knee. In *B. timori* infection lymph node pathology in the legs is often severe, sometimes with skin ulceration. Upper limb and breast lesions are common in diurnally subperiodic *W. bancrofti* infections in the Pacific, but they do occur elsewhere with other strains of this parasite.

Parasitological

Microfilariae (Fig. 9.2.6) are typically found in Giemsa-stained blood films, but also in aspirates from a lymph varix, hydrocele, or lymphocele of the cord, or in urine in chyluria patients. Blood should be taken to coincide with the expected microfilarial periodicity. For quantitative studies, measured 10- or 20-μl volumes are used to prepare thick blood films. For measuring changes in intensity, larger measured quantities of blood (60 μl) should be used to increase the sensitivity and accuracy of a key parameter. Counting chambers taking 100 μl of lysed blood can be used, or larger volumes may be lysed and the spun deposit examined. A sensitive method which allows quantitation of parasite density is filtration of 1–5 ml of heparinized venous blood through a nucleopore filter

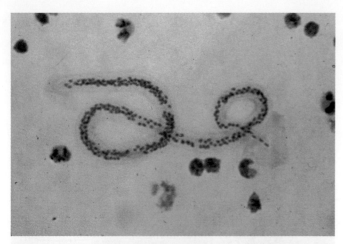

Fig. 9.2.6 Microfilaria of *W.bancrofti* on a Giemsa stained blood film showing sheath and row of terminal nuclei (right).

of pore size 5 microns; microfilariae on the filters can then be stained. Nocturnally periodic *W. bancrofti* microfilariae appear transiently in the blood 30 to 60 min after a 100-mg dose of diethylcarbamazine, which forms the basis of the provocation test. Species diagnosis of stained microfilariae is made by their sheath characteristics and the arrangement of caudal nuclei. The microfilariae of *Loa loa*, the tropical eye worm (found only in West and Central Africa) are diurnally periodic and also have a sheath; they must be distinguished from those of lymphatic filariasis.

Immunodiagnosis

Positive filarial antibody and skin tests are common in those exposed to infection, and may be of value in visitors to an endemic area. Several tests are now available for *W. bancrofti* antigen in serum, including a card test for field use. A positive test indicates persisting adult worms; antigen may be present in the absence of microfilaraemia. For *Brugia* infections, techniques for DNA detection by polymerase chain reaction (PCR) are available, and also specific IgG4 antibody tests.

Imaging of lymphatic vessels

Lymphangiography will delineate the anatomical details of abnormal lymphatic tissues, such as lymph varices and lymphatic connections to the urinary tract in chyluria. They are not usually diagnostic for filariasis. Scrotal ultrasonography can show nests of live worms—the 'filarial dance' sign; this can be used to assess the impact of chemotherapy on adult worms.

Lymphoscintigraphy using technetium-labelled dextran or albumin is a less invasive technique for demonstrating lymphatic pathology. Abnormal dermal lymphatics occur in many asymptomatic infected persons in endemic areas.

Drugs for the control and treatment of lymphatic filariasis

Filaricides may act against adult worms (macrofilaricides), against microfilariae (microfilaricides), or both. They often also act against other filarial infections such as *Onchocercaa volvulus* and *L. loa*; this may cause severe reactions in patients coinfected with these parasites. Side effects of filaricides are mainly due to immunological reactions to dying worms and the release of *Wolbachia* lipoproteins.

Diethylcarbamazine (DEC)

DEC was first introduced for treatment of lymphatic filariasis in 1948 and until 25 years ago it was the only drug available. It acts against both adult worms and microfilariae, but predominantly the latter; its mode of action is poorly understood but involves the arachidonic pathway. The resulting damage to the worm surface leads to vigorous immunological reactions that may be dangerous. A single dose of 6 mg/kg body weight greatly reduces the level of blood microfilariae for a year and kills some adult worms. In communities with low and declining endemicity many of the remaining adult worms are near the end of their lifespan and more easily killed with DEC.

Ivermectin

Ivermectin has a broad spectrum of antiparasitic activity. In lymphatic filariasis it acts only against microfilariae, and a dose of 100 to 200 µg/kg will clear microfilariae as well as DEC. Its action is rapid and side effects correlate with microfilaria load. Ivermectin immobilizes microfilariae by hyperpolarization of glutamate-sensitive channels.

Albendazole

Albendazole is a broadspectrum anthelminthic and is widely used to treat intestinal nematodes. It acts by inhibiting polymerization of β-tubulin and microtubules. A 400-mg dose will clear most intestinal nematode infections and will reduce microfilaria levels in lymphatic filariasis progressively over 6 to 12 months; greater reductions occur when it is given with either DEC or ivermectin, with which it acts synergistically against microfilariae. It does not kill adult worms.

Doxycycline

Doxycycline is a broad-spectrum antibiotic that kills the *Wolbachia* endosymbionts. A 100-mg or 200-mg dose given daily for 3 to 8 weeks will kill both adult worms and microfilarariae; its action is slow over 12 months and this greatly reduces the severity of side effects that occur in response to the rapidly dying worms and *Wolbachia* with other filaricides. Treated patients show a significant improvementof hydrocele, lymphoedema, and other clinical manifestations of lymphatic filariasis. Unfortunately the drug courses are contraindicated in children under 9 years of age and in pregnant women.

Filariasis at the community level

The Global Programme to Eliminate Lymphatic Filariasis

A World Health Assembly Resolution in 1997 launched a programme to eliminate lymphatic filariasis as a public health problem by 2020. This resolution was based on new evidence of the impact of two drug combinations on microfilaraemia, and the availability of a rapid antigen test (immunochromatographic card test) that allows mapping of the prevalence of disease and assessment of the impact of mass drug administration (MDA). Clinical studies had demonstrated that the annual distribution of diethylcarbamazine and albendazole, or albendazole and ivermectin, reduced microfilaraemia to levels that would interrupt transmission, provided that treatment with high coverage could be achieved.

The programme was backed by generous commitments by the manufacturers to donate albendazole and ivermectin (donated as Mectizan), for use with albendazole in Africa where diethyl-carbamazine cannot be used because of the risks in patients with onchocerciasis and loiasis. A global public–private partnership was formed in 2000, the Global Alliance to Eliminate Lymphatic Filariasis (GAELF). The extensive distribution of lymphatic filariasis required a regional approach to programme management and planning. According to GAELF strategy, countries launched programmes based on World Health Organization (WHO) recommendations on mapping, baseline data collection, and the establishment of evaluation and monitoring based on sentinel-site selection. Training drug distributors; selecting appropriate drug distribution systems; information, education, and communication; social mobilization needs; and reporting systems were recognized as being of great importance.

In 2010, having reviewed the global situation, WHO reported that 72 countries were endemic and 53 of these had implemented mass drug distribution to stop transmission; nine countries that were previously included in the list of endemic countries were deemed to be free of endemic disease. In 2010, a total of 622 million people were targeted for MDA, of whom 466 million received the recommended WHO two-drug combination of albendazole plus either ivermectin or diethylcarbamazine. The estimated numbers of cumulative treatments since the programme began in 2000 is around 2.8 billion treatments. These numbers suggest that conservatively at least some 310 million women of child-bearing age and school-age children have benefited from albendazole treatment reducing the burden of soil-transmitted helminths such as hookworm, *Trichuris*, and *Ascaris* and at least 25 million children have been born and will not be at risk of acquiring the diseases. Over 6.7 billion DEC tablets have been purchased, and 1.3 billion tablets of ivermectin (Mectizan) and 2 billion tablets of albendazole have been donated to date. The results of the 8 years of MDA programmes show that there have been significant public health gains as well as cost savings of around $24 million for the period 2000–2008. Apparent success in arresting transmission, based on several assessment measures, is now being reported from Egypt, Togo, Vanuatu, and Zanzibar. To assess the impact of MDA WHO has provided guidelines for Transmission Assessment Surveys (TAS) which are based on using immunochromatographic tests (ICT) in cohorts of children aged 6 to 10 years who were born shortly after the annual drug distributions began. Additional assessment of transmission or the existence of filarial parasites in the population can be achieved by a technique known as xenomonitoring when mosquitoes are caught and examined for the presence of filarial DNA.

The needs of patients already afflicted with lymphoedema and hydrocele must also be addressed. To this end WHO has issued guidelines for home-based care, whereby lymphoedema patients and their families are taught how to treat lymphatic filariasis -related lymphoedema and prevent acute attacks. WHO also aims to increase access to hydrocele surgery that uses new reconstructive techniques.

Despite resource constraints, particularly in sub-Saharan Africa, there are encouraging signs that the programme is reducing the prevalence of the disease. Egypt has reported the elimination of transmission in formerly endemic areas of the Nile delta. China has been certified by WHO as free of transmission in a population of some 350 million who were previously at risk. The Republic of Korea has also eliminated a focus of *Brugia malayi* and certified free of transmission. Several smaller countries previously demonstrated disease elimination following a range of different interventions. These are Suriname, Costa Rica, Trinidad and Tobago, and also the Solomon Islands, where vector control for malaria, using indoor residual spraying with dichlorodiphenyltrichloroethane (DDT) in the 1970s, appears to have been effective.

Population-based chemotherapy

In the past, different dosage regimens of diethylcarbamazine were used in many endemic areas. Drugs were given annually or 6 monthly, either to the whole population or to those found to be infected; medicated salt being the alternative. The main aim was to eliminate microfilaraemia and hence transmission, but with repeated doses many adult worms are eventually killed.

Ivermectin offers an effective alternative for reducing microfilaraemia, but does not kill adult worms. A single dose of 200 or 400 μg/kg of ivermectin is as effective as a 6 mg/kg dose of diethylcarbamazine. Both will virtually eliminate microfilaraemia for 6 or 12 months, adverse reactions are probably equally common with both drugs. Albendazole is also effective as a microfilaricide, and has some activity against adult worms. A 600 mg dose given annually can replace either diethylcarbamazine or ivermectin in a two-drug annual regimen. Annual dosage with either of these two drug combinations, continued for 4 to 6 years (the lifespan of nearly all adult worms), will interrupt transmission.

It is not recommended that diethylcarbamazine be given in areas where onchocerciasis or loiasis are endemic to avoid dangerous reactions. *Loa*-associated encephalopathy occurs especially in people with *Loa* microfilarial loads of more than 8000/ml of blood. Similarly, extreme caution needs to be exercised when community treatment with ivermectin and albendazole is implemented in areas where there is a high risk due to the prevalence of *L. loa* due to the risk of Loa-associated encephalopathy caused by the presence of high-intensity Loa microfilaraemia in some individuals. Maps have been produced of *L. loa* distribution. As there are few areas in sub-Saharan Africa where *Loa* and *Onchocerca* do not have potential overlap with *W. bancrofti*, the use of diethylcarbamazine has been discouraged or abandoned there in recent years.

In areas where population-based annual chemotherapy is in progress there is a reduced incidence of worm-related acute manifestations, and often reductions hydrocele size.

In *Brugia* areas recent studies have show that that mass drug administration programmes can reverse the subclinical lymphatic damage in children as well as providing what is termed 'beyond LF benefits' because the drugs have a wide spectrum of antihelminthic benefits as well as the impact of ivermectin on scabies. In addition, there is stabilization or regression in lymphoedema when this is managed by health education, skin hygiene, and antibiotics.

Vector control

The vector control method used depends on the habits of the local vector to be targeted: *Aedes* breeding sites, such discarded tins, tyres, or coconut shells, can be removed; *Culex* numbers can be reduced by improved sanitation, larvicides, and polystyrene beads applied to the water surface of latrines and cesspits. Bed nets and repellents are universally applicable.

However, vector control as part of the GAELF must be planned according to the cost of MDA, the collateral benefits from annual intervention with broad spectrum drugs, and the costs of vector control itself. Thus, vector control targeted specifically at the transmission of lymphatic filariasis itself has not been a major part of the global elimination programme. This is because a lymphatic filariasis specific vector control activity, whilst it may reduce the number of rounds of MDA, is not likely to be a sustainable or cost effective exercise. WHO promotes the principles of integrated vector management (IVM); hence in any country the vector control capacity must be assessed and opportunities for synergy and optimization of resources taken into account in initiating vector control. There is no doubt, however, that where there is vector control in *Anopheles* transmission areas to control malaria, i.e. bed nets, particularly long-lasting impregnated nets (LLINs) and indoor residual spraying, there will be an impact on the transmission of *W. bancrofti* which will likely reduce the number of rounds of MDA required. Evidence is emerging that LLINs alone at full coverage can arrest transmission. This strategy could be applied where *L. loa* is coendemic with *W. bancrofti* to reduce the risks of severe adverse reactions if ivermectin is used. There is also a case for implementation of vector control in settings where MDA has not not achieved the required reduction in prevalence (<1%) and intensity to reduce transmission below the threshold for parasite elimination.

Management of patients in clinics and hospitals

Chemotherapy

Individual chemotherapy with diethylcarbamazine or doxycycline is needed in some situations, including infected visitors, people leaving infected areas, and those with tropical pulmonary eosinophilia or other clinical features where elimination of adult worms is a priority. Doxycycline has the advantage that side effects are much less because of its much slower mode of action; it also has a significant morbidity reducing effect on both hydrocele and lymphoedema. Treatment with diethylcarbamazine may provoke both local and systemic reactions, and thus requires care and supervision in the initial stages, especially in *Brugia* infections. Coinfection with *L. loa* must be treated with great care as both ivermectin and diethylcarbamazine can cause encephalopathy when *Loa* microfilaria counts are high; patients coinfected with *Onchocera volvulus* should not be given diethylcarbamazine as serious ocular damage or systemic reactions may develop (see Chapter 9.1).

Diethylcarbamazine treatment should be started at 1 mg/kg on the first day, increasing over 3 days or more to 6 mg/kg daily. In the standard regimen 6 mg/kg is contnued for 12 days; alternatively this dose is given weekly for 12 weeks. These regimens are poorly evidenced based. Ultrasonography reveals the variable killing of adult worms, both within and between individuals, as even a single 600 mg dose will kill most worms in some patients. For tropical pulmonary eosinophilia a full 21 days of treatment is indicated, and may need to be repeated.

Doxycycline is given at a dose of 200 mg/kg daily for 4 weeks. Unless the patient is coinfected with L. loa a single dose of ivermectin 200 µg/kg is then given to clear microfilariae. For patients with hydrocele, and perhaps those with other morbidities, the doxycycline is given for 6 weeks. For Brugia infections, doxycycline 100 mg/kg for 6 weeks has been recommended.

Filarial worms harbour *Wolbachia* endosymbionts, which are antibiotic sensitive. In Tanzania an 8-week course of doxycycline 200 mg daily was effective against *Wolbachia bancrofti* adult worms, and reduced morbidity. More recently, in a study in India, a 3 week course produced a significant effect against adult worms and reduced lymphatic dilatation. Doxycycline clearly has therapeutic potential either combined with other filaricides, or alone when the latter are contraindicated; it is also effective against *O. volvulus* which harbour similar *Wolbachia*.

Surgical and supportive management

The acute manifestations of filariasis can mimic strangulated hernia and testicular torsion. The surgical treatment of filarial hydrocele is the same as that for nonfilarial disease. Scrotal lymphoedema can be treated surgically, usually with preservation of the testes. Lymphosaphenous anastomosis is being used for leg elephantiasis; many other procedures have been used in the past, often with disappointing results (Fig. 9.2.2).

Bacterial infection is common in those with lymphoedema, especially when skin integrity is breached. Early use of antibiotics, together with resting the affected limb, lessens the risk of increasing lymphoedema; supportive bandaging reapplied each morning reduces chronic oedema.

Further reading

Beaver PC (1970). Filariasis without microfilaremia. *Am J Trop Med Hyg*, **19**, 181–9.

Bockarie M, *et al* (2009). Role of vector control in the Global Programme to Eliminate Lymphatic Filariasis. *Ann Rev Ent*, **54**, 469–87.

Boggild AK, KeystoneJS, Kain KC (2004). Tropical pulmonary eosinophilia. *Clin Infect.Dis*, **39**, 1123–8.

Chu B, *et al*. (2010). The economic benefits resulting from the first 8 years of the Global Programme to Eliminate Lymphatic Filariasis (2000–2007). *PLOS Negl Trop Dis*, **4**, 708.

Critchley J, *et al*. (2005). Albendazole for lymphatic filariasis. *Cochrane Database Syst Rev*, **4**, CD003753.

Debrah AY, *et al*. (2009). Reduction in levels of plasma vascular endothelial factor-A and improvement in hydrocele patients by targeting endosymbiotic Wolbachia sp. in Wuchereria bancrofti with doxycycline. *Am J Trop Med Hyg*, **80**, 601–8.

Dreyer G, *et al*. (2006). Efficacy of co-administered diethylcarbamazine and albendazole against adult *Wuchereria bancrofti*. *Trans R Soc Trop Med Hyg*, **100**, 1118–25.

Dreyer G, *et al*. (1999). Acute attacks in the extremities of persons living in an area endemic for bancroftian filariasis: differentiation of two syndromes. *Trans R Soc Trop Med Hyg*, **93**, 413–17.

Dreyer G, *et al*. (2000). Pathogenesis of lymphatic disease in bancroftian filariasis: a clinical perspective. *Parasitol Today*, **16**, 544–8.

Dreyer G, *et al*. (2002). Progression of lymphatic vessel dilatation in the presence of living *Wuchereria bancrofti*. *Trans R Soc Trop Med Hyg*, **96**, 157–61.

Freedman DO, *et al*. (1994). Lymphoscintographic analysis of lymphatic abnormalities in symptomatic and asymptomatic human filariasis. *J Infect Dis*, **170**, 927–33.

Gyapong JO, Chinbuah MA, Gyapong M (2003). Inadvertent exposure of pregnant women to ivermectin and albendazole during mass drug treatment for lymphatic filariasis. *Trop Med Int Health*, **8**, 1093–101.

Helmy H, *et al*. (2006). Bancroftian filariasis: effect of repeated treatment with diethylcarmabazine and albendazole on microfilaraemia, antigenaemaia and antifilarial antbodies. *Trans Roy Soc Trop Med Hyg*, **100**, 656–62.

Jiraamonnimit C, *et al.* (2009). A cohort study of anti-filarial IgG4 and its assessment in good and uncertain MDA-compliant subjects in brugian filariasis endemic areas in southern Thailand. *J Helminthol*, **83**. 351–60.

Kim Y-J, *et al.* (2005). Genetic polymorphisms of eosinophil-derived neurotoxin and eosinophil cationic protein in pulmonary eosinophilia. *Am J Trop Med Hyg*, **73**, 125–30.

Langhammer J, Birk HW, Zahner H (1997). Renal disease in lymphatic filariasis: evidence for tubular and glomerular disorders at various stages of the infection. *Trop Med Int Health*, **2**, 875–84.

Liang JL, *et al.* (2008). Impact of five rounds of mass drug administration with diethylcarbamazine and albendazole on *Wuchereria bancrofti* in American Samoa. *Am J Trop Med Hyg*, **78**, 924–8.

Mand S, *et al.* (2009) Macrofilaricidal activity and amelioration of lymphatic pathology in bancroftian filariasis after 3 weeks of doxycycline followed by a single dose of diethylcarbamazine. *Am J Trop Med Hyg*, **81**, 702–11.

Molyneux DH (2006). Elimination of transmission of lymphatic filariasis in Egypt. *Lancet*, **367**, 966–8.

Norões J, *et al.* (1996). Occurrence of living adult *Wuchereria bancrofti* in the scrotal area of men with microfilaraemia. *Trans R Soc Trop Med Hyg*, **90**, 55–6.

Nuchprayoon S (2009). DNA-based diagnosis of lymphatic filariasis. *Southeast Asian J Trop Med Health*, **40**, 904–13.

Nutman TB (ed.) (2000). *Lymphatic filariasis*. Imperial College Press, London.

Ong RG, Doyle RL (1998). Tropical pulmonary eosinophilia. *Chest*, **113**, 1673–9.

Ottesen EA (2006). Lymphatic filariasis: treatment, control and elimination. *Adv Parasitol*, **61**, 395–441.

Otteson EA, *et al.* (2008). The global programme to eliminate lymphatic filariasis: health impact after 8 years. *Plos NTD*. **2**, e317, 1–12.

Shenoy RK, Bockarie M (2011). Lymphatic filariasis in children: clinical features, infection burdens and future prospects for elimination. *Parasitology*, **138**, 1559–68.

Supali T, *et al.* (2008) Doxycycline treatment for *Brugia* infected persons reduces microfilaraemia and adverse reactions after diethylcarbamazine and albendazole treatment. *Clin Infect Dis*, **46**, 1385–93.

Taylor MG, *et al.* (2005). Macrofilaricidal activity after doxycycline treatment for *Wuchereria bancrofti*: double-blind randomised placebo-controlled trial. *Lancet*, **365**, 2116–21.

Taylor MJ, *et al.* (2010). Lymphatic filariasis andonchocerciasis. *Lancet*, **376**, 1175–85.

Tisch DJ, *et al.* (2011). Reduction in acute filariasis morbidity during a mass drug administration trial to eliminate lymphatic filariais in Papua New Guinea. *PLOS Negl Trop Dis*, **5**, e1241.

Vijayan VK (2007). Tropical pulmonary eosinophilia: pathogenesis, diagnosis and treatment. *Curr Opin Pulm Med*, **13**, 28–33.

Weil GJ, Lammie PJ, Weiss N (1997). The ICT filariasis test: a rapid format antigen test for the diagnosis of bancroftian filariasis. *Parasitol Today*, **13**, 401–4.

Weil GJ, Ramzy RMR (2007). Diagnostic tools for filariasis elimination prgrammes. *Trends Parasitol*, **23**, 78–82.

Wongkamchai S, *et al.* (2006). Diagnostic value of IgG isotype responses against *Brugia malayi* antifilarial antibodies in the clinical spectrum of brugian filariasis. *J Helminthol*, **80**, 363–7.

World Health Organisation (2011). Global Programme to Eliminate Lymphatic Filariasis: progress report on mass drug administration, 2010. *Wkly Epidemiol Rec*, **86**, 377–8.

9.3 Guinea worm disease (dracunculiasis)

Richard Knight

Essentials

Guinea-worm disease (dracunculiasis)—now limited to sub-Saharan Africa—is caused by the nematode *Dracunculus medinensis*, whose life cycle involves water-borne copepod crustaceans and humans, who acquire the infection when they drink water containing infective larvae. Clinical presentation is usually with a skin blister, most often on the leg, sometimes preceded by allergic prodromal symptoms. Bacterial infection is a common complication. Most patients in endemic areas recognize their condition, but irrigation of ulcers can reveal larvae. Treatment is by physical removal of the worm; anthelmintics have no role in management. Provision of safe water for drinking is the key to prevention.

Introduction

The clinical manifestations of Guinea worm and its surgical removal were known in antiquity. Attention was drawn to the seasonal occurrence of painful limb blisters that broke down to reveal a 'worm' in the floor of an ulcer. *Dracunculus medinensis* is the longest nematode infecting humans; in the Bible it is described as the 'fiery serpent'. It was the first human parasite to be shown to have an arthropod intermediate host: in 1870 the Russian naturalist Fedtschenko described the worm's early development in *Cyclops*, a 'water flea'. Eradication programmes based on public health measures alone have been very successful. In 1986 3.2 million cases were reported from a total of 20 countries, but by 2010 this had been reduced to 1793 in five African countries. During the first 6 months of 2010 the provisional case count was 812 from four African countries.

Aetiology: the biology of the parasite

The life cycle of the Guinea worm is shown in Fig. 9.3.1. Mature female worms, 70 to 120 cm in length, migrate along fascial planes and subcutaneous tissue to reach the skin, usually below the knee. Tissue damage caused by worm products produces a blister that soon ulcerates (Fig. 9.3.2). Immersion of the affected part in water causes the worm to contract and expel numerous rhabditiform first-stage larvae from the uterus at the ruptured anterior end of the worm (Fig. 9.3.3). The larvae swim vigorously in water for up to 7 days, and some are ingested by predatory copepod crustaceans of the genus *Cyclops*. They penetrate the gut of the intermediate host, and develop with two moults in the haematocele over a period of 14 days to become infective third-stage larvae.

When water containing infected *Cyclops* is swallowed, the released infective larvae burrow though the wall of the duodenum to reach retroperitoneal tissue. After about 60 to 90 days the worms mate, and the females begin their migration towards the limbs; the male worms die and may later calcify. Ten months after infection most female worms, containing fully formed larvae, have reached

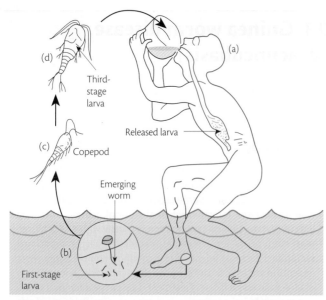

Fig. 9.3.1 Life cycle of Guinea worm in humans: (a) copepods infected with third-stage larvae are ingested in drinking water; larvae are released in the intestine, migrate to the body cavity, mature, and mate; (b) gravid female worms migrate to the limbs, cause a blister to form, and release first-stage larvae into water; (c) first-stage larvae are ingested by copepods; and (d) larvae undergo two moults in the copepod and are infective after 2 weeks.

their destination; within the next month they will rupture through the skin to begin the cycle anew.

Epidemiology

Guinea worm transmission is predominantly rural, with an annual cycle that often coincides with the planting or harvesting season. Usually, young adults and farmers are most at risk, and there is no immunity. The seasonal morbidity causes great economic hardship. Water sources containing *Cyclops* are easily contaminated by infected persons, including those seeking relief by immersing their painful lesion. In semiarid areas transmission occurs in temporary ponds during the rainy season; in wetter areas flooding and water turbidity limits transmission during the rains, and infection occurs

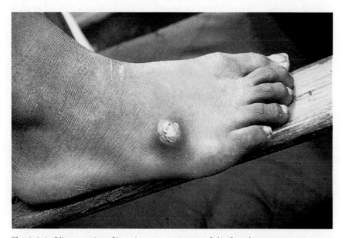

Fig. 9.3.2 Blister at site of imminent emergence of the female worm.
(Courtesy of the late P E C Manson-Bahr.)

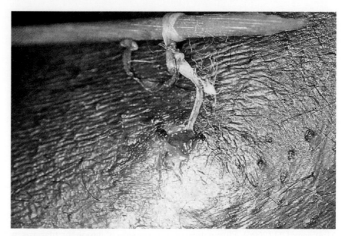

Fig. 9.3.3 Emergent female worm being wound out on a stick.
(Copyright D A Warrell.)

in shallow wells during the dry season. For practical purposes there is no zoonotic reservoir, although infected dogs have been found in endemic areas, and primates can be experimentally infected. Related *Dracunculus* spp. are found in mink, raccoons, and otters in North America.

Geographical distribution

This infection was previously endemic over wide areas of the Middle East and the Indian subcontinent. Largely as a result of improved and protected water sources the infection disappeared from the central Asian republics between 1926 and 1933, from Iran in the 1970s, and from Saudi Arabia in the 1980s. It was eradicated from Pakistan in 1996 and India in 2000. It is now limited to sub-Saharan Africa within the Sahel and Guinea savannah, between latitudes 2° north and 18° north (Fig. 9.3.4). It was also present in the Americas, having been introduced with the slave trade, but by the 1880s it had disappeared.

Clinical features

The blister (Fig. 9.3.2) is the first sign of infection in most patients. In others, pre-emergent worms may be seen or felt under the dermis; some are actively motile (Fig. 9.3.5). Allergic prodromal symptoms, with urticaria, facial oedema, dyspnoea, and gastrointestinal manifestations, may precede the blister by a few days and disappear when the blister ruptures. Most patients have one or two worms each season, but up to 50 have been recorded. Most gravid worms emerge from the lower limb, but other sites include the buttocks, trunk, arms, scrotum, and vulva.

Uncomplicated cases resolve within 4 weeks. Local complications derive from sensitization to worm products, inappropriate self-treatment, and bacterial infection; these can cause severe pain and prolonged disability. Gravid worms failing to reach the skin release larvae within the host's body, inducing vigorous tissue reactions and abscesses, sometimes presenting as buboes, epididymo-orchitis, or acute arthritis. Joint involvement, often with secondary bacterial infection, is also common near the site of emergence; this leads to ankylosis and tendon contractures, with deformities and permanent disability. Immature female worms may die before reaching the skin and become encapsulated by host tissue; some calcify. They may also enter ectopic sites, including the orbit,

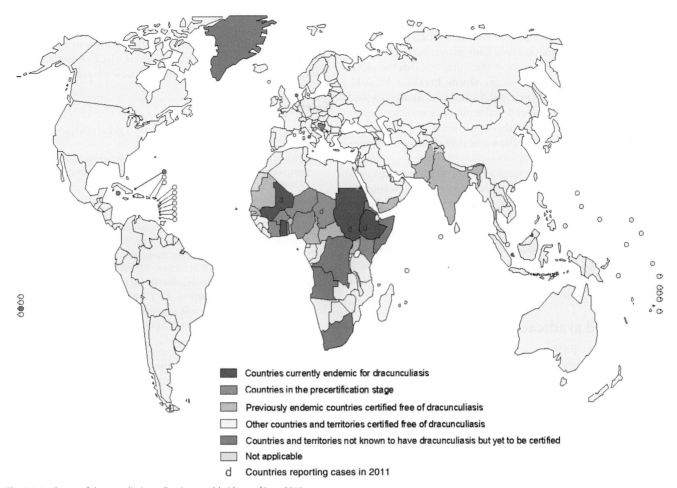

Countries currently endemic for dracunculiasis

Countries in the precertification stage

Previously endemic countries certified free of dracunculiasis

Other countries and territories certified free of dracunculiasis

Countries and territories not known to have dracunculiasis but yet to be certified

Not applicable

d   Countries reporting cases in 2011

Fig. 9.3.4a Status of dracunculiasis eradication, worldwide, as of June 2011.
(Reproduced with kind permission of the World Health Organization.)

pericardium, and central nervous system. Mortality is usually less than 1% and results from systemic or local bacterial infection. Tetanus is a significant risk when spores contaminate open lesions.

Diagnosis

Most patients in endemic areas recognize their condition. Worms release larvae on contact with water, and these can be seen as a milky cloud. When the worm is not visible, ulcers may be irrigated with saline and the centrifuged deposit examined for larvae.

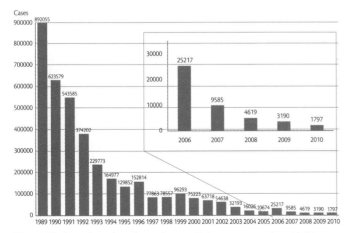

Fig. 9.3.4b Annual number of new dracunculiasis cases reported worldwide, 1989–2010.
(Reproduced with kind permission of the World Health Organization.)

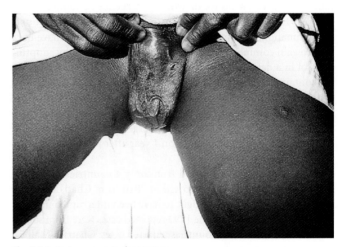

Fig. 9.3.5 Guinea worm in the scrotum.
(Copyright D A Warrell.)

Patient management

Local treatment can be very painful and must often be repeated. Warm moist packs should be applied for several hours, followed by gentle massage along the tract of the worm towards the ulcer. Light traction is then applied to the worm; breakage must be avoided as this greatly aggravates the situation. Analgesics and antibacterial soaks are useful, and oral antibiotics are often necessary. Between local treatments the lesion must be bandaged to reduce the risk of bacterial infection and contamination of water sources.

Pre-emergent worms can be surgically removed, a practice originating in India. A small incision is made adjacent to the worm near its midpoint, and a loop of worm is lifted out with a blunt curved probe. Massage is applied along the length of the worm towards the incision, and by gentle traction the whole worm can usually be removed. In the event of breakage the worm ends should be ligated to minimize contact between host tissue and worm antigens. Deep abscesses require surgical treatment. Anthelmintics have no role in the treatment of Guinea worm.

Control and eradication

Several factors facilitate control: Guinea worm is recognized by local communities as a major health problem, there are no carriers beyond the annual cycle, and there is no animal reservoir. The provision of safe water for drinking is the key to control; it is unrealistic to expect piped water supplies in most endemic areas, but covered tube wells or hand-dug wells provided with parapets are appropriate. Additional measures are filtration of household water with finely woven cloth, and the application of temephos to ponds to kill copepods.

National programmes have played a major role in many endemic areas. Case-detection surveys and health education can be integrated into existing primary health care systems. Unhygienic local treatments such as mud or leaf poultices and crude methods of worm extraction must be discouraged.

Several international health agencies took up the challenge of Guinea worm eradication in the mid 1980s, with an initial target eradication date of 1995. Much has been achieved, but the target was missed. The initial expensive hydrological programmes were later replaced by the training of local cadres who could recruit patients within 24 hours of worm emergence to 'containment centres' for treatment and education to prevent water source contamination. In some areas, private-sector initiatives have been able to gain commercially from the publicity achieved by adopting control in a defined area. Transmission from a patient is reported as 'contained' when it is detected less than 24 h after emergence, the patient has not entered a water source since emergence, and has been properly managed by the volunteer worker and seen by the supervisor with 7 days of worm emergence. Countries reach the precertification stage of eradication 1 year after reporting their last indigenous case.

In 2009, cases were reported from only 4 countries. However, 10 indigenous cases were reported in 2010 from Chad, a country where transmission was thought to have been interrupted in 2000.

In 2010, 1698 (95%) of the 1793 reported cases were from southern Sudan. Only 4 other countries reported cases: Ghana 8, Mali 57, Ethiopia 20, and Chad 10, and 76% of the 2010 total were reported as 'contained'. During the first 6 months of 2011 the provisional case count was 812: southern Sudan 801, Mali 3, Ethiopia 6, and

Chad 2. The last stages of eradication will be the most difficult, as vertical programmes then become inefficient. Unfortunately, some of the major residual foci are in situations of civil disorder where there are mobile refugees; in others a lack of resources or an absence of democratic institutions may slow progress.

Further reading

Berry M (2007). The tail end of Guinea worm – global eradication without a vaccine. *New Eng J Med*, **356**, 2561–4.

Cairncross S, Muller R, Zagaria N (2002). Dracunculiasis (Guinea worm disease) and the eradication initiative. *Clin Microbiol Rev*, **15**, 223–46.

CDC (2010). Progress towards global eradication of dracunculiasis January 2009 – June 2010. *MMWR Morb Mort Mortal Wkly Rep*, **59**, 1239–42.

CDC (2010). Renewed transmission of dracunculiasis in Chad, 2010. *MMWR Morb Mort Mortal Wkly Rep*, **60**, 744–8.

CDC (2011). Progress towards global eradication of dracunculiasis January 2010–June 2011. *MMWR Morb Mort Mortal Wkly Rep*, **60**, 1450–3.

Glenshaw MT, *et al.* (2009). Guinea worm disease outcomes in Ghana: determinants of broken worms. *Am J Trop Med Hyg*, **81**, 305–12.

Hochberg N, *et al.* (2008). The role of containment centres in the eradication of dracunculiasis in Togo and Ghana. *Am J Trop Med Hyg*, **79**, 722–8.

Muller R (1971). Dracunculus and dracunculiasis. *Adv Parasitol*, **9**, 73–151.

Rhode JE, *et al.* (1993). Surgical extraction of Guinea worm: disability reduction and contribution to disease control. *Am J Trop Med Hyg*, **48**, 71–6.

Ruiz Tiben E, Hopkins DR (2006). Dracunculiasis (Guinea worm disease) eradication. *Adv Parasitol*, 61, 275–309.Fig. 9.3.4a Status of dracunculiasis eradication, worldwide, as of June 2011.

9.4 Strongyloidiasis, hookworm, and other gut strongyloid nematodes

Michael Brown

Essentials

Strongyloides stercoralis and hookworms are common soil-transmitted nematodes in tropical and subtropical regions. After the organisms penetrate exposed skin, most infections are asymptomatic, but heavy infections can result in significant morbidity.

Strongyloidiasis

The roundworm S. *stercoralis* infects an estimated 30 million to 100 million people. Clinical manifestations include: (1) skin—often the only clinical manifestation, commonly in the form of larva currens, a serpiginous, pruritic, erythematous eruption at the site of migrating larvae; (2) lungs—cough and tracheal irritation; less commonly wheeze; patchy infiltrates on chest radiography with eosinophilia; (3) intestinal—epigastric pain and diarrhoea; (4) *Strongyloides* hyperinfection—occurs in patients who are immunosuppressed; severe diarrhoea is a common feature; mortality is high. Infection is persistent and may present decades after exposure. Diagnosis is usually by microscopy or culture of stool; serology is useful as a screening test. Treatment is typically with ivermectin or albendazole. Improved sanitation and appropriate footwear may reduce the acquisition of infection.

Hookworms

Hookworm infections, mainly caused by *Ancylostoma duodenale* and *Necator americanus*, affect more than 500 million people, predominantly in sub-Saharan Africa and Asia. Clinical manifestations include: (1) migratory/larval—ground itch (a pruritic, papular, and erythematous rash on the feet or hands); occasionally pneumonitis with eosinophilia; (2) intestinal—occasionally profuse watery diarrhoea, but most people are asymptomatic excepting for iron-deficiency anaemia (sometimes with haemoglobin <2 g/dl) in those with heavy infections, which are a particular problem in infants and pregnant women, in whom it affects pregnancy adversely. Diagnosis of acute infection is clinical and of chronic infection by discovering eggs in the stool by microscopy. A single dose of albendazole will reduce the worm load to levels below those likely to cause disease; complete eradication can be achieved with repeated doses.

Population-based control programmes, using single-dose anti-helmintic therapies, aim to reduce anaemia and improve childhood growth and cognitive development in countries with high prevalence of soil-transmitted helminths. Integration with other helminth control programmes is most effective. Increasing attention is being paid to the effect of coinfection with hookworm on other diseases such as malaria, tuberculosis, HIV, and asthma.

Nonhuman hookworms

These cannot complete their life cycle in humans but are capable of causing significant morbidity, including: (1) cutaneous larva migrans—usually due to dog hookworms; presents as intensely pruritic lesions on exposed areas of the skin; diagnosis is clinical, although the worm may be visualized in skin biopsies; albendazole is effective; (2) *Ancylostoma caninum*-associated enteritis; (3) oesophagostomiasis; (4) trichostrongyliasis.

Strongyloides stercoralis

Pathogenesis and life cycle

Strongyloides stercoralis is a roundworm that has two alternative life cycles, producing either parasitic or free-living forms. It is one of the few helminths that can complete its life cycle in humans. Filariform larvae in moist soil penetrate exposed skin, and pass via the bloodstream to the lungs and into the alveolar spaces. From there, the larvae ascend the trachea and are swallowed, reaching their final habitat in the crypts of Lieberkühn in the duodenum and upper jejunum, where they mature.

The adult males are rapidly eliminated from the intestine, leaving parthenogenetic adult parasitic females, 2.5 mm in length, attached to the mucosa, where they deposit eggs. One month after infection, the resulting rhabditiform larvae bore through the epithelium into the gut lumen. At this stage, most larvae follow an indirect developmental route—they are excreted in the faeces and develop into free-living adults, which produce eggs from which filariform larvae

develop. Some larvae by contrast develop directly via three moults into filariform larvae. These are usually passed in the faeces and can survive in the soil for many weeks. However, some may reinvade the host in the lower gastrointestinal tract or perianal skin before evacuation. It is this process of autoinfection that explains the persistence of chronic *S. stercoralis* infections for decades after exposure, and allows for the multiplication of worms that may lead to the phenomenon of hyperinfection seen in immunosuppressed patients.

Strongyloidiasis, like most helminth infections, is associated with a type 2 immune response, with raised IgE levels and increased circulating eosinophil numbers. In immunosuppressed patients, some elements of this immune response are lacking. The pathogenesis of hyperinfection is not well understood. A possible explanation is that immunosuppression facilitates the direct route of strongyloides development, leading to multiplicative autoinfection, increasing larval intensities, and ultimately, dissemination of larvae beyond the gut mucosa into other organs.

Epidemiology

S. stercoralis infects an estimated 30 to 100 million people, with a distribution throughout tropical and subtropical areas. Prevalence in rural areas of sub-Saharan Africa, South-East Asia, and Central and South America can reach 20%; a lower level of active transmission persists in temperate regions such as southern Europe and the southern United States of America. In highly endemic areas, infection intensities peak in childhood and then plateau or decline. Because of the chronicity of infection, prevalence remains high in immigrants from endemic areas, reaching 30 to 80% in South-East Asian immigrants screened in North America. A prevalence greater than 30% has been observed among former British servicemen who were prisoners of war in the Far East in 1941–5, screened 30 years or more after exposure.

Clinical features

Most infected individuals are asymptomatic. In such patients, diagnosis may only be considered as part of investigation for peripheral eosinophilia.

Cutaneous

Skin symptoms are often the only manifestation of infection, commonly in the form of larva currens, a serpiginous pruritic erythematous eruption on the legs, buttocks, and back, at the site of migrating larvae, that can advance as quickly as 15 cm/h (Fig. 9.4.1). The rash is more diffuse and migrates more rapidly than the cutaneous larva migrans associated with hookworm infections. It may occur with the initial infection, but also in people with chronic strongyloidiasis.

Pulmonary

The migratory phase may be associated with cough and tracheal irritation, and less commonly with wheeze, which may be persistent. Patchy infiltrates may be seen on chest radiographs. When larvae become trapped in the lung during migration, eosinophilic pneumonia occasionally occurs. Pulmonary manifestations, including pneumonia, bacterial lung abscesses, and acute respiratory distress syndrome are more prominent in hyperinfected patients (see below).

Intestinal

Intestinal symptoms are generally mild in people with light infection. Epigastric pain mimicking peptic ulcer disease may

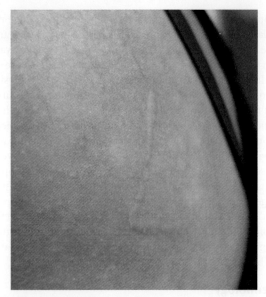

Fig. 9.4.1 Characteristic serpiginous rash of larva currens on the shoulder of a traveller with *Strongyloides stercoralis* infection acquired in India. The rash was transient, but recurrent and widespread.
(Courtesy of R H Behrens, Hospital for Tropical Diseases, London.)

occur within 3 weeks of infection and persist. Diarrhoea is usually chronic and mild, but may occur early and be associated with bloody stools. In more severe cases, usually associated with hyperinfection, intestinal oedema with malabsorption, mesenteric lymphadenopathy, and ascites may occur. An eosinophilic granulomatous enterocolitis resembling Crohn's disease is well described in older patients on corticosteroids. Subacute intestinal obstruction, biliary stenosis, and necrotizing enteritis are occasionally seen.

Strongyloides hyperinfection

Patients on long-term corticosteroids, and those undergoing chemotherapy or organ transplantation, are at risk from severe manifestations of strongyloidiasis. This also occurs in patients with lymphoma or leukaemia without chemotherapy, most commonly in those with T-cell leukaemia caused by human T-cell leukaemia virus (HTLV)-1 infection. It is also well described in HTLV-1-infected patients without overt malignancy, and less commonly in patients with AIDS. Disseminated disease has a very high mortality rate. Severe diarrhoea is a common feature. Gram-negative pneumonia, bacteraemia, or meningitis caused by enteric pathogens that have breached the mucosal barrier along with the strongyloides larvae are frequent manifestations. Petechial haemorrhages in the skin, especially around the umbilicus, and hepatitis may occur. Peripheral eosinophilia is often absent in disseminated disease.

Diagnosis

Microscopy of stool may reveal rhabditiform larvae, but the sensitivity of direct smears is low. Formol-ether concentration techniques are more useful, but multiple stool samples may be required to detect light infections. Culture techniques have been developed to enhance the diagnostic yield. Agar plate cultures have the highest yield; tracks made by larvae migrating across the plate can be seen. Charcoal culture and filter-paper methods make use of the indirect life cycle: stool is incubated for several days to allow the development of adults and second-generation filariform larvae.

Larvae may also be isolated by duodenal aspiration, or by the string test, although these are of limited sensitivity. Molecular techniques, such as real-time PCR on stool, perform well. In disseminated infection, larvae are found in the sputum and in biopsies from tissues such as the gastrointestinal tract and lung.

Enzyme-linked immunosorbent assays (ELISA) for strongyloides-specific IgG have high sensitivity for strongyloides infection. There is cross-reaction with filarial antibodies, and levels may remain elevated after treatment, so specificity may be limited. It is useful as a screening test, particularly before embarking on immunosuppressive therapy.

Treatment and prevention

Albendazole 400 mg once or twice daily for 3 days is reasonably effective in chronic infections, and is better tolerated than tiabendazole 25 mg/kg twice daily for 3 days. Currently, the treatment of choice is ivermectin 200 µg/kg as a single dose or for two doses 1 to 14 days apart. Prolonged courses of treatment are necessary in patients with severe or disseminated disease. Subcutaneous veterinary preparations have been used when parenteral treatment is required.

Improved sanitation and appropriate footwear may reduce the acquisition of infection. Once established, strongyloides should be eradicated in any patient being considered for immunosuppressive therapy, because of the potentially lethal consequences of hyperinfection.

Strongyloides fuelleborni

Strongyloides fuelleborni fuelleborni is a parasite of primates in tropical Africa and Asia, which can also infect human populations sharing similar habitats. Prevalence rates up to 20% have been reported among forest-dwelling communities. Infections are generally asymptomatic. Unlike *S. stercoralis*, eggs are passed in the stool, and may be confused with hookworm ova. Benzimidazole therapy is effective.

A phylogenetically distinct nematode, *Strongyloides fuelleborni kellyi*, has been found in rural communities in Papua New Guinea. Infection intensities are highest among young children. It is associated with 'swollen belly sickness' in 2-month-old infants, which is characterized by abdominal distension, respiratory distress, generalized oedema, and gastrointestinal disturbance.

Hookworm

Pathogenesis and life cycle

Hookworm infections are principally caused by the two species that can complete their life cycles in humans: *Ancylostoma duodenale* and *Necator americanus*. Their life cycles are similar. Larvae in moist soil penetrate exposed skin, usually on the feet or buttocks. They enter the circulation after 10 days, are carried to the lungs, and cross into the alveolae, from where they are transported to the pharynx and swallowed. The adults, approximately 10 mm in length, attach themselves to the small intestinal mucosa with their buccal cavities, which contain hooked teeth (ancylostoma) or cutting plates (necator). After 3 to 6 weeks the females produce up to 30 000 eggs per day, which are passed in the faeces. The eggs hatch within 48 h, but the larvae can remain viable for up to 6 weeks in appropriate soil conditions. Adult hookworms live for 1 to 9 years. Infection can also be acquired by the ingestion of contaminated soil, and the transmission of infective larvae via breast milk is well recognized.

Infection is associated with tissue and peripheral eosinophilia, and specific IgG and nonspecific IgE responses. Regulatory cytokine responses are probably crucial in limiting immunopathology in established infection. Equally important are a range of worm-derived immunomodulatory molecules that interfere with neutrophil migration and adhesion, inhibit complement, induce T-cell apoptosis, and prevent blood coagulation. Secreted anticoagulants, including serine protease inhibitors of factor Xa, are responsible for anaemia, the main consequence of infection. Radioisotope studies have demonstrated that hookworm infections produce a daily blood loss of up to 0.3 ml per worm per day. This translates into a loss of up to 100 ml per day in heavily infected people. The degree of anaemia is partly a function of worm burden, but also of iron stores. Variations in dietary iron intake, as well as coinfection with other parasites such as schistosomes and malaria, account for some of the geographical differences in the incidence of hookworm anaemia.

Epidemiology

Estimates suggest that more than 500 million people are infected with hookworm, predominantly in Asia and sub-Saharan Africa. Although significant overlap occurs, the distribution of *A. duodenale* is more restricted geographically than that of *N. americanus*. Necator is more widespread in sub-Saharan Africa, the Americas, South-East Asia, and India; ancylostoma is also widely distributed in South-East Asia, but is more common in temperate regions, North Africa, and the Middle East. As with other intestinal helminths, most infected people harbour a few adult worms, but a minority are heavily infected. Social, behavioural, and genetic factors determine which individuals within a community are most heavily infected. Unlike most other intestinal helminth infections, the prevalence and intensity of hookworm infection increases with age.

Clinical features

Migratory/larval

Repeated exposure to penetrating hookworm larvae results in ground itch, a pruritic papular erythematous rash on the feet or hands. Larval pulmonary migration is generally asymptomatic, but may result in a pneumonitis characterized by fever, cough, wheeze, haemoptysis, and peripheral eosinophilia. Symptoms may last several weeks, but are rarely severe. Oral ingestion of *A. duodenale* larvae can result in Wakana disease, which presents with nausea, vomiting, cough, pharyngeal irritation, and dyspnoea.

Intestinal

Recently acquired human hookworm infection occasionally causes profuse watery diarrhoea. Most people with established infection are asymptomatic. The major morbidity associated with hookworm infection is iron-deficiency anaemia in those with heavy infections. Haemoglobin concentrations of less than 2 g/dl are not uncommon. Hookworms were first identified in the investigation of anaemic miners in 19th century Europe, notably in Cornish tin mines, where an extreme form of anaemia (chlorosis or 'green disease') was prevalent. Now eradicated in developed countries, hookworm remains a major cause of anaemia in the developing world. It is particularly common among women of reproductive age, and a major contributor towards adverse outcomes in pregnancy, being responsible for 30 to 50% of cases of pregnancy-associated anaemia. Fatigue and listlessness are the principal symptoms, and probably have a significant economic impact in areas of high prevalence. High-output cardiac failure is a major cause of death in patients with severe anaemia. Malabsorption is not a frequent consequence of hookworm infection, but protein loss does occur and may contribute to the oedema seen in severe infections.

Dyspepsia, nausea, and a range of nonspecific symptoms are common in those with heavy worm burdens. Pica, a craving for eating soil, is well described in patients with hookworm anaemia.

Growth and cognitive development

There has been debate about the effect of chronic hookworm infection on growth and cognitive development in childhood. Seminal work in an impoverished community in the southern United States of America in the 1920s demonstrated an inverse association between IQ and hookworm intensity. The results of subsequent studies have been inconclusive. Intervention trials in East Africa have suggested a modest effect of heavy hookworm infection on growth, and the balance of evidence suggests that heavily infected subjects do have impairments of memory and other specific cognitive functions. It is not known to what extent these effects are mediated by or are independent of anaemia. Treatment results in improved cognitive performance and school attendance.

Diagnosis

The diagnosis of acute hookworm infection is clinical. Characteristic symptoms are usually associated with peripheral eosinophilia. The diagnosis of chronic infection is made by discovering eggs in the stool by microscopy. Symptomatic infection is readily diagnosed by direct microscopy of a single stool sample, as the worm burden is high in these patients. Where diagnosis of lighter infections is required, e.g. in the investigation of eosinophilia, the diagnostic yield is increased by examining multiple stool samples, using concentration methods, or by culture techniques. The latter allow for the development of third-stage larvae, which can be used to identify the infecting hookworm species and differentiate from related nematode species. Semiquantitative techniques, such as the modified Kato smear, can be used to estimate infection intensity. Hookworm eggs degenerate rapidly after excretion, and laboratory processing should be performed as soon as possible.

Treatment, prevention, and control

A single dose of albendazole 400 mg, will kill more than 80% of adult hookworms and thus reduce the worm load to a level below that likely to cause disease. Complete eradication can be achieved with repeated doses. Treatment is well tolerated, and can safely be given to children and in pregnancy (although not recommended in the first trimester). Single-dose mebendazole is much less effective. For patients with anaemia, anthelmintic treatment should be combined with iron replacement. Patients with heart failure or severe anaemia during pregnancy frequently require transfusion of packed red cells.

In developing countries where the prevalence of hookworm and other intestinal helminths is high, the increasing availability of safe, affordable, single-dose anthelmintics makes mass deworming programmes feasible (Fig. 9.4.2). The impact of empirical population-based treatment, e.g. in schools, can be sustained in the face of ongoing transmission by repeated treatment at 3- to 12-month intervals. These strategies can be integrated with control programmes for other helminthiases. The World Health Organization set a target date of 2010 for routine anthelmintic

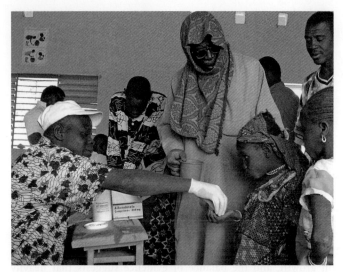

Fig. 9.4.2 School-based treatment as part of a mass anthelmintic treatment programme in Burkina Faso.
(Courtesy of A Gabrielli, Schistosomiasis Control Initiative.)

treatment to be provided to 75% of school-age children at risk of infection. However, this target was reached only in some countries, with a 30% coverage globally by 2009. The outcomes of national control programmes on anaemia have been mixed. School-based programmes miss the most vulnerable populations (preschool children and pregnant women); furthermore, programmes combining albendazole with antischistosomal treatment have had more impressive outcomes, suggesting that in coinfected populations both helminths contribute to anaemia.

The age–intensity distribution of hookworm infection is likely to limit any benefit of mass treatment programmes on hookworm transmission. The provision of better footwear and improved sanitation for infected communities probably has only a marginal role, at least in the medium term, in reducing transmission. Vaccines offer potential for better hookworm control but development has been hampered by challenges in generating relevant animal models and in eliciting safe immune responses in early clinical studies.

Consequences of immune modulation by hookworms

Helminth infections have a similar global distribution to other pathogens. Our understanding of the immune response to helminth infection has stimulated interest in the effect of helminths on subjects coinfected with other microorganisms, particularly malaria, tuberculosis, and HIV. Children with heavy hookworm infections mount a reduced febrile response to malaria. There may be effects of hookworm infection on immune responses to mycobacterial antigens, although hookworm does not appear to increase the incidence of tuberculosis or accelerate the progression of HIV infection.

There is evidence that childhood or maternal infection with some helminths, especially hookworm, may protect against the development of infantile eczema and/or atopy. These findings lend support to the 'hygiene hypothesis' that the increasing prevalence of allergy worldwide may partly be a result of reduced exposure to the immunosuppressive effects of helminths, and lead to concerns that mass deworming may have detrimental as well as beneficial effects. A recent trial of experimental hookworm infection as a treatment for asthma did not demonstrate a significant benefit.

Nonhuman hookworms

Nonhuman hookworms cannot complete their life cycle in the human host, but are capable of causing significant morbidity in the skin and gastrointestinal tract.

Cutaneous larva migrans

Cutaneous larva migrans presents as intensely pruritic lesions on exposed areas of the skin. The rash is commonly seen on the feet or buttocks, but may occur elsewhere (Fig. 9.4.3). Dog hookworms such as *Ancylostoma braziliense* are usually implicated. Like human hookworms these species thrive in sandy soil, and frequently infect travellers visiting beaches in the Caribbean, South-East Asia, and Africa. Untreated, the rash can persist for months, with gradual spread through the epidermis leaving serpiginous tracks. Secondary bacterial infection may sometimes occur. Diagnosis is clinical, although the worm may be visualized in biopsies taken from the leading edge of the lesion. Topical albendazole or tiabendazole are usually effective, although short courses of oral albendazole or ivermectin are more effective.

Ancylostoma caninum-associated gastroenteritis

First described in Australia in the 1980s, a distinctive eosinophilic enteritis has been linked to infection with *A. caninum*, a dog hookworm. The global distribution of this disease is unknown.

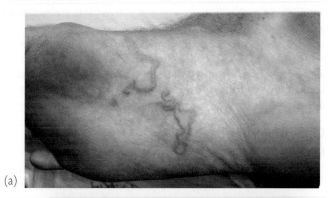

(a)

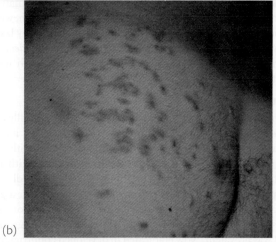

(b)

Fig. 9.4.3 Cutaneous larva migrans: (a) caused by probable *Ancylostoma braziliense* infection acquired on a beach in the Caribbean, and (b) heavy infection with *Ancylostoma braziliense* acquired in Brazil.
(a, courtesy of D Webster, Oxford Radcliffe Hospitals, United Kingdom; b, copyright D A Warrell.)

Oral ingestion may be the predominant route of infection. Manifestations range from a limited aphthous ileitis with tissue and peripheral eosinophilia, which may be asymptomatic, to a severe painful eosinophilic gastroenteritis with gut oedema, ascites, and regional lymphadenopathy. Immature hookworm larvae can be identified in the lesions, although the diagnosis may only be made at laparotomy. Benzimidazoles are effective.

Oesophagostomum spp.

Human oesophagostomiasis, usually caused by *Oesophagostomum bifurcum*, is common in forested areas of West Africa, but rare elsewhere. Prevalence in some areas of Togo and northern Ghana has reached 75%. The nematode can complete its life cycle in humans, and is distinct from related species in primates. Humans probably acquire the disease by ingesting infective third-stage larvae, although a percutaneous route of infection has not been excluded. The larvae migrate to and develop within the colonic wall before returning to the intestinal lumen, where they reach adulthood and excrete eggs.

Intense tissue reactions occur around the larvae, forming nodules along the wall of the (usually ascending) colon. Although these infections are generally asymptomatic, heavy infections may result in the development of multiple pea-sized nodules, with gross mucosal and serosal oedema, and microabscess formation (Fig. 9.4.4). Children are most commonly affected, and present with abdominal pain, diarrhoea, and weight loss. Solitary palpable painful inflammatory masses, known as Dapaong tumours, also occur within the bowel wall and in extraintestinal sites such as the mesentery or abdominal wall. Nodules can be detected ultrasonographically. Ova are morphologically indistinguishable from those of hookworm, but can be differentiated by culturing third-stage larvae. Treatment with short courses of albendazole is effective and may obviate the need for surgery. Mass treatment campaigns have reduced the burden of disease.

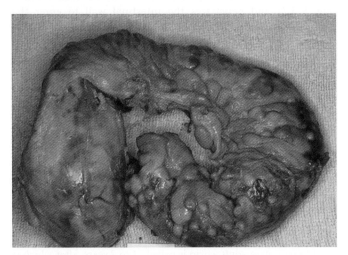

Fig. 9.4.4 Excised colon from a young Ghanaian adult with *Oesophagostomum bifurcum*-associated disease. Multiple nodules and serosal oedema are present. The diagnosis was made at laparotomy after the patient presented with abdominal pain and peritonism.
(Courtesy of A M Polderman, Leiden University Medical Center, Netherlands.)

Trichostrongylus spp.

Trichostrongylus spp. are ubiquitous nematode parasites of herbivores, particularly domesticated animals such as sheep, goats, cattle, and donkeys. Human infection occurs most commonly among herders, with a prevalence of more than 80% reported among Iranian nomads. Sporadic human infections occur in urban environments through contact with the faeces of domestic animals. Infective larvae hatch in the soil, and are ingested with contaminated vegetables. There is no migratory phase; the adults develop in the duodenal mucosa, and produce eggs after a long prepatent period. Most infected people are asymptomatic, although eosinophilia is common. Epigastric pain, diarrhoea, and rectal bleeding may occur. Diagnosis is made by finding eggs (which may be mistaken for hookworm ova) by stool microscopy. The adults are occasionally visualized at endoscopy. Benzimidazole anthelmintics may be effective, although resistance is increasing; a single dose of ivermectin 200 μg/kg is usually sufficient.

Further reading

Ashford RW, Barnish G, Viney ME (1992). *Strongyloides fuelleborni kellyi:* infection and disease in Papua New Guinea. *Parasitol Today*, **8**, 314–18.

Bethony JM, *et al.* (2011). Vaccines to combat the neglected tropical diseases. *Immunol Rev*, **239**, 237–70.

Croese J, *et al.* (1994). Human enteric infection with canine hookworms. *Ann Intern Med*, **120**, 369–74.

Elliott AM, *et al.* (2011). Treatment with anthelminthics during pregnancy: what gains and what risks for the mother and child? *Parasitology*, **138**, 1499–507.

Eziefula AC, Brown M, *et al*. (2008). Intestinal nematodes: disease burden, deworming and the potential importance of co-infection. *Curr Op Infect Dis*, **21**, 516–522.

Feary JR, *et al.* (2010). Experimental hookworm infection: a randomized placebo-controlled trial in asthma. *Clin Exp Allergy*, **40**, 299–306.

Gill GV, *et al.* (2004). Chronic *Strongyloides stercoralis* infection in former British Far East prisoners of war. *Q J Med*, **97**, 789–95.

Keiser J, Utzinger J. (2008). Efficacy of current drugs against soil-transmitted helminth infections: systematic review and meta-analysis. *JAMA*, **299**, 1937–48.

Marcos LA, *et al.* (2011). Update on strongyloidiasis in the immunocompromised host. *Curr Infect Dis Rep*, **13**, 35–46.

Polderman AM, *et al.* (2010). The rise and fall of human oesophagostomiasis. *Adv Parasitol*, **71**, 93–155.

Sangaré LR, *et al.* (2011). Species-specific treatment effects of helminth/HIV-1 co-infection: a systematic review and meta-analysis. *Parasitology*, **138**, 1546–58.

Smith JL, Brooker S (2010). Impact of hookworm infection and deworming on anaemia in non-pregnant populations: a systematic review. *Trop Med Int Health*, **15**, 776–95.

Verweij J, *et al.* (2009). Molecular diagnosis of Strongyloides stercoralis in faecal samples using real-time PCR. *Trans R Soc Trop Med Hyg*, **103**, 342–6.

World Health Organization (2011). Soil-transmitted helminthiases: estimates of the number of children needing preventive chemotherapy and number treated, 2009. Wkly Epidemiol Rec, N°25, 86, 257–68.

9.5 Gut and tissue nematode infections acquired by ingestion

David I. Grove

Ascariasis

Ascaris lumbricoides (the giant roundworm) is widespread in the tropics and subtropics where sanitation is poor and the soil is contaminated with its eggs. Ingested eggs hatch in the small bowel, cycle through the bloodstream and lungs, then return to the small bowel and develop into adult worms 15 to 30 cm long. Most infections are asymptomatic, but there may be pulmonary infiltrates with eosinophilia, abdominal discomfort and—in children with heavy infections—intestinal obstruction. Infection is diagnosed by finding eggs in the faeces. Treatment is with pyrantel, mebendazole, or albendazole.

Anisakidosis

This is caused by larvae of roundworms in the family *Anisakidae* which are parasites of marine mammals. After ingestion of larvae in uncooked fish or squid, immature larvae burrow into the gastric or intestinal mucosa and may cause abdominal pain. Diagnosis is usually made at endoscopy, with treatment by endoscopic removal (if possible) of the larvae, although symptoms resolve spontaneously in most cases.

Capillariasis

Intestinal capillariasis—caused by *Paracapillaria philippinensis*, this is acquired by ingestion of undercooked freshwater fish and may cause a severe diarrhoeal disease. Diagnosis is by finding eggs in the stool. Treatment is with mebendazole or albendazole. Prevention is by properly cooking fish.

Hepatic capillariasis—caused by *Capillaria hepatica*, a parasite of rats. Ingested eggs hatch and larvae pass to the liver and cause a syndrome similar to visceral larva migrans (see below). Diagnosis is made by identifying the parasite or eggs in a liver biopsy. Treatment is usually with thiabendazole or albendazole.

Enterobiasis

Enterobius vermicularis (the threadworm) is cosmopolitan. Ingested eggs develop directly into adult worms in the gut; fertilized female worms crawl out of the rectum at night and deposit eggs on the perianal skin. Most infections are asymptomatic, but pruritus ani may be troublesome at night. Diagnosis is made by finding eggs on clear adhesive tape applied to the perianal skin. Pyrantel, mebendazole, and albendazole are effective in combination with sanitary measures.

Toxocariasis

This is due to invasion by larvae of *Toxocara canis* and *T. cati*, acquired by ingestion of eggs from dog and cat stools. It occurs in two clinical forms—visceral and ocular larva migrans.

Visceral larva migrans—usually afflicts children; larvae migrate to the viscera and may be asymptomatic or cause protean manifestations including muscular pain, lassitude, anorexia, cough, urticarial

rashes, hepatomegaly, and (occasionally) splenomegaly, lymphadenopathy and skin lesions, and (rarely) central nervous system involvement (convulsions). Eosinophilia is prominent. Definitive diagnosis is by finding larvae on biopsy, usually of the liver; a negative serological test for toxocara antibody rules out the diagnosis. Most patients recover spontaneously; there is no proven therapy.

Ocular larva migrans—more commonly seen in older children and due to granuloma formation around a larva in the retina. Diagnosis depends upon positive serology together with consistent fundoscopic features. There is no proven anthelmintic therapy.

Trichinosis

This is acquired by ingestion of larvae of *Trichinella spiralis* in undercooked meat, usually pork. Adult worms in the small bowel produce larvae which seed the muscles and other tissues, where they develop. Most infections are asymptomatic, but heavy infections typically cause diarrhoea, followed by fever and myositis. Definitive diagnosis depends upon finding larvae in muscle biopsies, although this is usually unnecessary; serological tests become positive several weeks after infection. Treatment is symptomatic. Thorough cooking of pork is the best safeguard against infection.

Trichuriasis

Trichuris trichiura (whipworm) is most prevalent in the tropics and subtropics where sanitation is poor. Ingested eggs hatch in the small bowel and then develop within the gut into adult worms which become embedded in the large bowel mucosa. Very heavy infections may cause dysentery or rectal prolapse. Infection is diagnosed by finding eggs in the faeces. Treatment is with mebendazole or albendazole.

Ascariasis (giant roundworm infection)

Life cycle

Ascariasis is an infection caused by the giant roundworm, *Ascaris lumbricoides*. Infection is acquired when an egg is ingested (Fig. 9.5.1). The infective larva hatches out in the small intestine (Fig. 9.5.2) and penetrates the intestinal wall to enter the portal circulation. From here it enters the systemic circulation and reaches the lungs, where it breaks out of the capillaries into the alveoli and undergoes another moult to become a fourth-stage larva. From the lungs the larva moves up the bronchial tree to the mouth, and is then swallowed. In the intestine it moults again to become a sexually mature worm about 6 to 8 weeks after ingestion. The mature worm is cylindrical with tapering ends, and creamy white to light-brown in colour (Fig. 9.5.3). The female measures 20 to 35 cm in length and 3 to 6 mm in width, whereas the male is 12 to 31 cm long and 2 to 4 mm wide, and has a curved tail.

Normally, the adult worms live in the lumen of the small intestine, primarily the jejunum. The worm is able to maintain its position in the small intestine by the activity of its somatic muscles; if these are paralysed by anthelmintics it is expelled by peristalsis. The lifespan of an adult worm is usually 1 to 2 years, after which it is expelled spontaneously. The worms mate, and eggs are passed in the faeces, with gravid females producing 200 000 to 250 000 eggs daily. When freshly passed these eggs are not infective, and contain a single cell. This develops in the soil over the next 2 to 6 weeks

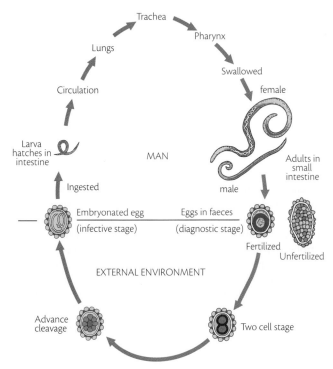

Fig. 9.5.1 Life cycle of *Ascaris lumbricoides*.

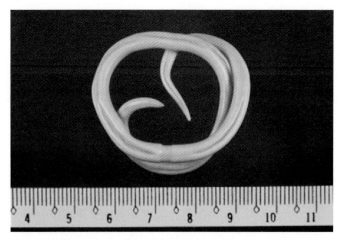

Fig. 9.5.3 Adult *Ascaris lumbricoides* (scale in mm).
(Copyright Viqar Zaman)

(faster in warmer temperatures) into an infective larva. The ova are resistant to chemicals and low temperatures, and may remain viable for years in moist soil.

Epidemiology and control

Ascariasis is cosmopolitan, and is probably the most common helminth infection. It is prevalent in areas where there is poor sanitation and contamination of the soil with eggs. Infection is more common in tropical climates, and is particularly prevalent in areas where human faeces are used to fertilize vegetable gardens. Infection is usually acquired by eating contaminated food, or from soil ingested by children when playing, and does not induce resistance to reinfection. It is relatively more common in children, who

also carry higher worm loads. In hyperendemic areas with constant warm temperatures and high humidity, children are continuously being infected, so that as some worms are being expelled, others are maturing to take their place. Transmission may only be associated with the rainy season in areas that are generally hot and arid. It has recently been suggested that the pig ascarid, *A. suum*, may be adapting to humans in Japan with maturation into adult worms. Environmental sanitation is the best control measure, but when this is not possible mass chemotherapy given at intervals of 6 months reduces the severity and intensity of infection.

Clinical features

The first passage of larvae through the lungs usually causes no symptoms or pathological changes, but subsequent infections may be associated with hypersensitivity reactions, causing ascaris pneumonia (Fig. 9.5.4). When this causes fever, cough, dyspnoea, bronchospasm, peripheral eosinophilia, and infiltrates on chest radiograph that are often migratory, this is known as Löffler's syndrome. The condition usually subsides after 7 to 10 days unless reinfection occurs. In areas where pig farming is common, the larvae of *A. suum* may also produce severe pneumonitis and bronchospasm.

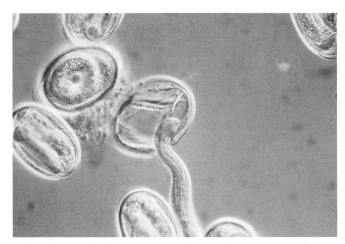

Fig. 9.5.2 Decorticated eggs of *Ascaris lumbricoides*, showing emergence of larvae.
(Copyright Viqar Zaman.)

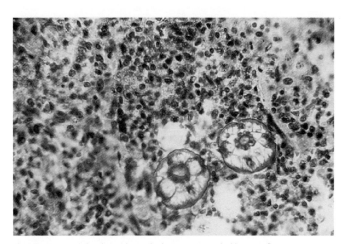

Fig. 9.5.4 *Ascaris lumbricoides* in the lungs, surrounded by an inflammatory reaction.
(Copyright Viqar Zaman.)

Most people with established infection with *A. lumbricoides* are asymptomatic, especially if the worm burden is small. Some may complain of anorexia, nausea, and abdominal discomfort or distension. Heavy infections in children may cause malnutrition, and hinder normal development in terms of both stature and cognitive performance. Mechanical complications probably occur in less than 1% of infected individuals. Occasionally, usually in children, large numbers of worms may become entangled to form a bolus that blocks the intestinal lumen, usually near the ileocaecal valve, producing signs and symptoms of acute intestinal obstruction. This may be complicated by perforation, intussusception, volvulus, and death. In unusual circumstances, such as fever, irritation caused by drugs, anaesthesia, or bowel manipulation during surgery, the worms may migrate to ectopic sites. Migration into the common bile duct may be complicated with cholangitis and liver abscesses, whereas entry into the pancreatic duct may precipitate acute pancreatitis. Worms may migrate into the appendix, occasionally come out through the mouth and nose, and are rarely found in other ectopic locations.

Diagnosis

Ascariasis is usually diagnosed by finding plentiful numbers of the characteristically oval fertilized eggs measuring 60 × 30 to 70 × 50 μm in the faeces (Fig. 9.5.5). Sometimes the patient brings developing or adult worms that have been passed in the faeces or have emerged from the anus or nose of a sick child. Occasionally, adult worms are outlined in the intestines during barium-meal examination, or are seen at upper gastrointestinal endoscopy.

Treatment

It is desirable to treat all infected individuals, even when the worm load is small. There are a number of effective drugs (listed below). None of them is recommended by its manufacturer for use in pregnancy, especially in the first trimester, or children under 1 to 2 years of age, although this has been disputed by some authorities.

- Pyrantel embonate (pyrantel pamoate) given in a single dose of 11 mg/kg body weight (maximum 1 g) is effective in curing more

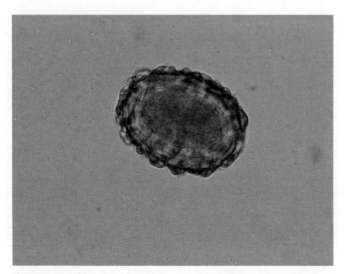

Fig. 9.5.5 Egg of *Ascaris lumbricoides*.

than 90% of cases of ascariasis. Side effects are mild, if any, and the drug is well tolerated.

- Mebendazole is given is given as 100 mg twice daily for 3 days in adults and children over 2 years of age. It should not be given to pregnant women.
- Albendazole is given as a single dose of 400 mg in adults and children over 2 years of age. It should not be given to pregnant women.

In cases of intestinal obstruction caused by an ascaris bolus, a piperazine salt given at a dose of 75 mg/kg (maximum 3.5 g) daily for two consecutive days has been recommended as it induces flaccid paralysis of the worms, which may relieve the obstruction. This should be supplemented with decompression of the bowel through an intestinal tube with constant suction, and rehydration and restoration of electrolyte balance with intravenous fluids. In most cases this conservative therapy will relieve the obstruction and the child will rapidly recover. If, however, the signs of obstruction persist and the child's general condition worsens, laparotomy is required. Acute obstructive jaundice or pancreatitis resulting from obstruction of the common bile duct by ascaris also requires urgent surgical intervention.

Anisakidosis

Life cycle

Anisakidosis is an infection caused by the larvae of various species of nematode belonging to the family Anisakidae, most commonly *Anisakis simplex* and *Peudoterranova decipiens*. Adults live in the lumen of the intestine of marine mammals (cetaceans: whales, dolphins, and porpoises). Eggs are passed in water, and second-stage larvae are ingested by crustaceans, which are then ingested by fish or squid, where they enter the muscles. Cetaceans and humans become infected by eating these saltwater fish or squid.

Epidemiology and control

The adult worms are commonly found in marine mammals in many parts of the world. Humans are infected when they eat raw or improperly cooked fish or squid. The incidence is highest in Japan, countries on the northern European seaboard, and the Pacific coast of the Americas, especially in the South. Infection is prevented by not eating raw, pickled, smoked, or undercooked fish and squid. Larvae are killed by cooking or freezing for 24 h before ingestion.

Clinical features

The larvae do not develop to maturity in humans, but attach themselves to and then burrow into the mucosa of the stomach (especially *Pseudoterranova* species) or small intestine (especially *Anisakis* species), and rarely the large bowel (Fig. 9.5.6). Symptoms often develop 4 to 24 h after eating infected fish. Gastric invasion produces severe epigastric pain, nausea, and vomiting, and sometimes haematemesis during the acute stage of the disease. Involvement of the intestine may cause severe lower abdominal pain, which may be misdiagnosed as appendicitis. If symptoms are mild and the patient is left untreated the infection can become chronic, with pseudotumour formation encompassing the parasite. Sometimes infection precipitates an allergic reaction, with urticaria, angio-oedema or anaphylaxis.

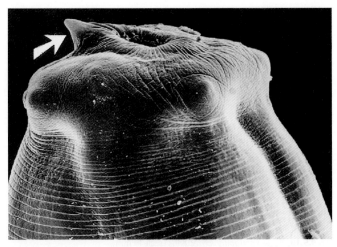

Fig. 9.5.6 Third-stage larva of *Anisakis simplex,* showing the tip of the boring tooth (arrow) (×400).

Diagnosis

A definitive diagnosis is made by upper gastrointestinal endoscopy, which reveals the lesion and the presence of white or yellow larvae up to 3 cm in size attached to the mucous membrane. Intestinal anisakidosis is more difficult to diagnose, but imaging studies may show thickening of the intestinal wall, and narrowing of the jejunum or ileum.

Treatment

In acute infection, an attempt should be made to remove all the larvae through an endoscope, although in most patients symptoms resolve spontaneously within 2 weeks. In chronic cases, surgical removal of the ulcerated areas or the tumour may be required. No chemotherapy has been proven to be effective, although of albendazole 400 mg daily for 3 days may be tried.

Capillariasis

There are two forms of capillariasis: intestinal capillariasis caused by *Paracapillaria philippinensis,* and hepatic capillariasis caused by *Capillaria hepatica.*

Intestinal capillariasis

This infection is caused by a worm still generally known as *Capillaria philippinensis* in medical circles, although it has been renamed *Paracapillaria philippinensis.* Fish-eating birds are the definitive reservoir. Adult *C. philippinensis* measure 2.5 to 4.3 mm in length and produce eggs that are deposited in water and ingested by fish, in which they develop into infective larvae. Humans are infected by eating undercooked freshwater or brackish-water fish. In humans, the parasite has the capacity to autoinfect; female worms produce eggs that hatch into larvae that reinvade the intestinal mucosa, resulting in prolonged infection, so that the original source and time of infection may be forgotten. There may be extremely heavy worm loads, especially in immunocompromised patients. The parasite is endemic in parts of South-East Asia, especially the Philippines and Thailand, and has more recently been found in Egypt. Infection is prevented by properly cooking fish.

Intestinal capillariasis may be a severe and even fatal disease. Patients often present with abdominal pain, diarrhoea, and borborygmi.

As the worm load increases, diarrhoea becomes more severe, with anorexia, nausea, and vomiting. Prolonged diarrhoea leads to cachexia. There may also be signs of hypotension and cardiac failure. The mortality rate in untreated cases approaches 20%. The diagnosis is made by finding eggs in the faeces, 36 to 45 µm in length by 19 to 21 µm in breadth (Fig. 9.5.7), which may superficially resemble those of *Trichuris trichiura.* Larvae or adult worms may also be present, and repeated stool examination may be required in some cases. The parasite may also be found in jejunal aspirate or biopsy. All cases should be treated with either mebendazole or albendazole 200 mg twice daily for 3 weeks. Stools should be re-examined to ensure the eradication of infection; if not, the course of treatment should be repeated. Supportive measures to overcome malnutrition and diarrhoea will be required in severely ill patients.

Hepatic capillariasis

The adults of *C. hepatica* measure 52 to 104 mm in length, and live in the liver of various mammals, especially rats. Eggs are produced that are retained in the liver parenchyma; they measure 28 × 48 to 36 × 66 µm, and have bipolar plugs. The ova eventually reach the soil and embryonate, either by decomposition of a carcass, or when the host is eaten by another animal and the eggs pass through the gut of that animal and are deposited in the faeces. Infective eggs are then ingested by another definitive host, the eggs hatch, and the larvae reach the liver via the portal system. *C. hepatica* is a rare human parasite, and infections occur when eggs in the soil are accidentally swallowed. Clinical features may resemble those of visceral larva migrans, with tender hepatomegaly, fever, and eosinophilia. The diagnosis is made by identifying the parasite or eggs in a liver biopsy (Fig. 9.5.8). The most effective treatment is unclear, although cases have been reported to respond to tiabendazole or albendazole; the latter is given as described for intestinal capillariasis.

Enterobiasis (threadworm infection)

Life cycle

Enterobiasis is an infection caused by the threadworm or pinworm, *Enterobius vermicularis.* Infection is acquired by the ingestion of eggs (Fig. 9.5.9). Larvae hatch in the upper intestine, and migrate to the region of the caecum, where they mature and copulate. Worms do not invade the tissues. About 1 month after infection, the white thread-like gravid female worms, about 10 to 13 mm long

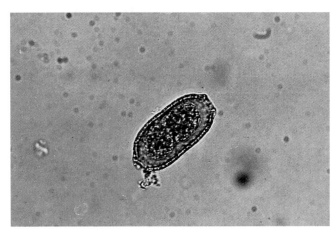

Fig. 9.5.7 *Capillaria philippinensis* egg (×1400).

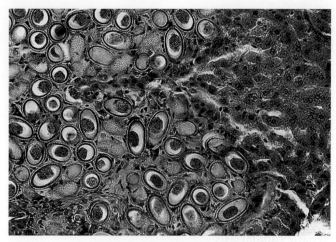

Fig. 9.5.8 *Capillaria hepatica* eggs in the liver (×250).

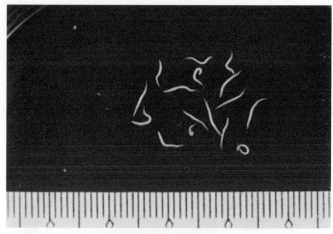

Fig. 9.5.10 Adult *Enterobius vermicularis* (scale in mm).
(Copyright Viqar Zaman)

by 0.3 to 0.5 mm in diameter, move down the bowel and pass out of the anus at night (Fig. 9.5.10). Each worm each night deposits approximately 10 000 eggs on the perianal skin. The worms then usually die, but sometimes they may re-enter the anus or migrate elsewhere. The eggs are infective within a few hours of deposition.

Epidemiology and control

This worm is found worldwide, and is extremely common, being found most frequently in children. Infections are commonly clustered in families and institutions. Humans are the only reservoir of infection. Eggs may remain viable for up to 3 weeks, and can be transmitted via contaminated clothing, bedding, and dust. Resistance to reinfection does not develop, and autoinfection may occur by contamination of the fingers.

Clinical features

Most infected people are asymptomatic. The most common presenting symptom is pruritus ani. This can be very troublesome, and

occurs more often during the night, causing restless sleep, especially in children. Persistent itching may lead to inflammation and secondary bacterial infection of the perianal region. Occasionally, adult worms migrate to aberrant sites such as the urinary tract. In females they may enter the female genital tract, causing vulvovaginitis or rarely salpingitis. *E. vermicularis* is sometimes found lodged in the lumen of the appendix (Fig. 9.5.11), but whether or not this causes appendicitis is controversial.

Diagnosis

The eggs are not usually found in the faeces. They are most easily found around the anus first thing in the morning by using cellulose adhesive tape applied with the sticky side against the perianal skin, which is then examined under the microscope; they are 33 × 55 μm in size, and flattened on one side (Fig. 9.5.12). Sometimes intact worms are passed in the faeces, and can easily be recognized by their size and shape.

Treatment

All the children and adults in a household should be treated at the same time. Several drugs are available, including mebendazole 100 mg in a single dose, albendazole 400 mg in a single dose, and

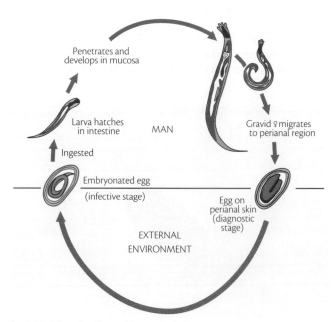

Fig. 9.5.9 Life cycle of *Enterobius vermicularis*.

Penetrates and develops in mucosa

Larva hatches in intestine   MAN   Gravid ♀ migrates to perianal region

Ingested

Embryonated egg (infective stage)

Egg on perianal skin (diagnostic stage)

EXTERNAL ENVIRONMENT

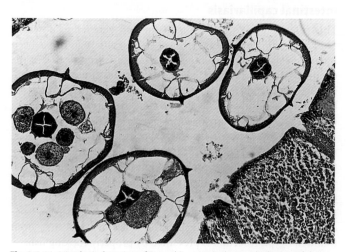

Fig. 9.5.11 Histological section of *Enterobius vermicularis* in the lumen of the appendix (×250).

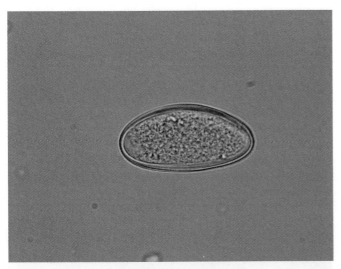

Fig. 9.5.12 *Enterobius vermicularis* egg.

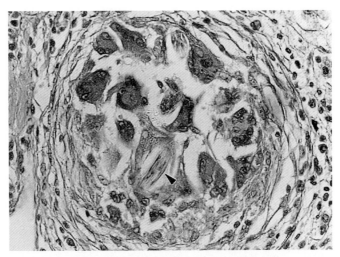

Fig. 9.5.13 Histological section. Granuloma formation in a monkey experimentally infected with *Toxocara canis*, showing a large number of giant cells and some fibroblastic reaction. The arrow marks the larva (×400).

pyrantel embonate 10 mg/kg in a single dose; pyrantel embonate is recommended for children under 2 years of age and pregnant women. The best results are achieved if the course is repeated after 2 weeks. Attention to personal hygiene is an important part of treatment and prevention. The patient should be instructed to keep fingernails short, and wash hands with soap and water after defecating. The bed cover and sleeping garments should be washed every day, and the floor in the bedroom kept clean.

Toxocariasis

Toxocariasis in humans occurs in two clinical forms, visceral larva migrans and ocular larva migrans, and is caused mainly by the migrating larvae of *Toxocara canis*, and to a lesser extent *T. cati*, and rarely other nematodes. *T. canis* and *T. cati* are parasites that live in the intestines of dogs and cats, which pass eggs in the faeces. Humans, usually young children, become infected by inadvertently ingesting embryonated eggs in the soil. The larvae hatch in the small intestine, and migrate to various organs of the body, including the liver, lungs, eye, and brain. The larvae, which are about 15 to 20 μm in length, do not mature in humans, but granulomas eventually develop around them (Fig. 9.5.13). In a fully formed granuloma the larvae are surrounded by layers of fibrous tissue, and inflammation subsides (Fig. 9.5.14). Eggs are never seen in human faeces. Toxocara infection occurs wherever there are large domestic dog and cat populations in close association with humans, and is more common in children. Deworming dogs, and stopping children from eating dirt (pica) when playing in areas frequented by dogs, are important control measures.

Visceral larva migrans

This disease is most often seen in young children, because of pica. Most people remain asymptomatic. In a minority, symptoms consist of muscular pain, lassitude, anorexia, cough, itching, and urticarial rashes. Physical signs may include wheezing and hepatomegaly. Occasionally there is splenomegaly, lymphadenopathy, and skin lesions. Central nervous system involvement may be manifested by convulsions. The acute phase generally lasts for 2 to 3 weeks, followed by recovery. Sometimes the resolution of all the signs may take up to 18 months. Rarely, the infection may end fatally if a massive dose of parasites has been ingested.

The hallmark of visceral larva migrans is marked eosinophilia, which may reach a level of 75%. Serological tests for toxocara antibody may be helpful; a negative test may rule out the diagnosis, but positive titres are often found in normal individuals. The definitive diagnosis is by finding larvae on biopsy, usually of the liver, but this is not often done because of the large sampling error. Most patients recover spontaneously; the larvae cannot multiply, and they eventually die. There is no proven therapy. Anthelmintics, including mebendazole, albendazole, and diethylcarbamazine, have been tried, but may be ineffective or precipitate an inflammatory reaction. Corticosteroids and nonsteroidal anti-inflammatory agents have been suggested in order to suppress inflammation.

Ocular larva migrans

This condition is caused by granuloma formation around a larva in the eye, and is most commonly seen in older children. If this is near the macula, impairment of vision or even blindness may result.

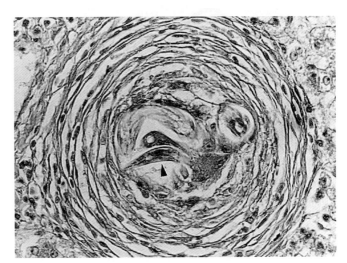

Fig. 9.5.14 Histological section. Granuloma formation in the same animal as Fig. 9.5.13, at a later stage when the larva is completely surrounded by fibroblasts (×400).

A rounded swelling, often near the optic disc, may be detected on fundoscopy. The features of visceral larva migrans are usually lacking. There is usually no marked peripheral eosinophilia. Diagnosis depends upon positive serology with consistent fundoscopic features; the major differential diagnosis is retinoblastoma. Antibody titres in vitreous or aqueous fluid may be higher than those found in serum. There is no proven anthelmintic therapy, but the agents used in visceral larva migrans may be tried. Visible larvae can be photocoagulated by laser. Vitrectomy has been used in some cases, and local and intraocular steroids also appear to be of some value.

Trichinosis (trichinellosis)

Life cycle

Trichinosis is an infection usually caused by *Trichinella spiralis* and related species. Humans become infected by eating undercooked meat, usually pork or pork products from domestic and wild pigs (boars) (Fig. 9.5.15). After ingestion the larvae are liberated in the stomach, then pass into the small bowel, where they invade the columnar epithelium and develop into adult worms living in the cytoplasm of a row of enterocytes. Male trichinellae are about 1.5 × 0.05 mm in size, and female worms measure 3.5 × 0.06 mm. Over 2 to 3 weeks or so before they are expelled, female worms release about 500 newborn larvae (Fig. 9.5.16), which enter the bloodstream and seed the skeletal muscles. Over the next few weeks these larvae in the muscles increase in size, moult, coil, usually develop a cyst wall, and become capable of infecting a new host (Fig. 9.5.17); they may remain viable for several years.

Epidemiology and control

Trichinella species are widely distributed in many geographical areas among a large number of carnivorous hosts found in three classes of vertebrate host: mammals, birds, and reptiles (Table 9.5.1). Domestic pigs become infected by eating infected scrap from slaughterhouses or farms. Humans are incidental hosts, and are usually infected with *T. spiralis*, but are occasionally infected

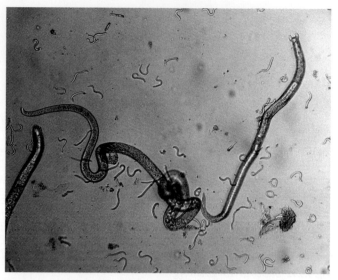

Fig. 9.5.16 *In vitro* preparation of infected mouse small bowel, showing adult worms of *Trichinella spiralis* surrounded by newborn larvae. (Courtesy of D I Grove.)

with other species, depending upon the animal eaten. Infection is best prevented by properly cooking meat.

Clinical features

Most people with light infections are asymptomatic. In heavy infections, diarrhoea develops in the first week and is associated with abdominal discomfort and vomiting. Fulminating enteritis may develop in patients with extremely heavy infections. Symptoms of larval invasion develop during the second week, and include fever, myositis with pain, swelling, and weakness, usually first involving the extraocular muscles, then the masseters, neck muscles, limb flexors, and lumbar muscles. Some patients may develop one or more of cough, dyspnoea, headache, periorbital oedema, subconjunctival haemorrhages, and a petechial rash. These symptoms slowly subside over several weeks, although symptoms persist longer in a minority of patients. In fulminant infections a potentially fatal myocarditis or meningoencephalitis may develop.

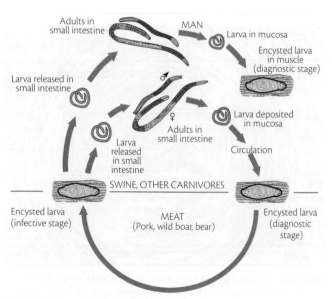

Fig. 9.5.15 Life cycle of *Trichinella spiralis*.

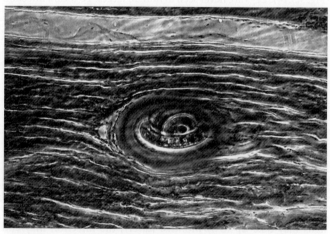

Fig. 9.5.17 *Trichinella spiralis* third-stage larvae in human muscle (×100).

Table 9.5.1 Major *Trichinella* spp. and their epidemiology

Species	Code	Distribution	Most common hosts	Cyst wall
T. spiralis	T1	Worldwide except Australasia	Pig, horse, bear, rodent, fox	Yes
T. nativa	T2	Arctic, subarctic	Bear, fox, dog	Yes
T. britovi	T3	Temperate, subarctic	Dog, bear, cat, boar	Yes
T. pseudospiralis	T4	Cosmopolitan	Bird	No
T. murrelli	T5	North America	Bear, coyote, dog	Yes
Uncertain	T6	Subarctic	Bear	Yes
T. nelsoni	T7	Sub-Saharan Africa	Hyena, cat	Yes
Uncertain	T8	Southern Africa	Lion, panther	Yes
Uncertain	T9	Japan	Bear	Yes
T. papuae	T10	Papua New Guinea	Pig, crocodile	No
T. zimbabwensis	T11	Central Africa	Crocodile, mammals	No
Uncertain	T12	Argentina	Cougars	No

Diagnosis

The diagnosis is suggested by a combination of fever, periorbital oedema, myositis, and eosinophilia in a patient who gives a history of eating undercooked meat, often in the context of an outbreak. Elevated creatine kinase and lactate dehydrogenase levels indicate considerable muscle involvement. Serological tests become positive several weeks after infection. A definitive diagnosis depends upon finding larvae in muscle biopsies, although this is usually unnecessary.

Treatment and prevention

Therapy is often unsatisfactory. If the diagnosis is made very early in the illness the administration of mebendazole 5 mg/kg or albendazole 5 mg/kg daily for 1 week may expel adult worms from the gut, and reduce the load of larvae seeding the tissues. In established infections these benzimidazole agents may be tried, but usually have little influence on the course of the disease. In established infections the mainstays of treatment are bed rest and the administration of nonsteroidal anti-inflammatory agents. Corticosteroids may be used in conjunction with anthelmintics in critically ill patients, but evidence of benefit is equivocal. Trichinosis in the pig population can be greatly reduced or eliminated by hygienic rearing methods. Larvae in pork can be killed by freezing at −18 C for 1 week. Since this cannot be relied upon, thorough cooking of pork is the best safeguard against infection in all endemic areas.

Trichuriasis (whipworm infection)

Life cycle

Trichuriasis is an infection caused by *Trichuris trichiura*. Infection is acquired when an egg is ingested (Fig. 9.5.18). The infective larva hatches in the small intestine and enters the mucosal crypts of the caecum, where it moults several times to become an adult worm 30 to 50 mm long. The anterior three-fifths of the worm are thin and elongated, and the posterior two-fifths bulbous and fleshy. The thin end is embedded in a syncytial tunnel in the large-bowel epithelium (Fig. 9.5.19). Nearly 3 months after infection the fertilized female worms begin to produce about 10 000 eggs per day. Adult worms live for 1 to 3 years. After passage in the faeces,

eggs embryonate in the soil and become infective after several weeks.

Epidemiology and control

Trichuriasis has a worldwide distribution, particularly in the warmer parts, and is most common in areas where sanitation is poor, especially where human faeces are used as fertilizer in vegetable gardens. Environmental sanitation is the best control measure. Ground-growing fruits and vegetables should be carefully washed.

Clinical features

Most infections are light and asymptomatic. In heavy infections there is colitis and/or proctitis, with the passage of blood and mucus in the faeces. In some cases prolapse of the oedematous

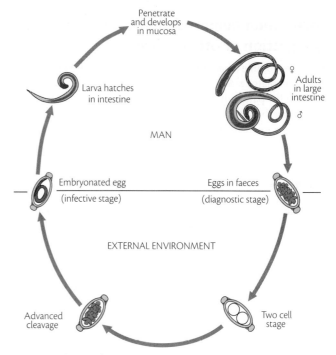

Fig. 9.5.18 Life cycle of *Trichuris trichiura*.

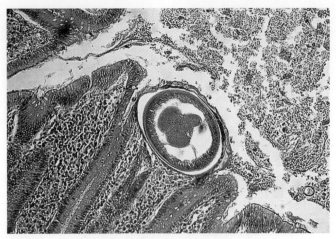

Fig. 9.5.19 Histological section. Anterior end of an adult *Trichuris trichiura* embedded superficially in the large bowel mucosa (×250).

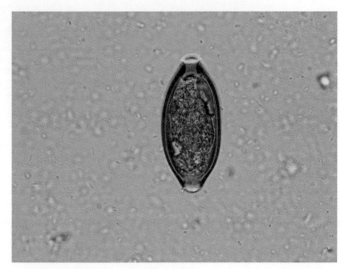

Fig. 9.5.20 Egg of *Trichuris trichiura*.
(Courtesy of A R Butcher.)

parasitized rectum occurs. Chronic heavy infection may be associated with iron-deficiency anaemia and growth retardation.

Diagnosis

This is based on finding characteristically barrel-shaped eggs 50×20 mm in size (Fig. 9.5.20) in the faeces. Sigmoidoscopy, proctoscopy, or colonoscopy may show worms attached to the mucous membrane, and sometimes intact worms may be passed in the faeces.

Treatment

Benzimidazole anthelmintics are effective when given for between 3 and 5 days, depending upon the severity of infection. Mebendazole is given is given as 100 mg, and albendazole as 400 mg, to both adults and children. Ivermectin in a dose of 200 μg/kg orally gives similar results.

Uncommon nematode infections acquired by ingestion or other routes

From time to time a patient may be encountered who harbours an unusual nematode. Some of these organisms are free-living parasites, and the patient has a spurious infection, usually as the result of ingesting the worm, or following the *in vitro* contamination of a clinical specimen such as faeces or urine. Other individuals may

have true infections, with worms being found in either the gastrointestinal tract or the tissues. Many of these infections are with parasites that are poorly adapted to the human host, and are unable to complete their development in humans. Thus worms in varying stages of development, including larvae, adults, and eggs, may be found in specimens. Some parasites may be recovered from fluids and are viewed intact; if there is uncertainty in identifying the worm help may often be obtained from a veterinary parasitologist, who may be more used to dealing with the species concerned. Sometimes parasites are seen only in histological sections; in these, definitive diagnosis may be very difficult, but the texts by Connor *et al.* and Orihel and Ash may be helpful. A summary of rarely reported nematodes, indicating geographical distribution, usual host, mode of acquisition, stage of development, clinical features, and suggested treatment, is shown in Table 9.5.2.

Nematodes found in the gastrointestinal tract may respond to a benzimidazole agent such as mebendazole (100 mg orally twice daily for up to 3 days) or albendazole (10 mg/kg orally daily for up to 1 week). Tiabendazole (25 mg/kg twice daily for several days) has been used traditionally for the treatment of systemic larval infections, but its effectiveness is very variable; albendazole may be more active than tiabendazole, and is absorbed better from the gut than mebendazole. If these drugs fail, ivermectin (0.15 mg/kg orally

Table 9.5.2 A summary of rarely reported nematodes found infecting humans, acquired by various routes

Nematode	Geographical distribution	Usual host	Mode of acquisition	Stage of development	Clinical features	Suggested treatment
Agamomermis spp.	?	Free living Grasshoppers	Ingestion?	Larvae, adults	Spurious; worms in mouth, faeces, urethra	Manual removal if necessary
Anatrichosoma spp.	Asia, Africa	Monkeys	?	Larvae	Cutaneous larva migrans	Tiabendazole Albendazole
Ancylostoma caninum	Widespread	Dogs	Cutaneous penetration	Larvae Adults?	Cutaneous larva migrans, myositis, pulmonary infiltrates, eosinophilic enteritis	Mebendazole (enteritis) Tiabendazole (other)

(Continued)

Table 9.5.2 *(Cont'd)* A summary of rarely reported nematodes found infecting humans, acquired by various routes

Nematode	Geographical distribution	Usual host	Mode of acquisition	Stage of development	Clinical features	Suggested treatment
Ancylostoma malayanum	Asia	Bear	?	?	?	Mebendazole
Ascaris suum	Widespread	Pigs	Ingestion of eggs	Larvae Adults?	Pneumonitis, abdominal discomfort	Albendazole
Baylisascaris procyonis	North America	Raccoons	Ingestion of eggs in soil	Larvae	Visceral and ocular larva migrans, eosinophilic meningoencephalitis	Albendazole
Bunostomum trigonocephalum	Widespread	Sheep	Cutaneous penetration	Larvae	Cutaneous larva migrans	Albendazole
Brugia spp. (not *malayi*, *timori*)	Widespread	Monkeys, raccoons, rabbits	Mosquito bite	Larvae, adults	Lymph node swelling	Excision
Cheilospirura spp.	Widespread	Birds	Ingestion of arthropods?	Larvae	Conjunctival nodule	Excision
Contracaecum spp.	Widespread	Fish, birds	Ingestion of undercooked fish	Larvae	See 'Anisakidosis'	See 'Anisakidosis'
Cyclodontostomum purvisi	Asia	Rats	?	Adults	Worms in faeces	Mebendazole
Dioctophyma renale	Widespread	Mammals	Ingestion of aquatic annelids, amphibians, crustaceans, fish	Larvae, adults	Haematuria, retroperitoneal mass, subcutaneous nodule	Excision
Diploscapter coronata	Widespread	Free living	Ingestion with vegetation	Adults	Spurious; worms in stomach contents, urine	Unnecessary
Dirofilaria immitis	Widespread	Dog	Mosquito bite	Larva	Nodule in lung, subcutaneous tissue	Excision
Dirofilaria repens	Europe, Asia	Dog, cat	Mosquito bite	Larva	Nodule in lung, subcutaneous tissue, eye, abdominal cavity	Excision
Dirofilaria tenuis	North America	Raccoon	Mosquito bite	Larva	Nodule in subcutaneous tissue, eye	Excision
Dirofilaria ursi	North America	Bear	Blackfly bite	Larva	Nodule in subcutaneous tissue	Excision
Eustrongylides spp.	Widespread	Fish, birds	Ingestion of undercooked fish	Larvae	Peritonitis	Laparotomy and surgical removal
Gongylonema pulchrum	Worldwide	Ruminants, swine	Ingestion of beetles, cockroaches etc.	Adult	Migrating worm, especially in the oral cavity	Surgical removal
Haemonchus contortus	Widespread	Sheep, cattle	Ingestion of larvae with vegetation?	Adults	?	Mebendazole
Lagochilascaris minor	Central and South America	?	?	Adults, eggs, larvae	Subcutaneous abscess in head and neck, nasopharyngeal or sinus lesions, encephalitis	Surgical removal Levamisole, diethylcarbamazine, tiabendazole
Mammomonogamus (Syngamus) laryngeus	Central and South America	Cattle, felines	?	Adults	Cough, pharyngeal lesion	Endoscopic removal
Meloidogyne (Heterodera) spp.	Widespread	Plant parasite	Ingestion of vegetation; contamination of faecal specimen	Eggs, larvae	Spurious; eggs and larvae in faeces	Unnecessary
Meningonema peruzzii	Africa	Monkeys	?	Larvae	Meningoencephalitis	Albendazole
Mermis nigrescens	North America	Grasshoppers	Ingestion of adult worm?	Adult	Worm in mouth	Manual removal
Metastrongylus elongatus	Widespread	Pigs	Ingestion of earthworms	Adult	Worm in gut or respiratory tract	Albendazole
Metastrongylid nematode	Italy	?	?	Larvae, adults	Pulmonary arteritis	Anthelmintics?
Micronema (syn. Halicephalobus) deletrix	Widespread	Free living Horses	Trauma or skin lesions	Adults, larvae, eggs	Meningoencephalitis; generalized spread	Albendazole

(Continued)

Table 9.5.2 *(Cont'd)* A summary of rarely reported nematodes found infecting humans, acquired by various routes

Nematode	Geographical distribution	Usual host	Mode of acquisition	Stage of development	Clinical features	Suggested treatment
Muspiceoid nematode	Australia	?	?	Larvae, adults	Polymyositis	Albendazole
Necator suillus	Central America	Pigs	Percutaneous	Adults	?	Mebendazole
Onchocerca spp. (not *O. volvulus*)	Widespread	Cattle, horses	Insect borne	Adults	Subcutaneous nodule, eye lesions	Surgical excision
Ostertagia spp.	Widespread	Cattle, sheep	Ingestion of adult worms in undercooked abomasums?	Adults	Spurious? Worms in gut	Mebendazole
Pelodera (Rhabditis) strongyloides	Widespread	Free living	Cutaneous	Larvae	Papular dermatitis	Albendazole, topical corticosteroid
Philometra spp.	Widespread	Fish	Cutaneous injury	Adults	Worms in laceration	Manual removal
Phocanema spp.	Widespread	Fish	Ingestion of undercooked fish	Larvae	See 'Anisakidosis'	See 'Anisakidosis'
Physaloptera caucasica	Europe, Africa	Primates	Ingestion of beetles, cockroaches?	Adults, eggs	Sometimes spurious; abdominal pain, small bowel gangrene	Mebendazole Surgical removal
Rhabditis spp.	Widespread	Free living	Ingestion	Adults	Spurious; worms in faeces, urine, skin	Unnecessary
Rictularia spp.	Widespread	Mammals, birds	Ingestion?	Adult	Found in an appendix	
Spirocerca lupi	Widespread	Dogs, wolves	Ingestion of beetle?	Adults	Intestinal obstruction and peritonitis in a baby	Surgery
Spiruroid nematode	Japan	Fish, squid	Ingestion of undercooked food	Larvae	Creeping eruption Ileal granuloma	Excision Anthelmintics?
Syphacia spp.	Widespread	Mice	Ingestion	Eggs, adults	Spurious?; worms in faeces	Mebendazole if necessary
Terranova spp.	Widespread	Fish	Ingestion of undercooked fish	Larvae	See 'Anisakidosis'	See 'Anisakidosis'
Tetrameres fissispina	Widespread	Birds	Ingestion of grasshoppers, cockroaches?	Adults	Spurious?; worms in gut	Mebendazole
Thelazia californiensis	North America	Mammals	Deposition on eye by fly	Adults	Conjunctivitis	Manual removal
Thelazia callipaeda	Asia	Dogs, rabbits	Deposition on eye by fly	Adults	Conjunctivitis	Manual removal
Trichuris suis	Widespread	Pigs	Ingestion of eggs	Eggs, larvae, adults	Usually asymptomatic	Mebendazole
Trichuris vulpis	Widespread	Dogs	Ingestion of eggs	Eggs, larvae, adults	Usually asymptomatic	Mebendazole
Turbatrix (Anguillula) aceti	Widespread	Free living (including vinegar, acetic acid)	Accidental inoculation	Larvae, adults	Spurious; urine, vaginal discharge, blood smears (in stains)	Unnecessary
Uncinaria stenocephala	Widespread	Dogs, cats	Cutaneous penetration	Larvae	Cutaneous larva migrans	Tiabendazole Albendazole

daily for several days) may be tried. Other drugs that have been used in these unusual nematode infections include levamisole and diethylcarbamazine. Unfortunately, some infections are refractory to all to anthelmintics. Nevertheless, these worms generally cannot multiply in humans, and the parasites will die spontaneously after months or years.

Further reading

Bethony J, *et al.* (2006). Soil-transmitted helminth infections: ascariasis, trichuriasis and hookworm. *Lancet*, **367**, 1521–32.

Connor DH, *et al.* (eds) (1997). *Pathology of infectious diseases*, vol 2, pp. 1305–588. Appleton and Lange, Stamford, CT.

Fuehrer HP, *et al.* (2011). Capillaria hepatica in man—an overview of hepatic capillariosis and spurious infections. *Parasitol Res*, **109**, 969–79.

Gottstein B, *et al.* (2009). Epidemiology, diagnosis, treatment, and control of trichinellosis. *Clin Microbiol Rev*, **22**, 127–45.

Hochberg NS, Hamer DH (2010). Anisakidosis: perils of the deep. *Clin Infect Dis*, **51**, 806–12.

Lu LH, *et al.* (2006). Human intestinal capillariasis (*Capillaria philippinensis*) in Taiwan. *Am J Trop Med Hyg*, **74**, 810–13.

Orihel TC, Ash LR (1995). *Parasites in human tissues.* American Society of Clinical Pathologists, Chicago.

Ok KS, *et al.* (2009). Trichuris trichiura infection diagnosed by colonoscopy: case reports and review of literature. *Korean J Parasitol*, **47**, 275–80. [This article is free at http://www.ncbi.nlm.nih.gov/pubmed and has excellent images of whipworms seen at colonoscopy.]

Rubinsky-Elefant G, *et al.* (2010). Human toxocariasis: diagnosis, worldwide seroprevalence and clinical expression of the systemic and ocular forms. *Ann Trop Med Parasitol*, **104**, 3–23.

Wani I, *et al.* (2010). Intestinal ascariasis in children. *World J Surg*, **34**, 963–8.

Websites

Centers for Disease Control and Prevention. *Laboratory investigation of parasites of public health concern.* http://www.dpd.cdc.gov/DPDx/

Korean Society for Parasitology. *Web atlas of medical parasitology.* http://www.atlas.or.kr

9.6 Parastrongyliasis (angiostrongyliasis)

Richard Knight

Essentials

Parastrongylus cantonensis

The rat lungworm causes outbreaks of eosinophilic meningitis in parts of South-East Asia, east Asia, Oceania, and the Caribbean. Elsewhere the condition is usually seen in travellers. Human infections follow ingestion of uncooked molluscs, the primary intermediate hosts, or one of several paratenic hosts. Clinical manifestations include headache, meningism, vomiting, cranial nerve lesions, and (less commonly) other neurological features such as seizures. Ocular lesions are quite common. Diagnosis is made by lumbar puncture revealing eosinophilic meningitis, with larval or immature adult worms sometimes seen. Treatment is with albendazole together with prednisolone, or with prednisolone alone. Mortality is usually below 2%. Prevention is by avoidance of raw high-risk dietary items and unwashed salads.

Parastrongylus costaricensis

The cotton rat is the principal reservoir host. Unwitting ingestion of slugs, the intermediate hosts, in salads or fruit leads to human infections, especially in Costa Rica, Nicaragua, Guatemala, and Honduras. The organism causes granulomatous lesions of the right colon and sometimes the liver: most patients present with right-sided or right iliac fossa pain, with tenderness and sometimes a palpable mass. Diagnosis is usually made histologically on resected material. Surgery may be necessary, but the value of anthelminthics is uncertain. Preventive measures include washing and careful inspection of vegetables, and hand washing before meals by children and those preparing salads.

Introduction

Human disease is caused by two nematode species of the genus *Parastrongylus*. Both parasites normally infect rodents, and molluscs are the primary intermediate hosts. They were previously placed in the genus *Angiostrongylus* but it is now recognized that angiostrongylid worms with rodent hosts belong to the genus *Parastrongylus*. Infection follows accidental or deliberate ingestion of molluscs or paratenic hosts. The epidemiology is complex because of multiple potential routes of transmission.

Parastrongylus cantonensis

This is the rat lungworm. The first known case, reported in 1944, was a 15-year-old Taiwanese boy with meningoencephalitis, in whose cerebrospinal fluid an immature adult worm was found. Detailed clinicopathological studies were made in 1962 during epidemics of eosinophilic meningitis in Tahiti.

Aetiology: the biology of the parasite

Adult worms live in the pulmonary arteries of rats; larvae from hatched eggs ascend the airways, are swallowed, and so reach the faeces. Molluscs ingest these larvae, and after two moults they are infective when eaten by a rodent. In the rat, infective larval worms migrate to the cerebral grey matter, where they start to mature. They then move to the meninges and enter the venous sinuses, thereby reaching the pulmonary arteries, where maturation is completed. Infective larvae from a mollusc can also enter a second or third intermediate host, in which they undergo no further development until they enter a mammalian host. Such supernumerary hosts are termed paratenic hosts, and are important sources of infection in humans.

Development in humans reaches the immature adult stage, measuring 11 to 15 mm in length. Nearly all will die in the superficial cortex, brainstem, and meninges, causing vigorous tissue reactions; very few reach the lungs.

Epidemiology

The parasite is endemic and causes human outbreaks in South-East Asia, east Asia, Oceania, and the Caribbean. Sporadic cases are reported in many other countries, usually in travellers. Most recent outbreaks have been in mainland China, Taiwan, Thailand, and Japan. In the Pacific epidemics have occurred in Hawaii, Samoa, and the Solomon Islands. In the Caribbean most cases are reported from Cuba, Costa Rica, and Jamaica. All ages can be affected, and outbreaks have occurred after weddings and feasts; infections are often seasonal. The modes of transmission differ geographically, by age and social group, and with time.

The principal rodent hosts are *Rattus rattus*, *R. norvegicus*, *R. alexandrinus*, and *R. exulans*. The prevalence in rats in endemic areas may be 40% or more. The geographical spread and population increase of these peridomestic rodents has increased the zoonotic reservoir; wildlife is now infected in the southern United States of America. Another factor leading to the increase in human infection has been the dispersal by human agency of the edible giant African land snail *Achatina fulica*, from Madagascar in 1800, eastwards across the Indian Ocean and the Pacific, to reach Hawaii in 1936. The freshwater golden apple snail *Pomacea canaliculata*, which is highly susceptible to the parasite, was recently introduced into Asia, where it has colonized paddy fields and caused disease when served raw in restaurants in China, Taiwan, and Japan. The popularity of heliculture, the cultivation of exotic snails for food, and keeping them as pets, facilitates the spread of the parasite. Raw snails are eaten as a delicacy and for medicinal purposes; salads may contain small undetected molluscs, their slime trails, or planarians. An outbreak in Taiwan followed the drinking of raw vegetable juice. In Thailand, *Pila* spp. snails are a seasonal delicacy eaten by all the family, but only young men take them raw with alcohol.

Paratenic hosts include freshwater prawns, land and coconut crabs, frogs, and land planarians, which cause infection if eaten raw; drinking-water may contain tiny immature prawns, especially after heavy rains. In Thailand, the yellow tree monitor lizard is an important paratenic host. In the Ryukyu islands of Japan, patients are usually infected by eating raw snails or toad liver for medicinal purposes.

The modes of transmission differ geographically, by age and social group, and with time. In Thailand, *Pila* spp. snails are a seasonal delicacy eaten by all the family, but young men take them raw with alcohol; another edible snail, *Ampullaria canaliculatus*, is infected in Taiwan and Japan. In the Ryukyu islands of Japan, patients are usually infected by eating raw snails or toad liver for medicinal purposes.

Pathology

Inflammatory granulomatous lesions, sometimes track-like, occur predominantly in the cortical grey matter and the meninges, but also in the brain stem and cerebellum; nerve roots and the spinal cord may also be affected. Live worms are occasionally found at autopsy, and dead worms are found in many lesions. The number of worms found varies greatly, and may reach several hundred; worm tracks in the tissue and meninges are surrounded by a cuff of eosinophils; Charcot–Leyden crystals derived from eosinophils are numerous. Rarely, adult worms have been found in human lung at autopsy. Ocular infection derives from worms that have migrated across the cribriform plate.

Clinical features

After an incubation period of 1 to 4 weeks the onset is acute, with headache (intermittent at first), together with nausea and vomiting. There is constitutional upset and frequently menigism; fever is unusual. The illness is often self limiting over a period of 4 weeks. Cranial nerve lesions are seen in the optic, abducens, and facial nerves. Less common are seizures, confusion, and radiculopathy (with paraesthesia, root pains, or weakness). Long-tract signs and impaired consciousness are uncommon, except in severe cases, but spinal cord damage can cause sphincter disturbance.

Ocular complications include retinitis, retinal haemorrhages, optic neuritis, and larval worms in the vitreous, anterior chamber, or beneath the conjunctiva (Fig. 9.6.1). Rarely, migration to the lungs produces clinical evidence of pneumonitis. Numerous eosinophils occur in the cerebrospinal fluid, and there is blood eosinophilia.

Diagnosis

Lumbar puncture reveals high opening pressure, with a clear or lightly turbid cerebrospinal fluid containing 500 to 2000 cells/mm^3 (of which 10–>90% are eosinophils); protein levels are usually elevated, with normal or less commonly reduced glucose. Detailed examination at low power reveals larval or immature adult worms in up to 25% of cases, measuring 5 to 15 mm in length. Cerebrospinal fluid changes may persist for up to 3 months. CT or MRI may reveal focal cortical abnormalities. Serology using antigens from fourth-stage larvae is useful, but cross-reactions with other nematodes can cause difficulty. Commercial serological tests are not yet available. Techniques to detect worm antigens in cerebrospinal fluid and serum have also been developed.

Differential diagnosis is from other helminth infections affecting the nervous system, as eosinophils are otherwise rare in cerebrospinal fluid. A detailed geographical and dietary history is essential; conditions to be considered include gnathostomiasis,

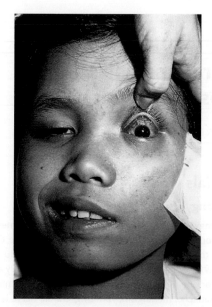

Fig. 9.6.1 Parastrongylus under the conjunctiva in a Thai girl with a left facial nerve palsy.
(Copyright D A Warrell.)

paragonimiasis, schistosomiasis, and neurocysticercosis. A particular problem in Thailand is confusion with *Gnathostoma spinigerum*, which more commonly causes long-tract signs, bloody or xanthochromic cerebrospinal fluid, neck stiffness, and clouding of consciousness.

Treatment, prognosis, and control

Although worm death might aggravate the clinical condition, clinical studies support the use of the anthelmintics albendazole or mebendazole together with prednisolone. However, in a recent prospective trial prednisolone alone was as effective as prednisolone plus albendazole. Prednisolone alone is now often the recommended treatment, although prednisolone plus albendazole is still used in China and probably elsewhere. Such treatment hastens recovery and relieves headache; it probably improves the prognosis in severe cases. Ocular disease may require laser therapy and larvae in the eye chambers should be removed surgically.

Mortality rates are generally low in uncomplicated cases, and depend mainly on the number of infective larvae ingested; some patients develop encephalitis and pass into coma after about 2 weeks, and their prognosis is then very poor. Most patients improve in 2 to 4 weeks, but focal neurological deficits can persist for longer; partial relapse after 2 months of illness may represent a reaction to dying worms. Some cases are relatively mild and can be discharged within a few days; during epidemics, mild cases may need only outpatient care.

Control measures include health education to limit the ingestion of raw high-risk dietary items, and unwashed salads. Warnings may be necessary regarding raw molluscs, amphibians, and reptiles used for medicinal purposes. Rodents in vegetable gardens and the peridomestic environment should be controlled.

Parastrongylus costaricensis

This was first recognized in Costa Rica in 1950 in surgical specimens simulating bowel malignancy. The parasite was described from such specimens in 1967, and the complete life cycle in rodents was elucidated during the next 3 years.

Aetiology: the biology of the parasite

In both the rodent and human hosts the worms are located in the ileocaecal mesenteric arteries. The cotton rat *Sigmodon hispidus* is the principal reservoir host, but other species of rodent (including the coatimundi) are also involved, and even dogs and marmosets. In the rodent hosts worm eggs embolize to gut-wall capillaries, and the hatched larvae pass into the gut lumen. Veronicellid slugs, especially *Vaginulus plebeius*, eat rodent faeces containing larvae, and these develop into infective larvae in the fibromuscular tissue of the mollusc after two moults over a period of 18 days. Infective larvae can persist in the slug for several months or be shed in slime trails. The prepatent period in rats eating infected slugs is 24 days.

In human infections the worms reach maturity, but the embryonated eggs do not hatch.

Epidemiology

Infections occur especially in Costa Rica, Nicaragua, Guatemala, and Honduras, but also sporadically elsewhere in the Americas from the United States of America to Argentina, and some Caribbean islands. Recently, infections have been increasingly recognized from southern Brazil. Small veronicellid slugs and their slime trails are the source of infection in man; infection rates in these hosts can reach 85%. Small or chopped slugs may be unnoticed on fallen fruits or in salads; their mucus also contains infective larvae. Many cases are in schoolchildren, but infants and older persons are also affected. Seropositivity in endemic areas suggests that there are unrecognized infections.

Pathology and clinical features

Lesions primarily affect the small arteries, producing subacute or chronic granulomatous inflammatory masses in the wall of the caecum, right colon, and less often the small intestine or elsewhere in the colon. Rarely, the predominant feature is ischaemic infarction. The finding of an adult nematode measuring 18 to 42 mm in length within a gut arterial vessel is diagnostic of infection; eggs may be seen in vessels or in tissue, where they are surrounded by eosinophil granulomas. Lesions also occur in regional abdominal lymph nodes or the omentum. Some larvae enter the hepatic artery and cause granulomatous or necrotic lesions in the liver; others enter testicular arteries causing similar lesions of the testis. In a recently reported case an adult worm was shown histologically within a hepatic arteriole.

Clinically, most patients present with right-sided or right iliac fossa pain, with tenderness and sometimes a palpable mass in this region. Other features are eosinophilia, fever, diarrhoea, or rectal bleeding. Tender hepatomegaly with high blood eosinophilia occurs in some patients. Serious complications are bowel obstruction and perforation, and rarely testicular infarction.

Diagnosis and treatment

The confirmation of diagnosis is usually made histologically on resected material. The condition can mimic appendicitis, bowel neoplasm, Meckel's diverticulitis, testicular torsion, or other surgical problems. Parasite eggs are not found in faeces, but serology using enzyme immunoassay or latex agglutination is useful. Contrast radiology reveals filling defects and altered motility of the terminal ileum, caecum, or ascending colon. Laparoscopy can reveal the bowel and hepatic lesions; biopsy may be diagnostic.

The value of anthelmintic treatment remains unproven; tiabendazole or high doses of mebendazole have been used. Surgery is often necessary, but can sometimes be deferred in uncomplicated cases when the diagnosis is strongly suspected, as spontaneous remission is common.

Preventive measures include washing and careful inspection of vegetables, and hand washing before meals by children and those preparing salads. Rinsing salads in 1.5% bleach kills larvae.

Further reading

Chotmongkol V, *et al.* (2004). Treatment of eosinophilic meningitis with a combination of albendazole and corticosteroid. *Southeast Asian J Trop Med Public Health*, **35**, 172–4.

Chotmongkol V, *et al.* (2006). Treatment of eosinophilic meningitis with a combination of prednisolone and mebendazole. *Am J Trop Med Hyg*, **74**, 1122–4.

Chotmongkol V, *et al.* (2009). Comparison of prednisolone plus albendazole with prednisolone alone for treatment of patients with eosinophilic meningitis. *Am J Trop Med Hyg*, **81**, 443–5.

Graeff-Teixeira C, *et al.* (1997). Seroepidemiology of abdominal angiostrongyliasis: the standardization of an immunoenzymatic assay and prevalence of antibodies in two localities in southern Brazil. *Trop Med Int Health*, **2**, 254–60.

Kramer MH, *et al.* (1998). First reported outbreak of abdominal angiostrongyliasis. *Clin Infect Dis*, **26**, 365–72.

Lo Re V 3rd, Gluckman SJ (2003). Eosinophilic meningitis. *Am J Med*, **114**, 217–23.

Mackerras MJ, Sandars DF (1995). The life history of the rat lungworm, *Angiostrongylus cantonensis* (Chen). *Aust J Zool*, **3**, 1–25.

Mota EM, Lenzi HL (2005). *Angiostrongylus costaricensis*: complete redescription of the migratory pathways based on experimental *Sigmodon hispidus* infection. *Mem Inst Oswaldo Cruz*, **100**, 407–20.

Pien FD, Pien BC (1999). *Angiostrongylus cantonensis* eosinophilic meningitis. *Int J Infect Dis*, **3**, 161–3.

Punyagupta S, Juttijudata P, Bunnag T (1975). Eosinophilic meningitis in Thailand. Clinical studies of 484 typical cases probably caused by *Angiostrongylus cantonensis*. *Am J Trop Med Hyg*, **24**, 921–31.

Quiros JL, *et al.* (2011). Abdominal angiostrongyliasis with involvement of liver histopathologically confirmed: a case report. *Rev Inst Trop S Paulo*, **53**, 219–22.

Quao-Ping W, *et al.* (2008). Human angiostrongyliasis. *Lancet Infect Dis*, **8**, 621–30.

Rambo PR, *et al.* (1997). Abdominal angiostrongylosis in southern Brazil—prevalence and parasitic burden in mollusc intermediate hosts from eighteen endemic foci. *Mem Inst Oswaldo Cruz*, **92**, 9–14.

Sawanyawisuth K, Sawanyawisuth K (2008). Treatment of angiostrongyliasis. *Trans R Soc Trop Med Hyg*, **102**, 990–6.

Sawanyawisuth K, *et al.* (2009). Clinical features predictive of encephalitis caused by Angiostrongylus cantonensis. *Am J Trop Med Hyg*, **81**, 608–701.

Slom TJ, *et al.* (2002). An outbreak of eosinophilic meningitis caused by *Angiostrongylus cantonensis* in travelers returning from the Caribbean. *N Engl J Med*, **346**, 668–75.

Tsai HC, *et al.* (2003). Eosinophilic meningitis caused by *Angiostrongylus cantonensis* associated with eating raw snails: correlation of brain magnetic resonance imaging scans with clinical findings. *Am J Trop Med Hyg*, **68**, 281–5.

Tsai HC, *et al.* (2004). Outbreak of eosinophilic meningitis associated with drinking raw vegetable juice in southern Taiwan. *Am J Trop Med Hyg*, **71**, 222–6.

Ubelaker JE (1986). Systematics of species referred to the genus *Angiostrongylus*. *J Parasitol*, **72**, 237–44.

Wan KS, Weng WC (2004). Eosinophilic meningitis in a child raising snails as pets. *Acta Tropica*, **90**, 51–3.

9.7 Gnathostomiasis

Valai Bussaratid and Pravan Suntharasamai

Essentials

Gnathostomiasis is an extraintestinal infection with larval or immature nematodes of the genus Gnathostoma (order Spirurida), the most common mode of human infection being consumption of undercooked freshwater fish. Clinical manifestations include recurrent cutaneous migratory swellings (common), creeping eruption (rare), and neurological deficits (occasional). Definitive diagnosis is by identification of the worm in surgical specimens; serological testing for antibody against gnathostoma antigen can confirm a presumptive diagnosis. Treatment of choice is albendazole or if possible, surgical removal of the worm in accessible areas and when the parasite can be located. Prevention is by avoiding all dishes that contain raw or poorly cooked flesh of animals or fish in or imported from endemic areas.

Acknowledgement: The authors thank Associate Professor Paron Dekumyoy for the use of unpublished data on serodiagnosis.

Aetiology, genetics, pathogenesis, and pathology

Five species of *Gnathostoma* are known to infect humans. Adult parasites live in the upper gastrointestinal tract of the definitive hosts: dogs, cats, and other mammals for *Gnathostoma spinigerum*, the most common infection in Thailand; pigs for *G. hispidum* and *G. doloresi*; weasels for *G. nipponicum*; and canines for *G. binucleatum*. Larvae from ova shed with the host's faeces hatch in water and are ingested by *Cyclops* spp. copepods. These are eaten by freshwater fish, amphibians, reptiles, crustaceans, birds, or mammals; third-stage larvae are found in the walls of the viscera and in the muscles of these second intermediate hosts. Unless the second intermediate hosts are eaten by definitive hosts, the parasites cannot develop into reproductive adults, but they remain infectious to humans and other paratenic hosts.

Consumption of the raw or undercooked flesh of second intermediate and paratenic hosts is the most common mode of transmission. Skin penetration after contact with infected material is less important. Prenatal transmission can occur, as larvae have been recovered in neonates as young as 3 days old.

Genetics

The nucleotide sequence analysis of the gnathostoma genome is incomplete. The 5.8S ribosomal DNAs are almost identical among species, whereas the internal transcribed spacer 2 region is a potential candidate as a genetic marker for the identification of gnathostoma species, because it varies considerably among species. The gene for a 24-kDa diagnostic glycoprotein of *G. spinigerum* has been identified.

Pathogenesis

The ingested larva penetrates the gut wall and migrates to the liver before wandering through almost any tissue except bone. Symptoms and signs vary according to the site and size of the inflammatory or haemorrhagic lesions induced intermittently along the migratory route.

Histopathology

Histopathological findings include mixed eosinophils and other inflammatory cell infiltration, areas of necrosis or haemorrhage, and occasionally parasite tracts. Occasionally, eosinophilic vasculitis or flame figures may be seen in skin biopsy. These findings are not characteristic for gnathostomiasis. The only diagnostic finding is the identification of a parasite. If the biopsy cuts through the bulb or cervical part of the worm, diagnostic features of *G. spinigerum* may be visible: a head bulb bearing eight transverse rows of spines or a cuticle bearing three-toothed spines.

Epidemiology

Isolated *G. spinigerum* infections are reported frequently in Thailand, and sporadically in Japan, China, Bangladesh, India, Sri Lanka, South-East Asia, Cameroon, Zambia, Ecuador, Peru, and Australia. Infections with *G. doloresi*, *G. nipponicum*, and *G. hispidum* have been reported from Japan. In Mexico and Ecuador, *G. binucleatum* is the most common infection.

Gnathostomiasis can present in places far away from these endemic areas as a result of migration of the latently infected human host, or importation of the infective flesh of paratenic hosts. Consumption of a raw fish dish at a party can result in an outbreak.

Prevention

All dishes that contain the raw or poorly cooked flesh of animals in or imported from endemic areas must be avoided. Those who prepare potentially infected flesh should use gloves if prolonged exposure is likely.

Clinical features

Nausea, vomiting, and epigastric pain may develop within 1 or 2 days of consumption of the infective food. Fever, pain in the right upper quadrant of the abdomen, chest pain, dry cough, and hypereosinophilia may develop within 1 to 2 weeks.

The primary invasive illness usually passes unnoticed, and so the incubation period is not known in most cases. General health is scarcely impaired, and fever is uncommon. The illnesses can be categorized according to the affected organs as below.

Cutaneous forms

Gnathostomal creeping eruption

This is rare in *G. spinigerum* infection, but more frequent with the other three species that are prevalent in Japan. The serpiginous track is similar to that caused by dog or cat hookworm larvae, but bigger and more variable in depth. A trail of subcutaneous haemorrhage is sometimes observed.

Cutaneous migratory swelling

The most common manifestation of human gnathostomiasis is intermittent swelling (Fig. 9.7.1). The first swelling may develop 3 to 4 weeks after infection, and can occur anywhere; it may recur close to or distant from the original site. The swelling develops rapidly, and usually lasts for about 1 to 2 weeks. Frequently it is extensive, e.g. involving the whole wrist or hand. Swelling of the digits or plantar surfaces can be very painful and incapacitating. Itching is the main associated symptom. Regional lymphadenitis is usually absent. When swelling involves the eyelid, chemosis and conjunctival haemorrhage may be observed.

The worms can escape spontaneously through the skin or the conjunctiva. The interval between episodes of swelling varies from a few days to a few months, and rarely 1 to 2 years. Intermittent cutaneous migratory swelling can persist for more than 5 years.

Visceral forms

Visceral invasion, as described below for *G. spinigerum* infection, has not been reported in infections with other *Gnathostoma* species.

Spinocerebral gnathostomiasis

Involvement of the spinal cord commonly starts with intermittent agonizing shooting pains in a limb or a segment of the trunk, followed by paraplegia with urinary retention, and rarely, quadriplegia. Sensation is correspondingly impaired, and Brown–Séquard syndrome is sometimes seen. A few patients with haematoma and inflammation caused by brain invasion present with severe headache and vomiting, followed very quickly by coma, cranial nerve palsies, and/or hemiplegia. A rapidly advancing or changing pattern of neurological deficits is characteristic. Subarachnoid

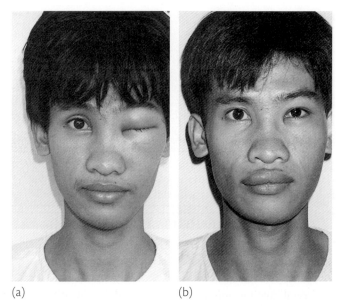

Fig. 9.7.1 Migratory swelling in a 23-year-old man. (a) In the left orbital region for 5 days when seen on 5 June 1986. (b) At the right side of the upper lip on 9 June 1986, when the larva was picked out by needle puncture and squeezing.

haemorrhage or eosinophilic meningitis without focal neurological deficit occasionally occurs.

The cerebrospinal fluid can be bloody, xanthochromic, or slightly turbid, with a minor increase in protein content. The proportion of eosinophils is higher than expected from haemorrhage *per se*.

Ocular gnathostomiasis

The parasite can be found in the anterior chamber (Fig. 9.7.2) and the vitreous, having migrated through the sclera or the cornea. It can induce uveitis, iritis, intraocular haemorrhage, retinal detachment and scarring, and blindness.

Auditory, pulmonary, intra-abdominal, and genitourinary gnathostomiasis

These uncommon forms can present with hearing loss, productive cough, pleurisy, intestinal obstruction, a painful intra-abdominal mass, and abnormal genital discharge.

Differential diagnosis

The diagnosis of cutaneous forms is based on clinical characteristics, geographical and dietary history, and by excluding other causes. Differential diagnoses include contact dermatitis, angio-oedema and urticaria, Calabar swellings (caused by *Loa loa*), fascioliasis, paragonimiasis, sparganosis, dirofilariasis, and noninfectious causes.

Gnathostoma infection is highly likely if rapidly advancing myelitis follows root pain, or if features of cerebral or subarachnoid haemorrhage occur in a person who is healthy apart from a history of cutaneous migratory swelling. Eosinophil pleocytosis is essential for the diagnosis, as is the exclusion of eosinophilic meningoencephalitis caused by *Angiostrongylus cantonensis*, *Baylisascaris procyonis*, or nonhelminthic encephalomyelitis.

In intraocular infections, the larvae of *A. cantonensis* can be distinguished from Gnathostoma species, as they are thinner, longer, and folding. They usually appear in the eyeball 2 to 3 weeks after the manifestation of eosinophilic meningoencephalitis.

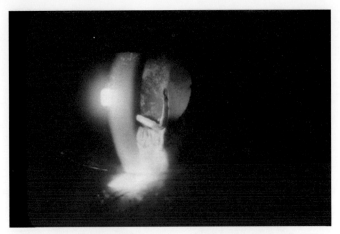

Fig. 9.7.2 Gnathostoma larva in the anterior chamber of the eye.
(Courtesy of Professor Tiam Lawtiamtong.)

Visceral gnathostomiasis usually depends on identifying the worm in surgical specimens (at autopsy the worms may have migrated away from the site of the main pathological lesion), or in secretions such as sputum, urine, or vaginal discharge.

Clinical investigation

The diagnosis is definitive if the worm can be identified in sections of surgical specimens, as described previously. The whole worm may be available if it emerges through the skin, in excretions and discharges, or from eye operations. Their sizes range from 0.34×2.2 mm to 1.0×16.25 mm. Their stage of development does not correlate with the duration of clinical illness. Infections with more than one worm are uncommon.

At present, there is no common serodiagnostic test available for all *Gnathostoma* species. Two serodiagnostic methods are currently used: enzyme immunoassay for *G. binucleatum* infection in Mexico, and immunoblot tests for *G. spinigerum* infection in Thailand and an immunblot test targeting a 40 kDa antigen for *G. binucleatum* has been developed in Mexico. A test using a recombinant 24 kDa antigen of advanced third-stage larvae of *G. spinigerum* is under development.

Blood eosinophilia count (7–76%) occurs irregularly in about 60% of cases, and therefore is not necessary for presumptive diagnosis.

MRI can show tortuous tracks and haemorrhage in cerebral gnathostomiasis.

Criteria for diagnosis

Since the identification of the worm is not always possible, and clinical manifestations overlap with other illnesses, the diagnosis of gnathostomiasis requires the following criteria: (1), clinical presentation described above, and evidence of exposure to gnathostoma larvae, or (2), serological test positive for antibody against gnathostoma antigen, confirming the presumptive diagnosis.

Treatment

Surgical removal is curative, but advisable only in accessible areas such as the eye or skin. Blind exploration of subcutaneous tissues in areas of diffuse swelling is not productive.

Oral therapy with albendazole at an adult dosage of 400 mg twice daily for 2 to 3 weeks induces migration of the parasite to the skin. The worms are frequently recovered between days 2 and 14 of treatment, picked out with a needle, excisional biopsy, or even scratched out by the patient's fingernails. However, the success rate is only 6 to 7%. Recurrence of swelling in patients whose worms do not migrate to the skin is less frequent after albendazole treatment. Aminotransferases should be measured before this treatment, even though hepatotoxicity at this dosage is usually mild and reversible. Oral therapy with a single dose of ivermectin at 200 µg/kg is not superior to placebo or albendazole, but may be considered in patients in whom albendazole treatment fails.

Prognosis

Cerebral gnathostomiasis can be fatal, and blindness is frequent after intraocular infection. Patients can be reassured that central nervous system or intraocular involvement occurs in less than 1% of cases with cutaneous migratory swelling.

Further reading

Bussaratid V, et al. (2006). Efficacy of ivermectin treatment of cutaneous gnathostomiasis evaluated by placebo-controlled trial. *Southeast Asian J Trop Med Public Health*, **37**, 433–40.

Bhaibulya M, Charoenlarp P (1983). Creeping eruption caused by *Gnathostoma spinigerum*. *Southeast Asian J Trop Med Public Health*, **14**, 226–8.

Caballero-Garcia M d L, et al. (2007). Protein profile analysis from advanced third-stage larvae (AdvI.3) and adult worms of Gnathostoma binucleatum (Nematoda: Spirurida). *Parasitol Res*, **100**, 555–60.

Inkatanuvat S, et al. (1998). Changes of liver functions after albendazole treatment in human gnathostomiasis. *J Med Assoc Thai*, **81**, 735–40.

Kraivichian K, et al. (2004). Treatment of cutaneous gnathostomiasis with ivermectin. *Am J Trop Med Hyg*, **7**, 623–8.

Laummaunwai P, et al. (2010). Gnathostoma spinigerum: molecular cloning, expression and characterization of the cyclophilin protein. *Exp Parasitol*, **126**, 611–16.

Miyazaki I (1991). *An illustrated book of helminthic zoonoses*, pp. 368–409. International Medical Foundation of Japan, Tokyo.

Nopparatana C, et al. (1991). Purification of *Gnathostoma spinigerum* specific antigen and immunodiagnosis of human gnathostomiasis. *Int J Parasitol*, **21**, 677–87.

Rusnak JM, Lucey DR (1993). Clinical gnathostomiasis: case report and review of the English language literature. *Clin Infect Dis*, **16**, 33–50.

Sirikulchayanonta V, Viriyavejakul P (2001). Various morphologic features of *Gnathostoma spinigerum* in histologic sections: Report of 3 cases with reference to topographic study of the reference worm. *Southeast Asian J Trop Med Public Health*, **32**, 302–7.

Suntharasamai P, et al. (1992). Albendazole stimulates outward migration of *Gnathostoma spinigerum* to the dermis in man. *Southeast Asian J Trop Med Public Health*, **23**, 716–22.

Swanson VL (1971). Gnathostomiasis. In: Marcial-Rojas RA (ed). *Pathology of protozoal and helminthic diseases with clinical correlation*, pp. 871–9. Williams and Wilkins, Baltimore.

Uparanukraw P, et al. (2001). Cloning and expression of Gnathostoma spinigerum recombinant protein: matrix metalloproteinase. *Parasitol Res*, **87**, 273–6.

Cestodes (tapeworms)

Contents

10.1 Cystic hydatid disease (*Echinococcus granulosus*)

Armando E. Gonzalez, Pedro L. Moro, and Hector H. Garcia

Essentials

Cystic hydatid disease, caused by *Echinococcus granulosus*, is a zoonotic disease principally transmitted between dogs and domestic livestock, particularly sheep. Humans are infected when they ingest tapeworm eggs, with disease occuring in most parts of the world where sheep are raised and dogs are used to herd livestock.

Clinical features, diagnosis, and treatment—the most common clinical manifestations are cysts in the liver (typically presenting with hepatomegaly) and/or lung (presenting with cough, haemoptysis, and dyspnoea). Diagnosis is usually made on the basis of serological tests in combination with imaging techniques. Treatment options include surgery, chemotherapy with anthelminthic agents, or—for liver cysts—PAIR (puncture–aspiration–injection–reaspiration).

Prevention—echinococcosis is a major public health problem in several countries. Control programmes have been aimed at educating dog owners to prevent their animals from having access to infected offal. Vaccines against sheep hydatidosis and the dog tapeworm stage are promising alternatives.

Introduction

Cystic hydatid disease is a zoonotic disease caused by infection with the larval stage (hydatid cyst) of the tapeworm *Echinococcus granulosus*. Hydatid cysts in liver and lung are frequent causes of human morbidity in endemic zones.

Aetiology

The lifecycle of *E. granulosus* requires two hosts. The adult tapeworm is found in the small intestine of the definitive host, usually dogs or other canids. It consists of only three to five proglottids, and measures between 3 and 7 mm long when fully mature. *E. granulosus* has remarkable biological potential; there may be as many as 40 000 worms in a heavily infected dog, each one of which sheds about 1000 eggs every 2 weeks. Dogs infected with echinococcus tapeworms pass eggs in their faeces that contaminate the soil and vegetation and remain viable for long periods in cold humid places. Intermediate hosts (sheep, cattle, horses, pigs, and other mammals, including humans) acquire hydatid disease by ingesting viable eggs of *E. granulosus*. Eggs hatch in the intestine, freeing oncospheres which penetrate the intestinal mucosa and are transported by the blood and lymphatic systems to the liver, lungs, and other organs, where they develop into cysts.

Molecular studies using mitochondrial DNA sequences have identified 10 distinct genetic types within *E. granulosus*. These include two sheep strains (G1, G2), two bovid strains (G3, G5), a horse strain (G4), the camelid strain (G6), a pig strain (G7) and the cervid strain (G8). A ninth genotype (G9) has been described in swine in Poland, and a tenth genotype (G10) in cervids. The sheep strain (G1) is the most cosmopolitan form that is most commonly associated with human infections. The other strains appear to be genetically distinct. The presence of distinct strains of *E. granulosus* affects clinical aspects and control strategy. The risk of human infection differs as does its localization, clinical expression, and geographical distribution. Shorter maturation time of a given strain in dogs would reduce the duration of infection by the adult intestinal form so that shorter intervals are required between rounds of administration of antiparasite drugs for control.

Epidemiology

Hydatid disease is an important cause of human morbidity, requiring costly surgical treatment. The infection is widely distributed in most parts of the world where sheep are raised and dogs are used to herd livestock. In the Americas, most cases have been reported from Argentina, Chile, Uruguay, Peru, and southern Brazil. Recent studies in Peru have revealed prevalences of hydatid disease ranging from 5.7 to 8.9% in highland villagers, and as high as 32 and 89% in dogs and sheep, respectively. High prevalence of liver hydatid disease, with rates of up to 5.6%, have also been reported in north-western Turkana in Kenya. *Echinococcus* is widespread in the Old World, particularly in Greece, Cyprus, Bulgaria, Lebanon, and Turkey. In the United States of America, most infections are seen in immigrants from endemic countries; however, sporadic autochthonous transmission is currently recognized in Alaska, California, Utah, Arizona, and New Mexico.

Communities at higher risk of infection include those where sheep are raised extensively and where dogs are used to care for large flocks of livestock. Known risk factors for infection include feeding dogs with raw offal and access of dogs to sheep that die in the field (Fig. 10.1.1). The risk of infection is also linked to poor hygiene and intimate contact with dogs. In north-western Turkana, dogs are allowed to stay within the house, and are used to clean up women's menses and lick vomit from faces and diarrhoea from the anal regions of their children.

Pathogenesis

The incubation period of human hydatid infections is highly variable and often prolonged for several years. Cysts have been reported to grow continuously. However, recent studies suggest that cyst growth is highly variable. Some cysts grow as much as 1 cm per year while other viable cysts showed no growth during 3 to 12 years of follow-up.

Most human infections remain asymptomatic; hydatid cysts are found incidentally at autopsy much more frequently than the

reported local morbidity rates. The locality of the cysts, their size, and their condition determine the particular manifestations.

Clinical features

Hydatid cysts are most frequently seen in the liver (60–70%) followed by the lungs (30–40%). Signs of hepatic hydatid disease include hepatomegaly with or without the presence of a mass in the upper right quadrant. Obstructive jaundice, mild epigastric pain, indigestion, and nausea may occur occasionally. Hydatid cysts may become secondarily infected with bacteria presenting as a hepatic abscess. Features of lung involvement (Fig. 10.1.2) are cough, haemoptysis, dyspnoea, and fever. The ratio of liver to lung cysts may vary from one geographical region to another: a liver to lung ratio of 1.4:1 has been observed in Peru, in contrast to the 3:1 to 13:1 ratio reported in Argentina and Uruguay. Differences in echinococcus strains may account for this variation. Brain cysts produce intracranial hypertension and epilepsy. Vertebral cysts compress the spinal cord causing paraplegia; bone cysts produce spontaneous fractures (Figs. 10.1.3 and 10.1.4) and deformity. Sudden rupture of cysts in the peritoneal cavity may result in peritonitis (Fig. 10.1.4), and rupture in the lungs may cause pneumothorax and empyema. Rupture may also cause allergic manifestations such as pruritus, oedema, dyspnoea, anaphylactic shock, and even death.

Diagnosis

Clinical findings such as a space-occupying lesion and residence in an endemic region are suggestive of hydatid disease. Abdominal ultrasonography is an important aid to the diagnosis of abdominal cysts. Portable ultrasonography machines are used with good results in field surveys. Chest radiography is useful for diagnosis of lung cysts. CT scanning is very helpful, especially for diagnosis of nontypical lesions (Fig. 10.1.4b).

Serology

A number of serological tests have been developed for diagnosis of hydatid disease, including an enzyme immunoassay, which identifies antibodies against antigen B or components of this antigen.

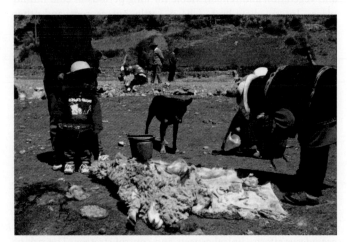

Fig. 10.1.1 Epidemiological conditions for completion of the life cycle of echinoccocus: stray dogs waiting for sheep offal outside a slaughterhouse in Peru.

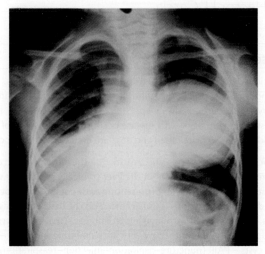

Fig. 10.1.2 Plain chest radiograph showing a lung hydatid cyst displacing the heart.

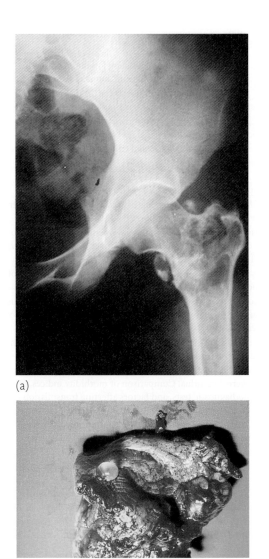

(a)

(b)

Fig. 10.1.3 (a) Pathological fracture of the femur caused by hydatid infection. (b) Hydatid cyst in muscle excised from around the femoral head (same case as shown in (a)).
(Copyright D A Warrell.)

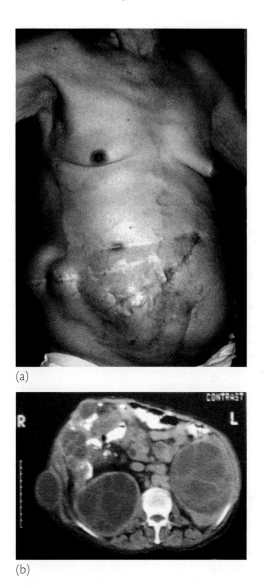

(a)

(b)

Fig. 10.1.4 (a) Numerous subcutaneous, peritoneal, and renal hydatid cysts in an Argentine patient. (b) Contrast CT scan of the same patient.(Courtesy of Professor Olindo Adriano Martino, Buenos Aires.)

A western blot assay based on the identification of three specific antigens of 8, 16, and 21 kDa is currently used. Major drawbacks in serological diagnosis are low sensitivity for detection of lung hydatid cysts and cross-reactivity with sera of patients with *Taenia solium* infection. Cyst rupture or secondary infection are strongly associated to a positive result in hydatid serology. In field surveys, serological tests should be used in combination with imaging techniques in order to detect most cases of hydatid disease.

Parasitological diagnosis

Although uncommon, this can be done from sputum samples of patients whose lung cysts have recently ruptured. Scolices have four spherical suckers and a rostellum with two rows of hooks.

Treatment

Surgery

Surgical removal of hydatid cysts remains the treatment of choice in many countries. The usual surgical approach involves aspiration

of cyst fluid and injection of a protoscolicidal agent into the cyst, usually 20% hypertonic saline solution or 90% alcohol, followed by evacuation of the fluid, prior to surgical excision. Major risks of surgical treatment include accidental spillage of fluid and scolices into the peritoneal cavity, which may lead to anaphylaxis or secondary peritoneal hydatidosis. Recurrence rates following surgery may be as high as 30%. Antihistamines are given as prophylaxis and suction cones have been used to prevent spillage. The efficacy of these methods is uncertain.

Chemotherapy

Benzimidazole compounds have been shown to be effective against hydatid disease. Courses of albendazole in a dose of 10 to 15mg/kg body weight per day for 28 days are interspersed with drug-free periods of 2 weeks. This regime cures approximately one-third of cases of liver hydatid disease and causes partial regression of cysts in another one-third of patients. However, many courses may be needed to achieve complete or partial cyst regression. Small liver or lung hydatid cysts should be treated with albendazole. Because of its high scolicidal activity, albendazole is recommended as a pro-phylactic agent 1 to 3 months before surgical intervention. Albendazole is indicated when surgery is contraindicated. Mebendazole may also be used, although it is less effective than albendazole. Albendazole, mebendazole, and other benzimidazole compounds should not be used in pregnant women because of their potentially teratogenic effects. The combination of praziquantel and albendazole seems to show a better efficacy than albendazole alone. Since benzimidazoles are potentially hepatotoxic, liver enzymes should be monitored before and during treatment.

Recent experimental studies in animals have shown that another benzimidazole compound, oxfendazole, has strong parasiticidal activity. Intermittent weekly therapy with oxfendazole was effective in sheep hydatid disease, suggesting the possibility that daily therapy as currently used with albendazole may not be needed. Current studies are exploring the effect of oxfendazole in the treatment of human hydatid disease.

Percutaneous aspiration, injection, reaspiration (PAIR)

PAIR consists of percutaneous puncture using sonographic guidance, aspiration of substantial amounts of the cyst fluid, and injection of a protoscolicidal agent, usually hypertonic saline for at least 15 min, followed by reaspiration of cyst contents. Albendazole should be administered before PAIR treatment, and antihistamines should be given to reduce the risk of allergic reactions if there is spillage of fluid. Good results have been reported with this procedure with no major complications. A metaanalysis comparing the use of PAIR and surgical treatment for liver hydatid cysts found less complications and a shorter hospital stay in the PAIR-treated group.

Prevention and control

The earliest successful programme against echinococcosis was carried out in Iceland. It was based on a health educational campaign that eradicated the parasite. Control programmes have been aimed at educating dog owners to prevent their animals from having access to infected offal. This approach includes periodic treatment of sheepdogs with praziquantel (every 45 days), reduction in the dog population, close veterinary inspection of slaughterhouse facilities for the presence of dogs, and cremation of infected offal. Control programmes are in force in Argentina, Chile, and Uruguay. Partial success has been achieved. Control programmes in New Zealand and Tasmania have reduced the number of infected animals and the incidence of human infection.

Serological tests such as the western blot for diagnosis of sheep hydatidosis and the coproantigen enzyme-linked immunosorbent assay (ELISA) for canine echinococcosis are potentially useful for measuring the burden of disease and monitoring control programmes in endemic regions. A recent major advance has been the development of a recombinant vaccine (EG95) which seems to confer 96 to 98% protection against challenge infection. Recent trials in Australia and Argentina using this vaccine have reported that 86% of immunized sheep were completely free of viable hydatid cysts when examined 1 year later. The number of viable cysts was reduced by 99.3%. Similarly, a vaccine against the dog tapeworm stage has been developed and conferred 97 to 100% protection against worm growth and egg production in immunized dogs. Although the results of these initial trials seem promising, further research is needed to assess the cost benefit of using these vaccines.

Further reading

Allan JC, et al. (1992). Coproantigen detection for immunodiagnosis of echinococcosis and taeniasis in dogs and humans. *Parasitology*, **104**, 347–55.

Brunetti E, et al. (2010). Expert consensus for the diagnosis and treatment of cystic and alveolar echinococcosis in humans. *Acta Trop*, **114**, 1–16.

Brunetti E, et al. (2011). Cystic echinococcosis: chronic, complex, and still neglected. *PLoS Negl Trop Dis*, **5**, e1146.

Craig PS, et al. (2007). Prevention and control of cystic echinococcosis. *Lancet Infect Dis*, **7**, 385–94.

Frider B, Larrieu E, Odriozola M (1999). Long-term outcome of asymptomatic liver hydatidosis. *J Hepatol*, **30**, 228–31.

Gavidia CM, et al. (2008). Diagnosis of cystic echinococcosis, central Peruvian Highlands. *Emerg Infect Dis*, **14**, 260–6.

Junghanss T, et al. (2008). Clinical management of cystic echinococcosis: State of the art, problems, and perspectives. *Am J Trop Med Hyg*, **79**, 301–11.

McManus DP, Thompson RCA (2003). Molecular epidemiology of cystic echinococcosis. *Parasitology*, **127**, S37–51.

Macpherson CNL, et al. (1987). Portable ultrasound scanner versus serology in screening for hydatid cysts in a nomadic population. *Lancet*, **ii**, 259–91.

Moro PL, et al. (1997). Epidemiology of *Echinococcus granulosus* infection in the Central Andes of Peru. *Bull World Health Org*, **75**, 553–61.

Schantz PM, Williams JF, Posse CR (1973). Epidemiology of hydatid disease in southern Argentina. Comparison of morbidity indices, evaluation of immunodiagnostic tests, and factors affecting transmission in southern Rio Negro Province. *Am J Trop Med Hyg*, **22**, 629–41.

Smego RA, et al. (2003). Percutaneous aspiration-injection-reaspiration-drainage plus albendazole or mebendazole for hepatic cystic echinococcosis: a meta-analysis. *Clin Infect Dis*, **27**, 1073–83.

Thompson RCA, McManus DP (2002). Towards a taxonomic revision of the genus *Echinococcus*. *Trends Parasitol*, **18**, 452–7.

Verastegui M, et al. (1992). Enzyme-linked immunoelectrotransfer blot test for the diagnosis of human hydatid disease. *J Clin Microbiol*, **30**, 1557–61.

Zhang W, et al. (2006). Vaccination of dogs against *Echinococcus granulosus*, the cause of cystic hydatid disease in humans. *J Infect Dis*, **194**, 966–74.

10.2 Cyclophyllidian gut tapeworms

Richard Knight

Essentials

The cyclophyllidean tapeworms are cestodes that maintain anchorage to the host small-gut mucosa by means of a scolex bearing four suckers; mature reproductive proglottids develop at the end of the worm. The life cycle involves a cystic larval stage, usually in a nonhuman host species. Humans are an obligatory part of the life cycle in four gut species; in the rest they are an accidental host.

Taenia saginata

The beef tapeworm is common in Africa, the Middle East, Asia, and South America. It remains endemic, although now rare, in the United States of America and western Europe. Transmission occurs where cattle have access to human faeces and where humans eat undercooked beef containing cysts. Many people who are infected have no symptoms, except that they experience active exit of single proglottids through the anus. Diagnosis is by finding typical eggs in perianal swabs. Treatment is with niclosamide or praziquantel. Prevention is by health education concerning production and cooking of meat, also by proper sewage treatment and disposal. Mass treatment of selected or whole adult populations is the most effective short-term measure when endemicity is high.

Taenia asiatica

Adult worms resemble *T. saginata* but the cysts are much smaller and occur in the liver of pigs and wild boar. First recognized in 1973 and now known to be quite widespread in east Asia and South-East Asia. Cattle are not involved in the life cycle.

Taenia solium

Adult pork tapeworm infections occur when cysts in undercooked pig meat are eaten. High prevalences occur in Africa, parts of Asia, and Central and South America. Symptoms, diagnosis and treatment are similar to those of *T.saginata*. The potentially dangerous condition of cysticercosis occurs when eggs from the faeces of persons harbouring adult worms are ingested; this produces cysts in striated muscle, subcutaneous tissue, nervous system and the eye. See Chapter 10.3 for further discussion.

Other tapeworms

Several species are recognized as accidental human parasites, but *Hymenolepis nana*, the dwarf tapeworm, is common; the life cycle involves only humans. Heavy infection can lead to anorexia, abdominal pain, and malabsorption. Diagnosis is by finding eggs in the faeces. Treatment is with praziquantel or niclosamide.

Introduction

The cyclophyllidean tapeworms are cestodes that maintain anchorage to the host small-gut mucosa by means the scolex, a holdfast structure bearing a circlet of four suckers and usually a central evertible rostellum with one or more circlets of minute hooks (Figs. 10.2.1a, b, c). The rest of the body forms the strobila and consists of a chain of flattened proglottids, which bud behind the scolex. The worms change their site of attachment regularly, and are surprisingly motile. Gravid proglottids are lost from the end of the worm and are replaced by others that have grown and matured as they pass down the strobila. Each proglottid possesses a complete set of hermaphroditic sex organs and marginal genital openings. Eggs accumulate in the uterus of gravid proglottids and only enter the faecal stream if the proglottids are disrupted. In many species the eggs enter the environment within intact proglottids. In either case the eggs are embryonated and contain a six-hooked hexacanth embryo. The egg shells have two membranes, but in *Taenia* the outer is lost early and the inner forms the thick embryophore.

After ingestion by the intermediate host, eggs hatch and the released hexacanth embryo bores its way into the mucosa. The larval stages of the parasite ('metacestode') are generally cystic with an invaginated embryonic scolex—the protoscolex. The cycle is completed when the larval stage, within the intermediate host or its tissues, is eaten by the definitive host; the protoscolex evaginates and attaches to the gut mucosa.

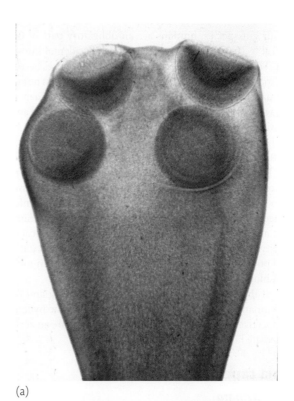
(a)

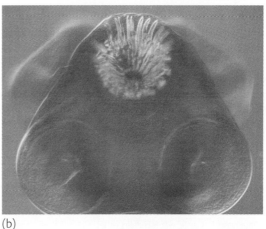
(b)

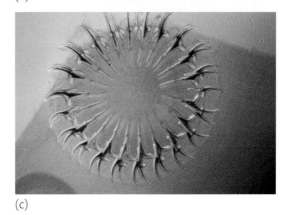
(c)

Fig. 10.2.1 (a) *Taenia saginata* showing scolex with four suckers and no hooks. (b *Taenia solium* showing scolex with four suckers and a double row of hooks. (c) *Taenia solium* detail of hooks. (Courtesy of Professor Viqar Zaman.)

In four gut species, humans are an obligatory part of the life-cycle (Table 10.2.1), in the rest they are an accidental host (Table 10.2.2). The three *Taenia* species are anthropozoonoses because the cycle is maintained by an obligatory alternation between human and nonhuman hosts. Phylogenetic studies suggest that *Taenia* tapeworms were acquired, before humans domesticated cattle and pigs, by hominid hunters intruding into predator–prey cycles involving perhaps lions and hyenas. Patients with *Taenia* infections pass proglottids in their faeces or experience their active migration per anum. The clinical importance the pork tapeworm relates mainly to cysticercosis, the occurrence of larval forms in human tissue (see Chapter 10.3). The dwarf tapeworm *Hymenolepis nana* infects an estimated 9 million people; there is normally no intermediate host.

With any gut cestode, symptoms also result from local hypersensitivity reactions to the worm and its scolex, altered gut motility, and poorly defined systemic symptoms with an immunological basis. A blood eosinophilia up to 10% can occur.

Eggs of the cyclophyllidian tapeworms of the dog and fox can infect humans to produce hydatid and multilocular hydatid disease respectively (see Chapter 10.1), here humans are an accidental intermediate host.

Taenia tapeworms

Taenia saginata

Geographical distribution
The beef tapeworm *T. saginata* is prevalent where cattle have access to human faeces and where humans eat undercooked beef. The highest prevalence is in Africa, particularly in eastern and northeastern parts; it is also common in many countries in the Middle East, South America, and South-East Asia. Prevalence is now very low in the United States of America, Canada, and Australia. It still persists endemically in Europe; but prevalence increases progressively eastwards and into the former Soviet Union.

Epidemiology
Most worms are solitary. Multiple worms are smaller and typically occur in high-transmission areas, probably by simultaneous infection. Viable eggs from human faeces persist on pasture for many months and can survive most forms of sewage treatment. Cattle have access to human faeces on farms, at camp sites and recreation areas, and on railway lines. Infected herdsmen can initiate epizootics. Eggs may be dispersed by flies and dung beetles, and seabirds can ingest proglottids in refuse or estuarine waters and deposit them in their faeces on inland pastures.

In cattle the whitish, ovoid, cysticerci become infective within 12 weeks and remain viable in the living host for 2 years; they are viable in stored, chilled meat for several weeks but are killed at −20°C within 1 week. The prepatent period in man is 3 months and worms may live 30 years. Cattle develop protective immunity to new infection.

Clinical features
The whitish mature proglottids, approximately 2 to 3 cm long, are actively motile, elongating and contracting (Fig. 10.2.2). Most patients experience active exit of single proglottids through the anus, others pass proglottids at defecation, often in short chains; free eggs also occur in faeces. Many have no other symptoms, but others complain of nausea and upper abdominal pains, often relieved by food. In children, impaired appetite can have nutritional consequences. Some patients have symptoms suggestive of hypoglycaemia, namely dizziness and sweating. Pruritus ani is common. The worm may be visible on small-bowel barium studies.

Proglottids have been found in a variety of surgical specimens, including resected appendices, but a pathogenic role is usually

Table 10.2.1 Major gut cestodes that infect humans

	Taenia saginata **Beef tapeworm**	*Taenia asiatica* **Asian tapeworm**	*Taenia solium* **Pork tapeworm**	*Hymenolepis nana* **Dwarf tapeworm**
Larval tapeworm				
Intermediate hosts	Cattle, water buffalo, other bovids, reindeer	Pig, wild boar	Pig, wild boar; also in humans (cysticercosis)	None but human and murine subspecies perhaps cross-infect
Type and size	Cysticercus 7–10 × 4–6 mm	Cysticercus 2 × 2 mm	Cysticercus 5–8 × 3–6 mm	Minute tailless cysticercoid 50 μm
Location	Muscle, viscera, brain (reindeer only)	Viscera, mainly liver	Muscle, brain, subcutaneous, eye, tongue	Villi of small intestine
Adult tapeworm				
Length	4–12 m	4–12 m	3–5 m	25–40 mm
Number of proglottids	2000 (mean)	2000 (mean)	700–1000	200 (mean)
Gravid proglottid	Longer than wide; 20–30 × 5–7 mm	Longer than wide; 20–30 × 5–7 mm	Longer than wide; 18–25 × 5–7 mm	Wider than long; 0.8 × 0.2 mm
Scolex	No rostellum, no hooks	Rostellum; no hooks	Rostellum with double circlet of hooks	Rostellum with single circlet of minute hooks
Gravid uterus	15–20 lateral branches	15–20 lateral branches	7–12 lateral branches	Bilobed
Egg (contains hexacanth embryo)	Embryophore shell is radially striated and 31–40 μm in diameter	Embryophore shell is radially striated and 31–40 μm in diameter	Embryophore shell is radially striated and 31–40 μm in diameter	Oval, 30–47 μm long; two shell membranes; 4–8 filaments arise from each pole of inner membrane

Table 10.2.2 Uncommon gut cestodes that infect humans

Species	Geographic distribution	Definitive hosts	Intermediate hosts	Length and width of tapeworm	Shape of gravid proglottid	Other features
Bertiella mucronata	South America, Cuba	Primates	Oribatid mites	15–45 cm × 5–10 mm	Wider than long	Inner eggshell bears bicornuate knob
B.studeri	South and South-East Asia, Africa, Cuba	Primates	Oribatid mites	27–30 cm × 6–10 mm	Much wider than long	As above
Dipylidium caninum	Worldwide	Dog, cat	Fleas and dog louse	10–70 cm × 2.5–3 mm	Elongate, wider in middle	Double set of sex organs. Egg capsules with 8–15 eggs
Hymenolepis diminuta (rat tapeworm)	Worldwide	Rat	Fleas, beetles, cockroaches	20–60 cm × 3–4 mm	Much wider than long	Egg like *H. nana* but yellow outer membrane and no filaments; 60–85 μm
Inermicapsifer madagascariensis	Madagascar, Africa, Central America, Cuba	Rats	Arthropod	26–42 cm × 2.6 mm	Slightly elongate, white and opaque	Egg capsules with 6–11 eggs
Mathevotaenia symmetrica	Thailand	Rodents	Beetles	13 cm × 1–2 mm	Elongate, wider in middle	Capsule surrounds individual eggs
Mesocestoides lineatus	China, Japan, Korea	Carnivores	Mites (1st host); amphibia, reptiles, birds, rodents (2nd hosts)	40 cm × 1.5–2 mm	Longer than broad	Single medioventral genital opening
Mesocestoides variabilis	Greenland, USA	Carnivores	Mites (1st host); amphibia, reptiles, birds, rodents (2nd hosts)	40 cm × 1.5–2 mm	Longer than broad	Single medioventral genital opening
Raillietina celebensis	East Asia, Polynesia, Australia	Rats	Ant	16–60 cm × 3 mm	As above	Egg capsules with 1–4 eggs
R. demerariensis	Guyana, Cuba, Ecuador	Rats	Cockroach	16- 60 cm × 2–3 mm	As above	Egg capsule with 8–10 eggs

difficult to establish. They occasionally obstruct the small intestine, pancreatic duct, or bile duct. Proglottids are recorded in the gallbladder, and eggs have been found in gallstones.

Diagnosis

The typical eggs (Fig. 10.2.3) may be found in faeces, but this is an insensitive method; perianal swabs are more useful. Eggs are indistinguishable from those of *T. solium* and *T asiatica*; patients should be asked to bring worm specimens. Unless the proglottid is fully gravid the number of uterine branches is an unreliable diagnostic character. A better morphological distinction is the presence of a vaginal sphincter; this is absent in *T. solium*. In human surveys

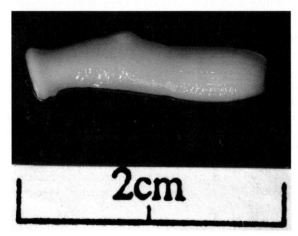

Fig. 10.2.2 Actively mobile, contracting proglottid of *Taenia saginata* found by a patient in the stool.
(Copyright D A Warrell.)

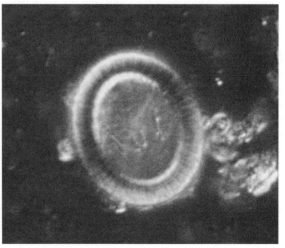

Fig. 10.2.3 Egg of *Taenia*.
(Courtesy of Professor Viqar Zaman.)

in endemic areas a 24-h faecal collection after an anthelmintic will give the most reliable prevalence.

Treatment

Niclosamide, 2 g, is given to adults and older children as a single morning dose on an empty stomach; the tablets should be chewed. Children aged 2 to 6 years should receive 1 g, and those below 2 years 500 mg. The alternative is praziquantel, 5 to 20 mg/kg as a single dose after a light breakfast. After either drug the proximal part of the worm disintegrates in the gut and the scolex cannot be found. Failure of proglottids to reappear within 3 to 4 months indicates cure.

Control

This includes health education concerning raw beef, meat inspection, sanitation and hygiene on cattle farms, and proper sewage treatment and disposal. Mass treatments of herd contacts, or whole adult populations, are the most effective short-term measures when endemicity is high. *T. saginata* causes great economic loss to the beef industry in some developing countries. Vaccines may soon become available for use in cattle.

Taenia asiatica

This was first described in 1973 as a subspecies *T. saginata* from rural Taiwan, where raw pig or wild boar liver, but no beef, was eaten. It is now recognized as a separate species and known also to occur in Korea, China, northern Sumatra, Indonesia, and Thailand. The cysticerci in pig viscera are very small. In immunodeficient mice *T. asiatica* eggs, but not those of *T. saginata*, produce cysticerci with hooked protoscolices. Eating uncooked pork with viscera from home-killed pigs is a recognized risk factor. Symptoms and treatment are the same as for *T. saginata*. It does not cause cysticercosis in humans.

Taenia solium (see also Chapter 10.3)

Generally less common than the beef tapeworm, the pork tapeworm *T. solium* is now very rare in North America and western Europe, but it remains common in much of sub-Saharan Africa, and in China, India, and other parts of Asia. It is highly prevalent in Mexico and other Latin American countries. Two genotypes are now recognized: the European type that has been introduced into the Americas and Africa since the 1500s, and the Asian type. Both types can produce neurocysticercosis, but only the latter causes subcutaneous cysticercosis.

Epidemiology

In pigs, muscle cysticerci produce 'measly pork' (Fig. 10.2.4). The cysts are most numerous in the tongue, masseter, heart, and diaphragm, but also occur in the brain. When eaten by humans in undercooked pork, the worms mature in 5 to 12 weeks. The eggs have the same resistant qualities as those of *T. saginata*.

Human cysticercosis arises when eggs from the faeces of people infected with adult worms are ingested and hatch in the upper gut; humans thus become an accidental intermediate host.

Conditions favouring cysticercosis include poor personal hygiene, which facilitates external autoinfection, and contaminated fingers among food handlers. Faecal pollution of the peridomestic environment, irrigation water, or cultivated vegetables is also important. In parts of Africa, tapeworm proglottids are used in traditional medicine. In the absence of these factors,

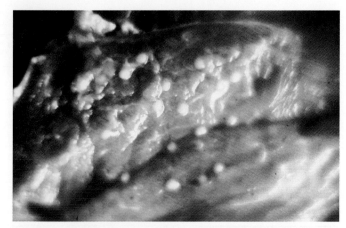

Fig. 10.2.4 'Measly pork' showing numerous cysts in the pig's muscle. (Copyright Sornchai Looareesuwan.)

cases of cysticercosis may be very sporadic even when *T. solium* is common. Cysticercosis is a major health problem in Mexico, some South American countries, and to a lesser extent in Africa and Asia. In 1969, *T. solium* was introduced from Bali into the highlands of Indonesian New Guinea, where the disease is now of great importance.

Pathology of human cysticercosis

Cysts occur especially in striated muscle, subcutaneous tissue (Asian genotype), the nervous system, and the eye. Many remain clinically silent until the parasite dies after 3 to 5 years, when vigorous inflammatory and hypersensitivity reactions can occur; later lesions may calcify. In the brain, particularly in the subarachnoid and the ventricular system, atypical racemose cysts may occur. They appear as irregular or grape-like clusters of cysts that have no protoscolex; they can be mistaken pathologically for nonparasitic cysts.

Clinical features

Symptoms, if any, due to the adult worms are similar to those of *T. saginata* but are often milder and not associated with pruritus ani. The proglottids do not migrate actively *per anum*.

Diagnosis

Adult worm infection is detected as for *T. saginata*. Methods for detecting faecal antigen are available and have great potential use in epidemiological studies. Proglottid fragments can be identified using DNA probes.

Treatment and control

Adult worms are treated as for *T. saginata*. Because of the potential risk of internal autoinfection vomiting must be avoided and an antiemetic is often recommended before treatment, together with a laxative 2 h after the medication. It should be remembered that the faeces will be potentially highly infective for several days, for both the patient and the attendants. Control measures include meat inspection, health education, and population-based chemotherapy. Local risk factors for human cysticercosis must receive special attention. Pigs can be treated with a single dose of oxfendazole and perhaps in the future given recombinant hexacanth vaccines.

Hymenolepis nana

The dwarf tapeworm, sometimes now placed in the genus *Rodentolepis*, is the most common cestode in humans; it is also the smallest. When worm loads are high, it causes more gut pathology than any other species. It is common in most developing and tropical countries. The life cycle normally involves only humans. Fully embryonated infective eggs are passed in the faeces; gravid proglottids normally disintegrate completely in the gut. Infection is commonly direct, but also by the other faeco-oral routes. Eggs hatch in the jejunum and the hexacanth embryo bores into a villus where it transforms into a cysticercoid larva. After 4 to 6 days it re-enters the gut, everts the scolex, and attaches to the mucosa; eggs appear in the faeces within 12 days. The lifespan is 3 months. The eggs are delicate and survive less than 10 days in the environment. Prevalence is usually much higher in children than adults; outbreaks can occur in families and institutions. External autoinfection is common in high-risk groups and enables high worm loads to build up. In addition, internal autoinfection occurs when there is gut stasis or retroperistalsis. Because of the importance of direct transmission, this infection may be common even in arid environments such as Western Australia.

A similar parasite, recognized as a subspecies *H. nana fraterna*, occurs in the mouse but this has normally has the flour beetle tribolium as intermediate host, although direct mouse-to-mouse transmission can occur. Both human and murine subspecies will infect these beetles. The zoonotic potential of the murine subspecies is uncertain, as at least Australian human strains will not infect mice.

Clinical features

Heavily infected people, especially children, may harbour up to 1000 or more worms. Mucosal damage caused by both larval and adult worms leads to protein loss and sometimes malabsorption. Abdominal pains and anorexia are common.

Immunosuppressant or steroid therapy, particularly in lymphoma patients, can lead to the development of bizarre cystic larval forms in the gut wall, mesenteric nodes, liver, and lungs. A similar condition can be produced in immunosuppressed mice.

Diagnosis and treatment

Eggs can be detected in faeces using concentration methods. Proglottids are rarely found in faeces, except after treatment.

Praziquantel in a single dose of 25 mg/kg is the most effective drug. If niclosamide is used, a 7-day course is needed to ensure that larval stages are killed when they re-enter the gut lumen. The dose on the first day is as for *T. saginata*; on the remaining days one-half of this dose is given. Relapses often result from persistence of eggs in the patient's environment.

Uncommon gut cestodes

Several species have been recorded in humans (Table 10.2.2). All have arthropods as intermediate hosts, the larval cysticercoid stage being in the haemocele; the full life cycles of some species are still uncertain. The normal definitive host becomes infected by eating the arthropod, intentionally or accidentally. The means by which humans become infected is sometimes not clear, but fleas, small beetles, and mites are easily overlooked in food. *Dipylidium caninum* infection occurs in children who have groomed their pets. Infections with *Bertiella* are mostly in owners of pet monkeys, but oribatid mites are common in fallen fruit especially mangoes.

Children may eat insects deliberately, and this appears to be the mode of infection by *Raillietina* in Bangkok. Beetles are used for medicinal purposes in parts of Thailand and Malaysia, and this is the most likely route by which *Mathevotaenia* is acquired.

In many of these species the eggs are in capsules that are released when the proglottid disintegrates in the gut, or more commonly, in the faecal mass. *Mesocestoides* is unique among these parasites in that two intermediate hosts are required and the genital opening is medioventral. Human *Mesocestoides* infections follow ingestion of raw viscera or blood from game, including birds, or from chickens.

Many patients will present because they have passed proglottids. *D. caninum* actively migrates out of the anus, like *T. saginata*. Faecal examinations of people with abdominal complaints may reveal unusual eggs or egg capsules. Poorly defined systemic and allergic complaints are common. Treatment is as for *T. saginata*.

Recognition of these parasites is of epidemiological interest and may indicate potential transmission of other zoonotic pathogens. It is certain that all these parasites are under-reported. Unusual proglottids or eggs should be preserved in formol saline and sent to a parasitologist.

Further reading

Alexander A, *et al.* (2011). Economic implications of three strategies for the control of taeniasis. *Trop Med Int Health*, **16**, 1410–16.

Chitchang S, *et al.* (1985). Relationship between the severity of the symptom and the number of *Hymenolepis nana* after treatment. *J Med Assoc Thailand*, **68**, 424–6.

Eom KS, Jeon H-K, Rim H-J (2009). Geographical distribution of Taenia asiatica and related species. *Korean J Parasitol*, **47**, S115–124.

Fuentes MV, Galan-Puchades MT, Malone JB (2003). Short report: a new case report of human *Mesocestoides* infection in the United States. *Am J Trop Med Hyg*, **68**, 566–7.

Hoberg EP (2006). Phylogeny of *Taenia*: Species definitions and origins of human parasites. *Parasitol Int*, **55** Suppl, 23–30.

Hoberg EP, *et al.* (2001). Out of Africa: origins of the *Taenia* tapeworms in humans. *Proc Roy Soc London B*, **268**, 781–7.

Ito A, Craig PS (2003). Immunodiagnostic and molecular approaches for the detection of taeniid cestode infections. *Trends Parasitol*, **19**, 377–81.

Ito A, Nakao M, Wandra T (2003). Human taeniasis and cysticercosis in Asia. *Lancet*, **362**, 1918–20.

Liu YM, *et al.* (2005). Acute pancreatitis caused by tapeworm in the biliary tract. *Am J Trop Med Hyg*, **73**, 377–80.

Macnish MG, *et al.* (2002). Failure to infect laboratory rodent hosts with human isolates of *Rodentolepis* (= *Hymenolepis*) *nana*. *J Helminthol*, **76**, 37–43.

Mason PR, Patterson BA (1994). Epidemiology of *Hymenolepis nana* in primary school children in urban and rural communities in Zimbabwe. *J Parasitol*, **80**, 245–50.

Olson PD, *et al.* (2003). Lethal invasive cestodiasis in immunosuppressed patients. *J Infect Dis*, **187**, 1962–6.

Pawlowski Z, Schultz MG (1972). Taeniasis and cysticercosis (*Taenia saginata*). *Adv Parasitol*, **10**, 269–343.

Subianto DB, Tumada LR, Morgono SS (1978). Burns and epileptic fits associated with cysticercosis in mountain people of Irian Jaya. *Trop Geogr Med*, **30**, 275–8.

10.3 **Cysticercosis**

Hector H. Garcia and Robert H. Gilman

Essentials

Cysticercosis, infection by larvae of the pork tapeworm *Taenia solium* (see Chapter 10.2), is the commonest helminthic infection of the human central nervous system. It accounts for up to 30% of all seizures and epilepsy in endemic countries, and travel and immigration now lead to its more frequent presentation in industrialized countries. Ingestion of raw or undercooked pork can lead to infection with the *T. solium* cysticercus, formerly known as 'Cysticercus cellulosae', which is an immature tapeworm. Once attached to the person's small intestine, the cysticercus develops segments (proglottids) to become an adult tapeworm. Proglottids discharged in the faeces contain tens of thousands of ova that can autoinfect the human host or pigs and other susceptible mammals. Ingestion of *T. solium* ova, for example by the faecal-oral route in those infected with adult tapeworms or their close contacts, or by eating food contaminated with raw sewage, can result in development of cysticerci in various tissues, but not an adult tapeworm. The ingested ova release embryos that penetrate the intestinal mucosa and migrate in the blood stream to the brain (causing neurocysticercosis), muscles, and subcutaneous tissues. Only by ingesting *T. solium* ova can humans develop cysticercosis.

Clinical features and diagnosis—manifestations of neurocysticercosis depend on the number, location, size, and stage of the parasite cysts in the brain, as well as on the immunological response of the host. The commonest syndromes are late-onset epilepsy or intracranial hypertension. Diagnosis is based on brain imaging studies (CT or MRI) and supported by highly specific serology.

Treatment and prognosis—treatment is (1) symptomatic—e.g. anticonvulsants; shunts for intracranial hypertension in patients with hydrocephalus; and (2) antiparasitic—albendazole or praziquantel, which are generally given with steroids to control cerebral oedema; but there is no role for these drugs in inactive neurocysticercosis (i.e. calcifications with or without enhancement on CT scan). Prognosis depends mainly on whether the cysts are intraparenchymal (better prognosis) or extraparenchymal (subarachnoid or intraventricular, poorer prognosis).

Introduction

Known since the Hippocratic era, cysticercosis is the commonest helminthic infection of the human central nervous system. It is probable that the suspicion of its origins led some religions expressly to forbid the consumption of pork. Socioeconomic improvements eradicated the infection in Europe and North America. However, endemic *Taenia solium* taeniasis/cysticercosis persists in most developing countries, where human cysticercosis is an important cause of epilepsy and other neurological morbidity, and porcine infections cause considerable economic losses to peasant farmers.

Aetiology

Cysticercosis is infection with the larval stage (cysticercus) of *T. solium*, the pork tapeworm (Chapter 10.2). In the life cycle of this two-host zoonotic cestode(Fig. 10.3.1), humans are the only definitive host and harbour the adult tapeworm, whereas pigs are intermediate hosts. The hermaphroditic adult *T. solium* inhabits the small intestine. Its head or scolex bears four suckers and a double crown of hooks, connected by a narrow neck to a large body (strobila) between 2 and 4 m long, composed of several hundred proglottids (Chapter 10.2, Fig. 10.3.1b, c). Gravid proglottids, each containing 50 000 to 60 000 fertile eggs, detach from the distal end of the worm and are excreted in the faeces. The cycle is completed when pigs ingest stools contaminated with *T. solium* eggs. Once ingested by the pig, the invasive oncospheres in the eggs are liberated by the action of gastric acid and intestinal fluids and actively penetrate the bowel wall, enter the bloodstream, and are carried to the muscles and other tissues where they develop into larval cysts (Chapter 10.2, and see Fig. 10.3.5). When humans ingest undercooked pork containing cysticerci, the larva evaginates in the small intestine, its scolex attach to the intestinal mucosa, and it begins forming proglottids. By accidentally ingesting taenia eggs, humans may also act as intermediate hosts for *T. solium* and develop cysticercosis.

Epidemiology

The availability of neuroimaging studies and the subsequent development of specific serodiagnostic tests has resulted in the identification of neurocysticercosis as a frequent neurological disorder in Latin America, Africa, and Asia, where the prevalence of active epilepsy is almost twice that in Western countries. Cysticercosis was introduced from Bali to the highlands of Papua, Indonesia nearly 40 years ago. Its seroprevalence is more than 20% in many communities. Neurocysticercosis is also an emerging problem in industrialized countries, seen mainly in immigrants from endemic areas, some of whom may spread the infection as tapeworm carriers. This applies to California and other southern areas of United States of America bordering Mexico.

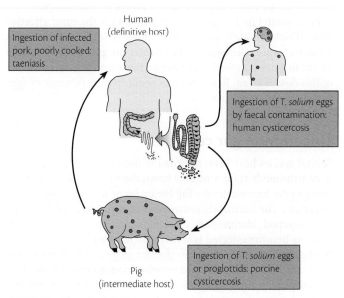

Fig. 10.3.1 Life cycle of *T. solium*.

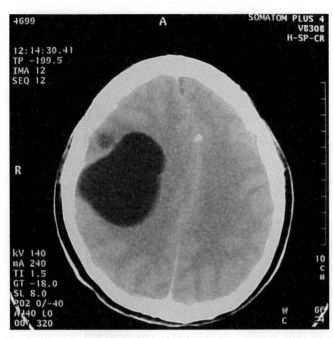

Fig. 10.3.2 Giant cysticercotic cyst (brain CT).

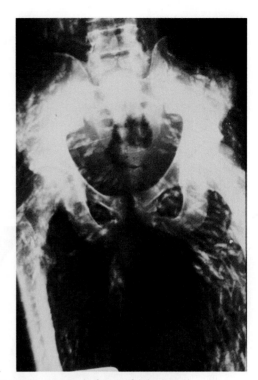

Fig. 10.3.4 Heavy cysticercal infection of skeletal muscles.
(Courtesy of the late Professor Sornchai Looareesuwan.)

The main sources of human cysticercosis are faecal–oral contamination in those carrying the tapeworm or their contacts and ingestion of food contaminated with *T. solium* eggs. Epidemiological studies suggest that almost every newly diagnosed patient with cysticercosis has been infected by someone in their close environment who is harbouring a *T. solium* and the tendency is to dismiss the role of environment or water in transmission. Airborne transmission of *T. solium* eggs and internal autoinfection by regurgitation of proglottids into the stomach have been suggested but not proved.

Pathogenesis

Any organ may be infected, but parasites survive more frequently in the nervous system, possibly because the immune response there is limited. Signs and symptoms are caused by perilesional

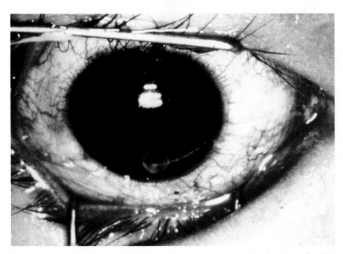

Fig. 10.3.3 Intraocular cysticercosis: cysticercus in the anterior chamber of a Thai patient.
(Courtesy of the late Prof Sornchai Looareesuwan.)

inflammation and oedema, mass effect, or obstruction of cerebrospinal fluid circulation. Although complete development of cysts takes 2 to 3 months, symptoms usually develop years after the initial infection. This clinically silent period, and finding inflammation around cysts in symptomatic cases, suggests that in many cases symptoms are due to inflammatory processes associated with the recognition of the parasite by the immune system of the host (presumably progressing towards the death of the parasite) rather than to the presence of the parasite itself.

Subarachnoid cysticerci elicit an intense inflammatory reaction causing thickening of basal leptomeninges. The optic chiasma and other cranial nerves are usually entrapped within this dense exudate, resulting in visual field defects and other cranial nerve dysfunctions. The foramens of Luschka and Magendie may be occluded by the thickened leptomeninges, leading to hydrocephalus. Blood vessels may be affected by the inflammatory reaction. The walls of small penetrating arteries are invaded by inflammatory cells, leading to a proliferative endarteritis with occlusion of the lumen, and which may result in cerebral infarction.

Clinical features

Neurocysticercosis is a pleomorphic disease, whose manifestations vary with the number, size, and topography of the lesions and the intensity of the host's immune response to the parasites. Patients can be classified by the number, stage, and location of the cysticerci, and the presence or absence of associated inflammation or calcifications.

Epilepsy, the most common presentation of neurocysticercosis, is usually the primary or sole manifestation of the disease. Seizures occur in 50 to 80% of patients with parenchymal brain cysts or calcifications but are less common in other forms of the disease. Other focal signs are less frequent and include pyramidal tract

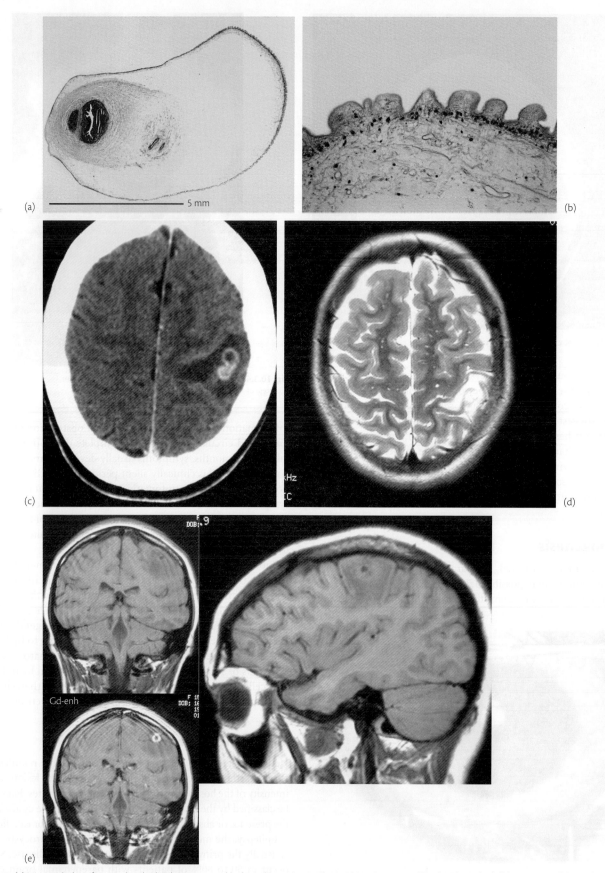

Fig. 10.3.5 (a) Histopatholgy of a complete hydatid cyst removed by brain biopsy in a patient with recent onset of focal epilepsy (×4). (b) Structure of the cyst wall (×40). (c) Cerebral imaging CT enhanced. (d) MRI T_2-weighted. (e) MRI T_1-weighted with and without gadolinium enhancement. (Copyright DA Warrell.)

signs, sensory deficits, signs of brainstem dysfunction, and involuntary movements. These manifestations usually follow a subacute or chronic course, making neurocysticercosis difficult to differentiate clinically from neoplasms or other infections of the central nervous system. Focal signs may occur abruptly in patients who develop a cerebral infarct as a complication of subarachnoid neurocysticercosis. Subarachnoid cysticerci may reach 10 cm or more in diameter ('giant' cysticercosis, Fig. 10.3.3), and exert a mass effect.

Neurocysticercosis may present with increased intracranial pressure, usually from hydrocephalus secondary to basal subarachnoid cysticercosis or intraventricular cysts, cysticercotic arachnoiditis, or granular ependymitis. In these cases, intracranial hypertension develops subacutely and progresses slowly. An encephalitic picture may result from overwhelming inflammation around many parasitic cysts, a syndrome that occurs more frequently in younger people, especially women. In contrast, some patients may tolerate hundreds of intraparenchymal cysticerci with only minor symptoms. Ocular cysticercosis can involve the posterior segment, retina, vitreous, subconjunctiva, orbit or eyelid (Fig. Fig. 10.3.3).

Muscular pseudohypertrophy, a rare presentation, is caused by heavy cysticercal infection of skeletal muscles (Fig. 10.3.4) giving a 'Herculean' appearance. The few cases reported are all from India. Other apparent differences in clinical manifestations between Asia and Latin America include a high frequency of subcutaneous cysts and single degenerating brain lesions in Asia.

Pathology

The cysticerci are liquid-filled vesicles consisting of vesicular wall and scolex (Fig. 10.3.5). The vesicular wall is composed of an outer or cuticular layer, a middle or cellular layer with pseudoepithelial structure, and an inner or reticular layer. The invaginated scolex has a head or rostellum armed with suckers and hooks, and a rudimentary body or strobila that includes the spiral canal.

The macroscopic appearance of cysticerci varies in different locations within the central nervous system. Cysticerci within the brain parenchyma are usually small and tend to lodge in the cerebral cortex or basal ganglia (Fig. 10.3.6). Subarachnoid cysts may be small if located in the depths of cortical sulci, or grow to 5 cm or more in the basal cisterns or sylvian fissures. Ventricular cysticerci are usually single, may or may not have a visible scolex, and may be attached to the choroid plexus or float freely in the ventricle. Spinal cysticerci are usually located in the subarachnoid space (rarely intramedullary). Their morphology is similar to cysts located within the brain.

Basal cysticerci may undergo a disproportionate growth of their membrane, with extension processes, resembling a brunch of grapes (racemose cysticercosis, Fig. 10.3.7). In these cases, the scolex is frequently unidentifiable even by microscopy.

Viable vesicular cysticerci elicit little inflammatory change in surrounding tissues because of active immune evasion mechanisms. The appearance of symptoms is interpreted as the result of immunological attack from the host, in a process of degeneration that ends with the death of the parasite. Inflammatory changes in the parasite membrane and increased density of cyst fluid mark the transition between four defined stages: viable, colloidal, granular nodular, and calcified cyst. Viable cysts may coexist with degenerating cysts or calcifications.

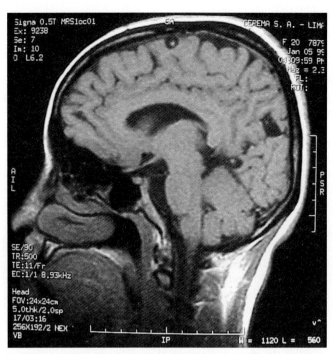

Fig. 10.3.6 Uncontrasted T_1 MR image showing two intraparenchymal cysticerci with visible scolices.

Laboratory/imaging diagnosis

The pleomorphism of neurocysticercosis makes it impossible to diagnose on clinical grounds alone. In endemic regions, late-onset seizures in otherwise healthy individuals are highly suggestive of neurocysticercosis. Most of these patients are normal on neurological examinations. Routine neuroimaging and serological studies are therefore mandatory. Finding cysticerci outside the central nervous system (eye, subcutaneous tissue, muscle) assists the diagnosis of neurocysticercosis. Muscular and subcutaneous cysticerci are far less common in American than in African or Asian patients with neurocysticercosis.

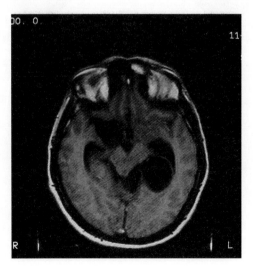

Fig. 10.3.7 Basal 'racemose' cysticercosis.

Neuroimaging

CT and MRI have drastically improved diagnostic accuracy by providing objective evidence about the topography of the lesions and the degree of the host inflammatory response to the parasite. Imaging findings in parenchymal neurocysticercosis depend on the stage of involution of cysticerci. Viable cysticerci appear as rounded cystic lesions on CT (Fig. 10.3.3), hypointense on T_1 and FLAIR sequences on MRI (Fig. 10.3.6), without associated enhancement, whereas degenerating parasitesare seen as focal enhancing lesions surrounded by oedema (Fig. 10.3.5c–e), and calcifications as hyperdense dots or nodules (Fig. 10.3.8). Disappearance of cyst fluid signals the degenerative phase and calcified nodules the residual phase. Single or multiple ring-like or nodular enhancing lesions are non-specific and present a diagnostic challenge. Pyogenic brain abscesses, fungal abscesses, tuberculomas, toxoplasma abscesses, and primary or metastatic brain tumours may produce similar findings on CT or MRI.

CT and MRI findings in subarachnoid neurocysticercosis are less specific. They include hydrocephalus, abnormal meningeal enhancement, and subarachnoid cysts. Cerebral angiography may show segmental narrowing or occlusion of major intracranial arteries in patients with cerebral infarcts secondary to parasitic vasculitis. In neurocysticercosis there is rarely fever or signs of meningeal irritation; glucose levels in cerebrospinal fluid are usually normal. MRI is generally better than CT for the diagnosis of neurocysticercosis, particularly in patients with basal lesions, brainstem or intraventricular cysts, and spinal lesions. MRI is, however, less sensitive than CT for the detection of calcifications.

Immunological tests

Immunoblot (western blot) using purified antigens is the best available serological test for *T. solium* antibodies. It performs well with serum samples and is 98% sensitive in cases with more than one active lesion, and 100% specific. Its sensitivity may drop in patients with a single cyst. Other assays using unfractionated

antigens (e.g. enzyme immunoassay, ELISA) suffer from poor specificity but are more reliable when performed with cerebrospinal fluid than serum. Antigen-detection tests may provide a tool for serological monitoring of antiparasitic therapy. Although results of serology and imaging studies may be similar, they evaluate different aspects of the disease and may be discordant in some patients. Intestinal tapeworm carriers, naturally cured patients, or non-neurological infections may have normal brain images but be positive serologically. Those with only inactive lesions or a single cerebral lesion may be seronegative.

Parasitological diagnosis

A proportion (c.10–15%) of patients with neurocysticercosis are tapeworm carriers at the time of diagnosis, and in another 10% or so a carrier can be detected in the household. Parasitological diagnosis is difficult: eggs and proglottids are shed only intermittently in stool and are usually missed by routine stool examination. Stool assays to detect parasite antigens are more sensitive than microscopy, but are not widely available. A recently described serological test for tapeworm carriers may improve detection.

Diagnostic criteria

A set of diagnostic criteria based on neuroimaging studies, serological tests, clinical presentation, and exposure history has been proposed by Del Brutto and colleagues. Besides absolute demonstration of the presence of the parasite, 'major' criteria (including typical findings on neuroimaging, demonstration of specific anticysticercal antibodies, or the presence of typical cigar-shaped calcifications in muscle) are combined with 'minor' criteria and epidemiological data to suggest a probable or possible diagnosis. Application of these criteria should improve the consistency of diagnosis.

Treatment

Because of the clinical and pathological pleomorphism of neurocysticercosis, precise assessment of the viability and size of cysts, the location of parasites, and the severity of the host's immune response is important before planning treatment.

Symptomatic treatment is very important. Seizures secondary to parenchymal neurocysticercosis can usually be controlled with anticonvulsants. However, the optimal duration of anticonvulsant therapy in patients with neurocysticercosis has not been determined, and it is difficult to withdraw this treatment. Prognostic factors associated with recurrence of seizures include the development of parenchymal brain calcifications, and occurrence of recurrent seizures or multiple brain cysts before starting antiparasitic therapy.

Antiparasitic agents destroy viable cysts and are associated with fewer seizures (particularly seizures with generalization) in the long term follow up. Antiparasitic or steroid treatments in patients with a single enhancing lesion seem to independently improve radiological resolution and decrease the chance of seizure relapses, albeit the magnitude of this effect is small. Albendazole is the drug of choice for antiparasitic treatment of cerebral cysticercosis (15 mg/kg per day for 7 days, with steroids), although a recently described single-day praziquantel regimen (75–100 mg/kg, in three doses at 2-h intervals, followed by steroids 6 h later)

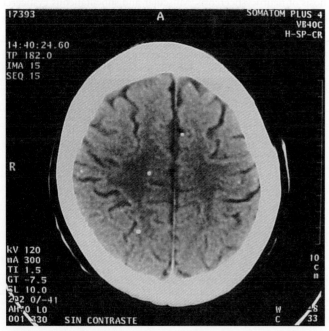

Fig. 10.3.8 Calcified neurocysticercosis.

demonstrated similar cestocidal activity in patients with few cysts. Longer courses may be required in patients with many lesions or subarachnoid cysticercosis. Transient worsening of neurological symptoms can be expected during antiparasitc therapy, secondary to the perilesional inflammatory reaction. There is no role for antiparasitic drugs in inactive neurocysticercosis (i.e. calcifications with or without enhancement on CT scan) since the parasites are dead.

Between the second and fifth day of antiparasitic therapy there is usually an exacerbation of neurological symptoms, attributed to local inflammation caused by the death of the larvae. For this reason, albendazole or praziquantel is generally given simultaneously with steroids in order to control the oedema and intracranial hypertension. Serum levels of praziquantel decrease when steroids are administered simultaneously, an effect that does not occur with albendazole. However, there is no evidence that cysticidal efficacy is decreased. Serum levels of praziquantel or albendazole may be lowered by simultaneous antiepileptic drug (phenytoin or carbamazepine) administration.

Some forms of neurocysticercosis should not be treated with antiparasitic agents. In patients with severe cysticercotic encephalitis, these drugs may result in worsening cerebral oedema and fatal herniation. In this case, the mainstay of therapy is high doses of corticosteroids or mannitol to decrease the inflammatory response. In patients with both hydrocephalus and parenchymal brain cysts, antiparasitic drugs should be started only after placement of a ventricular shunt in case the intracranial pressure increases as a result of drug therapy. Antiparasitic drugs must be used with caution in patients with giant subarachnoid cysticerci. In such patients, concomitant steroid administration is mandatory to avoid cerebral infarction. Albendazole can successfully destroy ventricular cysts, but the surrounding inflammatory reaction may cause acute hydrocephalus if the cysts are located within the fourth ventricle or near the foramens of Monro and Luschka.

Surgery is limited to ventriculoperitoneal shunts to relieve obstructive hydrocephalus, and excision of single cysts (in the fourth ventricle or giant intraparenchymal cysts). However, shunts frequently dysfunction. The protracted course in these patients and their high mortality rates (up to 50% in 2 years) is directly related to the number of surgical interventions required to change the shunts. Recently, neuroventriculoscopy has been employed as a less invasive option for resection of ventricular cysticerci.

Prognosis

Parenchymal cysticercosis has a good prognosis. Appropriately managed, seizures usually subside in time without sequelae. In contrast, extraparenchymal cysticercosis and especially racemose cysticercosis have a poor prognosis, responding poorly to antiparasitic therapy, and leading to progressively deteriorating disease and death. Multiple courses of antiparasitic treatment and careful, prolonged follow-up are crucial in this type of patients.

Prevention and control

Cysticercosis would not exist if pigs had no access to human faeces. However, this approach is hampered in endemic zones by the lack of sanitary facilities and veterinary inspection, and more importantly, because farmers tend to raise pigs under free-range conditions in order to reduce the cost of feeding them. Intervention programmes have concentrated on mass chemotherapy to eliminate

human taeniasis, but their results have not been sustained. New tools for control are oxfendazole, an effective and cheap single-dose therapy for porcine cysticercosis, and the candidate porcine vaccines under trial by several groups. TSOL18, an oncosphere-based vaccine developed in Australia, may provide over 99% protection.

Monitoring the effect of an intervention requires suitable indicators. Human seroprevalence does not reflect changes in infection patterns because antibodies persist for years, even after successful treatment. Studies in Peru have shown that serological monitoring of porcine infection is a useful marker for both prevalence and changes in infection intensity over time. Similarly, the rate of infection in uninfected (sentinel) pigs over time can be used to estimate intensity of *T. solium* infection in the community. The prevalences of human and porcine infection are strongly correlated.

Possible future developments

Although most cysts disappear after antiparasitic treatment, the antiparasitic efficacy of currently available regimes is incomplete. Data is missing on whether new drugs, combination therapy, or different schemes of albendazole of praziquantel can improve this efficacy.

Schemes and doses of antiparasitic and steroid therapy need to be assessed in controlled trials targeted to specific types of neurocysticercosis. Some authors suggested an association between brain calcifications secondary to cysticercosis and glial neoplasms. This has not yet been confirmed or rejected. Systematic long-term evaluation is needed to determine whether hydrocephalus is a late complication of anti-parasitic therapy. The efficacy and costs of comprehensive human–porcine eradication programmes must be assessed.

Further reading

Del Brutto OH, *et al.* (2001). Proposed diagnostic criteria for neurocysticercosis. *Neurology*, **57**, 177–83. [A guide to systematic diagnosis.]

Del Brutto OH, *et al.* (2006). Albendazole and praziquantel therapy for neurocysticercosis: a meta-analysis of randomized trials. *Ann Intern Med*, **145**, 43–51.

Evans C, *et al.* (1997). Controversies in the management of cysticercosis. *Emerg Infect Dis*, **3**, 403–5.

Garcia HH, *et al.* (2003). *Taenia solium* cysticercosis. *Lancet*, **362**, 547–56.

Garcia HH, *et al.* (2004). A trial of anti-parasitic treatment to reduce the rate of seizures due to cerebral cysticercosis. *N Engl J Med*, **350**, 249–58.

Garcia HH, *et al.* (2005). Neurocysticercosis: updated concepts about an old disease. *Lancet Neurol*, **4**, 653–61.

Garcia HH, *et al.* (2011). Cysticercosis of the central nervous system: how should it be managed? *Curr Opin Infect Dis*, **24**, 423–7.

Gonzalez AE, *et al.* (1997). Treatment of porcine cysticercosis with oxfendazole: a dose–response trial. *Vet Record*, **141**, 420–2.

Gonzalez AE, *et al.* (2005). Vaccination of pigs to control human neurocysticercosis. *Am J Trop Med Hyg*, **72**, 837–9.

Montano SM, *et al.* (2005). Neurocysticercosis: association between seizures, serology and brain CT in rural Peru. *Neurology*, **65**, 229–33.

Nash TE, *et al.* (2006). Treatment of neurocysticercosis—current status and future research needs. *Neurology*, **67**, 1120–7.

Salim L, *et al.* (2009). Seroepidemiologic survey of cysticercosis-taeniasis in four central highland districts of Papua, Indonesia. *Am J Trop Med Hyg*, **80**, 384–8.

Wender JD, *et al.* (2011). Intraocular cysticercosis: case series and comprehensive review of the literature. *Ocul Immunol Inflamm*, **19**, 240–5.

10.4 **Diphyllobothriasis and sparganosis**

David I. Grove

Essentials

Diphyllobothriasis—procercoid larvae of *Diphyllobothrium latum* develop in the gut of people infected by eating undercooked freshwater fish, especially in Scandinavia and Russia (other species cause disease in Japan, Korea, and South America). Adult worms cause mild gastrointestinal symptoms and urticaria, and compete with the host for vitamin B_{12}, occasionally leading to pernicious anaemia. Diagnosis is by finding characteristic ova in the stool. Treatment is with niclosamide or praziquantel.

Sparganosis—infection by animal *Spirometra* spp. is by ingestion of water containing infected crustaceans or uncooked meat (frog, snake, poultry, pork). The worm migrates through tissues, often presenting as a lump in subcutaneous tissue or muscle, and more notably in the brain (typically leading to presentation with epilepsy). Diagnosis and treatment is by surgical excision.

Diphyllobothriasis

Life cycle

Diphyllobothriasis is an infection usually caused by adult tapeworms belonging to the genus *Diphyllobothrium*. The broad tapeworm first described was *D. latum* which was acquired from ingesting undercooked fish. In recent years other species have been recognized, some of which are listed in Table 10.4.1. When undercooked fish are ingested by humans, larvae (known as plerocercoids or spargana) develop in the small intestine into adult worms up to 8 m long and consisting of a string of individual components called proglottids. Eggs begin to be passed in the faeces after about 1 month and large numbers of eggs are excreted each day. If the faeces are deposited in fresh water, the egg embryonates and releases

a larva called a coracidium which is ingested by various species of small crustacean copepods in which it further develops into a procercoid larva. When the copepod is ingested by a fish; the procercoid larvae migrates to the muscles and develops further into a plerocercoid larva up to 2 cm in length.

Epidemiology and control

Human infections occur where there is a coexistence of infected definitive hosts, susceptible intermediate hosts, deposition of infected faeces in fresh water, and a cultural practice of eating uncooked. Some species, especially *D. latum*, are acquired from freshwater fish such as perch, pike, and burbot in Europe and pike-perch and walleye in North America. Others follow consumption of anadromous fish such as salmon (*Oncorhynchus* species) which spend part of their lives in the sea but return to fresh water to spawn. The most important of these is *D. nihonkainse*, which was first found in Japan but is increasingly being seen in Europe, North America, and other parts of the world that import fresh or frozen wild Pacific salmon for consumption in sushi and sashimi. Rare infections with *D. cameroni*, *D. cordatum*, *D. hians*, *D. lanceolatum*, *D. orcini*, *D. scoticum*, and *D. stemmacephalum* (syn. *D. yonagoense*) have been seen in Japan, Greenland, and Alaska following ingestion uncooked marine fish, the precise nature of which is usually not known. More common is *D. pacificum* from seawater fish in the South American littoral, for which seals and sealions are the usual definitive hosts. Other than cooking, prevention is most reliably achieved by freezing fish for 7 days at -20°C or lower.

Clinical features

Infection usually causes no or few symptoms. Abdominal discomfort, fatigue, diarrhoea, and urticaria may be the vague presenting symptoms. Individual proglottids or a strip of gravid segments may pass out through the anus. Pernicious anaemia may be associated with *D. latum* infection because of competition for vitamin B_{12} in the bowel lumen. In these patients, elimination of the tapeworm results in improvement of the anaemia.

Diagnosis

The diagnosis can be confirmed by identifying eggs in the stool by microscopy (Fig. 10.4.1) or examination of a discharged proglottid.

Table 10.4.1 Species of *Diphyllobothrium* acquired from freshwater and andromadous fish and their epidemiology

Diphyllobothrium species	Distribution	Definitive host
Freshwater fish		
D. latum	Europe, Asia, North America	Humans
D dalliae	Alaska	Dog, Arctic fox
D dendriticum	Circumpolar regions	Birds, mammals
Anadromous fish		
D. nihonkainse, probable synonym *D. klebanovskii*	Northern Pacific rim	Brown bear, humans
D alascense	Alaska	Dog
D ursi	Alaska	Bear

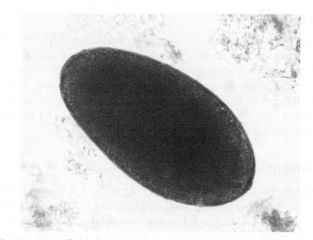

Fig. 10.4.1 Egg of *Diphyllobothrium* latum.
(Courtesy of A R Butcher.)

In endemic areas, all patients with pernicious anaemia should have their stools examined. These worms have been seen at colonoscopy or visualized by capsule endoscopy.

Treatment

Praziquantel in a single dose of 10 mg/kg body weight is usually effective. If it fails, the dose should be repeated at 25 mg/kg. The concurrent administration of a laxative is often helpful when treating young children as it aids in expulsion of the worm. An alternative drug (if available) is niclosamide in a single dose of 2 g for adults and 1 g for children aged more than 6 years. If anthelmintic therapy fails, the intraduodenal instillation of Gastrografin may be effective.

Sparganosis

Sparganosis is an infection usually caused by larval tapeworms belonging to the genus *Spirometra* which are unable to complete their development in humans. *Spirometra* and *Diphyllobothrium* are both classified as pseudophyllidean tapeworms. The usual definitive hosts for *S. mansoni*, *S. mansonoides*, and *S. erinacei* are dogs and cats, with adult worms living in the small bowel and passing eggs. When these are deposited in fresh water, the egg embryonates and releases a larva called a coracidium which is ingested by various species of small crustacean copepods in which it further develops into a procercoid larva. When the copepod is ingested by amphibians (tadpoles and frogs), reptiles (lizards and snakes), birds and some mammals (mice, rats, and humans), it develops further into a white, slender, plerocercoid larva 1 to 30 cm long, otherwise known as a sparganum, in the muscles or connective tissues (Fig. 10.4.2). Furthermore, this stage can be transferred from one host to another, e.g. when a snake eats a frog.

Epidemiology and control

Human sparganosis occurs sporadically worldwide. Human infection can be acquired by ingestion of water containing infected crustaceans or infected uncooked tadpole, frog, snake, poultry, or pork meat where this is a traditional habit. Some people believe that eating raw meat is a tonic or is beneficial for patients with tuberculosis. Rural people in some countries practise applying poultices of infected frog or snake skin to an inflamed eye, in which case a sparganum can directly penetrate the conjunctiva, or to a wound or skin ulcer. Infection is prevented by ingesting only treated water or properly cooked meats.

Clinical features

When larvae of *S. mansoni*, *S. mansonoides*, and *S. erinacei* are ingested, they penetrate the intestinal wall and migrate systemically. The worm usually lodges in subcutaneous tissue or muscle of the chest or abdominal walls, breast, limbs, or scrotum. A lump may appear and then spontaneously disappear, only to reappear some weeks or months later at a site remote from the first. Sparganosis of the central nervous system may present with seizures. A granuloma with eosinophilic infiltration is formed along the tortuous migration track (Fig. 10.4.3). Suppuration may complicate sparganosis. Ocular infection is the most common presentation of sparganosis in Thailand. Spargana can survive for more than 5 years. In general, one or only a few worms infect each patient.

Sparganum proliferum is a branched, proliferating larva for which the adult worm is unknown. Rare human infections have been described from Japan and the Americas. Thousands of small egg-like larvae may be found in subcutaneous tissues and internal organs.

Diagnosis

The diagnosis of sparganosis is usually made after operative excision. Preoperative diagnosis of cerebral sparganosis is suggested with high confidence when CT or MRI of the brain shows an enhancing nodule with changing shape or position in the sequential images. Serology may be available in some countries.

Treatment

Excision of the mass or removal of the worm from the lesion is curative. Repeated surgery is necessary when the patient has multiple lesions. Drugs are usually ineffective in sparganosis but, when surgery is not possible, albendazole 10 to 15 mg/kg daily for 20 days or praziquantel 25 mg/kg daily for 3 days may be tried. All cases of *S. proliferum* infection have proved fatal.

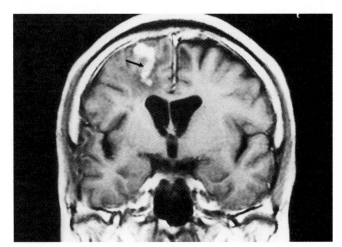

Fig. 10.4.3 MRI scan of cerebral sparganosis. Coronal contrast-enhanced T_1-weighted image shows a tortuous curvilinear enhancing lesion (arrows) with surrounding low density of oedema and degeneration in the right frontal lobe.

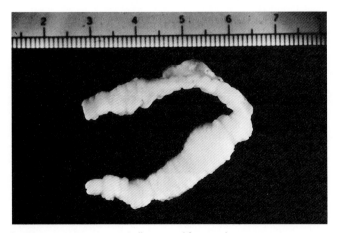

Fig. 10.4.2 A sparganum surgically removed from a subcutaneous mass.

Further reading

Anantaphruti MT, *et al.* (2011). Human sparganosis in Thailand: an overview. *Acta Trop*, **118**, 171–6.

Arizono N, *et al.* (2009). Diphyllobothriasis associated with eating raw Pacific salmon. *Emerg Infect Dis*, **15**, 866–70.

Kim JH, Lee JH. (2010). Images in clinical medicine. Diphyllobothrium latum during colonoscopy. *N Engl J Med*, **362**, e40. [This article is free at http://www.ncbi.nlm.nih.gov/pubmed and has an excellent image of a broad tapeworm seen at colonoscopy.]

Scholz T, Garcia HH, Kuchta R, Wicht B (2009). Update on the human broad tapeworm (Genus *Diphyllobothrium*), including clinical relevance. *Clin Microbial Rev*, **22**, 146–160.

Soga K, *et al.* (2011). Long fish tapeworm in the intestine: an in situ observation by capsule endoscopy. *Intern Med*, **50**, 325–7. [This article is free at http://www.ncbi.nlm.nih.gov/pubmed and has excellent images of a broad tapeworm seen at colonoscopy.]

Websites

Centers for Disease Control and Prevention. http://www.dpd.cdc.gov/DPDx/HTML/Image_Library.htm

Korean Society for Parasitology. http://www.atlas.or.kr

Trematodes (flukes)

Contents

11.1 Schistosomiasis

D.W. Dunne and B.J. Vennervald

Essentials

Schistosomiasis is caused by trematode worms *Schistosoma* spp., whose life cycle requires a definitive vertebrate host and an intermediate freshwater snail host. Transmission to humans occurs through exposure to fresh water containing infectious larvae, which can penetrate intact skin before developing into blood-dwelling adult worms. The disease is patchily distributed in parts of South America, Africa, the Middle East, China, and South East Asia, with about 200 million people infected and 20 million suffering severe consequences of infection.

Clinical features

Most infected people living in endemic areas have few (if any) overt symptoms, but clinical manifestations (when present) depend on the stage of infection.

Stage of invasion—larval invasion causes a transient immediate hypersensitivity reaction with intense itching ('swimmer's itch') and rash (cercarial dermatitis).

Stage of maturation (acute schistosomiasis or Katayama fever)—most marked in primary infections in nonimmune adults; an acute pyrexial illness associated with many non-specific symptoms and signs, and which can (rarely) be fatal. Eosinophilia is almost always present.

Established infection—(1) Urinary schistosomiasis (*Schistosoma haematobium*)—active disease most commonly presents with painless, terminal haematuria; chronic disease is associated with calcification, ulceration, and the development of papillomas in the bladder, and with ureteric fibrosis. (2) Intestinal schistosomiasis (*S. mansoni* and *S. japonicum*)—clinical features are generally encountered in those with high-intensity infections, including diarrhoea, hepatomegaly and splenomegaly; liver disease may progress to presinusoidal periportal fibrosis with portal hypertension. (3) Other manifestations—these include (a) nervous system—myelopathy and radiculopathy; (b) lungs—pulmonary hypertension and/or cor pulmonale; (c) renal—glomerulonephritis.

Diagnosis

A history of exposure to potentially contaminated water in geographically defined areas is important, especially in travellers and immigrants. Definitive diagnosis depends on direct microscopic detection of eggs in urine or stool samples, biopsies or (rarely) secretions such as seminal fluid. Serodiagnosis is not useful within endemic areas, but demonstration of schistosome-specific antibodies is helpful in travellers with a history of exposure and suspected schistosomiasis in whom eggs have not been detected.

Treatment and prognosis

Praziquantel is the drug of choice, with corticosteroids added in cases of Katayama fever to suppress the hypersensitivity reaction. Acute schistosomiasis responds well to early drug therapy, leaving little residual damage: chronic disease responds less well, although some improvement can occur. However, rapid re-exposure and reinfection are common, particularly in young children, unless control measures are implemented at the community level.

Prevention

In areas of high transmission, population-based chemotherapy or treatment of schoolchildren (who have the heaviest worm burdens

and contribute most to ongoing transmission) can reduce the prevalence and severity of morbidity. In areas of less intense transmission,
treatment can be restricted to diagnosed cases. Health education
should be aimed at improving practices of water use and preventing
indiscriminate urination and defecation.

Introduction

Schistosomiasis, also known as bilharzia, is caused by infection
with parasitic trematode worms (flukes) of the genus *Schistosoma*.
Disease is usually associated with chronic infections contracted by
exposure to fresh water containing infective cercarial larvae that
penetrate intact skin and develop into blood-dwelling worms.
Most human infections are caused by one of three species,
S. mansoni, *S. haematobium*, or *S. japonicum*. Two species,
S. intercalatum and *S. mekongi*, are less significant. Schistosomiasis
is patchily distributed in parts of South America, Africa, the Middle
East, China, and South-East Asia (Fig. 11.1.1). An estimated
779 million people are at risk of schistosomiasis worldwide, of
whom 207 million are infected (Steinmann *et al.*, 2006). Although
simple diagnosis and effective drug treatment is available for individual uncomplicated cases, the world disease burden caused by
these parasites has increased from an estimated 114 million human
infections in 1947. Diagnosis and treatment are often not available
to exposed rural populations, and drug-based control programmes
are hampered by the continued susceptibility to reinfection of
those who have been treated, particularly children. Human schistosomiasis is most often an insidious and chronic disease with a
range of pathological manifestations involving the intestine and
liver, or the urogenital tract. Mortality estimates are difficult, but
20 000 to 200 000 deaths may be directly associated with schistosomiasis each year.

Parasite life cycle

The schistosome life cycle requires two host species: a definitive
vertebrate host, in which adult male and female worms develop

and sexual reproduction occurs, and an intermediate freshwater
snail host, in which the parasite multiplies asexually. Transmission
between these hosts is achieved by two different free-swimming
larval stages. For species that infect humans, miracidia hatch from
eggs excreted in the faeces or urine of the vertebrate host, and then
seek out and infect snails. Cercariae are released from the snail and
are able actively to penetrate intact human skin. Different schistosome species have their own, often very restricted, range of snail
hosts. Schistosomiasis is thus closely associated with particular
freshwater habitats, and its geographical distribution is restricted
by the availability of particular snail species. *S. mansoni* and
S. haematobium are confined to aquatic snails (genera *Biomphalaria*
and *Bulinus* respectively) that inhabit ponds, lakes, irrigation
canals, slow-flowing streams, and rivers. *S. japonicum* is transmitted by amphibious snails of the genus *Oncomelania* that, in addition to a variety of freshwater habitats, are also present in damp
soil and vegetation, such as paddy fields.

Schistosomes that infect humans can also infect other mammals.
This is important in the transmission of *S. japonicum*, a zoonotic
infection in which cattle, water buffalo, pigs, dogs, and rodents can
act as reservoir hosts of the human parasite. *S. mansoni* infects a
narrower range of mammals, and only a few rodent species and
baboons have any potential to act as occasional reservoirs. In nature
S. haematobium is essentially specific to humans. The sites of maturation of the adult worms vary between schistosome species, affecting both the transmission of the infection and its clinical sequelae.

Once shed from freshwater snails, cercariae (Fig. 11.1.2) live
for about 24 h, but their effective period of infectivity is probably shorter under field conditions. Cercarial behaviour and the
timing of their release enhance their chance of contacting their
vertebrate host of choice. Light and increasing temperature trigger the release of *S. mansoni* and *S. haematobium* cercariae during
the day, and they use their tails actively to maintain their position
near the water surface. *S. japonicum* cercariae are shed late in the
day and are closely associated with the meniscus, perhaps reflecting their wider host range, as species specific for rodents are shed
at night. Contact with skin triggers adherence mechanisms, and
proteolytic enzymes and muscular movements allow penetration
of the skin in minutes. Penetration initiates transformation into
a schistosomular larva, with loss of the tail and of the protective

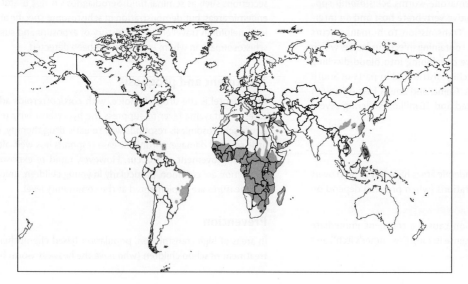

Fig. 11.1.1 Global distribution of the
schistosomes that affect humans.

outer glycocalyx layer, and the addition of an extra lipid bilayer to the surface membrane of the parasite's syncytial outer tegument. This tegument now forms the main parasite–host interface and so has physiological and immunological functions vital to long-term survival in the mammalian bloodstream. These include uptake of nutrients, response to injury, and surface adsorption of host antigens to provide an immunological disguise.

Newly transformed schistosomula remain in the epidermis for several days before migrating, via the bloodstream, lungs, and systemic circulation, to the hepatic portal system. Here the schistosomula mature and differentiate into adult worms, pair, and migrate against the portal blood flow to the small venules draining the genitourinary tract (*S. haematobium*) or the large and, to a lesser extent, small intestine (*S. mansoni*, *S. japonicum*, *S. intercalatum*, *S. mekongi*). Male and female worms are 1 to 2 cm long and morphologically distinct. Paired worms remain permanently coupled, with the shorter, flatter, more muscular male gripping the female in its gynaecophoric canal (Fig. 11.1.3). Worms ingest blood cells into their blind-ending bifurcated gut, producing a haematin-like pigment that is regurgitated into the blood. Adult worms have average lifespans in humans of 3 years (*S. haematobium*) to 7 years (*S. mansoni*), although active infections are reported in individuals who have left endemic areas more than 20 years previously. Female worms start to produce eggs between 5 and 12 weeks after infection, at rates of 300 (*S. mansoni*) to 3000 (*S. japonicum*) per day. A few days after an egg is laid, a single miracidium develops within the rigid eggshell, the shape and size of which is characteristic for each species. *S. mansoni* (Fig. 11.1.4) and *S. haematobium* eggs are ellipsoid, 65 × 150 μm, the former having a lateral spine and the latter a terminal spine. *S. japonicum* eggs are more spherical, 70 × 90 μm, with a small lateral knob that is not always apparent

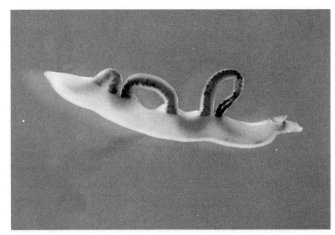

Fig. 11.1.3 Adult worms of *S. mansoni*. The shorter male encloses the female in its gynaecophoric canal, the characteristic haematin-like pigment can be seen in the female worm's gut.

microscopically. Embryonated eggs pass from the venules into the gut or bladder lumen. This is facilitated by host immune responses to secreted egg antigens, as egg excretion is inhibited in immuno-suppressed experimental hosts and HIV infected individuals. The passage of the eggs causes tissue damage, as does the granulomatous reactions to eggs that fail to escape from the bloodstream and get swept into the liver by the portal blood flow.

Eggs deposited in fresh water rapidly hatch in response to osmotic changes, releasing the miracidium. This ciliated and actively swimming larva lives for about 6 h, and can chemically detect the proximity of snails, modifying its swimming behaviour as it approaches a potential host. The parasite actively penetrates the snail's tissues and transforms into a primary sporocyst. Asexual replication gives rise to daughter sporocysts that migrate to the snail's hepatopancreas where cercariae are asexually generated within each sporocyst. Thus, snails infected with a single miracidium release cercariae that are all of the same sex. Cercariae are first released from snails 3 to 6 weeks after infection, depending on parasite species and ambient temperature. Infected snails can shed hundreds of cercariae daily over several months.

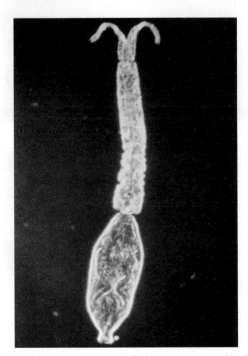

Fig. 11.1.2 The infective larva (cerceria) of *Schistosoma mansoni*, length approximately 200 μm. The head region has characteristic suckers; the muscular forked tail propels the free-swimming larva, but is discarded during skin penetration. This larva will develop into an adult worm in a human host.

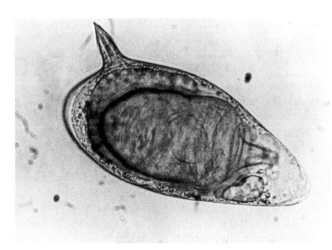

Fig. 11.1.4 Egg of *S. mansoni* containing a fully developed miracidium and showing the characteristic lateral spine of this species.

Schistosomiasis is associated with poor living conditions and inadequate sanitation and water supply. Its distribution has changed over the last 50 years. In some areas sustained control strategies have been successful. However, environmental changes, development of water resources, population increases, and migration, have led to its spread into previously nonendemic areas or areas with a low rate of infection. *S. japonicum* and *S. haematobium* have decreased, whereas *S. mansoni* has increased to become the most prevalent and widespread species. *S. japonicum* has been controlled effectively in many areas and is now endemic only in China, where it is much reduced, Indonesia, the Philippines, and Thailand. *S. mekongi* is found in Cambodia and Laos, and *S. intercalatum* is found in 10 countries within the rainforest belt of central Africa. *S. mansoni* is present in most countries of sub-Saharan Africa, and in Madagascar, the Nile delta and valley, as well as Saudi Arabia, Yemen, Oman, Libya, northern and eastern Brazil, Suriname, Venezuela, and some Caribbean islands. *S. haematobium* is widespread in sub-Saharan Africa and Madagascar, and is more prevalent than *S. mansoni* in North Africa and the Middle East.

Clinical features

Stage of invasion: cercarial dermatitis or 'swimmer's itch'

When cercariae penetrate the skin they can cause a skin reaction, called cercarial dermatitis or 'swimmer's itch'. This is frequently seen after exposure to avian schistosomes, and is associated with the death of cercariae in the skin. It is seen both in areas endemic for human schistosomiasis and in non-endemic areas. In people exposed for the first time, the invasion causes a transient immediate hypersensitivity reaction with intense itching. Within 12 to 24 h it is followed by a delayed reaction characterized by a small, red, pruritic, macular rash progressing to papules after 24 h. The rash may persist for up to 15 days and residual pigmentation may persist for months. Following repeated exposure, the signs and symptoms increase dramatically and start earlier. A similar reaction can be seen after re-exposure to human cercariae, predominantly *S. mansoni* and *S. japonicum*. Treatment, if needed, is symptomatic.

Stage of maturation: acute schistosomiasis or Katayama fever

The early stages of a primary infection can be associated with a severe systemic reaction that resembles serum sickness. This acute illness, called acute toxaemic schistosomiasis or Katayama fever, can occur following initial infection with any schistosome infecting humans, although it is more common in *S. japonicum* and *S. mansoni* infections. Acute schistosomiasis is most marked in primary infections in nonimmune adults, but acute *S. japonicum* infection can occur in re-exposed individuals. Symptoms appear 2 to 6 weeks after exposure. The clinical picture resembles an acute pyrexial illness with fever as a prime characteristic. The patient feels ill, and may have rigors, sweating, headache, malaise, muscular aches, profound weakness, weight loss, and a nonproductive irritating cough. Anorexia, nausea, abdominal pain, and diarrhoea can occur. Physical examination may reveal a generalized lymphadenopathy, an enlarged tender liver, and, sometimes, a slightly enlarged spleen and an urticarial rash (Fig. 11.1.5). Eosinophilia is almost always present. Patients may become

confused or stuporose or present with visual impairment or papilloedema. Severe cerebral or spinal cord manifestations may occur, and this is an indication for urgent investigative measures. Even light infections may cause severe illness and the syndrome can, in rare cases, be fatal.

Differential diagnoses include infections such as typhoid (leucopenia, no eosinophilia), brucellosis, malaria, infectious mononucleosis, miliary tuberculosis, leptospirosis, and other conditions with fever of unknown origin. Fever and eosinophilia occur in trichinosis, tropical eosinophilia, invasive ankylostomiasis, strongyloidiasis, visceral larva migrans, and infections with *Opisthorchis* and *Clonorchis* species.

Established infections

Urinary schistosomiasis (*Schistosoma haematobium*)

The signs and symptoms of *S. haematobium* infection relate to the worms' predilection for the veins of the genitourinary tract, and

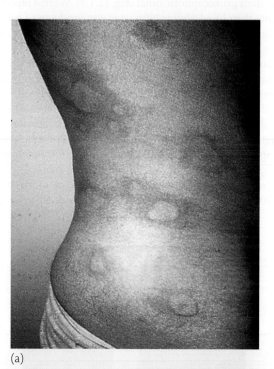
(a)

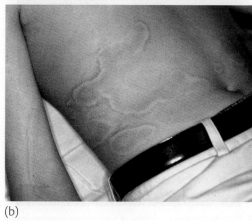
(b)

Fig. 11.1.5 Katayama fever (*S. mansoni* infection): (a) giant urticarial rash; (b) rash in a traveller.
(Courtesy of Dr Tom Doherty, London Hospital for Tropical Diseases.)

result from deposition of eggs in the bladder, ureters, and to some extent the genital organs. In the phase of established infection two stages can be recognized:

- an active stage mainly in children, adolescents, and younger adults with egg deposition in the urinary tract, egg excretion in the urine with proteinuria and macroscopic or microscopic haematuria

- a chronic stage in older patients with sparse or absent urinary egg excretion but the presence of urogenital tract pathology

In the active stage many patients will have minimal symptoms. The most frequently encountered complaint is a painless, characteristically terminal, haematuria, the prevalence and severity of which is related to the intensity of infection. In communities where *S. haematobium* is highly endemic, macroscopic haematuria among boys is considered a natural sign of puberty. Dysuria, frequency, and suprapubic discomfort or pain is associated with schistosomal cystitis and may continue throughout the course of active infection. Initially the eggs may give rise to an intense inflammatory response in the mucosa. This may cause ureteric obstruction leading to hydroureter and hydronephrosis. Cytoscopy reveals friable masses or polyps extending into the bladder, petechiae, and granulomas. These early inflammatory lesions, including the obstructive uropathy, are usually reversible after treatment with antischistosomal drugs. The bladder lesions and obstructive uropathy can be visualized by ultrasonography (Fig. 11.1.6).

As the infection progresses, the inflammatory component decreases, possibly due to modulation by the host immune response, and fibrosis increases. Various changes occur in the bladder, including calcification, ulceration, and the development of papillomas. Cytoscopy reveals 'sandy patches' composed of large numbers of calcified eggs surrounded by fibrous tissue and an atrophic mucosal surface. The bladder lesions may lead to nocturia, precipitancy, retention of urine, dribbling, and incontinence. Calculus formation is common, as is secondary bacterial infection, usually due to *Escherichia coli*, pseudomonas, klebsiella, enterobacter, or salmonella. the ureters are less commonly involved, but ureteric fibrosis can cause irreversible obstructive uropathy which can progress to uraemia. Bilateral ureteric involvement is common, although lesions may predominate on one side. Despite damage to the ureters, symptoms may be absent or minimal.

Egg deposition may also cause granulomas and lesions to develop in the genital organs, most commonly in the cervix and vagina in women and the seminal vessels in men leading to syndromes termed female and male genital schistosomiasis, respectively. This may result in dyspareunia, contact bleeding, and lower back pain in women, and perineal pain and painful ejaculation in men. Symptoms such as haematospermia and perineal discomfort have been described in travellers returning from Malawi. In some of these patients, eggs have been demonstrated in seminal fluid but not in urine. An association between female genital schistosomiasis and HIV infection has been demonstrated but the impact of genital lesions caused by *S. haematobium* infection on the spread of HIV needs to be elucidated. Although small numbers of *S. haematobium* eggs are frequently detected in faeces and rectal biopsies, intestinal symptoms are uncommon.

An association between *S. haematobium* infection and squamous cell carcinoma of the urinary bladder has been described and *S. haematobium* has been classified as definitely carcinogenic to humans (group 1 carcinogens). The aetiological significance of the parasite in the causation of this cancer is not proven, but is suggested by the finding that the prevalence of squamous cell carcinoma of the bladder is correlated with intensity of *S. haematobium* infection. In the established stage, *S. haematobium* should be distinguished from renal tuberculosis with haematuria, haemoglobinuria, and cancer of the urogenital tract.

Intestinal schistosomiasis

In most early *S. mansoni* and *S. japonicum* infections, symptoms are mild or absent. Clinical features are generally encountered in those with high-intensity infections. They include diarrhoea, sometimes with blood or mucus in the surface of the stool, abdominal discomfort, and hypogastric pain or colicky cramps. Severe dysentery is rare, but can occur. The liver, especially the left lobe, may be enlarged and tender; the spleen may also be enlarged, but is usually soft. At this stage, the condition is entirely reversible by antischistosomal treatment, but the relative lack of symptoms may cause it to pass unnoticed until irreversible complications set in. Later stages present as intestinal or hepatosplenic disease. Intestinal schistosomiasis is associated with granuloma formation (Fig. 11.1.7), inflammation, and fibrosis, primarily in the large intestine. Focal dense deposits of *S. mansoni* or *S. japonicum* eggs in the large intestine can induce the formation of inflammatory polyps. The major clinical manifestation is intermittent diarrhoea with or without passage of blood or mucus, occasionally associated

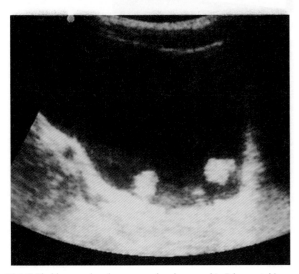

Fig. 11.1.6 Bladder pseudopolyps as seen by ultrasound in *S. haematobium* infection.
(Courtesy of Ms Hilda Kadzo, Kenyatta National Hospital, Nairobi, Kenya.)

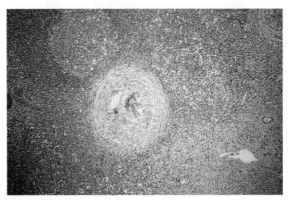

Fig. 11.1.7 Schistosomal granuloma in the appendix.

with protein-losing enteropathy and anaemia. Intestinal schisto-somiasis in *S. japonicum* infection may also involve the stomach, with gastric bleeding and pyloric obstruction.

Differential diagnosis includes irritable bowel syndrome, amoe-biasis, giardiasis, intestinal helminth infection, ulcerative colitis, Crohn's disease, and tuberculosis.

Hepatosplenic schistosomiasis is a chronic manifestation of *S. mansoni* and *S. japonicum* infection. The term covers two dis-tinct clinical entities: early inflammatory and late hepatosplenic disease with periportal fibrosis. Early inflammatory hepatosplenic schistosomiasis is the main cause of hepatosplenic schistosomiasis in children and adolescents. The liver is enlarged, especially the left lobe, and is smooth and firm. The spleen is enlarged, often extending below the umbilicus and firm or hard. Generally no hepatic fibrosis can be demonstrated by ultrasonography. Early inflammatory hepatosplenic schistosomiasis may be found in up to 80% of infected children and the severity is related to inten-sity of infection (Fig. 11.1.8). This type of hepatosplenomegaly may also be associated with concomitant chronic exposure to malaria.

Presinusoidal periportal fibrosis (clay pipe stem or Symmers' fibrosis) (Figs. 11.1.9 and 11.1.10) develops later in life, gener-ally in young and middle-aged adults with long-standing intense exposure to infection. Patients with periportal fibrosis may excrete very few or no eggs in faeces. During the early stages the liver is enlarged, especially the left lobe; it is smooth, firm, and sometimes tender. Later, in many cases, it becomes small firm and nodular. The spleen is enlarged, often massively, due to passive congestion and reticuloendothelial hyperplasia (Fig. 11.1.9). The patient may be asymptomatic or may complain of a left hypochondrial mass with discomfort and anorexia. Anaemia may be present. There may be reduced growth, infantilism, and amenorrhoea, especially in *S. japonicum* infection. Severe hepatosplenic schistosomiasis

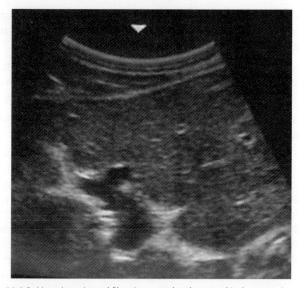

Fig. 11.1.9 Hepatic periportal fibrosis as seen by ultrasound in *S. mansoni* infection.

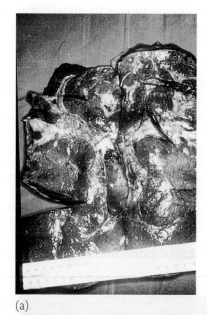

(a)

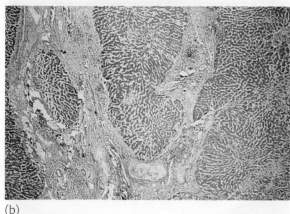

(b)

Fig. 11.1.10 The liver in *S. mansoni* infection in South Africa. Clay pipe stem fibrosis: (a) macroscopic views; (b) microscopic view.
(Copyright Gareth Turner.)

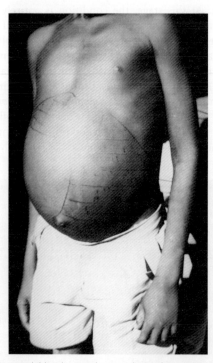

Fig. 11.1.8 Kenyan child with severe hepatosplenic schistosomiasis mansoni.

may lead to portal hypertension, but hepatic function usually remains normal. Ascites, attributable both to the portal hypertension and to hypoalbuminaemia, may be seen, especially in *S. japonicum* infection. Patients with severe hepatosplenic disease and portal hypertension may develop oesophageal varices detectable by endoscopy or ultrasound (Fig. 11.1.11). These patients may experience repeated bouts of haematemesis, melaena, or both. This is the most severe, potentially fatal, complication of hepatosplenic schistosomiasis, and death may result from massive loss of blood.

Differential diagnoses of hepatosplenic schistosomiasis include kala-azar (visceral leishmaniasis), tropical splenomegaly syndrome associated with malaria, leukaemia, lymphoma, alcoholic, or viral cirrhosis, and some of the haemoglobinopathies. Some regression of periportal fibrosis may occur after specific antischistosomal therapy, as judged by ultrasonography examination of the liver, but in most individuals with periportal fibrosis and clinical manifestations of hepatosplenic disease, regression does not occur.

In comparison with *S. japonicum* and *S. mansoni* infections, clinical symptoms of disease in *S. intercalatum* infection are commonly mild or absent, and it is not regarded as a serious public health problem. Active infection is seen in children and adolescents and pathology is detected only in those with egg excretion exceeding 400 eggs/g faeces. The usual clinical presentation is one of diarrhoea, often with blood in the stool and lower abdominal pain or discomfort. *S. mekongi* infections are usually asymptomatic but may produce a clinical picture similar to that of *S. japonicum*, although the infections are usually milder. Hepatosplenomegaly can occur.

Other manifestations

Nervous system manifestations

Nervous system involvement in *S. mansoni* and *S. haematobium* infections most frequently affect the spinal cord following acute infection. This manifestation is not related to the intensity of infection. A myelopathy and radiculopathy results from the inflammatory reaction, caused by the deposition of eggs around the spinal cord, and presents as an ascending flaccid paralysis with sensory level and sphincter involvement. The lesion is usually in the region of the cauda equina. Although paraparesis is seen most commonly

during acute schistosomiasis, it may also be a late-stage complication of *S. mansoni* infection in endemic areas with high rates of transmission. Myelography, CT, and MRI are of diagnostic value. In acute cases lesions are seen on MRI scans as a diffuse swelling of the lumbar cord with central softening or cyst formation.

The brain is the major site of central nervous system involvement in *S. japonicum* infections. About 2% of acutely infected patients experience symptoms that mimic acute encephalitis or a focal neurological process. CT shows multiple enhancing lesions. In chronic infections, patients may present with focal brain lesions that can resemble tumours and present as focal epilepsy. These lesions contain masses of eggs and granulomas. Antischistosomal drugs, corticosteroids, and surgery are the types of treatment available for neuroschistosomiasis, and uncontrolled studies suggest that treatment with a combination of praziquantel and corticosteroids is effective. However, a consensus regarding the best treatment of the different presentations of neuroschistosomiasis has not been reached.

Pulmonary manifestations

Eggs may be deposited in the lungs. Granulomatous reactions and fibrosis develop in the pulmonary vasculature leading to pulmonary hypertension and/or cor pulmonale (Fig. 11.1.12). This is normally seen secondary to hepatosplenic schistosomiasis in patients with portal fibrosis and portal hypertension, but pulmonary hypertension may also result from accumulation of *S. haematobium* eggs in the lungs. A syndrome of cough with multiple small radiographic lesions and eosinophilia has been described. Symptoms include fatigue, palpitations, dyspnoea, cough, and sometimes haemoptysis. Patients may progress to decompensation with congestive cardiac failure. In endemic areas schistosomiasis must always be considered as a possible cause of pulmonary hypertension and cor pulmonale.

Renal manifestations

Glomerulonephritis is common in chronic *S. mansoni* infection in Brazil, especially in patients with hepatosplenic disease. Immunoglobulins, complement components, and schistosome antigens are deposited in the mesangial area. The condition is manifested clinically as proteinuria and/or nephrotic syndrome, sometimes with hypertension.

Miscellaneous manifestations

Patients infected with any of the three major schistosome species and subsequently infected with salmonella may develop a prolonged intermittent febrile illness. Prolonged excretion of

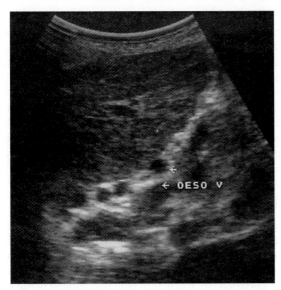

Fig. 11.1.11 Oesophageal varices as seen by ultrasound in *S. mansoni* infection.

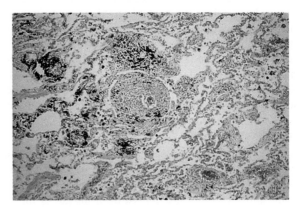

Fig. 11.1.12 Schistosomal granuloma in the lung.
(Copyright Gareth Turner.)

salmonella in the urine and intermittent bacteraemia has been demonstrated in *S. haematobium* infection. Treatment for the salmonella infection alone is often not effective without treatment of the underlying schistosome infection.

Diagnosis and investigations

Information about geographical area and history of exposure by wading, bathing, washing, or showering in potentially contaminated fresh water is important for diagnosis of schistosomiasis, especially in travellers and immigrants. This can indicate the likelihood of infection and point to the schistosome species involved. A definitive diagnosis is made by the direct demonstration of schistosome eggs by microscopy of urine or stool samples, biopsies or, on rare occasions, secretions such as seminal fluid. In epidemiological studies it is usually important to obtain quantitative estimates of egg output to provide information about intensity of infection within a population.

Direct parasitological methods

In *S. haematobium* infection, eggs can be detected in urine after filtration, sedimentation, or centrifugation followed by microscopy. Ideally, urine should be passed around midday and the terminal part of the stream examined. The most commonly used method in epidemiological studies in endemic areas is filtration of 10 to 20 ml of urine using a syringe and a polycarbonate (e.g. Nucleopore), polyamide (e.g. Nytrel), or paper filter. Infection intensity is expressed as eggs/10 ml of urine. This may not be sufficiently sensitive for detection of low-intensity infections in travellers. In such cases, diagnosis is often based on filtration of 24-h urine samples.

For *S. mansoni*, *S. japonicum*, *S. mekongi*, and *S. intercalatum* eggs in the faeces, sedimentation of the eggs followed by microscopy is a useful and simple technique. However, the Kato thick smear technique is the most widely used method in epidemiological studies. This is based on microscopic examination of a smear of a small but fixed amount of faecal sample (usually 20–50 mg). Coarse particles and fibrous material are first removed from the sample by passing it through a sieve. A fixed sample volume is obtained by the use of a template. This is placed on a microscope slide and squashed with either a piece of cellophane soaked in glycerol or a glass coverslip. After leaving the slide for 6 to 24 h to allow the preparation to clear, the eggs are counted and the level of infection expressed as eggs/g faeces. Unfortunately, watery or diarrhoeal stools cannot be processed this way, and low-intensity infections may not be detected, since only small faecal samples are examined and eggs may be clumped unevenly in the stool. Increased sensitivity is obtained by increasing the number of samples examined. For diagnosis of light infections in previously unexposed travellers, microscopic examination of a rectal tissue snip crushed between glass slides is often the most sensitive direct diagnostic method. This method can also be used for biopsies. The crushed tissue sample is far better than a sectioned biopsy for the detection and identification of eggs.

Other direct methods

Sensitive enzyme immune assays (ELISA) have been developed to detect circulating schistosome antigens in serum or urine. These antigens, circulating anodic antigen (CAA) and circulating cathodic antigen (CCA), are derived from the gut of the adult schistosomes. The assays have almost 100% specificity and high sensitivity, and are excellent epidemiological tools as they provide a direct estimate of worm burden and can be used to monitor the efficacy of chemotherapy. They are less well suited for diagnosis of light infections in travellers. A rapid point-of-care test for CCA in urine is now commercially available. Recently, a multiplex real-time PCR for detection of schistosome DNA in stool samples has proven to be a useful tool in epidemiological studies and may prove valuable in evaluation of control programmes since samples can be stored at room temperature. It is foreseen that the use of PCR-based methods in diagnosis of schistosomiasis will increase in future.

Indirect diagnostic techniques

In *S. haematobium* infections, chemical reagent strips for detection of microhaematuria are widely used in endemic areas as a diagnostic measure. The method can be used in areas of both high and low transmission and there is a consistent significant correlation between microhaematuria and intensity of infection. In intestinal schistosomiasis, blood may be found in the stools, but it is not as useful an indicator of infection. In urinary schistosomiasis, eosinophiluria, with high numbers of eosinophil granulocytes in the urine, is a characteristic finding. Recently, detection of the eosinophil granule protein ECP (eosinophil cationic protein) in urine has been used for the qualitative assessment of eosinophil infiltration of the bladder mucosa, and hence local inflammation. Measurement of ECP in urine has proved useful in following post-treatment resolution of urinary tract morbidity in endemic areas. Eosinophilia is often found in acutely infected travellers. In cases where eggs are difficult to find, eosinophilia plus a history of exposure may suggest the need for further examination for schistosomiasis including serodiagnosis.

Immunodiagnosis

In cases of suspected schistosomiasis in which eggs have not been detected, serology can be used to demonstrate specific antibodies. An indirect immunofluorescence test using sections of adult worms for detection of specific immunoglobulins (IgM and IgG) is widely used. For travellers, a positive antibody result combined with a history of exposure should lead to treatment. Serodiagnosis is not useful in endemic areas because of the high levels of specific antibodies found in naturally exposed populations.

Ultrasonography

Ultrasonography is noninvasive, portable, has no biological hazards for the patient, and can be used to either complement or replace many invasive diagnostic techniques. It is the technique of choice for grading schistosomal periportal fibrosis, portal hypertension, hydronephrosis, and urinary bladder lesions. A protocol for standardized investigations and methods of reporting has been produced by the World Health Organization (http://www.who.int/tdr/publications/publications/ultrasound.htm). Ultrasonography is especially useful for monitoring decreases in morbidity after chemotherapy programmes.

Pathophysiology/pathogenesis

Schistosome eggs can be trapped in the tissues, often the walls of the intestines or, depending on species, the urinary bladder or ureters. They may be seen in cone biopsies of the uterine cervix. The eggs of *S. mansoni* and *S. japonicum* are swept into the liver via the portal system, where they embolize into the portal radicles and give rise to vascular and granulomatous changes (Fig. 11.1.7).

Granulomatous pyelophlebitis and peripyelophlebitis is responsible for development of portal hypertension, while granulomata with subsequent fibrosis may be responsible for the periportal fibrosis. The characteristic lesion in the liver is a presinusoidal periportal fibrosis (Symmers' fibrosis, Fig. 11.1.10). There is typically no bridging between the fibrous tracts, no nodule formation, and no hepatic cell damage. Increased portal pressure can result in the development of portosystemic collaterals and eggs may pass directly from the portal vein to the pulmonary circulation (Fig. 11.1.12). Here the combination of vascular and granulomatous changes is responsible for pulmonary hypertension.

Treatment

Today the drug of choice is praziquantel, available as 600 mg tablets. It is administered orally, normally in a single dose, 40 mg/kg body weight and is effective against all schistosome species infecting humans. It is also effective for most other trematode infections and against adult cestodes. The drug is safe and well tolerated. After a single dose of 40 mg/kg up to 85% of those treated cease to excrete eggs, and egg counts are reduced by 95% or more in those not cured. In endemic areas, this level of efficacy is generally acceptable since very light residual infections do not lead to severe morbidity. In patients who are not cured by the initial treatment, the same dose can be repeated at weekly intervals for 2 weeks. A repeat dose 6–12 weeks later can be administered to cure prepatent infections, especially if eosinophilia or symptoms persist despite treatment.

Praziquantel has not been shown to be teratogenic in animals and it is now judged to be safe to use for the treatment of pregnant and lactating women and young children. Any side effects are generally mild, resolving spontaneously over a few hours and rarely requiring medication. Gastrointestinal side effects include abdominal pain or discomfort and sometimes vomiting. They occur more frequently in individuals with high infection intensities. Urticarial skin reactions and periorbital oedema may occur in about 2% of treated individuals. General side effects including headache, dizziness, fever, and fatigue can also occur, but less frequently.

As a general principle, all patients with acute schistosomiasis should be treated with praziquantel. Corticosteroids can be added in case of Katayama fever to suppress the hypersensitivity reaction. Since immature schistosomes are not susceptible to praziquantel, treatment should be repeated 4–6 weeks later. Use of praziquantel for cerebral *S. japonicum* infections is effective, resulting in rapid dissipation of cerebral oedema and resolution of cerebral masses. However, corticosteroids and anticonvulsants are sometimes needed in addition to praziquantel in cases with neuroschistosomiasis. Praziquantel should be administered with great caution in the case of concurrent neurocysticercosis. Chemotherapy is only part of the management of schistosomiasis-associated portal hypertension, since the main complications are due to obstructive pathology. Management of portal hypertension and prevention of bleeding from oesophageal varices is beyond the scope of this chapter. Praziquantel has largely replaced other drugs for treatment of schistosomiasis. Oxamniquine (marketed as Mansil in South America) is only effective against *S. mansoni* and is mainly used in Brazil. Artemisinin derivatives are effective against immature stages (schistosomulae) of *S. japonicum*, *S. mansoni*, and *S. haematobium* and clinical trials in China has shown that repeated oral doses of artesunate or artemether prevented patent *S. japonicum* infections. In order to reduce the risk of inducing drug-resistant malaria parasites, artemisinin-based combination therapies (ACTs) are used in treatment of malaria. So far two large-scale trials have examined the effect of ACTs on *S. haematobium* in Mali and *S. mansoni* in Kenya, respectively. Taken together, the evidence suggests that the efficacy of ACTs against the two major schistosome species is only moderate and inferior to a single dose of praziquantel and ACTs should be reserved for the management of malaria.

Prognosis

Most infected people have few, if any, overt symptoms. Acute schistosomiasis can be fatal or can lead to severe residual damage to the nervous system if not treated, but responds well to antischistosomal therapy if started early. Early infections respond extremely well to treatment and the pathological lesions regress leaving little residual damage. However, in endemic areas individuals, particularly young children, are rapidly re-exposed and reinfected unless control measures are taken at the community level. Chronic infections with severe periportal fibrosis respond less well to specific antischistosomal treatment, although some regression of hepatosplenic disease with periportal fibrosis has been seen after treatment. The lifetime prognosis is worst in patients with severe hepatosplenic schistosomiasis and oesophageal varices. Previous episodes of haematemesis indicate a 70%t risk of rebleeding.

Transmission and epidemiology

Each successful cercarial penetration of human skin has the potential to give rise to a single male or female adult worm, but it is probable that many cercariae die naturally in the epidermis. People tend to accumulate worms with continued exposure to infection. However, human populations in endemic areas do not just continue to accumulate worms with age. Intensities of infection increase in children during their younger years (as estimated by numbers of excreted eggs), peaking around the age of 12 years, before falling to lower levels in adulthood (Fig. 11.1.13a). This is probably due to the death of older worms, which are not replaced at a similar rate in older people. This age–infection intensity profile is more pronounced if study populations are given chemotherapy to remove existing infections and then monitored for levels of reinfection over several subsequent years. In these circumstances, it is clear that young children are much more susceptible to reinfection than older children or adults, and that a striking change in susceptibility to reinfection occurs after 12 years of age. The slower acquisition of worms in adulthood could be due to reduced exposure to infection or to age-dependent changes in innate resistance or acquired immunity. In many endemic areas children have more contact with water than adults, but careful observation of water-associated behaviour has shown that age profiles of water contact are variable between communities, whereas profiles of reinfection intensities are remarkably consistent (Fig. 11.1.13b). This suggests that host-related factors other than exposure influence susceptibility to reinfection. This has been most convincingly shown in fishing communities in areas with high *S. mansoni* transmission on Lake Albert, Uganda. Here occupational water contact results in adults having greater exposure to infection than their children, yet, within 12 months of treatment, it is the children under 12 years of age that suffer much higher reinfection intensities.

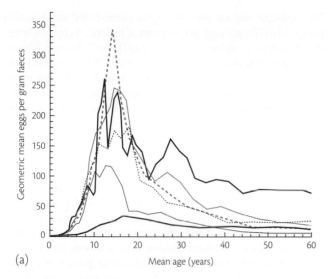

(a)

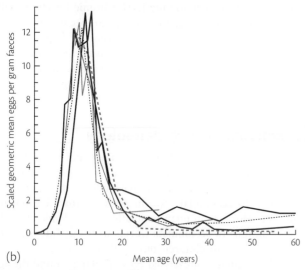

(b)

Fig. 11.1.13 (a) Age–intensity profiles of *S. mansoni* infection from six communities in Kenya. (b) Age–reinfection intensity profiles of *S. mansoni* after chemotherapy in the same six communities in Kenya, assessed between 12 and 36 months after treatment.

(a, from Fulford, AJ, *et al.* (1992). On the use of age-intensity data to detect immunity to parasitic infections, with special reference to *Schistosoma mansoni* in Kenya. *Parasitology* **105**: 219–227.)

Current research is focused on assessing the relative roles of innate resistance and acquired immunity in this age-dependent resistance and whether the onset of puberty or the length of time spent living in endemic areas might be important. For example, it is not known if this age-dependent resistance to infection holds true for travellers exposed to infection for the first time. Immune responses to schistosomes also differ between children and adults. Specific IgE and other characteristically Th2-type responses against the parasite are associated with resistance to reinfection. Whatever mechanisms underlie the contrasting susceptibilities of children and adults, continued exposure can be expected to result in reinfection, especially amongst younger children.

Prevention and control

Despite the high risk of reinfection, chemotherapy is usually highly beneficial at both the individual and population levels, as those suffering high intensities of infection are at greatest risk of the more severe forms of schistosomiasis. Furthermore, even low-intensity infections may lead to anaemia and have a negative impact on the well-being of the infected individual. This is especially important among vulnerable groups such as children and pregnant women. Various chemotherapy-based control strategies can be employed depending on intensity of transmission and the available resources. In the Nile delta region of Egypt, injections of tartar emetic were used for mass treatment from the 1960s to the 1980s. Tragically, the needles were not adequately sterilized and, as a result, hepatitis C virus was widely spread in this population to reach its highest recorded prevalence. In areas of high transmission, population-based chemotherapy can avoid the time and expense required for diagnosis and reduce the prevalence and severity of morbidity. Alternatively, schoolchildren can be targeted for treatment, as they invariably have the heaviest worm burdens and contribute most to ongoing transmission. In areas of less intense transmission, treatment can be restricted to diagnosed cases. The provision of safe water supplies and sanitation, where it can be achieved, will make an important additional contribution. Mortality can be prevented and morbidity best controlled by a combination of health education, chemotherapy, provision of safe water supplies and sanitation, and, where appropriate, snail control. Health education should be aimed at improving practices of water use and preventing indiscriminate urination and defecation. The role of molluscicides in control programmes depends on the local epidemiological and ecological circumstances and the resources available. Within the context of a larger concerted intervention, focal mollusciciding of major transmission sites can be useful. Eradication of host snail species is not usually feasible, although modification of the environment to eliminate snails has been successful in parts of China. In general, it has only been through sustained effort with integrated control strategies that disease control has been achieved.

In May 2001 the World Health Assembly passed Resolution 54.19, which called for efforts to reduce morbidity caused by schistosomiasis and soil-transmitted helminths in school-aged children. As a response to this call, the Schistosomiasis Control Initiative (SCI), supported by the Bill and Melinda Gates Foundation, with the objective of encouraging the development of sustainable schistosomiasis control programmes throughout sub-Saharan Africa, was launched in Uganda in March 2003. Eight additional countries have now been enrolled: Zambia, Tanzania, Mali, Burkina Faso, Niger, Rwanda, Burundi, and Yemen. The goal is to reduce the level of morbidity in schistosomiasis endemic areas throughout sub-Saharan Africa with praziquantel treatment. While the mass drug treatment of school-aged children in endemic areas is a very important and promising development, recent studies indicate that many infants and preschool-aged children have schistosomiasis and they are not presently targeted to receive praziquantel within current mass drug administration. A long-term solution for schistosomiasis control could be provided by a protective vaccine. Currently, one vaccine, Bilhvax (Sh28GST), is in phase III clinical trials in Senegal.

Further reading

Danso-Appiah A, *et al.* (2008). Drugs for treating urinary schistosomiasis. *Cochrane Database Syst Rev*, **3**, CD000053. [Review.].

Fairley J (1991). *Bilharzia. A history of imperial tropical medicine.* Cambridge University Press, Cambridge. [A detailed history of schistosomiasis, including developments in research and control up to the 1970s.]

Ferrari TC, Moreira PR (2011). Neuroschistosomiasis: clinical symptoms and pathogenesis. *Lancet Neurol*, **10**, 853–64.

Graham BB, *et al.* (2010). Schistosomiasis-associated pulmonary hypertension: pulmonary vascular disease: the global perspective. Chest, **137**(6 Suppl), 20S–29S.

Gryseels B, *et al.* (2006). Human schistosomiasis. *Lancet*, **368**, 1106–18. [Comprehensive review of various aspects of human schistosomiasis.]

Jordan P, Webbe G, Sturrock RF (eds) (1993). *Human schistosomiasis.* CAB International, Wallingford. [The definitive text on human schistosomiasis. Including: A comprehensive review of pathology and clinical aspects of *Schistosoma mansoni* infection by Lambertucci; of *S. haematobium* and *S. intercalatum* by Farid; and of *S. japonicum* and *S. japonicum*-like infections by Gang.]

King CH, Dickman K, Tisch DJ (2005). Reassessment of the cost of chronic helmintic infection: a meta-analysis of disability-related outcomes in endemic schistosomiasis. *Lancet*, **365**, 1561–9. [A systematic review of data on disability-associated outcomes for all forms of schistosomiasis.resulting in an evidenced-based reassessment of schistosomiasis-related disability.]

Mahmoud A (ed.) (2001). *Tropical medicine: science and practice*, Vol. 3 *Schistosomiasis.* Imperial College Press, London. [Reviews on various aspects of clinical and experimental schistosomiasis.]

Olds GR (2003). Administration of praziquantel to pregnant and lactating women. *Acta Tropica*, **86**, 185–95. [A summary of praziquantel toxicology with data from various studies that suggest that both the pregnant woman and her unborn fetus may suffer consequences from schistosome infection, and the very important conclusion is that pregnant and lactating women should no longer be systematically excluded from praziquantel treatment.]

Richter J (2003). The impact of chemotherapy on morbidity due to schistosomiasis. *Acta Tropica*, **86**, 161–83. [A comprehensive review of the impact of chemotherapy on schistosomiasis morbidity with several tables providing a useful overview of a large number of studies using different treatment regimes and assessment methods.]

Roca C, *et al.* (2002). Comparative, clinico-epidemiologic study of *Schistosoma mansoni* infections in travellers and immigrants in Spain. *Eur J Clin Microbiol Infect Dis*, **21**, 219–23.

Saconato H, Atallah ÁN (2005). Interventions for treating schistosomiasis mansoni. *Cochrane Database Syst Rev*, **3**, CD000528.

Silva LC, *et al.* (2004). Treatment of schistosomal myeloradiculopathy with praziquantel and corticosteroids and evaluation by magnetic resonance imaging: a longitudinal study. *Clin Infect Dis*, **39**, 1618–24.

Steinmann P, *et al.* (2006). Schistosomiasis and water resources development: systematic review, meta-analysis, and estimates of people at risk. *Lancet Infectious Diseases*; **6**, 411–425.

Stothard JR, *et al.* (2011). Closing the praziquantel treatment gap: new steps in epidemiological monitoring and control of schistosomiasis in African infants and preschool-aged children. Parasitology, **138**, 1593–606.

Vennervald BJ, Dunne DW (2004). Morbidity in schistosomiasis: an update. *Curr Opin Infect Dis*. **17**, 439–47. [A review of the factors that affect the level of schistosomiasis morbidity in populations living schistosomiasis endemic areas.]

Whitty CJ, *et al.* (2000). Presentation and outcome of 1107 cases of schistosomiasis from Africa diagnosed in a non-endemic country. *Trans R Soc Trop Med Hyg*, **94**, 531–4.

WHO (2011). *IARC monograph on the evaluation of carcinogenic risks to humans. Volume 100. A review of human carcinogens. Part B: Biological agents.* Schistosoma haematobium. International Agency for Research on Cancer, Lyon, France, pp. 377–90.

11.2 Liver fluke infections

David I. Grove

Essentials

Clonorchiasis and related flukes

Clonorchis (syn. *Opisthorchis*) *sinensis* is a fluke (flatworm) acquired by ingestion of undercooked freshwater fish in eastern Asia. Larvae in the duodenum enter the biliary tree through the sphincter of Oddi and mature. Most patients are asymptomatic, but there may be right upper abdominal discomfort, and infection can be complicated by bacterial cholangitis and there is an increased risk of cholangiocarcinoma. Diagnosis is suggested by finding eggs in faeces or in duodenal aspirates, but can only be confirmed by examination of adult flukes. Treatment is with praziquantel.

Opisthorchis viverrini in South-East Asia and *O. felineus* in Eurasia, also acquired from undercooked fish, cause similar infections. Praziquantel is the treatment of choice.

Fascioliasis

Fasciola hepatica and its relative *F. gigantica* are acquired by eating watercress contaminated with cysts. These hatch in the duodenum, from which larvae pass through the peritoneum and track through the liver parenchyma, causing considerable damage before they mature in the bile ducts. This produces a hepatitis-like syndrome followed months or years later by features of biliary obstruction. Diagnosis is made by finding eggs in stool or duodenal fluid. Triclabendazole and and artenusate are the treatments of choice.

Other liver flukes

Dicrocoelium dendriticum is a rare infection acquired by accidental ingestion of infected ants; *Metorchis conjunctus* infection follows consumption of infected freshwater fish. The clinical features of these infections and diagnostic approaches to them are similar to those of other liver fluke infections. Praziquantel is the treatment of choice.

Introduction

Liver flukes, otherwise known as trematodes, are leaf-like hermaphroditic flatworms. The hepatobiliary system of humans is commonly infected by flukes of the genera *Clonorchis* and *Opisthorchis* and occasionally by other species (Table 11.2.1). In addition, *Eurytrema pancreaticum* has been found rarely in the pancreatic duct. These infections are usually diagnosed by finding eggs in the faeces. Unfortunately, eggs of many of these species cannot be differentiated from each other, nor can they be distinguished reliably from the eggs of certain intestinal trematodes. In such cases, definitive diagnosis can only be made if adult worms are recovered from the stools after anthelmintic treatment, at surgery or at autopsy; parasitological texts should be sought for diagnostic details.

Table 11.2.1 Liver flukes infecting humans

Species	Geographical distribution	Source of infection	Size of eggs (μm)
Clonorchis sinensis	Eastern Asia	Freshwater fish	28–35 × 12–19[a]
Dicrocoelium dendriticum	Widespread	ants accidentally ingested with food	38–45 × 22–30[b]
Eurytrema pancreaticum	Eastern Asia	Grasshoppers	38–45 × 22–30[b]
Fasciola gigantica	Asia, Africa	Vegetation, e.g. watercress	130–150 × 60–90[c]
Fasciola hepatica	Widespread	Vegetation, e.g. watercress	130–150 × 60–90[c]
Metorchis conjunctus	Canada	Freshwater fish	28–35 × 12–19[a]
Opisthorchis felineus	Europe, Asia	Freshwater fish	28–35 × 12–19[a]
Opisthorchis guayaquilaris	Ecuador	Freshwater fish	28–35 × 12–19[a]
Opisthorchis viverrini	Indochina	Freshwater fish	28–35 × 12–19[a]

[a, b, c] Superscripts indicate that eggs within each group are indistinguishable

Clonorchiasis

Life cycle

Clonorchis (syn. *Opisthorchis*) *sinensis* adult worms, 10 to 25 mm long by 3 to 5 mm wide, are found in the bile ducts or occasionally the gallbladder, attached to the mucosa. They may live for up to 40 years. They produce eggs which are passed in the faeces. The miracidium within the egg hatches after ingestion by a suitable species of aquatic snail; nine species belonging to the families Hydrobidae, Melanidae, Assimineidae, and Thiaridae are known to be susceptible. *Parafossarulus manchouricus* is perhaps the most common. The miracidia develop into sporocysts then in turn become rediae which produce larvae known as cercariae. After 6 to 8 weeks, the cercariae emerge from the snail, swim about in the water until they encounter certain freshwater fishes (>100 species, mostly of the family Cyprinidae, i.e. carp, are susceptible). They attach to the surface of the fish, lose their tails, penetrate under the scales, encyst in the skin or flesh, and develop into infective metacercariae over several weeks. When raw or undercooked infected fish is eaten by humans, the metacercariae excyst in the stomach, enter the common bile duct through the ampulla of Vater and ascend into the biliary passages where they mature in 1 month (Fig. 11.2.1).

Epidemiology and control

Fish-eating mammals including humans, dogs, cats, and rats may be infected with *C. sinensis*. Human clonorchiasis is endemic in Japan, Korea, China, and Vietnam where the first and second intermediate hosts are found and where the population is accustomed to consume raw fish. In endemic areas, fish are kept in ponds and fertilized with human and animal faeces. Over 20 million people are thought to be infected in China. Control programmes include proper waste disposal, measures to control snail numbers, and mass treatment with praziquantel, but the most important is health education to discourage the habit of eating raw or undercooked fish.

Pathology

Pathological changes are related to the intensity and duration of infection. They are produced by mechanical irritation, toxin production, immunological responses, and secondary bacterial infection. Inspection of the cut surface of the liver often reveals dilated, thick-walled bile ducts with adult worms visible within the lumen. Adult flukes may be found in the gallbladder but they are usually killed by bile. Histologically, there is desquamation and hyperplasia of epithelial cells, formation of adenomatous tissue and proliferation of periductal connective tissue, and infiltration with eosinophils and mononuclear cells. This may be complicated by epithelial metaplasia then mucinous cholangiocarcinoma. Recurrent pyogenic cholangitis is a common complication and the worms and eggs act as a nidus for gallstone formation (Fig. 11.2.2). Some patients have flukes in the pancreatic duct which may cause pancreatitis.

Clinical features

Most patients are asymptomatic and are diagnosed incidentally on stool examination. Symptoms are more common in older patients with heavy worm burdens. It is difficult to differentiate these symptoms from other conditions but they include right hypochondrial

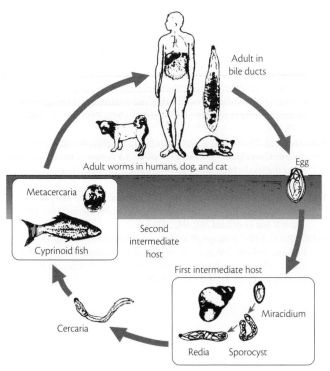

Fig. 11.2.1 Life cycle of *Clonorchis* and *Opisthorchis*.

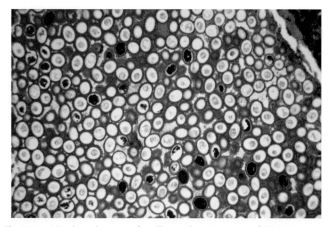

Fig. 11.2.2 Histological section of a gallstone showing masses of degenerate *Clonorchis/Opisthorchis* eggs.

or epigastric pain or discomfort, lassitude, anorexia, and flatulence. Some patients complain of a peculiar, hot sensation on the skin of the abdomen or back. Cholangitis causes fever, right upper quadrant pain, and jaundice. Cholangiocarcinoma is associated with pain, jaundice, and weight loss.

Diagnosis

The diagnosis is suggested by finding eggs in faeces or in duodenal aspirates. They are yellow-brown, 25 to 35 μm long by 12 to 19 μm wide and have a seated operculum with a small knob at the other end (Fig. 11.2.3). They cannot be differentiated from ova of *Opisthorchis* species. Furthermore, they are extremely difficult to differentiate from eggs of flukes in the family Heterophyidae (see intestinal trematode infections) although the latter tend to have a smoother egg shell, a less prominent shoulder at the operculum and the knob may be absent. The diagnosis can only be confirmed by examination of adult flukes. Serological tests are not routinely used for diagnosis. Imaging techniques including ultrasonography, CT, and MRI may disclose adult worms or sludge in the gallbladder. The bile ducts are often dilated and contain sludge or calculi and there may be 'too many ducts' on MRI or increased periductal

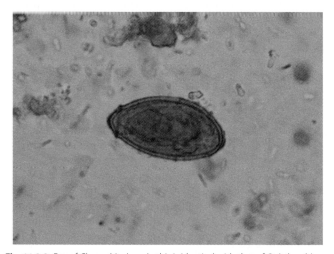

Fig. 11.2.3 Egg of *Clonorchis sinensis*: this is identical with that of *Opisthorchis viverrini*.
(Courtesy of A R Butcher.)

echogenicity on ultrasonography. Liver function tests may be abnormal, often with an obstructive picture.

Treatment

Praziquantel is the treatment of choice and in a dose of 25 mg/kg three times daily after meals for 2 days has a cure rate of close to 100%; eggs should disappear from the stool within 1 week. Biliary tract abnormalities sometimes reverse after treatment. Tribendimidine (see 'Opisthorchiasis') has recently been shown to be effective in experimental animals infected with *C. sinensis* and may eventually prove to be a useful alternative in human infections. Triclabendazole (see 'Fascioliasis') may prove to be useful, but there is insufficient documentation at present. Bacterial cholangitis is treated with antibiotic therapy such as a combination of amoxicillin, gentamicin, and metronidazole. Surgery or biliary extraction at enteric retrograde cholangiopancreatography may be required in some patients with obstructive jaundice.

Opisthorchiasis viverrini

This infection is very similar to clonorchiasis. The adult *O. viverrini* is smaller than *C. sinensis*, measuring 7 to 12 mm by 1.5 to 3 mm. It may live for over 10 years. The life cycle is similar to that of *Clonorchis*, with various species of snails of the genus *Bithynia* being the first intermediate host. Many species of carp serve as the second intermediate host. Humans, dogs, cats, and other fish-eating mammals are definitive hosts. This parasite is endemic in northern Thailand and adjacent Laos and Cambodia where 10 million people are estimated to be infected because of the popularity of chopped raw cyprinoid fish as a foodstuff.

The pathology and clinical features are similar to those induced by *C. sinensis*. The association with cholangiocarcinoma may be even more striking with this infection. The diagnosis is made as discussed under clonorchiasis. Praziquantel is the drug of choice; 25 mg/kg three times after meals for 1 day gives close to 100% cure rates. A recent preliminary study in Laos has compared the antimalarials mefloquine and artesunate (see 'Fascioliasis') with tribendimidine or praziquantel in patients infected with *O. viverrini*. Mefloquine and artenusate, alone or in combination, had only a modest effect on egg excretion and a negligible cure rate. On the other hand, the majority of patients were cured with either praziquantel or tribendimidine with near complete elimination of ova from the stools. Mebendazole (30 mg/kg daily) or albendazole (400 mg twice daily) may be effective if given for several weeks. Triclabendazole may prove to be useful but there is insufficient documentation at present. Control programmes depend heavily on intensive health education.

Opisthorchiasis felineus

This infection is very similar to clonorchiasis. The adult *O. felineus* is morphologically very similar if not identical to *O. viverrini* (the two species have been distinguished by the pattern of flame cells in the cercariae and more recently by molecular biological techniques). The life cycle is similar, with *Bithynia leachi* being the only known molluscan intermediate host. Many species of carp serve as the second intermediate host. Humans, dogs, cats, rats, foxes, seals, and other fish-eating mammals are definitive hosts. Infection is acquired by eating raw or undercooked fish; in Siberia, raw, slightly salted and frozen fish is often consumed. This parasite is endemic particularly in Russia and adjacent countries but also in parts of southern Europe and eastern Asia, with several million people probably being infected overall. Eggs are indistinguishable from those of *O. viverrini* and *C. sinensis*. The pathology, clinical features, and diagnosis are similar to *O. viverrini* and *C. sinensis* infections. Praziquantel 25 mg/kg three times in one day or albendazole 5 mg/kg twice daily for 7 days are both effective.

Fascioliasis

Life cycle

Fascioliasis is due to infection with the sheep liver fluke *Fasciola hepatica* or with *F. gigantica*. Adult *F. hepatica* flukes 20 to 30 mm by 8 to 13 mm in size live in the large bile ducts and produce eggs which are passed in the stools. The eggs require a period of 9 to 15 days for the miracidia to develop and hatch in water at 22 to 25°C but remain viable for up to 9 months if kept moist and cool. The miracidia penetrate the tissues of various species of amphibious snails of the family Lymnaeidae and develop over the following 4 to 5 weeks through the stages of sporocyst, rediae, daughter rediae, and cercariae. The cercariae emerge from the snails and encyst on various kinds of aquatic vegetation to become metacercariae. A wide range of mammals is susceptible to infection but sheep and cattle are the most important. Human infections are usually acquired by eating watercress or by drinking water contaminated with metacercariae. Metacercariae excyst in the duodenum, penetrate the intestinal wall, and pass into the peritoneal cavity. They then invade the liver capsule and migrate through the hepatic parenchyma to the bile ducts where they mature in about 3 to 4 months. The life span of these flukes is several years.

F. gigantica is large, attaining a size of up to 7.5 cm. The eggs are difficult to distinguish from those of *F. hepatica* and the life cycles of the two parasites are similar.

Epidemiology and control

Because of the wide range of susceptible definitive and intermediate hosts, the infection is geographically widespread. Human infections with *F. hepatica* have been reported from all continents. Fascioliasis gigantica is less frequent and has been seen mostly in Africa and Asia. Infection is prevented by not eating fresh aquatic plants, particularly watercress (*Nasturtium officinale*) and by boiling drinking-water. Veterinary control measures include elimination of the snail intermediate hosts by drainage of pastures and treatment with molluscicides and by eradication of infection from infected herds.

Pathology

In the early stages of infection, larvae migrating through the liver parenchyma may cause considerable destruction with necrosis, abscess formation, and haemorrhage. The number of tunnels lined by ragged walls of necrotic, bleeding and inflamed liver tissue is proportional to the number of worms. In the chronic stages, the walls of the bile ducts become thickened by fibrous tissue and inflammatory infiltration, the epithelium becomes hyperplastic, and the bile ducts dilate. Occasionally the lumina of the bile ducts may become obliterated causing obstructive jaundice. These structural changes predispose to secondary bacterial infection which exacerbates the problem. Sclerosing cholangitis and biliary cirrhosis may follow prolonged heavy infection. There is no apparent association with cholangiocarcinoma.

Clinical features

Human fascioliasis is usually mild and related to the phase of infection. There are three phases.

- Migratory phase—symptoms usually begin about 1 month after infection. Patients may develop abdominal discomfort or pain (especially in the epigastrium and right upper quadrant), anorexia, nausea, vomiting, fever, headache, tender hepatomegaly and urticaria. These initial symptoms may persist for several months.

- Latent phase—this phase is asymptomatic and may last for months to years.

- Obstructive phase—this phase is characterized by the recurrence or appearance for the first time of epigastric and right upper quadrant abdominal pain, biliary colic, anorexia, nausea, vomiting, tender hepatomegaly, fever, and jaundice. These features are frequently due to complicating bacterial cholangitis or cholecystitis and may be associated with bacteraemia.

Flukes occasionally migrate to other sites, especially the anterior abdominal wall, but have also been recovered from the breast, pleural cavity, lymph nodes, and subcutaneous tissue. Acute oedematous nasopharyngitis may be an allergic response to larval flukes which attach to the pharyngeal wall after ingestion of infected raw sheep or goat liver (see Chapter 13).

Diagnosis

In enzootic areas, early fascioliasis is suspected in patients with fever, tender hepatomegaly, and eosinophilia who give a history of consuming freshwater plants. If available, serological tests may be useful early in the illness before egg production begins. Liver biopsy may be helpful in some cases.

Chronic fascioliasis is diagnosed by finding the characteristic eggs in stools or fluid obtained by duodenal or biliary drainage but unfortunately egg excretion is often intermittent. The eggs of *F. hepatica* and *F. gigantica* cannot be distinguished reliably from each other or from those of the intestinal fluke, *Fasciolopsis buski*; differentiation of these two infections requires identification of adult flukes. Liver function tests are often abnormal and may show an obstructive picture. Radiolucent shadows of flukes may be seen by cholangiography. Ultrasonography and CT are useful in the demonstration of lesions in the liver and biliary tracts. If the patient has recently consumed infected liver, spurious infection (ingestion of eggs) should be ruled out by placing the patient on a liver-free diet for a few days and repeating the stool examination.

Treatment

Triclabendazole is the drug of choice but its safety in pregnant women has not been proven and resistance has developed in some veterinary populations that may be the source of infection. It is given in a single oral dose of 10 mg/kg although some patients require a second dose after a few weeks. This drug appears to have few side effects. It is available in some countries but not others; further information can be sought from the manufacturer (Novartis, Basle, Switzerland). Flukes are evacuated through the intestinal tract. If triclabendazole is unavailable or ineffective, the antimalarial artenusate may prove to be a useful alternative. A preliminary comparative trial found that artenusate 4 mg/kg once daily for 10 days produced a similar improvement in clinical symptoms to that seen with triclabendazole. Unfortunately, there have not yet been any studies reported in humans to correlate this observation with parasite eradication although studies in infected sheep and rats are encouraging. Nitazoxanide administered in a dose of 100 mg orally twice daily for 7 days cures approximately 50% of patients with fascioliasis; its safety in pregnancy has not yet been established. Good results have been claimed by some for oleo-resin of myrrh (mirazid) in a dose of 10 mg/kg per day for 6 consecutive days but others have reported that this drug is ineffective. Praziquantel, which is active against many trematodes, is usually ineffective in fascioliasis but may be tried if other agents are not available.

Dicrocoeliasis

Dicrocoelium dendriticum adult worms measuring 5 to 15 mm by 1.5 to 2.5 mm live in the biliary passages. Eggs passed in the stools are ingested by certain land snails (e.g. species of *Zebrina* and *Helicella*,) in which they develop through two stages of sporocysts with the eventual production of cercariae. The snail leaves slime balls of cercariae on the ground and these are ingested by ants (*Formica* species) in which they develop into metacercariae.

This organism is primarily an infection of sheep, goats, deer, and other herbivores which ingest ants on vegetation. Humans are rarely infected and are usually accidental. Cases have been reported from Europe, Asia, and Africa. Spurious infections result from the consumption of raw, infected liver, in which case ova disappear from the stools within several days. Patients may be asymptomatic but may complain of dyspepsia, flatulence, right upper quadrant pain and diarrhoea. The diagnosis is made by finding the eggs in faeces, bile, or duodenal fluid (Fig. 11.2.4); they cannot be differentiated from those of *Eurytrema pancreaticum*. Definitive diagnosis is made by identification of adult worms. Rare ectopic sites for adult worms include the peritoneal and pleural cavities and subcutaneous tissue. Treatment is with praziquantel 25 mg/kg three times after meals for 1 day. Triclabendazole (see 'Fascioliasis') has also been reported to be effective.

Metorchiasis

Many fish-eating mammals of North America serve as definitive hosts for *Metorchis conjunctus*. The aquatic snail *Amnicola limosa* is

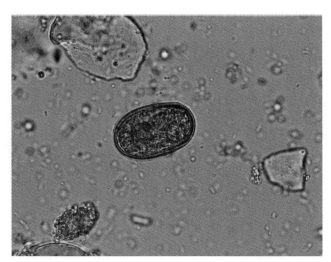

Fig. 11.2.4 Eggs of *Dicrocoelium dendriticum*.
(Courtesy of A R Butcher.)

the first intermediate host; eggs are ingested and hatch miracidia and ultimately release cercariae. Metacercariae develop in the flesh of several species of freshwater fish. Ingested metacercariae hatch in the duodenum and migrate up the biliary tree.

A point source outbreak of this disease has been reported in 19 people who ate raw fish prepared from the white sucker *Catostomus commersoni* caught in a river north of Montreal. The illness was characterized by upper abdominal pain, low-grade fever, eosinophilia, and abnormal liver function tests. Ten days after ingestion of infected fish, eggs indistinguishable from those of *O. viverrini* were seen in the stools. The patients responded to treatment with praziquantel.

Further reading

Ezzat RF, *et al.* (2010). Endoscopic management of biliary fascioliasis: a case report. *J Med Case Reports*, **4**, 83–6. [This article is free at http://www.ncbi.nlm.nih.gov/pubmed and has excellent images of F. hepatica seen at duodenoscopy in the duodenum and coming out of the bile duct.]

Hong ST, Fang Y. (2012). *Clonorchis sinensis* and clonorchiasis: an update. *Parasitol Int*, **61**, 17–24.

Keiser J, Itzinger J. (2009). Food-borne trematodiases. *Clin Microbiol Rev*. **22**, 466–83.

Lim JH. (2011). Liver flukes: the malady neglected. *Korean J Radiol*, **12**, 269–29. [This article is free at http://www.ncbi.nlm.nih.gov/pubmed and has excellent illustrations of the parasite, histopathology, and radiology.]

Sripa B, *et al* (2010). Food-borne trematodiases in Southeast Asia epidemiology, pathology, clinical manifestation and control. *Adv Parasitol*, **72**, 305–50.

Websites

Centers for Disease Control and Prevention. http://www.dpd.cdc.gov/DPDx/HTML/Image_Library.htm

Korean Society for Parasitology. http://www.atlas.or.kr

11.3 Lung flukes (paragonimiasis)

Udomsak Silachamroon and Sirivan Vanijanonta

Essentials

Paragonimiasis is an infection by flukes of the genus *Paragonimus*, with foci of disease in Asia, Africa, and Central and South America. Humans acquire infection by eating metacercariae in improperly cooked freshwater crabs or crayfish. Acute inflammatory and allergic symptoms are rarely serious and usually resolve spontaneously. Chronic manifestations may be (1) pulmonary—most remarkably with a chronic, productive cough with jam-like, brownish-red sputum; and (2) extrapulmonary—most importantly in the central nervous system, often presenting with seizures. Diagnosis is by demonstrating ova in sputum, stool, or pleural fluid. Serology can be used to support the diagnosis, especially in extrapulmonary paragonimiasis. Treatment with praziquantel is almost always effective. Prevention is by health education and the mass treatment of infected people in an endemic area.

Introduction

Lung fluke infection is caused by *Paragonimus* spp. of which there are more than 40 that cause disease in mammals and about 16 species causing human disease. *Paragonimus westermani* is the most common and widespread. Other species prevalent in some region are *P. heterotremus* in South-East Asia, *P. africanus* and *P. uterobilateralis* in West Africa, *P. skrjabini* in China, and *P. mexicanus* and *P. kellicotti* in Central and South America.

Aetiology and life cycle

Adult flukes are reddish-brown and pea-shaped. They are 0.8 to 1.6 cm in length, 0.4 to 0.8 cm in width, and 0.3 to 0.5 cm thick (Fig. 11.3.1). Typically, they are encapsulated in cysts adjacent to the bronchi. Ova (Fig. 11.3.2) are expelled through the bronchi and expectorated with sputum or swallowed and passed in the faeces. They hatch in fresh water after a few weeks. The resulting miracidia then infect various species of freshwater snail in which they form sporocysts, rediae, and daughter rediae. Metacercariae develop in susceptible freshwater crabs and crayfish (Fig. 11.3.3). Human infection results from ingestion of viable metacercariae in raw or insufficiently cooked crabs and crayfish. Metacercariae excyst in the intestine, then pass through the peritoneal cavity, diaphragm, and pleural cavity, before finally encysting in the lung. Tunnels may be formed during their migration. Encysted flukes mature over a period of 6 to 8 weeks and eggs are produced in 10 to 12 weeks. The circuitous routes of migration allow young flukes to lodge and mature in ectopic locations. The reservoir hosts are wild and domestic mammals. Pigs and wild boars are paratenic hosts in which the flukes remain immature and reside in the muscles. When human consume these meats raw, the young flukes mature into adult worms.

Pathogenesis and pathology

While they migrate, larvae cause irritation, acute inflammatory reactions, traumatic tracts, pressure effects, haemorrhage, and necrosis in affected tissues. Acute, diffuse, fibrinoexudative peritonitis may also occur. Abscess cavities containing young flukes are then formed and become enclosed in a fibrous capsule. Mature cysts adjacent to the bronchi may rupture and their contents then drain into the bronchial system. Single or multiple cysts may occur, usually in the lower lobes of the lungs.

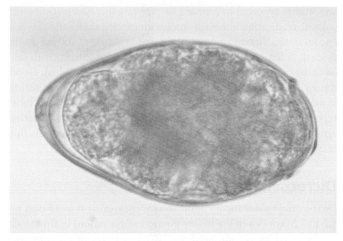

Fig. 11.3.2 Ovum of *Paragonimus westermani*, approximately 100 μm long.
(Courtesy of Mr Prayong Radamyos, Faculty of Tropical Medicine, Mahidol University, Bangkok.)

Extrapulmonary pathological changes may be caused by aberrant migratory flukes. Cysts, abscesses, and granulomas may be found in the abdominal viscera, subcutaneous tissue, muscles, genital organs, and brain.

Epidemiology

Paragonimiasis is an important zoonosis. Humans enter the life cycle accidentally. However, in some areas, human paragonimiasis may be common enough for person-to-person transmission. Human infection is limited in its distribution to places where there are contributory factors that facilitate the life cycle: reservoir hosts, suitable environment, intermediate hosts, and permissive dietary habits. The three major foci of this disease are Asia, Africa, and Central and South America. Human paragonimiasis is uncommon in North America but, both imported and endemic cases have been reported recently. *Paragonimus kellicotti* is considered an emerging pathogen in Missouri (United States of America) where there have been several cases of paragonimiasis following ingestion of raw freshwater crayfish.

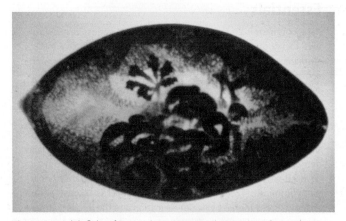

Fig. 11.3.1 Adult fluke of *Paragonimus westermani*, approximately 1 cm long.
(Courtesy of Mr Prayong Radamyos, Faculty of Tropical Medicine, Mahidol University, Bangkok.)

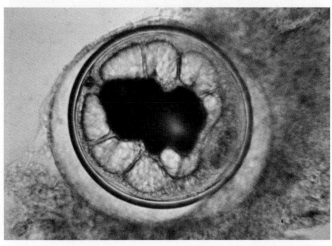

Fig. 11.3.3 Metacercaria of *Paragonimus westermani* in a freshwater crab.
(Courtesy of Mr Prayong Radamyos, Faculty of Tropical Medicine, Mahidol University, Bangkok.)

Clinical features

The clinical manifestations are divided into acute and chronic phases. The acute phase occurs after consumption of metacercariae. The incubation period varies from a few days to weeks. The severity of symptoms usually correlates with the worm load. Invasion and migration by young flukes cause inflammatory and allergic responses such as fever, rashes, urticaria, migratory swelling, abdominal pain, cough, and chest pain. Acute symptoms are rarely serious and usually resolve spontaneously.

Chronic manifestations may be pulmonary and extrapulmonary.

Pulmonary paragonimiasis

The most remarkable clinical feature is a chronic, productive cough with jam-like, brownish-red sputum (Fig. 11.3.4). Other symptoms include breathlessness and chest pain. Pleural effusion, empyema, or hydropneumothorax may occur. Occasionally, patients may experience haemoptysis following heavy work or exertion. Physical examination usually shows few abnormalities.

Extrapulmonary paragonimiasis

Aberrant migration of young flukes to other organ causes extrapulmonary paragonimiasis. The most common and important site is the central nervous system. Presentation of cerebral paragonimiasis depends on the site of the lesion. Seizures are common. Increased intracranial pressure induces persistent intense headache, nausea, vomiting, papilloedema, diplopia, and loss of visual acuity. Mental disturbances of the schizoid and paranoid type may develop. Involvement of the basal meninges results in increased intracranial pressure, hydrocephalus, arterial thrombosis, and stroke.

Involvement of intrabdominal organs such as spleen, liver, and small and large intestine causes nonspecific symptoms and signs. Migratory subcutaneous nodules may occur. Spinal involvement presents with back pain, paralysis, and sensory impairment of the lower extremities.

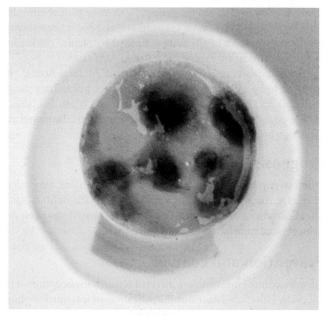

Fig. 11.3.4 Typical appearance of sputum coughed up by a patient with pulmonary paragonimiasis.
(Courtesy of the late Professor Sornchai Looareesuwan.)

Differential diagnosis

Pulmonary paragonimiasis should be differentiated from other conditions presenting with chronic cough productive of bloody or rusty sputum, notably pulmonary tuberculosis, bronchiectasis, lung abscess, and tumour. Paragonimiasis is frequently misdiagnosed as tuberculosis but does not respond to antituberculosis treatment. Patients usually look relatively healthy. A careful history of residence or travel to endemic areas and eating habits aids diagnosis.

Cerebral paragonimiasis should be differentiated from cerebral cysticercosis, hydatidosis, meningoencephalitis, brain abscesses, and tumours. Subcutaneous paragonimiasis may resemble gnathostomiasis, sparganosis, loiasis, or onchocerciasis.

Clinical investigation

Blood counts typically show leucocytosis with eosinophilia. Sputum is thick, gelatinous, rust-coloured or bloody. Microscopic examination shows necrotic tissue, blood, leucocytes, Charcot–Leyden crystals and ova. In pleuropulmonary paragonimiasis, examination of the pleural fluid may be pathognomonic. It is an exudate with eosinophils in variable proportions (12–75%). Typically, it has an elevated protein (6–7 g/dl), low glucose level (<10 mg/dl), low pH (<7.10) and elevated lactic dehydrogenase (>1000 U/litre). Parasite ova may be found in the pleural fluid.

A minority of symptomatic patients have normal chest radiographs. Abnormal findings include linear infiltrations, exudative pneumonia, localised pleural effusion, and nodular or cystic lesions. These lesions are found predominantly in the basilar and peripheral regions of both lower lung fields. Cysts may be single or multiple. The most characteristic radiographic feature is a ring shadow with a crescent-shaped opacity along one side of the heart shadow (Fig. 11.3.5). Multiple cysts may aggregate, producing a soap-bubble appearance. Other findings are pleural effusion, pleural thickening, and calcification. Fibroatelectasis resembling tuberculosis may occur.

CT is more sensitive for detecting these abnormalities. Cystic nodules are clearly seen even when they are invisible in plain radiographs (Fig. 11.3.6). Focal bronchiectasis is commonly found. Worm migration tracts may be identified. Paragonimiasis is one of the benign lesions that may give an increased uptake in a fluorodeoxyglucose positron emission tomography (FDG-PET) scan and can mimic malignant lung tumour.

Characteristic CT findings in cerebral paragonimiasis are conglomerate, multiple ring-shaped enhancing lesions with surrounding oedema (Fig. 11.3.7).

Demonstration of *Paragonimus* infection

Detection of characteristic eggs in sputum, stool, or pleural fluid confirms the diagnosis. *Paragonimus* eggs are golden brown in colour and ovoid in shape with an operculum at one end (size 80–120 × 50–60 μm) (see Fig. 11.3.2). Egg detection rate is low (28–62%) but repeating the examination results in a higher yield. *Paragonimus* eggs can be detected by Ziehl–Neelsen staining of sputum sample and this appears superior to the standard wet smear technique. Expectoration of the intact fluke is rare.

Various serological tests have been developed to aid the diagnosis. The complement fixation test is sensitive and can be used for evaluation of treatment response but it is now rarely available.

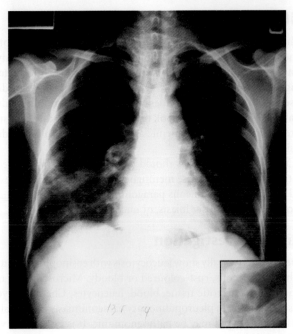

Fig. 11.3.5 Posteroanterior radiograph of a patient with pulmonary paragonimiasis showing thick-walled cystic lesions in the right perihilar area and left upper lobe. Patchy infiltration and pleural thickening are also seen in the right lower lobe. Insert, enlargement of the left upper lobe cystic lesion.
(Copyright Dr Udomsak Silachamroon.)

Currently enzyme-linked immunosorbent assay (ELISA) and immunoblot are commonly applied for various kinds of parasitic disease. These tests are highly sensitive (90–100%) and specific (>90%). Species differentiation could be achieved by these tests. They are essential for diagnosis of extrapulmonary paragonimiasis. Positive results persist for some time after successful treatment (4–24 months) so the response to treatment cannot be evaluated.

Criteria for diagnosis

Definitive diagnosis can be made by demonstrating ova in sputum, stool, pleural fluid, or tissue biopsy. In cases where eggs are not detected or paragonimiasis is extrapulmonary, compatible clinical findings with positive serology are accepted as diagnostic.

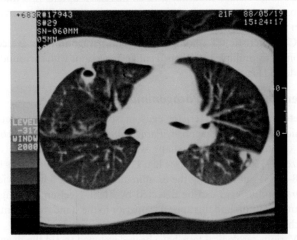

Fig. 11.3.6 CT scan of a patient with paragonimiasis, showing multiple cystic lesions in the subpleural region.
(Copyright Professor Sirivan Vanijanonta.)

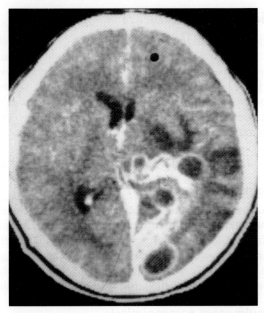

Fig. 11.3.7 Cerebral CT scan of a patient with paragonimiasis, showing multiple ring-shaped enhancing lesions with surrounding oedema.
(Courtesy of Professor Seung-Yull Cho, Suwon, Korea.)

Treatment

The drug of choice is praziquantel in a dose of 75 mg/kg per day in three divided doses for 2 to 3 days. A cure rate of nearly 100% has been reported in multicentre studies. Symptoms improve within a few days. Eggs disappear from the sputum in a few weeks. Radiological improvement takes months, depending on the extent and chronicity of the disease. Urticaria or transient increase in eosinophilia is occasionally seen, indicating a reaction to dead parasites. Convulsions, coma, and behavioural changes may develop during treatment of cerebral paragonimiasis as a result of brain oedema and increased intracranial pressure. Dexamethasone is suggested for this reaction. Repeated thoracentesis in combination with chemotherapy is required for patients with large pleural effusions. Chronic pleural effusion or empyema may resist chemotherapy because penetration of the drug is limited by pleural thickening. Surgical decortication may be indicated in such cases.

Triclabendazole, a drug for treatment of fascioliasis, was reported to be as effective as praziquantel for pulmonary paragonimiasis and better tolerated by the patients. When available, it may be considered as an alternative to praziquantel. Bithionol and niclofalan are also effective.

Prognosis

Pulmonary paragonimiasis is rarely fatal. The lesions may calcify or resolve completely in a few years. Cerebral paragonimiasis may cause chronic morbidity such as epilepsy, mental changes, and neurological sequelae.

Prevention and control

Effective control measures are directed towards interruption of the life cycle. However, control and eradication of intermediate hosts is impracticable; health education, changes in social and dietary customs, and the mass treatment of infected people in an endemic area are therefore more effective for prevention and control.

Further reading

Dekumyoy P, Waikagul J, Eom KS (1998). Human lung fluke *Paragonimus heterotremus*: differential diagnosis between *Paragonimus heterotremus* and *Paragonimus westermani* infection by EITB. *Trop Med Int Health*, **3**, 52–6. [Development of currently used immunoblot for diagnosis of paragonimiasis.]

Im JG, Chang K, Reeder M (1997). Current diagnostic imaging of pulmonary and cerebral paragonimiasis, with pathological correlation. *Semin Roentgenol*, **32**, 301–24. [A comprehensive review and demonstration of imaging in pulmonary and cerebral paragonimiasis.]

Keiser J, et al. (2005). Triclabendazole for the treatment of fascioliasis and paragonimiasis. *Expert Opin Invest Drugs*, **14**, 1513–26. [An overview of triclabendazole including phamacokinetics and phamacodynamics, toxicology and efficacy against the major food-borne trematodes.]

Keiser J, Utzinger J (2009). Food-borne trematodiases. *Clin Microbial Rev*, **22**, 466–483.

Kim TS, et al. (2005). Pleuropulmonary paragonimiasis: CT findings in 31 patients. *Am J Roentgenol*, **185**, 616–21. [A recent report of thin section CT scan findings in pleuropulmonary paragonimiasis.]

Kuroki M, et al. (2005). High-resolution computed tomography findings of *P. westermani*. *J Thorac Imaging*, **20**, 210–13. [A report of high-resolution CT findings, a useful technique for evaluating lung parenchyma in pulmonary paragonimiasis.]

Nakamura-Uchiyama F, Mukae H, Nawa Y (2002). Paragonimiasis: a Japanese perspective. *Clin Chest Med*, **23**, 409–20. [A comprehensive review of paragonimiasis from the main endemic zone.]

Procop GW (2009). North American paragonimiasis (caused by Paragonimus kellicotti) in the context of global paragonimiasis. *Clin Micobiol Rev*, **22**, 415–46. [A comprehensive review of North American paragonimiasis.]

Romeo DP, Pollock JJ (1986). Pulmonary paragonimiasis: diagnostic value of pleural fluid analysis. *South Med J*, **79**, 241–3. [A landmark study of characteristic of pleural fluid profile in pleuropulmonary paragonimiasis.]

Slesak G, et al. (2011). Ziehl–Neelsen staining technique can diagnose paragonimiasis. *PLoS Negl Trop Dis*, **5**, e1048. [A recent report on validation of Ziehl–Neelsen staining for diagnosis of paragonimiasis.]

Vanijanonta S, Bunnag D, Harinasuta T (1984). *Paragonimus heterotremus* and other *paragonimus* spp. in Thailand: pathogenesis, clinical and treatment. *Drug Res*, **34**, 1186–8. [A review of paragonimiasis caused by *P. heterotremus*, which is prevalent in South-East Asia.]

Velez ID, Ortega JE, Velasquez LE (2002). Paragonimiasis: a view form Columbia. *Clin Chest Med*, **23**, 421–31. [A recent review of paragonimiasis from South America.]

Watanabe S, et al. (2003). Pulmonary paragonimiasis mimicking lung cancer on FDG-PET imaging. *Anticancer Res*, **23**, 3437–40. [The first reported case of pulmonary paragonimiasis mimicking lung cancer on FDG-PET imaging.]

11.4 Intestinal trematode infections

David I. Grove

Essentials

Intestinal trematode infections are widespread, but most common in Asia as a reflection of cultural culinary factors.

Echinostomiasis and fasciolopsiasis—infection of the intestines with flukes (flatworms) of the family *Echinostomatidae* is acquired by the ingestion of undercooked freshwater fish, molluscs, frogs, or vegetation. Heavy infections with these worms (2–20 mm long) may cause abdominal discomfort and diarrhoea. *Fasciolopsis buski* is a similar fluke (20–70 mm long), acquired by ingestion of contaminated water plants. Diagnosis is by finding eggs in the stool, but ova of these different species are very difficult to differentiate from each other.

Heterophyiasis (including metagonimiasis)—caused by smaller flukes (1–2 mm long), belonging to the family *Heterophyidae*. Infection is acquired by ingestion of undercooked freshwater or coastal fish. Heavy infections may cause abdominal discomfort and diarrhoea. Diagnosis is by finding heterophyid eggs in the stool, but the various species cannot be easily differentiated from each other.

Treatment and prevention—praziquantel is the drug of choice for all of these infections, which can be prevented by thoroughly cooking potentially infected foodstuffs.

Introduction

This chapter is concerned with intestinal trematode infections of humans other than intestinal schistosomiasis. These infections are widespread but are most common in Asia. This is a reflection of cultural factors, particularly the consumption of raw, undercooked, smoked, pickled or dried vectors, most frequently freshwater fish and molluscs but also water plants which contain infective forms of worms called metacercariae that may remain viable for a few days. More than 50 million people are estimated to harbour one or more species of these hermaphroditic flukes. In many instances, the extent of morbidity due to these infections is uncertain.

Diagnosis

The diagnosis of intestinal fluke infections is usually based on recovery of eggs from stools. Unfortunately, ova from species within a given family often look very similar and it may only be possible when using routine laboratory methods to identify an infection to family level such as a heterophyid or echinostomatid egg. Definitive identification relies upon recovery of adult worms after anthelmintic treatment. Identifying characteristics are provided in parasitology texts. To make matters even more complex, many of these flukes have one or more synonyms which may be found by searching the internet or consulting one of the references by Chai given in the 'Further reading' section.

Treatment

Praziquantel has been shown to be effective with a number of these infections and is the drug of first choice. It is given in a dose of 20 mg/kg orally after a meal, perhaps repeated once or twice. Flukes are usually expelled the following day. The role of triclabendazole, perhaps in a dose of 10 mg/kg orally, in the treatment of intestinal trematodiases is not yet clear. Other alternatives which are less likely to be effective include niclosamide 150 mg/kg orally for 1 or 2 days and albendazole 200 mg orally for 2 days.

Prevention

These fluke infections can be prevented by thoroughly cooking potentially infected foodstuffs.

Echinostomiasis

This term may be conveniently used to include all infections with flukes of the family Echinostomatidae. There are more than 30 genera in this family and nearly 20 species have been reported to infect humans (Table 11.4.1). These species vary in size from 1 to 20 mm in length. Echinostomes live in the intestines of various birds and mammals. When eggs are passed in the stools and reach water, the miracidium develops, hatches and enters a snail, the first intermediate host. It then develops through the stages of sporocyst, mother rediae,

and daughter rediae to release cercariae. The cercariae in turn infect second intermediate hosts which include various species of gastropod snails, bivalves, tadpoles, frogs, and fish to become encysted metacercariae, or they encyst on vegetation. Humans are infected after ingestion of inadequately cooked food containing these metacercariae.

In humans, they live in the small bowel, particularly the jejunum, and attach to the mucosa where they may cause a variable amount of damage. Heavy worm loads may cause abdominal discomfort, flatulence and diarrhoea. Eggs (80–150 × 50–75 μm in size) are passed in the stools (Fig. 11.4.1). They are yellow-brown, ellipsoidal, thin-shelled and operculate and contain an immature embryo; they cannot be reliably differentiated from each other or from those of the intestinal fluke *Fasciolopsis buski* or the liver flukes *Fasciola hepatica* and *F. gigantica*.

Table 11.4.1 Intestinal trematodes belonging to the family Echinostomatidae that infect humans

Species	Geographical distribution	Definitive hosts other than humans	Source of infection	Size of adults (mm)	Size of eggs (μm)
Acanthoparyphium tyosenense	Korea	Birds	Freshwater molluscs	2–4 × 0.5–0.7	84–110 × 60–69
Artyfechinostomum mehrai malayanum	India, South East Asia	Rats, pigs	Freshwater snails	4.8–8.4 × –	96 × 64
Echinochasmus fujianensis	East Asia	Dogs. cats. foxes, pigs	Water, raw freshwater fish	1.5–2.1 × 0.47–0.56	
Echinochasmus japonicus	East Asia	Cats, dogs, rodents, chickens	Freshwater fish	0.6–0.9 × 0.16–0.18	77–90 × 51–57
Echinochasmus liliputanus	China, Middle East	Dogs, cats	Freshwater fish	1.5–2 × 0.5	66–80 × 43×46
Echinochasmus perfoliatus	Asia, Egypt	Cats, dogs, foxes, rats, pigs	Freshwater fish	4.0–5.5 0.85–1.1	99–125 × 58–74
Echinochasmus recurvatum	Egypt, East Asia	Birds, mammals	Amphibians, freshwater molluscs	1.9–7.3 × 0.4–0.9	88–111 × 54–75
Echinostoma cinetorchis	East Asia	Rats	Amphibians, freshwater snails	5.6–21.2 × 1.3–3.7	96–100 × 61–70
Echinostoma echinatum	Indonesia, Brazil	Rats, bird	Freshwater molluscs	13–22 × 2.5–3.0	92–124 × 65–76
Echinostoma hortense	East Asia	Dogs, rats	Freshwater fish, amphibians	8.2–14 × 0.9–1.6	110–126 × 61–70
Echinostoma ilocanum	South-East Asia, China	Dogs, rats, mice	Freshwater snails	4–8 × 0.55–1.0	86–116 × 52–72
Echinostoma melis (= Euparyphium jassyense)	Romania, China	Tadpoles		5.5–7.5 × 1.2	132–154 × 75–85
Echinostoma echinatum (=lindoense)	Indonesia, Brazil	Rats, birds	Freshwater molluscs	13–22 × 2.5–3.0	92–124 × 65–76
Echinostoma macrorchis	Japan	Rats	Freshwater snails	3.3–4.2 × 0.68–0.86	81–89 × 54–58
Echinostoma malayanum	South-East Asia, China	Rats	Freshwater snails, tadpoles, fish	5–10 × 2.5	137 × 75.5
Echinostoma revolutum (=paraulum)	Asia	Ducks, geese, chickens, rats	Amphibians, freshwater molluscs	21–26 × 2.0–3.5	104–112 × 64–72
Episthmium caninum	Thailand	Dogs	Fish	1.0–1.5 × 0.40–0.75	84 × 50–60
Himasthla muehlensi	USA	Birds	Molluscs	11–18 × 0.41–0.67	114–149 × 62–85
Hypoderaeum conoideum	Thailand	Ducks, fowl	Amphibians, freshwater molluscs	6–12 × 1.3–2.0	95–108 × 61–68
Isthmiophora melis	Romania, China	Rodents and carnivores	Tadpoles, fish	5.5–7.5 × 1.20	132–154 × 75–85

Other echinostomes described for which few details are available include *Echinochasmus jiufoensis* and *Echinostoma angustitestis* from China and *A. araoni* from India.

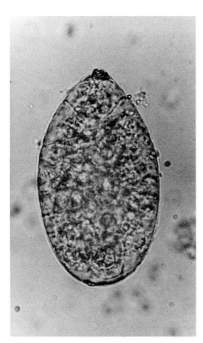

Fig. 11.4.1 Egg of *Echinostoma ilocanum*. All echinostome eggs look similar, as do those of *Fasciolopsis* and *Fasciola* species.
(Courtesy of P Radomyos.)

Fasciolopsiasis

This infection, caused by *Fasciolopsis buski*, is endemic in Asia. The adult fluke (20–70 × 8–20 mm in size; Fig. 11.4.2) is found in the small intestine of humans and pigs. When eggs are passed in the stools and reach water, the miracidium develops, hatches, and enters the first intermediate host which is a freshwater snail,

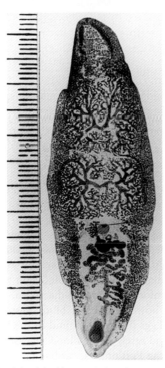

Fig. 11.4.2 Adult *Fasciolopsis buski*, 6.5 cm in length.
(Courtesy of P Radomyos.)

including species of *Segmentina*, *Hippeutis*, and *Gyraulis*. The miracidium then develops through the stages of sporocyst and rediae to release cercariae after 8 weeks or so. The cercariae swim out and encyst on water plants and develop into metacercariae over 4 weeks. Infection is acquired by ingestion of infected uncooked edible plants such as water caltrop (*Trapa* species), water chestnut *Eliocharis tuberosa*, water bamboo *Zizania aquatica*, and watercress *Neptunia oleracea*.

Fifty years ago it was estimated that 10 million people were infected with this parasite. The current prevalence is unknown. Fasciolopsiasis occurs most commonly in areas where people keep pigs and raise and eat freshwater plants.

The adult worms attach themselves to the mucosa of the upper small bowel where they may cause inflammation and erosion and provoke a mucous intestinal discharge. Light infections are generally asymptomatic but heavy worm burdens may be associated with anorexia, nausea, abdominal discomfort and diarrhoea, or even intestinal obstruction. Rarely, heavy infections may cause small bowel perforation. Stools may be foul-smelling and contain undigested food. In marked cases, a protein-losing enteropathy is associated with ascites, generalized oedema and prostration.

Eggs (130–140 × 80–85 μm in size) are passed in the stools (Fig. 11.4.3). They are yellow-brown, ellipsoid, thin-shelled and operculate and contain an immature embryo; they cannot be reliably differentiated from those of the intestinal echinostomes or of the liver flukes *F. hepatica* and *F. gigantica*.

Heterophyiasis

This term may be conveniently used to include all infections with flukes of the family Heterophyidae, although some infections are more precisely known by the generic name of the infecting organism, e.g. metagonimiasis. These are small flukes, generally less than 1 to 2 mm in length. Almost 30 species in this family have been reported to infect humans (Table 11.4.2). These infections are found in many places but are most common in Asia and Egypt. *Metagonimus yokogawai* is believed to be the most common heterophyid infection.

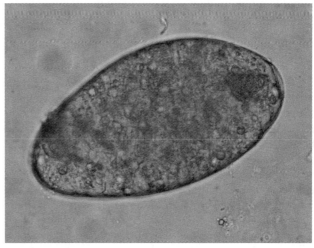

Fig. 11.4.3 Egg of *Fasciolopsis buski*. Note its similarity to ova of *Fasciola* species and echinostomes.
(Courtesy of A R Butcher.)

Table 11.4.2 Intestinal trematodes belonging to the family Heterophyidae that infect humans

Species	Geographical distribution	Definitive hosts other than humans	Source of infection	Size of adults (mm)	Size of eggs (μm)
Apophallus donicus	USA	Dogs, cats, rats, foxes, rabbits	Fish	1.1–1.3 × 0.58–0.72	35 × 25
Centrocestus armatus	East Asia	Cats, dogs, rodents, herons	Fish	0.35–0.63 × 0.18–0.29	28–32 × 16–17
Centrocestus caninus	Taiwan	Dogs, cats, rats	Fish	0.4–0.45 × 0.21–0.25	32–35 × 17–20
Centrocestus cuspidatus	Egypt, Taiwan	Chickens, rats	Fish	0.5–0.8 × 0.25–0.35	30–35 × 15–20
Centrocestus formosanus	East Asia	Rats, cats, dogs, chickens, ducks	Fish, frogs	0.42–0.47 × 0.21–0.25	0.24–0.42 × 0.21–0.25
Centrocestus kurokawai	Japan	Dogs, rodents (experimental)	Fish	0.35–0.51 × 0.18–0.23	33–40 × 17–21
Centrocestus longus	Taiwan	Dogs, cats (experimental)	Fish	0.6 × 0.15	41 × 22
Cryptocotyle lingua	Greenland	Cats, dogs, rats	Fish	1.2–2.0 × 0.4–0.9	42–48 × 20–22
Haplorchis plourolophocerca	Egypt	Cats	Fish	0.32–0.42 × 0.14–0.17	29–32 × 15–18
Haplorchis pumilio	South-East Asia, Egypt	Dogs, cats, birds	Fish	0.45–0.89 × 0.2–0.4	24–28 × 12–15
Haplorchis taichui	Asia	Dogs, cats	Fish	0.47–0.64 × 0.18–0.22	20–33 × 11–17
Haplorchis vanissimus	Philippines		Fish	0.38–0.51 × 0.25–0.31	25–30 × 18–21
Haplorchis yokogawai	Asia	Dogs, cats	Fish	0.47–0.64 × 0.18–0.22	20–33 × 10–17
Heterophyes heterophyes	Egypt, Asia	Cats, dogs, rats, foxes, weasels, birds	Fish	1.0–1.7 × 0.3–0.4	28–30 × 15–17
Heterophyes nocens	East Asia	Dogs, cats, rats	Fish	0.9–1.1 × 0.4–0.5	28 × 15.5
Heterophyopsis continua	East Asia	Dogs	Fish	2.0–2.1 × 0.24–0.28	25–26 × 14–16
Metagonimus minutus	Taiwan	Cats, mice	Fish	0.43–0.50 × 0.25–0.40	21–24 × 12–15
Metagonimus miyatai	Korea		Fish	0.9–1.3 × 0.4–0.6	28–32 × 16–19
Metagonimus takahashii	Korea	Dogs, cats, rats, birds	Fish	0.84–1.48 × 0.42–0.72	28–34 × 17–21
Metagonimus yokogawai	Asia, Europe	Dogs, cats, pigs, pelicans	Fish	1.0–2.5 × 0.40–0.75	26–28 × 15–17
Phagicola sp.	Brazil	Dogs	Fish		
Procerovum calderoni	Philippines	Cats, dogs	Fish	0.47–0.55 × 0.25–0.26	21–25 × 11–15
Procerovum varium	Japan	Cats, birds	Fish	0.26–0.38 × 0.13–0.16	25–29 × 12–18
Pygidiopsis summa	Korea	Birds, cats, dogs, rats	Fish	0.49–0.76 × 0.25–0.44	21–23 × 11–14
Stellantchasmus falcatus	Asia, Hawaii	Dogs, cats	Fish	0.59 × 0.23	21–23 × 12–13
Stellantchasmus formosanus	Taiwan	Cats, rats	Fish	0.32–0.56 × 0.13–0.21	18–24 × 20–22
Stellantchasmus pseudocirratus	Hawaii, Philippines	Dogs, cats	Fish	0.3–0.6 × 0.2–0.3	18–21 × 9–12
Stictodora fuscata	East Asia	Cats, birds	Fish	0.59 × 0.23	36–38 × 22–23
Stictodora lari	Korea	Seagulls	Fish	0.70–0.86 × 0.27–0.36	28–37 × 17–20

Heterophyids live in the intestines of various mammals and birds. When eggs are passed in the stools, they contain a ciliated miracidium which hatches when ingested by a freshwater or brackish-water snail, the first intermediate host. Snails susceptible to *Heterophyes* include *Pirenella conica*, *Cerithidea cingulata*, and *Tympanotonus micropterus* while *Semisulcospira libertina* and *Thiara granifera* are host to *Metagonimus*. The miracidium then develops through the stages of sporocyst and one or two generations of rediae to release cercariae. The cercariae in turn infect various species of freshwater or coastal salmonoid and cyprinoid fish as the second intermediate hosts. These include mullet (e.g. *Mugil cephalus*) and minnow (*Gambusia* species) for *Heterophyes* species, and carp (e.g. *Carassius carrasius*) and sweet fish *Plecoglossus altivelis* in the case of *Metagonimus* species.

Humans are infected after ingestion of inadequately cooked fish containing metacercariae, which mature in the flesh or scales of the fish.

The adult worms attach to or invade the mucosa of the upper small bowel where they may cause granulomatous inflammation and erosion. Light infections are generally asymptomatic but heavy worm burdens may be associated with anorexia, nausea, abdominal discomfort and mucous diarrhoea. Occasionally ova deposited in the bowel wall enter blood vessels and embolize to other tissues. Eggs have been found in the heart and central nervous system and rarely in the blood. In cases of heterophyiasis described in the Philippines, cardiac failure was associated with subepicardial haemorrhages, myocardial damage caused by occlusion of vessels by ova, and eggs stuck to a thickened,

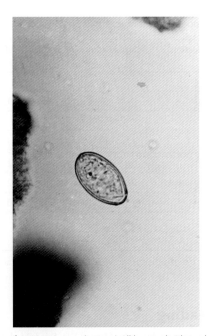

Fig. 11.4.4 Egg of *Metagonimus yokogawai*. All heterophyid eggs look similar, as do those of *Clonorchis sinensis* and *Opisthorchis viverrini*. (Courtesy of P Radomyos.)

calcified mitral valve. Neurological features include focal cerebral disturbances and transverse myelitis.

Eggs (20–40 × 10–20 μm in size) are passed in the stools (Fig. 11.4.4). They are yellow-brown, elongated, operculate, and contain a miracidium. Eggs of members of the family Heterophyidae cannot be reliably differentiated from each other. Furthermore, they are extremely difficult to differentiate from eggs of *Clonorchis sinensis* and *Opisthorchis* species although heterophyids tend to have a smoother egg shell and a less prominent shoulder at the operculum, and the abopercular knob may be absent.

Other intestinal fluke infections

There are another dozen or so species of intestinal flukes belonging to various families that have been reported to infect humans (Table 11.4.3). Diagnosis is suggested by finding eggs in the faeces (e.g. Fig. 11.4.5) but as with other fluke infections, definitive diagnosis depends upon recovery of the adult worms; this is most commonly achieved by treatment with praziquantel. *Gastrodiscoides hominis* is unusual in that it attaches to the mucosa of the large bowel.

Table 11.4.3 Families of intestinal trematodes containing species that are uncommon human pathogens

Species	Geographical distribution	Definitive hosts other than humans	Source of infection	Size of adults (mm)	Size of eggs (μm)
Brachylaimidae					
Brachylaima cribbi	South Australia	Mice, birds	Land snails	6–12 × 0.3–0.5	28–30 × 16–17
Gastrodiscidae					
Gastrodiscoides hominis	Asia, Nigeria	Pigs, rats, monkeys, deer	Water plants	4–8 × 3–4	150 × 72
Gastrothylacidae					
Fischoederius elongatus	China	Ruminants	Aquatic plants	9–20 × 3–6	110–140 × 60–80
Gymnophallidae					
Gymnophalloides seoi	Korea	Birds	Oysters	0.4–0.5 × 0.2–0.3	20–25 × 11–15
Lecithodendriidae					
Phaneropsulus bonnei	Thailand, Indonesia	Bats, monkeys	Dragonflies	0.48–0.78 × 0.22–0.35	27–29 × 10–12
Phaneropsulus spinicirrus	Thailand			0.55–0.76 × 0.43–0.63	27–33 × 13–16
Prosthodendrium molenkampi	Thailand, Indonesia	Bats, monkeys, rats	Dragonflies, damselflies		30 × 15
Microphallidae					
Gynaecotya squataroloe	Korea	Birds	Crabs	560–690 × 285–361	21 × 17
Spelotrema (=Carneophallus) brevicaeca	Philippines	Birds	Crabs	0.5–0.7 × 0.3–0.4	15–16 × 9–10
Nanophyetidae (= Troglotrematidae)					
Nanophyetus salmincola (=schickhobalowi)	Russia, North America	Dogs, foxes, birds	Fish	1–2 × 0.3–0.5	80 × 40
Neodiplostomidae					
Neodiplostomumseoulense	Korea	Freshwater snails	Frogs, snakes	0.8–1.2 × 0.4–0.5	86–99 × 55–63

(Continued)

Table 11.4.3 *(Cont'd)* Families of intestinal trematodes containing species that are uncommon human pathogens

Species	Geographical distribution	Definitive hosts other than humans	Source of infection	Size of adults (mm)	Size of eggs (μm)
Paramphistomatidae					
Watsonius watsoni	Southern Africa	Monkeys	Water plants?	8–10 × 4–5	120–130 × 75–80
Plagiorchidae					
Plagiorchis harinasutai	Thailand		Insect larvae	1.75–1.87 × 0.60–0.65	32–34 × 16–18
Plagiorchis javensis	Indonesia	Birds, bats	Insect larvae	1.8 × 0.7	36 × 22–24
Plagiorchis muris	Japan	Birds, dogs, rats	Snails, aquatic insects	0.8–2.0 × 0.24–0.84	36 × 21
Plagiorchis philippinensis	Philippines	Birds, rats	Insect larvae	1.5–2.0 × 0.39–0.44	28–30 × 19–21
Strigeidae					
Cotylurus japonicus	China	Birds	Snails		

Note: other human fluke infections for which few details are available are *Cathaemacia cabrerai* (Cathaemaciidae) in the Philippines, *Fischoederius elongates* (Paramphistomatidae) in China, *Plagiorchis vespertilionis* in Korea, and *Psilorchis hominis* (Psilomatidae) in Japan.

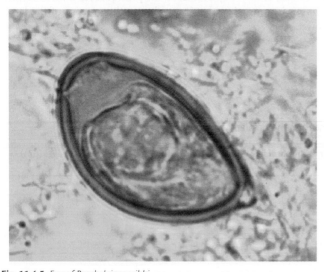

Fig. 11.4.5 Egg of *Brachylaima cribbi*.
(Courtesy of A R Butcher)

Further reading

Chai JY. (2007). Intestinal flukes. In: Murrell KD, Fried B (eds) *Food-borne parasitic zoonoses*, p. 429. Springer, New York.

Chai JY, *et al.* (2009). Foodborne intestinal flukes in Southeast Asia. *Korean J Parasitol*, **47**, Suppl S69–S102.

Fried B (2001). Biology of echinostomes except *Echinostoma*. *Adv Parasitol*, **49**, 163–210.

Fried B, Gradczyk TK, Tamang L (2004). Food-borne intestinal trematodiases in humans. *Parasitol Res*, **93**, 159–70.

Keiser J, Utzinger J (2009). Food-borne trematodiases. *Clin Microbial Rev*, **22**, 466–83.

Sripa B, *et al.* (2010).Food-borne trematodiases in Southeast Asia: epidemiology, pathology, clinical manifestation and control. *Adv Parasitol*, **72**, 305–50.

Websites

Centers for Disease Control and Prevention. http://www.dpd.cdc.gov/DPDx/HTML/Image_Library.htm

Korean Society for Parasitology. http://www.atlas.or.kr

12

Nonvenomous arthropods

J. Paul

Essentials

Most medically important arthropods are insects (including mosquitoes, midges, other flies, bedbugs and other true bugs, lice, fleas, and cockroaches) or arachnids (spiders, ticks, mites, scorpions).

Clinical features

Arthropod-related problems include the following: (1) injuries from direct contact (bites, stings, and other penetrating or crushing injuries from spines, bristles, or pincers) and the consequences of such contact (envenoming, allergic reactions, secondary infection of wounds, and transmission of infectious agents); (2) infestation of the patient's body, skin, hair, clothes, or immediate environment (myiasis, canthariasis, tungosis, pediculosis etc.); (3) inhalant allergy; (4) hygiene and aesthetic issues; and (5) the psychological phenomena of delusion and phobia.

Treatment and prevention—general aspects

Broad principles of management include: (1) Identification of the problem and the kind of arthropod involved. (2) The immediate treatment—if necessary—of allergic reactions or secondary infection. (3) Appreciation of consequences of exposure, such as transmission of infectious agents; many species of dipterans (flies)—including mosquitoes, blackflies, sand flies, tsetse flies, and horse flies—bite humans, and in some regions some of these are important vectors. (4) Use of antimalarials or vaccines and the development of strategies to avoid further contact, including eradication of infestations, changes in behavior, use of repellents and clothing that covers the skin, and bed nets. Travellers and their clinicians should be aware of the risks posed by arthropod-borne infections and ways to prevent them in particular geographical areas.

Particular conditions

True bugs (Hemiptera)—bedbugs infest dwellings and bite at night: patients may complain of mysterious skin lesions and sleeplessness, and a special search may be necessary to find the bugs. In South America, triatomine bugs bite at night and are vectors of trypanosomiasis.

Ticks (Ixodoidea)—these attach themselves while feeding and are noticed by the patient. They are important vectors of many infections, which are often specific to particular genera or species of tick and confined to particular geographical areas. In Europe, tick-related infections include Lyme borreliosis and tick-borne encephalitis.

Infestations—clinically important infestations include the following. (1) Scabies (infestation of the skin by scabies mites) and pediculosis (infestation of the hair or clothing by head or body lice)—these are cosmopolitan in distribution and usually managed by use of topical acaricides or insecticides, although resistance is a growing problem. (2) Fleas—the human flea is now rare in the developed world, but infestation of dwellings with cat fleas is commonly reported. Tungosis is a condition of tropical areas where jigger fleas (not to be confused with similarly named trombiculid mites) burrow into the feet or under the toenails of those who walk about barefoot. (3) Fly and beetle larvae—myiasis, which is the infestation of the body by the larvae (maggots) of dipteran flies, is classified as (a) benign when self-limiting or malign when there is destructive tissue invasion, (b) according to anatomical site (dermal, wound, orbital, ophthalmic, urogenital, intestinal), and (c) according to the species involved. Canthariasis—infestation of the body by beetles or beetle larvae—is clinically similar to myiasis and is rarely reported.

Other aspects—some synanthropic insects, especially certain species of fly, cockroach, and pharaoh's ants, have been implicated in the passive transmission of infections, e.g. shigellosis and hepatitis A. It is generally considered to be in the interests of good hygiene to control these insects in health care settings or where food is prepared.

Introduction

Most arthropods are harmless, but there is a select group of medically significant species. Invertebrates with jointed limbs belong to the phylum Arthropoda. Most of the medically important arthropods are in the classes Insecta (insects) or Arachnida (spiders, ticks, mites, scorpions). Some members of the class Chilopoda (centipedes) may bite humans, and some of the larger members of the Crustacea (crabs, lobsters) may cause injury with pincers or spines. Although they are classified as a separate group, phylum Pentastomida, there is some evidence that the parasitic tongueworms may actually be highly specialized crustaceans (Chapter 13). Categories of medical significance include: envenoming by bites or stings (Chapters 5.3 and 9.2); allergic reactions to bites, stings, hairs, or inhaled allergens; transmission of infectious agents; infestation; the pain and trauma from bites or penetrating spines; phobia and delusory parasitosis. Arthropods may cause nuisance by their presence or the noises they may make, or by being perceived as unhygienic. To allow a logical approach to the management of arthropod-related issues it is helpful to identify the species involved, although as this may not always be possible, generic approaches may be developed to the management of problems.

Bites

Arthropod bites are common and often trivial but bites may be important when associated with envenoming (Oxford Textbook of Medicine 5e Chapter 9.2), sensitization (leading to pruritus, excoration, and secondary infection), anaphylaxis, or the transmission of infectious agents. Biting insects may simply be a nuisance: e.g. it may be difficult to tolerate swarms of biting flies, making it difficult to work outdoors and dangerous to operate machinery. Immune response varies with age, past exposure, and other factors. Management may be directed towards treatment of the bite, if necessary (topical corticosteroids, systemic antihistamines), considering the risk of transmitted infection and prevention of further bites (eradication of ectoparasites, change in behaviour to avoid exposure, repellents, special clothing, insecticide-impregnated bed nets). It is often possible to associate bites with infesting ectoparasites, such as arthropods which remain attached (ticks) or predatory bloodsuckers that are highly visible (mosquitoes, midges, and blackflies, when swarming) and which cause immediately painful bites (tsetse flies, some mosquitoes, tabanid flies). In is harder to ascribe a cause to bites from arthropods which bite at night or when the patient is asleep (some mosquitoes, sand flies, bedbugs, triatomine bugs) or from arthropods that are inconspicuous and do not cause immediately painful bites (harvest mites, some fleas, some biting flies). Bites of larger arthropods typically have a central punctum and a surrounding area of inflammation and are pruritic. In cases of uncertainty it may be necessary to obtain a dermatological opinion to exclude other diagnoses, including organic disorders, artefact and delusion.

Blood-sucking flies (Diptera)

Many flies are haematophagous (Table 12.1). Most blood-sucking flies are in the suborder Nematocera (mosquitoes, sand flies, blackflies, biting midges) and family Tabanidae of the suborder Brachycera (horse flies, deer flies, clegs). The tsetse flies, *Glossina* spp., are in the suborder Cyclorrhapha. Parasitic louse-like flies known as keds, such as the deer ked *Lipoptena cervi*, have been

placed in a separate group, Pupipara, although they are considered by many authors to be specialized members of the Cyclorrhapha. All blood-sucking flies are at least a nuisance: the bites are often painful and associated with sensitization. More important, biting flies may transmit infection. Mosquitoes (Culicidae) are vectors of

Table 12.1 Blood-sucking flies

Family	Representative genera (and species)	Associated agent or condition
Suborder Nematocera		
Culicidae (mosquitoes)		
Subfamily Anophelinae	*Anopheles*	Malaria, brugian and bancroftian filariasis
Subfamily Culicinae	*Culiseta*	Western equine encephalitis
	Culex	Bancroftian filariasis
	Mansonia	Brugian filariasis
	Aedes	Eastern equine encephalitis, dengue fever, yellow fever, bancroftian filariasis
	Haemagogus	Yellow fever
	Sabethes	Yellow fever
Phlebotomidae (sand flies)	*Phlebotomus*	*Leishmania* spp.
	Lutzomyia	*Leishmania* spp., *Bartonella bacilliformis*
Simuliidae (blackflies)	*Simulium*	*Onchocerca volvulus*, *Mansonella ozzardi*, haemorrhagic syndrome of Altimira
Ceratopogonidae (biting midges)	*Culicoides*	*Dipetalonema perstans*, *Mansonella ozzardi*
Suborder Brachycera		
Tabanidae (horse flies, clegs)	*Haematopota*	
	Tabanus	
	Pangonia	
	Chrysops	*Loa loa*
Rhagionidae (snipe flies)	*Symphoromyia*	
	Atherix	
	Spaniopsis	
	Austroleptis	
Suborder Cyclorrhapha		
Glossinidae (tsetse flies)	*Glossina*	African trypanosomiasis
Calliphoridae (Congo floor maggot)	*Auchmeromyia luteola*	
Muscidae	*Stomoxys calcitrans* (stable fly)	
Hippoboscidae	*Melophagus ovinus* (sheep ked)	
	Lipoptena cervi (deer ked)	

filariasis and numerous viral diseases, including yellow fever and dengue fever. Mosquitoes of the genus *Anopheles* transmit malaria. Depending on species and location, mosquitoes bite at various times of the day. Mosquitoes may be controlled by reducing their access to stagnant water needed for development of their larval stages and by application of insecticides to dwellings. Use of permethrin-impregnated bed nets has been shown to reduce malaria transmission. Sand flies (Phlebotominae) are mainly tropical and subtropical in distribution and transmit leishmaniasis. In South America, sand flies of the genus *Lutzomyia* transmit *Bartonella bacilliformis*. Blackflies (Simuliidae) occur worldwide and are vectors of *Onchocerca volvulus* and *Mansonella ozzardi*. Blackfly larvae require well-oxygenated water. Female blackflies pierce the skin and suck blood from the edge of the puncture. Substances in blackfly saliva inhibit platelet aggregation, impair the final common pathway of the coagulation cascade, and encourage vasodilatation. The bites, oozing blood, have a characteristic appearance and may be associated with severe reaction, sometimes referred to as simuliosis or simuliotoxicosis. Puncture sites often become surrounded by a wide zone of haemorrhagic erythema and oedema (Fig. 12.1a). Rarely, haemorrhagic shock may occur. In Brazil, the haemor-

rhagic syndrome of Altimira has been epidemiologically associated with exposure to blackflies. Blackfly saliva appears to contain immunomodulating substances. In Brazil, the autoimmune condition 'fogo selvagem' (a form of pemphigus foliaceus) occurs in simuliid-infested areas (Fig. 12.2a). In Britain, blackflies are rarely troublesome to humans except in certain localities. In southern England, the Blandford fly, *Simulium posticatum* occurs on the river Stour, Dorset, on tributaries of the river Thames in Oxfordshire, and on other rivers. In 1993, 16% (22% female, 9% male) of Blandford's inhabitants reported bites. Use of the biological larvicide *Bacillus thuringiensis* as a control measure was associated with a marked drop in the number of people complaining of

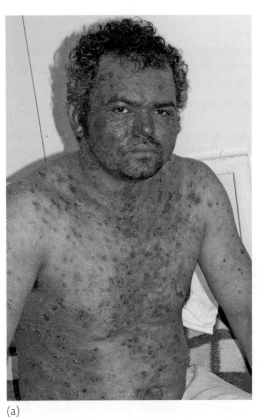

(a)

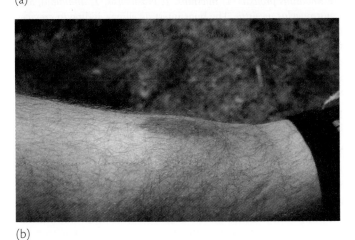

(a)

(b)

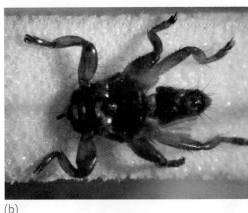

(b)

Fig. 12.1 (a) Reaction to blackfly (Simulium sp.) bites, 48 hours after exposure. Algonquin, Ontario. (b) Reaction to midge (Ceratopogonidae) bites, 24 hours after exposure. Sligachan, Isle of Skye.

Fig. 12.2 (a) Endemic Pemphigus foliaceus ('fogo selvagem' meaning 'wild fire') in a man from a rural area of São Paulo State, Brazil infested with Simulium flies. (b) Deer ked or deer fly without wings (*Lipoptena cervi* Diptera, Hippoboscidae). (a) (Copyright DA Warrell.) (b) (Copyright J Paul.)

bites. In Scotland, *S. reptans*, *S. argyreatum*, and other species may bite humans.

Biting midges (Ceratopgonidae) (Fig. 12.1b) are vectors of the filarial worms *Mansonella* (*Dipetalonema*) *perstans* and *M. ozzardi*. In Africa, tabanid flies transmit *Loa loa*. Tsetse flies are vectors of African trypanosomiasis (see Chapter 8.10). Deer keds *Lipoptena cervi* are highly evolved louse-like flies with biting mouth parts that feed on deer. Occasionally, deer keds bite people, such as forest workers, hunters, or entomologists (Fig. 12.2b). Deer ked dermatitis is a condition where itchy papules exist for weeks to months at the site of bites. Eventually, papules resolve without specific treatment. Recently, it has been suggested that *Bartonella schoenbuchensis* may have a role in the aetiology of the conditions as this agent has been detected in roe deer and in deer keds but not as yet from humans.

Prevention

When visiting locations where biting flies are troublesome, bites may be avoided to some extent by wearing clothing that covers the skin and by use of repellents.

True bugs (Hemiptera)

Bedbugs

The common bedbug *Cimex lectularius* (Fig. 12.3) is cosmopolitan. In recent years, reports of infestations in developed countries such as the United Kingdom and the United States of America have increased. The resurgence has been linked to the emergence of resistance to pyrethroid insecticides used for bedbug control. Deep sequencing has revealed a number of candidate genes likely to account for metabolic resistance. Infestation may be unrelated to lack of general hygiene but associated with translocation of personal effects or furniture. The tropical bedbug *C. hemipterus* occurs in tropical and subtropical countries. Epidemiological studies have failed to produce clear evidence of bedbugs as vectors of infections, such as hepatitis B. They are nocturnal, hiding during the day and feeding at night. Although in some cases bites may go unnoticed and there may be no allergic reaction, bedbugs may cause sleeplessness and the bites may cause pain and swelling and, exceptionally, disseminated bullous eruptions (Fig. 12.4). Rooms that are heavily infested may acquire an unpleasant odour. Bugs may be found by making special searches at night or by seeking their hiding places during the day. They resemble lentils superficially, being round and flat. Adults reach a length of about 5 mm. Nymphs pass through five instars to reach adulthood after about 4 months. Bedbugs can

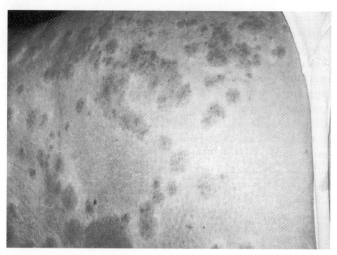

Fig. 12.4 Erythematous macules of bedbugs.
(Courtesy of D Hill, Adelaide, South Australia.)

live for 6 months without feeding, becoming paper-thin. Related bugs which occasionally bite humans derive from pigeons, bats, and martins (*C. columbarius*, *C. pipistrelli*, and *Oeciacus hirundinis* respectively). Infestation may be managed by restricting access of host species to dwellings, but in the United Kingdom, for example, bats are protected under the Wildlife and Countryside Act.

Prevention Bites are discouraged by keeping the light on all night, sleeping under a permethrin-impregnated mosquito net, and putting newspaper under the undersheet. Eradication is by thorough cleaning of the environment and application of residual insecticides. Sheets should be steam cleaned or exposed to the sun and treated with insecticide. However, insecticide resistance has developed and bedbugs are becoming more abundant.

Cone-nose bugs

Most of the 129 species of cone-nose bugs (family Reduviidae, subfamily Triatominae) occur in the Americas. Seven species occur in Asia and one species, *Triatoma rubrofasciata*, is cosmotropical. Many triatomines are obligate feeders on the blood of vertebrates. Triatomines transmit South American trypanosomiasis. Important vector species are *Rhodnius prolixus*, *T. infestans*, *T. brasiliensis*, *T. dimidiata*, and *Panstrongylus megistus*. The bugs infest dwellings, hiding in crevices during the day and biting at night. Dwellings may be heavily infested: in Columbia, 11 403 specimens of *R. prolixus* were reported from a house occupied by 9 people, all of whom were seropositive for trypanosomiasis. As well as transmitting trypanosomiasis, triatomines may cause significant blood loss to occupants of infested buildings.

Prevention Dwellings are deinfested with insecticides and constructed to offer few hiding places for the bugs (Chapter 8.11).

Ticks (Ixodoidea)

Hard ticks (Ixodidae) and soft ticks (Argasidae) occur worldwide. Stages of the life-cycle are egg, larva (six-legged), and nymph and adult (both eight-legged). Ticks attach and feed with a barbed hypostome and detach when engorged. Smaller stages and ticks in inconspicuous sites, such as the perineum may feed unobserved. Bites are usually painless but may result in local sensitization, secondary infection, and transmission of infectious agents, including numerous viruses, rickettsias, and Lyme disease (Table 12.2). Local reaction to bites may be confused with erythema migrans of Lyme

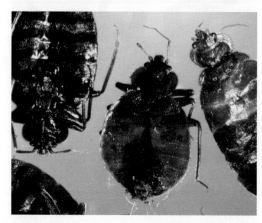

Fig. 12.3 Bedbugs *Cimex lectularus*.
(Copyright J Paul.)

Table 12.2 Ticks and tick-borne diseases

Genus and species	Geographical distribution	Associated infections
Argasidae (soft ticks)		
Ornithodoros spp.	Widely distributed	Endemic relapsing fever
Ixodidae (hard ticks)		
Amblyomma hebraeum	Africa	Tick typhus
Amblyomma cajennense	Americas	Rocky mountain spotted fever
Dermacentor andersoni	North America	Colorado tick fever, Rocky Mountain spotted fever
Dermacentor marginatus	Palaearctic	Tick typhus, Omsk haemorrhagic fever
Dermacentor silvarum	Eastern Palaearctic	Tick typhus, tick-borne encephalitis
Dermacentor variabilis	North America	Rocky Mountain spotted fever
Haemaphysalis concinna	Palaearctic	Tick typhus
Haemaphysalis spinigera	India	Kyasanur Forest disease
Haemaphysalis turturis	India	Kyasanur Forest disease
Hyalomma spp.	Old World	Crimean-Congo haemorrhagic fever
Ixodes scapularis	Eastern North America	Lyme disease
Ixodes pacificus	Western North America	Lyme disease
Ixodes ricinus	Western Palaearctic	Lyme disease, tick-borne encephalitis, louping ill
Ixodes persulcatus	Eastern Palaearctic	Tick-borne encephalitis, Omsk haemorrhagic fever
Rhipicephalus sanguineus	Cosmopolitan	Tick typhus

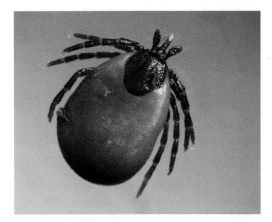

Fig. 12.5 Upperside of hedgehog tick *Ixodes hexagonus*, to show sucking mouthparts (hypostome).
(Copyright J Paul.)

disease, (which expands as a ring with a central punctum—see Chapter 6.32). Ticks may be removed by gripping with forceps (or, in the field, with finger and thumbnail), between the skin and the tick's head and pulling gently. Special tools for removing ticks have been made widely available by the pet industry and such devices should work just as well with humans. Toothed devices that work in the manner of combs or forceps that are curved in profile (tick tweezers) have the advantage of allowing removal while avoiding squeezing the tick. Careless removal may detach the head or hypostome, leaving a potential source of inflammation and secondary infection. In the United Kingdom, the ticks most often found on humans are the sheep tick *Ixodes ricinus* (a vector of Lyme disease) and the hedgehog tick *I. hexagonus* (Fig. 12.5).

Prevention
When visiting tick-infested places, bites may be avoided by tucking trousers into boots and wearing light-coloured clothing which makes ticks highly visible. After visiting tick-infested habitats, searches of the body allows prompt removal of ticks which reduces the chance of disease transmission.

Harvest mites (Trombiculidae)
In the United Kingdom, larvae of the harvest mite *Neotrombicula autumnalis* are a common cause of bites in late summer, especially in chalk downland. They are tiny and seldom noticed, crawling rapidly on to the body, attaching (often under tight-fitting clothes), injecting proteolytic enzymes, feeding on tissue fluid and then detaching, leaving pruritic, sometimes bullous lesions hours later. For many victims, the cause of irritation remains a mystery. Red bugs or chiggers (confusingly, a term also applied to the flea *Tunga penetrans*) are names given to trombiculids in the Americas. Bites to the penis, associated with swelling and dysuria, have been described in the paediatric literature as 'summer penile syndrome'. In Asia, trombilucids are vectors of scrub typhus.

Prevention
Where trombiculids are troublesome, tucking trousers into boots and applying diethyltoluamide or other repellents may be partially effective. Notorious 'mite islands' densely infested with trombiculids in cleared areas of jungle should be avoided.

Accidental bites
Arthropods which do not normally bite humans but can inflict painful but usually trivial bites when provoked by handling, e.g. by children and entomologists, include predatory true bugs such as the water boatman *Notonecta glauca* and the assassin bug *Reduvius personatus* in the United Kingdom and wheel bugs *Arilus* spp. in the Americas; larger beetles (Coleoptera); dragonflies (Odonata); and bush-crickets (Orthoptera) such as the wartbiter *Decticus verrucivorus*.

Spines used in defence by the great silver diving beetle *Hydrous piceus* and larger tropical grasshoppers of the subfamily Cyrtacanthridinae can cause penetrating injury when handled. Pincers of larger crabs and lobsters (Crustacea) can cause crushing injuries of digits and their spines may cause penetrating injury.

Infestation

Sites of infestation include the hair, body surface, and immediate environment (ectoparasites: lice, fleas); the skin and subdermis (scabies, tungosis, dermal myiasis); wounds, tissues and orifices (myiasis); and the gastrointestinal tract (myiasis, canthariasis). With ectoparasites, the main problems are related to their bites: diagnosis and management may be based on the identification of the ectoparasite.

Delusory parasitosis is a condition in which the patient becomes convinced of infestation by parasites despite reassurance by the doctor and absence of clinical or laboratory evidence.

Scabies

The agent of human scabies, a chronic infestation, is the human scabies mite *Sarcoptes scabiei* var. *hominis*. Scabies mites adapted to other hosts, such as *Sarcoptes scabiei* var. *canis*, cause a self-limiting pruritus in humans. Clinical manifestations of scabies are caused by the adult female mite that burrows through the epidermis. The adult female is oval and about 0.33 mm long (Fig. 12.6). The female lives for about 1 month, burrowing and ovipositing daily. The burrow may extend to 1 cm in length. Six-legged larvae hatch after a few days and moult to become eight-legged nymphs and later eight-legged adults. Adult males are smaller than females, do not burrow, and die after mating on the epidermis. Scabies is cosmopolitan in distribution. Prevalence rates vary but may be higher in conditions of overcrowding and following social disruption in wartime. Outbreaks may occur in nursing homes and hospitals. Most cases must be acquired by close contact, as the mites do not survive long away from the body. The main presenting symptom is pruritus which occurs with sensitization about 1 month after the onset of infestation. Symptoms may be worse at night and after a hot bath or shower. Burrows commonly occur in web spaces between the fingers and on the wrists but may be very widespread. There is often evidence of excoriation but the appearance of the skin is variable and may show secondary infection, eczematization, lichenification, and papulovesicles (Figs. 12.7 and 12.8). Careful examination may reveal burrows and mites. Diagnosis may be confirmed by microscopy of scrapings

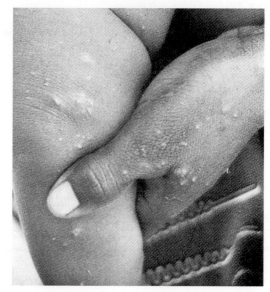

Fig. 12.7 Secondarily infected scabies in mother and child.

from affected areas, especially interdigital spaces, but many cases are atypical and a dermatological opinion may be required to exclude other causes. Immunosuppressed patients, including transplant recipients and patients with AIDS, are prone to crusting or so-called Norwegian scabies in which crusting lesions of scales and mites accumulate over the hands, feet, and other sites such as eyebrows, but the patient suffers relatively little discomfort. Such cases, and presumably their fomites, are highly contagious. Occasionally the mites *Dermanyssus gallinae* and *Ornithonyssus* spp., whose normal hosts are birds, bite humans, causing lesions that resemble scabies.

Treatment

Treatment of scabies is by topical application of acaricides. Aqueous lotions of 0.5% malathion or 5% permethrin are currently recommended in the United Kingdom, given as two treatments a week apart. γ-Benzene hexachloride is also effective. The lotion is applied to the whole body surface of all affected people and left on for 24 h before being washing off. Itching may persist for several weeks and requires a topical counter irritant and corticosteroid (e.g. crotamiton

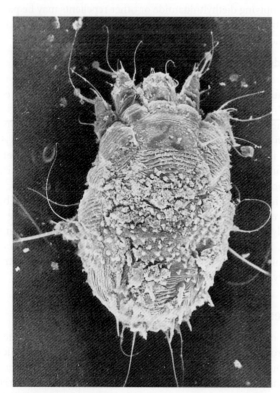

Fig. 12.6 Adult specimen of *Sarcoptes scabei*.
(Courtesy of R V Southcott, Adelaide, South Australia.)

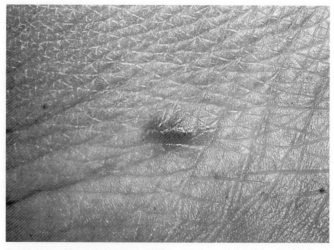

Fig. 12.8 Papulovesicular lesions of scabies.

and hydrocortisone) and a sedating antihistamine (chlorphenamine at night). Ivermectin (200 µg/kg single dose) is used for Norwegian scabies and in patients whose severe excoriations make topical treatment intolerably irritating and painful. During outbreaks, it may be necessary to treat whole cohorts of patients or health care teams.

Louse infestation

Lice are obligate parasites of animals. They bite using piercing mouthparts to feed on blood or tissue fluids. Three species, of cosmopolitan distribution, are associated with humans: the pubic louse *Pthirus pubis*, the body louse (or clothing louse) *Pediculus humanus* (Fig. 12.9), and the head louse *P. capitis*. Body and head lice are morphologically similar and are treated by some authors as subspecies or forms of *P. humanus*. Lice complete their life cycle on their host. Adult females deposit eggs (nits) on hair shafts (pubic and head lice) or on clothing (body louse). Larvae hatch after about 1 week, begin to feed and over the course of about 2 weeks, undergo several moults before reaching adulthood. Adult females live for about 1 month and may lay about 100 eggs. Egg cases remain where attached and may persist after successful treatment of infestation. Most infestations are probably acquired through close contact with an infested case, but some cases may result from contact with clothing, bedclothes, or hairbrushes containing living lice or their eggs, which may be attached to shed hairs. In addition to the aesthetic and social drawbacks of louse infestation, medical problems common to all three taxa relate to sensitization of the host to louse antigens from bites and the resulting pruritus which may lead to excoriation and secondary infection. Louse bites have a central punctum and surrounding small red macule. Body lice may transmit a number of agents, including those of endemic typhus (*Rickettsia prowazekii*), trench fever (*Bartonella quintana*), and relapsing fever (*Borrelia recurrentis*).

Pubic lice (crab lice)

The lice (*Pthirus pubis*) attach themselves to pubic hairs. Rarely, lice may be found on eyebrows, eyelashes (phthirosis palpebrarum), axillary, head, or chest hair. Eggs are deposited on hair shafts. Most infestations are probably acquired through sexual contact with an infested case. Children may acquire phthirosis at atypical sites through close contact with adults. Lice seldom stray from the body. Transmission is possible but unlikely without close contact with an

infested case. The main symptom is pruritus, sometimes with excoriation and secondary infection. Grey patches (maculae caeruleae) may occur on the skin. Diagnosis is by observation of the lice, which may be difficult to find, or of eggs or egg cases attached to hair shafts. Adults are 1 to 2 mm long. The anterior legs are smaller than the other two pairs. The body is squat and crablike (body length, excluding head, *c.*1.2 times body width) (Fig. 12.10). The original description contained a printing error (pthirus) for phthirus (Greek: louse).

Treatment

Aqueous carbaryl, permethrin, phenothrin, or malathion is applied to the whole body and left on for 1–2 days. This is repeated a week later to kill newly hatched larvae. Sexual contacts must be treated.

Head lice

Head lice infest the scalp and rarely other body sites. They lay their eggs at the base of hair shafts. Infestation is more common in children than in adults and more common in females than in males. Prevalence rates vary but may be very high in certain communities or institutions, such as schools. Prevalence rates may be high despite good standards of hygiene. Most cases probably occur as a result of close contact. The main symptom is pruritus which may be associated with excoriation, secondary infection and lymphadenopathy. Diagnosis is by observation of lice, which generally remain close to the scalp, or of eggs or egg cases, attached to hairs (Fig. 12.11). A fine comb (nit comb) may be used to collect material to make the diagnosis. Adults are 3 to 4 mm long.

Treatment

Insecticide lotion (malathion, permethrin, phenothrin, dimeticone, or carbaryl) is applied to the scalp overnight. This is repeated a week later to destroy newly hatched larvae. Permethrin failure has

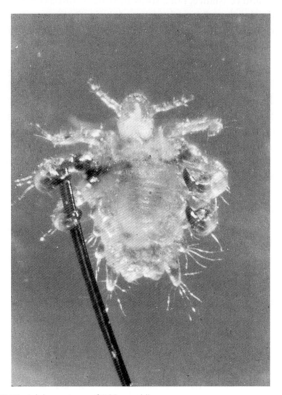

Fig. 12.10 Adult specimen of *Pthirus publis*.
(Courtesy of D Hill, Adelaide, South Australia.).

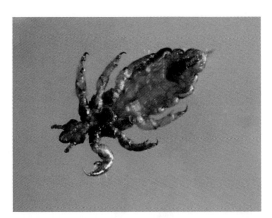

Fig. 12.9 Louse *Pediculus humanus*. Head lice and body lice are morphologically similar.
(Copyright J Paul.)

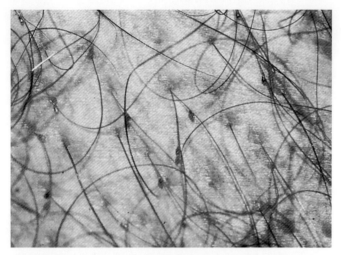

Fig. 12.11 Nits attached to hair. Photograph from a patient with pediculosis showing several hair fibres with numerous egg cases attached.
(Courtesy of D Hill, Adelaide, South Australia.)

been reported from many parts of the world. Compared with laboratory reference strains, lice collected from infestations failing to respond to permethrin have shown relative resistance to the agent. In Israel, there is evidence that permethrin resistance may be due to monooxygenase plus nerve insensitivity resistance mechanisms. Malathion resistance has been reported and may be due to a malathion-specific esterase. Pediculocides should be used with caution in children and asthmatics. Regular and fastidious use of a nit comb may be used (on its own or in combination with a pediculocide) to treat infestation. There is much anecdotal evidence, that combing can be effective, and it avoids concerns of pediculocide toxicity and resistance, but a study in Wales showed combing to be less effective that chemical treatment. In institutions, coordinated treatment campaigns may be required to prevent reinfestation.

Body lice

Body lice infest clothing and body hair. They lay their eggs on clothing, often along seams. Body lice are morphologically like head lice but slightly larger. Body louse infestation is associated with poor hygiene and social deprivation, as may occur in wartime. Transmission occurs as a result of close contact or through contact with infested clothing. Bites occur on the body, resulting in pruritus which may be associated with excoriation, eczematization, and secondary infection. Diagnosis is confirmed by finding lice, usually on clothing.

Treatment

Infestation may be treated by topical application of carbaryl or malathion to the whole body, repeated a week later to kill newly hatched larvae. Hot washing of clothing will destroy adults and early stages.

Fleas (Siphonaptera)

Fleas are bloodsucking ectoparasites. There are thousands of species, adapted to various host animals. Adults are a few millimetres long, brown, laterally compressed and typically very active. Adults move through the fur or under clothing but can survive in the environment for long periods without feeding. Eggs are dropped to the ground, where the larvae develop, feeding on organic matter. The pupa may remain in the environment for long periods before

the adult emerges. Increasing standards of hygiene in developed countries have made the human flea *Pulex irritans* a rarity. Most flea bites in Britain are now due to cat and dog fleas, *Ctenocephalides felis* (Fig. 12.12) and *C. canis*, either through direct exposure to an infested animal or to an environment exposed to an infested animal, possibly months previously. Flea bites result in intense pruritus at the bite site. There is a central punctum and there may be bulla formation (Fig. 12.13). Flea bites often occur in groups.

Although patients may not witness fleas, clues that bites have been caused by fleas include intense pruritus, the appearance of bites in small linear groups, and a history of exposure to a flea-ridden animal or its domain. Troublesome bites may be treated with topical corticosteroids and systemic antihistamines.

Prevention

Good domestic hygiene is important. Infested animals and environments should be treated with insecticides. Certain species of flea are vectors of a number of infectious diseases including plague and murine typhus.

Tungosis

Tungosis is infestation by a flea *Tunga penetrans*, known as the jigger, chigger, or chigoe (but popular names are shared with trombiculid mites) or sand flea. Tungosis is a zoonosis that affects a range of domestic animals as well as humans. The gravid female, about 1 mm long, burrows into exposed skin (usually the foot), or under a toenail, and swells to about 1 cm in diameter, causing local inflammation and discomfort. The wearing of footwear prevents infestation. In the developed world tungosis is regarded as an easily treatable condition that is occasionally seen in returning travellers. Lesions may be enucleated surgically and the diagnosis confirmed by histology. Local remedies in endemic areas (tropical Africa and the Americas) of shelling out fleas may leave cavities prone to secondary infection and lethal tetanus. In endemic areas of the tropics, such as in parts of Brazil and Uganda, high levels of infestation may cause significant disability and morbidity.

Myiasis

Myiasis is the infestation of living animals by the larvae of flies (Diptera). Useful schemes of classification of myiasis include those based on the anatomical site (dermal, subdermal, wound, nasopharyngeal, orbital, ophthalmic, aural, urogenital, pulmonary, intestinal) and on the species of fly involved. Myiasis caused by flies whose

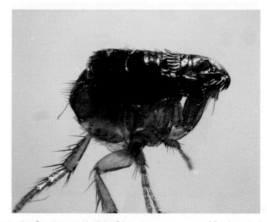

Fig. 12.12 Cat flea *Ctenocephalides felis*, a common cause of flea bites in humans.
(Copyright J Paul.)

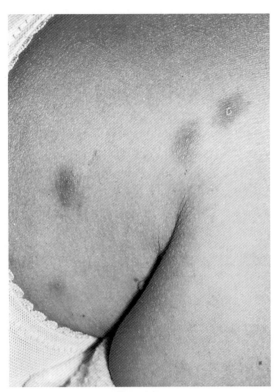

Fig. 12.13 Flea bites. Erythematous macropapule with central bite point visible. (Courtesy of D Hill, Adelaide, South Australia.)

larvae are obligate parasites of living tissues may be termed specific or primary myiasis. Myiasis associated with larvae which feed on decaying organic matter may be termed opportunistic or secondary myiasis. Myiasis due to larvae which find their way into the body (especially the gastrointestinal tract) by chance may be called accidental myiasis. Of the many species listed as possible agents (Table 12.3), most are opportunists whose saprophagous larvae feed on decaying organic matter, which might include necrotic wound tissue. Opportunists usually confine themselves to dead tissue and may even benefit the healing process. There is no dipterous obligate intestinal parasite of man.

Intestinal myiasis may be caused by coprophagous larvae which invade the rectum or by resilient maggots, such as those of the false stable fly *Muscina stabulans* and the cheese skipper *Piophila casei* which survive when swallowed in food and may cause intestinal disturbance and scarring. Intestinal myiasis may be spurious, following diagnosis based on observation of rapidly hatching larvae on freshly passed faeces. Rat-tailed maggots, larvae of drone flies *Eristalis* spp., are sometimes referred for identification to laboratories and numerous case reports link these maggots to intestinal myiasis. As the maggots naturally live in aqueous environments that are rich in organic matter, the finding of maggots in latrines may represent spurious association in some cases. Flies from several genera, notably *Fannia*, may cause urogenital myiasis. Scuttle flies (Phoridae) have been reported to cause pulmonary myiasis, possibly following inhalation of the gravid female fly. A small number of flies are obligate parasites of living tissues and a few species are closely associated with, but not specific to, humans. Many cases of myiasis are benign, self-limiting, and relatively harmless, but aural, nasopharyngeal, and malign wound myiasis are potentially lethal entities that may require removal of the larvae and possibly reconstructive surgery. Myiasis is diagnosed by observing dipteran larvae in a lesion. Identification of larvae may require entomological expertise but management of the patient, which depending on the type of lesion, may involve the removal of larvae, surgical exploration, debridement, or treatment of secondary infection, should be based on clinical assessment.

Table 12.3 Flies associated with myiasis in humans

Genus and species	Common name	Distribution	Type of myiasis
Psychodidae			
Telmatoscopus albipunctatus	Moth fly	Widely distributed	Intestinal, nasal
Phoridae			
Megasalia	Scuttle flies	Cosmopolitan	Wound, intestinal, urogenital, pulmonary
Syrphidae			
Eristalis tenax	Common drone fly	Widely distributed	Rectal
Piophilidae			
Piophila casei	Cheese skipper	Widely distributed	Intestinal
Muscidae			
Fannia canicularis	Lesser house fly	Cosmopolitan	Urogenital
Musca domestica	House fly	Cosmopolitan	Wound, intestinal
Muscina stabulans	False stable fly	Cosmopolitan	Intestinal
Stomoxys calcitrans	Stable fly	Cosmopolitan	Intestinal
Calliphoridae			
Auchmeromyia luteola	Congo floor maggot	Africa	Sanguinivorous
Calliphora spp.	Bluebottles	Widely distributed	Wound, intestinal

Table 12.3 (Cont'd) Flies associated with myiasis in humans

Genus and species	Common name	Distribution	Type of myiasis
Cochliomyia hominivorax	New World screw worm	Americas	Primary
Cochliomyia macelleria	Secondary screw worm	Americas	Wound
Cordylobia anthropophaga	Tumbu fly	Africa	Subdermal
Cordylobia rodhaini	Lund's fly	Africa	Subdermal
Chrysomya bezziana	Old World screw worm	Africa, Asia	Wound, auricular
Lucilia spp.	Green bottles	Widely distributed	Wound
Sarcophagidae			
Wohlfahrtia magnifica	Wohlfahrt's myiasis fly	Southern Palaearctic	Primary
Wohlfahrtia vigil	Grey flesh fly	North America	Dermal
Wohlfahrtia nuba		Southern Palaearctic	Wound
Sarcophaga spp.	Flesh flies	Widely distributed	Intestinal, wound
Gasterophilidae			
Gasterophilus spp.	Horse bot fly	Widely distributed	Dermal (creeping), tracheopulmonary
Cuterebridae			
Cuterebra spp.	Rabbit bot fly	Americas	Subdermal, nasal, tracheopulmonary
Dermatobia hominis	South American bot fly	Neotropics	Subdermal
Oestridae			
Oestrus ovis	Sheep nasal bot fly	Widely distributed	Ocular myiasis
Hypoderma spp.	Warble flies	Holarctic	Dermal (creeping), ophthalmic, oral

Dermal myiasis

The human bot fly *Dermatobia hominis* is a common cause of dermal myiasis in the American tropics. The female fly lays her eggs on biting arthropods, such as mosquitoes. The eggs hatch when in contact with skin into which the larva burrows. The larval stage lasts about 10 weeks, a boil with a small aperture forming as the larva grows. Such boils are not infrequently seen in Europeans returning from the neotropics. The larva may grow to more than 1 cm in length (Fig. 12.14). An early symptom is sporadic pain caused by the spiny larva. Unless in an unusual anatomical site, such as close to the eye, infestation is generally harmless. Secondary infection of the wound is the most common complication. Larvae may be removed through a simple incision. Alternatively, a commercially available snake venom extractor (*not* recommended for snake bite) has been shown to serve as a useful tool for removal of the larvae. Remedies which include application of raw meat or glue to the lesion may not be successful. Squeezing may rupture the larva to evoke a local granulomatous reaction.

The tumbu fly *Cordylobia anthropophaga* is widespread in the Afrotropical region. There have also been rare reports of apparent acquisition in Spain and Portugal. The female oviposits on sand and also on drying clothes. Ironing destroys eggs. Contact with viable ova on clothing leads to infestation. The larvae pierce the skin and grow rapidly. An uncomfortable boil forms which oozes serosanguinous fluid (Fig. 12.15). Fever and lymphadenopathy may occur. Larvae reach maturity in about 10 days. Larvae may be removed through a simple incision, but with care it may be possible to express larvae following application of petroleum jelly (Fig. 12.16).

The larvae of warble flies *Hypoderma* spp. occasionally cause dermal myiasis in humans. Larvae of horse bot flies *Gasterophilus* spp. cannot complete their life cycle in humans but they can pierce human skin, where they wander for a week or so, causing intense itching (creeping eruption).

Wound myiasis

Many dipterous species are known to cause wound myiasis, but most of them are facultative feeders on necrotic tissue and are rarely destructive to the host although the presence of maggots in

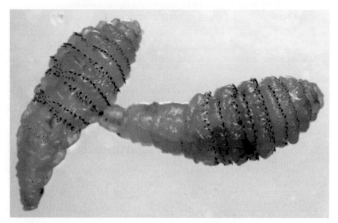

Fig. 12.14 Two third larval instars of the human bot fly *Dermatobia hominis* (c.13 mm long) extracted from a facial 'boil' in a European who had been visiting Guyana.

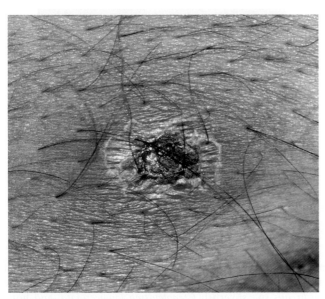

Fig. 12.15 Skin lesion caused by larva of the Tumbu fly *Cordylobia anthropophaga* in a Peruvian man who had been working in Zambia. (Copyright DA Warrell.)

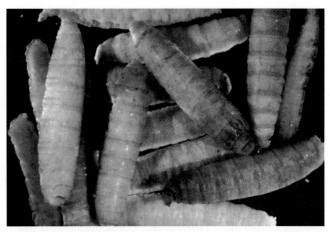

Fig. 12.17 Larvae of the New World screw-worm *Cochliomyia hominivorax* (*c.*8 mm long) extracted from the wound illustrated in Fig. 12.18. These were sent to the Natural History Museum in London where they were identified. Larvae of the second myiasis species (*C. macellaria*) were also found in the sample and were probably collected from the edges of the wound.
(Courtesy of Dr Martin J R Hall, Medical and Veterinary Division, Natural History Museum, London.)

a wound may cause distress. Debridement of nectrotic tissue will control such infestation. In contrast, under controlled conditions, clinicians may introduce maggots to promote healing.

Causes of malign myiasis include the New World screw-worm *Cochliomyia hominivorax* in the Americas and the Old World screw-worm, *Chrysomya bezziana* and Wohlfahrt's wound myiasis fly *Wohlfahrtia magnifica* in the Old World. Their larvae are obligate parasites of living tissue. Eggs are laid on wounds, in ears and on mucous membranes. The larvae (Fig. 12.17) burrow in groups into healthy tissue, causing widespread destruction which may be mutilating or fatal (Fig. 12.18). Secondary bacterial infection or secondary wound myiasis may ensue. All species may cause nasopharyngeal, aural, orbital, genital and malign wound myiasis. Infestation is best avoided by cleaning and dressing wounds as they occur. Treatment involves surgical removal of the larvae, debridement of affected tissue, and treatment of secondary infection. Reconstructive surgery may be required.

Ophthalmomyiasis (ocular myiasis)

Fewer than 5% of cases of human myiasis affect the eye. Usually only external structures such as the lids and conjunctivae are infested but some fly larvae can penetrate the conjunctiva or sclera, causing corneal ulceration and damage to anterior and posterior internal structures that may result in blindness. The usual cause of ophthalmomyiasis externa is *Oestrus ovis*, the cosmopolitan sheep and goat nasal botfly, whose natural host is herbivorous mammals.

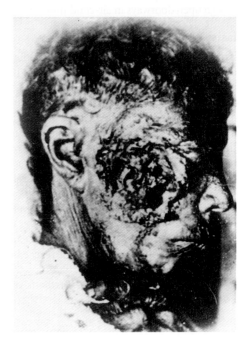

Fig. 12.18 Fatal myiasis (New World screw-worm). Historical illustration of a 50-year-old Honduran woman who complained of a small chronic ulcer on the right cheek; on admission to hospital she was found to have a huge ulcer exposing the bones of the face and forehead and destroying the tissues of the cheek and face, right eye, and orbit. More than 300 larvae were removed (see Fig. 12.17).
(From Harrison JHH (1908). A case of myiasis. *J Trop Med Hyg*, **XI**, 20.)

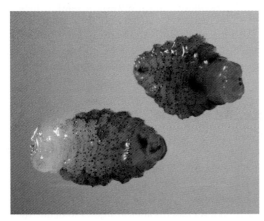

Fig. 12.16 Larvae of African tumbu fly *Cordylobia anthropophaga*, a common agent of dermal myiasis.

Although most common in tropical developing countries (especially North Africa, the Middle East, and the Caribbean) it still occurs rarely in Western cities. Female flies eject their larvae into the nostrils of the host, where they mature. Human victims may give a history of having been buzzed in the face or struck on the eye by an insect and later of developing irritation and redness of the eye, foreign body sensation, pain, lacrimation, palpebral oedema, and signs of purulent conjunctivitis or a stye (hordeolum). *O. ovis* larvae rarely develop beyond the first instar in humans and so symptoms are self-limiting, but they may be more rapidly relieved by slit lamp examination and removal of larvae which cling to the conjunctivae and may cause follicular conjunctival reaction and pseudomembrane formation. Other causes of human ophthalmomyiasis include *Rhinoestrus purpureum*, *Dermatobia hominis*, *Hypoderma* spp., (Oestridae); and *Cochlyomyia hominis*, *Lucilia* spp., *Phormia* spp. (Calliphoridae). Larvae of *Hypoderma*, *Cochlyomyia*, *Dermatobia*, and *Oedemagena tarandi* are more dangerous as they may burrow into the eye, resulting in pain, nausea, and destruction. They must be surgically removed.

Nosocomial myiasis

Hospitalized patients with exposed wounds, ulcers, or medical devices that breach the skin are susceptible to wound myiasis. Patients with impaired mobility or decreased levels of consciousness are also susceptible to infestation of the airways and urogenital tract. Cases of nosocomial myiasis have been reported from developed countries as well as from hospitals in resource-poor settings. Many reported cases involve infestation with opportunistic species including members of the genera Lucilia, Sarcophaga, and Musca. Cases of infestation with the New World screw-worm *Cochliomyia hominivorax* in hospitalized patients have been reported in the Americas. Flies are attracted to necrotic tissues and readily gain access through open windows but may even reach patients through open doorways in air-conditioned rooms.

Canthariasis

Infestation of the body by beetles (Coleoptera) or their larvae is called canthariasis. Clinically, it may resemble myiasis but is much rarer.

Larvae swallowed with food may dwell temporarilly in the intestines, causing discomfort and may be detected in excreta. Beetles occasionally invade orifices. In Sri Lanka, scarabid dung beetles have been reported to invade the rectum. A specimen of the Asian carabid ground beetle *Scarites sulcatus* was recovered from the vagina of a women complaining of vaginal discharge who had visited Pakistan (Fig. 12.19).

In Israel, the dung beetle *Maladera matrida* has been reported to invade the external auditory canal. In Oman, two cases of invasion of the external auditory canal by the ground beetle *Crasydactylus punctatus* were reported. In one case, the beetle reached the middle ear causing sensorineural hearing loss.

(See also venomous coleoptera, Oxford Textbook of Medicine 5e Chapter 9.2.)

Allergy

A wide range of immunological responses to arthropod bites has been described, from local pruritus to anaphylaxis. The dead remains, cast skins (exuviae), and faeces of many arthropods include sensitizing agents. They may act as contact or inhalant allergens, following domestic or occupational exposure resulting in dermatitis, conjunctivitis, rhinitis, and asthma. Allergic patients

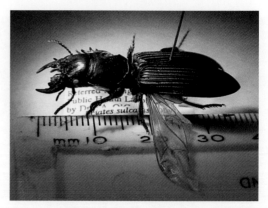

Fig. 12.19 An Asian carabid beetle *Scarites sulcatus*, from a patient complaining of vaginal discharge; a rare example of genital canthariasis.

may show specific IgE antibody to a wide range of domestic pests including house flies, clothes moths, cockroaches, carpet beetles *Anthrenus* sp., silverfish *Ctenolepisma longicaudata*, and house dust mites *Dermatophagoides* spp. *Dermatophagoides* spp. are a common cause of allergy in the United Kingdom and exposure to cockroach allergens in household dust has been associated with asthma in the United States of America.

Following mass emergence, nonbiting midges (Chironimidae) and the exuviae of mayflies (Ephemeroptera) and caddis flies (Trichoptera) may act as inhalant allergens. Chironimid midges occur worldwide and are especially troublesome in the Sudan, where *Cladotanytarsus lewisi* (green nimitti midge) breeds in dammed stretches of the Nile, causing seasonal epidemic allergy. Chironimid haemoglobin has been shown to be allergenic. The rearing of chironimid larvae as food for fish has been associated with occupational allergy.

Entomologists who collect insects by sucking them into pooters may develop inhalant allergy to their subject of study. Occupational exposure to deer keds *Lipoptena cervi* has been associated with allergic rhinoconjunctivitis in forest workers in Finland. Larvae of the beetles *Tenebrio molitor* (mealworm) and *Alphitobius diaperinus* (lesser mealworm), which are reared for fish bait and animal food, have been associated with rhinoconjunctivitis, contact urticaria, and asthma. Beetles which infest stored grain, including *Tenebrio molitor*, *Tribolium confusum* (confused flour beetle), *Sitophilus* sp. (grain weevil), and *Alphitobius diaperinus* have been associated with occupational allergy in grain workers or bakers. Allergy has been associated with other beetles, including *Dermestes peruvianus* (hide beetle), *Gibbium psylloides* (mite beetle), and *Harmonia axyridis* (Asian ladybird). Insect allergy can be investigated by skin prick tests, measurement of allergen-specific serum IgE, and monitoring of respiratory function following allergen exposure.

Insects and hygiene

Synanthropic insects which feed or wander over faeces, wounds, and food may serve as passive vectors of bacterial and viral diseases. Such insects include pharaoh's ants *Monomorium pharaonis*, flies, and cockroaches (Dictyoptera). Despite many reports of the isolation of pathogenic bacteria and viruses from these insects, there have been few epidemiological studies to define their importance as passive vectors, although is generally accepted that the presence of these insects in hospitals should be monitored and controlled.

Flies

Many species of fly (especially of the suborder Cyclorrhapha), frequent human and animal food, wounds, eyes, and faeces. Such flies vomit and defecate where they feed. Numerous pathogenic bacteria and viruses have been isolated from flies, suggesting that they may act as passive vectors of bacterial and viral diseases. A controlled study in the Gambia, where fly control was associated with fewer new cases of trachoma, suggested that flies may act as vectors of the trachoma agent *Chlamydia trachomatis*. In the Gambia, *Musca sorbens* is the most common eye-visiting fly. In Pakistan, a controlled study showed fly control to be significantly associated with a reduction in incidence of childhood diarrhoeal illness. In Israel, fly control was associated with a reduction in cases of shigellosis. Flies may be controlled by using insecticides or fly traps in dwellings and latrines.

Ants

Pharaoh's ants *Monomorium pharaonis* L. commonly infest hospitals, where they invade sterile packs and wound dressings. They are potential passive vectors: bacteria including salmonella and staphylococcus have been isolated from these ants, which should therefore be controlled with insecticides. In Iran, ants of the genus *Pheidole* have been associated with sudden localized hair loss from the scalp. Patients in different parts of the country reported awakening to find collections of hair on their pillows and ants on their beds or scalps.

Cockroaches

Cockroaches are omnivorous scavengers. A few of the 3500 described species have become cosmopolitan synanthropes. The main pest species are the common cockroach *Blatta orientalis*, the American cockroach *Periplaneta americana*, the German cockroach *Blattella germanica*, and the banded cockroach *Supella longipalpa*. Other species may be locally important, e.g. *Ectobius lapponicus*, described by Linnaeus as infesting dried fish in Lapland. The common pest species are mostly of tropical origin and require temperatures of 25 to 33°C, but *B. orientalis* will tolerate 20°C. In cooler climates they are restricted to permanently heated areas and can occur in large numbers in hospitals and in sewers. Many pathogenic viruses, including poliomyelitis virus and coxsackie A virus, and bacteria, including *Shigella* spp., have been isolated from cockroaches. There is evidence that cockroaches acted as vectors of hepatitis A during an outbreak in California and of *Salmonella typhimurium* on a paediatric ward in Belgium. Cockroaches are potential allergens, 7.5% of healthy individuals being skin-test positive in one study. Cockroaches wander over sleepers and are attracted to nasal and oral secretions. Herpes blattae is a dermatitis described from Réunion and attributed to cockroach allergy. Cockroaches sometimes wander into ears and nostrils, where they become trapped or reluctant to leave. Lignocaine (lidocaine) spray is reported to hasten the exit of such visitors.

Eye-frequenting moths and beetles

Like the oriental eye fly (*Siphunculina funicola*, Diptera, Chloropidae), some nocturnal moths of the families Pyralidae, Noctuidae, and Geometridae in Africa and South-East Asia habitually feed on the lachrymal secretions of animals. They may visit human eyes, causing a certain amount of discomfort, and may transmit eye infections, including trachoma and viral conjunctivitis. They may also cause mechanical damage to the cornea. The moths stimulate the flow of secretions by vibrating and probing with their proboscis. Implicated species include *Lobocraspis griseifulva*, *Arcyophora* spp., and *Filodes fulvidorsalis*. *Calyptra eustrigata* is a skin-piercing, blood-sucking noctuid moth from Malaya. Such Lepidoptera may be avoided by sleeping under a net. In Australia, a beetle, *Orthoperus* sp. has been associated with corneal erosion.

Further reading

Aguilera A, *et al.* (1999). Intestinal myiasis caused by *Eristalis tenax*. *J Clin Microbiol*, **37**, 3082.

Auerbach PS (ed.) (2012). *Wilderness medicine: management of wilderness and environmental emergencies,* 6th edition. Elsevier. Mosby, Philadelphia.

Baker AS (1999). *Mites and ticks of domestic animals: an identification guide and information source*. The Stationery Office, London.

Boggild A, *et al.* (2002). Furuncular myiasis: a simple and rapid method for extraction of intact Dermatobia hominis larvae. *Clin Infect Dis*, **35**, 336–8.

Feldmeier H, *et al.* (2003). Severe tungosis in underprivileged communities: case series from Brazil. *Emerg Infect Dis*, **9**, 949–55.

Liebold K (2003). Disseminated bullous eruption with systemic reaction caused by *Cimex lectularius*. *J Eur Acad Dermatol Vet*, **17**, 461–3.

Radmanesh M (1999). Alopecia induced by ants. *Trans Roy Soc Trop Med, Hyg*, **93**, 427.

Roberts DT (ed.) (2000). *Lice and scabies: a health professional's guide to epidemiology and treatment*. Public Health Laboratory Service, London.

Rosenstreich DL, *et al.* (1997). The role of cockroach allergy and exposure to cockroach allergen in causing morbidity among inner-city children with asthma. *N Engl J Med*, **336**, 1356–63.

Roth LM, Willis ER (1957). The medical and veterinary importance of cockroaches. *Smithsonian Miscellaneous Collection*, **134**, 1–147.

Smith KGV (ed.) (1973). *Insects and arthropods of medical importance*. British Museum (Natural History), London.

Zach A, *et al.* (2011). Deep sequencing of pyrethroid-resistant bed bugs reveals multiple mechanisms of resistance within a single population. *PLoS One*, **6**, e26228.

Zumpt, F. (1965). *Myiasis in man and animals in the Old World*. Butterworth, London.

Pentastomiasis (porocephalosis, linguatulosis/ linguatuliasis)

David A. Warrell

Essentials

Pentastomiases or porocephaloses are zoonotic infections caused by maxillopod crustacean parasites (subclass Pentastomida).

Linguatula serrata ('tongueworm')—this is cosmopolitan, infecting upper respiratory tracts of the definitive hosts, canids. Nymphs discharged in nasal secretions are taken up by herbivorous animals, the intermediate hosts, which pass on the infection when they are eaten. Humans may be infected by eating raw liver and other offal of sheep, goats, and other animals, soon after which acute allergic obstructive nasolaryngopharyngitis (halzoun or marrara syndrome) may develop. Larvae can be found in sputum and vomitus.

Armillifer spp.—these are confined to Africa and South-East Asia, where they infect the respiratory tracts of snakes. Humans are infected by drinking snake-polluted water or by eating raw snake, a common practice in some communities. Most infections are asymptomatic, but massive infections may produce symptoms of an acute abdomen and are rarely fatal by causing intestinal obstruction or enterocolitis. Nymphs are detected at laparotomy or autopsy and (calcified) on abdominal radiographs.

Treatment and prevention—aside from standard measures for hypersensitivity phenomena, there is no specific treatment, although mebendazole has been suggested. Prevention is by thoroughly cooking all meat of whatever origin.

Introduction

The Pentastomida are currently regarded as a subclass of maxillopod crustaceans. Common names are 'pentastomes'—because two pairs of hooks above the mouth give the impression of five stomata (Fig. 13.1) and 'tongueworms'—because some resemble an animal's tongue. They inhabit the respiratory tracts of vertebrates, feeding on blood and other tissues. There are about 100 living species in the orders Cephalobaenida (e.g. genus *Raillietiella*) and Porocephalida (e.g. genera *Linguatula, Armillifer, Porocephalus, Leiperia,* and *Sebekia*). About 10 species are recognized zoonotic parasites of humans, causing infections termed pentastomiasis, porocephalosis, linguatulosis, or linguatuliasis. In humans, visceral pentastomiasis is most often caused by *Linguatula serrata* or *Armillifer armillatus*. Nasopharyngeal pentastomiasis ('Halzoun' or 'Marrara syndrome') is caused by *L. serrata*. Phylogenetic trees have been constructed for all pentastome species infecting humans and animals from which sequence data were available. Pentastomes form their own branch close to the Branchiura (fish lice) and Remipedia (blind Crustacea). *Armillifer armillatus* is closest to *A. agkistrodontis* and *P. crotali* (Porocephalida), followed by *L. serrata* and Cephalobaenida (bird pentastomes). Pentastomes appear to have coevolved with other maxillopodan/branchiuran parasites and their vertebrate hosts: birds, snakes, mammals, and fish.

Aetiology

Linguatula species

Linguatula serrata occurs in Europe, the Middle East, Africa, and North, Central, and South America. The names 'linguatula' and 'tongueworm' describe the numerous annular grooves and flattened shape, particularly of the adult female. Dogs, foxes, and wolves, the definitive hosts, harbour adults and nymphs in their upper respiratory tract and shed them in their nasal secretions, saliva, and faeces. Herbivorous animals ingest the ova, which hatch in the lumen of the gut, releasing larvae that burrow into the tissues and encyst. When these intermediate hosts are eaten by the definitive host, nymphs hatch from the cysts and migrate to the lungs and nasopharynx where they mature.

Clinical features

When humans ingest ova of linguatula, larvae hatch in the gut, burrow through its wall, migrate through the tissues, and encyst especially in the liver. Second- or third-stage larvae cause symptoms only by obstruction or compression, e.g. in biliary, gastrointestinal or respiratory tracts, meninges, or brain. In the anterior chamber of the eye, larvae have caused iritis and secondary glaucoma in the United States of America and elsewhere.

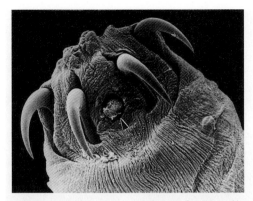

Fig. 13.1 Adult pentastomid showing mouth (arrowed) and lateral hooks giving the appearance of five stomata. Scanning electron micrograph, ×400. (Courtesy of Professor Viqar Zaman.)

Ingestion of cysts containing third-stage larvae in raw liver or lymph nodes from sheep, goats, cattle, camels, and lagomorphs can cause nasopharyngeal pentostomiasis, known as 'halzoun' (meaning "snail" in Arabic) in Lebanon and 'marrara syndrome' in the Sudan, and reported from Greece, Turkey, North Africa, Egypt, and Jordan. In the human stomach, larvae escape from the cysts and migrate up the oesophagus to the nasopharynx mucosa. Within minutes to a few hours of eating the infected viscera, there is intense irritation of the upper respiratory and gastrointestinal tracts causing coughing, sneezing, rhinorrhoea, retching, vomiting, lacrimation, haemoptysis, epistaxis, cervical lymphadenopathy, transient deafness, difficulty in speaking, dysphagia, wheezing, dyspnoea, and oedema of the face and oropharynx. The larvae, which are 5 to 10 mm long, can be found in sputum and vomitus. Patients usually recover in 1 or 2 weeks, but fatal acute upper airway obstruction is reported. Clinical features suggest a hypersensitivity reaction. Flukes (*Fasciola hepatica* and *Dicrocoelium dendriticum*) and nematodes (*Mammomonogamus laryngeus*) ingested in raw sheep and goat liver, and aquatic leeches (*Limnatis nilotica* and *Dinobdella ferox*) (see Oxford Textbook of Medicine 5e Chapter 9.2) have been implicated in halzoun but cannot explain the classic syndrome. Very rarely, larvae may mature to adulthood in the human nasal cavity, causing bleeding and obstruction.

Armillifer (Porocephalus) species

These are also annulated, nonsegmented parasites (Fig. 13.2a). Adult males and the much larger females (up to 20 cm long) inhabit the respiratory and digestive tracts of snakes (Fig. 13.3), especially those of the genera *Python*, *Lamprophis/Boaedon* (African house snakes), *Naja* (cobras) (Fig. 13.4), *Bitis* (African vipers) (Fig. 13.2b), *Bothrops* (Latin American lanceheads) (Fig. 13.5), and other vertebrates. Ova are shed in the snake's nasal secretions and are picked up by herbivorous mammals. Larvae encyst in the tissues of these intermediate hosts and will develop to the nymph stage if ingested by another animal, but develop to adults only in snakes. Humans may ingest ova by drinking water contaminated by snakes, or they may ingest living encysted larvae in raw or undercooked snake meat. This is eaten habitually or as part of *ju ju* rituals in Africa (Nigeria, Côte d'Ivoire, Benin, Cameroon, and the Democratic Republic of Congo (DRC)) and in South-East Asia, especially by the Temuan tribe of Malaysian aborigines. Ingested eggs hatch in the gut, releasing larvae which burrow into the tissues where they encyst as nymphs. The parasite species are *A. armillatus* and *A. grandis* in Africa and *A. moniliformis* in South-East Asia.

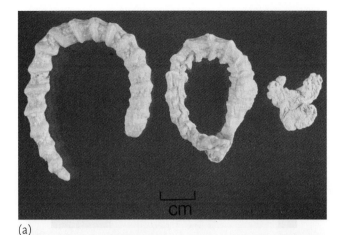

(a)

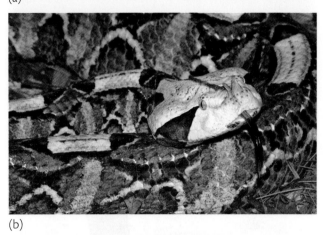

(b)

Fig. 13.2 *Armillifer armillatus*. (a) Left: two adults found in the lungs of (b) rhinoceros viper *Bitis rhinoceros*. Right: calcified nymph from the mesentery of a Ghanaian patient. (Copyright D A Warrell.)

Epidemiology

The prevalence of infection can be judged by discovering calcified nymphs (Fig. 13.2) on radiographs of the abdomen and chest (Fig. 13.6). These appear as discrete, crescent-shaped, soft tissue calcifications, 4 to 8 mm in size. In West Africa they are seen particularly in the right upper quadrant and are situated beneath the peritoneum covering the liver. In Ibadan, Nigeria, they were seen in 1.4% of randomly selected straight abdominal films (7% in men aged 50–59 years). However, the prevalence of encysted nymphs or larvae at autopsy was 22.5% in DRC, 8% in Cameroon, 5% in West Africa and 45% in Malaysian Orang Asli. Cysts are found most commonly in liver (Fig. 13.7), mesentery, gut wall, peritoneum,

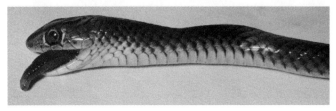

Fig. 13.3 Whip snake *Demansia atra* (Papua New Guinea) bringing up a pentastome. (Copyright Mark O'Shea.)

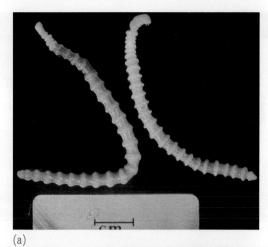

(a)

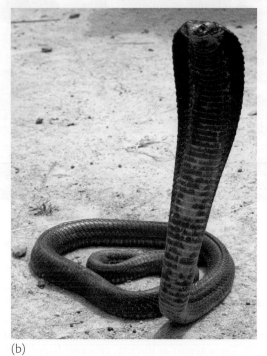

(b)

Fig. 13.4 (a) Pentastomes from the lungs of (b) an Egyptian cobra *Naja haje*.

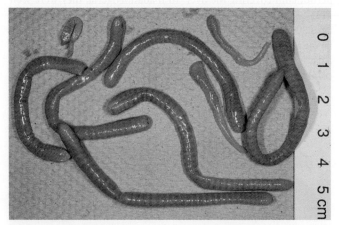

Fig. 13.5 Pentastomes found in the respiratory tract of lancehead vipers *Bothrops* spp., Manaus, Brazil.
(Copyright D A Warrell.)

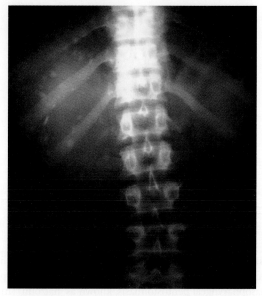

Fig. 13.6 Typical radiographic appearance of calcified nymphs of *Armillifer armillatus* in the abdominal cavity of a Ghanaian patient.
(Courtesy of Dr G M Ardran.)

spleen, kidneys, omentum and lungs. In Ibadan, pentastomiasis was the third most common cause of hepatic cirrhosis.

Human infections with the larvae or nymphs of the following species of *A. Armillifer* have been reported:

◆ *A. agkistrodontis*—China (in the snake *Deinagkistrodon acutus*)

◆ *A. armillatus* (18–22 annular rings)—Africa: Egypt, Senegal, the Gambia, Ghana, Benin, Nigeria, Cameroon, DRC, and Zimbabwe

◆ *A. grandis*—DRC, Côte d'Ivoire

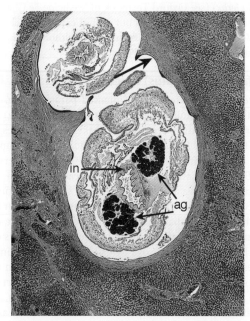

Fig. 13.7 Encysted nymph/larva of *Armillifer armillatus* in human liver. The outer layer of the parasite (arrowed) lines the cyst wall. Acidophilic glands (ag), intestine (in), ×21.
(Armed Forces Institute of Pathology photograph, negative number 75–2703.)

- *A. moniliformis* (30 annular rings)—Malaysia, Philippines, Indonesia, Tibet, and Australia

- *A. najae*—India

Clinical features

Most infections are entirely asymptomatic. Migration of large numbers of larvae from the gut into the tissue may produce abdominal pain and obstructive jaundice. Massive infection, perhaps following ingestion of a gravid female, can cause acute abdominal symptoms prompting laparotomy at which hundreds of wriggling nymphs may be discovered beneath the visceral peritoneum. Serious inflammatory and obstructive effects have been described in the gut, peritoneum, liver and biliary tract, lungs, pleura, pericardium, central nervous system, and anterior chamber of the eye. These may be due partly to hypersensitivity. The few reported fatal cases had intestinal obstruction or haemorrhagic enterocolitis complicated perhaps by secondary Gram-negative septicaemia.

There is no convincing evidence of an association between *Armillifer* infection and colonic or other malignancies.

Other pentastomid infections

Human infections with *Leiperia cincinnalis* have been described in Africa and by *Porocephalus crotali* (from rattlesnakes) in North America. Subcutaneous infections by *Raillietiella gehyrae* and *R. hemidactyli* occur in Vietnam and by *Sebekia* species in Costa Rica. In Vietnam, infection with *Raillietiella* spp. results from swallowing small live lizards for medicinal purposes.

Diagnosis

The radiographical appearances of calcified pentastomid nymphs are distinctive (Fig. 13.6). They are not found in muscle, distinguishing pentastomiasis from cysticercosis. Pentastomes may be discovered at surgery or autopsy. In the liver (Fig. 13.7), intestinal wall, mesentery, mesenteric lymph nodes, peritoneum, or lung, viable encysted larvae or granulomas containing necrotic pentastomes or their moulted cuticles may be identified. Initially, encysted larvae excite little or no tissue reaction, but the granulomas are surrounded by hyalinized or calcified fibrous tissue. In tissue sections, pentastomes can be distinguished from helminths. Some patients have mild blood eosinophilia. Antibodies to *Armillifer* spp. have been detected by fluorescence in infected patients. Pentastomids have also been identified by consensus PCR and immunological tests are being developed.

Treatment

There is no specific treatment, although ivermectin, praziquantel, and mebendazole have been suggested. Obstruction and compression should be relieved surgically. Hypersensitivity phenomena should be treated with adrenaline (epinephrine), antihistamines, and corticosteroids.

Prevention

Pentostomiasis can be prevented by thoroughly cooking all meat of any origin and boiling or filtering drinking-water. Eating sheep's lymph nodes is proscribed by the Shi'ite Muslims of Lebanon.

Other zoonoses transmitted from reptiles to humans

The most important of these is salmonellosis transmitted to humans by the faecal–oral route or by scratches and bites, from chelonians (tortoises, turtles, terrapins) and from snakes and lizards, especially iguanas. In the United Kingdom, 38% of imported tortoises (*Testudo* spp.) contain salmonella. In the United States of America, where 8 million reptiles are kept as pets, contact with reptiles and amphibians accounts for an estimated 74 000 (6%) of the approximately 1.2 million sporadic human salmonella infections that occur there annually. The banning by the United States Food and Drug Administration of commercial distribution of small turtles has prevented an estimated 100 000 cases of salmonellosis among children each year. Although salmonellosis usually causes self-limiting gastroenteritis, septicaemia or meningitis may occur especially in infants and immunocompromised people. Species associated with reptile salmonellosis include *S. enterica* serotype Typhimurium, *S. enterica* serotype Pomona, and *S. enterica* subspecies *diarizonae*.

Other infections transmissible from reptiles to humans include *Arizona hinshawii* (in snake powder, Pulvo de Vibora, made from rattlesnakes), *Plesiomonas shigelloides*, *Edwardsiella tarda*, leptospirosis, Q fever, sparganosis, capillariasis, strongyloidiasis, mesocestoidiasis, and infestation with the mite *Ophionyssus natricis*. Potential zoonoses include mycobacteria, pseudomonas, other aeromonas species, proteus, and some togaviruses (such as western equine encephalitis in garter snakes in western North America) and herpesviruses.

Further reading

Brookins MD, *et al.* (2009). Massive visceral pentastomiasis caused by *Porocephalus crotali* in a dog. *Vet Pathol*, **46**, 460–3. [Description of consensus PCR.]

Chen SH, *et al.* (2010). Multi-host model-based identification of *Armillifer agkistrodontis* (Pentastomida), a new zoonotic parasite from China. *PLoS Negl Trop Dis*, **4**(4), e647.

Drabick JJ (1987). Pentastomiasis. *Rev Infect Dis*, **9**, 1087–94.

Haugerud RE (1989). Evolution in the pentastomids. *Parasitol Today*, **5**, 126–32.

Lai C, *et al.* (2010). Imaging features of pediatric pentastomiasis infection: a case report. *Korean J Radiol*, **11**, 480–4.

Lavrov DV, *et al.* (2004). Phylogenetic position of the Pentastomida and (pan)crustacean relationships. *Proc Biol Sci*, **271**, 537–44.

Magnino S, Colin P, Dei Cas E, *et al.* (2009). Biological risks associated with consumption of reptile products. *Int J Food Microbiol*, **134**, 163–75.

Palmer PES, Reeder MM (eds) (2001). Pentastomida. In: *The imaging of tropical diseases with epidemiological, pathological and clinical correlation*, Vol. 2, pp. 389–95. Springer, Berlin.

Riley J (1986). The biology of pentastomids. *Adv Parasitol*, **25**, 45–128.

Schacher JF, Khalil GM, Salman S. (1965). A field study of Halzoun (parasitic pharyngitis) in Lebanon. *J Trop Med Hyg*, **68**, 226–30.

Tappe D, Büttner DW (2009). Diagnosis of human visceral pentastomiasis. *PLoS Negl Trop Dis*, **5**, e320.

Tappe D, *et al.* (2011). Transmission of Armillifer armillatus ova at snake farm, The Gambia, West Africa. *Emerg Infect Dis*, **17**, 251–4.

Warwick C, *et al.* (2001). Reptile-related salmonellosis. *J Roy Soc Med*, **94**, 124–6.

Yagi H, *et al.* (1996). The Marrara syndrome: a hypersensitivity reaction of the upper respiratory tract and buccopharyngeal mucosa to nymphs of *Linguatula serrata*. *Acta Trop*, **16**, 127–34.

Yao MH, Wu F, Tang LF (2008). Human pentastomiasis in China: case report and literature review. *J Parasitol*, **94**, 1295–8.

Yapo Ette H, *et al.* (2003). Human pentastomiasis discovered postmortem. *Forensic Sci Int*, **137**, 52–4.

Index

Page numbers in *italics* denote figures or tables that are separate from the text.